Textbook of Palliative Nursing

Textbook of Palliative Nursing

SECOND EDITION

EDITED BY

Betty R. Ferrell, RN, PhD, FAAN
Research Scientist
Department of Nursing Research and Education
City of Hope National Medical Center
Duarte, California

Nessa Coyle, RN, PhD, FAAN
Pain and Palliative Care Service
Memorial Sloan-Kettering Cancer Center
New York, New York

OXFORD
UNIVERSITY PRESS

2006

OXFORD
UNIVERSITY PRESS

Oxford University Press, Inc., publishes works that further
Oxford University's objective of excellence
in research, scholarship, and education.

Oxford New York
Auckland Cape Town Dar es Salaam Hong Kong Karachi
Kuala Lumpur Madrid Melbourne Mexico City Nairobi
New Delhi Shanghai Taipei Toronto

With offices in
Argentina Austria Brazil Chile Czech Republic France Greece
Guatemala Hungary Italy Japan Poland Portugal Singapore
South Korea Switzerland Thailand Turkey Ukraine Vietnam

Published by Oxford University Press, Inc.
198 Madison Avenue, New York, New York 10016
www.oup.com

Library of Congress Cataloging-in-Publication Data
Textbook of palliative nursing / edited by Betty R. Ferrell and Nessa Coyle.— 2nd ed.
p. ; cm.
Includes bibliographical references and index.
ISBN-13: 978-0-19-517549-3
ISBN 0-19-517549-2
1. Palliative treatment. 2. Nursing. 3. Terminal care.
[DNLM: 1. Nursing Care. 2. Palliative Care. 3. Terminal Care. WY 152 T355 2004] I. Ferrell, Betty.
II. Coyle, Nessa.
RT87.T45T49 2004
616'.029—dc22 2004020497

9 8 7 6 5 4 3 2
Printed in the United States of America
on acid-free paper

FOREWORDS

Dame Cicely Saunders, OM, DBE, FRCP
Chair
St. Christopher's Hospice
Syndenham, London
United Kingdom

Palliative care stems from the recognition of the potential at the end of life for discovering and for giving, a recognition that an important dimension of being human is the lasting dignity and growth that can continue through weakness and loss. No member of the interdisciplinary team is more central to making these discoveries possible than the nurse. Realizing how little had been written and even less studied in this field, Peggy Nuttall, a former nursing colleague and then editor of the *Nursing Times* in London, invited me to contribute a series of six articles on the care of the dying in the summer of 1959.[1] A registered nurse and qualified medical social worker, I had trained in medicine because of a compulsion to do something about the pain I had seen in patients and their families at the end of life. During 3 years as a volunteer nurse in an early home for such patients, I had persuaded the thoracic surgeon, Norman Barrett, for whom I was working, to follow up a few of his mortally ill patients both there and in their homes. "Go and read medicine," he said. "It's the doctors who desert the dying, and there's so much more to be learned about pain. You'll only be frustrated if you don't do it properly, and they won't listen to you." He was right and I obeyed. After 7 years' work, the first descriptive study of 1100 patients in St. Joseph's Hospice, London, from 1958 to 1965[2] was coupled with visits to clinical pain researchers such as Harry Beecher in Boston and many U.S. homes, social workers, and nurses in 1963. This visit included an all-important meeting with Florence Wald at Yale. A prodigious program of fundraising letters, professional articles, and meetings led to the opening of St. Christopher's Hospice in 1967, the first inpatient, home care, research, and teaching hospice. All of those early contacts and countless other interested people led to the hospice movement and the palliative care that developed within and from it.

Nurses were the first to respond to this challenge and remain the core of the personal and professional drive to enable people to find relief, support, and meaning at the end of their lives. All of the expertise described in this important collection is to this end. The window to suffering can be a window to peace and opportunity. The nurse, in her or his skilled competence and compassion, has a unique place to give each person the essential message, "You matter because you are you and you matter to the last moment of your life. We will do all we can to help you, not only to die peacefully but to live until you die."[3]

Dame Cicely Saunders died in July 2005. The editors and all nurses in hospice and palliative care are grateful for her life contributions.

REFERENCES

1. Saunders CM. Care of the dying. *Nursing Times* reprint. London: Macmillan, 1976.
2. Clark D. "Total pain," disciplinary power and the body in the work of Cicely Saunders, 1958–67. Soc Sci Med 1999;49:727–736.
3. Saunders C. Care of the dying. 1. The problem of euthanasia. Nurs Times 1976;72:1003–1005.

Florence Wald, RN, FAAN
Branford, Connecticut

Nurses of my generation in the second half of the twentieth century were fortunate to be part of the hospice movement and to respond to an eager public with an alternative way of care for the dying. Medical sociologists' studies of hospital culture showed what many nurses already knew, that when technological intervention failed to stop the course of disease, physicians could not see that the treatment was futile or join the patient in a willingness to cease.

By 1950, nurses began to carry out studies as principal investigators and were on their way to being respected by other disciplines. Two outstanding leaders were Hilde Peplau and Virginia Henderson, both educated nurses in clinical practice who established a foundation for the advanced nurse practitioner to be a valued member of an interdisciplinary team.

This surfaced first in psychiatric nursing, but as hospice care came into being, the nurse became a pivotal part of the interdisciplinary team. "Hospice nursing," Virginia Henderson said, "was the essence of nursing"; volunteers came quickly into hospice care, proving Henderson's precept and giving the lay individual "the necessary strength, will, and knowledge to contribute to a peaceful death."[1]

Physicians in the forefront of medical ethics, such as Edmund Pellegrino and Raymond Duff, encouraged physicians to recast their roles as decision makers and communicators so that the whole team could keep the patients' values and the families' wants the prime concern.

The works of those who have brought alternative therapies into use, for example, Martha Rogers and Barbara Dossey, have added to the spiritual dimensions of care. The growth of the religious ministry movement and the creative addition of the arts and environment round out the cast of contributors.

Reviewing the progress we nurses have made allows us to proceed more effectively.

REFERENCE

1. Henderson V. Basic Principles of Nursing Care. London: International Council of Nurses, 1961:42.

Jeanne Quint Benoliel, DNSc, FAAN
Professor Emeritus
Psychosocial and Community Health School of Nursing
University of Washington
Seattle, Washington

At the end of the Second World War in 1945, people in Western societies were tired of death, pain, and suffering. Cultural goals shifted away from war-centered activities to a focus on progress, use of technology for better living, and improvements in the health and well-being of the public. Guided by new scientific knowledge and new technologies, health care services became diversified and specialized and lifesaving at all costs became a powerful driving force. End-of-life care was limited to postmortem rituals, and the actual caregiving of dying patients was left to nursing staff. Palliative nursing in those days depended on the good will and personal skills of individual nurses, yet what they offered was invisible, unrecognized, and unrewarded.

Thanks to the efforts of many people across the years, end-of-life care is acknowledged today as an important component of integrated health care services. Much knowledge has accrued about what makes for good palliative care, and nurses have been in the forefront of efforts to improve quality of life for patients and families throughout the experience of illness. This book is an acknowledgment of the important part played by nurses in helping patients to complete their lives in a context of care and human concern.

PREFACE

For Every Nurse—A Palliative Care Nurse

Betty Rolling Ferrell, RN, PhD, FAAN
Research Scientist
City of Hope National Medical Center

Nessa Coyle, RN, PhD, FAAN
Pain and Palliative Care Service
Memorial Sloan Kettering Cancer Center

The first edition of *Textbook of Palliative Nursing* was published in 2001. Since that time the field of palliative nursing has evolved quite dramatically.

One major advance has been the extension of the principles of palliative care into all settings of care, as reflected in these pages. Initially found only in hospice units or oncology units, or in settings that focused on the care of individuals with HIV/AIDS, palliative nursing is now practiced in emergency departments, intensive care units, neonatal intensive care units, renal dialysis centers, pediatric care facilities, and many other settings.

In addition, much has happened since the first edition of this textbook to bring long-overdue attention to the area of pediatric palliative care. Of great importance has been the Report by the Institute of Medicine on Pediatric Palliative Care. This second edition of the *Textbook of Palliative Nursing* thus includes an expanded section on pediatric palliative care. This enhanced section includes new chapters on pediatric bereavement as well as care in the neonatal intensive care unit. The authors of these chapters are leaders in the field who have lived the work of caring for children and their families as well as contributed to the evolving literature, research, and model programs. We are greatly indebted to them for their leadership, and hope that this expanded section will be a valuable resource for all nurses in palliative care.

The basic assumptions of palliative nursing—the principles of attention to physical pain and suffering as well as existential distress; inclusion of the family as the unit of care; extension of care into bereavement; interdisciplinary care; and many other basic tenets of the field—are applicable across the very diverse profession of nursing. For this reason we believe that *every* nurse should be a palliative care nurse. We therefore dedicate this second edition of the *Textbook of Palliative Nursing* to every nurse, for each of us will have the opportunity to provide comfort and compassion to patients in our everyday practice. May we all strive to advance our knowledge and improve the quality of care in serving patients and families faced with serious illness.

About the Forewords

On the previous pages readers will find three Forewords, written for the first edition by three pioneers in the field of palliative nursing: Dame Cicely Saunders, founder of the modern hospice movement; Florence Wald, founder of the first hospice in America; and Jeanne Quint Beneliel, pioneer in psychosocial nursing and the role of nursing in caring for the terminally ill. We have reprinted the Forewords from these pioneers in the second edition because we believe that their legacy is an enduring contribution to all that has come to be known as palliative nursing care. We are indebted to these women and to the many other nurses who have brought the field of palliative care to the forefront, and whose dedication will provide a foundation for us in the future.

Acknowledgments

The editors acknowledge the assistance of Megan Grimm, MPH, who served as our research assistant throughout the process of this second edition. Her commitment and attention to detail were greatly appreciated and are reflected on every page of this text.

CONTENTS

CONTRIBUTORS

Paula R. Anderson, RN, MN
Clinical Trials Coordinator
University of Texas Southwestern
Moncrief Cancer Center
Fort Worth, Texas

Sanchia Aranda, RN, BApp Sci (Adv Nurs), MN, Cert Onc, PhD
Professor/Director of Cancer Nursing Research
Peter MacCallum Cancer Centre and School of Nursing
University of Melbourne
Melbourne, Victoria, Australia

Marie Bakitas, MS, ARNP, DNSc(c), FAAN
Adult Nurse Practitioner
Section of Palliative Medicine
Dartmouth Hitchcock Medical Center
Lebanon, New Hampshire

Barbara M. Bates-Jensen, PhD, RN, CWOCN
Adjunct Assistant Professor
University of California, Los Angeles, School of Medicine
Division of Geriatrics and Jewish Home for the Aged
Anna and Harry Borun Center for Gerontological Research
Los Angeles, California

Susan Berenson, RN, MSN, OCN
Clinical Nurse Specialist
Department of Integrative Medicine
Memorial Sloan-Kettering Cancer Center
New York, New York

Patricia Berry, PhD, APRN, BC-PCM
Assistant Professor
Co-Director, Geriatric Nursing Leadership Program
University of Utah
Salt Lake City, Utah

Marilyn Bookbinder, RN, PhD
Director of Nursing
Department of Pain Medicine and Palliative Care
Beth Israel Medical Center
New York, New York

Tami Borneman, RN, MSN, CNS
Senior Research Specialist
Department of Nursing Research and Education
City of Hope National Medical Center
Duarte, California

Carleen Brenneis, RN, MHSA
Program Director
Regional Palliative Care Program
Grey Nuns Community Hospital
Edmonton, Alberta, Canada

Pam Brown, RN, MSN
Director
Seniors Health and Palliative Care
Calgary Health Region
Calgary, Alberta, Canada

Katherine Brown-Saltzman, RN, MA
Executive Director
University of California, Los Angeles, Ethics Center
Assistant Clinical Professor
University of California, Los Angeles, Medical Center
University of California, Los Angeles, School of Nursing
Los Angeles, California

Eduardo Bruera, MD
Chair, Department of Palliative Care and Rehabilitation Medicine
University of Texas MD Anderson Cancer Center
Houston, Texas

Ira Byock, MD
Professor of Anesthesiology and Community and Family Medicine
Dartmouth Medical School
Director of Palliative Medicine
Dartmouth Hitchcock Medical Center
Lebanon, New Hampshire

Maura Byrnes-Casey, RN, MA, PNP-BC
Nurse Practitioner
Department of Pediatrics
Memorial Sloan-Kettering Cancer Center
New York, New York

Fern Campbell, RN, MSN, FNP
Pediatric Urology Nurse Practitioner
Department of Urology
University of Virginia
Charlottesville, Virginia

Margaret Campbell RN, PhD(c), FAAN
Nurse Practitioner
Palliative Care and Clinical Ethics
Detroit Receiving Hospital
Detroit, Michigan

Eleanor Canning, RN, BSN
Regional Director, Business Development
Visiting Nurse Service of New York
Jericho, New York

Nathan Cherny, MBBS, FRACP, FRCP
Director, Cancer Pain and Palliative Medicine
Shaare Zedek Medical Center
Jerusalem, Israel

Douglas Cluxton, MA, LPC
Project Coordinator
Ohio Hospice and Palliative Care Organization
Community Educator
HomeReach Hospice
Columbus, Ohio

John J. Collins, MBBS, PhD, FRACP
Head
Department of Pain Medicine and Palliative Care
Children's Hospital at Westmead
Sydney, Australia

Peggy Compton, RN, PhD
Associate Professor
University of California, Los Angeles, School of Nursing
Los Angeles, California

Inge B. Corless, RN, PhD, FAAN
Professor
Graduate Program in Nursing
MGH Institute of Health Professions
Boston, Massachusetts

Nessa Coyle, RN, PhD, FAAN (Editor)
Pain and Palliative Care Service
Memorial Sloan-Kettering Cancer Center
New York, New York

Patrick J. Coyne, MSN, APRN, FAAN
Clinical Nurse Specialist for Pain/Palliative Care
Clinical Director of Thomas Palliative Care Services
Virginia Commonwealth University Health Care Systems
Richmond, Virginia

Constance M. Dahlin, RN, MSN, APRN, BC, PCM
Palliative Care Specialist and Nurse Practitioner
Palliative Care Service
Massachusetts General Hospital
Boston, Massachusetts

Kathleen Daretany, MA, APRN, BC-PCM
Palliative Care Nurse Educator—Project ENABLE II
Dartmouth College/Dartmouth-Hitchcock Medical Center
Center for Psycho-Oncology Research
Lebanon, New Hampshire

Betty Davies, RN, PhD, FAAN
Professor
Department of Family Health Care Nursing
School of Nursing
University of California, San Francisco
San Francisco, California

Grace E. Dean, PhD, RN
Postdoctoral Fellow
School of Nursing
Center for Sleep and Respiratory Neurobiology
University of Pennsylvania
Philadelphia, Pennsylvania

Susan Derby, RN, MA, CGNP
Nurse Practitioner
Pain and Palliative Care Service
Memorial Sloan-Kettering Cancer Center
New York, New York

Ruth Yorkin Drazen
Filmmaker
New York, New York

Deborah Dudgeon, MD, FRCPC
W. Ford Connell Professor of Palliative Care Medicine
Queen's University
Kingston, Ontario, Canada

Anna R. Du Pen, ARNP, MN
Palliative Care Nurse Practitioner
Peninsula Pain Clinic
Bremerton, Washington

Lynne Early, RN, MSN, ONP, OCN, CWOCN
Oncology Nurse Practitioner
University of Southern California
Kenneth Norris, Jr., Cancer Center
Santa Barbara, California

Denice Caraccia Economou, RN, MN, AOCN
Manager, Pain and Symptom Management
Aptium Oncology
Los Angeles, California

Kathleen A. Egan, MA, BSN, CHPN
Vice President
Hospice Institute of the Florida Suncoast
Clearwater, Florida
Community Director
The Center for Hospice, Palliative Care and End-of-Life Studies
University of Southern Florida
Tampa, Florida

Nancy English, PhD, APRN
Clinical Faculty
University of Colorado Health Science Center
School of Nursing
Denver, Colorado

Mary Ersek, PhD, RN
Research Scientist
Pain Research Department
Swedish Medical Center
Seattle, Washington

Laura A. Espinosa, RN, MS, CS
Administrative Director of Heart and Vascular Services
Memorial Hermann Hospital
Houston, Texas

Betty R. Ferrell, RN, PhD, FAAN (Editor)
Research Scientist
Department of Nursing Research and Education
City of Hope National Medical Center
Duarte, California

Perry G. Fine, MD
Professor
Department of Anesthesiology
University of Utah
Pain Management and Research Center
Salt Lake City, Utah

Regina Fink, RN, PhD, FAAN, AOCN
Research Nurse Scientist
University of Colorado Hospital
Denver, Colorado

Wayne L. Furman, MD
Member
Department of Hematology-Oncology
St. Jude's Children's Research Hospital
Memphis, Tennessee

Rose Gates, RN, PhD(c), CNS/NP, AOCN
Oncology Nurse Practitioner
Rocky Mountain Cancer Center
Colorado Springs, Colorado

David F. Giansiracusa, MD
Co-Director, Pain and Palliative Care Service
Division of Psychosocial Oncology and Palliative Care
Dana Farber Cancer Institute and Brigham and Women's Hospital
Boston, Massachusetts

Elaine Glass, RN, MS, APRN, BC-PCM
Clinical Nurse Specialist
Palliative Care at Grant Medical Center
Columbus, Ohio

Tessa Goldsmith, MA, CCC/SLP
Clinical Specialist
Department of Speech-Language Pathology
Massachusetts General Hospital
Boston, Massachusetts

Mary Layman Goldstein, RN, MS, APRN, BC
Nurse Practitioner
Pain and Palliative Service
Memorial Sloan-Kettering Cancer Center
New York, New York

Marcia Grant, DNSc, RN, FAAN
Research Scientist and Director
Department of Nursing Research and Education
City of Hope National Medical Center
Duarte, California

Mikel Gray, PhD, FNP, PNP, CUNP, FAAN
Professor and Nurse Practitioner
Department of Urology and School of Nursing
University of Virginia
Charlottesville, Virginia

Julie Griffie, MSN, CS, AOCN
Clinical Nurse Specialist, Cancer Program
Froedtert Hospital
Milwaukee, Wisconsin

Debra E. Heidrich, MSN, RN, CHPN, AOCN
Consultant, Pain and Palliative Care
West Chester, Ohio

Melody Brown Hellsten MS, APRN-BC, PNP
Pediatric Nurse Practitioner
University of Texas Health Science Center, San Antonio
Program Coordinator
Pediatric Palliative and Supportive Care
CHRISTUS Santa Rosa Children's Hospital
San Antonio, Texas

Pamela S. Hinds, PhD, RN, CS
Director of Nursing Research
Division of Nursing Research
St. Jude Children's Research Hospital
Memphis, Tennessee

Marianne Jensen Hjermstad, RN, MPH, PhD
Associate Professor
University of Trondheim
Research Coordinator
Ulleval University Hospital HF
Oslo, Norway

Anne Hughes, APRN, MN, FAAN
Advance Practice Nurse, Palliative Care
Laguna Honda Hospital and Rehabilitation Center
San Francisco Department of Public Health
San Francisco, California

Juhye Jin, RN, MS
Doctoral Student
Department of Family Health Care Nursing
School of Nursing
University of California, San Francisco
San Francisco, California

Gloria Juarez, RN, PhD
Assistant Research Scientist
Department of Nursing Research and Education
City of Hope National Medical Center
Duarte, California

Marta H. Junin, RN
Palliative Care Service
Bonorino Udaondo Hospital
Palliative Care Nurse Educator
University of Buenos Aires
Buenos Aires, Argentina

Javier Kane, MD
Associate Professor, Department of Pediatrics
University of Texas Health Science Center, San Antonio
Medical Director, Pediatric Palliative Care Program
CHRISTUS Santa Rosa Children's Hospital
San Antonio, Texas

Stein Kaasa, MD, PhD
Professor
Pain and Palliation Research Group
Department of Cancer Research and Molecular Medicine
Faculty of Medicine
The Norwegian University of Science and Technology and The Palliative Medicine Unit
St. Olavs Hospital
Trondheim, Norway

David Kahn, PhD, RN
Associate Professor on Leave
School of Nursing
University of Texas at Austin
Austin, Texas
Visiting Scholar
Institute of Anthropology
Department of Human Development
Tzu chi Buddhist University
Haulien, Taiwan

Pamela Kedziera, RN, MSN, AOCN
Clinical Nurse Specialist
Pain Management Center
Fox Chase Cancer Center
Philadelphia, Pennsylvania

Charles Kemp, FNP, FAAN
Senior Lecturer
Baylor University
Dallas, Texas

Carole Kenner, DNS, RNC, FAAN
Dean/Professor
University of Oklahoma College of Nursing
Oklahoma City, Oklahoma

Cynthia King, PhD, NP, MSN, RN, FAAN
Program Director for Nursing Research
Assistant Professor
Public Health Services, Social Science and Public Policy
Wake Forest University Baptist Medical Center
Winston-Salem, North Carolina

Kenneth L. Kirsh, PhD
Assistant Professor
Assistant Director for Research
Symptom Management and Palliative Care Program
Division of Hematology/Oncology
Department of Internal Medicine
Markey Cancer Center
University of Kentucky
Lexington, Kentucky

Andrew Knight, RN, MA
Princess Alice Hospice
West End Land
Esher, Surrey, United Kingdom

Patti Knight, RN, MSN, CS, CHPN
Palliative Care Unit Patient Manager
Department of Palliative Care and Rehabilitation Medicine
University of Texas MD Anderson Cancer Center
Houston, Texas

Linda J. Kristjanson, RN, PhD
The Cancer Council of Western Australia
Chair of Palliative Care
School of Nursing & Public Health
Edith Cowan University
Churchlands, Western Australia

Kim K. Kuebler, MN, RN, ANP-CS
Regional Medical Scientist
Boehringer-Ingelheim Pharmaceuticals
Palliative Care Nurse Practitioner
Adjuvant Therapies, Inc.
Atlanta, Georgia

Mary J. Labyak, MSW, LCSW
President and Chief Executive Officer
The Hospice of the Florida Suncoast
Largo, Florida

Margaret Anne Lamb, PhD, RN
Adjunct Associate Professor
Department of Nursing
University of New Hampshire
Durham, New Hampshire

Marcia Levetown, MD, FAAP
Pain and Palliative Care Education Consultant
Houston, Texas

Laurie Lyckholm, MD
Associate Professor of Internal Medicine
Hematology/Oncology and Palliative Care Medicine
Virginia Commonwealth University School of Medicine
Richmond, Virginia

Polly Mazanec, MSN, APRN, BC, AOCN
Nurse Practitioner
Safe Conduct Team
University Hospitals of Cleveland
Ireland Cancer Center
Cleveland, Ohio

Ruth McCorkle, PhD, FAAN
Florence S. Wald Professor of Nursing and Director
Center for Excellence in Chronic Illness Care
Yale University School of Nursing
New Haven, Connecticut

Sylvia McSkimming, PhD, RN
Executive Director
Supportive Care of the Dying: A Coalition for Compassionate Care
Providence Health System
Portland, Oregon

Kathleen Michael, PhD, RN, CRRN
Program Manager
The Claude D. Pepper Center
Geriatric Research Education Clinical Center
University of Maryland
Veterans Administration Medical Center
Baltimore, Maryland

Paula Milone-Nuzzo, PhD, RN, FAAN, FHHC
Professor and Director
School of Nursing
Associate Dean for International Partnerships
College of Health and Human Development
Pennsylvania State University
University Park, Pennsylvania

Pamela A. Minarik, MS, APRN, BC, FAAN
Professor of Nursing
Professor, Office of International Affairs
Yale University School of Nursing
Psychiatric Consultation Liaison Clinical Nurse Specialist
Yale-New Haven Hospital
New Haven, Connecticut

Leslie Nield-Anderson, APRN, BC, PhD
Private Practice
Geropsychiatric Consultant
Sunhill Medical Center
Sun City Center, Florida

Kaye Norris, PhD
Private Consultant
Kaye Norris Consulting: Research and Evaluation
Missoula, Montana

Linda Oakes, MSN, RN, CCNS
Pain Clinical Nurse Specialist
St. Jude's Children's Research Hospital
Memphis, Tennessee

Sean O'Mahony, MBBCh, BAO
Medical Director
Palliative Care Service
Montefiore Medical Center
Assistant Professor
Albert Einstein College of Medicine
Bronx, New York

Judith A. Paice, PhD, RN, FAAN
Director, Cancer Pain Program
Division of Hematology-Oncology
Northwestern University
Feinberg School of Medicine
Chicago, Illinois

Joan T. Panke, RN, APRN, BC-PCM
Palliative Care Coordinator
Washington Cancer Institute
Washington Hospital Center
Washington, DC

Jeannie V. Pasacreta, PhD, FAAN
Private Practice
Adult and Family Integrated Mental Health Services
Newtown, Connecticut

Steven D. Passik, PhD
Associate Attending Psychologist
Memorial Sloan-Kettering Cancer Center
New York, New York

Richard Payne, MD
Director and Esther Colliflower Professor
Duke Institute on Care at the End of Life
Duke University School of Divinity
Durham, North Carolina

Stacey Pejsa
Coordinator
Department of Nursing Research and Education
City of Hope National Medical Center
Duarte, California

Elizabeth Ford Pitorak, MSN, APRN, CHPN
Director of the Hospice Institute
Hospice of the Western Reserve
Cleveland, Ohio

Kathleen Puntillo, RN, DNSc, FAAN
Professor of Nursing
Department of Physiological Nursing
University of California, San Francisco
San Francisco, California

Patrice Rancour, MS, RN, CS
Prospective Health Care Program Manager
Ohio State University Faculty/Staff Wellness Program
Columbus, Ohio

Michelle Rhiner, RN, MSN, NP, CHPN
Patient Coordinator/Manager
Supportive Care, Pain and Palliative Medicine
City of Hope National Medical Center
Duarte, California

Jeanne Robison, RN, MN, ARNP
Director of Medical Oncology Services
Rockwood Clinic
Spokane, Washington

Ora Rosengarten, MD
Oncologist, Palliative Care Physician
Department of Medical Oncology
Shaare Zedek Medical Center
Jerusalem, Israel

Colleen Scanlon, RN, JD
Senior Vice-President, Advocacy
Catholic Health Initiatives
Denver, Colorado

Susie Seaman, MSN, NP, CWOCN
Nurse Practitioner
Grossmont Hospital Wound Healing Center
Sharp HealthCare
La Mesa, California

Denice K. Sheehan, RN, MSN, PhD(c)
Palliative Care Consultant
Twinsburg, Ohio

Deborah Witt Sherman, PhD, APRN, ANP, BC-PCM, FAAN
Associate Professor and Program Coordinator of the Advanced Practice Palliative Care Master's and Post Master's Programs
New York University
New York, New York

Neal E. Slatkin, MD, DABPM
Director
Supportive Care, Pain and Palliative Medicine
City of Hope National Medical Center
Duarte, California

Jean K. Smith, RN, MS, OCN
Lymphedema Clinical Nurse Specialist
Centura Health Penrose Cancer Center
Colorado Springs, Colorado

Thomas J. Smith, MD, FACP
Chairman of Hematology/Oncology and Palliative Care Medicine
Virginia Commonwealth University School of Medicine
Richmond, Virginia

Karen J. Stanley RN, MSN, AOCN, FAAN
Nursing Consultant
President, Oncology Nursing Society
Greenwich, Connecticut

Daphne Stannard, RN, PhD, CCRN, CCNS
Assistant Professor
San Francisco State University School of Nursing
San Francisco, California

Richard Steeves, PhD, RN, FAAN
Associate Professor
University of Virginia School of Nursing
Charlottesville, Virginia

Lizabeth H. Sumner, RN, BSN
Adjunct Faculty
University of Chicago, Illinois
School of Nursing
Consultant, Palliative Care
Vista, California

Virginia Sun, RN, MSN
Senior Research Specialist
Department of Nursing Research and Education
City of Hope National Medical Center
Duarte, California

Elizabeth Johnston Taylor, PhD, RN
Associate Professor
School of Nursing
Loma Linda University
Loma Linda, California

Jeanne Twohig, MPA
Deputy Director
Duke Institute of Care at the End of Life
Durham, North Carolina
Deputy Director
Promoting Excellence in End-of-Life Care
Missoula, Montana

Mary L. S. Vachon, RN, PhD
Psychotherapist and Consultant in Private Practice
Full Professor
Departments of Psychiatry and Public Health Science
University of Toronto
Toronto, Ontario, Canada

Catherine Vena, PhD, RN
Postdoctoral Fellow
Woodruff Postdoctoral Instititute
Nell Hodgson School of Nursing
Emory University
Atlanta, Georgia

Rose Virani, RNC, MHA, OCN
Senior Research Specialist
Department of Nursing Research and Education
City of Hope National Medical Center
Duarte, California

Deborah L. Volker, PhD, RN, AOCN
Assistant Professor
The University of Texas at Austin
School of Nursing
Austin, Texas

Ashby C. Watson, APRN, BC, OCN
Psychosocial Oncology Clinical Nurse Specialist
Virginia Commonwealth University Medical Center
Richmond, Virginia

Sarah A. Wilson, PhD, RN
Associate Professor
Director, Institute for End-of-Life Education
Marquette University College of Nursing
Milwaukee, Wisconsin

Robert Zalenski, MD, MA
Palliative Medicine Consultant
John D. Dingell Veterans Hospital
Director of Clinical Research
Professor, Emergency Medicine and Cardiology
Wayne State University School of Medicine
Detroit, Michigan

Laurie Zoloth-Dorfman, PhD, RN
Professor of Medical Humanities and Bioethics and of Religion
Director of Bioethics, Center for Genetic Medicine
Northwestern University
Feinberg School of Medicine
Chicago, Illinois

Textbook of **Palliative Nursing**

I

General Principles

1

Nessa Coyle

Introduction to Palliative Nursing Care

They said there was "nothing to do" for this young man who was "end stage." He was restless and short of breath; he couldn't talk and looked terrified. I didn't know what to do, so I patted him on the shoulder, said something inane, and left. At 7 AM he died. The memory haunts me. I failed to care for him properly because I was ignorant.—A young clinician who later became a palliative care expert

- ***Key Points***
- *Palliative nursing reflects "whole person" care.*
- *Palliative nursing combines a scientific approach with a humanistic approach to care.*
- *The caring process is facilitated through a combination of science, presence, openness, compassion, mindful attention to detail, and teamwork.*
- *The patient and family is the unit of care.*
- *The goal of palliative nursing is to promote quality of life across the illness trajectory through the relief of suffering, including care of the dying and bereavement follow-up.*

"I failed to care for him properly because I was ignorant"—these are haunting words, and they are as true today as they were several decades earlier. Clinicians cannot practice what they do not know. However, the opposite is also true: Individuals and their families, struggling to live in the face of progressive, symptomatic, and debilitating disease, can be well cared for and supported throughout this process and find meaning and peace in the face of death. This is the essence of skilled palliative nursing care—to facilitate the "caring" process through a combination of science, presence, openness, compassion, mindful attention to detail, and teamwork. Although we have both the knowledge and the art to control the majority of symptoms that occur during the last months, weeks, and days of life, we still have much to learn about how to alleviate the psychological and spiritual distress that comes with life-threatening illness.[1]

Shifting the Paradigm of End-of-Life Care to Palliative Care

Advances in health care have changed the trajectory of dying. Improved nutrition and sanitation, preventive medicine, widespread vaccination use, the development of broad-spectrum antibiotics, and an emphasis on early detection and treatment of disease have resulted in fewer deaths in infancy and childhood and fewer deaths from acute illness.[2,3] The combination of a healthier population in many developed countries and effective treatments for disease has resulted in the ability to prolong life. This has led to both benefits and challenges for society. For example, in the United States, more than 70% of those who die each year are 65 years of age or older. The majority of these deaths, however, occur after a long, progressively debilitating chronic illness, such as cancer, cardiac disease, renal disease, lung disease, or acquired immunodeficiency syndrome

(AIDS).[2] It is also now recognized that the palliative care needs and end-of-life needs of children have long been ignored.[4] The field of palliative care nursing has expanded in response to these challenges. It has built on the long tradition of hospice care and the models of excellent nursing care within hospice.

The Relationship of Hospice Care to Palliative Care

The hospice model of care was developed to address the specific needs of the dying and of their families, so long neglected by the medical system of care. The modern hospice movement started in England in 1967, through the work of Dame Cicely Saunders and colleagues at St. Christopher Hospice in London. The hospice movement came to the United States in the mid-1970s, when Dr. Florence Wald, a nursing pioneer, led an interdisciplinary team to create the first American hospice.[5]

Hospice care became a Medicare benefit in the 1980s. Patients traditionally followed in hospice programs could no longer receive life-prolonging therapy, and it was required that they be certified by a physician as having a life expectancy of 6 months or less. This presented a problem for patients living with a chronic debilitating disease, whose life expectancy was unclear or was greater than 6 months, or who, for a variety of reasons, did not want to be "identified" as a hospice patient. The palliative care and family-centered care provided through hospice programs was needed, but the barriers presented by the rationing of hospice programs (based on prognosis) and the requirement of denying life-prolonging therapies deprived many individuals of the benefit of such care.

The palliative care model evolved from the traditional hospice perspective to address quality-of-life concerns for those patients living for prolonged periods with a progressive, debilitating disease. It recognized the change in the trajectory of dying in many industrial countries, from that of a relatively short illness leading to death, to one involving a progressive and prolonged debilitating illness frequently associated with multiple factors affecting the quality of life. It recognized that such factors required skilled and compassionate palliative care interventions regardless of prognosis, life-prolonging therapy, or closeness to death. In looking at the relationship between hospice and palliative care, perhaps hospice can best be described as a program through which palliative care is intensified as an individual moves closer to death. Ideally, patients and families living with a chronic debilitating and progressive disease could receive palliative care throughout the course of their disease and its treatment, and as they come closer to death could transition seamlessly and without added distress into a hospice program of care.

World Health Organization Definition of Palliative Care

In recognition of the changing trajectory of dying and the implications for palliative care, the World Health Organization (WHO) has modified its 1982 definition of palliative care to the following: "Palliative care is an approach to care which improves quality of life of patients and their families facing life-threatening illness, through the prevention, assessment and treatment of pain and other physical, psychological and spiritual problems."[6]

The new WHO definition broadens the scope of palliative care beyond end-of-life care and suggests that such an approach can be integrated with life-prolonging therapy and should be enhanced as death draws near. In a similar vein, the National Comprehensive Cancer Network (NCCN) developed guidelines to facilitate the "appropriate integration of palliative care into anticancer therapy."[7] The focus of all these efforts is to change the standard practice of palliative care (identified as "too little, too late")—in which there is a distinct separation between diagnosis, treatment, and end-of-life care—to a vision of the future in which there is "front-loading" of palliative care.[8] This means, for example, that at the time of the cancer diagnosis and initiation of treatment the patient would also have access to psychological counseling, nutrition services, pain management, fatigue management, and cancer rehabilitation.[8] Such a model is appropriate for other chronic diseases as well. Medicaring, a national demonstration project spearheaded by the Center to Improve Care of the Dying, is an example of an attempt to integrate palliative care into the medical and disease management for seriously ill patients with cardiac and pulmonary disease, who have a life expectancy between 2 to 3 years. The intent is to make this program a Medicare benefit, as is the case with hospice care.[9]

The Distinctive Features of Palliative Care Nursing

It is useful to define the field of palliative care nursing and to recognize how it differs in essence from other areas of nursing care. In this way, nurses can be educated and trained appropriately, and the special nature of such education and training can be recognized. Palliative care nursing reflects a "whole person" philosophy of care implemented across the lifespan and across diverse health settings. The patient and family is the unit of care. The goal of palliative nursing is to promote quality of life along the illness trajectory through the relief of suffering, and this includes care of the dying and bereavement follow-up for the family and significant others in the patient's life. Relieving suffering and enhancing quality of life include the following: providing effective pain and symptom management; addressing psychosocial and spiritual needs of the patient and family; incorporating cultural values and attitudes into the plan of care; supporting those who are experiencing loss, grief, and bereavement; promoting ethical and legal decision-making; advocating for personal wishes and preferences; using therapeutic communication skills; and facilitating collaborative practice.

In addition, in palliative nursing, the "individual" is recognized as a very important part of the healing relationship. The nurse's individual relationship with the patient and family is seen as crucial. This relationship, together with knowledge and skills, is the essence of palliative care nursing and sets it apart from other areas of nursing practice. However, palliative care as a therapeutic approach is appropriate for all nurses to practice. It is an integral part of many nurses' daily practice, as is clearly demonstrated in work with the elderly, the neurologically impaired, and infants in the neonatal intensive care unit.

The palliative care nurse frequently cares for patients experiencing major stressors, whether physical, psychological, social, spiritual, or existential. Many of these patients recognize themselves as dying and struggle with this role, which they neither sought nor wanted. To be dying and to care for someone who is dying are two sides of a complex social phenomenon. There are roles and obligations for each person. To be labeled as "dying" affects how others behave toward an individual and how the individual behaves toward self and others.[10–12] The person is dying, is "becoming dead" (personal communication, Eric Cassell, January 1, 2000), with all that that implies at both an individual and a social level. A feeling of failure and futility may pervade the relationship between the patient and a nurse or physician not educated or trained in hospice or palliative care. They may become disengaged, and the potential for growth on the part of both patient and clinician may be lost—"I failed to care for him properly because I was ignorant . . . the memory haunts me."

The Palliative Care Nurse and the Interdisciplinary Palliative Care Team: Collaborative Practice

The composition of teams providing palliative care varies tremendously, depending on the needs of the patients and the resources available. The one common denominator is the presence of a nurse and a physician on the team. Regardless of the specific type of palliative care team, it is the nurse who serves as a primary liaison between the team, patient, and family and who brings the team plan to the bedside, whether that is in the home, the clinic, or the inpatient setting. Because of the close proximity of the nurse to the patient and family through day-to-day observation and care, there is often a shift in the balance of decision-making at the end of life from physician to nurse.[13] However, continued involvement of the physician in palliative care should still be fostered and encouraged; it is a myth that the physician need be less involved as the goal of care shifts from cure to comfort. However, a physician oriented toward life-prolonging therapies who has provided care for a given patient over a number of years may feel lost, helpless, overwhelmed, and uncertain of his or her role in the care of the dying; yet, the patient and family may feel very close to that physician and have a great need for him or her at this time. Fear of abandonment by the patient, and the desire of the physician to "do everything" rather than abandon the patient, may result in inappropriate and harmful treatment's being offered and accepted. A nurse who is educated and trained in palliative care and end-of-life care can do much to guide and support the physician during this transition and to redirect or reframe the interventions from "doing everything" toward doing everything to provide comfort and healing.

There may be other reasons why patients want to continue aggressive, life-prolonging interventions in the face of impending death. Understanding why at times aggressive medical care and life-prolonging measures are sought is an integral part of the role of the nurse on the palliative care team. This is illustrated in the following case example:

CASE STUDY

Mr. Ray, a Patient with Prostate Cancer

Mr. Ray, a 57-year-old man with far advanced prostate cancer and rapidly failing pulmonary status, wanted every measure to be used to maintain life, including a tracheostomy and respirator. He had a wonderful and caring family who wanted whatever he wanted. Staff members felt that they were doing harm by introducing these extraordinary measures but complied with the patient's wishes. Mr. Ray had fought "the odds" on several previous occasions and expected to do so again. He remained on a respirator for 6 weeks, during which time he was alert and cognitively intact. What the staff did not realize was that during this time the man was completing important work. He sold his business, which he wanted to do before he died so that his wife would not be burdened with this task after his death. Once this goal was completed, Mr. Ray gave his physician the "thumbs up" sign and indicated that he was ready to come off the respirator. The family was at peace with this decision, but the young physician who was responsible for his care and had become very close to the patient and family over the weeks struggled with the concept of prolonging death versus hastening death if the respirator was withdrawn. Some of the nursing staff were similarly troubled. It would have been easier not to have started the treatment than to start and then withdraw it. An experienced palliative care nurse mentored the young physician and nurses through their personal ethical struggles and stayed by the physician's side as he administered the sedative drug and withdrew the respirator. The patient died 2 days later; a family member was with him all the time. The young physician expressed relief that the patient had not died "right away" and said he felt more comfortable for having "not crossed the line."

Although other members of the interdisciplinary team, including the chaplain and social worker, were involved with this patient and family's care and in family and staff "debriefing" and bereavement follow-up sessions, the palliative care nurse played a central coordinating and mentoring role in meeting the needs of the patient, family, physician, and nursing staff. However, no single discipline can meet the needs of most patients and their families; an interdisciplinary team greatly enhances such care.[13]

How little is known about patients and their families, and their aspirations, is also illustrated in this case. What seems to be an irrational choice to health care providers may be eminently sensible to the patient and family. The frequent struggle and suffering of nurses and physicians as they grapple with their own mortality and with being asked to provide care they think is inappropriate or harmful for dying patients is also demonstrated. Assessment and communication skills, as well as a firm foundation in the ethical principles of palliative care and end-of-life care when treating such patients, are clearly important.

End-of-Life Care in the United States Today: Improving But Still a Long Way To Go

The inadequacy of care for the dying, who are among the most voiceless and vulnerable in our society, came into national focus during the debates over the past decade surrounding physician-assisted suicide and euthanasia. The national dialogue was fueled by the actions of Dr. Jack Kevorkian and his suicide machine; the rulings of two United States Appeals Courts on the right to die[14,15]; findings from the Study to Understand Prognoses and Preferences for Outcomes and Risks of Treatments (SUPPORT)[16]; interviews with family caretakers[17]; a review of end-of-life content in nursing and medical texts,[18,19] which reflected minimal to no such content; and the Institute of Medicine's reports on end-of-life care, with its series of recommendations to address deficiencies in care of the chronically ill and dying, both children and adults.[2,4]

Means to a Better End, a report card generated by Last Acts (a Robert Wood Johnson–funded coalition created with almost 1000 national partner organizations dedicated to end-of-life reform), was the first attempt at a comprehensive report on the state of end-of-life care in the United States.[20] Between August 30 and September 1, 2002, slightly more than 1000 Americans were surveyed by telephone and asked their opinions regarding the quality of health care at the end of life. Three quarters of those surveyed had suffered the loss of a family member or close friend in the last 5 years. Each of the 50 states and the District of Columbia were represented in the survey and were rated on eight criteria: state advance directive policies, location of death, hospice use, hospital end-of-life care services, care in intensive care units at the end of life, pain among nursing home residents, state pain policies, and the presence of palliative care–certified nurses and doctors.

The findings suggested that, "despite many recent improvements in end-of-life care and greater public awareness about it, Americans had no better than a fair chance of finding good care for their loved ones or for themselves when facing a life-threatening illness." For example, nationally only 25% of deaths occur at home, although 70% of Americans say that they would prefer to die at home; about half of all deaths occur in hospitals, but fewer than 60% of the hospitals in any given state offer specialized end-of-life services, and most states have only "fair" hospice use.[20] In 2000, there were approximately 3100 hospice programs in the United States, caring for 700,000 patients and their families. Of these patients, more than 50% had a cancer diagnosis, 10% had end-stage cardiac disease, 6% had dementia, 3% had end-stage kidney disease, and 2% had end-stage liver disease.[21]

Although the state report card measures were very disturbing, activities at the federal, state, and community levels continue to work toward improving access to skilled palliative care and end-of-life care. Some broad examples of these initiatives by professional organizations supported through philanthropic funding include the following:

- Promoting Excellence in End-of-Life Care, a program of the Robert Wood Johnson Foundation that provides grants and technical support to innovative programs throughout the United States to improve care of the dying[22]
- The End-of-Life Nursing Education Consortium (ELNEC), a national education program to improve end-of-life care[23]
- The Education on Palliative and End-of-Life Care (EPEC) project, a national program for physicians to improve end-of-life care[24]
- The pain standards supported by the Joint Commission on Accreditation of Healthcare Organizations (JCAHO), which hold institutions accountable for assessment and management of pain among the patients in their care[25]

In addition, philanthropically supported programs to improve care of the dying have been developed at a community level to meet the needs of specific populations (e.g., the Missoula Demonstration Project[26]) or underserved communities (e.g., the Harlem Palliative Care Network[27]). There are also a growing number of palliative care programs being developed within institutions and long-term care facilities, as well as end-of-life pathways and critical care pathways for the dying.[28] Home hospice programs that offer palliative care consultation services to the broader patient population are a recent innovation that may improve access to palliative care in nonhospice patients. Board certification in palliative nursing and palliative medicine are also important milestones in recognizing the specific body of knowledge and expertise necessary to practice with competence in this specialty.

Many of these professional, state, and community initiatives address the barriers identified by the National Cancer Policy Board that keep individuals with progressive cancer from receiving excellent palliative care.[29] These barriers include

- The separation of palliative and hospice care from potentially life-prolonging treatment within the health care system, which is both influenced by and affects reimbursement policy
- Inadequate training of health care personnel in symptom management and other end-of-life skills
- Inadequate standards of care and lack of accountability in caring for dying patients
- Disparities in care, when available, for African Americans and other ethnic and socioeconomic segments of the population
- Lack of information and resources for the public dealing with end-of-life care
- Lack of reliable data on the quality of life for patients dying of cancer (as well as other chronic diseases)
- Low public sector investment in palliative care and end-of-life care research and training

The National Institute of Medicine Report on improving care at the end of life[2] suggested that people should be able to achieve a "decent" or "good" death—"one that is free from avoidable distress and suffering for patients, families, and caregivers; in general accord with patients' and families' wishes; and reasonably consistent with clinical, cultural and ethical standards" (p. 24). The report and recommendations focused on the interdisciplinary nature of palliative care, of which nursing is the core discipline. Traditionally, nursing has been at the forefront in the care of patients with chronic and advanced disease, and recent advances in symptom management, combined with the growing awareness of palliative care as a public health issue, have provided the impetus for bringing together this compendium of nursing knowledge.

The general public and the health care community, of which nurses are the largest group, have been confronted with facts about care for the dying and with the task of determining how to achieve quality of life even at the end of life. In December 2001, a consortium of five national palliative care organizations came together in New York because of the identified need to expand access to palliative care for patients and families; to increase the number of reliable, high-quality programs; and to ensure quality.[30] Participants from these organizations were nominated by their peers, with palliative care nursing leadership well represented by Connie Dahlin, Betty Ferrell, Judy Lentz, and Deborah Sherman.

The National Consensus Project for Quality Palliative Care

The National Consensus Project consists of five key national palliative care organizations: American Academy of Hospice and Palliative Medicine, Center to Advance Palliative Care, Hospice and Palliative Nurses Association, National Hospice and Palliative Care Organization, and Partnership in Caring: America's Voice for the Dying. The consensus project has five goals: (1) to build national consensus concerning the definition, philosophy, and principles of palliative care through an open and inclusive process that includes the array of professionals, providers, and consumers involved in and affected by palliative care; (2) to create voluntary clinical practice guidelines for palliative care that describe the highest quality services to patients and families; (3) to broadly disseminate the clinical practice guidelines to enable existing and future programs to define better their program organization, resource requirements, and performance measures; (4) to help clinicians provide the key elements of palliative care in the absence of palliative care programs; and (5) to promote recognition, stable reimbursement structure, and accreditation initiatives.

The clinical practice guidelines cover in detail eight domains identified as being crucial to the delivery of comprehensive palliative care: the structure and process of care; the physical domain; the psychological and psychiatric domain; the social domain; the spiritual, religious, and existential domain; the cultural domain; the imminently dying patient; and ethics and the law. The guidelines were released in April 2004 and are outlined in Appendix 1–1.

The Scope and Aims of the Second Edition of the *Textbook of Palliative Nursing*

Palliative nursing is a world of many connections. To see the world of the individual, a multidimensional, multilens perspective is needed. Often, this complexity is best conveyed through simple stories.[31–33] This duality of complexity and simplicity is incorporated into the structure of the current and expanded second edition of the *Textbook of Palliative Nursing*. Each chapter is introduced by a quotation from a patient or family member, to illustrate the content of the chapter. Key Points are included as a quick reference and also as an overview of the chapter content. In addition, brief case examples are used to anchor the theoretical and practical content of the chapter in real-life situations.

The textbook, which includes an international perspective, is intended as a comprehensive resource for nurses in the emerging field of palliative care. The approach has been to incorporate the principles of palliative care nursing throughout the course of a chronic, progressive, incurable disease rather than only at the end of life. The scope is broad. The content, contributed by more than 100 national and international nurse experts and divided into 67 chapters in ten parts, covers the world of palliative care nursing.

Part I provides a general introduction to palliative nursing care and includes an in-depth discussion of hospice care as a model for quality of end-of-life care, the principles of family assessment, and the principles of communication in palliative care. Part II moves into the critical area of symptom assessment and management. Each of the 21 chapters in this section addresses the assessment and pathophysiology of the symptom, pharmacologic interventions, nondrug treatments, and patient/family teaching within the goals of palliative care. The chapter on complementary and alternative medicine has been greatly expanded, and a chapter on sedation for intractable symptoms has been added.

Part III addresses psychosocial support in palliative care and at the end of life. Here the focus is on the meaning of hope at the end of life, bereavement, family support, and planning for the death and death rituals. Spiritual care and meaning in illness are addressed in Part IV. The impact of spiritual distress on quality of life at the end of life has become increasingly clear, and the ability of the nurse to recognize such distress in patients and their families, and to make appropriate interventions and referrals, is an essential component of palliative care. Much remains to be learned in this area. An addition to this section is a chapter written by a family caregiver that gives a very personal perspective.

In Part V, the needs of special populations and cultural considerations in palliative care are addressed. Included here are the elderly, the poor and underserved, and individuals with AIDS; a new chapter covers care for the drug-addicted patient at the end of life. Part VI focuses on improving the quality of end-of-life care across settings. After a practical overview on monitoring quality and development of pathways and standards in end-of-life care, subsequent chapters discuss long-term care, home care, hospital care, intensive care, rehabilitation, and care in the outpatient or office setting. Additions to this section are chapters on palliative care in the emergency department, palliative surgery, and palliative chemotherapy and clinical trials.

It is with enormous pleasure, and in recognition of the need, that Part VII is entirely devoted to pediatric palliative care across care settings. Part VIII moves into special issues for nurses in end-of-life care and includes ethics, public policy, requests for assistance in dying, nursing education, and nursing research. Part IX explores models of excellence and innovative community projects. International models of excellence are represented here, replacing the international chapters found in the first edition of this textbook. Part X gives voice to the patient and family, exploring the concept of "a good death" through a detailed case discussion. The appendix provides a very comprehensive and useful list of community and professional resources.

The purpose of the *Textbook of Palliative Nursing* is to organize and disseminate the existing knowledge of experts in palliative care nursing and to provide a scientific underpinning for practice. The focus is on assessment and management of the wide range of physical, psychosocial, and spiritual needs of patients, their families, and staff in palliative care across clinical settings. Topics frequently cited as challenges in nursing care at the end of life—including palliative sedation, communication, ethics, research, and providing care for the underserved and homeless—are specifically addressed. As illustrated throughout, the world of palliative care nursing is complex, scientifically based, and immensely rewarding.

REFERENCES

1. Kuhl D. What dying people want: Practical wisdom for the end of life. New York: Public Affairs, 2002.
2. Field M, Cassel C. Approaching Death: Improving Care at the End of Life. Committee on Care at the End of Life, Institute of Medicine. Washington, DC: National Academy Press, 1997.
3. Corr C. Death in modern society. In: Doyle D, Hanks WC, MacDonald N, eds. Oxford Textbook of Palliative Medicine, 2nd ed. Oxford: Oxford University Press, 1998:31–40.
4. Institute of Medicine. When children die: Improving palliative and end-of-life care for children and their families. Washington, DC: National Academy Press, 2003.
5. Wald FS. Hospice care in the United States: A conversation with Florence S. Wald. JAMA 1999;281:1683–1685.
6. World Health Organization. Palliative care. Available at: http://www.who.int/hiv/topics/palliative/care/en/index.html (accessed October 23, 2004).
7. National Comprehensive Cancer Network (NCCN). Practice guidelines in oncology: Palliative care, version 1.2004. Available at: http://www.nccn.org (accessed October 23, 2004).
8. Oncology Roundtable. Culture of Compassion: Best Practices in Supportive Oncology. Washington, DC: The Advisory Board Company, 2001:98–99.
9. Washington Home Center for Palliative Care Studies (CPCS). Medicaring. Available at: http://www.medicaring.org (accessed October 23, 2004).
10. Cassell EJ. Diagnosing suffering: A perspective. Ann Intern Med 1999;131:531–534.
11. Aries P. Western attitudes towards death: From the Middle Ages to the present. Baltimore, Md.: Johns Hopkins University Press, 1974.
12. Cherny N, Coyle N, Foley KM. Suffering in the advanced cancer patient. Part I: A definition and taxonomy. J Palliat Care 1994; 10:57–70.
13. Ingham J, Coyle N. Teamwork in end-of-life care: A nurse-physician perspective on introducing physicians to palliative care concepts. In: Clark D, Hockley J, Ahmedzai S. New Themes in Palliative Care. Buckingham: Open University Press, 1997: 255–274.
14. United States Court of Appeals for the Ninth Circuit. Compassion in Dying v. State of Washington. Fed Report. 1996 Mar 6 (date of decision);79:790–859.
15. United States Court of Appeals for the Second Circuit. Quill v. Vacco. Fed Report. 1996 Apr 2 (date of decision);80:716–743.
16. SUPPORT principal investigators. A controlled trial to improve care for seriously ill hospitalized patients: The Study to Understand Prognoses and Preferences for Outcomes and Risks of Treatments (SUPPORT). JAMA 1995;274:1591–1598.
17. Lynn J, Teno JM, Phillips RS, Wu AW, Desbiens N, Harrold J, Claessens MT, Wenger N, Kreling B, Connors AF Jr. for SUPPORT investigators. Perceptions by family members of the dying experience of older and seriously ill patients. Study to Understand Prognoses and Preferences for Outcomes and Risks of Treatments. Ann Intern Med 1997;126:97–106.
18. Ferrell BR, Virani R, Grant M, Juarez G. Analysis of palliative care content in nursing textbooks. J Palliat Care 2000; 16: 39–47.
19. Rabow MW, Hardie GE, Fair JM, McPhee SJ. End-of-life care content in 50 textbooks from multiple specialties. JAMA. 2000; 283:771–778.

20. Last Acts. Means to a better end: A report card on dying in America today. November 2002. http://www.lastacts.org/files/misc/meansfull.pdf (accessed April 7, 2003).
21. National Hospice and Palliative Care Organization. NHPCO facts and figures. Available at: http://www.NHPCO.org/files/public/Facts%20Figures%20Feb04.pdf (accessed October 23, 2004).
22. Promoting Excellence in End-of-Life Care website. Available at: http://www.promotingexcellence.org (accessed October 23, 2004).
23. American Association of Colleges of Nurses. End-of-Life Nursing Education Consortium (ELNEC) website. Available at: http://www.aacn.nche.edu/ELNEC/ (accessed October 23, 2004).
24. The Education on Palliative and End-of-Life Care (EPEC) project website. Available at: http://www.epec.net (accessed October 23, 2004).
25. Joint Commission on Accreditation of Healthcare Organizations and National Pharmaceutical Council, Inc. Improving the quality of pain management through measurement and action. Available at: http://www.jcaho.org/news+room/health+care+issues/pain+mono_jc.pdf (accessed October 23, 2004).
26. Life's End Institute. Missoula demonstration project. Available at: http://www.missoulademonstration.org (accessed October 23, 2004).
27. Payne R, Payne TR. The Harlem Palliative Care Network. J Palliat Med 2002;5:781–792.
28. Coyle N, Schacter S, Carver AC. Terminal care and bereavement. Neurol Clin 2001;19:1005–1025.
29. Institute of Medicine and National Research Council. Improving Palliative Care for Cancer: Summary and Recommendations. Washington, DC: National Academy Press, 2001:5–9.
30. National Consensus Project for Quality Palliative Care. Available at: http://www.nationalconsensusproject.org (accessed October 23, 2004).
31. Steeves RH. Loss, grief and the search for meaning. Oncol Nurs Forum 1996;23:897–903.
32. Ferrell BR. The quality of lives: 1525 voices of cancer. Oncol Nurs Forum 1996;23:907–915.
33. Coyle, N. Suffering in the first person. In: Ferrell BF, ed. Suffering. Boston: Jones and Bartlett, 1996:29–64.

APPENDIX 1–1

Summary of the National Consensus Project Clinical Practice Guidelines

Domain 1: Structure and Practice of Care

- Care starts with a comprehensive interdisciplinary assessment of the patient and family.
- Addresses both identified and expressed needs of the patient and family.
- Education and training available.
- Team in commitment to quality improvement.
- Emotional impact of work on team members is addressed.
- Team has a relationship with hospice.

Domain 2: Physical

- Pain, other symptoms, and treatment side effects are managed using best practice.
- Team documents and communicates treatment alternatives, permitting patient/family to make informed choices.
- Family is educated and supported to provide safe/appropriate comfort measures to the patient.

Domain 3: Psychological and Psychiatric

- Psychological and psychiatric issues are assessed and managed based on best available evidence.
- Team employs pharmacologic, non pharmacologic and CAM as appropriate.
- Grief and bereavement program is available to patients and families.

Domain 4: Social

- Assessment includes family structure, relationships, medical decision-making, finances, sexuality, caregiver availability, access to medications and equipment.
- Individualized comprehensive care plans lessens caregiver burden and promotes well-being.

Domain 5: Spiritual, Religious, and Existential

- Assesses and addresses spiritual concerns.
- Recognizes and respects religious belief—provides religious support.
- Makes connections with community and spiritual religious groups or individuals as desired by patient/family.

Domain 6: Cultural

- Assesses and aims to meet cultural-specific needs of patients and families.
- Respects and accommodates range of language, dietary, habitual, and religious practices of patients and families.
- Team has access to/uses translation resources.
- Recruitment and hiring practices reflect cultural diversity and community.

Domain 7: The Imminently Dying Patient

- Team recognizes imminence of death and provides appropriate care to the patient and family.
- As patient declines, team introduces hospice referral option.
- Team educates the family on signs/symptoms of approaching death in a developmentally, age, and culturally appropriate manner.

Domain 8: Ethics and Law

- Patient's goals, preferences, and choices are respected and form basis for plan of care.
- Team is knowledgeable about relevant federal and state statutes and regulations.

(*Source:* National Consensus Project, reference 30.)

2

Kathleen A. Egan and Mary J. Labyak

Hospice Palliative Care: A Model for Quality End-of-Life Care

It made me proud that I was able to take care of my loved one at home like we wanted to do for each other. With the help and advice from hospice we were able to do it. I will never regret the time I spent caring for my husband. Sure, there were hard times, but there were also really close times. Hospice helped us prepare together and allowed us some quality time for closure. This experience has given us a sense of satisfaction and our lives more meaning. We learned to cherish each moment and memory we had and enjoy our time together. They really understood his needs as well as mine. We experienced the true meaning of unconditional love from hospice.—Spouse of a hospice patient

- ***Key Points***
- *Nurses must understand and honor each patient's and family's unique experiences near life's end, addressing the physical, emotional, and spiritual dimensions of the experience through holistic care guided by what is most important to the patient and family at this time in their lives.*
- *Hospice blends compassion and skill to support patients and families through life-limiting illnesses and caregiving, so that they may experience life and relationship completion and closure with dignity and comfort.*
- *Hospice care models are expanding to serve people across the lifespan with a variety of services that are helpful from the time of diagnosis of a life-limiting condition through bereavement, including preventive approaches of a public health model.*
- *Hospice palliative care services can be provided in all care settings or in the patient's and family's home throughout the disease process.*
- *Nurses working with the dying and bereaved can experience cumulative loss while finding great meaning and purpose in their work.*

Hospice is a program of care provided across a variety of settings, based on the understanding that dying is part of the normal life cycle. As people experience this last phase of life, hospice provides comprehensive palliative medical and supportive services, compassion, and care with the goals of comfort and quality of life closure. A hospice supports the patient through the dying process and the family through the experience of caregiving, the patient's illness, dying, and their own bereavement. Understanding that the last phase of life is as individual as each person who experiences it, a hospice advocates so that people may live the remainder of their lives with dignity and die in a manner that is meaningful to them.

Instead of asking the patient and family members to fit into a caregiving system, hospice extends services according to their unique situation and values focusing on compassionate care. Compassionate care by its very nature is shaped to fit the individual needs and values of the people involved. Hospice allows the patient and family to direct the services received, rather than having professionals direct the lives of the patient and family. Hospice focuses on the individual's and family's world and encourages personal choices and meaningful experiences concerning the process of illness, dying, and death.

Hospice's unique blend of compassion and skill helps patients and their families deal with life-limiting illnesses and caregiving so that they may (1) live each day with comfort and dignity, (2) retain control over their lives, and (3) discover renewed meaning and purpose in this time of their lives.[1]

"Family Perspectives on End-of-Life Care at the Last Place of Care," an article published in the *Journal of the American Medical Association* in January 2004, revealed that the physical and emotional needs of the dying in this country continue to be poorly met, particularly for those who die in institutions. Home-based hospice care received the highest levels of overall satisfaction from respondents in this study. The authors reported that "bereaved family members of patients with home hospice services [in contrast to other settings of care] reported higher satisfaction, fewer concerns with care and fewer unmet needs."

The study stated that "high quality end-of-life care results when health care professionals ensure desired physical comfort and emotional support, promote shared decision making, treat the dying person with respect, provide information and emotional support to family members, and coordinate care across settings." These characteristics of quality end-of-life care are integral to the interdisciplinary hospice philosophy of care.[2]

Hospice in the United States

Hospice began in the United States as a grassroots effort to improve the quality of the dying experience for patients and their families. Historically, health care delivery systems have been disease driven, with the focus on cure and rehabilitation. Approaches have focused on scientific knowledge of diseases, which drives the care processes. However, approaches to care are different when cure is the goal and when cure is no longer possible. End-stage disease progression and resulting symptoms produce different physiological responses as well as different emotional responses. Hospice care began as a grassroots effort in communities where the traditional medical model fell short of addressing those differences.

The *Standards of Practice for Hospice Programs* of the National Hospice and Palliative Care Organization (NHPCO) describes palliative care as follows:

- Palliative care is treatment that enhances comfort and improves the quality of an individual's life during the last phase of life. No specific therapy is excluded from consideration. The test of palliative care lies in the agreement between the individual, his or her physicians, the primary caregiver, and the hospice team that the expected outcome is relief from distressing symptoms, the easing of pain, and/or enhancement of the quality of life. The decision to intervene with active palliative care is based on an ability to meet stated goals rather than affect the underlying disease. An individual's needs must continue to be assessed, and all treatment options must be explored and evaluated in the context of the individual's values and symptoms. The individual's choices and decisions regarding care are paramount and must be followed.[3]
- Palliative care is considered to be the model for quality, compassionate care at the end of life. Hospice care involves a team-oriented approach to expert medical care, pain management, and emotional and spiritual support expressly tailored to the patient's needs and wishes. Support is extended to the patient's family as well. At the center of hospice is the belief that each of us should be able to live and die free of pain, with dignity, and that our families should receive the necessary support to allow us to do so.[4]

According to National Hospice Foundation research, 80% of Americans wish to die at home. Of the 2.4 million Americans who die each year, fewer than 25% actually die at home. Of the 700,000 patients who received hospice care, more than 75% died at home.[4] Hospice programs provide state-of-the-art palliative care and supportive services to individuals who are near the end of their lives, and to their family members and significant others; 24 hours a day, 7 days a week; in private homes, facility-based care settings, or wherever the patient may reside, including acute care settings. Physical, social, spiritual, and emotional care are provided by a medically directed interdisciplinary team (IDT) consisting of patients and their families, professionals, and volunteers during the last phase of an illness, the dying process, and the bereavement period.[3]

Hospice Palliative Care: A Holistic Approach Focusing on the Experience of the Patient and Family

Understanding the need for a better way to care for the dying, the hospice movement began to provide alternatives to the traditional curative model. Hospice expanded the traditional model, not only to address end-stage disease and symptom management but also to provide for the emotional, social, and spiritual dimensions of the patient's and family's illness, dying, and caregiving experiences.

The beginning of the contemporary hospice movement is credited to Dame Cicely Saunders. Beresford[5] described her pioneering work as follows: "Her concept of hospice was to combine the most modern medical techniques in terminal care with the spiritual commitment of the medieval religious orders that had once created hospices as way stations for people on pilgrimages."

The experience of the last phase of life is an individual journey involving one's mind, body, and spirit. Cassell[6] described a theory of personhood whereby each person is a holistic being with dynamic, interrelated dimensions that are affected by the changes and adaptations experienced with progressive illness and dying. These dimensions involve the physical experience of end-stage disease, the emotional experience of one's relationships, and the way in which one defines spiritual existence.[7] As the disease progresses and the physical dimensions decline, the other dimensions (i.e., interpersonal and spiritual) take on added meaning and purpose. What one defines as quality of life changes substantially for people with life-limiting illnesses. Life perspectives, goals, and needs change. It is a time of reflection on a broader sense of meaning, purpose, and relationships, based on each individual's values.

Hospice grew from this understanding of full personhood; it is designed to offer expert end-of-life care to patients and families that addresses all of these dimensions through an IDT approach. Each patient and family is supported by an IDT consisting of physicians, nurses, social workers, counselors, chaplains, therapists, home health aides, and volunteers. These disciplines reflect the expertise needed to address the varied dimensions that are affected through the course of illness, caregiving, dying, and bereavement.

Aging in the United States and End-of-Life Care

The aging of America has changed the nature and needs of people who are in their last years of life. The Medicare Hospice Benefit (MHB) was designed to provide substantial professional and material support (e.g., medications, equipment) to families caring for dying individuals at home during their last 6 months of life. The benefit was designed for, and lends itself well to, the predictable trajectory of end-stage cancers but not as well to unpredictable chronic illnesses such as congestive heart failure, chronic lung disease, stroke, and dementing illnesses.[8] An examination of hospice care and the delivery of quality end-of-life services must reflect the societal change in aging demographics and the resulting varied needs in end-of-life care models.

In our society, the overwhelming majority of dying people are elderly, and they typically die of a slowly progressing, chronic disease or of multiple coexisting problems that result in multisystem failure. Their final phase of life, which often lasts several years before death, is marked by a progressive functional dependence and associated family and caregiver burden. Hospice programs in demographic areas that represent the future of our aging society, such as Florida, have expanded their care and service options well beyond the original definition of the (MHB) to more fully respond to the frail elderly in their communities who are dying of chronic, progressive illnesses. These expanded hospice delivery models (Table 2–1) are applying hospice philosophy and services in the care of patients and their families throughout the lifespan, long before the last 6 months of life; recognizing the variable dying process; and providing an array of services and intensities of service so that individuals may age in place and stay in their own homes or wherever they choose until death. Hospice, therefore, neither hastens nor postpones death but, rather, affirms life. The focus is on quality of life closure, which begins with the patient's and family's definitions of what is most important to them for their remaining time together and is guided by their values, choices, goals, and dreams.

Hospice Palliative Care Philosophy

Hospice philosophy supports the long-term objective of creating a personalized experience with each patient and family at the end of life, whereby in the face of suffering there is opportunity to find meaning, growth, and quality end of life and relationship closure. Promoting quality of life and relationships as well as death with dignity, hospice assists the patient and family to live each day as fully as possible for the remaining time together.

Honoring the Patient's and Family's Experience

The experiences of advanced illness, dying, and caregiving have significant and profound effects on both the patient and the family. Therefore, hospice philosophy supports both patient

Table 2–1
Hospice Palliative Care Services Across the Lifespan

Community Programs	Palliative Care Programs	Home Care	Hospice	Bereavement/ Bridges
Prenatal	Decision Making Consultation	Home Care Volunteers	Medicare Hospice Benefit	Emergency Response
Early Childhood Education	Palliative Care Consulting	Counseling	Caregiver	Victims of Crime Seminars
Teen Programs	Palliative Care Units in Hospitals/NHs	Spiritual Care	Residential Care	Education
Education	Supportive Care	Children's Program	Independent Living	Camps
Information/Referral	Pain Team	HIV Programs	Inpatient	Retreats
Patient/Caregiver Support Groups	Disease State Management		Jewish Hospice	CISD
Advance Directive Consulting	Case Management		Children's Hospice	Grief Counseling
Counseling	HIV Program		HIV Programs	Peer Counseling
HIV Program	Children's Program		Long-Term Care	
Children's Program	PACE		ALF	
Long-Distance Case Management	Community-Based Chronic Care Partners		Prison Hospice	
Peer Care	Caregiver Support and Resources		Catholic Hospice	
Community Mobilization				

PACE, program of all-inclusive care for the elderly; NH, nursing home; ALF, adult living facilities; CISD, critical incident stress debriefing
Source: The Hospice of the Florida Suncoast, Largo, Florida, copyright January 2004.

and family as the unit of care. Family is defined as not only the biological relatives but also those people who are identified by the patient as significant.

Patients and families face many changes and losses during the last years of life. Patients often become concerned about the burden they may cause their family and how their family will survive after they are gone. Families become concerned about how to care for the patient, how to adapt to role changes, their reactions to their losses, and how their lives will change after the death. Families provide varying degrees and types of support, love, and compassion during times of change and crisis. As the patient becomes more dependent on others for care, families become even more significant in this process. Yet, many families have never experienced caring for a loved one who is dying, and many lack the experience of their own losses.

With understanding of the importance of these relationships and family dynamics, patient and family suffering can be minimized and experiences can be enhanced through education, support, and services. Hospice honors the intimate and important role of the family in caregiving and offers resources, education, and support so that family members can be involved in a meaningful way with the care of their loved one.

Hospice philosophy, therefore, promotes the patient and family as a single unit of care. Care does not stop after the death of the patient. Just as the patient's death experience involves the physical, emotional, spiritual, and social dimensions, survivors' reactions to caregiving and loss are experienced through the same dimensions. Bereavement-support services are continued for family caregivers for 1 year or longer after the death of the patient, assisting them through bereavement and reintegration to a different life.

Care Is Directed by Patient and Family Choices and Values

Hospice philosophy supports the understanding that dying is the patient's and family's experience. Nurses are challenged to approach the hospice care process differently from other situations. Hospice care begins and continues with ongoing facilitated discussions with the patient and family, to discern what is most important to them—their values, choices, wishes, and needs for the remaining life and death. This information becomes the foundation that directs the team in the provision of care and services. Goals become patient- and family directed rather than nurse directed. It is not about what nurses feel is best but about what the patient and family choose and decide. The care plan becomes the "patient/family care plan," and the care process is defined by what the patient and family decide is important for this time. A care process directed by patient and family values begins to differentiate the specialty of hospice nursing, with an overall goal of quality of life and relationship closure as defined by the patient and family. This goal is achieved when the patient and family are given opportunities to identify what is most important to completion of their life and relationships, finding meaning in closure, and reaching personal goals before and after the death.

Hospice Care, Palliative Care, and Curative Care

Hospice is a defined, integrated model of palliative care, which can be as aggressive as curative care, with a focus on comfort, dignity, quality of life/relationship closure, and patient/family choice. Palliative care extends the principles of hospice care to a broader population that could benefit from receiving this type of care earlier in their illness or disease process. Palliative care, ideally, would segue into hospice care as the illness progresses.

Palliative care is most appropriate when it is applied throughout the care continuum, even concurrently with curative approaches if appropriate. A patient receiving curative chemotherapy or radiation therapy could certainly benefit from palliative symptom management. From a psychological and spiritual perspective, patients and their families begin to think about the aspects of life and relationship closure from the time they recognize that the patient has an incurable disease. Emotional and spiritual support from the time of diagnosis, including preparation for remaining life, advancing illness, caregiving, death, and bereavement, creates optimal experiences. When a patient's disease process is no longer curable or reversible, aggressive curative treatment becomes increasingly inappropriate. An aggressive curative approach to care may actually cause more suffering if cure is no longer possible, or it may simply extend the period of suffering needlessly. As a patient advocate, the hospice nurse is responsible for understanding the differences between curative and palliative interventions, to avoid futile care and prevent unnecessary suffering.

The curative model of care has an inherent problem orientation. Practitioners are often trained to assess and identify "problems" and then determine how to reverse the problem and its effects. Palliative care moves beyond problem identification. The specialty of hospice nursing involves the expert management of end-stage disease symptomatology as a prerequisite to providing the opportunity for patients and families to experience life and relationship closure in ways that are personally meaningful. Hospice expands the traditional disease- and problem-orientated model to a proactive, preventive, quality of life/relationship closure orientation that reflects the full scope of the patient's and family's illness, dying, and caregiving experiences.

Through anticipation and prevention of the negative effects of physical symptoms, suffering can be decreased; this allows the patient and family the time and personal resource energy to attend to what is most important for their life and relationship closure. Moving beyond a simple problem orientation, the focus has become one of prevention of suffering and opportunity for growth rather than simply the physical reaction to disease.

A search for meaning and purpose in life is a common experience for people in their last years of life and for their families. From the individual experience of suffering, death can be a time for personal growth, deepening or reconnecting interpersonal and spiritual relationships, and preparing for death and afterlife with enrichment of meaning.

Autonomy and Choice

Hospice philosophy promotes patient and family autonomy in which illness, caregiving, and dying are in accordance with the patient's and family's desires. Hospice philosophy strongly believes in patient choice regarding all aspects of living, caregiving, dying, and grieving, including where they will die, how they will die, and with whom they will die. Respecting the patient's and family's choices is paramount to quality hospice palliative care.

One of the dying patient's and family's greatest concerns is the fear of loss of control. Many losses are anticipated and experienced by terminally ill patients and their families, including loss of bodily functions, loss of independence and self-care, loss of income with resulting financial burdens, loss of the ability to provide for loved ones, loss or lack of time to complete tasks and mend relationships, and loss of decision-making capacity. Dying patients have a right to remain in control of their lives and their deaths. They are often concerned that their wishes will not be honored, that their requests will not be answered, and that, when they are too ill to prevent it, control of their lives will be taken from them. It is critical to provide continued opportunities for choice, input, informed decision making, and the ability to change decisions as situations change.

National Hospice Foundation research shows that the top four services Americans feel are most important for a loved one who has less than 6 months to live are (1) someone to be sure that the patient's wishes are honored, (2) choice among the types of services the patient can receive, (3) pain control tailored to the patient's wishes, and (4) emotional support for the patient and family.[4]

Informed Decisions and Autonomy

Hospice philosophy has been built on the ethical principle of veracity, or truth-telling. Patients' wishes for information about their condition are respected. Patients and families have the right to be informed about their condition, treatment options, and outcomes so that they can make autonomous, informed choices and spend the rest of their life the way they choose.

Truth-telling is the essence of open, trusting relationships. A sense of knowing often relieves the burden of the unknown. Knowing and talking about diagnosis and prognosis aids in making informed decisions. Patients who have not been told about their illness naturally suspect that something is wrong or being hidden from them, which can result in frustrating, unanswered questions. When patients and families are not told the truth or information is withheld, they can no longer make informed choices about the end of life.

Autonomy results in empowerment of the patient and family to make their own informed decisions regarding life and death. Hospice encourages the discussion of advance directives but does not influence those decisions. Hospice nurses educate on these issues and offer support while the patient and family discuss and choose what is best for them. Their choices may change over time, as the disease progresses, the patient becomes more dependent, or they accomplish their life and relationship closure goals.

When advance directives such as living wills, health care surrogacy, durable power of attorney, and do-not-resuscitate orders are honored, the patient's wishes are carried out even if he or she is no longer able to communicate or to make health care decisions. With advance preparation, these directives can act in place of the patient's verbal requests to ensure that her or his wishes are honored. When patient and family members discuss advance directives together, there is often less conflict over decisions and family members are more comfortable supporting the patient's choices. When advance directives are combined with hospice philosophy, they can serve as preventive measures to ensure that patient's choices will be communicated, supported, and carried out, avoiding ethical dilemmas. It is critical to provide continued opportunities for choice, input, informed decision-making, and ability to change decisions as situations change. Hospice team members are trained to facilitate personal and family decision-making regarding care, service, and life closure issues. Often, simply having professionals comfortable enough to approach these issues allows patients and families to express their inner feelings, desires, and wishes.

Hospice care supports sensitivity in truth-telling to the degree that the patient and family choose, encouraging open communication among the patient, the family, physicians, and the hospice team. Preparation for death becomes difficult if communication is not open and truthful. With a truthful understanding and freedom of informed choice, patients are more able to control their own living and dying instead of being controlled by the disease or by the treatment plans of others. They can put their affairs in order, say their good-byes, and prepare spiritually in a way that promotes quality and dignity.

Dignity and Respect for Patients and Families

Quality end-of-life care is most effective from the patient and family perspective when the patient's lifestyle choices are maintained and his or her philosophy of life is respected. Individual patient's and family's needs vary depending on values, cultural orientation, personal characteristics, and environment. Dignity is provided when individual lifestyles are supported and respected. This requires respect for ethnicity, cultural orientation, social and sexual preferences, and varied family structures. Hospice nursing requires the provision of nonjudgmental, unconditional, positive regard when caring for patients and families, treating each person's experience as unique.

Each person and family has individual coping skills, varied dynamics, and strengths and weaknesses. It is our responsibility to accept patients and families "where they are," approaching living and dying in their own way. Patients and families should be encouraged to express any emotion, including anger, denial, or depression. By listening without being judgmental, the hospice nurse accepts the patient's and family's coping mechanisms as real and effective.

Dying patients have their own needs and wants, and hospice nurses must be open to accept direction from the patient. A patient's focus may include saving all of one's energy for visits from loved ones, loving and being loved, sharing with others one's own philosophy of life and death, reviewing one's life and family history, and sharing thoughts and prayers with one's family or caregivers. Patients' goals may include such things as looking physically attractive or intrinsically exploring the purpose and meaning of their lives. Hospice workers' openness and being prepared to accept and support the patient's and family's direction on any given visit helps facilitate and respect their goals. The patient's and family's own frame of reference for values, preferences, and outlook on life and death is considered and respected without judgment.

Respecting patients requires hospice nurses to communicate a sense of what is important to the patient and family by ensuring that they express their values and opinions, participate in care planning, make decisions regarding care and how they choose to spend their time, and participate in their own care. Fostering an environment that allows the patient and family to retain a sense of respect, control, and dignity is the foundation of hospice care and services.

The Hospice Nurse as Advocate

Enhancing quality of life and relationships is the primary goal of hospice and palliative care. Patients who, in the later stages of their life, have chosen to receive palliative care have a right to have their wishes honored and respected at all points of entry into and across the health care continuum. Optimizing quality of life and respecting patient's and family's wishes involve a great deal of commitment, collaboration, and communication. In promoting patient autonomy, hospice nurses participate as patient advocates across all care settings, supporting the choices and goals that the patient and family have selected for the remainder of their lives.

By integrating the hospice philosophies and values, the hospice nurse acts as advocate for the patient and family, to preserve their rights and protect the goals of their palliative care plan. The hospice nurse's role of professional advocacy involves collaboration with patients, families, physicians, health care institutions, and health care systems. She or he may be involved in advocating for appropriate symptom management, identifying valuable resources, gaining access to these resources, and coordinating the utilization of resources and services.

The patient, family, hospice IDT, physician, hospice organization, other health and human service providers, and legal institutions are all affected by patient choices. It is the responsibility of every care provider to respect and ensure the rights of dying patients and their families. The services provided by hospice care are what Americans want, yet 83% of Americans do not know about hospice care. Rather than reinforcing their fears about death, it is the nurse's responsibility to advocate so that every patient and family understands that hospice care provides the compassion and dignity that they want at the end of life.[2]

Hospice Palliative Care Delivery Systems

Hospice care is not defined by a distinct physical setting or individual organizational structure. It is provided in a variety of settings. Although 90% of hospice patient time is spent in a personal residence, some patients live in long-term care facilities, assisted-living facilities, hospice care centers, or other group settings. In addition, some hospices provide day care programs.[9] In 2002, approximately 3200 hospice programs were in existence in the United States. As identified by the NHPCO, the following organizational structures of hospice programs exist, with ever-expanding care and service designs to meet the needs of varied communities:

Free-standing entities represent approximately 50% of hospice programs. Free-standing is defined as being independent of affiliation to a hospital, home health care agency, or other care agency.

Hospices affiliated with hospitals are managed as departments or divisions of a hospital or health system. Approximately 31.5% of hospice programs are of this type.

Hospices affiliated with home health agencies represent approximately 18% of hospice programs.[10]

Expanded Hospice Palliative Care Models

Although hospice appears to add value to end-of-life care, and although it probably does not cost government payers significantly more, the Medicare Hospice Benefit alone is not meeting all the needs of communities for comprehensive high-quality hospice and palliative end-of-life care.[11] The most prevalent model of U.S. hospice care, the "Medicare hospice model," is not viewed as the answer to the challenge of just or equitable access to hospice care nationwide.[12] Hospices compatible with this model provide all or almost all of their care within the eligibility requirements and funding parameters of the Medicare (and Medicaid) hospice benefit; this creates numerous access barriers. These hospice models are much less likely to admit individuals who do not meet Medicare hospice eligibility requirements (i.e., those without a 6-month terminal prognosis and those who do not choose to relinquish all curative care options); they are also less able to admit individuals whose palliative care treatments and medications are costly, although the receipt of costly beneficial palliative care treatment has become increasingly more frequent.[13]

With the understanding that the Medicare hospice model needs to expand to meet the growing needs for palliative care, hospice programs nationally are developing expanded models. The NHPCO *2004 Facts and Figures* report states that more than 60% of hospice programs nationally already have services beyond those outlined in the MHB model.[10] Jennings and colleagues[12] described two models of hospice care that provide care beyond the Medicare hospice model (Table 2–2). The first of these is the *Community Hospice*;

Table 2–2
Services Provided by the Medicare Hospice Model and Extended Hospice Models

Medicare Hospice Model	Community Hospice Model (in Addition to All Medicare Hospice Model Services)	Comprehensive Hospice Model (in Addition to All Medicare Hospice Model and Community Hospice Model Services)
Core services, required by law: Florida Statutes Section 400.609(1)	Services and care for patients and families	Research/Academic endeavors
Physician	Community support groups/programs	Structured sharing of knowledge through presentations and publications
Nursing	Palliative care treatments	
Social work	General palliative care	Best practice protocols and services—designing, assessing, and educating staff
Pastoral or counseling	Caregiver programs	
Dietary counseling	Specialized staff in hospitals for supportive palliative care and pain and symptom control	Academic-based research affiliations
Bereavement counseling		Research on end-of-life care
As needed services, provided or arranged for patient	Special hospice therapy programs	Community advocacy
Physical therapy	Veteran's initiative	Partner in a community coalition on end-of-life issues
Occupational therapy	Telephone installation in patient's home	
Speech therapy	Assistance with home renovation or modification	
Massage therapy	Caregiver/Companion funded program	
Home Health Aide services	Durable medical equipment	
Infusion therapy	Pharmacy	
Medical supplies	Specialized HIV/AIDS care teams	
Durable medical equipment	Services and programs for communities at large	
Day care	Community education programs	
Homemaker/Chore services	Workplace initiatives and support	
Funeral services	Community support groups and programs	
	Community programs to youth	
	Community programs for crisis/emergency	
	Professional education	
	Faith-based initiatives	
	Cultural/Diversity initiatives	
	Community programs for the needy	

Source: Jennings et al., 2003, reference 12.

hospices compatible with this model rely on Medicare hospice revenue but also provide services that reach beyond the Medicare hospice patient to individuals who may not meet the eligibility requirements of the MHB or who do not wish to choose Medicare hospice. However, although the community hospice model is considered superior to the Medicare hospice model, a third form—the *Comprehensive Hospice Center* model—was believed by Jennings and colleagues to be better for addressing the hospice and palliative care needs of communities. Comprehensive hospices provide all the care and services provided by community hospices, but, in addition, they also have a dedicated academic mission.[12] Considering this, comprehensive hospices are "centers of excellence" for hospice and palliative care.

Hospice Palliative Care and Service Sites

Private Homes. Encompassing the philosophical principle of autonomy, hospice supports patients and families wherever they choose to live and die. The majority of hospice care is provided in the patient's private home setting. According to a Gallup poll commissioned by the NHPCO and released in 1996, hospice care coupled with a wish to die at home has widespread support among the public. In perhaps the most striking response in the survey, 88% of those polled said that they would prefer to die in the comfort of their own home, surrounded by family and friends, rather than in any health care institution.[14] Therefore, hospice supports patients' staying at home until death, if that is where they choose to die.

With so many people choosing to stay at home with family, hospice emphasizes the need to empower families so they may participate in meaningful ways in the care of their loved one. Hospice's ability to involve the family in caregiving often improves the family's perspectives and experiences. Research has shown significant differences in favor of hospice in four measures used to evaluate the quality of life of the primary caregiver (family). Primary family caregivers for hospice patients were found to be less anxious and more satisfied with their involvement in care, compared with their nonhospice counterparts.[15]

Long-Term Care Settings. As the population ages, health care professionals are challenged to provide care and services in different ways. Hospices are increasingly serving elderly people, many older than 75 years of age, who live alone or with a frail family caregiver. As evidenced by the recent expansion of elder care communities, the definition of "home" has also changed for many elderly persons and can include a variety of residential settings with various levels of assistance.

Hospice seeks to affirm life while ensuring continuity of palliative care in long-term care settings. Some hospice patients are referred while residing in long-term care, whereas others are transferred into long-term care after being served by a hospice program at home. As patient and family needs change at the end of life, hospice home care patients may find long-term care placement a chosen, necessary alternative care setting.

There are many potential benefits to a joint approach and partnership between hospices and nursing homes, but key is the experience of the resident and family as a result of coordinated resources and efforts. The potential benefits of partnership to residents and their families or significant others are detailed in Table 2–3.

Research on the benefits of hospice care in nursing homes has focused on medical dimensions of support. This research has shown that hospice residents, compared to nonhospice residents, experience fewer hospitalizations near the end of life, have fewer invasive treatments (e.g., enteral tubes, intravenous fluids, intramuscular medications), and receive analgesic

Table 2–3
Benefits of Hospice and Long-Term Care Collaboration

Benefits to Patient/Family	Benefits to Long-Term Care Facility and Staff	Benefits to Hospice Provider
Access to care expertise in both long-term care and hospice care	Additional professionals to help with care planning and provision	Professionals expert in chronic residential care
Additional attention from the increased number of people involved in care	Interdisciplinary team expertise in the specialty of palliative care	Nursing home staff who know and support the resident as their extended family
Access to counseling and spiritual care disciplines to meet the intense and varied needs that surround the end-of-life experience	Shared expertise in pain and symptom management	Extended team to help in care of resident 24 hr/day, 7 days/wk
Access to hospice volunteers who spend time with residents and provide diversional and quality-of-life activities that nursing home staff do not have time to provide	Ethical decision-making consulting services	Clinical expertise in chronic care
Access to hospice volunteers who assist and support families and significant others so they can spend more quality time with residents	Family decision-making counseling	More people to provide services near life's end
Continuity of care team providers	Hospice nursing assistant visits to supplement the increasing intensity of hands-on care	
Coverage of medications, medical supplies, and equipment related to terminal illness	Validation of residents' palliative care (and care outcomes) needs to an outside reviewer (such as federal government quality indicator outcomes that, if observed for nonpalliative care patients, would be considered negative outcomes)	
Access to professionals who specialize in supporting residents and families to a more meaningful life closure	Expertise in documenting palliative care assessment, interventions, and expected outcomes that differ from restorative/rehabilitative outcomes	
Additional support for family members providing care and anticipating life without their loved one	Volunteers to sit with residents so they are not alone	
Bereavement support for family members for up to 12 months after the resident has died	Grief support for other residents	
	Grief support for nursing home staff who experience cumulative loss with the deaths of many residents	
	Education for staff on palliative care	

Miller SC, Egan KA (In Press), reference 42.

management for daily pain that is more in agreement with guidelines for management of chronic pain in long-term care settings.[11,16,17] Family members of persons who died in nursing homes perceived improvements in care after hospice admission; they cited fewer hospitalizations and lower levels of pain and other symptoms after hospice admission.[18] Nonhospice residents in nursing homes also appeared to benefit from hospice presence in the nursing home. Nonhospice residents residing in nursing homes with a greater hospice presence (i.e., a greater proportion of residents enrolled in hospice), compared with those in homes with limited or no hospice presence, were less frequently hospitalized at the end of life and more frequently had a pain assessment performed.[19,20] Considering the cited potential and actual benefits, collaboration seems to be a care alternative worthy of pursuit.

Many hospice programs also have arrangements to admit hospice home patients into long-term care facilities for respite care. *Respite care* is care for a limited period of time that provides a break for the family while the patient is cared for in another setting. Wherever the patient resides, hospice philosophy can be incorporated and care provided by the full IDT in collaboration with the long-term care staff.

The hospice IDT again advocates and supports autonomy in decision-making by providing information on many alternative care options to the patient and family when home care is no longer appropriate. The hospice nurse and team have the responsibility to educate the family about patient care needs and to respect and support the family's ability to set limits and acknowledge their own needs in placing their loved ones in other care settings.

Assisted-Living Settings. With the aging of the population, there are a variety of elder care living settings in which people may be dying. Recent expansion of adult living facilities (ALFs) has presented the challenge to care for people while allowing them to "age in place" and to "die in place." In the past, facilities licensed as ALFs were required to transfer a resident out of their facility if they could not independently provide care. For many people, this removed them from their home environment as they came closer to death, often resulting in loss of all sense of control over their lives. These residents were prevented from aging in place and dying in place.

Recognizing the detrimental effects of moving people at this time in their lives, residents in ALFs in many parts of the country are now able to stay in the ALF until death, as long as hospice is involved in their care. The end result supports patient autonomy related to where and how the patient chooses to live until life's end. Just as in other care settings, the hospice team remains the care manager in collaboration with the family and ALF staff to advocate for the patient's and family's palliative care goals.

Hospice Residences. Emerging as another alternative setting for people who can no longer stay in their own home is hospice residential care. Residential hospice care refers to the care provided in a facility that is staffed and owned by hospice programs. Patients and their families are given the choice of admission to a hospice residential setting if they are no longer able to care for themselves at home or do not have a caregiver, the caregiver is frail, or the caregiver is working and is unable to provide care at home. Patients may also be admitted to hospice residential care when needs for care (especially highly skilled technical care) are more than the family can manage at home. The same hospice services are available at the residence as in private homes. Family of patients at hospice residences are encouraged to participate in their care to their level of comfort, but hospice staff and volunteers are available 24 hours a day to provide needed care, support, and assistance. The number of hospice residences is growing as communities are realizing their value in filling a care need not provided in the same way in other settings.

Children, adolescents, young adults, and the elderly can be cared for in hospice residential settings. Consistent with hospice philosophy, admittance to residential care should not depend on race, color, creed, or ability to pay. Admission to hospice residences is based on the needs and preferences of the patient and family. Some hospice programs have admission guidelines that restrict their residential care option to those who are closer to death (e.g., within 2 months). However, most programs have found this option of care to be beneficial for many different reasons and have not limited its use or length of stay to a specific time frame.

Hospice seeks to create a community of caring within its residences, striving to be flexible and home-like. Patients may follow their own personal schedule, and their visitors have unlimited access. Patients are usually free to come and go as they please and are encouraged to bring some of their belongings to create an environment that is most comforting to them. The residential setting promotes community and affirms life by offering group activities, group meals, events, and celebrations that promote socialization. Patient choice in participation is respected.

Palliative Care Units. More recently in the United States, hospice programs have created partnerships with acute and long-term care settings to open or manage palliative care units. These units offer a range of services within those facilities, including palliative care consultation, palliative case management, caregiver support and counseling services, and full MHB services. The expertise of acute care professionals coupled with that of hospice professionals allows for the combined benefits of both systems in care of patients at the end of life. Generally, there are patients in palliative care units who are placed there as hospice patients needing acute care interventions or as transfers from the acute care hospital settings, when a transition to hospice may be beneficial or the palliative care expertise of hospice will be beneficial earlier in the disease progression, before Medicare model hospice services are instituted.

Many people access acute care settings during an episode of exacerbated symptomatology related to an end-stage or chronic disease process. Depending on the response to care and prognostic indicators, patients, families, and physicians begin to realize that conventional curative care may no longer be beneficial or that a combination of curative and palliative care is optimal. Palliative care units provide an option that allows attention to acute symptomatology by expert end-of-life clinicians while encouraging comfort and dignity for the patient's and family's experience. Palliative care units provide the opportunity for a smooth transition from the curative model of care to a palliative model for these patients and families. The advantage for the patient and family is that they are cared for by staff and volunteers who are competent in skilled medical care and end-of-life supportive care.

Hospital Settings and Hospice. In addition to inpatient palliative care consultation and case management services, inpatient hospital care is an option for hospice patients and families, usually to meet their acute care needs. Most hospice patients admitted to the hospital setting are considered to be inpatients, as defined by the Medicare levels of care, receiving skilled care. Although most patients prefer to live out the remainder of their lives in their home, there are times when inpatient hospitalization is requested or necessary to meet the changing needs of patients and families.

The reasons for hospitalization can vary. For some patients, the physician may request hospitalization for acute problems, including exacerbation of symptoms that are difficult to control in a home care setting. The patient may also require hospitalization for palliative surgical intervention. At times, hospice patients are admitted to the hospital for a condition that is not related to their terminal diagnosis. Physical needs resulting in hospitalization vary from patient to patient and should be an option in response to patient need and choice.

Some patients may request hospitalization for a fracture repair, whereas others may request to stay at home with medication for pain control. In situations involving possible hospitalization, it is important for the hospice nurse and the IDT to be available to explore with the patient the available choices in care and care setting before hospitalization. The patient and family should also remain involved in the plan of care, to determine how to best meet their changing needs. It is vital that the team provide the patient and family with other available services and care options, to prevent hospitalization if that is their wish.

While assessing the changing needs of patients and families, it is also important that the hospice nurse and IDT support patient and family choice regarding care setting and that they continue to honor the patient's and family's requests.

Other population groups receiving hospice care are the homeless and those in prison. These groups have posed challenges for hospice programs to expand service delivery options and provide care in all of these "homes."

The Hospice Nurse's Responsibilities in Facility-Based Care Settings

Regardless of the type of setting, the hospice nurse and IDT are responsible for continuity of the patient's and family's palliative plan of care. When a patient is admitted to a facility, the hospice IDT remains the patient's care manager. Regulations also require collaborative care planning as well as documentation of mutually developed goals and interventions in some settings (e.g., between long-term care facilities and hospice).

To ensure the highest level of patient and family autonomy, hospice nurses have a responsibility to educate the facility staff about the philosophy, principles, and practices of hospice care. The staff should be able to integrate into their practice a dying patient's rights and their responsibility in allowing the patient to make his or her own decisions. The specialty of end-of-life symptom management and support of the emotional and spiritual aspects of life closure are still elusive to most nurses; therefore, hospice nurses are often involved in nonhospice settings, educating staff about protocols for pain and symptom management, as well as ways to assist patients and families with the emotional and spiritual aspects of closure of their life and relationships. Education of the staff improves the delivery of palliative care and makes the staff feel more confident and comfortable in caring for dying patients and their families, in contrast to the avoidance that sometimes comes from feelings of inadequacy.

To provide continuity of care, the hospice nurse should be in contact with the facility staff to ensure the patient's and family's physical, psychosocial, and spiritual status; their goals and wishes; and that their decisions regarding advance directives are communicated. While respecting the policies and procedures of each setting, the hospice IDT must communicate and collaborate with the patient, family, physician, and facility staff to ensure continuity of the plan of care formulated by the patient and family.

Hospice Care Provided Through an Interdisciplinary Team

The Hospice Experience Model: A Patient/Family Value-Directed End-of-Life Care Model

Nurses caring for patients and their families at the end of life need to first comprehend the basic differences between curative approaches and palliative end-of-life approaches that honor the unique experiences of patients and families.

Within the foundation of hospice philosophy, one of the significant differences in hospice nursing is the concept that the patient and family direct care, based on their personal values, culture, wishes, and needs. Such issues as dignity and quality can be defined only subjectively, by those who are experiencing life changes associated with illness, caregiving, dying, and bereavement.

The *Hospice Experience Model,*[21] an end-of-life model based on patient/family values, is founded on the following principles that apply to both the patient and family caregivers:

Illness, caregiving, dying, and bereavement are unique personal experiences.

People experience the last phase of their relationships and lives through many related dimensions.

The last phase of life and relationships provides continued opportunity for positive growth and development in the face of suffering.

Principle 1: Illness, caregiving, dying, and bereavement are unique personal experiences.

Respecting patients' individuality is the foundation of humane care. It requires confronting the fullness of the human context in which illness and aging occur. Individual patients must be the focus of attention, and their particular values, concerns, and goals must be recognized and addressed.[22]

Just as earlier stages of life for each individual are different, so is dying and end-of-life caregiving. How one adapts to changes brought on as a result of an end-stage disease process or by the normal slowing of systems associated with aging is a very personal response. This response reflects the diversity of an individual's life experience, beliefs, culture, and values. Looking to the future in end-of-life care and understanding the vast differences among individuals who are in the final phase of life, nurses must provide care that results in individualized, customized relationships that respect the values, preferences, and expressed needs of the patient and family in the final phase of life and relationships.

What one person defines as quality of life in the final phase may differ drastically from the next person's definition or differ at points in the life continuum. For one patient, self-determined life closure may mean not being dependent on life-sustaining machines or having a living will. For another patient, it may mean being able to die at home, with family at the bedside. For the patient who has spent the last 3 years confined to a wheelchair, it may involve dying on the screened porch of a mobile home.

The hospice philosophy of care most closely attends to respecting and honoring the individual experiences of caregiving for the family and of illness and dying for the patient. Nurses providing quality end-of-life care must use the guiding principles of autonomy or choice, advocacy, and acceptance to best meet the goal of supporting individualized dying experiences.

Principle 2: People experience the last phase of their relationships and lives through many related dimensions.

The caregiving and dying experience is one that affects all dimensions of a person. To comprehend the nature of suffering among the dying, it is essential to know and understand the person. Eric Cassell[23] described a model for understanding suffering in his "topology" of personhood. In his multidimensional model of personhood, each person exists as a dynamic matrix of dimensions, or realms, of the self. Each dimension has a significant and dynamic impact on and relationship with the other dimensions. Application of this dynamic relationship of dimensions to the last phase of life can guide the nurse in providing excellence in service and an optimal end-of-life experience for the patient and family.

Ira Byock and Melanie Merriman,[24] authors of the Missoula-VITAS Quality of Life Index (the only assessment tool designed to evaluate quality of life closure as an interdimensional, subjective experience of the patient), have developed an end-of-life construct based on Cassell's topology of personhood. The basis for this construct is that people experience the last phase of life as multidimensional beings. As a person's physical and functional dimensions decline, quality of life can be enhanced by attention to their interpersonal, well-being, and transcendent dimensions. Each dimension is briefly described as follows.

Physical Dimension: a patient's experience of the physical discomfort associated with progressive illness, perceived level of physical distress; also, caregivers' experience of their physical response to caregiving, which may include fatigue or altered health as a result of the effects of caregiving or the lack of attention to their own health status

Function Dimension: a patient's and family's perceived ability to perform accustomed functions and activities of daily living (ADLs), experienced in relation to expectations and adaptations to declining functionality; may include functional ADLs such as bathing, transfer, and feeding, but also includes the expanded aspects of those things that one does to "function" within the social context, such as childcare, paying bills, maintaining a household, and maintaining employment

Interpersonal Dimension: degree of investment in personal relationships and perceived quality of one's relations with family, friends, and others; quality of relationships between the patient and others as well as the caregiver and others; from the caregivers experience, this specifically refers to the changes in their relationship with the patient as a result of the illness as well as the anticipated changes in the caregiver's life after the patient's death

Well-being Dimension: self-assessment of internal condition, subjective sense of "wellness" or "dis-ease," contentment or lack of contentment, personal sense of well-being, how individuals feel within themselves; may include anxiety, sadness, restlessness, depression, fears, sense of peace, readiness, mindfulness, acceptance

Transcendent Dimension: one's experienced degree of connection with an enduring construct; one's relationship on a transpersonal level, which may involve, but does not have to involve, spiritual or religious values; may involve one's perception of the meaning of life, caregiving, suffering, death, and afterlife

Nurses must approach end-of-life care and caregiving with the understanding that a change in one of these dimensions affects the other dimensions. Examining pain as a physical dimension without being prompted to determine how this has affected all of the other dimensions of that person's experience would not attend to the full dying experience. Examining fatigue of a family caregiver as a physical experience alone would not allow us to understand the full experience of the caregiver. In both of these cases, by not examining the experiences from an interdimensional perspective, we miss the opportunity to affect the quality of the experience.

An example of a hospice nurse's assessment of a patient's pain from an interdimensional perspective is illustrated in the following case study.

CASE STUDY

Mrs. Little, a Patient with Chronic Obstructive Pulmonary Disease

Mrs. Little is having increasing difficulty with breathing at a self-rated level of 4 on a scale of 0 to 10 *(physical dimension)*. She can no longer walk from her bedroom to the kitchen *(functional dimension)* and is becoming more isolated from family and friends *(interpersonal dimension)*. Mrs. Little becomes anxious just thinking about being alone at night and not being able to catch her breath *(well-being dimension)*. She begins asking God, "Why is this happening to me?" "What did I do to deserve this?" *(spiritual dimension)*.

Continuing with the understanding that hospice cares for the patient and the family, the nurse's interdimensional assessment of the family (Mrs. Little's daughter, Goldie, who is her primary caregiver) may be illustrated in the following.

Mrs. Little awakens her daughter several times a night when she gets anxious and feels short of breath, so Goldie is becoming exhausted *(physical dimension)* and can no longer work out of the home and care for her mother *(functional dimension)*. She misses her friends and coworkers, begins to resent her mother's demands, and sometimes lashes back at her *(interpersonal dimension)*. At the same time, she feels inadequate and states, "I just don't know what else to do for her, sometimes I don't feel very adequate as a caregiver" *(well-being dimension)*. She turns to prayer for her strength to make it through the next day *(spiritual dimension)*.

Referred to as interdimensional care, this approach respects the full scope of the dying and caregiving experience and is the basis for optimally affecting quality of life and relationship closure. The challenge within hospice nursing is to approach all interactions with patients and families with an understanding of this dynamic, dimensional relationship. If this patient's and family's situation were approached and assessed from a singular symptom dimension and medical/physical perspective, opportunities to improve the quality of life and relationship closure for the patient and family in all of the other dimensions would be neglected.

When all dimensions are assessed and the patient or family member is able to direct her or his own care and support, an extraordinary possibility for growth, healing, dignity, and positive life and relationship closure can occur. There is opportunity for review, restitution, amends, exploration, development, insight affecting all dimensions, and, therefore, end-of-life and relationship growth.

Family caregivers also experience this phase of their lives through these related dimensions. With so many people choosing to stay at home with family, hospice emphasizes the importance of empowering families so that they can participate to the level they are able in providing care to the patient. In order to understand and honor the family's experience, it is important not to "take over" the care but instead to provide resources, assistance and support so family members may find the potential for deep meaning and purpose in caregiving and the last phase of their relationship with the care-receiver. Hospice's ability to involve the family in caregiving often improves family members' perspectives and experiences. Research has shown significant differences in favor of hospice in four measures used to evaluate the quality of life of the primary caregiver (family). Primary caregivers for hospice patients were found to be less anxious and more satisfied with their involvement in care than were their nonhospice counterparts.[15]

Principle 3: The last phase of life and relationship provides continued opportunity for positive growth and development in the face of suffering.

In his book, *Dying Well: The Prospect for Growth at the End of Life*, Ira Byock[25] wrote about the opportunities for growth and development at the end of life. As a hospice physician, he shared his observations of patients and families at the end of life. He explained how people in the face of suffering are able to personally develop a sense of completion, to find meaning in their lives, to experience love of self and others, to say their good-byes, and to surrender to the unknown.

Application of the Hospice Experience Model

Hospice nursing involves incorporating the first two principles of the Hospice Experience Model. Illness, caregiving, dying, and bereavement are unique individual and interdimensional experiences of the patient and caregiver, with life and relationship developmental landmarks and tasks for completion and closure (Table 2–4). The ultimate goal is to provide the opportunity for growth and to improve the quality of life and relationship closure for patients and families as they attend to what is most important to them before the patient dies, through the accomplishment of these life closure tasks.

In addition to the potential for physical distress and suffering, terminal illness presents a final opportunity to complete landmarks and tasks of lifelong development. Quality of life is enhanced as the tasks are completed and the landmarks achieved. Hospice protects and amplifies the opportunity for personal growth in the final stage of life, thereby enhancing quality of life among patients and families.[26]

Dying is a part of living. The period of time referred to as dying can be considered a stage in the life of the individual person and the family. Developmental psychology involves the study of life stages and the related tasks to be accomplished and opportunities for growth associated with each stage. Within our current culture, there seems to be an assumption that, once a terminal diagnosis has been given, meaningful life has ended—yet dying and end-of-life caregiving are specific stages with related growth tasks and accomplishments.

As reflected in *The Quest to Die with Dignity: An Analysis of Americans' Values, Opinions and Attitudes Concerning End-of-Life Care,*[27] people tend to see the last phase of life as one of awaiting death, hoping minimally for some measure of comfort and not being a burden to others. This limited perspective devalues and separates this last stage of life from the continuum of a person's existence while minimizing hopes and goals. Hospice professionals have learned differently from patients and families, and the Hospice Experience Model integrates those lessons by incorporating the framework for life and relationship closure.

Byock[26] conceptualized dying as a stage of the human life cycle that inherently holds opportunities to broaden the personal experience, determine "what matters most," influence the outcome for improved quality of life closure, and, in so doing, reveal new sources of hope. He believes that individuality extends through the very end of life, characteristic challenges and meaningful developmental landmarks can be discerned, and representative tasks toward the achievement of goals for life completion and life closure can be identified.[26]

Byock[26] elucidated the opportunity, during this last phase of life, for uncovering new or deeper sources of meaning in people's

Table 2–4
Developmental Landmarks and Task Work for Life Completion and Life Closure

Landmark	Task Work
Sense of completion with worldly affairs	Transfer of fiscal, legal, and formal social responsibilities
Sense of completion in relationships with community	Closure of multiple social relationships (employment, business, organizational, congregational) Components include expressions of regret, expressions of forgiveness, acceptance of gratitude and appreciation Leave-taking, saying good-bye
Sense of meaning about one's individual life	Life review The telling of "one's stories" Transmission of knowledge and wisdom
Experience of love of self	Self-acknowledgment Self-forgiveness
Experience of love of others	Acceptance of worthiness Acceptance of forgiveness
Sense of completion in relationships with family and friends	Reconciliation, fullness of communication, and closure in each of one's important relationships Component tasks include expressions of regret, expressions of forgiveness and acceptance, expressions of gratitude and appreciation, expressions of affection Leave-taking, saying good-bye
Acceptance of the finality of life, of one's existence as an individual	Acknowledgment of the totality of personal loss represented by one's dying and experience of personal pain of existential loss Expression of the depth of personal tragedy that dying represents Decathexis (emotional withdrawal) from worldly affairs and cathexis (emotional connection) with an enduring construct Acceptance of dependency
Sense of new self (personhood) beyond personal loss	Acceptance of new definition of self Acknowledgement of the value of that new self
Sense of meaning about life in general	Achieving a sense of awe Recognition of transcendent realm Developing/achieving a sense of comfort with chaos
Surrender to the transcendent, to the unknown, "letting go"	Will to die Acceptance of death Saying good-bye Withdrawal from family, friends, and professional caregivers

Source: Byock (1996), reference 26.

Table 2–5
Aspects of Completion and Closure for the Caregiver

Aspect	The Caregiver's Experience
Life affairs	Transfer of knowledge or responsibility from care-receiver to caregiver (or to others such as family members or legal guardian) concerning financial matters, legal matters, and/or health care decision-making Respect for and advocacy of care-receiver's wishes at the end of life
Relationships with community	Changes and/or closure in multiple formal social relationships, including employment, business, organizational, congregational, and educational roles Expressing feelings regarding these changes, such as regret, gratitude, appreciation, and loss Maintaining connections for care-receiver and self
Personal relationships	Life review—facilitating the telling of "one's story; "the telling of "our story," including expression of meaning in the care-receiver's life and relationships with caregiver, family, friends Acceptance of transmission of knowledge and wisdom from care-receiver Reconciliation of conflicts with care-receiver and other personal relationships Open, honest communication in each important relationship Expressions of regret, forgiveness and acceptance, gratitude and appreciation, affection and love with family, friends Being present with the care-receiver throughout the dying process
Experience of love of self and others	Acknowledgment—affirmation and appreciation of self as a caregiver and as an individual Forgiveness—self-forgiveness; forgiveness to care-receiver, others, a higher power or spiritual entity; and acceptance of forgiveness from care-receiver, others, spiritual entity/higher power Worthiness—worthy of giving and receiving love, of assistance with caregiving, of self-care Acceptance of strengths, limitations; realistic expectations of new role as caregiver and value of that role, of self beyond caregiving, of self as individual
Acceptance of the finality of life	Acknowledgment of the personal loss and personal tragedy represented by care-receiver's dying Anticipatory grief—experience pain of loss (all losses, loss of care-receiver) Acknowledgement and/or acceptance of care-receiver's impending death Letting go—giving permission to die, assurance of caregiver's well-being, saying good-bye Understanding and/or acceptance of care-receiver's withdrawal from worldly affairs, family, friends, and caregivers and transition to the unknown Closure of relationship with care-receiver
Meaning of life	Achieving a sense of awe about the journey, death and life Attending to the spiritual elements, including recognition of life after death, recognition of a higher power, a connectedness with something greater than oneself, and/or spiritual growth, spiritual peace Acceptance of constant changes in life, growth in experiences Sense of meaning and purpose as a caregiver and in life
Bereavement—loss, mourning, and grief; renewal, resocialization	Loss of role as caregiver Tasks of grief New self beyond caregiver role New definition of self Acknowledge, value, and accept the new self Readiness for new life New self in personal relationships and community Moving on

Source: The Hospice Institute of the Florida Suncoast (2003), reference 43.

lives and in their dying. It is important that a developmental approach to the end of life not be misconstrued as a set of prescribed requirements. Rather, these landmarks and tasks can become part of a conceptual framework in which to approach end-of-life care processes, systems, and relationships. They can provide a common language and common approaches to ensure patient/family value–directed care that optimizes quality of life and relationship closure. How each patient and family chooses to attend to or accomplish these tasks will be specific to what is most important to them at this time in their lives, as reflected by their values, goals, and needs.

The developmental landmarks and task work for life completion and life closure that Byock[26] defined provide direction for care in the final phase of life (Table 2–4). They reflect the gradual process of life transition from worldly and social affairs, to individual relationships, and to intrapersonal and transcendent dimensions. In a landmark national research project, *Caregiving at Life's End*, a national needs assessment of hospice family caregivers confirmed the hypothesis that family caregivers also experience these aspects of completion and closure (Table 2–5), and the more they experience these aspects, the greater gain they have in the end-of-life caregiving experience.[28] What was also learned was that the more caregivers feel they can have an impact on the life closure aspects for the care-receiver, the more meaning they themselves find in the experience of caregiving. The aspects of completion and closure are closely interrelated for the patient and family caregiver, as illustrated in case examples shown in Table 2–6.

These tasks and landmarks can offer a guide for professionals caring for patients and families in the last years of life. By first opening dialogue about the possibility of meaningful experiences related to these landmarks and tasks, we acknowledge and validate the patient's and family's experience. As with other developmental stages in life, developmental tasks are best accomplished with optimal interventions and in a supportive environment. As with a toddler who is learning to walk or talk, a safe, encouraging, and nurturing environment is essential to safe accomplishment of these tasks. The hospice approach to the relationships among the patient and the family or other caregivers becomes one of providing interventions that create optimal, safe, nurturing environments to facilitate work on life and relationship closure tasks to the extent that they choose, are interested, and are able to engage.

As nurses, we have the responsibility to attend to the physical and functional dimensions of care while supporting issues of life closure in the other dimensions so that patients and families can accomplish the end-of-life developmental landmarks to the extent that they choose. Accordingly, the hospice nurse's initial role in end-of-life care is to work with the patient and family to prevent or minimize the suffering that results from the physical and functional decline of advancing age or from end-stage disease progression. It is after these dimensions are addressed and managed that the patient and family can attend to life- and relationship-closure tasks and landmarks that they feel are important and that involve the interpersonal, well-being, and transcendent dimensions of their experiences.

Although each patient approaches these landmarks and associated task work in his or her own way, there are some common aspects. Generally, patients first accomplish the few landmarks or tasks that relate to separating from and settling worldly affairs and community relationships, before the tasks involving moving away or separating from friends and family and, finally, those tasks marked by introspection. As people get closer to death, it is common to observe a gradual withdrawal from worldly relationships, friends, and family as they begin the transition on their individual journey from life to death. The nurse's goal is to explain and normalize this experience, thereby recruiting the IDT and family members to help preserve the patient's and family's opportunities to experience peace and comfort within themselves during their personal encounter with illness, caregiving, death, and bereavement.

Salmon and colleagues[28] confirmed the positive aspects of caregiver relationship closure through their research with hospice family caregivers. They found that hospice family caregivers did the following:

- Indicated that they want practical information about caregiving, such as information that helps them to understand the illness, know how to give medications, make end-of-life decisions, communicate with health care professionals, and give hands-on care.
- Valued and felt comfortable with tasks such as understanding the illness and giving medications.
- Wanted to know what to expect at the time of death.
- Experienced greater caregiver gain when comfortable with what are known as the transformative tasks of caregiving—finding meaning and purpose, feeling closure, and self-acceptance.

These results support the principle of opportunity for gain and positive experiences in the face of suffering and clearly indicate the unique value of hospice services for family caregivers.

The Experience of Illness and Dying: Nursing Process from a Hospice Perspective

Hospice nursing involves three broad areas: (1) approaching care from a patient- and family-based, interdimensional care focus, as described earlier; (2) expertise in end-stage disease and symptom management; and (3) applying the nursing process as a member of the hospice IDT through a critical thinking approach that supports the Hospice Experience Model.

End-stage disease and symptom management present a unique challenge for many nurses when they begin hospice nursing. This challenge involves incorporating norms for disease progression and symptom management different from those applied in a curative model. Symptoms that are considered abnormal in a curative approach may become the expected norm for a person who is dying.

Pharmacological interventions for pain and symptom management are emerging as a body of knowledge that has not yet been integrated well into the nursing curriculum. Nonpharmacological interventions that are considered appropriate for a patient on a curative path may actually increase suffering for a patient who is dying. An example may be encouraging intake of food and fluids. For a curative approach, this is appropriate to increase strength and healing. When a patient approaches death, however, the body's systems are slowing. This slowing results in a decreased caloric requirement as well as a slowing of fluid perfusion. By forcing food and fluids, we could increase the demands on the gastrointestinal and circulatory systems, thereby creating increased discomfort. It becomes the

Table 2–6
Interrelatedness of Care-receiver and Caregiver Tasks

Care-receiver and Caregiver Tasks	Example of Interrelatedness (see Tables 2–4 and 2–5)
Care-receiver: Sense of completion with worldly affairs • Transfer of social responsibilities *Caregiver:* Life affairs • Transfer of knowledge and/or responsibility • Advocacy of care-receiver's wishes	*Care-receiver:* Mr. Kent, the patient, wants his son (caregiver) to have power of attorney to manage his wife's financial accounts. Mrs. Kent has dementia, and he is concerned about having money available for her continued care after he dies. *Caregiver:* Mr. Kent, an only child, does not want his dad to worry. He is willing to be the primary caregiver for his mother after his dad dies. He knows he will need to be able to manage the family money so that it is available for her care at home if he must hire additional help or if he needs to place her in a long-term care facility.
Care-receiver: Sense of completion in relationships with community • Closure of multiple social relationships • Expression of feelings • Leave-taking *Caregiver:* Relationships with community • Changes and/or closure in multiple social relationships • Expressing feelings • Maintaining connections	*Care-receiver:* Mr. Jay wants to sell his business to his partner, because he can no longer attend to the clients. *Caregiver:* Mrs. Jay does not want the business to be sold, especially because her husband worked so hard to make it successful. She was employed in the business until her spouse got very sick and could no longer care for himself. She feels she lacks some of the skills to be a partner but could learn. She is hesitant to ask her husband about it, because he is so ill. She very much wants to spend time with her husband right now and has no time to attend to work. She feels she is losing both her husband and the family business.
Care-receiver: Sense of meaning about one's individual life • Life review • Telling "one's story" • Transmission of knowledge and wisdom *Care-receiver:* Sense of completion in relationships with family and friends • Reconciliation, fullness of communication, and closure • Expression of feelings • Leave-taking *Caregiver:* Personal relationships • Facilitating the life review • Acceptance of transmission of knowledge and wisdom • Reconciliation of conflicts • Open, honest communication • Expression of feelings	*Care-receiver:* Mrs. Thomas is widowed and lives alone on the family farm. She has two daughters, both living in distant cities, having left the state for college, started careers, and seldom returned to the family home. When Mrs. Thomas became bed bound, her daughter, Judy, came to care for her and intends to share the caregiving with her sister. Mrs. Thomas tells stories about the girls' childhoods, trying to understand what she did to make her children want to leave the farm. She also tells stories about her own childhood and growing up on the family farm, her fame as the best cook in the county, and her willingness to take in stray animals. Judy is a successful corporate lawyer. Mrs. Thomas feels the need to relay to her daughter that success is not measured by money but by being "good to all creatures great and small." *Caregiver:* Judy has taken a leave of absence from work to care for her mother for a month. She is very concerned about her job and corporate clients while she is away. When Judy returned home, she noticed the peace and quiet of her family home. As her mother told stories about her life and raising her and her sister, Judy realized how little she knew about the family tree and family history. She began to ask other questions about the family. As her mother provided advice about success and felt such accomplishment in what Judy considered "little things," Judy began questioning her own accomplishments and whether they really made a difference in anyone else's life. She began to examine her role as a caregiver and the difference it was making in her mother's life.

(*continued*)

Table 2–6
Interrelatedness of Care-receiver and Caregiver Tasks *(continued)*

Care-receiver and Caregiver Tasks	Example of Interrelatedness (see Tables 2–4 and 2–5)
Care-receiver: Experience of love of self • Self-acknowledgment • Self-forgiveness *Care-receiver:* Experience of love of others • Acceptance of worthiness • Acceptance of forgiveness *Care-receiver:* Sense of a new self beyond personal loss • Acceptance of new definition of self • Acknowledgment of the value of that new self *Caregiver:* Experience of love of self and love of others • Acknowledgment • Forgiveness	*Care-receiver:* Mrs. Snider is dying from breast cancer, and her husband is her caregiver. Their son died when he was 4 years old; he drowned in the backyard pool while in her care. She was never able to forgive herself for the death of her son, and she believes her husband never really forgave her in the 50 years they have been together since that awful time. He grieved hard, and he punished her for her son's death by never really letting go of the grief. She feels she missed life because of her guilt and her husband's grief. With the help of the chaplain, Mrs. Snider has been able to forgive herself for her son's death, and she is glad that after death she will be reunited with him. She also realizes that her love of her husband allowed him to stay a shut-in, because she did not want to hurt him any more by leaving him. She only wishes he could forgive her. She did the best she could, and that is worth something. *Caregiver:* After the death of his son, Mr. Snider felt he had no other reason to live. His legacy was gone, and he and his wife could not have any other children. They were so grief-stricken that he felt the need to protect both of them from the outside world, which became a lifelong pattern. They depended on each other for everything, never asking for help and never socializing with anyone. Since he lost his son, he has had difficulty loving anyone for fear he would lose them. Now he is losing his wife. Even though he tried not to love her for not being there when his son fell into the pool, he finds he still loves her. For the past 50 years, however, he has not shown his love to her. He also did not know he could care for anyone the way he has been able to care for his wife throughout this illness. The chaplain who visits is helping him feel better. He realizes that his grief filtered down to his relationships, and that it was okay to miss his son. He feels he had no right to punish his wife for this long; holding onto her so tightly to keep from losing someone else was not intentional and was a sign of love. Could she ever forgive him? He needs to show her his love and ask her forgiveness for his past actions. He is worried about life without her—he will have no one if he doesn't act now. Perhaps he will call his sister to help.
Care-receiver: Acceptance of the finality of life • Acknowledgment of personal loss • Expression of the depth of personal tragedy that dying represents • Decathexis and cathexis • Acceptance of dependency *Care-receiver:* Surrender–"letting go" • Will to die • Acceptance of death • Saying good-bye • Withdrawal from family, friends, and professional caregivers *Caregiver:* Acceptance of the finality of life • Acknowledgment of personal loss/tragedy • Anticipatory grief	*Care-receiver:* Here she was, dying. She was so saddened to be leaving her kids, her husband, and her mother and father behind. There had been so much she wanted to do, such as seeing her children grow up and become mothers and fathers. She wanted to hold her grandchildren. She wanted to take care of her husband forever and her parents in their old age, not have her husband and parents take care of her. She wanted to learn how to play the piano. She would never be able to do any of these things. She could not even bathe or dress herself. The pain had become unbearable, and watching herself deteriorate was even more difficult. Flo counted on her faith and put all her troubles, the care of her children, and the care of her parents into God's hands. There was no turning back, and she began to welcome death. She said her good-byes and wrote letters to her children to be opened on special occasions after her death. She even wrote her memoirs so they would know the kind of person she was. She hired a nanny for the kids so that her husband could focus on his

(continued)

Table 2–6
Interrelatedness of Care-receiver and Caregiver Tasks *(continued)*

Care-receiver and Caregiver Tasks	Example of Interrelatedness (see Tables 2–4 and 2–5)
• Acknowledgment and/or acceptance of the care-receiver's impending death • Letting go–acceptance of care-receiver's withdrawal • Closure of relationship with care-receiver	work and grief, and she gave him permission to remarry. As she became more ill, she withdrew and focused more on God and on the possibility of heaven and life after death. She was ready to die and wished God would take her now. *Caregiver:* Michael was grieving the loss of his wife, his high school sweetheart. He had loved her forever. He had no idea how to raise the kids without her, how to go on without her. He had lost his future. He knew there was nothing more that could be done, and he was trying to support her as she prepared for her death. She was quickly withdrawing from everyone, including him, as she moved closer to death. She had asked him if he would be okay without her, and he had always said not to say that, because he would love her forever. He knew he had to say good-bye and tell her that he and the kids would be okay. But would he be okay? He did not think so, but perhaps she would help him from wherever she was. He said good-bye, and she died 3 hours later.
Care-receiver: Sense of meaning about life in general • Achieving a sense of awe • Recognition of transcendent realm • Developing/achieving a sense of comfort with chaos *Caregiver:* Meaning of life • Achieving a sense of awe • Attending to the spiritual elements • Acceptance of constant changes in life, growth in experiences • Sense of meaning and purpose as a caregiver and in life	*Note:* The care-receiver and the caregiver usually do not go through this stage at the same time. The care-receiver usually finds meaning in life before he or she dies, whereas the caregiver may not find meaning in life until after the death, sometimes as a result of paralleling the care-receiver's journey and observing him or her make sense of death and look to the unknown with comfort. The care-receiver finds comfort with the chaos that surrounds dying, whereas the caregiver realizes after the death that change is constant, that it is still affecting him or her, and that growth can result from change. In addition, while the care-receiver's focus becomes death, the caregiver's focus becomes one of life—a sense of awe about life, a new-found appreciation for life, a purpose in life (possibly a feeling of connectedness between this world and the next or between the self and a higher power or the universe). The caregiver may also find spiritual peace as he or she begins to feel that everything is connected, that there is meaning and purpose in caregiving and in life. *Care-receiver:* Fred's health was declining rapidly. He became weaker and slept more. He was not eating and was taking only sips of fluids. He felt as though there was nothing more to do, nothing more to say, and he had somehow accepted death. He was comfortable with who he was and what he had accomplished. He felt in awe about life and what a wonderful gift it was to be able to live, but he also sensed that there was something greater, something beyond this place. While his daughter was running around and fretting about her job, her income, how much she had to do, and managing all his care and the community services he received, he found himself relaxing and actually trying to comfort her. He thought she was dumbfounded by how calm he was about dying. He was not sure he even knew why he was so calm, except that he knew there was nothing more he could do or had to do, and he instinctually felt that there was something beyond this world, something waiting for him, someone waiting for him. He hoped it was his wife and his favorite dog.

(continued)

Table 2–6
Interrelatedness of Care-receiver and Caregiver Tasks *(continued)*

Care-receiver and Caregiver Tasks	Example of Interrelatedness (see Tables 2–4 and 2–5)
	Caregiver: Katie missed her dad terribly, but she was glad her dad had died comfortably and peacefully. She felt as though he had somehow resigned himself to death a few weeks before he actually died. He tried to explain to her that he was not afraid and that she should take life less seriously, but she did not quite understand what he was saying, or perhaps she was too busy to think about it. She now felt privileged to have been a part of his life, his care, and his death. She never thought she could do it, but she had, and she very much wanted to tell other caregivers about how special it could be. Death was not as bad as she had thought it would be, either. It seemed so natural, and she felt such a sense of relief when her dad began talking to her mother, who had been deceased for 5 years. She felt a sense of hope about life after death, and a sense that life had a purpose even if she was not sure what that meant for her in the future. It would come to her; she just needed some time to grieve first. She also felt a renewed appreciation for life and hoped to enjoy it more fully when she felt physically and emotionally able.
Caregiver: Bereavement–loss, mourning, and grief; renewal, resocialization • Loss of role as caregiver • Tasks of grief • New self beyond caregiver role • New definition of self • Acknowledge, value, and accept the new self • Readiness for new life • New self in personal relationships and community • Moving on	*Note:* Although the care-receiver is not physically present, the caregiver still honors and respects the memory of the deceased. *Caregiver:* After the death of her partner, Joanne went through the stages of grief. It took her almost a year before she realized she was no longer a caregiver or the same person she had been before Susan died. She was partly her old self and partly someone stronger, more self-sufficient, and more appreciative of life. She now volunteers with the local branch of the Red Cross. She would never have given volunteering a thought before Susan died, but now she wants to make a difference in the lives of others. She still thinks about Susan frequently, especially during holidays and their anniversary, and when she is on the beach. The beach was where she and Susan met and where they shared their favorite activity of windsurfing. Just a few weeks ago, Joanne began windsurfing again. She hadn't done that since Susan became ill and she began caregiving. She also changed jobs to one she enjoyed. She likes her "new self." She still visits the gravesite every month to change the flowers and to honor the memory of her loved one. Lately, she has been thinking about dating again. She feels as though she will never find anyone like Susan and isn't sure she could love that deeply again, but she would enjoy some companionship.

Source: Adapted from Hospice Institute of the Florida Suncoast (2003), reference 43.

responsibility of any nurse caring for patients at the end of life to gain specific knowledge and competence in end-stage disease and symptom management.

Critically Thinking Through the End-of-Life Nursing Process

Illness, caregiving, suffering, dying, and bereavement evoke many interdimensional changes and reactions for both the patient and the family. By looking at the patient and family from this perspective, we begin to move away from a traditional, problem-oriented approach to a quality-of-life and relationship closure–oriented approach. All of the care processes and tools must therefore prompt a different critical thought process.[29]

Each step of the hospice interdimensional care process (assessment, care planning, goal setting, interventions, and evaluation) must involve three critical questions:

> Are we approaching care based on the patient's and family's experience, values, goals, and choices?

How does an issue, problem, or opportunity in one dimension affect the other dimensions of the patient and family?
How does an issue, problem, or opportunity affect the patient's or family's quality of life and relationship closure?

The main steps of the hospice interdimensional care process are similar to the nursing process but with a focus on preventing and managing suffering and on quality of life and relationship closure rather than rehabilitation or cure. Nurses must also look beyond problem identification as they apply the interdimensional care process and anticipate changes to prevent suffering while preserving opportunity for growth. At each step of the care process (assessment, planning, intervention, and evaluation), the three critical thinking questions must be applied.

Integrating the Nursing Process with the Hospice Interdimensional Care Process

Incorporating the nursing process into an interdimensional care process further defines the specialty of hospice nursing in that it involves the nurse working as a collaborative member of the IDT and expands the picture of the nursing process to an interdisciplinary interdimensional care process. All disciplines on the hospice team are valued, and their expertise is combined to apply the hospice interdimensional care process. The steps of the hospice interdimensional care process are outlined in the following paragraphs.

Step 1: Performing Interdimensional Assessment

Assessment begins with discussion soliciting information about the patient's and family's situation, including the values, wishes, and dreams that they identify as important. Data collection assesses all dimensions of a person and family as well as how changes in those dimensions affect the quality of life closure. Traditional nursing physical assessment is accomplished during this step, using norms for end-stage disease and symptom management.

Subjective and objective data are collected from a palliative, comfort care perspective and based on what patients and families define as important to them at this time. Their identified goals become the focus and driving force for the hospice team.

The focus of a palliative care assessment is to ask the question, "What is happening that is helping or hindering this patient and family from reaching their end-of-life goals?" From that perspective, the IDT supports integrated family systems theory, supporting the strengths of the patient and family while providing options for resources in areas of challenge.

Step 2: Identifying Specific Issues, Problems, and Opportunities and Their Causes

The next step involves identifying specific issues, which is comparable to developing the nursing diagnosis. A specific issue, problem, or opportunity is defined from a palliative perspective, and the cause is identified. In this step, hospice differentiates between definitions of problems that are expected norms for the dying process and those that are unexpected or may cause secondary suffering for the patient or family.

For example, a patient may become incontinent as her or his systems fail and death is imminent. This is an expected physical change during the dying process. Assessment of this using an interdimensional approach might determine that the problem is the potential for skin breakdown (with the cause being incontinence), rather than incontinence as the primary problem secondary to advanced disease. Another problem or issue may be that the "spouse is exhausted from being awake all day and night changing the patient's linens secondary to incontinence of the patient." What a nurse may instinctively identify as a problem in a curative model often becomes the cause of a problem in end-of-life care.

Another important difference in hospice nursing is that problems, issues, or opportunities are assessed and identified beyond the physical and functional dimensions, including the following for both patient and family:

- Physical symptoms and prevention of related suffering
- Psychosocial symptoms and prevention of related suffering
- Spiritual symptoms and prevention of related suffering
- Accomplishment of developmental tasks of life and relationship completion and closure to the extent that the patient and family choose to participate
- Issues and opportunities in the family dynamics and relationships
- Issues of grief, loss, and bereavement
- Functional status and environmental status

This step also involves determining the cause of the problem, issue, or opportunity. The cause of a medical problem can often be identified through physiological changes, but nurses must also take into consideration other causes related to all of the dimensions. For example, a patient with end-stage chronic obstructive pulmonary disease (COPD) may complain of shortness of breath. Initial reactions would be to identify the problem as shortness of breath "secondary to ineffective air exchange in the lung." Again, in end-stage COPD, this is an expected norm. With further interdimensional assessment, the patient identifies episodes of shortness of breath secondary to "anticipated fear of being alone at night." Obviously, the interventions are different if the full dimensions are assessed and the patient's and family's experiences direct the process.

The cause of a problem that is not physiologically based can often be attributed to the patient's or family's adaptation to the current situation or unfinished personal conflict. In this step, opportunities can also be identified for prevention of problems or issues, or situations can be presented that would enhance personal growth and completion of life and relationship closure tasks.

For example, a patient with COPD who was imminently dying was becoming progressively anxious, with increased episodes of shortness of breath despite all medical interventions. On assessment of this problem, the patient shared that he had a son to whom he had not spoken in more than 20 years. The patient was afraid of dying before mending that relationship, apologizing to his son, and letting him know he loved him. The hospice team assisted in locating his son and arranging for a visit. The patient and son were able to spend time together, give and receive forgiveness, and, in so doing, mend their relationship. The patient's unfinished relationship issues and related anxieties were the cause of his physical episodes of shortness of breath. Hospice nursing involves a holistic approach that realizes the potential effect of one dimension (e.g., interpersonal) on all other dimensions and ensures that the nursing assessment gathers and uses all dimensional changes for optimal interventions.

Step 3: Planning Interdisciplinary Team Care

Interdisciplinary care planning is a process that occurs from the time the patient is referred through the family's bereavement period. It occurs both in formal IDT care planning meetings and, between meetings, as patient and family needs change and members of the IDT collaborate on care. Patients and families are assessed by the nurse and by a psychosocial professional on admission. As the care plan is developed, each discipline blends its own area of expertise with those of other team members to formulate shared interventions that support the patient's and family's goals.

Similar to the nursing process, this step involves planning the care, including identifying patient and family goals and the appropriate staff and facilities; determining the best interventions; and devising a team plan for providing services. The key components in this process are collaboration, patient/family-directed goal setting, and IDT planning of interventions.

Collaboration. Collaboration builds an interdisciplinary awareness of interdependence with a common mission, values, and patient/family goals for optimal care. Collaboration is essential for all hospice professionals as they stimulate each other and innovative ideas and interventions are formulated. One of the key reasons for IDT collaboration is to share assessment data and feedback that each member was able to solicit from the patient and family so that a comprehensive interdimensional care plan can be established and mutually understood by all team members caring for that patient and family. The hospice nurse therefore collaborates first with the patient and family to determine their goals, and then with other IDT members to ensure a holistic approach to continuity of care. If the patient is residing in a facility, the nurse must also include the staff of that facility in care planning. Collaboration ensures continuity of care.

Patient/Family-Directed Goal Setting. A comprehensive plan is developed according to three types of goals: (1) patient/family goals, (2) life and relationship-closure goals, and (3) clinical obligation goals.

Primarily, the care plan should be directed by what the patient and family have defined as their goals. The hospice plan of care belongs to the patient and family; therefore, goals should be articulated from their perspective, not the nurse's perspective of how things "should happen." Goals articulated by hospice patients and families may include such things as being able to care for a spouse while he or she is bedridden or ranking pain as 2 or less out of 10 at meal times so that the patient can join the family at the table. Articulating goals from the perspective of the patient and family makes it apparent what direction each member of the IDT should take to collaboratively help them meet their goals. It also becomes apparent that the IDT as a group, not one discipline alone, is equipped to deal with complex issues associated with dying and bereavement.

Life and relationship completion and closure goals relate to the end-of-life accomplishments, the completion of unfinished business, landmarks and tasks of dying, the emotional and spiritual separation between family and patient, and anticipated changes for the caregiver after the death. Hospice nurses, as part of the IDT, add their expertise to support the patient and family in accomplishing life and relationship closure goals through disease and symptom management as well as emotional and spiritual support. An example of a life-closure goal as defined by the patient may be to take one last trip to visit and say good-bye to family and friends. The nurse may be involved by teaching energy conservation, the use of portable oxygen, transfer techniques for car transportation, or titration of medications to ensure comfort. Life and relationship-closure goals may also include "creating a memory book for my grandchildren to have when I'm gone" or being forgiven by a spouse for a life transgression. Again, the focus becomes the patient's and family's goals as they relate to life and relationship-closure tasks; the nurse collaborates with other team members, such as the psychosocial counselor or chaplain, to help the patient and family accomplish these goals.

Clinical obligation goals are identified by the IDT only in those situations in which the patient or family is unable to identify the problem or issue. These goals are strictly related to clinical obligation situations such as neglect or suicide, in which the team must establish goals to ensure the patient's or family's safety.

Interdisciplinary Team Planning of Interventions. Interventions are based on interdimensional assessment, with the overall goals of reducing or preventing suffering and accomplishing life and relationship closure in a way that is important and meaningful to the patient and family. Directed by the goals of the patient and family, and with their input and approval, the hospice nurse and the other IDT members collaborate to determine the optimal interventions that would move the patient and family closer to their goals.

The interdisciplinary planning process involves determining which discipline, or combination of disciplines, is most appropriate to assist patients and families in accomplishing their goals. Some patients and families may allow only one or two disciplines to be involved in their care. Some individuals expect nurses to provide care and are not always open to visits from social workers or chaplains. The nurse in these situations may be the sole team representative, incorporating the expertise of all disciplines. If this happens, it becomes crucial that members of the IDT collaborate and share expertise so that interdisciplinary care can still be delivered and the patient's and family's goals can still be addressed. The nurse's role may then include facilitating the involvement of the team to the degree that the patient and family are comfortable.

Step 4: Providing Interventions to Meet Patient and Family Goals

The hospice care plan involves interventions in four areas: palliative therapeutic interventions, educational interventions, collaboration interventions, and assessment interventions.

Palliative Therapeutic Interventions. Palliative therapeutic interventions include those that have been identified to be conducive to meeting the patient's and family's goals. These include both pharmacological and nonpharmacological interventions to best address the interdimensional adaptation and goals of the patient and family.

Hospice nurses must always be aware of not only the traditional medical interventions but also those interventions specific to the specialty of end-of-life care that support quality of life and relationship closure. An example is a patient who had a stroke that left him aphasic of both spoken and written word. During his lifetime, he had kept a scrapbook of national newspaper articles, including articles and current events journals. In the scrapbook, he had written his perceptions of how an event may have been significant to his daughter's life. To assist this patient in finding meaning and purpose in his life, the nurse requested a volunteer to help the patient engage in life review. The volunteer visited the patient, reading the articles and the patient's philosophical messages to his daughter related to each event in the history of their life together. Through the reading of these scrapbooks, the patient was able to sense his contribution and value as a parent.

Again, hospice nursing is based on a holistic approach and the understanding that life closure is an interdimensional experience for both the patient and the family.

Educational Interventions. As with all nursing practice, patient and family education is a cornerstone of hospice nursing. Because most patients followed by hospice do stay in their homes until death, the primary role of the hospice team is to empower the patient and family caregivers so that they can develop the skills to comfortably provide care and find meaning and purpose in the experience.

The nurse becomes involved in education of the patient and family as it relates to personal care, prevention of problems such as skin breakdown, administration and management of medications, nonpharmacological interventions such as therapeutic touch, application of heat, breathing exercises, and functional assistance with ADLs. As the patient's disease progresses, the hospice nurse is also involved in educating the family about expected changes. Common responses to each stage of the disease and related interventions to decrease suffering are taught so that the patient and family are optimally prepared before the changes occur. When patients and families know what to expect, hospice can help to prevent or reduce anxiety related to the unknown. Critical to the specialty of hospice nursing is the ability to be comfortable having conversations with patients and families about the aspects of life and relationship closure, offering opportunities for them to identify what is most important and finding ways to support their goals in these aspects.

Another crucial goal of education is to provide information and support so that patients and families can advocate for themselves in all care settings, with other providers, and with other family members.

Collaboration Interventions. Crucial to ensuring unified delivery of care to patients and families is the practice of collaboration. In planning interventions, it is crucial to ensure that the patient, the family, and the professional caregivers are all involved. Caregivers include IDT members, facility staff, attending and consulting physicians, therapists, and the family. For example, the hospice nurse collaborates with the attending physician about the need for medication for symptom management or with facility nurses to educate and ensure around-the-clock administration of pain medications. If a hospice patient is residing in a nursing facility, the hospice nurse must collaborate with the nursing facility staff, communicating and documenting the outcome of that collaboration. Communication of these interventions is paramount to ensure continuity of care among team members, caregivers, and care settings.

Assessment Interventions. The final type of hospice nursing intervention is ongoing assessment necessary to determine whether continuation of the care plan is effective or optimal. For hospice nursing, this may include closely monitored titration of opioids for pain control or respiratory status to determine effective doses as symptoms change or the patient's needs change throughout the trajectory of illness.

Step 5: Evaluating Interventions and Continuation or Revision of the Care Plan

With the patient and family as the core of the hospice team, evaluation begins with their perspective of the effectiveness of the care plan interventions in meeting their end-of-life and relationship closure goals. Do the interventions help them to reach their goals? What has been most beneficial from their perspective? What do they want to continue or discontinue? As with all other steps in the care process, the patient and family direct the care. Therefore, it is crucial that the hospice nurse involve the patient and family in evaluating the effectiveness of the care plan interventions on an ongoing basis.

By evaluating and documenting the effects of interventions, the hospice nurse shares his or her expertise as a valued member of the IDT. If the current care plan is effective at meeting the patient's and family's palliative care goals, then interventions continue. If interventions do not meet the patient's and family's goals, then the hospice nurse collaborates with the patient, family, and IDT for additional assessment and identification of meaningful goals.

Illness, caregiving, dying, death, and bereavement are experienced in unique, personal ways. Hospice care allows for the patient and family to direct the care based on their own values, goals, and needs. A significant difference between traditional nursing and hospice care is the involvement of the patient and the family as they guide the hospice IDT in providing palliative care and services that are most meaningful to them.

Key Elements of a Hospice Palliative Care Program

Purpose and Process of Interdisciplinary Team Care Management

In *The Hospice Handbook*, Larry Beresford stated, "The glue that holds together this hospice approach to care is the interdisciplinary team."[5] The primary purpose of the IDT model of care management is to build a caring community between the patient, the family, and the hospice team. This integrated community is responsible for responding to the patient's and family's dynamic needs 24 hours a day, 7 days a week. The entire IDT is accountable for the physical, psychosocial, spiritual, and bereavement needs of both the patient and the family, ensuring that the palliative care plan is carried out across all care settings.

Because the physical, psychosocial, spiritual, and bereavement needs of patients and families are inseparable, the interdisciplinary approach is also the hospice approach to care. The team, not just the hospice nurse, becomes the care manager. The patient, family, and IDT are equally important in problem solving and goal formulation, collaborating with each other for expertise and input into care planning. The hospice approach is a holistic care process that is directed by the patient and family to best meet their interdimensional needs.

Care management by the IDT is a process, not an event. This process begins at the time the patient is admitted to the hospice program and continues until well after the death of the patient, through bereavement services for the survivors. Effective IDT care management promotes daily, ongoing collaborative practice that incorporates shared goals, care planning, role blending, and shared leadership.

Interdimensional Care Delivered by an Interdisciplinary Team

Chronic illness, aging, and terminal illness affect patients and families not only physically but psychologically, emotionally, spiritually, and financially. To provide effective, quality hospice care, all of these dimensions of the dying experience should be addressed. An IDT, incorporating the expertise of members from several disciplines who are trained to meet these varied needs of patients and families, provides the most effective holistic approach to end-of-life care.

In a traditional multidisciplinary approach to patient care, a member representing each discipline visits the patient and formulates goals depending on his or her own area of expertise. The patient and family may not always be considered together as a unit of care, and the specific goals of one discipline are not always shared by the other disciplines caring for the patient. Often, one discipline is the "case manager," having more direction and input than the others in the care-planning process. This lack of collaborative care planning and goal setting can create an inconsistent approach that lacks cohesion and continuity and often frustrates those receiving care. The focus is on the "discipline" (e.g., nurse, social worker) rather than the patient and family. In the interdisciplinary approach to care, the nurse coordinates the plan of care with the patient, family, and other members of the IDT to "effectively mobilize each other's skills to meet patients' needs in a variety of healthcare settings.[30]

The hospice IDT model improves on the multidisciplinary approach with a process that allows for the following:

- Patient and family direction of care and services and involvement in decision-making in all aspects of care
- Determination of patient/family value–directed care plan goals
- Collaboration of expertise from varied disciplines to meet patient/family goals
- Identification of interventions that support patient/family goals
- Role blending of expertise among disciplines toward common patient/family goals and outcomes

The IDT model provides optimal interdimensional care by jointly assessing and determining goals and sharing ideas for interventions with the patient, the family, and all team members working toward common goals and interventions. The success of the hospice IDT model lies in the partnership between patient/family and care professionals that best reflects the full scope and experience of illness, caregiving, dying, and bereavement—focusing on the choices, goals, wishes, and experiences of the patient and family.

The Hospice Interdisciplinary Team Structure and Role Blending

The structure of the hospice IDT is designed to meet the interdimensional needs of patients and families. To be most effective, care teams must be designed to honor the experience of the patients and families they serve. End-of-life care teams, the disciplines that comprise the IDT, and how they function as a collaborative team mirror the patient's and family's complex experience of life-limiting illness, caregiving, dying, death, and bereavement. Collaboration as an IDT focuses on transforming the patient's and family's end-of-life experience. The critical components of this interdisciplinary model can and should be offered in all settings of care for patients and families near the end of life.[31]

As previously discussed, a number of dimensions define the full experience of patients and families. The related dimensions and the corresponding staff that form an effective hospice/palliative care team include the following:

- *Physical dimension:* physician, nurse, pharmacist, therapists, nutritionist, and volunteers
- *Functional dimension:* nurse, nursing assistant, therapists, and volunteers
- *Interpersonal dimension:* counselors, social worker, psychologist, and volunteers
- *Well-being dimension:* counselors, social worker, psychologist, chaplain, and volunteers
- *Transcendent dimension:* chaplain, counselors, social worker, psychologist, and volunteers

Interdimensional care provided by an IDT focuses on the experience of those served and the core disciplines that can best support that experience. By changing from a singular discipline to an interdimensional approach, all disciplines attend to all dimensions of the patient's and family's experience.[31]

Whereas each discipline of the IDT involves special areas of expertise, responsibilities, and duties, the IDT approach to care management requires that each team member expand and blend the traditional roles with those of other disciplines to provide a holistic approach to patient and family care.

One must be an expert in her or his own discipline and have the basic competence to provide physical, psychosocial, spiritual, and bereavement care. Assessment, planning, intervention, and evaluation are ongoing responsibilities of all team members, implying that each is attentive to all dimensions of patient and family care. Role blending is essential for providing coordinated, comprehensive hospice services. As such, roles need to be dynamic, changing, growing, and overlapping.

Direct Responsibilities of Patient/Family Care Team Members

Nurses, Including Advanced Registered Nurse Practitioners and Registered Nurses. In the MHB model, the registered nurse is primarily responsible for physical care, including the patient's physical condition and comfort, yet must also possess some level of expertise in psychosocial and spiritual aspects of care, to address the patient and family from a holistic perspective. She or he must be highly skilled in end-stage physical assessment, disease progression, and pain and symptom management. The nurse is also responsible for educating the patient and family regarding physical care, which includes such things as medication administration, equipment use, skin care, nutrition, catheter care, and transfers.

For those hospice programs that are MHB certified, regulations require the coordination of care by a registered nurse and primary physician. As a member of the IDT, the nurse's expertise related to disease and symptom management is one of the critical aspects of providing competent end-of-life care. The nurse's primary role involves managing and preventing the physical and functional decline, to reduce suffering so that the patient and family can attend to activities that promote quality of life and relationship closure.

The hospice nurse is also responsible for supervising related nursing personnel, including licensed practical nurses, certified nursing assistants, and home health aides. Communicating care plan goals and interventions and monitoring and evaluating the care provided by these other IDT members are the responsibilities of the hospice registered nurse.

Advanced registered nurse practitioners are most often used as collaborative primary care practitioners, providing palliative care consultation and care management for the expanded hospice palliative care programs (e.g., pain consultation in hospital and long-term care settings). Advanced registered nurse practitioners and clinical nurse specialists are also involved as consultants to the primary hospice team.

Psychosocial Professionals. Psychosocial professionals may include social workers and counselors who are competent in psychosocial assessment, family dynamics, social/emotional therapeutic interventions, grief and bereavement, and group work. They provide support to patients and families, assisting with psychological issues, emotional responses, and the overall adaptation of the patient, family, and significant others through counseling and utilization of community resources. They may also be involved with financial issues, legal issues, advance directives, and funeral arrangements. Overall, the psychosocial professional helps the patient and family as they adapt to and cope with a terminal illness and the survivors as they adjust to life during the bereavement process. It is also crucial for nurses to possess expertise in end-of-life psychosocial issues because they, too, will be involved in addressing and supporting the patient's and family's psychosocial needs as members of the IDT. Both the psychosocial and the spiritual care team members are experts in addressing many of the aspects of care relating to life and relationship closure.

Spiritual Care Professionals. Spiritual care is a significant component in end-of-life care. The spiritual caregiver, also known as the chaplain, clergy person, or pastoral care worker, can be a paid hospice professional or a resource volunteer from the community. Hospice spiritual care is nonsectarian, nondenominational, and all-inclusive, with the goal of supporting the patient's and family's spiritual and/or religious practices. The hospice philosophy in terms of spiritual care is nonjudgmental and focuses on healing, forgiveness, and acceptance. Spiritual care is provided through direct spiritual counseling and support by collaboration with the patient's and family's own clergy or by working with patients who do not have a clergy person but request spiritual care. Spiritual interventions can include prayer, rites, rituals, assistance in planning and performing funerals and memorial services, and assistance with ethical dilemmas. Again, the nurse must have some level of expertise in the spiritual aspects of care to address the patient's and family's spiritual needs.

Patient's Primary Physician. The patient's primary physician is also part of the IDT. The primary physician is responsible for overseeing patient care. The physician often refers the patient to hospice; certifies the patient's terminal condition; and collaborates throughout the care process, providing the admitting diagnosis and prognosis, current medical findings, dietary orders, and orders for medications, treatments, and symptom management.

Hospice Medical Director. The hospice medical director is a member of the IDT. She or he is responsible for the overall medical management of all patients. Depending on the structure of the hospice program, the medical director may also become a patient's primary physician. The role of the hospice medical director is to participate in the team care planning process as a collaborative member of the IDT. The director may also be responsible for the oversight of medical services provided by the hospice.

Certified Nursing Assistant or Home Health Aide. Certified nursing assistants provide basic physical and functional care if there is a need, as well as patient and family support. They provide and educate caregivers on personal care assistance with ADLs, which may include bathing, grooming, mouth care, skin care, transfers, and repositioning, and sometimes with light housekeeping, shopping, cooking, and laundry. Visits vary depending on patient and family needs and what is most important to the patient at each visit. At times, a walk in the garden is more therapeutic than a bath.

Homemaker/Companion. The homemaker/companion assists the patient and family by doing light housekeeping, meal planning and preparation, laundry, and shopping and by acting as a companion to the patient. The homemaker/companion does not provide direct, hands-on care. For elderly patients living alone, it is often the addition of a homemaker/companion that allows them to remain independent in their homes until they die.

Patient Care Volunteer. Volunteers play an integral role in providing hospice care and are fundamental to the hospice philosophy. Hospice patient care volunteers are trained to work in a variety of roles. The most common role is working with a single patient and family in providing support through companionship, listening, diversion, delivering medications, running errands, taking patients to appointments or on outings, shopping, or preparing a special meal. They may provide companionship to patients in extended care facilities or respite time for the home patient's caregiver. Specialized volunteer roles may include bereavement volunteers, who work exclusively with grieving families and friends, or those who sit at the bedside during the dying process. The scope of volunteers' duties is all-inclusive, depending on the needs of the patient and family and their quality-of-life goals.

Roles and Responsibilities of Consultative Team Members

Consultative team members participate in direct patient care as needed to meet the palliative care goals of the care plan. Consultative team members may include the hospice team medical director; consulting physician; psychologist or psychiatrist; nutritional counselor; community clergy; clinical pharmacist; occupational, physical, respiratory, speech, and language therapists; intravenous infusion nurse; and members of pharmacy, radiology, laboratory, and durable medical equipment services.[31]

Coping with Cumulative Loss: The Nurse as Caregiver

The hospice philosophy of care, which emphasizes intense interpersonal care and active involvement with the patient and family, creates more intense and more intimate relationships among the nurse, patient, and family than exist in traditional health care settings. Like families who grieve the loss of their loved ones, the hospice nurse also grieves the loss and, in fact, may need to grieve on a continuous basis due to the number of deaths that occur. As the hospice nurse adjusts to caring for dying patients and their families, the stress of coping with death on a daily basis can trigger many emotional feelings, reactions, and behaviors.

Other factors may also influence a nurse's successful adaptation to caring for dying patients and their families. If the nurse has experienced death on a personal level or has experienced life changes that signify loss (e.g., children leaving home, divorce), caring for dying patients and families may trigger issues of unresolved grief. The nurse's ability to verbalize his or her feelings regarding death and loss with other members of the IDT is important for support and for normalizing these feelings.

Hospice nurses who are unable to process these losses through appropriate grief and personal death awareness may begin to distance themselves from emotional involvement with patients and families. This withdrawal may negatively affect not only the coping ability of the professional but also the quality of compassionate delivery of care and the ability to meet the needs of dying patients and their families during the terminal phases of an illness.

Stages of Adaptation for the Hospice Nurse

Hospice nurses go through many stages when they begin caring for dying patients and their families. Successful progression through these stages and the support systems in place to facilitate successful progression are vitally important in determining whether the nurse will be comfortable and effective in caring for the dying.

As proposed by Bernice Harper,[32] an expert in anxiety issues in the professional caregiver, there are six stages of adaptation

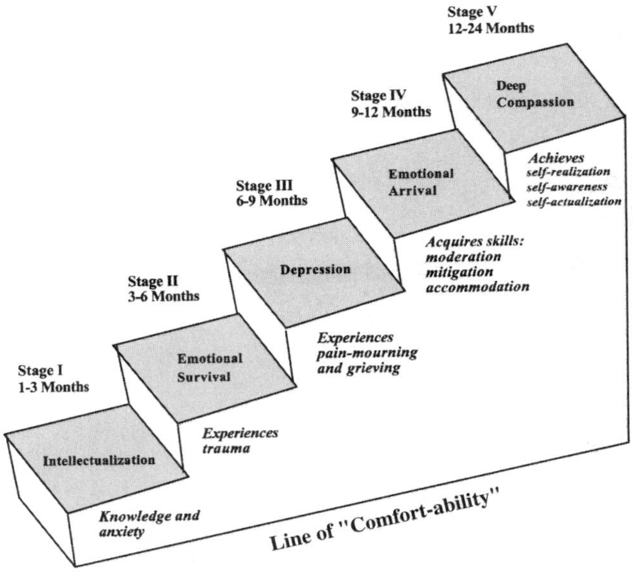

Figure 2–1. Cumulative loss and the caregiver: Five stages experienced by the hospice nurse while caring for the dying. (*Source:* Harper [1994], reference 32.)

that characterize the hospice nurse's normal progression, adaptation, and coping in caring for the dying: intellectualization, emotional survival, depression, emotional arrival, deep compassion, and The Doer. Five of these stages and the emotions, behaviors, and reactions of each stage are shown in Figure 2–1 and Table 2–7.

Intellectualization. Intellectualization usually occurs during the first 1 to 3 months of caring for the dying. During this time, professional caregivers are usually confronted with their first experience of a hospice death. Nurses in this initial stage spend much of their energy learning the facts, tasks, policies, and procedures of the job. Emotional involvement in the dying and death of the patient may be inadvertently avoided, and the hospice nurse seldom reacts on an emotional level to the death.

Emotional Survival. Emotional survival generally occurs within 3 to 6 months of employment. Emotional involvement and a deeper connection with the patient and family occur. The nurse begins to confront the reality of the patient's death, to face her or his own mortality, and to feel sadness about the patient's situation and/or the loss of the patient. Often during this stage, the nurses begin to fully understand the magnitude of their roles and responsibilities and to question their abilities and desire to continue caring for dying patients and their families. This is a crucial time, and the nurse needs to be reassured and given support and resources to feel competent and confident so that he or she can progress successfully in the field.

Depression. Depression occurring at 6 to 9 months is often a time when hospice nurses process the losses rather than avoid them or remain emotionally detached. They begin to explore their own feelings about death, accept their own mortality, and accept death as a natural part of life.

It is in this stage that hospice professionals positively move toward resolution of death and loss and accept the reality of death and dying, or negatively resolve death and loss by choosing to avoid the emotional pain. In positive resolution, hospice professionals emotionally arrive at a comfortable place in caring for dying patients and their families.

Emotional Arrival. Emotional arrival occurs within 9 to 12 months of caring for the dying. With positive resolution of the last stage, hospice professionals become sensitive to the emotional needs and issues associated with dying and death. They can now cope with and accept loss, participate in healthy grieving, experience and conceptually work within the principles of hospice philosophy by advocating for the patient and family, and become involved with patients and families on a deeper level.

Deep Compassion. Deep compassion occurs after the first year as a hospice nurse. In this stage, hospice professionals begin to refine their knowledge and skills and are comfortable in providing compassionate, physical, psychosocial, and spiritual care to dying patients and their families. This stage is characterized by personal and professional growth and development.

The Doer. The final stage, the doer, is the culmination of nurses' experiencing the first five stages in a healthy and balanced manner; this outcome is characterized by hospice professionals who are efficient, vigorous, knowledgeable, and able to understand and comprehend humankind. Death has an inner meaning embedded in caring. Doers have grown and developed personally and professionally through the experiences of caring for the terminally ill.

Support Systems

In caring for dying patients and their families, the hospice nurse is vulnerable to emotions, reactions, and behaviors that can ultimately affect his or her personal well-being and the delivery of quality palliative care. To effectively care for patients and families, the nurse must also be responsible for attending to her or his own emotional, physical, and spiritual needs. Successfully coping with and adapting to dying, death, and cumulative loss is possible only if a system is in place that provides support to the nurse. Support systems may include personal death awareness exercises, time to verbalize in one-on-one counseling or with the IDT or both, supervisor support, preceptors or mentors, spiritual support, funeral or memorial services for closure, joint visits with members of other disciplines, and educational opportunities. The nurse should also explore individually facilitated support systems through journal writing, exercise, relaxation, meditation, and socialization with family and friends. By exploring and accessing support systems, hospice nurses can find satisfaction, fulfillment, and growth and development in their personal and professional lives as they provide compassionate end-of-life care to patients and their families.

Table 2–7
Cumulative Loss and the Professional Caregiver

Stage I (0–3 mo) *Intellectualization*	**Stage II** (3–6 mo) *Emotional Survival*	**Stage III** (6–9 mo) *Depression*	**Stage IV** (9–12 mo) *Emotional Arrival*	**Stage V** (12–24 mo) *Deep Compassion*
Professional knowledge	Increasing professional knowledge	Deepening professional knowledge	Acceptance of professional knowledge	Refining professional knowledge
Intellectualization	Less intellectualization	Decreasing intellectualization	Normal intellectualization	Refining intellectual base
Anxiety	Emotional survival	Depression	Emotional arrival	Deep compassion
Some uncomfortableness	Increasing uncomfortableness	Decreasing uncomfortableness	Increasing comfortableness	Increased comfortableness
Agreeableness	Guilt	Pain	Moderation	Self-realization
Withdrawal	Frustration	Mourning	Mitigation	Self-awareness
Superficial acceptance	Sadness	Grieving	Accommodation	Self-actualization
Providing tangible services	Initial emotional involvement	More emotional involvement	Ego mastery	Professional satisfaction
Use of emotional energy in understanding the setting	Increasing emotional involvement	Overidentification with the patient	Coping with loss of relationship	Acceptance of death and loss
Familiarizing self with policies and procedures	Initial understanding of the magnitude of the area of practice	Exploration of own feelings about death	Freedom from concern about own death	Rewarding professional growth and development
Working with families rather than patients	Overidentification with the patient's situation	Facing own death	Developing strong ties with dying patients and families	Development of ability to give of one's self
		Coming to grips with feelings about death	Development of ability to work with, on behalf of, and for the dying patient	Human and professional assessment
			Development of professional competence	Constructive and appropriate activities
			Productivity and accomplishments	Development of feelings of dignity and self-respect
			Healthy interaction	Ability to give dignity and self-respect to dying patient
				Feeling of comfortableness in relation to self, patient, family, and the job

Source: Harper (1994), reference 32.

Access Barriers to Hospice Care

In the national dialogue about improving care at the end of life, access to hospice services has been raised as a public policy and public health concern. There is acknowledgment of the value of hospice care for patients who need palliative care, with the recognition that there are barriers to its full utilization. Often patients are referred for hospice care just a few days or even hours before their deaths. Hospice demonstration projects are now underway testing how to care for patients who have an extended life expectancy or are receiving experimental or disease-modifying treatments. Policy proposals have been offered to allow for hospice programs to receive reimbursement for providing palliative care consultations to recently diagnosed patients and how to define alternative eligibility criteria that could be substituted for the 6-month prognosis requirement.[33] Many factors contribute to late referrals and access barriers, and communities are collaborating to ensure that palliative care is available across settings throughout the disease trajectory.[12]

A Death-Defying Society

The prevailing attitude of society toward death continues to be "death-defying." Unquestionable acceptance of innovation, efficiency, science, technological advances, and the ability to prolong life reflects the current perspective on health care. Therefore, acceptance of death as a natural process is difficult and offensive. Even with the growing hospice movement, most deaths happen in hospitals, often with uncontrolled pain.[34] As experts in the care of patients and families at the end of life, hospice workers will continue to shape the way in which people view dying and death.

Access Barriers

As a result of dissatisfaction with care afforded the dying more than 25 years ago, community members introduced the vision of hospice care. Congress adopted this vision through the creation of the MHB in 1982. Millions of Americans have benefited from care under this act, but it has fallen short of meeting current needs of the dying.

At the request of the NHPCO, the Committee on the Medicare Hospice Benefit and End-of-Life Care spent almost a year addressing issues related to hospice and end-of-life care. As part of the committee's review and recommendations, barriers to achieving the characteristics of the ideal future hospice and extending hospice to more Americans were identified. The specific recommendations of the report were wide-ranging, from improving the MHB to changing the education of health and human service professionals to raising the expectations for performance by hospice programs. All are important, but the following steps were identified as having the highest priority:

- Eliminating the 6-month prognosis under the MHB and identifying alternative eligibility specifications;
- Collecting and analyzing comprehensive data on the cost of meeting patient and family needs through hospice, with the intent to address inadequacies in Medicare payments;
- Developing outcome measures for assessing the quality of end-of-life care;
- Engaging the public in a campaign to create wider understanding and utilization of hospice care.[35]

Prognostic Limitations

One of the significant factors limiting access to hospice care is the determination of when hospice care should begin. There is mounting clinical evidence of the appropriateness of palliative care but few documented, valid, and reliable prognostic indicators of when palliative care should begin, especially for patients with diagnoses of chronic noncancer disease or aging and multisystem failure. This ambiguity can cause delay in referral to hospice or toward any palliative care focus. Further development and research on practice protocols for the care of patients with terminal disease is needed.

Terminally ill persons, given physician-certified prognosis of 6 months or less to live, represent patients who are potentially eligible for the MHB model. From historical,[36] contemporary,[37] and scientific perspectives,[38] however, determination of terminal status is notoriously elusive.

In an effort to implement criteria to identify when hospice should begin, the Centers for Medicare and Medicaid (formerly the Health Care Financing Administration) implemented Medicare prognostic criteria called Local Medical Review Policies (LMRPs) through the national Fiscal Intermediaries in the mid-1990s. The appropriateness of the Medicare prognostic criteria (LMRPs) has been contested on several points. First, mounting quantitative evidence shows little association between the LMRPs and short-term survival outcomes in hospice.[39,40] Second, although Medicare hospice was founded on the value of holistic, physical, psychosocial, and spiritual treatment of dying individuals, the LMRP criteria exclude nonphysical markers of disease progression. Third, although the consequences of regulatory reform have yet to be fully understood, the LMRPs appear to disadvantage those who are less obviously and imminently terminally ill. Sets of criteria to reliably distinguish terminally individuals (i.e., those with 6 months or less of life expectancy) from persons with severe and progressive disease would serve important clinical, practical, and humanitarian goals in hospice and in many other health care settings.[34] However, the LMRP criteria appear to have limited scientific merit.[41]

As is apparent from the findings of the largest project testing the validity of the LMRPs as prognostic criteria, application of the LMRP criteria can yield considerable misclassification. Moore observed a consistent pattern of relatively low rates of false-positive error and much higher corresponding rates of false-negative error. The practical consequence of high false-negative errors is erroneous classification of individuals who would survive less than 6 months as ineligible for the MHB. The consequence of false-positive errors is erroneous classification of individuals who will survive longer than 6 months as MHB-eligible. Relative to the costs and benefits of regulatory innovation, false-negative errors most disadvantage patients, families, and providers, whereas false-positive errors most disadvantage payers of public services.[41] These results further support those of previous smaller studies, which also indicated that prognostication is not a clear and concise science. The MHB was initially implemented with the understanding that the IDT in collaborative assessment would be the ideal way to identify when someone is eligible for the MHB.

Eliminating Barriers and Improving Access

Hospice programs have begun to respond to these barriers and are now providing a broader range of services by using more liberal internal eligibility criteria, flexible state hospice licensing provisions, home health agency licensure, no-fee volunteer support programs, counseling centers, and other approaches. Many hospice programs have extended their services to incorporate new palliative treatments, eliminated access barriers by admitting patients who live alone or lack a family caregiver or stable home setting, and cared for more patients with diagnoses other than cancer, including children with life-threatening illnesses. Other hospice agencies have pursued a somewhat different path to the same goal of expanded access by labeling their broader service offerings as "palliative care." Some have changed their services and their names to include palliative care components through discrete programs or separately incorporated subsidiaries, integrating those initiatives with traditional hospice care.[32]

The Comprehensive Hospice Center model, described earlier, aligns care and services with the needs of an aging population; these centers are compatible with a public health paradigm reflecting the preventive and care needs of youth, middle-aged, and older persons—a birth-to-death public health paradigm (Figure 2–2). Comprehensive hospices provide primary prevention services to the community by offering education on terminal disease trajectories and end-of-life care and caregiving and by providing bereavement support to communities. Through such activities, these hospices have the potential to contribute to the occurrence of lower survivor morbidity and mortality—to contribute to the public's health.[12]

Comprehensive hospices provide educational programs and services in schools and universities, in workplaces, and in other public places within communities (e.g., churches); they sponsor culturally diverse initiatives and help in the creation and dissemination of new knowledge.

Figure 2–2. Elements of a birth-to-death public health paradigm: an extension of an integrated public health and aging model by Andersen and Pourat. (*Sources:* Andersen R, Pourat N. Toward a synthesis of a public health agenda for an aging society. In: Hickey T, Speers MA, Prohaska TR, eds. Public Health and Aging. Baltimore: Johns Hopkins University Press, 1997, pp 311–324; Miller and Lima [2004], reference 11.)

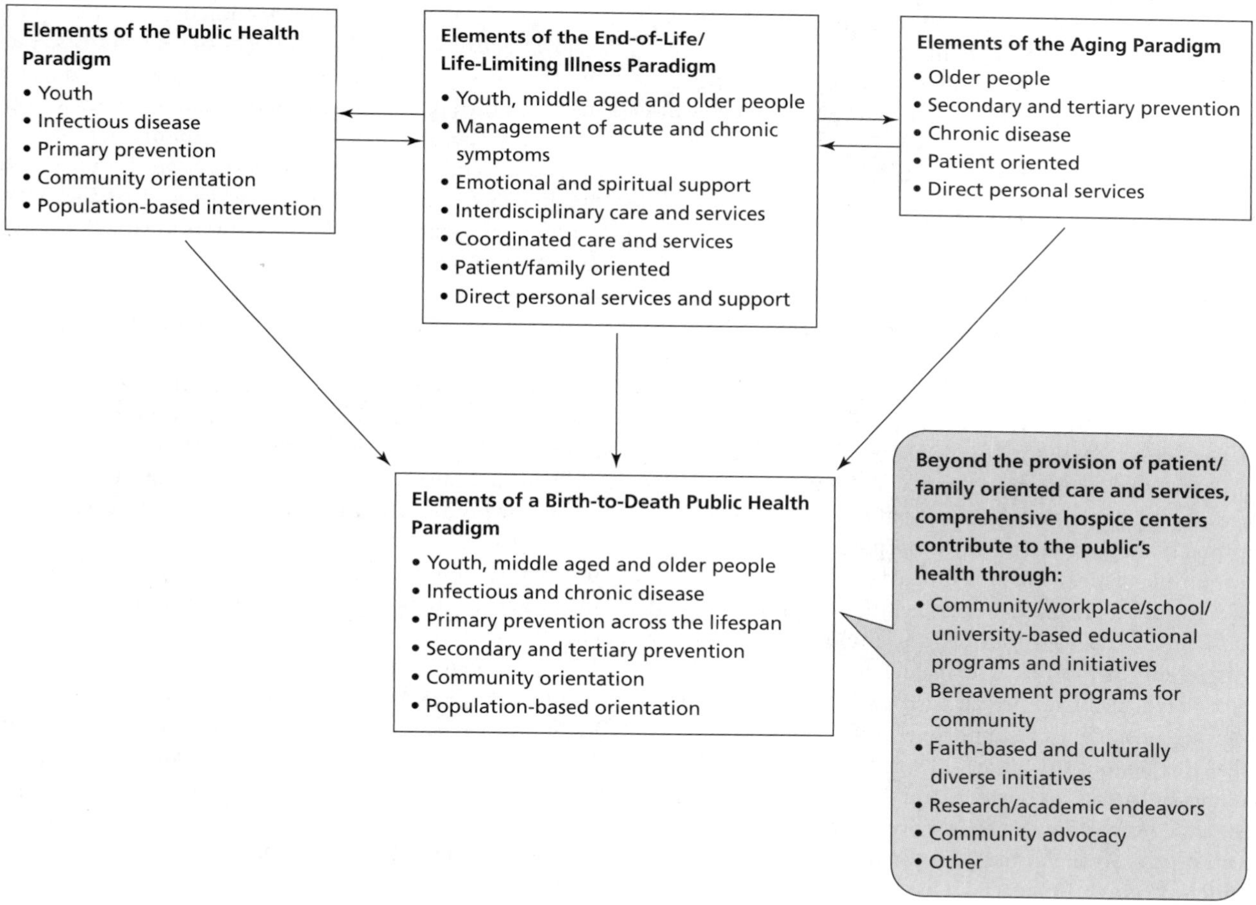

Hospice–Hospital Collaborations

A growing number of people in acute care settings are recognized as being in need of palliative care. It is now recognized that palliative care should not be an alternative to curative or life-prolonging treatment but should be offered in conjunction with such medical treatment. It is also recognized that this type of care is increasingly important as the health care system faces the need to find ways to treat the growing number of older adults with complex chronic illness.[33]

One approach to meeting the expanding needs of patients and families is evident in the growing number of partnerships between hospital systems and hospice programs. A study conducted by the NHPCO and the Center to Improve Palliative Care identified various structures currently in place to meet the palliative care needs of patients in acute care. Their report, *Hospice–Hospital Collaborations: Providing Palliative Care Across the Continuum of Services*, offers glimpses of how some models of collaboration are contributing to the expansion of palliative care in the hospital setting. Hospital–hospice collaboration is generally proceeding on two tracks. The first overall direction lies in enhanced use of the MHB for appropriate patients by promoting closer relationships between hospice programs and hospitals, offering education, developing specialized units, and encouraging the direct admission of hospitalized patients to hospice. The second track involves development of new, nonhospice benefit services, such as hospice palliative care management and consultation services.[33]

When Nurses Should Consider Hospice for Their Patients

All nurses must be familiar with the benefits and services of their local hospice programs, so that they can effectively educate and advocate for palliative care when their patients and families could benefit from this approach and scope of supportive services. Considering the expanding hospice models, there are many myths and misperceptions that must be eliminated—such as the need to be within 6 months of death to receive hospice services—so that patients and families can be optimally supported. The most common comment nationally on hospice family satisfaction surveys is, "I wish we had hospice sooner." The voices of these families support the need for earlier referral to hospice. It is important for nurses providing end-of-life care to consider when to think about hospice. Table 2–8 lists practical scenarios to guide nurses in offering hospice as a supportive service to patients and families throughout the lifespan. Hospice teams are expert at assessing palliative care needs and are available to assist nurses in determining which services may benefit a given patient. A call to collaborate with the local hospice provider can initiate this assessment.

The Funding of Hospice Programs

The original hospices, which began as grassroots community efforts, were funded almost exclusively by charitable support, grants, and volunteer efforts. Some components of care were supported by Medicare or insurance, such as skilled nursing visits, medications, or durable medical equipment on a per-unit fee-for-service basis allowed under an acute care model. In 1980, the U.S. Congress authorized a 2-year demonstration program in 27 hospices around the nation to study the outcomes of hospice care and the costs associated with it. The demonstrations included researchers at each site who collected both field data from patients and families and cost data from each organization. Ultimately, the demonstration was continued for an additional year. Based on very preliminary findings, Congress created the MHB as a 2-year endeavor and then subsequently approved it as a permanent part of the Medicare program in August of 1982.

The MHB was a landmark event under Medicare in that it was the first formal recognition of the unique needs of dying patients and their families. It was also the first form of what ultimately became managed care. It included provisions never before included as health care benefits, such as spiritual support, volunteers, and bereavement support for family members. It was an all-inclusive benefit in which all services related to the terminal illness were to be provided, coordinated, and paid for through the hospice program. Although this approach is now frequently viewed as a strategy to control costs, it was at the time designed in this manner because surviving family members cited the complexity of bills and the financial toll of a terminal illness as one of the greatest stressors.

The benefit included the following core hospice services: nursing care, medical and social services, physician services, counseling/pastoral services, short-term inpatient and respite care, medical appliances and supplies including drugs and biologicals, home health aide and homemaker services, therapies (physical, occupational, speech), bereavement counseling, and drugs for symptom management and pain control.[15] It also had a provision for four levels of care depending on the intensity and place of care rendered on any given day. Continuity across all care settings with hospice professional management of care was and continues to be a strong underpinning of the benefit.

Following the MHB demonstration and benefit development, Medicaid and private insurance hospice benefits began to emerge. Ultimately, most states developed Medicaid benefits, which are mandated to be no less than the Medicare benefit. Private insurers frequently model their benefit on the MHB, although they are under no mandate to do so.

Most hospices are committed to providing care regardless of ability to pay, and they continue to be dependent on charitable dollars to provide such care. Additional supportive services, beyond the benefit, such as children's programs, in-home caregiver programs, hospice residences, and community bereavement and education programs, are provided in many hospice communities.

Table 2–8
When to Call Hospice

Call for a Consultation When	How Hospice May Help
Your patients and family members are calling more and more to ask questions about care	Hospice can provide support for the patient and family to help lessen their anxieties, normalize their feelings, connect them to community caregiver resources, and teach caregiving skills.
You would not be surprised by this patient's death within the next year	The number one comment made by hospice families after the death of a loved one is, "I wish we had hospice services earlier. We needed the help." Hospice can outline ways to support your patient and family earlier.
You see a sudden decline in the patient's condition	Hospice admissions staff and medical directors are experts at assessing for needed care and services. If the patient is not eligible for the Medicare Hospice Benefit, the patient and family may be offered other services, such as palliative care or counseling.
There is progressive loss of function	Loss of function is a key prognostic indicator for a life-limiting condition. Hospice can provide durable medical equipment, personal care, and other assistance.
Your patient has been hospitalized twice in the past year due to symptom exacerbation from a chronic illness	Two hospitalizations for the same chronic disease within 12 months is often an indicator of less than 1 year to live. Hospice interdisciplinary teams can assess the progression of the disease and help determine whether it a good time for hospice support.
There is an onset of multiple comorbidities and/or an increase in symptoms associated with comorbidities	Especially for the elder population, a rapid change in condition or progressive decline of functional abilities indicate it may be time for hospice. Call for an assessment and identification of support services.
Your patient would benefit from help with advance directive/care planning	Hospice staff are experienced in clarifying the various options for advance directives. They can assist patients and family members in having discussions to clarify end-of-life goals and make informed choices.
Your patient could benefit from palliative symptom management while still pursuing curative therapy	Through an array of programs, hospice may be able to provide palliative care coordination to patients along the care continuum. Physicians, nurse practitioners, and the hospice interdisciplinary team can help control side effects and other symptoms.

(*continued*)

Table 2–8
When to Call Hospice *(continued)*

Call for a Consultation When	How Hospice May Help
A patient is making decisions about transitioning to palliative care	Hospice counselors and peer volunteers can help your patients/families address options and fears and advocate for their wishes. Hospice staff assist patients and families in identifying and defining quality of life, so that decisions can be made with peace of mind.
Someone needs information about any end-of-life or related health care issues	Hospice has an extensive resource center with a broad range of topics including end of life, wellness, complementary therapies, and advance directives.
Your patient is in the intensive care unit and is considering comfort measures only	Hospice can provide family support in decision-making, resources on alternative placement options if the patient cannot be cared for at home, and the option for hospice residence placement.
The family or other caregivers are unable to care for the patient at home	Hospice can help patients and families to determine caregiving resources available through personal support systems, community groups/agencies and hospice. The hospice residence expands the available options.
At the time of diagnosis of a life-limiting illness	Someone to talk to may be the best support you can offer. Hospice reassurance volunteers are trained to help in these difficult situations.
It is time to have a difficult discussion	Hospice counselors can be present during these conversations or can meet with families afterward and provide resources to patients and families to guide conversations.

Although a small portion of all people receiving health care are at the end of life and receiving terminal care, the terminally ill consume a disproportionate percentage of all health care expenditures. There are several studies on the cost savings in hospice versus traditional health care at the end of life. Hospice has remained a positive example of integrating a managed care model with proven cost savings while meeting patients' and families' needs and receiving high quality scores.

Initially, hospices were slow to seek certification for Medicare status, but this connection has grown steadily as hospices have become more comfortable with assuming the risk of total costs of care. There were also financial reimbursement and other utilization caps in the program that concerned many. Today, most hospices are Medicare certified, and the number of recipients of hospice care in America has grown commensurately, from approximately 500,000 patients and families in 1998 to more than 885,000 in 2002.[10]

The Medicare Hospice Benefit

The levels of care outlined in the MHB reflect the variations in care intensity that are required to meet patient and family needs in the last phase of life. Medicare provides coverage for hospice care to Medicare beneficiaries who have elected the hospice benefit and who have been certified as terminally ill with a prognosis for a life expectancy of 6 months or less. Once elected, Medicare pays one of four prospective, per diem rates for hospice care: routine home care, continuous home care, respite care, general inpatient care. Each of these payment categories is defined later. Changing the level of care is determined through a collaborative effort by the hospice IDT, patient, family, and primary physician.

Routine Home Care. Routine home care is provided in the patient's home, nursing home, or residential care setting or wherever the patient and family reside. The hospice core services provided at this level include nursing care, home health aide care, social services, therapies, medical appliances and supplies, and drugs.

Continuous Care. Continuous care covers patients in brief periods of crisis, during which 8 or more hours per day of care is provided to the patient at home, with at least 50% of the care being delivered by a registered nurse or licensed practical nurse.

Inpatient Respite Care. Inpatient respite care covers patients in an approved inpatient facility for the relief of the patient's primary caregiver, for a maximum of 5 days per episode. It includes coverage of drugs, supplies, and equipment as well.

General Inpatient Care. General inpatient care covers patients in a participating hospice inpatient unit of a hospital, skilled nursing facility, intermediate care facility, or free-standing hospice for medically necessary days for the control of pain or acute or chronic symptom management that cannot be managed in other settings. It includes coverage for ancillary services (e.g., oxygen, laboratory, pharmacy).[15]

The Medicaid Hospice Benefit

Medicaid coverage for hospice is patterned after the Medicare benefit, including both patient eligibility requirements and coverage for specific services. States do have some flexibility in developing their hospice benefit.

Private Insurance Reimbursement and Managed Care

Private insurance companies have begun to realize the benefits of hospice care and are including a hospice benefit in their services. As with Medicaid, many private insurers pattern their benefit after Medicare. Some insurers have negotiated services with hospices, including those palliative care consultation and care management services of the Community Hospice Model, before the MHB services begin. Many managed care companies have also reflected the Medicare benefit in services provided to their members either through their own hospice programs or under contract with programs serving the patient's community.

Conclusion

Hospice is more than a program of health services. It is an approach and philosophy of care and services that strive to encompass and support the full experience of illness, aging, caregiving, dying, and bereavement for both the patient and the family. Although the last phase of life and relationship is a difficult time, with sensitive support it can be a time of tremendous growth and opportunity for the person who is dying and for loved ones—such as in the finding of meaning and purpose in one's suffering, the value of one's life accomplishments, the deepening of relationships, and the personal spiritual significance of the experience.

Nurses can positively affect this experience for others by allowing the patient's and family's personal values and goals to direct the support and care they offer as they are invited to share in this intimate time of life. Regardless of the site of care or type of program or services, nurses providing end-of-life care must be proficient in end-stage disease and symptom management. They also have a responsibility to be knowledgeable about the services a hospice program can offer their patients and families and to know when to consider offering hospice care. Nurses must be guided by dignity, compassion, love, and individual acceptance of patient and family values and choices to ensure quality end-of-life care.

REFERENCES

1. Panke J, Coyne P. Conversations in Palliative Care. Pensacola, Fla.: Pohl Publishing Company, 2004.
2. Teno JM, Cartridge BR, Casey V, Welch LC, Wetle T, Shield R, Moor V. Family perspectives on end-of-life care at the last place of care. JAMA 2004;7:291:88–93.
3. Standards and Accreditation Committee. Standards of Practice for Hospice Programs. Arlington, Va.: National Hospice and Palliative Care Organization, 2000.
4. National Hospice and Palliative Care Organization. Keys to Quality Care. Arlington, Va.: NHPCO, 2004:2. Available at: http://www.nhpco.org in the section entitled "Hospice and Palliative Care Information" (accessed October 18, 2004).
5. Beresford L. The Hospice Handbook: A Complete Guide. Boston: Little, Brown, 1993.
6. Cassell EJ. The nature of suffering and the goals of medicine. N Engl J Med 1982;306:639–642.
7. Cassell EJ. The Nature of Suffering and the Goals of Medicine. Oxford: Oxford University Press, 1991.
8. Meier DE, Morrison RS. Old age and care near the end of life. J Am Soc Aging 1999;23:7.
9. Lattanzi-Licht M, Mahoney JJ, Miller GW. The Hospice Choice: In Pursuit of a Peaceful Death. New York: Simon and Schuster, 1998.
10. National Hospice and Palliative Care Organization. NHPCO Facts and Figures. Updated February 2004. Available at: http://www.nhpco.org/files/public/Facts%20Figures%20Feb04.pdf (accessed October 18, 2004).
11. Miller SC, Lima J. The Florida Model of Hospice Care: A Report for Florida Hospices and Palliative Care, Inc, pp 8–9. Tallahasee, FL: Florida Hospices & Palliative Care, Inc., 2004.
12. Jennings B, Ryndes R, D'Onofrio C, Baily MA. Access to Hospice Care: Expanding Boundaries, Overcoming Barriers. Hastings Center Report. March 1, 2003.
13. Huskamp HA, Buntin MB, Wang V, Newhouse JP. Providing care at the end of life: Do Medicare rule impede good care? Health Affairs 2001;20:204–211.
14. Mooney B. Hot topics in hospice management: Poll shows Americans prefer to die at home. Hospital Management Advisor (Atlanta, Ga.), 1997:167–170.

15. Manard B, Perrone C. Hospice Care: An Introduction and Review of the Evidence. Arlington, Va.: National Hospice Organization, 1994.
16. Miller SC, Mor V. The emergence of Medicare hospice in U.S. nursing homes. Palliat Med 201;15:471–480.
17. Miller SC, Mor V, Wu N, et al. Does receipt of hospice care in nursing homes improve the management of pain at the end-of-life? J Am Geriatr Soc 2002;50:507–515.
18. Baer WM, Hanson LC. Families' perception of the added value of hospice in the nursing home. J Am Geriatr Soc 2000;48: 879–882.
19. Miller SC, Gozalo P, Mor V. Hospice enrollment and hospitalization of dying nursing home patients. Am J Med 2001;111:38–44.
20. Wu N, Miller SC, Lapane K, Gozalo P. The problem of assessment bias when measuring the hospice effect on nursing home residents' pain. J Pain Symptom Manage 2003;26: 998–1009.
21. Labyak M, Egan K, Brandt K. The experience model: Transforming the end-of-life experience. Hospice and Palliative Care Insights 2002;2:9–14.
22. Gerteis M, Edgman-Levitan S, Daley J, Delbanco TL, eds. Through the Patient's Eyes: Understanding and Promoting Patient-Centered Care. San Francisco: Jossey-Bass, 1993:20.
23. Cassell EJ. The Nature of Suffering and the Goals of Medicine, 2nd ed. Oxford: Oxford University Press, 2004.
24. Byock I, Merriman MP. Measuring quality of life for patients with terminal illness: The Missoula-VITAS® Quality of Life Index. Palliat Med 1998;12:231–244.
25. Byock I. Dying Well: The Prospect for Growth at the End of Life. New York: G. P. Putnam's Sons, 1997.
26. Byock I. The nature of suffering and the nature of opportunity at the end-of-life. Clin Geriatr Med 1996;2:237–251.
27. Tyler BA, Perry MJ, Lofton TC, Millard F. The Quest to Die with Dignity: An Analysis of Americans' Values, Opinions and Attitudes Concerning End-of-Life Care. Atlanta, Ga.: American Health Decisions, 1997.
28. Salmon JR, Deming AM, Kwak J, Acquaviva K, Brandt K, Egan K. Caregiving at Life's End: The National Needs Assessment and Implications for Hospice Practice. Executive Summary, to The Hospice Institute of the Florida Suncoast. Tampa, Fla.: Florida Policy Exchange Center on Aging, University of South Florida, June 2003:2–7.
29. Egan KA. The hospice experience model: A framework for peaceful life closure. Presented at American Society on Aging, Chicago, 2003.
30. Sherman DW. Training advanced practice palliative care nurses. J Am Soc Aging 1999;23:88.
31. Connor SR, Egan KA, Wilosz DK, Larson DG, Reese DJ. Interdisciplinary approaches to assisting with end-of-life care and decision making. Am Behav Sci 2002;46:340–356.
32. Harper BC. Death: The Coping Mechanism of the Health Professional. Greenville, S.C.: Swiger Associates, Inc., Southeastern University Press, 1994.
33. Hospital–Hospice Partnerships in Palliative Care: Creating a Continuum of Service. National Hospice and Palliative Care Organization and The Center to Advance Palliative Care in Hospitals and Health Systems. Arlington, Va.: NHPCO, 2002.
34. SUPPORT Principal Investigators. A controlled trial, to improve care for seriously ill hospitalized patients. JAMA 1995;274: 1591–1598.
35. Committee on the Medicare Hospice Benefit and End-of-Life Care. Final Report to the Board of Directors. Arlington, Va.: National Hospice Organization, 1998:23–25.
36. Christakis NA, Lamont EB. Extent and determinants of error in doctors' prognoses in terminally ill patients: Prospective cohort study. BMJ 2000;320:469–473.
37. Lynn J, Harrell FE, Cohn F, Wagner D, Conners AF Jr. Prognoses of seriously ill hospitalized patients on the days before death: Implications for patient care and public policy. New Horizons 1997;5:56–61.
38. Pearlman RA. Variability in physician estimates of survival for acute respiratory failure in chronic obstructive pulmonary disease. Chest 1987;91:515–521.
39. Schonwetter RS, Robinson BE, Ramirez G. Prognostic factors for survival in terminal lung cancer patients. J Gen Intern Med 1994; 9:366–371.
40. Fox E, Landrum-McNif K, Zhong Z, Dawson NV, Wu AW, Lynn J. Evaluation of prognostic criteria for determining hospice eligibility in patients with advanced lung, heart or liver disease. JAMA 1999;282:1638–1645.
41. Moore HD. Evaluation of the Prognostic Criteria for Medicare Hospice Eligibility. A dissertation submitted in partial fulfillment of the requirements for the degree of Doctor of Philosophy, School of Aging Studies, College of Arts and Sciences, University of South Florida. March 2004.
42. Miller SC, Egan KA. How can clinicians with diverse backgrounds and training collaborate with one another to care for patients at the end of life? Nursing home and hospice partnerships. In: Pruchno R. Ethical Issues at the End of Life. Baltimore, Md.: Johns Hopkins University Press. In press.
43. The Hospice Institute of the Florida Suncoast. Caregiving at Life's End: The National Train-the-Trainer Curriculum. Module 3: Life Affairs. Key Largo, Fla.: The Hospice Institute of the Florida Suncoast, 2003:M3HO1–M3HO2.

3

Elaine Glass, Douglas Cluxton, and Patrice Rancour

Principles of Patient and Family Assessment

The question is not what you look at, but what you see.—Henry David Thoreau

- ***Key Points***
- *Comprehensive assessment of the patient and family is essential to planning palliative care.*
- *Assessment involves input from the interdisciplinary team with information shared verbally as well as in the patient record.*
- *Detailed and comprehensive assessment is needed to identify the complex and changing needs of patients and families facing advanced disease.*

An effective assessment is key to establishing an appropriate nursing care plan for the patient and family. The initial palliative care nursing assessment varies little from a standard nursing assessment.[1] In order to assess effectively, members of the health care team need to maximize their listening skills and minimize quick judgments. Medical experts contend that during a medical assessment interview, in which a physician mostly listens and gently guides the patient's story, the physician can accurately diagnose the patient's problem 70% to 80% of the time.[2]

The goals of the palliative care plan that evolve from the initial and ongoing nursing assessments focus on enhancing quality of life. Ferrell's quality-of-life framework[3] is used to organize the assessment. The four quality-of-life domains in this framework are physical, psychological, social, and spiritual well-being. For the purpose of this chapter, the psychological and social domains are combined into one, the psychosocial domain.

Because the needs of patients and families change throughout the course of a chronic illness, these quality-of-life assessments are examined at four times during the illness trajectory: at the time of diagnosis, during treatments, after treatments (long-term survival or terminal phase), and during active dying.

CASE STUDY

Ghedi, a Man with Colon Cancer

Ghedi, a fictitious patient from Somalia, serves as a case example throughout his illness experience with colon cancer. He is a 68-year-old man who emigrated to the United States in 1998. He lives with his older brother, Asad; his sister-in-law, Laila; and their adult son and daughter. Asad and his family have lived in the United States for 15 years; they have developed ease with English and are sensitive to many American customs and norms. Ghedi came to this country after losing his wife and son in the war in his native land in 1991. He has continued to speak Somali exclusively, retaining his affiliation with his native land, and has avoided assimilation into American culture. He understands some spoken English. Ghedi and Asad have no other family members in the United States, but they are well integrated within the Somali community that is located in their city. Ghedi is a devout Sunni Muslim who believes that God will protect him, that good health is a gift from God, and that illness can be a result of the presence of spirits in one's life.

Malignant versus Nonmalignant Terminal Diseases

Because the authors of this chapter work primarily with oncology patients, much of the assessment content is based on the cancer experience. The experiences of terminally ill patients with diseases other than cancer can be equally dynamic in terms of the continuous or episodic declines they face throughout the illness trajectory.

A primary difference between patients with malignant and nonmalignant illness lies in the current acceptance by the medical establishment that efforts toward cure are unavailable for many nonmalignant diseases. Thus, from the start, the focus of medical care for these patients is palliative rather than curative: reduction of symptoms, improvement of quality of life, and optimization of the highest level of wellness. Examples of these kinds of illness today include acquired immune deficiency syndrome (AIDS); refractory cardiovascular, hepatic, and renal diseases; brittle diabetes; and neurological disorders such as multiple sclerosis, cerebral palsy, amyotrophic lateral sclerosis, Parkinson's disease, and Alzheimer's disease. For some of these diseases, the focus of medical care may include attempting to extend life through research with the hope of finding a cure.

In contrast, medical professionals and the public are continually looking and hoping for a cure for cancer. As a result, the oncology patient may repeatedly alter his or her expectations about the future. Words describing the status of the disease during a cancer illness include "no evidence of disease," "remission," "partial remission," "stable disease," "recurrence," "relapse," and "metastasis." Patients report experiencing a "roller-coaster ride," in which the hopeful points in remission are often followed by a crisis with relapse or disease progression. Patients may be told, more than once, that they are likely to die within a short time. Then, they may recover and do well for awhile. As a result, the reality of death may be more difficult when it does occur.

Introduction to Physical Assessment

Before beginning the assessment interview and physical examination, it is important for the nurse to establish a relationship with the patient by doing the following:

- Introducing himself or herself to the patient and others in the room.
- Verifying that this is the correct patient.
- Determining how the patient would like to be addressed: first name? last name? a nickname?
- Explaining the purpose of the interaction and the approximate length of time that he or she intends to spend with the patient.
- Asking the patient's permission to proceed with the assessment, giving the patient an opportunity to use the restroom, and excusing others whom the patient does not wish to be present during the interview and examination. (Some patients may want significant others to be present during the interview, to assist with recall, but not during the examination. The nurse needs to modify the assessment routine to accommodate the patient's preferences.)
- Taking a seat near the patient, being respectful of the patient's cultural norms for physical closeness and eye contact.
- Inviting the patient to tell about how he or she learned of the illness.
- Taking care not to interrupt the patient too often; using communication techniques such as probing, reflecting, clarifying, responding empathetically, and asking open-ended questions to encourage greater detail if the patient's account is brief or sketchy.

Refer to Figure 3–1 for a sample physical symptom assessment charting form that includes a severity measurement scale.

Introduction to Psychosocial Assessment

Tables 3–1 through 3–3 provide a framework for three key elements of assessment: conducting a psychosocial assessment, distinguishing normal grief from depression, and doing a general mental status assessment. Throughout the illness trajectory, the nurse can use these tools to monitor the patient's response to illness and treatment.

Anyone diagnosed with a serious or life-threatening illness experiences many losses. However, responses to illness vary tremendously among individuals. In addition, the same person may respond differently at various times during an illness. How a particular patient copes depends on the severity of the illness, the patient's history of coping with stressful life events, and available supports. Some individuals develop coping styles that are more helpful than others when facing a life-threatening illness.

The nurse needs to assess two very important parameters in order to assist the patient in coping in the most functional way possible. These parameters are the patient's need for information and her or his need for control in making decisions. Observers of "exceptional" patients, such as Bernie Siegel,[4] have

Name Preference:		**DOB:**	**Age:**
Referring Physician:	**Service:**	**Reason:**	
Diagnoses:			

Communication: ☐ Capacity to make decisions Surrogate: Relationship:

Constitutional: ☐ Wt ↑ ↓ ______# ☐ Fatigue __/3 Activity: ☐ Bed ☐ Chair ☐ Walk ☐ Run

Ht: ____' ____" Dependent ADLs: ☐ Eating ☐ Toileting ☐ Bathing ☐ Dressing ☐ Transferring ☐ Walking

Review of Systems: ☐ According to pt ☐ According to: ☐ Unable to obtain **Appearance:**

System	**Neg**	**Positive Responses:** 0= None 1= Mild 2= Moderate 3= Severe				**Other:**
Eyes	☐	☐ Wears glasses	☐ ∅ read labels	☐ ∅ see TV	☐ Legally blind	☐
Ear, Nose, & Throat	☐	☐ Hard of hearing __/3	☐ Dysphasia	☐ Aspiration	☐ Sinus problems	☐
	☐	☐ Poor dentition	☐ Dentures	☐ Mouth sores__/3	☐ Aphasia	☐
Cardiovascular	☐	☐ Edema __/3	☐ Palpitations	☐ Orthopnea __/3	☐ DOE __/3	☐
Respiratory	☐	☐ Dyspnea __/3	☐ Cough __/3	☐ Smokes now / hx	☐ 02:	☐
Gastrointestinal	☐	☐ Vomiting __/3	☐ Nausea __/3	☐ ↓ Appetite__/3	☐ Dyspepsia __/3	☐
BMs q __ days	☐	☐ Constipation __/3	☐ Diarrhea __/3	☐ Hemorrhoids	☐ Incontinent	☐
Genitourinary	☐	☐ Difficulty U.O.	☐ Hematuria	☐ Nocturia	☐ Incontinent	☐
Musculoskeletal	☐	☐ Muscle weakness __/3		☐ ROM ↓	☐ Arthritis __/3	☐
Skin	☐	☐ Pruritis__/3	☐ Dehydration	☐ DPUs		☐
Neurological	☐	☐ Paresthesia__/3	☐ Dizziness	☐ Headaches	☐ Insomnia__/3	☐
Hem/Lymphatic	☐	☐ + Bruises __/3	☐ Anemia	☐ Bleeding:		☐
Immune	☐	☐ Colds/yr:_____	☐ Flu hx	☐ Non drug allergies:		☐

PAIN Location	**0-10**	**Pattern**	**Descriptors**	**↑s Pain**	**↓s Pain**
		☐ Intermittent ☐ Constant			
		☐ Intermittent ☐ Constant			

Pain priority: ☐ Alertness even if less comfortable ☐ Comfort even if a little sleepy

Priority Symptoms Wanting to Minimize:	**Recommendations/Plan**
cc:	

Perception of illness:

Health Care Goals: ☐ Cure at all costs ☐ Quality of life > Length of life ☐ Length of life > quality of life ☐ Comfort Care

Information preference if bad news: ☐ Truth with details ☐ Soften truth ☐ Tell:

Things important in health care decision making: ☐ What family thinks ☐ What religion says ☐ Being in control ☐ Cost

If illness is terminal: Wants to know if dying ☐ Yes ☐ No Wants family to know if dying ☐ Yes ☐ No ☐ N/A

Talking about end of life: ☐ Comfortable ☐ Uncomfortable but willing ☐ Does not want to discuss

Name: ______________________________ **Pager:** ______________ **Date:** ________

Grant Medical Center

Palliative Care at Grant Physical Assessment

614-566-Pall (7255)

Addressograph

3002514 GMC PAL (3/29/04)

Figure 3–1. Sample physical assessment charting form. (*Source:* © Grant Medical Center, Columbus, Ohio. Reprinted with permission; all rights reserved.)

(*continued*)

Drug Allergies: ☐ NKDA			
Prescription coverage? ☐ Co-Pay of:______per script ☐ None ☐ Could use assistance		IV Access:	
Local Pharmacy:		Knowledge of Medicines: None=0 Poor=1 Fair=2 Good=3	
Current Medications in Hospital	Home?	Knowledge of? / Comments	Cost/Month
Other Medications at Home + Supplements & Vitamins:			

Use of Complementary Therapies:		
☐ Acupuncture	☐ Dietary Program	☐ Music
☐ Aromatherapy	☐ Guided Imagery	☐ Pet Therapy
☐ Art Therapy	☐ Hypnosis	☐ Relaxation
☐ Biofeedback	☐ Journaling	☐ Other:

Impression:

Recommendations/Plan:

Name: ______________________ **Pager:** ____________ **Date:** ________

Grant Medical Center

Palliative Care at Grant Physical Assessment

614-566-Pall (7255)

Page 2 of 2

Addressograph

300XXXX (9/15/03)

Figure 3–1. *(continued)*

Table 3–1
Framework for Psychosocial Assessment

Determining the types of losses

Physical	Psychosocial	Spiritual
Energy	Autonomy	Illusion of predictability/certainty
Mobility	Sense of mastery	Illusion of immortality
Body parts	Body image alterations	Illusion of control
Body function	Sexuality	Hope for the future
Freedom from pain and other forms of physical dysfunction	Relationship changes	Time
Sexuality	Lifestyle	
	Work changes	
	Role function	
	Money	
	Time	

Observing emotional responses

Anxiety, anger, denial, withdrawal, shock, sadness, bargaining, depression

Identifying coping styles

Functional: normal grief work and problem-solving

Dysfunctional: aggression, fantasy, minimization, addictive behaviors, guilt, psychosis

Assessing the need for information

Wants to know details

Wants the overall picture

Wants minimal information

Wants no information, but wants the family to know

Assessing the need for control

Very high

High

Moderate/average

Low

Absent, wants others to decide

noted that patients who are proactive, assertive information-seekers often appear to have better outcomes than patients who are passive in making decisions. Indicators of a person's need for control may include the following:

- Comfort in asking questions
- Willingness to assert own needs and wishes relative to the plan of care
- Initiative taken to research print and Internet resources on the illness and treatment

Table 3–1 provides details for doing a psychosocial assessment. More detailed information on the psychosocial aspects of oncology can be found in Holland's *Psycho-oncology.*[5]

Grief is a normal reaction to loss, especially a major loss such as one's health. In chronic illness, grief is likely to be recurrent as losses accumulate. This does not make it pathological, but it does form the basis of the "roller-coaster" phenomenon that many patients describe. Some patients with advanced disease have been able to integrate their losses in a meaningful way, managing to reconcile and transcend them. An example of such a person is Morrie Schwartz, who wrote about his illness in *Letting Go: Morrie's Reflections on Living While Dying.*[6]

Table 3–2 contrasts and compares normal grief with depression, to assist the nurse in determining when a patient needs to be referred for counseling. For further information, consult John Schneider's classic work, "Clinically Significant Differences between Grief, Pathological Grief and Depression."[7]

In some cases, patients may appear to be having difficulties in coping but the nurse cannot easily identify the specific

Table 3–2
Differentiating Normal Grief from Depression

Normal Grief/Response to Loss of Health	Depression
Self-limiting but recurrent with each additional loss	Frequently not self-limited, lasting longer than 2 months
Preoccupied with loss	Self-preoccupied, rumination
Emotional states variable	Consistent dysphoria or anhedonia (absence of pleasure)
Episodic difficulties sleeping	Insomnia or hypersomnia
Lack of energy, slight weight loss	Extreme lethargy, weight loss
Identifies loss	May not identify loss or may deny it
Crying is evident and provides some relief	Crying absent or persists uncontrollably
Socially responsive to others	Socially unresponsive, isolated
Dreams may be vivid	No memory of dreaming
Open expression of anger	No expression of anger
Adaptation does not require professional intervention	Adaptation requires professional treatment

problem. The nurse may need to make a more thorough mental health assessment to determine the most appropriate referral. Key elements in such an assessment are found in Table 3–3. For more detailed psychosocial information, consult Holland's *Psycho-oncology*.[5]

Table 3–3
General Mental Health Assessment

Appearance	**Psychomotor Behavior**
Hygiene	Gait
Grooming	Movement
Posture	Coordination
Body language	Compulsions
Mood and Affect	Energy
Interview behavior	Observable symptoms (tics, perseveration)
Specific feelings expressed	**Speech**
Facial expressions	Pressured, slow, rapid
Intellectual Ability	Goal-oriented, rambling, Incoherent, fragmented, coherent
Attention	Relevant, irrelevant
Concentration	Poverty of speech
Concrete/abstract thinking	Presence of latencies (delayed ability to respond when conversing)
Comprehension	**Thought Patterns**
Insight	Loose, perseverating
Judgment	Logical, illogical, confused
Educational level	Oriented, disoriented
Sensorium/Level of Consciousness	Tangential, poorly organized, well-organized
Alert	Preoccupied
Somnolent	Obsession
Unresponsive	Paranoid ideas of reference
	Delusions
	Hallucination, illusions
	Blocking, flight of ideas
	Neologisms (made-up words)
	Word salad (meaningless word order)
	Presence of suicidal or homicidal ideation

Introduction to Spiritual Assessment

Although Chapter 30 provides a more detailed discussion of spiritual assessment, the following discussion illustrates the importance of assessing the spiritual domain as a component of a comprehensive evaluation.

Attempts to define spirituality can often result in feelings of dismay and inadequacy. It is like trying to capture the wind or grasp water. Therefore, assessing and addressing the spiritual needs of patients can be a formidable challenge. Spirituality may include one's religious identity, beliefs, and practices, but it involves much more. The person without an identified religious affiliation is no less spiritual. Indeed, the desire to speak one's truth, explore the meaning of one's life and illness, and maintain hope are fundamental human quests that reflect the depth of the spirit. Haase and colleagues[8] concluded that the spiritual perspective is "an integrating and creative energy based on belief in, and feeling of interconnectedness with, a power greater than self." Amenta[9] viewed spirituality as "the life-force springing from within that pervades our entire being." Hay[10] defined it as "the capacity for transcending in order to love or be loved, to give meaning, and to cope." Doyle[11] wrote, "Spiritual beliefs may be expressed in religion and its hallowed practices, but a person can and often does have a spiritual dimension to his or her life that is totally unrelated to religion and not expressed or explored in religious practice." He further noted that "a prerequisite to discussion of spiritual issues with a patient is to create a situation which permits speaking of spiritual problems, i.e. environment, ambiance, and attitude."[11]

The spiritual issues that arise after the diagnosis of a serious or life-threatening illness are abundant and varied. As a person progresses through the phases of an illness (diagnosis, treatment, posttreatment, and active dying), he or she is confronted with mortality, limitations, and loss. This frequently leads to questions such as, "What is my life's purpose?," "What does all this mean?," "What is the point of my suffering?," "Why me?," and "Is there life after death?" Indeed, Victor Frankl,[12] in his classic work, *Man's Search for Meaning*, affirmed that the quest to find meaning is one of the most characteristically human endeavors. To find meaning in suffering enhances the human spirit and fosters survival.

According to Abraham Maslow's[13] theory, human needs can be placed on a hierarchy that prioritizes them from the most basic physical and survival needs to the more transcendent needs. Thus, a patient's ability and willingness to engage in dialogue about issues of meaning, to discuss successes and regrets, and to express his or her core values may occur only after more fundamental needs are addressed. This reality in no way diminishes the spiritual compared with the physical; rather, it supports the need for an interdisciplinary approach that provides holistic care of the entire person. For example, if a physician relieves a young woman's cancer pain and a social worker secures transportation for her to treatments, she and her family may be more able to address the vital concerns of her soul.

The sensitivity of the nurse to a patient's spiritual concerns improves the quality of palliative care throughout the illness trajectory. When members of the health care team serve as "companions" to a patient and family during their journey with an illness, they offer vital and life-affirming care.

Responding to the spiritual needs of patients and families is not solely the domain of the chaplain, clergy, or other officially designated professionals. All members of the health care team share the responsibility of identifying and being sensitive to spiritual concerns.

It is vital that a patient be viewed not in isolation but in the context of those who are affected by the illness. Thus, the focus of spiritual assessment includes both the patient and the family or significant others. This perspective affirms the power of a systems view, which sees the patient and family as interdependent and connected. Providing support to family members not only assists them directly but may also contribute to the patient's comfort secondarily, as she or he sees loved ones being cared for as well.

The purpose of a spiritual assessment is to increase the health care team's knowledge of the patient's and family's sources of strength and areas of concern, in order to enhance their quality of life and the quality of care provided. The methods of assessment include direct questioning, acquiring inferred information, and observing. This is most effectively accomplished when a basis of trust has been established. Fitchett[14] noted that spiritual assessments consist of both "substantive" and "functional" information. Table 3–4 examines these categories of spiritual assessment.

Table 3–4
Categories of Spiritual Assessment

Substantive Information: The "What" of Spiritual Life
Present religious affiliation or past religious background
Beliefs about God, the transcendent, an afterlife
Present devotional practice and spiritual disciplines, like praying, attending worship services, meditation, yoga, etc.
Significant religious rituals
Identification of membership in a faith community and the degree of involvement and level of support
Functional Information: The "How" of Spiritual Life
Making meaning
Retaining hope
Securing a source of inner strength and peace
Exploring the relationship between beliefs, practices, and health
Surviving losses and other crises

One of the fundamental principles underlying spiritual assessment and care is the commitment to the value of telling one's story. Alcoholics' Anonymous, a very successful program with spiritual tenets, acknowledges the power of story. This might be paraphrased as follows: in the hearing is the learning, but in the telling is the healing. Similarly, Thompson and Janigan[15] developed the concept of "life schemes," which provide a sense of order and purpose for one's life and promotes a perspective on the world, oneself, events, and goals. Simple, open-ended questions, such as, "How is this illness affecting you?" and "How is the illness affecting the way you relate to the world?" provide the opportunity for validation and exploration of the patient's life scheme.

Cultural Competence

It is unrealistic to expect that health care professionals will know all of the customs, beliefs, and practices of patients from every culture. There are useful reference sources to assist in gaining cultural competence.[16] However, all providers should strive for some degree of cultural competence, which has been defined as "an educational process, which includes the ability to develop working relationships across lines of difference. This encompasses self-awareness, cultural knowledge about illness and healing practices, intercultural communication skills and behavioral flexibility."[17]

The members of the health care team can increase their cultural competence by concentrating on the following:

- Being aware of one's own ethnocentrism.
- Assessing the patient's and family's beliefs about illness and treatments.

Table 3–5
Meeting the Need for Interpreter Services

A child or family member should not be used as an interpreter for major explanations or decision-making about health care. Even adult children may feel uncomfortable speaking with their parents or grandparents about intimate topics. Furthermore, many lay people do not know or understand medical terms in their own language. Informed consent requires that the patient receive accurate information that he or she can understand, before making a health care decision.

It is recommended that the health care team obtain the services of a certified medical interpreter, if possible.

In the absence of an on-site certified translator, use AT&T interpreters. In the United States or Canada, call 1-800-752-6096 to set up an account and obtain a password.

- Conveying respect, such as saying, "I am unfamiliar with your culture. Please help me understand why you think you got sick and what you think will make you better."
- Soliciting the patient and family as teachers and guides regarding cultural practices.
- Asking about the patient's personal preferences and avoiding expectations for any individual to represent his or her whole culture.
- Respecting cultural differences regarding personal space and touch, such as requesting, "Whom do I ask for permission to examine you?" and "May I touch you here?"
- Determining needs and desires regarding health-related information, such as asking, "When I have information to tell you, how much detail do you want to know and to whom do I give it?"
- Noting and affirming the use of complementary and integrative health care practices.
- Incorporating the patient's cultural healing practices into the plan of care.
- Responding to resistance from the patient and family about the recommended treatment plan with understanding, negotiation, and compromise.
- Being sensitive to the need for interpreter services (Table 3–5).

Assessment at the Time of Diagnosis

The goals of a palliative care nursing assessment at the time of diagnosis are as follows:

1. Determine the baseline health of the patient and family.
2. Document problems and plan interventions with the patient and family to improve their quality of life.
3. Identify learning needs to guide teaching that promotes optimal self-care.
4. Recognize patient and family strengths to reinforce healthy habits and behaviors for maximizing well-being.
5. Discern when the expertise of other health care professionals is needed (e.g., social worker, registered dietitian).

Physical Assessment at Diagnosis

When the patient has finished telling his or her story about the illness, the nurse needs to do a head-to-toe physical assessment. This assessment uses the general categories of head and neck, shoulders and arms, chest and spine, abdomen, pelvis, legs and feet, and overall evaluation. The nurse obtains data by observing, interviewing, and examining the patient. The forms, policies, procedures, and expectations of the health care agency in which the assessment occurs guide the specific details that are collected and documented. Figure 3–2 shows cues to guide the physical assessment.

Because the family is so important to the palliative care focus on quality of life, the overall health of other family members needs to be documented. Identification of the major health problems, physical limitations, and physical strengths of family members serves as a basis for planning. The physical capabilities and constraints of the caregivers available to assist and support the patient may affect the plan of care, especially in relation to the most appropriate setting for care. This information also provides direction for the types of referral that may be needed to provide care.

Psychosocial Assessment at Diagnosis

The primary psychosocial feature of a new diagnosis is anticipatory grief. Patients' responses to receiving bad news range from shock, disbelief, and denial to anger and fatalism. As further losses occur along the illness continuum, this grief mechanism is retriggered, and losses become cumulative. Statements such as, "I can't believe this is happening to me" or "Why is this happening to us?" are signals to the health care professional that the patient and family are grappling heavily with this threat to their equilibrium. There is already a sense that life will be forever changed. A longing emerges to return to the way things were.

In response to these emotional states, the health care team is most helpful when they do the following:

- Normalize the patient's and family's experiences: "Many people share similar reactions to this kind of news."
- Use active listening skills to facilitate grief work: "Of all that is happening to you right now, what is the hardest part to deal with?"

Head & Neck:

Hair- Texture, fullness, shine, dandruff, well-kept, bald? Complexion- Skin condition? Scars? Make-up?

Mind- Alert & Oriented x3? MMSE needed? Capacity for decision-making? Speech, language, vocabulary? Education? Ability to read? Memory & attention span? General mood? Stress level? Hx of anxiety, depression, phobias? Hx headaches? Seizures? Knowledge & experience with illness? Perception of illness? Meds?

Senses-Sight - PERRLA? Visual acuity? Glasses/contacts? Redness, itching, puffiness, icterus? Eye drops?
Hearing - Deficits? Use of aids? Tinnitus? Dizziness? Pain? Inspect for excess wax, signs of infection.
Smell - Ability? Sensitivities? Taste - Flavor dislikes?

Nose- Hx of sinusitis or other sinus problems? Nose bleeds? Frequency of URIs? Pain? Meds?

Mouth-Inspect condition of teeth, gums, & mucous membranes? Dryness? Sores? Infection? Brushing & flossing habits? Semi-annual cleanings & dental exams? Dentures, bridges? Hx of sore throats? Pain?

Lips- Dry or cracked? Hx of fever blisters?

Neck- Quality & clarity of voice? Full ROM? Hx of problems- swallowing, laryngitis, esophagitis, reflux? Swollen lymph nodes? Venous distension? Carotid pulses? Pain?

Shoulders & Arms:

Full ROM? Strength? Dexterity? Coordination? Crepitus? Deformities? Swelling? Joint/muscle pain or stiffness? Neuropathies? Changes in sensation? Reflexes? Venous access?

Chest & Spine:

Lungs-Respiratory rate; SOB? DOE? Orthopnea? Lung sounds? Cough? Sputum? CXR? Shape of chest? Smoking hx? Hx of infections, asthma, or night sweats? Pain? Meds?

Heart-Heart rate & rhythm? Murmurs? BP? EKG? Hx of palpitations, CP, MI? CAD/CHF? Pedal edema? Meds?

Breasts-Appearance, lumps, discharge? BSE? Mammogram? Regular HCP Exam? Pain/tenderness?

Spine-Hx back pain, problems, or injuries? Flexibility? Deformities?

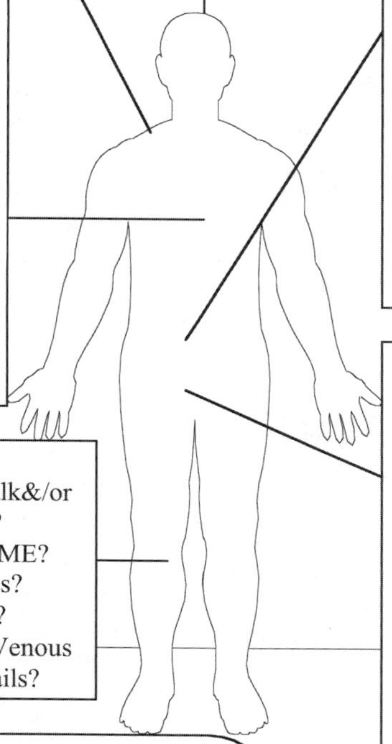

Abdomen:

General- Appearance? Ascities? Masses? Tenderness? Surgery scars?

Stomach- Usual diet? Appetite? Caffeine intake? Vitamin use? Hx of problems?- PUD? Belching? Pain? Motion sickness? N & V with pregnancy?

Liver- Alcohol intake? Hx hepatitis? LFTs?

GB- Hx of indigestion? Pain?

Pancreas- Hx of diabetes?

Bowels- Normal habits? Recent changes? Color, form? Diarrhea? Incontinence? Constipation? Laxative use? Gas? Pain? Fat & fiber diet? Hemorrhoids? Rectal bleeding? Hemocult tests? Regular HCP rectal exams? Sigmoidoscopy?

Pelvis:

Kidneys- /Urine Color, frequency? Nocturia? Pain? Hx of UTIs? Incontinence? Other problems?

Male= TSE? DRE? PSA? Hx BPH? Meds? Hernia? Sexually active? Hx STDs? Contraception? Circumcised? Sexual function concerns? Impotence? Importance to self concept, relationships, & quality of life?

Female= Gx Px? Contraception? LMP? Menarche age? Usual menses cycle? Break through bleeding? Menses pain or problems? Menopause - age? ERT? Pelvic exam & PAP smear? Vaginal discharge, dryness, odor, infection? Sexually active? Sexual function concerns? Importance to self concept, relationships, & quality of life?

Legs & Feet:

Full ROM? Strength? Crepitus? Ability to walk&/or run? How far? Gait? Coordination? Balance? Weakness? Paralysis? Deformities? Use of DME? Hx of problems? Muscle/joint pain or stiffness? Reflexes? Change in sensation? Temperature? Edema? Pedal pulses? Dryness? Cellulitis? Venous stasis? Skin discoloration? Condition of toenails?

General:

Allergies? Temperature? Height? Weight? -loss, gain, ideal?
Functional Status? Exercise tolerance? Needs related to ADLs?

Appearance- Personal hygiene, dress, posture, body language, sweating? Intolerance to heat or cold?

Skin- Color, turgor, bruising, rashes, itching? Moles? - ABCD? Wounds? Previous surgical sites healed?

General- Aches, pains? Muscle twitching, tingling, cramps? Hx broken bones? Hx of major illness, injuries, surgeries? Family hx of illnesses? Past health & well-being? Sleep patterns/problems? Prevention habits? Rest, relaxation, recreation? Immunizations? Use of alternative therapies?

Figure 3–2. Assessment at the time of diagnosis: obtaining a baseline of the patient's health status. Abbreviations: ABCD = How to assess a skin mole (Asymmetry; Borders, regular or irregular; Color, multicolored; Diameter, generally >6 mm); ADLs = activities of daily living; BP = blood pressure; BPH = benign prosatic hyperplasia; BSE = breast self-exam; CAD = coronary artery disease; CHF = congestive heart failure; CP = chest pain; CXR = chest x-ray; DOE = dyspnea on exertion; DME = durable medical equipment (e.g., wheelchairs, walkers, hospital beds, etc.); DRE = digital rectal exam; EKG = electrocardiogram; ERT = estrogen replacement therapy; Gx = gravida (number of pregnancies), Px = parity (number of deliveries past 20 weeks, number of abortions,

(*continues on p. 56*)

- Create a safe space for self-disclosure, and build a trust relationship: "No matter what lies ahead, you will not face it alone."
- Develop a collaborative partnership to establish a mutual plan of care: "What would help you the most right now?"
- Respect the patient's or family's use of denial in the service of coping with harsh realities: "It must be hard to believe this is happening."
- Assess the patient's and family's coping styles: "When you have experienced difficult times in the past, how did you get through them?"
- Reinforce strengths.
- Maximize a sense of control, autonomy, and choice.
- Assess the patient's need for information: "What do you know about your illness?," "Are you the kind of person who likes to know as much as possible, or do you function on a need-to-know basis only?," "What would you like to know about your illness now?"
- Check the need for clarification: "What did you hear?" or "Summarize in your own words how you understand your situation now."
- Avoid "medspeak," which is medical terminology unfamiliar to the average person.
- Mentor patients and families who have had little experience with the health care system, including coaching them in conversations with their physicians and teaching them ways to be wise healthcare consumers.

The nurse must remember that, while the patient is feeling strong emotions, the family is also experiencing intense feelings. Similar assessments of family members will help to mobilize resources at critical times. Family members experience their grief reactions at their own individual rates throughout the course of the illness. Each family member has his or her own particular coping style and need for information.

The nurse and other members of the health care team assist the patient and family when they do the following:

- Observe changes in family members' roles and responsibilities (e.g., the breadwinner becomes a caregiver, the homemaker begins working outside the home).
- Identify external community support systems.
- Assist the patient and family in identifying coping strategies to use while awaiting test results, which is one of the most stressful times and which recurs throughout the illness.

Table 3–6
Common Responses of Children to Serious Illness in the Family

Magical thinking that results in feelings of guilt (e.g., "I once told Mommy I wished she were dead.")
Fears of abandonment, especially in younger children
Fears of contracting the disease
Anger, withdrawal, being uncooperative, especially in adolescents
Acting-out behavior with lack of usual attention
Frustrations with an altered lifestyle because of decreased financial resources, less family fun activities because of the ill person's inability to participate, etc.
Inability to concentrate and focus, especially regarding schoolwork

- Help the patient and family explore the benefits and burdens of various treatment options when changes are needed in the plan of care.
- Assess parental readiness to assist children with their adaptation needs: "How do you plan to tell your children?"
- Identify family communication ground rules and seek to improve communication among family members: "Is it OK if we discuss this subject with you and your family?"

Assess the coping of children within the family by being aware of their fears and concerns. Table 3–6 describes some common responses of children to having an adult loved one who is ill.

Assisting in the process of making initial treatment decisions can be an opportunity to begin a relationship that will continue to grow. Members of the health care team may ask questions such as, "What is most important to you in life?" and "Is quality of life or quantity of life most meaningful?" Assisting the patient and family in identifying and expressing their values will guide them in subsequent decision-making.

Spiritual Assessment at Diagnosis

The diagnosis of a serious illness generally brings with it a sense of shock to the patient and family. It may threaten many of their assumptions about life, disrupt their sense of control, and cause them to ask "Why?" The health care team can be most helpful at this time if they do the following:

number of premature deliveries, number of living children); GB = gallbladder; HCP = health care provider/professional; Hx = history; LFTs = liver function tests; LMP = last menstrual period; Meds = medications; MI = myocardial infarction; MMSE = Mini Mental Status Exam; N & V = nausea and vomiting; PAP = Papanicolaou test for cervical cancer; PERRLA = pupils equal, round, react to light, accommodation; PSA = prostate-specific antigen; PUD = peptic ulcer disease; ROM = range of motion; SOB = shortness of breath; STD = sexually transmitted disease; TSE = testicular self-exam; URIs = upper respiratory infections; UTIs = urinary tract infections. *Source:* Courtesy of Elaine Glass, APRN, BC-PCM.

- Determine the patient's and family's level of hopefulness about the future: "What are you hoping for?" or "How do you see the future at this time?"
- Inquire about how the patient and family have dealt with past crises of faith, meaning, or loss: "What helped you get through that?"
- Determine the patient's and family's comfort level in talking about the spiritual life: "Some people need or want to talk about these things; others don't. How is it for you?"
- Inquire about spiritual support persons available to the patient and family (e.g., pastor, rabbi, counselor, spiritual advisor).
- Determine the patient's or family's need or desire to speak with a spiritual support person.
- Ask about spiritual self-care practices to promote healthy coping: "How are you taking care of yourself at this time?"
- Listen for comments from the patient and family regarding the importance of their religious traditions and practices.

Spiritual goals at this phase are to normalize initial concerns, to provide information that fosters positive coping, and to encourage the patient and family to seek supportive spiritual resources.

CASE STUDY
Ghedi at the Time of Diagnosis of Colon Cancer

Ghedi was reluctant to seek medical attention for his increasing gastrointestinal problems. He found American health care confusing and did not want to rely too heavily on his brother, Asad, to navigate the system for him. He did not want to appear weak and in need of assistance. Initially, Ghedi relied on traditional treatments provided by one of the elders in their community. As his gastrointestinal problems persisted, he finally agreed to allow his brother to make an appointment for him with Asad's primary care physician. At this point, Ghedi was experiencing severe diarrhea and pain in the lower abdomen. An x-ray film revealed an apparent mass in the colon; a colonoscopy and biopsy were performed. Ghedi was referred to Dr. Yang, a surgical oncologist, for further evaluation and treatment. This specialist recommended complete removal of the mass, which would probably necessitate a colostomy. After much ambivalence and discussion, Ghedi agreed.

The ostomy nurse, Mindy, met with Ghedi before the operation to identify the best stoma site. As she explained what she was going to do, Ghedi refused to let her touch him. Asad explained to Mindy that his brother would not allow a woman to examine him. Remaining sensitive to Ghehi's cultural background, Mindy called the male resident and guided him in marking the correct stoma placement.

The goals at this phase of care are to

- Use a certified medical interpreter for information-giving, decision-making, and completion of consent forms.
- Build trust with Ghedi and Asad by encouraging the integration of their native healing practices into the plan of care and by respecting their cultural boundaries.
- Determine who among his male support network Ghedi would allow to assist him in learning how to care for his colostomy after surgery. (Ghedi would not permit his sister-in-law, Laila, to assist him in any way.)
- Communicate Ghedi's cultural preferences to other members of the health care team.

Assessment During Treatments

The goals of a palliative care assessment during active treatment are as follows:

1. Assess the patient's systems in all domains that are at risk for problems, considering both the patient's baseline problems and any side effects of the treatments.
2. Record the current and potential problems and plan early interventions with the patient and family.
3. Ascertain the need for teaching to prevent, minimize, and manage problems with the goal of maximizing quality of life.
4. Reinforce patient and family strengths, healthy habits, and behaviors to maximize well-being.
5. Recognize when other health care professionals' expertise is needed and make appropriate referrals (e.g., physical therapist, pharmacist).

Physical Assessment During Treatments

Reassessments during treatment determine the changes that have occurred since the initial assessment. Knowledge of the usual disease process and the side effects of treatment assists the nurse in focusing reassessments on those body systems most likely to be affected.

In addition to the patient's physical assessment, the nurse should make periodic observations and inquiries about the health of other family members. It is important to document any changes in their health problems or physical limitations and physical strengths that might have an impact on the patient's care and the family's overall quality of life.

Psychosocial Assessment During Treatments

Once a treatment plan has been initiated, patients often express relief that "something is finally being done." Taking action frequently reduces anxiety. The most important psychosocial intervention at this stage is the amelioration of as many treatment side effects as possible. After basic needs for physical well-being are assessed and symptoms are controlled, the patient is able to explore and meet higher needs, including the needs for belonging, self-esteem, and self-actualization.[13] Patients who are preoccupied with pain and nausea or vomiting have no energy or ability to explore the significance of their illness or their feelings about it. Effective management of physical symptoms is mandatory before the patient can begin to work on integrating the illness experience into the tapestry of his or her life.

After several months or years of treatment, the effects of having a chronic illness may exhaust even the hardiest person. Patients may begin to weigh the benefits versus the burdens of continuing aggressive therapies. Initially, patients will endure almost anything if they believe a cure is possible. As time unfolds, their attitudes may change as they watch their quality of life erode with little prospect of a more positive outcome. Patients may also reprioritize what is most important to them. For example, the workaholic may find less satisfaction at the office, or the homemaker may experience less fulfillment from daily routines around the house. Change, transition, and existential questioning characterize this phase.

The nurse and other members of the health care team will assist the patient and family when they do the following:

- Inquire about the patient's newly emerging identity as a result of the illness: "What activities and which relationships bring you the most joy and meaning?" or "Have you been able to define a new purpose for yourself?"
- Assess for signs of anxiety and depression, which remain the two most common psychosocial problems associated with severe illness (Table 3–7); for more information contrasting anxiety and depression, consult Holland's *Psycho-oncology.*[5]
- Screen for suicidal ideation in cases of depression: "Have you been feeling so bad that you've been thinking of a way to hurt yourself?" and "Do you have a plan for how to do it?"
- Refer for counseling and possible psychotropic medication to enhance positive coping and comfort.

Spiritual Assessment During Treatments

With the treatment of a serious illness comes the introduction of an additional stressor to the patient and family. It is important to assess how they incorporate the demands of treatment into their daily routine and how these changes have affected the meaning of their lives.

The nurse and other members of the care team will be helpful to the patient and family if they normalize the stress of treatment and do the following:

- Inquire about the patient's and family's hopes for the future.
- Assess the level and quality of support they are receiving—for instance, from other family members, faith community, and neighbors.
- Explore expressions of anxiety and fear by asking, "What is concerning you the most at this time?"
- Assess how the patient and family are coping with the rigors of treatment: "What is the most challenging part of this for you?" and "What is helping you day by day?" Consider referrals to a chaplain or faith community as needed.

Table 3–7
Assessment of Anxiety and Depression

Signs and Symptoms of Anxiety	Signs and Symptoms of Depression
Excessive worry	Depressed mood
Trouble falling or staying asleep	Insomnia and hypersomnia
Irritability, muscle tension	Anhedonia (absence of pleasure)
Restlessness, agitation	Psychomotor retardation
Unrealistic fears (phobias)	Feelings of worthlessness or inappropriate guilt
Obsessions (persistent painful ideas)	Diminished ability to concentrate, make decisionsor remember
Compulsions (repetitive ritualistic acts)	Recurrent thoughts of death, suicidal ideation (lethality assessed by expressed intent, presence of a plan and the means to carry it out, previous attempts, and provision for rescue)
Frequent crying spells, headaches, gastrointestinal upsets, palpitations, shortness of breath	Marked weight loss or weight gain
Self-medication	Fatigue
Anorexia or overeating	
Interference with normal activities of daily living	

- Inquire about the patient's and family's definitions of quality of life and the impact of treatment on these aspects of their lives: "What is most important to you in life now?"
- Determine their use of spiritual practices and offer assistance in developing these (e.g., meditation, relaxation, prayer).
- Ask how the patient or family members feel about their current practices: "Are these helpful or not?"

The health care team's goals are to reinforce positive coping, mobilize existing spiritual resources, invite the patient and family to develop new skills for self-care, and continue disclosures in an atmosphere of trust.

CASE STUDY
Ghedi During Treatments for Colon Cancer

A few weeks after surgery and the colostomy, Ghedi started on the recommended regimen of chemotherapy. He experienced side effects of diarrhea, nausea, and vomiting. He insisted on the addition of traditional "fire burning" from the Somali elder, who was also the community's traditional Somali physician. Ghedi took several herbal preparations designed to ease his digestive problems. The clinic pharmacist determined that the herbs were compatible with Ghedi's chemotherapy drugs. Between treatments, Ghedi received follow-up care from a home care agency. Asad specifically requested a male nurse and male aide to provide Ghedi's personal care.

Throughout Ghedi's treatment, Asad and the elder were in attendance and Ghedi increasingly depended on them to assist with decision-making. He exhibited a stoic demeanor, and although the medical team believed he might have been experiencing pain, Ghedi insisted he was not.

The goals at this phase of care are to

- Ask Asad and the Somali elder to assist the health care team in assessing Ghedi's degree of pain and discomfort from the side effects of the chemotherapy. Suggest that the health care team encourage Asad and the elder to give Ghedi permission to take the pain medication.
- Continue to respect Ghedi's cultural modesty and try to accommodate his request for male health care providers.

Assessment After Treatments (Long-Term Survival or Terminal Phase)

The goals of a palliative care assessment after treatments are as follows:

1. Examine the benefits and burdens of all interventions to manage the residual symptoms remaining from the treatments and/or the disease process.
2. Determine the current physical problems that are most distressing to the patient and family, and plan rehabilitative interventions.
3. Assess learning needs and provide teaching to aggressively manage problems with the goal of maximizing quality of life.
4. Continue to reinforce patient and family strengths, healthy habits, and behaviors to enhance well-being and to prevent problems.

Survivors are defined as those patients whose diseases are cured, who go into long remissions, or who become chronically ill. These individuals may require some degree of palliative care for the rest of their lives. Examples of survivors likely to require palliative care include those with graft-versus-host disease (GVHD), irreversible peripheral neuropathies, or structural alterations of the integumentary, gastrointestinal, and genitourinary systems (e.g., mastectomies, amputations, colostomies, ileostomies, laryngectomies).

Psychosocial issues for survivors include fear of recurrence as well as practical considerations such as insurance and job discrimination. Many patients make major life changes regarding work and relationships as a result of their illness experiences. These patients, even if cured, live with the ramifications of the disease and its treatment for the rest of their lives.

Some patients begin to explore, in new ways, the spiritual foundations and assumptions of their lives. Often, patients relate that in spite of the crisis of an illness and its treatment, the experience resulted in a deepened sense of meaning and gratitude for life. Examples of such growth experiences as a result of surviving cancer can be found in *Cancer as a Turning Point: A Handbook for People with Cancer, Their Families and Health Professionals*[20] and *Silver Linings: The Other Side of Cancer.*[21]

Physical Assessment After Treatments

The patient is reassessed after treatments are finished to determine the changes that have occurred since previous assessments; the focus is on the systems that have been affected and altered by the treatments. Thorough assessment of the residual problems and changes in the patient's body are critical to successful symptom management. Effective management of symptoms with rehabilitative interventions achieves the goal of maximizing the patient's and family's quality of life, whether in long-term survival or during the terminal phase. Two examples of functional assessment tools used in physical rehabilitation are the Functional Assessment of Cancer Therapy (FACT) Scale[22] and the Rotterdam Symptom Checklist.[23]

In addition to the patient's physical assessment, the nurse should continue to make periodic observations and inquiries about the health of other family members. Noting changes in family members' health, physical limitations, and physical strengths is important to ascertain any impact on the patient's care and the family's lifestyle.

An emerging issue that relates to family members' health is genetic testing for familial diseases. The health care team needs to ask patients with diseases that could have a genetic origin whether they would be interested in receiving more information. Patients or family members who desire more facts will benefit from written materials and referral to an experienced genetic counselor. Table 3–8 provides resource information on genetic counseling.

Psychosocial Assessment After Treatments

For those patients who are free of disease, palliative care focuses on posttreatment-related symptoms and fears of recurrence. For others, recurrence is most often signaled by the appearance of advancing physical symptoms. When this happens, the patient's worst nightmare has been realized. A recurrence is experienced differently from an initial diagnosis, because the patient is now a "veteran" of the patient role and may understand all too well what the recurrence means.

Attention to concerns at this phase of illness include the following:

- Revisiting the quality versus quantity of life preferences as the patient and family weigh the benefits and burdens of treatment.
- Being sensitive to the patient's readiness to discuss a transition in emphasis from curative to palliative care. The patient often signals his or her readiness by statements such as, "I'm getting tired of spending so much time at the hospital" or "I've had it with all of this." Ask: "What has your physician told you that you can expect now?" or "How do you see your future?"
- Exploring readiness to set new goals of treatment: "I know you understand that your illness has not responded to the treatments as we had hoped. I'd like to talk with you about changing your care plan goals."
- Beginning to discuss the patient's preferences for resuscitation: "If your heart or lungs should stop, have you thought about whether or not you would want us to try to revive you? This means that we would shock your heart, put you on a breathing machine, and transfer you to an intensive care unit. You need to think about your desire to have such life support treatments."
- Considering a discussion about hospice if the patient begins to question the efficacy of treatments.
- Presenting hospice as the gold standard for end-of-life care. A hospice referral should never be made as a gesture indicating that "There is nothing more that we can do for you." The benefits of increased availability and services, such as bereavement care for the family, should be emphasized.
- Discussing the completion of advance directives: "Who would you want to make your health care decisions for you if you were not able to make them yourself?"
- Determining the patient's and family's interest or need for education about death and dying.
- Discerning risk factors for complicated bereavement in family members, as described in Table 3–9.

Spiritual Assessment After Treatments

After treatment, the patient embarks on a journey leading to long-term survival, chronic illness, or recurrence and the terminal phases of the illness. The nurse and other caregivers can provide valuable spiritual support at these junctures when they do the following:

- Determine the quality and focus of the patient's and family's hopes for the future. Listen for a transition

Table 3–8
Genetic Counseling Information

To locate a genetic counselor in a particular region of the United States, contact
National Society of Genetic Counselors
610-872-7608 www.nsgc.org

Table 3–9
Assessment of Family Members' Risk Factors for Complicated Bereavement

Concurrent life crises
History of other recent or difficult past losses
Unresolved grief from prior losses
History of mental illness or substance abuse
Extreme anger or anxiety
Marked dependence on the patient
Age of the patient and the surviving loved ones, developmental phases of the patient and family members
Limited support within the family's circle or community
Anticipated situational stressors, such as loss of income, financial strain, lack of confidence in assuming some of the patient's usual responsibilities
Illnesses among other family members
Special bereavement needs of children in the family
The patient's dying process is difficult (e.g., poorly controlled symptoms such as pain, shortness of breath, agitation, delirium, anxiety)
Absence of helpful cultural and/or religious beliefs

from hoping for a cure to another kind of hope (e.g., hope for a remission, hope to live until a special family event occurs). For an in-depth, practical, and inspiring discourse on hope, refer to *Finding HOPE: Ways to See Life in a Brighter Light*.[24]

- Listen for comments that suggest a crisis of belief and meaning. For example, at recurrence, a patient may feel abandoned or experience an assault on his or her faith. Questions such as "Why?" and "Where is God?" and "Why are my prayers not being answered?" are very common. The nurse can best respond to these questions by normalizing them and emphasizing that to question God or one's faith can indicate a vitality of faith, not its absence.
- Assess the patient's and family's use of spiritual practices: "What are you doing to feel calmer and more peaceful?" Consider a chaplain referral if the patient or family are interested and open to such an intervention.
- Inquire regarding the desire for meaningful rituals, such as communion or anointing. Consult with local clergy or a hospital chaplain to meet these needs.
- Assess the level and quality of community supports: "Who is involved in supporting you and your family at this time?"
- Encourage referral to hospice for end-of-life care.
- Listen for indicators of spiritual suffering (e.g., unfinished business, regrets, relationship discord, diminished faith, fears of abandonment): "What do you find yourself thinking about at this time?" and "What are your chief concerns or worries?"
- Assess the need and desire of the patient and family to talk about the meaning of the illness, the patient's declining physical condition, and possible death.
- Ask questions to foster a review of critical life incidents, to allow grieving, and explore beliefs regarding the afterlife: "What do you believe happens to a person at the time of death?"

Table 3–10
Assessment of Funeral Plans and Preferences

Has the patient and/or family selected a funeral home?
Has the patient and/or family decided about the disposition of the body: organ, eye, and/or tissue donation; autopsy; earth burial (above ground or below ground); cremation; simple disposition?
Has the decision been made regarding a final resting place?
Does the patient want to make his or her wishes known regarding the type of service, or will the family decide this?

- Determine the need and desire for reconciliation: "Are there people with whom you want or need to speak?" and "Do you find yourself having any regrets?"
- Invite a discussion of the most meaningful, celebratory occurrences in life to foster integrity, life review, and a sense of meaning.
- Assess the patient's and/or the family's readiness to discuss funeral preferences and plans and desired disposition of the body, as noted in Table 3–10.

The main spiritual goal of this phase of illness is to provide the patient and family a "place to stand" in order to review the past and look toward the future. This encourages grieving past losses, creating a sense of meaning, and consolidating strengths for the days ahead.

CASE STUDY

Ghedi After Completion of Treatments for Colon Cancer

After his chemotherapy was completed, Ghedi was able to return to work in the housekeeping department of his neighborhood elementary school. He was in remission for 2 years before he began exhibiting jaundice. He immediately resumed traditional Somali treatments with his elder, who prescribed habakhedi and fire-burning. Because colostomy care had been challenging for him, Ghedi wanted to avoid returning to Dr. Yang. Ghedi told Asad that Dr. Yang was too direct about his future and was offering no hope of recovery. Ghedi observed ritual prayers imploring God to heal him and relieve his suffering.

A few months after he became jaundiced, Ghedi began to complain of severe itching. He lost a great deal of weight as he experienced more frequent episodes of nausea and vomiting. One day, Ghedi passed out on the bathroom floor. Laila called Asad at work. Asad immediately came home and took Ghedi to the emergency department. Ghedi was severely dehydrated and had several abnormal electrolyte results. The emergency department physician began administering intravenous fluid and admitted Ghedi to the palliative care service. The palliative care team provided comfort medications to relieve Ghedi's pain and symptoms. They also offered integrative therapies to relieve Ghedi's distress. He agreed to aromatherapy, massage by a male licensed massage therapist, and music. The palliative care team worked with Ghedi, Asad, and the Somali elder to develop a plan of care after discharge. After much discussion and consideration, Ghedi and Asad agreed to hospice care at home.

The goals of this phase of care are to:

- Solicit the Somali elder's help in determining how best to support Asad's family in caring for Ghedi at home.
- Assist Ghedi in applying for Medicaid, because he cannot return to work.

- Inform the hospice team of Ghedi's desire for male health care providers and the need to include the Somali elder's traditional healing practices in Ghedi's hospice plan of care.

Assessment During Active Dying

The goals of a palliative care assessment when the patient is actively dying are as follows:

1. Observe for signs and symptoms of impending death, aggressively managing symptoms and promoting comfort (Table 3–11).
2. Determine the primary source of the patient's and family's suffering and plan interventions to provide relief.
3. Identify the primary sources of strength for the patient and family members so that they can be used to provide support.
4. Ascertain the patient's and family's readiness and need for teaching about the dying process.
5. Look for ways to support the patient and family to enhance meaning during this intense experience.
6. Determine whether the family members and friends who are important to the patient have had the opportunity to visit in person or on the telephone, as desired by the patient and family.

Physical Assessment During Active Dying

Physical assessment during the active dying process is very focused and is limited to determining the cause of suffering and identifying sources of comfort. Figure 3–3 shows common areas to assess in the last few days of a person's life.

Table 3–11
Common Physical Symptoms Experienced by People Who Are Actively Dying

Pain from the illness and/or immobility
Dyspnea
Sleepiness
Confusion
No interest in eating or drinking
Gurgling sounds in the back of the throat from not being able to swallow saliva
Agitation/restlessness/delirium
Coolness in extremities
Incontinence
Skin breakdown from immobility

In addition to the patient's physical assessment, the nurse should monitor the health of other family members to prevent and minimize problems that could compromise their health during this very stressful time.

Hospice team members have excellent skills in making palliative care assessments at the end of life. The goal of hospice is to support the terminally ill patient and family at home, if that is their wish. Many hospice teams also provide palliative care in acute care settings and nursing homes. Unfortunately, many patients die without the support of hospice services in any of these settings.

Psychosocial Assessment During Active Dying

Many people believe that the transition from life to death is as sacred as the transition experienced at birth. Keeping this in mind, the nurse can help to create a safe environment in which patients and families are supported in their relationships and the creation of meaningful moments together. The patient may also still be reviewing his or her life. Common psychosocial characteristics of the person who is actively dying include social withdrawal, decreased attention span, and decreasing ability to concentrate, resulting in gradual loss of consciousness. Experiences normally considered to be psychotic in Western culture, such as visions and visitations, are often viewed as transcendent—and normal—at this stage of life by those with strong spiritual beliefs.

Members of the health care team can assist the patient and family in the following vital ways:

- Normalize the patient's reports of seeing deceased loved ones or visions of another world.
- Encourage continued touching and talking to the patient, even if he or she is unconscious.
- Assist communication among the patient, family members, and close friends.
- Invite family members to "give permission" to the patient "to let go," providing reassurance that the family will remain intact and learn to deal effectively with the person's absence.
- Assess the patient's and family's need for continued education about death and dying.
- Observe family members for evidence of poor coping and consider making referrals for additional support.
- Encourage family members to consider "shift rotation" in the face of lengthy, exhausting vigils at the bedside.

Spiritual Assessment During Active Dying

When the patient enters the phase of active dying, spiritual realities often increase in significance. The nurse and other members of the care team will facilitate adaptation during the process of dying and provide much valuable support when they do the following:

Head & Neck:

Mind- How important is level of alertness versus control of pain and anxiety which may cause sedation?

Senses-Sight - What objects at the bedside provide comfort when seen by the patient? Family photos? Children's drawings? Special objects? Pets? Loved ones sitting nearby? What degree of lighting does the patient prefer? Does darkness increase anxiety? Would scented candles provide solace?

Hearing - What sounds most comfort the patient? Music? Family chatting nearby? The TV or radio on in the back-ground? Someone reading to him or her? Silence?

Smell - What scents does the patient enjoy? Would aromatic lotions be soothing?

Taste - What are the patient's favorite flavors? Would mouth care to relieve dryness be more acceptable with fruit punch or apple juice?

Mouth/Lips - Does the family/caregiver understand how to provide good, frequent mouth and lip care, especially if the patient is a mouth-breather?

Shoulders & Arms:

Does the family/caregiver understand good body alignment and several ways to position the patient comfortably? Are they following good body mechanics when repositioning the patient?

Would applying aromatic lotion to hands and arms comfort the patient and give family members some-thing meaningful to do?

Abdomen:

Bowels- If the patient is incontinent of stool, do family members know how to provide personal hygiene?

Do family members know how to use protective pads, adult diapers, pull sheets to keep the patient clean?

Does the family know how to make an occupied bed, using good body mechanics?

Are protective ointments needed to decrease skin breakdown if the incontinence is frequent?

If stools are frequent, can anti-diarrheals be given?

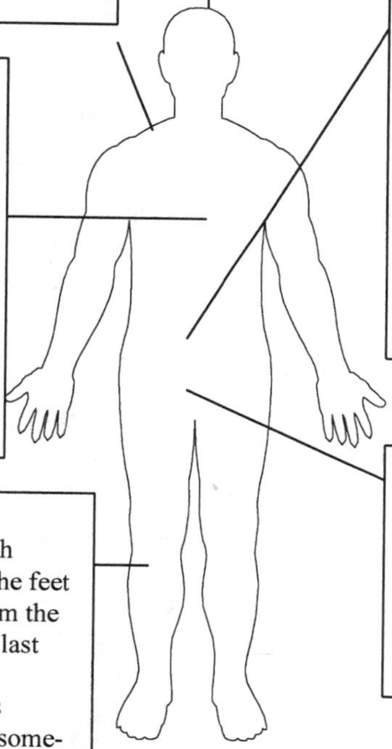

Chest & Spine:

Lungs-Is the patient at high risk for death rales? Is there a Scopolamine Patch or Atropine Eye Drops in the home for immediate use if noisy respirations begin? Would oxygen help the patient breathe easier?

Heart-If pt at home, is the family prepared for the moment of death? E.g., do they know NOT to call 911? Do they have a neighbor close by to come and be with them until a HCP arrives?

Pelvis:

Kidneys/Urine -If incontinence is present, would inserting a Foley catheter prevent skin irritation & conserve the patient's & family's energies?

Legs & Feet:

Are family members interested/concerned with learning the assessment technique of feeling the feet and limbs for coolness slowly progressing from the periphery to the center of the body during the last few hours of life?

Would applying aromatic lotion to feet & legs comfort the patient and give family members some-thing meaningful to do?

General:

- Are the patient's pain & other symptoms well-controlled?
- Are family members capable & comfortable with continuing to provide physical care for the patient? Are family members getting enough sleep and rest to maintain their own health? Are additional resources needed to support the family?
- Is the home the best place for the patient to die? Has the family thought about their comfort in living in the house if their loved one dies there?
- Does the family know whom to call on a 24-hour basis for advice and support?

Figure 3–3. Assessment when the patient is actively dying: determining causes of pain and discomfort and identifying sources of comfort. HCP = health care professional; pt = patient. (*Source*: Courtesy of Elaine Glass, APRN, BC-PCM.)

- Determine the need for different or more frequent visits by the patient's or family's spiritual support person: "Is there anyone I can call to be with you at this time?" and "Are there any meaningful activities or rituals you want to do?"
- Inquire about dreams, visions, or unusual experiences (e.g., seeing persons who have died). Normalize these if they are disclosed. Ask if these experiences are sources of comfort or fear. Encourage further discussion if the patient is interested.
- Foster maintenance of hope by asking, "What are you hoping for at this time?" Reassure the patient and family that they can be hopeful and still acknowledge that death is imminent. Moving toward a transcendent hope is vital. Observe that earlier the focus of hope may have been on cure, remission, or an extension of time. Now, hope may be focused on an afterlife, the relief of suffering, or the idea of living on in loved ones' memories.
- Listen for and solicit comments regarding the efficacy of spiritual practices. For instance, if the patient is a person who prays, ask, "Are your prayers bringing you comfort and peace?"
- Realize that expressions of fear, panic attacks, or an increase in physical symptoms such as restlessness, agitation, pain, or shortness of breath may indicate intense spiritual distress. A chaplain's intervention may provide spiritual comfort and assist the patient in reaching peace. This may reduce the need for medications.
- Determine the need and desire of the patient and family to engage in forgiveness, to express feelings to one another, and to say their good-byes.
- Recognize that a prolonged dying process may indicate that the patient is having difficulty "letting go," perhaps due to some unfinished business or fears related to dying. Assist the patient and family in exploring what these issues might be. A referral to a chaplain may be very helpful.
- Encourage celebration of the life of the loved one by acknowledging his or her contributions to family members, close friends, and the community.
- Explore the need and desire for additional comfort measures in the environment, such as soothing music, devotional readings, gazing out a window at nature, or increased quiet.
- Ask the family about their anticipated needs and preferences at the time of death: "Is there anyone you will want us to call for you?" "What can the health care team do to be most supportive?" "Are there specific practices regarding the care of the body that you want the team to carry out?"

The goals of spiritual care at this phase of illness are as follows:

- Facilitate any unfinished business among the patient and significant others (e.g., expressions of love, regret, forgiveness, gratitude).
- Promote the integrity of the dying person by honoring his or her life. One way to do this is by encouraging reminiscence at the bedside of the patient, recalling the "gifts" the patient bestowed on the family—that is, his or her legacy of values and qualities passed on to survivors.
- Assist the patient and family in extracting meaning from the dying experience.
- Provide sensitive comfort by being present and listening.
- Provide information regarding bereavement support groups and/or counseling if indicated.

CASE STUDY
Ghedi's Death

The Somali community rallied around Ghedi and his brother to assist in offering support to supplement the care provided by the local hospice agency. Ghedi died at home, as he wanted, with his elder reciting Yasin prayers from the Quran as he lay dying. Asad's family remained quiet at the bedside without overt expressions of grief. A male sheik prepared Ghedi's body for burial by washing, perfuming, and wrapping it in a white cloth. Asad, Ghedi's nephew, and two male elders from the community dug his grave. (This required special arrangements with the local funeral service.)

Because the hospice team was so effective in caring for Ghedi and his family, the Somali elder was receptive to endorsing hospice services for other terminally ill people in their community.

The goal of the final phase of family care was as follows:

- Encourage Asad's family to accept bereavement services for the family.

Summary of a Comprehensive Palliative Care Assessment

A comprehensive assessment of the patient and family provides the foundation for mutually setting goals, devising a plan of care, implementing interventions, and evaluating the effectiveness of care. Reassessments are done throughout the patient's illness, to ensure that quality of life is maximized (Table 3–12). Further sources of information are listed in Appendix 3–1.

Finally, as Colleen Scanlon[25] reminds us, two of the most important assessment questions that nurses and other health care team members can ask the patient and family, regardless of the phase or focus of the assessment, are, "What is your greatest concern?" and "How can I help?"

Table 3–12 Best Practice Tip
Clinicians may find the use of an abbreviated symptom assessment form helpful to track the efficacy of palliative care interventions. Whereas pain is usually plotted along the familiar 0–10 scale, other symptoms such as nausea, vomiting, diarrhea, constipation, fatigue, anxiety, and depression can be quickly evaluated on a flow sheet as 0, mild, moderate, or severe. These kinds of tools assist in interdisciplinary evaluation of symptoms without requiring paging through lengthy progress notes. In this way, treatment can be highly individualized and always evidence based.

REFERENCES

1. Bickley LS, Szilagyi PG. Bates' Guide to Physical Examination and History Taking, 8th ed. Philadelphia: Lippincott Williams & Wilkins, 2002.
2. Cassell EJ, Coulehan JL, Putnam SM. Making good interview skills better. Patient Care 1989;3:145–166.
3. Ferrell BR. The impact of pain on quality of life: A decade of research. Nurs Clin North Am 1995;30:609–624.
4. Siegel BS. Love, Medicine and Miracles. New York: Harper and Row, 1986.
5. Holland J, ed. Psycho-oncology. New York: Oxford University Press, 2001.
6. Schwartz M. Letting Go: Morrie's Reflections on Living While Dying. New York: Delta, 1997.
7. Schneider JM. Clinically significant differences between grief, pathological grief and depression. Patient Counsel Health Educ 1980;4:267–275.
8. Haase J, Britt T, Coward D, Leidy N, Penn P. Simultaneous concept analysis of spiritual perspective, hope, acceptance, and self-transcendence. Image J Nurs Sch 1992;24:143.
9. Amenta M. Nurses as primary spiritual care workers. Hospice J 1988;4:47–55.
10. Hay MW. Principles in building spiritual assessment tools. Am J Hospice Care 1989;6:25–31.
11. Doyle D. Have you looked beyond the physical and psychosocial? J Pain Symptom Manage 1992;7:303.
12. Frankl V. Man's Search for Meaning. Boston: Beacon Press, 1959.
13. Maslow AH. Motivation and Personality, 3rd ed. Hummelstown, PA: Scott Foresman-Addison Wesley, 1987.
14. Fitchett G. Assessing Spiritual Needs. Minneapolis, Minn.: Augsburg, 1993.
15. Thompson S, Janigan A. Life schemes: A framework for understanding the search for meaning. J Soc Clin Psychol 1988; 7: 260–280.
16. Lipson J, Dibble SL, Minarik PA, eds. Culture and Nursing Care: A Pocket Guide. San Francisco: University of California Nursing Press, 1996.
17. Andrews M, Boyle J. Competence in transcultural nursing care. Am J Nurs 1997;8:16AAA–16DDD.
18. Noyes R, Holt CS, Massie MJ. Anxiety disorders. In: Holland J, ed. Psycho-oncology. New York: Oxford University Press, 1998: 548–563.
19. Massie MJ. Depressive disorders. In: Holland J, ed. Psycho-oncology. New York: Oxford University Press, 1998:518–540.
20. Shehan L. Cancer as a Turning Point: A Handbook for People with Cancer, Their Families and Health Professionals. Long Beach, Calif.: Plume, 1994.
21. Gullo S, Glass E, Gamiere M. Silver Linings: The Other Side of Cancer. Pittsburgh, Pa.: Oncology Nursing Press, 1997.
22. Cella DF, Tulsky DS, Gray G, et al. The Functional Assessment of Cancer Therapy Scale: Development and Validation of the General Measure. J Clin Oncol 1984;11:570–579.
23. de Haes JCJM, van Knippenberg FCE, Neijt JP. Measuring psychological and physical distress in cancer patients: Structure and application of the Rotterdam Symptom Checklist. Br J Cancer 1990;62:1034–1038.
24. Jevene RF, Miller JE. Finding Hope: Ways to See Life in a Brighter Light. Fort Wayne, Ind.: Willowgreen, 1999.
25. Scanlon C. Creating a vision of hope: The challenge of palliative care. Oncol Nurs Forum 1989;16:491–496.

BIBLIOGRAPHY

Back AL, Arnold RM, Quill TE. Hope for the Best, and Prepare for the Worst. Ann Intern Med 2003;138:439–443.

Bolen JS. Close to the Bone: Life Threatening Illness and the Search for Meaning. New York: Scribner, 1996.

Byock I. Dying Well: Peace and Possibilities at the End of Life. New York: Riverhead Books, 1998.

Carroll-Johnson R. Psychosocial Nursing Care Along the Cancer Continuum. Pittsburgh, Pa.: Oncology Nursing Press, 1998.

Davis L, Keller A. At the Close of Day: A Person Centered Guide Book on End-of-Life Care. Charleston, NC: Streamline Press, 2004.

Glass E, Cluxton D. Truth-telling: ethical issues in clinical practice. J Hosp Pall Care 2004;6:232–242.

Hutchinson J, Rupp J. May I Walk You Home? Courage and Comfort for Caregivers of the Very Ill. Notre Dame, Ind.: Ave Maria Press, 1999.

Kramp E, Kramp D. Living with the End in Mind: A Practical Checklist for Living Life to the Fullest by Embracing Your Mortality. New York: Three Rivers Press, 1998.

Lo B, Quill T, Tulsky J. Discussing palliative care with patients. American College of Physicians–American Society of Internal Medicine End-of-Life Care Consensus Panel. Ann Intern Med 1999;130: 744–749.

Lynn J, Harrold J. Handbook for Mortals: Guidance for People Facing Serious Illness. New York: Oxford University Press, 1999.

Miller JE. One You Love Is Dying: 12 Thoughts to Guide You On the Journey. Fort Wayne, Ind.: Willowgreen Publishing, 1997.

Miller JE. When You Know You're Dying: 12 Thoughts to Guide You Through the Days Ahead. Fort Wayne, Ind.: Willowgreen Publishing, 1997.

National Family Caregivers Association website. Available at: http://www.thefamilycaregiver.org (accessed October 23, 2004).

National Selected Morticians. Arranging a funeral; A friend's guide to funeral services; Funeral services by religion. Available at: http://www.nsm.org (assessed October 23, 2004).

Ohio State University Medical Center, Columbus, Ohio. Patient education materials are available at: http://medicalcenter.osu.edu/patientcare/healthinformation/ (accessed October 23, 2004). (For information on purchasing the rights to use or adapt these materials for your organization, contact Diane Moyer, Consumer Health Education, 13–5–522 BTL, 1375 Perry Street, Columbus OH 43201/614-293-3191.)

Rancour, P. Those tough conversations. American Journal of Nursing: Critical Care Supplement, 2000;100:24HH–24LL.

Rancour P. Catapulting through life stages: When young adults are diagnosed with life-threatening illness. In: Psychosocial Nursing and Mental Health Services 2002;40(2):32–37.

Robertson C. Let the Choice Be Mine: A Personal Guide to Planning Your Own Funeral. Standpoint, Idaho: MCR, 1995. (Available from MCR, P.O. Box 1922, Sandpoint, ID 83864, telephone 208-263-8960.)

Stoll R. Guidelines for spiritual assessment. Am J Nurs 1979;79: 1574–1577.

Taylor R. Check your cultural competence. Nurs Manage 1998; 3: 30–32.

Warm E, Weissman D. Fast fact and concept #21: Hope and truth telling. EPERC: Educational Materials Fast Facts Print Preview. August 2000. Available at: http://www.eperc.mcw.edu/fastFact/ff_021.htm (accessed October 23, 2004).

4

Constance M. Dahlin and David F. Giansiracusa

Communication in Palliative Care

Talking about all the issues made his last few days and nights for him and our family better, as we felt a great deal of love and compassion.—Wife of 56-old-man with cancer

- ***Key Points***
- *Effective communication is essential to all aspects of palliative care.*
- *Listening is a valuable component of communication and is a skill that requires practice and mastery.*
- *Nonverbal communication is as critical as verbal communication.*

A nurse uses a myriad of tools in working with patients. For patients with heart disorders, a nurse uses blood pressure cuffs, scales, and stethoscopes as tools to promote optimal pressure. For patients with diabetes, a nurse teaches how to use glucometers and interpret laboratory test values as tools for maintaining blood sugars. For patients in the intensive care unit (ICU), a nurse employs various monitoring devices to measure jugular venous pressure, oxygen saturation, and vital signs, as well as ventilators and other tubes and machines as tools to maintain vital functions. However, for palliative care patients, the fundamental tool is communication.

Communication is the foundation from which assessments are ascertained, goals of care are developed, and relationships are established. A patient with an uncertain future needs honest disclosure, to pursue realistic hopes, and the most current information, to reorganize priorities and to make adaptations in coping with his or her disease process. Effective communication is critically important to elicit the patient's and family's needs, to negotiate goals of care, and to help patients and family members address concerns.[1] Good communication sets the tone for all aspects of care at this time of life, allowing patients to paint a picture of themselves and their priorities, values, and needs in the last stages of life. Ongoing discussion facilitates expression of feelings by patients and family members, including their sense of issues and problems surrounding a life-threatening disease and their concerns about care. This in turn creates a framework that serves as a guide for health care providers to establish priorities in care at the end of life, from which the plan of care is developed. Without effective communication, the patient's experience of suffering is unknown, and effective symptom control is impossible.[2]

According to the American Nurses Association, nurses have a duty to educate patients and families about end-of-life issues, to encourage the discussion of life preferences, to communicate relevant information for any decision, and to advocate for the patient.[3] However, many nurses are uncomfortable communicating with dying patients. Various studies have identified a lack of communication in addressing care wishes and inadequate knowledge and skill in end-of-life-care communication.[4,5] The barriers to communication are multidimensional. Patients often avoid talking about their pain, anger, sense of loss, sense of guilt, and fears due to embarrassment, shyness, confusion, and cultural prohibitions. Families may be unable to talk about the advanced nature of their loved one's illness. They may have no knowledge of the patient's preferences for types of care. Not surprisingly, families tend to overestimate the possibility of cure and to fear experiencing future regrets if they do not pursue or demand further curative treatment.

Nursing issues in communication include fear and medical and legal issues. One concern is the supposition that bringing up issues related to dying or advanced care planning will cause emotional distress. Nurses may anticipate conflict between patient and family. They may have concerns about medical and legal issues related to their scope of practice. Yet, nurses are often the first health care providers to identify problems in regard to advanced care planning, goals of care, conflict between patient and family wishes, and use of life-sustaining measures. Moreover, Fallowfield[6] suggested that some physicians believe nurses are more capable than they are of talking with distressed patients and families. However, many nurses feel uncomfortable with their communication skills, feel the pressure of too little time, or feel threatened by such conversations. Yet, in our experience, the majority of palliative care consultation is spent on discussions of care goals.

Across the palliative care spectrum, communication occurs at critical junctures. Depending on the prognosis of the patient, these communications may occur over a long or a short period of time. The initial communication consists of introduction of the nurse and patient, perhaps at the time of the initial diagnosis of a potentially life-threatening illness. During this time, the patient and nurse get to know each other. The tasks of the nurse at this stage are to elicit personality and coping styles and to explore the patient's understanding of his or her illness. Additionally, the nurse identifies any existing advanced care planning and determines priorities and goals of the patient. The task of the patient is getting to know the nurse as a member of the health care team. This communication may proceed smoothly until the patient's condition changes, at which time the focus of care may change. At this point, the patient seeks trust and reassurance from the nurse, including continued involvement. Later, there may be a discussion of bad news, in which the reality of the situation is addressed and mutual goals are established. During this time, conflicts may be negotiated or life-sustaining treatments discussed. The nurse may be a part of these discussions; if not, the nurse may later serve to reinforce the information. Finally, as the patient is dying, communication with the patient and family often focuses on such issues as support of decisions, continued reassurance that comfort will be maintained, and anticipatory grieving. Communication with family members continues during anticipatory grief and, after the death of the patient, during bereavement.

Within the spectrum of health care, nurses are trusted members of the health care team at the time of diagnosis, during treatment, and in the final stages of life. Through effective communication, the nurse has a pivotal role in supporting the patient. Indeed, the nurse may have the best opportunity to learn the patient's hopes, fears, dreams, and regrets and to create a healing environment. Many nurses have not had either the training in communication as part of their education nor the luxury to work collaboratively with other health disciplines to learn these skills. This chapter reviews the fundamental elements of communication and the roles of the nurse in communicating with patients, facilitating the communication process in advanced care planning, helping to set goals, and delivering bad news. A discussion of the nursing role in collaborative care and conflict resolution is also included.

Historical Perspective

Communication about the end of life has changed dramatically since the 1960s, when death and dying were closed, unacknowledged topics. Field and Copp[7] described an interesting movement in communication with dying patients. Initially, the topic of death was avoided with patients and was discussed only among health care providers. Moreover, communication skills were considered to be intuitive or inherited traits. Practitioners either had empathetic and effective communication skills, or they did not.[2] For patients being cared for by an uncommunicative or ineffective clinician, dying could be an isolating, anxious, fearful, mistrustful experience that translated into a sense of abandonment. In such a situation, families experience complex grief and bereavement and increased stress. For nurses, this indirect communication and lack of truth-telling in the dying process results in greater stress, anxiety, and inauthentic communication, which translates to guilt, internal conflict, and a sense of failure.

From the 1960s to the 1980s, the principles of informed consent and autonomy became valued in health care. In the 1990s, as truth-telling became a central focus of terminal care, death became a more open topic of discussion for patients. For better or worse, without any consideration to the uniqueness of patient/family systems, patients and families were informed of death and dying irrespective of their wishes to know such information. Active participation of patients in their care became the underlying value that led to a greater sense of control and diminished anxiety. However, this shift did not necessarily allow for the individual issues of patients to be discussed, such as whether they wanted to be involved in making decisions. Currently, the trend is a conditional process that supports the patient's individual coping style. This allows for care to follow the patient's individual personality, particularly in terms of the patient's level of acceptance or denial of the dying process.

Given this need to identify and treat each patient individually, communication skills are essential to provide optimal nursing care. Interestingly, a shift in communication theory has simultaneously occurred. The research has demonstrated that communication skills, like any other skills, can be acquired by health care providers.[2] Therefore, communication education should be initiated at every level of education for nursing, regardless of the degree with which nurses are entering practice—associate's degree, bachelor's, master's, or post-master's education. However, there is also a need to provide continuing education in communication for nurses currently in practice.

Importance of Communication

In the health care environment, communication, whether intentional or not, occurs all the time between nurses and patients in every aspect of care. Patients consider communication skills to be very important. Bailey and Wilkinson[8] performed a qualitative study that evaluated patients' perceptions of nurses' communication skills and attributes of a good nurse. Twenty-nine patients were surveyed about communication. Patients specified that nurses must have good verbal and nonverbal skills and be approachable, sympathetic, and nonjudgmental as well as caring. Patients also felt that a good nurse has the personal characteristic of being a good listener and the professional quality of being a good communicator. All of these are important characteristics of general nursing. Clearly, nursing and communication at the end of life go hand in hand.

Communication needs of the nurse include skill acquisition, credible knowledge in the area of end-of-life care, empowerment to participate and communicate in death and dying discussions, and appropriate communication behaviors.[8,9] Moreover, communication skills affect the success of the nurse in her various therapeutic roles, including advocacy, support, information-sharing, empowerment, validation, and ventilation.[10]

There are two levels of necessary communication skills based on education and expertise. At the registered nurse or generalist level, critical communication skills include, but are not limited to, listening and supporting patients in coping with their disease, providing information to patients so that they can make important decisions, being present at the delivery of bad news, being present in family meetings, reinforcing information to give consistent content, reviewing options of care, supporting decision-making, advocating for the patient and family, reviewing signs and symptoms of dying, facilitating communication between the patient and family, being present in the dying process, providing postdeath care and direction, and providing support in grief and bereavement. Some generalist nurses consider the role of information sharing and any discussion of diagnosis and treatment to be outside their scope of practice. However, from the perspective of the advocacy role in nursing, information sharing empowers the patient to make informed decisions. Moreover, the very proximity of the nurse in the direct bedside caregiving role affords the nurse many opportunities to create positive communication encounters. The plethora of opportunities to begin dialogue about death and dying include, in addition to planned meetings, moments of privacy between nurse and patient during bathing, feeding, and self-care activities.

At the master's or advanced practice level, critical nursing communication skills include discussions of diagnosis, treatment options, and prognosis; delivery of bad news when disease progresses; transition into palliative care; discussions of life-sustaining treatment; facilitation of family meetings; discussion of postdeath options such as autopsy or organ donation; and grief and bereavement support. However, the issue of which consultation is used is important to the APN. In the medical model primarily used in the academic setting, the focus is on expertise in palliative care. In the nursing model, the focus is on coaching or mentoring, depending on the culture and environment of the work setting.

Lack of education or training or lack of personal and professional experience with death and dying[11,12] results in little exposure to end-of-life communication. Unless nurses are mentored or coached by colleagues, lack of confidence in performing these tasks leads to avoidance of participation in difficult communication encounters. Other nurses may have discomfort with communication in such circumstances due to personal struggles of unresolved grief, fear of their own mortality, or fear of being emotional in front of a patient.[13,14] Nevertheless, in order to be effective in dealing with patients at the end of life, nurses must examine their own feelings about death and dying, receive support for their personal grief, and seek mentoring to improve communication skills.

Communication during the end-of-life period is critical. The players involved in the communication process include the patient, the nurse and health care providers, and the family or support people. Each person has different needs, related to personal communication styles and learning styles. Communication styles vary by speech, tone, intensity, amplitude, and speech patterns. Learning styles include seeing, hearing, doing, or a mixture of all three. Therefore, it may be necessary to use a variation of verbal discussion, written materials, and videos.

There are several needs of the patient, including management of symptoms, support from family and friends, fulfillment of family or cultural expectations, attaining meaning, and maintaining dignity and control.[15] Discrete communication needs of the patient related to these issues include obtaining information, synthesizing the information, making decisions, and trying to maintain some sense of control. The nurse serves to assess these areas, particularly in times of stress, when information processing may be impaired. As Pasacreta and colleagues[16] described, a person who is mildly anxious may be able to process information and, in fact, may be quite creative. Indeed, mild anxiety helps most people do their work by being alert to issues, identifying problems, and facilitating creative solutions. Some patients experience mild anxiety simply by participating in a preventive health encounter. In this situation, the nurse may provide basic health information. However, as anxiety increases toward a moderate level, as often occurs with receiving news about disease progression, information processing becomes selective. In terms of patients, this means that when something scary or threatening is communicated, the patient may not be able to take in much information. For instance, a patient may be told that an x-ray film looks abnormal. At that point, the patient has a heightened awareness and may be thinking of possible issues. In this case, the nurse provides support to the patient in allowing the patient to ventilate fears and concerns and reiterating information that the team has provided.

In cases of severe anxiety and panic, such as when hearing bad news in the form of a short prognosis or lack of options, a patient's information processing may be totally impaired.[16] This occurs when a patient is given a terminal diagnosis. As soon as the physician or the advanced practice nurse (APN) gives bad news of such gravity, the patient may then not be able to hear anything else. He or she may have gone into shock or panic about the news and cannot comprehend other information. This is important for the timing of further communication and follow-up of such an event. Nurses have an important role in validating the patient's reactions and offering support in determining what further information the patient may need.

The existential aspects of end-of-life communication include disclosure, searching for meaning, and responding to grief reactions to the received information.[17,18] Exploration surrounding life-threatening illnesses can help a patient live while dying, lessen fear, and achieve quality of life during this process.[19]

The communication needs of the family and other supportive people depend on their role in the family system, age, decision-making ability, and other rules within and specific to the family. Families are often very involved in care, but they may also have multiple home and work responsibilities. Therefore, it may be a challenge for family members to be present at the bedside. Families may experience a high level of frustration from the need for constant updating of information in order to organize and prioritize other activities around their caregiving role. In an attempt to balance their self-care issues, they may not be present for important informal information sharing unless a meeting is scheduled.

To facilitate participation in the patient's care, families need communication regarding several issues: understanding what is the care plan is, what is currently being done, and how they can be helpful; reassurance of the patient's comfort; support in coping with the patient's condition; and support in being with the patient.[15] Correspondingly, the communication needs for the patient include information, ongoing explanations of the rationale for care, the need to be listened to, and the opportunity to participate in important discussions.[20] For both the patient and the family, the nurse is the pivotal clinician in fostering the communication processes.

Communication Framework

Communication comprises both verbal expression, including various words and language, and nonverbal expression or the use of body language. Other aspects of communication include the educational level of content, the emotional expression, and the nature of the relationship between the sender and receiver, or between the patient and the health care provider.[21] Communication can be affected by myriad factors including, but not limited to, education of the patient and family; literacy of the patient and family; cultural issues of the patient and family; English as first language; stress, coping, and anxiety of patient and family; use of medical jargon, particularly three-letter acronyms; and assumed common understanding of vocabulary.[21,22]

Nurses often act as translators between the various health disciplines and providers and the patient/family. By the virtue of their constant bedside presence, nurses must create the optimal method of interaction with a patient. This includes assessing the patient's coping and learning styles and discerning the patient's ability to understand simple requests to promote healing, as influenced by his or her mental status and severity of illness. The process itself varies according to the age and cognitive development of the patient. For children and some older adults, the family or support unit is primarily involved in the information process. Their intimate proximity allows nurses to broach sensitive topics based on the hours they spend at the bedside. More specifically, according to Pierce,[23] nurses fulfill three critical communication tasks in end-of-life care: (1) they create an environment conducive to communication, (2) they ease interaction between physician and patient, and (3) they facilitate interaction between family and patient. The case study is an example of opening dialogue.

CASE STUDY
Mr. L, a Man with End-Stage Cardiac Disease

Mr. L, a 70-year-old man with end-stage cardiac disease, has been treated with a number of medications but has been having more angina. The cardiac team has told him there is no further treatment. They said they will try to keep him comfortable but that he was to expect more pain. They are planning on sending him home with various medications and home health services in the next day or so.

NURSE: Hi, Mr. Jones. I will be your nurse today. How are you feeling?

MR. L: I am okay, but I am in pain. So many people have been poking at me.

NURSE: Can you tell me a little about your pain?

MR. L: My chest hurts like they said it would. But there is nothing more they can do. I guess I should just forget about it and try to make the best of it.

NURSE: What did the doctors tell you?

MR. L: They said it would hurt. My heart isn't working well.
NURSE: Hmm, what do you understand about your heart?
MR. L: The heart doctors said my heart is broken and not working right. There is nothing to be done. I just have to wait till it stops.
NURSE: Well, that is a lot to take in. Let me help you understand better. It is true your heart is not working well. And it is true we cannot get it back to normal. But we can use medicines to keep you comfortable. We are not just waiting for it to stop. I could give you some medicine to help your pain now.
MR. L: You can? I thought there were no more medicines that would help.
NURSE: I can give you medicine to help the pain. It won't fix your heart, but it will make you feel better.
MR. L: That would be good. I thought they were just waiting for me to die and didn't want to give me pain medication until I was close to dying.

Here the nurse promotes an open environment for the patient to ask questions and clarifies communication that has occurred between the patient and the physician.

Elements of Communication

There are four basic elements to communication: imparting information, listening, information gathering, and presence and sensitivity. Realistically, these elements do not occur in a linear fashion but may occur concurrently. However, for the sake of simplicity, they are discussed separately here.

Imparting Information

As nurses, our role is to impart information. This often includes teaching, educating about illness, and providing general information about treatments. APNs may offer other information, including diagnosis and treatment options. Imparting information is complex, because information alone is not enough. Rather, information must be provided within the appropriate context of educational level, developmental level, stress level, and time constraints. The patient's educational level and understanding of medical language affects his or her information processing. Many patients have not finished high school; they may not understand complex words, or they may not understand many English words if it is their second language. Developmental language refers to the age of the patient and his or her ability to reason. Younger children do not have complex reasoning abilities, whereas adolescents do. Information for pediatric patients and families must meet their particular needs, and the same is true for those patients with developmental delays or cognitive deficits. The stress of being in a health care setting impairs a person's ability to process in information. The more anxious a person is, the less able she or he is to process information. Therefore, imparting information usually means providing information at a fifth or sixth grade education level and at small intervals, to allow patients and families to best hear and process what is being said.

CASE STUDY
JQ, a Young Woman with Recurrent Melanoma

JQ is a 19-year-old young adult with recurrent melanoma. She was originally diagnosed when she was 16 years of age. She underwent surgical excision and aggressive chemotherapy. She is struggling with her diagnosis.

JQ: I can't believe this. I want to go out with my friends. I can't be sick now. I have too much going on. They did the tests too quickly and didn't read them properly. They will just have to redo everything as I don't believe it.
NURSE: It must be hard to go through this.
JQ: Go through what? They just didn't do the tests right. I plan on leaving here and I will come back when they can focus on me. There have been too many people. Besides, my parents told me not to worry.
NURSE: Can you tell me what your doctor told you?
JQ: My cancer doctor told me I was cured of cancer. But I just have a little spot on my stomach. They just need to work on it. It is no big deal.
NURSE: What is your understanding of your type of cancer?
JQ: I have melanoma, which they can cut out and give me chemotherapy. They just need to figure out what to cut.
NURSE: This must be hard to take in. Would it be helpful to set a time to talk with your doctor again?

Here the nurse listens to the patient to hear what she understands and to assess her ability to process new information. Because the young woman is having difficulty processing the news, the nurse allows her to vent and validates her feelings.

Listening

Listening is an active process that requires full presence and attention. Specifically, one both listens to the words and interprets nonverbal gestures. Often it is very helpful to hear the patient's story in his or her own words. This allows better understanding of the patient's journey within the disease trajectory and of how the patient is processing information. The nurse must perceive the verbal content of the patient's responses as well as the words left unsaid. Concurrently, the nurse perceives the nonverbal expressions of emotion and of psychological or spiritual distress.[24] In this process, the nurse listens to the patient's words and concerns without interrupting. The use of silence is paramount. The nurse must not be mentally preparing answers or replies; rather, the nurse uses self-reflection and conveys empathy. The nurse clarifies what has been heard by such comments as, "Hmm" or, "Tell me more." By acknowledging the patient's comments and emotions and exploring their meaning in a compassionate and supportive way, the nurse encourages the patient to explain difficult issues and concerns.[25] There may be times when the patient is silent. In this circumstance, it may appropriate for the nurse to just sit quietly, letting the patient reflect on the moment and the current situation.

CASE STUDY
PM, a 21-Year-Old with a Neurogenerative Disease

PM is a 21-year-old woman with a progressive neurodegenerative disorder that has left her quadriplegic. She has developed respiratory weakness necessitating ventilatory support. Although she did not want treatment, PM was convinced to undergo a tracheostomy with mechanical ventilatory support. She went to a rehabilitation hospital for 2 months then returned home. She is now at home and has asked the palliative care nurse (PCN) to talk with her about her situation. After introductions, the nurse and the patient begin talking.

PCN: PM, how are you doing?

PM: I am stuck. I am on the breathing machine. I had this trach done because they told me I would have a better life. Nothing has changed. I cannot leave this room. I am not going to get better, I will only get worse. I can still talk a little now, but for how long? How long do I have to suffer like this?

PCN: PM, you have been thinking a lot about treatment. You said you are suffering. Can you tell me more?

PM: This is suffering. I have nothing to look forward to. I will never be able to walk. I cannot eat; I need this tube. Soon I will not be able to talk. This is not what life is about.

PCN: Hmmm.

PM: My parents are exhausted because they must do everything for me. Can you imagine what it is like to be in my body? There is no pleasure or joy. I cannot go on like this. I do not want to live by machines. I want to be able to do more. However, I cannot. I was talked into having this trach. But it has brought more grief. It is the big monster that controls my life. I want to take control. I want to be the one who shuts down the machine, not the other way around. (Tears roll down her face.)

PCN: (Silence)

PM: I am tired of living like this. Please help me take control by withdrawing the vent.

PCN: I can hear your suffering. This must be very difficult. When you talk about withdrawing the vent, do you understand what it means?

PM: It means I will die. I have thought about it. This is not quality of life. Can you understand that?

PCN: (Nods yes)

PM: Could you live like I am and think it is quality of life? I don't want to be like this. Please help me.

Here the nurse listens to the patient and her language. She shows that she is really listening by using the patient's own words and having the patient define what she means. The nurse also provides support by not trying to have all the answers and by letting the patient guide the conversation.

Information Gathering

To gather information from patients, the use of open-ended questions is most effective. This allows the patient to tell his or her story in narrative. During this process, the nurse therapeutically uses open-ended questions rather than "yes-or-no" questions or closed-ended questions. Open-ended questions allow the patient to tell his or her story, whereas closed-ended questions limit the patient's answer and thereby inhibit elaboration, explanations, and clarifications from the patient. Open-ended questions promote a richness in hearing the patient's words and nonverbal cues, which express issues of importance and priorities of care.[26] Open-ended questions may take many directions in terms of coping, life priorities, and spiritual concerns.

A nurse may not be able to ask many questions. However, a few key questions can set a tone of a caring relationship with the nurse. See Table 4–1 for a list of questions. Once such a question is asked, it is essential to listen to the answer. Often important questions are asked, but, as the patient starts to answer, the conversation moves on, with no time or attention being given to hearing what the patient is expressing, no further elaboration, and no response to the patient's verbal and nonverbal messages. This can cause resentment in the patient if he

Table 4–1
Sample of Open-Ended Questions to Begin Discussions About Life-threatening Illness

What concerns do you have about your illness?
How are you doing with your illness?
How is treatment going for you?
What are your worries?
What are your hopes?
Who is important to you?
Who provides support to you?
What gives you meaning in your life?
What gives you joy in your life?
What provides you with the strength to live each day?
Do you consider yourself spiritual or religious?
What rituals are important to you?
Is there any unfinished business you need to attend to?
What relationships are the most important to you?

Source: Adapted from City of Hope National Medical Center and the American Association of Nursing (2003), reference 10, and Quill (2000), reference 27.

or she has shared something intimate without acknowledgment as to its significance. The following is a sample of the use of open-ended questions.

CASE STUDY

Ms. M, a Woman with Metastatic Ovarian Cancer

Ms. M is a 50-year-old woman with metastatic ovarian cancer. She has no further treatment options. However, she has come in for thoracentesis and paracentesis.

NURSE: How are things going at home?

MS. M: It is really hard. I am in more pain. I can't get around as much. I hate staying in bed. I feel like a burden to my family.

NURSE: In what way are you a burden?

MS. M: I have to ask them for everything. They must bring me my pills, bring me meals. They must even help me to the bathroom. It is so embarrassing. I used to take care of them. Now they must help me. It doesn't seem fair. How can I keep doing this to them?

NURSE: What do you feel you are doing to them?

MS. M: I am making them focus on me instead of their lives. It is not fair.

NURSE: What is giving you strength?

MS. M: I am not sure. I used to think my religion did. Now I don't know, because it makes no sense.

NURSE: What makes no sense?

MS. M: This disease. How did this happen?

NURSE: (Quiet)

MS. M: This disease stinks and it is making me rethink all sorts of things I took for granted.

NURSE: Like what?

MS. M: All the things I thought I would do and can't.

NURSE: What were those things?

MS. M: Getting my family in order.

NURSE: How can we help you to still do some of those things?

MS. M: I am not sure, but I will think about it.

Here the nurse promotes open dialogue by asking open-ended questions to learn more about the patient and her coping.

Sensitivity

Sensitivity, another term for cultural competence, includes issues pertaining to religious, spiritual, cultural, ethnic, racial, gender, and language issues and is a very important element of communication. Not only is it important to appreciate verbal cues, but also it is critical to interpret nonverbal cues. Communication varies in different cultures. In many situations, beneficence takes precedence over autonomy. Disclosure and nondisclosure must be viewed within the context of the patient and the family, with understanding of and respect for their values and beliefs.

Table 4–2
Useful Cultural Assessment Questions

Where were you born and raised?
What do you want to know about your medical condition/illness?
How do you describe your medical condition/illness?
How have you treated your medical condition/illness?
Who else, if anyone, do you want to know about your medical condition/illness?
Who else, if anyone, should we talk to about your medical condition/illness, treatment options, and the disease process?
Who is responsible for your health care decisions?
Who are important people in your community?
What do you fear most about your condition and its treatment?

Source: Adapted from Lapine et al. (2001), reference 28; Kagawa-Singer and Blackhall (2001), reference 29; and Buchwald et al. (1994), reference 30.

In these situations, nurses must first examine their own cultural backgrounds and be aware of their own ethical values and beliefs. Then, they can assess the communication patterns of the patient and the family, using questions from Table 4–2. For example, the nurse may ask the patient how she wants to receive medical information. The patient may state she wants to hear it directly, or she may defer to family members. Next, the nurse helps the patient identify others whom she wishes to be told about her medical issues. The nurse then may help the patient state who she wants to make health care and treatment decisions.

If the patient and family do not speak English as a first language, it is incumbent to use an interpreter for any discussions. Too often, family members are asked to interpret from English to another language, which puts them in a double bind. Culturally, although they may be translators, they must also act within their family roles and may need to protect the patient from information depending on cultural norms. Translating family members may withhold information if they are not comfortable with another family member knowing it. As a result, it may be very unclear what the patient has actually been told.[28] For this reason, a translator not known by the family must always be used. The following example demonstrates how a nurse may facilitate appropriate cultural care.

CASE STUDY

Mrs. C, a Woman with End-Stage Renal Disease

Mrs. C is a 75-year-old Chinese woman with end-stage renal disease who is starting dialysis. She was admitted for weakness, pain, and anorexia. Her dialysis nurse meets her when she comes to start dialysis while still in the hospital.

NURSE: Mrs. Chen, I am going to be your nurse when you come to see Dr. Lee. May I ask what you know about your condition?
MRS. C: I know I am sick, but I don't want to know any details. I want my family to know and make decisions for me.
NURSE: Is there anyone in particular in your family who is making these decisions?
MRS. C: My son.
NURSE: If you need further therapies, do you want us to discuss this with you or your son?
MRS. C: I want my son to make all decisions for me.
NURSE: Do you have any questions?
MRS. C: No, I know everything I need to know.
NURSE: If you have any questions or want to know anything, you can always ask. Even though you want your son to make decisions, I would like you to feel as much a part of the process as you feel comfortable with.
MRS. C: Thank you.

Here the nurse clarifies and validates the patient's information preferences while promoting allowance for these to change if the patient desires.

In addition to these aspects of communication, there are general behaviors that facilitate good communication and general behaviors that inhibit communication. Facilitating behaviors include open-ended questions as discussed earlier, questions with a psychological focus, clarification of psychological issues, empathy, summarization, and hypotheses about how the patient may be feeling. Inhibiting behaviors include closed-ended questions, leading questions, physically focused questions that do not address affect or coping, and advice-giving.[31]

The Scope of Communication

Communication among nurse, patient, and family is a continuous process throughout the spectrum of the disease. A powerful therapeutic intervention in and of itself, communication creates a dialogue[32] for the exchange of information and understanding throughout the course of care. At the time of diagnosis, discussions include the anticipated course of the illness and treatment options. As the disease progresses, discussions focus on symptom assessment and additional diagnostic and therapeutic interventions. Later, when the patient reaches the point at which further curative options are no longer appropriate, the focus of care changes to comfort, anticipating the dying process, and family bereavement. Thus, in addition to serving as the tool for exchange of information, communication serves to facilitate human relationships and connections among nurses, patients, and families.

Methods and Techniques of Communications

The context in which communications occur, including the verbal and nonverbal content of messages, the tone, and the emotional affect of the participants, influences the process and outcomes of interactions. Important information is best conveyed face-to-face, allowing observation of verbal as well as nonverbal communication by various team members. Scheduled meetings are good for both patients and health care providers. For the interdisciplinary health care team, scheduled meetings allow for preparation of the important information to be shared, including medical facts, prognosis, treatment options, and sources of support and guidance. They promote collaborative care by allowing the team (nurse, physician, social worker, and other clinicians) to review the information in order to provide a unified and consistent message to the patient and family. They also allow the bedside nurse to organize his or her day so as to be part of these important discussions.

The timing of communication is important. Quill and colleagues[33] defined the following "urgent" situations that necessitate immediate communication: (1) the patient is facing imminent death; (2) the patient is talking about wanting to die[34]; (3) the patient or family is inquiring about hospice; (4) the patient has recently been hospitalized for severe, progressive illness; and (5) the patient is experiencing severe suffering and poor prognosis. Less urgent situations that require more routine planned meetings include (1) the discussion of prognosis, particularly if life expectancy is thought to be between 6 and 12 months; (2) the discussion of treatment options with low probability of success; and (3) the discussion of hopes and fears. End-of-life communication in more "routine" circumstances, when stability or recovery is predicted, normalizes the discussion of advanced care planning. These discussions assist the determination of the patient's values, goals, fears, and concerns while also developing the core issues for patient education, including the right to high-quality pain control and symptom management.[27]

Scheduled meeting times are critical in allowing the patient to prepare emotionally and psychologically for any potential news. This includes allowing for the presence of the patient's support network to hear and validate information conveyed. Nurses play a vital role in these meetings because they are often responsible for arranging the meeting and securing a comfortable space. Before the meeting, the nurse may assess the patient's physical, emotional, and psychological concerns. This information can assist the team in planning discussion points at the scheduled meetings.

When such a meeting occurs, several steps are important. After introductions have been done, the goals of the meeting can be stated. Then the patient can be asked about his or her understanding of the medical condition and situation. This is followed up by ascertaining the patient's worries and fears, how much information the patient wishes to know,[35] and which other people the patient wishes to be informed or involved in his or her care. A patient who is hesitant to express emotional concerns may need prompting or an invitation to speak. With overbearing families, it may be important to reinforce the goals of the meeting and to restate that the focus of care is on the patient.[36] The nurse may facilitate the initial conversation by serving as a reference point for the patient and family in conveying important conversations and concerns at the beginning of the meeting and personalizing the discussions to the specific needs of the patient and family. In addition, the nurse may act as a translator between the medical team and the patient, facilitating information sharing, interpreting information and medical jargon in language the patient understands, and also ensuring that the members of the care team understand the patient's words and language.

CASE STUDY

KZ, a Woman with Metastatic Nerve Sheath Tumor

KZ is a 30-year-old woman with metastatic nerve sheath tumor. She has undergone multiple surgeries, various chemotherapy regimens, and some radiation. KZ is cared for at home by an extended family. Her oncology nurse practitioner (ONP) was called to the home by the home health nurse because KZ's condition was declining. KZ is bedbound, with lower extremity paralysis and left hip pain. After much discussion and consideration, she is brought to the hospital for symptom management and transition of care. A meeting is scheduled by the ONP with the oncologist, the primary nurse, and the palliative care nurse practitioner. The goal of the meeting is to discuss code status and further treatment. At the meeting, KZ is in her bed surrounded by her many family members and the health care team. The oncologist reviews her cancer and treatment to date. Then the ONP begins her part of the discussion.

ONP: K, I have been concerned about you. I brought you into the hospital because you were in so much pain. I am wondering how you are doing.

KZ: Well, it has been okay. But this pain is incredible. Do you think you can make it better?

ONP: I think we can. We will have you evaluated by a team that specializes in pain control. However, I am wondering how you are doing with your cancer?

KZ: Well, I know it is still there, and I would like to continue treatment.

ONP: When we saw you last time, we discussed that the common chemotherapies were not working. We discussed some experimental treatment. Do you remember that?

KZ: I do, and I want to continue treatment.

ONP: Do you remember when we discussed further chemotherapy, we also discussed functional status? I am concerned because you are hardly able to get out of bed.

KZ: I will be okay soon. I can do it.

ONP: K, do you remember when we met you said you wanted me to be direct and honest with you.

KZ: Yes.

ONP: Well, I need to be honest now. I am not sure you will be able to tolerate more treatment. I think things are changing.

KZ: What do you mean?

ONP: K, remember that the last time you were here your cancer had grown. I am sorry but I have to tell you it is still growing. We are concerned that giving you more chemotherapy would do more harm than good now. Is that true, Dr. J?

DR. J: K, I know you want to be cured. But as we discussed last time, when the other chemo didn't work, we don't have very many options. None of the chemotherapies we give you now will cure you. It may have a very small chance as slowing the growth.

KZ: I can still do it. I will be okay.

DR. J: K, you are weak and having so many side effects that I can't offer it right now. If you get stronger, we may be able to do it. But right now, you have to take an ambulance to get here.

ONP: Dr. J and I have been discussing this, and we are afraid the side effects are too great. We would like to focus on your comfort.

KZ: If I get better, would you still give me chemo?

ONP: If you got better we would still give you chemotherapy, but we don't think that will happen. We would like to have palliative care work with us to focus on your comfort.

KZ: I just want you to stay involved in my care.

Here the ONP builds on her strong relationship with the patient as well as referring to previous conversations to convey bad news and to reassure the patient of nonabandonment.

Effective communication, as viewed by terminally ill patients, their families, and health care professionals, primarily consists of providing accurate information in a sensitive, simple, and straightforward manner and in understandable language. Studies indicate that patients want their physicians to be honest and straightforward as well as hopeful, and this also can be applied to nurses. Therefore, the nurse should encourage questions from the patient and be responsive to his or her readiness to talk about death[37]; this can best be achieved by discussing outcomes other than cure, such as improved functional status or independence in care needs. Focusing on quality of life offers hope and meaning to the patient, helping the patient prepare for losses and leaving open the possibility of "miracles."[38] It is helpful to have a nurse present at conversations between physician and patient at which bad news or other important information is conveyed. The nurse can then reinforce the information provided and promote optimal coping. If the nurse is not able to participate in the delivery of difficult information, it is helpful to ask for specifics about the conversation, in terms of what and how information was conveyed as well as the patient's response. This allows the nurse to follow up with the patient's perception of the information and his or her understanding of the next steps.

The actual process of conducting a meeting at which important information is to be conveyed has seven steps[9]: (1) confirming medical facts and establishing an appropriately private place and sufficient time for discussions, (2) using open-ended questions to establish what the patient (and family) knows, (3) determining how the patient wishes the information to be presented, (4) presenting information in a straightforward manner, using understandable language, in small quantities and with pauses for processing and questions to assess understanding, (5) responding to emotions, (6) clarifying goals of care and treatment priorities, and (7) establishing a plan.

Quill[27] emphasized the importance of these end-of-life conversations in their early, systematic occurrence. He described how the early introduction of such conversations in the disease process promotes better outcomes. These outcomes include more informed choices, better palliation of symptoms, and more opportunity for resolution of important issues.[27] Such questions as, "Are there things that would be left undone if you were to die sooner rather than later?" stimulate thought and discussion about dying and important life closure issues such as healing relationships and completing financial transactions. However, a nurse may ask this in a different way, such as, "Are there things you need to do in case things do not go as well as we hope?"[39] Encouraging patients to hope for the best outcome while preparing for the possibility that treatment may not work is helpful in guiding the patient.[40] Again, the nurse advocate role facilitates the essential process of providing the patient with all the necessary information to make choices.

CASE STUDY

Mrs. D, a Woman in Respiratory Distress

Mrs. D, a 40-year-old woman, was in the ICU for respiratory distress. Her history included obesity, chronic obstructive pulmonary disease, emphysema, and cardiomyopathy. She was taking four inotropes to stabilize her blood pressure and multiple medications for respiratory support. Her breathing was so compromised that it was difficult for her to talk for long. The cardiac team had offered her the surgical option of a heart repair. She had consented, but it was very clear that she did not understand the risks. First, she might not be able to undergo intubation, and that would preclude surgery. Second, she might be intubated and not be able to be extubated. Third, anesthesia might go well, but the cardiac team might find that they could not help her. Fourth, she might die during the procedure. Fifth, even with the procedure, the inotropic and respiratory support might not make her situation better, and she might not make it home. The palliative care team was called in to see this woman. Her room was dark, and it was clear that she was afraid, depressed, and anxious.

NURSE: Mrs. D, I am a nurse with the pain and symptom team. Your physician asked that I come talk to you to make sure we were keeping you comfortable. Is this an okay time to talk?

MRS. D: (Nods "yes")

NURSE: I don't want to increase your work of breathing while we talk, so I am going to ask simple questions. To begin with, I notice you have been in the ICU awhile. It must be hard to be here and not at home.

MRS. D: (Nods yes and then tears up).

NURSE: Is getting home really important?

MRS. D: Yes, I need to take care of my children.

NURSE: What have the doctors told you about going home?

MRS. D: They told me I need an operation, and then I can go home.

NURSE: How do you feel about that?

MRS. D: I am scared.

NURSE: What are you scared about?

MRS. D: That I won't make it.

NURSE: That must be hard.

MRS. D: I am so scared. I don't know what to do.

NURSE: How can I help you?

MRS. D: Tell me about the operation.

NURSE: What do you know about the operation?

MRS. D: They said they would repair my heart.

NURSE: Yes, that is true.

MRS. D: But they said it was complicated, but I don't know why. What is wrong?

NURSE: You are right about the operation. It is very complicated. Would you like me to explain it all?

MRS. D: Yes.

NURSE: You understand your heart is not working correctly, right?

MRS. D: (Nods yes).

NURSE: But they want to fix it. However, there are other parts to the operation. Did they tell you about the process of the operation?

MRS. D: No (shaking her head).

NURSE: Do you want to know?

MRS. D: Yes. My children keep asking me.

NURSE: Well, they will need to put you to sleep. That may be hard with your breathing issues.

MRS. D: What else . . .

NURSE: Then they will need to get to your heart. They may find they can't repair the problem.

MRS. D: They didn't tell me that there was a possibility they may not be able to fix it. That is a risk.

NURSE: Yes it is. Then they also need to get you back awake and off the breathing machine, which may be difficult to do.

MRS. D: So this is not an easy operation.

NURSE: No, it is not. And there are no guarantees.

MRS. D: Oh my. I really need to reconsider all this. With what you are telling me, I could have the operation and still never get home.

NURSE: That is true.

MRS. D: And without the operation, I will never get home. So I am in a hard spot.

NURSE: That is correct. There is not a clear answer. Are there more things you have questions about?

MRS. D: No, I just want to think about this and talk it over later.

NURSE: Please feel free to write down any questions you think of, and I will come back later to answer anything else you need.

Often nurses understand that a patient is facing a choice but either does not understand all the information or is being given an unrealistic option. Here, the nurse realizes that the patient does not understand the complexities of the surgery and has unrealistic expectations that the surgery will cure her. She provides this information in accordance with Mrs. D's information preferences.

Sometimes nurses, in their fear of communicating difficult issues at the end of life, employ several mechanisms to avoid discussion. When discussing bad news, nurses and physicians may focus more on the biomedical aspects, and thereby avoid eliciting and responding to patients' thoughts and feelings.[41] A nurse may focus only on the present time, thereby preventing the patient from expressing concerns about a previous time. For example, rather than listening to the patient relate concerns from an earlier time, the nurse may stop the conversation by saying, "But how are you now?" Another way of avoiding discussion is to change the focus or the subject. For example, if the patient says, "I am nauseated," the nurse may nurse divert the conversation by saying, "So, how is your family?" Sometimes the nurse cuts off the conversation by offering advice: "Of course, you will get over this in time. It won't last for too long." Another avoidance technique is responding to a patient's expressed difficulties by stating, "Clearly you need to talk to the social worker about your issues."[31] Finally, nurses and physicians may collude with patients in avoiding discussions of death and dying.[27,55]

Delivering Bad News

Bad or unfavorable medical news may be defined as "any news that drastically and negatively alters the patient's view of her or his future."[42] In palliative care, bad news includes, but is not limited to, disease diagnosis, recurrence, disease progression, lack of further curative treatments, transition to comfort care, and a terminal prognosis for a patient's condition. Nurses, particularly APNs, along with their physician colleagues, generally have the responsibility of communicating unfavorable news to a patient. The decision as to who delivers the news may depend on the relationship of the patient with the team, whom the patient trusts, as well as the APN's scope of practice within the institution and state practice guidelines.

Two recent survey studies of oncology physicians conducted by Baile and colleagues are insightful. One study reported that 22% of oncology physicians had no consistent manner of communicating bad news, and 51.9% used several techniques or tactics without having an overall plan.[43] The second study revealed considerable variability in disclosing diagnoses and prognoses, reporting the absence of further curative treatments, discussing resuscitation, and making recommendations for hospice services.[44] There have been no such surveys among nurses, but, given the lack of education in this area, there is a high probability that the findings would be similar.

Coyle and Sculco beautifully described the emotional setting of giving bad news for the clinician and the patient (p. 212):[45]

> Is it possible for any news, transmitted by a doctor [or nurse] to a patient, to be "good news" in the face of advancing disease that is not responsive to chemotherapy? The doctor [or nurse] is in a position of having to give information that the patient does not want to hear, and yet the patient needs to have the information in order to make necessary life decisions. Does it matter how the information is given when medical information itself can remove hope for continued existence? . . . In a way, both parties—the doctor and the patient—are engaged in a communication dance of vulnerability. The physician is vulnerable because he/she must deliver the facts, whatever they may be, and the patient is vulnerable because he/she doesn't want to hear any more bad news.

From Coyle and Sculco's perspective, patients with advanced disease generally do want to have the information. Additionally, both physicians and nurses can be part of this communication dance. In a report by Yun and colleagues,[46] 96% of 380 cancer patients and 76.9% of 280 family members stated that patients should be informed of a terminal illness. Not surprisingly, some discrepancy was apparent between the opinions of patients and those of family members regarding disclosure. Another study of cancer patients' perspectives concluded that the most important factors when receiving bad news were the expertise of the physician and being given pertinent information about their condition and treatment options. Patients also rated other lesser, but still important, aspects of bad news delivery related to content, setting, and supportive aspects of the meetings.[38]

It should be noted that, although patients may want to have the information, they may be reluctant to initiate such a discussion.[47] Moreover, patients may not be actively invited to express their feelings and concerns. One study showed that patients not provided with an opportunity to disclose concerns before the information is provided tended to remain silently preoccupied with the information and were more likely to develop a pessimistic sense of their situation, compared with patients who were invited to share and discuss their concerns.[47]

CASE STUDY
PE, a Young Man with Metastatic Sarcoma

PE is a 20-year-old Spanish-speaking man with new diagnosis of metastatic sarcoma after having had back pain for 6 months. He was brought to the emergency department, where radiographs and computed tomography scans confirmed the diagnosis. A family meeting is called with a Spanish interpreter.

APN: P, I wanted to meet today to discuss your pain and your tests.
PE: (Quiet)
APN: Can you tell me how you are feeling?
PE: Okay.
APN: Are you having any pain?
PE: Some.
NURSE: How much, if 1 is none and 10 is the most pain you have ever had?
PE: A 3.
APN: And the cause of your pain, do you have any idea of that?
PE: Well I hurt my back and they couldn't find anything.
APN: Well, do you remember that when you came here we did more tests? That was because the pain was worse.
PE: Yes.
APN: Well, I am afraid I have bad news about the tests.
PE: (Quiet)
APN: They do not look normal. We are having the experts on x-rays and the specialists look at them.
PE: (Still quiet)
APN: Can you tell me what you are thinking?
PE: My mind is cloudy right now. I am not thinking well. How can you be sure?
APN: We did several tests that showed a possible cancer in the pictures. In order to confirm the diagnosis, we would like to take a test of some of the tissue. Would you be okay with that?
PE: I want to be sure of the diagnosis, too. Cancer is bad. When would you do the test?
APN: Tomorrow. Is that okay? The results would take a couple of days. Then we could meet again with a cancer specialist to discuss these results.
PE: Yes.
APN: When we meet again, who would you want to be there?
PE: My family and my minister.
APN: Okay, we will do the test tomorrow and meet again in 3 days. I am hoping that perhaps I can give you better news. But I want to prepare you that it may still be bad news. In the meantime, other people are also available to be of support, such as our social worker. And we will continue to work on getting you more comfortable.

Here the nurse gives a warning shot of bad news but offers the follow-up meeting with test results and the specialist.

Behaviors used in presenting unfavorable information may be grouped into four domains: (1) preparation, (2) delivering the content of the message, (3) dealing with the responses of the patient (and family), and (4) closing the encounter.[48] Critically important in the preparation for giving bad news is attention to one's own emotional stress. This may include acknowledgment of possible feelings of guilt, lack of control, failure, loss, fear, or resentment.[49] Awareness of these feeling can allow for a more objective encounter and clarity in ownership of issues. Nurses need to deal with their own sense of anxiety that results from empathizing with the patient.[50]

Recommended guidelines have been developed for delivering unfavorable or bad news. Based on a review of the literature and a consensus panel of patients and physicians, Girgis and Sanson-Fisher[51] recommended the following: (1) ensuring privacy and adequate time, (2) assessing patients' understanding, (3) providing information about diagnosis and prognosis simply and honestly, (4) avoiding the use of euphemisms, (5) encouraging patients to express their feelings, (6) being empathetic, (7) giving a broad but realistic time frame regarding prognosis, and (8) arranging review or follow-up. Other points are summarized in Table 4–3.

Nurses perform a number of critically important functions when the patient is given bad news. First, the nurse may need to interpret, for the patient and the family, the medical information and jargon in a way that is understandable. Second, the nurse may need to restate information that the patient may not have heard due to the emotional impact of the bad news. Third, the nurse may need to investigate and support the patient's emotional and psychological reactions to hearing the bad news.

In response to presenting bad news, patients may express comments or so-called dreaded questions, such as, "Why me?", which many clinicians find very difficult to respond to. One approach is to maintain a sense of openness and curiosity,[56] and not to assume that one knows want the patient really means. An acknowledgment, such as "That is a tough question," allows the nurse to comment and explore further without feeling the need to solve or "fix" the assumed source of the patient's question or comment. This can be followed up by, "Please tell me what you are concerned about." The nurse, by acknowledging and normalizing the patient's feelings, invites the patient to voice his or her thoughts. It also reduces the patient's sense of aloneness, and by sharing the patient's distress, reduces suffering.

Another "dreaded question," one that is particularly common when a patient has been informed of a terminal diagnosis or the lack of curative therapy, is the question, "How long do I have to live?" The nurse may choose to answer in several ways, depending on his or her comfort in these discussions. One response is, "How long do you think you have to live?" This allows the patient to voice his or her concern about time. The patient may say, "Not long, but I wanted to see how long you thought," as if to compare input from different members of the team. Another response is, "Are you asking something specific?" Here the nurse is trying to ascertain whether the patient is asking about dying or is thinking of a certain event

Table 4–3
Main Teaching Points Regarding Delivering Bad News

1. Create a physical setting consisting of a quiet, comfortable room with all participants sitting and free of interruptions.
2. Determine who should be present. Ask whom the patient wishes to have present and clarify the relationship to the patient. Clarify how much the patient wants to know. Decide whether other professionals (nurse, consultants, social worker, case manager, chaplain) should attend, and obtain patient/family permission.
3. Clarify and clearly state your goals and the patient's goals for the meeting.
4. Be knowledgeable about the patient's medical condition/illness, prognosis, and treatment options.
5. If the patient is not competent, arrange to have the legal decision-maker present.
6. If the patient or family does not speak English, use a skilled interpreter.
7. Determine what the patient and family know about the patient's condition and what they have been told.
8. Provide a brief overview of the patient's course and condition as a foundation for understanding for the entire group.
9. Speak slowly, deliberately, and clearly. Provide information in small units. Frequently ask the patient for understanding and emotional responses.
10. Give a warning: "Unfortunately, I have some bad news to share with you." Others[33] have suggested stating, "I wish things were different," followed by a pause.
11. Present bad news in a concise and direct manner. Present information at the patient's and family's pace. Provide an initial overview. Assess understanding. Answer questions. Provide the next level of detail or repeat more general information in response to the patient's and family's needs. Provide truthful, hopeful statements, but avoid false assurances.
12. Sit quietly and allow the patient and family to absorb the information. Wait for the patient to respond. After being silent, check in with the patient such as by saying, "I have just told you some pretty serious news. Do you feel comfortable sharing your thoughts about this?" This may help the patient verbalize concerns.[52]
13. Listen carefully and acknowledge the patient's and family's emotions, such as by reflecting on both the meaning and the affect of their responses. A study of patients' perceptions to receiving bad news (about cancer) indicated the importance, to the patient, of a comfortable environment, adequate time for the meeting, attempts to empathize with the patient's experiences.[53]
14. Normalize and validate emotional responses, such as feeling numb, angry, sad, fearful. Using the pneumonic, *NURSE* (*n*ame, *u*nderstand, *r*espect, *s*upport, and *e*xplore), facilitate the sharing of emotions and reactions.[54]
15. Give an opportunity for questions and comments.
16. Assess thoughts of self-harm.
17. Agree on a specific follow-up plan, such as a date and time for the next meeting, while inviting telephone contact in the interim. Treatment should be provided at the time of closure that meets the patient's immediate needs, including treatment of any distressing symptoms. By the end of the meeting, the patient should feel supported. Conversation addressing aloneness and referral to other resources such as support groups, counselors, and pastoral care providers may help minimize a sense of isolation and abandonment.

that he or she wishes to live to experience. A third response is, "Why do you ask?" This invites the patient to share his or her concerns about dying. Finally, if the anticipated survival time is short or the nurse is uncomfortable, the reply, "What has the team told you?" may be used. In this case, the patient may state that the team has given a certain estimate of time, or the patient may be seeking validation of the prediction.

Nonetheless, responding to and acknowledging such questions normalizes the discussion. It promotes further exploration of thoughts and feelings, resulting in reduced suffering through addressing of the patient's fears and concerns. The nurse reflects on difficult information with, "I imagine it is very frightening not knowing what will happen and when. Do you have particular fears and concerns?"

After listening to the patient's and family members' fears and concerns, it is critically important to provide accurate, hopeful information while deliberately addressing the issue of nonabandonment. This can be done with such words as, "I wish things were different. But no matter what, I will be there to support you in your decisions and focus on your quality of life."

Advanced Care Planning

The American Nurses Association stated that nurses "have a responsibility to facilitate informed decision-making, including but not limited to advance directives."[57] Studies have been performed of patients', families', physicians', and other caregivers' preferences regarding preparing for the end of life. All agree on the importance of (1) naming someone to make decisions, (2) knowing what to expect about one's physical condition, (3) having financial affairs in order, (4) having treatment preferences in writing, and (5) knowing that one's physician is comfortable talking about death and dying. Patients, more than others, want to have funeral plans made and to know the timing of death. Patients were less inclined to talk about personal fears than were families, physicians, and other caregivers.[58] Identified as the most important factors in achieving quality at the end of life were the relief of pain and other distressing symptoms, communication with one's physician, preparation for death, and the opportunity to achieve a sense of completion.[1] In spite of widespread agreement about the importance of preparation, such discussions often are not included in clinical encounters.[58]

Both nurses and physicians perform advanced care planning discussions with patients and their families. Advanced care planning involves setting goals of therapy, developing advanced care directives, and making decisions about specific forms of medical therapy. For chronically ill, debilitated, and terminally ill patients, advanced care planning includes making decisions about life-sustaining therapies (code status), artificial feeding and hydration, and palliative and hospice care. Performing advanced care planning prepares for both incapacity and death, relieves burdens on others, solidifies relationships,[59] and identifies appropriate surrogates and delineates their authority.[60,61] For the terminally ill patient, the health care provider may begin the discussion about planning for the future by asking any of a number of questions, as described in Table 4–4.

Advanced care planning may be regarded differently depending on one's perspective. For the health care provider, advanced care planning prepares for the possibility that the patient may become incapable of making decisions. Advanced care planning is based on the ethical principle of autonomy and exercise of patient control, focuses on completing written advance directive forms, and occurs in the context of the provider–patient relationship. For the patient, advanced care planning may be regarded as a mechanism to prepare for death. Advanced care planning is a social process based on relationships and relief of burdens on others. It involves previous experience with poor health and death of family members, and it occurs in the context of relationships with close loved ones, not just with the health care system.[59] As such, the nurse has a role in advocating the implementation of the patient's wishes.[57]

Because survival estimates affect the decisions patients make, patients need accurate prognostic information. Interviews of 56 terminally ill patients concluded that all patients wanted their physicians to be honest about the prognoses conveyed.[63] However, physicians often do poorly at estimating and reporting accurate survival times to patients.[64,65] The patient's wish to hear optimistic information and the physician's reluctance to present information on disease progression may impair accurate portrayal of the patient's condition.[55] Therefore, it is very helpful for nurses to be in attendance when such information is delivered. Nurses may then attempt to temper some of the overly optimistic survival times, given their knowledge from working with colleagues in various other professions. The disparity of the estimated survival times may confuse patients, particularly with other references such as the Internet readily available. Discussions between patients and providers about complementary treatments is essential to promote realistic outcomes.[66] Some of this information, including complementary and alternative treatments, may be inaccurate, harmful, or inapplicable when put in context of the patient's situation.

Advanced care planning discussions are best completed over time, allowing the patient opportunity for reflection and discussion with family and friends. The process of advanced care planning allows discussion about possible scenarios, which in

Table 4–4
Questions to Begin an Advanced Care Planning Conversation

How can we help you live in the best way possible for you?
How do you wish to spend what ever time you have left?
What activities or experiences are most important for you to do to maximize the quality of your life?
What fears or worries do you have about your illness, or about medical care? Do you have other worries or fears?
What do you hope for your family?
What needs or services would you like to talk about?
What do you now find particularly challenging in your life?
Do you have religious or spiritual beliefs that are important to you?
What would make this time especially meaningful for you?
What makes life worth living for you?
Can you image any situation in which life would not be worth living?[62]
How would you describe your priorities with regard to prolongation of life, maintenance of function, and comfort?[52]

itself may prepare the patient for the course of disease. This includes potential circumstances of death and sharing of values. The result may be a sense of control, a sense of trust with health care providers, and a sense of resolution in aspects of one's life. Patients tend to express their preferences for care after they understand their condition and options for therapy. Advanced care planning promotes the ability to evaluate such information in the context of the patient's values and goals. A change in focus from future cure-oriented treatments to goals of current living may facilitate meaning and purpose.[67] Having the patient consider such questions as, "What if we are not sure whether we will be able to get you off the breathing machine?" can help facilitate thought and decision about how much chance of success a patient needs to have to make certain decisions.[68]

Nurses at all levels provide important assistance in helping patients define their goals and wishes and express their cultural and religious practices and preferences. Nurses also help patients clarify both emotional reactions to their clinical situations and information about treatment options. Nurses play a critical role in advocating for the patient's wishes and preferences and communicating these to family members and other health care providers.

Although patients may differ in the extent to which they wish to participate in treatment decisions, a number of studies have indicated preference to take a collaborative role. Being provided with adequate information is critical. However, simply being offered choices, particularly without any direction, can cause a patient to feel excessively burdened and responsible. The weight of these decisions can cause patients and families to feel a sense of self-blame or to lose confidence in the physician, particularly if the outcome is poor. Therefore, it is critically important to identify how much the patient wishes to be involved in decision-making at all stages of disease.[69]

It is widely agreed that discussions about advanced care planning and completion of advance directives should occur before acute, disabling events and hopefully before the end stage of a terminal illness. However, these conversations may not occur earlier, for a number of reasons: reluctance to initiate such discussions due to time constraints, lack of comfort with such discussions, lack of skills in such communications, and fear of upsetting the patient even though she or he may wish to have the conversation. A study of patients 50 years of age and older who had at least one chronic, morbid medical condition (ischemic heart disease, chronic heart failure, chronic obstructive pulmonary disease, cerebrovascular disease, cancer, chronic renal disease, or chronic liver disease) found that greater satisfaction with the primary care physician was expressed if advance directives were discussed during outpatient visits.[70]

Nurses may be particularly helpful in advocating for patients' wishes and preferences when they are unable to speak for themselves. The nurse, working with the surrogate, may assist the surrogate to convey the patient's wishes. If the surrogate is not certain about the patient's wishes or if no advance directive is available, the nurse, by posing questions as those recommended by Harlow in "Family Letter Writing,"[71] can be very helpful. Such questions include, "What type of person was the patient?" "Did she/he ever comment on another person's situation when they were incapacitated or on life support?" "Did she/he relate those experiences to her/his own personal views of her/himself?" and "What vignettes can you recall from his/her life that illustrate her/his values?"[71] In addition to helping to clarify a patient's wishes, addressing these questions may also serve as a healing review of the person's life and help identify what has brought them meaning. The nurse is often the best person to engage the family in such reflections and discussions as they have ample opportunity to talk during patient care.[72]

Communications About the Use of Life-Sustaining Therapies

One aspect of advanced care planning is often referred to as defining the code status of the patient. In the ideal collaborative process, nurses and physicians are jointly involved in these discussions. Nurses are heavily invested in clarification, because they often are the ones who find the patient in respiratory or cardiac arrest and must initiate a code. The nurse has a 24-hour presence with the patient, including bathing and being with the patient in the middle of the night and at off-hours; for this reason, the nurse may be the one to whom the patient and family turn for explanations and support. The nurse may be asked to explain what medical jargon such as "DNR/DNI" actually means, particularly in the context of the patient. The patient and family may also seek reassurance from the nurse about the appropriateness of their preferences and decisions or about pressure or responsibility they may feel concerning the way in which information was presented and the decisions they are being asked to make. Patients may very well ask the nurse, "Do you feel I made the right decision?" or "What would you do?" Patients may also need reassurance—for instance, that, by forgoing cardiopulmonary resuscitation (CPR), they are not denying themselves an intervention that could be beneficial. They may need reassurance that the nurses will continue to provide care. By educating the patient about the actual intervention and likely outcome, a nurse may be able to reassure the patient.[72]

"Code status" is commonly defined as the use, or limitation of use, of life-sustaining therapy in the event of clinical deterioration of respiratory function and/or cardiac arrest. Life-sustaining measures include nasotracheal intubation and mechanically assisted ventilation and cardiac resuscitation, the combination of which is called CPR. Other measures may include pressors to help the heart pump more efficiently and effectively, dialysis for kidney failure, and antibiotics for infections. If a patient in a hospital or nursing home or in the community experiences a cardiac arrest and/or respiratory failure and medical personnel are called to respond, CPR is performed *unless* the patient, or the patient's surrogate, has indicated the patient's desire not to be resuscitated (DNR) and/or not to be intubated and supported with mechanical ventilation (DNI).

When patient's wishes for or against application of these medical interventions or treatments are being discussed and documented in the medical record, the process is often referred to as "getting the code status" or discussing "Do-Not-Resuscitate" orders.[73]

As in all other discussions with patients and their families about preferences for care, communications about code status should follow the same multiple-step process as described for communication on other topics of end-of-life care.[9] In discussing a DNR order, Dr. Charles von Gunten[74] recommended the steps of (1) establishing an appropriate setting, (2) inquiring of patient and family what they understand of the patient's condition, (3) finding out what the patient expects for the future, (4) discussing the DNR order with the patient in the context of the patient's understanding of present condition and thoughts of the future, including the context in which resuscitation would be considered, (5) responding to the patient's emotions, and (6) developing a plan.[74] Again, it is essential to place the conversation in the context of the patient's wishes for goals of therapy.

In developing appropriate goals of care for the patient's condition, the patient or health care proxy must understand the very low likelihood of survival after CPR in the presence of terminal illness.[75] Patients are less likely to opt for CPR knowing that almost no patients with severe, multiple, chronic illnesses who receive CPR in hospital survive to discharge.[68,76]

For nurses to discuss code status, there are several issues. First, just discussing code status in and of itself is worthless. Alone, a code status guides the health care team in deciding whether or not to perform a procedure. Use of medical vernacular, such as "full code" or "no code" and "Do you want everything done?" is ambiguous at best, and offers little guidance. Use of language that the patient understands and review of the broad topic of life-sustaining treatments can guide the health care team to a better understanding of the patient's values and preferences about quality of life. Von Gunten[77] identified the key elements and offered particular language for such discussions. Table 4–5 lists questions that may be helpful in facilitating communications about advance directives.

The goal of these discussions is to review the anticipated benefits and burdens of interventions without placing any responsibility on the patient and family. Often the patient and family look for recommendations and validation of choices from the nurse. This may include queries from the patient and family such as, "What do you think?" or "What should I do?" The nurse can offer the facts and reflect back the patient's values and preferences such as, "Mr. X, you told me you want to be comfortable and not return to the hospital. We can get support at home to keep you comfortable and aggressively treat any symptoms." Important elements of this discussion include sensitivity to, acknowledgment of, and response to emotions of the patient, family, and surrogate.

Sometimes, the responsibility of making such a decision is too great for patients and families. They may feel that by making a choice to refuse resuscitation, they are "pulling the plug." In these situations, the nurse can offer a plan and then ask for agreement from the patient and family. By saying, "We would like to focus on comfort and maximal pain and symptom management. That would include medications to treat symptoms with nurses to manage these medications. We will not do any procedures that would cause more pain than benefit. And because we anticipate your decline, we will try to keep you home with hospice and not to do anything to prolong your dying. Is that okay?" It may still be the same plan, but the family doesn't have to make the decision. The burden of the decision is removed from the family and placed on the care team, but the patient and family agree to the plan.

To dispel concerns of abandonment, it is particularly important to reassure the patient, family, and surrogate that even though CPR will not be performed, all beneficial care will be actively provided. The final task is to develop and document a plan and share this information with other health care professionals caring for the patient.[77] This may be done through documenting the conversation and completing state-recognized comfort care/DNR order forms.

Table 4–5
Questions for Advance Directive Conversations

Normalizing comments/questions:
I'd like to talk with you about possible health care decisions in the future.
I'd like to discuss something I discuss with all patients admitted to the hospital.
Inquiries of patient's understanding:
What do you understand about your current health situation?
What do you understand from what the doctors have told you?
Inquiries to elicit hopes and expectations:
What do you expect in the future?
Have you ever thought about how you want things to be if you were much more ill?
Inquiries to elicit thoughts regarding cardiopulmonary resuscitation:
If you should die despite all our efforts, do you want us to use "heroic measures" to bring you back?
How do you want things to be when you die?
If you were to die unexpectedly, would you want us to try to bring you back?[77]

Conversations About Artificial Hydration and Nutrition

Decisions about resuscitation are just one of the many decisions that patients and families need to make regarding end-of-life care. Both nurses and physicians discuss specific treatment options and develop a plan of care with the patient, but it is often the nurse who facilitates a peaceful death[78] by talking with the patient about his or her goals, wishes, and preferences; being cognizant of the patient's suffering; and conveying this information to other health care providers.

When patients are not able to take food or fluid by mouth, artificial hydration and nutrition may be provided through the gastrointestinal tract with a nasogastric or gastric tube or intravenously. The rationale for and against these procedures is discussed in the Chapter 12. The discussion points regarding artificial hydration and nutrition with the patient and/or the patient's surrogate include (1) their perception of the benefits and the suffering with or without these interventions; (2) the values, beliefs, and culture of the patient and family along with the goals; (3) the available data regarding the benefits and burdens of the interventions; and (4) collaborative decision-making about these interventions to meet the patient's goals.

Many cultures place great social and cultural importance on drinking and eating. Many people believe that not eating and drinking causes great physical suffering. Therefore, it is necessary to discuss the potential benefits and burdens of instituting artificial hydration and nutrition, as well as the benefits and burdens of withholding artificial hydration and nutrition. Nurses can stress ways of maintaining social contact associated with eating and drinking. A speech and language pathologist or a swallowing therapist can assist in promoting maximal safe and appropriate intake. If the patient is unable to take any food or fluid by mouth, providing human contact on a regular basis, similar to that while feeding, may address this concern. The concern of "suffering" or of "starving the patient to death" may be minimized by education regarding dry mouth or oral discomfort. Families can be taught to provide relief with sips of water, ice chips, and conscientious mouth and lip care.[73]

The risks and burdens of artificial hydration and nutrition include lung congestion and increased respiratory tract secretions, increased edema with its attendant pain at sites of tumors and inflammation, more urine production, more peripheral swelling (particularly in the setting of liver or kidney disease), and skin breakdown. Feeding tubes and intravenous lines may be painful, carry risks of infections, and may be fraught with complications. These may include restraint of the patient to prevent removal, which can cause secondary agitation and may also result in accelerated skin breakdown from less turning in bed. Ultimately, the use or avoidance of such interventions as artificial hydration and/or nutrition depends on the patient's goals of care.[79–82]

Conversations about the Transition to Palliative Care or Hospice

The hospice and palliative care movement has promoted discussions of the benefits and burdens of medical interventions. The patient and family are helped to prepare for death in as comfortable and meaningful a way as possible by focusing on various physical, psychological, and spiritual aspects of care.[73,83,84] The nurse has a central role in palliative and hospice care by implementing the plan of care. The APN may assist the patient in this transition and develop orders for the treatment plan. The nurse, together with the interdisciplinary health care team, empowers family and friends to support and care for the patient. The constant presence of the nurse reassures patients and families that abandonment is not an issue.

The transition from curative to palliative care is often a challenge for clinicians, patients, and families alike. It signals the recognition of loss from various perspectives. Patients may feel a sense of sadness, anger, denial, and loss of control to the disease. Physicians may feel a sense of failure for not curing the disease, a lack of confidence in not knowing what else they can do for the patient, and perhaps worry about their own personal reactions as well as patients' emotions.[48] Nurses may be frustrated if a patient is not well informed to accomplish life closure. Moreover, nurses involved in direct bedside care may dread the possibility of having to provide resuscitation measures in such a circumstance. Nurses may dread situations in which the primary physician, who knows the patient, is not available, and the nurse must deal with a covering physician who may employ inappropriately aggressive and burdensome interventions because he or she has not been involved in the patient's care and does not know the patient and the family.

As in other end-of-life conversations, talking about the transition to palliative care or hospice care should be guided by the patient's overall goals. As previously explained, these goals are stated in terms of the relative value of prolonging life compared with focusing on quality of life and comfort. In addition to advance directives, health care proxy documentation and living wills, resuscitation orders (code status), and use of other life-sustaining therapies, other important facets of end-of-life discussions include use of antibiotic therapy; use of hemodialysis; management of pain and other distressing symptoms; relief of psychological, emotional, spiritual, and existential suffering; completion of unfinished business; and anticipatory grief.[27]

Strategies recommended by Larson and Tobin[85] for initiating end-of-life conversations during the last phase of life include (1) focusing on the patients' unique experiences of illness, (2) helping patients confront their fears, (3) helping patients address practical issues, (4) facilitating the shift to palliative care, and (5) helping the patient achieve a peaceful and dignified death. This means that each situation is individual and cannot be determined by an algorithm or recipe approach. To facilitate such end-of-life discussions, which focus on the realities of advancing illness and changing treatment goals, Larson and Tobin propose specific questions and comments, which are listed in Table 4–6.

After the patient has been referred to palliative care, the nurse may reinforce the reason for end-of-life care and the involvement of new specialized health care providers. The focus on quality of life continues in its multidimensionality determined by the patient. Both patients and physicians display reluctance to discuss psychosocial issues unless the other party initiates the discussion.[36] It behooves nurses, along with social work colleagues, to initiate such conversations, because the evidence suggests that little time is devoted to quality-of-life issues

Table 4–6
Questions to Facilitate the Goals and Focus of Care in the Last Phases of Life

Tell me about the history of your illness.
What do you understand as your treatment options?
What are some of the concerns you have at this time?
What, if anything, are you worried about or afraid of?
Have you had family members or other loved ones die? How was their death? And what was that like for you?
What practical problems is your illness creating for you?
Are there any family members or loved ones who need to know what's going on?
There is a lot I can do for you at this time to control your pain, keep you comfortable, and help you live each day to the fullest extent that you can.[85]
Given the severity of your illness, what is most important for you to achieve?
How do you think about balancing quality of life with length of life in terms of your treatment?
What are your most important hopes?
What are your biggest fears?
What makes life most worth living for you?
Would there be any circumstances under which you would find life not worth living?
What do you consider your quality of life to be like now?
Have you seen or been with someone who had a particularly good death or particularly difficult death?
Have you given any thought to what kinds of treatment you would want(and not want) if you become unable to speak for yourself in the future?
If you were to die sooner rather than later, what would be left undone?
How is your family handling your illness? What are their reactions?
Are there any spiritual issues you are concerned about at this point?
Has religion been an important part of your life?[27]

during outpatient palliative care visits.[86] Table 4–7 lists open-ended questions that may help facilitate quality-of-life discussions with patients.[86,87]

Von Gunten[77,88,89] recommended a step-wise approach of establishing the setting, eliciting the patients' understanding of their condition and their expectations for the future, discussing what hospice care is, responding to emotions, and developing a plan. Conducting a family meeting to respond to patient and family concerns, to discuss the patient's wishes with other family members and health care professionals, to have the hospice team provide information, and to collaboratively develop a plan may serve to help communicate what hospice care is.[77,88,89]

A number of strategies may be used to address feelings of powerlessness, uncertainty, isolation, and helplessness that otherwise could lead to a sense of hopelessness in the patient. These strategies include explaining what to expect regarding the patient's decline and the patient's involvement in decision-making, as well as encouraging relationships and connections with important people.[90] Such discussions lend themselves to strategies for life closure in identifying patient goals and purposes, preparation for death, leaving a legacy for loved ones, and often legal and financial issues. Completing these tasks frees the patient to concentrate on emotional and spiritual matters and to enjoy the company of loved ones.[32]

Table 4–7
Questions to Facility Quality-of-Life Discussions

Which symptoms bother you the most?
How has your disease interfered with your daily activities?
How are you getting along with family and friends?
Have you been feeling worried, sad, or frightened about your illness?
How have your religious or spiritual beliefs been affected by your illness?
Do you question the meaning of all this?

Source: Detmar et al. (2001), reference 86; Brunelli et al. (1998), reference 87.

Communications as the Patient Is Dying

> When curing is no longer viable and this message is communicated to or intuited by the patient, a pregnant moment for healing arises for both physician and patient. The focus and fight for life can give way to a new alliance based on sharing the inevitability of the human contract. . . . The smallest, most humble act of a change to more generic reaching out can have exponential benefit to the patient's subjective sense of well-being.[91]

Nurses' communications with the patient and family, when death becomes inevitable, may facilitate comfort and healing in a number of ways. Using patient wishes to review treatment options, advanced care planning issues, and use of life-sustaining measures, nurses can promote comfort in a patient's final days. Treatment issues include pain management while respecting a patient's preferences for pain alleviation versus desired level of alertness, and addressing eating, drinking, and artificial hydration and nutrition. The nurse should review the actual physiological and biological process of dying in language that also addresses the benefits and burdens of various interventions. This includes discussions with the patient, family, and other health care professionals about withdrawing ineffective and/or burdensome medical treatments that may not yet have been discontinued. Simple presence, listening, and attending to the basic humanity of the dying patient may be one of the nurse's most powerful contributions.

> The simple act of visitation, of presence, of taking the trouble to witness the patient's process can be in itself

> a potent healing affirmation—a sacramental gesture received by the dying person who may be feeling helpless, diminished, and fearful that they have little to offer others. The patient may also fear that he or she has failed. . . . I and many dying persons would agree that beyond pain control, the three elements we most need are feeling cared about, being respected, and enjoying a sense of continuity, be it in relationships or in terms of spiritual awareness.[91]

The communication skills required include being present with the patient in his or her state of vulnerability and decline, and consciously and nonjudgmentally listening and bearing witness to the patient, encouraging the patient to express all feelings while resisting defensiveness if the patient voices anger or disappointment about dying.

> The willingness to extend to the patient with freshness, innocence, and sincere concern far outweighs any technique or expertise in the art of listening. Practice and exposure hone these skills and deepen one's personal awareness, which in itself is the fertile soil for end-of-life completion work for both parties.[91]

Nurses, by communicating physical and behavioral signs of the dying process, may help prepare patients and families and thereby reduce anxiety and ease the bereavement process. Nurses, in response to patients' desires to appreciate the purpose and meaning in their lives as they face death, may use interventions to help relieve spiritual suffering. Being present with the patient and encouraging a life review by recalling and talking about memories and past conflicts may help patients and loved ones to recognize purpose, value, and meaning. Performing a life review also helps patients achieve resolution of past conflicts, forgiveness, reconciliation, a sense of personal integration, and inner peace. Goals may be reframed into short-term activities that can be accomplished. Meditation, guided imagery, music, reading, and art that focuses on healing may be comforting.[24]

Role modeling the art of being present to the dying person for families is important. Engaging in loving, physical contact, such as holding hands, embracing, or lying next to the patient, may help the patient in his or her transition and may help the survivors in their anticipatory grieving. For families who want to be present at the time of death, explaining that patients often wait until they are alone to die may prevent the family from feeling a sense of guilt if they are away from the patient at the time of death. Allowing the family to be with the patient after death may help the surviving family members grieve the loss of their loved one.

Nurses' awareness of anticipatory grief and bereavement and communications with family members and other loved ones may help them through these painful times. Bereaved families are often in most need of having someone to listen to them. One of the nurses' most important roles in working with grieving patients and bereaved families is active, compassionate listening. Encouraging the bereaved to tell stories of their loss, including details of the days and weeks around the death of their loved one; encouraging the sharing of memories of the person; asking about how things are different now; and helping to identify sources of support, of coping, and of accomplishing practical daily activities may be of great assistance.[92]

Family Communication

In 1995, Zerwekh[93] suggested a family hospice caregiving model whereby communication, in particular the nurse's communication, sets the tone for all care. In this model, the role of the nurse is to help guide the care. Speaking the truth enables the nurse to connect with family members and empower them to make choices, but also to be collaborative, to comfort, to guide the dying process, and to provide spiritual support.

Nurses, by the nature of their practice, understand that the focus of care is on patients and their families. Because the essence of nursing is to care for actual and potential health problems of the patient and family, the scope of care is broad. Challenges arise when the patient and the family are in conflict. In these times of nursing shortages, interference from family members at the bedside may overwhelm the nurse in her best efforts to provide care for the patient.

Within the spectrum of the patient's illness, the family has various communication needs. First of all, because of caregiving demands, family members feel a part of the illness.[19] Therefore, they want to be included in any communication pertaining to disease progression, treatment options, and goals of care. Additionally, family members, because of their knowledge of the patient, may serve as the best advocates for their ill family member.[19] This is well illustrated in pediatrics, where parents are considered to be the experts on their children. Family members carry the burden of caregiving—an exhausting task that may include scheduling appointments related to care, arranging transportation for these appointments, attending to the ill person, and providing direct care.[19]

One challenge for the nurse is to decipher the patient's important relationships and determine who should get what information. Another challenge is to help family members with the issues of caregiving. The very logistics of caregiving can be overwhelming with respect to demands of time and energy. Families need assistance in rallying support to care for loved ones and to identify and access community services. Additionally, families need support in dealing with the emotional burden of caring for the loved one alone while at the same time dealing with other aspects of their own lives, demands that may include a full or part-time job and financial stresses. For some families, it may be necessary to continue working in order to maintain insurance coverage. Families may need to hire extra help that is considered custodial and is not covered by insurance. Moreover, lack of education about providing direct care may create a tremendous sense of inadequacy in the caregiver. Families often need education in aspects of physical caregiving, including transfers and personal care.[94]

Moreover, there may be a number of challenges within the family itself related to family functioning, coping strategies, and processes of communication.[95] In an attempt to negotiate the health care system and advocate for a loved one, a family member can intentionally or unintentionally create havoc by rejecting assistance or accepting too much help. In an attempt to seek a cure at all costs, too many health care providers may be consulted for a case. This can be a set-up for failure due to splitting or absence of a lead person to make decisions. Family members, intentionally or unintentionally, may work at cross-purposes or cause health team members to work at cross-purposes. This may serve to undermine care and to prevent addressing important aspects of terminal care. However, there may be clear informational issues that need to be addressed. To successfully ascertain the situation, the nurse needs to know about the communication style of the family. Duhamel and Dupuis[96] offered the following questions:

What is helping you the most?
Where are you getting support?
What information do you need right now?

Other challenges for the nurse are a mismatch of patient and family needs for information and communication and differences in coping styles. A patient may need little communication, whereas certain family members may need constant updates, partially because they are unable to attend appointments with the patient. In other settings, a patient may have a need to communicate but the family member is comfortable being quiet. Being at different places in coping may also create tension between a patient and his or her family. A patient may be coping well and adjusting to the physical changes, whereas a family member may just be beginning to deal with the diagnosis of a life-threatening illness and not be able to even conceptualize a prognosis. On the other hand, a patient may be too overwhelmed by symptoms to deal with psychological aspects of care, whereas a family member may be more objective.

To best work with families, the nurse can use several strategies. First, frequent interaction with family members can help the family feel included and not avoided. Second, understanding of the family's communication styles can help in these interactions. As part of the nursing assessment, a determination of the family's understanding of the patient's condition helps facilitate communication. In collaboration with the patient, the nurse can clarify the family's roles and responsibilities and support their efforts and sacrifices as caregivers. This is critically important when working in partnership with patients and their families.[97] The nurse may also be of great assistance to the family in helping them with anticipatory grieving and bereavement. Eliciting the coping mechanisms of the patient and family is an important part of patient assessment, as the patient transitions in care and later progresses to dying, and also of family assessment during these times and during bereavement. Particular questions may help clinicians and other members of the palliative care and hospice teams address and support patients' and families' coping mechanisms (Table 4–8).

Table 4–8
Questions to Address Patients' and Families' Coping

Have you/your family been through something like this before? How did you/your family react/cope?
Do you have a belief in a higher power that supports you?
Is there anyone you'd like us to call?
Can you anticipate any potential areas of concern for you and your family?
Who could you call if you started to feel really sad?
Did the patient ever tell you what he/she wanted for himself/herself?
Is there anyone you think the patient would like to see?
Who can support you when the patient dies?

Source: Braveman et al. (2003), reference 98.

Communication with family members is as important as communication with the patient. The family may not understand as much as the patient does, or the family may understand more than the patient. The family's questions and comments may focus on their coping and coming to terms with the patient's potential death. Sometimes, a nurse needs to interact with many family members, which can be exhausting and can ultimately require one family member to serve as the spokesperson. This work is very labor intensive, because different family members have varying needs for information and reassurance. Nevertheless, this communication is essential, because the nurse may coach the family as to how to communicate effectively and compassionately with the patient.

CASE STUDY
Mr. T, an Elderly Man with Complications After a Fall

Mr. T is an 85-year-old man who was living without family and was fiercely independent. One day, he fell down the flight of stairs in his house. He crawled back up to bed. Three days later, he tried to move and could not. He called 911 and was brought to the hospital by emergency responders. There he underwent spinal cord surgery and then spinal fusion. During his recovery from surgery, he suffered a stroke. He was treated with heparin and then suffered an intracranial bleed. He is now limited to movement in only his left upper extremity. Mr. T is awake and alert, but is nonverbal and does not follow commands. His sister, Mrs. O, is distraught over his care. A meeting is held with the neurosurgeon and the palliative care nurse.

NURSE: Mrs. O, I am the palliative care nurse. I was asked by Dr. Q and Dr. P to help out with your brother's care. We decided it would be best to meet with you together to figure out a plan of care.

MRS. O: Dr. P , please tell me if my brother will get better.

DR. P: Well your brother suffered major injury to the spine when he fell. He was brought here, and we tried to fix his spinal cord so that he would be able to move. We were somewhat successful in giving him a little movement. However, then he suffered a stroke. The neurologists have treated him and believe that this is the best he will get. As you can see, he is alert and awake.

MRS. O: But he doesn't seem to understand anything and he can't talk to me.

DR. P: Well, he seems to enjoy watching TV and could do well with some rehabilitation. However, he will probably never be able to live alone again.

MRS. O: What do you expect from rehabilitation?

DR. P: He may gain a little strength and some vocalization. But he will never be able to move more than his arm.

MRS. O: So this is the best he will get?

DR. P: Yes, we managed to save him. Although, he won't be able to do much, he can get satisfaction from being with people and watching TV.

MRS. O: But he was very independent and never wanted any help. In addition, he always told me he would never want to go into a nursing home. He thought that was a horrible way to live, and he said it every time we passed a nursing home.

DR. P: But he could still get a little better with some rehabilitation.

MRS. O: For what, to be like that? That is no quality of life. What choices does he have?

DR. P: Well, if you don't want rehabilitation for him, you could have the palliative care service start a morphine drip. (He then leaves)

MRS. O: Is that what you do?

NURSE: No, we focus on the preferences of the patient and the family. Tell me about your brother and what he was like.

MRS. O: Well he lived alone all his live. He loved my sons like his own. He taught them woodworking. They would go up and see him once a week to check up on him and make sure he had enough food. We asked him to live with us, but he would have none of it.

NURSE: What are your thoughts about his care?

MRS. O: He would never want to be like this. If he could look at himself, he would die from embarrassment. He hated TV. Having only the quality of life to watch TV would be awful for him. He was a doer. He never sat for long.

NURSE: So you are thinking this would not be the type of life he would want?

MRS. O: No. It seems like getting him rehabilitation would serve no purpose. But I don't want to kill him. You wouldn't do that, would you?

NURSE: No, we only treat a patient's symptoms. He does not seem to have any physical pain or distress.

MRS. O: Then I just have to wait for him to die? Where will he go?

NURSE: No, there are some considerations about his treatment you can make. First of all, he has been in bed a long time. He is deconditioned and he could get pneumonia. You can decide not to treat that.

MRS. O: I can?

NURSE: Yes. You can also decide that if he has any other events, such as if his heart or his breathing stops, he would not undergo shock to restart his heart or be put on a breathing machine.

MRS. O: I definitely don't want him put on any machines to keep him alive.

NURSE: You can also decide that you don't want to give him artificial nutrition and hydration. Instead, he can eat what he can with the assistance of other people. And we could keep his mouth and lips moist so he doesn't feel thirsty. He could still taste food, but we would let him enjoy eating while knowing he may get pneumonia. Is that something you would consider?

MRS. O: Yes. My brother would have hated all this. I just want to let nature take its course, but not see him suffer.

NURSE: Then we will not do any aggressive life-prolonging treatment. Instead, we will focus on his comfort and quality of life. Only if he seems uncomfortable—is restless, agitated, or in pain—would we use medicines to help him be comfortable. Does that seem like the right plan for him?

MRS. O: Oh yes. Thank you so much. My brother would be so relieved to know all this. I just can't go against his character.

Here the nurse allows the family member to describe her loved one. This facilitates the decision-making by the sister on her brother's behalf.

Often, family communication is best done within a family meeting, a wonderful but greatly underutilized tool. Most clinicians, with the exception of social workers, have not been taught how to effectively run a family meeting. Family meetings help the family understand the involvement of various health care providers, the disease process, and options of care. They also reassure families that a plan is in place and everyone is working toward a consistent goal. The family meeting also provides clinicians an opportunity to collaboratively formulate a plan of care that is consistent with the goals and wishes of the patient and family.

Before calling a family meeting, it is important to clarify the goal for the meeting, to maximize the effective use of time. This can range simply from an update of care to discussing withdrawal of technological interventions. Consideration should be given to the attendance of key and central health care providers, who should meet at least a few minutes before the meeting to clarify the messages to be conveyed. For more complex or contentious families, having a meeting specifically to plan strategies to deal with a difficult family is time well spent.

The actual family meeting is fairly easy and is based on common sense. The patient may or may not attend depending on his or her condition, decision-making capacity, and preference for involvement. One person should take the lead, ensuring that everyone in the room is introduced, and review of the goal of the meeting. Often the family has not met various providers, even if the patient has, and not all health care providers know each other. At that point, depending on what the team has decided ahead of time, another person may ask for the family's understanding of the patient's current condition. This speaker may offer a summary of the care. The next part of the meeting addresses questions and issues that require clarification. It is helpful to have the health care team present to hear the concerns and clarify issues in their areas of expertise. After this discussion, the lead person can summarize the issues and collaboratively develop a plan of care. If the family agrees to the plan, the meeting can end with a synopsis of the meeting and the decisions made. If the family disagrees, another meeting can be suggested. One of the most important tasks after the meeting is documentation. The names and titles of the people who attended, the issues discussed, and the decisions made should be documented in the medical record, as outlined in Table 4–9.

Table 4–9
The Family Meeting

Calling a Family Meeting

1. Clarify goals of meeting
2. Decide the appropriate people to attend—patient, family, and health care providers
3. Providers should meet beforehand to ensure consistency of message and process

The Actual Meeting

4. Arrange appropriate setting
5. Introductions of everyone in room and their relationships to patient
6. Review goal of meeting
7. Elicit patient/family understanding of care to date
8. Review current medical condition
9. Questions
10. Options for care
11. Elicit response from patient if decisional
12. Elicit response from family in terms of what patient would choose if she/he could

Summary

13. Review plan
    If agreement—then decision
    If no agreement—what follow-up is planned
14. Document meeting—who attended, what was discussed, and plan

Source: Adapted from Rabow et al. (2004), reference 94; Quill & Townsend (1991), reference 49; and Buckman (2001), reference 2.

Team Communication

It is commonly agreed that palliative care is best delivered in an interdisciplinary fashion. The underlying reasoning is that well-functioning interdisciplinary teams can share responsibility for care, are able to balance multiple perspectives in care, can support each other in the provision of care, and can provide more comprehensive care, compared with a sole individual clinician.[99] More simply put, a team is more capable of achieving better results than are individuals working in isolation.[100] Good teams promote the establishment of effective communication, cooperation, and competence.[15] The essential elements that make effective and efficient teams include coordination of services, shared responsibility, and, not surprisingly, good communication.[101]

The diversity that gives the interdisciplinary team its effectiveness is dependent on good communication among its members.[102] Witnessing good communication among health care professionals is also reassuring to patients and their families.[103]

Nurses must work closely with physicians at various levels, depending on their role and practice.[104] Nurses find that working in different environments dictate interactions with physicians that may be characterized by deference or by true collaboration. Communication skills with colleagues vary from those used with patients; mutual respect and understanding, rather than hierarchy, lead to the best results. However, nurses and physicians may differ in their communication styles. Whereas physicians often want facts and numbers, nurses often emphasize process, leading to conflict in information styles. It is best if nurses are clear about the purpose of any communication, and it is important for them to have the appropriate supporting evidence. If the contact is about information sharing, the nurse should be brief. If a treatment change is warranted, the nurse should have the supporting evidence. For example, if calling about pain and symptoms, the nurse should know the medications the patient is taking, when they were last taken, and the patient's pain scores, and should offer a suggested plan. Without this information, it can be frustrating for physicians to offer any treatment changes.

A struggle often occurs because much of palliative care is care that nurses have historically provided. Indeed, the central caregiver in hospice is the nurse. In palliative care, the more academic aspect of end-of-life care, physicians now are taking on many aspects of the nursing role. Because of the interdependence of the members of the team, interdisciplinary roles may become blurred. This can result in a favorable collaboration, but it may also result in tension and competition among members of the interprofessional team. Tension may exist due to the fact that much of palliative care is still the 24-hour care provided by the bedside nurse.[105] Therefore, it is important to work out the conflicts and to recognize the role of each team member in the care of the patient.

Understandably, there can be some darker sides of team interactions. According to Kane,[106] stress and tension can arise from ethical conflicts among team members and conflicting goals regarding patient care. Eight problems may occur within a team: (1) overwhelming the patient, (2) making the patient part of the team, (3) squelching of individual team members, (4) lack of accountability, (5) team process trumping client outcome, (6) orthodoxy and groupthink, (7) overemphasis on health and safety goals, and (8) squandering of resources. All of these issues can occur at various times within the palliative care team and necessitate good communication and conflict resolution. Examples of these problems include the following:

1. Overwhelming the patient—This occurs often at a family meeting, where there may be the patient, one family member, and many health care professionals. The patient or family may feel outnumbered and hesitant to talk about the goals of care.
2. Making the client part of the team—Patients are told that they are part of the decision-making team and are asked for input. However, the fact is that patients who are dying may not have the energy to advocate for themselves. Rather, they want other people to advocate for them.
3. Squelching of individual team members—The team may explicitly say that everyone's input is equal when implicitly that is not the case. Nonphysician voices may be dismissed. The nurse must often work hard to be heard.
4. Lack of accountability—This is often a challenge when there is a primary team working with other consultants such as palliative care teams. The team is consulted to do a certain thing. There can be tension if they see other things that should be done but they have not been asked to address these issues.
5. Team process trumping client outcome—Often, in providing end-of-life care, health care providers have certain ideas or feelings about what is right or wrong. The challenge is to allow an open process to occur and not to limit it to one particular pathway simply because that is the way it is always done.
6. Orthodoxy and groupthink—A group can become insular and not incorporate new ideas. The team becomes unable to assess itself, and obvious problems are overlooked. In end-of-life situations, this often happens in relation to the dying process. Nurses may see that the patient is dying, but other health professionals look for a specific symptom and treat it. The fact that the patient is dying is overlooked.
7. Overemphasis on health and safety goals—The care plan takes over, in preference to the patient's needs.
8. Squandering of resources—Needs of patients are missed, and high-cost interventions are implemented.

In summary, interdisciplinary teams have much to offer patients and families. Together, the various disciplines can meet the needs of the whole person.[107] However, teams have their own dynamics, just as a family does, because they are, in effect, social systems. With good leadership, role delineation, and flexibility, interdisciplinary teams work well, creating a synergy that promotes positive outcomes.[107] There are inherent issues that may make teams less helpful if they do not take the time to reflect on their process. To look at its effectiveness, a team needs to assess its process. First, the participation of all members is essential; the degree of involvement may depend on the issues of the patient and family. Second, each team member should have a voice in the process. Third, the mission and goals should be a periodically reviewed so that all members are working on the same premise. Finally, each team member should understand his or her role in patient care and maintain the process of the group. With a periodic review of these issues, the group will work more effectively and efficiently as a team. Reflection helps a team mature, avoiding some of the pitfalls of teamwork.

Conflict Resolution

Conflict is a situation in which the concerns of two or more people or parties appear to clash.[108] This may occur between a patient and a nurse, between a nurse and a doctor, or between two health care teams. Conflict is inevitable and healthy. If managed well, it helps people look at different perspectives and can allow for creativity and positive movement. If dismissed or ignored, it can breed decreased productivity, decreased quality and commitment, and negativity. Nurses on the front line deal with conflict all the time. The challenge is to recognize the conflict and the nature of the conflict. Often, two teams have different ideas, and the nurse is caught in the middle. In this situation, it is best if the nurse expresses the need for the teams to talk to each other. Sometimes, patients and families split staff. Here it is best if the team speaks with consistency and frequency.

There are several methods to resolve conflict between team members, or between a colleague and a patient. The two extremes are conflict avoidance and continued conflict. Between the extremes on this spectrum are negotiation, accommodation, and collaboration. What differentiates these processes is the perceived power differences. Nurses, depending on their level of practice, practice site, and experience, may deal with conflict differently. Even within nursing, there may be tension between generalists and APNs. Historically, an imbalance of power has existed between attending physicians and nurses. However, with social work colleagues, nurses have felt equal, with a balanced or similar power. Often, nurses avoid conflict if they constantly have difficulty dealing with a team member who will not talk about disagreements. However, in palliative care, the goal should be collaboration in which all problems are discussed and mutual solutions are reached. In order to best solve conflict, there are several strategies. Common issues of team conflict include information, common goals, values, role expectations, and differences in underlying values.[101]

Conflict resolution occurs through a process (Table 4–10). First, the nurse identifies the source of the conflict. This includes reviewing the conflict in terms of what happened, what the impact was, and what emotions contributed to the conflict. Second, the nurse reflects on the goal of conflict resolution in terms of what she or he hopes to accomplish. Then the nurse addresses the conflict. In doing so, the two parties share their common purposes and differing interests. This leads to exploration of the conflict and letting each party tell his or her perspective while acknowledging feelings and each party's version of the events. Finally, the two parties problem solve and decide on a tack of resolution.[109,110]

Table 4–10
Approaches to Effective Conflict Negotiation

Reflection of the conflict
1. Identify source of conflict
What happened?
What emotions contributed to conflict?
What impact has the situation had on you?
What did you contribute to the problem?
2. Identify the goal of conflict resolution
What do you hope to accomplish?
What is best way to raise issue?
What's at stake for you?
Negotiation of the conflict
3. Address the conflict
When and how is the best way to raise the issue and achieve the purpose?
4. Identify each individual's purpose in conflict resolution
Where do the individuals share purposes?
Where do the individuals' interests differ?
5. Explore the conflict
Listen to other individual and explore the story
Acknowledge feelings behind story and paraphrase them
Ask other individual to listen to you as you share your version of events and your intentions
6. Problem solving
Invent options to meet each side's most important concerns and interests
Decide tack of resolution—avoidance, collaboration, compromise
Use objective criteria or gold standard of palliative care for what should happen
Include approach for future communication

Source: Adapted from Stone et al. (1999), reference 109, and Fisher et al. (1991), reference 110.

Achieving Expertise in Communication

Achieving expertise in communication requires a long-term commitment. First, a nurse must assess her own strengths and weaknesses in communication, and specifically in the area of death and dying. Completing a death awareness questionnaire helps identify areas of comfort and discomfort regarding discussions of death and dying. Often, it is helpful for the nurse to ask colleagues to observe how he or she talks with patients and to give honest feedback. It may also be helpful to spend some time with hospice and palliative nurses who can discuss more about the communication process. Reflection of a nurse's own areas of strength and style of communication is helpful, because language and words are individual to one's experience and practice. It is also helpful to have a place to develop and acquire skills. This may occur in a formal preceptorship, formal education, or mentoring with expert nurse colleagues. Sometimes, this can be done by writing a narrative about a difficult case, doing a case review, or participating in peer supervision of all cases of patients with life-threatening illnesses.

Conclusion

Communication is the cornerstone of end-of-life care. Good communication sets the trust and the tone for all aspects of care. Effective communication allows patients to paint a picture of themselves and their priorities, values, and needs in the last stages of life. Communication facilitates the expression of feelings by the patient and family members, including their sense of issues and problems surrounding a life-threatening disease and their concerns about care.

Properly developed and used, communication holds all the essentials of end-of-life care together. If it is improperly used, the care and care plan of the patient can fall apart. Nurses, by the virtue of their close proximity to patients, have the potential to participate in myriad communications with their patients. It is incumbent on nurses to acquire the skills necessary to make their communications effective.

REFERENCES

1. Steinhauser KE, Christakis NA, Clipp EC, et al. Factors considered important at the end of life by patients, family, physicians, and other care providers. JAMA 2000;284:2476–2482.
2. Buckman R. Communication skills in palliative care. Neurol Clin 2001;19:989–1004.
3. American Nurses Association. Position Statement on Nursing Care and Do-Not-Resuscitate (DNR) Decisions. Revised 2003.

Washington, DC. Available at: http://nursingworld.org/readroon/position/ethics.
4. SUPPORT Principal Investigators. A controlled trial to improve care for seriously ill patients. JAMA 1995;274:1591–1598.
5. Marvel MK, Epstein RM, Flowers K, Beckman HB. Soliciting the patient's agenda: Have we improved? JAMA 1999;281:283–287.
6. Fallowfield L. Communication and palliative medicine: Communication with the patient and family in palliative medicine. In: Doyle D, Hanks G, Cherny N, and Calman K, eds. The Oxford Textbook of Palliative Medicine, 3rd ed. Oxford, England: Oxford University Press, 2004:101–115.
7. Field D, Copp G. Communication and awareness about dying in the 1990s. Palliat Med 1999;13:459–468.
8. Bailey E, Wilkerson S. Patients' views on nurses' communication skills: A pilot study. Int J Palliat Nurs 1998;4:300–305.
9. von Gunten CF, Ferris FD, Emanuel LL. Ensuring competency in end-of-life care: Communication and relational skills. JAMA 2000;284:3051–3057.
10. City of Hope National Medical Center and the American Association of Nursing. End-of-Life Nursing Education Consortium (ELNEC) Graduate Curriculum. (Suppported by a grant from the National Cancer Institute.) Duarte, CA: Authors, 2003.
11. White K, Coyne P, Patel DW. Are nurses adequately prepared for end-of-life care? J Nurs Scholarship 2001;33:147–151.
12. Ferrell B, Virani R, Grant M. Review of communication and family caregivers content in nursing texts. J Hospice Palliat Nurs 1999;1:97–100.
13. Kruijver IP, Kerkstra A, Bensing JM, van de Wiel HB. Nurse-patient communication in cancer care: A review of the literature. Cancer Nurs 2000;23:20–31.
14. Andershed B, Ternestedt BM. Being a close relative of a dying person: Development of concepts "involvement in the light and the dark." Cancer Nursing 2000;23:151–159.
15. Cist A, Truog R, Brackett S, Hurford W. Practical guidelines on the withdrawal of life-sustaining therapies. Int Anesth Clin 2001;39(3):87–102.
16. Pasareta JV, Minarik PA, Nield-Anderson L. Anxiety and depression. In: Ferrell B, Coyle N, eds. Textbook of Palliative Nursing. New York: Oxford University Press, 2001:269–289.
17. Vachon MLS. Caring for the caregiver in oncology and palliative care. Semin Oncol Nurs 1998;14:152–157.
18. Greisinger A, Lorimor R, Aday, Winn R, Baile W. Terminally ill cancer patients: Their most important concerns. Cancer Pract 1997;5:147–154.
19. McSkimming S, Hodges M, Super A, Driever M, Schoessler FS, Lee M. The experience of life-threatening illness: Patients' and their loved ones' perspectives. J Palliat Med 1999;2:173–184.
20. Wilkerson S, Mula C. Communication in care of the dying. In: Ellershaw J, Wilkerson S, eds. Care of the Dying: A Pathway to Excellence. New York: Oxford University Press, 2003.
21. Kristjanson L. Establishing goals of care: Communication traps and treatment lane changes. In: Ferrell BR, Coyle N, eds. Textbook of Palliative Nursing. New York: Oxford University Press, 2001:331–338.
22. Fischberg D. Talking to Families. In session: Do Everything! Responding to Request for Non Beneficial Treatment. Annual Assembly. AAHPM and HPNA. January 22, Phoenix, AZ, 2004.
23. Pierce SF. Improving end-of-life care: Gathering questions from family members. Nurs Forum 1999;34:5–14.
24. Rousseau P. Spirituality and the dying patient. J Clin Oncol 2003;21(Supplement):54s–56s.
25. Fogarty LA, Curbow BA, Wingard JR, McDonnell K, Somerfield MR. Can 40 seconds of compassion reduce patient anxiety? J Clin Oncol 1999;17:371–379.
26. City of Hope National Medical Center and the American Association of Nursing. End-of-Life Nursing Education Consortium (ELNEC) Oncology Curriculum. (Supported by a grant from the National Cancer Institute.) Duarte, CA: Authors, 2004.
27. Quill TE. Initiating end-of-life discussions with seriously ill patients: Addressing the "elephant in the room." JAMA 2000;284: 2502–2507.
28. Lapine A, Wang-Cheng R, Goldstein M, Nooney A, Lamb G, Derse A. When cultures clash: Physicians, patient, and family wishes in truth disclosure for dying patients. J Palliat Med 2001;4:475–480.
29. Kagawa-Singer M, Blackhall LJ. Negotiating cross-cultural issues at end of life. JAMA 2001;286:2993–3001.
30. Buchwald D, Panagiota C, Gany F, Hardt E, Johnson T, Muecke M, Putsch R. Caring for patient in a multicultural society. Patient Care 1994;June 15:105–120.
31. Heaven C, Magure P. Communication issues. In: Lloyd-Williams M, Ed. Psychosocial Issues in Palliative Care. Oxford: Oxford University Press, 2003:13–34.
32. Schapira L, Eisenberg PD, MacDonald N, Mumber MP, Loprinzi C. A revisitation of "Doc, how much time do I have?" J Clin Oncol 2003;21(Supplement):8s–11s.
33. Quill TE, Arnold RM, Platt F. "I wish things were different": Expressing wishes in response to loss, futility, and unrealistic hopes. Ann Intern Med 2001;135:551–555.
34. Block SD, Billings JA. Patient requests to hasten death: Evaluation and management in terminal care. Arch Intern Med 1994; 154:2039–2047.
35. Neff P, Lyckholm L, Smith T. Truth or consequences: What to do when the patient doesn't want to know. J Clin Oncol 2002;20: 3035–3037.
36. Detmar SB, Aaronson NK, Wever LD, Muller M, Schornagel JH. How are you feeling? Who wants to know? Patients' and oncologists' preferences for discussing health-related quality-of-life issues. J Clin Oncol 2000;18:3295–3301.
37. Wenrich MD, Curtis JR, Shannon SE, et al. Communicating with dying patients within the spectrum of medical care from terminal diagnosis to death. Arch Intern Med 2001;161:868–874.
38. Parker PA, Baile WF, de Moor C, et. al. Breaking bad news about cancer: Patient preferences for communication. J Clin Oncol 2001;19:2049–2056.
39. Lo B, Quill T, Tulsky J, for the ACP-ASIM End-of-Life Care Consensus Panel. Discussing palliative care with patients. Ann Intern Med 1999;130:744–749.
40. Back AL, Arnold RM, Quill TE. Hope for the best, and prepare for the worst. Ann Intern Med 2003;138:439–443.
41. Maguire P. Breaking bad news. Eur J Surg Oncol 1998;24:188–191.
42. Buckman R. How to Break Bad News: A Guide for Health Care Professionals. Baltimore, Md.: The Johns Hopkins University Press, 1992.
43. Baile WF, Buckman R, Lenzi R, et al. SPIKES: A six-step protocol for delivering bad news—Application to the patient with cancer. Oncologist 2000;5:302–311.
44. Baile WF, Lenzi R, Parker PA, Buckman R, Cohen L. Oncologists' attitudes toward and practices in giving bad news: An exploratory study. J Clin Oncol 2002;20:2189–2196.
45. Coyle N, Sculco L. Communication and patient/physician relationship: Phenomenological inquiry. J Support Oncol 2003; 1:206–215.

46. Yun YH, Lee CG, Kim S-Y, Heo DS, Kim JS, Lee KS, Hong YS, Lee JS, You CH. The attitudes of cancer patients and their families toward disclosure of terminal illness. J Clin Oncol 2004;22:307–314.
47. Buchanan J, Borland R, Cosolo W, Millership R, Haines I, Zimet A, Zalcberg J. Patient's beliefs about cancer management. Supportive Care Cancer 1996;4:110–117.
48. Fischer GS, Tulsky JA, Arnold RM. Communicating a poor prognosis. In: Portenoy RK, Bruera E, eds. Topics in Palliative Care 2000;Vol. 4. New York: Oxford University Press.
49. Quill TE, Townsend P. Bad news: Delivery, dialogue, and dilemmas. Arch Intern Med 1991;151:463–468.
50. Friedrichsen MJ, Strong PM, Carlsson ME. Breaking news in the transition from curative to palliative cancer care: Patients' view of doctors giving the information. Supportive Care Cancer 2000; 8:472–478.
51. Girgis A, Sanson-Fisher RW. Breaking bad news: Consensus guidelines for medical practitioners. J Clin Oncol 1995;13: 2449–2456.
52. Tulsky JA, Arnold RM. Communications at the end of life. In: Berger AM, Portenoy RK, Weissman DE, eds. Principles and Practice of Palliative Care and Supportive Oncology, 2nd ed. Philadelphia: Lippincott Williams & Wilkins, 2002:675–677.
53. Ptacek JT, Ptacek JJ. Patients' perceptions of receiving bad news about cancer. J Clin Oncol 2001;19:4160–4164.
54. Herth K. Fostering hope in terminally ill people. J Adv Nurs 1990;15:1250–1259.
55. The A-M, Hak T, Koeter G, van der Wal G. Collusion in doctor-patient communication about imminent death: An ethnographic study. BMJ 2000;321:1376–1381.
56. Faulkner A. ABC of palliative care: Communication with patients, families, and other professionals. BMJ 1998;316:130–132.
57. American Nurses Association. Position Statement on Nursing and the Patient Self-Determination Acts. Revised 1991. Washington, DC. Available at: http://nursingworld.org/readroom/position/ethics (accessed December 15, 2004).
58. Steinhauser KE, Christakis NA, Clipp EC, McNeilly M, Grambow S, Parker J, Tulsky JA. Preparing for the end of life: Preferences of patients, families, physicians, and other care providers. J Pain Sympt Manage 2001;22:727–737.
59. Singer PA, Martin DK, Lavery JV, Thiel EC, Kelner M, Mendelssohn DC. Reconceptualizing advance care planning from the patient's perspective. Arch Intern Med 1998;158:879–884.
60. Hammes B. What does it take to help adults successfully plan for future medical decisions? J Palliat Med 2001;4:453–456.
61. Barnard D. Advanced care planning is not about "getting it right." J Palliat Med 2002;5:475–481.
62. Pearlman RA, Cain KC, Patrick DL et al. Insights pertaining to patient assessments of states worse than death. J Clin Ethics 1993;4:33–41.
63. Kutner JS, Steiner JF, Corbett KK, Jahnigen DW, Barton PL. Information needs in terminal illness. Soc Sci Med 1999;48: 1341–1352.
64. Christakis NA, Lamont EB. Extent and determinants of error in doctors' prognoses in terminally ill patients: Prospective cohort study. BMJ 2000;320:469–472.
65. Lamont EB, Christakis NA. Prognostic disclosure to patients with cancer near the end of life. Ann Intern Med 2001;134:1096–1105.
66. Cassileth BR. Enhancing doctor-patient communications. J Clin Oncol (Suppl) 2001;19(18s):61s–63s.
67. Fischer GS, Arnold RM, Tulsky JA. Talking to the older adult about advanced directives. Clin Geriatr Med 2000;16:239–254.
68. Weeks SC, Cook EF, O'Day SJ et al. Relationship between cancer patients' predictions of prognosis and their treatment preferences JAMA 1998;279:1709–1714.
69. Maguire P. Improving communications with cancer patients. Eur J Cancer 1999;35:1415–1422.
70. Tierney WM, Dexter PR, Gramelspacher GP, Perkins AJ, Zhou X-H, Wolinsky FD. The effect of discussions about advance directives on patients' satisfaction with primary care. J Gen Intern Med 2001;16:32–40.
71. Family letter writing: An interview with Nathan Harlow. Innovations in end of life care: An international on-line forum for leaders in end of life care (1999). [on-line] Available: http://www2.edc.org/lastacts/featureinn.asp.
72. Matzo ML, Sherman DW, eds. Palliative Care Nursing: Quality Care to the End of Life. New York: Springer Publishing Company, 2001.
73. Dunn H. Hard Choices for Loving People: CPR, Artificial Feeding, Comfort Care, and the Patient with a Life-Threatening Illness, 4th ed. Herndon, Va.: A&A Publishers, 2001.
74. von Gunten CF. Discussing hospice care. J Clin Oncol (Suppl) 2003;21(9):31s–36s.
75. Saklayen M, Liss H, Markert R. In-hospital cardiopulmonary resuscitation: Survival in 1 hospital and literature review. Medicine (Baltimore) 1995;74:163–175.
76. Waisel DB, Truog RD. The cardiopulmonary resuscitation-not-indicated order: Futility revisited. Ann Intern Med 1995;122: 304–308.
77. von Gunten CF. Discussing do-not-resuscitate status. J Clin Oncol 2003;21(9)(Supplement), 21(9):20s–25s (May 1).
78. Stein C. Ending a life. Boston: Boston Globe Magazine, 1999; March 14;13,24,30–34,39–42.
79. Zerwekh J. Do dying patients really need IV fluids? Am J Nurs 1997;97:26–30.
80. Sullivan RJ. Accepting death without artificial nutrition or hydration. J Gen Intern Med 1993;8:220–223.
81. Gillick M. Rethinking the role of tube feeding in patients with advanced dementia. N Engl J Med 2000;342:206–210.
82. Finucane T, Christmas C, Travis K. Tube feedings in patients with advanced dementia: A review of the evidence. JAMA 1999; 282:1365–1370.
83. Weissman DE. Consultation in palliative medicine. Arch Int Med 1997;157:733–737.
84. Task Force on Palliative Care, Last Acts Campaign, and Robert Wood Johnson Foundation. Precepts of palliative care. J Palliat Med 1998;1:109–112.
85. Larson DG, Tobin DR. End-of-life conversations: Evolving practice and theory. JAMA 2000;284:1573–1578.
86. Detmar SB, Muller MJ, Wever LD et al. The patient-physician relationship. Patient-physician communication during outpatient palliative treatment visits: An observational study. JAMA 2001; 285:1351–1357.
87. Brunelli C, Constantini M, DiGiulio P et al. Quality of life evaluation: When do terminal cancer patients and health-care providers agree? J Pain Symptom Manage 1998;15:151–158.
88. von Gunten CF. Discussing hospice care. J Clin Oncol 2002;20: 1419–1424.
89. Emanual LL, von Gunten CF, Ferris FD, eds. The EPEC Curriculum. 1999. The EPEC Project www.epec.net.
90. van Servellen G. Communicating with patients with chronic and/or life-threatening illness. In: Communication for the

Health Care Professional: Concepts and Techniques. Gaithersburg, MD: Aspen, 1997, Chapter 13.
91. Fahnestock DT. Partnership for good dying. JAMA 1999;282: 615–616.
92. Cassett D, Kutner JS, Abrahm J, for the End-of-Life Care Consensus Panel. Life after death: A practical approach to grief and bereavement. Ann Intern Med 2001;134:208–215.
93. Zerwekh J. A family caregiving model for hospice nursing. The Hospice Journal 1995;10:27–44.
94. Rabow M, Hauser J, Adams J. Supporting family caregivers at the end of life. JAMA 2004;291:483–489.
95. Hudson P, Sanchia A, Kristjianson L. Meeting the supportive needs of family caregivers in palliative care: Challenges for health professionals. J Palliat Med 2004;7:19–25.
96. Duhamel F, Dupuis F. Families on palliative care: Exploring family and healthcare professional's beliefs. Int J Palliat Nurs 2003; 9:113–119.
97. Levine C, Zuckerman C. The trouble with families: Toward an ethic of accommodation. Ann Intern Med 1999;130: 148–152.
98. Braveman C, Cunningham R, Masi V, Kennedy P, Pace C, Turner M. Best Practice Protocols: Short Length of Stay, Admitting, Assessment Practice. A Report of the Standards/Best Practices Committee, Hospice and Palliative Care Federation of Massachusetts, 2003.
99. Billings J, Dahlin C, Dungan S, Greenberg D, Krakauer E, Lawless N, Montgomery P, Reid C. Psychosocial training in a palliative care fellowship. J Palliat Med 2003;6:355–263.
100. Long DM, Wilson NL, eds. American Congress on Rehabilitation Medicine. Houston Geriatric Interdisciplinary Team Training Curriculum. Houston, TX: Baylor College of Medicine, Huffington Center on Aging, 2001.
101. Hyer K, Flaherty S, Fairchild S, Bottrell M, Mezey M, Fulmer T. Geriatric Interdisciplinary Team Training Program (GITT) Curriculum Guide. New York: New York University, 2001.
102. Mystakidou K. Interdisciplinary working: A Greek perspective. Palliat Med 2001;15:67–68.
103. Hill A. Multiprofessional teamwork in hospital palliative care teams. Int J Palliat Nurs 1998;4:214–221.
104. Lockhart-Wood K. nurse-doctor collaboration in cancer pain management. Int J Palliat Nurs 2001;7:6–16.
105. Coyle N. Interdisciplinary collaboration in hospital palliative care: Chimera or goal? Palliat Med 1997;11:265–266.
106. Kane R. Avoiding the dark side of geriatric teamwork. In: Mezey MD, Cassel CK, Bottrell MM, Hyer K, Howe JL, Fuher TT, eds. Ethical Patient Care: A Casebook for Geriatric Health Care Teams. Baltimore: John Hopkins Press, 2002:187–207.
107. Crawford G, Price S. Team working: Palliative care as a model of interdisciplinary practice. Med J Aust 2003;6(179) Supplement S32–S34.
108. Thomas K. Introduction to Conflict Management. Palo Alto, CA: CPP, 2002.
109. Stone D, Patton B, Heen S. Difficult Conversations: How to Discuss What Matters Most. New York: Penguin Books, 1999.
110. Fisher R, Ury W, Patton B. Getting to Yes: Negotiating Agreement Without Giving In, 2nd ed. New York: Penguin, 1991.

II

Symptom Assessment and Management

5

Regina Fink and Rose Gates

Pain Assessment

Pain—has an Element of Blank—
It cannot recollect
When it began—or if there were
A time when it was not—

It has no Future—but itself—
Its Infinite realms contain
Its Past—enlightened to perceive
New Periods—of Pain.

—*Emily Dickinson, 1955*[1]

- ***Key Points***
- *Pain is multifactorial and affects the whole person.*
- *Pain prevalence at the end of life is high and can be acute, chronic, or both.*
- *Patients or residents should be asked whether they have pain (screened for pain) on admission to a hospital, clinic, nursing home, hospice, or home care agency.*
- *If pain or discomfort is reported, a comprehensive pain assessment should be performed at regular intervals, whenever there is a change in the pain, after analgesic administration, and after any modifications in the pain management plan.*
- *The patient's self-report of pain is the gold standard, even for those patients who are nonverbal or cognitively impaired.*
- *Standard pain scales should be used in combination with clinical observation and information from health care professionals and family caregivers.*
- *Multiple barriers to pain assessment exist.*

Pain is a common companion of birth, growth, death, and illness; it is intertwined intimately with the very nature of human existence. Most pain can be palliated, and patients can be relatively pain free. To successfully relieve pain and suffering, accurate and continuous pain assessment is mandatory. However, evidence demonstrates that pain is undertreated in the palliative care setting, contributing significantly to patient discomfort and suffering at the end of life. Studies suggest that as many as 30% of newly diagnosed cancer patients, 40% of those undergoing treatment, and 75% of those in the terminal phase of disease have unrelieved pain.[2–9] One study reported that more than 50% of cancer patients have increased suffering requiring sedation in the last days of life.[9] Coyle and colleagues[10] reported that 100% of their patients had pain and 37% had increased opioid requirements of 25% or more during the last month of life. In the Palliative Care Consultation Service at the Medical College of Wisconsin, pain and end-of-life decisions were the most frequent reasons for consultation.[11] Although nursing homes are increasingly becoming the most common site of death for the elderly,[12,13] pain relief in long-term care facilities varies widely, with 45% to 80% of residents having substantial pain with suboptimal pain management.[14–20]

This chapter considers various types of pain, describes barriers to optimal pain assessment, and reviews current clinical practice guidelines for the assessment of pain in the palliative care setting. A multifactorial model for pain assessment is proposed, and a variety of instruments and methods that can be used to assess pain in patients at the end of life are discussed.

Types of Pain

According to the International Association for the Study of Pain (IASP), *pain* is defined as "an unpleasant sensory or emotional experience associated with tissue damage. The inability to communicate verbally does not negate the possibility that an individual is experiencing pain and is in need of appropriate pain-relieving treatment."[21] Pain has also been clinically defined as "whatever the experiencing person says it is, existing whenever the experiencing person says it does."[22]

Pain is commonly described in terms of categorization along a continuum of duration. Acute pain is usually associated with tissue damage, inflammation, a disease process that is relatively brief, or a surgical procedure. Regardless of its intensity, acute pain is of relatively brief duration: hours, days, weeks, or a few months.[23] Acute pain serves as a warning that something is wrong and is generally viewed as a time-limited experience. In contrast, chronic or persistent pain worsens and intensifies with the passage of time, lasts for an extended period (months, years, or a lifetime), and adversely affects the patient's function or well-being.[24] Chronic pain has been further subclassified into chronic malignant and chronic nonmalignant pain. Chronic pain may accompany a disease process such as cancer, human immunodeficiency virus (HIV) infection and acquired immune deficiency syndrome (AIDS), arthritis or degenerative joint disease, osteoporosis, chronic obstructive pulmonary disease, neurological disorders (e.g., multiple sclerosis, cerebrovascular disease), fibromyalgia, sickle cell disease, cystic fibrosis, and diabetes. It may also be associated with an injury that has not resolved within an expected period of time, such as low back pain, trauma, spinal cord injury, reflex sympathetic dystrophy, or phantom limb pain.

Additionally, the American Geriatric Society (AGS) Panel on Persistent Pain in Older Persons[18] has classified persistent pain in pathophysiological terms that assist the health care professional to determine the cause of pain and select the appropriate pain management interventions. The four pain subcategories that have been delineated are nociceptive pain (visceral or somatic pain resulting from stimulation of pain receptors), neuropathic pain (pain caused by peripheral or central nervous system stimulation), mixed or unspecified pain (having mixed or unknown pain mechanisms), and pain due to psychological disorders.

Barriers to Optimal Pain Assessment

Inadequate pain control is not the result of a lack of scientific information. Over the last two decades, a plethora of research has generated knowledge about pain and its management. Reports that document the inability or unwillingness of health care professionals to use knowledge from research and advances in technology continue to appear in the nursing and medical literature. The armamentarium of knowledge is available to assist professionals in the successful assessment and management of pain; the problems lie in its misuse or lack of use. Undertreatment of pain often results from clinicians' failure or inability to evaluate or appreciate the severity of the patient's problem. Although accurate and timely pain assessment is the cornerstone of optimal pain management, studies of nurses and other health care professionals continue to demonstrate the contribution of suboptimal assessment and documentation to the problem of inadequate pain management.[2,24–27]

Multiple barriers to the achievement of optimal pain assessment and management have been identified (Table 5–1).[25,29–35] The knowledge and attitudes of health care professionals toward pain assessment are extremely important, because these factors influence the priority placed on pain treatment.[36]

Recognition of the widespread inadequacy of pain assessment and management has prompted corrective efforts within many health care disciplines, including nursing, medicine, pharmacy, and pain management organizations. Representatives

Table 5–1
Barriers to Optimal Pain Assessment

Health care professional barriers
Lack of identification of pain assessment and relief as a priority in patient care
Inadequate knowledge about how to perform a pain assessment
Perceived lack of time to conduct a pain assessment
Failure to use validated pain measurement tools
Inability of clinician to empathize or establish rapport with patient
Prejudice and bias in dealing with patients
Health care system barriers
A system that fails to hold health care professionals accountable for pain assessment
Lack of criteria or availability of instruments for pain assessment in health care settings
Lack of institutional policies for performance and documentation of pain assessment
Patient/family/societal barriers
The highly subjective and personal nature of the pain experience
Lack of patient and family awareness about the importance of pain assessment
Lack of patient communication with health care professionals about pain
Patient reluctance to report pain
Patient not wanting to bother staff
Patient fears of not being believed
Patient age-related stoicism
Patient not reporting pain because "nothing helps"
Patient concern that curative therapy might be curtailed with pain and palliative care
Lack of a common language to describe pain
Presence of unfounded beliefs and myths about pain and its treatment

from various health care professional groups have convened to develop clinical practice guidelines and quality assurance standards for the assessment and management of acute, cancer, and end-of-life pain.[5,6,18,19,37–42] The establishment of a formal monitoring program to evaluate the efficacy of pain assessment and interventions has been encouraged. The Agency for Health Care Policy and Research (AHCPR) Acute and Cancer Pain Practice Guidelines, The American Pain Society (APS) Quality Assurance Standards, The Oncology Nursing Society (ONS) Position Paper on Cancer Pain Management, the APS Position Statement on Treatment of Pain at the End of Life, the AGS Panel on Persistent Pain in Older Persons, the American Medical Directors Association (AMDA) Pain Guidelines, APS Guidelines for the Management of Cancer Pain in Adults and Children, and the National Comprehensive Cancer Network (NCCN) Guidelines are reflective of the national trend to assess quality of care in high-incidence patients by monitoring outcomes as well as assessing and managing pain. The AHCPR recommends the following "ABCDE" mnemonic list as a summary of the clinical approach to pain assessment and management:

A—*A*sk about pain regularly. *A*ssess pain systematically.
B—*B*elieve the patient and family in their reports of pain and what relieves it.
C—*C*hoose pain control options appropriate for the patient, family, and setting.
D—*D*eliver interventions in a timely, logical, and coordinated fashion.
E—*E*mpower patients and their families. *E*nable them to control their course to the greatest extent possible.

Members of the Joint Commission on Accreditation of Healthcare Organizations (JCAHO) routinely inquire about pain assessment and management practices and quality assurance activities designed to monitor patient satisfaction and outcomes within institutions. Revised JCAHO standards[43] for assessing and managing pain in hospital, ambulatory, home care, and long-term care have been released. The JCAHO supports "institutionalizing pain management" and using an interdisciplinary approach to effect change in health care organizations. It also recommends that culturally sensitive pain rating scales appropriate to a patient's age be available and that new or existing assessment forms include pain. Additionally, the APS has created the phrase "Pain: The Fifth Vital Sign" to heighten health care provider awareness of pain assessment and treatment.[44] The continuous quality improvement (CQI) process is continuous, with the achievement of low levels of reported pain severity and of pain-related behaviors as an appropriate objective.[45] Providing health care systems within a CQI perspective of patient-centered care requires that health care professionals seek opportunities to improve pain management by improving assessment processes to produce the desired outcome of decreased pain for patients.

Health care reform processes such as managed care require that patients be discharged sooner, without adequate time to assess pain or to evaluate newly prescribed pain management regimens. Therefore, the prevalence of inadequate pain assessment and management may be even greater than reported, because more persons may be suffering silently in their homes. An adequate pain assessment may not have been done or documented. Health care professionals may not believe patients' reports of pain and may not take time to communicate, care, or understand the meaning of the pain experience for the patient. With the influences and increasing demands of managed care and changes in the delivery of health care, pain assessment and management may not be a priority.

Process of Pain Assessment

Accurate pain assessment is the basis of pain treatment; it is a continuous process that encompasses multidimensional factors. In formulating a pain management plan of care, an assessment is crucial to identify the pain syndrome or the cause of pain. A comprehensive assessment addresses each type of pain and includes the following: a detailed history, including an assessment of the pain intensity and its characteristics (Figure 5–1); a physical examination with pertinent neurological examination, particularly if neuropathic pain is suspected; a psychosocial and cultural assessment; and an appropriate diagnostic workup to determine the cause of pain.[5,40] Attention should be paid to any discrepancies between patients' verbal descriptions of pain and their behavior and appearance. The physical examination should focus on an examination of the painful areas as well as common referred pain locations. In frail or terminally ill patients, physical examination maneuvers and diagnostic tests should be performed only if the findings will potentially change or facilitate the treatment plan. The burden and potential discomfort of any diagnostic test must be weighed against the potential benefit of the information obtained.[46] Ongoing and subsequent evaluations are necessary to determine the effectiveness of pain relief measures and to identify any new pain.

Patients or residents should be asked whether they have pain (screened for pain) on admission to a hospital, clinic, nursing home, hospice, or home care agency. If pain or discomfort is reported, a comprehensive pain assessment should be performed at regular intervals, whenever there is a change in the pain, after analgesic administration, and after any modifications in the pain management plan. The frequency of a pain assessment is determined by the patient's or resident's clinical situation. Pain assessment should be individualized and documented so that all multidisciplinary team members involved will have an understanding of the pain problem. Information about the patient's pain can be obtained from multiple sources: observations, interviews with the patient and significant others, reviews of medical data, and feedback from other health care providers.

Although pain is uniquely personal and subjective, its management necessitates certain objective standards of care and

PAIN ASSESSMENT GUIDE

TELL ME ABOUT YOUR PAIN

Words to describe pain

aching, stabbing, tender, tiring, numb, dull, crampy
throbbing, gnawing, burning, penetrating, miserable, radiating, deep
shooting, sharp, exhausting, nagging, unbearable, squeezing, pressure

Pain in other languages

itami	Japanese	dolor	Spanish
tong	Chinese	douleur	French
dau	Vietnamese	bolno	Russian

Intensity (0-10)
If 0 is no pain and 10 is the worst pain imaginable, what is your pain now? ... in the last 24 hours?

Location
Where is your pain?

Duration
Is the pain always there?
Does the pain come and go? (Breakthrough Pain)
Do you have both types of pain?

Aggravating and Alleviating Factors
What makes the pain better?
What makes the pain worse?

How does pain affect

sleep, appetite, energy, activity, relationships, mood

Are you experiencing any other symptoms?

nausea/vomiting, constipation, itching, sleepiness/confusion, urinary retention, weakness

Things to check

vital signs, past medication history, knowledge of pain, and use of noninvasive techniques

REFERENCES: Jacox A, Carr DB, Payne R, et al. Management of Cancer Pain. Clinical Practice Guideline No. 9. AHCPR Publication No. 94-0592. Rockville, MD. Agency for Health Care Policy and Research, U.S. Department of Health and Human Services, Public Health Service, March 1994. — Wong, D, and Whaley, L: Clinical Handbook of Pediatric Nursing, ed. 2, The C.V. Mosby Company, St. Louis, 1986, p. 373.

0 2 4 6 8 10

0-10 Numeric Pain Intensity Scale

0 No Pain — 1 — 2 Mild Pain — 3 — 4 Moderate Pain — 5 — 6 Severe Pain — 7 — 8 Very Severe — 9 — 10 Worst Possible

Figure 5–1. A pocket pain assessment guide (front and back) for use at the bedside. The health care professional can use this guide to help the patient identify the level and intensity of pain and to determine the best approach to pain management in the context of overall care. *Sources*: © 1996 Regina Fink, University of Colorado Health Science Center, used with permission; and Wong D, Whaley L. Clinical Handbook of Pediatric Nursing, 2nd ed. St. Louis: CV Mosby, 1986, p. 373.

practice. The first opportunity to understand the subjective experience is at the perceptual level. Perception incorporates the patient's self-report and the results of pain assessment accomplished by the health care provider. *Perception* is "the act of perceiving, to become aware directly in one's mind, through any of the senses; especially to see or hear, involving the process of achieving understanding or seeing all the way through"; *assessment* is defined as "the act of assessing, evaluating, appraising, or estimating by sitting beside another."[47] Perception is an abstract process in which the person doing the perceiving is not just a bystander but is immersed in understanding of the other's situation. Perception is influenced by "higher-order" processes that characterize the cognitive and emotional appraisal of pain—what people feel and think about their pain and their future with the pain. Perception also includes the interpersonal framework in which the pain is experienced (with family or friends or alone), the meaning or reason for the pain, the person's coping pattern or locus of control, the presence of additional symptoms, and others' concerns (e.g., family members' depression or anxiety). Alternatively, assessment is a value judgment that occurs by observing the other's experience.

Assessment and perception of the pain experience of a patient at the end of life is essential before planning interventions. However, the quality and usefulness of any assessment is only as good as the ability of the assessor to be thoroughly focused on the patient. This means listening empathetically, maintaining open communication, and validating

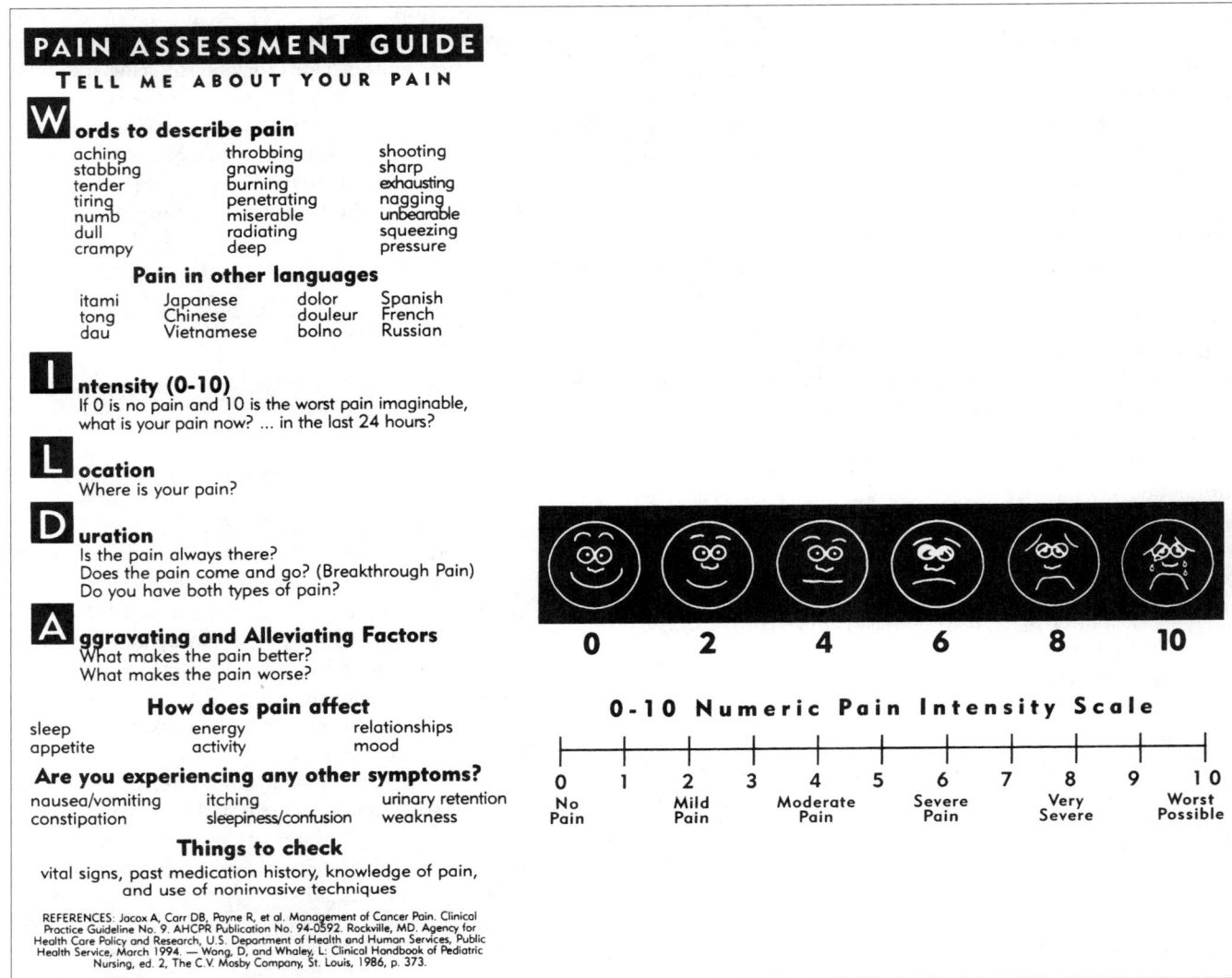

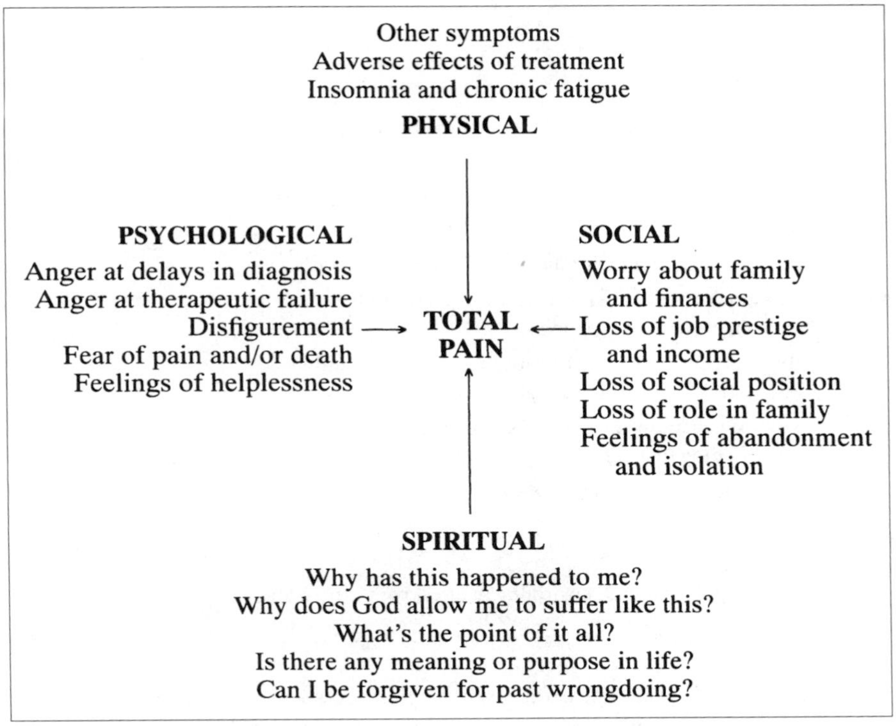

Figure 5–2. Factors influencing the perception of pain. Pain intensity is modulated by psychological, social, and spiritual factors as well as by tissue damage and other physical influences. *Source:* Reproduced with permission from Twycross (1997), reference 48.

and legitimizing the concerns of the patient and family or significant others. A clinician's understanding of the patient's pain and accompanying symptoms confirms that there is genuine personal interest in facilitating a positive pain management outcome.

Pain does not occur in isolation. Other symptoms and concerns experienced by the patient compound the suffering associated with pain. Total pain has been described as the sum of all of the following interactions: physical, emotional/psychological, social, spiritual, bureaucratic, and financial (Figure 5–2).[48] At times, patients describe their whole life as painful. The provision of palliative care to relieve pain and suffering is based on the conceptual model of the whole person experiencing "total pain."

It is not always necessary or relevant to assess all dimensions of pain in all patients or in every setting. At the very least, both the sensation of pain and the response to pain must be considered during an assessment. The extent of the assessment should be dictated by its purpose, the patient's condition or stage of illness, the clinical setting, feasibility, and the relevance of a particular dimension to the patient or health care provider. For example, a comprehensive assessment may be appropriate for a patient in the early stage of palliative care, whereas only a pain intensity score is needed when evaluating a patient's response to an increased dose of analgesic. Incorporation of the multidimensional factors described in the following paragraphs into the pain assessment will ensure a comprehensive approach to understanding the patient's pain experience.

Multifactorial Model for Pain Assessment

Pain is a complex phenomenon involving many interrelated factors. The multifactorial pain assessment model is based on the work of a number of researchers over the last three decades.[49–54] An individual's pain is unique; it is actualized by the multidimensionality of the experience and the interaction among factors both within the individual and in interaction with others.

Melzack and Casey[50] suggested that pain is determined by the interaction of three components: the sensory/discriminative (selection and modulation of pain sensations), the motivational/affective (affective reactions to pain via the brain's reticular formation and limbic system), and the cognitive (past or present experiences of pain). Evidence presented by Ahles and coworkers[51] supported the usefulness of a multidimensional model for cancer-related pain by describing the following theoretical components of the pain experience: physiologic, sensory, affective, cognitive, and behavioral. McGuire[53,55] expanded the work of Ahles and colleagues by proposing the integration of a sociocultural dimension to the pain model. This sociocultural dimension, comprising a broad range of ethnocultural, demographic, spiritual, and social factors, influences an individual's perception of and responses to pain. Bates[52] proposed a biocultural model, combining social learning theory and the gate control theory, as a useful framework for studying and understanding cultural influences on human pain perception, assessment, and response. She believed that different social communities (ethnic groups) have different cultural experiences,

Table 5–2
Multifactorial Pain Assessment

Factors	Question
Physiologic/sensory	What is happening in the patient's body to cause pain?
	How does the patient describe his or her pain?
Affective	How does the patient's emotional state affect the patient's report of pain?
	How does pain influence the patient's affect or mood?
Cognitive	How do the patient's knowledge, attitudes, and beliefs about pain affect the pain experience?
	How does the patient's past experience with pain influence the pain?
Behavioral	How do you know the patient is in pain and what is the patient doing that tells you that pain is being experienced?
	What is the patient doing to decrease his or her pain?
Sociocultural	How does the patient's sociocultural background affect pain expression
Environmental	How does the patient's environment affect pain expression?

attitudes, and meanings for pain that may influence pain perception, assessment, tolerance, and neurophysiological, psychological, and behavioral responses to pain sensation. Hester[54] proposed an environmental component, referring to the setting, environmental conditions, or stimuli that affect pain assessment and management. Excessive noise, lighting, or adverse temperatures may be sources of stress for individuals in pain and may negatively affect the pain experience.

Given the complexity of the interactions among the factors, if a positive impact on the quality of life of patients is the goal of palliative care, then the multifactorial perspective provides the foundation for assessing and ultimately managing pain. Some questions that can guide the nurse's multifactorial pain assessment are reviewed in Table 5–2.

Physiological and Sensory Factors

The physiological and sensory factors of the pain experience explain the cause and characterize the person's pain. Patients should be asked to describe their pain, including its quality, intensity, location, temporal pattern, and aggravating and alleviating factors. The five key factors included in the pain assessment are outlined in Figure 5–1. In the palliative care setting, the patient's cause of pain may have already been determined. However, changes in pain location or character should not always be attributed to these preexisting causes but should instigate a reassessment. Treatable causes, such as infections or fractures, may be the cause of new or persistent pain.

Words. Patients are asked to describe their pain using words or qualifiers. Neuropathic or deafferentation pain may be described as burning, shooting, numb, radiating, or lancinating pain; visceral pain is poorly localized and may be described as squeezing, cramping, or pressure; somatic pain is described as achy, throbbing, and well-localized. Additionally, some patients may not actually complain of pain but may say they feel discomfort. Identifying the qualifiers enhances understanding of the pain's cause and should optimize pain treatment. Not doing so may result in an incomplete pain profile. Table 5–3 summarizes various pain types, qualifiers, etiological factors, and choice of analgesia based on pain type.

Intensity. Although an assessment of intensity captures only one aspect of the pain experience, it is the most frequently used parameter in clinical practice. Asking for the patient's or resident's pain intensity or pain score will objectively measure how much pain a person is experiencing. Pain intensity should be evaluated not only at the present level, but also at its least or best, worst, and with movement. Patients should also be asked how their pain compares with yesterday or with their worst day. A review of the amount of pain after the administration of analgesics, adjuvant drugs, and/or nonpharmacological approaches can also add information about the patient's level of pain. Pain intensity can be measured quantitatively with the use of a visual analog scale, numeric rating scale, verbal descriptor scale, faces scale, or pain thermometer. In using these tools, patients typically are asked to rate their pain on a scale of 0 to 10: no pain = 0; mild pain is indicated by a score of 1 to 3; moderate pain, 4 to 6; and severe pain, 7 to 10.[6] No single scale is appropriate for all patients. During instrument selection, the nurse must consider the practicality, ease, and acceptability of the instrument's use by terminally ill patients (for a description of these instruments, refer to Table 5–5). To ensure consistency, staff should carefully document which scale worked best for the patient, so that all members of the health care team will be aware of the appropriate scale to use.

Table 5–3
Pain Descriptors

Pain Type	Qualifiers	Etiological Factors	Analgesic of Choice
Neuropathic (deafferentation)	Burning, shooting, numb, tingling, radiating, lancinating, "fire-like," electrical sensations, "pins and needles"	Nerve involvement by tumor (cervical, brachial, lumbosacral plexi), postherpetic neuralgia, diabetic neuropathies, poststroke pain	Antidepressants, anticonvulsants, local anesthetics, benzodiazepines ± opioids, ± steroids
Visceral (poorly localized)	Squeezing, cramping, pressure, distention, deep, stretching, bloated feeling	Bowel obstruction, venous occlusion, ischemia, liver metastases, ascites, thrombosis, postabdominal or thoracic surgery, pancreatitis	Opioids (caution must be used in the administration of opioids to patients with bowel obstruction) ± nonsteroidal antiinflammatory drugs (NSAIDs)
Somatic (well localized)	Dull, achy, throbbing, sore	Bone or spine metastases, fractures, arthritis, osteoporosis, injury to deep musculoskeletal, structures or superficial cutaneous tissues	NSAIDs, steroids, muscle relaxants, bisphosphonates ± opioids and/or radiation therapy (bone metastasis)
Psychological	All-encompassing, everywhere	Psychological disorders	Psychiatric treatments, support, non-pharmacological approaches

Location. More than 75% of persons with cancer have pain in two or more sites[56,57]; therefore, it is crucial to ask questions about the location of a patient's pain. Using an assessment sheet with a figure demonstrating anterior and posterior views or encouraging the patient to point or place a finger on the area involved will provide more specific data than verbal self-report does. Separate pain histories should be acquired for each major pain complaint, since their causes may differ and the treatment plan may need to be tailored to the particular type of pain. For example, neuropathic pain may radiate and follow a dermatomal path; pain that is deep in the abdomen may be visceral; and when a patient points to an area that is well-localized and nonradiating, the pain may be somatic indicating bone metastasis. Metastatic bone pain is the most common pain syndrome in cancer patients, with up to 79% of patients experiencing severe pain before palliative therapy. For further information, visit the website, http://www.whocancerpain.wisc.edu.

Duration. Learning whether the pain is persistent, intermittent, or both will guide the nurse in the selection of interventions. Patients may experience "breakthrough" pain—an intermittent, transitory flare of pain.[58] This type of pain requires a fast-acting opioid, whereas persistent pain is usually treated with long-acting, continuous-release opioids. Patients with progressive diseases such as cancer and AIDS may experience chronic pain that has an ill-defined onset and unknown duration.

Aggravating and Alleviating Factors. If the patient is not receiving satisfactory pain relief, inquiring about what makes the pain better or worse—the alleviating and aggravating factors—will assist the nurse and other health care professionals in determining which diagnostic tests need to be ordered or which nonpharmacological approaches can be incorporated into the plan of care. This is also an important aspect of the initial pain assessment, because it helps to determine the cause of the pain. Pain interference with functional status can be measured by determining the pain's effects on activities such as walking, sleeping, eating, energy, activity, relationships, sexuality, and mood. Researchers have found that pain interference with functional status is highly correlated with pain intensity scores; for example, a pain intensity score greater than 4 has been shown to significantly interfere with daily functioning.[2,59]

Affective Factor

The affective factor includes the emotional responses associated with the pain experience and, possibly, such reactions as depression, anger, distress, anxiety, decreased ability to concentrate, mood disturbance, and loss of control. A person's feelings of distress, loss of control, or lack of involvement in the plan of care may affect outcomes of pain intensity and patient satisfaction with pain management.

Cognitive Factor

The cognitive factor of pain refers to the way pain influences the person's thought processes; the way the person views himself or herself in relation to the pain; the knowledge, attitudes, and beliefs the person has about the pain; and the meaning of the pain to the individual. Past experiences with pain may influence one's beliefs about pain. Whether the patient feels that another person believes in his or her pain also contributes to the cognitive dimension. Bostrom and colleagues[60] interviewed 30 palliative care patients with cancer-related pain to examine their perceptions of the management of their pain. Patients expressed a need for open communication with health care professionals about their pain problem and a need for being involved in the planning of their pain treatment. Those who felt a trust in their health care organization, their nurse, and their doctor described an improved ability to participate in their pain management plan.

Patients' knowledge and beliefs about pain play an obvious role in pain assessment, perception, function, and response to treatment. Patients may be reluctant to tell the nurse when they have pain; they may attempt to minimize its severity, may not know they can expect pain relief, and may be concerned about taking pain medications for fear of deleterious effects. A comprehensive approach to pain assessment includes evaluation of the patient's knowledge and beliefs about pain (Table 5–4) and its management and common misconceptions about analgesia.[29,35,61,62]

Behavioral Factor

Pain behaviors may be a means of expressing pain or a coping response.[63,64] The behavioral factor describes actions the person exhibits related to the pain, such as verbal complaints, moaning, groaning, crying, facial expressions, posturing, splinting, lying down, pacing, rocking, or suppression of the expression of pain. Other cues can include anxious behaviors, insomnia, boredom, inability to concentrate, restlessness, and fatigue.[65] Unfortunately, some of these behaviors or cues may relate to causes or symptoms other than pain. For example, insomnia caused by depression may complicate the pain assessment.

Nonverbal expression of pain can complement, contradict, or replace the verbal complaint of pain[66] (see later discussion). Observing a patient's behavior or nonverbal cues, understanding the meaning of the pain experience to the patient, and collaborating with family members and other health care professionals to determine their thoughts about the patient's pain are all part of the process of pain assessment.

The behavioral dimension also encompasses the unconscious or deliberate actions taken by the person to decrease the pain. Pain behaviors include, but are not limited to, using both prescribed and over-the-counter analgesics; seeking medical assistance; using nonpharmacological approaches; and other coping strategies such as removing aggravating factors (e.g., noise and light). Behaviors used to control pain in patients with advanced-stage disease include assuming special positions, immobilizing or guarding a body part, rubbing, and adjusting pressure to a body part.

Sociocultural Factor

The sociocultural factor encompasses all of the demographic variables of the patient experiencing pain. The impacts of these factors (e.g., age, gender, ethnicity, spirituality, marital status, social support) on pain assessment, treatment, and outcomes have been examined in the literature. Although many studies have promoted each individual dimension, few have concentrated on their highly interactive nature. Ultimately, all of these factors can influence pain assessment.

Table 5–4
Common Patient Concerns and Misconceptions About Pain and Analgesia

Pain is inevitable. I just need to bear it.
If the pain is worse, it must mean my disease (cancer) is spreading.
I had better wait to take my pain medication until I really need it or else it won't work later.
My family thinks I am getting too "spacey" on pain medication; I'd better hold back.
If it's morphine, I must be getting close to the end.
If I take pain medicine (such as opioids) regularly, I will get "hooked" or addicted.
If I take my pain medication before I hurt, I will end up taking too much. It's better to "hang in there and tough it out."
I'd rather have a good bowel movement than take pain medication and get constipated.
I don't want to bother the nurse or doctor; they're busy with other patients.
If I take too much pain medication, it will hasten my death.
Good patients avoid talking about pain.

Sources: Ward et al. (1993), reference 33; Jones et al. (2005), reference 35; Fink (1997), reference 61; Gordon and Ward (1995), reference 62.

Age. Much of the pain literature has called attention to the problem of inadequate pain assessment and management in the elderly in a palliative care setting. Elderly patients suffer disproportionately from chronic painful conditions and have multiple diagnoses with complex problems and accompanying pain. Elders have physical, social, and psychological needs distinct from those of younger and middle-aged adults, and they present particular challenges for pain assessment and management. Pain assessment may be more problematic in elderly patients because their reporting of pain may differ from that of younger patients due to their increased stoicism.[35] Elderly people often present with failures in memory, depression, and sensory impairments that may hinder history taking; they may also underreport pain because they expect pain to occur as a part of the aging process.[67,68] Moreover, dependent elderly people may not report pain because they do not want to bother the nurse or doctor and are concerned that they will cause more distress in their family caregivers.[69]

Studies have documented the problem of inadequate pain assessment in the elderly.[70] Cleeland and colleagues[2] studied 1308 outpatients with metastatic cancer and found that those 70 years of age or older were more likely to have inadequate pain assessment and analgesia. Approximately 40% of elderly nursing home patients with cancer experience pain every day, according to Bernabei and colleagues,[71] who reviewed Medicare records of more than 13,625 cancer patients aged 65 years or older who were discharged from hospitals to almost 1500 nursing homes in five states. Pain assessment was based on patient self-report and determined by a multidisciplinary team of nursing home personnel involved with the patients. Of the more than 4000 patients who complained of daily pain, 16% were given a nonopioid drug, 32% were given codeine or another weak opioid, 26% received morphine, and 26% received no analgesic medication at all. As age increased, a greater proportion of patients in pain received no analgesic drugs (21% of patients aged 65 to 74 years, 26% of those aged 75 to 84 years, and 30% of those 85 years of age and older; $P = 0.001$). Therefore, it is imperative to pay particular attention to pain assessment in the elderly patient, so that the chance of inadequate analgesia is decreased. Dementia, cognitive and sensory impairments, and disabilities can make pain assessment and management more difficult. Also, residents in long-term care facilities are likely to have multiple medical problems that can cause pain.

Gender. Gender differences affect sensitivity to pain, pain tolerance, pain distress, willingness to report pain, exaggeration of pain, and nonverbal expression of pain.[72–75] Multiple studies have demonstrated that men show more stoicism than women do, women exhibit lower pain thresholds and less tolerance to noxious stimuli than men, women become more upset when pain prevents them from doing things they enjoy, and women seek care of the pain sooner and respond better to κ-opioid analgesics than do men.[75–79] The mechanism of pain was studied in 181 men and women with advanced cancer.[80] Women experienced more visceral pain, whereas men had more somatic pain (bone metastases). Neuropathic pain was observed in both women and men yet was more severe than the other pain types. Whether women are more willing to report pain than men or experience pain differently from men is unclear. However, beliefs about gender differences may affect nurses' interpretation and treatment of patients' pain. Nurses and other health care professionals need to be mindful of possible gender differences when assessing pain and planning individualized care for persons in pain.

Ethnicity. Despite controversies and uncertainties, the relationship between ethnicity and pain is an important area for study. The term *ethnicity* refers to one or more of the following[81]: (1) a common language or tradition, (2) shared origins or social background, and (3) shared culture and traditions that are distinctive, passed through generations, and create a sense of identity. Ethnicity may be a predictor of pain expression and response. While assessing pain, it is important to remember that certain ethnic groups and cultures have strong beliefs about expressing pain and may hesitate to complain of unrelieved pain.[82] The biocultural model of Bates and associates[83] proposed that culturally accepted patterns of ethnic meanings of pain may influence the neurophysiological processing of nociceptive information that is responsible for pain threshold, pain tolerance, pain behavior, and expression. Thus, the manner in which a person reacts to the pain experience may be strongly related to cultural background. The biocultural model also hypothesizes that social learning from family and group membership can influence psychological and physiological processes, which in turn can affect the perception and modulation of pain. Bates and colleagues[83] stressed that all individuals, regardless of ethnicity, have basically similar neurophysiological systems of pain perception. Early clinical studies of pain expression and culture concluded that the preferred values and traditions of culture affected an individual's handling and communication of pain.[84–86]

Other studies have reported that members of minority groups are at risk for undertreatment of pain.[2,87,88] However, caution must be used when interpreting the results of these studies, because the findings may be due to variations in the pain experience, pain behavior, the language of pain, or staff perception and subsequent pain management.[89] When caring for any patient who is experiencing pain, it is important for the nurse to avoid cultural stereotyping and to provide culturally sensitive assessment and educational materials, enlisting the support of an interpreter when appropriate.

Marital Status and Social Support. The degree of family or social support in a patient's life should be assessed, because these factors may influence the expression, meaning, and perception of pain and the ability to comply with therapeutic recommendations. Few studies have examined the influence of marital status on pain experience and expression. Dar and coworkers[90] studied 40 patients (45% women, 55% men) with metastatic cancer pain and found that patients minimized their pain when their spouses were present. When asked if and how their pain changed in the presence of spouses, 40% of the patients said the pain was better and 60% reported no change; none reported that the pain was worse. The majority (64%) of patients agreed that they conceal their pain so that their spouses will not be upset, even though spouses were generally accurate in their estimates of the patients' pain levels. Almost all patients reported a very high degree of satisfaction with the way their spouses helped them cope with pain.

Spirituality. Spross and Wolff Burke[91] believed that the spiritual dimension mediates the person's holistic response to pain and pain expression and influences how the other aspects of pain are experienced. Whereas pain refers to a physical sensation, suffering refers to the quest for meaning, purpose, and fulfillment. Although pain is often a source of suffering, suffering may occur in the absence of pain. Many patients believe that pain and suffering are meaningful signs of the presence of a higher being and must be endured; others are outraged by the pain and suffering they must endure and demand alleviation. The nurse must verify the patients' beliefs and give them permission to verbalize their personal points of view. Assessing a patient's existential view of pain and suffering is important because it can affect the processes of healing and dying. Understanding patients' use of spiritual comfort strategies is also an area to explore. Dunn and Horgas[92] found that elderly women and older patients of minority background reported using religious coping strategies (prayer or spiritual comfort) to manage their pain more often than did older Caucasian men. Spiritual assessment is covered in greater detail in Chapter 30.

Environmental Factor

The environmental factor refers to the context of care, the setting, or the environment in which the person receives pain management. Creating a peaceful environment free from bright lights, extreme noise, and excessive heat or cold may assist in alleviating the patient's pain.

Additionally, particular nurse or physician specialists may perceive an individual's pain differently. A review of the literature suggests that nurses and other health care professionals are inconsistent in their reliance on patient self-report as a major component in the assessment process. Agreement between patients' perceptions and health care professionals' perceptions was relatively low and was generally an inadequate substitute for patients' reports of pain.[93,94] Ferrell and colleagues[95] found that 91% of nurses surveyed reported asking patients about the intensity of their pain, yet only 45% believed that a patient's report of pain was the most important factor in determining pain intensity. It is not apparent whether this belief resulted from a deficiency of information, lack of time to perform an assessment, or interference of values or bias in the decision-making process. Health care providers' ratings corresponded more with patients' ratings when pain was severe.[94,96] Additionally, when nurses' pain assessment was documented over time, early assessments were more accurate than later ones.[97] Werner and colleagues[98] suggested that patients who are cognitively intact might have better pain assessments.

A multifactorial framework describing the influences of all of these factors on the assessment of pain and the pain experience is desirable to attain positive pain outcomes. The factors comprising the framework are assumed to be interactive and interrelated. Use of this framework for pain assessment has clear implications for clinical practice and research.

Quantitative Assessment of Pain

Although pain is a subjective, self-reported experience of the patient, the ability to quantify the intensity of pain is essential to monitoring a patient's responsiveness to analgesia.

Pain Intensity Assessment Scales

The most commonly used pain intensity scales—the visual analog scale (VAS), the numeric rating scale (NRS), the verbal descriptor scale (VDS), the Wong-Baker FACES pain scale, the Faces Pain Scale (FPS), Faces Pain Scale-Revised (FPS-R), and the pain thermometer—are illustrated in Figure 5–3 and reviewed in Table 5–5 with advantages and disadvantages delineated. These scales have proved to be very effective, reproducible means of measuring pain and other symptoms, and they can be universally implemented and regularly applied in many care settings. How useful these tools are in the assessment of pain in the palliative care patient is a question that still needs to be answered.

Although no one scale is appropriate or suitable for all patients, Dalton and McNaull[123] recommended universal adoption of a 0-to-10 scale, rather than a 0-to-5 or a 0-to-100 scale, for clinical assessment of pain intensity in adult patients. Jensen and colleagues[124] examined the maximum number of levels needed to measure pain intensity in patients with chronic pain and concluded that an 11-point scale (0 to 10) provided sufficient levels of discrimination when compared with a 0-to-100 scale. Standardization may promote collaboration and consistency in evaluation among caregivers in multiple settings (i.e., inpatient, outpatient, and home care or hospice environments). It would facilitate multiple studies of pain across sites. Collection of comparative data would be enabled, allowing for simplification of the analytical process when conducting research. Detailed explanation of how to use the pain scales is necessary before use by patients in any clinical care area.

Another area deserving attention is health care professionals' inconsistent use of word anchors on pain intensity scales. The intention behind the use of a word anchor to discriminate pain intensity is to provide a common endpoint; although that point may have not been reached by a patient, it would provide a place for any pain experienced to date or pain that may be experienced in the future. Some of the common endpoint word anchors that have been used are "worst possible

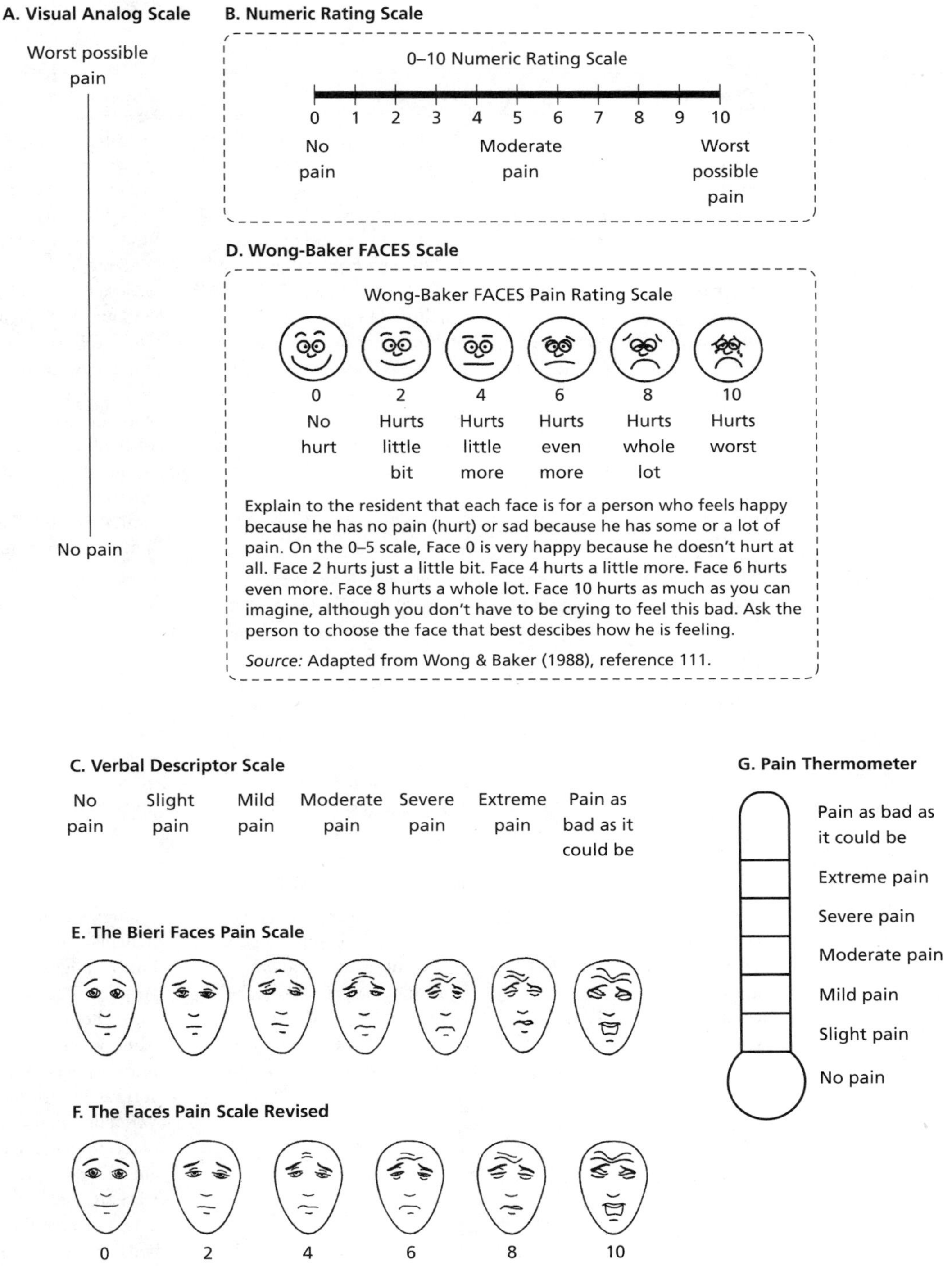
A. Visual Analog Scale
Worst possible pain
No pain
B. Numeric Rating Scale
0–10 Numeric Rating Scale
0 1 2 3 4 5 6 7 8 9 10
No pain
Moderate pain
Worst possible pain
D. Wong-Baker FACES Scale
Wong-Baker FACES Pain Rating Scale
0 2 4 6 8 10
No hurt
Hurts little bit
Hurts little more
Hurts even more
Hurts whole lot
Hurts worst
Explain to the resident that each face is for a person who feels happy because he has no pain (hurt) or sad because he has some or a lot of pain. On the 0–5 scale, Face 0 is very happy because he doesn't hurt at all. Face 2 hurts just a little bit. Face 4 hurts a little more. Face 6 hurts even more. Face 8 hurts a whole lot. Face 10 hurts as much as you can imagine, although you don't have to be crying to feel this bad. Ask the person to choose the face that best descibes how he is feeling.
Source: Adapted from Wong & Baker (1988), reference 111.
C. Verbal Descriptor Scale
No pain
Slight pain
Mild pain
Moderate pain
Severe pain
Extreme pain
Pain as bad as it could be
G. Pain Thermometer
Pain as bad as it could be
Extreme pain
Severe pain
Moderate pain
Mild pain
Slight pain
No pain
E. The Bieri Faces Pain Scale
F. The Faces Pain Scale Revised
0 2 4 6 8 10

Figure 5–3. Commonly used pain intensity scales. Refer to table 5–5 for descriptions, advantages, and disadvantages.

pain," "pain as bad as it can be," "worst pain imaginable," "worst pain you have ever had," "most severe pain imaginable," and "most intense pain imaginable." Inconsistent or different word anchors may yield different pain reports. Therefore, it is important to come to some consensus about consistent use of word anchors.

Comparison of Pain Scales

Several studies have been systematically reviewed,[125,126] and although many are limited in sample size and population, a positive correlation was demonstrated among the VAS, VDS, NRS, Wong-Baker FACES scale, and Bieri FPS. Each of the commonly

Table 5–5
Pain Intensity Assessment Scales

Scale	Description	Advantages	Disadvantages
A. Visual Analog Scale (VAS)	A vertical or horizontal line of 10 cm (or 100 mm) in length anchored at each end by verbal descriptors (e.g., no pain and worst possible pain). Patients are asked to make a slash mark of X on the line at the place that represents the amount of pain experienced.	Positive correlation with other self-reported measures of pain intensity and observed pain behaviors.[99,100] Sensitive to treatment effects and distinct from subjective components of pain.[101,102] Qualities of ratio data with high number of response categories make it more sensitive to changes in pain intensity.[100,103] Parametric statistics can be used to analyze data.	Scoring may be more time-consuming and involve more steps.[99] Patients may have difficulty understanding and using a VAS measure.[104] Too abstract for many adults, and may be difficult to use with geriatric patients/residents, non–English-speaking patients, and patients with physical disability, immobility, or reduced visual acuity, which may limit their ability to place a mark on the line.[104–106]
B. Numeric Rating Scale	The number that the patient gives represents his/her pain intensity from 0 to 10 with the understanding that 0 = no pain and 10 = worst possible pain.	Validity and demonstrated sensitivity to treatments that affect pain intensity.[107] Verbal administration to patients allows those by phone or who are physically and visually disabled to quantify pain intensity.[108] Ease in scoring, high compliance, high number of response categories.[99,108] Scores may be treated as interval data and are correlated with VAS.[109]	Lack of research comparing sensitivity with that of VAS.
C. Verbal Descriptor Scale (VDS)	Adjectives reflecting extremes of pain are ranked in order of severity. Each adjective is given a number which constitutes the patient's pain intensity.	Short, easily administered to patients, easily comprehended, high compliance.[99] Easy to score and analyze data on an ordinal level.[64] Validity is established.[101] Sensitivity to treatments that are known to affect pain intensity.[100]	Less reliable among illiterate patients and persons with limited English vocabulary.[109] Patients must choose one word to describe their pain intensity even if no word accurately describes it.[99] Variability in use of verbal descriptors is associated with affective distress.[104] Scores on VDS are considered ordinal data; however, the distances between its descriptors are not equal but categorical. Thus, parametric statistical procedures may be suspect.[108]
D. FACES Scale (Wong-Baker[111])	The scale consists of six cartoon-type faces. The "no pain" (0) face shows a widely smiling face and the "most pain" (5) face shows a face	Validity is supported by research reporting that persons from many cultures recognize facial expressions and identify them in similar	Presence of tears on the "most pain" face may introduce cultural bias if the scale is used by adults from cultures not sanctioning crying in

(continued)

Table 5–5
Pain Intensity Assessment Scales *(continued)*

Scale	Description	Advantages	Disadvantage
	with tears.[110,111] The scale is treated as a Likert scale and was originally developed by Wong and Baker to measure children's pain intensity or amount of hurt. It has also been used in adults.	ways.[112] Simplicity, ease of use, and correlation with VAS makes it a valuable option in clinical settings.[113,114] Short; requires little mental energy and little explanation for use.[115]	response to pain.[116]
E. Faces Pain Scale (FPS)[117]	Developed by Bieri and colleagues to measure pain intensity in children. Based on drawings made by children, the FPS consists of seven oval faces ranging from a neutral face (no pain) to a grimacing, sad face without tears (worst pain).	Neutral face represents no pain. Incorporates facial expressions associated with pain in adults—furrowed brow, tightened lids/cheek raising, nose wrinkling/lip raising, and eye closure. Oval-shaped faces without tears are more adult-like in appearance, possibly making the scale more acceptable to adults.[117]	Facial expressions may be difficult to discern by patients who have visual difficulties. The FPS may measure other constructs (anger, distress, and impact of pain on functional status) than just pain intensity.[118,119]
F. Faces Pain Scale–Revised (FPS-R)[120]	Adapted from the FPS to make it compatible with a 0–10 metric scale. The FPS-R measures pain intensity by using six drawings of faces.	Easy to administer, uses realistic facial expressions.[121] Has been used in children as young as 4 years of age. The FPS-R uses faces without tears or smiles to avoid affect (depression or mood) instead of pain intensity.	Facial expressions may be difficult to discern by patients who have visual difficulties.
G. Pain Thermometer[122]	Modified vertical verbal descriptor scale that is administered by asking the patient to point to the words that best describe his/her pain.		

used rating scales appear to be adequately valid and reliable as a measure of pain intensity in both cancer patients and elders.

The VAS has been evaluated comprehensively by many researchers over the years and has usually been found to be valid and reliable.[127,128] However, some patients find it difficult to convert a subjective sensation into a straight line.[129] Herr and Mobily[106] studied 49 senior citizens 65 years of age with reported leg pain to determine the relationships among various pain intensity measures, to examine the ability of patients to use the tools correctly, and to determine elderly people's preferences. The VAS consisted of 10-cm horizontal and vertical lines; the VDS had six numerically ranked choices of word descriptors, including "no pain," "mild pain," "discomforting," "distressing," "horrible," and "excruciating"; the NRS had numbers from 1 to 20; and the pain thermometer had seven choices, ranging from "no pain" to "pain as bad as it could be." The scale preferred by most respondents was the VDS. Of the two VAS scales, the vertical scale was chosen most often because the elderly subjects had a tendency to conceptualize the vertical presentation more accurately. Elderly patients may have deficits in abstract ability that make the VAS difficult to use.[130] Other researchers have noted that increased age is associated with an increased incidence of incorrect response to the VAS.[126,129]

Paice and Cohen[108] used a convenience sample of 50 hospitalized adult cancer patients with pain to study their preference in using the VAS, the VDS, and the NRS. Fifty percent of the patients preferred using the NRS. Fewer patients preferred the VDS (38%), and the VAS was chosen infrequently (12%). Twenty percent of the patients were unable to complete the VAS or had difficulty in doing so. Problems included needing assistance with holding a pencil, making slash marks that were too wide or not on the line, marking the wrong end of the line, and asking to have instructions read repeatedly during the survey.

Additional problems exist with use of the VAS. When multiple horizontal scales are used to measure different aspects or dimensions (e.g., pain intensity, distress, depression), subjects tend to mark all of the scales down the middle. Pain intensity has been noted to be consistently higher on each scale for depressed and anxious patients compared with nondepressed, nonanxious patients.[130] Photocopying of VAS forms may result in distortion so that the scales may not be exactly 10 cm long and the reliability of measurement may be in question. Physical disability or decreased visual acuity may limit the ability of the palliative care patient to mark the appropriate spot on the line. The VAS also requires pencil and paper and requires the patient to be knowledgeable about various English pain adjectives. In conclusion, a VAS is more difficult to use with elderly patients and has a higher failure rate, compared with an NRS or a VDS, in addition, the failure rate is slightly greater with an NRS compared with a VDS.

The use of a faces pain scale to measure pain intensity avoids language and may cross cultural differences.[131] Several faces pain scales have been used[110,111,117,120] to assess pain in both pediatric and adult populations. Jones and associates[132] asked elderly nursing home residents to choose which of three pain intensity scales (NRS, VDS, and FPS) they preferred to use to rate their pain. Of those able to choose, the VDS was the most commonly selected (52%); 29% chose the NRS; 19% preferred the FPS. More men than women and those residents with moderate to severe pain preferred the NRS; a higher percentage of minority (Hispanic) residents preferred the FPS.

Findings from various studies indicated that patients used the FPS to measure pain appropriately and that the FPS should be considered an alternative to the NRS or VAS in various populations. However, the literature regarding choice of scale among ethnic groups is equivocal. Carey and colleagues[133] asked hospitalized patients which of several scales they preferred to use: a modified Wong-Baker FACES scale (tears were removed), an NRS, or a vertical VAS. They found that less educated adults, both African American and Caucasian American, preferred the Wong-Baker FACES scale; more educated patients preferred the NRS. Stuppy[115] also found that patients preferred the FPS to the NRS, VAS, or VDS, with no significant differences noted between African American and Caucasian American participants. Taylor and Herr[119,131] discovered that both cognitively impaired and intact African American elders preferred the FPS to the NRS or the VDS, and they found support for the ordinal nature of the FPS. Participants clearly agreed that the FPS represented pain but also agreed that the FPS may represent other constructs, such as sadness or anger, depending how they were cued; this suggests that the FPS may be measuring pain affect, not just intensity. Jensen and coworkers[118] examined six pain rating scales, including the seven-point FPS, in persons with cerebral palsy and also found that the FPS measured more than just pain intensity; it may be reflective of a distress dimension associated with pain and its impact on functioning.

In summary, a variety of scales have been used to assess pain in many different patient populations. Each has been widely used in clinical research and practice. Little research has been done on the appropriateness of pain scales in the palliative care setting. Intellectual understanding and language skills are prerequisites for such pain assessment scales as the VAS and VDS. These scales may be too abstract or too difficult for patients in the palliative care setting. Because most dying patients are elderly, simple pain scales, such as the NRS or a faces scale, may be more advantageous.

Multifactorial Pain Instruments

There are several pain measurement instruments that can be used to standardize pain assessment, incorporating patient demographic factors, pain severity scales, pain descriptors, and other questions related to pain.[134] Four instruments have been considered short enough for routine clinical use with cancer patients. All of these instruments provide a quick way of measuring pain subjectively; however, their use in seriously ill, actively dying patients needs further study (see the AHCPR Acute and Cancer Pain Guidelines[5] for a more comprehensive description of many of these instruments).

Short Form McGill Pain Questionnaire. A short form of the McGill Pain Questionnaire[135] (SF-MPQ) has been developed and includes 15 words to describe pain. Each word or phrase is rated on a four-point intensity scale (0 = none, 1 = mild, 2 = moderate, and 3 = severe). Three pain scores are derived from the sum of the intensity rank values of the words chosen for sensory, affective, and total descriptors. Two pain measures are also included in the SF-MPQ: the Present Pain Intensity Index (PPI) and a 10-cm VAS. The SF-MPQ has demonstrated reliability and validity and is available in multiple languages.

Brief Pain Inventory. The Brief Pain Inventory[136] (BPI) is a multifactorial instrument that address pain etiology, history, intensity, quality, location, and interference with activities. Patients are asked to rate the severity of their pain at its worst, least, and average and at present. Using an NRS (0 to 10), patients are also asked for ratings of how much their pain interferes with walking ability, mood, general activity, work, enjoyment of life, sleep, and relationships with others. The BPI also asks patients to represent the location of their pain on a drawing and asks about the cause of pain and the duration of pain relief.

Memorial Pain Assessment Card. The Memorial Pain Assessment Card[137] (MPAC) is a simple valid tool consisting of three VAS, for pain intensity, pain relief, and mood, and one VDS to describe the pain. The MPAC can be completed by patients in 20 seconds or less and can distinguish between pain intensity, relief, and psychological distress.

City of Hope Patient and Family Pain Questionnaires. The City of Hope Patient and Family Pain Questionnaires[138] were designed to measure the knowledge and experience of patients with chronic cancer pain and their family caregivers. The 16-item surveys use an ordinal scale format and can be administered in inpatient or outpatient settings.

Because terminally ill patients have multiple symptoms, it is impossible to limit an assessment to only the report of pain. Complications or symptoms related to the disease process may exacerbate pain, or interventions to alleviate pain may cause side effects that result in new symptoms or a worsening of other symptoms, such as constipation or nausea. Symptoms such as fatigue and anxiety are distressful and may affect quality of life in seriously ill cancer and noncancer patients.[139,140] Therefore, pain assessment must be accompanied by assessment of other symptoms. Various surveys or questionnaires not only assess pain but also incorporate other symptoms into the assessment process. Many of these instruments are discussed in other chapters.

Pain Assessment in Nonverbal or Cognitively Impaired Patients

The gold standard or primary source of pain assessment is the patient's self-report. However, pain instruments that rely on verbal self-report and are very useful in the early stages of palliative care may not be practical for dying patients who cannot verbalize pain or for patients with advanced disease if delirium or cognitive failure is prevalent. The IASP notes that "pain is always subjective," that "each individual learns about pain through experiences related to injury in early life," and that "the inability to communicate verbally does not negate the possibility that an individual is experiencing pain and is in need of appropriate pain-relieving treatment."[21]

The potential for unrelieved and unrecognized pain is greater in patients who cannot verbally express their discomfort. Older, nonverbal, and cognitively impaired patients are at increased risk for pain,[139,141–143] as well as underassessment and undertreatment of pain.[95,144–148] Patients who are nonverbal or have dementing conditions such as Alzheimer's disease are usually excluded from pain studies, and pain assessment and treatment in this group are poorly understood.[149]

The inability to communicate effectively due to impaired cognition and sensory losses is a serious problem for many patients with terminal illnesses. Cognitive failure develops in the majority of cancer patients before death, and agitated delirium is frequently observed in patients with advanced cancer.[150,151] Loss of consciousness occurs in almost half of dying patients during the final three days of life.[152] These complications have been shown in part to be significantly correlated with a higher dose requirement of opioids and the presence of icterus.[153] Clearly, pain assessment techniques and tools are needed that apply to patients, whether mentally incompetent or nonverbal, who communicate only through their unique behavioral responses. Interpretation of the meaning of specific biobehavioral response patterns during episodes of pain could potentially reduce barriers to optimal pain assessment and management in nonverbal patients.[154] An instrument that could detect a reduction in pain behaviors could assess the effectiveness of a pain management plan. However, because pain is not just a set of pain behaviors, the absence of certain behaviors would not necessarily mean that the patient was pain free.[155]

It is important for nurses and other health care professionals to remember that pain is communicated through both verbal and nonverbal behaviors. Verbal self-reports, whenever possible, are still important to reflect the individual's perception of pain. Because nonverbal pain behaviors may or may not concur with verbal reports, caution is necessary when assessing pain based solely on any single parameter. In addition to the appropriate use and selection of pain assessment instruments, the following points recommended by Taylor and Herr[131] should be remembered when assessing pain in cognitively impaired older individuals: allow enough time for patients to understand questions and formulate answers; avoid overstimulation; ensure adequate lighting and hearing aids (if needed); and provide large print for ease of reading.

Pain Behaviors

It may be more complicated to assess nonverbal cues in the palliative care setting because terminally ill patients with chronic pain, in contrast to patients with acute pain, may not demonstrate any specific behaviors indicative of pain. It is also not satisfactory and even erroneous to assess pain by reliance on involuntary physiological bodily reactions, such as increases in blood pressure, pulse, or respiratory depth. Elevated vital signs may occur with sudden, severe pain; but they usually do not occur with persistent pain after the body reaches physiological equilibrium.[156] However, the absence of behavioral or involuntary cues does not negate the presence of pain.[5] Assessment of behavior for signs of pain during rest and movement provides a potentially valid and reliable alternative to verbal and physiological indices of pain.[157,158] Examples of pain behaviors in cognitively impaired or nonverbal patients or residents are displayed in Table 5–6.[159–161]

Pain indicators in elderly patients with dementia identified by nursing home staff members included specific physical repetitive movements, vocal repetitions, physical signs of pain, and changes in behavior from the norm for that person.[162] Four distinct facial actions that have been consistently identified in pain expression are brow lowering, eye narrowing or closure, and raising the upper lip.[157] Although facial expressions are related to pain intensity ratings on sensory and affective scales,[163,164] facial assessment tools such as the Facial Action Coding System (FACS)[165] are too time-consuming and laborious for use in the clinical setting. Furthermore, observations of facial expressions may not be valid in those patients with conditions that result in distorted facial expressions, such as Parkinson's disease or stroke. Cultural influences on behavioral expressions and interpretation of behavior must also be considered.[90]

The Pain Experience in Patients with Cognitive Failure

The experience or behavior of pain in individuals with cognitive failure or dementia may be altered or different from that of patients or residents who are cognitively intact. There is a tendency for patients with increased levels of cognitive impairment to report less severe pain.[131,144,166–169] Lapalio and Sakla[170] suggested some impairment of affective pain perception in patients

Table 5–6
Possible Pain Behaviors in Nonverbal and Cognitively Impaired Patients or Residents

Behavior Category	Possible Pain Behaviors
Facial expressions	Grimace, frown, winces, sad or frightened look, wrinkled forehead, furrowed brow, closed or tightened eyelids, clenched teeth or jaw
Body movements	Restless, agitated, jittery, "can't seem to sit still," fidgeting, pacing, rocking, constant or intermittent shifting of position, withdrawing
Protective mechanisms	Bracing, guarding, rubbing or massaging a body part, splinting; clutching or holding onto side rails, bed, tray table, or affected area during movement
Verbalizations	Saying common phrases, such as, "Help me," "Leave me alone," "Get away from me," "Don't touch me," or "Ouch," cursing, verbally abusive, praying
Vocalizations	Moaning, groaning, crying, whining, oohing, aahing, calling out, screaming, breathing heavily
Mental status changes	Confusion, disorientation, distress
Changes in activity patterns, routines, or interpersonal interactions	Decreased appetite, sleep alterations, decreased social activity participation, change in ambulation, immobilization

Sources: Adapted from American Geriatrics Society Panel on Persistent Pain (2002), reference 18; American Medical Directors Association (2003), reference 19; and references 132, 145, 159, 160, and 161.

with Lewy body dementia, because the Lewy bodies have been shown to occupy the hypothalamus and frontal cortex. Significantly increased pain tolerance in patients with mild dementia,[171–173] reported by several experimental studies, implies that motivational-affective and cognitive-evaluative, not sensory-discriminative pain systems are affected: "In other words, mildly demented individuals seem to experience the same nociceptive sensations as nondemented individuals, but they fail to interpret these sensations as painful"[149] (p. 103). If the patient's anxiety and expectation of pain are decreased, impaired memory may reduce pain. The individual with memory impairments may also be unable to adapt to pain due to a loss of habituation to painful stimuli.[174] Studies suggesting that pain reports in cognitively impaired individuals are decreased in intensity and frequency are probably related to a decreased capacity to report pain.[175]

Behavior or responses caused by noxious stimuli in a cognitively impaired or demented individual may not necessarily reflect classic pain behaviors. In a study of 26 patients with painful conditions from a nursing home Alzheimer's unit, Marzinski[176] reported diverse responses to pain that were not typical of conventional pain behaviors. For example, with pain, a patient who normally moaned and rocked became quiet and withdrawn. Pain in another nonverbal patient caused rapid blinking. Other patients who normally exhibited disjointed verbalizations could, when experiencing pain, give accurate descriptions of their pain. Parmelee[167] and Huffman[177] and their colleagues also found that verbal pain reports by patients with dementia are accurate and valid.

The questions and suggestions in Table 5–7 can be used as a template for assessment of pain in the nonverbal or cognitively impaired patient or resident. A summary of instruments used to assess pain in nonverbal or cognitively impaired patients is found in Table 5–8. One of these instruments, the Pain Assessment in Advanced Dementia (PAINAD), is presented in Table 5–9.

Table 5–7
Assessment and Treatment of Pain in the Nonverbal or Cognitively Impaired Patient/Resident

Is there a reason for the patient to be experiencing pain?
Was the patient being treated for pain? If so, what regimen was effective (include pharmacologic and nonpharmacologic interventions)?
How does the patient usually act when he or she is in pain? (Note: the nurse may need to ask family/significant others or other health care professionals.)
What is the family/significant others' interpretation of the patient's behavior? Do they believe the patient is in pain? Why do they feel this way?
Try to obtain feedback from the patient; for example, ask patient to nod head, squeeze hand, move eyes up or down, raise legs, or hold up fingers to signal presence of pain.
If appropriate, offer writing materials or pain intensity charts that patient can use or point to.
If there is a possible reason for or sign of acute pain, treat with analgesics or other pain-relief measures.
If a pharmacologic or nonpharmacologic intervention results in modifying pain behavior, continue with treatment.
If pain behavior persists, rule out potential causes of the behavior (delirium, side effect of treatment, symptom of disease process); try appropriate intervention for behavior cause.
Explain interventions to patient and family/significant other.

Table 5–8
Pain Assessment Tools for the Cognitively Impaired or Nonverbal Patient/Resident

Tool	Goal	Dimensions/Parameters
Discomfort Scale for Dementia of the Alzheimer Type (DS–DAT)[187]	Measure discomfort in elders with advanced dementia who have decreased cognition and verbalization	Noisy breathing Negative vocalizations Content facial expression Sad facial expression Frightened facial expression Frown Relaxed body language Tense body language Fidgeting
Assessment of Discomfort in Dementia Protocol (ADD)[188–190]	Evaluate persons with difficult behaviors that may represent discomfort and develop a treatment plan for physical and affective discomfort	Facial expression Mood Body language Voice Behavior Other
Checklist of Nonverbal Pain Indicators (CNPI)[144,145]	Measure pain behaviors in cognitively impaired elders	Nonverbal vocalizations Facial grimaces/winces Bracing Rubbing Restlessness Verbalizations
Noncommunicative Patient's Pain Assessment Instrument (NOPPAIN)[191]	Assess pain behaviors in patients with dementia by nursing assistants	Activity Behaviors and intensity • Pain words • Pain noises • Pain faces • Bracing • Rubbing • Restlessness Location Pain thermometer
Pain Assessment for the Dementing Elderly (PADE)[192]	Assess pain behaviors in patients with advanced dementia	Physical • Facial expression • Breathing pattern • Posture Global • Proxy pain intensity Functional • Dressing • Feeding oneself • Wheelchair-to-bed transfers
Pain Assessment Tool in Confused Older Adults (PATCOA)[193]	Observe nonverbal cues to assess pain in acutely confused older adults	Quivering Guarding Frowning Grimacing Clenching jaws Points to where it hurts Reluctance to move Vocalizations of moaning Sighing

(*continued*)

Table 5–8
Pain Assessment Tools for the Cognitively Impaired or Nonverbal Patient/Resident *(continued)*

Tool	Goal	Dimensions/Parameters
Pain Assessment in Advanced Dementia (PAINAD)[194] Adapted from DS-DAT[187] and FLACC[195]	Assess pain in patients with advanced dementia	Breathing Negative vocalization Facial expression Body language Consolability
Pain Assessment Checklist for Seniors with Limited Ability to Communicate (PACSLAC)[196]	Assess common and subtle behaviors in seniors with advanced dementia	Facial expressions Activity and body movements Social/personality/mood indicators Physiological indicators/eating and sleeping/vocal behaviors
Abbey Pain Scale[197]	Assess pain in patients with late-stage dementia in nursing homes	Vocalization Facial expression Change in body language Behavioral change Physiological change Physical change

Table 5–9
Pain Assessment in Advanced Dementia (PAINAD)

Items	0	1	2
Breathing independent of vocalization	Normal	Occasional labored breathing Short period of hyperventilation	Noisy labored breathing Long period of hyperventilation Cheyne-Stokes respirations
Negative vocalization	None	Occasional moan or groan Low-level speech with a negative or disapproving quality	Repeated troubled calling out Loud moaning or groaning Crying
Facial expression	Smiling or inexpressive	Sad Frightened Frown	Facial grimacing
Body language	Relaxed	Tense Distressed Pacing Fidgeting	Rigid Fists clenched Knees pulled up Pulling or pushing away Striking out
Consolability	No need to console	Distracted or reassured by voice or touch	Cannot be consoled, distracted, or reassured

Source: Warden et al. (2003), reference 194.

Instruments Used to Assess Pain in Nonverbal or Cognitively Impaired Patients

The following are examples of pain scales and tools being used or tested in the non-verbal or cognitively impaired population.

Pain Intensity Scales

Recent research[131,132,141,144,167,178–180] indicates that the verbal descriptor scale (VDS), the numeric rating scale (NRS), the faces pain scale (FPS), the Iowa pain thermometer (IPT), and the 21-point box pain intensity scales are reliable and valid in older adults with mild to moderate degrees of cognitive impairment. The IPT is a modified VDS that provides more options between words and is aligned with a pain thermometer to improve the conceptualization of pain.[106] The horizontal 21-point box scale has a row of 21 boxes labeled from 0 (no pain) to 100 (pain as bad as it could be) in increments of five; respondents indicate the box that best represents their pain.[180] Cognitively impaired older adults are able to accurately complete one or more pain intensity scales;[131,144,179–182] however, there is concern about the reliability of their short-term pain reports.[183] Taylor & Herr[131] recommend consideration of the FPS when repeat assessments are indicated. While the FPS is generally favored for both cognitively intact and cognitively impaired older adults, particularly minorities,[119,131,132] it should be noted that the FPS may not clearly represent pain intensity only but may represent a broader construct "pain affect." [118,119,131] Because the FPS is easy to use and easily understood, it can be offered to minority older adults as an alternative if other validated tools, such as the VDS and NRS, are not usable by this population because of language barriers. Further research is needed to determine whether preference for pain intensity scales is influenced by specific cognitive level and disability, gender, age, education, race, and ethnicity/culture.

Pain Behavior Tools

Assessing pain in patients/residents who are nonverbal or cognitively impaired and are unable to verbally self-report pain presents a particular challenge to clinicians. There have been a variety of instruments that have been used by chronic pain programs to systematically observe and measure the frequency of pain behaviors,[184–186] but their use has been limited in the palliative care setting. Many health care providers and researchers[187–197] have attempted to develop an easy-to-use yet valid and reliable instrument for the assessment of pain in this vulnerable population (see Table 5–8). Herr and colleagues[198] have performed an extensive and critical evaluation of many of these existing tools (conceptualization, subject/setting, reliability and validity, administration/scoring methods, strengths/weaknesses) with the intent of providing up-to-date information to clinicians and researchers. The findings from the Herr and colleagues review is available at http://prc.coh.org; it is anticipated that this web site will be updated regularly with the most current data on pain assessment tools. Brief descriptions of pain behavior tools follow.

Discomfort Scale for Dementia of the Alzheimer Type (DS–DAT). Hurley and colleagues,[187] based on behaviors observed by nurses, developed an objective scale for assessing discomfort in nonverbal patients with advanced Alzheimer's disease. The investigators defined discomfort as "a negative emotional and/or physical state subject to variation in magnitude in response to internal or environmental conditions." The negative state to which they referred could be a condition other than pain, such as anguish and suffering. After testing for reliability, a scale of 9 items was retained from an original list of 26 behavioral indicators for discomfort. Items retained were noisy breathing, negative vocalization, absence of a look of contentment, looking sad, looking frightened, having a frown, absence of relaxed body posture, looking tense, and fidgeting. Scoring of the DS–DAT is based on evaluation of frequency, intensity, and duration of the behaviors and may be cumbersome, requiring more training and education than is feasible or realistic for clinicians in hospital or long term care settings. Although the DS–DAT has been criticized for being too complex for routine nursing care,[199] it has been revised[194] and offers potential for use in the palliative care setting.

The Assessment of Discomfort in Dementia Protocol (ADD).[188] The ADD was developed to improve the recognition and treatment of pain and discomfort in patients with dementia who cannot report their internal states, with the added goal of decreasing inappropriate use of psychotropic medication administration. This protocol is "based upon the assumption that behaviors associated with dementia are symptoms of unmet physiologic and/or nonphysiologic needs"[189](p.193). In addition to the DS–DAT items, the ADD protocol includes more overt symptoms, such as physical aggression, crying, calling out, resisting care, and exiting behaviors. Implementation of the protocol when basic care interventions failed to ameliorate behavioral symptoms resulted in significant decreases in discomfort, significant increases in the use of pharmacologic and nonpharmacologic comfort interventions,[188] and improved behavioral symptoms.[189,190] Use of a combined assessment and treatment protocol appears promising for the palliative care setting.

Checklist of Nonverbal Pain Indicators (CNPI).[144,145] Feldt[145] developed the CNPI specifically for cognitively impaired elders. Modified from the University of Alabama-Birmingham Pain Behavior Scale for chronic pain patients, [184] the CNPI is a six-item tool that rates the absence or presence of the following behaviors, at rest and on movement: nonverbal vocalizations (moans, groans, sighs), facial grimaces (furrowed brow, narrowed eyes, clenched teeth), bracing (clutching or holding onto furniture or affected area), rubbing (massaging affected area), restlessness (constant or intermittent shifting of position, rocking, inability to keep still), and verbal complaint (saying "ouch," "don't touch me," "that's enough," or cursing during movement). A summed score of the number of nonverbal pain indicators observed at rest and on movement is calculated (total possible score = 0–12). It should be noted that an increased score does not reflect actual pain severity nor does it compare to other numeric scales measuring pain. In a study of elderly hip fracture inpatients in which 60% were cognitively impaired, the CNPI demonstrated face validity and interrater reliability (93% agreement by two gerontologic nurse practitioners), although internal consistency was low ($\alpha = .54$ and .64, at rest and movement).[144] It was also reported to be easy to use by nursing staff.[64] Further research is needed on this tool's validity, reliability, and appropriateness for cognitively impaired patients.

Non-communicative Patient's Pain Assessment Instrument (NOPPAIN).[191] The NOPPAIN was developed as a nursing assistant–administered instrument. Pain is observed at rest and on movement while nursing assistants perform resident care (bathing, dressing, transferring). Pain behaviors are observed and pain intensity is scored using a pain thermometer.

Pain Assessment for the Dementing Elderly (PADE).[192] The PADE was designed to help caregivers assess patient/resident behavior indicating pain. PADE items (n = 24) were developed after a literature review, interviews with nursing staff, and observations of residents in a dementia unit. The PADE consists of three parts: physical (facial expressions, breathing, and posture); global (caregiver-rated pain); functional (activities of daily living).

Patient Assessment Tool in Confused Older Adults (PATCOA).[193] The PATCOA was evaluated in an initial study of 116 older adults (60 to 80 years of age) undergoing orthopedic surgery.[193] Patients with Alzheimer's disease were excluded from the study. The PATCOA is an ordinal scale which includes 9 items of nonverbal pain cues rated as absent or present while the patient is at rest; higher scores indicate higher pain intensity. A vertical VAS was used in the study to meet the sensory needs of the older age group. Several nonverbal cues consistent with the CNPI[144] included clenching jaws, frowning, grimacing, and vocalizations of moaning and sighing. The internal consistency reliability was below 0.70 which the investigators related to measurement of multiple dimensions of the pain experience, low interrater reliability for several nonverbal cues, and the small number of items in the tool. The study showed no significant differences between self-report of pain and demonstration of nonverbal cues with acute confusion. However, this initial study was limited by the predominance of a cognitively intact sample (only 3.5% of the patients were confused and 12% at high risk for confusion), making it too difficult to differentiate between nonverbal cues of pain from acute confusion. Further reliability and validity testing of the PATCOA is planned.

The Pain Assessment in Advanced Dementia Scale (PAINAD).[194] Warden, Hurley, & Volicer[194] derived the PAINAD from the behaviors and categories of the FLACC,[195] a behavioral scale used to measure pain severity in postoperative children; the DS-DAT[187]; and pain descriptors of dementia by experienced clinicians. The intent of the PAINAD is to simply measure pain using a 0–10 score in noncommunicative individuals. This tool, tested on Caucasian male veteran residents with advanced dementia (n = 19) who were not able to communicate their pain intensity, was compared with the DS–DAT and two VAS by trained raters/expert clinicians, and was shown to have good construct validity and reliability; internal consistency was lower than what is desired for a new scale. Future research using this tool with a more diverse population (long-term care or palliative setting) is warranted.

Pain Assessment Checklist for Seniors with Limited Ability to Communicate (PACSLAC).[196] Fuchs-Lacelle and Hadjistavropoulos[196] developed and preliminarily evaluated an observational tool to assess pain in severely demented seniors. To validate the tool, forty nurses were asked to recall patients under their care who were experiencing pain, distress, and calm, and to rate those experiences using the 60-item checklist, taking approximately 5 minutes per administration. Four subscales of the tool were derived: Social/Personality/Mood Indicators, Facial Expressions, Activity/Body Movement, and Physiological Indicators/Eating/Sleeping Changes/Vocal Behaviors. Preliminary evidence suggests that the PACSLAC can differentiate between pain and distress; scores were positively correlated with cognitive impairment level. This tool may be appropriate for use in the cognitively impaired palliative care patient. However, further research is needed on clinicians who complete the checklist while observing the patient in pain.

Abbey Pain Scale.[197] A tool based on Hurley's[187] and Simon & Malabar's[200] work was developed for use with residents with end or late stage dementia unable to express their needs. Six behavioral indicators were identified and scored with three grades of severity (0 = absent through 3 = severe) for a total possible score of 18. Further testing is warranted to establish reliability and validity.

Proxy Pain Assessment in the Nonverbal or Cognitively Impaired Patient/Resident

Just as the experience of pain is subjective, "witnessing another in pain is a subjective experience."[201] Without verbal validation from the patient, the clinician must rely not only on behavioral observations but on intuition and personal judgment. It is also particularly important to elicit the opinions of the individuals closest to the patient, which are also subjective.

Nurses and other health care providers reflect the difficulty of accurately assessing pain in nonverbal or cognitively impaired patients in studies that show low concurrence between patients' self-ratings of pain and clinicians' ratings.[202–204] Other findings are equivocal, with some studies suggesting that family caregivers or significant others accurately estimate the amount of pain cancer patients experience[89] and others proposing that family caregivers overestimate patients' pain.[205–207] Bruera and colleagues[208] studied relatives and the nurses who cared for 60 unresponsive, dying patients. Both were asked to rate a patient's discomfort level, six observed behaviors (grimacing, groaning, shouting, touching or rubbing an area, purposeless movement, labored breathing), and the suspected reason for the discomfort. Although the mean levels of perceived discomfort were similar, relatives reported significantly more observed behaviors and more often indicated pain as a reason for discomfort than did the nurse caregivers. According to Cohen-Mansfield,[209] relatives of cognitively impaired nursing home residents are better able to interpret facial expressions and other pain behaviors if they visit their loved ones at least once a week and have a close relationship. Additionally, higher levels of cognitive functioning were related to improved ability of relatives to assess pain and to higher levels of perceived pain.

The Edmonton Symptom Assessment System (ESAS) is a validated tool for use in the palliative care setting (Figure 5–4). It was originally tested in 101 consecutive palliative care inpatients; 83% of symptom assessments were done by nurses or patients' relatives.[210] The ESAS is a brief and reproducible scale consisting of separate visual analog or numeric scales that

Capital Health | CARITAS HEALTH GROUP

Edmonton Symptom Assessment: Numerical Scale

Please circle the number that best describes:

No Pain	0	1	2	3	4	5	6	7	8	9	10	Worst Possible Pain
Not Tired	0	1	2	3	4	5	6	7	8	9	10	Worst Possible Tiredness
Not Nauseated	0	1	2	3	4	5	6	7	8	9	10	Worst Possible Nausea
Not Depressed	0	1	2	3	4	5	6	7	8	9	10	Worst Possible Depression
Not Anxious	0	1	2	3	4	5	6	7	8	9	10	Worst Possible Anxiety
Not Drowsy	0	1	2	3	4	5	6	7	8	9	10	Worst Possible Drowsiness
Best Appetite	0	1	2	3	4	5	6	7	8	9	10	Worst Possible Appetite
Best Feeling of Wellbeing	0	1	2	3	4	5	6	7	8	9	10	Worst Possible Feeling of Wellbeing
No Shortness of Breath	0	1	2	3	4	5	6	7	8	9	10	Worst Possible Shortness of Breath
Other Problem	0	1	2	3	4	5	6	7	8	9	10	

Name: ____________
Date: ____________
Time: ____________
Assessed By: ____________

A

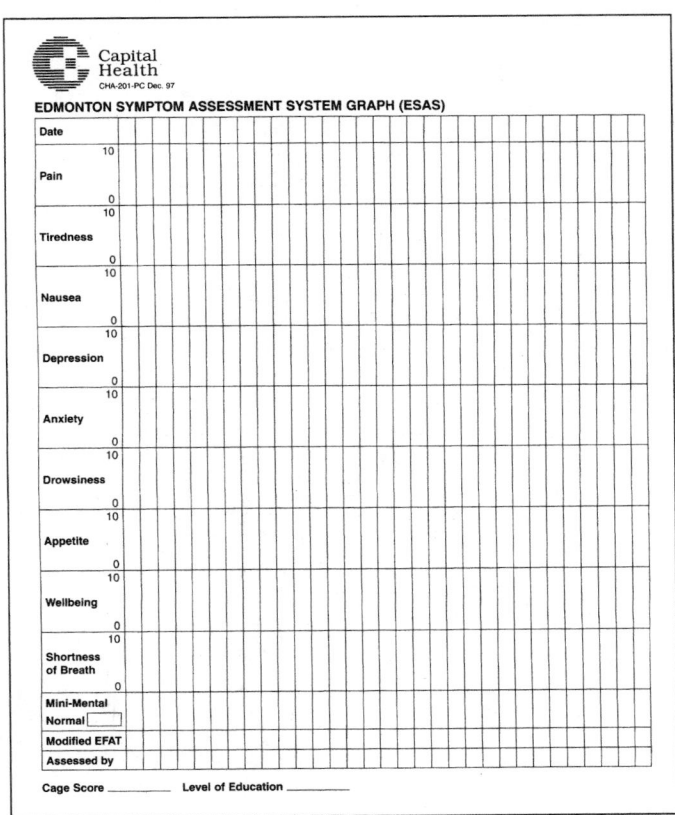

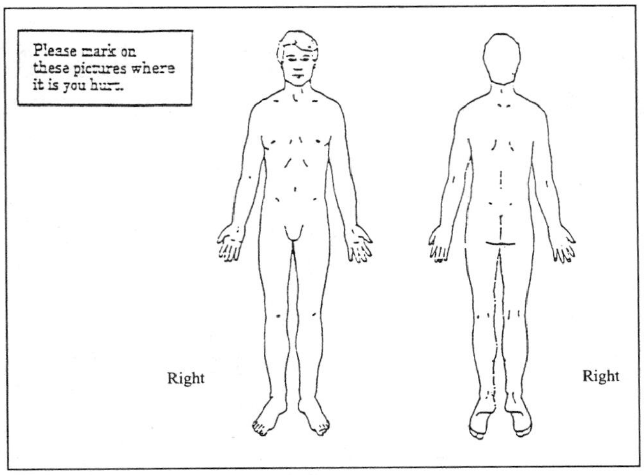

B

Figure 5–4. The Edmonton Symptom Assessment System (ESAS). (A) Visual analog scale. (B) Graphic for self-report of pain locations. (C) ESAS graph. (D) Edmonton Comfort Assessment Form (ECAF). (E) ECAF graph. Instructions for the use of this multipart form are presented in Appendix 5–1. *Source*: Reprinted with permission of Carleen Brenneis, Capital Health, Edmonton, Alberta, Canada.)

Capital Health
CHA-201-PC Dec. 97

EDMONTON SYMPTOM ASSESSMENT SYSTEM GRAPH (ESAS)

Date		
Pain	10 / 0	
Tiredness	10 / 0	
Nausea	10 / 0	
Depression	10 / 0	
Anxiety	10 / 0	
Drowsiness	10 / 0	
Appetite	10 / 0	
Wellbeing	10 / 0	
Shortness of Breath	10 / 0	
Mini-Mental Normal ☐		
Modified EFAT		
Assessed by		

Cage Score ________ **Level of Education** ________

C

Capital Health
CARITAS HEALTH GROUP

Edmonton Comfort Assessment Form (ECAF)

(Please ask caregivers to complete first) Date Completed: ______________ Time: ______________

Regular Family Caregiver (if present) ______________________________ ☐ Not Applicable

1. How comfortable has the person been during the last day? *(Please circle the appropriate number)*

Very comfortable 0 1 2 3 4 5 6 7 8 9 10 Very Uncomfortable

2. Why do you think the patient is uncomfortable today? (Check the reason-You may check more than one)

☐ Pain ☐ Nausea ☐ Confusion / Restlessness ☐ Need to Urinate / Defecate

☐ Shortness of Breath ☐ Hunger / Thirst ☐ Unknown

☐ Other *(please specify)* ______________________________

Nurse Score:					
1. Behaviour Observed Today *(Please check only 1 scale for Behaviour)*	Not Observed During Shift 0	Observed only upon Stimulation 1	Occasional Spontaneous 2	Frequent *(most of the time)* 3	Continuous 4
A. Grimacing					
B. Groaning-Isolated Words					
C. Shouting					
D. Touching-Rubbing Area					
E. Purposeless Movements					
F. Laboured Noisy Breathing					
SCORE					
				TOTAL SCORE (0-24)	

2. Suspected Reason *(Check more than one)*

☐ Pain ☐ Nausea ☐ Confusion / Restlessness ☐ Urinary Retention / Defecation

☐ Dyspnea ☐ Hunger / Thirst ☐ Unknown

☐ Other *(please specify)* ______________________________

3. RN Global Comfort Assessment Score: 0 - 10 scale ______________ *(0 = very comfortable; 10 = very uncomfortable)*

D

Capital Health
CARITAS HEALTH GROUP

Edmonton Comfort Assessment Form (ECAF)
GRAPH

DATE		
ADMISSION DAY		
HOUR (End of Shift)		
1. Caregiver Comfort VAS	10 9 8 7 6 5 4 3 2 1 0	
Caregiver VAS		
2. Caregiver Reason (✓)	Pain	
	Nausea	
	Confusion / restlessness	
	Urinate / defecate	
	Shortness of breath	
	Hunger / thirst	
	Unknown	
	Other	
1. Nurse Score (0-24)		
2. Nurse Reason (✓)	Pain	
	Nausea	
	Confusion / restlessness	
	Urinate and / or defecate	
	Dyspnea	
	Hunger / Thirst	
	Unknown	
	Other	
3. RN VAS		
4. MD VAS		

E

Figure 5–4. *(continued)*

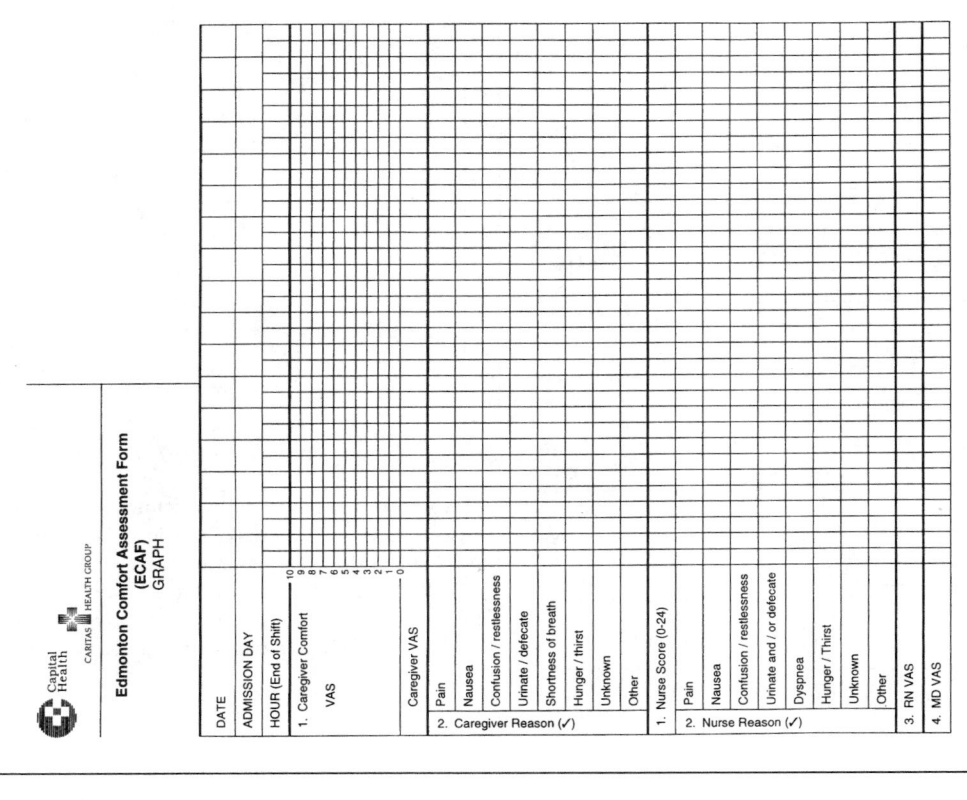

evaluate nine symptoms (pain, activity, nausea, depression, anxiety, drowsiness, appetite, sensation of well-being, and shortness of breath). The tool is completed twice a day by palliative care unit patients, daily by hospice patients, and several times a week by home care patients. If patients are unable to complete the form, a space is provided for the person completing the assessment. If patients or residents are unresponsive and incapable of reporting their own pain (e.g., during the final days of life), observer judgments of pain become necessary. In this situation, the main caregiver or nurse completes the Edmonton Comfort Assessment Form (ECAF). The scores on either assessment can be transferred to a graph to present a visual display of trends in a patient's symptoms and discomfort. Lower scores designate better symptom control (the highest possible score is 900 on the ESAS). Although the ESAS has been considered useful to display the incidence of symptoms, some investigators have found it to be impractical in patients with a poor performance status.[211] To evaluate pain and other symptoms, an individualized approach may be a more appropriate practice than completing health-related checklists.

Implications for Treatment

Although pain assessment in the nonverbal or cognitively impaired patient or resident presents a challenge to clinicians, it should not pose a barrier to optimal pain management. If patients are no longer able to verbally communicate whether they are in pain or not, the best approach is to assume that their underlying disease is still painful and to continue pain interventions.[212] Nonverbal patients should be empirically treated for pain if there is preexisting pain or evidence that an individual in a similar condition would experience pain.[213] Likewise, palliative measures should be considered in nonverbal patients with behavior changes potentially related to pain. Studies demonstrate that pain behaviors are modified or decreased by pain interventions and adjustments in analgesia.[190,200]

Summary

In summary, multiple factors should be incorporated into the assessment of the pain experience. The following case examples include some of the pain assessment techniques discussed in this chapter and may prove beneficial in applying this content for nurse clinicians.

CASE STUDY

Paul, a Hospice Patient with Pain

Paul is an 88-year-old man with prostate cancer metastatic to the bone that is unresponsive to hormonal manipulation, chemotherapy, and radiation therapy. Paul has new left hip and low back pain; a recent bone scan shows widespread metastatic disease. Paul's past medical history includes arthritis and stroke with residual left-sided weakness. Paul has had difficulty walking due to increased pain and disuse syndrome due to his previous stroke. He recently fell and is now bedridden. It is extremely uncomfortable for him to be moved from side to side because of the pain. He also has a stage II pressure ulcer on his coccyx that seems to be worsening.

Paul describes his pain as achy, throbbing, and gnawing as he points to his left hip and lower back. He rates his persistent pain as a 4 (on a scale of 0 to 10), worsening to an 8 with movement and activity. His pain has interfered with his ability to sleep throughout the night and with his movement; his appetite has decreased significantly over the past month, and he has had some constipation. Paul's family is concerned about his taking pain medication because of fears of dependence and side effects (constipation, sedation). Paul is a stoic man who does not openly complain about pain to his wife, daughters, nurses, or doctor. He does not want to be a burden on his family, and realizes his prostate cancer is incurable. He has accepted hospice care.

1. What type of pain is Paul experiencing?
2. How do you know he is having pain?
3. What pharmacological approaches would you suggest?
4. What nonpharmacological strategies would you incorporate into the pain management plan?
5. What other symptoms or side effects would you be concerned about?

CASE STUDY

June, a Cognitively Impaired Resident with Pain

June is an 87-year-old woman with a history of pneumonia, degenerative joint disease, osteoporosis, diabetes, Alzheimer's dementia, and myelodysplastic disorder who has been admitted to your facility. June is extremely depressed. The certified nursing assistants caring for June report that she moans and groans when they bathe and change her (she is incontinent of bowel and bladder) and screams, "You're so mean to me!" She often is tearful, has a sad facial expression, and is very restless.

1. What kind of pain might June be having?
2. What can be done for her pain?
3. Did she take any pain medication previously?
4. What does her family think?
5. How can her caregivers tell if the pain has been controlled?

REFERENCES

1. Dickinson E. Pain—Has an Element of Blank [poem]. Available at: http://www.americanpoems.com/poets/emilydickinson/10602 (accessed November 5, 2004).

2. Cleeland CS, Gonin R, Hatfield AK, Edmonson JH, Blum RH, Stewart JA, Pandya KJ. Pain and its treatment in outpatients with metastatic cancer. N Engl J Med 1994;330:592–596.
3. Desbiens NA, Wu AW, Broste SK, Wenger NS, Connors AF Jr, Lynn J, Yasui Y, Phillips RS, Fulkerson W. Pain and satisfaction with pain control in seriously ill hospitalized adults: Findings from the SUPPORT research investigations. Crit Care Med 1996;24:1953–1961.
4. Desbiens NA, Wu AW, Yasui Y, Lynn J, Alzola C, Wenger NS, Connors AF Jr, Phillips RS, Fulkerson W. Patient empowerment and feedback did not decrease pain in seriously ill hospitalized adults. Pain 1998;75:237–246.
5. Jacox A, Carr DB, Payne R, et al. Management of Cancer Pain: Clinical Practice Guideline No. 9. AHCPR Publication 94-0592. Rockville, Md.: Agency for Health Care Policy and Research, U.S. Department of Health and Human Services, Public Health Service, March 1994.
6. National Comprehensive Cancer Network. Cancer Pain. Clinical Practice Guidelines in Oncology, version 1.2004. Jenkintown, Pa.: NCCN, 2004.
7. Weiss SC, Emanuel LL, Fairclough DL, Emanuel EJ. Understanding the experience of pain in terminally ill patients. Lancet 2001;357:1311–1315.
8. Bruera E, Kim HN. Cancer pain. JAMA 2003;290:2476–2479.
9. Ventafridda V, Ripamonti C, DeConno F, Tambarini M, Cassileth BR. Symptom prevalence and control during cancer patient's last days of life. J Palliat Care 1990;6:3–4.
10. Coyle N, Adelhardt J, Foley KM, Portenoy RK. Character of terminal illness in the advanced cancer patient: Pain and other symptoms during the last four weeks of life. J Pain Symptom Manage 1990;5:83–93.
11. Weissman DE, Griffie J. The palliative care consultation service of the Medical College of Wisconsin. J Pain Symptom Manage 1994;9:474–479.
12. Miller SC, Mor V, Teno J. Hospice enrollment and pain assessment and management in nursing homes. J Pain Symptom Manage 2003;26:791–799.
13. Sloane PD, Zimmerman S, Hanson L, Mitchell CM, Riedel-Leo C, Custis-Buie V. End-of-life care in assisted living and related residential care settings: Comparison with nursing homes. J Am Geriatr Soc 2003;51:1587–1594.
14. Bernabei R, Gambassi G, Lapane K, Landi F, Gatsonis C, Dunlop R, Lipsitz L, Steel KL, Mor V. Management of pain in elderly cancer patients. JAMA 1998;279:1877–1882.
15. Ferrell BA. Pain management. In: Hazzard WR, Blass JP, Ettinger WH Jr, Halter JB, Ouslander JG, eds. Principles of Geriatric Medicine and Gerontology, 4th ed. New York: McGraw-Hill, 1999:413–433.
16. Won A, Lapane K, Gambassi G, Bernabei R, Mor V, Lipsitz LA. Correlates and management of nonmalignant pain in nursing homes. J Am Geriatr Soc 1999;47:936–942.
17. Teno JM, Weitzen S, Wetle T, Mor V. Persistent pain in nursing homes: Validating a pain scale for the Minimum Data Set. Gerontologist 2001;41:173–179.
18. American Geriatrics Society (AGS) Panel on Persistent Pain in Older Persons. Clinical practice guideline: The management of persistent pain in older persons. J Am Geriatr Soc 2002;50 (6 Suppl):S205–S224.
19. American Medical Directors Association. Pain Management in the Long-Term Care Setting: Clinical Practice Guideline. Columbia, Md.: AMDA, 2003;1–33.
20. Won A, Lapane K, Vallow S, Schein J, Morris J, Lipsitz L. Persistent nonmalignant pain and analgesic prescribing patterns in elderly nursing home residents. J Am Geriatr Soc 2004;52: 867–874.
21. Merskey H, Bogduk N (eds.). Classification of Chronic Pain, 2nd ed. International Association for the Study of Pain, Task Force on Taxonomy. Seattle, Wash.: IASP Press, 1994:209–214.
22. McCaffery M. Nursing Practice Theories Related to Cognition, Bodily Pain, and Man–Environment Interactions. Los Angeles: UCLA Press, 1968:95.
23. Turk DC, Melzack R. The measurement of pain and the assessment of people experiencing pain. In: Turk DC, Melzack R, eds. Handbook of Pain Assessment. New York: Guilford Press, 1992:3–14.
24. Chodosh J, Solomon D, Roth C, Chang JT, MacLean CH, Ferrell BA, Shekelle PG, Wenger NS. The quality of medical care provided to vulnerable older patients with chronic pain. J Am Geriatr Soc 2004;52:756–767.
25. Ferrell BR, Dean GE, Grant M, Coluzzi P. An institutional commitment to pain management. J Clin Oncol 1995;13:2158–2165.
26. Fink RM, Gates RA, Slover R. A Comprehensive Multidisciplinary Education and Research Program to Assess and Improve Outcomes of Patients with Pain. Abstract submitted and poster presented at the 14th Annual American Pain Society Scientific Meeting, Los Angeles, Calif., 1995.
27. Jones K, Fink R, Hutt E, Pepper G, Hutt E, Vojir CP, Scott J, Clark L, Mellis K. Improving nursing home staff knowledge and attitudes about pain. The Gerontologist 2004;44: 469–478.
28. Weissman DE, Dahl JL. Attitudes about cancer pain: A survey of Wisconsin's first year medical students. J Pain Symptom Manage 1990;5:345–349.
29. Cleeland CS. Documenting barriers to cancer pain management. In: Chapman CR, Foley KM, eds. Current and Emerging Issues in Cancer Pain: Research and Practice. New York: Raven Press, 1993:321–330.
30. Coyle N. In their own words: Seven advanced cancer patients describe their experience with pain and the use of opioid drugs. J Pain Symptom Manage 2004;27:300–309.
31. Paice J, Toy C, Shott S. Barriers to cancer pain relief: Fear of tolerance and addiction. J Pain Symptom Manage 1998;16:1–9.
32. Weiner DK, Rudy TE. Attitudinal barriers to effective treatment of persistent pain in nursing home residents. J Am Geriatr Soc 2002;50:2035–2040.
33. Ward S, Goldberg N, Miller-McCauley V, Mueller C, Nolan A, Pawlik-Plank D, Robbins A, Stormoen D, Weissman DE. Patient-related barriers to management of cancer pain. Pain 1993;52:319–324.
34. Gunnarsdottir S, Donovan HS, Serlin RC, Voge C, Ward S. Patient-related barriers to pain management: The Barriers Questionnaire II (BQ-II). Pain 2002;99:385–396.
35. Jones K, Fink R, Clark L, et al. Nursing home resident barriers to effective pain management: Why nursing home residents may not seek pain medication. JAMDA 2005;6:10–17.
36. Cleeland CS. The impact of pain on the patient with cancer. Cancer 1984;58:2635–2641.
37. Acute Pain Management Guidelines Panel. Acute Pain Management: Operative or Medical Procedures and Trauma. Clinical Practice Guideline. AHCPR Publication 92-0032. Rockville, Md.: Agency for Health Care Policy and Research, U.S. Department of Health and Human Services, Public Health Service, February 1992.

38. American Pain Society. Principles of Analgesic Use in the Treatment of Acute Pain and Cancer Pain, 5th ed. Glenview, Ill.: APS, 2003.
39. American Pain Society Quality of Care Committee. Quality improvement guidelines for the treatment of acute pain and cancer pain. JAMA 1995;1874–1880.
40. Miakowski C, Cleary J, Burney R, et al. Guideline for the Management of Cancer Pain in Adults and Children. APS Clinical Practice Guidelines, Series No. 3. Glenview, Ill.: APS, 2005.
41. Spross JA, Curtiss CP, Coyne P, McGuire D, Fink RS. Oncology Nursing Society position paper on cancer pain management (revised). Oncology Nursing Forum 1998;25:817–818.
42. Max M, Cleary J, Ferrell BR, Foley K, Payne R, Shapiro B. Treatment of pain at the end of life: A position statement from the American Pain Society. American Pain Society Bulletin 1997;7:1–3.
43. Joint Commission on Accreditation of Healthcare Organizations. Available at: http://www.jcaho.org/news+room/health+care+issues/pain+mono_npc.pdf (accessed 12/15/04).
44. American Pain Society. Pain: The Fifth Vital Sign. Available at: http://www.ampainsoc.org/advocacy/fifth.htm (accessed November 5, 2004).
45. Miaskowski C. Pain management: Quality assurance and changing practice. In: Gebhardt GF, Hammond DL, Jensen TS, eds. Proceedings of the 7th World Congress on Pain: Progress in Pain Research and Management, Vol. 2. Seattle, Wash.: IASP Press, 1994:75–96.
46. Peyerwold M. Pain assessment. In: Coluzzi PH, Volker B, Miashowski C, eds. Comprehensive Pain Management in Terminal Illness. Sacramento: California State Hospice Association, 1996:29–34.
47. Morris W, ed. American Heritage Dictionary of the English Language. Boston: Houghton Mifflin, 1996:79, 428, 972.
48. Twycross RG. Oral Morphine in Advanced Cancer, 3rd ed. Beaconsfield, Bucks, UK: Beaconsfield Publishers, 1997:1–42.
49. McGuire D. The multiple dimensions of cancer pain: A framework for assessment and management. In: McGuire D, Yarbro CH, and Ferrell BR, eds. Cancer Pain Management, 2nd ed. Boston: Jones and Bartlett, 1995:1–17.
50. Melzack R, Casey KL. Sensory, motivational, and central control determinants of pain: A new conceptual model. In: Kenshalo D, ed. The Skin Senses. Springfield, Ill.: Charles C Thomas, 1968:423–439.
51. Ahles TA, Blanchard EB, Ruckdeschel JC. The multidimensional nature of cancer-related pain. Pain 1983;17:277–288.
52. Bates MS. Ethnicity and pain: A biocultural model. Soc Sci Med 1987;24:47–50.
53. McGuire DB. The multidimensional phenomenon of cancer pain. In: McGuire DB, Yarbro CH, eds. Cancer Pain Management. Philadelphia: WB Saunders, 1987:1–20.
54. Hester NO. Assessment of acute pain. Baillieres Clin Paediatr 1995;3:561–577.
55. McGuire DB. Comprehensive and multidimensional assessment and measurement of pain. J Pain Symptom Manage 1992;7:312–319.
56. Twycross RG, Fairfield S. Pain in far-advanced cancer. Pain 1982;14:303–310.
57. Banning A, Sjogren P, Henriken H. Pain causes in 200 patients referred to a multidisciplinary cancer pain clinic. Pain 1991;45: 45–48.
58. Portenoy RK, Hagen NA. Breakthrough pain: Definition, prevalence, and characteristics. Pain 1990;41:273–281.
59. Twycross R, Harcourt J, Bergl S. A survey of pain in patients with advanced cancer. J Pain Symptom Manage 1996;12:273–282.
60. Bostrom B, Sandh M, Lundberg D, Fridlund B. Cancer-related pain in palliative care: Patients' perceptions of pain management. J Adv Nurs 2004;45:410–419.
61. Fink RM. Pain assessment: The cornerstone to optimal pain management. Analgesia 1997;9:17–25.
62. Gordon DB, Ward SE. Correcting patient misconceptions about pain. Am J Nurs 1995;95:43–45.
63. Keefe FJ, Dunsmore J. Pain behavior: Concepts and controversies. American Pain Society Journal 1992;1:92–100.
64. McGuire D, Kim HJ, Lang X. Measuring pain. In: Frank Stromberg M, Olsen SJ, eds. Instruments for Clinical Health Care Research, 3rd ed. Boston: Jones and Bartlett, 2004;603–644.
65. Turk DC, Matyas TA. Pain-related behaviors: Communication of pain. American Pain Society Journal 1992;1:109–111.
66. Craig KD. The facial expression of pain: Better than a thousand words? American Pain Society Journal 1992;1:153–162.
67. Ferrell BA. Overview of aging and pain. In: Ferrell BR, Ferrell BA, eds. Pain in the Elderly. Seattle, Wash.: IASP Press, 1996: 1–10.
68. Miaskowski C. The impact of age on a patient's perception of pain and ways it can be managed. Pain Manage Nurs 2000;1(Suppl 1): 2–7.
69. Ferrell BR. Patient education and nondrug interventions. In: Ferrell BR, Ferrell BA, eds. Pain in the Elderly. Seattle, Wash.: IASP Press, 1996;35–44.
70. Cleeland CS. Undertreatment of cancer pain in elderly patients. JAMA 1998;279:1914–1915.
71. Bernabei R, Gambassi G, Lapane K, Landi F, Gatsonia C, Dunlop R, Lipsitz L, Steel K, Mor V. Management of pain in elderly patients with cancer. SAGE Study Group. JAMA 1998;279: 1877–1882.
72. Vallerand AH. Gender differences in pain. Image J Nurs Sch 1995;27:235–237.
73. Miaskowski C. Women and pain. Crit Care Nurs Clin North Am 1997;9:453–458.
74. Berkley KJ. Sex, drugs and. . . . Nat Med 1996;2:1184–1185.
75. Unruh AM. Gender variations in clinical pain experience. Pain 1996;65:123–167.
76. Miaskowski C, Levine JD. Does opioid analgesia show a gender preference for females? Pain Forum 1999;8:34–44.
77. Vallerand AH, Polomano RC. The relationship of gender to pain. Pain Manage Nurs 2000;1(Suppl 1):8–15.
78. Dubreuil D, Kohn P. Reactivity and response to pain. Person Indiv Diff 1986;7:907–909.
79. Robin O, Vinard H, Varnet-Maury E, Saumet JL. Influence of sex and anxiety of pain threshold and tolerance. Func Neurol 1987; 2:73–179.
80. Mercadante S, Casuccio A, Pumo S, Fulfaro F. Factors influencing opioid response in advanced cancer patients with pain followed at home: The effects of age and gender. Support Care Cancer 2000;8:123–130.
81. Senior PA, Bhopal R. Ethnicity as a variable in epidemiological research. BMJ 1994;309:327–330.
82. Fink RS, Gates R. Cultural diversity and cancer pain. In: McGuire DB, Yarbro CH, Ferrell BR, eds. Cancer Pain Management, 2nd ed. Boston: Jones and Bartlett, 1995:19–39.
83. Bates MS, Edwards WT, Anderson KO. Ethnocultural influences on variation in chronic pain perception. Pain 1993;52:101–112.
84. Lipton JA, Marbach JJ. Ethnicity and the pain experience. Soc Sci Med 1984;19:1279–1298.
85. Zborowski M. People in Pain. San Francisco: Jossey-Bass, 1969.

86. Zola IK. Culture and symptoms: An analysis of patients' presenting complaints. Am Soc Rev 1996;31:615–630.
87. Martin ML. Ethnicity and analgesic practices [editorial]. Ann Emerg Med 2000;35:77–79.
88. Anderson KO, Richman SP, Hurley J, Palos G, Valero V, Mendoza TR, Gning I, Cleeland CS. Cancer pain management among underserved minority outpatients: Perceived needs and barriers to optimal control. Cancer 2002;94:2295–2304.
89. Dar R, Beach CM, Barden PL, Cleeland CS. Cancer pain in the marital system: A study of patients and their spouses. J Pain Symptom Manage 1992;7:87–93.
90. Lasch KE. Culture, pain, and culturally sensitive pain care. Pain Manage Nurs 2000;1(Suppl 1):16–22.
91. Spross J, Wolff Burke M. Nonpharmacological management of cancer pain. In: McGuire DB, Yarbro CH, Ferrell BR, eds. Cancer Pain Management, 2nd ed. Boston: Jones and Bartlett, 1995: 159–205.
92. Dunn KS, Horgas AL. Religious and nonreligious coping in older adults experiencing chronic pain. Pain Manag Nurs 2004; 5:19–28.
93. Brunelli C, Costantini M, Di Giulio P, Gallucci M, Fusco F, Miccinesi G, Paci E, Peruselli C, Morino P, Piazza M, Tamburini M. Quality of life evaluation: When do terminally ill cancer patients and health-care providers agree? J Pain Symptom Manage 1998;15:151–158.
94. Grossman SA, Sheidler VR, Swedeen K, Mucenski J, Piantadosi S. Correlation of patient and caregiver ratings of cancer pain. J Pain Symptom Manage 1991;6:53–57.
95. Ferrell BR, Eberts M, McCaffery M, Grant M. Clinical decision making and pain. Cancer Nurs 1991;14:289–297.
96. Carpenter JS, Brockopp D. Comparison of patients' ratings and examination of nurses' responses to pain intensity rating scales. Cancer Nurs 1995;18:292–298.
97. Puntillo KA, Miaskowski C, Kehrle K, Stannard D, Gleeson S, Nye P. Relationship between behavioral and physiological indicators of pain, critical care patients, self-reports of pain, and opioid administration. Crit Care Med 1997;25:1159–1166.
98. Werner P, Cohen-Mansfield J, Watson V, Pasis S. Pain in participants of adult day care centers: Assessment by different raters. J Pain Symptom Manage 1998;15:8–17.
99. Jensen MP, Karoly P. Self-report scales and procedures for assessing pain in adults. In: Turk DC, Melzak R, eds. Handbook of Pain Assessment. New York: Guilford Press, 1992: 135–151.
100. Ohnhaus EE, Adler R. Methodological problems in the measurement of pain: A comparison between the verbal rating scale and the visual analogue scale. Pain 1975;1:379–384.
101. Ahles TA, Ruckdeschel JC, Blanchard EB. Cancer-related pain: II. Assessment with visual analogue scales. J Psychosom Res 1984; 28:121–124.
102. Scott J, Huskisson EC. Graphic representation of pain. Pain 1976; 2:175–184.
103. Revill SI, Robinson JO, Rosen M, Hogg MIJ. The reliability of a linear analogue for evaluating pain. Anaesthesia 1976;31:1191–1998.
104. Kremer E, Atkinson J. Pain language: Affect. J Psychosom Res 1984;28:125–132.
105. Shannon MM, Ryan MA, D'Agostino N, Brescia FJ. Assessment of pain in advanced cancer patients. J Pain Symptom Manage 1995;10:274–278.
106. Herr KA, Mobily PR. Comparison of selected pain assessment tools for use with the elderly. Appl Nurs Res 1993;6:39–49.
107. Wallenstein SL, Heidrich G, Kaiko R, Houde RW. Clinical evaluation of mild analgesics: The measurement of clinical pain. Br J Clin Pharmacol 1980;10:319S–327S.
108. Paice JA, Cohen FL. Validity of a verbally administered numeric rating scale to measure cancer pain intensity. Cancer Nurs 1997;20:88–93.
109. Ferraz MB, Quaresma MR, Aquino LRL, Atra E, Tugwell P, Goldsmith CH. Reliability of pain scales in the assessment of literate and illiterate patients with rheumatoid arthritis. J Rheumatol 1990;17:1022–1024.
110. Wong DL, Baker CM. Pain in children: comparison of assessment scales. Pediatr Nurs 1988;14:9–17.
111. Wong DL, Hockenberry-Eaton M, Wilson D, Winkelstein ML, Schwartz P. Wong's Essential of Pediatric Nursing, 6th ed. St. Louis: Mosby, 2001:1301.
112. Matsumoto D. Ethnic differences in affect intensity, emotion judgments, display rule attitudes, and self-reported emotional expression in an American sample. Motiv Emot 1993;17: 107–123.
113. Frank AJM, Moll JMH, Hort JF. A comparison of three ways of measuring pain. Rheumatol Rehabil 1982;21:211–217.
114. Wilson JS, Cason CL, Grissom NL. Distraction: An effective intervention for alleviating pain during venipuncture. J Emerg Nurs 1995;21:87–94.
115. Stuppy DJ. The Faces Pain Scale: Reliability and validity with mature adults. Appl Nurs Res 1998;11:84–89.
116. Casas JM, Wagenheim BR, Banchero R, Mendoza-Romero J. Hispanic masculinity: Myth or psychological schema meriting clinical consideration. Hisp J Behav Sci 1994;16:315–331.
117. Bieri D, Reeve R, Champion GD, Addicoat L, Ziegler JB. The Faces Pain Scale for the self assessment of the severity of pain experienced by children: Development, initial validation, and preliminary investigation for ratio scale properties. Pain 1990;41: 139–150.
118. Jensen MP, Engel JM, McKearnan KA, Hoffman AJ. Validity of pain intensity assessment in persons with cerebral palsy: A comparison of six scales. J Pain 2003;4:56–63.
119. Taylor LJ, Herr K. Evaluation of the faces pain scale with minority older adults. J Gerontol Nurs 2002;27:15–23.
120. Hicks CL, von Baeyer CL, Spafford P, van Korlaar I, Goodenough B. The Faces Scale—Revised: Toward a common metric in pediatric pain measurement. Pain 2001;93:173–183.
121. Spagrud LJ, Piira T, von Baeyer C. Children's self-report of pain intensity: The Faces Pain Scale—Revised. Am J Nurs 2003;103: 62–64.
122. Herr K. Assessment of pain intensity in older adults: Is there a better way? Paper presented at the 19th Annual American Pain Society Scientific Meeting, Atlanta, GA, 2001.
123. Dalton JA, McNaull F. A call for standardizing the clinical rating of pain intensity using a 0 to 10 rating scale. Cancer Nurs 1998; 21:46–49.
124. Jensen MP, Turner JA, Romano JM. What is the maximum number of levels needed in pain intensity measurement. Pain 1994;58:387–392.
125. Rodriguez CS. Pain measurement in the elderly: A review. Pain Manage Nurs 2001;2:38–46.
126. Jensen M. The validity and reliability of pain measures in adults with cancer. J Pain 2003;4;2–21.
127. Gift AG. Visual analogue scales: Measurement of subjective phenomena. Nurs Res 1989;38:286–288.
128. Grossman SA, Sheidler VR, McGuire DB, Geer C, Santor D, Piantadosi S. A comparison of the Hopkins Pain Rating

Instrument with standard visual analogue and verbal descriptor scales in patients with cancer pain. J Pain Symptom Manage 1992;7:196–203.
129. Jensen MP, Karoly P, Braver S. The measurement of clinical pain intensity: a comparison of six methods. Pain 1986;27:117–126.
130. Kremer E, Hampton Atkinson J, Ignelzi RJ. Measurement of pain: Patient preference does not confound pain measurement. Pain 1981;10:241–248.
131. Taylor LJ, Herr K. Pain intensity assessment: A comparison of selected pain intensity scales for use in cognitively intact and cognitively impaired African American older adults. Pain Manage Nurs 2003;4:87–95.
132. Jones K, Fink R, Hutt E, Vojir C, Clark L, et al. Unpublished data, University of Colorado Health Sciences Center, 2004.
133. Carey SJ, Turpin C, Smith J, Whatley J, Haddox D. Improving pain management in an acute care setting: The Crawford Long Hospital of Emory University experience. Orthopaedic Nursing 1997;16:29–36.
134. Cleeland CS, Syrjala KL. How to assess cancer pain. In: Turk DC, Melzack R, eds. Handbook of Pain Assessment. New York: Guilford Press, 1992:362–390.
135. Melzak R. The short-form McGill Pain Questionnaire. Pain 1987;30:191–197.
136. Daut RL, Cleeland CS, Flanery R. Development of the Wisconsin Brief Pain Inventory to assess pain in cancer and other diseases. Pain 1983;17:197–210.
137. Fishman B, Pasternak S, Wallenstein SL, Houde RW, Holland JC, Foley KM. The Memorial Pain Assessment Card: A valid instrument for the evaluation of cancer pain. Cancer 1987;60: 1151–1158.
138. Ferrell B. Patient pain questionnaire. Available at: http://www.cityofhope.org/prc/res_inst.asp (accessed 2/15/05).
139. Desbiens NA, Wu AW. Pain and suffering in seriously ill hospitalized patients. J Am Geriatr Soc 2000;48:S183–S186.
140. Tranmer J, Heyland D, Dudgeon D, Groll D, Squires-Graham M, Coulson K. Measuring the symptom experience of seriously ill cancer and noncancer hospitalized patients near the end of life with the Memorial Symptom Assessment Scale. J Pain Symptom Manage 2003;25:420–429.
141. Ferrell BA, Ferrell BR, Rivera L. Pain in cognitively impaired nursing home patients. J Pain Symptom Manage 1995;10:591–598.
142. Thomas M, Roy R. Epidemiology of chronic pain in the elderly. In: The changing nature of pain complaints over the lifespan. New York: Plenum Press, 1999:143–154.
143. Weiner D, Peterson BL, Ladd K, McConnell E, Keefe FJ. Pain in nursing home residents: An exploration of prevalence, staff perspectives, and practical aspects of measurement. Clin J Pain 1999;15:92–101.
144. Feldt KS, Ryden MB, Miles S. Treatment of pain in cognitively impaired compared with cognitively intact elder patients with hip fracture. J Am Geriatr Soc 1998;46:1079–1985.
145. Feldt KS. The Checklist of Nonverbal Pain Indicators (CNPI). Pain Manage Nurs 2000;1:13–21.
146. Klopfenstein CE, Herrman FR, Mamie C, Van Gessel E, Forster A. Pain intensity and pain relief after surgery: A comparison between patients' reported assessments and nurses' and physicians' observations. Acta Anaesthesiol Scand 2000; 44:58–62.
147. Lee DS, McPherson ML, Zuckermann IH. Quality assurance: Documentation of pain assessment in hospice patients. Am J Hospice Palliat Care 1992;9:38–43.
148. Tucker KI. A new risk emerges: Provider accountability for inadequate treatment of pain. Ann Long-Term Care 2001;9: 52–55.
149. Bachino C, Snow AL, Kunik ME, Cody M, Wristers K. Principles of pain assessment in non-communicative demented patients. Clin Gerontol 2001;23:97–115.
150. Bruera E, Fainsinger RL, Miller MJ, Kuehn N. The assessment of pain intensity in patients with cognitive failure: A preliminary report. J Pain Symptom Manage 1992;7:267–270.
151. Stiefel F, Fainsinger R, Bruera E. Acute confusional states in patients with advanced cancer. J Pain Symptom Manage 1992;7: 94–98.
152. Lynn J, Teno JM, Phillips RS, Wu AW, Desbiens N, Harrold J, Claessens MT, Wenger N, Kreling B, Connors AF Jr. Perceptions by family members of the dying experience of older and seriously ill patients. SUPPORT Investigators. Study to Understand Prognoses and Preferences for Outcomes and Risks of Treatment. Ann Intern Med 1997;126:97–106.
153. Morita T, Tei Y, Inoue S. Impaired communication capacity and agitated delirium in the final week of terminally ill cancer patients: Prevalence and identification of research focus. J Pain Symptom Manage 2003;26:827–834.
154. Anand KJS, Craig KD. New perspectives on the definition of pain. Pain 1996;67:3–6.
155. Keefe FJ, Dunsmore J. Pain behavior: Concepts and controversies. American Pain Society J 1992;1:92–100.
156. McCaffery M, Ferrell BR. How vital are vital signs? Nursing 1992;22:43–46.
157. Prkachin KM, Berzins S, Mercer SR. Encoding and decoding of pain expressions: A judgment study. Pain 1994;58:253–259.
158. Wilkie DJ, Keefe FJ, Dodd MJ, Copp LA. Behavior of patients with lung cancer: Description and associations with oncologic and pain variables. Pain 1992;51:231–240.
159. Argoff CE, Cranmer KW. The pharmacological management of chronic pain in long-term care settings: Balancing efficacy and safety. Consulting Pharmacist 2003;Suppl C:4–24.
160. Jones K, Fink R, Hutt E, Clark L, Pepper G, Scott J, et al. Improving Pain Management in Nursing Homes. Staff Training Workbook—Nursing Edition. OTR04054-0404. Denver, Colo.: University of Colorado Health Sciences Center, School of Nursing, 2003.
161. Herr K, Decker S. Assessment of pain in older adults with severe cognitive impairment. Ann Long-Term Care 2004;12:46–52.
162. Cohen-Mansfield J, Creedon M. Nursing staff members' perceptions of pain indicators in persons with severe dementia. Clin J Pain 2002;18:64–73.
163. LeResche L, Dworkin SF. Facial expressions of pain and emotions in chronic TMD patients. Pain 1988;35:71–78.
164. Prkachin KM, Mercer SR. Pain expression in patients with shoulder pathology: Validity, properties and relationship to sickness impact. Pain 1989;39:257–265.
165. Ekman P, Friesen WV. Facial Action Coding System: A technique for the measurement of facial movement. Palo Alto, Calif.: Consulting Psychologists Press, 1978.
166. Cohen-Mansfield J, Marx MS. Pain and depression in the nursing home: Corroborating results. J Gerontol 1993;48:96–97.
167. Parmelee PA, Smith B, Katz IR. Pain complaints and cognitive status among elderly institution residents. J Am Geriatr Soc 1993;41:517–522.
168. Fisher-Morris M, Gellatly A. The experience and expression of pain in Alzheimer patients. Age Aging 1997;26:497–500.

169. Werner P, Cohen-Mansfield J, Watson V, Pasis S. Pain in participants of adult day care centers: Assessment by different raters. J Pain Symptom Manage 1998;15:8–17.
170. Lapalio LR, Sakla SS. Distinguishing Lewy body dementia. Hospice Practice (Office Edition) 1998;33:93–108.
171. Beneditti F, Vighetti S, Ricco C, Lagna E, Bergamasco B, Pinessi L, Rainero I. Pain threshold and tolerance in Alzheimer's disease. Pain 1999;80: 377–382.
172. Porter FL, Malortra KM, Wolf CM, Morris JC, Miller JP, Smith MC. Dementia and response to pain in the elderly. Pain 1996;68: 413–421.
173. Scherder E, Bouma A, Borkent M, Rahman O. Alzheimer patients report less pain intensity and pain affect than non-demented elderly. Psychiatry 1999;62:265–272.
174. Kovach CR, Noonan PE, Griffie J, Muchka S, Weissman DE. Use of the assessment of discomfort in dementia protocol. Appl Nurs Res 2001;14:193–200.
175. Farrell MJ, Katz B, Helm RD. The impact of dementia on the pain experience. Pain 1996;67:7–15.
176. Marzinski LR. The tragedy of dementia: Clinically assessing pain in the confused nonverbal elderly. J Gerontol Nurs 1991;17: 25–28.
177. Huffman JC, Kinik ME. Assessment and understanding of pain in patients with dementia. Gerontologist 2000;40:574–581.
178. Herr KA, Mobily PC, Kohart FJ, Wagenaar D. Evaluation of the faces pain scale for use with the elderly. Clin J Pain 1998;14: 29–38.
179. Manz BD, Mosier R, Nusser-Gerlach MA, Bergstrom N, Agrawal S. Pain assessment in the cognitively impaired and unimpaired elderly. Pain Manage Nurs 2000;1:106–115.
180. Chibnall JT, Tait RC. Pain assessment in cognitively impaired and unimpaired older adults: A comparison of four scales. Pain 2001;92:173–186.
181. Kamel H, Phlavan M, Malekgoudarzi B, Gogel P, Morley JE. Utilizing pain assessment scales increases the frequency of diagnosing pain among elderly nursing home residents. J Pain Symptom Manage 2001;21:450–455.
182. Closs SJ, Barr B, Briggs M, Cash K, Seers K. A comparison of five pain assessment scales for nursing home residents with varying degrees of cognitive impairment. J Pain Symptom Manage 2004;27:196–205.
183. Buffum M, Miaskowski C, Sands L, Brod M. A pilot study of the relationship between discomfort and agitation in patients with dementia. Geriatr Nurs 2001;22:80–85.
184. Richards JS, Neopomuceno C, Riles M, Suer Z. Assessing pain behavior: The UAB Pain Behavior Scale. Pain 1982;14: 393–398.
185. Kerns RD. Turk DC, Rudy TE. The West Haven–Yale Multidimensional Pain Inventory (WHYMPI). Pain 1985;23:345–356.
186. Vlaeyen JW, Pernot DF, Kole SA, Schuerman JA, Van EH, Groenman NH. Assessment of the components of observed chronic pain behavior: The Checklist for Interpersonal Behavior (CHIP). Pain 1990;43:337–347.
187. Hurley AC, Volicer BJ, Hanrahan PA, Houde S, Volicer L. Assessment of discomfort in advanced Alzheimer patients. Res Nurs Health 1992;15:369–377.
188. Kovach CR, Weissman D, Griffie J, Matson S, Muchka S. Assessment and treatment of discomfort for people with late-stage dementia. J Pain Symptom Manage 1999;18:412–419.
189. Kovach CR, Noonan PE, Griffie J, Muchka S, Weissman DE. Use of the Assessment of Discomfort in Dementia protocol. Appl Nurs Res 2001;14:193–200.
190. Kovach CR, Noonan PE, Griffie J, Muchka S, Weissman DE. The Assessment of Discomfort in Dementia protocol. Pain Manage Nurs 2002;3:16–27.
191. Snow AL, Weber JB, O'Malley KJ, Cody M, Beck C, Bruera E, Ashton C, Kunik ME. NOPPAIN: A nursing assistant-administered pain assessment instrument for use in dementia. Dement Geriatr Cogn Disord 2004;17:240–246.
192. Villanueva MR, Smith TL, Erickson JS, Lee AC, Singer C. Pain Assessment for the Dementing Elderly (PADE): Reliability and validity of a new measure. J Am Med Dir Assoc 2003;4:1–8.
193. Decker SA, Perry AG. The development and testing of the PATCOA to assess pain in confused older adults. Pain Manage Nurs 2003;4:77–86.
194. Warden V, Hurley AC, Volicer L. Development and psychometric evaluation of the Pain Assessment in Advanced Dementia (PAINAD) scale. J Am Med Dir Assoc 2003;9–15.
195. Merkel SI, Voepel-Lewis T, Shayevitz JR, Malviya S. The FLACC: A behavioral scale for scoring postoperative pain in young children. Pediatr Nurs 1997;23:293–297.
196. Fuchs-Lacelle S, Hadjistavropoulos T. Development and preliminary validation of the Pain Assessment Checklist for Seniors with Limited Ability to Communicate (PACSLAC). Pain Manage Nurs 2004;5:37–49.
197. Abbey J, Piller N, De Bellis A, Esterman A, Parker D, Giles L, Lowcay B. The Abbey Pain Scale: A 1 minute numerical indicator for people with end-stage dementia. Int J Palliat Nurs 2004;10: 6–13.
198. Herr K, Decker S, Bjoro K. State of the art review of tools for assessment of pain in nonverbal older adults. Iowa City, Iowa: University of Iowa, College of Nursing, 2004. Available at: http://www.nursing.uiowa.edu/centers/gnirc/state%20of%20art%20review.htm (accessed November 5, 2004).
199. Miller J, Neelson V, Dalton J, Ng'andu N, Bailey DJ, Layman E, Hosfeld A. The assessment of discomfort in elderly confused patients: A preliminary study. J Neurosci Nurs 1996;28: 175–182.
200. Simons W, Malabar R. Assessing pain in elderly patients who cannot respond verbally. J Adv Nurs 1995;22:663–669.
201. Cunningham N. Primary requirements for an ethical definition of pain. Pain Forum 1999;8:93–99.
202. Choiniere M, Melzack R, Girard N, Rondeau J, Paquin MJ. Comparisons between patients' and nurses' assessments of pain and medication efficacy in severe burn injuries. Pain 1990;40: 143–152.
203. Teske K, Daut RL, Cleeland CS. Relationships between nurses' observations and patients' self-reports of pain. Pain 1983;16: 289–296.
204. Weiner D, Peterson B, Keefe F. Chronic pain associated behaviors in the nursing home: Resident versus caregiver perceptions. Pain 1999;80:577–588.
205. Clipp EC, George LK. Patients with cancer and their spouse caregivers. Cancer 1992;69:1074–1079.
206. Madison JL, Wilkie DJ. Family members' perceptions of cancer pain: Comparisons with patient sensory report and by patient psychologic status. Nurs Clin North Am 1995;30: 625–645.
207. Yeager KA, Miaskowski C, Dibble SL, Wallhagen M. Differences in pain knowledge and perceptions of the pain experience between outpatients with cancer and their family caregivers. Oncol Nurs Forum 1995;22:1235–1241.
208. Bruera E, Sweeney C, Willey J, Palmer JL, Strasses F, Strauch E. Perception of discomfort by relatives and nurses in unresponsive

terminally ill patients with cancer: A prospective study. J Pain Symptom Manage 2003;26:818–826.

209. Cohen-Mansfield J. Relatives assessment of pain in cognitively impaired nursing home residents. J Pain Symptom Manage 2002;24:562–571.

210. Bruera E, Kuehn N, Miller MJ, Selmser P, MacMillan K. The Edmonton Symptom Assessment System (ESAS): A simple method for the assessment of palliative care patients. J Palliat Care 1991;7:6–9.

211. Rees E, Hardy J, Ling J, Broadley K, A'Hearn R. The use of the Edmonton Symptom Assessment Scale within a palliative care unit in the UK. Palliat Med 1998;12:75–82.

212. Levy M. Pain management in advanced cancer. Semin Oncol 1985;12:394–410.

213. Coluzzi PH, Volker B, Miaskowski C. Comprehensive Pain Management in Terminal Illness. Sacramento: California State Hospice Association, 1996.

APPENDIX 5–1
Instructions for Use of the Edmonton Comfort Assessment Form (ECAF)

Capital Health

Regional Palliative Care Program Guideline

Title: Edmonton Comfort Assessment Form (ECAF) - Instructions for Use

Date: June 8, 1998 **Approved By:** Program Director

Purpose: Patient assessment is required throughout the palliative care process. The majority of patients will experience confusion and delirium before death. In these patients, who are unable to communicate, primary caregivers, and staffs input is important for assessment and for the opportunity to explain to the caregiver how to interpret the discomfort of the patient. This evaluation may decrease the caregivers concerns regarding the comfort of their family/friend

Procedure:

1. ECAF vs. ESAS: When to use: All patients admitted to all the palliative programs within the Edmonton region are assessed using the ESAS. When patients reach the unresponsive state of their illness, the ESAS will be discontinued and replaced by the ECAF. If patients present with brief periods of confusion or somnolence, then expect it to be reversible. The assessment should continue with ESAS. When the patient is considered to have reached the last hours or days of life the assessment will be changed to the ECAF.

   The decision to change the assessment system will be determined by the physicians and/or team leaders in the Acute Palliative Care Unit, it will be written by the Unit Managers in the 3 hospices, by the physician or nurse consultants at the Regional Palliative Care Program, and the Referral Centre palliative care program. In Home Care, the decision to change from ESAS to ECAF will be made by the Palliative Home Care Coordinator.

2. Frequency of Completion: At the end of the day/evening shift in the (Acute Palliative Care Unit), day shift in the (Hospices) or the nursing visit for patients assessed at home or in the referral centres.

3. Method of Completion: Please note that the form has two parts.

   a) Main Caregiver: This part should only be completed by the caregiver that is at the bedside most of the time; at home, in hospice, or in the palliative care unit. If no caregiver is present most of the time at the bedside checkmark not applicable . If there is a caregiver, he or she should be presented with the upper portion of the form and asked to circle the item #1 (comfort) and to check the appropriate reasons under item #2.

b) Nurse Score: The nurse will complete the form regarding behaviors. Please notice that these also have three items:
   i) Observed behavior: Rate the observed behavior according to the graph by placing an X in the appropriate box. Calculate the total score by adding the corresponding number for each X together. Maximum score is 24.
   ii) Checkmark the suspected reason(s).
   iii) Enter the global comfort assessment score from 0-10 (same as caregiver scale above).

4. After completing the form the information will be transcribed to the ECAF Graph. The ECAF Graph has the following components:

a) Date and admission day: Please notice that there is enough room for two daily assessments (Acute Palliative Care Unit). Patients admitted to the hospices will undergo one assessment a day. Patients seen by the other teams will have one assessment done on occasion of each visit.

b) Caregiver VAS (Item 1): Fill the bar up to the number across by the caregiver in the same way as we graph the results of the ESAS. If no caregiver enter N for not applicable.

c) Caregiver Reason (Item 2): Simply check the reason(s) that have been checked in the ECAF form by the caregiver.

d) Nurse Score (0-24): Write down on the space the number that results from adding each of the 6 line items for the observed behaviour (Item 1 of the Nursing Score).

e) Nurse Reason: Check the suspected reason(s) identified by the nurse during the assessment.

f) RN VAS: Enter the number of the nurse's assessment of the level of comfort (0-10).

g) Physician VAS: Upon every visit (once a day on acute unit), on each visit in acute care, hospice and home) the physician assesses the level of comfort and enters the global comfort assessment score (0-10).

GUIDELINES FOR USING THE EDMONTON SYMPTOM ASSESSMENT SHEET (ESAS VISUAL ANALOGUE, NUMERICAL SCALE AND GRAPH)

1. This tool is designed to assist the patient in the assessment of his/her symptoms. Those symptoms include pain, activity, nausea, depression, anxiety, drowsiness, appetite, wellbeing and shortness of breath. The patient and family should be taught how to complete the scales. It is the patients opinion of the severity of the symptoms that is the "gold standard" for symptom assessment.

2. There are two formats for the ESAS. The first is a visual analogue scale (ESAS) that is 100mm long. The patient marks the line to indicate where the symptom is between the two extremes. (See Tool) This tool is used on the acute palliative care units, and referral hospital sites.

3. The other format, ESAS numerical is a scale from 0 to 10 where the patient circles the most appropriate number to indicate where the symptom is between the two extremes. This tool is used in all other settings, such as home care and continuing care. This tool is considered easier for a patient to complete with minimal assistance.

No pain	0	1	2	3	4	5	6	7	8	9	10	worst possible pain

The circled number on the continuum is then transcribed onto the symptom assessment graph. (ESAS graph) (See #12)

4. Synonyms for words that may be difficult for the patients to comprehend include the following:

Depression	-	blue or sad
Anxiety	-	nervous or restless
Drowsy	-	sleepy
Wellbeing	-	overall comfort both physical and psychological, truthfully answering the question, how are you?

5. For Home Care, during each telephone or personal contact, the ESAS scale should be completed and the values transferred to the ESAS graph. If the patient's symptoms are in good control, and there are no predominant psychosocial issues, the ESAS can be completed 2 to 3 times a week.

In continuing care settings the ESAS should be completed daily. Referral hospital site consultants will utilize the tool in their assessment on every visit. The ESAS is completed twice (~1000h, 1800h) on the acute palliative care unit.

6. In the home, or hospice, if the patient's symptoms are not in good control (>5/10), the nurse should be notifying the family doctor, and visiting the patient on a daily basis, until the symptoms are back within good control. (See #8)

7. If symptom management is not attained, or consultation about possible care options is needed, a consult to the Regional Palliative Care Program should occur. (***Family doctor must agree***). Informal consultation with the Regional program nurses and physicians can occur at any time.

8. A patient may consistently score high on an isolated symptom, and treatment has been actively pursued, until no resolution is possible. If at this point, consensus is reached between the coordinator and the family practitioner and/or consultant that a symptom cannot be modified, visits may return to their normal pattern for that patient.

9. Ideally, the patient should fill out their own assessment (ESAS). However, if there is cognitive impairment (ie: patient's mini-mental score below normal for their age and education) or lack of understanding on how to mark the continuum, the assessment becomes family assisted, or nurse.

10. The person who did the assessment must be identified on the symptom control graph. (ESAS graph)

P	=	Patient
N	=	Nurse/Health Care Worker
NA	=	Nurse/Health Care Worker Assisted
F	=	Family/Primary Caregiver

11. If the assessment is done by the nurse and she/he is unable to communicate with the patient (ie: cognitively impaired and cognition level might be reversible) she/he assesses the following areas only: pain, activity, nausea, drowsiness, appetite and shortness of breath.

NB: **ACTIVITY IS A PURPOSEFUL VOLUNTARY ACTION BY THE PATIENT. CONSIDER THE PATIENT NOT ACTIVE IF HE/SHE IS RESTLESS OR AGITATED**

APPETITE BECOMES THE ABSENCE OR PRESENCE OF EATING

NAUSEA BECOMES THE ABSENCE OR PRESENCE OF RETCHING, VOMITING, ETC.

12. The nurse can document her assessment directly on the Symptom Assessment Graph (ESASII). She does not have to fill out the ESAS scale. The ESAS graph is kept in the patient home envelope, and a copy on the patient chart. The chart copy should be brought to the home and updated with the home copy, on each visit.

13. A patient has the right to refuse the symptom assessment or any question on it. In the event the patient refuses to do his/her own assessment, it becomes a nurse assessment (see # 10,11)

15. The ESAS is available in Cantonese, German, French and in faces, for those patients who do not read.

16. The ESASII (graph) provides an excellent clinical "picture" or "snapshot" of how a patient is feeling in various physical or psychological areas. You may see a symptom increase or decrease over time. On rare occasions, a patient may score everything as 9 or 10 out of 10. The graph looks very black and shows a picture of total pain or total suffering. A patient with this picture requires interdisciplinary support.[1]

17. The Graph also contains space to add the patient's mini mental state exam score. The "normal" box refers to the normal range for the patient, based on age and education level (see Instructions for MMSE).

18. Modified EFAT score can be entered on this form (as applicable).

19. A new assessment tool for patients who are not able to complete their own ESAS is currently being developed. (Edmonton Discomfort Assessment Tool).

6

Judith A. Paice and Perry G. Fine

Pain at the End of Life

"How much I suffered last night . . . there are no words to express it, only howls of pain could do so."
—Alphonse Daudet[1]

- ***Key Points***
- *Pain is highly prevalent in palliative care, yet the majority of individuals can obtain good relief with available treatment options.*
- *An awareness of barriers to adequate pain care allows palliative care nurses to assess for and to plan interventions to overcome these obstacles when caring for patients. Advocacy is a critical role of the palliative care nurse.*
- *Assessment of pain, including a thorough history and comprehensive physical exam, guides the development of the pharmacological and nonpharmacological treatment plan.*
- *Pharmacological therapies include nonopioids, opioids, coanalgesics, cancer therapies, and in some cases, interventional techniques.*
- *Intractable pain and symptoms, although not common, must be treated aggressively. In some cases, palliative sedation may be warranted.*

Of the many symptoms experienced by those at the end of life, pain is one of the most common and most feared.[1a,2] However, this fear is largely unfounded because the majority of patients with terminal illness can obtain relief. Nurses are critical members of the palliative care team, particularly in providing pain management. The nurse's role begins with assessment and continues through the development of a plan of care and its implementation. During this process, the nurse provides education and counsel to the patient, family, and other team members. Nurses also are critical for developing institutional policies and monitoring outcomes that ensure good pain management for all patients within their palliative care program. To provide optimal pain control, all health care professionals must understand the frequency of pain at the end of life, the barriers that prevent good management, the assessment of this syndrome, and the treatments used to provide relief.

Prevalence of Pain

The prevalence of pain in the terminally ill varies by diagnosis and other factors. Approximately one third of persons who are actively receiving treatment for cancer and two thirds of those with advanced malignant disease experience pain.[3–6] Individuals at particular risk for undertreatment include the elderly, minorities, and women.[7,8] Almost three quarters of patients with advanced cancer admitted to the hospital experience pain upon admission.[9] In a study of cancer patients very near the end of life, pain occurred in 54% at 4 weeks and 34% at 1 week before death.[10] In other studies of patients admitted to palliative care units, pain often is the dominant symptom, along with fatigue and dyspnea.[1a] Children dying of cancer also are at risk for pain and suffering.[11]

More recently, an attempt has been made to characterize the pain experience of those with human immunodeficiency virus (HIV) disease, a disorder frequently seen in palliative care settings.[12,13] Headache, abdominal pain, chest pain, and neuropathies are the most frequently reported types of pain. Lower CD4 cell counts and HIV-1 RNA levels are associated with higher rates of neuropathy.[14] Numerous studies have reported undertreatment of persons with HIV disease, including those patients with a history of addictive disease.[15,16]

Unfortunately, there has been little characterization of the pain prevalence and experience of patients with other life-threatening disorders. However, those working in palliative care are well aware that pain frequently accompanies many of the neuromuscular and cardiovascular disorders, such as multiple sclerosis and stroke, seen at the end of life.[17–19] Furthermore, many patients in hospice and palliative care are elderly and more likely to have existing chronic pain syndromes, such as osteoarthritis or low back pain.[20]

Additional research is needed to fully characterize the frequency of pain and the type of pain syndromes seen in patients at the end of life. This information will lead to improved detection, assessment, and, ultimately, treatment. Unfortunately, pain continues to be undertreated, even when prevalence rates and syndromes are well understood. The undertreatment is largely due to barriers related to health care professionals, the system, and patients and their families.

Barriers to Pain Relief

Barriers to good pain relief are numerous and pervasive. Often, because of lack of education, misconceptions, or attitudinal issues, these barriers contribute to the large numbers of patients who do not get adequate pain relief.[21,22] Careful examination of these barriers provides a guide for changing individual practice, as well as building an institutional plan within the palliative care program to improve pain relief (Table 6–1). Most studies address the barriers associated with cancer pain. Therefore, barriers facing individuals with other disorders commonly seen in palliative care are not well characterized. One might suggest that these individuals are affected to an even greater extent as biases may be more pronounced in those with noncancer diagnoses.

Table 6–1
Barriers to Cancer Pain Management

Problems related to health care professionals
Inadequate knowledge of pain management
Poor assessment of pain
Concern about regulation of controlled substances
Fear of patient addiction
Concern about side effects of analgesics
Concern about patients' becoming tolerant to analgesics
Problems related to the health care system
Low priority given to cancer pain treatment
Inadequate reimbursement
Restrictive regulation of controlled substances
Problems of availability of treatment or access to it
Problems related to patients
Reluctance to report pain
Concern about distracting physicians from treatment of underlying disease
Fear that pain means disease is worse
Concern about not being a "good" patient
Reluctance to take pain medications
Fear of addiction or of being thought of as an addict
Worries about unmanageable side effects
Concern about becoming tolerant to pain medications

Adapted from References 222, 223.

Health Care Providers

Fears related to opioids held by professionals lead to underuse of these analgesics. Numerous surveys have revealed that physicians, nurses, and pharmacists express concerns about addiction, tolerance, and side effects of morphine and related compounds.[23] Inevitability of pain is also expressed, despite evidence to the contrary.[24] Not surprisingly, lack of attention to pain and its treatment during basic education is frequently cited.[24–27] Those providing care at the end of life must evaluate their own knowledge and beliefs, including cultural biases, and strive to educate themselves and colleagues.[28]

Health Care Settings

Lack of availability of opioids is pervasive, affecting not only sparsely populated rural settings but also inner-city pharmacies reluctant to carry these medications.[29–31] Pain management continues to be a low priority in some health care settings, although the Joint Commission on Accreditation of Healthcare Organizations (JCAHO) standards on pain management are helping to alleviate this problem.[32,33] All JCAHO-certified clinical settings must evaluate their procedures to ensure that pain is appropriately assessed, treated, and documented.

Patients and Families

Understanding these barriers will lead the professional to better educate and better counsel patients and their families.[34] Since these fears are pervasive, patients and family members or support persons should be asked if they are concerned about addiction and tolerance (often described as becoming "immune" to the drug by laypersons).[35] Studies have suggested that these fears lead to undermedication and increased intensity of pain.[36] Concerns about being a "good" patient or belief in the inevitability of cancer pain lead patients to hesitate in reporting pain.[22,37,38] In these studies, less educated and older patients were more likely to express these beliefs.[39–41] Patients seeking active treatment may believe that admitting to pain or other symptoms may reduce their eligibility for clinical trials.

At the end of life, patients may need to rely on family members or other support persons to dispense medications. Each person's concerns must be addressed or provision of medication may be inadequate. Studies suggest that little concordance exists between patients' and family members' beliefs regarding analgesics.[42,43] The interdisciplinary team is essential, with nurses, social workers, chaplains, physicians, volunteers, and others providing exploration of the meaning of pain and possible barriers to good relief. Education, counseling, reframing, and spiritual support are imperative. Ersek[22] provided an excellent review of the assessment and interventional approaches indicated for specific patient barriers.

Effects of Unrelieved Pain

Although many professionals and laypersons fear that opioid analgesics lead to shortened life, there is significant evidence to the contrary. Inadequate pain relief hastens death by increasing physiological stress, potentially diminishing immunocompetence, decreasing mobility, worsening proclivities toward pneumonia and thromboembolism, and increasing work of breathing and myocardial oxygen requirements.[44,45] Furthermore, pain may lead to spiritual death as the individual's quality of life is impaired.[46,47] Therefore, it is the professional and ethical responsibility of clinicians to focus on and attend to adequate pain relief for their patients and to properly educate patients and their caregivers about opioid analgesic therapies.

Assessment and Common Pain Syndromes

Comprehensive assessment of pain is imperative. This must be conducted initially, regularly throughout the treatment, and during any changes in the patient's pain state.[48] A randomized controlled trial using algorithms found that the comprehensive pain assessment integral to these algorithms contributed to reduced pain intensity scores.[49] For a complete discussion of pain assessment, see Chapter 5.

Pharmacological Management of Pain in Advanced and End-Stage Disease

A sound understanding of pharmacotherapy in the treatment of pain is of great importance in palliative care nursing. First, this knowledge allows the nurse to contribute to and fully understand the comprehensive plan of care. Thorough understanding also allows the nurse to recognize and assess medication-related adverse effects, to understand drug–drug and drug–disease interactions, and to educate patients and caregivers regarding appropriate medication usage. This will assure a comfortable process of dying for the well-being of the patient and for the sake of those in attendance.

This section provides an overview of the most commonly used agents and some of the newer pharmaceutical agents available in the United States for the treatment of unremitting and recurrent pain associated with advanced disease. The intent of this section is to arm the reader with a fundamental and practical understanding of the medications that are (or should be) available in most contemporary care settings, emphasizing those therapies for which there is clear and convincing evidence of efficacy. For an extensive review of mechanisms of pain and analgesia, pharmacological principles of analgesics, and more-detailed lists of all drugs used for pain control throughout the world, the reader is referred to recent comprehensive reviews.[13,50–57] Since patients or family members are not always aware of the names of their medications, or they may bring pills to the hospital or clinic that are not in their original bottles, several web-based resources provide pictures that can assist the nurse in identifying the current analgesic regimen. These can be found at http://www.healthsquare.com/drugmain.htm or http://www.drugs.com.

Nonopioid Analgesics

Acetaminophen

Acetaminophen has been determined to be one of the safest analgesics for long-term use in the management of mild pain or as a supplement in the management of more intense pain syndromes. It is especially useful in the management of nonspecific musculoskeletal pains or pain associated with osteoarthritis, but acetaminophen (also abbreviated as APAP) should be considered an adjunct to any chronic pain regimen. It is often forgotten or overlooked when severe pain is being treated, so a reminder of its value as a "coanalgesic" is warranted. However, acetaminophen's limited antiinflammatory effect should be considered when selecting a nonopioid. Reduced doses or avoidance of acetaminophen is recommended in the face of renal insufficiency or liver failure, and particularly in individuals with significant alcohol use.[58,59]

Nonsteroidal Antiinflammatory Drugs

Nonsteroidal antiinflammatory drugs (NSAIDs) affect analgesia by reducing the biosynthesis of prostaglandins, thereby inhibiting the cascade of inflammatory events that cause, amplify, or maintain nociception. These agents also appear to reduce pain by influences on the peripheral or central nervous system independent of their antiinflammatory mechanism of action. This secondary mode of analgesic efficacy is poorly understood. The "classic" NSAIDs (e.g., aspirin or ibuprofen) are relatively nonselective in their inhibitory effects on the enzymes that convert arachidonic acid to prostaglandins.[60] As a result, gastrointestinal (GI) ulceration, renal dysfunction, and impaired platelet aggregation are common.[61,62] The cyclooxygenase-2 (COX-2) enzymatic pathway is induced by tissue injury or other inflammation-inducing conditions.[63] It is for this reason that there appears to be less risk of GI bleeding with short-term use of the COX-2 selective NSAIDs.[64] However, although several studies demonstrate prolonged GI-sparing effects[65], others suggest that these benefits may not extend beyond 6 to 12 months, and there may be a risk of cardiovascular events with prolonged COX-2 selective NSAID use.[66–69] Additionally, because there is cross-sensitivity, patients allergic to sulfa-containing drugs should not be given celecoxib (Table 6–2).

The NSAIDs, as a class, are very useful in the treatment of many pain conditions mediated by inflammation, including those caused by cancer.[61,70] There are insufficient data to determine whether the newly available COX-2 agents have any specific advantages over the nonselective NSAIDs in the management of pain due to conditions such as metastatic bone pain. The NSAIDs do offer the potential advantage of causing minimal nausea, constipation, sedation, or other effects on mental functioning, although there is evidence that short-term memory in older patients can be impaired by them.[71] Therefore, depending on the cause of pain, NSAIDs may be useful for moderate to severe pain control, either alone or as an adjunct to opioid analgesic therapy. The addition of NSAIDs to opioids has the benefit of potentially allowing the reduction of the opioid dose when sedation, obtundation, confusion, dizziness, or other central nervous system effects of opioid analgesic therapy alone become burdensome.[72] As with acetaminophen, decreased renal function and liver failure are relative contraindications for NSAID use. Similarly, platelet dysfunction or other potential bleeding disorders contraindicate use of the nonselective NSAIDs due to their inhibitory effects on platelet aggregation, with resultant prolonged bleeding time. Proton pump inhibitors can be given to prevent GI bleeding.[73]

Opioid Analgesics

As a pharmacological class, the opioid analgesics represent the most useful agents for the treatment of pain associated with advanced disease. The opioids are nonspecific insofar as they decrease pain signal transmission and perception throughout the nervous system, regardless of the pathophysiology of the pain.[74] Moderate to severe pain is the main clinical indication for the opioid analgesics. Despite past beliefs that opioids were ineffective for neuropathic pain, these agents have been found to be useful in the treatment of this complex pain syndrome.[75] Other indications for opioid use include the treatment of dyspnea, use as an anesthetic adjunct, and as a form of prophylactic therapy in the treatment of psychological dependence to opioids (e.g., methadone maintenance for those with a history of heroin abuse).[76,77]

The only absolute contraindication to the use of an opioid is a history of a hypersensitivity reaction (rash, wheezing,

Table 6–2
Acetaminophen and Selected Nonsteroidal Antiinflammatory Drugs

Drug	Dose If Patient >50 kg	Dose If Patient <50 kg
Acetaminophen*†	4000 mg/24 h q 4–6 h	10–15 mg/kg q 4 h (oral) 15–20 mg/kg q 4 h (rectal)
Aspirin*†	4000 mg/24 h q 4–6 h	10–15 mg/kg q 4 h (oral) 15–20 mg/kg q 4 h (rectal)
Ibuprofen*†	2400 mg/24 h q 6–8 h	10 mg/kg q 6–8 h (oral)
Naproxen*†	1000 mg/24 h q 8–12 h	5 mg/kg q 8 h (oral/rectal)
Choline magnesium trisalicylate*§	2000–3000 mg/24 h q 8–12 h	25 mg/kg q 8 h (oral)
Indomethacin†	75–150 mg/24 h q 8–12 h	0.5–1 mg/kg q 8–12 h (oral/rectal)
Ketorolac‡	30–60 mg IM/IV initially, then 15–30 mg q 6 h bolus IV/IM or continuous IV/SQ infusion; short-term use only (3–5 days)	0.25–1 mg/kg q 6 h short-term use only (3–5 days)
Celecoxib§¶	100–200 mg PO up to b.i.d.	No data available

*Commercially available in a liquid form.
†Commercially available in a suppository form.
‡Potent antiinflammatory (short-term use only due to gastrointestinal side effects).
§Minimal platelet dysfunction.
¶Cyclooxygenase-2-selective nonsteroidal antiinflammatory drug.

edema). Allergic reactions are almost exclusively limited to the morphine derivatives. In the rare event that a patient describes a true allergic reaction, one might begin therapy with a low dose of a short-acting synthetic opioid (e.g., IV fentanyl) or try an intradermal injection as a test dose. The rationale for using a synthetic opioid (preferably one without dyes or preservatives since these can cause allergic reactions) is that the prevalence of allergic reactions is much lower. If the patient does develop a reaction, using a low dose of a short-acting opioid will produce a reduced response for a shorter period of time when compared to long-acting preparations.

Because misunderstandings lead to undertreatment, it is incumbent upon all clinicians involved in the care of patients with chronic pain to clearly understand and differentiate the clinical conditions of tolerance, physical dependence, addiction, pseudoaddiction, and pseudotolerance (Table 6–3).

It is also critically important for clinicians who are involved in patient care to be aware that titration of opioid analgesics to affect pain relief is rarely associated with induced respiratory depression and iatrogenic death.[78,79] In fact, the most compelling evidence suggests that inadequate pain relief hastens death by increasing physiological stress, decreasing immunocompetence, diminishing mobility, increasing the potential for thromboembolism, worsening inspiration and thus placing the patient at risk for pneumonia, and increasing myocardial oxygen requirements.[44,45] Furthermore, in a recent survey of high-dose opioid use (299-mg oral morphine equivalents) in a hospice setting, there was no relationship between opioid dose and survival.[80]

Table 6–3
Definitions

Addiction:

Addiction is a primary, chronic, neurobiological disease, with genetic, psychosocial, and environmental factors influencing its development and manifestations. It is characterized by behaviors that include one or more of the following: impaired control over drug use, compulsive use, continued use despite harm, and craving.

Physical Dependence:

Physical dependence is a state of adaptation that is manifested by a drug-class-specific withdrawal syndrome that can be produced by abrupt cessation, rapid dose reduction, decreasing blood level of the drug, and/or administration of an antagonist.

Tolerance:

Tolerance is a state of adaptation in which exposure to a drug induces changes that result in a diminution of one or more of the drug's effects over time.

Pseudoaddiction:

Pseudoaddiction is the mistaken assumption of addiction in a patient who is seeking relief from pain.

Pseudotolerance:

Pseudotolerance is the misconception that the need for increasing doses of drug is due to tolerance rather than disease progression or other factors.

Adapted from references 223, 224.

In a study of patients with advanced cancer, no reliable predictors for opioid dose were identified.[9] There is significant inter- and intraindividual variation in clinical responses to the various opioids, so in most cases, a dose-titration approach should be viewed as the best means of optimizing care. This implies that close follow-up is required to determine when clinical end points have been reached. Furthermore, idiosyncratic responses may require trials of different agents to determine the most effective drug and route of delivery for any given patient. Table 6–4 lists more specific suggestions regarding optimal use of opioids.

Another factor that needs to be continually considered with opioid analgesics is the potential to accumulate toxic metabolites, especially in the face of decreasing drug clearance and elimination as disease progresses and organ function deteriorates.[81] Due to its neurotoxic metabolite, normeperidine, meperidine use is specifically discouraged for chronic pain management.[82] Propoxyphene (e.g., Darvocet N-100) also is discouraged for use in palliative care due to the active metabolite, norpropoxyphene, its weak analgesic efficacy, and the significant acetaminophen dose found in some formulations.[48] As well, the mixed agonist–antagonist agents, typified by butorphanol, nalbuphine, and pentazocine, are not recommended for the treatment of chronic pain. They have limited efficacy, and their use may cause an acute abstinence syndrome in patients who are otherwise using pure agonist opioid analgesics.[57]

Morphine

Morphine is most often considered the "gold standard" of opioid analgesics and is used as a measure for dose equivalence (Table 6–5).[48] Although some patients cannot tolerate morphine due to itching, headache, dysphoria, or other adverse effects, common initial dosing effects such as sedation and nausea often resolve within a few days.[57] In fact, one should anticipate these adverse effects, especially constipation, nausea, and sedation, and prevent or treat appropriately (see below). One metabolite of morphine, morphine-3-glucuronide (M3G) is active and may contribute to myoclonus, seizures and hyperalgesia (increasing pain), particularly when patients cannot clear the metabolite due to renal impairment.[81,83] Side effects and metabolic effects can be differentiated by the time course. Side effects generally occur soon after the drug has had time to absorb, whereas there usually is a delay in metabolite-induced effects by several days. If adverse effects exceed the analgesic benefit of the drug, convert to an equianalgesic dose of a different opioid. Because cross-tolerance is incomplete, reduce the calculated dose by one third to one half and titrate upward

Table 6–4
Guidelines for the Use of Opioids

Clinical studies and experience suggest that adherence to some basic precepts will help optimize care of patients who require opioid analgesic therapy for pain control:

- Intramuscular administration is highly discouraged except in "pain emergency" states when nothing else is available. (Subcutaneous delivery is almost always an alternative.)
- Noninvasive drug delivery systems that "bypass" the enteral route (e.g., the transdermal and the oral transmucosal routes for delivery of fentanyl for treatment of continuous pain and breakthrough pain, respectively) may obviate the necessity to use parenteral routes for pain control in some patients who cannot take medications orally or rectally.
- Anticipation, prevention, and treatment of sedation, constipation, nausea, psychotomimetic effects, and myoclonus should be part of every care plan for patients being treated with opioid analgesics.
- Changing from one opioid to another or one route to another is often necessary, so facility with this process is an absolute necessity. Remember the following points:
  - Incomplete cross-tolerance occurs, leading to decreased requirements of a newly prescribed opioid.
  - Use morphine equivalents as a "common denominator" for all dose conversions in order to avoid errors.

Adapted from Reference 48.

Table 6–5
Approximate Equianalgesic Doses of Most Commonly Used Opioid Analgesics

Drug	Parenteral Route	Enteral Route
Morphine†	10 mg	30 mg
Codeine	130 mg	200 mg (not recommended)
Fentanyl‡††	50–100 mcg	OTFC available‡
Hydrocodone	Not available	30 mg
Hydromorphone§	1.5 mg	7.5 mg
Levorphanol¶	2 mg acute, 1 chronic	4 mg acute, 1 chronic
Methadone¶	See text & Table 6–7	See text & Table 6–7
Oxycodone††	Not available	20–30 mg

*Dose conversion should be closely monitored since incomplete cross-tolerance may occur.

†Available in continuous and sustained-release pills and capsules, formulated to last 12 or 24 hours. Interindividual variation in duration of analgesic effect is not uncommon, signaling the need to increase the dose or shorten the dose interval.

‡Also available in transdermal and oral transmucosal forms, see package insert materials for dose recommendations. OTFC = oral transmucosal fentanyl citrate.

§Available as a continuous-release formulation lasting 24 hours.

¶These drugs have long half-lives, so accumulation can occur; close monitoring during first few days of therapy is very important.

**Available in several continuous-release doses, formulated to last 12 hours. Interindividual variation in duration of analgesic effect is not uncommon, signaling the need to increase the dose or shorten the dose interval.

††Fentanyl 100 mcg patch ≈4 mg IV morphine/h.

Adapted from References 48, 97, 98, 105, 107, 117.

based on the patient's pain intensity scores (see Chapter 18 for more information on the neurotoxicity of opioids).[48]

Morphine's bitter taste may be prohibitive, especially if "immediate-release" tablets are left in the mouth to dissolve. When patients have dysphagia, several options are available. The 24-hour, long-acting morphine capsule can be broken open and the "sprinkles" placed in applesauce or other soft food.[84] Oral morphine solution can be swallowed, or small volumes (0.5–1 mL) of a concentrated solution (e.g., 20 mg/mL) can be placed in the mouth of patients whose voluntary swallowing capabilities are more significantly limited.[85,86] Transmucosal uptake of morphine is slow and unpredictable due to its hydrophilic chemical nature. In fact, most of the analgesic effect of a morphine tablet or liquid placed buccally or sublingually is due to drug trickling down the throat and the resultant absorption through the GI tract. Furthermore, again due to the hydrophilic nature of morphine, creams and patches that contain morphine provide little if any analgesic effect. Another useful route of administration when oral delivery is unreasonable is the rectal route.[87] Commercially prepared suppositories, compounded suppositories, or microenemas can be used to deliver the drug into the rectum or stoma.[88] Sustained-release morphine tablets have been used rectally, with resultant delayed time to peak plasma level and approximately 90% of the bioavailability achieved by oral administration.

Fentanyl

Fentanyl is a highly lipid soluble opioid that has been administered parenterally, spinally, transdermally, transmucosally, and by nebulizer for the management of dyspnea.[70,89] Because of its potency, dosing is usually conducted in micrograms.

Transdermal Fentanyl. Transdermal fentanyl (Duragesic®), often called the fentanyl patch, is particularly useful when patients cannot swallow, do not remember to take medications, or have adverse effects to other opioids.[90] Opioid-naive patients should start with a 25-mcg/h patch (currently the lowest available dose) after evaluation of effects with immediate-release opioids (Table 6–6). Patients should be monitored by a responsible caregiver for the first 24 to 48 hours of therapy until steady-state blood levels are attained. Fever, diaphoresis, cachexia, morbid obesity, and ascites may have a significant impact on the absorption, predictability of blood levels, and clinical effects of transdermal fentanyl; thus, this form of administration may not be appropriate in those conditions.[91,92] The specific effects of body mass and temperature on absorption have not been studied. Some believe the changes in fat stores (seen with cachexia) alter the fat depot needed for absorption of this lipid-soluble compound. There is some suggestion that transdermal fentanyl may produce less constipation when compared to long-acting morphine.[90] Further study is needed to confirm these findings.

Some patients experience decreased analgesic effects after only 48 hours of applying a new patch; this should be accommodated by determining if a higher dose is tolerated with increased duration of effect or a more frequent (q 48 h) patch change should be scheduled. As with all long-acting preparations, breakthrough pain medications should be made available to patients using continuous-release opioids such as the fentanyl patch. Several reports have documented the safe and effective use of subcutaneous fentanyl when the transdermal approach could no longer provide relief or side effects occurred with other opioids.[90] However, parenteral fentanyl is commercially available in a 50-mcg/mL concentration. Higher doses may preclude the subcutaneous route. When this occurs, the intravenous (IV) route is warranted.

Oral Transmucosal Fentanyl Citrate. Oral transmucosal fentanyl citrate (OTFC or Actiq) is composed of fentanyl on an applicator that patients rub against the oral mucosa to provide rapid absorption of the drug.[93] This formulation of fentanyl is particularly useful for breakthrough pain, described later in this chapter. One example of OTFC use would be pain relief of rapid onset or during a brief but painful dressing change. Adults should start with the 200-mcg dose and monitor efficacy, advancing to higher dose units as needed.[94] Clinicians must be aware that, unlike other breakthrough pain drugs, the around-the-clock dose of opioid does not predict the effective dose of OTFC. Pain relief can usually be expected in about 5 minutes after beginning use.[95] Patients should use OTFC over a period of 15 minutes because too-rapid use will result in more of the agent being swallowed rather than being absorbed transmucosally. Any remaining partial units should be disposed

Table 6–6
Fentanyl Patch Instructions to Patients and Caregivers

1. Place patch on the upper body in a clean, dry, hairless area (clip hair, do not shave).
2. Choose a different site when placing a new patch, then remove the old patch.
3. If a skin reaction consistently occurs despite site rotation, spray inhaled steroid (intended for inhalational use in asthma) over the area, let dry and apply patch (steroid creams prevent adherence of the patch).
4. Remove the old patch or patches and fold sticky surfaces together, then flush down the toilet.
5. Wash hands after handling patches.
6. All unused patches (patient discontinued use or deceased) should be removed from wrappers, folded in half with sticky surfaces together, and flushed down the toilet.

Adapted from References 90, 92.

of by placing under hot water or inserting the unit in a child-resistant temporary storage bottle provided when the drug is first dispensed.

Oxycodone

Oxycodone is a synthetic opioid available in a long-acting formulation (OxyContin, generic long-acting oxycodone), as well as immediate-release tablets (alone or with acetaminophen) and liquid. It is approximately as lipid soluble as morphine, but has better oral absorption.[96] The equianalgesic ratio is approximately 20–30:30 of oral morphine. Side effects appear to be similar to those experienced with morphine; however, one study comparing these two long-acting formulations in persons with advanced cancer found that oxycodone produced less nausea and vomiting.[97] Despite significant media attention to OxyContin and its role in opioid abuse, it does not appear to be inherently "more addicting" than other opioids used in palliative care. Because of this attention, however, several states have restricted the number of tablets that will be distributed to an individual per month.

Methadone

Methadone has several characteristics that make it useful in the management of severe, chronic pain.[98–100] The half-life of 24 to 36 hours or longer allows prolonged dosing intervals.[101] Methadone may also bind as an antagonist to the *N*-methyl-D-aspartate (NMDA) receptor, believed to be of particular benefit in neuropathic pain.[102] Furthermore, methadone is much less costly than comparable doses of proprietary continuous-release formulations, making it potentially more available for patients without sufficient financial resources for more costly drugs.

Despite these advantages, much is unknown about the appropriate dosing ratio between methadone and morphine, as well as the safest and most effective time course for conversion from another opioid to methadone.[103] Early studies suggested the ratio might be 1:1, and this appears to be true for individuals without recent prior exposure to opioids. Newer data suggest the dose ratio increases as the previous dose of oral opioid equivalents increases.[104–106] (Table 6–7) Furthermore, although the long half-life is an advantage, it also increases the potential for drug accumulation before achieving steady-state blood levels, putting patients at risk for oversedation and respiratory depression. This might occur after 2 to 5 days of treatment with methadone. Close monitoring of these potentially adverse or even life-threatening effects is required.[107] Myoclonus has been reported with methadone use.[108] Finally, recent studies suggest high doses of methadone may lead to QT wave changes (also called torsade de pointes), although it is not clear whether this is due to the methadone or to preservatives in the parenteral formulation.[109,110]

Methadone is metabolized primarily by CYP3A4, but also by CYP2D6 and CYP1A2. As a result, drugs that induce CYP enzymes accelerate the metabolism of methadone, resulting in reduced serum levels of the drug. This may be demonstrated clinically by shortened analgesic periods or reduced overall pain relief. Examples of these drugs often used in palliative care include several antiretroviral agents, dexamethasone,

Table 6–7
Rotation to Methadone from Other Opioids in Oral Morphine Equivalents

Bruera E. & Sweeney, C.[99]	Manfredi, P.L. & Houde, R.W.[225]	Gazelle, G. & Fine PG.[226]
If oral morphine < 100 mg, change to methadone 5 mg every 8 hours. If oral morphine > 100 mg, use 3-day rotation period: Day 1—Reduce oral morphine dose by 30%–50% and replace opioid using a 10:1 ratio. Administer methadone every 8 hours. Day 2—Reduce oral morphine by another 35%–50% of original dose and increase methadone if pain is moderate to severe. Supplement with short-acting opioids. Day 3—Discontinue oral morphine and titrate methadone dose daily.	Conversion can be accomplished in one step using the following ratios: 30–90 mg—4:1* 91–300 mg—8:1 > 300 mg—12:1 Higher doses require higher ratio.	No recommendations for speed of rotation < 100-mg oral morphine—3:1* 101–300 mg—5:1 301–600 mg—10:1 601–800 mg—12:1 801–1000 mg—15:1 > 1001 mg—20:1 Do not increase methadone dose more frequently than every 4 days.

*Morphine: methadone

carbamazepine, phenytoin, and barbiturates.[111] Drugs that inhibit CYP enzymes slow methadone metabolism, potentially leading to sedation and respiratory depression. These include ketoconazole, omeprazole, and SSRI antidepressants such as fluoxetine, paroxetine, and sertraline.[99,101]

Patients currently receiving methadone as part of a maintenance program for addictive disease will have developed cross tolerance to the opioids, and as a result, will require higher doses than naive patients.[112] Prescribing methadone for addictive disease requires a special license in the United States. Therefore, prescriptions provided for methadone to manage pain in palliative care should include the statement "for pain."

Hydromorphone

Hydromorphone (Dilaudid) is a useful alternative when synthetic opioids provide an advantage. It is available in oral tablets, liquids, suppositories, and parenteral formulations, and it is now also available in the United States in a long-acting formulation. As a synthetic opioid, hydromorphone provides an advantage when patients have true allergic responses to morphine, or when inadequate pain control or intolerable side effects occur. Recent experience suggests that the metabolite hydromorphone-3-glucuronide (H3G) may lead to the same opioid neurotoxicity seen with morphine metabolites: myoclonus, hyperalgesia, and seizures.[83,113] This is of particular risk in persons with renal dysfunction.[114,115]

Other Opioids

Codeine, hydrocodone, levorphanol, oxymorphone and tramadol are other opioids available in the United States for treatment of pain. Their equianalgesic comparisons are included in Table 6–5.

Alternative Routes of Administration for Opioid Analgesics

Many routes of administration are available when patients can no longer swallow or when other dynamics preclude the oral route or favor other routes. These include transdermal, transmucosal, rectal, vaginal, topical, epidural, and intrathecal. In a study of cancer patients at 4 weeks, 1 week, and 24 hours before death, the oral route of opioid administration was continued in 62%, 43%, and 20% of patients, respectively. More than half of these patients required more than one route of opioid administration. As patients approached death and oral use diminished, the use of intermittent subcutaneous injections and IV or subcutaneous infusions increased.[10]

Thus, in the palliative care setting, nonoral routes of administration must be available. Enteral feeding tubes can be used to access the gut when patients can no longer swallow. The size of the tube should be considered when placing long-acting morphine "sprinkles," to avoid obstruction of the tube. The rectum, stoma, or vagina can be used to deliver medication. Thrombocytopenia or painful lesions preclude the use of these routes. Additionally, delivering medications via these routes can be difficult for family members, especially when the patient is obtunded or unable to assist. Because the vagina has no sphincter, a tampon covered with a condom or an inflated urinary catheter balloon may be used to prevent early discharge of the drug.[116] As previously discussed, transdermal fentanyl is a useful alternative to these techniques.

Parenteral administration includes subcutaneous and IV delivery (intramuscular opioid delivery is inappropriate in the palliative care setting). The IV route provides rapid drug delivery but requires vascular access, placing the patient at risk for infection. Subcutaneous boluses have a slower onset and lower peak effect when compared with IV boluses.[48] Subcutaneous infusions may include up to 10 mL/h (although most patients absorb 2 to 3 mL/h with least difficulty).[117,118] Volumes greater than these are poorly absorbed. Hyaluronidase has been reported to speed absorption of subcutaneously administered drugs.

Intraspinal routes, including epidural or intrathecal delivery, may allow administration of drugs, such as opioids, local anesthetics, and/or α-adrenergic agonists. A recent randomized controlled trial demonstrated benefit for cancer patients experiencing pain.[119] However, the equipment used to deliver these medications is complex, requiring specialized knowledge for health care professionals and potentially greater caregiver burden. Risk of infection is also of concern. Furthermore, cost is a significant concern related to high-technology procedures. See Chapter 22 for a review of high-technology procedures for pain relief.

Preventing and Treating Adverse Effects of Opioid Analgesics

Constipation. Patients in palliative care frequently experience constipation, in part due to opioid therapy.[1a,120] Always begin a prophylactic bowel regimen when commencing opioid analgesic therapy. Avoid bulking agents (e.g., psyllium) since these tend to cause a larger, bulkier stool, increasing desiccation time in the large bowel. Furthermore, debilitated patients can rarely take in sufficient fluid to facilitate the action of bulking agents. Fluid intake should be encouraged whenever feasible. Senna tea and fruits may be of use. For a more comprehensive review of bowel management, refer to Chapter 11.

Sedation. Excessive sedation may occur with the initial doses of opioids. If sedation persists after 24 to 48 hours and other correctable causes have been identified and treated if possible, the use of psychostimulants may be beneficial. These include dextroamphetamine 2.5 to 5 mg PO q morning and midday or methylphenidate 5 to 10 mg PO q morning and 2.5 to 5 mg midday (although higher doses are frequently used).[121,122] Adjust both the dose and timing to prevent nocturnal insomnia and monitor for undesirable psychotomimetic effects (such as agitation, hallucinations, and irritability). Interestingly, in a recent study, as-needed dosing of methylphenidate in cancer patients did not result in sleep disturbances or agitation, even though most subjects took doses in the afternoon and evening.[122] Modafinil, a newer agent approved to manage narcolepsy, has been reported to relieve opioid-induced sedation with once-daily dosing.[123]

Respiratory Depression. Respiratory depression is rarely a clinically significant problem for opioid-tolerant patients in pain.[48] When respiratory depression occurs in a patient with advanced disease, the cause is usually multifactorial.[78,79] Therefore, other factors beyond opioids need to be assessed, although opioids are frequently blamed for the reduced repirations. When undesired depressed consciousness occurs along with a respiratory rate less than 8/min or hypoxemia (O_2 saturation < 90%) associated with opioid use, cautious and slow titration of naloxone should be instituted. Excessive administration may cause abrupt opioid reversal with pain and autonomic crisis. Dilute 1 ampule of naloxone (0.4 mg/mL) in 10 mL of injectable saline (final concentration 40 mcg/mL) and inject 1 mL every 2 to 3 minutes while closely monitoring the level of consciousness and respiratory rate. Because the duration of effect of naloxone is approximately 30 minutes, the depressant effects of the opioid will recur at 30 minutes and persist until the plasma levels decline (often 4 or more hours) or until the next dose of naloxone is administered.[48]

Nausea and Vomiting. Nausea and vomiting are common with opioids due to activation of the chemoreceptor trigger zone in the medulla, vestibular sensitivity, and delayed gastric emptying, but habituation occurs in most cases within several days.[124] Assess for other treatable causes. In severe cases or when nausea and vomiting are not self-limited, pharmacotherapy is indicated. The doses of nausea-relieving medications and antiemetics listed below are to be used initially but can be increased as required. See Chapter 9 for a thorough discussion of the assessment and treatment of nausea and vomiting.

Myoclonus. Myoclonic jerking occurs more commonly with high-dose opioid therapy.[125] If this should develop, switch to an alternate opioid, especially if using morphine, since evidence suggests this symptom is associated with metabolite accumulation, particularly in the face of renal dysfunction.[83,108,113,126] A lower relative dose of the substituted drug may be possible, due to incomplete cross-tolerance, which might result in decreased myoclonus. Clonazepam 0.5 to 1 mg PO q 6 to 8 hours, to be increased as needed and tolerated, may be useful in treating myoclonus in patients who are still alert, able to communicate, and take oral preparations.[127] Lorazepam can be given sublingually if the patient is unable to swallow. Otherwise, parenteral administration of diazepam is indicated if symptoms are distressing. Grand mal seizures associated with high-dose parenteral opioid infusions have been reported and may be due to preservatives in the solution.[128] Preservative-free solutions should be used when administering high-dose infusions. (See Chapter 18 for more specific information).

Pruritus. Pruritus appears to be most common with morphine, in part due to histamine release, but can occur with most opioids. Fentanyl and oxymorphone may be less likely to cause histamine release.[48] Most antipruritus therapies cause sedation, so this side effect must be viewed by the patient as an acceptable trade-off. Antihistamines (such as diphenydramine) are the most common first-line approach to this opioid-induced symptom when treatment is indicated. Ondansetron has been reported to be effective in relieving opioid-induced pruritus, but no randomized controlled studies exist.[129]

Coanalgesics

A wide variety of nonopioid medications from several pharmacological classes have been demonstrated to reduce pain caused by various pathological conditions (Table 6–8). As a group, these drugs have been called analgesic 'adjuvants,' but this is something of a misnomer since they often reduce pain when used alone. However, under most circumstances, when these drugs are indicated for the treatment of severe neuropathic pain or bone pain, opioid analgesics are used concomitantly to provide adequate pain relief.

Antidepressants

The mechanism of the analgesic effect of tricyclic antidepressants appears to be related to inhibition of norepinephrine and serotonin.[130] Despite the absence of positive controlled clinical trials in cancer pain or other palliative care pain conditions, the tricyclic antidepressants are generally believed to provide relief from neuropathic pain.[131] A recent consensus panel listed this category as one of five first-line therapies for neuropathic pain.[132] Side effects often limit the use of these agents in palliative care. Cardiac arrhythmias, conduction abnormalities, narrow-angle glaucoma, and clinically significant prostatic hyperplasia are relative contraindications to the tricyclic antidepressants. The delay in onset of pain relief, from days to weeks, may preclude the use of these agents for pain relief in end-of-life care. However, their sleep-enhancing and mood-elevating effects may be of benefit.[133] A newer, atypical antidepressant, venlafaxine, has been shown to reduce neuropathy associated with cisplatin-induced neuropathy[134] and following treatment for breast cancer.[135]

Anticonvulsants

The older anticonvulsants, such as carbamazepine and clonazepam, relieve pain by blocking sodium channels.[133] Often referred to as membrane stabilizers, these compounds are very useful in the treatment of neuropathic pain, especially those with episodic, lancinating qualities. Gabapentin is believed to have several different mechanisms of action, including having

Table 6–8
Adjuvant Analgesics

Drug Class	Daily Adult Starting Dose* (Range)	Routes of Administration	Adverse Effects	Indications
Tricyclic antidepressants	Nortriptyline 10–25 mg Desipramine 10–25 mg	PO	Anticholinergic effects	Neuropathic pain, such as burning pain, poor sleep
Anticonvulsants	Clonazapam 0.5–1 mg hs, bid or tid Carbamazapine 100 mg q day or tid Gabapentin 100 mg tid	PO PO PO	Sedation	Neuropathic pain, such as shooting pain
Corticosteroids	Dexamethasone 2–20 mg q day; may give up to 100 mg IV bolus for pain crises Prednisone 15–30 mg tid, qid	PO/IV/SQ PO	"Steroid psychosis," dyspepsia	Cerebral edema, spinal cord compression, bone pain, neuropathic pain, visceral pain
Local anesthetics	Mexiletine 150 mg tid Lidocaine 1–5 mg/kg hourly	PO IV or SQ infusion	Lightheadedness, arrhthymias	Neuropathic pain
N-Methyl-D-aspartate antagonists	Dextromethorphan, effective dose unknown Ketamine (see Pain Crises)	PO IV	Confusion	Neuropathic pain
Bisphosphonates	Pamidronate 60–90 mg over 2 h every 2–4 wk	IV infusion	Pain flare	Osteolytic bone pain
Calcitonin	25 IU/day	SQ/nasal	Hypersensitivity reaction, nausea	Neuropathic pain, bone pain
Capsaicin	0.025–0.075%	Topical	Burning	Neuropathic pain
Baclofen	10 mg q day or qid	PO	Muscle weakness, cognitive changes	
Calcium channel blockers	Nifedipine 10 mg tid	PO	Bradycardia, hypotension	Ischemic pain, neuropathic pain, smooth muscle spasms with pain

*Pediatric doses for pain control not well established.
Adapted from References 132, 133, 135–137, 142–152.

NMDA antagonist and other analgesic activities. The analgesic doses of gabapentin reported to relieve pain in non-end-of-life pain conditions ranged from 900 to 3600 mg/day in divided doses.[136,137] A common reason for inadequate relief is failure to titrate upward after prescribing the usual starting dose of 100 mg po three times daily. Additional evidence supports the use of gabapentin in neuropathic pain syndromes seen in palliative care, such as thalamic pain, pain due to spinal cord injury, cancer pain, along with restless leg syndrome.[138–140] Withdrawal from gabapentin should be gradual to prevent possible seizures.[141] Other anticonvulsants have been used with success in treating neuropathies, including lamotrigine, levetiracetam, tiagabine, topiramate, and zonisamide, yet no randomized controlled clinical trials are currently available.[132]

Corticosteroids

Corticosteroids inhibit prostaglandin synthesis and reduce edema surrounding neural tissues.[142] This category of drug is particularly useful for neuropathic pain syndromes, including plexopathies and pain associated with stretching of the liver capsule due to metastases.[142,143] Corticosteroids are also highly effective for treating bone pain due to their antiinflammatory effects, as well as relieving malignant intestinal obstruction.[144] Dexamethasone produces the least amount of mineralocorticoid effect, leading to reduced potential for Cushing's syndrome. Dexamthasone is available in oral, IV, subcutaneous, and epidural formulations. The standard dose is 16 to 24 mg/day and can be administered once daily due to the long half-life of this drug.[48] Doses as high as 100 mg may be given with severe pain crises. IV bolus doses should be pushed slowly, to prevent uncomfortable perineal burning and itching.

Local Anesthetics

Local anesthetics work in a manner similar to the older anticonvulsants, by inhibiting the movement of ions across the neural membrane.[145] They are useful for relieving neuropathic pain. Local anesthetics can be given orally, topically, intravenously, subcutaneously, or spinally.[145] Mexiletine has been reported to be useful when anticonvulsants and other adjuvant therapies have failed. Doses start at 150 mg/day and increase to levels as high as 900 mg/day in divided doses.[146,147] Local anesthetic gels and patches have been used to prevent the pain associated with needlestick and other minor procedures. Both gel and patch (Lidoderm) versions of lidocaine have been shown to reduce the pain of postherpetic neuropathy.[148] IV lidocaine at 1 to 5 mg/kg (maximum 500 mg) administered over 1 hour, followed by a continuous infusion of 1 to 2 mg/kg/hour has been reported to reduce intractable neuropathic pain in patients in inpatient palliative care and home hospice settings.[149] Epidural or intrathecal lidocaine or bupivacaine delivered with an opioid can reduce neuropathic pain.[150]

N-Methyl-D-Aspartate Antagonists

Antagonists to NMDA are believed to block the binding of excitatory amino acids, such as glutamate, in the spinal cord. Ketamine, a dissociative anesthetic, is believed to relieve severe neuropathic pain by blocking NMDA receptors (see the section 'Pain Crisis,' below). A recent Cochrane review found insufficient trials conducted to determine safety and efficacy in cancer pain.[151] Routine use often is limited by cognitive changes and other adverse effects. Oral compounds containing dextromethorphan have been tested. Unfortunately, dextromethorphan was ineffective at relieving cancer pain.[152]

Bisphosphonates

Bisphosphonates inhibit osteoclast-mediated bone resorption and alleviate pain related to metastatic bone disease and multiple myeloma.[153,154] Pamidronate disodium reduces pain, hypercalcemia, and skeletal morbidity associated with breast cancer and multiple myeloma.[155–157] Dosing is generally repeated every 4 weeks and the analgesic effects occur in 2 to 4 weeks. Interestingly, a recent randomized, controlled trial of pamidronate in men experiencing pain due to prostate cancer failed to demonstrate any benefit.[158] Zoledronic acid is a newer bisphosphonate that has been shown to relieve pain due to metastatic bone disease.[159] It is somewhat more convenient because it can be infused over a shorter duration of time. Clodronate and sodium etidronate appear to provide little or no analgesia.[160]

Calcitonin

Subcutaneous calcitonin may be effective in the relief of neuropathic or bone pain, although studies are inconclusive.[161] The nasal form of this drug may be more acceptable in end-of-life care when other therapies are ineffective. Usual doses are 100 to 200 IU/day subcutaneously or nasally.

Radiation Therapy and Radiopharmaceuticals

Radiotherapy can be enormously beneficial in relieving pain due to bone metastases or other lesions.[162,163] In many cases, single-fraction external beam therapy can be used to facilitate treatment in debilitated patients.[163] Goals of treatment should be clearly articulated so that patients and family members understand the role of this therapy. Radiolabeled agents such as strontium-89 and samarium-153 have been shown to be effective at reducing metastatic bone pain.[164–166] Thrombocytopenia and leukopenia are relative contraindications since strontium-89 causes thrombocytopenia in as many as 33% of those treated and leukopenia up to 10%.[164] Because of the delayed onset and timing of peak effect, only those patients with a projected life span of greater than 3 months should be considered for treatment. Patients should be advised that a transitory pain flare is reported by as many as 10% of individuals treated, and additional analgesics should be provided in anticipation.

Chemotherapy

Palliative chemotherapy is the use of antitumor therapy to relieve symptoms associated with malignancy. Patient goals, performance status, sensitivity of the tumor, and potential toxicities must be considered.[167] Examples of symptoms that may improve with chemotherapy include hormonal therapy in breast cancer to relieve chest wall pain due to tumor ulceration, or chemotherapy in lung cancer to relieve dyspnea.[168]

Other Adjunct Analgesics

Topical capsaicin is believed to relieve pain by inhibiting the release of substance P. This compound has been shown to be useful in relieving pain associated with postmastectomy syndrome, postherpetic neuralgia, and postsurgical neuropathic pain in cancer.[142] A burning sensation experienced by patients is a common reason for discontinuing therapy.

Baclofen is useful in the relief of spasm-associated pain. Doses begin at 10 mg/day, increasing every few days.[169] A generalized feeling of weakness and confusion or hallucinations often occurs with doses above 60 mg/day. Intrathecal baclofen has been used to treat spasticity and resulting pain, primarily due to multiple sclerosis and spinal cord injury, although a case report describes relief from pain due to spinal cord injury.[170,171]

Calcium channel blockers are believed to provide pain relief by preventing conduction. Nifedipine 10 mg orally may be useful to relieve ischemic or neuropathic pain syndromes.[172]

Interventional Therapies

In addition to previously discussed spinal administration of analgesics, interventional therapies to relieve pain at end of life can be beneficial, including nerve blocks, vertebroplasty, radiofrequency ablation of painful metastases, procedures to drain painful effusions and other techniques.[48,173–175] Few of these procedures have undergone controlled clinical studies. One technique, the celiac plexus block, has been shown to be superior to morphine in patients with pain due to unresectable pancreatic cancer.[176] A complete review of these procedures can be found in a variety of sources. Choosing one of these techniques is dependent upon the availability of experts in this area who understand the special needs of palliative care patients, the patient's ability to undergo the procedure, and the patient's and family's goals of care.

Nonpharmacological Therapies

Nondrug therapies, including cognitive–behavioral techniques and physical measures, can serve as adjuncts to analgesics in the palliative care setting. This is not to suggest that when these therapies work the pain is of psychological origin.[177] The patient's and caregivers' abilities to participate must be considered when selecting one of these therapies, including their fatigue level, interest, cognition, and other factors.[178]

Cognitive–behavioral therapy often includes strategies to improve coping and relaxation, such as relaxation, guided imagery, music, prayer, and reframing.[177,179,180] In a randomized clinical trial of patients undergoing bone marrow transplantation, pain was reduced in those patients who received relaxation and imagery training and in those who received cognitive–behavioral skill development with relaxation and imagery.[181] Patients who received treatment as usual or those randomized to receive support from a therapist did not experience pain relief.

Physical measures, such as massage, reflexology, heat, chiropractic and other techniques, produce relaxation and relieve pain.[182–186] In a study of massage in hospice patients, relaxation resulted as measured by blood pressure, heart rate, and skin temperature.[187] A 10-minute back massage was found to relieve pain in male cancer patients.[188] Rhiner and colleagues[189] employed a comprehensive nondrug program for cancer patients that included education; physical measures such as heat, cold, and massage; and cognitive–behavioral strategies such as distraction and relaxation. All therapies were rated as useful, with distraction and heat scoring highest. More research is needed in the palliative care setting regarding nondrug therapies that might enhance pain relief.

Difficult Pain Syndromes

The above therapies provide relief for the majority of patients (Table 6–9). Unfortunately, complex pain syndromes may require additional measures. These syndromes

Table 6–9
Guidelines for Pain Management in Palliative Care

- Sustained-release formulations and around-the-clock dosing should be used for continuous pain syndromes.
- Immediate-release formulations should be made available for breakthrough pain.
- Cost and convenience (and other identified issues influencing compliance) are highly practical and important matters that should be taken into account with every prescription.
- Anticipate, prevent, and treat predictable side effects and adverse drug effects.
- Titrate analgesics based on patient goals, requirements for supplemental analgesics, pain intensity, severity of undesirable or adverse drug effects, measures of functionality, sleep, emotional state, and patients'/caregivers' reports of impact of pain on quality of life.
- Monitor patient status frequently during dose titration.
- Discourage use of mixed agonist–antagonist opioids.
- Be aware of potential drug–drug and drug–disease interactions.
- Recommend expert pain management consultation if pain is not adequately relieved within a reasonable amount of time after applying standard analgesic guidelines and interventions.
- Know the qualifications, experience, skills, and availability of pain management experts (consultants) within the patient's community before they may be needed.

These basic guidelines and considerations will optimize the pharmacologic management of all patients with pain, particularly those in the palliative care setting.

Adapted from References 48, 51, 223.

include breakthrough pain, pain crises, and pain control in the patient with a past or current history of substance abuse.

Breakthrough Pain

Intermittent episodes of moderate to severe pain that occur in spite of control of baseline continuous pain are common in patients with advanced disease.[190] Studies suggest that although breakthrough pain in cancer patients at home is common, short-acting analgesics are frequently not provided and patients do not take as much as is allowed.[191,192] Mostly described in cancer patients, there is evidence that patients with other pain-producing and life-limiting diseases commonly experience breakthrough pains a few times a day, lasting moments to many minutes.[193,194] A recent prospective study of patients with noncancer diagnoses at end of life experienced an average of 5 breakthrough episodes per day (range 1–13), with 56% of these episodes occuring without any warning.[195] The risk of increasing the around-the-clock or continuous-release analgesic dose to cover breakthrough pains is that of increasing undesirable side effects, especially sedation, once the more short-lived, episodic breakthrough pain has remitted. Guidelines for categorizing, assessing, and managing breakthrough pain are described below:

Incident Pain. Incident pain is predictably elicited by specific activities. Use a rapid-onset, short-duration analgesic formulation in anticipation of pain-eliciting activities or events. Use the same drug that the patient is taking for baseline pain relief for incident pain whenever possible. In 1998, OTFC was approved specifically for this indication in cancer patients.[94] Clinical experience is being gained on its efficacy in other clinical situations. Adjust and titrate the breakthrough pain medication dose to the severity of anticipated pain or the intensity and duration of the pain-producing event. Past experience will serve as the best prescriptive guide.

Spontaneous Pain. Spontaneous pain is unpredictable and not temporally associated with any activity or event. These pains are more challenging to control. The use of adjuvants for neuropathic pains may help to diminish the frequency and severity of these types of pain (see Table 6–8). Otherwise, immediate treatment with a potent, rapid-onset opioid analgesic is indicated.

End-of-Dose Failure. End-of-dose failure describes pain that occurs toward the end of the usual dosing interval of a regularly scheduled analgesic. This results from declining blood levels of the around-the-clock analgesic before administration or uptake of the next scheduled dose. Appropriate questioning and use of pain diaries will assure rapid diagnosis of end-of-dose failure. Increasing the dose of around-the-clock medication or shortening the dose interval to match the onset of this type of breakthrough pain should remedy the problem. For instance, a patient who is taking continuous-release morphine every 12 hours and whose pain "breaks through" after about 8 to 10 hours is experiencing end-of-dose failure. The dose should be increased by 25% to 50%, if this is tolerated, or the dosing interval should be increased to every 8 hours.

Bone Pain

Pain due to bone metastatis or pathological fractures can include extremely painful breakthrough pain, often associated with movement, along with periods of somnolence when the patient is at rest.[172] In one study of cancer patients admitted to an inpatient hospice, 93% had breakthrough pain, with 72% of the episodes related to movement or weight bearing.[196] Treatment of bone pain includes the use of corticosteroids, bisphosphonates if indicated, radiotherapy or radionuclides if consistent with the goals of care, long-acting opioids, along with short-acting opioids for the periods of increasing pain.[162] Vertebroplasty may stabilize the vertabrae if tumor invasion leads to instability.[173]

Pain Crisis

Most nociceptive (i.e., somatic and visceral) pain is controllable with appropriately titrated analgesic therapy.[197] Some neuropathic pains, such as invasive and compressive neuropathies, plexopathies, and myelopathies, may be poorly responsive to conventional analgesic therapies, short of inducing a nearly comatose state. Widespread bone metastases or end-stage pathological fractures may present similar challenges.[172,198] When confronted by a pain crisis, the following considerations will be helpful:

- Differentiate terminal agitation or anxiety from "physically" based pain, if possible. Terminal symptoms unresponsive to rapid upward titration of an opioid may respond to benzodiazepines (e.g., diazepam, lorazepam, midazolam).
- Make sure that drugs are getting absorbed. The only route guaranteed to be absorbed is the IV route. Although invasive routes of drug delivery are to be avoided unless necessary, if there is any question about absorption of analgesics or other necessary palliative drugs, parenteral access should be established.
- Preterminal pain crises that respond poorly to basic approaches to analgesic therapy merit consultation with a pain management consultant as quickly as possible. Radiotherapeutic, anesthetic, or neuroablative procedures may be indicated.[172]

Management of Refractory Symptoms at the End of Life

Sedation at the end of life is an important option for patients with intractable pain and suffering. The literature describing the use of sedation at the end of life, however, is largely anecdotal

Table 6–10
Protocol for Using Ketamine to Treat a Pain Crisis

1. Bolus: ketamine 0.1 mg/kg IV. Double the dose if no clinical improvement in 5 minutes. Repeat as often as indicated by the patient's response. Follow the bolus with an infusion. Decrease opioid dose by 50%.
2. Infusion: ketamine 0.015 mg/(kg/min) IV (about 1 mg/min for a 70 kg individual). Subcutaneous infusion is possible if IV access is not attainable. In this case, use an initial IM bolus dose of 0.3–0.5 mg/kg. Decrease opioid dose by 50%.
3. It is advisable to administer a benzodiazapine (e.g., diazapam, lorazapam) concurrently to mitigate against the possibility of hallucinations or frightful dreams because moribund patients under these circumstances may not be able to communicate such experiences.
4. Observe for problematic increases in secretions; treat with glycopyrrolate, scopolomine, or atropine as needed.

Adapted from Reference 205.

and refers to the use of opioids, neuroleptics, benzodiazepines, and barbiturates.[199–201] The anesthetic propofol is also used.[202] In the absence of controlled relative efficacy data, guidelines for drug selection are empirical. Irrespective of the agent or agents selected, administration initially requires dose titration to achieve relief, followed by ongoing therapy to maintain effect. The depth of sedation necessary to control symptoms varies greatly. Once adequate relief is obtained, the parameters for ongoing monitoring are determined by the goal of care. If the goal of care is to ensure comfort until death, the salient parameters to monitor are those pertaining to comfort of the patient, family, and staff. See Chapter 24 for additional discussion regarding palliative sedation.

Parenteral administration of ketamine is also useful for some patients with refractory pain at the end of life. Ketamine is a potent analgesic at low doses and a dissociative anesthetic at higher doses.[203] Its use under conditions of terminal crescendo-type pain may not only provide greatly improved pain relief but also allow a significant decrease in the dose of concurrent analgesics and sedatives, allowing in some cases increased interactive capability. Ketamine is usually reserved for terminal situations, due to rapidly developing tolerance and psychotomimetic effects (hallucinations, dysphoria, nightmares) that may occur with higher doses and drug accumulation (Table 6–10).[204,205] Long-term IV or subcutaneous use of ketamine (e.g., over 2 months) has been reported to be effective in intractable pain states not relieved by large doses of opioids and other adjuncts.[205] Haloperidol can be used to treat the hallucinations, and scopolamine may be needed to reduce the excess salivation seen with this drug. Research is needed regarding the efficacy of and adverse effects associated with the use of ketamine for intractable pain.

Pain Control in People with Addictive Disease

The numbers of patients entering palliative care with a current or past history of addictive disease are unknown, yet thought to be significant.[13,206] As approximately one third of the U.S. population has used illicit drugs, it would logically follow that some of these individuals will require palliative care. In one uncontrolled survey of people with cancer or HIV, more than half of those with HIV considered themselves to be recovering addicts.[207] Therefore, all clinicians must be aware of the principles and practical considerations necessary to adequately care for these individuals (see Chapter 38 for a complete discussion of care for the addicted patient at the end of life).

The underlying mechanisms of addiction are complex, including the pharmacological properties of the drug, personality and psychiatric disorders, as well as underlying genetic factors.[208] Caring for these patients can be extremely challenging. Thorough assessment of the pain and their addictive disease is critical. Defensive behavior is to be expected, therefore the interview should begin with general questions about the use of caffeine and nicotine and gradually become more specific about illicit drug use.[209] Patients should be informed that the information will be used to help prevent withdrawal from these drugs, as well as ensure adequate doses of medications used to relieve pain.

Patients can be categorized in the following manner: (1) individuals who used drugs or alcohol in the past but are not using them now; (2) patients in methadone maintenance programs who are not using drugs or alcohol; (3) persons in methadone maintenance programs but who continue to actively use drugs or alcohol; (4) people using drugs or alcohol occasionally, usually socially; and (5) patients who are actively abusing drugs.[210,211] Treatment is different for each group.

A frequent fear expressed by professionals is that they will be 'duped,' or lied to, about the presence of pain. One of the limitations of pain management is that pain, and all its components, cannot be proven. Therefore, expressions of pain must be believed. As with all aspects of palliative care, an interdisciplinary team approach is indicated. This may include inviting addiction counselors to interdisciplinary team meetings. Realistic goals must be established. For example, recovery from addiction is impossible if the patient does not seek this rehabilitation. The goal in that case may be to provide a structured and safe environment for patients and their support persons. Comorbid psychiatric disorders are common, particularly depression, personality disorders, and anxiety disorders. Treatment of these underlying problems may reduce relapse or aberrant behaviors and may make pain control more effective.[212]

The pharmacological principles of pain management in the person with addictive disease are not unlike those in a person without this history. Nonopioids may be used, including antidepressants, anticonvulsants, and other adjuncts. However, psychoactive drugs with no analgesic effect should be avoided in the treatment of pain. Tolerance must be considered;

thus, opioid doses may require more rapid titration and may be higher than for patients without previous exposure to opioids.[213] Requests for increasing doses may be due to psychological suffering, so this possibility must also be explored.

Consistency in the treatment plan is essential. Inconsistency can increase manipulation and lead to staff frustration. Setting limits is a critical component of the care plan, and medication contracts may be indicated.[214] In fact, one primary clinician may be designated to handle the pharmacological management of pain. Prescriptions may be written for 1-week intervals if patients cannot manage an entire month's supply. The prescriptions may be delivered to one pharmacy to reduce the potential for altered prescriptions or prescriptions from multiple prescribers. Writing out the number for the dose and the total number of tablets will prevent alterations of the prescription (e.g., increasing the number of tablets from 10 to 100). Use long-acting opioids whenever possible, limiting the reliance upon shortacting drugs.[209] Avoid bolus parenteral administration, although at the end of life, infusions can be effective and diversion limited by keeping no spare cassettes or bags in the home. Weekly team meetings provide a forum to establish the plan of care and discuss negative attitudes regarding the patient's behavior. Family meetings may be indicated, particularly if they are also experiencing addictive behaviors.

Withdrawal from drugs of abuse must be prevented or minimized. These may include cocaine, benzodiazepines, and even alcohol. Alcoholism in palliative care has been underdiagnosed.[215] Thus, a thorough assessment of recreational drug use, including alcohol, must be conducted. This provides evidence for adherence to the treatment plan.[216] Urine toxicology studies may be necessary. An excellent monograph detailing the clinical use of urine toxicology can be found at www.familydocs.org. Another resource is the *Fast Fact Urine Drug Testing for Opioids and Marijuana* available at http://www.eperc.mcw.edu.

Patients in recovery may be extremely reluctant to consider opioid therapy. Patients may need reassurance that opioids can be taken for medical indications, such as cancer or other illnesses. If patients currently are treated in a methadone maintenance program, continue the methadone but add another opioid to provide pain relief. Communicate with the program to ensure the correct methadone dose. Nondrug alternatives may also be suggested. An excellent resource for information about addiction treatment is http://www.opiateaddictionrx.info.

Nursing Interventions: Outcomes and Documentation

Quality-improvement measures to relieve pain in the palliative care setting include setting outcomes, developing strategies to maintain or meet these outcomes, and then evaluating effectiveness.[217,218] Some suggested goals and outcome measures that can be used in each patient's care plan are listed in Table 6–11.

Table 6–11
Outcome Indicators for Pain Control in the Palliative Care Setting

- *Initial Evaluation:* Pain that is not well controlled (patient self-report of 3 out of 10 or greater than the patient's acceptable comfort level) is brought under control within 48 hours of a patient's initial evaluation.
- *Ongoing Care:* Pain that is out of control is assessed and managed with effective intervention(s) within a predetermined time frame in all patients (set an appropriate time limit).
- *Terminal Care:* No patient dies with pain out of control.
- *Adverse Effects:* Analgesic adverse effects and side effects are prevented or effectively and quickly managed in all patients

Adapted from References 218, 219.

Documentation is also essential to ensure continuity of care. Recommendations for documentation in the medical record include the following:

- Initial assessment, including findings from the comprehensive pain assessment; the current pain management regimen; prior experience with pain and pain control; patient and caregiver understanding of expectations and goals of pain management; elaboration of concerns regarding opioids; and a review of systems pertinent to analgesic use, including bowels, balance, memory, function, etc.[219]
- Interdisciplinary progress notes, including ongoing findings from recurrent pain assessment; baseline pain scores; breakthrough pain frequency and severity with associated causes and timing of episodes; effect of pain and pain treatment on function, sleep, activity, social interaction, mood, etc.; types and effects (outcomes) of intervention, including adverse effects (bowel function, sedation, nausea/vomiting assessments); documentation of specific instructions, patient/caregiver understanding, and compliance; and patient/caregiver coping.[219]

Comprehensive strategies to improve pain outcomes in the hospice setting have included improving professional education, developing policies and procedures, enhancing pain documentation, and instituting other performance-improvement measures.[217,218,220,221] These have resulted in reduction of pain-intensity scores and other changes. More research is needed in the development of quality-improvement strategies that most accurately reflect the needs of patients and families in palliative care settings.

CASE STUDY

Ms. Matthews, a Patient with Pathological Fracture of the Femur

Ms. Matthews is a 38-year-old woman who was diagnosed with a pathological fracture of the femur due to advanced breast cancer. Her husband is very supportive, although financial difficulties require that he work two jobs. She has two school-aged children at home. The Palliative Care Consult Service (including a nurse and a physician) was asked to see her on the inpatient oncology unit to assist in pain management, because she could not tolerate lying flat to receive radiotherapy treatments. A thorough pain assessment revealed minimal to moderate (3–5/0–10 intensity scale) pain in the right femur at rest, with severe (10+) sharp, shooting pain when lying flat or weight bearing. She denied other sites of pain. Oral hydrocodone 5 mg in admixture with 500 mg of acetaminophen was given up to 8 doses per day with minimal relief. Other symptoms included difficulty sleeping due to the pain, with frequent waking through the night, and constipation (her last bowel movement was 4 days ago and her normal pattern was daily defecation). She admitted to feeling sad that she could not see her children and worried that they were not coping well with her illness. Her goals of care were to return home with good pain control.

After assessing Ms. Matthews and discussing her case with the medical and radiation oncologist, plus the advanced practice nurse who had been seeing her in the outpatient clinic, her analgesic regimen was changed to include long-acting oxycodone 20 mg every 12 hours, supplemented with oral short-acting oxycodone 5 mg for breakthrough pain every hour as needed. An additional dose of short-acting oxycodone was ordered to be given 1 hour before radiotherapy treatments. Daily oral dexamethasone 12 mg also was added, along with omeprazole for GI protection. A stimulant laxative and softener were ordered to regulate the bowels.

The team reassessed Ms. Matthews' pain during the next few days and titrated the opioids to achieve improved relief. They requested the physical therapy department to assist with teaching her family about transferring and occupational therapy to provide information regarding assistive devices. The expressive arts therapist was consulted to explore Ms. Matthews' sadness, and to work with her children during their visits. The social worker was contacted to discuss equipment that might be needed in the home, safety issues, and support that might be offered to address financial concerns. She also offered to contact the childrens' school to alert the teachers regarding their mother's illness as a source of stress for the children, yet Ms. Matthews declined this suggestion. The chaplain was asked to see Ms. Matthews to address potential spiritual issues. A family meeting was called to discuss goals of care and preparation for home. Ms. Matthews returned home safely and with good pain relief, with ongoing follow-up from the palliative care clinic.

Conclusion

Pain control in the palliative care setting is feasible in the majority of patients. For patients whose pain cannot be controlled, sedation is always an option. Understanding the barriers that limit relief will lead to improved education and other strategies to address these obstacles. Developing comfort and skill with the use of pharmacological and nonpharmacological therapies will enhance pain relief. Quality improvement efforts within a palliative care setting can improve the level of pain management within that organization and ultimately the pain relief experienced by these patients. Together, these efforts will reduce suffering, relieve pain, and enhance the quality of life of those at the end of life.

REFERENCES

1. Daudet A. In the Land of Pain. New York: Alfred A. Knopf, 2002.

1a. Ng K, von Gunten CF. Symptoms and attitudes of 100 consecutive patients admitted to an acute hospice/palliative care unit. J Pain Symptom Manage 1998;16:307–316.

2. Caraceni A, Weinstein SM. Classification of cancer pain syndromes. Oncology (Huntingt) 2001;15:1627–1640, 1642; discussion 1642–1623, 1646–1627.

3. Chang VT, Hwang SS, Feuerman M, Kasimis BS. Symptom and quality of life survey of medical oncology patients at a veterans affairs medical center: a role for symptom assessment. Cancer 2000;88:1175–1183.

4. Meuser T, Pietruck C, Radbruch L, Stute P, Lehmann KA, Grond S. Symptoms during cancer pain treatment following WHO guidelines: a longitudinal follow-up study of symptom prevalence, severity and etiology. Pain 2001;93:247–257.

5. Wells N. Pain intensity and pain interference in hospitalized patients with cancer. Oncol Nurs Forum 2000;27:985–991.

6. Morita T, Ichiki T, Tsunoda J, Inoue S, Chihara S. A prospective study on the dying process in terminally ill cancer patients. Am J Hosp Palliat Care 1998;15:217–222.

7. Cleeland CS, Gonin R, Baez L, Loehrer P, Pandya KJ. Pain and treatment of pain in minority patients with cancer. The Eastern Cooperative Oncology Group Minority Outpatient Pain Study. Ann Intern Med 1997;127:813–816.

8. Cleeland CS, Gonin R, Hatfield AK, Edmonson JH, Blum RH, Stewart JA, et al. Pain and its treatment in outpatients with metastatic cancer. N Engl J Med 1994;330:592–596.

9. Brescia FJ, Portenoy RK, Ryan M, Krasnoff L, Gray G. Pain, opioid use, and survival in hospitalized patients with advanced cancer. J Clin Oncol 1992;10:149–155.

10. Coyle N, Adelhardt J, Foley KM, Portenoy RK. Character of terminal illness in the advanced cancer patient: pain and other symptoms during the last four weeks of life. J Pain Symptom Manage 1990;5:83–93.

11. Wolfe J, Grier HE, Klar N, Levin SB, Ellenbogen JM, Salem-Schatz S, et al. Symptoms and suffering at the end of life in children with cancer. N Engl J Med 2000;342:326–333.

12. Vanhems P, Dassa C, Lambert J, Cooper DA, Perrin L, Vizzard J, et al. Comprehensive classification of symptoms and signs

reported among 218 patients with acute HIV-1 infection. J Acquir Immune Defic Syndr 1999;21:99–106.
13. Breitbart W, Dibiase L. Current perspectives on pain in AIDS. Oncology (Huntingt) 2002;16:964–968, 972; discussion 972, 977, 980, 982.
14. Simpson DM, Haidich AB, Schifitto G, Yiannoutsos CT, Geraci AP, McArthur JC, et al. Severity of HIV-associated neuropathy is associated with plasma HIV-1 RNA levels. AIDS 2002;16: 407–412.
15. Vogl D, Rosenfeld B, Breitbart W, Thaler H, Passik S, McDonald M, et al. Symptom prevalence, characteristics, and distress in AIDS outpatients. J Pain Symptom Manage 1999;18:253–262.
16. Swica Y, Breitbart W. Treating pain in patients with AIDS and a history of substance use. West J Med 2002;176:33–39.
17. Ehde DM, Gibbons LE, Chwastiak L, Bombardier CH, Sullivan MD, Kraft GH. Chronic pain in a large community sample of persons with Mult Scler. Mult Scler 2003;9:605–611.
18. Svendsen KB, Jensen TS, Overvad K, Hansen HJ, Koch-Henriksen N, Bach FW. Pain in patients with Mult Scler: a population-based study. Arch Neurol 2003;60:1089–1094.
19. Kong KH, Woon VC, Yang SY. Prevalence of chronic pain and its impact on health-related quality of life in stroke survivors. Arch Phys Med Rehabil 2004;85:35–40.
20. Woolf AD, Pfleger B. Burden of major musculoskeletal conditions. Bull World Health Organ 2003;81:646–656.
21. Soares LG. Poor social conditions, criminality and urban violence: Unmentioned barriers for effective cancer pain control at the end of life. J Pain Symptom Manage 2003;26:693–695.
22. Ersek M. Enhancing effective pain management by addressing patient barriers to analgesic use. J Hospice Palliat Nurs 1999;1:87–96.
23. Lasch K, Greenhill A, Wilkes G, Carr D, Lee M, Blanchard R. Why study pain? A qualitative analysis of medical and nursing faculty and students' knowledge of and attitudes to cancer pain management. J Palliat Med 2002;5:57–71.
24. Weinstein SM, Laux LF, Thornby JI, Lorimor RJ, Hill CS, Jr., Thorpe DM, et al. Physicians' attitudes toward pain and the use of opioid analgesics: results of a survey from the Texas Cancer Pain Initiative. South Med J 2000;93:479–487.
25. O'Brien S, Dalton JA, Konsler G, Carlson J. The knowledge and attitudes of experienced oncology nurses regarding the management of cancer-related pain. Oncol Nurs Forum 1996;23: 515–521.
26. Von Roenn JH, Cleeland CS, Gonin R, Hatfield AK, Pandya KJ. Physician attitudes and practice in cancer pain management. A survey from the Eastern Cooperative Oncology Group. Ann Intern Med 1993;119:121–126.
27. Singh RM, Wyant SL. Pain management content in curricula of U.S. schools of pharmacy. J Am Pharm Assoc 2003;43:34–40.
28. Cornelison AH. Cultural barriers to compassionate care—patients' and health professionals' perspectives. Bioethics Forum 2001;17:7–14.
29. Anderson KO, Richman SP, Hurley J, Palos G, Valero V, Mendoza TR, et al. Cancer pain management among underserved minority outpatients: perceived needs and barriers to optimal control. Cancer 2002;94:2295–2304.
30. Baltic TE, Whedon MB, Ahles TA, Fanciullo G. Improving pain relief in a rural cancer center. Cancer Pract 2002;10(Suppl 1): S39–44.
31. Morrison RS, Wallenstein S, Natale DK, Senzel RS, Huang LL. "We don't carry that"—failure of pharmacies in predominantly nonwhite neighborhoods to stock opioid analgesics. N Engl J Med 2000;342:1023–1026.
32. Berry PH, Dahl JL. The new JCAHO pain standards: implications for pain management nurses. Pain Manage Nurs 2000;1:3–12.
33. Cohen MZ, Easley MK, Ellis C, Hughes B, Ownby K, Rashad BG, et al. Cancer pain management and the JCAHO's pain standards: an institutional challenge. J Pain Symptom Manage 2003;25:519–527.
34. Keefe FJ, Ahles TA, Porter LS, Sutton LM, McBride CM, Pope MS, et al. The self-efficacy of family caregivers for helping cancer patients manage pain at end-of-life. Pain 2003;103(1–2):157–162.
35. Paice JA, Toy C, Shott S. Barriers to cancer pain relief: fear of tolerance and addiction. J Pain Symptom Manage 1998;16:1–9.
36. Potter VT, Wiseman CE, Dunn SM, Boyle FM. Patient barriers to optimal cancer pain control. Psychooncology 2003;12:153–160.
37. Gunnarsdottir S, Donovan HS, Serlin RC, Voge C, Ward S. Patient-related barriers to pain management: the Barriers Questionnaire II (BQ-II). Pain 2002;99:385–396.
38. Ward SE, Goldberg N, Miller-McCauley V, Mueller C, Nolan A, Pawlik-Plank D, et al. Patient-related barriers to management of cancer pain. Pain 1993;52:319–324.
39. Anderson KO, Mendoza TR, Valero V, Richman SP, Russell C, Hurley J, et al. Minority cancer patients and their providers: pain management attitudes and practice. Cancer 2000;88:1929–1938.
40. Weiner DK, Rudy TE. Attitudinal barriers to effective treatment of persistent pain in nursing home residents. J Am Geriatr Soc 2002;50:2035–2040.
41. Davis GC, Hiemenz ML, White TL. Barriers to managing chronic pain of older adults with arthritis. J Nurs Scholarsh 2002;34: 121–126.
42. Ward SE, Berry PE, Misiewicz H. Concerns about analgesics among patients and family caregivers in a hospice setting. Res Nurs Health 1996;19:205–211.
43. Berry PE, Ward SE. Barriers to pain management in hospice: a study of family caregivers. Hosp J 1995;10:19–33.
44. Page GG. The immune-suppressive effects of pain. Adv Exp Med Biol 2003;521:117–125.
45. Page GG, Blakely WP, Ben-Eliyahu S. Evidence that postoperative pain is a mediator of the tumor-promoting effects of surgery in rats. Pain 2001;90(1–2):191–199.
46. Chang VT, Thaler HT, Polyak TA, Kornblith AB, Lepore JM, Portenoy RK. Quality of life and survival: the role of multidimensional symptom assessment. Cancer 1998;83:173–179.
47. Hwang SS, Chang VT, Kasimis B. Dynamic cancer pain management outcomes: the relationship between pain severity, pain relief, functional interference, satisfaction and global quality of life over time. J Pain Symptom Manage 2002;23:190–200.
48. American Pain Society. Principles of analgesic use in the treatment of acute pain and cancer pain, 5th ed. Glenview, IL: American Pain Society, 2003.
49. Du Pen SL, Du Pen AR, Polissar N, Hansberry J, Kraybill BM, Stillman M, et al. Implementing guidelines for cancer pain management: results of a randomized controlled clinical trial. J Clin Oncol 1999;17:361–370.
50. Portenoy RK, Conn M. Cancer pain syndromes. In: Bruera E, Portenoy RK, eds. Cancer Pain: Assessment and Management Cambridge: Cambridge University Press, 2003:89–108.
51. Bruera E, Kim HN. Cancer pain. JAMA 2003;290:2476–2479.
52. Mantyh PW. A mechanism based understanding of cancer pain. Pain 2002;96(1–2):1–2.
53. Foley KM, Gelband H. Improving palliative care for cancer. Washington, D.C.: Institute of Medicine and National Research Council, 2001.

54. Cherny NI. The management of cancer pain. Ca 2000;50:70–116; quiz 117–120.
55. Portenoy RK, Lesage P. Management of cancer pain. Lancet 1999;353(9165):1695–1700.
56. McCaffery M, Pasero C. Pain: Clinical manual, 2nd ed. St. Louis: Mosby, 1999.
57. Ripamonti C. Pharmacology of opioid analgesia: clinical principles. In: Bruera E, Portenoy RK, eds. Cancer Pain: Assessment and Management, Cambridge: Cambridge University Press, 2003: 124–149.
58. Schiodt FV, Rochling FA, Casey DL, Lee WM. Acetaminophen toxicity in an urban county hospital. N Engl J Med 1997;337:1112–1117.
59. Tanaka E, Yamazaki K, Misawa S. Update: the clinical importance of acetaminophen hepatotoxicity in non-alcoholic and alcoholic subjects. J Clin Pharm Thera 2000;25:325–332.
60. Vane JR, Botting RM. Anti-inflammatory drugs and their mechanism of action. Inflamm Res 1998;47(Suppl 2):S78–87.
61. Mercadante S. The use of anti-inflammatory drugs in cancer pain. Cancer Treat Rev 2001;27:51–61.
62. Perez Gutthann S, Garcia Rodriguez LA, Raiford DS, Duque Oliart A, Ris Romeu J. Nonsteroidal anti-inflammatory drugs and the risk of hospitalization for acute renal failure. [comment]. Arch Intern Med 1996;156:2433–2439.
63. Cryer B, Feldman M. Cyclooxygenase-1 and cyclooxygenase-2 selectivity of widely used nonsteroidal anti-inflammatory drugs. Am J Med 1998;104:413–421.
64. Simon LS, Weaver AL, Graham DY, Kivitz AJ, Lipsky PE, Hubbard RC, et al. Anti-inflammatory and upper gastrointestinal effects of celecoxib in rheumatoid arthritis: a randomized controlled trial. JAMA 1999;282:1921–1928.
65. Silverstein FE, Faich G, Goldstein JL, Simon LS, Pincus T, Whelton A, et al. Gastrointestinal toxicity with celecoxib vs nonsteroidal anti-inflammatory drugs for osteoarthritis and rheumatoid arthritis: the CLASS study: a randomized controlled trial. Celecoxib Long-term Arthritis Safety Study. JAMA 2000; 284:1247–1255.
66. Juni P, Rutjes AW, Dieppe PA. Are selective COX 2 inhibitors superior to traditional nonsteroidal anti-inflammatory drugs? [see comment] [erratum appears in BMJ 2002 Jun 29;324(7353):1538]. BMJ 2002;324:1287–1288.
67. Juni P, Dieppe P, Egger M. Risk of myocardial infarction associated with selective COX-2 inhibitors: questions remain. Arch Intern Med 2002;162:2639–2640; author reply 2630–2632.
68. Wright JM. The double-edged sword of COX-2 selective NSAIDs. CMAJ 2002;167:1131–1137.
69. Peterson WL, Cryer B. COX-1-sparing NSAIDs—is the enthusiasm justified? JAMA 1999;282:1961–1963.
70. Lucas LK, Lipman AG. Recent advances in pharmacotherapy for cancer pain management. Cancer Pract 2002;10(Suppl 1):S14–20.
71. Hoppmann RA, Peden JG, Ober SK. Central nervous system side effects of nonsteroidal anti-inflammatory drugs. Aseptic meningitis, psychosis, and cognitive dysfunction. Arch Intern Med 1991; 151:1309–1313.
72. Mercadante S, Fulfaro F, Casuccio A. A randomised controlled study on the use of anti-inflammatory drugs in patients with cancer pain on morphine therapy: effects on dose-escalation and a pharmacoeconomic analysis. Eur J Cancer 2002;38: 1358–1363.
73. Wolfe MM, Lichtenstein DR, Singh G. Gastrointestinal toxicity of nonsteroidal antiinflammatory drugs. [comment] [erratum appears in N Engl J Med 1999 Aug 12;341:548]. N Engl J Med 1999; 340:1888–1899.
74. Inturrisi CE. Pharmacology of Analgesia: Basic Principles. In: Bruera E, Portenoy RK, eds. Cancer Pain: Assessment and Management, pp 111–123. Cambridge: Cambridge University Press, 2003.
75. Rowbotham MC, Twilling L, Davies PS, Reisner L, Taylor K, Mohr D. Oral opioid therapy for chronic peripheral and central neuropathic pain. N Engl J Med 2003;348:1223–1232.
76. Thomas JR, von Gunten CF. Clinical management of dyspnoea. Lancet Oncol 2002;3:223–228.
77. Jennings AL, Davies AN, Higgins JP, Broadley K. Opioids for the palliation of breathlessness in terminal illness. Cochrane Database Syst Rev 2001:CD002066.
78. Sykes N, Thorns A. Sedative use in the last week of life and the implications for end-of-life decision making. Arch Intern Med 2003;163:341–344.
79. Sykes N, Thorns A. The use of opioids and sedatives at the end of life. Lancet Oncol 2003;4:312–318.
80. Bercovitch M, Waller A, Adunsky A. High dose morphine use in the hospice setting. A database survey of patient characteristics and effect on life expectancy. Cancer 1999;86:871–877.
81. Andersen G, Jensen NH, Christrup L, Hansen SH, Sjogren P. Pain, sedation and morphine metabolism in cancer patients during long-term treatment with sustained-release morphine. Palliat Med 2002;16:107–114.
82. Kaiko RF, Foley KM, Grabinski PY, Heidrich G, Rogers AG, Inturrisi CE, et al. Central nervous system excitatory effects of meperidine in cancer patients. Annals of Neurology 1983;13:180–185.
83. Smith MT. Neuroexcitatory effects of morphine and hydromorphone: evidence implicating the 3-glucuronide metabolites. Clin Exp Pharmacol Physiol 2000;27:524–528.
84. O'Brien T, Mortimer PG, McDonald CJ, Miller AJ. A randomized crossover study comparing the efficacy and tolerability of a novel once-daily morphine preparation (MXL capsules) with MST Continus tablets in cancer patients with severe pain. Palliat Med 1997;11:475–482.
85. Coluzzi PH. Sublingual morphine: efficacy reviewed. J Pain Symptom Manage 1998;16:184–192.
86. Zeppetella G. Sublingual fentanyl citrate for cancer-related breakthrough pain: a pilot study. Palliat Med 2001;15:323–328.
87. Walsh D, Tropiano PS. Long-term rectal administration of high-dose sustained-release morphine tablets. Support Care Cancer 2002;10:653–655.
88. Du X, Skopp G, Aderjan R. The influence of the route of administration: a comparative study at steady state of oral sustained release morphine and morphine sulfate suppositories. Ther Drug Monit 1999;21:208–214.
89. Coyne PJ, Viswanathan R, Smith TJ. Nebulized fentanyl citrate improves patients' perception of breathing, respiratory rate, and oxygen saturation in dyspnea. J Pain Symptom Manage 2002; 23:157–160.
90. Muijsers RB, Wagstaff AJ. Transdermal fentanyl: an updated review of its pharmacological properties and therapeutic efficacy in chronic cancer pain control. Drugs 2001;61:2289–2307.
91. Menten J, Desmedt M, Lossignol D, Mullie A. Longitudinal follow-up of TTS-fentanyl use in patients with cancer-related pain: results of a compassionate-use study with special focus on elderly patients. Curr Med Res Opin 2002;18:488–498.
92. Radbruch L, Sabatowski R, Petzke F, Brunsch-Radbruch A, Grond S, Lehmann KA. Transdermal fentanyl for the management of

cancer pain: a survey of 1005 patients. Palliat Med 2001;15: 309–321.
93. Egan TD, Sharma A, Ashburn MA, Kievit J, Pace NL, Streisand JB. Multiple dose pharmacokinetics of oral transmucosal fentanyl citrate in healthy volunteers. Anesthesiology 2000;92:665–673.
94. Coluzzi PH, Schwartzberg L, Conroy JD, Charapata S, Gay M, Busch MA, et al. Breakthrough cancer pain: a randomized trial comparing oral transmucosal fentanyl citrate (OTFC) and morphine sulfate immediate release (MSIR). Pain 2001;91:123–130.
95. Payne R, Coluzzi P, Hart L, Simmonds M, Lyss A, Rauck R, et al. Long-term safety of oral transmucosal fentanyl citrate for breakthrough cancer pain. J Pain Symptom Manage 2001;22:575–583.
96. Davis MP, Varga J, Dickerson D, Walsh D, LeGrand SB, Lagman R. Normal-release and controlled-release oxycodone: pharmacokinetics, pharmacodynamics, and controversy. Support Care Cancer 2003;11:84–92.
97. Lauretti GR, Oliveira GM, Pereira NL. Comparison of sustained-release morphine with sustained-release oxycodone in advanced cancer patients. Br J Cancer 2003;89:2027–2030.
98. Shaiova L, Sperber KT, Hord ED. Methadone for refractory cancer pain. J Pain Symptom Manage 2002;23:178–180.
99. Bruera E, Sweeney C. Methadone use in cancer patients with pain: a review. J Palliat Med 2002;5:127–138.
100. Bruera E, Palmer JL, Bosnjak S, Rico MA, Moyano J, Sweeney C, et al. Methadone versus morphine as a first-line strong opioid for cancer pain: a randomized, double-blind study. J Clin Oncol 2004;22:185–192.
101. Davis MP, Walsh D. Methadone for relief of cancer pain: a review of pharmacokinetics, pharmacodynamics, drug interactions and protocols of administration. Support Care Cancer 2001;9:73–83.
102. Morley JS, Bridson J, Nash TP, Miles JB, White S, Makin MK. Low-dose methadone has an analgesic effect in neuropathic pain: a double-blind randomized controlled crossover trial. Palliat Med 2003;17:576–587.
103. Mercadante S, Casuccio A, Fulfaro F, Groff L, Boffi R, Villari P, et al. Switching from morphine to methadone to improve analgesia and tolerability in cancer patients: a prospective study. J Clin Oncol 2001;19:2898–2904.
104. Watanabe S, Tarumi Y, Oneschuk D, Lawlor P. Opioid rotation to methadone: proceed with caution. J Clin Oncol 2002;20: 2409–2410.
105. Moryl N, Santiago-Palma J, Kornick C, Derby S, Fischberg D, Payne R, et al. Pitfalls of opioid rotation: substituting another opioid for methadone in patients with cancer pain. Pain 2002;96:325–328.
106. Santiago-Palma J, Khojainova N, Kornick C, Fischberg DJ, Primavera LH, Payne R, et al. Intravenous methadone in the management of chronic cancer pain: safe and effective starting doses when substituting methadone for fentanyl. Cancer 2001;92:1919–1925.
107. Hanks GW, Conno F, Cherny N, Hanna M, Kalso E, McQuay HJ, et al. Morphine and alternative opioids in cancer pain: the EAPC recommendations. Br J Cancer 2001;84:587–593.
108. Sarhill N, Davis MP, Walsh D, Nouneh C. Methadone-induced myoclonus in advanced cancer. Am J Hosp Palliat Care 2001;18:51–53.
109. Kornick CA, Kilborn MJ, Santiago-Palma J, Schulman G, Thaler HT, Keefe DL, et al. QTC interval prolongation associated with intravenous methadone. Pain 2003;105:499–506.
110. Krantz MJ, Kutinsky IB, Robertson AD, Mehler PS. Dose-related effects of methadone on QT prolongation in a series of patients with torsade de pointes. Pharmacotherapy 2003;23:802–805.
111. Bernard SA, Bruera E. Drug interactions in palliative care. J Clin Oncol 2000;18:1780–1799.
112. Doverty M, Somogyi AA, White JM, Bochner F, Beare CH, Menelaou A, et al. Methadone maintenance patients are cross-tolerant to the antinociceptive effects of morphine. Pain 2001;93: 155–163.
113. Wright AW, Mather LE, Smith MT. Hydromorphone-3-glucuronide: a more potent neuro-excitant than its structural analogue, morphine-3-glucuronide. Life Sci 2001;69:409–420.
114. Fainsinger R, Schoeller T, Boiskin M, Bruera E. Palliative care round: cognitive failure and coma after renal failure in a patient receiving captopril and hydromorphone. J Palliat Care 1993;9:53–55.
115. Lee MA, Leng ME, Tiernan EJ. Retrospective study of the use of hydromorphone in palliative care patients with normal and abnormal urea and creatinine. Palliat Med 2001;15:26–34.
116. McCaffery M, Martin L, Ferrell BR. Analgesic administration via rectum or stoma. J ET Nurs 1992;19:114–121.
117. Nelson KA, Glare PA, Walsh D, Groh ES. A prospective, within-patient, crossover study of continuous intravenous and subcutaneous morphine for chronic cancer pain. J Pain Symptom Manage 1997;13:262–267.
118. Watanabe S, Pereira J, Hanson J, Bruera E. Fentanyl by continuous subcutaneous infusion for the management of cancer pain: a retrospective study. J Pain Symptom Manage 1998;16:323–326.
119. Smith TJ, Staats PS, Deer T, Stearns LJ, Rauck RL, Boortz-Marx RL, et al. Randomized clinical trial of an implantable drug delivery system compared with comprehensive medical management for refractory cancer pain: impact on pain, drug-related toxicity, and survival. J Clin Oncol 2002;20:4040–4049.
120. Potter J, Hami F, Bryan T, Quigley C. Symptoms in 400 patients referred to palliative care services: prevalence and patterns. Palliat Med 2003;17:310–314.
121. Breitbart W, Rosenfeld B, Kaim M, Funesti-Esch J. A randomized, double-blind, placebo-controlled trial of psychostimulants for the treatment of fatigue in ambulatory patients with human immunodeficiency virus disease. Arch Intern Med 2001;161:411–420.
122. Bruera E, Driver L, Barnes EA, Willey J, Shen L, Palmer JL, et al. Patient-controlled methylphenidate for the management of fatigue in patients with advanced cancer: a preliminary report. J Clin Oncol 2003;21:4439–4443.
123. Webster L, Andrews M, Stoddard G. Modafinil treatment of opioid-induced sedation. Pain Med 2003;4:135–140.
124. Cole RM, Robinson F, Harvey L, Trethowan K, Murdoch V. Successful control of intractable nausea and vomiting requiring combined ondansetron and haloperidol in a patient with advanced cancer. J Pain Symptom Manage 1994;9:48–50.
125. Nunez-Olarte J. Opioid-induced myoclonus. European J Palliat Care 1995;2:146–150.
126. Sjogren P, Thunedborg LP, Christrup L, Hansen SH, Franks J. Is development of hyperalgesia, allodynia and myoclonus related to morphine metabolism during long-term administration? Six case histories. Acta Anaesthesiol Scand 1998;42:1070–1075.
127. Eisele JH, Jr., Grigsby EJ, Dea G. Clonazepam treatment of myoclonic contractions associated with high-dose opioids: case report. Pain 1992;49:231–232.
128. Hagen N, Swanson R. Strychnine-like multifocal myoclonus and seizures in extremely high-dose opioid administration: treatment strategies. J Pain Symptom Manage 1997;14:51–58.
129. Larijani GE, Goldberg ME, Rogers KH. Treatment of opioid-induced pruritus with ondansetron: report of four patients. Pharmacotherapy 1996;16:958–960.

130. Max MB, Lynch SA, Muir J, Shoaf SE, Smoller B, Dubner R. Effects of desipramine, amitriptyline, and fluoxetine on pain in diabetic neuropathy. N Engl J Med 1992;326:1250–1256.
131. Hammack JE, Michalak JC, Loprinzi CL, Sloan JA, Novotny PJ, Soori GS, et al. Phase III evaluation of nortriptyline for alleviation of symptoms of cis-platinum-induced peripheral neuropathy. Pain 2002;98:195–203.
132. Dworkin RH, Backonja M, Rowbotham MC, Allen RR, Argoff CR, Bennett GJ, et al. Advances in neuropathic pain: diagnosis, mechanisms, and treatment recommendations. Arch Neurol 2003;60:1524–1534.
133. Farrar JT, Portenoy RK. Neuropathic cancer pain: the role of adjuvant analgesics. Oncology (Huntingt) 2001;15:1435–1442, 1445; discussion 1445, 1450–1433.
134. Durand JP, Goldwasser F. Dramatic recovery of paclitaxel-disabling neurosensory toxicity following treatment with venlafaxine. Anti-Cancer Drugs 2002;13:777–780.
135. Tasmuth T, Hartel B, Kalso E. Venlafaxine in neuropathic pain following treatment of breast cancer. Eur J Pain 2002;6:17–24.
136. Backonja M, Beydoun A, Edwards KR, Schwartz SL, Fonseca V, Hes M, et al. Gabapentin for the symptomatic treatment of painful neuropathy in patients with diabetes mellitus: a randomized controlled trial. JAMA 1998;280:1831–1836.
137. Rowbotham M, Harden N, Stacey B, Bernstein P, Magnus-Miller L. Gabapentin for the treatment of postherpetic neuralgia: a randomized controlled trial. JAMA 1998;280: 1837–1842.
138. Garcia-Borreguero D, Larrosa O, de la Llave Y, Verger K, Masramon X, Hernandez G. Treatment of restless legs syndrome with gabapentin: a double-blind, cross-over study. Neurology 2002; 59:1573–1579.
139. Pandey CK, Bose N, Garg G, Singh N, Baronia A, Agarwal A, et al. Gabapentin for the treatment of pain in guillain-barre syndrome: a double-blinded, placebo-controlled, crossover study. Anesth Analg 2002;95:1719–1723.
140. Ahn SH, Park HW, Lee BS, Moon HW, Jang SH, Sakong J, et al. Gabapentin effect on neuropathic pain compared among patients with spinal cord injury and different durations of symptoms. Spine 2003;28:341–346.
141. Barrueto F, Jr., Green J, Howland MA, Hoffman RS, Nelson LS. Gabapentin withdrawal presenting as status epilepticus. J Toxicol Clin Toxicol 2002;40:925–928.
142. Mercadante S, Fulfaro F, Casuccio A. The use of corticosteroids in home palliative care. Support Care Cancer 2001;9:386–389.
143. Wooldridge JE, Anderson CM, Perry MC. Corticosteroids in advanced cancer. Oncology (Huntingt) 2001;15:225–234; discussion 234–236.
144. Feuer DJ, Broadley KE. Corticosteroids for the resolution of malignant bowel obstruction in advanced gynaecological and gastrointestinal cancer. Cochrane Database Syst Rev 2000:CD001219.
145. Mao J, Chen LL. Systemic lidocaine for neuropathic pain relief. Pain 2000;87:7–17.
146. Sloan P, Basta M, Storey P, von Gunten C. Mexiletine as an adjuvant analgesic for the management of neuropathic cancer pain. Anesth Analg 1999;89:760–761.
147. Wallace MS, Magnuson S, Ridgeway B. Efficacy of oral mexiletine for neuropathic pain with allodynia: a double-blind, placebo-controlled, crossover study. Reg Anesth Pain Med 2000;25:459–467.
148. Galer BS, Rowbotham MC, Perander J, Friedman E. Topical lidocaine patch relieves postherpetic neuralgia more effectively than a vehicle topical patch: results of an enriched enrollment study. Pain 1999;80:533–538.
149. Ferrini R, Paice JA. Infusional lidocaine for severe and/or neuropathic pain. J Support Oncol 2004;2:90–94.
150. Deer TR, Caraway DL, Kim CK, Dempsey CD, Stewart CD, McNeil KF. Clinical experience with intrathecal bupivacaine in combination with opioid for the treatment of chronic pain related to failed back surgery syndrome and metastatic cancer pain of the spine. Spine J 2002;2:274–278.
151. Bell R, Eccleston C, Kalso E. Ketamine as an adjuvant to opioids for cancer pain. Cochrane Database Syst Rev 2003:CD003351.
152. Mercadante S, Casuccio A, Genovese G. Ineffectiveness of dextromethorphan in cancer pain. J Pain Symptom Manage 1998; 16:317–322.
153. Walker K, Medhurst SJ, Kidd BL, Glatt M, Bowes M, Patel S, et al. Disease modifying and anti-nociceptive effects of the bisphosphonate, zoledronic acid in a model of bone cancer pain. Pain 2002;100:219–229.
154. Wong R, Wiffen PJ. Bisphosphonates for the relief of pain secondary to bone metastases. Cochrane Database Syst Rev 2002: CD002068.
155. Groff L, Zecca E, De Conno F, Brunelli C, Boffi R, Panzeri C, et al. The role of disodium pamidronate in the management of bone pain due to malignancy. Palliat Med 2001;15:297–307.
156. Lipton A, Theriault RL, Hortobagyi GN, Simeone J, Knight RD, Mellars K, et al. Pamidronate prevents skeletal complications and is effective palliative treatment in women with breast carcinoma and osteolytic bone metastases: long term follow-up of two randomized, placebo-controlled trials. Cancer 2000; 88:1082–1090.
157. Hultborn R, Gundersen S, Ryden S, Holmberg E, Carstensen J, Wallgren UB, et al. Efficacy of pamidronate in breast cancer with bone metastases: a randomized, double-blind placebo-controlled multicenter study. Anticancer Res 1999;19:3383–3392.
158. Small EJ, Smith MR, Seaman JJ, Petrone S, Kowalski MO. Combined analysis of two multicenter, randomized, placebo-controlled studies of pamidronate disodium for the palliation of bone pain in men with metastatic prostate cancer. J Clin Oncol 2003;21:4277–4284.
159. Lipton A, Small E, Saad F, Gleason D, Gordon D, Smith M, et al. The new bisphosphonate, Zometa (zoledronic acid), decreases skeletal complications in both osteolytic and osteoblastic lesions: a comparison to pamidronate. Cancer Invest 2002;20(Suppl 2):45–54.
160. Jagdev SP, Purohit P, Heatley S, Herling C, Coleman RE. Comparison of the effects of intravenous pamidronate and oral clodronate on symptoms and bone resorption in patients with metastatic bone disease. Annals of Oncology 2001;12:1433–1438.
161. Martinez MJ, Roque M, Alonso-Coello P, Catala E, Garcia JL, Ferrandiz M. Calcitonin for metastatic bone pain. Cochrane Database Syst Rev 2003:CD003223.
162. Janjan N. Bone metastases: approaches to management. Semin Oncol 2001;28(4 Suppl 11):28–34.
163. Jeremic B. Single fraction external beam radiation therapy in the treatment of localized metastatic bone pain. A review. J Pain Symptom Manage 2001;22:1048–1058.
164. Serafini AN. Therapy of metastatic bone pain. J Nucl Med 2001;42:895–906.
165. Kraeber-Bodere F, Campion L, Rousseau C, Bourdin S, Chatal JF, Resche I. Treatment of bone metastases of prostate cancer with strontium-89 chloride: efficacy in relation to the degree of bone involvement. European J Nucl Med 2000;27:1487–1493.
166. Sciuto R, Festa A, Pasqualoni R, Semprebene A, Rea S, Bergomi S, et al. Metastatic bone pain palliation with 89-Sr and 186-Re-HEDP in breast cancer patients. Breast Cancer Res Treat 2001;66:101–109.

167. Prommer E. Guidelines for the use of palliative chemotherapy. AAHPM Bulletin 2004;5:1–4.
168. Geels P, Eisenhauer E, Bezjak A, Zee B, Day A. Palliative effect of chemotherapy: objective tumor response is associated with symptom improvement in patients with metastatic breast cancer. J Clin Oncol 2000;18:2395–2405.
169. Fromm GH. Baclofen as an adjuvant analgesic. J Pain Symptom Manage 1994;9:500–509.
170. Thompson E, Hicks F. Intrathecal baclofen and homeopathy for the treatment of painful muscle spasms associated with malignant spinal cord compression. Palliat Med 1998;12:119–121.
171. Schapiro RT. Management of spasticity, pain, and paroxysmal phenomena in Mult Scler. Curr Neurol Neurosci Rep 2001; 1:299–302.
172. Fine PG. Analgesia issues in palliative care: bone pain, controlled release opioids, managing opioid-induced constipation and nifedipine as an analgesic. J Pain Palliat Care Pharmacother 2002; 16:93–97.
173. Alvarez L, Perez-Higueras A, Quinones D, Calvo E, Rossi RE. Vertebroplasty in the treatment of vertebral tumors: postprocedural outcome and quality of life. Eur Spine J 2003;12:356–360.
174. Brubacher S, Gobel BH. Use of the Pleurx Pleural Catheter for the management of malignant pleural effusions. Clin J Oncol Nurs 2003;7:35–38.
175. Goetz MP, Callstrom MR, Charboneau JW, Farrell MA, Maus TP, Welch TJ, et al. Percutaneous image-guided radiofrequency ablation of painful metastases involving bone: a multicenter study. J Clin Oncol 2004;22:300–306.
176. Wong GY, Schroeder DR, Carns PE, Wilson JL, Martin DP, Kinney MO, et al. Effect of neurolytic celiac plexus block on pain relief, quality of life, and survival in patients with unresectable pancreatic cancer: a randomized controlled trial. JAMA 2004;291:1092–1099.
177. Spiegel D, Moore R. Imagery and hypnosis in the treatment of cancer patients. Oncology (Huntingt) 1997;11:1179–1189; discussion 1189–1195.
178. Kwekkeboom KL, Kneip J, Pearson L. A pilot study to predict success with guided imagery for cancer pain. Pain Manage Nurs 2003;4:112–123.
179. Magill L. The use of music therapy to address the suffering in advanced cancer pain. J Palliat Care 2001;17:167–172.
180. Sahler OJ, Hunter BC, Liesveld JL. The effect of using music therapy with relaxation imagery in the management of patients undergoing bone marrow transplantation: a pilot feasibility study. Altern Ther Health Med 2003;9:70–74.
181. Syrjala KL, Donaldson GW, Davis MW, Kippes ME, Carr JE. Relaxation and imagery and cognitive-behavioral training reduce pain during cancer treatment: a controlled clinical trial. Pain 1995;63:189–198.
182. Ernst E. Manual therapies for pain control: chiropractic and massage. Clin J Pain 2004;20:8–12.
183. Post-White J, Kinney ME, Savik K, Gau JB, Wilcox C, Lerner I. Therapeutic massage and healing touch improve symptoms in cancer. Integr Cancer Ther 2003;2:332–344.
184. Stephenson N, Dalton JA, Carlson J. The effect of foot reflexology on pain in patients with metastatic cancer. Appl Nurs Res 2003;16:284–286.
185. Zappa SB, Cassileth BR. Complementary approaches to palliative oncological care. J Nurs Care Qual 2003;18:22–26.
186. Stephenson NL, Weinrich SP, Tavakoli AS. The effects of foot reflexology on anxiety and pain in patients with breast and lung cancer. Oncol Nurs Forum 2000;27:67–72.
187. Meek SS. Effects of slow stroke back massage on relaxation in hospice clients. Image—the J Nurs Scholarsh 1993;25:17–21.
188. Weinrich SP, Weinrich MC. The effect of massage on pain in cancer patients. Appl Nurs Res 1990;3:140–145.
189. Rhiner M, Ferrell BR, Ferrell BA, Grant MM. A structured nondrug intervention program for cancer pain. Cancer Pract 1993; 1:137–143.
190. Mercadante S, Radbruch L, Caraceni A, Cherny N, Kaasa S, Nauck F, et al. Episodic (breakthrough) pain: consensus conference of an expert working group of the European Association for Palliative Care. Cancer 2002;94:832–839.
191. Ferrell BR, Juarez G, Borneman T. Use of routine and breakthrough analgesia in home care. Oncol Nurs Forum 1999;26: 1655–1661.
192. Miaskowski C, Dodd MJ, West C, Paul SM, Tripathy D, Koo P, et al. Lack of adherence with the analgesic regimen: a significant barrier to effective cancer pain management. J Clin Oncol 2001;19:4275–4279.
193. Caraceni A, Portenoy RK. An international survey of cancer pain characteristics and syndromes. IASP Task Force on Cancer Pain. International Association for the Study of Pain. Pain 1999;82: 263–274.
194. Portenoy RK, Hagen NA. Breakthrough pain: definition, prevalence and characteristics. Pain 1990;41:273–281.
195. Zeppetella G, O'Doherty CA, Collins S. Prevalence and characteristics of breakthrough pain in patients with non-malignant terminal disease admitted to a hospice. Palliat Med 2001;15: 243–246.
196. Swanwick M, Haworth M, Lennard RF. The prevalence of episodic pain in cancer: a survey of hospice patients on admission. Palliat Med 2001;15:9–18.
197. Hagen NA, Elwood T, Ernst S. Cancer pain emergencies: a protocol for management. J Pain Symptom Manage 1997;14:45–50.
198. Clohisy DR, Mantyh PW. Bone cancer pain. Cancer 2003;97 (3 Suppl):866–873.
199. Braun TC, Hagen NA, Clark T. Development of a clinical practice guideline for palliative sedation. J Palliat Med 2003;6: 345–350.
200. Fainsinger RL, Waller A, Bercovici M, Bengtson K, Landman W, Hosking M, et al. A multicentre international study of sedation for uncontrolled symptoms in terminally ill patients. Palliat Med 2000;14:257–265.
201. Hanks-Bell M, Paice J, Krammer L. The use of midazolam hydrochloride continuous infusions in palliative care. Clin J Oncol Nurs 2002;6:367–369.
202. Golf M, Paice JA, Feulner E, O'Leary C, Marcotte S, Mulcahy M. Refractory status epilepticus. J Palliat Med 2004;7:85–88.
203. Hocking G, Cousins MJ. Ketamine in chronic pain management: an evidence-based review. Anesth Analg 2003;97:1730–1739.
204. Bell RF, Eccleston C, Kalso E. Ketamine as adjuvant to opioids for cancer pain. A qualitative systematic review. J Pain Symptom Manage 2003;26:867–875.
205. Fine PG. Low-dose ketamine in the management of opioid nonresponsive terminal cancer pain. J Pain Symptom Manage 1999; 17:296–300.
206. Katz N. Neuropathic pain in cancer and AIDS. Clin J Pain 2000;16(2 Suppl):S41–48.
207. Passik SD, Kirsh KL, McDonald MV, Ahn S, Russak SM, Martin L, et al. A pilot survey of aberrant drug-taking attitudes and behaviors in samples of cancer and AIDS patients. J Pain Symptom Manage 2000;19:274–286.

208. Cami J, Farre M. Drug addiction. N Engl J Med 2003;349: 975–986.
209. Whitcomb LA, Kirsh KL, Passik SD. Substance abuse issues in cancer pain. Curr Pain Headache Rep 2002;6:183–190.
210. Newshan G. Pain management in the addicted patient: practical considerations. Nurs Outlook 2000;48:81–85.
211. Kirsh KL, Whitcomb LA, Donaghy K, Passik SD. Abuse and addiction issues in medically ill patients with pain: attempts at clarification of terms and empirical study. Clin J Pain 2002;18 (4 Suppl):S52–60.
212. Passik SD, Theobald DE. Managing addiction in advanced cancer patients: why bother? J Pain Symptom Manage 2000;19: 229–234.
213. Kaplan R, Slywka J, Slagle S, Ries K. A titrated morphine analgesic regimen comparing substance users and non-users with AIDS-related pain. J Pain Symptom Manage 2000;19:265–273.
214. Fishman SM, Kreis PG. The opioid contract. Clin J Pain 2002;18(4 Suppl):S70–75.
215. Bruera E, Moyano J, Seifert L, Fainsinger RL, Hanson J, Suarez-Almazor M. The frequency of alcoholism among patients with pain due to terminal cancer. J Pain Symptom Manage 1995; 10:599–603.
216. Fishman SM, Wilsey B, Yang J, Reisfield GM, Bandman TB, Borsook D. Adherence monitoring and drug surveillance in chronic opioid therapy. J Pain Symptom Manage 2000;20:293–307.
217. Braveman C, Rodrigues C. Performance improvement in pain management for home care and hospice programs. [see comment]. Am J Hosp Palliat Care 2001;18:257–263.
218. Higginson IJ. Clinical and organizational audit in palliative medicine. In: Doyle D, Hanks G, Cherny N, Calman K, eds. Oxford Textbook of Palliative Medicine, 3rd ed., Oxford: Oxford University Press, 2004:183–196.
219. Gordon DB, Pellino TA, Miaskowski C, McNeill JA, Paice JA, Laferriere D, et al. A 10-year review of quality improvement monitoring in pain management: recommendations for standardized outcome measures. Pain Manage Nurs 2002; 3:116–130.
220. Hall P, Schroder C, Weaver L. The last 48 hours of life in long-term care: a focused chart audit. J Am Geriatr Soc 2002;50:501–506.
221. Oderda GM. Outcomes research: what it is and what it isn't. J Pain Palliat Care Pharmacother 2002;16:83–89.
222. Ersek M, Kraybill BM, DuPen A. Factors hindering patients' use of medications for cancer pain. Cancer Pract 1999; 7: 226–232.
223. Jacox A, Carr DB, Payne R, Berde CB, Brietbart W, Cain JM, et al. Management of cancer pain. Rockville, MD: Agency for Health Care Policy and Research, Public Health Service, 1994.
224. Definitions related to the use of opioids for the treatment of pain. American Academy of Pain Medicine, American Pain Society, and American Society of Addiction Medicine, 2001.
225. Manfredi PL, Houde RW. Prescribing methadone, a unique analgesic. J Support Oncol 2003;1:216–220.
226. Gazelle G, Fine PG. Fast Facts and Concepts #75 Methadone for the treatment of pain. End-of-Life Physician Education Resource Center 2002;http://www.eperc.mcw.edu (accessed October 21, 2004).

7

Paula R. Anderson and Grace E. Dean

Fatigue

The deadening fatigue which invades the very bones of cancer patients is totally unlike even the most profound fatigue experienced by a well person.—M.J. Poulson[1]

- ***Key Points***
- *The patient with fatigue symptomatology requires thorough ongoing assessment and intervention, just as with other symptoms of chronic debilitating illness.*
- *Psychosocial factors such as depression, anxiety, and stress of life exhaust personal energy reserves, contributing to the underestimation of fatigue.*
- *Pharmacological as well as nonpharmacological measures to combat fatigue have met with encouraging results.*

Patients do not have the energy, words, or language that would make doctors, nurses, and other health care professionals understand just how tired they feel.[1] Fatigue is a devastating symptom that deserves the same attention that pain and other well-recognized symptoms of chronic illness receive. Fatigue is the symptom that has the greatest potential for hindering the optimism of patients that they will one day be well again.[1]

Definitions of Fatigue

I sit down in a chair and cannot will myself to get up . . . I tell my husband, "If you want to eat dinner, then you'll have to get it for us, I'm not doing it." He tells me how this has happened to "both of us," but I only see that I'm the one who cannot function the way that I used to.—A patient

Fatigue is an example of a complex phenomenon that has been studied by many disciplines but has no widely accepted definition.[2] The discipline of nursing is no exception. Even within different specialties of nursing, there has been little agreement on a definition of fatigue. In oncology, for example, patients perceive fatigue differently depending on where in the disease trajectory fatigue occurs. Fatigue is often the symptom that causes the patient with an undiagnosed cancer to seek medical treatment. Once diagnosed, the cancer patient experiences fatigue as a side effect of treatment. The patient who has finished treatment and is in recovery discovers a "new normal" level of energy. The patient who has experienced a recurrence of cancer considers fatigue to be as much an enemy as the diagnosis itself. Finally, the patient who is in the advanced stages of cancer interprets fatigue as the end of a very long struggle to be endured. It is not surprising then that a unifying definition has not been adopted.

The National Comprehensive Cancer Network (NCCN) Fatigue Practice Guidelines Panel, charged with synthesizing research on fatigue to develop recommendations for care, defines fatigue as "an unusual, persistent, subjective sense of tiredness related to cancer or cancer treatment that interferes with usual functioning."[3] This definition is similar to that of a multiple sclerosis panel that defined fatigue as a subjective lack of physical and/or mental energy perceived by individuals that interferes with usual and desired activities.[4] While other definitions have been proposed, two key elements in most definitions appear to be the subjective perception as well as interference with functioning.[5–8]

As with adults, no universal definition for fatigue in children has been agreed upon, but two definitions were identified. Fatigue derived from a group of 7- to 12-year-old pediatric oncology patients consisted of "a profound sense of being weak or tired, or of having difficulty with movement such as using arms or legs, or opening eyes."[9] In the same study, 13- to 18-year-old pediatric oncology patients' fatigue was described as "a complex, changing state of exhaustion that at times seems to be a physical condition, at other times a mental state, and still other times to be a combination of physical and mental tiredness."[9] The children's definition emphasizes a physical sensation (weakness), whereas the adolescents' definition accentuated both physical and mental exhaustion. These researchers concluded that fatigue existed within the greater context of the child's developmental stage and that the developmental stage might have a greater impact when evaluating fatigue than has yet been appreciated.

More recently, researchers identified three different types of fatigue in a study of pediatric oncology patients, 5 to 15 years of age: typical tiredness (normal ebb and flow of energy), treatment fatigue (energy loss greater than replenishment), and shutdown fatigue (profound, sustained loss of energy).[10] Additional exploratory research is needed to confirm the findings of these pioneers in pediatric cancer fatigue.

Table 7–1
Prevalence and Populations at Risk

Populations at Risk	Description and Prevalence Rates
Cancer	Patients consistently report that fatigue is more distressing than other symptoms, with prevalence rates ranging from 78%–96%, depending on type of treatment and stage of disease.[12,24,68–72] Prevalence rates for survivor fatigue range from 17%, when strict ICD-10 diagnostic criteria are applied, to as high as 80%, when less stringent criteria are applied.[73,74]
Cardiac	Coronary artery disease (CAD) affects nearly 13 million Americans and continues as the leading cause of death in the United States.[75] Fatigue is a significant side effect of CAD.[75,76,77]
Chronic fatigue syndrome (CFS)	CFS has a prevalence rate of 0.52% in women and 0.29% in men in the United States.[78]
Chronic obstructive pulmonary disease (COPD)	In the few studies that have examined fatigue in patients with COPD, fatigue is an extremely prevalent symptom, second only to dyspnea.[79,80]
End-stage renal disease (ESRD)	Fatigue and tiredness are prevalent symptoms in ESRD. For patients undergoing hemodialysis, the prevalence rate for fatigue ranges from 87%–100%, and for peritoneal dialysis, the rate is 82%.[81,82]
HIV/AIDS	Fatigue often precedes the diagnosis of HIV infection. For patients with AIDS, the prevalence rates range from 43%–70%.[83]
Multiple sclerosis (MS)	Fatigue is common and one of the most disabling symptoms of multiple sclerosis (MS). It has affected between 75% to 90% of these patients, and at least half experience fatigue on a daily basis.[84] Currently, there is no pharmacological treatment that is widely accepted to treat this fatigue. In patients with MS, fatigue can easily be misinterpreted as a cognitive disturbance, a psychological effect, or as part of respiratory–cardiovascular symptoms that are prevalent within the MS disease process.[85]
Parkinson's disease (PD)	Fatigue has not been well documented in PD. One study reported a 44% prevalence rate.[86] Two studies documented higher fatigue levels in patients with PD compared with control subjects.[86,87]

Source: Adapted from Piper (2003), reference 88.

Prevalence

During my radiation treatment I remember sitting in my car in the cancer center parking lot without moving for quite some time. I remember the social worker tapping on the window and asking me if I needed help. I could only say, "Please call my son to pick me up, I don't have the energy to put the car in gear."—A patient

Research in the palliative care arena has focused primarily on adults.[11–13] One prospective study of fatigue compared advanced cancer patients to age- and sex-matched controls. The control group had a moderate excess of women (57%), with 49% (48/98) who were overweight and 50% having at least one concomitant medical problem, such as arthritis, airflow limitation, or hypertension.[12] Although both patients and controls complained of a degree of fatigue, the severity of symptoms in patients was much worse. The prevalence of severe subjective fatigue (defined as a score on the fatigue scale of greater than the 95th percentile of controls) was 75% in the advanced cancer group. In this patient group, there were a variety of cancer diagnoses (breast, lung, and prostate) and many of the patients were also taking opioid medications.[12]

Another relevant study, conducted by the World Health Organization, included 1840 palliative care patients.[14] The prevalence of nine symptoms (pain, nausea, dyspnea, constipation, anorexia, weakness, confusion, insomnia, and weight loss) was examined in seven palliative care centers from the United States, Europe, and Australia. With the exception of moderate to severe pain, weakness was the most common symptom, reported by 51% of patients.[14]

Cancer is only one of many diseases in which fatigue is a common symptom. Table 7-1 presents prevalence rates for a variety of common chronic illnesses. Of note, 11% to 25% of patients present with chronic fatigue as their chief complaint in primary care settings.[15] Of these, 20% to 45% will have a primary organic cause and 40% to 45% will have a primary psychiatric disorder diagnosed. The remaining patients will either meet the CDC criteria for CFS or remain undiagnosed.[15]

The amount of research conducted on the symptom of fatigue has been increasing steadily over the past 2 decades.[16] However, the majority of this research has been conducted on adults. Fatigue research in children and adolescents has received little attention.[17] The prevalence of fatigue in children is difficult to gauge from the general lack of research, but one study in 75 school-aged children receiving cancer treatments reported a prevalence rate of 50%.[18] Fatigue was expressed by the children as being tired, not sleeping well, and not being able to do the things they wanted to do. More than half the children were not as active as before the illness and reported playing less. No studies on fatigue in children with advanced cancer were identified.

Pathophysiology

I had a dream that my sister wanted me to take a walk with her. In the dream, I remember clearly that I told her that we would have to walk another time as I was too tired to go with her. It is really strange, that even in my dreams, I'm fatigued.—A patient

Models to explain the causes of fatigue have been developed by different disciplines in the basic sciences and by clinicians. Table 7–2 represents a variety of theories, models, or frameworks to explain cancer-related fatigue that have been reported in the literature. The two most prominent theories are presented in more detail below. While these models were developed with the cancer patient in mind, the depletion model may also be applied to end-stage renal disease and the central peripheral model may be applied to multiple sclerosis.

Anemia, a deficiency of red blood cells or lack of hemoglobin that leads to a reduction in oxygen-carrying capacity of the blood, is an example of the depletion theory. Anemia is a common occurrence in patients with advanced disease or those receiving aggressive therapy.[19] Multiple studies evaluating recombinant erythropoietin in patients with end-stage renal failure, orthopedic surgery, and those receiving chemotherapy for cancer have demonstrated an improvement in fatigue, exercise capacity, muscle strength, and performance of daily activities.[20] Although there is reliable evidence that fatigue can be caused by anemia,[21] little is known about the relationship between the degree or rate of hemoglobin loss and the development of fatigue. One study described results of a new questionnaire that was tested on a sample of 50 patients with either solid tumors or hematological malignancies.[22] The fatigue subscale, a new addition to the Functional Assessment of Chronic Illness Therapy Measurement System, was able to distinguish patients with a hemoglobin level greater than 12 g/dL from those with a level less than 12 g/dL. Research on patients with end-stage renal disease indicates no relationship between hematocrit and subjective fatigue, even though anemia is a major side effect of the disease.[23,24] While one study demonstrated some association between subjective fatigue and anemia, it is by no means conclusive and suggests that further research is needed.[24]

Recent studies have linked inflammatory processes to central nervous system-mediated fatigue.[25–27] Proinflammatory cytokines may be released as part of the host response to the tumor or in response to tissue damage (from injury) or depletion of immune cells associated with cancer treatments.[28] These inflammatory stimuli can signal the central nervous system (CNS) to generate fatigue, as well as changes in sleep, appetite reproduction and social behavior.[27]

The search for foundational causes of fatigue continues because no one theory thoroughly explains the basis for fatigue in the patient with advanced disease. The search for such a theory is complicated. Fatigue, like pain, is not only explained by physiological mechanisms, but must be understood as

Table 7–2
Fatigue Theories, Models, and Frameworks

Theory/Model/Framework	Description
Accumulation hypothesis	Accumulated waste products in the body result in fatigue.
Depletion hypothesis	Muscular activity is impaired when the supply of substances such as carbohydrate, fat, protein, adenosine triphosphate, and protein is not available to the muscle. Anemia can also be considered a depletion mechanism.
Biochemical and physiochemical phenomena	Production, distribution, use, equalization, and movement of substances such as muscle proteins, glucose, electrolytes, and hormones may influence the experience of fatigue.
Central nervous system control	Central control of fatigue is placed in the balance between two opposing systems: the reticular activating system and the inhibitory system, which is believed to involve the reticular formation, the cerebral cortex, and the brain stem.
Adaptation and energy reserves	Each person has a certain amount of energy reserve for adaptation, and fatigue occurs when energy is depleted. This hypothesis incorporates ideas from the other hypotheses but focuses on the person's response to stressors.
Psychobiological entropy	Activity, fatigue, symptoms, and functional status are associated based on clinical observations that persons who become less active as a result of disease or treatment-related symptoms lose energizing metabolic resources.
Aistar's organizing framework	This framework is based on energy and stress theory and implicates physiologic, psychologic, and situational stressors as contributing to fatigue. Aistar attempts to explain the difference between tiredness and fatigue within Selye's general adaptation syndrome.
Piper's integrated fatigue model	Piper suggests that fatigue mechanisms influence signs and symptoms of fatigue. Changes in biological patterns such as host factors, metabolites, energy substrates, disease, and treatment, along with psychosocial patterns, impact a person's perception and lead to fatigue manifestations. The fatigue manifestations are expressed through the person's behavior.
Attentional fatigue model	The use of attentional theory is linked to attentional fatigue. When increased requirements or demands for directed attention exceed available capacity, the person is at risk for attentional fatigue.

Source: Barnett (1997), reference 89. Copyright © 1997, with permission from Elsevier.

a multicausal, multidimensional phenomenon that includes physical, psychological, social, and spiritual aspects. As such, factors influencing fatigue are beginning to be addressed.

Factors Influencing Fatigue

Keep talking to me and hold my hand . . . I know you're there and I want to open my eyes and talk with you, but I just don't have the energy to keep my eyelids open.—A patient

Characteristics that may predispose patients with advanced disease to develop fatigue have not been comprehensively studied. Oncology research has placed importance on patient characteristics in treatment-related fatigue. Table 7–3 provides a list of factors that have been associated with cancer-related fatigue. Several of these factors have been studied and are presented in some detail below.

Age is one factor that has been examined in several studies of treatment-related fatigue in oncology. The majority of completed research indicates that younger adult patients with cancer report more fatigue than older patients with cancer.[22,24] This suggests that reported fatigue may be influenced by the developmental level of the adult. For example, young adults may have heavy responsibilities of balancing career, marriage, and child-rearing, while older adults may be at the end of their careers or retired with empty nests. Additionally, the older adult often has more than one medical condition and may even attribute the fatigue to advancing age, thereby not viewing it as abnormal. These may partially explain why younger adults have reported fatigue more frequently.

Psychological depression has been linked to patients with cancer-related fatigue.[29–31] Depression and fatigue are two related concepts. Fatigue is part of the diagnostic criteria for depression,[32] and depression may develop as a result of being fatigued.[33] While depression is less frequently reported than fatigue, feelings of depression are common in patients with cancer, with a prevalence rate in the range of 20% to 25%.[34,35] One study exploring correlates of fatigue found a fused relationship between depression and fatigue. This research indicated that fatigued women scored twice as high on the depression scale as those who were not fatigued and also that depression was the strongest predictor of fatigue.[36] Additionally, depression and fatigue may coexist with cancer without having a causal relationship, because each can originate from the same pathology.[33,37]

Recent information derived from the scientific literature supports the notion that advanced stage of disease compounds the level of fatigue. Evidence demonstrates that the more advanced the cancer, the greater the occurrence of subjective fatigue.[38] Fobair and colleagues[38] interviewed 403 long-term survivors of Hodgkin's disease who had completed their initial therapy between 1 and 21 years before. Patients were asked if their energy had changed, and, if it had changed, how long it took to return to normal. Patients whose energy level had not returned to normal were more frequently found to be in the later stages of the disease. Additional research by Wang and colleagues[39] that examined fatigue severity and fatigue interference in hematological malignancies, indicated that patients with acute leukemia reported more severe fatigue when compared with chronic leukemia or non-Hodgkin's lymphoma. Their research also indicated that nausea was the clinical predictor of severe fatigue.

As illustrated by the following case reports, patient perceptions may be influenced by other symptoms.

Table 7–3
Predisposing Factors in Developing Fatigue

Personal Factors
Age (youth vs. aged)
Marital status (home demands)
Menopausal status
Psychosocial factors (depression, fear, anxiety, unfinished business, unresolved family/friend conflicts, unmet goals)
Culture/ethnicity
Income/insurance
Physical living situation
Spiritual factors
Disease-Related Factors
Anemia
Stage of disease/presence of metastases
Pain
Sleep patterns/interruptions
Permanent changes in energy "new normal"
Continency
Cachexia
Dyspnea
Treatment-Related Factors
Radiation related side effects (skin reaction, urinary or bowel changes, temporary altered energy level, temporary increase in physical demands)
Medication side effects (nausea, vomiting, diarrhea, weight loss or gain, taste changes)
Permanent physiologic consequences (altered energy or sleep pattern)
Care Factors
Number/cohesiveness of caregivers
Commitment of doctor/nurse (involvement and availability)

CASE STUDY

Mrs. Patterson, a Patient with Stage III Breast Cancer

Mrs. Patterson is a 65-year-old retired postal inspector. She attends night school, taking economics and international business classes, plays golf a couple of times a week, and has a rigorous walking routine for exercise. She was recently diagnosed with stage III breast cancer, and had surgery and radiotherapy. She participated in a fatigue study to help identify physiological indicators of fatigue. At baseline and midradiation treatment, her fatigue intensity was "0" or no fatigue.

At the end of treatment, Mrs. Patterson rated her fatigue as an "8," severe fatigue. She had been able to play golf 2 weeks before and had to cut her walking time from 45 minutes to 15 minutes. She was studying for a test and could not comprehend what she had read. When she sat and read, she would fall asleep. She used to watch her husband fall asleep while reading shortly before he died. He had non–small-cell lung cancer and died 2 years ago. His tendency to fall asleep like that was incomprehensible to her until now.

At 2 months' postradiation therapy, Mrs. Patterson rated her fatigue as a "9." She was forcing herself to attend night classes, two evenings a week from 7 to 10 PM. When not in school, she would go to bed between 8 and 9 PM and wake up in the morning between 5 and 6 AM. She was also taking 2½-hour naps every day. She started to play golf again once a week, but was exhausted after only nine holes. She continued to walk but not as far or as long as before. She received a B on her exam (previously a straight-A student), but felt her concentration was improving.

One month later, Mrs. Patterson was contacted by phone at home. She was obviously short of breath, but remarked that she had just crawled up the side of a hill where she had been installing a sprinkler system for her flowers. On further discussion, she reported that her family and friends had been commenting on her shortness of breath for weeks. She never really gave it much thought, except that she was still quite fatigued.

Case Study Assessment

When considering postradiation patient assessment, this case study illustrates the importance of evaluating symptoms and obtaining analysis of the patient's condition over time. At end of treatment, the patient indicated a fatigue level at "8." Two months later, her self-rated fatigue advanced to a "9." At the 3-month postradiation check, the patient experienced severe dyspnea, yet she had not deduced that this experience was other than a normal response to treatment. A thorough assessment and management of the fatigued patient is illustrated in the algorithm depicted in Figure 7–1.[40] It succinctly describes likely perpetrators of fatigue and potential management scenarios for medicine and nursing. Mrs. Patterson was encouraged to seek medical attention and was eventually diagnosed with radiation pneumonitis. She was prescribed corticosteroid treatment, and her symptoms, dyspnea, and fatigue improved with therapy.

Fatigue in patients undergoing cancer treatment has been closely linked with other distressing symptoms, such as pain, dyspnea, anorexia, constipation, sleep disruption, depression, anxiety, and other mood states.[41–43] Research on patients with advanced cancer has demonstrated that fatigue severity was significantly associated with similar symptoms.[12]

Like patients with cancer, patients with end-stage renal disease on chronic dialysis complained of a high level of fatigue that was associated with other symptoms.[44] The other symptoms identified were headaches, cramps, itching, dyspnea, sleep disruption (highest mean score), nausea, chest pain, and abdominal pain. However, there was no relationship found between other symptoms and any of the demographic variables.

One hundred patients with rheumatoid arthritis (RA) were asked to identify factors that contributed to their fatigue.[45] Results indicated that the rheumatoid disease process itself was the primary cause of fatigue, with specific mention of joint pain. Disturbed sleep was the second most frequent factor, and physical effort to accomplish daily tasks ranked third. Patients with RA indicated that they had to exert twice the effort and energy to accomplish the same amount of work. Another study of patients with RA reported that women experienced more fatigue than men.[46] The authors explained this variance as a result of the female patients' higher degrees of pain and poor quality of sleep.

Various physical symptoms were also identified as affecting fatigue in a study of 80 women with congestive heart failure.[47] Women were interviewed 12 months after hospitalization for heart failure. A second interview occurred 18 months later. Sleep difficulties, chest pain, and weakness accounted for a unique variance in fatigue during the first interview. By the second interview, dyspnea was the only symptom that explained the variance in fatigue level.[47]

Fatigue in children and adolescents with advanced cancer has not been addressed. However, research has begun on pediatric oncology patients' reports of factors influencing their fatigue.[9,48] In one study, for example, 7- to 12-year-old patients with cancer viewed hospital noises, new routines, changing sleep patterns, getting treatment, and low blood counts as contributing factors to the development of fatigue.[48] In the same study, 13- to 18-year-old patients reported that going for treatment, noisy nurses and inpatient children, changes in sleep position, boredom, being fearful or worried, and treatment side effects led to their fatigue. In another pediatric study on end-of-life symptoms and suffering, parents related that 89% of their children experienced substantial suffering from fatigue, pain, or dyspnea. When asked whether treatment for these symptoms was successful, parents indicated success in 27% of those with pain and only 16% of those with dyspnea.[49]

Little research on factors influencing fatigue in patients with advanced cancer has been conducted. However, results from treatment-related fatigue research do give direction for assessment and management of fatigue in the palliative care setting.

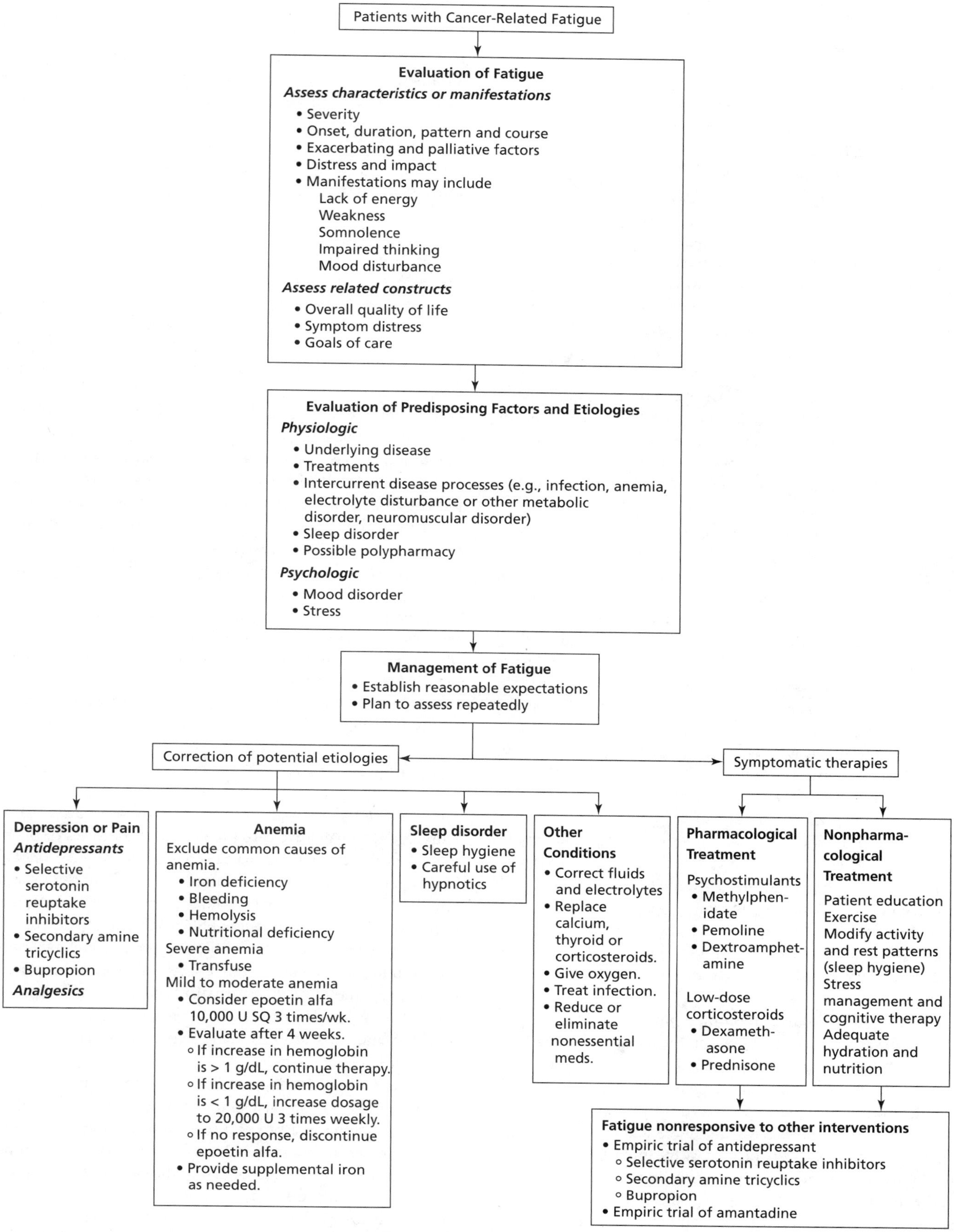

Figure 7–1. Algorithm for the evaluation and management of cancer-related fatigue. (*Source:* Portenoy RK, Itri LM. Cancer-related fatigue: guidelines for evaluation and management. Oncologist 1999;4:5. Copyright 1999 AlphaMed Press. Reprinted with permission.)

Assessment

They told me that I might experience fatigue. But I thought, "who cares about that, I have cancer." Now I know what they meant. I could have never anticipated how completely consuming the fatigue would be.—A patient

Fatigue assessment of the whole person remains paramount and includes the consideration of the body as well as the mind and spirit (Figure 7–1). When assessing fatigue, one may refer to the current literature regarding pain assessment for assistance. In pain assessment, the patient is the one whose opinion is most highly regarded. Pain is whatever the patient says it is; so, too, it should be with fatigue. Caregiver or staff perceptions may be quite different from those of the person experiencing fatigue. There is no agreement as to the perfect definition for fatigue; therefore, it is most efficient to use an individual patient's definition or description of fatigue. This personal fatigue may include any reference to or decrease in energy, weakness, or feeling tired or 'wiped out.'

There are numerous methods of assessing fatigue. Many scales have been developed to measure fatigue in the adult, with varying levels of research-related validity and reliability. Current fatigue measurement tools include the Multidimensional Assessment of Fatigue, the Symptom Distress Scale, the Fatigue Scale, the Fatigue Observation Checklist, and a Visual Analogue Scale for Fatigue.[50] These scales are available for use in research and may be used in the clinical area. One scale that has been used extensively in the oncology population is the Piper Fatigue Scale.[51] This questionnaire has 22 items that measure four dimensions of fatigue: affective meaning, behavioral/severity, cognitive/mood, and sensory. This scale measures perception, performance, motivation, and change in physical and mental activities.[52]

In clinical practice, however, a verbal rating scale may be the most efficient. Fatigue severity may be quickly assessed using a "0" (no fatigue) to "10" (extreme fatigue) scale. As with the use of any measure, consistency over time and a specific frame of reference are needed. During each evaluation, the same instructions must be given to the patient. For example, the patient may be asked to rate the level of fatigue for the past 24 hours.

Fatigue, as with any symptom, is not static. Changes take place daily and sometimes hourly in the patient with advanced disease. As such, fatigue bears repeated evaluation on the part of the health care provider. One patient, noticing the dramatic change in his energy level, remarked 'Have I always been this tired?' He seemed unsure whether there had ever been a time when he did not feel overwhelmed by the impact of fatigue. The imperative for palliative care nursing is simply to ask the patient and continue to ask, while keeping in mind that the ultimate goal is the patient's comfort. An example of a thorough assessment of the symptom of fatigue is found in Table 7–4.

Fatigue assessment tools for use in the pediatric population are in the developmental stages. Additionally, many questionnaires developed for the adult patient with cancer may provide a framework for use in pediatrics. Until then, a simple assessment of fatigue severity may be incorporated.

Management/Treatment

I fall into bed exhausted. I can't wait one minute longer or speak one more sentence. But within a couple of hours, I'm wide awake. My eyes will not rest, my mind will not rest. It's horrible not being able to sleep when I know I'm completely spent. What is wrong with me? I need to be knocked out so I can get some sleep.—A patient

When considering palliative care, the management of fatigue is extremely challenging. By its very definition, palliative care may encompass a prolonged period before death, when a person is still active and physically and socially participating in life, to a few weeks before death, when participatory activity may be minimal. With fatigue interventions, the wishes of the patient and family are paramount. One must consider management in the context of the extent of disease, other symptoms (pain, nausea, diarrhea, etc.), whether palliative treatment is still in process, age and developmental stage, and the emotional "place" of the patient.

Interventions for fatigue have been suggested to occur at two levels: managing symptoms that contribute to fatigue and the prevention of additional or secondary fatigue by maintaining a balance between restorative rest and restorative activity.[53] Fatigue interventions have been grouped into two broad categories: medical interventions and nursing interventions.

Medical Intervention

Pharmacological approaches to treat fatigue have been sparse with regard to palliative care (Table 7–5). Categories of pharmacological therapies that have been used in limited numbers in this patient population are stimulants, antidepressants and low-dose steroids.[54] Methylphenidate, a psychostimulant, has been shown to improve quality of life when given to depressed, terminally ill patients. It has also been shown to counteract opioid somnolence, enhance the effects of pain medication, improve cognition, and increase patient activity level.[55,56] Appropriate dosing for this drug is between 5 mg–10 mg orally at breakfast and 5 mg at lunch daily. The elderly may require a downward dose adjustment.

Another stimulant that has been used in the past to treat fatigue is Pemoline. Liver toxicities have caused concern with this drug, and, subsequently, its use tends to be avoided. Dextroamphetamines are a potent CNS stimulant that may also be used. They are quickly absorbed from the gastrointestinal tract with high concentrations in the brain.

Antidepressants have shown effectiveness when a patient experiences both fatigue and depression. Efficacy has been shown with both nortriptyline and amitriptyline.[54] Corticosteroids have been used to increase energy levels at a dose of

Table 7–4
Fatigue Assessment

Location: Where on the body is the fatigue located: Upper/lower extremities? All muscles of the body? Mental/attentional fatigue? Total body fatigue?
Intensity/severity: Does the fatigue interfere with activities (work, role/responsibilities at home, social, things the patient enjoys)?
Duration: How long does the fatigue last (minutes, hours, days)? Has it become chronic (more than 6 months' duration)? What is the pattern (wake up from a night's sleep exhausted, evening fatigue, transient, unfading, are circadian rhythms affected)?
Aggravating factors: What makes it worse (rest, activity, other symptoms, environmental heat, noise)?
Alleviating factors: What relieves it (a good night's rest, food, listening to music, exercise)?
Patient's knowledge of fatigue: What meaning does the patient assign to the symptom of fatigue (getting worse, disease progression, dying)?
Medications: Is the patient taking any medications that could cause the fatigue (for pain or sleep)?
Physical exam based on subjective symptom: Is there anything obvious on exam that could account for the fatigue (nerve damage, malnourished, dehydrated)?
Muscle strength: Tests to elicit muscle strength are available (Jamar grip strength, nerve conduction studies).
General appearance: Often, there is nothing in a patient's general appearance to indicate how fatigued he or she is; however, some patients do exhibit signs such as appearing pale or having a monotone voice, slowed speech, short of breath, obvious weight loss, dull facial expression.
Vital signs: Anything out of the ordinary to explain their fatigue (fever, low blood pressure, weak pulse)?
Laboratory results: Oxygenation status (blood gases, hemoglobin, hematocrit), electrolytes, other hormones such as thyroid?
Level of activity: Have usual activities changed?
Affect: What is the patient's mood (anxious, depressed, flat)?

about 20 mg–40 mg/day. Prednisone has been shown to decrease the degree of fatigue experienced in some patients. Results from one study indicated an increase in activity level when palliative care patients were treated with methylprednisolone.[57] The side effects that may occur with these drugs are always a concern.

Anemia as a result of chemotherapeutic regimens has been the most responsive to intervention. Erythropoietin alpha has been critical in increasing hemoglobin levels to obtain the highest quality of life possible for cancer patients. Doses vary in timing from 10,000 U subcutaneously given three times per week, to 40,000 U once a week, with a similar increase in hemoglobin level.[58] In one study of 4382 anemic cancer patients, the highest quality of life was experienced when hemoglobin was maintained between 11 g–13 g/L with the use of epoetin alfa.[59]

Nonpharmacological Nursing Interventions

Historically, nurse clinicians and researchers have been the trailblazers in assessing and managing fatigue in the clinical setting. Research has been conducted on all of the fatigue management strategies listed below, but sample sizes have often been small and homogeneous. Much more research is needed, but the beginning evidence is encouraging (Table 7–6).

Several investigators have reported the benefits of a consistent exercise regime in breast cancer patients.[60–62] They have found that exercise decreased perceptions of fatigue, and they indicated that those patients who exercised reported half the fatigue level of those not exercising. Whether these findings can be generalized to palliative care is unknown.

When attention-restoring interventions were used with cancer patients, it was found that attention capacity was enhanced and fatigue was reduced.[63,64] These activities are based on a program that required patients to select and engage in a favorite activity for 30 minutes three times a week. The use of this technique seemed to provide restorative distraction and replace boredom and understimulation. Included in the activities were spending time in a natural environment, participating in favorite hobbies, writing, fishing, music, and gardening. Regardless of the limitations of the patients with advanced disease, incorporation of some of these activities may prove helpful.

Another broad category for fatigue intervention includes taking advantage of every educational opportunity during the advanced disease course. With education of both the patient and the family as a constant theme, every attempt should be made to forewarn of changes in disease progression, procedures, treatment, medication side effects, or scheduling. Even

Table 7–5
Pharmacologic Agents Used in Fatigue Management

Author	Medication	Diagnosis	N	Result
Bruera[57]	Methylprednisolone	Palliative care	40	Increased activity
Bruera[90]	Methylphenidate	Advanced cancer	48	Improved pain Improved somnolence
Bruera[91]	Methylphenidate	Advanced cancer pain	20	Improved cognition
MacLeod[92]	Methylphenidate 17.7 mg QD	Major depressive disorder Hospice inpatients	26	46% therapeutic response, 7% significant response
Myers[93]	Methylphenidate 10 mg bid	Brain tumor	30	Increased stamina, energy, cognition, mood
Sarhill[94]	Methylphenidate	Advanced cancer	11	Beneficial effect on fatigue
Rammohan[84]	Modafinil (Provigil®) 200 mg/day	Multiple sclerosis	72	Significantly improves fatigue
Gillson[95]	Histamine phosphate/caffeine citrate transdermal patch	Multiple sclerosis	29	37% improvement in fatigue
Cleare[96]	Hydrocortisone 5–10 mg QD (limited use due to possible side effects)	Chronic fatigue syndrome	32	Enhance mood, appear to improve fatigue for limited period of time
Crawford et al.[59]	Epoetin alfa	Review of data from two community trials of anemic cancer patients	4382	Maximum improvement in QOL w/Hgb. 11–13 g/dL
Schwartz et al.[97]	Exercise plus methylphenidate 20 mg SR Q am	Patients w/melanoma taking interferon	12 (pilot)	Appeared to reduce fatigue and increase cognitive function

Source: Adapted from "Palliative Uses of Methylphenidate In Patients with Cancer: A Review," by M. Rozans, A. Dreisbach, J. Lertora, M. Kahn, J Clin Oncol 2001; 20: 338.[98] Copyright 2001 by American Society of Clinical Oncology. Reprinted with permission.

a personnel change can be enough to impact the physical and emotional energy reserves. Nurse-initiated and planned educational sessions with both the patient and family give a forum in which to field forgotten questions, reinforce nutritional information, and together manage symptoms.

Sleep disruption is a common problem encountered by the patient with advanced cancer. Sleep cycles may be negatively affected by innumerable internal and external factors, whose effect should not be underestimated. Simple changes in environment and habits may improve sleep distress tremendously. One study evaluated the feasibility of sleep interventions while patients underwent adjuvant chemotherapy.[65] Components of the intervention included sleep hygiene, relaxation therapy, stimulus control and sleep-restriction techniques. For those situations where pharmacological intervention is necessary, a thorough assessment of past and current sleep habits is essential. The temporary use of sleep medications such as Ambien (zolpidem tartrate) may be used to minimize sleep deprivation enough to energize the patient into trying nonpharmacological measures.

Psychosocial techniques are the last broad category of fatigue intervention. One review of 22 studies of psychosocial treatment with cancer patients reported findings that indicate that psychosocial support and individualized counseling have a fatigue-reducing effect.[66] If deemed appropriate, encourage the patient and/or family to participate in disease-specific support groups, using the telephone or the Internet if unable to travel. Individual counseling by professionals in nursing, social work, or psychology are also helpful to many.

Fatigue-management interventions need to be considered within the cultural context of the patient and family. For some cultures, this may include only the "nuclear" family, whereas in other cultures, there are ritual or extended relatives. When information is shared and decisions are made regarding intervention, the "family" is acknowledged formally, and care should be made inclusive of these variations.[67]

Management of and interventions for fatigue in pediatric oncology in general have not yet been defined. Additionally, what helps the pediatric patient with fatigue depends on his or her developmental stage.[9] Children up to 13 years old with cancer view fatigue-alleviating factors as taking a nap or sleeping, having visitors, and participating in fun activities. Adolescent patients with cancer add their perceptions of what helps their fatigue by including going outdoors, protracted rest time, keeping busy, medication for sleep, physical therapy, and receiving blood transfusions.[9] Regardless of the perceptions of the contributing or alleviating factors in the younger patient, knowing the results of this research emphasizes the importance of including all members of the team (patient, parent, and staff) in designing approaches to intervene in solving the problem of fatigue.

Table 7–6
Nursing Management of Cancer-Related Fatigue

Problem	Intervention	Rationale
Lack of information/lack of preparation	Explain complex nature of fatigue and importance of communication with health care professionals. Explain causes of fatigue in advanced cancer: • Fatigue can increase in advanced disease. • Cancer cells can compete with body for essential nutrients. • Palliative treatments, infection, and fever increase body's need for energy. • Worry or anxiety can cause fatigue as well as depression, sadness, or tension. • Changes in daily schedules, new routines, or interrupted sleep schedules contribute to the development of fatigue. Prepare patients for all planned activities of daily living (eating, moving, bath).	Preparatory sensory information reduces anxiety and fatigue. Realistic expectations decrease distress and decrease fatigue.
Disrupted rest/sleep patterns	Establish or continue regular bedtime and awakening. Obtain as long sleep sequences as possible, plan uninterrupted time. Rest periods or naps during the day, if needed, but do not interfere with nighttime sleep. Use light sources to cue the body into a consistent sleep rhythm. Pharmacological management of insomnia should be used only when behavioral and cognitive approaches have been exhausted.	Curtailing time in bed, unless absolutely necessary, helps patient feel refreshed and avoids fragmented sleep, strengthens circadian rhythm.
Deficient nutritional status	Recommend nutritious, high-protein, nutrient-dense food to make every mouthful of food "count". Suggest more small, frequent meals. Use protein supplements to augment diet. Encourage adequate intake of fluids, recommend 8–10 glasses or whatever is comfortably tolerated unless medically contraindicated to maintain hydration. Frequent oral hygiene. Corticosteroids may be prescribed to assist with appetite stimulation.	Food will help energy levels; less energy is needed for digestion with small, frequent meals.
Symptom management	Control contributing symptoms (pain, depression, nausea, vomiting, diarrhea, constipation, anemia, electrolyte imbalances, dyspnea, dehydration). Assess for anemia and evaluate for the possibility of medications or transfusion.	Managing other symptoms requires energy and may interfere with restful sleep.
Distraction/restoration	Encourage activities to restore energy: spending time in the natural environment, listening to music, praying, meditating, engaging in hobbies (art, journaling, reading, writing, fishing), spending time with family and friends, joining in passive activities (riding in car, being read to, watching meal preparation).	Pleasant activities may reduce/relieve mental (attentional) fatigue.

(continued)

Table 7–6
Nursing Management of Cancer-Related Fatigue *(continued)*

Problem	Intervention	Rationale
Decreased energy	Plan/schedule activities: • Choose someone to be in charge (fielding questions, answering the phone, organizing meals). • Determine where energy is best spent and eliminate or postpone other activities. Use optimal times of the day: • Save energy for most important events. • Learn to listen to the body; if fatigued, rest. Let things go around the house.	Energy conservation helps to reduce burden and efficiently use energy available.
Physical limitations	Engage in an individually tailored exercise program approved by the health care team. Enjoy leisure activities (sitting outside, music, gardening, etc) Be receptive to the patient's pace, and move slowly when providing care. Mild physical therapy may be helpful in maintaining joint flexibility and preventing potential pain from joint stiffness.	Exercise reduces the deleterious effects of immobility and deconditioning.

Summary

This chapter has provided an overview of fatigue as it spans the illness trajectory and end-of-life experience. While fatigue is a complex phenomenon that has been widely studied, there is no universally accepted definition. Fatigue is experienced by individuals with various chronic diseases; is influenced by many factors such as age, depression, stage of disease and other concurrent symptoms; and has numerous causes. The authors have provided a fatigue-assessment checklist that can be used to identify potential sources and/or antecedents for the patient's fatigue. Because there is no instant cure for fatigue, the patient experiencing it may be frustrated and reluctant to use the practical interventions. Nurses are challenged to provide current information about fatigue, its reversible causes, and its normal occurrence with various illnesses and to encourage patients to actively participate in fatigue-management strategies.

REFERENCES

1. Poulson MJ. Not just tired. J Clin Oncol 2001;19:4180–4181.
2. Nail LM. Fatigue in patients with cancer. Oncol Nurs Forum 2002;537–546.
3. Mock V. Fatigue management: evidence and guidelines for practice. Cancer 2001;92(6 Suppl):1699–1707.
4. Multiple Sclerosis Council for Clinical Practice Guidelines. Fatigue and multiple sclerosis: evidence-based management strategies for fatigue in multiple sclerosis. Washington, DC 1998.
5. Busichio K, Tiersky LA, Deluca J, Natelson BH. Neuropsychological deficits in patients with chronic fatigue. J Int Neuropsych Soc 2004;10:278–285.
6. North American Nursing Diagnosis Association. NANDA nursing diagnoses: definitions and classification 2001–2002. Philadelphia: NANDA; 2001.
7. Piper B. Fatigue. In: Carrieri-Kohlman V, Lindsey A, West C, eds. Pathophysiological Phenomena in Nursing: Human Responses to Illness, 2nd ed. Philadelphia: W.B. Saunders, 1993: 279–302.
8. Richardson A, Ream E. Fatigue in patients receiving chemotherapy for advanced cancer. Int J Palliat Nurs 1996;2:199–204.
9. Hinds PS, Hockenberry-Eaton M, Gilger E, et al. Comparing patient, parent, and staff descriptions of fatigue in pediatric oncology patients. Cancer Nurs 1999;22:277–289.
10. Davies B, Whitsett SF, Bruce A, McCarthy P. A typology of fatigue in children with cancer. J Ped Oncol 2002;19:12-21.
11. Maltoni M, Nannie O, Pirovano M, et al. Successful validation of the palliative prognostic score in terminally ill cancer patients. J Pain Symptom Manage 1999;17:240–247.
12. Stone P, Hardy J, Broadley K, Tookman A, Kurowska A, Hern R. Fatigue in advanced cancer: a prospective controlled cross-sectional study. Br J Cancer 1999;79:1479–1486.
13. Priovano M, Maltoni M, Nanni O, et al. A new palliative prognostic score: a first step for the staging of terminally ill cancer patients. J Pain Symptom Manage 1999;17:231–239.
14. Vainio A, Auvinen A. Prevalence of symptoms among patients with advanced cancer: an international study. J Pain Symptom Manage 1996;12:3–10.

15. Epstein KR. The chronically fatigued patient. Med Clin North Am 1995;79:315–327.
16. Fu M, LeMone P, McDaniel RW, Bausler C. A multivariate validation of the defining characteristics of fatigue. Nurs Diagnosis 2001;12:15–27.
17. Erickson JM. Fatigue in adolescents with cancer: a review of the literature. Clin J Oncol Nurs 2004;8:139–145.
18. Bottomly S, Teegarden C, Hockenberry-Eaton M. Fatigue in children with cancer: clinical considerations for nursing. J Pediatr Oncol Nurs 1996;13:178.
19. Bosanquet N, Tolley K. Treatment of anaemia in cancer patients: implications for supportive care in the National Health Service Cancer Plan. Curr Med Res Opin 2003;19:643–650.
20. Carson JL, Terrin ML, Jay M. Anemia and postoperative rehabilitation. Can J Anaesth 2003;50(6suppl):S60–64.
21. Cella D. The Functional Assessment of Cancer Therapy–Anemia (FACT-An) Scale: a new tool for the assessment of outcomes in cancer anemia and fatigue. Semin Hematol 1997;3(Suppl 2):13–19.
22. Ashbury FD, Findlay H, Reynolds B, McKerracher K. A Canadian survey of cancer patients' experiences: are their needs being met? J Pain Symptom Manage 1998;16:298–306.
23. Cardenas D, Kutner N. The problem of fatigue in dialysis patients. Nephron 1982;30:336–340.
24. Woo B, Dibble SL, Piper BF, Keating SB, Weiss MC. Differences in fatigue by treatment methods in women with breast cancer. Oncol Nurs Forum 1998;25:915–920.
25. Bower JE, Ganz PA, Aziz N, Fahey JL. Fatigue and proinflammatory cytokine activity in breast cancer survivors. Psychosom Med 2002;64:604–611.
26. Bower JE, Ganz PA, Aziz N, Fahey JL, Cole SW. T-cell homeostasis in breast cancer survivors with persistent fatigue. J Natl Cancer Institute 2003;95:1165–1168.
27. Kent S, Bluthe RM, Kelley KW, Dantzer R. Sickness behavior as a new target for drug development. Trends Pharmacol Sci 1992;13: 24–28.
28. Herskind C, Bamberg M, Rodemann H. The role of cytokines in the development of normal-tissue reactions after radiotherapy. Strahlenther und Onkol 1998;174(suppl III):12–15.
29. Hardman A, Maguire P, Crowther D. The recognition of psychiatric morbidity on a medical oncology ward. J Psychosom Res 1989;33:235–239.
30. Kathol RG, Noyes R, Williams J. Diagnosing depression in patients with medical illness. Psychosomatics 1990;31:436–449.
31. Valente SM, Saunders JM, Cohen MZ. Evaluating depression among patients with cancer. Cancer Pract 1994;2:65–71.
32. American Psychiatric Association. Diagnostic and Statistical Manual of Mental Disorders, 4th ed. Washington DC: American Psychiatric Association, 1994:317–391.
33. Visser MRM, Smets EMA. Fatigue, depression and quality of life in cancer patients: how are they related? Support Care Cancer 1998;6:101–108.
34. Hayes JR. Depression and chronic fatigue in cancer patients. Prim Care 1991;18:327–339.
35. Ibbotson T, Maguire P, Selby P, Priestman T, Wallace L. Screening for anxiety and depression in cancer patients: the effects of disease and treatment. Eur J Cancer 1993;30:37–40.
36. Bower JE, Ganz PA, Desmond KA, Rowland JH, Meyerowitz BE, Belin TR. Fatigue in breast cancer survivors: occurrence, correlates, and impact on quality of life. J Clin Oncol 2000;18:743–753.
37. Redd WH, Jacobson PB. Emotions and cancer. Cancer 1988; 62:1871–1879.
38. Fobair P, Hoppe RT, Bloom J, Cox R, Varghese A, Spiegel D. Psychosocial problems among survivors of Hodgkin's disease. J Clin Oncol 1986;4:805–814.
39. Wang XS, Giralt SA, Mendoza TR, Engstrom MC, Johnson BA, Peterson N, Broemeling LD, Cleeland CS. Clinical factors associated with cancer-related fatigue in patients being treated for leukemia and non-Hodgkin's lymphoma. J Clin Oncol 2002;20: 1319–1328.
40. Portenoy RK, Itri LM. Cancer-related fatigue: guidelines for evaluation and management. Oncologist 1999;4:1–10.
41. Aaronson LS, Teel CS, Cassmeyer V, et al. Defining and measuring fatigue. Image–J Nurs Sch 1999;31:45–50.
42. Blesch K, Paice J, Wickman R, et al. Correlates of fatigue in people with breast or lung cancer. Oncol Nurs Forum 1991;18:81–87.
43. Gift A, Pugh G. Dyspnea and fatigue. Nurs Clin North Am 1993;28:373–384.
44. Brunier G, Graydon J. The influence of physical activity on fatigue in patients with ESRD on hemodialysis. Am Nephrol Nurses Assoc J 1993;20:457–461.
45. Crosby L. Factors which contribute to fatigue associated with rheumatoid arthritis. J Adv Nurs 1991;16:974–981.
46. Belza B, Henke C, Yelin E, Epstein W, Gilliss C. Correlates of fatigue in older adults with rheumatoid arthritis. Nurs Res 1993;42:93–109.
47. Friedman M, King K. Correlates of fatigue in older women with heart failure. Heart Lung 1995;24:512–518.
48. Hinds PS, Hockenberry-Eaton M, Quargnenti A, et al. Fatigue in 7- to 12-year old patients with cancer from the staff perspective: an exploratory study. Oncol Nurs Forum 1999;26:37–45.
49. Wolfe J, Holcombe GE, Klar N, Levin SB, Ellenbogen JM, Salem-Schatz S, Emanuel EJ, Wees JC. Symptoms and suffering at the end of life in children with cancer. N Engl J Med 2000;342 326–333.
50. Aaronson LS, Teel CS, Cassmeyer V, Neuberger GB, Pallikkathayil L, Pierce J, Press AN, Williams PD, Wingate A. Defining and measuring fatigue. Image—J Nurs Scholarship, 1999;31:45–50.
51. Piper BF, Dibble SL, Dodd MJ. The revised Piper Fatigue Scale: confirmation of its multidimensionality and reduction in number of items in women with breast cancer [abstract]. Oncol Nurs Forum 1996;23:352.
52. Piper B. Fatigue. In: Carrieri-Kohlman V, Lindsey A, West C, eds. Pathophysiological Phenomena in Nursing: Human Responses to Illness, 2nd ed. Philadelphia: WB Saunders, 1993:279–302.
53. Winningham ML. Strategies for managing cancer-related fatigue syndrome: a rehabilitation approach. Cancer 2001;92(4 Suppl): 988–997.
54. Escalante CP. Treatment of cancer-related fatigue: an update. Support Care Cancer 2003;11:79–83.
55. Rozans M, Dreisbach A, Lertora JJ, Kahn MJ. Palliative uses of methylphenidate in patients with cancer: a review. J Clin Oncol 2002;20:335–339.
56. Barnes EA, Bruera E. Fatigue in patients with advanced cancer: a review. Int J Gynecol Cancer 2002;12:424–428.
57. Bruera E, Roca E, Cedaro L, Carraro S, Chacon R. Action of oral methylprednisolone in terminal cancer patients: a prospective randomized double-blind study. Cancer Treat Report 1985;69: 751–754.
58. Gabrilove JL, Einhorn LH, Livingston RB, Sarokhan B, Winer E, Einhorn LH. Once weekly dosing of epoetin alfa is similar to three times weekly dosing in increasing hemoglobin and quality of life. Proc Am Soc Clin Oncol 1999;18:574A.
59. Crawford J, Cella D, Cleeland CS, Cremieux PY, Demetri GD, Sarokhan BJ, Slavin MB, Glaspy JA. Relationship between changes

in hemoglobin level and quality of life during chemotherapy in anemic cancer patients receiving epoetin alfa therapy. Cancer 2002;95:888–895.

60. Mock V, Dow KH, Meares CJ, et al. Effects of exercise on fatigue, physical functioning, and emotional distress during radiation therapy for breast cancer. Oncol Nurs Forum 1997;24:991–1000.
61. Pickett M, Mock V, Ropka ME, Cameron L, Coleman M, Podewils L. Adherence to moderate-intensity exercise during breast cancer therapy. Cancer Pract 2002;10:284–292.
62. Winningham M, MacVicar M, Burke C. Exercise for cancer patients: guidelines and precautions. Physician Sportsmed 1986; 14:125.
63. Cimprich B. Attentional fatigue following breast cancer surgery. Res Nurs Health 1992;15:199–207.
64. Cimprich B, Ronis DL. An environmental intervention to restore attention in women with newly diagnosed breast cancer. Cancer Nurs 2003;26:284–292.
65. Berger AM, VonEssen S, Kuhn BR, Piper BF, Farr L, Agrawal A, Lynch JC, Higginbotham P. Feasibility of a sleep intervention during adjuvant breast cancer chemotherapy. Oncol Nurs Forum 2002;29:1431–1441.
66. Trijsburg R, van Knippengerg F, Rijpma S. Effects of psychological treatment on cancer patients: a comparison of strategies. Psychosom Med 1992;54:489–517.
67. Kagawa-Singer M. A multicultural perspective on death and dying. Oncol Nurs Forum 1998;25:1752–1756.
68. Stone P, Richardson A, Ream E, Smith AG, Kerr DJ, Kearney N. Cancer-related fatigue: inevitable, unimportant, and untreatable? Results of a multi-centre patient survey. Annals Oncol 2000;11:971–975.
69. Vogelzang N, Breitbart W, Cella D, Curt GA, Groopman JE, Horning SJ, et al. Patient, caregiver and oncologist perceptions of cancer-related fatigue: results of a tri-part assessment survey. Semin Heme 1997;34:4–12.
70. Hickok JT, Morrow GJ, McDonald S, Bellg AJ. Frequency and correlates of fatigue in lung cancer patients receiving radiation therapy: implications for management. J Pain Symptom Manage 1996;11:370–377.
71. Donnelly S, Walsh D. The symptoms of advanced cancer. Semin Oncol 1995;22:67–72.
72. Vanio A, Auvinen A. Prevalence of symptoms among patients with advanced cancer: an international collaborative study, symptom prevalence group. J Pain Symptom Manage 1996;2:3–10.
73. Cella D, Davis K, Breitbart W, Curt G. Fatigue Coalition. Cancer-related fatigue: prevalence of proposed diagnostic criteria in a United States sample of cancer survivors. J Clin Oncol 2001; 19:3385–3391.
74. Knobel H, Havard Loge J, Brit Lund M, Forfang K, Nome O, Kaasa S. Late medical complications and fatigue in Hodgkin's disease survivors. J Clin Oncol 2001; 19:3226–3233.
75. Miller CL. A review of symptoms of coronary artery disease in women. J Adv Nurs 2002;39:17–23.
76. Friedman M, King K. Correlates of fatigue in older women with heart failure. Heart Lung 1995;24:512–518.
77. Redberg RF. Coronary artery disease in women: understanding the diagnostic and management pitfalls. Medscape Womens Health 1998;3:1.
78. Jason LA, Richman JA, Rademaker AW, Jordan KM, Plioplys AV, Taylor RR, McCready W, Huang CF, Plioplys S. A community-based study of chronic fatigue syndrome. Arch Intern Med 1999; 159:2129–2137.
79. Gift AG, Shepard CE. Fatigue and other symptoms in patients with chronic obstructive pulmonary disease; do women and men differ? J Obstet Gynecol Neonatal Nurs 1999;28:201–208.
80. Janson-Bjerklie S, Carrieri VK, Hudes M. The sensations of pulmonary dyspnea. Nurs Res 1986;35:154–159.
81. Merkus MP, Jager KJ, Dekker FW, de Haan RJ, Boeschoten EW, Krediet RT. Physical symptoms and quality of life in patients on chronic dialysis: results of The Netherlands Cooperative Study on Adequacy of Dialysis (NECOSAD) Nephrol Dial Transplant 1999;14:1163–1170.
82. McCann K, Boore JR. Fatigue in persons with renal failure who require maintenance haemodialysis. J Adv Nurs 2000;32: 1132–1142.
83. Piper BF. Fatigue. In: Ropka ME, Williams A. eds. Handbook of HIV nursing symptom management. Boston: Jones & Bartlett, 1998:449–470.
84. Rammohan KE, Rosenberg JH, Lynn DJ, Blumenfled AM, Pollak CP, Nagaraja HN. Efficacy and safety of modafinil (Provigil) for the treatment of fatigue in multiple sclerosis: a two centre phase 2 study. J Neurol Neurosurg Psychiatry 2002;72:179–183.
85. Costello K, Harris C. Differential diagnosis and management of fatigue in multiple sclerosis: considerations for the nurse. J Neuroscience Nurs 2003;35:139–148.
86. Karlsen K, Larsen JP, Tandberg E, Jorgensen K. Fatigue in patients with Parkinson's disease. Mov Disord 1999;14:237–241.
87. Lou JS, Kearns G, Oken B, Sexton G, Nutt J. Exacerbated physical fatigue and mental fatigue in Parkinson's disease. Mov Disord 2001;16:190–196.
88. Piper BF. Fatigue. In: Carriere-Kohlman V, Kindsey A, and West C, eds. Pathophysiological Phenomena in Nursing: Human Responses to Illness, 3rd ed. Philadelphia: W.B. Saunders, 2003; 209–234.
89. Barnett ML. Fatigue. In: Otto SE, ed. Oncology Nursing, 3rd ed. St. Louis: Mosby, 1997;670.
90. Bruera E, Brenneis C, Paterson AH, MacDonald RN. Use of methylphenidate as an adjuvant to narcotic analgesics in patients with advanced cancer. J Pain Symptom Manage 1989;4:3–6.
91. Bruera E, Miller MJ, Macmillan K, Kuehn N. Neuropsychological effects of methylphenidate in patients receiving a continuous infusion of narcotics for cancer pain. Pain 1992;48:163–166.
92. Macleod AD. Methylphenidate in terminal depression. J Pain Symptom Manage 1998;16:193–198.
93. Myers CA, Weitzner MA, Valentine AD, Levin VA. Methylphenidate therapy improves cognition, mood, and function of brain tumor patients. J Clin Oncol 1998;16:2522–2527.
94. Sarhill N, Walsh D, Nelson KA, Homsi J, Lerand S, Davis MD. Methylphenidate for fatigue in advanced cancer: a prospective open-label pilot study. Am J Hospice Palliat Care 2001; 8:187–192.
95. Gillson G. A double-blind pilot study of the effect of Prokarin on fatigue in multiple sclerosis. Mult Scler 2002;8:30–35.
96. Cleare AJ, Heap E, Malhi GS, Wessely S, O'Keane V, Miell J. Low dose hydrocortisone in chronic fatigue syndrome: a randomized crossover trial. Lancet 353:455–458.
97. Schwartz AL, Thompson JA, Masood N. Interferon-induced fatigue in patients with melanoma: a pilot study of exercise and Methylphenidate. Oncol Nurs Forum Online Exclusive 2002;29: E85–E90.
98. Rozans M, Dreisbach A, Lertora J, Kahn M. Palliative uses of methylphenidate in patients with cancer: a review. J Clin Oncol 2001;20:338.

8

Charles Kemp

Anorexia and Cachexia

When you can't eat, you're just no longer a part of your family. There's no need for me to go to the dinner table but sometimes I go so my family won't feel so sad. They try all the time to help me eat but I just can't. I know it adds to their suffering. I think it's worse than the pain.—A woman with lung cancer

- ***Key Points***
- *Anorexia and cachexia are a distressing part of advanced illness.*
- *They are distinct syndromes but clinically difficult to differentiate.*
- *Metabolic alterations are the primary cause of anorexia/cachexia syndrome.*
- *Assessment and treatment of anorexia and cachexia include determining whether exogenous etiologies such as nausea and pain are involved and vigorous treatment of any such etiologies if present.*

Anorexia, the "lack or loss of appetite, resulting in the inability to eat," and resulting weight loss are common in many illnesses.[1] In the early stages, anorexia usually resolves with resolution of the illness, and any weight lost may be replaced with nutritional supplements or increased intake.[2–4] Unchecked, anorexia (or decreased nutritional intake from other causes such as lack of available food) leads to protein calorie malnutrition (PCM) and weight loss, primarily of fat tissue but also of lean muscle mass. These conditions are common among patients with advanced cancer and acquired immune deficiency syndrome (AIDS).[3,5]

Cachexia, a condition distinct from anorexia or simple starvation from decreased food intake, also is common in cancer and AIDS, as well as other advanced conditions, including congestive heart failure, severe sepsis, tuberculosis, rheumatoid arthritis, and malabsorption.[6–9] The word "cachexia" is derived from the Greek *kakos*, meaning bad, and *hexis*, meaning condition. Cachexia is defined as a state of "general ill health and malnutrition, marked by weakness and emaciation"; it occurs in more than 80% of patients with cancer before death and is the main cause of death in more than 20% of such patients.[4,10] In contradistinction to anorexia or starvation, in cachexia, there is approximately equal loss of fat and muscle, significant loss of bone mineral content, and no response to nutritional supplements or increased intake. Weight loss, regardless of etiology, has a decidedly negative effect on survival, and loss of lean body mass has an especially deleterious effect.[4,10]

In patients with cancer, weight loss is most common in cancers of digestive organs (stomach, pancreas, colon) and is also common in (but not limited to) solid tumors. However, even in digestive organ cancers, the weight loss is not due solely to decreased digestive function but also to other metabolic processes, as described below.[10–13]

Cachexia was previously considered to result from tumor energy demands and/or an advanced state of anorexia, but

Table 8–1
Mechanisms and Effects of Anorexia/Cachexia Syndrome

Mechanisms	Effect
Loss of appetite	Generalized host tissue wasting, nausea or "sick feeling," loss of socialization and pleasure at meals
Reduced voluntary motor activity (fatigue)	Skeletal muscle wasting and inanition (fatigue)
Reduced rate of muscle protein synthesis	Skeletal muscle wasting and asthenia (weakness)
Decreased immune response	Increased susceptibility to infections
Decreased response to therapy	Earlier demise and increased complications of illness

Sources: Bistrian (1999), reference 25; Grant & Rivera (1995), reference 26; Seligman et al. (1998), reference 27.

there is now convincing evidence that in advanced diseases, such as cancer and AIDS, anorexia is a common characteristic of cachexia and that cachexia develops from a low-level, lengthy, systemic inflammatory response (metabolic imbalance) related especially to the presence of proinflammatory cytokines. In other cases, however, anorexia results from, or is a symptom of, exogenous processes such as primary eating disorders, psychiatric illnesses, or unpleasant aspects of illness like pain or nausea.[10,11]

The basic etiologies of primary anorexia/cachexia syndrome (ACS, or in the case of cancer-related anorexia/cachexia, CACS) are (1) metabolic abnormalities, (2) the actions of proinflammatory cytokines, (3) systemic inflammation, (4) decreased food intake, (5) tumor by-products, and (6) the catabolic state. These result in derangement of function with negative effects on survival and quality of life. There is within some of these mechanisms a mutually reinforcing aspect; for example, anorexia leads to fatigue, fatigue increases anorexia, anorexia increases fatigue, and so on. Table 8–1 summarizes the mechanisms and effects of ACS.

Etiologies and Process

Common causes of anorexia and/or ACS are described below. Anorexia or ACS may be considered primary if resulting from endogenous metabolic abnormalities such as cytokine production stimulation and secondary if resulting from symptoms or exogenous etiologies such as pain, depression, nausea, or obstruction.

Metabolic Alterations as the Primary Cause of Anorexia/Cachexia Syndrome

Metabolic alterations are common (and in many respects similar) in cancer and AIDS and are thought to be due in large part to the systemic inflammatory response and stimulation of cytokine production (principally tumor necrosis factor alpha [TNF-]), prostaglandins [PG], interleukin-1 [IL-1], interleukin-6 [IL-6], interferon α [IFN-α], and interferon β [IFN-β]). Other catabolic tumor-derived factors thought to play a role in cachexia include proteolysis-inducing factor (PIF) and lipid mobilizing factor (LMF). Note, however, that cachexia is incompletely understood and a clear cause-and-effect link has been established only with TNF-α, LMF, and PIF.[7,10] At least initially, the metabolic alterations cause the anorexia rather than the anorexia causing the metabolic alterations. Major metabolic alterations include glucose intolerance, insulin resistance, increased lipolysis, increased skeletal muscle catabolism, negative nitrogen balance, and, in some patients, increased basal energy expenditure.[7,10] Table 8–2 lists metabolic abnormalities in ACS.

Paraneoplastic Syndromes

Metabolic paraneoplastic syndromes, such as hypercalcemia or hyponatremia (syndrome of inappropriate antidiuretic hormone) may also cause anorexia or symptoms such as fatigue that contribute to anorexia. Paraneoplastic gastrointestinal tract syndromes, such as esophageal achalasia or intestinal pseudoobstruction, result in decreased intake and, thus, PCM.[6,14]

Physical Symptoms

A number of physical symptoms of advanced disease may contribute to or cause anorexia, including pain, dysguesia (abnormalities in taste, especially aversion to meat), ageusia (loss of taste), hyperosmia (increased sensitivity to odor), hyposmia (decreased sensitivity to odor), anosmia (absence of sense of smell), stomatitis, dysphagia, odynophagia, dyspnea, hepatomegaly, splenomegaly, gastric compression, delayed emptying, malabsorption, intestinal obstruction, nausea, vomiting, diarrhea, constipation, inanition, asthenia, various infections (see below), and early satiety. Alcoholism or other substance dependence may also contribute to or cause anorexia. Primary or metastatic disease sites have an effect on appetite, with cancers, such as gastric and pancreatic, having direct effects on organs of alimentation.[15]

Each of these should be ruled out as a primary or contributing cause of anorexia and, if present, treated as discussed elsewhere in this book. In general, people who are seriously ill and/or suffering distressing symptoms have poor appetites. Many cancer or human immunodeficiency virus (HIV) treatments have deleterious effects on appetite or result in side effects leading to anorexia and/or weight loss (see

Table 8–2
Metabolic Abnormalities in Cachexia

Metabolic Dimension	Parameter	Usual Effect
Carbohydrate	Body glycogen mass	Decreased
	Glucose tolerance	Decreased
	Glucose production	Increased
	Glucose turnover	Increased
	Serum glucose level	Unchanged
	Insulin resistance	Increased
	Serum insulin level	Unchanged
Protein	Body (lean) muscle mass	Decreased
	Body protein synthesis	Increased
	Nitrogen balance	Negative
	Urinary nitrogen excretion	Unchanged
Lipid	Body lipid mass	Decreased
	Lipoprotein lipase activity	Decreased
	Fat synthesis	Decreased
	Fatty acid oxidation	Increased
	Serum lipid levels	Increased
	Serum triglyceride levels	Increased
Energy	Voluntary motor activity	Decreased
	Energy expenditure	Increased or decreased
	Energy stores	Decreased
	Energy balance	Negative

Sources: Ma and Alexander (1997), reference 13; Rivandiera et al. (1998), reference 20; Bistrian (1999), reference 25; Tisdale (1997), reference 28.

Medication Side Effects, below). Patients with HIV disease may also develop primary muscle disease, leading to weight loss.

Medication Side Effects

Side effects of medications (especially those used to treat HIV infection, such as acyclovir, ethambutol, foscarnet, ganciclovir, isoniazid, interferon, pyrimethamine, zidovudine, and others) may directly result in anorexia or have side effects such as nausea, taste changes, and diarrhea that lead to anorexia and PCM. While aggressive curative treatment is seldom appropriate for patients with terminal illness, it is not always possible to discern who is terminal, who is not terminal, and, if terminal, how much time remains. Moreover, palliative care is not restricted to patients who are expected to die. Cytotoxic drugs that tend to be most emetic are cisplatin, dacarbazine, cyclophosphamide, carboplatin, and streptozocin. Moderate emetic effects occur after the administration of adriamycin, methotrexate, and cytarabine.[16]

Psychological and/or Spiritual Distress

Psychological and/or spiritual distress is an often overlooked cause of anorexia. The physical effects of the illness and/or treatment coupled with psychological responses (especially anxiety and/or depression) and/or spiritual distress, such as feelings of hopelessness, may result in little enthusiasm or energy for preparing or eating food. As weight is lost, changes in body image occur, and as energy decreases, changes in self image occur. Moreover, appetite and the ability to eat are key determinants of physical and psychological quality of life.[15] In some cultures, for example, Southeast and East Asian, some degree of obesity is perceived as a sign of good health and weight loss is seen as a clear sign of declining health.[17] For many patients, the net result of ACS and the resulting weight loss constitute a negative-feedback loop of ever-increasing magnitude and increased suffering in multiple dimensions. Clinicians evaluating patients with anorexia are encouraged to review basic principles for the assessment and management of depression as covered in detail in Chapter 19. Treatment of underlying depression can improve appetite considerably.

Other Physical Changes

The fit of dentures may change with illness, or already poorly fitting dentures may not be as well tolerated in advanced disease. Dental pain may be overlooked in the context of terminal illness. Oral (and sometimes esophageal) infections and complications increase with disease progression and immunocompromise. Aphthous ulcers, mucositis, candidiasis, aspergillosis, herpes simplex, and bacterial infections cause oral or esophageal pain and, thus, anorexia.[15,18]

Assessment

Assessment parameters in anorexia and ACS are summarized in Table 8–3.

Anorexia and weight loss may begin insidiously with slightly decreased appetite and slight weight loss characteristic of virtually any illness. As the disease progresses and comorbid conditions increase in number and severity, anorexia and PCM increase and a mutually reinforcing process may emerge. For example, along with the metabolic abnormalities of ACS, fatigue leads to more pronounced anorexia and PCM, which, in turn, leads to increased fatigue and weakness that may accelerate the metabolic processes of ACS.

With ACS common, and in many cases inevitable among patients with terminal illness, identifying specific causes is an extremely challenging and, in far advanced disease, an ultimately futile task. Moreover, there are no clear and widely accepted diagnostic criteria for ACS. Nevertheless, anorexia from some etiologies is treatable; hence, assessment of the possible presence of etiologies noted above is integral to quality palliative care. Other assessment parameters are used according to the patient's ability to tolerate and benefit from the assessment. At some point in the illness, even basic assessments, such as weight, serve only to decrease the patient's quality of life. Assessment parameters of nutritional status include decreased intake, decreased weight, muscle wasting, decreased fat, loss of strength, and changes in laboratory values. The patient is likely to report anorexia and/or early satiety and to experience a decline in mental acuity.

The following laboratory values are of significance in ACS[15]:

- Serum albumin is influenced by a number of stressors, such as infection, hydration, and kidney or liver disease, and hence is not an accurate measure of nutritional status. Decreased serum albumin is prognostic of increased morbidity and/or mortality.
- Serum thyroxin-binding prealbumin (transtyretin) levels are indicative of visceral protein stores and nutritional status. Decreased levels indicate under-nutrition.
- Changes in other laboratory values, such as electrolyte and mineral levels, may also show changes in nutritional status.

Assessment also includes determining usual intake patterns, food likes and dislikes, and the meaning of food or eating to the patient and family. Too often, a family member attaches huge significance to nutritional intake and exerts

Table 8–3
Assessment Parameters in Anorexia and Cachexia

The patient is likely to report anorexia and/or early satiety.
Weakness (asthenia) and fatigue are present.
Mental status declines, with decreased attention span and ability to concentrate. Depression may increase concurrently.
Inspection/observation may show progressive muscle wasting, loss of strength, and decreased fat. There often is increased total body water, and edema may thus mask some wasting.
Weight may decrease. Weight may reflect nutritional status or fluid accumulation or loss. Increased weight in the presence of heart disease suggests heart failure.
Triceps skinfold thickness decreases with protein calorie malnutrition (PCM, skinfold thickness and mid-arm circumference vary with hydration status).
Mid-arm muscle circumference decreases with PCM.
Serum albumin concentrations decrease as nutritional status declines. Albumin has a half-life of 20 days; hence, it is less affected by current intake than other measures.
Other lab values associated with anorexia/cachexia syndrome include anemia, increased triglycerides, decreased nitrogen balance, and glucose intolerance.[13,32]

Sources: Ottery et al. (1998), reference 3; Rivadeniera et al. (1998), reference 20; Casciato (1995), reference 29.

pressure on the patient to increase intake . . . "If he would just get enough to eat." Giving sustenance is a fundamental means of caring and nurturing, and it is no surprise that the presence of devastating illness often evokes an almost primitive urge to give food.

Interventions

There are few credible reports of nutritional interventions that reverse ACS in advanced disease. Nevertheless, the process may be slowed to some extent in early and even late disease stages, especially with the use of multimodal approaches (nutritional, combined drug therapy, exercise, psychological/social, and spiritual). There are, of course, interventions that are efficacious in treating anorexia from exogenous etiologies such as nausea or esophageal stricture. Interventions are divided into exogenous symptom management, nutritional support, enteral and parenteral nutrition, pharmacological management, and multimodal approaches.

(Exogenous) Symptom Management

The presence or absence of symptoms that may cause or contribute to anorexia and weight loss should be evaluated. If anorexia is due to an identifiable problem or problems, such as pain, nausea, fatigue, depression, or taste disorder, for example, then intervene as discussed elsewhere in this book.

Nutritional Support

Nutritional support, especially oral, to increase intake overall or to maximize nutritional content may be helpful to some extent, especially early in the disease process.[4,15] As noted earlier, some degree of obesity is thought by some cultures to be a sign of good health and any weight loss to be a sign of ill health. Helping family members understand nutritional needs and limitations in terminal situations is essential. General guidelines for altering diet include the following:[4,15,17–19]

The nutritional quality of intake should be evaluated and, if possible and appropriate, modified to improve the quality. Patients who are not moribund may benefit from supplementary sources of protein and calories, though "taste fatigue" may result from too frequent intake of these. See "Multimodal Approach" later in this chapter.

Determine the meaning to the patient and family of giving, taking, and refusing food. In families in which dying is experienced to some extent as a time of personal growth or closeness, redirection of food-related personal values from symbolic nurturing to actual sharing is possible. Thus, even half a bite of food shared in "sacred meals" eaten with loved ones is a kind of victory over the disease or hopelessness. Usually, however, strong and even unconscious beliefs about food are difficult to modify, and many families require education and frequent support in the face of helplessness and frustration related to ever-diminishing intake.

Culturally appropriate or favored foods should be encouraged. In some cases, certain traditional foods may be thought especially nutritious and some foods with good nutritional content, harmful. Some commercial supplements (called "milk"), for example, are thought by many Southeast Asians to have highly desirable, almost magical healing properties.

Small meals, on the patient's schedule and according to the taste and whims of the patient, are helpful, at least emotionally, and should be instituted early in the illness so that eating does not become burdensome.

Foods with different tastes, textures, temperatures, seasonings, degrees of spiciness, degrees of moisture, and colors, for example, should be tried, but the family should be cautioned against overwhelming the patient with a constant parade of foods to try. Room temperature and less spicy foods are preferred by many patients.

Different liquids should also be tried. Cold, clear liquids are usually well tolerated and enjoyed, though cultural constraints may exist. For example, patients with illnesses that are classified as "cold" by some Southeast Asians and Latinos are thought to be harmed by taking drinks or foods that are either cold in temperature or thought to have "cold" properties.

Measures as basic as timing intake may also be instituted. Patients who experience early satiety, for example, should take the most nutritious part of the meal first (usually without fluids other than nutritional supplements).

Oral care may be considered an integral part of nutritional support. Hygiene and management of any oral pain are essential in nutritional support. Procedures, treatments, psychological upsets (negative or positive), or other stresses or activities should be limited prior to meals.

Enteral and Parenteral Nutrition

Enteral feeding (via nasoenteral tube, gastrostomy, jejunostomy) is indicated in a few terminally ill patients, including those with weight loss due to, or exacerbated by, fistulas, mechanical bowel obstruction, dysphagia, odynophagia, vomiting, or malabsorption due to tumor or treatment. For short-term feeding (< 4 weeks), nasoenteral feeding is commonly used, while for long-term enteral feeding (> 4 weeks), gastrostomy or jejunostomy is the preferred means.[20] A wide variety of feeding formulas exist, with many providing complete nutrition. The primary sources of nutrients are usually as follows:

- Calories from carbohydrates
- Protein from casein or whey
- Fat from triglycerides or vegetable oils
- Various nutrients (fish oil, glutamine, arginine, and RNA are sometimes added)

Specific formulas are based on various body functions (usually decreased), for instance, heart, liver, kidneys, as well as other factors.

Total parenteral nutrition (TPN) clearly has a place early in the process of cancer, for example, during some treatment regimes such as bone marrow transplantation and under circumstances noted above (dysphagia, etc.). It has greater potential for complications than does enteral nutrition, seldom improves outcome, and thus is very seldom indicated in terminally ill patients with advanced disease.[4]

Pharmacological Interventions

Pharmacological options to address ACS in the palliative setting are useful in early stages of illness, but futile in the final stages of terminal illness. Pharmacological options with indications and notable side effects are presented in Table 8–4.

Medications under investigation for the treatment of ACS[10] include:

- Nonsteroidal antiinflammatory drugs (NSAIDs), especially cyclooxygenase-2 (COX-2) inhibitors such as celecoxib, but also COX-1 inhibitors such as ibuprofen affect the systemic inflammatory response inherent in ACS. COX-2 inhibitors also block angiogenesis and suppress tumor growth.
- Melatonin may decrease circulating levels of TNF-α.
- N-3 polyunsaturated fatty acids (PUFA) such as found in fish oil decrease TNF-α, IL-1, IL-6, and IFN-β.
- β_2-adrenergic agonists (clenbuterol, salbutamol, salmeterol) given in low doses improve muscle mass status.
- Thalidomide inhibits TNF-α production and neoangiogenesis.
- Anabolic agents such as growth hormone (GH), insulin-like growth factor (IGF-1), testosterone, dihydrotestosterone, and testosterone analogs may maintain or improve lean body mass through enhanced protein synthesis.
- Anabolic androgens (synthetic derivatives of testosterone) also improve body weight, muscle mass, and performance status in wasting diseases.
- Branched-chain amino acids (BCAAs) such as leucine, isoleucine, and valine improve protein and albumin synthesis.

Medications that have not shown efficacy in the treatment of ACS include cyproheptadine, pentoxifylline, and hydrazine sulfate.[21]

Multimodal Approach

The devastating consequences, complexities, and resistance to the treatment of ACS lead inevitably to consideration of a multimodal approach.[5,10,15,22] Such an approach could include some or all of the following:

- Prevention or early recognition and treatment of exogenous symptoms that may contribute to anorexia

Table 8–4
Pharmacological Options in Anorexia/Cachexia Syndrome

Medication and Common Dosing	Effects and/or Indications	Side Effects and Other Considerations
Progestational agents, especially megestrol acetate 160–800 mg/24 h; up to 1600 mg/24 h	Improves appetite, weight gain, sense of well-being	Thromboembolic events, glucorticoid effects, heart failure, GI upset, menstrual irregularities, dyspnea, tumor flare, hyperglycemia, hypertension, mood changes
Corticosteroids, e.g., dexamethasone 0.75–9 mg/24 h	Improves appetite, sense of well-being	Immunosuppresion, masks infection, hypertension, myopathy, GI disturbances, dermal atrophy, increased intracranial pressure, electrolyte imbalances, decreased muscle strength, increased protein requirements; short-term; avoid abrupt cessation
Cannabinoids (dronabinol) 5–20 mg/24 h; marijuana	Increased appetite, decreased anxiety	Somnolence, confusion (especially if taken orally and in elderly), smoked form illegal
Metoclopramide 10 mg 30 min ac and at bedtime	Improved gastric motility, decreased early satiety, improved appetite	Diarrhea, restlessness, drowsiness, fatigue, extrapyramidal effects, antagonized by opioids
Thalidomide 200–300 mg/24 h	Weight gain	Sedative, category X in pregnancy
Melatonin 20 mg hs	Decreased weight loss, decreased depression, improved performance	No known toxicities

Sources: Van Halteren et al. (2003), reference 4; Inui (2002), reference 11; Cunningham (2004), reference 15; Monthly Prescribing Reference (2004), reference 24.

- Recognition and early intervention in the nutritional needs of patients with potentially life-threatening illnesses or illnesses associated with ACS
- Pharmacological therapy that combines oral progestagen (medroxyprogesterone 500 mg/24 hours) with the following (note that this approach is under investigation):
  - A diet high in polyphenol content (green tea, red wine, apples, oranges, onions) or supplements to increase antioxidant activity
  - Oral pharmaconutritional support high in N-3 PUFA
  - Antioxidant treatment with alpha lipoic acid, carbocysteine lysine salt, vitamin E, vitamin A, and vitamin C
  - Celecoxib 200 mg daily
  - With or without antiTNF-α monoclonal antibody (mAb)
- Resistance training to increase lean muscle mass is effective at least early in the disease process.

Clearly, the involvement of several disciplines (medicine, nursing, nutrition, physical therapy, and perhaps others) is required in this approach. The following case study illustrates some of the issues commonly associated with ACS.

CASE STUDY

A 58-Year-Old Woman with ACS and Alcohol Addiction

A 58-year-old woman with a diagnosis of advanced cervical carcinoma was cared for at home by family and the services of a home care agency. Despite careful symptom management and nutritional support, she continued to lose weight and suffer from increasing weakness and fatigue. She had refused several opportunities for inpatient treatment, but when she developed fever, diarrhea, and dehydration, she agreed to go to the hospital.

Within several hours of admission, she became agitated and disoriented. Her condition deteriorated rapidly; she developed chest pain and became extremely fearful and paranoid, and she began hallucinating. She was started on intravenous haloperidol with little effect. A consulting psychiatrist, called from the emergency department, determined that she was experiencing acute alcohol withdrawal. Although the patient and family had previously denied alcohol use, when confronted with her deteriorating condition, the family admitted that the patient was a heavy drinker.

She was switched to intravenous diazepam and within several days was lucid. She also was septic, requiring hospitalization for 6 weeks for treatment of her sepsis and nutritional status. In the 3rd week, she began to gain weight. She continued to gain weight throughout the hospitalization and experienced a slight increase in strength. Within a few weeks of discharge, she, unfortunately, began losing weight, and it was clear that she was again drinking. She died in an emaciated state at home several months later.

Summary

Increasingly, ACS is recognized as a serious aspect of advanced or terminal illness and as an area requiring further research, especially with respect to (1) the pathophysiology of cachexia and (2) increasing treatment options. Current understanding of ACS includes the following:

- Anorexia and cachexia are distinct syndromes but clinically are difficult to differentiate.
- Anorexia is characterized by decreased appetite that may result from a variety of causes (including unmanaged symptoms such as nausea and pain), it results primarily in loss of fat tissue, and resultant weight loss is reversible.
- Cachexia is a complex metabolic syndrome thought to result from the production of proinflammatory cytokines such as TNF and IL-1. In cachexia, there is approximately equal loss of fat and muscle and significant loss of bone mineral content. Weight loss from cachexia does not respond to nutritional interventions.
- Assessment and treatment of ACS include determination of whether exogenous etiologies such as nausea or pain are involved, the vigorous treatment of any such etiologies, and nutritional support if indicated.
- Treatment of cachexia is unsatisfactory, but some temporary gains may occur with progestational agents, especially megestrol acetate and a multimodal approach such as discussed above. Other pharmacological measures are also helpful.

Progress is being made in understanding and treating the problem, but ACS is neither yet completely understood nor is treatment optimized.

REFERENCES

1. Mosby's Medical, Nursing, and Allied Health Dictionary, 6th ed. St. Louis: Mosby, 2002.
2. Finley JP. Management of cancer cachexia. AACN Clin Issues 2000;11:590–603.
3. Ottery FD, Walsh D, Strawford A. Pharmacologic management of anorexia/cachexia. Semin Oncol 1998; 25(suppl 6):35–44.
4. Van Halteren HK, Bongaerts GPA, Wagener DJ. Cancer cachexia: what is known about its etiology and what should be the current treatment approach? Anticancer Res 2003;23: 5111–5116.

5. Zinna EM, Yarasheski KE. Exercise treatment to counteract protein wasting of chronic diseases. Curr Opin Clin Nutr Metab Care 2003;6:87–93.
6. Anker SD, Sharma R. The syndrome of cardiac cachexia. Int J Cardiol 2002;85:51–66.
7. Sanchez OH. Insights into novel biological mediators of clinical manifestations in cancer. AACN Clin Issues 2004;15:112–118.
8. Thomas L, Kwok Y, Edelman MJ. Management of paraneoplastic syndromes in lung cancer. Curr Treat Opt Oncol 2004;5:51–62.
9. Walsmith J, Roubenoff R. Cachexia in rheumatoid arthritis. Int J Cardiol 2002;5:89–99.
10. Mantovani G, Macciò A, Madeddu C, Massa E. Cancer-related cachexia and oxidative stress: beyond current therapeutic options. Expert Rev Anticancer Ther 2003;3:381–392.
11. Inui A. Cancer anorexia-cachexia syndrome: current issues in research and management. CA Cancer J Clin 2002;52:72–91.
12. Palesty JA, Dudrick SJ. What we have learned about cachexia in gastrointestinal cancer. Dig Dis 2003;21:198–213.
13. Ma G, Alexander HR. Prevalence and pathophysiology of cancer cachexia. In: Bruera E, Portenoy RK, eds. Topics in Palliative Care, vol 2. New York: Oxford University Press, 1997:91–129.
14. Thomas L, Kwok Y, Edelman MJ. Management of paraneoplastic syndromes in lung cancer. Curr Treat Options Oncol 2004;5:51–62.
15. Cunningham RS. The anorexia-cachexia syndrome. In: Yarbro CH, Frogge MH, Goodman M, eds. Cancer Symptom Management, 3rd ed. Boston: Jones and Bartlett, 2004:137–167.
16. Tohgo A, Kumazawa E, Akahane K, Asakawa A, Inui A. Anticancer drugs that induce cancer-associated cachectic syndromes. Expert Rev Anticancer Ther 2002;2:121–129.
17. Kemp C, Rasbridge L. Refugee & Immigrant Health. Cambridge: Cambridge University Press, 2004.
18. Holder, H. Nursing management of nutrition in cancer and palliative care. Br J Nrsg 2003;12:667–674.
19. Brown JK. A systematic review of the evidence on symptom management of cancer-related anorexia and cachexia. Oncol Nurs Forum 2002;29:517–530.
20. Rivadeneira DE, Evoy D, Fahey TJ, Lieberman MD, Daly JM. Nutritional support of the cancer patient. CA Cancer Clin 1998; 48:69–80.
21. Bruera E, Fainsinger RL. Clinical management of cachexia and anorexia. In: Doyle D, Hanks GWC, MacDonald N, eds. Oxford Textbook of Palliative Medicine, 2nd ed. Oxford: Oxford University Press, 1998:548–557.
22. Cerchietti LCA, Navigante AH, Peluffo GD, Diament MJ, Stillitani I, Klein SA, Cabalar ME. Effects of celecoxib, medroxyprogesterone, and dietary intervention on systemic syndromes in patients with advanced lung adenocarcinoma: a pilot study. J Pain Symptom Manage 2004;27:85–95.
23. Slaviero KA, Read JA, Clarke SJ, Rivory LP. Baseline nutritional assessment in advanced cancer patients receiving palliative chemotherapy. Nutr Cancer 2003;46:148–157.
24. Monthly Prescribing Reference. 2004;20(4).
25. Bistrian BR. Clinical trials for the treatment of secondary wasting and cachexia. J Nutr 1999;129(suppl):290S–294S.
26. Grant MM, Rivera LM. Anorexia, cachexia, and dysphagia: the symptom experience. Semin Oncol Nurs 1995;11:266–271.
27. Seligman PA, Fink R, Massey-Seligman EJ. Approach to the seriously ill or terminal cancer patient who has a poor appetite. Semin Oncol 1998;25(suppl):33–34.
28. Tisdale MJ. Biology of cachexia. J Natl Cancer Inst 1997;89: 1763–1773.
29. Casciato DA. Symptom care. In: Casciato DA, Lowitz BB, eds. Manual of Clinical Oncology, 3rd ed. Boston: Little, Brown, 1995:76–97.
30. Kemp CE. Terminal Illness: A Guide to Nursing Care, 2nd ed. Philadelphia: Lippincott Williams & Wilkins, 1999.
31. Fainsinger R. The modern management of cancer related cachexia in palliative care. Prog Palliat Care 1997;5:191–195.
32. Brant JM. The art of palliative care: living with hope, dying. Oncol Nurs Forum 1998;25:995–1004.
33. Waller A, Caroline NL. Handbook of Palliative Care in Cancer. Boston: Butterworth-Heinemann, 1996.

9

Cynthia King

Nausea and Vomiting

Queasiness and heaving have been my worst symptoms these last few weeks. These feelings are relentless. I am scared to eat or drink anything, but I long to taste some of my favorite foods and drink lemonade before I die. I just pray every day that I can get comfortable before I die.
—C. B., a patient 3 weeks before dying

- ***Key Points***
- *Nausea and vomiting are common and significant symptoms experienced by patients with advanced diseases.*
- *There still remains a lack of knowledge specifically related to assessing and managing nausea and vomiting in terminally ill patients, yet there are many pharmacological and nonpharmacological therapies that can be used.*
- *All nurses in all settings can play an important role in advancing the knowledge and skills related to nausea and vomiting in palliative care.*

Nausea and vomiting are symptoms commonly experienced by patients with advanced disease. Currently, the majority of available research about nausea and vomiting deals with cancer patients. Thus, this chapter will use advanced cancer patients as a model for assessment and treatment of nausea and vomiting, but these principles can also be applied to other patients with advanced disease. For cancer patients, these symptoms may be experienced secondary to the underlying malignancy as well as to the frequent side effects of the medications used to treat the cancer. To date, most research has focused on treatment-induced nausea and vomiting in patients receiving chemotherapy for cure or control of disease. Unfortunately, there is a paucity of literature about nausea and vomiting in cancer patients who are not receiving chemotherapy or who are in the terminal phase of their illness.[1]

Nausea and vomiting are frequent and distressing symptoms experienced by patients with advanced cancer who are receiving palliative care. Research has shown that 40% to 60% of patients with advanced cancer experience nausea and/or vomiting. Additionally, research has shown that these symptoms are more common in patients under 65 years old, in women, and in patients with cancer of the stomach or breast. For stomach cancer, the high frequency may be due to local causes such as obstruction. For breast cancer, the causes may be multifactorial and include hypercalcemia, brain metastases, medications, and gender.[2–4] Ross and Alexander[4] describe the 11 Ms of nausea and vomiting in terminally ill patients. These include: (1) metastases (cerebral or liver), (2) meningeal irritation, (3) movement (causing vestibular stimulation), (4) mentation (e.g., cerebral cortex), (5) medications (e.g., opioids, chemotherapy), (6) mucosal irritation (e.g., hyperacidity, gastroesophageal reflux), (7) mechanical obstruction (e.g., constipation, obstipation, tumor), (8) motility (e.g., ileus), (9) metabolic imbalance (e.g., hypercalcemia, hyponatremia), (10) microbes (e.g., esophagitis), and (11) myocardial dysfunction (e.g., ischemia, congestive heart failure). Sadly, this symptom complex of nausea and vomiting in advanced cancer has not been reduced in the past decade.

The level of distress and sense of treatment burden associated with nausea and vomiting may be profound.[5] If these symptoms are left untreated, they can interfere with usual daily activities, increase anxiety and other symptoms, and impair quality of life (QOL).[6–9] It is essential that these symptoms be adequately treated throughout the trajectory of cancer care and across all settings. As more palliative care is provided in outpatient settings, homes, and hospices, it is important to involve the patient and family in the management of nausea and vomiting. Nurses who provide palliative care to cancer patients of any age and in any setting need to adequately assess for nausea and vomiting, provide appropriate drug and nondrug interventions, provide essential teaching of self-care to patients and families, and evaluate all interventions and self-care. The approach must be practical, with the goal being relief of symptoms as soon as possible. The treatment may be directed at the cause, at the symptom, or at both. This disruption in QOL can be of particular significance to patients facing the end of life.

Nausea and Vomiting and Quality Of Life

The distress and disruption in daily activities caused by nausea and vomiting can impair QOL for patients with advanced disease. Although there is controversy over the number and exact dimensions of QOL, the City of Hope National Medical Center QOL model includes the four dimensions of physical well-being, psychological well-being, social well-being, and spiritual well-being.[10] The distress caused by nausea and vomiting can affect one or all of the four dimensions of QOL (Figure 9–1).[11] Adequate management of nausea and vomiting can positively affect all dimensions of a patient's QOL. The control of nausea and vomiting can provide patients with a sense of control over their body and life; decrease anxiety and fear; decrease caregiver burden; decrease fatigue, anorexia, and insomnia; increase physical, social, and cognitive functioning; and allow patients to carry out some of their usual daily activities.[9,11]

Figure 9–1. The effect of nausea and vomiting on the domains of quality of life (QOL). *Source:* Grant (1997), reference 11, with permission.

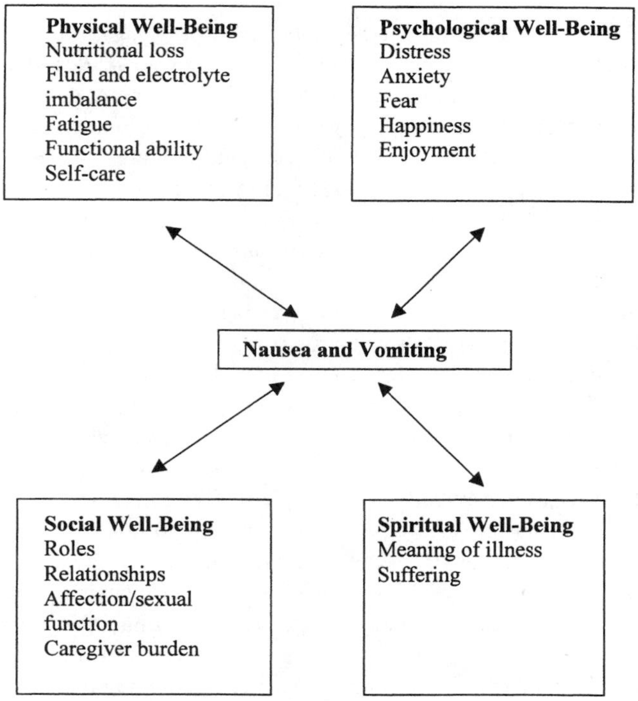

Conceptual Concerns Related to Nausea and Vomiting

To thoroughly examine the problem of nausea and vomiting in palliative care, it is important to be clear about certain concepts. Symptoms such as nausea and vomiting are composed of subjective components and dimensions unique to each patient. Symptoms are different from signs, which are objective and can be observed by the health care professional.[12,13] Symptom occurrence is comprised of the frequency, duration, and severity with which the symptom presents.[13] Symptom distress involves the degree or amount of physical and mental or emotional upset and suffering experienced by an individual. This is different from symptom occurrence.[12,13] Lastly, symptom experience involves the individual's perception and response to the occurrence and distress of the symptom.[12,13]

The terms "nausea" and "vomiting" represent clearly distinct concepts. Unfortunately, terms used to describe them are frequently used interchangeably. This may result in confusion during assessment, measurement, treatment, or patient and family education. Nausea is a subjective symptom involving an unpleasant sensation experienced in the back of the throat and the epigastrium, which may or may not result in vomiting.[12–15] Other terms used by patients include "sick at my stomach," "butterflies," and "fish at sea." The symptoms of increased salivation, dizziness, light-headedness, difficulty swallowing, and tachycardia may accompany the feeling of nausea. Patterns of nausea include acute, delayed, and anticipatory. Acute nausea occurs within minutes or hours after such events as having chemotherapy. Delayed nausea generally occurs at least 24 hours after events like chemotherapy and may last for several days. Anticipatory nausea occurs before the actual stimulus and develops only after an individual has had a previous bad experience with an event such as chemotherapy that resulted in nausea or vomiting.[12,13,15–17]

Vomiting is often confused with nausea but is, in fact, a separate phenomenon and may or may not occur in conjunction with nausea. It is a self-protective mechanism by which the body attempts to expel toxic substances and involves the expulsion of gastric contents through the mouth, caused by forceful contraction of the abdominal muscles. Vomiting is frequently described as "throwing up," "pitching," "barfing," or "upchucking." Retching involves the spasmodic contractions of the diaphragm and abdominal muscles.[12–16]

Physiological Mechanisms of Nausea and Vomiting

After thoroughly understanding the concepts of nausea and vomiting, it is important to understand the physiological mechanisms and causes of this symptom complex. Vomiting is controlled by stimulation of the vomiting center (VC) or emetic center, which is an area of the brainstem. There are multiple central and peripheral pathways that can stimulate the VC. It is important for nurses to understand these pathways to determine a cause and to select appropriate treatments. The various pathways include the peripheral pathways of the vagal afferents, the pharyngeal afferents, and the vestibular system. The central pathways include the midbrain afferents and the chemoreceptor trigger zone (CTZ) (Figure 9–2).[14,16,18–20]

The vagal afferent pathway involves fibers located in the wall of the stomach and proximal small intestine, which sense mechanical or chemical changes in the upper gastrointestinal tract. The pharyngeal afferent pathway involves mechanical irritation of the glossopharyngeal nerve. Excessive coughing may irritate this. The vestibular system involves stimulation starting in the inner ear. This involves nausea and vomiting resulting from such causes as motion sickness. If a patient has a prior history of motion sickness, he or she may have an increased incidence of nausea and vomiting with treatments such as chemotherapy.[16,18,19]

The central pathways include the midbrain and the CTZ. Intracranial pressure, stress, anxiety, sights, sounds, or tastes may stimulate the midbrain afferent pathway. The CTZ is located at the area postrema of the fourth ventricle of the brain. Once the CTZ is exposed to various neurotransmitters, such as serotonin, dopamine, histamine, or prostaglandins, nausea and vomiting may result. The vagal afferents also enter the CTZ.[16–20]

In the past, it was hypothesized that chemotherapy-induced nausea and vomiting occurred as a result of stimulation of the CTZ by the chemotherapy or other drugs. Although it is now known that exposure of the CTZ to the neurotransmitters is the most important factor, there is more emphasis being placed on understanding other mechanisms, such as the 5-hydroxytryptamine$_3$ (5-HT$_3$) receptor sites in the small intestine. In newer theories, it appears that for patients receiving chemotherapy, radiation to the duodenum, or other drugs, the enterochromaffin cells of the mucosa of the duodenum lead to the release of 5-HT$_3$. When 5-HT$_3$, or serotonin, is released from these cells, it binds to specific 5-HT$_3$ receptors and these afferent impulses travel to the VC.[16,21]

More recently, a new ligand-receptor pair has been described as having an important role in nausea and vomiting. The three neurokinin receptors are called neurokinin-1 (NK-1), neurokinin-2, and neurokinin-3 receptors. Their preferred ligands are known as neurokinins or tachykinins. These are 11-amino acid peptides including substance p, neurokinin A, and neurokinin B. The NK-1 receptor is stimulated by substance p and is thought to be involved with emesis.[13,22]

Figure 9–2. Physiological mechanisms of nausea and vomiting.

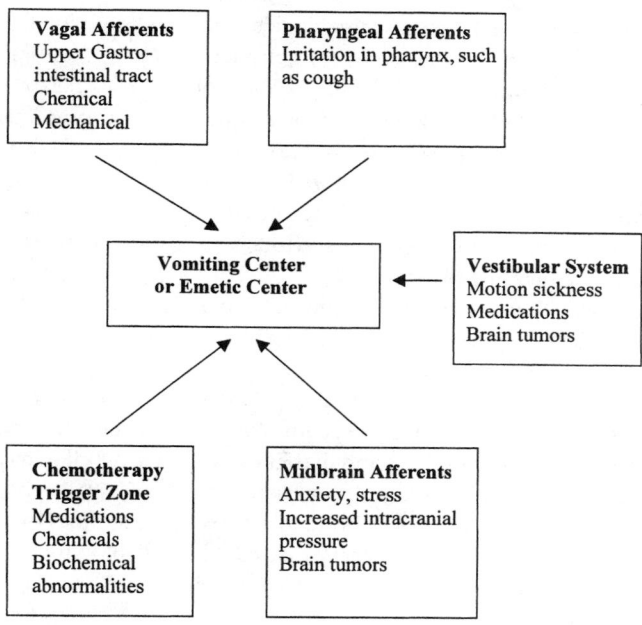

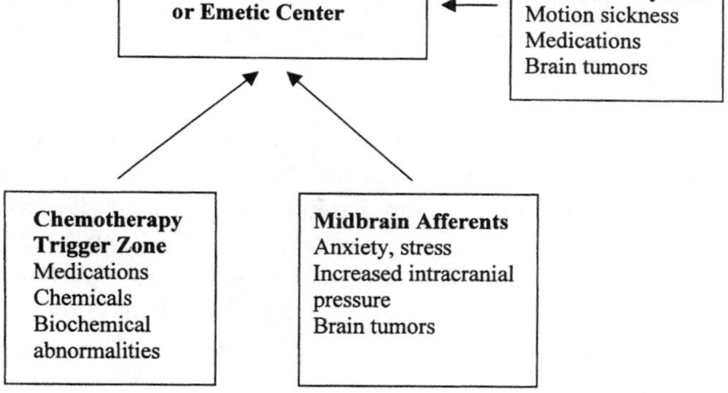

Causes of Nausea and Vomiting

There are numerous potential causes of nausea and vomiting in terminal cancer patients requiring palliative care. These are presented in Table 9–1 and are useful to remember when dealing with advanced disease. Reversible causes (e.g., constipation) may be found, and it is crucial to abolish nausea and vomiting as quickly as possible. Often, the cause for nausea and vomiting is multifactorial.[3,4,16,20,23,24] For instance, there may be a physiological imbalance, such as a fluid and electrolyte imbalance, occurring at the same time as nausea is provoked by addition of opioids or nonsteroidal antiinflammatory drugs (NSAIDs) to control pain. In the 2-year experience of the World Health Organization with the analgesic ladder in cancer pain, nausea and vomiting were present in 22% of the days during the three-step treatment.[25] It has recently been hypothesized that patients' expectations may affect their expectations of symptom distress and experience of nausea and vomiting. One study examined chemotherapy-related nausea and vomiting in treatment-naïve patients and found a statistically significant relationship ($p = 0.015$) between the patient's expectations of the symptom occurrence and their expectations of symptom distress.[13,26] Roscoe and colleagues[27] described two studies that found significant relationships between patients' expectations for nausea development measured before their first chemotherapy treatment and their mean postchemotherapy nausea severity. Additionally, when considering nausea and vomiting from a QOL perspective (see Figure 9–1),[11] psychological, social, and spiritual distress can cause or exacerbate nausea and vomiting.

Table 9–1
Causes of Nausea and Vomiting

Irritation/Obstruction of Gastrointestinal	Biochemical Abnormalities
Cancer	Hypercalcemia
Chronic cough	Hyponatremia
Esophagitis	Fluid and electrolyte imbalances
Peptic ulcer	Volume depletion
Gastric distention	Adrenocorticol insufficiency
Gastric compression	Liver failure
Delayed gastric emptying	Renal failure
Bowel obstruction	
Constipation	**Drugs**
Hepatitis	Chemotherapy
Biliary obstruction	Opioids
Chemotherapy	Digoxin
Radiation	Antibiotics
Sepsis	Anticonvulsants
Metastases	Aspirin and NSAIDs
CNS	
Brain	**Increased Intracranial Pressure**
Meninges	Cerebral edema
Liver	Intracranial tumor
Psychological	Intracranial bleeding
Fear	Skull metastases
Anxiety	

CNS = central nervous system; NSAIDs = nonsteroidal antiinflammatory drugs.

Assessment of Nausea and Vomiting

Assessment is an important process and the foundation of all treatment-related decisions. It should be an ongoing process that begins with the initial patient contact regarding nausea and vomiting. Without a complete and ongoing assessment, nausea and vomiting may be mismanaged. This can result in unnecessary anxiety, suffering, and a decrease in QOL for the patient and family. Nurses working in all settings and with all age ranges of patients need to use skillful observation along with effective data collection techniques during assessment. It is rare that patients present with nausea and vomiting as a first sign of advanced cancer. Generally, patients who complain of this symptom complex have a well-documented history of their disease, including diagnosis, prior treatment, and sites of metastases. If this information is not available, nurses should obtain a complete medical/surgical history, including previous episodes of nausea and vomiting, effectiveness of previous treatments for this symptom complex, and any current treatment that might be contributing to these symptoms. Information obtained by questionnaires or self-report tools such as diaries, journals, or logs is crucial for the identification and management of this symptom complex and for improving the patient's QOL.[12,18,20]

Assessment and evaluation of nausea and vomiting also must include the pattern, what triggers the symptom complex, assessment of the mouth, assessment of the abdomen and bowel sounds, assessment of the rectum, possible laboratory studies (e.g., renal and liver function, ionized calcium, electrolytes, white blood cell count and differential, serum drug levels), and possible radiographic studies (e.g., computed tomography, magnetic resonance imaging scan, abdomen flat plate). Specifically, nurses should try to determine if there is a pattern to the nausea after certain drugs, after meals, on movement, in certain situations, or with certain smells. It is also important to ask if there is epigastric pain (possibly indicating gastritis), pain on swallowing (oral thrush), pain on standing (mesenteric traction), thirst (hypercalcemia), hiccups (uremia), heartburn (small stomach syndrome), or constipation.[28]

There are several measurement tools that may be used to assess one or more of the components of nausea and vomiting. Some tools measure multiple components, while others measure a single component or a global measure of the nausea/vomiting. Instruments may involve checklists, visual analogue scales, patient interviews, or Likert scales. Almost all involve self-report by the patient.[14,15,29–33] The most commonly used tools with reliability and validity are shown in Table 9–2.[13,15,29,34,35]

Whatever tool nurses use should be evaluated and chosen carefully. The words on the tools should have the same meaning to all participants. It is also important not to burden the patient or family with lengthy or intrusive questions.[13] Rhodes[12] recommends the following points when using an instrument to measure nausea and vomiting: (1) use self-report tools instead of observational assessments; (2) determine and describe the symptoms and components; (3) consider the clarity, cultural sensitivity, and understandability of the tool; (4) check reliability and validity; (5) use an instrument with an easy-to-read format; (6) consider the purpose of the tool, the target population, and whether it is for acute, delayed, or anticipatory nausea and vomiting or for patients with advanced cancer; and (7) consider the type of score obtained (total versus subscale scores) and the ease of scoring.

Self-report tools such as journals, logs, or diaries can be especially helpful for assessing nausea and vomiting. The patient, family, or caregiver can complete this tool. By using these tools, patients and families can develop experience in problem-solving and a sense of control. For health care providers, journals, logs, and diaries can offer useful information on patterns of symptom occurrence, self-care strategies, and situational events.[13] Goodman[36] provided examples of a chemotherapy treatment diary that could be adapted for use with terminally ill patients to record nausea and vomiting (Figure 9–3).

Table 9–2
Tools to Measure Nausea and Vomiting

Instrument	Type	Reliability/Validity
Visual Analog Scale (VAS)	100-mm line, with anchor descriptors at each end	Reliability is a strength.
Morrow Assessment of Nausea and Emesis (MANE)	16 item, Likert scale (onset, severity–intensity)	Test/retest reliability 0.61–0.78
Rhodes Index of Nausea and Vomiting Form 2 (INV-2)	8 item, Likert scale	Split-half reliability 0.83–0.99 Cronbach's alpha 0.98 Construct validity 0.87
Functional Living Index Emesis (FLIE)	18 item, Likert scale	Content and criterion validity Internal consistency

Name

Medications to take for Nausea & Vomiting

Medication	Time to take	How to take

Special instructions:

If you have difficulty drinking fluids or your nausea and/or vomiting does not go away, you must call your doctor or hospice.

Doctor's phone ____________________

Hospice phone ____________________

Nausea Log

Date	Drug	Time	Degree of Nausea*	Vomiting (# of times)	Effect of Drug**

*0 = no nausea; 1 = slight nausea; 2 = moderately severe nausea, interferes with activities and eating; 3 = severe nausea, intolerable.
** Effect of drug: 1 = very effective, 2 = moderately effective, 3 = not effective

Figure 9–3. Nausea diary. *Source*: Goodman (1997), reference 36. Copyright 1997 by Oncology Nursing Society. Reproduced by permission.

CASE STUDY 1

Teresa, a Patient with Acute Onset of Nausea

Teresa, a 34-year-old mother of two young children, is a hospice patient with metastatic ovarian cancer. She tells you she has had mild intermittent "stomach upset" with her pain medication but now states she has severe nausea. She feels like she will vomit but only has dry heaves. She currently has three 100 mcg/h transdermal fentanyl patches that are changed every 48 hours. She also uses oral transmucosal fentanyl citrate four times per day as needed for pain. She recently had to increase her dose from 400 mcg to 800 mcg four times per day. Teresa does not want to eat or drink fluids because of the nausea and dry heaves. You perform a thorough assessment of this new symptom by (1) asking the patient/family about the severity/intensity of the nausea, duration of nausea, frequency of nausea, pattern of nausea, triggers (e.g., with movement, after eating or drinking), and presence of vomiting; (2) asking the patient/family about epigastric pain, pain on swallowing, pain on standing, thirst, hiccups, heartburn, constipation, and any changes in medications; and (3) performing a thorough assessment of the abdomen and bowel sounds, and of the rectum.

Through your assessment you discover that bowel sounds are decreased in all quadrants, and the abdomen is firm and distended. The patient states that she stopped taking the stool softener and laxative because she thought it was causing her nausea and she does not remember the last time she had a stool.

You decide to prepare and give Teresa an enema of molasses, skim milk, and warm water and follow this by 8 ounces of warm water. The patient has a large bowel movement and agrees to restart a bowel regimen with Senokot-S. You choose this product because it has a stool softener and mild stimulant in one pill rather than the multiple pills the patient was taking previously. The hospice physician also prescribes 10 mg of metoclopramide every 6 hours, with additional 10-mg doses as needed for severe nausea. Within 3 days Teresa's nausea and dry heaves are under control, she is having regular bowel movements, and she is able to take some fluids, food, and medications by mouth.

Pharmacological Palliative Management of Nausea and Vomiting

Progress has been made in managing chemotherapy-induced nausea and vomiting but not necessarily in nausea and vomiting experienced by patients with advanced disease requiring end-of-life care. The challenge is to provide appropriate antiemetic protocols for these patients in the setting in which they are receiving palliative care, while appreciating the demand for cost containment in health care delivery. Individuals with advanced cancer range from pediatric patients to elderly patients and receive end-of-life care in many health care settings (e.g., home, hospitals, inpatient hospice units, hospice houses, and outpatient and ambulatory units). The array of antiemetics available has increased (Table 9–3),[3,12,20,36–39] allowing for individualized protocols. Thus, it is important for nurses to continually ask the patient and family about nausea and vomiting and the effectiveness of the treatment. Additionally, it is essential that nurses use nonpharmacological methods to prevent and decrease nausea and vomiting.

In recent years, health care associations and groups of health care providers have developed recommendations or guidelines for the use of antiemetics in clinical practice. However, only a few of these mention the use of antiemetics for terminally ill patients.[22,37,40–42]

According to Kaye[28] the overall plan of management for palliative care of nausea and vomiting should be as follows:

1. Make an assessment.
2. Consider the causes.
3. Choose the antiemetic(s).
4. Choose the route.
5. Change the protocol if it is not working.
6. Consider steroids.
7. Consider ranitidine.
8. Decrease or change the opioid for pain.
9. Remember that anxiety can cause nausea.

Woodruff[19] adds that pharmacological management should include adequate doses of antiemetics, combinations of antiemetics, and use of intravenous (IV) and rectal routes if necessary. If nausea and vomiting continue, consider psychological factors, reassess for missed physical causes, and try different combinations of antiemetics.

Successful pharmacological management of nausea and vomiting in advanced cancer is related to the frequency, dose, and type of antiemetic. Successful management is also related to providing antiemetics around the clock.

Classes of Antiemetics

There are currently 10 classes of drugs used as antiemetics in palliative care: butyrophenones, prokinetic agents, cannabinoids, phenothiazines, antihistamines, anticholinergics, steroids, benzodiazepines, 5-HT_3 receptor antagonists, and NK1 receptor antagonists.

Mannix[3] recommends seven steps to choosing an appropriate antiemetic protocol for palliative care. The first step involves identifying the likely cause(s) of the symptoms. In the second step, the health care professional should try to identify the pathway by which each cause is triggering nausea and vomiting (see Figure 9–3). In step three, it is helpful to identify the neurotransmitter receptor that may be involved in the pathway, such as the 5-HT_3 receptor. Once the receptor is identified, step four requires selection of the most potent antagonist to that receptor. Step five involves selecting a route of administration that will ensure that the drug will reach the site of action. Once the route is chosen, step six is to titrate the dose carefully and give the antiemetic around the clock. Lastly, in step seven, if symptoms continue, review the likely cause(s) and consider additional treatment that may be required for an overlooked cause.

The clinical practice guidelines developed by the American Society of Clinical Oncologists (ASCO)[40] provides levels and grades of evidence for the guidelines. The five levels of evidence include:

- Level I: Evidence is obtained from meta-analysis of multiple, well-designed, controlled studies.
- Level II: Evidence is obtained from at least one well-designed experimental study
- Level III: Evidence is obtained from well-designed, quasi-experimental studies such as nonrandomized, controlled, single-group, pre-post, cohort, time, or matched case-control studies
- Level IV: Evidence is from well-designed, nonexperimental studies, such as comparative and correlational descriptive and case studies
- Level V: Evidence is from case reports and clinical examples

Table 9–3
Antiemetic Drugs in Palliative Care

Drug	Indication	Dosage, Route, and Schedule	Side Effects	Comments
Butyrophenones				
Haloperidol	Opioid-induced nausea, chemical and mechanical nausea	Oral: 0.5–5 mg every 4–6 h IM: 5 mg/mL every 3–4 h IV: 0.5–2 mg every 3–4 h	Dystonias, dyskinesia, akathisia	Side effects are less at low doses. Butyrephenones may be as effective as phenothiazines, may have additive effects with other CNS depressants. Use when anxiety and anticipatory symptoms aggravate intensity of nausea and vomiting.
Droperidol		IV, IM: 1.25–2.5 mg every 2–4 h		
Prokinetic agents				
Metoclopramide	Gastric stasis, ileus	Oral: 5–10 mg every 2–4 h IV: 1–3 mg/kg every 2–4 h	Dystonias, akathisia, esophageal spasm, colic if gastrointestinal obstruction, headache, fatigue, abdominal cramps, diarrhea	Infuse over 30 min to prevent agitation and dystonic reactions; use diphenhydramine to decrease extrapyramidal symptoms.
Domperidone		Oral: 10–30 mg every 2–4 h PR: 30–90 mg every 2–4 h		
Cannabinoids				
Dronabinol	Second-line anti-emetic	Oral: 2–10 mg every 4–6 h	CNS sedation, dizziness, disorientation, impaired concentration, dysphoria, hypo-tension, dry mouth, tachycardia	More effective in younger adults
Phenothiazines				
Prochlorperazine	General nausea and vomiting. Not as highly recommended for routine use in palliative care	Oral: 5–25 mg every 3–4 h PR: 25 mg every 6–8 h IM: 5 mg/mL every 3–4 h IV: 20–40 mg every 3–4 h	Drowsiness, irritation, dry mouth, anxiety hypotension, extra-pyramidal side effects	May cause excessive drowsiness in elderly, IM route is painful
Thiethylperazine		Oral: 10 mg every 3–4 h IM: 10 mg/2 mL every 3–4 h PR: 10 mg every 6–8 h		
Trimethobenzamide		Oral: 100–250 mg every 3–4 h PR: 200 mg every 3–4 h IM: 200 mg/2 mL every 3–4 h		

(continued)

Table 9–3
Antiemetic Drugs in Palliative Care *(continued)*

Drug	Indication	Dosage, Route, and Schedule	Side Effects	Comments
Antihistamines				
Diphenhydramine	Intestinal obstruction, peritoneal irritation, vestibular causes, increased ICP	Oral: 25–50 mg every 6–8 h IV: 25–50 mg every 6–8 h	Dry mouth, blurred vision, sedation	Cyclizine is the least sedative, so it is a better choice.
Cyclizine		Oral: 25–50 mg every 8 h PR: 25–50 mg every 8 h SQ: 25–50 mg every 8 h		
Anticholinergics				
Scopolamine	Intestinal obstruction, peritoneal irritation, increased ICP, excess secretions	Sublingual: 200–400 mcg every 4–8 h SQ: 200–400 mcg every 4–8 h Transdermal: 500–1500 mcg every 72 h	Dry mouth, ileus, urinary retention, blurred vision, possible agitation	Useful if nausea and vomiting co-exist with colic.
Steroids				
Dexamethasone	Given alone or with other agents for nausea and vomiting	Oral: 2–4 mg every 6 h IV: 2–4 mg every 6 h	Insomnia, anxiety, euphoria, perirectal burning	Compatible with 5-HT_3 receptor antagonists or metoclopramide. Taper dose to prevent side effects.
Benzodiazepine				
Lorazepam	Effective for nausea and vomiting as well as anxiety	Oral: 1–2 mg every 2–3 h IV: 2–4 mg every 4–8 h	Sedation, amnesia, pleasant hallucinations	Use with caution with hepatic or renal dysfunction or debilitated patients.
5-HT_3 receptor antagonists				
Ondansetron	Chemotherapy, abdominal radiotherapy, postoperative nausea and vomiting	Oral, IV: 0.15–0.18 mg/kg every 12 h	Headache, constipation, diarrhea, minimal sedation	Indicated for moderate to highly emetogenic chemotherapy. Ideal for elderly and pediatric patients. Effectiveness is increased if used with dexamethasone.
Granisetron		Oral: 1 mg every 12 h IV: 10 mcg/kg every 12 h		
Miscellaneous				
Octreotide acetate	Nausea and vomiting associated with intestinal obstruction	SQ (recommended), IV bolus (emergencies): 100–600 mcg SQ in 2–4 doses/day	Diarrhea, loose stools, anorexia, headache, dizziness, seizures, anaphylactic shock	May interfere as others with insulin and β-adrenergic blocking agents; watch liver enzymes.
Dimenhydrinate	Nausea, vomiting, dizziness, motion, sickness	Oral: 50–100 mg q 4 h, not >400 mg/day IM, IV: 50 mg prn	Dry mouth, blurred vision, sedation	Geriatric clients may be more sensitive to dose.

IM = intramuscular; SQ = subcutaneous; IV = intravenous; PR = per rectum; ICP = intracranial pressure; prn = as required; 5-HT = 5-hydroxytryptamine.

Sources: Baines (1997), reference 2; Mannix (2004), reference 3; Rhodes & McDaniel (2001), reference 13; Fallon (1998), reference 20; Enck (1994), reference 23; Goodman (1997), reference 36; Gralla et al. (1999), reference 39; Gralla et al. (1999), reference 40.

There are four grades in the ASCO guidelines. They are:

A: There is evidence of Level I or consistent findings from multiple studies of Levels II, III, and IV.
B: There is evidence of Level II, III, and IV, and findings are generally consistent.
C: There is evidence of types II, III, and IV, but findings are inconsistent.
D: There is little or no systematic empirical evidence.

Butyrophenones are dopamine antagonists (D2 subtype) and are rated by the ASCO guidelines as Level I and grade A. Haloperidol and droperidol are the drugs in this class, and they are most potent at the CTZ (see Figure 9–3). Butyrophenones are major tranquilizers, whose mode of action, other than dopamine blockade, is not well understood. In general, these drugs are less effective at controlling nausea and vomiting than other drugs, except for the phenothiazines. They are effective, however, when used in combination with other drugs, especially with the 5-HT_3 receptor antagonists. Butyrophenones can be effective when anxiety and anticipatory symptoms aggravate the intensity of a patient's nausea and vomiting. They can have severe side effects, including dystonic reactions, akathisia, sedation, and postural hypotension.[3,13,19,22,36,40]

Prokinetic agents (see Table 9–3) include metoclopramide and domperidone. ASCO rates these agents as Level I and grade A for nausea and vomiting. They are also called 'substituted benzamides.' Metoclopramide is the most commonly used drug in this category. It has some antidopaminergic activity at the CTZ and stimulates 5-HT_4 receptors, which helps to bring normal peristalsis in the upper gastrointestinal tract and to block 5-HT_3 receptors in the CTZ and gut. Extrapyramidal side effects are common. Infusing the drug over 30 minutes and administering diphenhydramine 25 mg to 50 mg at the same time may lessen these side effects. Metoclopramide also enhances gastric emptying, decreases the sensation of fullness caused by gastric stasis, decreases the heartburn caused by chemotherapy, and slows the colonic transit time caused by the 5-HT_3 receptor antagonists. Although initially used as a single agent, metoclopramide is now the main component of several combination protocols.[13,22,40]

Cannabinoids (see Table 9–3), such as dronabinol, are options for patients who are refractory to other antiemetics. These drugs presumably target higher CNS structures to prevent nausea and vomiting. According to the ASCO guidelines, there is Level I and grade A evidence that cannabinoids have antiemetic activity when used alone or in combination with other agents. Marijuana is the best known cannabinoid, but dronabinol is the plant extract preparation available for prescriptive use. The semisynthetic agents are nabilone and levonantradol. Marijuana, however, may be more effective. The actual site of action is not known but thought to be at the cortical level. Cannabinoids are especially helpful in younger adults who do not have a history of cardiac or psychiatric illness. Younger patients may have a more positive experience. Older adults tend to have more hallucinations, feeling 'high' and sedated, though these side effects may be decreased by low-dose phenothiazines. Because the central sympathomimetic activity may increase with the use of cannabinoids, these drugs should be used with caution in patients with hypertension or heart disease or in those who are receiving psychomimetic drugs.[3,13,19,22,36,40,43,44]

Phenothiazines (see Table 9–3) were once considered the mainstay of antiemetic therapy. The level of evidence for their use is rated I by ASCO and the grade is A. These drugs, like prochlorperazine and thiethylperazine, are primarily dopamine antagonists. They have tranquilizing as well as antiemetic effects. They have been used as single agents and in combination protocols. One advantage has been that they are available in several preparations (oral, rectal suppository, parenteral, and sustained-release preparation). The phenothiazines are especially effective for acute or delayed nausea. Because they have a different mechanism of action, they may be combined with 5-HT_3 receptor antagonists and dexamethasone. There is a high risk for extrapyramidal side effects (e.g., dystonia, akathisia, dyskinesia, akinesia). These symptoms appear to be greater in patients who are less than 30 years old. Frequently, 25 mg to 50 mg of diphenhydramine is given to prevent the extrapyramidal side effects.[3,13,19,22,36,40,43]

Antihistamines act on histamine receptors in the VC and on the vestibular afferents. Diphenhydramine is often used in combination protocols to minimize the development of extrapyramidal side effects. Cyclizine is less sedative than scopolamine (an anticholinergic) and can be given subcutaneously (SQ). These are rarely used as single agents for nausea and vomiting in palliative care, and the ASCO guidelines rate the level of evidence as II and grade as B.[3,13,19,40,43]

Anticholinergics currently are not used as frequently in antiemetic therapy. They do have an advantage in that they can be given sublingually, SQ, and transdermally. They have an anticholinergic effect at or near the VC. Parasympathetic side effects, like drying secretions, may sometimes be beneficial or troublesome because they cause dry mouth, ileus, urinary retention, and blurred vision. These drugs are effective at reducing peristalsis and inhibiting exocrine secretions and, thus, contribute to the palliation of colic and nausea.[3,19]

Corticosteroids, especially dexamethasone, are frequently a component of aggressive antiemetic regimens.[13,22,45–47] The use of steroids remains controversial. They appear to exert their antiemetic effect as a result of their antiprostaglandin activity. Dexamethasone has an advantage because it is in oral and parenteral forms and is compatible in solution with 5-HT3 receptor antagonists and metoclopramide. In general, corticosteroids are most effective in combination with other agents. The efficacy of ondansetron, granisetron, and metoclopramide can be enhanced by adding dexamethasone.[48] Use of corticosteroids for 4 to 5 days can prevent delayed nausea and vomiting. However, the dose should be tapered after several days to decrease or prevent insomnia, anxiety, euphoria, and other side effects common to corticosteroids. A trial of high-dose steroids should be considered if there is increased intracranial pressure, hypercalcemia, or malignant pyloric stenosis. They also should be tried for advanced cancer when nausea is resistant to other antiemetics.[13,19,28,36,43,49] The ASCO guidelines suggest that the level of evidence is II and grade is B for the use of single doses of corticosteroids.[40]

The site of action for benzodiazepines, like lorazepam (see Table 9–3), is the central nervous system. Lorazepam may be used alone but is more commonly used in combination protocols. The ASCO guidelines recommend that benzodiazepines be used in combination regimens (level of evidence II and grade B).[40] Additionally, lorazepam is a potent anxiolytic and amnesic. The temporary amnesic effect may be useful in patients with anticipatory nausea and vomiting.[3,13,19,22,36,43] Malik and Khan[50] found that lorazepam decreased the incidence of anticipatory nausea and vomiting as well as acute emesis. Pediatric patients may experience sedation and pleasant hallucinations. Lorazepam should be used with caution in debilitated patients or those with hepatic or renal dysfunction.

Since 1986, when the selective blockade of 5-HT 'm' receptors was shown to block vomiting associated with cisplatin, there has been a rapid creation of new drugs and increased knowledge of the sites and roles of 5-HT receptors. The 5-HT_3 receptors have been discovered in the CTZ, in the VC (centrally), and in the terminals of the vagal afferents in the gut (peripherally). The activities of these 5-HT_3 receptor antagonists (see Table 9–3), like ondansetron, granisetron, and dolasetron mesylate appear to be limited to serotonin inhibition. Therefore, the extrapyramidal side effects associated with dopamine antagonists are eliminated. Ondansetron was the first of these agents to become available in 1991, followed by granisetron in 1994, and dolasetron mesylate in 1997. Each of these drugs may be given orally or intravenously. The oral route is preferred when feasible for ease of use and cost. Granisetron is the most specific 5-HT_3 receptor antagonist and has the highest potency and a longer duration of action than ondansetron. All of these medications can be given to children and the elderly and have few side effects.[3,13,19,22,36,38,40] The ASCO guidelines state the level of evidence for these medications as effective single agents is I and the grade is A.[40] Many clinicians feel that there are no major differences in the efficacy and toxicity of the three approved drugs in this category.[22] Palonosetron is a pharmacologically distinct 5-HT_3 antagonist that has recently been approved by the FDA. It appears to have 100-fold higher affinity for the receptor compared to ondansetron, granisetron and dolasetron.[22]

As previously discussed, there is a new ligand-receptor pair which has been described as having an important role in nausea and vomiting. This new class of drugs are called substance p antagonists or neurokinin-1 antagonsists.[22] Aprepitant is an oral drug that acts as an NK-1 antagonist. It has been shown to be effective with ondansetron and dexamethasone to prevent acute and delayed nausea and vomiting.[22]

There are some additional miscellaneous agents that may be helpful for terminally ill patients. Octreotide acetate is a somatostatin analogue. Thus, it mimics the actions of the natural hormone somatostatin and is long-acting. It may be helpful for nausea and vomiting associated with intestinal obstruction. Specifically, it inhibits gastric, pancreatic, and intestinal secretions and reduces gastrointestinal motility. Another agent is dimenhydrinate, which contains both diphenhydramine and chlorotheophylline. It is not known how dimenhydrinate alleviates nausea and vomiting. It is helpful for nausea, vomiting, and dizziness. There have been a few studies conducted with olanzapine for the relief of nausea in patients with advanced cancer and patients with delayed nausea[51,52] Olanzapine is currently indicated for schizophrenia and bipolar mania. Further research is needed to efficacy of this drug with terminally ill patients.

Combination Protocols

Currently, combining antiemetic drugs appears to improve efficacy, decrease side effects, and increase QOL. This practice is based on the theory that blocking different types of neurotransmitter receptors may offer better management of nausea and vomiting. In some instances, single agents, such as granisetron, ondansetron, and prochlorperazine, may be used for this symptom complex. However, the combination of a 5-HT_3 receptor antagonist and a corticosteroid may be the most effective antiemetic regimen.[3,13,36,43,53,54] The various agents used in combination are adjusted according to the individual's tolerance to specific agents.

Routes of Administration

Nausea and vomiting may be treated with a combination of oral medications. If tolerated by the patient, this may be the most cost-effective treatment and provide the best prophylaxis because different drugs can attack from several sites and mechanisms of action.[22] Unfortunately, other routes are needed if the patient has severe vomiting or is unable to swallow. If the patient has IV access, IV medications are appropriate. Some drugs may be given by intramuscular (IM) injection, but this can be painful and, thus, is usually avoided. Other options are to give drugs by a continuous SQ infusion, rectal suppository or tablet in the rectum, sublingually, or by a transdermal patch. A continuous SQ infusion is useful for severe nausea and vomiting, to avoid repeated injections. It is also important to remember non-drug methods in combination with antiemetic agents.[28]

Nonpharmacological Palliative Management of Nausea and Vomiting

Some literature exists related to nonpharmacological management of chemotherapy-induced nausea and vomiting,[13,55,56] but there is little current literature concerning nonpharmacological techniques for patients receiving end-of-life care. Nonpharmacological management of nausea and vomiting may involve simple self-care techniques (Table 9–4)[18,23] or uniting the body and mind using psychological interventions to control physiological responses.[57] There are many different nonpharmacological techniques available today that could be used for palliative management of nausea and vomiting.

Many nonpharmacological techniques used to control nausea and vomiting in patients with advanced cancer are classified

Table 9–4
Nonpharmacological Self-Care Activities for Nausea and Vomiting

Provide oral care after each episode of emesis.
Apply a cool damp cloth to the forehead, neck, and wrists.
Decrease noxious stimuli such as odors and pain.
Restrict fluids with meals.
Eat frequent small meals.
Eat bland, cold, or room-temperature food.
Lie flat for 2 hours after eating.
Wear loose-fitting clothes.
Have fresh air with a fan or open window.
Avoid sweet, salty, fatty, and spicy foods.
Limit sounds, sights, and smells that precipitate nausea and vomiting.

Sources: Ladd (1999), reference 18; Enck (1994), reference 23.

as behavioral interventions. This involves the acquisition of new adaptive behavioral skills. These techniques may include relaxation, biofeedback, self-hypnosis, cognitive distraction, guided imagery, and systematic desensitization. Other therapies that are gaining in popularity are acupuncture, acupressure, and music therapy (Table 9–5).[13,55,56,58]

Behavioral interventions can be used alone or in combination with antiemetic drugs to prevent and control nausea and vomiting. All of these techniques attempt to induce relaxation as a learned response. They differ only in the manner in which they induce relaxation.[55]

Behavioral interventions have been found to be effective for the following reasons: (1) they produce relaxation, which can decrease nausea and vomiting; (2) they serve as a distraction from the stimulus causing nausea and vomiting; (3) they enhance feelings of control and decrease feelings of helplessness as patients are actively involved in decreasing nausea and vomiting; (4) they have no side effects; (5) they are easily self-administered; and (6) they can be cost effective because they require limited time by a health care professional to teach these interventions.[10,55,58–60] There is currently no definitive research that indicates which method is most effective; rather, it appears to depend on individual preference.

Self-Hypnosis

Self-hypnosis was the first behavioral technique tested to control the symptom complex of nausea and vomiting. This used to be considered a psychoanalytical approach in psychotherapy, but more recently has been categorized as a behavioral intervention. With this intervention, individuals learn to invoke a physiological state of altered consciousness and total-body relaxation. This results from the individual's intensified attention receptiveness, and increased receptiveness to a specific idea.[55,56] As with many of the behavioral techniques, there have been few controlled studies on self-hypnosis. Most of the research has been performed with children and adolescents because they are more easily hypnotized than adults.[61–66] Additionally, this research has been with individuals receiving chemotherapy and not individuals with advanced cancer receiving palliative care.[13] The results of the research have been mixed, with only some patients having a decrease in the frequency, severity, amount, and duration of vomiting as well as duration of nausea. Unfortunately, hypnotic methods are not standardized, but all include relaxation and relaxation imagery. The advantages include an absence of side effects, no need for equipment, minimal physical effort, and minimal training. Health care professionals, including nurses, have successfully taught patients self-hypnosis techniques.[61,62] In a study by Marchioro and associates,[66] all subjects showed a complete remission of anticipatory nausea and vomiting and major responses regarding postchemotherapy nausea and vomiting; however, these were not terminal patients. Research is desperately needed to evaluate which behavioral interventions are most effective in patients of all ages with advanced disease receiving end-of-life care.

Progressive Muscle Relaxation

Progressive muscle relation (PMR), also called active relaxation, involves individuals learning to relax by progressively tensing and then relaxing different muscle groups in the body. Passive relaxation is considered relaxation that does not involve active tensing of the muscles. Often, PMR is used in combination with guided imagery, and research has shown that it can decrease chemotherapy-induced nausea and vomiting as well as depression and anxiety.[55,58,59,67–69] However, research has not been conducted on terminally ill patients receiving palliative care.[13] When reviewing the research that has been performed on chemotherapy-induced nausea and vomiting, PMR has been shown to decrease the following: anxiety and nausea during chemotherapy, physiological indices of arousal (e.g., heart rate and blood pressure), anxiety after treatment, depression after treatment, and the occurrence of vomiting.[69] One study[70] was conducted with 60 Japanese cancer patients receiving chemotherapy protocols similar to those used in the United States. The subjects were randomly assigned to the PMR intervention or a control group. The findings verified the effectiveness of PMR in reducing the total scores used to measure nausea, vomiting and retching, and subjective feelings of anxiety. Another study[71] was performed with Chinese breast cancer patients receiving chemotherapy to evaluate the use of PMR as an adjuvant intervention to pharmacological antiemetic treatment. The use of PMR significantly decreased the duration of nausea and vomiting in the experimental group as compared to the control group.

Interestingly, as many as 65% of patients who learned PMR while undergoing chemotherapy continued to use it even after chemotherapy.[72] It can also be easily taught to health care professionals and to patients to apply on their own.[59,73] However, there remains much to learn about the use of PMR with terminally ill cancer patients suffering from nausea and vomiting.

Table 9–5
Nonpharmacological Interventions for Nausea and Vomiting

Techniques	Description	Comments
Behavioral interventions		
Self-hypnosis	Evocation of physiological state of altered consciousness and total body relaxation. This technique involves a state of intensified attention receptiveness and increased receptiveness to an idea.	Used to control anticipatory nausea and vomiting Limited studies, mostly children and adolescents No side effects Decreases intensity and duration of nausea Decreases frequency, severity, amount, and duration of vomiting
Relaxation	Progressive contraction and relaxation of various muscle groups	Often used with imagery Can use for other stressful situations Easily learned No side effects Decreases nausea during and after chemotherapy Decreases duration and severity of vomiting Not as effective with anticipatory nausea and vomiting
Biofeedback	Control of specific physiological responses by receiving information about changes in response to induced state of relaxation	Two types: electromyographic and skin temperature Used alone or with relaxation Easily learned No side effects Decreases nausea during and after chemotherapy More effective with progressive muscle relaxation
Imagery	Mentally takes self away by focusing mind on images of a relaxing place	Most effective when combined with another technique Increases self-control Decreases duration of nausea Decreases perceptions of degree of vomiting Feel more in control, relaxed, and powerful
Distraction	Learn to divert attention away from a threatening situation and toward relaxing sensations	Can use videos, games, and puzzles No side effects Decreases anticipatory nausea and vomiting Decreases postchemotherapy distress
Desensitization	Three-step process involving relaxation and visualization to decrease sensitization to aversive situations	Inexpensive Easily learned No side effects Decreases anticipatory nausea and vomiting
Other interventions		
Acupressure	Form of massage using meridians to increase energy flow and affect emotions	Inconclusive literature support Acupressure wrist bands may be helpful to decrease nausea and vomiting
Music therapy	Use of music to influence physiological, psychological, and emotional functioning during threatening situations	Often used with other techniques No side effects Decreases nausea during and after chemotherapy Decreases perceptions of degree of vomiting

Biofeedback

Biofeedback is a behavioral technique by which patients learn to control a specific physiological response (e.g., muscle tension) by receiving information about moment-to-moment changes in that response. Two specific types of biofeedback include electromyography (EMG) and skin temperature (ST). The purpose of EMG biofeedback is to induce a state of deep muscle relaxation from tense muscles. The purpose of ST is to prevent skin temperature changes that precede nausea and vomiting.[55,59,62]

Recently, research has shown that biofeedback may help individuals achieve a state of generalized relaxation.[59,62,74,75] However, research has not shown EMG or ST biofeedback to be as effective as PMR alone or biofeedback with PMR at decreasing chemotherapy-induced nausea and vomiting.[74] Therefore, little definitive data exist regarding biofeedback as a behavioral technique for chemotherapy-induced nausea and vomiting and even fewer data to demonstrate that either EMG or ST is effective at decreasing this symptom complex with terminally ill patients.

Guided Imagery

Guided imagery allows individuals with nausea and vomiting to mentally take themselves away from their current site to a place that is relaxing. Individuals may choose a vacation spot, a safe place, a specific place at home, or any pleasant place. It is believed that when individuals imagine what they would usually feel, hear, see, taste, and smell at their pleasant spot, they can mentally block the negative conditioned stimuli from the cerebral cortex and prevent nausea and vomiting. It is possible that the body physiologically responds to the created image rather than to the negative conditioned stimuli.[55–57,76]

Research has suggested that guided imagery, or visualization, can facilitate relaxation, decrease anxiety, decrease anticipatory nausea and vomiting, and increase self-control.[77–79] Guided imagery has also been assessed in combination with music therapy.[79] When the results were compared to the pretest measures of nausea and vomiting, the duration of nausea was shorter with music therapy combined with guided imagery than preintervention. Interestingly, the subjects' perceptions of the occurrence of nausea remained unchanged. The degree of vomiting was also reduced significantly, and there was a trend toward a decreased duration of vomiting observed with the music therapy/guided imagery intervention. In a more recent study,[80] patients who received guided imagery plus the standard antiemetic therapy exhibited a significantly more positive response to chemotherapy. Unfortunately, guided imagery did not have an effect on patients' perceptions of the frequency of nausea and vomiting or the distress associated with these symptoms. The subjects did, however, express that they felt more prepared, in control, powerful, and relaxed when using guided imagery.

From the limited research, it appears that guided imagery may be most effective at decreasing nausea and vomiting associated with chemotherapy and only when it is combined with another nonpharmacological technique, such as PMR or music therapy. There is little research that has examined guided imagery alone or in combination with another behavioral technique for patients receiving palliative care. Certainly, oncology nurses could instruct patients with advanced cancer in all settings regarding guided imagery alone or with another technique.

Cognitive Distraction

Cognitive distraction is also known as attentional diversion. This behavioral technique is thought to act by focusing an individual's attention away from nausea, vomiting, and the stimuli associated with these phenomena.[55,56,58,59,62,81] Research has shown that simply distracting children and adolescents by video games can decrease anticipatory nausea and vomiting.[81,82] Research with adults has demonstrated that cognitive distraction can significantly decrease postchemotherapy nausea, whether patients have low or high anxiety.[83] Whether cognitive distraction, such as video games, would be effective at decreasing nausea and vomiting in patients receiving end-of-life-care requires further research. Certainly, it is worth discussing this technique with patients.

Systematic Desensitization

Systematic desensitization is a standardized intervention that has been used to counteract anxiety-laden maladaptive responses such as phobias.[58] There are three key steps to the desensitization process. First, the individual is taught a response, such as PMR, that is incompatible with the current maladaptive response (e.g., chemotherapy-induced nausea and vomiting). After this first step, the individual and teacher create a hierarchy of anxiety-provoking stimuli related to the feared situation (events related to receiving chemotherapy such as driving to the clinic, entering the treatment room, and seeing the chemotherapy nurse). This hierarchy of anxiety-provoking stimuli range from the least to the most frightening. In the last step, the individual uses the alternative response while systematically visualizing the increasingly aversive scenes related to chemotherapy and nausea and vomiting.[55,58,62,84–86]

Early studies demonstrated that systematic desensitization can be effective with anticipatory nausea and vomiting associated with chemotherapy.[73,84,87,88] Specifically, systematic desensitization has decreased the frequency, severity, and duration of anticipatory nausea and vomiting. Additionally, systematic desensitization significantly decreased the duration and severity of posttreatment nausea. Research has also shown that this particular behavioral technique can be effectively implemented by a variety of trained health care professionals (e.g., nurses, physicians, and clinical psychologists).[84] Currently, research supports the use of this technique as an inexpensive, effective, nonpharmacological treatment for chemotherapy-induced nausea and vomiting; but there is little research with health care professionals effectively implementing this as a palliative care technique. It is important for trained nurses to begin to teach this technique to patients who might benefit when terminally ill and suffering from nausea and vomiting.

Other Nonpharmacological Interventions

Acupuncture and acupressure are Eastern health care therapies that are gaining awareness in oncology nursing and palliative care. Acupressure is a form of massage that uses specific energy channels known as meridians. *Tsubos* are acupuncture/acupressure points. Tsubos are points of decreased electrical resistance running along the body's energy pathways that form the meridian system. It is believed that stimulating the tsubo improves energy flow, affects organs distant from the area being stimulated, and positively affects emotions.[55,89] Most studies have been performed with chemotherapy-induced nausea and vomiting and not as palliative care techniques for nausea and vomiting.[90–94] Some studies have shown acupuncture on P6 (Neiguan point) to be effective at decreasing nausea and vomiting for 8 hours, and if acupressure is applied immediately after P6 acupuncture, there is a prolonged antiemetic effect.[91–93] Aglietti and colleagues[95] treated women receiving cisplatin with metoclopramide, dexamethasone, and diphenhydramine with and without acupuncture. Patients had a temporary acupuncture needle for 20 minutes during the infusion of chemotherapy and then a more permanent needle 24 hours after chemotherapy. Acupuncture did decrease the intensity and duration of nausea and vomiting, but the investigators commented that it was difficult to perform acupuncture in daily practice. Dibble and associates[96] conducted a pilot study with women undergoing chemotherapy for breast cancer and reported that finger acupressure decreased nausea. An NIH Consensus Conference has stated that acupuncture for adult postoperative and chemotherapy-related nausea and vomiting is efficacious.[97] Additionally, several reviews of acupuncture and acupressure have concluded that these are efficacious methods for relieving nausea and vomiting.[98,99] One study has been conducted on terminally ill patients. Unfortunately, the investigators found that acupressure wristbands were ineffective at decreasing the intensity or frequency of nausea and vomiting.[100] The investigators experienced difficulty in obtaining complete data and found subject recruitment a problem. Thus, studies on terminally ill patients need to be repeated and extended to confirm the usefulness of acupuncture or acupressure, even though research with terminally ill patients is difficult to conduct.

Music therapy has been used with patients to prevent or control nausea or vomiting. This involves the application of music to produce specific changes in behavior. The main objective in the past has been to influence the patient's physiological, psychological, emotional, and behavioral well-being.[101] Music therapy has most often been used in combination with other nonpharmacological techniques. Few studies have been conducted on the ability of music therapy to decrease nausea and vomiting in cancer patients.[13] Most of the studies have not used music therapy as a single intervention and have assessed nausea and vomiting only related to chemotherapy. Frank[79] combined music therapy with guided imagery. The duration of nausea and the patients' perceptions of the degree of vomiting were decreased; however, the patients' perceptions of nausea did not change, and there was only a slight decrease in the duration of vomiting. Standley[102] used music therapy alone as an intervention and assessed the effects on the frequency and degree of anticipatory nausea and vomiting, as well as vomiting during and after chemotherapy. The individuals who received the music intervention reported less nausea and a longer time before nausea began. Ezzone and colleagues[103] evaluated whether a music intervention would decrease bone marrow transplant patients' perceptions of nausea and number of episodes of vomiting while receiving high-dose chemotherapy. Significant differences were found, with the music therapy patients having less nausea and fewer episodes of vomiting. Generally, music such as classical, folk, pop, or jazz is best. The music should be quiet and should create a calm background rather than being disruptive.[104] Music therapy is an intervention that can be initiated independently by nurses in all settings for all oncology patients and individualized for each patient. Additionally, music as an intervention for patients with advanced cancer receiving end-of-life care would require less time and energy to implement than relaxation or guided imagery and, therefore, may be less taxing for the terminally ill patient. Certainly, music therapy in combination with antiemetic therapy warrants further study as a way to significantly decrease the distressing symptoms of nausea and vomiting.

Nursing Interventions

Palliative care is by definition active total care, thus, it is essential that nurses provide active care to relieve nausea and vomiting for terminally ill patients. Some of the important palliative care interventions recommended by the National Comprehensive Cancer Network (NCCN) palliative care guidelines are to provide adequate symptom management, to let the patient know that comfort is one of the primary concerns, to anticipate patient and family needs, to involve the family in care, and to educate the patient and family.[41] As discussed in this chapter, the NCCN guidelines include the need to continue to assess and to treat symptoms and quality of life to determine if the status warrants changes in interventions. This is a key role that nurses should play related to nausea and vomiting in terminally ill patients.

Based on the current lack of literature on palliative care for symptoms such as nausea and vomiting,[1,13] it is vital that nurses in all settings (e.g., administrators, clinicians, educators, and researchers) lead the way in learning how to manage these symptoms appropriately for terminally ill patients. From a clinical perspective, nurses need to provide initial and ongoing assessment of the patient's symptom experience, implement appropriate drug and nondrug interventions, evaluate all interventions, and provide patient and family education. Administrators play a key role in providing the resources necessary for clinical nurses to give quality, but cost-effective, palliative care in all settings (hospitals, inpatient hospice units, hospice houses, homes, and outpatient/ambulatory units).

Family caregivers are also involved with managing nausea and vomiting, as with all aspects of end-of-life care. They often are responsible for overall symptom management, emotional support, support of daily activities, administering medications, providing nutrition, and performing other aspects of care. Additionally, the family is frequently the communication link between the patient and the nurse. Nurses depend heavily on family members for information about patients, especially when patients deteriorate. Thus, it is essential that family be involved in any education given to the patient. Education is an important tool for family members to have if they are to function effectively as a team.[105]

First, patients and family need to be taught how to systematically assess the patient's nausea and vomiting. They may use a log, such as the one developed by Goodman[36] (see Figure 9–3).

It is helpful to teach the patient and family members to rate the distress caused by these symptoms on a scale of 0 to 10. This provides more accurate information regarding the intensity and/or relief of symptoms. The patient and family need to be taught problem-solving skills for specific situations (e.g., when they can give an extra dose of antiemetic) and self-care activities (see Table 9–4). The importance of taking antiemetics on a schedule and as prescribed should be reinforced. Information regarding medications and instructions for self-care should be provided in written form. Specific instruction should be given as to when to call the physician or nurse. Lastly, it is helpful to teach nonpharmacological methods for decreasing nausea and vomiting (e.g., music therapy or relaxation).

Nurse educators must begin to incorporate end-of-life issues and symptom management for terminally ill patients into the nursing curriculum and into textbooks. Educators can work collaboratively with clinicians to develop educational tools for patients and families (pamphlets, videos, and audiotapes). Additional research is desperately needed regarding appropriate antiemetic regimens, nonpharmacological interventions, appropriate self-care activities, and QOL issues for patients receiving palliative care. Nurse researchers can be actively involved in this research and in the dissemination of the results to clinicians and educators. Nurse researchers should design studies using prospective, longitudinal models, adequate sample sizes, and appropriate control groups. Findings should be reported in terms of clinical and statistical significance. Through collaborative efforts, nurse administrators, clinicians, educators, and researchers can help to decrease the incidence of nausea and vomiting and improve the QOL of terminally ill patients.

CASE STUDY 2

VA, a 62-Year-Old Man Who Wants to Be at Home

VA, a 62-year-old man with metastatic lung cancer, is admitted to a palliative care unit because his family 'can no longer care for him at home.' He has severe bone pain, severe nausea, anorexia, anxiety, and panic attacks. He has told the hospice team and his family that he wants to be at home when he dies. He currently has three 100-mcg fentanyl patches placed every 3 days and takes two hydrocodone (7.5-mg hydrocodone with 750-mg acetaminophen) tablets every 3 to 4 hours for breakthrough pain. VA takes one prochloraperazine every 8 hours as needed for nausea. He has nothing prescribed for anxiety. You do a thorough assessment of his pain, nausea, and anxiety and learn the following: (1) his persistent pain is a 6 to 9 out of 10, his breakthrough pain level is 8 to 10 out of 10, his fentanyl patches give pain relief for 48 to 52 hours (pain level decreases to 2 to 3 out of 10 for the first 40 hours of the patch), his nausea is a 10 out of 10; (2) many years ago, he had learned transcendental meditation but has not practiced in 20 years; (3) his anxiety and panic attacks are precipitated by planning his funeral and will; (4) he is 'allergic' to morphine; and (5) he refuses anything for pain, nausea, or anxiety that will involve needles or invasive procedures.

After a hospice-team discussion and talking to the patient and family, several changes are made. The order for the fentanyl transdermal patch is changed to three 100-mcg patches every 48 hours. The hyrocodone tables are changed to fentanyl oral transmucosal fentanyl citrate (Actiq). This is started at 200 mcq orally four times per day as needed for breakthrough pain and titrated upward to 600 mcg. Prochlorperazine is changed to metoclopramide 10 mg P.O. every 6 hours around the clock, with an additional 10 mg as needed for severe nausea. Dexamethasone is added at 4 mg P.O. three times per day to help with nausea and anorexia. Lorazepam is ordered at 1 mg P.O. every 6 hours as needed for anxiety. Additionally, you teach VA and his family how to use PMR with imagery. After 3 days, the patient's persistent pain level has decreased to 2 to 4 out of 10, breakthrough pain level has decreased to 1 to 3 out of 10, nausea has decreased to 3 to 4 out of 10, and he is taking lorazepam only once per day for anxiety. Additionally, VA is using PMR and imagery with the help of his family three times per day, and his family decides to take him home.

Conclusion

A major goal of palliative care is to improve QOL by decreasing undue suffering. This can be achieved through symptom management, such as adequate treatment of nausea and vomiting in terminally ill patients. It is often difficult for nurses to meet the challenge of providing palliative care when there is a limited amount of research or literature to guide interventions for symptom management. This body of research and literature is growing but significantly less than the information available related to symptom management for patients receiving active cancer treatment. Nurses in all settings (e.g., administrators, clinicians, educators, and researchers) need to help increase our knowledge base and skills in the areas of symptom management and QOL issues for patients receiving end-of-life care. Vigilant assessment, appropriate use and evaluation of pharmacological and nonpharmacological interventions, appropriate patient and family education and support, and further research can accomplish this. Nausea and vomiting profoundly affect all aspects (physical well-being, psychological well-being, social well-being, and spiritual well-being) of an individual's QOL, especially at the end of life. It is essential that nurses meet the challenge to improve QOL for patients with advanced disease by decreasing or abolishing nausea and vomiting.

REFERENCES

1. Ferrell B, Virani R, Grant M. Analysis of end-of-life-content in nursing textbooks. Oncol Nurs Forum 1999;26:869–876.
2. Baines M. ABC of palliative care: nausea, vomiting and intestinal obstruction. BMJ 1997;315:1148–1150.

3. Mannix KA. Palliation of nausea and vomiting. In: Doyle D, Hanks G, Cherny N, Calman K, eds., Oxford Textbook of Palliative Medicine. New York: Oxford University Press, 2004: 459–468.
4. Ross D, Alexander C. Management of common symptoms in terminally ill patients: Part I. Am Fam Physician 2001;64:807–814.
5. Maibach B, Thurlimann B, Sessa C, Aapro M. Patients' estimation of overall treatment burden: why not ask the obvious? J Clin Oncol 2002;20:65–72.
6. Bosnjack S, Radulovic S, Neskovic-Konstantinovic. Patient statement of satisfaction with antiemetic treatment is related to quality of life. Am J Clin Oncol 2000;23:575–578.
7. Grunberg S, Boutin N, Ireland A, Miner S, Silveira J, Ashikaga T. Impact of nausea/vomiting on quality of life as a visual analogue scale-derived utility score. Support Care Cancer 1996;4: 435–439.
8. Morrow G, Roscoe J, Hickock J, et al. Initial control of chemotherapy-induced nausea and vomiting in patient quality of life. Oncology 1998;3(suppl 4):32–37.
9. Osoba D, Zee B, Warr D, Latreille J, Kaizer L, Pater J. Effect of postchemotherapy nausea and vomiting on health-related quality of life. Support Care Cancer 1997;5:307–313.
10. Ferrell B, Grant M, Padilla G, Vemuri S, Rhiner M. The experience of pain and perceptions of quality of life: validation of a conceptual model. Hospice J 1991;7:9–24.
11. Grant M. Nausea and vomiting, quality of life and the oncology nurse. Oncol Nurs Forum 1997;24:5–7.
12. Rhodes V. Criteria for assessment of nausea, vomiting and retching. Oncol Nurs Forum 1997;24:13–19.
13. Rhodes V, McDaniel R. Nausea, vomiting, and retching: complex problems in palliative care. CA Cancer J Clin 2001;51:232–248.
14. Rhodes V, Watson P, Johnson M, Madsen R, Beck N. Patterns of nausea and vomiting and distress in patients receiving antineoplastic drug protocols. Oncol Nurs Forum 1987;14:35–44.
15. Rhodes V, McDaniel R. The index of nausea, vomiting, and retching: a new format of the index for nausea and vomiting. Oncol Nurs Forum 1999;26:889–894.
16. Hogan C, Grant M. Physiologic mechanisms of nausea and vomiting in patients with cancer. Oncol Nurs Forum 1997; 24:8–12.
17. Nausea and vomiting. National Cancer Institute. Available at: http://www.cancer.gov/cancerinfo/pdq/supportivecare/nausea/HealthProfessional (accessed October 28, 2004).
18. Ladd L. Nausea in palliative care. J Hospice & Palliative Nursing 1999;1:67–70.
19. Woodruff R. Symptom Control in Advanced Cancer. Melbourne: Asperula, 1997.
20. Fallon B. Nausea and vomiting unrelated to cancer treatment. In: Berger A, Portenoy R, Weissman D, eds. Principles and Practice of Supportive Oncology. Philadelphia: Lippincott Williams & Wilkins, 1998:179–189.
21. Andrews P, CJ Davis. The mechanism of induced anticancer therapies. In: Andrews P, Sanger G, eds. Emesis in Anticancer Therapy: Mechanisms and Treatment. New York: Chapman and Hall, 1993:113–161.
22. National Comprehensive Cancer Network. Practice guidelines in oncology: antiemesis. National Comprehensive Cancer Network Available at: http://www.nccn.org (accessed October 28, 2004).
23. Enck R. The Medical Care of Terminally Ill Patients. Baltimore: Johns Hopkins University Press; 1994.
24. Nausea, vomiting, constipation, and bowel obstruction in advanced cancer. National Cancer Institute. Available at: http://www.cancer.gov/cancerinfo/pdq/supportivecare/nausea/HealthProfessional (accessed October 28, 2004).
25. Ventrafridda, VM, Tamruini A, Caraceni F, DeConno F, Naldi F. A validation study of the WHO method for cancer pain relief. Cancer 1987;59:850–856.
26. Rhodes V, Watson P, McDaniel R, Hanson B, Johnson M. Expectation and occurrence of postchemotherapy side effects. Cancer Pract 1995;3:247–253.
27. Roscoe J, Hickock J, Morrow G. Patient expectations as predictor of chemotherapy-induced nausea. Ann Behav Med 2000;22: 121–126.
28. Kaye P. Symptom control in hospice and palliative care. Essex, CT: Hospice Education Institute, 1997.
29. Zhou Q, O'Brien B, Soeken K. Rhodes index of nausea and vomiting—Form 2 in pregnant women. Nurs Res 2001;50:251–257.
30. McDaniel R, Rhodes V. Symptom experience. Semin Oncol Nurs 1995;11:232–234.
31. Del Favero A, Tonato M, Roila F. Issues in the measurement of nausea. Br J Cancer 1992;66(suppl 19):S69–S71.
32. Rhodes V, McDaniel R, Homan S, Johnson M, Madsen R. An instrument to measure symptom experience. Cancer Nurs 2000; 23:49–54.
33. Heedman P, Strang P. Symptom assessment in advanced palliative home care for cancer patients using the ESAS: clinical apsects. Anticancer Res 2001;21:4077–4082.
34. Morrow G. A patient report measure for the quantification of chemotherapy induced nausea and emesis: psychometric properties of the Morrow assessment of nausea and emesis (MANE). Br J Cancer 1992;19(suppl):S72–S74.
35. Martin A, Pearson J, Cai B, Elmer M, Horgan K, Lindley C. Assessing the impact of chemotherapy-induced nausea and vomiting on patients' daily lives: a modified version of the Functional Living Index-Emesis (FLIE) with 5-day recall. Support Care Cancer 2003;11(8):522–527.
36. Goodman M. Risk factors and antiemetic management of chemotherapy-induced nausea and vomiting. Oncol Nurs Forum 1997;26:20–32.
37. Koeller J, Aapro M, Gralla R, et al. Antiemetic guidelines: creating a more practical treatment approach. Support Care Cancer 2002;10:519–522.
38. Lucarelli C. Formulary management strategies for type 3 serotonin receptor antagonists. Am J Health Syst Pharm 2003;60(suppl 1): S4–S11.
39. Engstrom C, Hernandez I, Haywood J, Lilenbaum R. The efficacy and cost effectiveness of new antiemetic guidelines. Oncol Nurs Forum 1999;26(9):1453–1458.
40. Gralla R, Osoba D, Kris M, et al. Recommendations for the use of antiemetics: evidence-based, clinical practice guidelines. J Clin Oncol 1999;17:2971–2994.
41. National Comprehensive Cancer Network. Practice Guidelines in Oncology: Palliative Care. National Comprehensive Cancer Network. Available at: http://www.nccn.org (accessed October 28, 2004).
42. Finnish Medical Society Duodecim. Palliative treatment of cancer. Duodecim Medical Publications Ltd. Available at: http://www.duodecim.fi/ (accessed December 30, 2004).
43. Hogan C. Advances in the management of nausea and vomiting. Nurs Clin North Am 1990;25:475–497.
44. Gonzalea-Rosales F, Walsh D. Intractable nausea and vomiting due to gastrointestinal mucosal metastases relieved by tetrahydrocannabinol (dronabinol). J Pain Symptom Manage 1997;14:311–314.

45. Kris M, Gralla R, Clark R. Antiemetic control and prevention of side effects of anticancer therapy with lorazepam or diphenydramine when used in combination with metoclopramide plus dexamethasone. Cancer 1987;60:2816–2822.
46. Fox S, Einhorn L, Cox E, Powell N, Abdy A. Ondansetron versus onansetron, dexamethasone and chlorpromazine in the prevention of nausea and vomiting associated with mutliple-day cisplatin chemotherapy. J Clin Oncol 1993;11:2391–2395.
47. Roila F, Tonato M, Cognetti F, al. Prevention of cisplatin-induced emesis: a double-blind multicenter randomized crossover study comparing ondansetron and ondansetron plus dexamethasone. J Clin Oncol 1991;9:675–678.
48. Joss R, Bacchi M, Buser K. Ondansetron plus dexamethasone is superior to ondansetron alone in the prevention of emesis in chemotherapy naive and previously treated patients. Ann Oncol 1994;5:253–258.
49. Levy M, Catalano R. Control of common physical symptoms other than pain in patients with terminal disease. Semin Oncol 1985;12:411–430.
50. Malik I, Khan W. Clinical efficacy of lorazepam prophylaxis of anticipatory, acute and delayed nausea and vomiting induced by high doses of cisplatin. Am J Clin Oncol 1995;18:170–175.
51. Passik S, Kirsh K, Theobald D, et al. A retrospective chart review of the use of olanzapin for the prevention of delayed emesis in cancer patients. J Pain Symptom Manage 2003;25:485–489.
52. Passik S, Lundberg J, Kirsh K, et al. A pilot exploration of the antiemetic activity of olanzapine for the relief of nausea in patients with advanced cancer and pain. J Pain Symptom Manage 2002;23:526–532.
53. Ettinger D. Preventing chemotherapy induced nausea and vomiting: an update and review of emesis. Semin Oncol 1995; 22:6–18.
54. Bartlett N, Koczwara B. Control of nausea and vomiting after chemotherapy: what is the evidence? Intern Med J 2002;32: 401–407.
55. King C. Nonpharmacologic management of chemotherapy-induced nausea and vomiting. Oncol Nurs Forum 1997; 24(suppl):41–48.
56. Redd W, Montgomery G, DuHamel K. Behavioral intervention for cancer treatment side effects. J Nat Cancer Inst 2001;93:810–823.
57. Yasko J. Holistic management of nausea and vomiting caused by chemotherapy. Top Clin Nurs 1985;7:26–38.
58. Matteson S, Roscoe J, Hickock J, Morrow G. The role of behavioral conditioning in the development of nausea. Am J Obstet Gynecol 2002;186:S239–S243.
59. Burish T, Tope D. Psychological techniques for controlling the adverse side effects of cancer chemotherapy: findings from a decade of research. J Pain Symptom Manage 1992;7:287–301.
60. Fallowfield L. Behavioral interventions and psychological aspects of care during chemotherapy. Eur J Cancer 1992;28A (suppl 1):S39–S41.
61. Cotanch P, Hockenberry M, Herman. Self-hypnosis as an antiemetic therapy in children receiving chemotherapy. Oncol Nurs Forum 1985;12:41–46.
62. Morrow G, Hickok J. Behavioral treatment of chemotherapy-induced nausea and vomiting. Oncol Nurs Forum 1993;7:83–89.
63. Redd W, Andresen G, Minagawa R. Hypnotic control of anticipatory emesis in patients receiving chemotherapy. J Consult Clin Psychol 1982;50:14–19.
64. Zeltzer L, LeBaron S, Zeltzer P. The effectiveness of behavioral interventions for reducing nausea and vomiting in children receiving chemotherapy. J Clin Oncol 1984;2:683–690.
65. Jacknow D, Tschann J, Link M, Boyce T. Hypnosis in the prevention of chemotherapy-related nausea and vomiting in children: a prospective study. J Dev Behav Pediatr 1994;15:258–264.
66. Marchioro G, Azzarello G, Vivani F, et al. Hypnosis in the treatment of anticipatory nausea and vomiting in patients receiving cancer chemotherapy. Oncology 2000;59:100–104.
67. Burish T, Carey M, Krozely M, Greco A. Conditioned side effects induced by cancer chemotherapy. Prevention through behavioral treatment. J Consult Clin Psychol 1987;55:42–48.
68. Burish T, Snyder S, Jenkins R. Preparing patients for cancer chemotherapy. Prevention through behavioral treatment. J Consult Clin Psychol. 1991;59:518–525.
69. Lyles J, Burish T, Krozely M, Oldham R. Efficacy of relaxation training and guided imagery in reducing the aversiveness of cancer chemotherapy. J Consult Clin Oncol 1982;50:509–526.
70. Arakawa S. Relaxation to reduce nausea, vomiting, and anxiety induced by chemotherapy in Japanese patients. Cancer Nurs 1997;20:342–349.
71. Molassiotis A, Yung H, Yan B, Chan F, Mok T. The effectiveness of progressive muscle relaxation training in managing chemotherapy-induced nausea and vomiting in Chinese breast cancer patients: a randomized controlled trial. Support Care Cancer 2002;10:237–246.
72. Burish T, Vasterling J, Carey M, Matt D, Krozely M. Posttreatment use of relaxation training by cancer patients. Hospice J 1988;4:1–8.
73. Morrow GC, Asbury R, Hamon S, Dobkin P, Caruso L, Pandya K, Rosenthal S. Comparing effectiveness of behavioral treatments for chemotherapy-induced nausea and vomiting when administered by oncologists, oncology nurses, and clinical psychologists. Health Psychology 1992;11(4):250–256.
74. Burish T, Jenkins R. Effectiveness of biofeedback and relaxation training in reducing the side effects of cancer chemotherapy. Health Psychol 1992;11:17–23.
75. Morrow G, Angel C, DuBeshter B. Autonomic changes during cancer chemotherapy induced nausea and emesis. Br J Cancer 1992;66(suppl 19):S42–S45.
76. Mundy E, DuHamel K, Montgomery G. The efficacy of behavioral interventions for cancer treatment-related side effects. Semin Clin Neuropsychiatry 2003;8:253–275.
77. LaBaw W, Holton C, Tewell K, Eccle D. The use of self-hypnosis by children with cancer. Am J Clin Hypn 1975;17:233–238.
78. Achterberg J, Lawlis F. Imagery and health intervention. Top Clin Nurs 1982;3:55–60.
79. Frank J. The effects of music therapy and guided visual imagery on chemotherapy induced nausea and vomiting. Oncol Nurs Forum 1985;12:47–52.
80. Troesch L, Rodehaver C, Delaney E, Yanes B. The influence of guided imagery on chemotherapy-related nausea and vomiting. Oncol Nurs Forum 1993;20:1179–1185.
81. Redd W, Jacobsen, PB, Die-Trill M, Dermatis H, McEvoy M, Holland J. Cognitive-attentional distraction in the control of conditioned nausea in pediatric cancer patients receiving chemotherapy. J Consult Clin Psychol 1987;55:391–395.
82. Kolko D, Rickard-Figueroa J. Effects of video games in the adverse corollaries of chemotherapy in pediatric oncology patients: a single case analysis. J Consult Clin Psychol 1985;53:223–225.
83. Vasterling J, Jenkins R, Tope D. Cognitive distraction and relaxation training for the control of side effects due to cancer chemotherapy. J Behav Med 1993;16:65–80.
84. Morrow G, Asbury R, Hammon S, et al. Comparing the effectiveness of behavioral treatment for chemotherapy-induced nausea

and vomiting when administered by oncologists, oncology nurses, and clinical psychologists. Health Psychol 1992;11: 250–256.
85. Morrow G, Dobkin P. Anticipatory nausea and vomiting in cancer patients undergoing chemotherapy treatment. Prevalence, etiology, and behavioral interventions. Clin Psychol Rev 1988;8:517–556.
86. Redd W. Behavioral intervention for cancer treatment side effects. Acta Oncol 1994;33:113–117.
87. Hailey B, White J. Systematic desensitization for anticipatory nausea associated with chemotherapy. Psychosomatics 1983;24: 287–291.
88. Hoffman M. Hypnotic desensitization for the management of anticipatory emesis in chemotherapy. Am J Clin Hypn 1983;25: 173–176.
89. Hare M. Shiatsu acupressure in nursing practice. Holistic Nurs Pract 1988;2:68–74.
90. Dundee J, Ghaly R, Fitzpatrick K. Randomized comparison of the antiemetic effects of metoclopramide and electroacupuncture in cancer chemotherapy. Br J Clin Pharmacol 1988;25: 678P–679P.
91. Dundee J, Ghaly R, Fitzpatrick K, Abram W, Lynch G. Acupuncture prophylaxis of cancer chemotherapy-induced sickness. J R Soc Med 1989;82:268–271.
92. Dundee J, Yang J. Acupressure prolongs the antiemetic action of P6 acupuncture. Br J Clin Pharmacol 1990;29:644P–645P.
93. Dundee J, Yang J. Prolongation of the antiemetic action of P6 acupuncture by acupressure in patients having cancer chemotherapy. J R Soc Med 1990;83:360–362.
94. Dundee J, Yang J, Macmillan C. Non-invasive stimulation of the P(6) (Neiguan) antiemetic acupuncture point in cancer chemotherapy. J R Soc Med 1991;84:210–212.
95. Aglietti L, Roila F, Tonato M, et al. A pilot study of metoclopramide, dexamethasone, diphenhydramine and acupuncture in women treated with cisplatin. Cancer Chemother Pharmacol 1990;26:239–240.
96. Dibble S, Chapman J, Mack K, Shih A. Acupressure for nausea: results of a pilot study. Oncol Nurs Forum 2000;27:41–47.
97. Anonymous. NIH Consensus Conference. Acupunture. JAMA 1998;280:1518–1524.
98. Roscoe J, Matteson S. Acupressure and acustimulation bands for control of nausea: a brief review. Am J Obstet Gynecol 2002;188: S244–S247.
99. Vickers A. Can acupunture have specific effects on health? A systematic review of acupuncture antiemesis trials. J Royal Soc Med 1996;89:303–311.
100. Brown S, North D, Marvel M, Fons R. Acupressure wrist bands to relieve nausea and vomiting in hospice patients. Do they work? Am J Hospice Palliat Care 1992;9:26–29.
101. Dossey B. Psychophysiologic self-regulation interventions. In: Dossey B, ed. Essentials of Critical Care Nursing: Body, Mind, Spirit. Philadelphia: J.B. Lippincott, 1990:42–54.
102. Standley J. Clinical applications of music and chemotherapy: the effects on nausea and emesis. Music Ther Perspect 1992;10:27–35.
103. Ezzone S, Baker C, Rosselet R, Terepka E. Music as an adjunct to antiemetic therapy. Oncol Nurs Forum 1998;25:1551–1556.
104. Pervan V. Practical aspects of dealing with cancer therapy induced nausea and vomiting. Semin Oncol Nurs 1990;6(suppl):3–5.
105. Weitzner M, Moody L, McMillan S. Symptom management issues in hospice care. Am J Hospice Palliat Care 1997;14: 190–195.

10

Constance M. Dahlin and Tessa Goldsmith

Dysphagia, Xerostomia, and Hiccups

It seems ridiculous that with everything else going on, that what bothers me the most is my difficulty swallowing and my dry mouth. Can you help this?—Mark, 53-year-old ALS patient

- ***Key Points***
- *Dysphagia, dry mouth, and hiccups affect social interaction and cause unnecessary suffering.*
- *Dysphagia has many etiologies and a multitude of management options.*
- *Xerostomia is a common complaint.*
- *Hiccups, though seemingly harmless, can be extremely frustrating for patients and can be difficult to treat.*
- *Comprehensive and regular mouth care relieves suffering and promotes comfort.*

Dysphagia and dry mouth are disturbing symptoms that occur frequently in progressive terminal illness. Hiccups, while less frequent, can be as distressing, adversely affecting quality of life. These problems impact the essence of pleasurable activities such as food, communication, intimacy, social interaction, as well as nutrition.

In a culture where food is both the core of life and a central focus of one's daily structure, disinterest in food and lack of the ability to eat can cause distress for both patients and families. Patients lose interest and then withdraw from social interaction. Families, with all good intentions, keep focusing on food. This creates a tension that may make the situation worse because the focus shifts from the patient to the importance of food. Thus, care for patients with terminal illnesses who are experiencing dysphagia, hiccups, or dry mouth should focus on the following principles: (1) the patient and family are the unit of care, (2) relief of suffering is the primary goal, and (3) care is best delivered with a plan that reflects the underlying aspect of the life-threatening disease.[1]

DYSPHAGIA

CASE STUDY

TM, a Patient with Advanced Parkinson's Disease

TM, a 74-year-old retired chef, was diagnosed with Parkinson's disease in his mid 60s. His symptoms began with the classic small-amplitude intention tremor of his right hand, which was successfully treated with levodopa. Over the years, his overall status declined slowly, to the point that he developed a shuffling, festinating gait, with difficulty getting up from a chair and walking unassisted. His speech and voice function became increasingly marked by overall weakness of the muscles of articulation, with hypokinetic dysarthria and impaired speech intelligibility, hypophonia (reduced vocal loudness), and a masked facial appearance. He gradually lost his independence with activities of daily living and required assistance for dressing, bathing, and even feeding himself. Furthermore, the weakness of the oral articulators had an impact on chewing and swallowing. Over the past year, TM began to hold food in his mouth for extended periods of time before he would begin the process of mastication. His chewing was slow and deliberate paired with his weak tongue muscles, and increasingly he would drool while eating. TM gradually began to lose weight, became more sedentary, and was markedly depressed at the loss of his functional independence.

TM's wife became increasingly concerned about her husband's declining status, especially the onset of coughing and choking while drinking and eating. Her concern was amplified by the need for a hospital admission for the third pneumonia in 6 months. This last admission prompted a referral to the speech language pathologist to evaluate TM's swallowing safety. The evaluation findings revealed a cachectic and reserved gentleman who displayed considerable weakness of the lips, jaw, and tongue muscles, with drooling at rest. His face was expressionless and his voice was low in volume and gurgly in quality. He was unable to control liquids in his mouth, and mastication of solid foods was slow and disorganized. He coughed weakly and inconsistently while drinking thin liquids—both signs highly suspicious for aspiration. It was clear TM had been struggling with eating and swallowing for a long time. Swallowing inefficiency and aspiration of liquids were confirmed on videofluorographic examination. TM showed a moderate decrease in aspiration on thicker consistencies of liquids and soft foods, but it was clear that the effort it would take to meet his nutritional needs would be immense for both he and his family. This episode of pneumonia had increased the rigidity of his extremities and exacerbated his oral weakness. He was minimally communicative. The findings of the examination were discussed with TM and his family. Given his poor pulmonary clearance, there was a high likelihood that the aspiration pneumonia would recur if he were to continue to eat by mouth, perhaps even requiring a repeat hospitalization. An alternative was artificial nutrition and hydration.

During the months preceding his latest functional decline, TM and his family had discussed his wishes for nonoral nutrition, wishes that he had communicated with his primary care team. He wanted to proceed with eating by mouth, understanding the risks. He did not wish to have a gastrostomy tube placed. A plan was devised with TM's wife to continue to feed him by mouth, acknowledging the inherent risks. The goal was to keep him comfortable: small, frequent meals with favorite foods; small sips of water before and between meals to decrease oral dryness; crushed medications given in applesauce or with thickened liquids; upright positioning during "mealtimes." His wife was taught how to complete these tasks. Eventually, TM's oral intake diminished to a teaspoon of pureed foods here and there, although he lost his desire for water. Over the next few weeks, TM's pulmonary status deteriorated, so much so that supplemental oxygen and morphine were required because of difficulty breathing. The family opted not to treat the recurrent pneumonias, and eventually TM passed away at home in the care of his family, who upheld his wishes to avoid artificial hydration and nutrition.

Definition

Dysphagia is defined as difficulty swallowing food or liquid. Typically, chronic difficulty swallowing affects the efficiency with which oral alimentation is maintained. In addition, airway protection or swallowing safety can be threatened. Patients may complain of food getting caught along the upper digestive tract anywhere from the throat to the esophagus. In addition, diversion of food or liquid into the trachea may occur, causing aspiration, choking, or, in severe cases, asphyxiation. Chronic difficulty swallowing can be both frustrating and frightening for patients. Because nutrition is compromised, generalized weakness, appetite loss, and weight loss may ensue. In severe cases, malnutrition may occur. Aspiration pneumonia may also occur, causing fevers, malaise, shortness of breath, and, rarely, death.

The psychological impact of dysphagia cannot be underestimated. Eating or eating enough becomes a focus of care in the chronically ill patient and is more evident in terminally ill patients with dysphagia. Since the essence of nurturing is intertwined with the ability to provide and receive nourishment, the chronically ill patient, isolated from social interactions that take place around the consumption of food, becomes increasingly depressed. Caregivers often feel that nourishment is the one area in which they have had some opportunity to nurture their loved one in the past. When this is no longer available to them, the palliative care challenge in managing dysphagia is how to ensure comfort, even at the expense of optimal nutrition and hydration. Understanding the physiology of normal and aberrant swallowing is critical to meeting this challenge.

Physiology and Pathophysiology of Swallowing

Normal Swallowing

Swallowing involves the passage of food or liquid from the oral cavity through the esophagus and into the stomach, where the process of digestion begins. Swallowing is an extremely complex physiological act, and demands exquisite timing and coordination of more than 30 pairs of muscles under both voluntary and involuntary nervous control. Because humans swallow hundreds of times per day and are largely unaware of the activity, it is remarkable that difficulties do not occur more frequently.

For purposes of discussion, the act of swallowing is divided into three stages (Figure 10–1). In reality, these stages occur simultaneously. The act of swallowing takes less than 20 seconds from the moment of bolus propulsion into the pharynx until the bolus reaches the stomach. The longest phase comprises the transit of the bolus through the esophagus.

The first stage of swallowing (see Figure 10–1A), the oral stage, is responsible for readying the bolus for swallowing. Bolus preparation is under voluntary control and can be halted or changed at any point. The primary activities of mastication include gathering and placement of semisoft and liquid boluses on the tongue. It is during this stage that one takes pleasure from the flavor and texture of food through the chemoreceptors of the tongue and palate. The duration of the oral stage is variable, depending on the viscosity or consistency of the food bolus and individual chewing styles. During mastication, the tongue moves the bolus to the dental arches to grind into smaller pieces. Opening the jaw as well as rotary and lateral movements achieves the masticatory process. Cohesive solid bolus formation is dependent on several factors: the presence of enzyme-rich saliva to bind the material together, the ability of the tongue to gather particles from the sulci of the cheek and the mouth floor, the prevention of food falling out of the oral cavity anteriorly, and the premature spilling into the pharynx.[2]

Once the bolus is prepared and ready for swallowing, it is positioned on the blade of the tongue and propelled into the pharynx (see Figure 10–1B). Contact with the tongue occurs laterally on the hard palate and anteriorly on the central incisors. The soft palate then elevates, permitting the bolus to enter the pharynx, while closing off the nasopharynx, to prevent regurgitation of the bolus into the nose. The floor muscles of the mouth contract as the tongue base depresses, forming a chute down which the bolus can flow. Through a series of contractions by the intrinsic tongue muscles pressed against the hard palate, the torpedo-shaped bolus is propelled

Figure 10–1. Stages of swallowing, beginning with voluntary initiation of the swallow by the tongue (A), oral transit (B), pharyngeal stage of swallowing with airway protection (C) and (D), and esophageal stage (E). *Source:* Logemann (1998), reference 2.

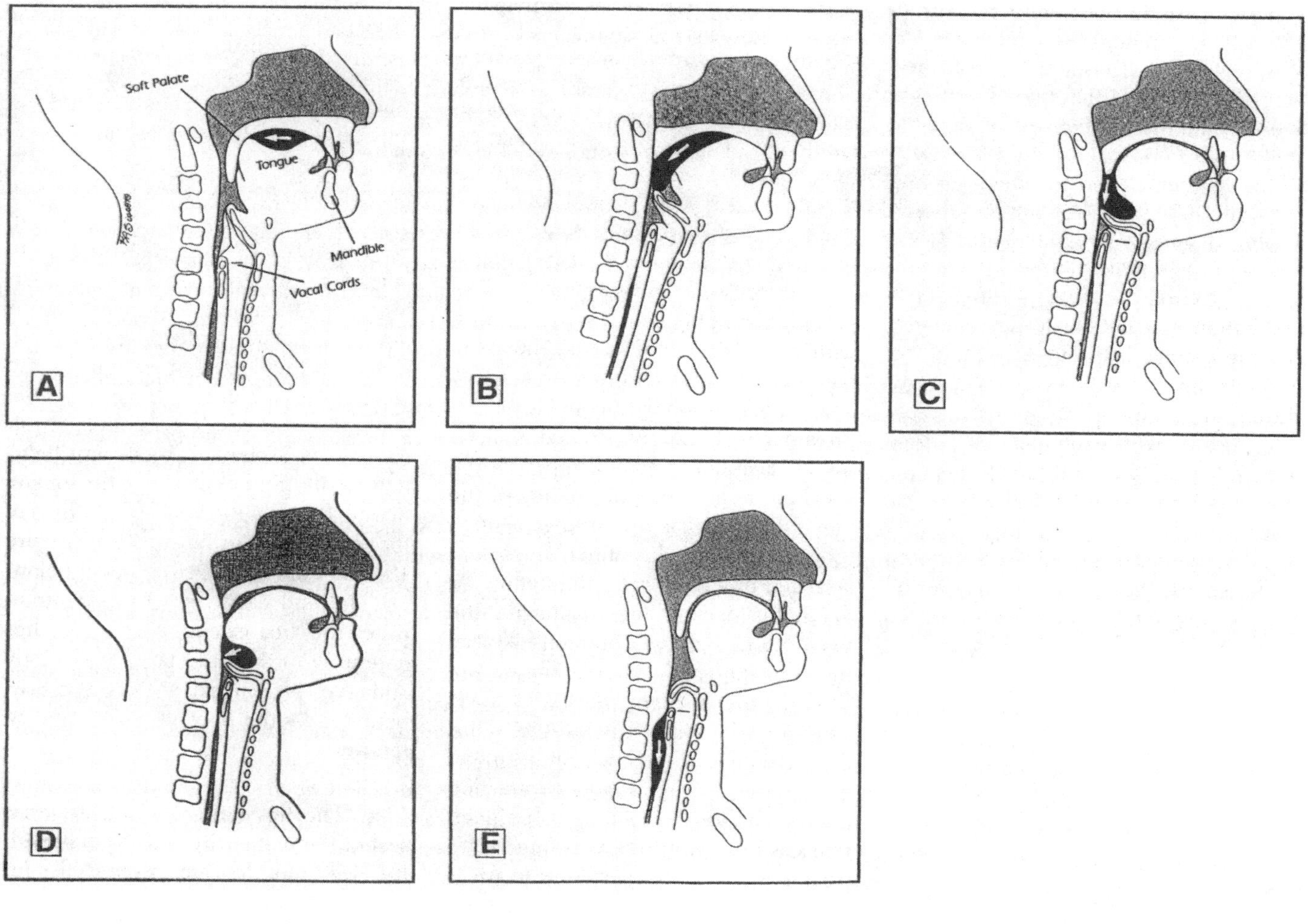

in a rolling motion from anterior to posterior into the pharynx. Depending on the consistency of the bolus, this stage lasts approximately 1 second.

The second stage of swallowing, the pharyngeal stage (see Figure 10–1C/D), is elicited as the posterior movement of the tongue and passage. The bolus passage stimulates the sensory impulses of the glossopharyngeal and vagus nerves, which travel to the afferent swallowing center located in the lower medulla of the brain stem and then to the cortex. The pharyngeal and oral transit stages are closely associated. The oral cavity and the pharynx become one continuous tube with the entrance to the larynx closed off.[2] The pharyngeal stage of swallowing is the most complex, requiring the most precise timing and coordination. It is during this stage that the airway is protected and the upper esophagus opens to accept the bolus.

The process of airway protection, that is, closure of the airway, is quite remarkable and intricate. There are several aspects of airway protection. Respiration ceases for up to 2.5 seconds, with an average of 0.3 to 0.6 second for a single sip of liquid.[2,3,4] Swallowing usually occurs during the expiratory stage of the respiratory cycle, with expiration preceding and following the swallow. Laryngeal closure occurs from inferior to superior so that if material is present in the laryngeal entrance, it will be extruded into the hypopharynx during the swallow. As the floor of the mouth/tongue muscles contract to propel the bolus from the oral cavity, the larynx moves upward, closing the laryngeal vestibule. The vocal folds adduct simultaneously, and the epiglottis begins to invert over the entrance of the larynx, further protecting the airway. Opening of the upper esophageal segment is the result of traction of the cricoid cartilage and larynx away from the posterior pharyngeal wall as the suprahyoid muscles contract, pulling the larynx upward and forwards.[5–8,10] The greater the excursion of the larynx, the larger the diameter of the opening of the upper esophagus becomes.[7] This movement creates a negative pressure in the esophagus, helping to propel the bolus toward the distal esophagus.

As the bolus enters the pharynx, its tail is driven toward the hypopharynx and esophagus by the positive pressure generated from the base of the tongue contacting the pharyngeal walls. The pharyngeal constrictor muscles contract sequentially, and their topographic arrangement has the effect of stripping the bolus through the hypopharynx and clearing the pharyngeal recesses.

The duration of the pharyngeal stage of swallowing is approximately 1 second. The order of contraction of muscles is invariant, but the timing of contraction depends on the viscosity and size of the bolus.[3,5] The biomechanical events involved in this stage of swallowing are under involuntary control and carefully sequenced in a pattern by the central swallowing center in the lower medulla. In the medulla, sensory feedback continually modulates the motor response. For example, if the bolus is dense, the firing of a particular group of muscles of the tongue may be increased, or the opening of the upper esophagus may last longer with a large bolus volume. If the sensory feedback loop is disturbed, the onset of the pharyngeal stage of swallowing may be delayed or, in severe cases, absent.[2,3,6]

The esophageal stage or final stage of swallowing (see Figure 10–1E) involves transport of the bolus from the upper esophageal segment, through the lower esophageal segment, and into the stomach, a distance of approximately 25 cm.[2,10] The esophageal stage is coordinated with the pharyngeal stage, with continued sequential contraction of muscles in the cervical esophagus. Like the pharyngeal phase of swallowing, the esophageal stage is under involuntary neuromuscular control. Unlike the pharyngeal stage, however, the speed of propagation of the bolus is much slower, with a rate of 3 to 4 cm/second compared to 12 cm/second in the pharynx.[7] The upper esophagus consists of approximately 8 cm of striated skeletal muscle, beginning at the upper esophageal segment. The outer fibers of the cervical esophagus are arranged longitudinally, while the inner fibers are arranged in a circular configuration. As the bolus reaches the esophagus, the longitudinal muscles contract, followed by contraction of the circular fibers, constituting the primary peristaltic wave. The primary wave carries the bolus through the lower esophageal sphincter in a series of relaxation–contraction waves. The lower esophageal sphincter remains open until the peristaltic wave passes. A secondary peristaltic wave is generated where the striated muscle meets the smooth muscle and clears the esophagus of residue. This wave is reflexive in nature and initiated by distention of the esophagus during the primary peristaltic wave.[3,9]

After passage of the bolus, the upper and lower esophageal sphincters contract to their baseline tonic posture. This contains the gastric contents within the stomach and prevents regurgitation of material into the hypopharynx and airway.[6]

Pathophysiology of Swallowing

Difficulty swallowing can occur during, within, or across any of the above-described stages, depending on the underlying disease. Evaluation and treatment of dysphagia is dependent on a thorough understanding of the underlying aberrant anatomical and physiological components. It is helpful to conceptualize the process of bolus transfer through the oral cavity according to a piston–chamber model proposed by McConnell and Cerenko in 1988.[8] The oral cavity, or chamber, comprises the area extending from the lips anteriorly to the hard palate superiorly and the pharyngeal wall posteriorly, bounded by the floor of the mouth inferiorly.

The tongue acts as the piston that creates pressure on the bolus to drive it into the esophagus. The ability of the oral cavity to fulfill its function as a closed chamber depends on the integrity of a number of muscular contractions, which form valves that open and close and are illustrated in Figure 10–2.

Bolus flow, and, hence swallowing, is affected if there is dysfunction in the chamber or the piston. If the chamber leaks, residue, regurgitation, or aspiration may occur. Inefficient bolus flow results from weakness in the tongue-driving force on the bolus or reduced contraction of the pharynx. Patients with muscle weakness due to stroke, degenerative neuromuscular disease, or neoplastic lesions involving motor and sensory function of the lips and face may experience difficulty containing the

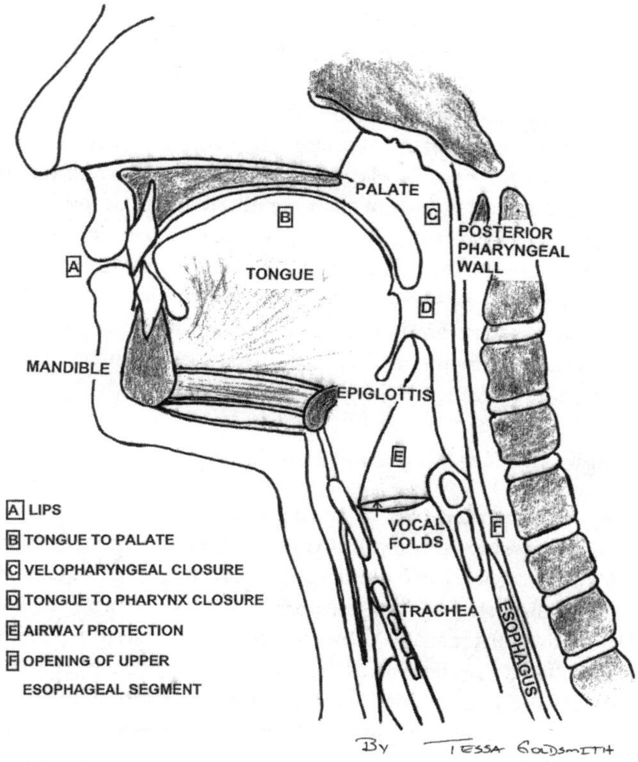

Figure 10–2. Valves of the oral cavity illustrating twin function.

bolus in the oral cavity, producing drooling. Patients with severe dementia who are not aware of food in their mouth may fail to close their lips. In the presence of facial weakness, for example, patients with Parkinson's disease or ALS, the boluses may pocket in the lateral buccal sulci, making retrieval difficult, especially if buccal and lingual weakness coexist. In cases of reduced sensation, pocketed food may remain in the oral cavity for several hours, possibly increasing the risk of aspiration. Nasal regurgitation of liquids and particles of solids occurs when the velopharyngeal port is dysfunctional. This is common in both palate cancer if treatment has involved resection and in patients with progressive neuromuscular disease. Weak tongue-driving force during swallowing results in a significant amount of residue in the pharyngeal recesses, loss of control over the bolus, or incomplete laryngeal closure, causing aspiration before, during, or after the swallow.

Valving of the larynx during the swallow is important for prevention of aspiration into the tracheobronchial tree. Failure of the larynx to close due to timing or muscular incompetence can result in aspiration of liquids or solid materials. Reduced sensory function and weakened laryngeal musculature impair expectoration of aspirated material. Functional and reliable laryngeal valving is crucial not only during oropharyngeal swallowing but also during periods of gastroesophageal reflux, regurgitation, or emesis. Failure of the upper esophagus to open completely results in residue in the pyriform sinuses superior to the pharyngoesophageal segment and, if abundant, may spill over into the unprotected larynx and trachea.[10]

Prevalence and Impact

A multitude of diseases can affect the "chamber–piston" relationship, causing dysphagia, particularly in patients receiving palliative care. These include degenerative neuromuscular diseases, progressive cognitive decline disorders, recurrent or fatal neoplastic nervous system or gastrointestinal obstructive lesions, or pervasive debilitation from multisystem decline. In some cases, side effects of treatment including radiation therapy or chemotherapy, are the precipitating causative factors of dysphagia, whereas in other cases, the progressive nature of the disease leads to unsafe and inefficient swallowing.

Understanding the physiological impact of the illness is critical in evaluation of the swallowing disorder and the method of management. For example, generalized weakness of the oropharyngeal musculature may be evident in two patients, one with a diagnosis of ALS who requires mechanical ventilation, and one who has undergone further chemoradiation therapy for a recurrent neck squamous cell carcinoma. In the patient with ALS, the likely rapid progression would avoid the suggestion of effortful swallows as a compensatory strategy to clear boluses through the pharynx while swallowing due to fatigue. On the other hand, in the patient with neck cancer, encouraging effortful swallows to preserve motor flexibility may assist in protecting his airway to enable him to take some food by mouth in the short term. The proceeding recommendations describe some commonly encountered etiological categories and their impact on swallowing.

Neoplasms

Tumors involving the nervous system as well as the head and neck and upper aerodigestive tract can interfere with swallowing.

Brain Tumors. Brain tumors are classified into primary and secondary types. Primary brain tumors are a diverse group of neoplasms arising from different cells of the central nervous system. In contrast, secondary tumors originate elsewhere in the body and metastasize to the brain.

It has been estimated that 34,000 new cases of primary brain tumors, malignant or benign, are diagnosed each year.[11] Although dysphagia is rarely the presenting symptom, swallowing problems can develop as the tumor increases in size and compresses surrounding structures. The corticobulbar tracts involved in coordinating both the oral and pharyngeal stages of swallowing may be affected.

Extrinsic tumors located around the brain stem, such as acoustic neuromas and meningiomas, as well as those originating in the skull base, such as glomus jugulare, glomus vagale tumors, and chordomas, may compress or invade the lower medulla. Hence, the cranial nerves and their nuclei that are critical for swallowing will be affected, with the specific swallowing impairment dependent upon which cranial nerves are affected. Compromise of the glossopharyngeal, vagus, and hypoglossal cranial nerves singly or in combination results in the greatest swallowing dysfunction. The relative inaccessibility of these tumors for treatment is associated with recurrence, which, in turn, can result in increased cranial nerve and swallowing impairment.[12] In addition to direct tumor effects, swallowing may be indirectly affected by depressed levels of consciousness and reduced awareness that is associated with tumor progression and treatment effects.

Head and Neck Cancer. Oropharyngeal dysphagia is almost synonymous with advanced stage head and neck cancer because the vital structures involved in swallowing can be impaired by the tumor, as well as by treatment. Head and neck tumors are located in a variety of sites in the oral cavity, including the bony structures, the lips, floor of the mouth, tongue, palate, and tonsillar fossa, as well as the hypopharynx, larynx, and nasopharynx. Treatment of head and neck neoplasms varies according to cell type, location, tumor size, and presence of neck metastases. In the past decade, treatment for locally advanced head and neck cancer has shifted from primary surgical resection to an "organ-sparing" approach whereby chemoradiation therapy is the primary treatment and salvage surgery is reserved for recurrent disease.[13] This is most evident in patients with laryngeal cancer because of the morbidity associated with surgical resection of the larynx or laryngectomy.[14] However, even with the goal of organ preservation, significant speech and swallowing dysfunction can occur.

Many patients with advanced head and neck cancer are unable to resume oral nutrition as a result of the surgical resection or secondary radiation or chemotherapy treatment. Subsequent side effects include mucositis in the acute stage, as well as muscle fibrosis, scarring, and dry mouth, even after the completion of treatment. Some patients manage to compensate for their dysphagia with changes in posture or diet consistencies suggested by speech language pathologists or nutritionists. Other patients rely on oral nutritional supplements delivered by mouth or gastrostomy tube. In any case, by the time the patient with advanced head and neck cancer reaches the terminal stage, he or she has already been coping with dysphagia and its very visible consequences for many months.[15]

Malignant Esophageal Tumors. The incidence of malignant esophageal tumors is approximately 3 to 4 per 100,000.[16] Symptomatic presentation of dysphagia usually occurs late in the disease, resulting in diagnosis of advanced malignancy. Esophageal carcinoma can arise either from squamous cells of the mucosa or as adenocarcinomas of the columnar lining of Barrett's epithelium.[16] Patients commonly complain of weight loss and progressive dysphagia with solid foods rather than liquids. In some cases, intractable cough may indicate extension of the tumor to the mediastinum or trachea. The presence of local extension to the aorta, trachea, or other mediastinal structures eliminates the possibility of surgical resection. Survival rates are reported to be between 10% and 20% at 5 years,[16,17] and thus, palliative care is the foundation of management for this disease.

If diagnosed early, esophagectomy or esophagogastrectomy may be the treatment of choice. However, in cases of unresectable advanced disease, symptomatic relief of dysphagia can be accomplished by radiation therapy, esophageal dilation, yttrium-argon-garnet (YAG) laser electrocautery, chemotherapy, or placement of an esophageal stent to open the lumen of the esophagus.[17–20] Each of these treatments is associated with considerable side effects, including radiation-induced esophagitis and chemotherapy-induced mucositis. Esophageal perforation during laser surgery or dilation and migration of the esophageal stents are potential complications from palliative procedures.[21] Frequently, jejunostomy tubes must be placed for nonoral feeding.

Progressive Neuromuscular Diseases

Amyotrophic Lateral Sclerosis. Amyotrophic lateral sclerosis, or ALS, is encountered with unfortunate regularity in patients on a palliative care service. A rapidly progressive degenerative disease of unknown etiology, ALS involves the motor neurons of the brain and spinal cord.[22,23] One quarter of ALS patients present with difficulty swallowing as their initial complaint, while other patients begin with distal weakness that travels proximally to involve the bulbar musculature. As the disease progresses, there is involvement with upper and lower motor neurons and the respiratory system in the later stages. Respiratory failure is the usual cause of death in patients with ALS because of weakness in diaphragmatic, laryngeal, and lingual function.[23]

Typically, patients with ALS also experience a reduction in tongue mobility, affecting the ability to lateralize food for chewing and to control material in the mouth. With disease progression, heavier foods, even pureed, are difficult to manipulate, resulting in significant residue in the oral cavity and hypopharynx. With oral musculature weakening, several conditions occur: nasal regurgitation of fluids and loss of control over liquids, resulting in aspiration and coughing before the swallow is triggered. Speech impairment parallels swallowing difficulty, affecting communication as well as alimentation. Diet modifications with calorie-dense foods and postural alterations are necessary if oral intake is to continue. However, many patients reach a point where the effort involved in eating is too great and the pleasure is lost. If the patient chooses, a gastrostomy tube is placed percutaneously to provide nutrition, and sometimes supplemental oral intake for pleasure is possible.[2,22,23,24]

Parkinson's Disease. Parkinson's disease is a relatively common, slowly progressive disease of the central nervous system, marked by an inability to execute learned motor skills automatically.[17,18] A classic triad of symptoms, resting tremor, bradykinesia, and rigidity, accompanies Parkinson's disease. An imbalance between dopamine-activated and acetylcholine-activated neural pathways in the basal ganglia causes the symptoms.[18,20] The largest etiological group is idiopathic, however, Parkinson-like symptoms may occur as a result of medications, toxins, head trauma, or degenerative conditions.[22]

Dysphagia in Parkinson's disease is related to changes in striated muscles under dopaminergic control and in smooth muscles under autonomic control.[23] The oral stage is associated with rigidity of the lingual musculature rather than weakness. Small-amplitude, ineffective tongue-rolling movements are observed as patients attempt to propel the boluses into the pharynx. As a result, pharyngeal swallow responses are delayed, with aspiration occurring before and during the swallow. Expectoration of cough-aspirated material is weak because of rigidity of the laryngeal musculature. Incomplete opening of the upper esophageal sphincter and esophageal dysmotility are also commonly observed in patients with Parkinson's disease.[23,25]

In the early stages, antiparkinsonian medications such as levodopa improve flexibility and speed during swallowing.[26] However, pharmacotherapy has only a limited amount to offer dysphagic patients with severe symptoms and sometimes nonoral feeding is necessary.[27] Pneumonia is one of the most prevalent causes of death in patients with Parkinson's disease, irrespective of whether the patients are fed orally or via a feeding tube.[23]

Multiple Sclerosis. Swallowing difficulty is uncommon in the early stages of multiple sclerosis.[2,23,28,29] The scattered inflammatory white- matter lesions observed in the central nervous system result in varying combinations of motor, sensory, and cognitive deficits, which usually run a remitting–relapsing course.[2,23,28] Swallowing problems are less common in this disease, occurring in the end stages in approximately 10% to 33% of cases.[29] Difficulties arise with respect to the feeding process because of hand tremors and spasticity. Sclerosed plaques can be found in the cortex and the brain stem and can affect cranial nerves. Therefore, swallowing dysfunction will depend on the location of the lesions.

Sometimes the swallowing dysfunction is mild and goes unnoticed by the patients.[2,23] In patients who complain of dysphagia, the most commonly observed symptoms are delayed oropharyngeal swallowing initiation, reduced tongue strength, and weak pharyngeal contractions. These result in pharyngeal residue after the swallow and a sense of food getting caught in the throat.

A coexisting feature of multiple sclerosis in the later stages is cognitive decline and dementia.[23,29] Patients may be unaware of the act of eating and may be dependent on being fed. Family and caregivers require specific information to help patients compensate for reduced awareness.

Dementia

Dementia can result from several causes, including cumulative brain damage from multiple small cerebral infarcts in patients with hypertension and diabetes, Alzheimer's disease, advanced stages of other diseases such as Parkinson's or Huntington's disease, or multiple sclerosis. In addition, patients can demonstrate cognitive decline from chronic metabolic derangement, sedating medications, and/or depression.[2,22,25] Patients with dementia frequently encounter pneumonia, particularly in the advanced stages of the disease.

Dementia causes fluctuating attention span, inactivity, agitation, confusion, and memory loss. These symptoms may necessitate medications to calm the wandering, agitation, and somnolence. Decreased consciousness predisposes patients to aspirate food and liquid.[25] For additional information on dementia, consult Chapter 20 of this textbook.

No single dysphagia profile exists for demented patients because of the variety of causes of the disease. However, common observations include the inability to feed self independently and to remain focused for the duration of the meal. Some patients do not engage in the task of eating and swallowing. They may hold food in their mouth for prolonged periods without mastication or bolus formation, especially with uniformly textured foods such as pureed items or bland foods. As a result of sensory impairments and lack of attention, the patient may fail to control the bolus in the mouth and lose it prematurely over the tongue base and into the larynx before the pharyngeal swallow has been elicited, resulting in aspiration. Moreover, their distractible or agitated behavior may prolong the feeding time and hence reduce the amount of nutrition and hydration received. Malnutrition and dehydration can produce medical complications that in turn exacerbate the cognitive decline even further.[2]

Systemic Dysphagia

The broadest category of causes of dysphagia includes inflammatory and infectious factors, which affect oral, pharyngeal, and esophageal stages of swallowing. Candida esophagitis can occur in an immunocompromised host, such as in patients with AIDS or patients who have undergone chemotherapy. Dysphagia for solids is greater than for liquids, and patients frequently complain of food getting caught. Heartburn, nausea, and vomiting are other common complaints.[16]

Autoimmune inflammatory disorders can affect swallowing in either specific organs or the immune system as a whole. This category of diseases includes polymyositis, scleroderma, and secondary autoimmune diseases. Patients with HIV/AIDS have been shown to have aspiration on videofluoroscopy.[30] Sometimes intrinsic obstruction is observed, such as in Wegener's granulomatosis. With other disorders, there is external compression, abnormal esophageal motility as in scleroderma, or inadequate lubrication as in Sjögren's syndrome. Pharyngeal and esophageal symptoms are common. Poor esophageal motility restricts patients to small meals of pureed or liquid substances, and eating duration is long and drawn out. Patients report the sensation of solid foods getting caught in the esophagus. Weight loss is frequent. Gastroesophageal reflux results from poor esophageal peristalsis.[16,31,32]

General Deconditioning

Multisystem diseases, including the more frequently encountered progressive diseases such as end-stage chronic obstructive pulmonary disease, coronary artery disease, and chronic renal failure, cause insidious weakness. Weight loss in these patients is a common consequence because of reduced endurance for activities of daily living, including eating and swallowing. Patients with emphysema have difficulty coordinating swallowing and respiration, and may be unable to tolerate the obligatory cessation of breathing required for airway protection during the swallow. General immobility impairs spontaneous pulmonary clearance, resulting in an inability to expectorate material if it is aspirated. Patients are often discouraged and depressed by their loss of independence and declining health.

Medications can play a major role in causing dysphagia. The number of medications increases proportionally to the number of disorders to be treated, but their reactions may be exponential. Medications can affect lubrication of the oral cavity and pharynx, reduce coordination or motor function, and cause local mucosal toxicity.[33] This is discussed further under xerostomia. Antipsychotic or neuroleptic medications can produce extrapyramidal motor disturbances, resulting in impaired function of the striated musculature of the oral cavity, pharynx, and esophagus. Long-term use of antipsychotics may result in tardive dyskinesia, with choreiform tongue movements affecting the coordination of swallowing. Delayed swallow initiation is a reported side effect of some neuroleptic medications.[34]

Assessment

Approaching the evaluation of swallowing in the terminally ill patient demands a holistic view and reaches beyond the physiology of deglutition. While aspiration of food or liquid could realistically evolve into aspiration pneumonia, paradoxically, committing a patient to nonoral feeding or non per os (NPO) is also fraught with complications. It therefore behooves caregivers to carefully consider the multiple parameters in decision-making about oral nutrition in the terminally ill patient. The matter is not a simple decision of "if the patient is aspirating food he or she should not receive nutrition orally."

For the patient with a life-threatening illness, the goals of the clinical swallowing evaluation are to (1) identify the underlying physiological nature of the disorder; (2) determine whether any short-range interventions can alleviate the dysphagia; and (3) collaborate with the patient, family, and caregivers on the safest and most efficacious method of nutrition and hydration.

Evaluation of dysphagia in patients receiving palliative care is best accomplished within a multidisciplinary framework where the patient's needs and wishes are held paramount. The patient may report coughing or choking sensations while eating or drinking. A number of patients underestimate their swallowing difficulty, having accommodated to the gradually increasing dysphagia. Nurses and family caregivers usually report symptoms of difficulty swallowing when the problems are witnessed regularly at meals and while administering medications. In some cases, there may be no overt coughing spells when the patient is eating or drinking, and the question of aspiration is entertained because of recurrent pneumonias. Speech language pathologists who are skilled at identifying causes of oropharyngeal swallowing and who understand the complications of dysphagia can be consulted to evaluate the swallowing behavior and to suggest compensatory management strategies for alleviating the dysphagia. In terminally ill patients, it may be possible to determine the least restrictive diet that will provide the patient with safe and efficient oral intake while at the same time preserving a small amount of pleasure associated with eating by mouth. The assistance of a gastroenterologist may be required in cases requiring palliative dilation of the esophagus.

Clinical History

A comprehensive understanding of the difficulties involved in swallowing depends in large part on a detailed history from the patient and caregivers. Eliciting a description of the patient's complaints about swallowing is critical to painting a picture of the physiological basis of the problem and to integrating these hypotheses with attitudes and wishes about eating and not eating. Details of disease progression along with the accompanying emotional and psychological impact on the patient and the family should also be considered when determining the aggressiveness of a swallowing work-up and its treatment.

The swallowing history may indicate a mechanical obstruction etiology or an underlying neuromuscular cause. Asking the patient which foods are easier and which are avoided, with special focus on liquids versus solids, provides clues about the location of the disorder. For example, patients who complain of solid food dysphagia and localize the area of difficulty to the throat may present with bolus propulsion problems, whereas those who choke on liquids may have a sensory deficit with mistiming of airway protection. It is important to note low diagnostic specificity regarding the patient's localization of the problem with radiographic or endoscopic findings.[35]

Information about the patient's current eating habits and diet should be elicited. Does the patient choke on all consistencies of solid foods and fluids? Can the patient feed himself or herself? How have meal times changed since the illness? What is the total calorie intake the patient receives on a daily basis, and how far short does this fall from the patient's nutritional requirements? Length of meal times and effort required are indicators of eating efficiency. Additional areas of concern include appetite, factors that appear to alleviate or exacerbate the problem such as positioning, time of day, ability to swallow medication, and the presence of pain on swallowing.

The current complaints with respect to the physiology of swallowing are as important as the patient's previous attitudes toward eating. These attitudes form the foundation on which management strategies are implemented. The patient with a poor appetite, fatigue, and a sense of hopelessness will understandably be less compliant and less motivated to engage in

Table 10–1
Patient Complaints of Swallowing Difficulty and Their Possible Physiological Correlates

Patient's Complaint	Physiological Impairment
Choking on fluids	Poor tongue control for oral manipulation
	Impaired laryngeal closure
	Delayed onset of pharyngeal swallow
Protracted meal times	Weak chewing
	Diminished endurance
Nasal regurgitation of fluids	Incompetent velopharyngeal mechanism
Difficulty getting swallow started	Reduced oral and hypopharyngeal sensation
Dry mouth	Reduced or impaired saliva production
Solids caught in throat	Weak tongue-driving force
	Impaired laryngeal excursion fails to open upper esophageal segment
Regurgitation or emesis after swallowing	Poor esophageal motility or esophageal obstruction
Sour taste in mouth after eating	Gastroesophageal reflux
Pain on swallowing	Esophagitis, mucositis, esophageal obstruction

a complex treatment program. Additionally, the patient and caregivers should understand and consider the competing benefits and risks regarding nutrition, with attention to the patient's preferences.

Table 10–1 lists frequently encountered complaints by patients regarding swallowing and their potential physiological counterparts.

Examination of Swallowing by Direct Observation

Direct observation by a perceptive clinician of the patient while eating, drinking, or taking medications can yield valuable information about the underlying disorder. As discussed previously, the speech-language pathologist is vigilant for indications of chewing inefficiencies, aspiration, or obstruction. Table 10–2 lists warning signs that can alert caregivers to possible swallowing problems.

Usually, the clinician assesses the patient's oral motor sensory function and cognitive communicative function, while observing the partaking of a variety of liquid and solid foods (e.g., semisolid, soft solid, and, where appropriate, food requiring mastication). Speech and voice are analyzed, (bearing in mind the piston–chamber model described earlier) to determine the underlying physiology of the swallowing disorder. Since aspiration may be silent in up to 40% of patients with dysphagia, close attention is paid to occult signs of aspiration, including wet vocal quality or gurgliness, frequent throat clearing, delayed coughing, and oral/pharyngeal residue.[2]

Assessment of Oral Hygiene. The status of the oral mucosa and general oral hygiene reflect a patient's ability to manage secretions and swallowing. As mentioned earlier, xerostomia may exacerbate, and in some cases even cause, difficulty swallowing. Patients who require supplemental oxygen delivered via a nasal cannula frequently experience dryness in the oral cavity. It is not uncommon to find dry secretions crusted along the tongue, palate, and pharynx in patients who have not eaten orally in some time. Dental caries and dentures that are not well cared for can also contribute to a state of poor oral hygiene as well as poor quality of life. Before giving the patient food or liquids, even for assessment purposes, it is vital to clear the oral cavity of extraneous secretions, using mouth swabs, tongue scrapers, toothbrushes, and oral suction if necessary. Dried oral secretions may loosen during trials of fluid and inadvertently obstruct the airway.

Evaluation of the Gag Reflex. A word of caution is needed regarding the gag reflex and oropharyngeal swallowing. Health care professionals routinely assess the gag reflex as a predictor of swallowing behavior. The gag reflex and the pattern of neuromuscular events comprising the swallow are very different, both in their innervation and in their execution. The gag reflex is a protective reflex that prevents noxious substances arising from the oral cavity or digestive tract from entering the airway. It involves simultaneous constriction of the pharyngeal and laryngeal muscles closing the airway and the pharyngeal lumen and results in anterior movement of the tongue.[36] A gag reflex is not elicited during the normal swallow.[37] Unlike the pattern of events in the swallow, the gag reflex can be extinguished or reduced by a nasogastric feeding tube, endotracheal intubation, or repeated stimulation. The pharyngeal swallow response, which closes the airway and opens the

Table 10–2
Indications of a Swallowing Disorder

Reduced alertness or cognitive impairment
Coma, heavy sedation, dementia, delirium
Impulsivity with regard to eating, playing with food, inattention during eating
Alterations in attitudes toward eating
Refusal to eat in the presence of others
Avoidance of particular foods or fluids
Protracted meal times, incomplete meals, large amounts of fluids to flush solids
Changes in posture or head movements during eating
Laborious chewing, multiple swallows per small bites
Signs of oral–pharyngeal dysfunction
Dysarthria or slurred, imprecise speech
Dry mouth with thick secretions coating the tongue and palate
Wet voice with "gurgly" quality
Drooling or leaking from the lips
Residual in the oral cavity after eating
Frequent throat clearing
Coughing or choking
Nasal regurgitation
Specific patient complaints
Sensation of food getting caught in the throat
Coughing and choking while eating
Regurgitation of solids after eating
Pain on swallowing
Food or fluid noted in tracheotomy tube
Inability to manage secretions
Drooling
Shortness of breath while chewing or after meals
Regurgitation of food or fluid through the nose
Difficulty initiating the swallow
Unexplained weight loss

upper esophagus, cannot be extinguished once it begins, and it continues in a predetermined progression until the sequence of events is completed. These inherent differences highlight the need to examine the gag reflex and the swallow separately. Only evaluation of the biomechanical events of the swallow, not the gag reflex, can predict the safety of airway protection.

Assessment of Airway Protection. Functional airway protection is a critical predictor of safe swallowing and, thus, an important element of the clinical swallowing evaluation. Effective airway protection entails timely and complete laryngeal closure during swallowing and the efficient expectoration of material in response to aspiration. Audible strong cough at the glottis and pharyngeal contraction, which is necessary for bringing up a sputum sample, are required for functional airway protection. Patients who have weak voices and weak respiratory force for coughing and pulmonary clearance are at risk for pulmonary compromise. Airway protection cannot be definitively discerned from a clinical evaluation alone. Although the clinician may palpate moderate superior and anterior laryngeal elevation on swallowing, may perceive a normal vocal quality, and may not observe cough on swallowing, the patient may in fact be silently aspirating. Silent aspiration can only be confirmed definitively with an instrumental examination. Previous radiation therapy, as well as cranial nerve IX (glossopharyngeal) and X (vagus) deficits, may all contribute to the picture of silent aspiration. Depending on the stage of progression of the patient's illness and overall management goals, it may be prudent to identify silent aspiration with the aim of limiting progression with behavioral strategies.

Instrumental Evaluation

The clinical examination of swallowing is not conclusive regarding location of the swallowing disorder or the underlying physiology. Radiographic or endoscopic evaluation of swallowing are functional examinations providing valuable information for management. Sometimes disease progression with its sequelae, including inability to travel, inability to sit upright, wakefulness, pain and/or somnolence, preclude instrumental examination. Management shifts from maintenance to comfort, with compensatory behaviors being inappropriate.

Videofluorographic Evaluation of Swallowing. Radiographic swallowing studies are helpful in understanding the underlying physiology of swallowing.[2] The videofluorographic swallowing study (commonly known as modified barium swallow study) examines oropharyngeal swallowing with the patient positioned upright while swallowing a variety of consistencies of barium-coated foods (liquids, semisolids, and solids) in controlled volumes. Speech pathologists and radiologists perform these studies together. The goal of this study is not only to determine the presence or absence of aspiration but also to evaluate the effectiveness of compensatory swallowing strategies (described below) that may decrease the risk of aspiration and increase swallowing efficiency. The test is not invasive, takes a short time to administer, and provides valuable information that can be used in managing the dysphagia.[2,38]

A barium swallow study examines esophageal function during swallowing in contrast to the videofluoroscopic swallowing study, which focuses on the oropharyngeal mechanism. The barium swallow identifies mucosal abnormalities, esophageal strictures, esophageal motility, and gastroesophageal reflux. This test is conducted with the patient positioned upright and supine position while swallowing liquid barium or in some cases a barium tablet. If necessary, gastric emptying can also be assessed.[16] Since the esophagus is under involuntary neural control, compensatory swallowing strategies cannot be assessed with this procedure. However, recommendations can be made for changing to liquid consistencies in a patient with an esophageal stricture.

Endoscopic examination of oropharyngeal swallowing can be performed at the bedside by a trained speech-language pathologist. The oropharynx and larynx can be visualized transnasally while the patient is swallowing food substances dyed with food coloring and the presence of laryngeal penetration, aspiration, and pharyngeal retention can be observed. As in the videofluoroscopic swallowing study, compensatory swallowing strategies such as postural modifications or swallowing maneuvers can be evaluated for their efficacy.[39] Endoscopic evaluation of the esophagus and stomach while the patient is sedated can confirm the presence of strictures and mucosal anomalies.[16]

Assessment of Compensatory Swallowing Strategies

The physiologic information obtained from the clinical and instrumental swallowing facilitates on-line assessment of intervention strategies aimed at increasing swallowing safety and efficiency. These include alterations in head and neck posture, consistency of food, sensory awareness, and feeding behaviors. The chief advantage of these strategies is that they are simple for the patient to learn and to perform. In addition, once their effectiveness is determined, the patient can use the intervention during meals to improve swallowing function.

Postural Modifications. Postural changes during swallowing often have the effect of diverting the food or liquid to prevent aspiration or obstruction but do not change the swallowing physiology.[2,38] A commonly used strategy is the chin tuck posture. This posture has the advantage of increasing the pressure on the bolus and restricting the opening of the laryngeal inlet during swallowing, thus potentially reducing the risk of laryngeal penetration and aspiration. However, in select cases a chin tuck may exacerbate the aspiration, underscoring the need for radiographic evidence of its clinical value, if at all possible. Head rotation to the weak side in a patient with head and neck cancer is another postural change that may assist bolus flow down the intact side by obstructing the weak side and, hence, preventing residue or aspiration. These strategies may be used in isolation or in combination depending on the nature of the underlying swallowing pathophysiology.

Although it is not possible to detect the effectiveness of these strategies with complete certainty at the bedside, they may have empiric benefit that could be tested with an instrumental procedure, if that is deemed appropriate or necessary in the future. Table 10–3 lists some of the postural strategies that may be introduced and their potential benefits on bolus flow.

Changes in Texture and Consistency of Food. Underlying physiological constraints, such as reduced tongue control or strength, may affect the safety of swallowing certain solids or liquids. The patient with advanced ALS or Parkinson's disease with profound tongue weakness may exhibit signs of aspiration on thin liquids but may have sufficient control to drink liquids thickened to a nectar-like or honey-like consistency in small sips. Patients debilitated by chronic disease and who lack endurance to complete a meal may benefit from ground or pureed moist foods that require limited mastication. In certain circumstances, altered food consistency is the only way a patient

Table 10–3
Compensatory Postural Changes that Improve Bolus Flow and Reduce Aspiration and Residue During Swallowing

Postural Strategy	Effects on Bolus Flow
Chin tuck	Closes laryngeal vestibule, pushes tongue closer to posterior pharyngeal wall, and promotes epiglottic deflection
Head back	Promotes posterior bolus movement with assistance of gravity
Head tilt to stronger side	Directs bolus down stronger side with assistance of gravity
Head turned to weaker side	Diverts bolus away from weaker side by obstruction of weaker pharyngeal channel, promotes opening of upper esophagus
Head tilt plus chin tuck	Directs bolus down stronger side while increasing closure of laryngeal vestibule
Head rotation plus chin tuck	Diverts bolus away from weaker side while facilitating closure of laryngeal vestibule and vocal folds

Source: Logemann (1998), reference 2.

can continue to eat orally, for example, in the patient with esophageal carcinoma or a severe esophageal motility disorder. Some nutritional supplement drinks are both thicker liquids and calorically fortified, providing a safer alternative to more solid consistencies.

Changes in the consistency of food and liquid are frequently difficult for patients because they often lack appeal. Thus, this management strategy should be used as a last resort and reserved for patients who are unable to follow directions to use postural changes or for whom other compensatory strategies are not feasible.[2]

Increased Sensory Awareness. Sensory enhancement techniques include increasing downward pressure of a spoon against the tongue when presenting food in the mouth and presenting a sour bolus, a cold bolus, a bolus requiring chewing, or a large-volume bolus. These techniques may elicit a quicker pharyngeal swallow response while reducing the risk of aspiration. Some patients benefit from receiving food or liquid at a slower rate, while others are more efficient with larger boluses. Enhancing the bolus characteristics to include more texture can sometimes induce mastication and bolus formation more readily than a bolus that is both flavorless and homogenous in texture. This is particularly evident in patients with advanced dementia. Patient responses to these behaviors can be evaluated at the bedside, and the findings can be easily communicated to the caregivers.[2]

Secondary Behaviors. Attention is focused on the secondary behaviors that have an impact on the efficiency of swallowing. For example, the patient's attitude toward eating, endurance, efficiency of swallowing, and the length of time it takes to eat a meal influence the overall nutritional picture and, ultimately, quality of life.

Management

Effortless, efficient, and safe swallowing are important criteria for continued oral nutrition. Experience has shown that most patients prefer oral alimentation even if it means they do not receive sufficient nutrition. Patient autonomy in shared decision-making is a critical ethical principle to respect but should be accompanied by a clear understanding of the risks involved in eating by mouth. Specifically, families and patients should be informed about the risks and consequences of developing aspiration pneumonia and malnutrition. Health care professionals must present the information in as objective a manner as possible, taking the patient's wishes or the wishes of the surrogate decision-maker into consideration. If the decision is to continue with oral intake, the safest diet should be suggested and aspiration precautions introduced, using assessment of the swallowing problem as a guide.

The decision to pursue the option of nonoral nutritional support has significant ramifications for both the patient and the family. The family may feel that they have neglected their obligation to nourish their loved one safely and may be overwhelmed by the practical obligations demanded by the nonoral route, for example, frequent nocturnal feedings, monitoring of gastric residuals, etc. However, tube feeding may provide the patient with several more months of improved quality of life afforded by strength and endurance. Patients and families may also feel a sense of reduced pressure to eat by mouth because of the tube feeding.

Pharmacological Management. There are no pharmacological agents that directly act on swallowing function. However, there are agents for concurrent issues, which can exacerbate an underlying mucosal problem.

Candida esophagitis requires oral antifungal agents such as nystatin topical every 4 hours for 2 to 3 weeks.[40] Other antifungal medications include ketoconazole, miconazole, fluconazole, and amphotericin B. Immunocompromised patients with candidiasis require potent systemic antifungal medications. Resistance can occur, however, in patients with long-term prophylaxis. Patients who fail the above regimen may be considered for antiviral agents.[41] The prokinetic agent or ranitidine may be prescribed for poor esophageal motility, and proton pump inhibitors have been found to be effective in patients with gastroesophageal reflux disease.[42]

Dietary Changes. Evaluation results highlight the most appropriate nutritional method for the patient. If oral alimentation has been determined as safe, the guiding principle for diet is to ingest the maximum amount of calories for the least amount of effort. Examples of modified diets are listed in Table 10–4.

Nutritionists can provide individualized suggestions for calorie-dense foods or high-calorie liquid supplements, depending on the patient's metabolic status. Patients with oropharyngeal dysphagia may require thickened liquids. Commercial thickening agents from modified food starch can be used to thicken liquids. These release the fluid in the gastrointestinal tract and provide water for hydration requirements.[43]

Feeding the Patient. While there is no cure for a swallowing disorder in the terminally ill patient, continued ability to eat by mouth may be facilitated by careful hand-feeding techniques and strategies employed by family and caregivers. These techniques will vary depending on the underlying swallowing/feeding difficulty. Compliance with feeding strategies is often related to understanding of the rationale. Family members are more likely to feed a patient a particular diet and in a particular manner if they understand the physiological and psychological reasons for the recommendation and if they have been included in the decision-making.[2] Although hand feeding is time consuming, it allows for continued intimate contact between patient and caregiver. Interestingly, hand feeding has been shown in some cases to equal duration of survival compared with patients who have gastrostomy tubes placed.[44]

Table 10–4
Diet Modifications for Patients with Dysphagia

Diet	Definition	Example	Indication
Pureed diet	Blenderized food with added liquid to form smooth consistency	Applesauce, yogurt, moist mashed potatoes, puddings	Reduced tongue function for chewing, impaired pharyngeal contraction, esophageal stricture
Mechanically altered diet	Ground, finely chopped foods that form a cohesive bolus with minimal chewing	Pasta, soft scrambled eggs, cottage cheese, ground meats	Some limited chewing possible but protracted due to impaired tongue control
Soft diet	Naturally soft foods requiring some chewing; food is cut in small pieces	Soft meats, canned fruits, baked fish; avoid raw vegetables, bread, and tough meats	Reduced endurance for prolonged meal due to tongue weakness for chewing, reduced attention span

Additional suggestions for feeding the patient include the following:

1. Remove distractions at mealtime. This is appropriate for patients who need to concentrate on swallowing to increase safety, such as patients with head and neck cancer who are using compensatory swallowing strategies, and for patients who easily lose their focus and need to be fed, such as patients with Alzheimer's dementia.[44]
2. Emphasize heightened awareness of sensory clues, such as feeding patients larger boluses, increasing downward pressure of the spoon on the tongue to alert the patient that food is in the mouth, or feeding patients cold or sour boluses or foods requiring some mastication. Some patients with Alzheimer's disease demonstrate the most efficient swallow when offered finger foods that require chewing. These foods allow them to tap into the automatic motor rhythm of chewing and swallowing that is reminiscent of the patterns they have used all their life.
3. Provide feeding utensils. Patients with multiple sclerosis who have feeding difficulties associated with hand tremors may be aided with devices such as weighted cuffs that reduce the intention tremor. These may also be useful in patients with Parkinson's disease. Occupational therapists are often able to provide individualized assistive devices to patients.
4. Position the patient. Ensure optimal posture of the patient at meals, that is, reduce the tendency to slump forward, causing loss of food from the oral cavity, or head extension, making the airway vulnerable to aspiration.
5. Schedule meal times. Some medications enhance swallowing function. For example, patients with Parkinson's disease may become more alert and flexible after their medications.[18] Thus, timing of meals to coincide with increased function may enhance swallowing efficiency and safety. In contrast, some medications, particularly benzodiazepines such as valium, may increase somnolence and produce bradykinesia, affecting the efficiency of swallowing. In such cases, withholding oral intake may reduce the risk of aspiration.

Nonoral Nutrition. Some patients require primary nonoral feeding, and gastrostomy or jejunostomy tubes are placed endoscopically or in open surgical procedures. Some patients, such as those with esophageal cancer, head and neck cancer, or ALS, have had their feeding tubes in place for several months prior to the terminal period. For other patients, families and caregivers may have recently decided to pursue the nonoral feeding option. Irrespective of the scenario, the following should be considered:

1. The presence of a feeding tube does not imply NPO, or nothing by mouth. Some patients are able to take small amounts of food for their pleasure. Restrictions to reduce the risk of aspiration may apply during these "trials" of oral intake, such as texture of the food, postural requirements, and length of the trial.
2. Patients who are fed nonorally remain at risk for aspiration of either oral secretions or refluxed gastric contents, including tube feeding and aspiration pneumonia. A long-term study by Langmore and associates[45] examined the predictors of aspiration pneumonia in 189 elderly patients, including such factors as oropharyngeal and esophageal dysphagia, medical and dental status, feeding status, and functional status. They found that the dominant risk factor for aspiration pneumonia was dependence

for feeding, that is, inability to feed oneself. This variable included those patients who were tube-fed as well as those who were fed orally by a caretaker. This study found that patients who were tube-fed had a significantly increased risk of developing aspiration pneumonia. The authors posited that oral hygiene is frequently neglected in tube-fed patients, promoting colonization of bacteria, and aspiration of these secretions can result in pneumonia.

3. Inserting a form of nonoral nutrition in a patient with a terminal illness is controversial and is the subject of numerous recent publications, particularly in relation to institutionalized adults with advanced cognitive impairment due to dementia. Continued careful hand feeding over artificial nutrition is the overwhelming recommendation by the geriatricians who have conducted studies comparing multiple outcome parameters including survival, cost, and quality-of-life ratings.[46]

Gastroesophageal Reflux Precautions. Poor esophageal motility or reduced tone of the lower esophageal sphincter can be managed either pharmacologically with the pro-motility agents described above or nonpharmacologically. Ideally, a combination approach is most efficacious. Gastroesophageal reflux precautions include elevation of the head of the bed to 45 degrees at night, inexpensively and effectively accomplished by placing blocks under the head of the bed; frequent small meals; upright posture for 45 to 60 minutes after eating; monitoring of gastric residuals in tube-fed patients, and avoidance of spicy foods, coffee, tea, chocolate, and alcohol.[47]

Administration of Medication. Oral medications can present enormous challenges to patients with dysphagia. Patients who take pills with fluid complain that they can swallow the water but the pills get caught in the throat. This phenomenon is explained by the differences in speed of transit of the fluid and the pill: the water travels more rapidly than the pill. Patients with delayed pharyngeal swallow initiation, reduced tongue strength, and/or pharyngeal contractions are unable to coordinate propulsion of the entire bolus. Crushing medications or burying them whole in a semisolid such as applesauce or ice cream creates a similar consistency and makes swallowing easier. Alternately patients can be offered their medications in elixir form. A recent development is a new technology that packages the widely used compounds used in medications into tablets that disintegrate and dissolve on the tongue (RapiTab Technology, Schwarz-Pharma, Milwaukee WI). This type of medication delivery would be most helpful for the dysphagic patient having difficulty swallowing tablets.

Tracheostomy Tubes and Oral Intake. The presence of a tracheotomy tube does not preclude oral intake. In fact, access to the upper respiratory tract improves pulmonary toilet in patients who have chosen to eat in spite of aspiration. Contrary to common thinking, an inflated tracheotomy cuff is not fully protective against aspiration.[2,47] The seal in the trachea is not complete, and material sitting above the cuff can be aspirated. Tracheal suctioning should be performed after meals in patients with dysphagia who have chosen to eat. Ideally, the cuff should be deflated and the patient encouraged to cough, clearing material that may have been aspirated.

DRY MOUTH (XEROSTOMIA)

CASE STUDY
Mrs. M, a Patient with Abdominal Pain

Mrs. M was an 80-year-old woman with a history of dementia, end-stage cardiac disease, and peripheral vascular disease. One weekend she developed abdominal pain and was admitted to the hospital. Work-up revealed a blockage with probable toxic colon. She was made NPO and placed on multiple antibiotics to prevent further infection. She became more agitated and was given round-the-clock haloperidol. She was started on an IV morphine drip. However, she complained of constant thirst. The nurses provided her with frequent mouth swabs. They also painted artificial saliva in her mouth and applied lip balm to her lips. They brushed her teeth several times a day to stimulate saliva.

Definition

Xerostomia is the sensation of oral dryness, which may or may not be accompanied by decreased salivary secretions. Although patients receiving palliative care commonly experience oral dryness,[48,49] it may be difficult to identify the exact underlying cause and contributing factors. Decreased salivary function and prolonged xerostomia cause myriad oral/esophageal problems in the mouth, including dental caries, gum, tongue, and oral mucosal irritations and lesions, mouth infections, taste changes, bad breath, swallowing problems, and speech problems. Thus, treatment offers much comfort to patients by moisturizing dry lips and mouth, but also by eliminating these long-term sequelae. Ultimately, sleep, rest, and nutrition are secondary issues arising out of these problems.[50,51]

Incidence

Due to lack of studies outside of the cancer population, it is difficult to estimate the incidence of xerostomia. In a prevalence study of palliative care admissions, 55% experienced xerostomia.[52] Other authors estimate that xerostomia affects

30% of palliative care patients.[53] In the population at large, it increases with age and medical problems because medication therapy increases incidence. In palliative care, it is listed as a major source of discomfort in patients with cancer. In noncancer, patients, there has not been much research except for Sjögren's disease.

Pathophysiology

Xerostomia results from four causes. First, it may result from reduced salivary secretion. Common causes include surgery performed on head and neck areas, radiation aimed at head and neck regions, medication side effects, infections, hypothyroidism, autoimmune processes, and sarcoidosis. Second, xerostomia may be caused by buccal erosion. Potential factors are cancer and cancer treatment, particularly chemotherapy and radiation. Additionally, immunocompromised conditions such as AIDS, arthritis, or lupus may exacerbate dry mouth. Third, local or systemic dehydration may induce xerostomia. Factors contributing to dehydration include anorexia, vomiting, diarrhea, fever, drying oxygen therapies, mouth breathing, polyuria, diabetes, hemorrhage, and swallowing difficulties. Fourth, other miscellaneous disorders such as mental health issues including depression, coping reactions, anxiety, and pain can cause xerostomia.[48–50,54] There has been a long-standing assumption that as one ages, dry mouth naturally occurs as part of the process. In fact, age is not a factor;[50,51] rather, as one ages, the chance of dry mouth increases due to increasing comorbid conditions that occur in the older adult, along with the higher probability of the necessity to take more medications.[50]

Although saliva is necessary for oral nutrition, it also facilitates chewing, swallowing, tasting, and talking. For these functions, its properties allow lubrication, repair, food-bolus formation, and food breakdown. Additionally, saliva breaks down bacterial substances, offering immunoprotection for oral mucosa and dental structures.[50,51] In this way, it has antimicrobial properties, buffering properties, and liquid properties to help with gustation. Saliva thereby inhibits dental caries and infections, while providing protection against extreme temperatures of food and drink.[50,51,55–57]

The function of saliva production is regulated by the nervous system. After experiencing smell, sight, or taste of food, the salivary glands are stimulated to produce saliva within 2 to 3 seconds.[57] There is a two-step process to saliva secretion; production at the acinar level of the cells, and secretion where saliva is actually secreted into the mouth via the ducts.[50] Saliva is comprised of several elements. Ninety-nine percent of saliva is fluid composed of water and mucus, providing a lubricative element. The remaining 1% of saliva is solid, containing salts, proteins, minerals such as calcium bicarbonate ions, and enzymes such as pytalin, antibodies, and other antimicrobial agents.[48–51,55]

Saliva is produced by numerous glands in the oropharynx,[50,55] where the average healthy adult produces up to 1.5 liters of saliva a day. The parotid glands, the submandibular glands, and the sublingual glands produce 90% of saliva, with the rest produced in the oral pharynx. Parotid glands, located below and in front of each ear, produce a serous and watery saliva.[57] Therefore, damage to the parotid gland will produce a thicker saliva. Submandibular glands, located in the lower jaw, secrete mostly serous saliva with some mucinous elements.[57] Sublingual glands produce purely mucous saliva.[55,58] The overall viscosity of saliva is dependent on the functioning of the various glands.

There are numerous causes of xerostomia. Medications are notorious culprits of dry mouth, particularly several categories commonly used in palliative care.[50,58] These medications include sedatives, tranquilizers, antihistamines, anti-Parkinsonian medications, antiseizure medications, skeletal muscle relaxants, cytoxic agents, tricyclic antidepressants, and anticholinergics. Oral dryness may result from oral diseases such as acute and chronic parotitis, or partial or complete salivary obstruction. Other diseases such as Sjögren's syndrome, diabetes mellitus, HIV/AIDS, scleredema, sarcoidosis, lupus, Alzheimer's disease, and graft versus host disease can cause dry mouth.[50,58] Radiation to the head and neck can produce a 50% to 60% reduction of saliva within the 1st week of treatment because of inflammation.[58] Chemotherapy may also cause dry mouth, particularly in advanced disease.[58] Usually, dry mouth sensations are worse at night. Salivary secretions may be further reduced due to the duration of radiation and/or greater radiation doses.[58,59] However, it eventually may become a more persistent issue the longer radiation continues or as disease progresses.[54]

Assessment

Xerostomia may be accompanied by discomfort of the oral mucosa and the tongue, such as burning, smarting, and soreness with or without the presence of ulcers. Additionally, there may be difficulty with mastication, swallowing, and speech. Taste alterations, difficulty with dentures, and an increase in dental caries may also be associated with xerostomia. Additionally, sleep may be altered because of dry mouth. Therefore, a thorough history should review these problem areas along with the subjective distress of xerostomia (Table 10–5). Reviewing onset of oral dryness correlation with medication initiation may be insightful in assessment.[58]

An oral exam will reveal clear indications of dry mucosa. Extraoral examination is noted for dry, cracked lips, often with angular cheilitis or candida at the corners of the mouth.[50] Intraoral examination includes inspection of both mucosal and buccal dryness, noting whether the mouth is pale and dry, the presence of a dry and fissured tongue, the absence of salivary pooling, and the presence of oral ulcerations, gingivitis, or candidiasis.[49,55] Finally, salivary glands should be noted for swelling, indicating obstruction, and dentition should be examined for caries.[50]

Table 10–5
Assessment Questions for Xerostomia

Does oral dryness bother you?
Is your sleeping interrupted by a dry mouth?
Do you need to take increase fluids?
Is your mouth sore?
Do you experience altered taste sensations?
Is it difficult to speak?
Do you use tobacco? If so, what type and how much?
Do you drink alcohol or caffeine? If so, how much?
Are you taking any medications, including over-the-counter preparations, prescriptions, or herbs?

Sources: Sreebny and Valdini (1987), reference 49; Cooke et al. (1996), reference 55; Ship (2002), reference 50; Jensen et al., (2003), reference 51.

Two quick bedside tests are the cracker biscuit test and the tongue blade test. The cracker biscuit test involves giving a patient a dry cracker or biscuit. If the patient cannot eat the cracker without extra fluids, xerostomia is present.[49] The tongue blade test is an extension of mouth inspection. After inspection is complete, the tongue blade is placed on the tongue. Since dry mouth makes a ropey, pasty saliva, the tongue blade will stick to the tongue of a patient with xerostomia.[55]

Another, more aggressive test is unstimulated or stimulated sialometric measurement of saliva. This test measures the amount of saliva collected by spitting into a container, swabbing the mouth with a cotton-tipped applicator, or salivating into a test container at a set time.[49,55] However, for most palliative care patients, this may be a burdensome and unnecessary test.

To document the extent of xerostomia, it may be helpful to use rating scales specifically designed for this purpose. Two scales, contained in Table 10–6, rates xerostomia in a four-point system.[60,61]

Table 10–6
Dry Mouth Rating Scales

Oncology Nursing Society Documentation for Xerostomia	
0	No dry mouth
1	Mild dryness, slightly thickened saliva; little change in taste
2	Moderate dryness, thick and sticky saliva, markedly altered taste
3	Complete dryness of mouth
4	Salivary necrosis
Salivary Gland Changes: National Cancer Institute Documentation of Dry Mouth	
0	None
1	Slightly thickened
2	Thick, ropey, sticky saliva
3	Acute salivary necrosis
4	Disabling

Sources: National Cancer Institute (2003), reference 61; Oncology Nursing Society (2002), reference 60.

Management

Much of xerostomia management focuses on interventions to alleviate rather than interventions to eradicate or to prevent the symptom. This is because there is little to offer patients to ward off oral dryness. Therefore, the goal becomes protecting patients from further complications, which may be more problematic.[62] Medical treatment of xerostomia, as summarized in Table 10–7, would involve the following stepwise approach:

1. Treat underlying infection or disease. Candidiasis can cause xerostomia. Treating it with nystatin swish-and-swallow or with fluconazole 150 mg PO can improve xerostomia.[48,50,54,55]
2. Review and alter current medications as appropriate. There are some 500 medications that may cause oral dryness as a side effect.[50,58] Specifically, anticholinergics, antihistamines, phenothiazines, antidepressants, opioids, ß-blockers, diuretics, anticonvulsants, sedatives, and tobacco all may cause oral dryness. Thus, patients with heart conditions, mental health issues, depression, anxiety, neurological disorders, and pain disorders may be at risk for dry mouth. It is important to first evaluate the necessity of specific xerostomia-inducing drugs. If eliminating possible culprits is not possible, other possible strategies include decreasing the dosage to decrease dryness, or altering the schedule to assure that the peak effect of medication does not coincide with nighttime peak of decreased salivary production.[48–50,55]
3. Stimulate salivary flow. Salivary stimulation can occur with both nonpharmacological and pharmacological interventions.
4. Replace lost secretions with saliva substitutes.

Table 10–7
Stepwise Process for Managing Xerostomia

Treat underlying infections.
Review and alter current medications.
Stimulate salivary flow.
Replace lost secretions with saliva substitutes.
Protect teeth.
Rehydrate.
Modify diet.

Nonpharmacological Interventions

Nonpharmacological use of gustatory stimulation includes simple measures. Table 10–8 summarizes possible procedures. All of these interventions, except acupuncture, are inexpensive and may be as efficacious as medications for some patients, without uncomfortable side effects. However, relief is not long lasting.[55]

- Peppermint water. Peppermint stimulates saliva and can be taken as needed. However, it should not be used with metoclopramide as they have opposing actions.[48–50]
- Vitamin C. Use in lozenges or other forms as preferred. Disrupts salivary mucins to reduce viscosity of saliva.[56] Although inexpensive, vitamin C may be irritating to the mouth, particularly if the patient has mouth sores.[54] Also, there is a need to be careful as continual vitamin C can erode dental enamel.[56]
- Citric acids. Present in malic acid or in sweets. Citric acids can act similar to vitamin C in causing a burning sensation.[54]
- Chewing gum, mints. Preferably sugarless, to prevent caries and infections, as an immunocompromised state can hasten cavities and infections. These are most preferred by patients, are cheap, and have no side effects. May create a buffer system to compensate for dietary acids.[54,56]
- Acupuncture. Effective with a variety of types of xerostomia, although mechanism not understood. It occurs as a single treatment with eight needles placed in three places: bilaterally in the ears and a single distal point in the radial aspect of the index finger.[57] One study showed that 6 weeks of twice-weekly treatment increased salivation for up to 1 year.[63] Another study used a 3-to-4 weekly regimen, with monthly maintenance visits to relieve xerostomia.[64]

Pharmacological Interventions

- Pilocarpine. Pilocarpine is a parasympathetic agent that increases exocrine gland secretion and stimulates residual functioning tissue in damaged salivary gland. Saliva production is greatest after a dose and response lasts for about 4 hours.[56] Dose is 5 mg PO tid or QI, not to exceed 10 mg per dose.[57] Response varies with severity of xerostomia. Side effects include mild to moderate sweating, visual disturbances, nausea, rhinitis, chills, flushing, dizziness, abdominal cramping, and asthenia,[54,55] but can be lessened if taken with milk.[56] Pilocarpine should not be used in patients with chronic obstructive pulmonary disease or bowel obstruction.[54,55,57] New studies have shown that pilocarpine given before and during radiotherapy can reduce xerostomia.[54,65,66]
- Bethanechol. Bethanechol relieves anticholinergic side effects of tricyclic antidepressants. Few studies

Table 10–8
Review of Interventions of Xerostomia

Intervention	Role/Effect	Benefit	Side Effect
Nonpharmacological			
Peppermint Water	Mucous saliva	Inexpensive	Interacts with metoclopromide
Vitamin C	Chemical reduction	Inexpensive Reduces viscosity	Can irritate mouth if sores present
Citric acid/Sweets	Mucous saliva	Inexpensive	Can irritate like vitamin C. In sweets, can cause caries.
Chewing gum, mints	Watery saliva	Inexpensive More volume Only dentate	No side effects if sugarless, otherwise can promote caries
Acupuncture	Increase production	Noninvasive	Expensive
Pharmacological			
Pilocarpine	Nonselective muscarinic	Increases saliva production	Sweating, nausea, flushing, cramping
Bethanechol	M-3 muscarinic	Relieves side effect of TCA	
Methacholine	Parasympathetics	Increases salivation	Hypotension
Yohimbine	Blocks α-2 adrenoreceptors	Increases saliva	Drowsiness, confusion, atrial fibrillation
Cevimeline	M-1 & M-3 muscarinic agonist	Increases saliva	Less effects than pilocarpine

Sources: Adapted from Amerongen (2003), reference 56; Ship (2002), reference 50.

have been done that focus specifically on xerostomia rather than the side effects of antidepressants.[54,55]

- Methacholine. Methacholine is a parasympathomimetic compound that increases salivation. Dose is 10 mg a day. One side effect is hypotension. It is short-acting.[54,55]
- Yohimbine. Yohimbine blocks α_2-adrenoreceptors. Side effects include drowsiness, confusion, and atrial fibrillation, lasting up to 3 hours. Dose is 14 mg a day.[54,66]
- Cevimeline. Cevimeline is a muscarinic agonist that acts to increase saliva by inhibiting acetylcholinesterase. It works on salivary glands and lacrimal glands. Used in a spray or mouthwash, it lasts up to 6 hours.[56,57]
- Water. Water is simple and inexpensive. It is usually well tolerated and easily accessible. There is no research on whether optimal relief results from either warm or cold. Thus, temperature is a personal choice.[54,55]
- Artificial saliva. Artificial saliva contains carboxymethylcellulose or mucin; dose 2 mL every 3 to 4 hours.[54,55] Some examples include Glandosane, Xero-Lube, Orex, and Saliment.[51,56]
- Protect teeth. Oral hygiene, such as frequent brushing with soft brushes, water jet, denture cleaning, fluoride rinses, mouthwash, and flossing, stimulate salivation. This can help prevent candidiasis, particularly since dentures can harbor infections.[50]
- Use of lip balm prevents cracked lips, and use of saliva moistens lips. Care should be taken not to use products with alcohol since these can be irritating.[54,57,60,61]
- Dentifrices. Several are manufactured for patients with dry mouth that contain antimicrobial enzymes to reduce oral infections and enhance mouth wetting. Examples are Biotene and Oral Balance.[50,56,57]
- Mouthwashes. Help rinse debris from mouth. Includes homemade mouthwashes made from saline, sodium bicarbonate, glycerin, and perhaps lemon.[50,56]
- Rehydrate. Replenish oral hydration by sipping water, spraying water, and increasing humidity in the air.[67] To assist in sleep, instituting these measures at night may help rest.
- Modify diet. Education regarding the avoidance of sugars, spicy foods, sometimes salt, and dry or piquant foods is important. Patients may sip such foods in milk, tea, or water to assist in swallowing. In addition, instruct patients to take fluids with all meals and snacks. The use of gravies and juices with foods can add moisture to swallowing. Again, preferred tastes may vary from one patient to the next regarding salt, sweet, and sour. For dry mouth without oral ulcerations, provide carbonated drinks such as ginger ale, as well as cider, apple juice, or lemonade. Fresh fruits, papaya juice, or pineapple juice may help some patients refresh their mouths,[54,66] however, citrus products may be too acidic and irritating for other patients.[56]

Nursing Interventions

Because the degree of xerostomia varies, nursing intervention will vary from one patient to the next. Little research has focused on dry mouth, and clear evidence of the efficacy of one treatment over another has not been demonstrated. The result is a lack of standardized oral care procedures, with protocol varying from one institution to the next.[57] Therefore, the nurse must assess how much distress xerostomia is causing and help patients find a suitable therapy within their financial means.

Both the financial and physical burden of therapy may be of concern for patients. Many patients choose nonpharmacological therapy because it is inexpensive and has fewer side effects.[54] Other patients may consider nonpharmacological interventions depending on how many other symptoms they are experiencing or how many other medications they are currently taking. If a pharmacological therapy is chosen, it is important to consider previous patient choice, as patients seem to prefer saliva stimulants to saliva substitutes.[54] If saliva substitutes are used, those with a mucin base appear to be better tolerated than those derived from carboxymethylcellulose.[68] However, both types of preparation bases are better tolerated as an oral spray than as a gel or rinse.[68] The issue of prophylactic antifungal therapy occasionally arises. The evidence thus far has not shown it to be beneficial.

Patient and family education focuses on the goal of treatment as palliative. The nurse may help a family systematically go through a variety of therapies to achieve relief. Helping patient and families to demonstrate good oral care maintains the comfort of the patient. As a patient weakens, provision of mouth care gives a family member a tangible role in care.

HICCUPS

CASE STUDY
MB, a Patient with Gastric Cancer

MB is a 70-year-old male with rapidly progressing gastric cancer. He was diagnosed 7 months earlier and underwent chemotherapy. He is fairly weak and has begun to get more pain and discomfort. His wife cares for him at home in a small guest room because he is bedridden and has no energy to climb the stairs. His family asks the nurse to evaluate him. Upon arrival, the nurse finds him moderately uncomfortable with pain. He is disheveled, lying flat on a twin bed facing against the wall. He complains of pain in his abdomen and constant hiccups. He has not eaten in several days due to his discomfort. He is washed and bathed. Morphine elixir is initiated for his pain. For the hiccups, the family is encouraged to use a bolster pillow or several pillows to decrease the pressure of his large abdomen on his diaphragm and lungs. Additionally, baclofen 15 mg tid is initiated. Over the next 2 days, he is much more comfortable. After several days, his hiccups continue. The baleen is increased without effect. Because he is declining and also feeling nauseous, haloperidol 1 mg q 4 to 6 hours is initiated, which resolves the hiccups.

Definition

Hiccup, or singultus, is defined as sudden, involuntary contractions of one or both sides of the diaphragm and intercostal muscles, terminated by an abrupt closure of the glottis, producing a characteristic sound of "hic."[69–74] Hiccup frequency is usually 4 to 60 per minute.[75] Prolonged hiccups can produce fatigue and exhaustion if sleep is interrupted. Additionally, anxiety, depression, and frustration may arise if the important daily activities of eating or sleeping are interrupted. The long-term effects are exhaustion, increasing distress from lack of rest, and wasting because of interference with eating. Therefore, although seemingly a mere disturbance with no long-term pathology, intractable hiccups affect the quality of life.[69,71,72,75]

Prevelence and Impact

Hiccups in palliative care have not been well studied. Estimates of prevalence of hiccups in cancer patients is about 10% to 20%.[76] Because of their perceived insignificance, the incidence and prevalence are not well known. Additionally, most discussion of the impact of hiccups occurs in case reports. Children are more at risk than adults.[76]

Pathophysiology

There are three categories of hiccups. First are benign, self-limiting hiccups, which occur frequently. Such a bout of hiccups can last from several minutes to 2 days. Benign hiccups are primarily associated with gastric distention.[66,77] However, sudden changes in temperature, alcohol ingestion, excess smoking, and psychogenic causes may also induce benign hiccups.[69,71–73] Second are persistent, or chronic, hiccups. These continue for more than 48 hours but less than 1 month. Third and last are intractable hiccups, which persist longer than 1 month.[67,69,71–73] However, for patients in palliative care, these times may not be the important issue; rather, the amplitude can cause much distress, depending on the patient's diagnosis.[73]

Intractable hiccups in the third category have more than 100 different causes, varying from simple metabolic disturbances to complex structural lesions of the central nervous system or infections.[67,69,71,73] Particular causes can be distilled into four conditions: structural, metabolic, inflammatory, and infectious disorders.[69] Specifically, structural conditions affect or irritate the peripheral branches of the phrenic and vagus nerves, such as in abdominal or mediastinal tumors, hepatomegaly, ascites, or gastric distention, and central nervous disorders in which persistent hiccups can signal serious underlying disorders, such as thoracic aneurysm, brainstem tumors, metabolic and drug-related disorders, infectious diseases, and psychogenic disorders.[73,74,78] Common causes in terminal illness include neurological disorders such stroke, brain tumors, and sepsis and metabolic imbalance; phrenic nerve irritation such as tumor compression or metastases, pericarditis, pneumonia, or pleuritis; and vagal nerve irritation such as esophagitis, gastric distention, gastritis, pancreatitis, hepatitis, and myocardial infarction.[71,72] Medications such as steroids, chemotherapy, dopamine antagonists, megestrol, methyldopa, nicotine, opioids, and muscle relaxants may also cause hiccups.[76]

The precise pathophysiology of hiccups is unknown, as is their physiological function. It is considered a primitive function, such as yawning or vomiting, that through evolution now serves no purpose.[69,72,79] The anatomical cause of hiccups is thought to be bimodal, with association either with the phrenic or vagus nerve,[75,78] or central nervous involvement, which causes misfiring.[72] There is thought to be a hiccup reflex arc located in the phrenic nerves, the vagal nerves, and T6–T12 sympathetic fibers, as well as a possible hiccup center in either the respiratory center, the brain stem, or the cervical cord between C3 and C5.[80] However, there is not a discrete hiccup center, such as the chemoreceptor trigger zone for nausea.[75,79,77]

Evidence suggests an inverse relationship between partial pressure of carbon dioxide (pCO_2) and hiccups; that is, an increased pCO_2 decreases the frequency of hiccups and a decreased pCO_2 increases frequency of hiccups.[67] Interestingly, hiccup strength or amplitude varies from patient to patient as well as among separate episodes in an individual.[73] Moreover, hiccups have a minimal effect on respiration.

Assessment

Extensive work-up for hiccups in palliative care may be impractical and more uncomfortable than the hiccups themselves, while revealing little. Indeed, a recent retrospective study revealed that laboratory studies neither assisted in treatment nor helped determine what treatment would be effective.[81] Nonetheless, assessment should include a subjective review of how much distress the hiccups cause the patient. For example, in a patient with an abdominal tumor, hiccups can cause excruciating pain, whereas in the obtunded patient in renal failure, hiccups may cause no distress at all.

History may give insight into to the distress of hiccups. Subjective assessment includes the history and duration of the current episode of hiccups, previous episodes, and interference with rest, eating, or daily routines. Inquiry into possible triggers of hiccups episodes may be helpful, including patterns in timing during the day or other activities proceeding the hiccups such as eating, drinking, positioning, or various procedures. In addition, a review of recent trauma, surgery, or acute illness and medication history is important to help focus on potential causes of the hiccups.[69,79]

Usually the presence of hiccups themselves is quite obvious. However, physical exam may not reveal the cause of the hiccups, but, rather, rules out other conditions. Oral examination may reveal signs of swelling or obstruction. Observation includes inspection of the patient's general appearance, observing for signs of a toxic or septic process. More specifically, it includes evaluating for tenderness of the temporal artery, foreign bodies in the ear, infection of the throat, goiter in the neck, pneumonia or pericarditis of the chest, abdominal distention or ascites, and signs of stroke or delirium.[69]

Specific testing may be warranted to eliminate other causes. Chest x-ray may rule out pulmonary or mediastinal processes as well as phrenic/vagal irritation from peritumor edema in the abdominal area.[76] In addition, blood work including a complete blood count with differential electrolytes may rule out infection as well as electrolyte imbalances and renal failure.[67,69,72,73]

Management

The lack of research to increase understanding on the nature of hiccups has resulted in anecdotal therapy and a lack of treatment consensus. The consequence is treatment bias based on previous success rather than a systematic, evidence-based approach. Similar to treatment of dysphagia or xerostomia, treatment for hiccups should be focused on the underlying disease. If the etiology questionably includes simple causes such as gastric distention or temperature changes, "empiric" treatment should be initiated. Both nonpharmacological and pharmacological interventions may be used.[69,71–73] Therapies include physical maneuvers, medications, and various other procedures to interfere with the hiccup arc.[80] Otherwise, treatment for more complex episodes of hiccups without clear etiology will focus on various pharmacological interventions.

Table 10–9
Nonpharmacological Interventions for Hiccups

Respiratory Measures
Breath holding
Rebreathing in a paper bag
Diaphragm compression
Ice application in mouth
Induction of sneeze or cough with spices or inhalants
Nasal and Pharyngeal Stimulation
Nose pressure
Stimulant inhalation
Tongue traction
Drinking from far side of glass
Swallowing sugar
Eating soft bread
Soft touch to palate with cotton-tipped applicator
Lemon wedge with bitters
Miscellaneous Vagal Stimulation
Ocular compression
Digital rectal massage
Carotid massage
Psychiatric Treatments
Behavioral techniques
Distraction
Gastric Distention Relief
Fasting
Nasogastric tube to relieve abdominal distention
Lavage
Induction of vomiting
Phrenic Nerve Disruption
Anesthetic block
Miscellaneous Treatments
Bilateral radial artery compression
Peppermint water to relax lower esophagus
Acupuncture

Sources: Lewis (1985), reference 69; Launois (1993), reference 79; Rousseau (2003), reference 73; Williams (2001), reference 72; Smith (2003), reference 71; and Kolodzik & Eilers (1991), reference 75.

Nonpharmacological Treatment

Nonpharmacological treatments can be divided into seven categories and are outlined in Table 10–9. First are simple respiratory maneuvers. These include breath holding, rebreathing in a bag, compression of the diaphragm, ice application in the mouth, and induction of sneeze or cough.[69,71–73] Second is nasal and pharyngeal stimulation. These techniques use pressure on the nose, inhalation of a stimulant, traction of the tongue, drinking from the far side of a glass, swallowing sugar, eating a lemon wedge with bitters, eating soft bread, or soft touch to the palate with a cotton-tipped applicator.[72,73,75] Third is miscellaneous vagal stimulation, which includes ocular compression, digital rectal massage, and carotid massage.

Fourth are psychiatric treatments, which focus on behavioral therapy. Fifth is gastric distention relief, which encompasses fasting, use of a nasogastric tube to decrease distention, lavage, and induction of vomiting.[69,72] Sixth is phrenic nerve disruption, such as an anesthetic injection or acupuncture.[69,80] Seventh are miscellaneous benign remedies, such as bilateral compression of radial arteries, peppermint water to relax the lower esophagus, use of distraction, or acupuncture.[67,69,71–73]

Table 10–10
Pharmacological Treatment Suggestions for Hiccups

Agents to Decrease Gastric Distention
Simethicone 15–30, mL PO q4h
Metoclopramide 10–20 mg PO/IV q4–6h (do not use with peppermint water)
Muscle Relaxants
Baclofen 5–10 mg PO q6-12 h up to 15–25 mg/d
Midazalom 5–10 mg
Anticonvulsants
Gabapentin 300–600 mg PO tid,
Carbamazepine 200 mg PO, QD—TID, titrate up as needed
Valproic acid 5–15 mg/kg/d PO, then increase by 250 mg/WK until hiccups stop
Corticosteroids
Dexamethazone 40 mg PO QD
Dopamine Agonists
Haloperidol 1–5 mg PO/SQ every 12h
Chlorpromazine 5–50 mg PO/IM/IV q6–8h
Calcium Channel Blockers/Antiarrythmics
Phenytoin 200 mg IV, 300 mg PO QD
Nefopam 10 mg IV QD-QID
Lidocaine bolus 1 mg/kg/h IV, then 2 mg/min until hiccups terminated
Quinidine 200 mg PO
Nifedipine 10–80 mg PO q d
Other Medications
Mephenesin 1000 mg PO q d
Amitriptyline 25–90 mg PO q d
Methyphenidate 5–20 mg IV, 5–20 mg QD
Sertaline 50 mg PO QD

Sources: Lierz & Felleiter (2002), reference 88; Rousseau (2003), reference 73; Marachal et al. (2003), reference 87; Regnaud (2004), reference 76; Petroinau et al. (2000), reference 83; Bilotta & Rosa (2000), reference 84; Viadya (2000), reference 85; Cersosimo & Brophy (1998), reference 86; and Williams (2001), reference 72.

Pharmacological Treatment

Initial therapy should attempt to decrease gastric distention, which is usually the problem in 95% of cases, hasten gastric emptying, and relax the diaphragm. This includes the use of simethicone and metoclopramide.[69,70,72,73] If ineffective, second-line therapy should focus on suppression of the hiccup reflex. Common pharmacological interventions, listed in Table 10–10, include the use of various classes of medications: muscle relaxants such as baclofen, midazolam, and chlordiazepoxide; anticonvulsants such as gabapentin, carbamazepine, and valproate[82,83]; corticosteroids such as dexamethasone and prednisone; dopamine antagonists such as haloperidol, droperidol, and chlorpromazine; calcium channel blockers/antiarrhythmics such as nifedipine, nimodipine, nefopam, phenytoin, lidocaine, quinidine[78,84]; SSRI antidepressants, specifically sertraline; and various other medications such as ketamine, THC, and methylphenidate.[76,85–87] Third-line therapy is the use of other drugs to disrupt diaphragmatic irritation or other possible causes of hiccups, which may include anesthesia and phrenic and cervical blocks.[78,88,89]

Nursing Interventions

Although hiccups appear to be a simple reflex, their specific mechanism of action is unclear due to myriad etiologies. Nurses are helpful in providing patients and families with a review of the nature of hiccups and their role as an annoyance rather than a pathological symptom. Thus, nursing interventions should focus on information sharing and comfort, with a goal of terminating the hiccups. The extent of aggressive treatment will depend on the degree of distress the hiccups cause on the patient's quality of life. In particular, what effect do the hiccups have on the daily routine, most particularly on sleep and on nutrition? Many patients have felt frustrated that little credence was given to their discomfort and disruption caused for intractable hiccups. Thus, the nursing role is one of advocate to promote initiation of some sort of therapy, empathetic listener, and educator. Nurses can provide patients with information on some nonpharmacological maneuvers such as respiratory maneuvers, nasal and pharyngeal stimulation, distraction, and peppermint waters. If unsuccessful, the nurse should provide education on the various classes of medications as prescribed as options. An example includes antacids to decrease gas, antiemetics to affect dopamine levels, and muscle relaxants to affect both gamma-aminobutyric acid channels and skeletal muscle.[71,73,76] Offering support to the patient is necessary since patients respond to different medications. If one class or type of medication fails, the nurse should suggest that another class of medication be tried, until all possible medications have been used. If all of these medications fail to induce hiccup reduction or cessation, the nurse should suggest a referral to a palliative care service, a pain service, or an anesthesia service to further explore treatment therapies. These services can review all attempts at treating hiccups and provide consideration for a nerve block or other types of infusions. However, as always, discussion with the patient should include their prognosis and the benefit and burden of any procedure. The nurse can help discuss with the patient their concerns about treatment and their desire for comfort. If hiccups become extremely burdensome and all therapies have failed, sedation may be a consideration. Again, the nurse may act as an advocate to provide the necessary information about the implications of sedation. For further discussion of palliative sedation, the reader is referred to Chapter 24.

SUMMARY

Dysphagia, xerostomia, and hiccups are common problems that often receive little attention. Since many health care providers consider them trivial, these symptoms are seemingly underreported and underestimated.[55] However, nurses at the bedside, whether in a facility or at home, may be the first to realize and witness the extent to which these symptoms cause discomfort and affect a patient's life. The mere act of a nurse listening to a patient's distress is an acknowledgment of his or her concerns. The patient feels she or he is taken seriously, as a unique individual. Moreover, the simple act of initiating treatment to manage these symptoms may promote psychological healing in itself because the patient feels respected about his or her concerns and experiences treatment as life-affirming.

The patient's preferences and desires form the basis of any interventions. These guide both the pharmacological and/or nonpharmacological treatment within the context of his or her definition of optimal management and goals. Having established that the patient and family is the unit of care, the family should be brought into discussions concerning decision-making. The nurse can elicit their concerns, promoting understanding and relief of anxiety and fears. Additionally, when death is imminent and aggressive treatment may not be warranted, specific discussion with the patient and family should focus on the individual circumstances that suggest comfort measures.

In summary, dysphagia, xerostomia, and hiccups are distressing symptoms that may affect nutrition, cause discomfort, and affect a person's sense of well-being. If left untreated, patients may experience physical suffering, lose a sense of dignity, and perhaps become isolated in their distress. Because patients talk differently to physicians and nurses, nurses may be the first to identify these symptoms, as well as evaluate the impact they have on a patient's daily routine. Therefore, nurses play a pivotal role in addressing these symptoms and initiating holistic management, providing relief, enhancing a patient's self-opinion, improving functional status, and promoting quality of life.

REFERENCES

1. Von Gunton C, Twaddle M. Terminal care in non-cancer patients. Clin Geriatr Med 1996;12:349–358.
2. Logemann JA. Evaluation and Treatment of Swallowing Disorders, 2nd ed, pp 135–189; 191–250. Austin, TX: Pro-Ed, 1998.
3. Shaker R, Hogan WJ. Normal physiology of the aerodigestive tract and its effect on the upper gut. Am J Med 2003;18(suppl 3A):2S–9S
4. Selley WG, Ellis RE, Flack FC, Bayliss CR, Pearce R. The synchronization of respiration and swallow sounds with videofluoroscopy during swallowing. Dysphagia 1994;9:162–167.
5. Miller AJ. The Neuroscientific Principles of Swallowing and Dysphagia, pp 36–48. San Diego: Singular Publishing, 1999.
6. Schindler JS, Kelly JH. Swallowing disorders in the elderly. Laryngoscope. 2002 Apr;112(4):589–602.
7. Dantas RO, Kern MK, Massey BT, et al. Effect of swallowed bolus variables on the oral and pharyngeal phases of swallowing. Am J Physiol 1990;258:G675–G681.
8. McConnel FM, Cerenko D, Mendelsohn MS. Manofluorographic analysis of swallowing. Otolaryngol Clin North Am 1988; 21:625–635.
9. Miller A, Bieger D, Conklin JL. Functional controls of deglutition. In: Perlman AL, Schulze-Delrieu K, eds. Deglutition and Its Disorders: Anatomy, Physiology, Clinical Diagnosis and Management. San Diego: Singular Publishing, 1997:43–98.
10. Cook IJ, Dodds WJ, Dantas RO, et al. Opening mechanism of the human upper esophageal sphincter. Am J Physiol 1989;257: G748–759.
11. Surawicz TS, McCarthy BJ, Kupelian V, et al. Descriptive epidemiology of primary brain and CNS tumors: results from the Central Brain Tumor Registry of the United States. Neuro-oncol 1999;1:14–25.
12. Newton HB, Newton C, Pearl D. Swallowing assessment in primary brain tumor patients with dysphagia. Neurology 1994;44:1927–1933.
13. Vokes EE, Kies MS, Haraf DJ et al. Concomitant chemoradiotherapy as primary therapy for locoregionally advanced head and neck cancer. J Clin Oncol 200;18:1652–1661.
14. Forastiere A, Goepfert H, Maor M, et al. Concurrent chemotherapy and radiotherapy for organ preservation in advanced laryngeal caner. N Engl J Med 2003;349:2091–2098.
15. Mittal BB, Pauloski BR, Haraf DJ, et al. Swallowing dysfunction—preventative and rehabilitation strategies in patient with head-and-neck cancers treated with surgery, radiotherapy and chemotherapy: a critical review. Int J Radiation Oncology Biol Phys 2003;57:1219–1230.
16. Murray JA, Rao SS, Schulze-Delrieu K. Esophageal diseases. In: Perlman AL, Schulze-Delrieu K, eds. Deglutition and Its Disorders: Anatomy, Physiology, Clinical Diagnosis and Management. San Diego: Singular Publishing, 1997:383–418.
17. Adler DG, Baron TH. Endoscopic palliation of esophageal malignancies. Mayo Clin Proc 2001;76:731–738.
18. Anand BS, Saeed ZA, Michaletz PA, et al. A randomized comparison of dilatation alone versus dilatation plus laser in patients receiving chemotherapy and external beam radiation for esophageal carcinoma. Dig Dis Sci 1998;43:2255–2260.
19. Cwikiel W, Tranberg KG, Cwiekel M, et al. Malignant dysphagia: palliation with esophageal stents—long term results with 100 Patients. Radiology 1998;207:513–518.

20. Adam A, Ellul J, Watkinson AF, et al. Palliation of inoperable esophageal carcinoma: a prospective randomized controlled trial of laser therapy and stent placement. Radiology 1997; 202:344–348.
21. Kozarek RA. Endoscopic palliation of esophageal malignancy. Endoscopy 2003;35:S9-S13.
22. Buchholz DW, Robbins JA. Neurologic diseases affecting oropharyngeal swallowing. In: Perlman AL, Schulze-Delrieu K, eds. Deglutition and Its Disorders: Anatomy, Physiology, Clinical Diagnosis and Management. San Diego: Singular Publishing, 1997:319–342.
23. Yorkston KM, Miller RM, Strand EA, Levesque RJ. Management of Speech and Swallowing in Degenerative Diseases, 2nd ed, pp 130–148; 200–206. Austin, TX: Pro-Ed, 2004.
24. Borasio GD, Voltz R, Miller RG. Palliative care in amyotrophic lateral sclerosis. Neurologic Clinics 2001;19:829–847.
25. Coyle JL, Rosenbek JC, Chignell KA. Pathophysiology of neurogenic oropharyngeal dysphagia. In: Carrau RL, Murry T, eds. Comprehensive Management of Swallowing Disorders. San Diego: Singular Publishing, 1999:93–108.
26. Clarke CE, Gullaksen E, Macdonald S, et al. Referral criterion for speech and language therapy assessment of dysphagia caused by idiopathic Parkinson's disease. Acta Neurologica Scandanavica 1998;97:27–35.
27. Deane KH, Whurr R, Clarke CE, et al. Non-pharmacological therapies for dysphagia in Parkinson's disease. The Cochrane Library 2004:1.
28. Dray TD, Hillel AD, Miller RM. Dysphagia caused by neurologic deficits. Otolaryngol Clin North Am 1998;31:507–524.
29. Hartelius L, Svensson P. Speech and swallowing symptoms associated with Parkinson's disease and multiple sclerosis. Folia Phoniatr Logop 1994;46:9–17.
30. Halvorsen RA Jr, Moelleken SM, Kearney AT. Videofluoroscopic evaluation of HIV/AIDS patients with swallowing dysfunction. Abdom Imaging. 2003 Mar-Apr;28(2):244–247.
31. Soliman AMS, Buchinsky FJ. Autoimmune disorders. In: Carrau RL, Murry T, eds. Comprehensive Management of Swallowing Disorders. San Diego: Singular Publishing, 1999:199–209.
32. Schechter GL. Systemic causes of dysphagia in adults. Otolaryngol Clin North Am 1998;31:525–535
33. Alvi A. Iatrogenic swallowing disorders: medications. In: Carrau RL, Murry T, eds. Comprehensive Management of Swallowing Disorders. San Diego: Singular Publishing, 1999:119–124.
34. Sokoloff LG, Pavlakovic R. Neuroleptic induced dysphagia. Dysphagia 1997;12:177–179.
35. Cooke IJ, Kahrilas PJ. AGA Technical Review on Management of Oropharyngeal Dysphagia. Gastroenterology 1999;116:455–478.
36. Leder SB. Gag reflex and dysphagia. Head Neck Surg 1996; 18:138–141.
37. Leder SB. Videofluoroscopic evaluation of aspiration with visual examination of the gag reflex and velar movement. Dysphagia 1997;12:21–23.
38. Rasley A, Logemann JA, Kahrilas PJ, Rademaker AW, Pauloski BR, Dodds WJ. Prevention of barium aspiration during videofluoroscopic swallowing studies: value of change of posture. Am J Roentgenol 1992;160:1005–1009.
39. Langmore SE. Normal swallowing: the endoscopic perspective. In: Endoscopic Evaluation and Treatment of Swallowing Disorders. NY: Thieme, 2001:37.
40. Ertekin C, Keskin A, Kiylioglu N, et al. The effect of head and neck positions on oropharyngeal swallowing: a clinical and electrophysiologic study. Arch Phys Med Rehabil 2001;82:1255–60.
41. Sullivan DJ, Moran GP, Pinjon E, et al. Comparison of the epidemiology, drug resistance mechanisms, and virulence of *Candida dubliniensis* and *Candida albicans*. FEMS Yeast Res 2004;4:369–76.
42. Maton PN. Profile and assessment of GERD pharmacotherapy. Cleve Clin J Med 2003;70(suppl 5):S51–70.
43. Lewis MM, Kidder JA. Nutrition Practice Guidelines for Dysphagia. Chicago: American Dietetic Association, 1996.
44. Mitchell SL, Buchanan JL, Littlehale S, Hamel MB. Tube-feeding versus hand-feeding nursing home residents with advanced dementia: a cost comparison. J Am Med Dir Assoc 2004;5(2 suppl):S22–9.
45. Langmore SE, Terpenning MS, Schork A, et al. Predictors of aspiration pneumonia: how important is dysphagia? Dysphagia 1998;12:69–81.
46. Gillick MR. Artificial nutrition and hydration therapy in advanced dementia. Lancet Neurol 2003;2:76.
47. Leonard R, Kendall K, McKenzie S, Goodrich S. The treatment plan. In: Leonard R, Kendall K, eds. Dysphagia Assessment and Treatment Planning; A Team Approach. San Diego: Singular Publishing, 1999:181.
48. Speilman A, Ben Aryad H, Gutman D, Szargel R, Duetsch E. Xerostomia—diagnosis and treatment. Oral Med 1981;51:144–147.
49. Sreebny L, Valdini A. Xerostomia. Arch Intern Med 1987;147: 1333–1337.
50. Ship JA, Pillemer, SR, Baum BJ. Xerostomia and the geriatric patient. Geriatrics Society 2002; 50:535–543.
51. Jensen SB, Pedersen AM, Reibel, Nauntofte B. Xerostomia and hypofunction of the salivary glands in cancer therapy. Supportive Cancer Care 2003;11:207–225.
52. Ng K, von Gunton, CF. Symptoms and attitudes of 100 consecutive patients admitted to an acute hospice/palliative care unit. J Pain Symptom Manage 1998;16:307–316.
53. Mercandante S, Calderone L, Villari P, Serretta R, Sapio M, Casuccio A, Fulfaro F. The use of pilocarpine in opioid-induced xerostomia. Palliat Med 2000;14:529–531.
54. Davies A. The management of xerostomia: a review. Eur J Cancer Care 1997;6:209–214.
55. Cooke C, Admedzel S, Mayberry J. Xerostomia—a review. Palliat Med 1996;10:284–292.
56. Amerongen AV, Veerman EC. Current therapies for xerostomia and salivary gland hypofunction associated with cancer therapies. Support Care Cancer 2003; 11:226–231.
57. Bruce S. Radiation-induced xerostomia: how dry is your patient. Clin J Oncol Nurs 2004;8:61–67.
58. Porter S, Scully C, Hegarty A. An update of the etiology and management of xerostomia. Oral Surg Oral Med Oral Pathol Oral Radiol Endod 2004;97:28–46.
59. Guchelaar H, Vermes A, Meerwaldt J. Radiation induced xerostomia: pathophysiology, clinical course, and supportive treatment. Support Care Cancer 1997;5:281–288.
60. Oncology Nursing Society. Radiation Therapy Patient Care Record. Pittsburgh: Oncology Nursing Society Press, 2002.
61. National Cancer Institute. Common terminology criteria for adverse events v3.0. Published December 12, 2003. http://www.ctep.cancer.gov/forms/CTCAEv3.pdf (accessed April 4, 2004).
62. Guggenheimer J, Moore P. Xerostomia: etiology, recognition and treatment. J Am Dental Asso 2003;134:61–69.
63. Blom M, Dawidson I, Angmar-Mansson B. The effect of acupuncture on buccal blood flow assessed by laser doppler flowmetry: a pilot study. Caries Res 1992;24:428.

64. Johnstone, P, Niemtzow R, Riffenburgh RH. Acupuncture for xerostomia. Cancer 2002;94:1151–1156.
65. Olasz L, Nyarady Z, Szentirmy M. Assessment of relieving symptoms of xerostomia with oral pilocarpine during irradiation in head-and-neck cancer patients. Cancer Detect Prev 2000;24 (suppl 1):489.
66. Chatelut E, Rispail Y, Berlan M, Montastruc J. Yohimbine increases human salivary secretion. Br J Clin Pharmacol 1989; 28:366–368.
67. Waller A, Caroline N. Handbook of Palliative Care in Cancer, 2nd ed, pp 136–137; 161–168. Boston: Butterworth-Heinemann, 2000.
68. Sweeney M, Bagg J, Baxter W, Aitchison T. Clinical trial of mucin-containing oral spray for treatment of xerostomia in hospice patients. Palliat Med 1997;11:225–232.
69. Lewis J. Hiccups: causes and cures. J Clin Gastroenterol 1985;7: 539–552.
70. Wilcock A, Twycross R. Midazolam for intractable hiccup. J Pain Symptom Manage 1996;12:59–61.
71. Smith H, Busracamwongs A. Management of hiccups in the palliative care population. Am J Palliat Care 2003;20:149–154.
72. Williams C. The unremitting hiccup. AAHPM Bulletin 2001; summer:6–7.
73. Rousseau P. Hiccups in patients with advanced cancer: a brief review. Prog Palliat Care 2003;11:10–12.
74. Pollack M. Intractable hiccups: a serious sign of underlying systemic disease. J Clin Gastroenterol 2003;37:272–273.
75. Kolodzik P, Eilers M. Hiccups (singulatus): review and approach to management. Ann Emerg Med 1991;20:565–573.
76. Regnaud C. Dysphagia, dyspepsia, and hiccup. In: Doyle D, Hanks G, Cherny N, Calman K, eds. Oxford Textbook of Palliative Medicine, 3rd ed, pp 468–482. Oxford University Press, 2004.
77. Pertel P, Till M. Intractable hiccups induced by the use of megestrol acetate. Arch Intern Med 1998;158:809–810.
78. Calvo E, Fernandez-Torre F, Brugarolas J. Cervical phrenic nerve block. J Nat Cancer Inst 2002; 94:1175–1176.
79. Launois S, Bizec J, Whitelaw W, Cabane J, Derenne J. Hiccups in adults: an overview. Eur Respir J 1993;6:563–575.
80. Schiff E, River Y, Oliven A, Odeh M. Acupuncture therapy for persistent hiccups. Am J Med Sciences 2002;323:166–168.
81. Cymet TC. Retrospective analysis of hiccups in patients in a community hospital from 1995–2000. J Nat Med Assoc 2002;94: 480–483.
82. Moretti R, Torre P, Antonello R, Ukmar M, Cazzato G, Bava A. Gabapention as a drug therapy of intractable hiccups because of vascular lesion: a three-year follow up. The Neurologist 2004;10: 102–106.
83. Petroianu P, Hein G, Stegmeier-Petroianu A, Bergler W, Rufer R. Gabapentin "Add-on Therapy" for idiopathic chronic hiccup (ICH). J Clin Gastroenterol 2000:30:321–324.
84. Bilotta F, Rosa G. Nefopam for severe hiccups. NEJM 2000;343: 1973–1974.
85. Vaidya V. Sertraline in the treatment of hiccups. Psychosomatics 2000;41:353–355.
86. Cersosimo R, Brophy M. Hiccoughs with high dose dexametasone administration. Cancer 1998;82:412–414.
87. Marechal R, Berghmans T, Sculier JP. Succcessful treatment of intractable hiccup with methylphenidate in a lung cancer patient. Support Care Cancer 2003;11:126–128.
88. Lierz P, Felleiter P. Anesthesia as therapy for persistent hiccups. Anesth Analg 2002;95:494–495.
89. Cohen SP, Lubin E, Stojanovic M. Intravenous lidocaine in the treatment of hiccups. South Med J 2001;94:1124–25.

11

Denice Caraccia Economou

Bowel Management: Constipation, Diarrhea, Obstruction, and Ascites

I feel like I am going to pop! This constipation is worse than the pain.—B. H., 58-year-old with pancreatic cancer

- ***Key Points***
- *Multiple factors contribute to constipation. Proactive management is essential for successful outcomes.*
- *Treating diarrhea requires a thorough assessment and therapy directed at the specific cause.*
- *Palliative care should allow for a thoughtful and realistic approach to management of symptoms within the goals of care.*

CONSTIPATION

Constipation affects 2% to 10% of the general population, but the incidence may be as high as 20% to 50% in older or ill persons.[1–3] Constipation is a major problem in cancer patients, with as many as 70% to 100% of cancer patients having this distressing symptom.[2,4] The use of opioids for pain is a contributory factor to constipation, and this side effect is the principal reason for their discontinuation.[1–3,5] Constipation is common and yet undertreated by both physicians and nurses.[2]

Definitions

Constipation is subjective to many patients, making assessment much more difficult. Constipation is defined as "a decrease in the frequency of passage of formed stools and characterized by stools that are hard and small and difficult to expel." Understanding the normal functioning of the bowel can provide insight into the contributing factors leading to constipation, diarrhea, and obstruction. Associated symptoms of constipation vary but may include excessive straining, a feeling of fullness or pressure in the rectum, the sensation of incomplete emptying, abdominal distention, and cramps.[7] The subjective experience of constipation may vary for different individuals, underscoring the importance of individualized patient assessment and management.

Prevalence and Impact

Prevalence among cancer patients is common.[1,2] The impact of constipation on quality of life is substantial. Constipation causes social, psychological, and physical distress for patients, which additionally impacts the caregiver and health care staff. Failure to anticipate and manage constipation in a proactive way significantly affects the difficulty a patient will experience in attempting to relieve this problem.

Pathophysiology

Normal bowel function includes three areas of control: small intestinal motility, colon motility, and defecation. Small-intestinal activity is primarily the mixing of contents by bursts of propagated motor activity that are associated with increased gastric, pancreatic, and biliary secretion. This motor activity occurs every 90 to 120 minutes but is altered when food is ingested. Contents are mixed to allow for digestion and absorption of nutrients. When the stomach has emptied, the small intestine returns to regular propagated motor activity.[1]

The colon propels contents forward through peristaltic movements. The colon movement is much slower than that of the small intestine. Contents may remain in the colon for up to 2 to 3 days, whereas small-intestinal transit is 1 to 2 hours. Motor activity in the large intestine occurs approximately six times per day, usually grouped in two peak bursts. The first is triggered by awakening and breakfast, and a smaller burst is triggered by the afternoon meal. Contractions are stimulated by ingestion of food, psychogenic factors, and somatic activity. Sykes[8] found that 50% of the constipated patients in a hospice setting had a transit time between 4 and 12 days.

The physiology of defecation involves coordinated interaction between the involuntary internal anal sphincter and the voluntary external anal sphincter. The residual intestinal contents distend the rectum and initiate expulsion. The longitudinal muscle of the rectum contracts, and with the voluntary external anal sphincter relaxed, defecation can occur. Additional coordinated muscle activity also occurs and includes contraction of the diaphragm against a closed glottis, tensing of the abdominal wall, and relaxation of the pelvic floor.

The enteric nervous system plays an important role in the movement of bowel contents through the gastrointestinal (GI) tract as well. Smooth muscles in the GI tract have spontaneous electrical, rhythmic activity, resembling pacemakers in the stomach and small intestine, that communicate with the remainder of the bowel. There are both submucosal and myenteric plexuses of nerves. These nerves are connected to the central nervous system through sympathetic ganglia, splanchnic nerves, and parasympathetic fibers in the vagus nerve and the presacral plexus. Opioid medications affect the myenteric plexus, which coordinates peristalsis. Therefore, peristalsis is decreased and stool transit time is decreased, leading to harder, dryer, and less frequent stools, or constipation.[1,9]

Important factors that promote normal functioning of the bowel include the following:

1. *Fluid intake.* Nine liters of fluid (which includes 7 liters secreted from the salivary glands, stomach, pancreas, small bowel, and biliary system, and the average oral intake of 2 liters) are reduced to 1.5 liters by the time they reach the colon. At this point, water and electrolytes continue to be absorbed, and the end volume for waste is 150 mL. Therefore, decreased fluid intake can make a significant difference in the development of constipation.
2. *Adequate dietary fiber.* The presence of food in the stomach initiates the muscle contractions and secretions from the biliary, gastric, and pancreatic systems that lead to movement of the bowels. The amount of dietary fiber consumed is related to stool size and consistency.[10]
3. *Physical activity.* Colonic propulsion is related to intraluminal pressures in the colon. Lack of physical activity and reduced intraluminal pressures can significantly reduce propulsive activity.[11]
4. *Adequate time or privacy to defecate.* Changes in normal bowel routines, such as morning coffee or reading the paper, can decrease peristalsis and lead to constipation. Emotional disturbances are also known to affect gut motility.[10]

Primary, Secondary, and Iatrogenic Constipation

Cimprich[10] offered three classifications of constipation:

1. Primary constipation is caused by reduced fluid and fiber intake, decreased activity, and lack of privacy.
2. Secondary constipation is related to pathological changes. These changes may include tumor, partial intestinal obstruction, metabolic effects of hypercalcemia, hypothyroidism, hypokalemia, as well as spinal cord compression at the level of the cauda equina or sacral plexus.
3. Iatrogenically induced constipation is related to pharmacological interventions. Opioids are the primary medications associated with constipation. In addition, Vinca rosea alkaloid chemotherapies (vincristine), anticholinergic medications (belladonna, antihistamines), tricyclic antidepressants (nortriptyline, amitriptyline), neuroleptics (haloperidol and chlorpromazine), antispasmodics, anticonvulsants (phenytoin and gabapentin), muscle relaxants, aluminum antacids, iron, diuretics (furosemide), and antiparkinsonian agents cause constipation.[1,3,9]

Constipation Related to Cancer and Its Treatment

Multiple factors associated with cancer and its treatment cause constipation. When it primarily involves the GI system or is anatomically associated with the bowel, cancer itself causes constipation. Pelvic cancers, including, ovarian, cervical, and uterine cancers, are highly associated with constipation and mechanical obstruction.[10] Malignant ascites, spinal cord compression, and paraneoplastic autonomic neuropathy also cause constipation. Cancer-related causes include surgical interruption of the GI tract, decreased activity, reduced intake of both fluids and food, changes in personal routines associated with bowel movements, bed rest, confusion, and depression.[1–3,8,10,14]

Opioid-Related Constipation

Opioids affect bowel function primarily by inhibiting propulsive peristalsis through the small bowel and colon.[1,2] McMillan and Williams[12] found that 100% of the patients in their study who had received at least 30 mg of morphine in the previous 24 hours developed constipation. Opioids bind with the receptors on the smooth muscles of the bowel, affecting the contraction of the circular and longitudinal muscle fibers that cause peristalsis or the movement of contents through the bowel.[2,14] Colonic transit time is lengthened, contributing to increased fluid and electrolyte absorption and dryer, harder stools.[1–3] Peristaltic changes occur 5 to 25 minutes after administration of the opioid and are dose related. Patients do not develop tolerance to the constipation side effects even with long-term use of opioids.[5] There is new evidence, particularly associated with transdermal fentanyl use, that constipation severity may differ among opioids.[13] The use of laxatives and stool softeners with opioids represents a rational, proactive approach to opioid-induced constipation.

Assessment of Constipation

History

The measurement of constipation requires more than assessing the frequency of stools alone. Managing constipation requires a thorough history and physical examination.

The use of a quantifying tool can be helpful in understanding what the patient is experiencing and how different that may be from the usual or baseline bowel habit. A tool developed in 1989, the Constipation Assessment Scale (CAS), has been tested for validity and reliability and found to have a significant ability to measure constipation as well as its severity between moderate and severe constipation. It is a simple questionnaire that requires 2 minutes to complete (Figure 11–1). The CAS includes eight symptoms associated with constipation: (1) abdominal distention or bloating, (2) change in amount of gas passed rectally, (3) less frequent bowel movements, (4) oozing liquid stool, (5) rectal fullness or pressure, (6) rectal pain with bowel movement, (7) small volume of stool, and (8) inability to pass stool.[12] These symptoms are rated as 0, not experienced; 1, some problem; or 2, severe problem. A score between 0 and 16 is calculated and can be used as an objective measurement of subjective symptoms for ongoing management.

The CAS gives a good sense of bowel function.[12] Sykes[15] also outlines similar questions to use in taking a constipation history. It is important to start by asking patients when they moved their bowels last and to follow up by asking what their normal movement pattern is. Remember, what is considered constipated for one person is not for someone else. What are the characteristics of their stools and did they note any blood or mucus? Were their bowels physically difficult to move? This is especially important if they have cancer in or near the intestines or rectal area that may contribute to physical obstruction. Ovarian cancer patients usually complain of feeling severely bloated. They may say things like "If you stick a pin in me, I know I will pop!" Evaluating the abdomen or asking patients if they feel bloated or pressure in the abdomen is important. Does the patient feel pain when moving the bowels? Is the patient oozing liquid stool? Does the patient feel that the volume of stool passed is small? Many patients may experience unexplainable nausea.[1–3]

Medication- or Disease-Related History

The patient's medical status and anticipated disease process are important in providing insight into areas where early intervention could prevent severe constipation or even obstruction. Constipation may be anticipated with primary and secondary bowel cancer, as well as with pelvic tumors, peritoneal mesothelioma or spinal cord compression, previous bowel surgery, or a history of Vinca alkaloid chemotherapy. Changes in dietary habits related to the above medications or the addition of new medications may contribute to constipation.[1] Anticholinergic medications, antihistamines, tricyclic antidepressants, aluminum antacids, and diuretics can cause constipation. Hypercalcemia and hypokalemia contribute to constipation by slowing down motility. Ask patients if there are things they do to aid in defecation. Sometimes physical actions the patient may use can help causes related to rectocele, or rectal ulcer.[15] Table 11–1 outlines causes of constipation in cancer and other palliative care patients.

Physical Examination

Begin the physical examination in the mouth, to ensure that the patient is able to chew foods and that there are no lesions or tumors in the mouth that could interfere with eating. Does the patient wear dentures? Patients who wear dentures and have lost a great deal of weight may have dentures that do not fit properly, which would make eating and drinking difficult. Patients may choose to eat only what they are able to chew as a result of their dentures or other dental problems. Therefore, they may not be eating enough fiber and, thus, contributing to primary constipation.

Abdominal Examination. Inspect the abdomen initially for bloating, distention, or bulges. Distention may be associated with obesity, fluid, tumor, or gas. Remember, the patient should have emptied the bladder. Auscultation is important to evaluate the presence or absence of bowel sounds. If no bowel sounds are heard initially, listen continuously for a minimum of 5 minutes. The absence of bowel sounds may indicate a paralytic ileus. If the bowel sounds are hyperactive, it could indicate diarrhea. Percussion of the bowel may result in tympany, which is related to gas in the bowel. A dull sound is heard over intestinal fluid and feces. Palpation of the abdomen should

Directions: Circle the appropriate number to indicate whether, during the past three days, you have had NO PROBLEM, SOME PROBLEM or a SEVERE PROBLEM with each of the items listed.

Item	No Problem	Some Problem	Severe Problem
1. Abdominal distension or bloating	0	1	2
2. Change in amount of gas passed rectally	0	1	2
3. Less frequent bowel movements	0	1	2
4. Oozing liquid stool	0	1	2
5. Rectal fullness or pressure	0	1	2
6. Rectal pain with bowel movement	0	1	2
7. Smaller stool size	0	1	2
8. Urge but inability to pass stool	0	1	2

Patient's Name Date

Figure 11–1. Constipation Assessment Scale. *Source:* McMillan et al. (1989), reference 12. Reproduced with permission.

start lightly; look for muscular resistance and abdominal tenderness. This is usually associated with chronic constipation. If rebound tenderness is detected with coughing or light palpation, peritoneal inflammation should be considered. Deep palpation may reveal a "sausage-like" mass of stool in the left colon. Feeling stool in the colon indicates constipation.[2] Although Sykes[15] points out that the distinction between tumor and stool is hard to make, recognizing the underlying anatomy is helpful in distinguishing the stool along the line of the descending colon or more proximal colon, including the cecum. A digital examination of the rectum may reveal stool or possible tumor or rectocele. If the patient is experiencing incontinence of liquid stool, obstruction must be considered. Examining for hemorrhoids, ulcerations, or rectal fissures is important, especially in the neutropenic patient. Patients with a neutropenia can complain of rectal pain well before a rectal infection is obvious. Evaluating the patient for infection, ulceration, or rectal fissures is very important. Additionally, determine whether the patient has had previous intestinal surgery, alternating diarrhea and constipation, complaints of abdominal colic pain or nausea, and vomiting. Examining the stool for shape and consistency can also be useful. Stools that are hard and pellet-like suggest slow transit time, whereas stools that are ribbon-like suggest hemorrhoids. Blood or mucus in the stool suggests tumor, hemorrhoids, or possibly a preexisting colitis.[15] Elderly patients may experience urinary incontinence related to fecal impaction.[1,2,14] Abdominal pain may also be related to constipation. Patients will complain of colic pain related to the effort of colonic muscle to move hard stool. The history may be complicated by known abdominal tumors. Patients in pain should still be treated with opioids as needed.

Table 11–1
Causes of Constipation in Cancer/Palliative Care Patients

Cancer-Related

Directly related to tumor site. Primary bowel cancers, secondary bowel cancers, pelvic cancers.

Hypercalcemia. Surgical interruption of bowel integrity.

Etiology

Intestinal obstruction related to tumor in the bowel wall or external compression by tumor. Damage to the lumbosacral spinal cord, cauda equina, or pelvic plexus. High spinal cord transection mainly stops the motility response to food. Low spinal cord or pelvic outflow lesions produce dilation of the colon and slow transit in the descending and distal transverse colon. Surgery in the abdomen can lead to adhesion development or direct changes in the bowel.

Hypercalcemia

Cholinergic control of secretions of the intestinal epithelium is mediated by changes in intracellular calcium concentrations. Hypercalcemia causes decreased absorption, leading to constipation, whereas hypercalcemia can lead to diarrhea.

Secondary Effects Related to the Disease

Decreased appetite, decreased fluid intake, low-fiber diet, weakness, inactivity, confusion, depression, change in normal toileting habits

Etiology

Decreased fluid and food intake leading to dehydration and weakness. Decreased intake, ineffective voluntary elimination actions, as well as decreased normal defecation reflexes. Decreased peristalsis; increased colonic transit time leads to increased absorption of fluid and electrolytes and small, hard, dry stools. Inactivity, weakness, changes in normal toileting habits, daily bowel function reflexes, and positioning affect ability to use abdominal wall musculature and relax pelvic floor for proper elimination. Psychological depression can increase constipation by slowing down motility.

Concurrent Disease

Diabetes, hypothyroidism, hypokalemia, diverticular disease, hemorrhoids, colitis, chronic neurological diseases

Etiology

Electrolytes and therefore water are transported via neuronal control. Like hypercalcemia, abnormal potassium can affect water absorption and contribute to constipation. Chronic neurological diseases affect the neurological stimulation of intestinal motility.

Medication-Related

Opioid medications

Anticholinergic effects (hydroscine, phenothiazines)

Tricyclic antidepressants

Antiparkinsonian drugs

Iron

Antihypertensives, antihistamines

Antacids

Diuretics

Vinka alkaloid chemotherapy

Etiology

Opioids in particular suppress forward peristalsis and increase sphincter tone. Opioids increase electrolyte and water absorption in both the large and small intestine; this leads to dehydration and hard, dry stools. Morphine causes insensitivity of the rectum to distention, decreasing the sensation of the need to defecate. Vinca alkaloid chemotherapy has a neurotoxic effect that causes damage to the myenteric plexus of the colon. This increases nonpropulsive contractions. Colonic transit time is increased, leading to constipation. Antidepressants slow large bowel motility. Antacids (bismuth, aluminum salts) cause hard stools.

Sources: Levy (1991), reference 1; Sykes (1996), reference 9.

Management of Constipation

Preventing constipation whenever possible is the most important management strategy. Constipation can be extremely distressing to many patients and severely affects quality of life. The complicating factor remains the individuality of a patient's response to constipation therapy. Therefore, there is no set rule for the most effective way to manage constipation. Patients with primary bowel cancers, pelvic tumors such as ovarian or uterine cancers, or metastatic tumors that press on colon structures will experience a difficult-to-manage constipation. It is not unusual for those patients to be admitted to the hospital to manage constipation and to rule out obstruction. To minimize those admissions whenever possible, as Dame Cicely Saunders, the founder of hospice recommends, "Do not forget the bowels." Nurses are at the bedside most often and are the ones who see the cumulated number and types of medication a patient may be taking. Understanding which medications and disease processes put a patient at high risk for constipation is essential for good bowel management.

Assessing the patient's constipation as discussed earlier is the best place to start. The patient's problem list should reflect the risk for constipation and the need for aggressive constipation management. For example, diabetic patients who are taking opioids for pain are at extremely high risk for constipation. Diabetes damages the sensory fibers that are most important for temperature and pain sensation. The neuronal influence on intestinal motility is also affected through diabetes.[2,6,10]

In addition to assessing the extent of the patient's constipation, determining the methods the patient has used to manage the constipation in the past is essential. This can usually provide information regarding what medications the patient tolerates best and where to start with recommendations for management. According to Sykes,[8] using radiography to evaluate whether constipation has advanced to obstruction may be useful if there is indecision, but in palliative medicine the use of x-ray procedures should be limited. He also suggests that blood work be limited to corrective studies; for example, if hypercalcemia or hyperkalemia can be reversed to improve constipation, such blood work may be useful.

Improving three important primary causes of constipation is essential. Encouraging fluid intake is a priority. Increasing or decreasing fluid intake by as little as 100 mL can contribute to constipation.[1,15] Increase dietary intake as much as possible. This is a difficult intervention for many patients. Focusing on food intake for some patients can increase their anxiety and discomfort. If a patient feels that bowel movements are less frequent, think about dietary intake. The Western diet is fiber-deficient.[1,5,11,15] Caution is needed for patients who use bulk laxatives such as psyllium, especially if they also are taking other bowel medications. Increasing the fiber intake for patients in general may be helpful, but in palliative care, high fiber in the diet can cause more discomfort and constipation. Fiber without fluid absorbs what little liquid the patient may have available in the bowel and makes the bowels more difficult to move.[1,2,8] For example, an elderly patient who experiences reduced appetite and decreased fluid intake related to chemotherapy or disease, and whose symptoms are nausea or vomiting with reduced activity, is at extreme risk for constipation. Encouraging activity whenever possible, even in end-of-life care, can be very helpful. Increased activity helps to stimulate peristalsis and to improve mood.[1,7] Physical therapy should be used as part of a multidisciplinary bowel-management approach. Providing basic range of motion, either active or passive, can improve bowel management and patient satisfaction.[2,11]

Pharmacological Management

Types of Laxatives

Bulk Laxatives. Laxatives can be classified by their actions. Bulk laxatives do just that—they provide bulk to the intestines to increase mass, stimulating the bowel to move. Increasing dietary fiber is considered a bulk laxative. The recommended dose of bran is 8 g daily. Other bulk laxatives include psyllium, carboxymethylcellulose, and methylcellulose.[15] Bulk laxatives are more helpful for mild constipation. Because bulk laxatives work best when patients are able to increase their fluid intake, they may be inappropriate for end-stage patients. In palliative care, patients may not ingest enough fluid. It is recommended that the patient increase fluids by 200 to 300 mL when using bulk laxatives. Patients may have difficulty with the consistency of bulk laxatives and find this approach unacceptable. Patients using bulk laxatives without the additional fluid intake are at risk of developing a partial bowel obstruction or, if an impending one exists, may risk complete bowel obstruction. The benefits of bulk laxatives in severe constipation are questionable.

Additional complications include allergic reactions, fluid retention, and hyperglycemia.[1] Bulk laxatives produce gas as the indigestible or nonsoluble fiber breaks down or ferments. The result can be uncomfortable bloating and gas.

The recommended dosage of bulk laxatives is to start with 8 g daily, then stabilize at 3 to 4 g for maintenance.

Psyllium is recommended at 2 to 4 teaspoons daily as a bulk laxative. Action may take 2 to 3 days.

Lubricant Laxatives. Mineral oil is probably the most common lubricant laxative used. It can help by both lubricating the stool surface and softening the stool by penetration, leading to an easier bowel movement. Overuse of mineral oil can cause seepage from the rectum and perineal irritation. With chronic use it can lead to malabsorption of fat-soluble vitamins (vitamins A, D, E, and K). Levy[1] recommends caution when giving mineral oil at bedtime or giving it to patients at risk for aspiration. Aspiration pneumonitis or lipoid pneumonia is common in the frail and elderly patient. A complication should be noted when mineral oil is given with docusate. If patients are on daily docusate (Colace) and are given mineral oil in addition to assist with constipation, the absorption of mineral oil increases, leading to a risk of lipoid granuloma in the intestinal wall.[1]

The recommended dosage of mineral oil is 10 to 30 mL/day, and action may occur in 1 to 3 days.

Surfactant/Detergent Laxatives. Surfactant/detergent laxatives reduce surface tension, which increases absorption of water and fats into dry stools, leading to a softening effect. According to Levy[1] and others,[2,6,9] medications such as docusate exert a mucosal contact effect, which encourages secretion of water, sodium, and chloride in the jejunum and colon and decreases electrolyte and water reabsorption in the small and large intestine.[4] At higher doses, these laxatives may stimulate peristalsis. Docusate is used in a compounded or fixed combination with bowel stimulants like casanthranol (Peri-Colace) or senna (Senokot S). Castor oil also works like a detergent laxative by exerting a surface-wetting action on the stool and directly stimulates the colon, but Levy[1] discourages its use in cancer-related constipation because results are difficult to control.

The recommended dosage of surfactant/detergent laxatives includes docusate (Colace) starting at 300 mg daily and calcium salt (Surfak) at 240 mg daily to twice a day. (This may take 1 to 3 days to be effective.)

Combination Medications. Peri-Colace is a combination of a mild stimulant laxative, casanthranol, and the stool softener docusate (Colace). Combination softener/laxative medications have been shown to be more effective than softeners alone at a lower total dose.[9]

The recommended dosage of Senokot S is two tablets daily to twice a day (see Senokot S flow chart in Table 11–2). Senokot is a combination of senna as a laxative and a stool softener for smoother and easier evacuation. Results occur in 6 to 12 hours. Flexibility of dosing allows individual needs to be met.

Table 11–2
Senokot S Laxative Recommendations for Cancer-Related Constipation

Day 0

- Senokot S 2 tablets at bedtime

If no BM on day 1

- Senokot S 2 tablets Bid.

If no BM on day 2

- Senokot S 3 or 4 tablets Bid or Tid.

If no BM on day 3

- Dulcolax 2 or 3 tablets Tid and/or Hs.
- If no BM, rule out impaction
- If impacted:
  - Lubricate rectum with oil-retention enema
  - Medicate with opioid and/or benzodiazepine
  - Disimpact
  - Give enemas until clear.
  - Increase daily laxative therapy per above
- If not impacted:
  - Give additional laxatives:
    - Lactulose (45–60 mL PO)
    - Magnesium citrate (8 oz)
    - Dulcolax suppository (1 PR)
    - Fleet enema (1 PR)

At any step, if medication is ineffective, continue at that dose. If <1 BM per day, increase laxative therapy per steps. If >2 BM per day, decrease laxative therapy by 24% to 50%.

Source: Adapted from Levy (1991), reference 1.

Osmotic Laxatives. Osmotic laxatives are nonabsorbable sugars that exert an osmotic effect in both the small and, to a lesser extent, the large intestines. They have the additional effect of lowering ammonia levels. This is helpful in improving confusion, especially in hepatic failure patients. According to Levy,[1] 30 mL of lactulose can increase the colon volume by 400 to 600 mL within 1 to 3 hours. These laxatives can be effective for chronic constipation, especially when related to opioid use. Drawbacks of these agents are that effectiveness is completely dose-related and, for some patients, the sweet taste is intolerable. The bloating and gas associated with higher doses may be too uncomfortable or distressing to tolerate. Lactulose or sorbitol can be put into juice or other liquid to lessen the taste. Patients may prefer hot tea or hot water to help reduce the sweet taste. Lactulose is more costly than sorbitol liquid. A study that compared the two medications found that there was no significant difference, except with regard to nausea, which increased with lactulose ($P = 0.05$).[17]

The recommended dosage of lactulose/sorbitol is 30 to 60 mL initially for severe constipation every 4 hours until a bowel movement occurs. Once that happens, calculate the amount of lactulose used to achieve that movement, and then divide in half for recommended daily maintenance dose.[1] An example would be: it took 60 mL to have a bowel movement, therefore 30 mL daily should keep the bowels moving regularly. Action can occur within 4 hours, depending on the dose. Polyethylene glycol (MiraLax) is used frequently and can be sprinkled over food. Recommended dose is 1 tablespoon. Evacuation can take between 2 to 4 days. If bowel obstruction is suspected, do not use.[18] Osmotic rectal compounds include glycerin suppositories and sorbitol enemas. Glycerin suppositories soften stool by osmosis and act as a lubricant. In one study, bisacodyl (Dulcolax) suppositories were more effective for moving the bowel than glycerin suppositories in chronically ill and geriatric patients.[5]

Dulcolax acts directly on the mucous membrane of the large intestine, causing a reflex stimulation. Because it is not absorbed in the small intestine, it can pass through without side effects. It can be especially helpful for bowel training or bedridden patients with dyschezia, or an incomplete reflex for defecation.

Suppositories should never be used in patients with severely reduced white cell or platelet counts due to the risk of bleeding or infection.

Saline Laxatives. Magnesium hydroxide (milk of magnesia) and magnesium citrate are the most commonly used saline laxatives. They increase gastric, pancreatic, and small intestinal secretion, as well as motor activity throughout the intestine. Aluminum salts in many of the antacid medications counteract the laxative effect of magnesium. This laxative can also cause severe cramping and discomfort. This medication is recommended for use only as a last resort in chronically ill patients. Opioid-related constipation requires the use of aggressive laxatives earlier rather than later to prevent severe constipation, referred to as obstipation, which leads to obstruction.

The recommended dosage of milk of magnesia is 30 mL to initiate a bowel movement. For opioid-related constipation, 15 mL of milk of magnesia may be added to the baseline bowel medications either daily or every other day. Magnesium citrate comes in a 10-ounce bottle. For severe constipation, it is used as a one-time initial therapy. It can be titrated up or down, depending on patient response. For patients with abdominal discomfort or pain, it is recommended that obstruction be ruled out before using this medication. If the patient were obstructed, even only partially, this would only increase the discomfort or lead to perforation.[14]

Bowel Stimulants. Bowel stimulants work directly on the colon to increase motility. These medications stimulate the myenteric plexus to induce peristalsis. They also reduce the amount of water and electrolytes in the colon. They are divided into two groups: the diphenylmethanes and the anthraquinones. The diphenylmethanes are commonly known as phenolphthalein (Ex-Lax, Fen-a-Mint, Correctol, and Doxidan) and bisacodyl (Dulcolax). Phenolphthalein must be metabolized in the liver rather than in the colon. Levy[1] points out that because the effect is difficult to control and hepatic circulation is significant, this class of stimulants may not be appropriate for cancer-related constipation. The anthraquinones are bowel stimulants that include senna and cascara. They are activated in the large intestine by bacterial degradation into the large bowel, stimulating glycosides. The negative side of bisacodyl is its cramping side effect. This action causes a 6- to 12-hour delay when taken orally. Rectal absorption is much faster, at 15 to 60 minutes. It is recommended that bisacodyl be taken with food, milk, or antacids to avoid gastric irritation. One Senokot S can counter the constipation caused by 120 mg of codeine.[2] Senna is available in a liquid form called X-Prep Liquid. This is used for bowel cleansing before radiology procedures; 72 mL of X-Prep is equivalent to 10 Senokot tablets. Cascara, another anthraquinone, is commonly combined with milk of magnesia to make a mixture referred to as "Black and White." This is a mild combination that reduces colic pain. Casanthranol is derived from cascara and is used as the stimulant component in Peri-Colace.

Recommendations for use are senna 15-mg tablets used alone or as Senokot S. Starting dose is two tablets daily (see Table 11-2). These stimulating laxatives are the most effective management for opioid-related constipation. Bisacodyl comes in 10-mg tablets or suppositories and is used daily. The suppository medication has a faster onset that is much appreciated in the uncomfortable, constipated patient.

Suppository Medications. As discussed above, bisacodyl (Dulcolax) comes in a suppository. Although the thought of rectal medications is unpleasant for many patients, suppositories' quick onset of action makes them more acceptable. Bisacodyl comes in 10 mg for adults and 5 mg as a pediatric dose.

Liquid rectal laxatives or lubricants should be used infrequently. In severely constipated patients, they may be necessary. Most commonly, saline enemas are used to loosen the stool and to stimulate rectal or distal colon peristalsis. Repeated use can cause hypocalcemia and hyperphosphatemia, so it is important to use enemas cautiously. Enemas should never be considered part of a standing bowel regimen.

Oil retention enemas, however, are particularly helpful for severely constipated patients, for whom disimpaction may be necessary. They work best when used overnight, to allow softening. Overnight retention is effective only if the patient is able to retain it that long. The general rule is that the longer the enema is retained, the better the results. Bisanz[10] recommends a milk-and-molasses enema (Figure 11–2) for patients with low impaction to ease stool evacuation in a nonirritating way. It is a low-volume enema of 300 mL and therefore thought to cause less cramping.

Combining an enema with an oral saline-type cathartic (lactulose, Cephylac) is helpful when a large amount of stool is present.[1,10] This may help to push the stool through the GI tract.

If disimpaction is necessary, remember that it can be extremely painful; therefore, premedicate the patient with either opioid and/or benzodiazepine anxiolytics to reduce physical and emotional pain.[2,3,15]

There are few studies outlining the efficacy of one enema over another. The reported success rates for rectal enemas

Figure 11–2. Milk and molasses enema recipe. *Sources:* Bisanz (1997), reference 10; Lowell (2003), reference 23; Walsh (1989), reference 50.

MILK and MOLASSES ENEMA RECIPE

8 oz. warm water
3 oz. powdered milk
4.5 oz. molasses

- Put water and powdered milk in a plastic jar. Close the jar and shake until the water and milk appear to be fully mixed.
- Add molasses, and shake the jar again until the mixture appears to have an even color throughout.
- Pour mixture into enema bag. Administer enema high by gently introducing tube about 12 inches. Do not push beyond resistance. Repeat every 6 hours until good results are achieved.

within 1 hour includes phosphate enemas (100%), mini-enemas (Micralax) (95%), bisacodyl suppositories (66%), and glycerine suppositories (38%).[16] If none of the above enemas is effective, Sykes[9] recommends rectal lavage with approximately 8 liters of warmed normal saline. It is important to remember that if a patient's constipation requires this invasive intervention, you must change the usual bowel regimen once this bowel crisis is resolved. For severe constipation associated with opioids, Levy[1] suggests four Senokot S and three Dulcolax tablets three times a day and 60 mL of lactulose every other night for a goal of a bowel movement every other day (see Table 11–2).

New Approaches to Constipation Management

Oral naloxone has been studied for the treatment of opioid-related constipation resistant to other treatments. Culpepper-Morgan and colleagues[19] found that the majority of opioid effect on the human intestine is mediated peripherally rather than centrally. Naloxone, which is an opioid antagonist, has less than 1% availability systemically when given orally, due to the first-pass effect in the liver. Therefore, the risk of causing a withdrawal response when using naloxone orally is small. Although the risk is small, patients who are opioid-dependent must be monitored closely for signs of withdrawal.[2] It has been recommended that the dose start with 1 mg twice per day and be titrated as a percentage of the current morphine dose. Titration of dose to a maximum of 12 mg at least 6 hr apart may be needed to avoid adverse reactions.[19] The cost of oral naloxone also prohibits its use beyond rare circumstances. Using naloxone in the outpatient setting is not recommended because of the increased risk of withdrawal or dose-benefit behavior.[19] Future studies will look at alternative drugs from the same class that do not cross the blood–brain barrier and that may offer more effective results.[15]

Oral erythromycin has been shown to cause diarrhea in 50% of patients who use it as an antibiotic.[15] Currently, researchers are investigating its use to promote diarrhea. There is also interest in identifying a medication that would increase colon transit time without being antibacterial.

Many herbal medicines have laxative properties, such as mulberry and constituents of rhubarb, which are similar to senna. These herbs are being evaluated for use as laxatives. Patients have been known to develop rashes; in one patient, changes were found in warfarin (Coumadin) levels that were related to natural warfarin found in a laxative tea. Many patients prefer these options instead of pharmaceutical laxatives, but they should be cautious about where they purchase any herbal product and be alert to any unexplained side effects, as their content is unregulated.

Nursing Interventions for Constipation

Nurses should always be proactive in initiating laxative therapy. Bowel function requires continued evaluation to follow the trajectory of the disease and the changes that occur in normal activities that affect bowel function. Nurses should also be alert to medications that can increase the risk of constipation (see Table 11–1). Some patients, especially those on long-term opioid therapy, sometimes need at least two different regimens that can be interchanged when one or the other loses its effectiveness for a time. Like opioids, over time, a standing laxative regimen may be less effective if tolerance develops.[1,15] It is also important to be aware of medication dosing changes, as it is common to forget to increase anticonstipation therapy when there is an increase in opioid therapy. Patients generally have increased risk of constipation when opioids are increased. Positioning patients to allow gravity to assist with bowel movements is helpful. Assisting with oral fluid intake as well as dietary interventions are both helpful. Discuss patients' management needs as well as personal cultural perspectives and factors that may contribute to good bowel hygiene. Exercise within each patient's tolerance is recommended to aid in elimination. Fatigue, advanced disease, and decreased endurance all play a role in obstructing good bowel maintenance. The importance of effective bowel management cannot be stressed enough. It remains the most distressing symptom in end-stage cancer patients.

DIARRHEA

Diarrhea has been a major symptom and significant problem associated with newer chemotherapeutic and biological and radiation treatment regimens.[20,24] It is a main symptom of 7% to 10% of hospice admissions.[15] Overgrowth of GI infections such as *Candida* can cause diarrhea as well.[15] Treating diarrhea requires a thorough assessment and therapy directed at the specific cause. Diarrhea is usually acute and short-lived, lasting only a few days, as opposed to chronic diarrhea, which lasts 3 weeks or more.[24] Diarrhea can be especially severe in human immunodeficiency virus (HIV)–infected patients. Forty-three percent of bone marrow transplant patients develop diarrhea related to radiation or graft versus host disease (GVHD).[25] Similar to constipation, this symptom can be debilitating and can severely affect quality of life.[19,20] Diarrhea can prevent patients from leaving their homes, increase weakness and dehydration, and contribute to feelings of lack of control and depression. Nurses play a significant role in recognizing, educating, and managing diarrhea and its manifestations.

Definitions

Diarrhea is described as an increase in stool volume and liquidity resulting in three or more bowel movements per day.[1,24] Secondary effects related to diarrhea include abdominal cramps, anxiety, lethargy, weakness, dehydration, dizziness, loss of electrolytes, skin breakdown and associated pain, dry mouth, and weight loss. Diarrhea varies among patients depending on their bowel history. Acute diarrhea occurs within 24 to 48 hours of exposure to the cause and resolves in 7 to 14 days.

Chronic diarrhea usually has a late onset and lasts 2 to 3 weeks, with an unidentified cause.

Prevalence and Impact

Cancer patients may have multiple causes of diarrhea. It may be due to infections or related to tumor type or its treatment. A common cause of diarrhea is overuse of laxative therapy or dietary fiber. Additional causes include malabsorption disorders, motility disturbances, stress, partial bowel obstruction, enterocolic fistula, villous adenoma, endocrine-induced hypersecretion of serotonin, gastrin calcitonin, and vasoactive intestinal protein prostaglandins.[1,20,24] Treatment-related causes include radiation and chemotherapy, which cause overgrowth of bacteria, with endotoxin production that has a direct effect on the intestinal mucosa. Local inflammation and increased fluid and electrolyte secretion occur, resulting in interference with amino acid and electrolyte transport and a shift toward secretion by crypt cells with shortened villi.[20]

Diarrhea associated with radiation can occur by the 2nd or 3rd week of treatment and can continue after radiation has been discontinued.[15,20,21] Radiation-induced diarrhea is related to focus of radiation and total of radiation dose. Pelvic radiation alone has been shown to cause diarrhea of any grade in up to 70% of the patients receiving it. A grade 3 or 4 diarrhea is associated with approximately 20% of those patients.[21]

The risk is increased in acquired immunodeficiency syndrome (AIDS), GVHD, or HIV patients. The end result could be a change in the intestinal mucosa that results in a limited ability to regenerate epithelium, which can lead to bleeding and ileus. The damaged mucosa leads to increased release of prostaglandins and malabsorption of bile salts, increasing peristaltic activity.[15,24]

Surgical patients who have had bowel-shortening procedures or gastrectomy related to cancer experience a "dumping syndrome," which causes severe diarrhea. This type of diarrhea is related to both osmotic and hypermotile mechanisms.[1] Patients may experience weakness, epigastric distention, and diarrhea shortly after eating.[34] The shortened bowel can result in a decreased absorption capacity and an imbalance in absorptive and secretory function of the intestine.

Pathophysiology

Diarrhea can be grouped into four types, each with a different mechanism: osmotic diarrhea, secretory diarrhea, hypermotile diarrhea, and exudative diarrhea. Cancer patients rarely exhibit only one type. Understanding the mechanism of diarrhea permits more rational treatment strategies.[20,24,32]

Osmotic Diarrhea. Osmotic diarrhea is produced by intake of hyperosmolar preparations or nonabsorbable solutions such as enteral feeding solutions.[32] Enterocolic fistula can lead to both osmotic diarrhea from undigested food entering the colon and hypermotile diarrhea. Hemorrhage into the intestine can cause an osmotic-type diarrhea because intraluminal blood acts as an osmotic laxative. Osmotic diarrhea may result from insufficient lactase when dairy products are consumed.

Secretory Diarrhea. Secretory diarrhea is most associated with chemotherapy and radiation therapy. The cause is related to mechanical damage to the epithelial crypt cells in the GI tract.[21] The necrosis that results, along with the inflammation and ulceration of the intestinal mucosa, leads to further damage related to exposure to bile and susceptibility to opportunistic infections, atrophy of the mucosal lining, and fibrosis. This all contributes to loss of absorption due to damaged villi, causing an increase in water, electrolytes, mucus, blood, and serum to be pulled into the intestine from immature crypt cells, and increased fluid secretion, resulting in diarrhea.[20,21]

Secretory diarrhea is the most difficult to control. Malignant epithelial tumors producing hormones that can cause diarrhea include metastatic carcinoid tumors, gastrinoma, and medullary thyroid cancer. The primary effect of secretory diarrhea is related to the hypersecretion stimulated by endogenous mediators that affect the intestinal transport of water and electrolytes. This results in accumulation of intestinal fluids.[22,34] Diarrhea associated with GVHD results from mucosal damage and can produce up to 6 to 8 liters of diarrhea in 24 hours.[35] Surgical shortening of the bowel, which reduces intestinal mucosal contact and shortens colon transit time, causing decreased reabsorption, leads to diarrhea. Active treatment requires vigorous fluid and electrolyte repletion, antidiarrheal therapy, and specific anticancer therapy.[1,22]

Preventing diarrhea associated with chemotherapy and radiation is not always realistic, but being proactive in anticipating diarrhea and prompt management may be effective.[22,24] Initiation of medication with the first episode is suggested. The recommendation starts with loperamide 4 mg, then 2 to 4 mg q 2 to 4 hours (max 16 mg/24 h). If there is no response at 24 to 48 hours, then, based on grade, either increase the loperamide dose, then reevaluate in 24 hours, or start octreotide 100 to 500 mcg subcutaneously, three times a day for grades 3 to 4 diarrhea.[22] The somatostatin analogue octreotide is used for grades 3 to 4 diarrhea with success. A study done by Barbounis and colleagues in patients experiencing chemotherapy-induced diarrhea unresponsive to loperamide had a 92% response to octreotide SC 500 mcg three times daily.[26] A major trial known as the STOP trial (Sandostatin LAR Depot Trial for the Optimum Prevention of Chemotherapy-Induced Diarrhea) has been initiated to identify optimal dosing and timing schedules for the long-acting version of octreotide. The goal is to prevent high-grade diarrhea that results in dose reduction or cessation of chemotherapy regimens.[23] Cost is a major issue with this medication; the long-acting version can cost between $10,000 and $20,000 for a single monthly dose.

Hypermotile Diarrhea. Partial bowel obstruction from abdominal malignancies can cause a reflex hypermotility that may require bowel-quieting medications such as loperamide.[34] Enterocolic fistula can lead to diarrhea from irritative hypermotility and osmotic influence of undigested food entering the colon.

Biliary or pancreatic obstruction can cause incomplete digestion of fat in the small intestine, resulting in interference with fat and bile salt malabsorption, leading to hypermotile diarrhea, also called steatorrhea. Malabsorption is related to pancreatic cancer, gastrectomy, ileal resection or colectomy, rectal cancer, pancreatic islet cell tumors, or carcinoid tumors. Chemotherapy-induced diarrhea is frequently seen with 5-fluorouracil or N-phosphonoacetyl-L-aspartate. High-dose cisplatin and irinotecan (Camptosar™) cause severe hypermotility. Other chemotherapy drugs that cause diarrhea include cytosine arabinoside, nitrosourea, methotrexate, cyclophosphamide, doxorubicin, daunorubicin, hydroxyurea and biotherapy-2, interferon and topoisomerase inhibitors (capecitabine [5-FU prodrug]), oxaliplatin.[20,22]

Exudative Diarrhea. Radiation therapy of the abdomen, pelvis, or lower thoracic or lumbar spine can cause acute exudative diarrhea.[24] The inflammation caused by radiation leads to the release of prostaglandins. Treatment using aspirin or ibuprofen was shown to reduce prostaglandin release and decrease diarrhea associated with radiation therapy.[24] Bismuth subsalicylate (Pepto-Bismol) is also helpful for diarrhea caused by radiotherapy.[10]

According to Sykes,[15] there are multiple causes of diarrhea in palliative medicine. Concurrent diseases such as diabetes mellitus, hyperthyroidism, inflammatory bowel disease, irritable bowel syndrome, and GI infection (*C. difficile*) can contribute to the development of diarrhea. Finally, the dietary influences of fruit, bran, hot spices, and alcohol, as well as over-the-counter medications, laxatives, and herbal supplements, need to be considered as sources of diarrhea.[15,24]

Assessment of Diarrhea

Diarrhea assessment requires a careful history to detail the frequency and nature of the stools. The National Cancer Institute Scale of Severity of Diarrhea uses a grading system from 0 to 4. Stools are rated by (1) number of loose stools per day and (2) symptoms (Table 11–3). This scale permits an objective score to define the severity of diarrhea.

The initial goal of assessment is to identify and treat any reversible causes of diarrhea. If diarrhea occurs once or twice a day, it is probably related to anal incontinence. Large amounts of watery stools are characteristic of colonic diarrhea. Pale, fatty, malodorous stools, called steatorrhea, are indicative of malabsorption secondary to pancreatic or small-intestinal causes. If a patient who has been constipated complains of sudden diarrhea with little warning, fecal impaction with overflow is the probable cause.[15,24]

Evaluate medications that the patient may be taking now or in the recent past. Is the patient on laxatives? If the stools are associated with cramping and urgency, it may be the result of peristalsis-stimulating laxatives. If stools are associated with fecal leakage, it may be the result of overuse of stool-softening agents such as Colace.[15,24]

Depending on the aggressiveness of the treatment plan, additional assessment could include stool smears for pus, blood, fat, ova, or parasites. Stool samples for culture and sensitivity testing may be necessary to rule out additional sources of diarrhea through *C. difficile* toxin, *Giardia lamblia*, or other types of GI infection.[1] If patients have diarrhea after 2 to 3 days of fasting, secretory diarrhea should be evaluated. Osmotic and secretory causes are considered first; if ruled out, then hypermotility is the suspected mechanism.

Management of Diarrhea

A combination of supportive care and medication may be appropriate for palliative management of diarrhea. The goal of diarrhea management should focus on minimizing or eliminating the factors causing the diarrhea, providing dietary interventions, and maintaining fluid and electrolyte balance as appropriate. Quality-of-life issues include minimizing skin breakdown or infections, relieving pain associated with frequent diarrhea, and maintaining the patient's dignity.[24]

If the patient is dehydrated, oral fluids are recommended over the IV route.[15] Oral fluids should contain electrolytes and a source of glucose to facilitate active electrolyte transport (Figure 11–3).

Table 11–3
National Cancer Institute Scale of Severity of Diarrhea

	National Cancer Institute Grade				
	0	1	2	3	4
Increased number of loose stools/d	Normal	2–3	4–6	7–9	>10
Symptoms		None	Nocturnal stools and/or moderate cramping	Incontinence and/or severe cramping	Grossly bloody diarrhea and/or need for parenteral support

ADULT HOMEMADE ELECTROLYTE REPLACEMENT SOLUTION

1 tsp salt	6 oz. frozen orange juice concentrate
1 tsp baking soda	6 cups water
1 tsp corn syrup	47 kcal/cup, 515 mg Na^+, 164 mg K^+

Following diarrhea, the diet should start with clear liquids, flat lemonade, ginger ale, and toast or simple carbohydrates. It is recommended that the patient avoid milk if diarrhea is related to infection due to acute lactase deficiency. Protein and fats can be added to the diet slowly as diarrhea resolves. Dietary management may help minimize amount of diarrhea.

Figure 11–3. Homemade electrolyte replacement solution for adults. *Source:* Weihofen & Marino (1998), reference 25.

Medication Recommendations

There are many nonspecific diarrhea medications that should be used unless infections are suspected as the cause. If *Shigella* or *C. difficile* are responsible, nonspecific antidiarrheal medications can make the diarrhea worse.[15] Loperamide (Imodium) has become the drug of choice for the treatment of nonspecific diarrhea. It is a long-acting opioid agonist.[22] The 2-mg dose has the same antidiarrheal action as 5 mg, two tablets of diphenoxylate, or 45 mg of codeine.[1] The usual management of diarrhea begins with 4 mg of loperamide, with one capsule following each loose bowel movement. Most diarrhea is managed by loperamide 2 to 4 mg once to twice a day.[1,22] Diphenoxylate (Lomotil 2.5 mg with atropine 0.025 mg) is given as one or two tablets orally as needed for loose stools, maximum of eight/day. Diphenoxylate is derived from meperidine and binds to opioid receptors to reduce diarrhea. Atropine was added to this antidiarrheal to prevent abuse.[1] Diphenoxylate is not recommended for patients with advanced liver disease because it may precipitate hepatic coma in patients with cirrhosis.[1,22] Neither diphenoxylate nor loperamide is recommended for use in children under 12 years old.[1] Codeine as an opioid for the reduction of diarrhea can be helpful. It is also less expensive than some opioid medications. Most cancer-related diarrheas respond well to this drug. For specific mechanisms, other medications might be more beneficial. Tincture of opium works to decrease peristalsis, given at .6 mL every 4 to 6 hours. This is a controlled substance but may also provide some pain relief.[22] Absorbent agents such as pectin and methylcellulose may help provide bulk to increase consistency of the stools.[33]

Anticholinergic drugs such as atropine and scopolamine are useful to reduce gastric secretions and decrease peristalsis. Somatostatin analogues such as octreotide (Sandostatin) are also effective for secretory diarrhea that may result from endocrine tumors, AIDS, GVHD, or post-GI resection.[1,15,22] They may be helpful for patients who experience painful cramping.[1] Side effects of that class of drug can complicate their use: dry mouth, blurred vision, and urinary hesitancy.

Mucosal antiprostaglandin agents such as aspirin, indomethacin, and bismuth subsalicylate (Pepto-Bismol) are useful for diarrhea related to enterotoxic bacteria, radiotherapy, and prostaglandin-secreting tumors. Octreotide (Sandostatin) is also effective for patients with AIDS, GVHD, diabetes, or GI resection.[15,31] Octreotide is administered subcutaneously at a dose of 50 to 200 mg two or three times per day. Ranitidine is a useful adjuvant to octreotide for patients with Zollinger-Ellison syndrome with gastrin-induced gastric hypersecretion.[1] Side effects include nausea and pain at injection site. Patients may also experience abdominal or headache pain.[1] Clonidine is effective at controlling watery diarrhea in patients with bronchogenic cancer. Clonidine effects an α_2-adrenergic stimulation of electrolyte absorption in the small intestine.[1] Streptozocin is used for watery diarrhea from pancreatic islet cell cancer because it decreases intestinal secretions. Hypermotile diarrhea involves problems with fat absorption. The recommended treatment is pancreatin before meals. Pancreatin is a combination of amylase, lipase, and protease that is available for pancreatic enzyme replacement. Lactaid may also be helpful for malabsorption-related diarrhea.

Nursing Interventions for Diarrhea

Nursing interventions should include nonpharmacological interventions focused on diet and psychosocial support (Tables 11–4 and 11–5).

Table 11–4
Nutritional Management of Cancer-Related Diarrhea: Foods and Medication to Avoid

Medications
Antibiotics, bulk laxatives (Metamucil, methylcellulose), magnesium-containing medications (Maalox, Mylanta), promotility agents (propulsid, metoclopramide), stool softeners/laxatives (Peri-Colace, Dulcolax), herbal supplements (milk thistle, aloe, cayenne, saw palmetto, Siberian ginseng)
Foods
Milk and diary products (cheese, yogurt, ice cream), caffeine-containing products (coffee, tea, cola drinks, chocolate), carbonated and high-sugar or high-sorbitol juices (prune pear, sweet cherry, peach, apple, orange juice), high-fiber/gas-causing legumes (raw vegetables, whole-grain products, dried legumes, popcorn), high-fat foods (fried foods, high-fat spreads, or dressings), heavily spiced foods that taste "hot"
High risk foods—sushi, street vendors, buffets

Source: Adapted from Stern & Ippoliti (2003), reference 22; Engelking (2004), reference 24.

Table 11–5
Nursing Role in the Management of Diarrhea

Environmental Assessment

- Assess the patient's and/or caregiver's ability to manage the level of care necessary.
- Evaluate home for medical equipment that may be helpful (bedpan or commode chair).

History

- Frequency of bowel movements in last 2 wks
- Fluid intake (normal 2 quarts/d)
- Fiber intake (normal 30–40 g/d)
- Appetite and whether patient is nauseated or vomiting. Does diet include spicy foods?
- Assess for current medications the patient has taken that are associated with causing diarrhea (laxative use, chemotherapy, antibiotics, enteral nutritional supplements, nonsteroidal antiinflammatory drugs).
- Surgical history that may contribute to diarrhea (gastrectomy, pancreatectomy, bypass or ileal resection)
- Recent radiotherapy to abdomen, pelvis, lower spine
- Cancer diagnosis associated with diarrhea includes abdominal malignancies, partial bowel obstruction; enterocolic fistulae; metastatic carcinoid tumors; gastrinomas; medullary thyroid cancer
- Immunosuppressed, susceptible to bacterial, protozoan, and viral diseases associated with diarrhea
- Concurrent diseases associated with diarrhea: gastroenteritis, inflammatory bowel disease, irritable bowel syndrome, diabetes mellitus, lactose deficiency, hyperthyroidism

Physical Assessment

- Examine perineum or ostomy site for skin breakdown, fissures, or external hemorrhoids
- Gentle digital rectal examination for impaction
- Abdominal examination for distention of palpable stool in large bowel
- Examine stools for signs of bleeding
- Evaluate for signs of dehydration

Interventions

- Treatment should be related to cause (i.e., if obstruction is cause of diarrhea, giving antidiarrheal medications would be inappropriate).
- Assist with correcting any obvious factors related to assessment (e.g., decreasing nutritional supplements, changing fiber intake, holding or substituting medications associated with diarrhea).
- If bacterial causes are suspected, notify physician and culture stools as instructed. *Clostridium difficile* is most common.
- Educate patient and family on importance of cleansing the perineum gently after each stool, to prevent skin breakdown. If patient has a colostomy, stomal area must also be watched closely and surrounding skin protected. Use skin barrier such as Desitin ointment to protect the skin. Frequent sitz baths may be helpful.
- Instruct patient and family on signs and symptoms that should be reported to the nurse or physician: excessive thirst, dizziness, fever, palpitations, rectal spasms, excessive cramping, water or bloody stools.

Dietary Measures

- Eat small, frequent, bland meals.
- Low-residue diet—potassium-rich (bananas, rice, peeled apples, dry toast)
- Avoid intake of hyperosmotic supplements (e.g., Ensure, Sustacal)
- Increase fluids in diet. Approximately 3 liters of fluid a day if possible. Drinking electrolyte fluids such as Pedialyte may be helpful.
- Homeopathic treatments for diarrhea include: ginger tea, glutamine, and peeled apples.

Pharmacologic Management

- Opioids—codeine, paregoric, dihenoxylate, loperamide, tincture of opium
- Absorbents—pectin, aluminum hydroxide

(*continued*)

Table 11–5
Nursing Role in the Management of Diarrhea *(continued)*

- Adsorbents—charcoal, kaolin
- Antisecretory—aspirin, bismuth subsalicylate, prednisone, Sandostatin, ranitidine hydrochloride, indomethacin.
- Anticholinergics—scopolamine, atropine sulfate, belladonna
- α_2-Adrenergic agonists—clonidine

Report to nurse or physician if antidiarrheal medication seems ineffective

Psychosocial Interventions

Provide support to patient and family. Recognize negative effects of diarrhea on quality of life:

- Fatigue
- Malnutrition
- Alteration in skin integrity
- Pain and discomfort
- Sleep disturbances
- Limited ability to travel
- Compromised role within the family
- Decreased sexual activity
- Caregiver burden

Source: Levy (1991), reference 1; Bisanz (1997), reference 10; Hogan (1998), reference 49.

- Evaluate medications currently being used to identify polypharmacy, where multiple medication side effects may be contributing to the problem.
- Minimize or prevent diarrhea accidents in an effort to reduce patient anxiety. Anticipate obstacles between the patient and the bathroom. Assist with access plans and timing needs. Recommend commode chair at bedside to allow easiest access and prevent falls or additional problems.
- Protecting the bed with Chux can be better accepted than diapers. It may also be better for skin integrity but requires multiple layers of Chux and drawsheets for best results.
- Applying skin ointment protection after cleaning and drying the area is also important. Thick protectant creams that apply a barrier on the skin are most beneficial. Eucerin cream, zinc oxide, and bag balm are three that have been used anecdotally with success.
- The psychosocial impact of diapers can be devastating for some patients. Encourage a discussion with patient and family about patient needs, fears, and perceptions.
- Along with focus on diet/medications, skin integrity, and psychosocial needs, odor management must also be addressed. Perfumed air fresheners sometimes only make it worse. Concentrate on being sure the perineum or periostomy area is clean and the linens are not soiled. Also be sure that dirty linens or trash are removed from the room. Using aromatherapy such as lavender may be soothing.
- Remember that there may be times when adult diapers are essential and can help alleviate distress to the patient, for example, when traveling or on necessary outings. Remind families to check them frequently to prevent skin breakdown and, again, be sure there is skin barrier ointment applied before the diaper padding.

Conclusion

Managing diarrhea in the cancer patient is challenging at best. The nurse's role in helping the patient and caregivers talk about this difficult symptom is essential. It is important to respect comfort levels about the topic among nurse, patient, and caregiver to allow information sharing. Goals of diarrhea therapy should be to restore an optimal pattern of elimination, maintain fluid and electrolyte balance as desired, preserve nutritional status, protect skin integrity, and ensure the patient's comfort and dignity.[10,30]

MALIGNANT OBSTRUCTION

As primary tumors grow in the large intestine, they can lead to obstruction. Obstruction is related to the site and stage of disease.[33] Tumors in the splenic flexure obstruct 49% of the time, but those in the rectum or rectosigmoid junction only 6% of the time.[32] Obstruction can occur intraluminally related to primary tumors of the colon. Intramural obstruction is related to tumor in the muscular layers of the bowel wall. The bowel appears thickened, indurated, and contracted.[15] Extramural obstruction is related to mesenteric and omental masses and malignant adhesions. The common metastatic pattern, in relation to primary disease in the pancreas or stomach, generally goes to the duodenum, from the colon to the jejunum and ileum, and from the prostate or bladder to the rectum.[15]

Definition

Intestinal obstruction is occlusion of the lumen or absence of the normal propulsion that affects elimination from the GI tract.[16] Motility disruption, either impaired or absent, leads to a mechanical obstruction but without occlusion of the intestinal lumen. Mechanical obstruction results in the accumulation of fluids and gas proximal to the obstruction. Distention occurs as a result of intestinal gas, ingested fluids, and digestive secretions. It becomes a self-perpetuating phenomenon as when distention increases, intestinal secretion of water and electrolytes increases. A small-bowel obstruction causes large amounts of diarrhea. The increased fluid in the bowel leads to increased peristalsis, with large quantities of bacteria growing in the intestinal fluid of the small bowel.[32]

Obstruction is related to the surrounding mesentery or bowel muscle, such as in ovarian cancer. Additional factors include multiple sites of obstruction along the intestine to constipating medications (Table 11–6), fecal impaction, fibrosis, or change in normal flora of the bowel. The goal of treatment is to prevent obstruction from happening whenever possible.

Table 11–6
Sites of Intestinal Obstruction and Related Side Effects

Site	Side Effects
Duodenum	Severe vomiting with large amounts of undigested food. Bowel sounds: succussion splash may be present. No pain or distention noted.
Small intestine	Moderate to severe vomiting; usually hyperactive bowel sounds with borborygmi; pain in upper and central abdomen, colic in nature; moderate distention.
Large intestine	Vomiting is a late side effect. Borborygmi bowel sounds, severe distention. Pain central to lower abdomen, colic in nature.

Source: Baines (1998), reference 16.

Prevalance and Impact

The best treatment options for bowel obstruction in a patient with advanced cancer remain undetermined.[38] As obstruction increases, bacteria levels increase and can lead to sepsis and associated multisystem failure and death.[33] The difficulty is knowing which patients will truly benefit from surgical intervention. The impact of obstruction on the patient and family is overwhelming. The patient and caregivers have been aggressively trying to manage the patient's constipation in an effort to prevent this very problem. Obstruction for patients means failure to manage constipation or a sign of growing disease. New interventions have been developed in an effort to provide additional noninvasive approaches for the management of bowel obstruction.[27,28]

In a retrospective study, Jong and colleagues[36] found that palliative surgery for bowel obstruction in advanced ovarian cancer achieved successful alleviation, defined as patient survival longer than 60 days after surgery, the ability to return home, and relief of bowel obstruction for longer than 60 days. Past studies associated with ovarian or abdominal cancers found survival rates in general to be less than 6 months. In patients for whom a definitive procedure could take place, such as a resection, bypass, colostomy, or ileostomy, the mean survival was 6 months. For these patients, who were not surgical candidates, the mean survival rate was 1.8 months. Progressive cancer was the cause of obstruction in 86% of patients.[32] There was a postoperative complication rate of 49%, which included wound infection, enterocutaneous fistulae, and other septic sequelae. Median postoperative survival was 140 days. In general, the operative mortality rate for this group was 12% to 25%.[35]

Further research needs to be done similar to that of Jong and colleagues,[36] who evaluated the effects of surgical intervention on quality as well as quantity of life. The effect of unrelieved intestinal obstruction on quality of life for the patient and loved ones is devastating.

Assessment and Management of Malignant Obstruction

Patients may experience severe nausea, vomiting, and abdominal pain associated with a partial or complete bowel obstruction. In the elderly patient, fecal impaction may also cause urinary incontinence.[15] General signs and symptoms associated with different sites of obstruction are listed in Table 11–6. Providing thoughtful and supportive interventions may be more appropriate than aggressive, invasive procedures. The signs and symptoms of obstruction may be acute, with nausea, vomiting, and abdominal pain. A majority of the time, however, obstruction is a slow and insidious phenomenon, which may progress from partial to complete obstruction. Palliative care should allow for a thoughtful and realistic approach to management of obstruction within the goals of care. Radiological examination should be limited unless surgery is being considered. The use of self-expanding metallic stents has been highly effective for malignant colorectal obstruction and, in some cases, has prevented the need for colostomy.[28,33] It is done in interventional radiology and requires close clinical observation, since perforation is a potential complication. At the minimum, it has allowed emergent relief of obstruction for surgical intervention in the future. Putting a patient through an x-ray of the abdomen may be helpful to confirm the obstruction and identify where it is, but defining the goal of therapy is essential.[33] When patients exhibit signs of obstruction, a physical exam may be helpful to assess the extent of the problem. Asking the patient for a bowel history, last bowel movement, and a description of consistency can be helpful. Does the patient complain of constipation? Physical examination should include gentle palpation of the abdomen for masses or distention. A careful rectal exam can identify the presence of stool in the rectum or a distended empty rectum. An empty, or "ballooned," rectum may be a symptom of high obstruction. It is also difficult to distinguish stool from malignant mass.[10,16] The ability to assess whether an impaction is low or high in the intestinal tract is important to help guide the intervention planning. As discussed above, lack of stool noted in the rectum during a digital exam is usually indicative of a high impaction. Stool has not or cannot move down into the rectum. The goal then would be to use careful assessment to be sure the obstruction is not a tumor and to concentrate on softening the stool and moving it through the GI tract. Again, using a stimulant laxative for this type of patient would result in increasing discomfort and possible rupture of the intestinal wall.[10,16] Low impactions are uncomfortable, and patients may need more comforting measures. Patients may need to lie down to decrease pressure on the rectal area and avoid drinking hot liquids or eating big meals, which may increase peristalsis and discomfort until the impaction can be cleared.[10]

Radiological Examination

Bowel obstruction may be diagnosed on the basis of a plain abdominal x-ray, but contrast may help identify the site and extent of the obstruction. Barium is not recommended because it may interfere with additional studies.[33]

Surgical Intervention

A percentage of cancer patients may experience nonmalignant obstruction.[35] Therefore, assuming the obstruction is related to worsening cancer may prevent the health care team from setting realistic treatment goals. A thorough assessment should be done, with attention to poor prognostic factors.[15,38] These factors historically include general medical condition or poor nutritional status, ascites, palpable abdominal masses or distant metastases, previous radiation to the abdomen or pelvis, combination chemotherapy, and multiple small-bowel obstructions.[35]

A study on the palliative benefit of surgery for bowel obstruction in advanced ovarian cancer found that surgical intervention provided successful palliation in 51% of the patients studied.[38] Four prognostic factors for the probable success of palliative surgery were found: (1) absence of palpable abdominal or pelvic masses, (2) volume of ascites less than 3 liters, (3) unifocal obstruction, and (4) preoperative weight loss less than 9 kg. Sixty-eight percent of the patients survived longer than 60 days and recovered enough to be able to return home.[38]

Surgical interventions can involve resection and reanastomosis, decompression, either colostomy or ileostomy, gastroenterostomy or ileotransverse colostomy, or lysis of adhesions.[15,33] Prospective trials need to be done to further assess the success of surgical interventions and their effect on the quality as well as the quantity of life.[38] Gastrostomy has been shown to be well tolerated for moderate to long-term decompression.[33]

Surgical intervention should be a decision made between patient and physician within the established goals of care. The patient's right to self-determination is essential. As patient advocates, our role is to educate the patient and family. Helping them to understand physician recommendations, as well as considering their personal desires and options in an effort to develop the treatment plan, is essential. Surgical resection for obstructing cancers of the GI tract, pancreatic, or biliary tracts was found to have a 3- to 7-month survival.[34] This study pointed out the importance of nutritional status at baseline and assessment of performance status for its relationship to "reasonable quality of life."[34] The important conclusion of these studies was to leave the decision to operate with the patient. Mortality is possible. The need for additional surgeries remains high due to recurrence of the obstruction, wound infections, sepsis and further obstruction.[33] Survival rates with each subsequent surgery lessen.

Alternative Interventions

Nasogastric or nasointestinal tubes have been used to decompress the bowel and/or stomach. Use of these interventions, although uncomfortable for the patient, has been suggested for symptom relief while evaluating the possibility of surgery. Venting gastrostomy or jejunostomy can be a relatively easy alternative, which is especially effective for severe nausea and vomiting. It can be placed percutaneously with sedation and local anesthesia. Patients can then be fed a liquid diet, with the tube clamped for as long as tolerated without nausea or vomiting.[16]

Symptom Therapy

Providing aggressive pharmacological management of the distressing symptoms associated with malignant bowel obstruction (MBO) can prevent the need for surgical intervention.[15] The symptoms of intestinal colic, vomiting, and diarrhea can be effectively controlled with medications for most patients.

Depending on the location of the obstruction, either high or low, symptom severity can be affected. As accumulation of secretions increases, abdominal pain also increases. Distention, vomiting, and prolonged constipation occur. With high obstruction, onset of vomiting is sooner and amounts are larger. Intermittent borborygmi and visible peristalsis may occur.[32,33] Patients may experience colic pain on top of continuous pain from a growing mass. In chronic bowel obstruction, colic pain subsides.

As stated above, the goal of treatment is to prevent obstruction whenever possible. The use of subcutaneous (SQ) or intravenous (IV) analgesics, anticholinergic drugs, and antiemetic drugs can be effective for reducing the symptoms of inoperable and hard-to-manage obstruction.[38] Octreotide may be an option in early management to prevent partial obstructions from becoming complete.[32] Although octreotide is used for diarrhea because it decreases peristalsis, it also slows the irregular and ineffective peristaltic movements of obstruction, reducing the activity and balancing out the intestinal movement.[22,32] It reduces vomiting because it inhibits the secretion of gastrin, secretin, vasoactive intestinal peptide, pancreatic polypeptide, insulin, and glucagon. Octreotide directly blocks the secretion of gastric acid, pepsin, pancreatic enzyme, bicarbonate, intestinal epithelial electrolytes, and water.[22,38] It has been shown to be effective in 70% of patients for the control of vomiting.[15] Octreotide is administered by SQ infusion or SQ injection every 12 hours. A negative aspect of this drug is its cost. It is expensive and requires SQ injections or SQ or IV infusions over days to weeks. The recommended starting dose is 0.3 mg/day and may increase to 0.6 mg/day.[15] Hyoscine butylbromide is thought to be as effective as octreotide at reducing GI secretions and motility. Hyoscine butylbromide is less sedating since it is thought to cross the blood–brain barrier less due to its low lipid solubility.[40] A recent study compared octreotide and scopolamine butylbromide for inoperable bowel obstruction with nasogastric tubes.[42] Both medications relieve colicky pain; both reduce the continuous abdominal pain and distention. Although this was a small study done over 3 days, they were able to remove the nasogastric tube in three of the seven patients on the first dose of octreotide 0.3 mg/day subcutaneously; three more patients were able to have the nasogastric tube removed when the dose was doubled to 0.6 mg/day. Scopolamine was similar in results, but the octreotide regimen was felt to be overall more effective. The negative effect is associated with the cost of drug; a definite consideration for overall quality of life. Scopolamine is less expensive.

Analgesic Medications

Opioid medications have been used to relieve pain associated with obstruction.[15] Providing the opioid through SQ or IV infusion via a patient-controlled analgesic (PCA) pump is beneficial for two reasons: patients may receive improved pain relief over the oral route due to improved absorption, and by giving access to a PCA pump, patients are allowed some control over their pain management. Alternative routes of opioid administration, such as rectal or transdermal, may also be effective but usually are inadequate if the pain is severe or unstable or there are frequent episodes of breakthrough pain.

Antiemetic Medications

Some antiemetic medications can also be given SQ and combined with an opioid.[15] Haloperidol (Haldol) is the classic first-line antiemetic.[37] Phenothiazine, butyrophenone, and antihistamine antiemetics are the most helpful. Recent additions of the selective serotonin antagonists, the 5-hydroxytryptamine blockers (5-HT_3) have made a significant difference in the treatment of nausea, especially when combined with corticosteroids for chemotherapy-induced nausea (see also Chapter 9).[41] Metoclopramide at 10 mg q 4 hours is the drug of choice for patients with incomplete bowel obstruction.[37] It stimulates the stomach to empty its contents into the reservoir of the bowel. Once complete obstruction is present, metoclopramide is discontinued and haloperidol or another antiemetic medication is started. Haloperidol is less sedating than other antiemetic or antihistamine medications.[16,37] The usual dose ranges from 5 to 15 mg/day, and at some institutions, it is combined with cyclizine.[16] Corticosteroids are particularly helpful antiemetics, especially when related to chemotherapy.[37]

In practice, it is recommended that morphine, haloperidol, and hyoscine butylbromide be given together by continuous SQ infusion. If pain or colic increases, the dose of morphine and hyoscine butylbromide should be increased; if emesis increases, increase the haloperidol dose.[16]

Fluid and nutrient intake should be maintained as tolerated. Usually, patients whose vomiting has improved will tolerate fluids with small, low-residue meals. Dry mouth is managed with ice chips, although this has been suspected to wash out saliva that is present in the mouth. The use of artificial saliva may be more beneficial.[16]

Corticosteroid Medications. Corticosteroids have been helpful as antiemetic medications. The recommended dose of dexamethasone is between 6 and 16 mg/day; the prednisolone dose starts at 50 mg/day (injection or SQ infusion).[15] Twycross and Lack[4] recommend starting with 4 mg bid for 5 days, then decreasing to 4 mg daily. One possible side effect to this medication is oral candidiasis.[37]

Antispasmodic Medications

Colic pain results from increased peristalsis against the resistance of a mechanical obstruction. Analgesics alone may not be effective. Hyoscine butylbromide has been used to relieve spasm-like pain and to reduce emesis.[16] Dosing starts at 60 mg/day and increases up to 380 mg/day given by SQ infusion.[40] Side effects are related to the anticholinergic effects, including tachycardia, dry mouth, sedation, and hypotension.[40]

Laxative Medications

Stimulant laxatives are contraindicated due to increased peristalsis against an obstruction. Stool-softening medications may be helpful if there is only a single obstruction in the colon or rectum. If the obstruction is in the small bowel, laxatives will not be of benefit.[16]

Antidiarrheal Medications

Patients who experience a subacute obstruction or a fecal fistula may complain of diarrhea. Antidiarrheal medicine, such as codeine or loperamide, may be helpful. The benefit of these medications is that they may also help to relieve pain and colic. Octreotide may be helpful with bowel obstruction due to its mechanism of action. By inhibiting the release of certain secretions of the gastric, biliary, and intestine, intestinal motility decreases and increases absorption of water and electrolytes.[33]

Helping families cope with symptoms associated with obstruction is important. Historically, the management of obstruction involved aggressive surgical intervention or symptom management alone. The initial assessment should include: (1) evaluating constipation, (2) evaluating for surgery, (3) providing pain management, and (4) managing nausea with metoclopramide. If incomplete obstruction, use dexamethasone, haloperidol, dimenhydrinate, chlorpromazine, or hyoscine butylbromide.[37] The introduction of new medications, such as octreotide, and newer antiemetics has made a difference in the quality of life a patient with a malignant bowel obstruction may experience. The important thing to remember is that the treatment plan must always be in agreement with the patient's wishes. Discussing the patient's understanding of the situation and the options available are essential to effective and thoughtful care of bowel obstruction in the palliative care patient.

ASCITES

Ascites associated with malignancy results from a combination of impaired fluid efflux and increased fluid influx.[42] Ascites may be divided into three different types. Central ascites is the result of tumor-invading hepatic parenchyma, resulting in compression of the portal venous and/or the lymphatic system.[44] There is a decrease in oncotic pressure as a result of limited protein intake and the catabolic state associated with cancer.[44] Peripheral ascites is related to deposits of tumor cells found on the surface of the parietal or visceral peritoneum. The result is a mechanical interference with venous and/or lymphatic drainage.[44] There is blockage at the level of the peritoneal space rather than the liver parenchyma. Macrophages increase capillary permeability and contribute to greater ascites. Mixed-type ascites is a combination of central and peripheral ascites. Therefore, there is both compression of the portal venous and lymphatic systems, as well as tumor cells in the peritoneum. Chylous malignant ascites occurs when tumor infiltration of the retroperitoneal space causes obstruction of lymph flow through the lymph nodes and/or the pancreas.[44] Additional sources of ascites not related to malignancy include the following:

- Preexisting advanced liver disease with portal hypertension
- Portal venous thrombosis
- Congestive heart failure
- Nephrotic syndrome
- Pancreatitis
- Tuberculosis
- Hepatic venous obstruction
- Bowel perforation

Severe ascites is associated with poor prognosis (40% 1-year survival, less than 10% 3-year survival).[44] The pathological mechanisms of malignant ascites make the prevention or reduction of abdominal fluid accumulation difficult.[45] Invasive management of ascites is seen as appropriate whenever possible, in contrast to intestinal obstruction. Although survival is limited, the effects of ascites on the patient's quality of life warrant an aggressive approach.[45]

Tumor types most associated with ascites include ovarian, endometrial, breast, colon, gastric, and pancreatic cancers.[44,45] Less common sources of ascites include mesothelioma, non-Hodgkin's lymphoma, prostate cancer, multiple myeloma, and melanoma.[44]

Assessment of Ascites

Symptoms Associated with Ascites

Patients complain of abdominal bloating and pain. Initially, patients complain of feeling a need for larger-waisted clothing and notice an increase in belt size or weight. They may feel nauseated and have a decreased appetite. Many patients will complain of increased symptoms of reflux or heartburn. Pronounced ascites can cause dyspnea and orthopnea due to increased pressure on the diaphragm.[44,45]

Physical Examination

The physical examination may reveal abdominal or inguinal hernia, scrotal edema, and abdominal venous engorgement. Radiological findings show a hazy picture, with distended and separate loops of the bowel. There is a poor definition of the abdominal organs and loss of the psoas muscle shadows. Ultrasound and computed tomographic scans may also be used to diagnose ascites.[44]

Management of Ascites

Traditionally, treatment of ascites is palliative due to decreased prognosis.[44] Ovarian cancer is one of the few types where the presence of ascites does not necessarily correlate with a poor prognosis. In this case, survival rate can be improved through surgical intervention and adjuvant therapy.[45]

Medical Therapy

Advanced liver disease is associated with central ascites. There is an increase in renal sodium and water retention. Therefore, restricting sodium intake to 100 µmol/day or less along with fluid restriction for patients with moderate to severe hyponatremia (125 µmol/L) may be beneficial. Using potassium-sparing diuretics is also important. Spironolactone (100 to 400 mg/day) is the drug of choice.[44] Furosemide is also helpful at 40 to 80 mg/day to initiate diuresis. Over-diuresis must be avoided. Over-diuresis may precipitate electrolyte imbalance, hepatic encephalopathy, and prerenal failure. The above regimen of fluid and sodium reduction and diuretics may work for mixed-type ascites, which results from compression of vessels related to tumor and peripheral tumor cells of the parietal or visceral peritoneum as well. Because mixed-type ascites is associated with chylous fluid, adding changes to the diet, such as decreased fat intake and increased medium-chain triglycerides, may be important. Chylous ascites results from tumor infiltration of the retroperitoneal space, causing obstruction of lymphatic flow.[44]

Medium-chain triglyceride oil (Lipisorb) can be used as a calorie source in these patients. Because the lymph system is bypassed, the shorter fatty acid chains are easier to digest. For patients with refractory ascites and a shortened life expectancy, paracentesis may be the most appropriate therapy.[46]

Paracentesis for tense ascites associated with cirrhosis or nonmalignant ascites has been shown to shorten hospitalization by 60%.[43] Multiple studies have found that removing 4 to 6 liters/day was a safe and effective treatment.[47] This treatment has been altered to include albumin infusions, which prevent hypovolemia and renal impairment, as well as hyponatremia.[44]

It is recommended that a maximum of 6 liters of ascites fluid be taken off. This can be a safe and effective way to promptly relieve patients of discomfort associated with ascites and to improve quality of life.[43,44]

Peritoneovenous shunts (Denver or LeVeen shunt) are helpful for the removal of ascites in 75% to 85% of patients.[44] These shunts are used primarily for nonmalignant ascites. The shunt removes fluid from the site, and the fluid is shunted up into the internal jugular vein.[44]

Nursing Management

Ascites management involves initially understanding the mechanism, then using interventions appropriately. The reality of recurring ascites requiring repeated paracentesis is present. Acknowledging the risk/benefit ratio of repeated paracentesis is essential, especially in palliative care. Nurses need to remember good supportive care in addition to other resources. These include skin care, to help prevent breakdown, and comfort interventions, such as pillow support, and loose clothing whenever possible. Educating the patient and caregivers on the rationale behind fluid and sodium restrictions when necessary can help their understanding and compliance. The cycle of a patient who feels thirsty, receives IV fluids, and has more discomfort is difficult for the patient to understand. Careful explanations about why an intervention is or is not recommended can go a long way toward improving the quality of life for these patients.

REFERENCES

1. Levy MH. Constipation and diarrhea in cancer patients. Cancer Bull 1991;43:412–422.
2. McMillan SC. Assessing and managing narcotic-induced constipation in adults with cancer. Cancer Control 1999;6:198–204.
3. Massey RL, Haylock PJ, Curtiss C. Constipation. In: Yarbro CH, Frogge MH, Goodman M. eds. Cancer Symptom Management, Vol. 3. Boston: Jones and Bartlett, 2004:512–527.
4. Twycross RG, Lack SA. Diarrhea. In: Control of Alimentary Symptoms in Far Advanced Cancer. New York: Churchill Livingstone, 1986:208–229.
5. Agency for Health Care Policy and Research. In: Management of Cancer Pain (AHCPR Guidelines), AHCPR Publication 94-0592. Washington DC: US Department of Health and Human Services, 1994.
6. Faigel, DO. A clinical approach to constipation. Clin Cornerstone 2002;4:11–21.
7. Devroede G. Constipation. In: Sleisenger MH, Fordtran JS, eds. Gastrointestinal Disease. Philadelphia: WB Saunders, 1989: 331–381.
8. Sykes NP. A clinical comparison of laxatives in a hospice. Palliat Med 1991;5:307–314.
9. Sykes NP. A volunteer model for the comparison of laxatives in opioid-related constipation. J Pain Symptom Manage 1996; 11:363–369.
10. Bisanz A. Managing bowel elimination problems in patients with cancer. Oncol Nurs Forum 1997;24:679–688.
11. Cimprich B. Symptom management: constipation. Cancer Nurs 1985;8(suppl 1):39–43.
12. McMillan SC, Williams FA. Validity and reliability of the constipation assessment scale. Cancer Nurs 1989;12:183–188.
13. Radbruch L, Sabatowski R, Loick G, Kolbe C, Kasper M, Grond S, Lehmann KA. Constipation and the use of laxatives: a comparison between TDF & oral morphine. Palliat Med 2000; 13:159–160.
14. Adler HF, Atkinson AJ, Ivy AC. Effect of morphine and Dilaudid on the ileum and of morphine, Dilaudid and atropine on the colon of man. Arch Intern Med 1942;69:974–985.
15. Sykes NP. Constipation and diarrhea. In: Doyle D, Hanks GWC, Cherny N, Calman K., eds. Oxford Textbook of Palliative Medicine, Vol 3. New York: Oxford University Press, 2004:483–495.
16. Baines MJ. The pathophysiology and management of malignant intestinal obstruction. In: Doyle D, Hanks GWC, MacDonald N, eds. Oxford Textbook of Palliative Medicine, Vol 2. New York: Oxford University Press, 1998:526–534.
17. Lederle FA, Busch DL, Mattox KM, West MJ, Aske DM. Cost-effective treatment of constipation in the elderly: a randomized double-blind comparison of sorbitol and lactulose. Am J Med 1990;89:597–601.
18. Wilkes GM, Ingwersen K, Barton-Burke M. Oncology Nursing Drug Handbook. Boston: Jones and Bartlett, 2003:905–906.
19. Culpepper-Morgan JA, Inturrisi CE, Portenoy RK, et al. Treatment of opioid-induced constipation with oral naloxone: a pilot study. Clin Pharmacol Ther 1992;52:90–95.

20. Viele CS. Overview of chemotherapy-induced diarrhea. Semin Oncol Nurs 2003;19(suppl 3):2–5.
21. Gwede CK. Overview of radiation and chemoradiation-induced diarrhea. Semin Oncol Nurs 2003;19(suppl 3):6–10.
22. Stern J, Ippoliti C. Management of acute cancer treatment-induced diarrhea. Semin Oncol Nurs 2003;19(suppl 3):11–16.
23. Lowell A. New strategies for the prevention and reduction of cancer treatment-induced diarrhea. Semin Oncol Nurs 2003; 19(suppl 3):17–21.
24. Engelking C. Diarrhea. In: Yarbro CH, Frogge MH, Goodman M. eds. Cancer Symptom Management Vol. 3, Boston: Jones and Bartlett, 2004:528–557.
25. Weihofen DL, Marino C. Cancer Survival Cookbook, p 28. Los Angeles: John Wiley & Sons, 1998.
26. Barbounis V, Koumakis G, Vassilomanolakis M, et al. Control of irinotecan-induced diarrhea by octreotide after loperamide failure. Support Care Cancer 2001;9:258–260.
27. Aviv RI, Shyamalan G, Watkinson A, Tibballs J, Ogunbaye G. Radiological palliation of malignant colonic obstruction. Clin Radiol 2002;57:347–351.
28. Camunez F, Echenagusia A, Gonzalo S, Turegano F, Vazquez J, Barreiro-Meiro I. Malignant colorectal obstruction treated by means of self-expanding metallic stents: effectiveness before surgery and in palliation. Radiology 2000;216:492–497.
29. Cello JP, Grendell JH, Basuk P, et al. Effect of octreotide on refractory AIDS-associated diarrhea: a prospective, multicenter clinical trial. Ann Intern Med 1991;115:705–710.
30. Rutledge DN, Engelking C. Cancer-related diarrhea: selected findings of a national survey of oncology nurse experiences. Oncol Nurs Forum 1998;25:861–872.
31. Ippoliti C, Neumann J. Octreotide in the management of diarrhea induced by graft versus host disease. Oncol Nurs Forum 1998;25:873–878.
32. Mercadante S, Kargar J, Nicološi G. Octreotide may prevent definitive intestinal obstruction. J Pain Symptom Manage 1997; 13:352–355.
33. Ripamonti C, Mercadante S. Pathophysiology and management of malignant bowel obstruction. In: Doyle D, Hanks GWC, Cherny N, Calman K., eds. Oxford Textbook of Palliative Medicine, Vol. 3. New York: Oxford University Press, 2004: 496–507.
34. Clarke-Pearson DL, Chin NO, DeLong ER, Rice R, Creasman WT. Surgical management of intestinal obstruction in ovarian cancer. Gynecol Oncol 1987;26:11–18.
35. Turnbull ADM, Guerra J, Starnes HF. Results of surgery for obstructing carcinomatosis of gastrointestinal, pancreatic, or biliary origin. J Clin Oncol 1989;7:381–386.
36. Jong P, Sturgeon J, Jamieson CG. Benefit of palliative surgery for bowel obstruction in advanced ovarian cancer. J Crit Care 1995;38:454–457.
37. Fainsinger RL, Spachynski K, Hanson J, Bruera E. Symptom control in terminally ill patients with malignant bowel obstruction. J Pain Symptom Manage 1994;9:12–18.
38. Mercadante S, Maddaloni S. Octreotide in the management of inoperable gastrointestinal obstruction in terminal cancer patients. J Pain Symptom Manage 1992;7:496–498.
39. Forgas I, Macpherson A, Tibbs C. Percutaneous endoscopic gastrostomy. The end of the line for nasogastric feeding? Br Med J 1992;304:1395–1396.
40. DeConno F, Caraceni A, Zecca E, Spoldi E, Ventafridda V. Continuous subcutaneous infusion of hyoscine butylbromide reduces secretions in patients with gastrointestinal obstruction. J Pain Symptom Manage 1991;6:484–486.
41. Osoba D, MacDonald N. Principles governing the use of of cancer chemotherapy in palliative care. In: Oxford Textbook of Palliative Medicine, Doyle D, Hanks G, MacDonald N, eds. Vol. 2. Oxford: Oxford University Press, 1998:249–267.
42. Ripamont C, Mercadante S, Groff L, Zecca E, DeConno F, Casuccio A. Role of octreotide, scopolamine butylbromide, and hydration in symptom control of patients with inoperable bowel obstruction and nasogastric tubes: a prospective randomization trial. J Pain Symptom Manage 2000;19:23–34.
43. Lee CW, Bociek G, Faught W. A survey of practice in management of malignant ascites. J Pain Symptom Manage 1998; 16:96–101.
44. Kichian K, Bain VG. Jaundice, ascites, and hepatic encephalopathy. In: Doyle D, Hanks G, Cherny N, Calman K, eds. Oxford Textbook of Palliative Medicine, Vol 2. Oxford: Oxford University Press, 2004:507–520.
45. Mercadante S, La Rosa S, Nicolosi G, Garofalo SL. Temporary drainage of symptomatic malignant ascites by a catheter inserted under computerized tomography. J Pain Symptom Manage 1998; 15:374–378.
46. Abrahm J. Promoting symptom control in palliative care. Semin Oncol Nurs 1998;14:95–109.
47. Runyon B. Paracentesis of ascitic fluid: a safe procedure. Arch Intern Med 1986;146:2259–2261.
48. Panos M, Moore K, Vlavianos P, et al. Single, total paracentesis for tense ascites: sequential hemodynamic changes and right atrial size. Hepatology 1990;11:662–667.
49. Hogan CM. The nurse's role with diarrhea management. Oncol Nurs Forum 1998;25:879–886.
50. Walsh TB. Constipation. In Symptom Control, Walsh TD, ed. Cambridge, MA: Blackwell Scientific, 1989:69–80.

12

Pamela Kedziera and Nessa Coyle

Hydration, Thirst, and Nutrition

I don't feel like pushing him any more [to eat]. He's had a long fight and its time to rest. It's not a failure.—A dying patient's wife

- ***Key Points***
- *Advances in health care have changed the trajectory of dying and the way people die.*
- *The last year of life for someone with a progressive debilitating disease is frequently associated with multiple distressing symptoms, comorbidities, and loss of independent function.*
- *Difficulties with eating and drinking are common during this period.*
- *Decisions regarding hydration and nutrition are confronted by patients, families, and staff at this time.*
- *Discussions regarding artificial hydration and nutrition are frequently couched in terms of ethics, religious beliefs, and strongly held personal views.*
- *Nurses need to know their state laws concerning provision of artificial hydration and nutrition in the dying patient.*
- *Decisions regarding hydration and nutrition at end of life are guided by goals of care, benefit versus burden, and the wishes of the patient and family.*
- *Patients have the right to refuse hydration and nutrition, whether parenteral or oral.*

There is lack of consensus either in society or among experts as to whether it is physically, psychologically, socially, or ethically appropriate to provide artificial hydration and nutrition to a terminally ill person. Do these therapies improve the way an individual feels physically and emotionally? Do they cause harm? Can an individual die comfortably without these interventions? Decisions are usually made on the basis of whether the intervention will make the patient more comfortable and whether it will honor his or her wishes. These elements are illustrated in the following two case reports.

CASE STUDY

Two Patients Receiving Total Parenteral Nutrition

Mrs. S was a 70-year-old woman with advanced uterine cancer. She was a Holocaust survivor, as was her husband. Receiving and giving food were all-important to them both. Mrs. S was obstructed, had a draining percutaneous endoscopic gastrostomy tube, and was unable to take food by mouth. Total parenteral nutrition (TPN), which had originally been started as nutritional support during intensive chemotherapy, became an expression of nurturing and life in both their minds, when the focus of care became directed toward end-of-life care. Although discontinuing chemotherapy had been a difficult transition for the patient and family, to discontinue TPN was inconceivable. This attitude continued until the end of life. The patient continued to receive TPN up until the time of her death. The deep-seated horror of living through the Holocaust and the deprivation of food they had experienced strongly affected this patient and her family's unshakeable belief that food and water must be given until death.

A contrasting situation is illustrated through a man in his 40s, dying of gastric cancer, who had received TPN for nutritional support during chemotherapy. Administration of TPN had repeatedly been associated with increased pain. The patient had been willing to tolerate the increased pain when the goal of care was prolongation of life. After this goal was no longer possible, the patient associated the TPN with diminished quality of life and asked that it be discontinued.

The meaning of food and water, and the meaning of discontinuing food and water, need careful exploration and ongoing discussion of the benefits and burden for each individual. There are no absolutes. Nurses have reported that patients knowingly refuse food and fluids to hasten death.[1] The following pages provide basic information on hydration and nutrition as a framework for the nurse when guiding a patient and family who are considering the benefits and burdens of artificial hydration and nutrition in the setting of advanced, progressive disease. In addition, the following questions are explored: What are the current practices with regard to managing hydration at the end of life, and how are these clinical strategies justified? What problems and benefits are associated with fluid and electrolyte imbalance? How is dehydration clinically recognized? Should dehydration at end of life be treated and if so, how?

HYDRATION

Water is an essential component of the human body. Complex cellular functions, such as protein synthesis and metabolism of nutrients, are affected by hydration status. The maintenance of hydration depends on a balance between intake and output, which is regulated by neuroendocrine influences. Homeostasis is maintained through parallel neuroendocrine activity on excretion of fluid via the kidneys[2] and on intake via thirst. Increased osmotic pressure is the prime stimulus for thirst, stimulating the release of vasopressin. Renal excretion is mainly dependent on the action of vasopressin, which is secreted by the posterior pituitary gland. This hormone, known as antidiuretic hormone (ADH), increases water reabsorption in the collecting ducts of the kidneys.[3] Thirst stimuli include hypertonicity; depletion of the extracellular fluid compartment arising from vomiting, diarrhea, or hemorrhage; and renal failure, in which plasma sodium is low but plasma renin levels are high.[4]

Dehydration

Dehydration is a loss of normal body water. There are several types of dehydration.[3,5] *Isotonic* dehydration results from a balanced loss of water and sodium. This occurs during a complete fast and during episodes of vomiting and diarrhea with the loss of water and electrolytes in the gastric contents. Billings[6] theorized that terminally ill individuals have this type of balanced decrease in food and fluid intake, causing eunatremic dehydration (sodium levels in normal range) because of the simultaneous loss of salt and water. *Hypertonic* dehydration occurs if water losses are greater than sodium losses. Fever can cause this problem, by loss of water through the lungs and skin and a limited ability to take in oral fluids. *Hypotonic* dehydration occurs when sodium loss exceeds water loss. This typically occurs when water is consumed but food is not. Overuse of diuretics is a major factor. Osmotic diuresis (e.g., from hyperglycemia), salt-wasting renal conditions, third spacing (ascites), and adrenal insufficiency are other common causes of sodium loss.[7]

The methodology for assessing dehydration has not been well studied and tends to vary among practitioners. The clinical sensitivity of each method has not been determined. Clinical assessment should include mental status changes, thirst, oral/parenteral intake, urine output, and fluid loss. Physical findings, weight loss, dry mouth, dry tongue, reduced skin turgor, and postural hypotension should be noted. Laboratory test findings, including increased hematocrit, elevated serum sodium concentration, azotemia with a disproportionate rise in blood urea nitrogen in relation to creatinine, concentrated urine, and hyperosmolarity, are indicative of dehydration.

Physical findings (Table 12–1) are complicated to evaluate.[7] Comorbid conditions can be the cause of many of these symptoms in the chronically or terminally ill individual. Dry mouth, for example, can be associated with mouth breathing or anticholinergic medication. Skin turgor can be hard to evaluate in the cachexic individual and is unreliable. Obtaining weights may be impractical, but rapid weight loss of greater than 3% is indicative of dehydration.[5] Postural hypotension can be related to medications and cardiac pathology. Confusion is common in the patient with advanced cancer and may have many causes, including the disease state itself. Thirst may be absent or mild in patients with hyponatremic dehydration, although marked volume loss may stimulate ADH and water craving.

There is evidence that elderly individuals do not perceive thirst in the same manner as healthy young adults.[4] In a study comparing the role of thirst sensation and drinking behavior in young versus older adults, water was restricted for 24 hours. Only the young, healthy study group reported a dry, unpleasant mouth and a general sense of thirst; the healthy elders had a deficit in the awareness of thirst despite plasma osmolarity and sodium and vasopressin concentrations that were greater than those in the younger group. During the rehydration period, the younger group consumed enough fluid to correct their laboratory values. Elder subjects did not consume enough fluid to correct the laboratory values.[8] There is not, however, any evidence to support this observation in terminally ill patients. In hypernatremia, thirst is a powerful stimulus, and persons with access to water usually will take in sufficient amounts of fluid. Confused or somnolent individuals and those who are unable to drink are at risk because water losses may not be adequately replaced. Dehydrated, terminally ill patients usually present with mixed disorders of fluid and salt loss.

Dehydration causes confusion and restlessness in patients with nonterminal disease. These same symptoms are frequently reported in terminally ill persons and could be aggravated by dehydration.[9] Reduced intravascular volume caused

Table 12–1
Signs and Symptoms of Dehydration

Hyponatremic Dehydration	Hypernatremic Dehydration	Isotonic Dehydration
Volume depletion	Thirst	Morose
Anorexia, taste alteration, and weight loss	Fatigue	Aggression
Nausea and vomiting	Muscle weakness	Demoralized
Diminished skin turgor	Mental status changes	Apathetic
Dry mucous membranes	Fever	Uncoordinated
Reduced sweat		
Orthostatic hypotension		
Lethargy and restlessness		
Delirium		
Seizures (related to cerebral edema)		
Confusion, stupor and coma		
Psychosis (rare)		
Laboratory Results		
Azotemia	Increased sodium	Minor or no abnormalities
Disproportionate blood urea nitrogen compared to creatinine		
Hyponatremia		
Hemoconcentration		
Urine osmolarity with sodium concentration		

by dehydration can result in renal failure. Opioid metabolite accumulation can result from renal failure and cause confusion, myoclonus, and seizures.[10] Dehydration has been associated with an increased risk of bedsores and constipation, particularly in the elderly. Discomfort, especially problems with xerostomia and thirst, may result from dehydration.[11]

Dehydration may improve physical caregiving for some patients. For example, urinary catheters may be avoided if the frequency of urination decreases. With dehydration, there is less gastrointestinal fluid, with fewer bouts of vomiting, and a reduction in pulmonary secretions, with less coughing, choking, and need for suctioning. Some palliative care clinicians suggest that dehydration at the end of life causes suffering in some patients, which should be relieved. This suffering may include thirst, dry mouth, fatigue, nausea, vomiting, confusion, muscle cramps, and perhaps the hastening of death.[12,13] Dehydration as a cause of renal failure has been well documented.[14,15] A study of terminally ill cancer patients, however, showed that the group receiving intravenous fluids at a rate of 1 to 2 L/day consistently had more abnormal laboratory values of serum sodium, urea, and osmolarity than the group who were not hydrated.[16]

A study of 82 patients in the last 2 days before death showed no statistically significant relationship between the level of hydration, respiratory tract secretions, dry mouth, and thirst.[17] The researchers concluded that artificial hydration to alleviate symptoms may be futile. These results contrast with those of a study of 100 palliative care patients receiving hypodermoclysis; researchers in the latter investigation concluded that this therapy was useful for achieving better symptom control.[18] An anecdotal study of three patients being hydrated by hypodermoclysis reported that hydration may have contributed to improved cognitive function and allowed patients to deal with end-of-life issues.[19]

Some experts suggest that hydration may relieve symptoms other than thirst, such as confusion and restlessness.[14] Still others who have looked at the issue of dehydration-related suffering have stressed the role of inappropriate medical interventions that cause their own problems. They contend that hydrating a patient can be associated with repetitive needlesticks, decreased mobility, increased secretions, increased edema, and possibly congestive heart failure.[20,21] It is also suggested that improving the cognition of a dying patient with pain may make the patient more aware of the pain, with the possiblity of decreasing cognition once more through increased opioid requirements. Others state that comatose patients feel no symptoms; fluids may prolong dying, and dehydration may act as an anesthetic.[14]

In a descriptive study of symptoms of dehydration in the terminally ill, no association was found between fluid intake, serum sodium, osmolality, blood urea nitrogen, and symptom severity.[12] A survey of Swiss physicians found that there was no consensus with respect to the assessment of "suffering" from dehydration or thirst. The physicians who chose artificial hydration were more likely to perceive suffering and thirst as serious problems. Two thirds of the doctors did not believe that artificial hydration was the best way to respond to terminal dehydration.[22]

The decision to use artificial means of hydration comes more from tradition than from science. To avoid unnecessary interventions in the course of the dying process, some practitioners have avoided artificial fluid replacement secondary to its perceived negative effects. Their conclusion, that artificial hydration may cause harm to some dying patients, keeps them from offering this therapy. Palliative care clinicians have noted that some individuals are more comfortable without artificial fluids, which may prolong the dying process, whereas others are more comfortable when artificial hydration is used. Emotional issues are often the driving force in the decision to provide or withdraw artificial hydration. The need to provide fluids may be directed by very strong cultural, religious, and/or moral convictions on the part of patients, families, and some caregivers even if there is no certainty that the therapy does provide comfort.

Screening for Dehydration, Management, and Assessing the Effects of Interventions

Screening for dehydration in the palliative care setting may include recording intake and output, examining skin turgor and mucous membranes, and monitoring mental status and blood pressure. Subjective reports of fatigue, muscle weakness, anorexia, and taste alteration are correlated with these signs and laboratory values (see Table 12–1). The benefits and possible adverse effects of hydration should be discussed within a broad framework of goals of care and the wishes of the patient and family explored within that framework. Each situation has unique aspects that affect choices and the outcome of therapy. Finally, there is a need for regular reassessment to allow for changes in therapy and frequent discussions with patients and families to provide opportunities to reevaluate decisions.

The treatment of dehydration starts with a review of medications and elimination, if possible, of any agents (diuretics) that may be contributing to the dehydration. Mouth care should be provided regularly. Intervening or treating dehydration may include various routes of administration. A standard goal for fluid intake is 1500 to 3000 mL, or 8 to 10 glasses, of water daily.[7] The least invasive approach to replacing fluids is to offer liquid orally at regular intervals. For those able to swallow, this approach can help the patient as well as promote the emotional well-being of the caregivers. Those who are very weak, depressed, confused, agitated, or demented may need significant assistance in getting the fluids in on a regular basis.

The benefit/burden ratio for the patient in aggressively pursuing such a fluid intake approach must be carefully weighed. Care must be taken to avoid overhydration by a well-meaning but misdirected aggressive approach, and the patient should be monitored for new orthopnea, shortness of breath, increased emotional distress, or change in mental status. If the ability to swallow is diminished, there is a risk of aspiration and causing more distress to the patient. Small, frequent sips of fluid or ice chips can be provided. Choice of fluids should be patient driven. Some individuals find sports replacement fluids a good choice because they are easily absorbed by the stomach and can correct hypertonic dehydration.[5] Use of a fine mist spray can also help to keep mucous membranes moist.[23] Hot, humid weather conditions can add to the risk of dehydration, so the use of air conditioning and fans should be considered.

Alternative Routes of Hydration When the Oral Route Is No Longer Reliable

If there are days or weeks of life expected, and if it is appropriate to the goals of care and wishes of the patient and family, a more reliable route of fluid replacement may be chosen. Rehydration by *proctoclysis* is relatively risk-free and less expensive than parenteral means of administration.[24] Through a nasogastric tube placed rectally, tap water or saline is instilled, starting at about 100 mL/h. If there is no discomfort, leakage, or tenesmus (spasm of the anal sphincter), the rate can be increased to 400 mL/h. One liter of fluid can be instilled over 6 to 8 hours. Care must be taken, however, not to overhydrate. Side effects of this route of hydration can include pain, edema, rectal leakage of fluid, and pain during insertion of the tube. Researchers report that although proctoclysis is effective, safe, and economical, most patients prefer hypodermoclysis.[24] It is possible to foresee cultural and social reluctance to accept the rectal mode of fluid administration. In an inpatient setting, clinical staff would administer the fluids, but in a home setting, it may be impractical to use professional staff daily for this treatment. Family caregivers or patients may be uncomfortable with relatives or friends having to assume this type of care.

Standard methods for replacement of fluids can be achieved by the use of enteral feeding tubes and by parenteral methods, such as subcutaneously (hypodermoclysis) or intravenously. A feeding tube placed through the nose is often uncomfortable and may agitate the confused individual. Patients often extubate themselves when agitated. Endoscopic gastrostomy tubes have become more popular but are usually placed for decompression or feeding rather than for fluid replacement. If the individual has a feeding tube or a permanent intravenous access device (port or peripherally inserted central catheter), these may be used safely without any added burden for the patient. Placement of these devices, however, needs to be considered in the context of the overall goals of therapy.

Table 12–2
Potential Complications of Routes for Artificial Hydration

IV Peripheral	IV Central	SC Hypodermoclysis
Pain	Sepsis	Pain
Short duration of access	Hemothorax	Infection
Infection	Pneumothorax	Third spacing
Phlebitis	Central vein thrombosis	Tissue sloughing
	Catheter fragment thrombosis	Local bleeding
	Air embolus	
	Brachial plexus injury	
	Arterial laceration	

IV, intravenous; SC, subcutaneous

Hypodermoclysis (subcutaneous fluid administration) does not require special access devices. This method has the advantage over the intravenous route in people who have poor venous access. Use of this method may prevent transfer to an acute setting for line placement. Hypodermoclysis can also be initiated in the patient's home. It does not require monitoring for clotting in the line, and there is no fear of letting the line "run dry." There can be local irritation at the site of infusion, however, as well as minor bleeding. Sloughing of tissue is possible with overinfusion, and abscess formation may occur (Table 12–2). Hypotonic or isotonic solutions, with or without hyaluronidase or corticosteroids, are administered through needles inserted into the subcutaneous tissue of the abdomen or anterior or lateral thigh. Most individuals can tolerate 100 mL/h or more. Up to 1500 mL can be administered into a single site.[8,25] The following case report illustrates the use of hypodermoclysis.

CASE STUDY

Mr. G, a 55-Year-Old Man with Colon Cancer

Mr. G was a 55-year-old man with advanced colon cancer. He was obstructed and unable to take oral food or water. His goal was to remain alert and interactive with his wife and children for as long as possible. Enteral feedings were not feasible, and venous access for fluids was complicated by recurrent port and line infections. Maintaining hydration, however, was felt to be important for achieving the patient's goals. Because of the complications associated with his venous access, hypodermoclysis was chosen as the most appropriate route for fluid administration. Subcutaneous fluids at 100 mL/h were continued for the last 4 months of his life. This subcutaneous access also provided a parenteral route for opioid administration. Mr. G remained alert and interactive up until the last day of life. In this case, hypodermoclysis appeared to have been an appropriate use of technology and hydration in end-of-life care.

Replacement of fluids by the *intravenous* route is more technically complicated, and access to a competent vein must be available. Some patients have permanent-access devices, placed for therapy earlier in their treatment, that are more than adequate for this type of administration. Others may wish to have a device placed. Use of a regular intravenous line for ongoing hydration at home can be hard to maintain; if ongoing parenteral fluids are required, placement of a central catheter or peripherally inserted central catheter (PICC) line is the norm in these situations. Small, portable pumps to regulate fluid flow are available for hydration of a patient in the inpatient or home setting. Some individuals choose to run fluids via the permanent-access devices only at night. This allows for more mobility during the daylight hours. There needs to be a competent caregiver to monitor the therapy, and because caregivers accept many duties, this can be overwhelming to some.

Consensus on the appropriate volume or type of fluid replacement does not exist. Clinicians make choices based on their previous experience and knowledge of the patient's condition and wishes. Some practitioners allow the individual to have 1 L/day despite the fact that it is inadequate replacement. Considerations also include safety and reality of the care burden on all caregivers. Providing 1 L of fluid per day may only partially correct the patient's deficits, but it may relieve the emotional burden of needing to provide fluids. Administration of 1 L/day can often be worked into the patient's and family's schedule better. If fluids are given only at night, the patient may be more mobile during the day. Fluid administration can be scheduled to accommodate the goals of living. More aggressive fluid replacement requires monitoring of serum electrolytes and blood counts by regular laboratory testing. This type of approach requires monitoring of laboratory results and making adjustments every 24 to 48 hours.

Patients and family members can be taught to manage hydration techniques at home. An assessment of their concerns should precede the instruction about the actual procedures.

Adequate time must be allowed for education and return demonstration. Backup support should be provided, and repetitive sessions may be required. If possible, direct instruction to more than one caregiver should be provided, to allow them to help each other with the tasks required. Printed materials that are age and reading level appropriate should be given. In addition, video instructions can be helpful, if they are available. Follow-up visits or calls should be scheduled to assess level of functioning, to give support, and to reinforce teaching. These therapies may mean more home visits, to accommodate those who learn more slowly or are not able to master all or part of the procedure. Specific protocols vary among institutions and agencies; however, written policies and procedures should guide practice.

Dry Mouth and Thirst

Other symptoms related to dehydration can be assessed and treated. Thirst can be relieved by small amounts of fluid offered frequently. Dry mouth is treated with an intensive every-2-hour schedule of mouth care, including hygiene, lip lubrication, and ice chips or popsicles. Elimination of medications that cause dry mouth, such as tricyclic antidepressants and antihistamines, should be considered. Usually, however, the drugs that contribute to these symptoms are being administered to palliate other symptoms. Mouth breathing can also cause dry mouth. *Candida* infection, a frequent cause of dry mouth in the debilitated individual, can be treated. Agents such as pilocarpine (Salagen) can be used to increase salivation.

Whether or Not to Provide Artificial Hydration at End of Life

Controversy about providing hydration for terminally ill individuals stems from trying to balance the medical tradition of doing everything possible to heal and prolong life with the idea of allowing patients to die comfortably without unnecessary interventions. Empirical studies of clinical practice suggest that the setting of end-of-life care influences the use of artifical hydration at the end of life. Patients are more likely to receieve hydration if they are cared for in an acute care setting and are less likely to receive hydration if they are cared for in a hospice program.[26–30]

What is the role of medical intervention at the final stage of illness? In conventional medical management, dehydration is routinely avoided or reversed with fluid and electrolyte replacement. Similarly, whenever a terminal ill patient seeks to prolong life, and if the goal of care is to prolong life, maintaining hydration is accepted medical management. Conversely, if a terminally ill patient does not wish to delay death or even seeks to hasten dying, fluid replacement is generally inappropriate. Table 12–3 outlines the principles of ethical decision-making in regard to artificial hydration and nutrition in the terminally ill. Table 12–4 illustrates four clinical scenarios or paradigm cases that the nurse may encounter while caring for the terminally ill and that influence clinical decision-making.

Dehydration may aggravate or alleviate the discomfort of terminal disease (Table 12–5).[6] Current research does not clearly guide practice. Dehydration causes unpleasant symptoms, such

Table 12–3
Hydration and Nutrition in the Terminally Ill: Guiding Principles of Ethical Decision Making

- Everything in the terminal phase of an irreversible illness should be decided on the basis of whether it will make the patient more comfortable and whether it will honor his or her wishes.
- Treatments are evaluated principally according to their consequences—benefits and burdens, physical, psychosocial, and spiritual—weighed within the patient's value framework.
- Dehydration per se does not require treatment, but symptoms associated with dehydration do require palliation.
- When a patient is unable to express his or her wishes, advance directives or input from the health care proxy is followed.
- Although the focus is the patient, attention to the concerns and distress of the family is essential.

Table 12–4
Nutrition and Hydration at the End of Life: Four Paradigm Cases

Paradigm case 1

The dying patient who becomes too weak or too obtunded to maintain normal fluid intake, who will die soon but may die less comfortably and perhaps more quickly without rehydration.

Paradigm case 2

The terminally ill cancer patient who has an inoperable intestinal obstruction, feels hungry, and wants to be fed.

Paradigm case 3

The terminally ill patient whose inability to take oral food or fluid is precipitated by, or partially the result of, palliative medical management; for example, the patient who is sedated in an attempt to manage a refractory symptom such as pain, dyspnea, or agitated delirium.

Paradigm case 4

The dying patient who voluntarily stops eating and drinking in order to hasten death.

Table 12–5
Hydration and Rehydration at the End of Life: Potential Effects

Body System	Effects of Dehydration	Effects of Rehydration
General appearance	Sunken eyes	Improved appearance
Mouth	Decreased saliva	Oral comfort
	Thirst	Relief of thirst
	Bad taste	Improved taste
	Dry, cracked lips	
Pulmonary	Dry airway, viscous secretions	Facilitates productive cough
	Reduced death rattle	Easier suctioning
	Reduced secretions, cough	
	Reduced congestion, wheezing, dyspnea, pleural effusions	
Gastrointestinal tract	Constipation	More normal bowel function
	Decreased secretions	
	Less vomiting, diarrhea	
	Anorexia	
	Reduced ascites	Ascites
Urinary tract	Reduced renal function	Improved renal drug clearance
	Edema	Reduced toxic metabolites
	Possible drug accumulation	May need more drug administration

Source: Billings (1998), reference 6.

as confusion and restlessness, in nonterminally ill patients. These problems are common in the dying. Dehydration can cause renal failure with an accompanying accumulation of opioid metabolites, which causes further symptoms, such as myoclonus and even seizures. Dehydration is also associated with constipation and increased risk of bedsores. Clinicians report that these symptoms are mild and easily treated without hydration and that some symptoms, such as increased secretions, are actually made worse by rehydration.[6,12,20] Hospice nurses have reported that the dehydrated patient is not uncomfortable.[31,32] There is concern that artificial hydration diminishes quality of life by adding tubes, which create a physical barrier that separates the terminally ill from their loved ones. There is often fear that hydration unnecessarily prolongs dying. Patients and families may be making decisions based on inadequate knowledge or misconceptions about artificial hydration, such as the idea that it is helpful at any stage of disease or that it can increase strength.[33]

Those clinicians who support the use of hydration point to the prevention or relief of some symptoms, such as delirium.[13,16] Because food and fluids are viewed by many as a symbol of life, not to maintain fluids or to withdraw artificial hydration at the end of life may cause spiritual or emotional conflict. These issues are complex and involve not only physical, psychological, and social concerns but also individual ethical dilemmas.

NUTRITION

To observe an anorexic, fatigued, wasted, and debilitated patient is disheartening for the family. Food is more than nutrition; it plays an important role in maintaining hope. For those who are able to enjoy eating, every opportunity to offer nourishment should be taken. However, attempts at aggressive nutritional intervention for someone who is unable to eat may end up being frustrating for the family and add to the patient's suffering.[34]

Malnutrition is a common problem in patients with chronic, advanced debilitating illnesses such as acquired immunodeficiency syndrome (AIDS) or cancer. *Anorexia*, a loss of appetite, occurs in most patients during the last weeks of life. *Cancer cachexia* is a complex syndrome characterized by loss of appetite, generalized tissue wasting, skeletal muscle atrophy, immune dysfunction, and a variety of metabolic alterations.[35,36] It is likely that *asthenia*, mental and physical fatigue coupled with generalized weakness, is directly related to malnutrition.[37–39]

Administration of nutrition in the terminally ill is sometimes proposed as a medical intervention for nutrition-related symptoms or management of side effects such as weight loss, weakness, constipation, pressure sores, intestinal obstruction, and dehydration. Nutritional intervention is also recommended to prevent further morbidity and maintain to quality of life by controlling blood sugars or electrolyte imbalance. Lastly, nutritional therapy is offered to provide enough dietary intake to maintain energy.

Enteral and parenteral feedings are, however, interventions with the potential for associated morbidity and increased suffering (Table 12–6). The American Medical Directors Association (AMDA), a group that represents nursing home physicians, has published a white paper including a section that cautions against tube feeding in patients with advanced dementia unless they have clearly indicated their desire for such treatment. This group believes that there is no advantage to tube feeding and that less time is spent and fewer complications are encountered with hand feeding.[40] Until the literature is conclusive, the clinician must stay current with the research in this area.[41]

Anorexia is influenced by alterations in taste, alterations in the gastrointestinal system, changes in metabolism, and effects of the tumor itself. In addition, psychological factors such as depression or anxiety can change eating habits. Pain, fatigue, and nausea may also decrease the desire for oral intake. Many aspects of the cancer experience decrease caloric intake. Taste changes may result from the tumor itself or from various treatments such as chemotherapy, surgery, radiation, or antibiotics.[42] These taste changes may in turn decrease digestive enzymes and delay digestion.[43] The gastrointestinal tract may be altered by tumor, opportunistic infections such as *Candida,* or ulcerations resulting from chemotherapy or radiation that cause diarrhea. These alterations can interfere with ingestion, digestion, and absorption. Nausea and vomiting may ensue. Abnormalities in glucose metabolism, increases in circulating amino acids or lactic acid, and increases in free fatty acids can cause early satiety.[44] Increased blood sugar and serotonin levels in the brain may also decrease appetite.[45] In addition, cytokines such as interleukin-1 and tumor necrosis factor, released from tumors, may mediate anorexia and decrease gastric emptying.[46]

The patient with advanced chronic illness may have increased caloric needs due to changes in metabolism. The basal metabolic rate can be increased by infection or malignancy. Age, nutritional status, temperature, hormones, and trauma can also change the metabolic rate. Unlike healthy persons, these patients have no adaptation to a decrease in food intake; metabolism does not slow down. Cytokines increase resting energy expenditure and skeletal muscle wasting.[46] Nutrients that help to maintain immune function are decreased, and the resulting immunosuppression increases the risk of infection. Tumors invading the esophagus, stomach, or bowel can cause compression or obstruction and may limit oral intake. Surgery to remove tumors can remove all or part of the organs that produce digestive enzymes. This results in incomplete digestion. A shortened intestine reduces the number of villi available for absorption of nutrients.[44]

Nutritional Assessment

Within the framework of goals of care, disease status, and closeness to death, nutritional assessment starts with a diet history. The history should include the individual's usual dietary habits, current eating habits, and disease symptoms. Food preferences and aversions should be explored, as well as family support and the ability to obtain and prepare foods. The educational needs of the patient and of caregivers should also be assessed. A food diary may be helpful in this situation, and dietitians recommend a 72-hour history followed by weekly documentation. A physical examination to screen for changes in oral mucosa and dentition should be performed.

Anthropometric measurements are part of nutritional assessment. These are often limited in scope at the end stages of disease. A history of weight loss of 20% or greater is indicative of increased morbidity and mortality.[47] In the patient with advanced disease, weight gain may indicate the presence of

Table 12–6
Potential Complications of Enteral Support

Complication	Symptom	Cause
Aspiration	Coughing	Excess residual
	Fever	Large-bore tube
Diarrhea	Watery stool	Hyperosmotic solution
		Rapid infusion
		Lactose intolerance
Constipation	Hard, infrequent stools	Inadequate fluid
		Inadequate fiber
Dumping syndrome	Dizziness	High volume
		Hyperosmotic fluids

edema or ascites, and weight loss may indicate dehydration. Other anthropometric measurements, such as skinfold thickness and midarm circumference, assess muscle and fat stores and can be used to monitor progress. Laboratory values are also used to estimate protein stores. These biochemical measurements are the mainstay for determining TPN. The appropriateness of each of these assessment parameters is determined on a case-by-case basis in the terminally ill.

Nutritional therapy is aimed at improving intake and managing cachexia. Increasing appetite is sometimes possible with pharmacological therapy. Steroids have been known to increase appetite, but their long-term use can cause muscle weakness. High-dose megastrol acetate has been shown to increase appetite with subsequent weight gain.[48,49] Hydrazine sulfate did not improve appetite more than placebo.[50] Metoclopramide, tetrahydrocannabinol, and insulin have resulted in some improvement, but toxicities were problematic and the data were often insufficient. Exercise has been shown to stimulate appetite; however, few end-stage patients are able to participate in the type of exercise that is necessary to increase appetite.

Nursing measures to promote oral intake include managing other symptoms (e.g., constipation, pain, nausea) that negatively affect appetite. In addition, patients may require more seasoning than usual for food to taste good. Good oral care and unhurried meals should be encouraged. Suggesting that the patient allow others to cook may preserve energy for eating as well as decrease the negative effects of food odors. Wine or beer has been known to stimulate appetite but may be poorly tolerated by terminally ill patients or those receiving multiple medications with sedating properties.

Enteral feedings use the gastrointestinal tract for delivery of nutrients, and oral supplementation of nutrients can be tried in individuals who have the capacity to swallow. Care must be taken, however, to monitor the use of these supplements. Caregivers and patients sometimes feel a moral obligation to provide food and "push" the supplements at the risk of harm to the patient, such as aspiration pneumonia or increased distress and decreased quality of life. Feedings may also be given through a nasogastric tube, an esophagostomy tube, a gastrostomy tube, or a jejunostomy tube. In addition to the possibility of aspiration with enteral feedings, dumping syndrome, diarrhea, constipation, skin irritation at tube site insertion, and clogging of feeding tubes are potential complications. Finally, it is possible to provide nutrition parenterally. This approach may be useful for a small and carefully selected group of patients. However, TPN can be complicated by venous thrombosis, air embolism, infection, sepsis, hyperglycemia, hypoglycemia, and increased pain.

Summary

We inherit beliefs that govern our behavior. Among them are numerous contradictory notions that associate support with sustenance. Attitudes, preferences, and decisions may be influenced by race, gender, and culture.[51] The rites of family meals and celebrations provide bonding and sharing as well as food—fundamental components of personal and social life. The issues of hydration and nutrition at the end of life are complex and require a thoughtful, individualized approach.[52] Nurses and physicians are guided to institute or withdraw artificial nutrition or hydration based on the ethical principles of autonomy, beneficience and nonmaleficience.[53,54] Provision of accurate and complete information by the nurse can influence a patient's and family's decisions about these matters.

REFERENCES

1. Ganzini L, Goy E, Miller LL, Harvarth TA, Jackson A, Delorit MA. Nurses' experiences with hospice patients who refuse food and fluids to hasten death. N Engl J Med 2003; 349: 359–365.
2. Rolls BJ, Phillips PA. Aging and disturbances of thirst and fluid balance. Nutr Rev 1990;48:137–144.
3. Smith SA. Patient-induced dehydration: Can it ever be therapeutic? Oncol Nurs Forum 1995;22:1487–1491.
4. Rolls BJ, Wood RJ, Rolls ET. Thirst following water deprivation in humans. Am J Physiol 1980;8:R476–R482.
5. Weinberg AD, Minaker KL; Council on Scientific Affairs, American Medical Association. Dehydration evaluation and management in older adults. JAMA 1995;274:1552–1556.
6. Billings JA. Comfort measures for the terminally ill: Is dehydration painful? J Am Geriatr Soc 1985;33:808–810.
7. Billings JA. Dehydration. In: Billings JA, Berger A, Portenoy R, Weissman D, eds. Principles and Practice of Supportive Oncology. Philadelphia: Lippincott-Raven, 1998:589–601.
8. Phillips PA, Rolls BJ, Ledingham JG, et al. Reduced thirst after water deprivation in healthy elderly men. N Engl J Med 1984; 311:753–759.
9. MacDonald N. Ethical issues in dehydration and nutrition. In: Bruera E, Portenoy RK, eds. Topics in Palliative Care, Vol 2. New York: Oxford University Press, 1998:153–169.
10. Fassing R. Dehydration and palliative care. Palliative Care Review 7 (1):1995.
11. Twycross R, Lichter I. The terminal phase. In: Doyle D, Hanks GWC, MacDonald N, eds. Oxford Textbook of Palliative Medicine, 2nd ed. Oxford: Oxford University Press, 1998:977–994.
12. Burge FI. Dehydration symptoms of palliative care cancer patients. J Pain Symptom Manage 1993;8:454–464.
13. del Rosario B, Martin AS. Hydration for control of syncope in palliative care. J Pain Symptom Manage 1997;14:5–6.
14. Fainsinger RL, Bruera E. Hypodermoclysis for symptom control versus the Edmonton Injector. J Palliat Care 1991;7:5–8.
15. Fainsinger R, Bruera E. The management of dehydration in terminally ill patients. J Palliat Care 1995;10:55–59.
16. Waller A, Hershkowitz M, Adunsky A. The effect of intravenous fluid infusion on blood and urine parameters of hydration and on state of consciousness in terminal cancer patients. Am J Hospice Palliat Care 1994;11:22–27.
17. Ellershaw JE, Sutcliffe JM, Saunders CM. Dehydration and the dying patient. J Pain Symptom Manage 1995;10:192–197.
18. Fainsinger R, MacEachern T, Miller MJ, et al. The use of hypodermoclysis for rehydration in terminally ill cancer patients. J Pain Symptom Manage 1994;9:298–302.

19. Yan E, Bruera E. Parenteral hydration of the terminally ill. J Palliat Care 1991;7:40–43.
20. Zerwekh J. The dehydration question. Nursing 1983;13:47–51.
21. Printz LA. Is withholding hydration a valid comfort measure in the terminally ill? Geriatrics 1988;43:84–88.
22. Collard T, Rapin CH. Dehydration in dying patients: Study with physicians in French-speaking Switzerland. J Pain Symptom Manage 1991;6:230–240.
23. Kemp C. Dehydration, fatigue and sleep. In: Kemp C, ed. Terminal Illness: A Guide to Nursing Care, 2nd ed. Philadelphia: Lippincott, 1999:205–210.
24. Bruera E, Pruvost M, Schoeller T, Montejo G, Watanabe S. Proctoclysis for hydration of terminally ill cancer patients. J Pain Symptom Manage 1998;8:454–464.
25. Berger EY. Nutrition by hypodermoclysis. J Am Geriatr Soc 1984; 32:199–203.
26. Asch DA, Faber-Langendoen K, Shea JA, Christakis NA. The sequence of withdrawing life-sustaining treatment from patients. Am J Med 1999;107:153-156.
27. Faber-Langendoen K. A multi-institutional study of care given to patients dying in hospitals: Ethical and practical implications. Arch Intern Med 1996;156:2130–2136.
28. Wilson D. A report of an investigation of end-of-life care practices in health care facilities and the influences on those practices. J Palliat Care 1997;13:34–40.
29. Zerzan J, Stearns S, Hanson L. Access to palliative care and hospice in nursing homes. JAMA 2000;284:2489–2494.
30. Lanuke K, Fainsinger RL, deMoissac D. Hydration management at the end of life. J Palliat Care 2004;7:257–263.
31. Andrews M, Bell ER, Smith SA, Tischler JF, Veglia JM. Dehydration in terminally ill patients: Is it appropriate palliative care? Postgrad Med 1993;93:201–208.
32. Andrews MR, Levine AM. Dehydration in the terminal patient: Perception of hospice nurses. Am J Hospice Care 1989;1:31–34.
33. Chiu TC, Hu WY, Chuang RB, Cheng YR, Chen CY, Wakai S. Terminal cancer patients' wishes and influencing factors toward the provision of artificial nutrition and hydration in Taiwan. J Pain Symptom Manage 2004;27:206–214.
34. Cimino JE. The role of nutrition in hospice and palliative care of the cancer patient. Top Clin Nutr 2003;18:154–161.
35. Rivadeneira DE, Envoy D, Fahey TJ, Lieberman MD, Daly JM. Nutritional support of the cancer patient. CA Cancer Clin 1998; 48:69–80.
36. Costa G. Cachexia, the metabolic component of neoplastic diseases. Cancer Res 1977;37:2327–2335.
37. Neuenschwander H, Bruera E. Asthenia. In: Doyle D, Hanks GWC, MacDonald N, eds. Oxford Textbook of Palliative Medicine, 2nd ed. New York: Oxford University Press, 1998:573–581.
38. Bruera E. Clinical management of cachexia and anorexia in patients with advanced cancer. Oncology 1992;49(Suppl 2):35–42.
39. Storey P. Symptom control in advanced cancer. Semin Oncol 1994;21:748–753.
39a. American Medical Directors Association. White Paper on Surrogate Decision-Making and Advanced Care Planning In Long-Term Care, 2003, http://www.amda.com/library/whitepapers/surrogate (accessed December 30, 2004).
40. Miller S, Teno JM, Roy J, Kabumoto G, Mor V. Clinical and organizational factors associated with feeding tube use among nursing home residents with advanced cognitive impairment. JAMA 2003; 290:73–80.
41. Meares C. Nutritional issuses in palliative care. Semin Oncol Nurs 2000;16:135–145.
42. Bender CM. Taste alterations. In: Yasko JM, ed. Nursing Management of Symptoms Associated with Chemotherapy, 3rd ed. Columbus, Ohio: Adria Laboratories, 1993:67–74.
43. Kesner DL, DeWys WD. Anorexia and cachexia in malignant disease. In: Newell GR, Ellison NM, eds. Nutrition and Cancer: Etiology and Treatment. New York: Raven Press, 1981: 303–317.
44. Tait NS. Anorexia-cachexia syndrome. In: Groenwald SL, Frogge MH, Goodman M, Yarbro CH, eds. Cancer Symptom Management. Boston: Jones and Bartlett, 1997:171–185.
45. Grant M, Ropka ME. Alterations in nutrition. In: Baird S, McCorkle R, Grant M, eds. Cancer Nursing: A Comprehensive Textbook. Philadelphia: WB Saunders, 1991:717–741.
46. Moldawer LL, Rogy MA, Lowry SF. The role of cytokines in cancer cachexia. J Parenter Nutr 1992;16(Suppl):43s–49s.
47. Bernard M, Jacobs D, Rombeau J. Nutrient requirements. In: Bernard M, Jacobs J, Romeau D, eds. Nutritional and Metabolic Support of Hospitalized Patients. Philadelphia: WB Saunders, 1986:11–45.
48. Tchekmedyian NS, Hickman M, Siau J, Greco FA, Keller J, Browder H, Aisner J. Megastrol acetate in cancer anorexia and weight loss. Cancer 1992;69:1268–1274.
49. Schmoll E, Wilke H, Thole R, Preusser P, Wildfang I, Schmoll HJ. Megastrol acetate in cancer cachexia. Semin Oncol 1991;18(Suppl 2):32–34.
50. Loprinzi CL, Goldberg RM, Su JQ, Mailliard JA, Kuross SA, Maksymiuk AW, Kugler JW, Jett JR, Ghosh C, Pfeifle DM, et al. Placebo-controlled trial of hydrazine sulfate in patients with newly diagnosed non small-cell lung cancer. J Clin Oncol 1994; 11:1126–1129.
51. Phipps E, True G, Harris D, Cong U, Tester W, Chavin SI, Braitman LE. Approaching the end of life: Attitudes, preferences, and behaviors of African-American and white patients and their family caregivers. J Clin Oncol 2003;21: 549–554.
52. Daly B. Special challenges of witholding artificial nutrition and hydration. J Gerontol Nurs 2000;(Sept):25–31.
53. Day L, Drought T, Davis AJ. Principle-based ethics and nurses' attitudes towards artificial feeding. J Adv Nurs 1995;21: 295–298.
54. Slomka J. Witholding nutrition at the end of life: Clinical and ethical issues. Cleve Clin J Med 2003;70;548–552.

13 Dyspnea, Death Rattle, and Cough

Deborah Dudgeon

Air! I need air! I can't breath . . . I'm going to die!—A patient

Can you help her? It sounds like she's choking to death!—A family member

I'm worn out from coughing!—A patient

- ***Key Points***
- *Dyspnea is a subjective experience.*
- *Tachypnea is not dyspnea.*
- *Patients can be very frightened when breathless.*
- *Nursing and medical interventions are helpful for patients with dyspnea.*
- *Death rattle is common in dying patients.*
- *Death rattle is very distressing for people at the bedside.*
- *Family members need to receive good teaching and reassurance about death rattle.*
- *Anticholinergics are the drugs of choice for death rattle.*
- *Chronic cough can be very debilitating.*
- *Massive hemoptysis is very frightening and needs to be anticipated.*
- *Pharmacological and nonpharmacological interventions can help patients with chronic cough.*

DYSPNEA

Dyspnea is a very common symptom in people with advanced disease and can severely impair their quality of life. The presence of dyspnea correlates with the probability of dying in hospital.[1] In one international study, dyspnea prompted the use of terminal sedation in 25% to 53% of patients.[2] Management of breathlessness requires understanding and assessment of the multidimensional components of the symptom, knowledge of the pathophysiological mechanisms and clinical syndromes that are common in people with advanced disease, and knowledge of the indications and limitations of the available therapeutic approaches.

Definition

The American Thoracic Society has defined *dyspnea* as the "term used to characterize a subjective experience of breathing discomfort that consists of qualitatively distinct sensations that vary in intensity."[3] Dyspnea, like pain, is multidimensional in nature, with not only physical elements but also affective components, which are shaped by previous experience.[4,5] The neuropathways responsible for the sensation of dyspnea are poorly understood,[6] and no simple physiological mechanism or unique peripheral site can explain the varied circumstances that lead to the perception of breathlessness.[4,7] Stimulation of a number of different receptors (Figure 13–1) and the conscious perception this stimulation invokes can alter ventilation and result in a sensation of breathlessness.

Prevalence and Impact

The prevalence of the dyspnea varies according to the stage and type of underlying disease. Approximately 50% of a general outpatient cancer population describe some breathlessness,[8] with this number rising to as much as 70% in the terminal phases of

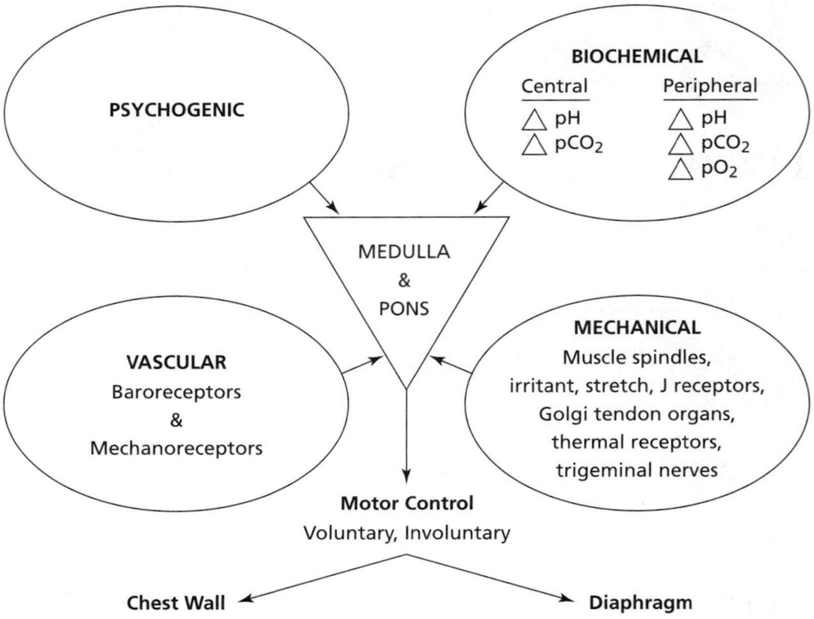

Figure 13–1. Schematic diagram of the neuroanatomic elements involved in the control of ventilation. *Source:* Dudgeon & Rosenthal (2000), reference 169.

the disease.[9–14] The prevalence of dyspnea is even more common in patients with lung cancer; almost 90% of them complain of breathlessness just before death.[15] In a study of patients with end-stage chronic obstructive pulmonary disease (COPD), extreme breathlessness was experienced by 95% of the participants and was the most distressing and debilitating symptom.[16] Dyspnea is also quite prevalent in the last year of life of people with congestive heart failure (CHF): 61% of these patients experience dyspnea, 72% of them having dyspnea for ≥6 months.[17] Likewise, dyspnea occurs in 37% of patients with cerebrovascular accident (of whom 57% were breathless for >6 months)[18]; in 47% to 50% of patients with amyotrophic lateral sclerosis (ALS); and in 70% of those with dementia.[19]

In a study of late-stage cancer patients, Roberts and associates[20] used patient self-report surveys, chart audits of patients under the care of a hospice program, and interviews of patients and nurses in a home-care hospice program to examine the occurrence of dyspnea during the last weeks of life. They found that 62% of the patients with dyspnea had been short of breath for >3 months. Various activities intensified dyspnea for these patients: climbing stairs, 95.6%; walking slowly, 47.8%; getting dressed, 52.2%; talking or eating, 56.5%; and at rest, 26.1%. The patients universally responded by decreasing their activity to whatever degree would relieve their shortness of breath. Most of the patients had received no direct medical or nursing assistance with their dyspnea, leaving them to cope in isolation. Brown and colleagues[21] found that 97% of lung cancer patients studied had decreased their activities, and 80% believed they had socially isolated themselves from friends and outside contacts to cope with their dyspnea. Studies in patients with COPD, CVA, or end-stage heart or neurological diseases have also demonstrated the presence of significant dyspnea and other symptoms, functional disability, and impaired quality of life in the last year of their lives.[16–19,22]

Patients with advanced disease typically experience chronic shortness of breath with intermittent acute episodes.[21,23] Acute attacks of breathlessness are usually accompanied by feelings of anxiety, fear, panic, and, if severe enough, a sensation of impending death.[23] Patients and family members who were participants in a qualitative study using narrative analysis consistently expressed fear of dying during a future acute episode of breathlessness, or of watching helplessly as a loved one became increasingly breathless and died before receiving any help.[24] Many dying persons are terrified of waking in the middle of the night with intense air hunger.[25] They need providers who will anticipate their fears and provide symptomatic relief of their breathlessness and anxiety as they approach death.[24,25]

Pathophysiology

Management of dyspnea of patients requires an understanding of its multidimensional nature and the pathophysiologic mechanisms that cause this distressing symptom. Exertional dyspnea in cardiopulmonary disease (Table 13–1) is caused by (1) increased ventilatory demand, (2) impaired mechanical responses, or (3) a combination of the two.[26] The effects of abnormalities of these mechanisms can also be additive.

Table 13–1
Pathophysiological Mechanisms of Dyspnea

Increased ventilatory demand
Increased physiological dead space
Thromboemboli
Tumor emboli
Vascular obstruction
Radiation therapy
Chemotherapy
Emphysema
Severe deconditioning
Hypoxemia
Change in V_{CO_2} or arterial P_{CO_2} set point
Psychological: anxiety, depression
Increased neural reflex activity
Impaired mechanical response/ventilatory pump impairment
Restrictive ventilatory deficit
Respiratory muscle weakness
Cachexia
Electrolyte imbalances
Peripheral muscle weakness
Neuromuscular abnormalities
Neurohumoral
Steroids
Pleural or parenchymal disease
Reduced chest wall compliance
Obstructive ventilatory deficit
Asthma
Chronic obstructive pulmonary disease
Tumor obstruction
Mixed obstructive/restrictive disorder (any combination of the above)

P_{CO_2}, partial pressure of carbon dioxide; V_{CO_2}, carbon dioxide output.

Increased Ventilatory Demand

Ventilatory demand is increased because of increased physiological dead space resulting from reduction in the vascular bed (from thromboemboli, tumor emboli, vascular obstruction, radiation, chemotherapy toxicity, or concomitant emphysema); hypoxemia and severe deconditioning with early metabolic acidosis (with excessive hydrogen ion stimulation); alterations in carbon dioxide output (V_{CO_2}) or in the arterial partial pressure of carbon dioxide (P_{CO_2}) set point; and nonmetabolic sources, such as increased neural reflex activity, or psychological factors such as anxiety and depression.

Impaired Mechanical Response/Ventilatory Pump Impairment

Impaired mechanical responses result in restrictive ventilatory deficits due to inspiratory muscle weakness,[27] pleural or parenchymal disease, or reduced chest wall compliance; airway obstruction from coexistent asthma or COPD, or tumor obstruction. Patients may also have a mixed obstructive and restrictive disorder.

Multidimensional Assessment of Dyspnea

Dyspnea, like pain, is a subjective experience that may not be evident to an observer. *Tachypnea,* a rapid respiratory rate, is not dyspnea. Medical personnel must learn to ask and accept the patient's assessments, often without measurable physical correlates. If patients say they are having discomfort with breathing, we must believe that they are dyspneic.

To determine whether dyspnea is present, it is important to ask more than the question, "Are you short of breath?" Patients often respond in the negative to this simple question because they have limited their activities so they won't become short of breath. It is therefore helpful to ask about shortness of breath in relationship to activities: "Do you get short of breath walking at the same speed as someone of your age?" "Do you have to stop to catch your breath when walking upstairs?" "Do you get short of breath when you are eating?"

Qualitative Aspects of Dyspnea

Dyspnea is not a single sensation. Recent work suggests that the sensation of breathlessness encompasses several qualities.[7] Just as the descriptions "burning" or "numb" suggest neuropathic pain, phrases such as "chest tightness," "exhalation," and "deep" were among a cluster of words associated with asthma.[7] It is possible that dyspnea mediated by similar receptors evokes common word descriptors. From the research to date, it is not known whether qualitative assessments of dyspnea in breathless patients permit any discrimination among the various cardiopulmonary disorders. O'Donnell and coworkers[28–30] found that, although descriptor choices were clearly different between health and disease states, they provided no discrimination among various diseases (e.g., COPD, restrictive lung disease, and CHF). Others have suggested that changes in the quality of dyspnea may prompt patients with heart failure to go to the emergency department.[31]

Clinical Assessment

Clinical assessments are usually directed at determining the underlying pathophysiology, to decide appropriate treatment, and at evaluating the response to therapy.

The clinical assessment of dyspnea should include a complete history of the symptom, including its temporal onset (acute or chronic), whether it is affected by positioning, its qualities, associated symptoms, precipitation and relieving events or activities, and response to medications. A past history of smoking, underlying lung or cardiac disease, concurrent medical conditions, allergy history, and details of previous medications or treatments should be elicited.[32,33]

Careful physical examination focused on possible underlying causes of dyspnea should be performed. Particular attention should be directed at signs associated with certain clinical syndromes that are common causes of dyspnea. Examples are the dullness to percussion, decreased tactile fremitus, and absent breath sounds associated with a pleural effusion in a person with lung cancer; an elevated jugular venous pressure (JVP), audible third heart sound (S_3), and bilateral crackles audible on chest examination associated with CHF; and elevated JVP, distant heart sounds, and pulsus paradoxus in people with pericardial effusions.[32,33]

Gift and colleagues[34] studied the physiological factors related to dyspnea in subjects with COPD and high, medium, and low levels of breathlessness. There were no significant differences in respiratory rate, depth of respiration, or peak expiratory flow rates at the three levels of dyspnea. There was, however, a significant difference in the use of accessory muscles between patients with high and low levels of dyspnea, suggesting that this is a physical finding that reflects the intensity of dyspnea.

Diagnostic tests helpful in determining the cause of dyspnea include chest radiography; electrocardiography; pulmonary function tests; arterial blood gases; complete blood counts; serum potassium, magnesium, and phosphate levels; cardiopulmonary exercise testing; and tests specific for suspected underlying pathologies, such as an echocardiogram for suspected pericardial effusion.[32] The choice of appropriate diagnostic tests should be guided by the stage of disease, the prognosis, the risk/benefit ratios of any proposed tests or interventions, and the desires of the patient and family.

Nguyen and colleagues[35] found that the ratings of intensity of dyspnea during laboratory exercise, clinical measures of dyspnea such as the Oxygen Cost Diagram, and pulmonary function tests captured distinctly different information in patients with moderate to severe COPD. It is therefore not surprising that results of pulmonary function tests do not necessarily reflect the intensity of a person's dyspnea. Individuals with comparable degrees of functional lung impairment may also experience considerable differences in the intensity of dyspnea they perceive.[4] Factors such as adaptation, differing physical characteristics, and psychological conditions can modulate both the quality and the intensity of the person's perception of breathlessness.

The Visual Analog Scale (VAS) is one of the most popular techniques for measuring the perceived intensity of dyspnea. This scale is usually a 100-mm vertical or horizontal line, anchored at each end by words such as "Not at all breathless" and "Very breathless." Subjects are asked to mark the line at the point that best describes the intensity of their breathlessness. The scales can be used as an initial assessment, to monitor progress, and to evaluate effectiveness of treatment in an individual patient.[36]

The modified Borg scale is a scale with nonlinear spacing of verbal descriptors of severity of breathlessness.[37] Patients are asked to pick the verbal descriptor that best describes their perceived exertion during exercise. It is usually used in conjunction with an exercise protocol with standardized power output or metabolic loads. When used in this manner, the slope of the Borg descriptors over time is very reproducible and reliable, permitting comparisons within individuals and across population groups.[38,39]

The Reading Numbers Aloud test was designed as an objective measure of the activity-limiting effect of breathlessness in people with cancer who were breathless at very low levels of exertion.[40,41] The test involves asking subjects to read a grid of numbers as quickly and clearly as possible for 60 seconds. The number of numbers read and the number read per breath are recorded.

Dyspnea and Psychological Factors

The person's perception of the intensity of his or her breathlessness is also affected by psychological factors. Anxious, obsessive, depressed and dependent persons appear to experience dyspnea that is disproportionately severe relative to the extent of their pulmonary disease.[4] Gift and colleagues[34] found that anxiety was higher during episodes of high or medium levels of dyspnea, compared with low levels of dyspnea. Kellner and associates[42] found in multiple regression analyses that depression was predictive of breathlessness. Studies in cancer patients by Dudgeon and Lertzman[27,43] and others[8,14,44] have also shown that anxiety is significantly correlated with the intensity of dyspnea ($r=0.3$) but explains only 9% of the variance in the intensity of breathlessness. These studies were done in people with chronic dyspnea and when the person was at rest. Carrieri-Kohlman and colleagues[45] found higher correlations between dyspnea intensity and anxiety associated with dyspnea at the end of exercise ($r=0.49$). It is also probable that anxiety is a more prominent factor during episodes of acute shortness of breath.

Management

The optimal treatment of dyspnea is to treat reversible causes. If this is no longer possible, then both nonpharmacological and pharmacological methods are used (Table 13–2).

Pharmacological Interventions

Opioids. Since the late 19th century, opioids have been used to relieve breathlessness of patients with asthma, pneumothorax, and emphysema.[46] Although most trials have demonstrated the benefit of opioids for the treatment of dyspnea,[46–56] some have been negative[57–60] or have produced undesirable side effects.[49,57]

In 2001, a systemic review examined the effectiveness of oral or injectable opioid drugs for the palliative treatment of breathlessness.[61] The authors identified 18 randomized, double-blind, controlled trials comparing the use of any opioid drug

Table 13–2
Management of Dyspnea

Sit upright supported by pillows or leaning on overbed table
Fan ± oxygen
Relaxation techniques and other appropriate non-pharmacological measures
Identify and treat underlying diagnosis (if appropriate)
Pharmacologic Management
Chronic
Opioids
Add phenothiazine (chlorpromazine, promethazine)
Acute
Opioids
Add anxiolytic

against placebo for the treatment of breathlessness in patients with any illness. In the studies involving nonnebulized routes of administration,[46,48,54,58,60,62–64] there was statistically strong evidence for a small effect of oral and parenteral opioids for the treatment of breathlessness.[61]

In recent years, there has been tremendous interest in the use of nebulized opioids for the treatment of dyspnea. Opioid receptors are present on sensory nerve endings in the airways[65]; therefore, it is hypothesized that if the receptors were interrupted directly, lower doses, with less systemic side effects, would be required to control breathlessness. The recent systemic review[61] identified nine randomized double-blind, controlled trials comparing the use of nebulized opioids or placebo for the control of breathlessness.[66–74] The authors concluded that there was no evidence that nebulized opioids were more effective than nebulized saline in relieving breathlessness.[61] It is hard to justify the continued use of nebulized opioids.

Physicians have been reluctant to prescribe opioids for dyspnea since the potential for respiratory failure was recognized in the 1950s.[75] The recent systematic review of opioids for breathlessness identified 11 studies that contained information on blood gases or oxygen saturation after intervention with opioids.[61] Only one study reported a significant increase in the arterial partial pressure of carbon dioxide ($PaCO_2$), but it did not rise above 40 mm Hg.[62] In studies of cancer patients, morphine did not compromise respiratory function as measured by respiratory effort and oxygen saturation[47,48,76] or respiratory rate and $PaCO_2$.[47] It is now known that the development of clinically significant hypoventilation and respiratory depression from opioids depends on the rate of change of the dose, the history of previous exposure to opioids, and possibly the route of administration.[77] Early use of opioids improves quality of life and allows the use of lower doses while tolerance to the respiratory depressant effects develops.[78] Twycross[79] suggested that early use of morphine or another opioid, rather than hastening death in dyspneic patients, might actually prolong survival by reducing physical and psychological distress and exhaustion.

Sedatives and Tranquilizers. Chlorpromazine decreases breathlessness without affecting ventilation or producing sedation in healthy subjects.[80] Woodcock and colleagues[81] found that promethazine reduced dyspnea and improved exercise tolerance of patients with severe COPD. O'Neill and associates[80] did not find that promethazine improved breathlessness in healthy people, nor did Rice and coworkers[57] find that it benefited patients with stable COPD. McIver and colleagues[82] found that chlorpromazine was effective for relief of dyspnea in advanced cancer.

The results of clinical trials to determine the effectiveness of anxiolytics for the treatment of breathlessness have also been quite variable. Two studies showed that diazepam was effective in treating dyspnea,[81,83] and one showed a reduction in dyspnea.[84] Greene and colleagues[85] reported an improvement in dyspnea with alprazolam; however, a randomized, placebo-controlled, double-blind study did not find any relief of dyspnea with alprazolam.[86] Clorazepate was not found to be effective for breathlessness.[87] Buspirone, a nonbenzodiazepine anxiolytic, had no effect on pulmonary function tests or arterial blood gases in patients with COPD but improved exercise tolerance and decreased dyspnea.[88] This drug warrants further study.

Combinations. In a double-blind, placebo controlled, randomized trial, Light and colleagues[63] studied the effectiveness of morphine alone, morphine and promethazine, and morphine and prochlorperazine for the treatment of breathlessness in patients with COPD. The combination of morphine and promethazine significantly improved exercise tolerance without worsening dyspnea, compared with placebo, morphine alone, or the combination of morphine and prochlorperazine.[63] Ventafridda and colleagues[89] also found the combination of morphine and chlorpromazine to be effective.

Other Medications. Indomethacin reduced exercise-induced breathlessness in a group of normal adults,[90] but no benefit was obtained in patients with diffuse parenchymal lung disease[91] or COPD.[92] Although inhaled bupivacaine reduced exercise-induced breathlessness in normal volunteers,[93] it failed to decrease breathlessness of patients with interstitial lung disease.[94] Inhaled lidocaine did not improve dyspnea in six cancer patients.[95] Dextromethorphan did not improve breathlessness of patients with COPD.[96] None of these medications can be recommended for the treatment of dyspnea at this time.

Nonpharmacological Interventions

Oxygen. The usefulness of oxygen for the terminally ill patient has been questioned.[97,98] Most authorities currently recommend oxygen for dyspneic hypoxic patients, even in the face of increasing hypercapnia to achieve and maintain a PaO_2 of 55 to 60 mm Hg and an oxygen saturation of 88% to 90%.[99,100] Bruera and colleagues[101,102] demonstrated the benefit of oxygen therapy in 20 hypoxic patients with terminal cancer. Rating of dyspnea by the patient, respiratory rate, oxygen saturation, and respiratory effort all improved with oxygen to

Table 13–3
Guidelines for Oxygen Therapy

Continuous oxygen
$PaO_2 \leq 55$ mm Hg or oxygen saturation $\leq 88\%$ at rest
PaO_2 of 56 to 59 mm Hg or oxygen saturation of 89% in the presence of the following:
Dependent edema, suggesting congestive heart failure
Cor pulmonale
Polycythemia (hematocrit > 56%)
Pulmonary hypertension
Noncontinuous oxygen is recommended during exercise:
$PaO_2 \leq 55$ mm Hg or oxygen saturation $\leq 88\%$ with a low level of exertion or during sleep
PaO_2 of ≤ 55 mm Hg or oxygen saturation $\leq 88\%$ associated with pulmonary hypertension, daytime somnolence, and cardiac arrhythmias

PaO_2, partial pressure of oxygen in alveoli.
Source: Tarsy and Celli. , reference 100.

a statistically significantly greater degree than with air. In hypoxic patients with COPD, oxygen supplementation improved survival, pulmonary hemodynamics, exercise capacity, and neuropsychological performance.[100] Guidelines for oxygen therapy are shown in Table 13–3.

The role of oxygen in the treatment of nonhypoxic dyspnea is less clear. Woodcock and coworkers[103] studied the effect of oxygen on breathlessness in nonhypoxic patients with COPD. Oxygen not only reduced breathlessness but also increased the distance that the patients were able to walk. However, in a study of nonhypoxic cancer patients with dyspnea, Bruera and colleagues[104] found no significant differences in dyspnea, fatigue, and distance walked between those who received oxygen or air during exercise.

Pleural Effusions. Whether a malignant pleural effusion requires treatment is determined by the degree of symptomatic compromise, the stage of the disease, the patient's life expectancy, and the patient's estimated tolerance for more aggressive therapeutic approaches.[105,106] At the time of initial diagnostic or therapeutic tap of the pleural effusion, the removal of 1000 to 1500 mL of pleural fluid helps predict response to further therapies.[106] If symptoms are not relieved and the lung does not reexpand, then further thoracenteses or insertion of a chest tube is unlikely to be of any benefit, and treatment should include medications to relieve symptoms. In 97% of cases, fluid reaccumulates within 1 month after thoracentesis alone.[107] Repeated thoracenteses increase the risk for pneumothorax, empyema, and pleural fluid loculation and therefore should be limited to people with a short life span. Traditionally, tube thoracostomy was performed with large-bore chest tubes connected to wall suction; this treatment necessitated hospitalization and limited mobility, with substantial discomfort and expense. Recent studies have shown the effectiveness of small-bore catheters and indwelling small pleural catheters in the outpatient setting.[108–110]

Instillation of any of several sclerosing agents into the pleural space after adequate drainage by tube thoracostomy creates a chemical pleuritis that obliterates the pleural space and prevents pleural fluid reaccumulation. Because pleurodesis is often painful, intrapleural lidocaine is administered before the instillation of the sclerosing agent to reduce local pain. Patients also should be premedicated and should have adequate analgesic available after the procedure.

Pericardial Effusion. As in all other situations, the approach to management of a pericardial effusion depends on the person's stage of disease, the prognosis, the potential benefits and complications, and the wishes of the patient and family. If pericardial tamponade with hemodynamic compromise is present and treatment is appropriate, an emergency pericardiocentesis is indicated, with aggressive intravenous fluid support and possible administration of a sympathomimetic agent to temporize.[111] Hemodynamic improvement usually occurs with removal of 50 to 100 mL of pericardial fluid. Continuous drainage can be achieved by placement of an indwelling pigtail catheter or creation of a pericardial window, or by percutaneous balloon pericardotomy.[112,113] Pericardial drainage can be followed by instillation of a sclerosing agent to obliterate the pericardial space.[113] Radiation or systemic chemotherapy could be considered if appropriate.[114]

Nursing Interventions

Many patients obtain relief of dyspnea by leaning forward while sitting and supporting their upper arms on a table. This technique is effective in patients with emphysema,[115] probably because of an improved length-tension state of the diaphragm, which increases efficiency.[116]

Pursed-lip breathing slows the respiratory rate and increases intraairway pressures, thus decreasing small airway collapse during periods of increased dyspnea.[117] Mueller and coworkers[51] found that pursed-lip breathing led to an increase in tidal volume and a decrease in respiratory rate at rest and during exercise in 7 of 12 COPD patients experiencing an improvement in dyspnea. Pursed-lip breathing reduces dyspnea in about 50% of patients with COPD.[118]

People who are short of breath often obtain relief by sitting near an open window or in front of a fan. Cold directed against the cheek[119] or through the nose[120,121] can alter ventilation patterns and reduce the perception of breathlessness, perhaps by affecting receptors in the distribution of the trigeminal nerve that are responsive to both thermal and mechanical stimuli.[119,120]

Randomized controlled trials support the use of acupuncture and acupressure to relieve dyspnea in patients with moderate to severe COPD.[122,123] Acupuncture provided marked symptomatic benefit in breathlessness and in respiratory rate in patients with cancer-related breathlessness.[124] Other randomized controlled trials support the use of muscle relaxation with breathing retraining to reduce breathlessness in COPD patients.[125,126]

Corner and colleagues[127] found that weekly sessions with a nurse research practitioner over 3 to 6 weeks, using counseling, breathing retraining, relaxation, and coping and adaptation strategies, significantly improved breathlessness and ability to perform activities of daily living compared with controls. Carrieri and Janson-Bjerklie[128] found that patients used self-taught relaxation to help control their breathlessness. Others have found that formal muscle relaxation techniques decrease anxiety and breathlessness.[129] Guided imagery[130] and therapeutic touch[131] resulted in significant improvements in quality of life and sense of well-being in patients with COPD and patients with terminal cancer, respectively, without any significant improvement in breathlessness.

Nursing actions that intubated patients thought helpful included friendly attitude, empathy, providing physical support, staying at the bedside, reminding or allowing patients to concentrate on changing their breathing pattern, and providing information about the possible cause of the breathlessness and possible interventions.[132]

Patient and Family Teaching

Carrieri and Janson-Bjerklie[128] identified strategies patients used to manage acute shortness of breath. These strategies could be taught to patients and their families. Patients benefited from keeping still with positioning techniques, such as leaning forward on the edge of a chair with arms and upper body supported, and using some type of breathing strategy, such as pursed-lip or diaphragmatic breathing. Some of the patients distanced themselves from aggravating factors, and others used self-adjustment of medications. Several subjects isolated themselves from others to gain control of their breathing and diminish the social impact. Others used structured relaxation techniques, conscious attempts to calm down, and prayer and meditation. The study of Carrieri and Janson-Bjerklie[128] and another by Brown and colleagues[21] demonstrated that most subjects reported some changes in activities of living, such as changes in dressing and grooming, avoidance of bending or stooping, advanced planning or reduction in activities, staying in a good frame of mind, avoidance of being alone, and acceptance of the situation.

Patients and families should be taught about the signs and symptoms of an impending exacerbation and how to manage the situation. They should learn problem-solving techniques to prevent panic, ways of conserving energy, how to prioritize activities, use of fans, and ways to maximize the effectiveness of their medications, such as using a spacer with inhaled drugs or taking an additional dose of an inhaled beta-agonist before exercise.[133] Patients should avoid activities in which their arms are unsupported, because these activities often increase breathlessness.[129]

Patients in distress should not be left alone. Social services, nursing, and family input need to be increased as the patient's ability to care for himself or herself decreases.[134]

CASE STUDY

Mrs. P, a 45-Year-Old Woman with Dyspnea

You are called to the room of Mrs. P and find her sitting at the bedside, gasping for breath. You know the Mrs. P is a 45-year-old woman with advanced ovarian carcinoma. She has known lung metastases and describes a progressive onset of worsening breathlessness with less and less activity. She says that she had gone to the washroom to have a sponge bath and while combing her hair got quite breathless and struggled to make it back to her bed. While getting an overbed table and pillow for her to rest on, you calmly instruct her to take slow, deep breaths and to use the breathing technique that you had previously taught her. You note that she is cyanosed and institute oxygen and fan to help relieve her breathlessness. On further examination, you find that her trachea is deviated to the right, there is dullness to percussion of her left chest, and there are decreased breath sounds in the left lung field. With institution of the oxygen, fan, and focused breathing, you note that she is slightly less distressed, but you ask her husband to stay with her while you prepare a dose of prn morphine. On your return 5 minutes later, Mrs. P's breathing has further improved but is still a little labored, so you administer the morphine. Her husband stays with her, and 15 minutes later, when you return, he has helped her back into bed, where she is resting comfortably.

Summary

Dyspnea is a very common symptom in people with advanced disease. The symptom is often unrecognized and therefore the patients receive little assistance in managing their breathlessness. Dyspnea can have profound effects on the person's quality of life, because even the slightest exertion may precipitate breathlessness.

DEATH RATTLE

Noisy, rattling breathing in patients who are dying is commonly known as death rattle. This noisy, moist breathing can be very distressing for the family, other patients, visitors, and health care workers, because it may appear that the person is drowning in his or her own secretions.[135] Management of death rattle can present health care providers a tremendous challenge as they attempt to ensure a peaceful death for the patient.[136]

Definition

Death rattle is a term applied to describe the noise produced by the turbulent movements of secretions in the upper airways that occur with the inspiratory and expiratory phases of respiration in patients who are dying.[137]

Prevalence and Impact

Death rattle occurs in 23% to 92% of patients in their last hours before death.[137–142] Studies have shown that there is an increased incidence of respiratory congestion in patients with primary lung cancer[139,142] or cerebral metastases,[142,143] with the symptom more likely to persist in cases with pulmonary pathology.[142] The incidence of death rattle increases closer to death[142]; the median time from onset of death rattle to death is 8 to 23 hours.[140–142] Most commonly this symptom occurs when the person's general condition is very poor, and most patients have a decreased level of consciousness.[142] If the person is alert, however, the respiratory secretions can cause him or her to feel very agitated and fearful of suffocating. Despite the identification of "noisy breathing" as a problem in 39% of patients dying in a long-term care setting, 49% of them received no treatment.[144] In one study of the attitudes of palliative care nurses, about the impact of death rattle, 13% thought that death rattle distressed the dying patient; 100% thought it distressed the dying person's relatives, with 52% indicating that bereaved relatives had mentioned death rattle as a source of distress; and 79% thought that death rattle distressed nurses.[136]

Pathophysiology

The primary defense mechanism for the lower respiratory tract is the mucociliary transport system. This system is a protective device that prevents the entrance of viruses, bacteria, and other particulate matter into the body.[145–147] The surface of the respiratory tract is lined with a liquid sol phase near the epithelium and a superficial gel phase in contact with the air.[145] Ciliated epithelial cells, located at all levels of the respiratory tract except the alveoli and the nose and throat, are in constant movement to propel the mucus up the respiratory tract, to be either subconsciously swallowed or coughed out. The mucus is produced by submucosal glands, which are under neural and humoral control. The submucosal glands are under parasympathetic, sympathetic, and noncholinergic nonadrenergic nervous control. Resting glands secrete approximately 9 mL/min., but mechanical, chemical, or pharmacological stimulation (via vagal pathways) of the airway epithelium can augment gland secretion. Surface goblet cells also produce mucus secretions, which can be increased with irritant stimuli (e.g., cigarette smoke). The secretory flow rate and amount, as well as the viscoelastic properties of the mucus, can be altered.[145]

The audible breathing of the so-called death rattle is produced when turbulent air passes over or through pooled secretions in the oropharynx or bronchi. The amount of turbulence depends on the ventilatory rate and airway resistance.[143] Mechanisms of death rattle include excessive secretion of respiratory mucus, abnormal mucus secretions inhibiting normal clearance, dysfunction of the cilia, inability to swallow, decreased cough reflex due to weakness and fatigue, and the supine recumbent position. Factors that may contribute to respiratory congestion include infection or inflammation, pulmonary embolism producing infarction and fluid leakage from damaged cells, pulmonary edema or CHF,[147] dysphagia, and odynophagia. Although it has been suggested that a state of relative dehydration decreases the incidence of problematic bronchial secretions,[148] Ellershaw and colleagues[139] found no statistically significant difference in the incidence of death rattle in a biochemically dehydrated group of patients, compared with a group of hydrated patients.

Bennett[143] proposed two types of death rattle. Type 1 involves mainly salivary secretions, which accumulate in the last few hours of life when swallowing reflexes are inhibited. Type 2 is characterized by the accumulation of predominantly bronchial secretions over several days before death as the patient becomes too weak to cough effectively. This characterization has been empirically supported by Morita and colleagues[142] and therefore may prove useful to determine appropriate treatment.

Assessment

Assessment of death rattle includes a focused history and physical examination to determine potentially treatable underlying causes. If the onset is sudden and is associated with acute shortness of breath and chest pain, it might suggest a pulmonary embolism or myocardial infarction. Physical findings consistent with CHF and fluid overload might support a trial of diuretic therapy; the presence of pneumonia indicates a trial of antibiotic therapy. The effectiveness of interventions should be included in the assessment. The patient's and family's understanding and emotional response to the situation should also be assessed so that appropriate interventions can be undertaken.

A recently developed and validated assessment tool, the Victoria Respiratory Congestion Scale (VRCS),[149] is clinically useful to determine the effectiveness of interventions. This instrument rates the congestion on a scale from 0 to 3 scale, with 0 indicating no congestion heard at 12 inches from the chest; 1 indicating congestion audible only at 12 inches from the chest; 2 indicating congestion audible at foot of patient's bed; and 3 indicating congestion audible at door of patient's room. This scale has demonstrated interrater reliability ($\kappa = 0.53$, $P < 0.001$) and concurrent validity with a noise meter ($P < 0.001$). It was weakly correlated with a caregiver distress scale ($\kappa = 0.24$, $P < 0.001$).

Management

Pharmacological Interventions

Primary treatment should be focused on the underlying disorder, if appropriate to the prognosis and the wishes of the patient and family. If this is not possible, then anticholinergics are the primary mode of treatment. Hyoscine hydrobromide (scopolamine), atropine sulfate, hyoscine butylbromide (Buscopan), and glycopyrrolate (Robinul) are the anticholinergic agents that are used to treat death rattle. Anticholinergic drugs can prevent vagally induced increased bronchial secretions, but they reduce basal secretions by only 39%.[145] A recent evidence-based guideline stated that there is insufficient evidence to support the use of one drug over another and that the decision should be based on the drug characteristics and the needs of the patient.[150]

Hyoscine hydrobromide (scopolamine) is the primary medication used for the treatment of death rattle. It inhibits the muscarinic receptors and causes anticholinergic actions such as decreased peristalsis, gastrointestinal secretions, sedation, urinary retention, and dilatation of the bronchial smooth muscle. It is administered subcutaneously, intermittently or by continuous infusion, or transdermally.[138,139,143,151] In one study,[152] hyoscine hydrobromide 0.4 mg subcutaneously was immediately effective and only 6% of the patients required repeated doses. In an open label study of the treatment of death rattle, 56% of patients who received hyoscine hydrobromide had a significantly reduced noise level after 30 minutes, compared with 27% of patients who had received glycopyrrolate ($P = 0.002$).[135] In other studies, between 22% and 65% of patients did not respond to hyoscine hydrobromide, and secretions recurred from 2 to 9 hours after the injection.[138] In a retrospective study of 100 consecutive deaths in a 22-bed hospice, 27% of patients received an infusion of hyoscine hydrobromide, with 5 of 17 requiring injections despite receiving an infusion.[143]

Atropine sulfate is another anticholinergic drug that is preferred by some centers for the treatment of respiratory congestion.[147] In a study of 995 doses of atropine, congestion was decreased in 30% of patients, remained the same in 69%, and increased in 1%.[147] Atropine is the drug of choice of this group, because it results in less CNS depression, delirium, and restlessness, with more bronchodilatory effect, than hyoscine hydrobromide. There is, however, the risk of increased tachycardia with atropine sulfate when doses >1.0 mg are given. Hyoscine hydrobromide is thought to have a more potent effect on bronchial secretions than atropine does,[137] but no comparative trials have been conducted in the palliative population.

Glycopyrrolate (Robinul) is also an anticholinergic agent. It has the advantages of producing less sedation and agitation and a longer duration of action than hyoscine hydrobromide. In two studies in which its effectiveness was compared with that of hyoscine hydrobromide, glycopyrrolate was not as effective in controlling secretions.[135,138] However, others have disputed this finding and suggest it is also more cost-effective.[153] Glycopyrrolate is available in an oral form and can be useful for patients at an earlier stage of disease, when sedation is not desired.

Table 13–4
Management of "Death Rattle"

Change position
Reevaluate if receiving intravenous hydration
Pharmacological management
Chronic
Glycopyrrolate or hyoscine hydrobromide patch
If treatment fails: subcutaneous hyoscine hydrobromide or subcutaneous atropine sulfate
Acute
Subcutaneous hyoscine hydrobromide or subcutaneous atropine sulfate

Hyoscine butylbromide (Buscopan) is another anticholinergic drug, but it has not been evaluated for its effectiveness in this condition. It is available in injection, suppository, and tablet forms.

Nonpharmacological Interventions

There are times when the simple repositioning of the patient may help him or her to clear the secretions (Table 13–4). Suctioning usually is not recommended, because it can be very uncomfortable for the patient and causes significant agitation and distress. Pharmacological measures are usually effective and prevent the need for suctioning. If the patient has copious secretions that can easily be reached in the oropharynx, then suctioning may be appropriate. In a study conducted at St. Christopher's Hospice, suctioning was required in only 3 of 82 patients to control the secretions.[139] In another study, 31% of the patients required only nursing interventions with reassurance, change in position, and occasional suctioning to manage respiratory congestion in the last 48 hours of life.[152]

Patient and Family Teaching

The patient and the family can be very distressed by this symptom. It is important to explain the process, to help them understand why there is a buildup of secretions and that there is something that can be done to help. The Victoria Hospice group suggests using the term "respiratory congestion" as opposed to "death rattle," "suffocation," or "drowning in sputum," because these terms instill strong emotional reactions.[147] When explaining to families the changes that can occur before death, this is one of the symptoms that should be mentioned. If the person is being treated at home, the family should be instructed as to the measures available to relieve death rattle and to notify their hospice or palliative care team if it occurs, so that appropriate medications can be ordered.

CASE STUDY

Mrs. S, a 60-year-old Woman with Metastatic Breast Cancer

When you start your shift and are walking down the hallway, you hear a loud gurgling noise as you pass Mrs. S's room. You enter and find her family surrounding the bed and looking extremely distressed. Mrs. S. has very advanced metastatic breast cancer to lung, bones, and brain. Her condition has deteriorated markedly over the past few days. She is very restless and is pulling at the intravenous line that is running at 125 mL/h. There are audible gurgling sounds as she breaths, with diffuse crackles throughout her chest, and 3+ pitting edema of all of her limbs. Her daughter, in tears, says, "It sounds like she is choking to death! Please do something!" While you help to reposition Mrs. S, you explain why this is happening and suction some of the mucus that has accumulated in her mouth. You go to the desk and get an order from the doctor for some furosemide, to change the intravenous line to a saline lock, and for an "as needed" dose of hyoscine hydrobromide subcutaneously. You administer the furosemide, but there is minimal improvement; therefore, you give Mrs. S an injection of hyoscine hydrobromide, and within 20 minutes she has settled.

Summary

Although death rattle is a relatively common problem in people who are close to death, very few studies have evaluated the effectiveness of treatment. Anticholinergics are the drugs of choice at this time. Death rattle can be a very distressing for family members at the bedside, and they need to receive good teaching and reassurance.

COUGH

Cough is a natural defense of the body to prevent entry of foreign material into the respiratory tract. In people with advanced disease, it can be very debilitating, leading to sleepless nights, fatigue, pain, and at times pathological fractures.

Definition

Cough is an explosive expiration that can be a conscious act or a reflex response to an irritation of the tracheobronchial tree. Cough lasting <3 weeks is considered acute, and that lasting >8 weeks is considered chronic.[154] A *dry cough* occurs when no sputum is produced; a *productive cough* is one in which sputum is raised. *Hemoptysis* occurs when the sputum contains blood. *Massive hemoptysis* is expectoration of at least 100 to 600 mL of blood in 24 hours.[155]

Prevalence and Impact

Chronic cough is a common problem; recurrent cough is reported by 3% to 40% of the population.[154] In population surveys, men report cough more frequently than women do, but women appear to have an intrinsically heightened cough response.[154] Cough is often present in people with advanced diseases such as bronchitis, CHF, uncontrolled asthma, human immunodeficiency virus infection, and various cancers. In a study of 289 patients with non–small cell lung cancer, cough was the most common symptom (>60%) and the most severe symptom at presentation.[15] Eighty percent of the group had cough before death. Over time, cough and breathlessness were much less well controlled than the other symptoms in this group of patients.

In a study of 25 advanced cancer patients designed to evaluate treatment of cough, 88% of patients rated their cough as moderate or severe and 68% coughed >10 times per day.[156] Cough was found to interfere with breathing, sleep, and speech and was associated with coughing spasms, pain, nausea, and vomiting.[156]

In patients with lung cancer, hemoptysis is the presenting symptom 7% to 10% of the time, 20% have it at some time during their clinical course, and 3% die of massive hemoptysis.[155] The mortality rate of massive hemoptysis in patients with lung cancer can be as high as 59% to 100%.[155]

Pathophysiology

Cough is characterized by a violent expiration, with flow rates that are high enough to sheer mucus and foreign particles away from the larynx, trachea, and large bronchi. The cough reflex can be stimulated by irritant receptors in the larynx and pharynx or by pulmonary stretch receptor, irritant receptor, or C-fiber stimulation in the tracheobronchial tree.[157] Different mechanisms are involved in isolation or together in patients with cough of various causes.[158] The vagus nerve carries sensory information from the lung that initiates the cough reflex. Infection can physically or functionally strip away epithelium, exposing sensory nerves and increasing the sensitivity of these nerves to mechanical and chemical stimuli. It is also thought that inflammation produces prostaglandins, which further increase the sensitivity of these receptors, leading to bronchial hyperreactivity and cough. When cough is associated with increased sputum production, it probably results from stimulation of the irritant receptors by the excess secretion.[157] Cough is associated with respiratory infection, bronchitis, rhinitis, postnasal drip, esophageal reflux, medications including angiotensin-converting enzyme inhibitors,[157] asthma, COPD, pulmonary fibrosis, CHF, pneumothorax, bronchiectasis, and cystic fibrosis.[98] In the person with cancer, cough may be caused by any of these conditions; however, direct tumor effects (e.g., obstruction), indirect cancer effects (e.g., pulmonary emboli), and cancer treatment effects (e.g., radiation therapy) could also be the cause.[159]

Hemoptysis can result from bleeding in the respiratory tract anywhere from the nose to the lungs. It varies from blood streaking of sputum to coughing up of massive amounts of blood. There are multiple causes of hemoptysis, but some of the more common ones are a tracheobronchial source, secondary to inflammation or tumor invasion of the airways; a pulmonary parenchymal source, such as pneumonia or abscess; a primary vascular problem, such as pulmonary embolism; a miscellaneous cause, such as a systemic coagulopathy resulting from vitamin K deficiency, thrombocytopenia, or abnormal platelet function secondary to bone marrow invasion with tumor, sepsis, or disseminated intravascular coagulation; or an iatrogenic cause, such as use of anticoagulants, nonsteroidal antiinflammatory drugs, or acetylsalicylic acid.[160]

Assessment

In assessing someone with cough, it is important to do a thorough history and physical examination. Because cough may arise from anywhere in the distribution of the vagus nerve, the full assessment of a patient with a chronic cough requires a multidisciplinary approach with cooperation between respiratory medicine, gastroenterology, and ear, nose, and throat (ENT) departments.[154] The assessment helps to determine the underlying cause and appropriate treatment of the cough. Depending on the diagnosis, the prognosis, and the patient's and family's wishes, it may be appropriate to perform diagnostic tests, including chest or sinus radiography, spirometry before and after bronchodilator and histamine challenge, and, in special circumstances in people with earlier-stage disease, upper gastrointestinal endoscopy and 24-hour esophageal pH monitoring. In patients with significant hemoptysis, bronchoscopy is usually needed to identify the source of bleeding.

In the history and physical examination, one should look for a link between cough and the associated factors listed in the previous section, whether the cough is productive, the nature of the sputum, the frequency and amount of blood, precipitating and relieving factors, and associated symptoms.

Management

It is important to base management decisions on the cause and the appropriateness of treating the underlying diagnosis, compared with simply suppressing the symptom. This decision is based on the diagnosis, prognosis, side effects, and possible benefits of the intervention, and the wishes of the patient and family. Management strategies also depend on whether the cough is productive (Table 13–5). Theoretically, cough suppressants, by causing mucus retention, could be harmful in conditions with excess mucus production.[157]

Pharmacological Interventions

Antitussive drugs can be divided into two categories: centrally acting agents (opioids and nonopioids) and peripherally acting agents (which directly or indirectly act on cough receptors).[156]

Table 13–5
Treatment of Nonproductive Cough

Nonopioid antitussive (dextromethorphan, benzonatate)
Opioids
Inhaled anesthetic (lidocaine, bupivacaine)

Centrally Acting Antitussives

Opioids suppress cough, but the dose is higher than that contained in the proprietary cough mixtures.[157] The exact mode of action is unclear, but it is thought that opioids inhibit the mu receptor peripherally in the lung; act centrally by suppressing the cough center in the medulla or the brainstem respiratory centers; or stimulate the mu receptor, thus decreasing mucus production or increasing mucus ciliary clearance.[157] Codeine is the most widely used opioid for cough; some authors claim that it has no advantages over other opioids and provides no additional benefit to patients already receiving high doses of opioids for analgesia,[161] whereas others state that the various opioids have different antitussive potencies.[156]

More than 200 synthetic *nonopioid antitussive agents* are available; most are less effective than codeine.[162] Dextromethorphan, a dextro isomer of levorphanol, is an exception; it is almost equiantitussive to codeine. Dextromethorphan acts centrally through nonopioid receptors to increase the cough threshold.[161] Benzonatate is a nonopioid antitussive with a sustained cough-depressing action[163] that provided excellent symptomatic relief for three cancer patients with opioid-resistant cough.[164] Opioid and nonopioid antitussives may act synergistically,[161] but further studies are needed to confirm this hypothesis.

Peripherally Acting Antitussives

Demulcents are a group of compounds that form aqueous solutions and help to alleviate irritation of abraded surfaces. They are often found in over-the-counter cough syrups. Their mode of action for controlling cough is unclear, but it is thought that the sugar content encourages saliva production and swallowing, which leads to a decrease in the cough reflex; stimulates the sensory nerve endings in the epipharynx, and decreases the cough reflex by a "gating" process; or the demulcents may act as a protective barrier by coating the sensory receptors.[157]

Benzonatate is an antitussive that inhibits cough mainly by anesthetizing the vagal stretch receptors in the bronchi, alveoli, and pleura.[156] Other drugs that act directly on cough receptors include levodropropizine, oxalamine, and prenoxdiazine.[156]

Inhaled anticholinergic *bronchodilators*, either alone or in combination with a β_2-adrenergic agonists, effectively decrease cough in people with asthma and in normal subjects.[165] It is thought that they decrease input from the stretch receptors, thereby decreasing the cough reflex, and change the mucociliary clearance.

The local anesthetic lidocaine is a potent suppressor of irritant-induced cough and has been used as a topical anesthetic for the airway during bronchoscopy. *Inhaled local anesthetics*, such as lidocaine and bupivacaine, delivered by nebulizer, suppress some cases of chronic cough for as long as 9 weeks.[157,166–168] Higher doses can cause bronchoconstriction, so it is wise to observe the first treatment. Patients must also be warned not to eat or drink anything for 1 hour after the treatment or until their cough reflex returns.

Productive Coughs

Interventions for productive coughs include chest physiotherapy, oxygen, humidity, and suctioning. In cases of increased sputum production, expectorants, mucolytics, and agents to decrease mucus production can be employed.[156] Opioids, antihistamines, and anticholinergics decrease mucus production and thereby decrease the stimulus for cough.

Massive Hemoptysis

In patients with massive hemoptysis, survival is so poor that patients may not want any kind of intervention to stop the bleeding; in such cases, maintenance of comfort alone becomes the priority. For those patients who want intervention to stop the bleeding, the initial priority is to maintain a patent airway, which usually requires endotracheal intubation. Management options include endobronchial tamponade of the segment, vasoactive drugs, iced saline lavage, neodymium/yttrium-aluminum-garnet (Nd/YAG) laser photocoagulation, electrocautery, bronchial artery embolization, and external beam or endobronchial irradiation.[155]

Nonpharmacological Interventions

If cough is induced by a sensitive cough reflex, then the person should attempt to avoid the stimuli that produce this. They should stop or cut down smoking and avoid smoky rooms, cold air, exercise, and pungent chemicals. If medication is causing the cough, it should be decreased or stopped if possible. If the cause is esophageal reflux, then elevation of the head of the bed may be tried. Adequate hydration, humidification of the air, and chest physiotherapy may help patients expectorate viscid sputum.[98] Radiation therapy to enlarged nodes, endoscopically placed esophageal stents for tracheoesophageal fistulas, or injection of Teflon into a paralyzed vocal cord may improve cough.[98]

Patient and Family Education

Education should include practical matters such as proper use of medications, avoidance of irritants, use of humidification, and ways to improve the effectiveness of cough. One such way is called "huffing." The person lies on his or her side, supports the abdomen with a pillow, blows out sharply three times, holds the breath, and then coughs. This technique seems to improve the effectiveness of a cough and helps to expel sputum.

If the patient is having hemoptysis and massive bleeding is a possibility, it is important to educate the family about this possibility, to prepare them psychologically and develop a treatment plan. Dark towels or blankets can help to minimize the visual impact of this traumatic event. Adequate medications should be immediately available to control any anxiety or distress that might occur. Family and staff require emotional support after such an event.

CASE STUDY

RM, a 67-Year-Old Man with Non–Small Cell Carcinoma of the Lung

RM is a 67-year-old man who presented to his family doctor 2 months ago with a 20-pound weight loss, hemoptysis, and shortness of breath. He was found to have an endobronchial adenocarcinoma of the lung with liver and bone metastases. He was treated with a course of radiotherapy, and the hemoptysis stopped. You are visiting him at home and find that he now has a dry, nonproductive cough that keeps him awake at night and is sometimes so forceful that he vomits. He is receiving hydromorphone 4 mg orally every 4 hours for pain. He has had a trial of demulcents, dextromethorphan, and opioids for his cough, with little effect. He has no evidence of pneumonia on physical examination but does have some scattered wheezes. You suggest a trial of inhaled Ventolin and Atrovent every 6 hours. When you next see him, he reports that his cough is much better and he has been able to get some rest.

Summary

Chronic cough can be a disabling symptom for patients. If the underlying cause is unresponsive to treatment, then suppression of the cough is the major therapeutic goal.

REFERENCES

1. Edmonds P, Higginson I, Altmann D, Sen-Gupta G, McDonnell M. Is the presence of dyspnea a risk factor for morbidity in cancer patients? J Pain Symptom Manage 2000;19:15–22.
2. Fainsinger R, Waller A, Bercovici M, Bengston K, Landman W, Hosking M, Nunez-Olarte JM, deMoissac D. A multicentre international study of sedation for uncontrolled symptoms in terminally ill patients. Palliat Med 2000;14:257–265.
3. American Thoracic Society. Dyspnea: Mechanisms, assessment, and management. A consensus statement. Am J Respir Crit Care Med 1999;159:321–340.
4. Cherniack NS, Altose MD. Mechanisms of dyspnea. Clin Chest Med 1987;8:207–214.
5. Tobin MJ. Dyspnea: Pathophysiologic basis, clinical presentation, and management. Arch Intern Med 1990;150:1604–1613.

6. Manning HL, Schwartzstein RM. Mechanisms of dyspnea. In: Mahler D, ed. Dyspnea. New York: Marcel Dekker, 1998:63–95.
7. Simon PM, Schwartzstein RM, Weiss JW, Fencl V, Teghtsoonian M, Weinberger SE. Distinguishable types of dyspnea in patients with shortness of breath. Am Rev Respir Dis 1990;142:1009–1014.
8. Dudgeon DJ, Kristjanson L, Sloan JA, Lertzman M, Clement K. Dyspnea in cancer patients: Prevalence and associated factors. J Pain Symptom Manage 2001;21:95–102.
9. Reuben DB, Mor V. Dyspnea in terminally ill cancer patients. Chest 1986;89:234–236.
10. Fainsinger R, MacEachern T, Hanson J, Miller MJ, Bruera E. Symptom control during the last week of life on a palliative care unit. J Palliat Care 1991;7:5–11.
11. Twycross RG, Lack SA. Respiratory symptoms. In: Twycross RG, Lack SA, eds. Therapeutics in Terminal Cancer. London: Churchill Livingstone, 1990:123–136.
12. Curtis EB, Krech R, Walsh TD. Common symptoms in patients with advanced cancer. J Palliat Care 1991;7:25–29.
13. Heyse-Moore LH, Ross V, Mullee MA. How much of a problem is dyspnoea in advanced cancer? Palliat Med 1991;5:20–26.
14. Heyse-Moore LH. On Dyspnoea in Advanced Cancer. Southampton, UK: Southampton University, 1993.
15. Muers MF, Round CE. Palliation of symptoms in non-small cell lung cancer: A study by the Yorkshire Regional Cancer Organisation thoracic group. Thorax 1993;48:339–343.
16. Skilbeck J, Mott L, Page H, Smith D, Hjelmeland-Ahmedzai S, Clark D. Palliative care in chronic obstructive airways disease: A needs assessment. Palliat Med 1998;12:245–254.
17. McCarthy M, Lay M, Addington-Hall J. Dying from heart disease. J R Coll Physicians Lond 1996;30:325–328.
18. Addington-Hall J, Lay M, Altmann D, McCarthy M. Symptom control, communication with health professionals, and hospital care of stroke patients in the last year of life as reported by surviving family, friends and officials. Stroke 1995;26:2242–2248.
19. Voltz R, Borasio GD. Palliative therapy in the terminal stage of neurological disease. J Neurol 1997;244(Suppl 4):S2–S10.
20. Roberts DK, Thorne SE, Pearson C. The experience of dyspnea in late-stage cancer: Patients' and nurses' perspectives. Cancer Nurs 1993;16:310–320.
21. Brown ML, Carrieri V, Janson-Bjerklie S, Dodd MJ. Lung cancer and dyspnea: The patient's perception. Oncol Nurs Forum 1986;13(5):19–24.
22. Gore JM, Brophy CJ, Greenstone MA. How well do we care for patients with end stage chronic obstructive pulmonary disease (COPD)? A comparison of palliative care and quality of life in COPD and lung cancer. Thorax 2000;55:1000–1006.
23. O'Driscoll M, Corner J, Bailey C. The experience of breathlessness in lung cancer. Eur J Cancer Care 1999;8:37–43.
24. Bailey PH. Death stories: Acute exacerbations of chronic obstructive pulmonary disease. Qual Health Res 2001;11:322–338.
25. Steinhauser KE, Clipp EC, McNeilly M, Christakis NA, McIntyre LM, Tulsky JA. In search of a good death: Observations of patients, families, and providers. Ann Intern Med 2000;132:825–832.
26. O'Donnell DE. Exertional breathlessness in chronic respiratory disease. In: Mahler D, ed. Dyspnea. New York: Marcel Dekker, 1998:97–147.
27. Dudgeon D, Lertzman M. Dyspnea in the advanced cancer patient. J Pain Symptom Manage 1998;16:212–219.
28. O'Donnell DE, Chau LL, Bertley J, Webb KA. Qualitative aspects of exertional breathlessness in CAL: Pathophysiological mechanisms. Am J Respir Crit Care Med 1997;155:109–115.
29. O'Donnell DE, Chau LKL, Webb KA. Qualitative aspects of exertional dyspnea in interstitial lung disease. J Appl Physiol 1998;84:2000–2009.
30. D'Arsigny C, Raj S, Abdollah H, Webb KA, O'Donnell DE. Ventilatory assistance improves leg discomfort and exercise endurance in stable congestive heart failure (CHF). Am J Respir Crit Care Med 1998;157:A451.
31. Parshall MB, Welsh JD, Brockopp DY, Heiser RM, Schooler MP, Cassidy KB. Reliability and validity of dyspnea sensory quality descriptors in heart failure patients treated in an emergency department. Heart Lung 2001;30:57–65.
32. Silvestri GA, Mahler DA. Evaluation of dyspnea in the elderly patient. Clin Chest Med 1993;14:393–404.
33. Ferrin MS, Tino G. Acute dyspnea. American Association of Critical-Care Nurses Clinical Issues 1997;8:398–410.
34. Gift AG, Plaut SM, Jacox A. Psychologic and physiologic factors related to dyspnea in subjects with chronic obstructive pulmonary disease. Heart Lung 1986;15:595–601.
35. Nguyen HQ, Altinger J, Carrieri-Kohlman V, Gormley JM, Paul SM, Stulbarg MS. Factor analysis of laboratory and clinical measurement of dyspnea in patients with chronic obstructive pulmonary disease. J Pain Symptom Manage 2003;25:118–127.
36. Gift AG. Validation of a vertical visual analogue scale as a measure of clinical dyspnea. Am Rev Respir Dis 1986;133(4, Part 2):A163.
37. Burdon J, Juniper E, Killian K, Hargeave F, Campbell E. The perception of breathlessness. Am Rev Respir Dis 1982;126:825–828.
38. O'Donnell DE, Lam M, Webb KA. Measurement of symptoms, lung hyperinflation, and endurance during exercise in chronic obstructive pulmonary disease. Am J Respir Crit Care Med 1998;158:1557–1565.
39. Tattersall MHN, Boyer MJ. Management of malignant pleural effusions. Thorax 1990;45:81–82.
40. Wilcock A, Crosby V, Clarke D, Corcoran R, Tattersfield AE. Reading numbers aloud: A measure of the limiting effect of breathlessness in patients with cancer. Thorax 1999;54:1099–1103.
41. Neff TA, Petty TL. Tolerance and survival in severe chronic hypercapnia. Arch Intern Med 1972;129:591–596.
42. Kellner R, Samet J, Pathak D. Dyspnea, anxiety, and depression in chronic respiratory impairment. Gen Hosp Psychiatry 1992;14:20–28.
43. Dudgeon D, Lertzman M. Etiology of dyspnea in advanced cancer patients. Program/Proceedings of the American Society of Clinical Oncology 1996;15:165.
44. Bruera E, Schmitz B, Pither J, Neumann CM, Hanson J. The frequency and correlates of dyspnea in patients with advanced cancer. Personal communication, 1997.
45. Carrieri-Kohlman V, Gormley JM, Douglas MK, Paul SM, Stulbarg MS. Differentiation between dyspnea and its affective components. West J Nurs Res 1996;18:626–642.
46. Woodcock AA, Gross ER, Gellert A, Shah S, Johnson M, Geddes DM. Effects of dihydrocodeine, alcohol, and caffeine on breathlessness and exercise tolerance in patients with chronic obstructive lung disease and normal blood gases. N Engl J Med 1981;305:1611–1616.
47. Bruera E, Macmillan K, Pither J, MacDonald RN. Effects of morphine on the dyspnea of terminal cancer patients. J Pain Symptom Manage 1990;5:6:341–344.

48. Bruera E, MacEachern T, Ripamonti C, Hanson J. Subcutaneous morphine for dyspnea in cancer patients. Ann Intern Med 1993;119:906–907.
49. Cohen MH, Anderson AJ, Krasnow SH, Spagnolo SV, Citron ML, Payne M, Fossiek BE Jr. Continuous intravenous infusion of morphine for severe dyspnea. South Med J 1991;84:2:229–234.
50. Light RW, Muro JR, Sato RI, Stansbury DW, Fischer CE, Brown SE. Effects of oral morphine on breathlessness and exercise tolerance in patients with chronic obstructive pulmonary disease. Am Rev Respir Dis 1989;139:126–133.
51. Mueller RE, Petty TL, Filley GF. Ventilation and arterial blood gas changes induced by pursed lip breathing. J Appl Physiol 1970;28:784–789.
52. Masood AR, Subhan MMF, Reed JW, Thomas SHL. Effects of inhaled nebulized morphine on ventilation and breathlessness during exercise in healthy man. Clin Sci 1995;88:447–452.
53. Robin ED, Burke CM. Single-patient randomized clinical trial: Opiates for intractable dyspnea. Chest 1986;90:888–892.
54. Johnson MA, Woodcock AA, Geddes DM. Dihydrocodeine for breathlessness in "pink puffers." Br Med J 1983;286:675–677.
55. Sackner MA. Effects of hydrocodone bitartrate on breathing pattern of patients with chronic obstructive pulmonary disease and restrictive lung disease. Mt Sinai J Med 1984;51:222–226.
56. Timmis AD, Rothman MT, Henderson MA, Geal PW, Chamberlain DA. Haemodynamic effects of intravenous morphine in patients with acute myocardial infarction complicated by severe left ventricular failure. Br Med J 1980;280:980–982.
57. Rice KL, Kronenberg RS, Hedemark LL, Niewoehner DE. Effects of chronic administration of codeine and promethazine on breathlessness and exercise tolerance in patients with chronic airflow obstruction. Br J Dis Chest 1987;81:287–292.
58. Eiser N, Denman WT, West C, Luce P. Oral diamorphine: Lack of effect on dyspnoea and exercise tolerance in the "pink puffer" syndrome. Eur Respir J 1991;4:926–931.
59. Boyd KJ, Kelly M. Oral morphine as symptomatic treatment of dyspnoea in patients with advanced cancer. Palliat Med 1997; 11:277–281.
60. Poole PJ, Veale AG, Black PN. The effect of sustained-release morphine on breathlessness and quality of life in severe chronic obstructive pulmonary disease. Am J Respir Crit Care Med 1998;157(6 Pt 1):1877–1880.
61. Jennings AL, Davies A, Higgins JPT, Broadley K. Opioids for the palliation of breathlessness in terminal illness. Cochrane Datbase Syst Rev. 2001;(4):CD002066.
62. Woodcock AA, Johnson MA, Geddes DM. Breathlessness, alcohol and opiates. N Engl J Med 1982;306:1363–1364.
63. Light RW, Stansbury DW, Webster JS. Effect of 30 mg of morphine alone or with promethazine or prochlorperazine on the exercise capacity of patients with COPD. Chest 1996;109:975–981.
64. Chua TP, Harrington D, Ponikowski P, Webb-Peploe K, Poole-Wilson PA, Coats AJ. Effects of dihydrocodeine on chemosensitivity and exercise tolerance in patients with chronic heart failure. J Am Coll Cardiol 1997;29:147–152.
65. Belvisi MG, Chung KF, Jackson DM, Barnes PJ. Opioid modulation of non-cholinergic neural bronchoconstriction in guinea-pig *in-vivo*. Br J Pharmacol 1988;95:413–418.
66. Beauford W, Saylor TT, Stansbury DW, Avalos K, Light RW. Effects of nebulized morphine sulfate on the exercise tolerance of the ventilatory limited COPD patient. Chest 1993;104:175–178.
67. Davis CL, Hodder C, Love S, Shah R, Slevin M, Wedzicha J. Effect of nebulised morphine and morphine 6-glucuronide on exercise endurance in patients with chronic obstructive pulmonary disease. Thorax 1994;49:393P.
68. Davis CL, Penn K, A'Hern R, Daniels J, Slevin M. Single dose randomised controlled trial of nebulised morphine in patients with cancer related breathlessness. Palliat Med 1996;10:64–65.
69. Harris-Eze AO, Sridhar G, Clemens RE, Zintel TA, Gallagher CG, Marciniuk DD. Low-dose nebulized morphine does not improve exercise in interstitial lung disease. Am J Respir Crit Care Med 1995;152:1940–1945.
70. Jankelson D, Hosseini K, Mather LE, Seale JP, Young IH. Lack of effect of high doses of inhaled morphine on exercise endurance in chronic obstructive pulmonary disease. Eur Respir J 1997; 10:2270–2274.
71. Leung R, Hill P, Burdon JGW. Effect of inhaled morphine on the development of breathlessness during exercise in patients with chronic lung disease. Thorax 1996;51:596–600.
72. Masood AR, Reed JW, Thomas SHL. Lack of effect of inhaled morphine on exercise-induced breathlessness in chronic obstructive pulmonary disease. Thorax 1995;50:629–634.
73. Noseda A, Carpiaux JP, Markstein C, Meyvaert A, de Maertelaer V. Disabling dyspnoea in patients with advanced disease: Lack of effect of nebulized morphine. Eur Respir J 1997;10:1079–1083.
74. Young IH, Daviskas E, Keena VA. Effect of low dose nebulised morphine on exercise endurance in patients with chronic lung disease. Thorax 1989;44:387–390.
75. Wilson RH, Hoseth W, Dempsey ME. Respiratory acidosis: I. Effects of decreasing respiratory minute volume in patients with severe chronic pulmonary emphysema, with specific reference to oxygen, morphine and barbiturates. Am J Med 1954;17: 464–470.
76. Mazzocato C, Buclin T, Rapin CH. The effects of morphine on dyspnea and ventilatory function in elderly patients with advanced cancer: A randomized double-blind controlled trial. Ann Oncol 1999;10:1511–1514.
77. Dudgeon D. Dyspnea, death rattle, and cough. In: Ferrell BR, Coyle N, eds. Textbook of Palliative Nursing. New York: Oxford University Press, 2001:164–174.
78. Dudgeon D. Dyspnea: Ethical concerns. Ethics in Palliative Care: Part II. J Palliat Care 1994;10(3):48–51.
79. Twycross R. Morphine and dyspnoea. In: Twycross R. Pain Relief in Advanced Cancer. New York: Churchill Livingstone, 1994:383–399.
80. O'Neill PA, Morton PB, Stark RD. Chlorpromazine: A specific effect on breathlessness? Br J Clin Pharmacol 1985;19:793–797.
81. Woodcock AA, Gross ER, Geddes DM. Drug treatment of breathlessness: Contrasting effects of diazepam and promethazine in pink puffers. Br Med J 1981;283:343–346.
82. McIver B, Walsh D, Nelson K. The use of chlorpromazine for symptom control in dying cancer patients. J Pain Symptom Manage 1994;9:341–345.
83. Sen D, Jones G, Leggat PO. The response of the breathless patient treated with diazepam. Br J Clin Pract 1983;37(June):232–233.
84. Mitchell-Heggs P, Murphy K, Minty K, Guz A, Patterson SC, Minty PS, Rosser RM. Diazepam in the treatment of dyspnoea in the "pink puffer" syndrome. Q J Med 1980;49:9–20.
85. Greene JG, Pucino F, Carlson JD, Storsved M, Strommen GL. Effects of alprazolam on respiratory drive, anxiety, and dyspnea in chronic airflow obstruction: A case study. Pharmacotherapy 1989;9:34–38.
86. Man GCW, Hsu K, Sproule BJ. Effect of alprazolam on exercise and dyspnea in patients with chronic obstructive pulmonary disease. Chest 1986;90:832–836.

87. Eimer M, Cable T, Gal P, Rothenberger LA, McCue JD. Effects of clorazepate on breathlessness and exercise tolerance in patients with chronic airflow obstruction. J Fam Pract 1985;21: 359–362.
88. Argyropoulou P, Patakas D, Koukou A, Vasiliadis P, Georgopoulos D. Buspirone effect on breathlessness and exercise performance in patients with chronic obstructive pulmonary disease. Respiration 1993;60:216–220.
89. Ventafridda V, Spoldi E, De Conno F. Control of dyspnea in advanced cancer patients. Chest 1990;98:1544–1545.
90. O'Neill PA, Stark RD, Morton PB. Do prostaglandins have a role in breathlessness? Am Rev Respir Dis 1985;132:22–24.
91. O'Neill PA, Stretton TB, Stark RD, Ellis SH. The effect of indomethacin on breathlessness in patients with diffuse parenchymal disease of the lung. Br J Dis Chest 1986;80:72–79.
92. Schiffman GL, Stansbury DW, Fischer CE, Sato RI, Light RW, Brown SE. Indomethacin and perception of dyspnea in chronic airflow limitation. Am Rev Respir Dis 1988;137:1094–1098.
93. Winning AJ, Hamilton RD, Shea SA, Knott C, Guz A. The effect of airway anaesthesia on the control of breathing and the sensation of breathlessness in man. Clin Sci 1985;68:215–225.
94. Winning AJ, Hamilton RD, Guz A. Ventilation and breathlessness on maximal exercise in patients with interstitial lung disease after local anaesthetic aerosol inhalation. Clin Sci 1988; 74:275–281.
95. Wilcock A, Corcoran R, Tattersfield AE. Safety and efficacy of nebulized lignocaine in patients with cancer and breathlessness. Palliat Med 1994;8:35–38.
96. Giron AE, Stansbury DW, Fischer CE, Light RW. Lack of effect of dextromethorphan on breathlessness and exercise performance in patients with chronic obstructive pulmonary disease (COPD). Eur Respir J 1991;4:532–535.
97. Shepard KV. Dyspnea in cancer patients. Palliat Care Lett 1990; 2:6(Insert 1).
98. Cowcher K, Hanks GW. Long-term management of respiratory symptoms in advanced cancer. J Pain Symptom Manage 1990;5:320–330.
99. Kaplan JD. Acute respiratory failure. In: Woodley M, Whelan A, eds. Manual of Medical Therapeutics: The Washington Manual. Boston: Little, Brown, 1992:179–195.
100. Tarpy SP, Celli BR. Long-term oxygen therapy. N Engl J Med 1995;333:710–714.
101. Bruera E, de Stoutz N, Velasco-Leiva A, Schoeller T, Hanson J. Effects of oxygen on dyspnoea in hypoxaemic terminal-cancer patients. Lancet 1993;342:13–14.
102. Bruera E, Schoeller T, MacEachern T. Symptomatic benefit of supplemental oxygen in hypoxemic patients with terminal cancer: The use of the *N* of 1 randomized controlled trial. J Pain Symptom Manage 1992;7:365–368.
103. Woodcock AA, Gross ER, Geddes DM. Oxygen relieves breathlessness in "pink puffers." Lancet 1981;1(8226):907–909.
104. Bruera E, Sweeney C, Willey J, Palmer JL, Strasser F, Morice RC, Pisters K. A randomized controlled trial of supplemental oxygen versus air in cancer patients with dyspnea. Palliat Med 2003;17:659–663.
105. Hausheer FH, Yarbro JW. Diagnosis and treatment of malignant pleural effusion. Semin Oncol 1985;1254–75.
106. Lynch TJ. Management of malignant pleural effusions. Chest 1993;4(Suppl):385S–389S.
107. Anderson CB, Philpott GW, Ferguson TB. The treatment of malignant pleural effusions. Cancer 1974;33:916–922.
108. Rauthe G, Sistermanns J. Recombinant tumour necrosis factor in the local therapy of malignant pleural effusion. Eur J Cancer 1997;33:226–231.
109. Grodzin CJ, Balk RA. Indwelling small pleural catheter needle thoracentesis in the management of large pleural effusions. Chest 1997;111:981–988.
110. Patz EF Jr. Malignant pleural effusions: Recent advances and ambulatory sclerotherapy. Chest 1998;113(1 Suppl):74S–77S.
111. Press OW, Livingston R. Management of malignant pericardial effusion and tamponade. JAMA 1987;257:1088–1092.
112. Vaitkus PT, Hermann HC, LeWinter MM. Treatment of malignant pericardial effusion. JAMA 1994;272:59–64.
113. Chong HH, Plotnick GD. Pericardial effusion and tamponade: Evaluation, imaging modalities, and management. Compr Ther 1995;21:378–385.
114. Mangan CM. Malignant pericardial effusions: Pathophysiology and clinical correlates. Oncol Nurs Forum 1992;19:1215–1223.
115. Barach AL. Chronic obstructive lung disease: Postural relief of dyspnea. Arch Phys Med Rehabil 1974;55:494–504.
116. Sharp JT, Drutz WS, Moisan T, Foster J, Machnach W. Postural relief of dyspnea in severe chronic obstructive pulmonary disease. Am Rev Respir Dis 1980;122:201–211.
117. Thoman RL, Stoker GL, Ross JC. The efficacy of pursed-lips breathing in patients with chronic obstructive pulmonary disease. Am Rev Respir Dis 1966;93:100–106.
118. Make B. COPD: Management and rehabilitation. Am Fam Physician 1991;43:1315–1324.
119. Schwartzstein RM, Lahive K, Pope A, Weinberger SE, Weiss JW. Cold facial stimulation reduces breathlessness induced in normal subjects. Am Rev Respir Dis 1987;136:58–61.
120. Burgess KR, Whitelaw WA. Effects of nasal cold receptors on pattern of breathing. J Appl Physiol 1988;64:371–376.
121. Burgess KR, Whitelaw WA. Reducing ventilatory response to carbon dioxide by breathing cold air. Am Rev Respir Dis 1984;129:687–690.
122. Jobst K, Chen JH, McPherson J. Controlled trial of acupuncture for disabling breathlessness. Lancet 1986;2:1416–1418.
123. Maa SH, Gauthier D, Turner M. Acupressure as an adjunct to a pulmonary rehabilitation program. J Cardiopulm Rehabil 1997;17:268–276.
124. Filshie J, Penn K, Ashley S, Davis CL. Acupuncture for the relief of cancer-related breathlessness. Palliat Med 1996;10:145–150.
125. Renfroe KL. Effect of progressive relaxation on dyspnea and state anxiety in patients with chronic obstructive pulmonary disease. Heart Lung 1988;17:408–413.
126. Rosser RM, Denford J, Heslop A. Breathlessness and psychiatric morbidity in chronic bronchitis and emphysema: A study of psychotherapeutic management. Psychol Med 1983;13:93–110.
127. Corner J, Plant H, A'Hern R, Bailey C. Non-pharmacological intervention for breathlessness in lung cancer. Palliat Med 1996;10:299–305.
128. Carrieri VK, Janson-Bjerklie S. Strategies patients use to manage the sensation of dyspnea. West J Nurs Res 1986;8:284–305.
129. van den Berg R. Dyspnea: Perception or reality. CACCN 1995;6:16–19.
130. Moody LE, Fraser M, Yarandi H. Effects of guided imagery in patients with chronic bronchitis and emphysema. Clin Nurs Res 1993;2:478–486.
131. Giasson M, Bouchard L. Effect of therapeutic touch on the well-being of persons with terminal cancer. J Holistic Nurs 1998;16:383–398.

132. Shih F, Chu S. Comparisons of American-Chinese and Taiwanese patients' perceptions of dyspnea and helpful nursing actions during the intensive care unit transition from cardiac surgery. Heart Lung 1999;28:41–54.
133. Tiep BL. Inpatient pulmonary rehabilitation: A team approach to the more fragile patient. Postgrad Med 1989;86:141–150.
134. Grey A. The nursing management of dyspnoea in palliative care. Nurs Times 1995;91:33–35.
135. Back IN, Jenkins K, Blower A, Beckhelling J. A study comparing hyoscine hydrobromide and glycopyrrolate in the treatment of death rattle. Palliat Med 2001;15:329–336.
136. Watts T, Jenkins K. Palliative care nurses' feelings about death rattle. J Clin Nurs 1999;8:615–616.
137. Wildiers H, Menten J. Death rattle: Prevalence, prevention and treatment. J Pain Symptom Manage 2002;23:310–317.
138. Hughes AC, Wilcock A, Corcoran R. Management of death rattle. J Pain Symptom Manage 1996;12:271–272.
139. Ellershaw JE, Sutcliffe JM, Saunders CM. Dehydration and the dying patient. J Pain Symptom Manage 1995;10:192–197.
140. Morita T, Ichiki T, Tsunoda J, Inoue S, Chihara S. A prospective study on the dying process in terminally ill cancer patients. Am J Hospice Palliat Care 1998;15:217–222.
141. Kass RM, Ellershaw JE. Respiratory tract secretions in the dying patient: A retrospective study. J Pain Symptom Manage 2003; 26:897–902.
142. Morita T, Tsunoda J, Inoue S, Chihara S. Risk factors for death rattle in terminally ill cancer patients: A prospective exploratory study. Palliat Med 2000;14:19–23.
143. Bennett MI. Death rattle: an audit of hyoscine (scopolamine) use and review of management. J Pain Symptom Manage 1996;12:229–233.
144. Hall P, Schroder C, Weaver L. The last 48 hours of life in long-term care: A focused chart audit. J Am Geriatr Soc 2002;50: 501–506.
145. Nadel JA. Regulation of airway secretions. Chest 1985;87(1 Suppl): 111S–113S.
146. Kaliner M, Shelhamer H, Borson B, Nadel JA, Patow C, Marom Z. Human respiratory mucus. Am Rev Respir Dis 1986;134: 612–621.
147. Victoria Hospice Society. Medical Care of the Dying, 3rd ed. Victoria, BC: Victoria Hospice Society, 1998.
148. Andrews MR, Levine AM. Dehydration in the terminal patient: Perception of hospice nurses. Am J Hosp Care 1989;6:31–34.
149. Downing M. Victoria Respiratory Congestion Scale. 2004. Personal Communication.
150. Bennett M, Lucas V, Brennan M, Hughes A, O'Donnell V, Wee B. Using anti-muscarinic drugs in the management of death rattle: Evidence-based guidelines for palliative care. Palliat Med 2002;16:369–374.
151. Dawson HR. The use of transdermal scopolamine in the control of death rattle. J Palliat Care 1989;5:31–33.
152. Lichter I, Hunt E. The last 48 hours of life. J Palliat Care 1990;6:7–15.
153. Murtagh FEM, Thorns A, Oliver DJ. Correspondence: Hyoscine and glycopyrrolate for death rattle. Palliat Med 2002;16:449–450.
154. Morice AH, Kastelik JA. Cough 1: Chronic cough in adults. Thorax 2003;58:901–907.
155. Kvale PA, Simoff M, Prakash UBS. Palliative care. Chest 2003;123:284S–311S.
156. Homsi J, Walsh D, Nelson KA. Important drugs for cough in advanced cancer. Support Care Cancer 2001;9:565–574.
157. Fuller RW, Jackson DM. Physiology and treatment of cough. Thorax 1990;45:425–430.
158. Lalloo UG, Barnes PJ, Chung KF. Pathophysiology and clinical presentations of cough. J Allergy Clin Immunol 1996;98(5, Part 2):S91–S97.
159. Dudgeon D, Rosenthal S. Pathophysiology and assessment of dyspnea in the patient with cancer. In: Portenoy RK, Bruera E, eds. Topics in Palliative Care. New York: Oxford University Press, 1999:237–254.
160. Ripamonti C, Fusco F. Respiratory problems in advanced cancer. Support Care Cancer 2002;10:204–216.
161. Hagen NA. An approach to cough in cancer patients. J Pain Symptom Manage 1991;6:257–262.
162. Eddy NB, Friebel H, Hahn KJ, Halbach H. Codeine and its alternatives for pain and cough relief. Potential alternatives for cough relief. Bull World Health Organ 1969;40:639–719.
163. Eddy NB, Friebel H, Hahn KJ, Halbach H. Codeine and its alternatives for pain and cough relief. Discussion and summary. Bull World Health Organ 1969;40:721–730.
164. Doona M, Walsh D. Benzonatate for opioid-resistant cough in advanced cancer. Palliat Med 1997;12:55–58.
165. Lowry R, Wood A, Johnson T, Higenbottam T. Antitussive properties of inhaled bronchodilators on induced cough. Chest 1988;93:1186–1189.
166. Louie K, Bertolino M, Fainsinger R. Management of intractable cough. J Palliat Care 1992;8:46–48.
167. Howard P, Cayton RM, Brennan SR, Anderson PB. Lignocaine aerosol and persistent cough. Br J Dis Chest 1977;71:19–24.
168. Sanders RV, Kirkpatrick MB. Prolonged suppression of cough after inhalation of Lidocaine in a patient with sarcoid. JAMA 1984;252:2456–2457.
169. Dudgeon D, Rosenthal S. Pathophysiology and treatment of cough. In: Portenoy R, Bruera E, eds. Topics in Palliative Care. New York: Oxford University Press, 2000:237–254.

14

Mikel Gray and Fern Campbell

Urinary Tract Disorders

As if being sick and dying isn't enough—it's all the indignity before you go. Losing control of my bladder and feeling like a baby in diapers has been the worst . . . when my daughter came and saw me like this (with the diaper), that's when she just lost it.—A patient

- ***Key Points***
- *The urinary system is frequently the cause of bothersome or deleterious symptoms that affect the patient receiving palliative care.*
- *A malignancy or systemic disease may affect voiding function and produce urinary incontinence, urinary retention, or upper urinary tract obstruction.*
- *Frequent lower urinary tract symptoms (LUTS) include intermittent or continuous urinary leakage, daytime voiding frequency, excessive nocturia, bothersome urgency, feelings of incomplete bladder emptying, and the abrupt cessation of urination.*
- *Upper urinary tract symptoms include flank or abdominal pain and constitutional symptoms related to acute renal insufficiency or failure.*
- *Significant hematuria leading to clot formation and catheter blockage is an uncommon but significant complication of pelvic radiation therapy. Bleeding may occur months to years following radiotherapy.*
- *Initial treatment of hematuria includes continuous bladder irrigation to evacuate clots from the bladder vesicle until the fragile bladder wall heals. If hematuria recurs, more aggressive treatment options include intravesical alum or prostaglandins. Intravesical formalin treatments are reserved for very severe cases of blood loss.*
- *Bladder spasms may be associated with urinary tract infection or catheter blockage, or they may be idiopathic. Any apparent underlying cause of bladder spasms, such as a urinary tract infection, should be treated initially.*
- *An antimuscarinic medication should be used for long-term relief of bladder spasms. Extended-release or transdermal agents are usually preferred because of their favorable side effect profiles and avoidance of the need for frequent dosing. However, classic anticholinergic drugs may be required if bladder spasms prove refractory to extended or transdermal formulations.*
- *A suprapubic catheter may be used as an alternative to urethral catheterization after urethral trauma or in the presence of urethral obstruction in cases of urethral injury, strictures, prostate obstruction, after gynecologic surgery, or for long-term catheterization.*

In many ways, the techniques used for management of urinary symptoms are similar to those used for patients in any care setting. However, in contrast to traditional interventions, the evaluation and management of urinary tract symptoms in the palliative care setting are influenced by considerations of the goals of care and closeness to death.

Urinary system disorders may be directly attributable to a malignancy, systemic disease, or a specific treatment such as radiation or chemotherapy. This chapter provides a detailed overview of the anatomy and physiology of the urinary system, which serves as a framework for understanding of the pathophysiology of bothersome symptoms and their management. This is followed by a review of commonly encountered urinary symptoms seen in the palliative care setting, including bothersome lower urinary tract symptoms (LUTS), lower urinary tract pain, urinary stasis or retention, and hematuria.

Lower Urinary Tract Disorders

Lower Urinary Tract Physiology

The lower urinary tract comprises the bladder, urethra, and supportive structures within the pelvic floor (Figures 14–1 and 14–2). Together, these structures maintain *urinary continence*, which can be simply defined as control over bladder filling and storage and the act of micturition. Continence is modulated by three interrelated factors: (1) anatomic integrity of the urinary tract, (2) control of the detrusor muscle, and (3) competence of the urethral sphincter mechanism.[1,2] Each may be compromised in the patient receiving palliative care, leading to bothersome LUTS, urinary retention, or a combination of these disorders.

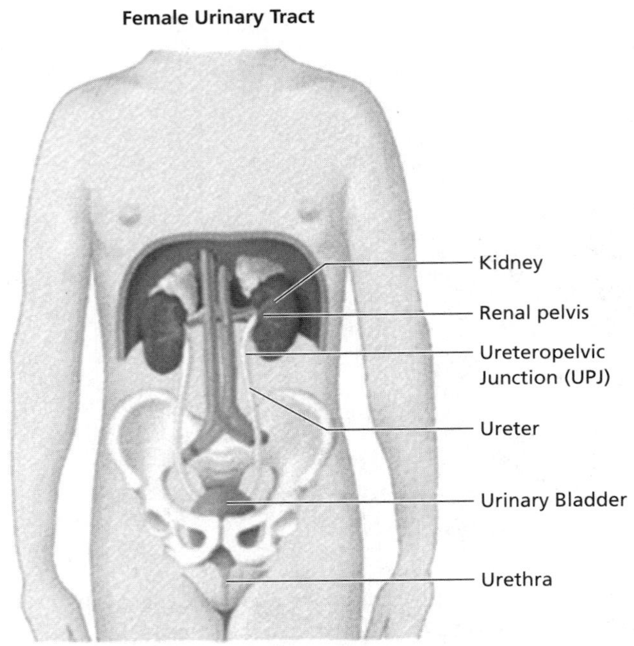

Figure 14–1. The female urinary tract.

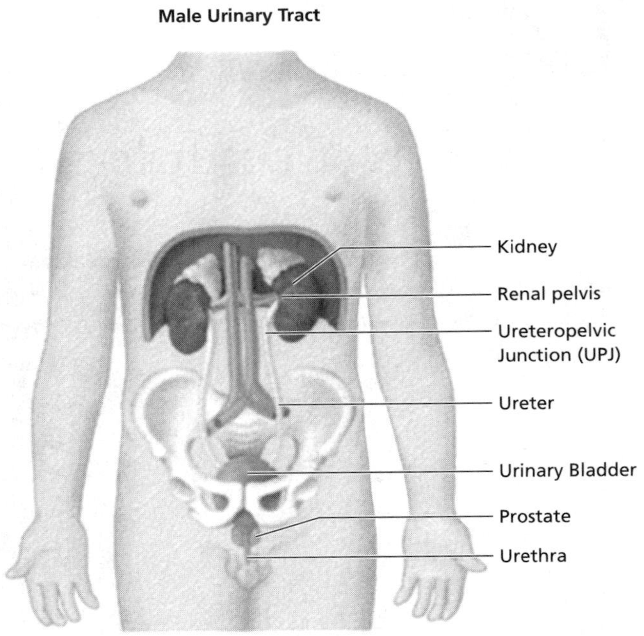

Figure 14–2. The male urinary tract.

Anatomic Integrity

From a physiological perspective, the urinary system comprises a long tube originating in the glomerulus and terminating at the urethral meatus. When contemplating urinary continence, anatomical integrity of the urinary system is often assumed, particularly because extraurethral urinary incontinence (UI) is uncommon. However, anatomical integrity may be lost in the patient receiving palliative care due to a fistula that bypasses the urethral sphincter. This epithelialized tract allows continuous urinary leakage, which varies from an ongoing dribble in a patient with otherwise normal urine elimination habits to total UI characterized by failure of bladder filling and micturition.[3]

Control of the Detrusor

In addition to a structurally intact urinary system, continence requires volitional control over detrusor contraction.[1,2] Control of this smooth muscle can be conceptualized on three levels. Multiple modulatory centers within the central nervous system modulate the detrusor reflex, allowing inhibition of detrusor activity until the person wishes to urinate. Detrusor control is also influenced by its histological characteristics.

The nervous control of the detrusor relies on input from multiple modulatory areas within the brain and spinal cord.[4] Bilateral detrusor motor areas are found within the lobes of the frontal cortex.[5] This modulatory center interacts with neurons in the thalamus,[6] hypothalamus,[7] basal ganglia,[8] and cerebellum[9] to modulate bladder filling and voiding. The net effect of these areas on continence is the maintenance of a stable detrusor that does not contract, even when provoked, until the person desires to urinate.[1,2]

Whereas modulatory centers within the brain are essential for continence, the primary integration centers for bladder filling and micturition are found within the brainstem.[10] Specific areas within the brainstem control bladder filling and storage under the influence of higher brain regions. These areas include the periaqueductal gray matter, which is responsible for coordinating multiple groups of neurons in the brainstem; the L and M regions, which modulate bladder filling and initiate the detrusor contraction; and the pontine micturition center, which coordinates the reflexive response of the urethral sphincter mechanism. Recognition of the significance of the brainstem micturition center is particularly important when providing palliative care, because a neurological lesion above the brainstem causes urge UI with a coordinated sphincter response, whereas lesions below this center affect bladder sensations and the coordination between the detrusor and the urethral sphincter.

The brainstem micturition center communicates with the bladder via spinal roots in the thoracolumbar and sacral segments.[4] Segments in the thoracolumbar spine (T10–L2) carry sympathetic nervous impulses that promote bladder filling and storage, whereas segments S2–S4 transmit parasympathetic impulses to the bladder wall, allowing micturition under modulation by the brain and brain-stem. These impulses are carried through several peripheral nerve plexi, including the pelvic and inferior hypogastric plexi.

Histological characteristics of the detrusor also contribute to its voluntary control.[11] Unlike the visceral smooth muscle of the bowel, stomach, or ureter, the detrusor muscle bundles are innervated on an almost one-to-one basis. The smooth muscle bundles of the detrusor also lack gap junctions, observed in other visceral organs, which allow propagation of a contraction independent of nervous stimulation. These characteristics promote urinary continence because they discourage spontaneous contractions of the detrusor in response to bladder filling, as is characteristic of other visceral organs.

On a molecular level, specific chemical substances, commonly called neurotransmitters, exert local control over the detrusor muscle.[12] Several neurotransmitters are released from the axons of neurons within the bladder wall and act at specific receptors to produce smooth muscle contraction or relaxation. Norepinephrine acts through β_3-adrenergic receptors, promoting detrusor muscle relaxation, and acetylcholine acts through muscarinic receptors, leading to detrusor contraction and micturition. Although it has long been known that the cholinergic receptors within the detrusor are muscarinic, physiological studies have identified at least five muscarinic receptor subtypes (M1 through M5).[13] Receptor subtypes M2 and M3 predominate within the bladder wall and are primarily responsible for the detrusor contraction that leads to micturition. Identification of these receptor subtypes is clinically relevant because it has facilitated the development of drugs that act on the bladder but produce fewer side effects than the older (nonselective) drugs traditionally used to manage urge UI or bladder spasms.

Competence of the Urethral Sphincter Mechanism

The urethral sphincter comprises a combination of compressive and tension elements to form a watertight seal against urinary leakage, even when challenged by physical exertion or sudden increases in abdominal pressure caused by coughing, laughing, or sneezing.[1,2] The soft urethral mucosa interacts with mucosal secretions and the submucosal vascular cushion to ensure a watertight seal that rapidly conforms to changes. Whereas the elements of compression provide a watertight seal for the urethra, striated and smooth muscle within the urethral wall and within the surrounding pelvic floor are necessary when sphincter closure is challenged by physical exertion. The muscular elements of the urethral sphincter comprise the smooth muscle of the bladder neck and proximal urethra (including the prostatic urethra in men), the rhabdosphincter, and the periurethral striated muscles. α_1-Adrenergic receptors in the smooth muscle of the bladder neck and proximal urethra promote sphincter closure when exposed to the neurotransmitter norepinephrine.[14] Innervation of the rhabdosphincter is more complex. Acetylcholine acts on nicotinic receptors in the rhabdosphincter to stimulate muscle contraction. In addition, norepinephrine and serotonin (5HT) act on neurons within Onuf 's nucleus (located at sacral spinal segments 2 through 4), modulating rhabdosphincter tone during bladder filling and storage.[15] A novel substance, duloxetine, is a balanced serotonin and norepinephrine reuptake inhibitor that is undergoing clinical investigation to determine its safety and efficacy for the management of stress urinary incontinence.

Pathophysiology of Urinary Incontinence

Urinary incontinence is defined as the uncontrolled loss of urine of sufficient magnitude to create a problem.[16] It is initially characterized as acute or chronic, according to its presentation and underlying pathophysiology. Causes of acute UI may be classified according to the DIAPERS mnemonic (Table 14–1). Several conditions, including acute delirium, restricted mobility, stool impaction, and specific medications, may occur in patients receiving palliative care and should be considered when assessing and managing UI.

Chronic UI is subdivided into types according to its presenting symptoms or underlying pathophysiology.[17] Stress UI occurs when physical stress (exertion) causes urine loss in the absence of a detrusor contraction. Two conditions lead to stress UI—urethral hypermobility (descent during physical activity) and intrinsic sphincter deficiency (incompetence of the striated or smooth muscle within the urethral sphincter mechanism).

Table 14–1
Causes of Acute Urinary Incontinence (DIAPERS Mnemonic)

Delirium	Acute delirium may cause functional UI, which resolves when underlying disease and related delirium subside.
Infection	A urinary tract infection may cause or exacerbate UI.
Atrophic urethritis	Although atrophic urethritis has been associated with irritative voiding symptoms and stress UI, systemic hormone replacement therapy has not been shown to alleviate associated UI.
Pharmacy	Multiple drugs may contribute to UI.
	Opioids, sedatives, antidepressants, antipsychotics, and antiparkinsonian drugs suppress detrusor contractility and increase the risk of urinary retention and overflow UI. α-Adrenergic blocking agents may cause stress UI in women. α-Adrenergic agonists increase smooth muscle tone in the male urethra and raise the risk of acute urinary retention.
Excessive urine production	Diabetes mellitus or insipidus causes polyuria and subsequent UI.
Restricted mobility	Restriction of mobility leads to UI when it prevents access to toileting facilities.
Stool impaction	Stool impaction increases the risk of UI, urinary retention, and urinary tract infection.

UI, urinary incontinence

Table 14–2
Causes of Intrinsic Sphincter Deficiency in the Patient Receiving Palliative Care

Urethral Surgery
Radical prostatectomy
Transurethral prostatectomy
Cryosurgery
Multiple urethral suspensions in women
Surgery Indirectly Affecting the Urethra via Local Denervation
Abdominoperineal resection
Pelvic exenteration
Radical hysterectomy
Neurological Lesions of the Lower Spine
Primary or metastatic tumors of the sacral spine
Pathological fracture of the sacral spinal column
Multiple sclerosis
Tertiary syphilis

Although urethral hypermobility is rarely the primary cause of significant stress UI in the patient receiving palliative care, intrinsic sphincter deficiency may compromise sphincter closure and lead to severe urinary leakage. Intrinsic sphincter deficiency occurs when the nerves or muscles necessary for sphincter closure are denervated or damaged.[18] Table 14–2 lists conditions that are likely to cause intrinsic sphincter deficiency in patients receiving palliative care.

Urge UI occurs when overactive detrusor contractions produce urinary leakage.[17] Urge UI has recently been defined as part of a larger symptom syndrome called the *overactive bladder*. Overactive bladder is characterized by bothersome urgency (a sudden and strong urge to urinate), and it is typically associated with daytime voiding frequency (more than every 2 hours) and nocturia (≥3 episodes per night). Reflex UI, in contrast, is caused by a neurological lesion below the brainstem micturition center.[19] It is characterized by diminished or absent sensations of bladder filling, overactive detrusor contractions associated with urinary leakage, and a loss of coordination between the detrusor and sphincter muscles (detrusor–sphincter dyssynergia).

Functional UI occurs when deficits in mobility, dexterity, or cognition cause or contribute to urinary leakage.[20] A variety of conditions may produce functional UI in the patient receiving palliative care. For example, neurological deficits or pain may reduce the patient's ability to reach the toilet in a timely fashion. Cognitive deficits caused by malignancies or diseases of the brain may predispose the patient to functional UI. In addition, sedative or analgesic medications may reduce awareness of bladder fullness and the need to urinate, particularly in the patient who experiences nocturia.

Extraurethral UI occurs when a fistula creates an opening between the bladder and the vagina or skin, allowing urine to bypass the urethral sphincter. Within the context of palliative care, fistulas are usually caused by invasive pelvic or gynecological malignancies, extensive pelvic surgery, or radiation treatment.[3]

Assessment and Management of Bothersome LUTS: Urinary Incontinence

The results of a focused history, physical assessment, urinalysis, and bladder log are essential for the evaluation of UI in the patient receiving palliative care. Urine culture and sensitivity testing, blood tests, urodynamic evaluation, or imaging studies also may be completed in specific cases.

The history focuses on the duration of the problem and the probable cause of bothersome symptoms. *Acute* UI is typically characterized by a sudden occurrence of urinary leakage or an acute exacerbation of preexisting symptoms. These symptoms are typically similar to those of urge or stress UI. In contrast, chronic or established UI usually evolves over a period of time, typically months or possibly years.

The history can also be used to provide clues about the type of chronic UI. Stress UI is characterized by urine loss occurring with physical exertion or a sudden increase in abdominal pressure caused by coughing or sneezing. It occurs in the absence of a precipitous and strong urge to urinate. Approximately 36% of patients with overactive bladder syndrome experience urge UI. (The diagnosis of overactive bladder is based on a combination of symptoms: diurnal voiding frequency, nocturia, bothersome urgency with or without the symptom of urge UI, and urinary leakage associated with a sudden desire to urinate).[21] A diagnosis of overactive bladder cannot be accurately inferred from a report of the symptom of urge UI alone.

Reflex UI is suspected in the patient who experiences a paralyzing neurological lesion that affects spinal segments below the brainstem and above S2. The patient frequently reports periodic urination with little or no warning and little or no associated urgency. The urinary stream may be intermittent (stuttering), and the patient may perceive a sensation of incomplete bladder emptying or report additional urinary leakage soon after completion of micturition.

Functional UI is suspected when a general evaluation of the patient reveals significant limitations in mobility, dexterity, or cognition. Continuous urinary leakage that is not associated with physical exertion raises the suspicion of extraurethral UI associated with a fistula, but it is also associated with severe stress UI caused by intrinsic sphincter deficiency.

A focused physical examination provides additional evidence concerning the UI type and its severity. A general examination is used to evaluate the presence of functional UI and to determine the influence of functional limitations on other types of UI. A pelvic examination is completed to assess perineal skin integrity, to identify the presence of obvious fistulas or severe sphincter incompetence, and to evaluate local neurological function. Altered skin integrity, particularly if accompanied by a monilial rash or irritant dermatitis, indicates high-volume (severe) urinary leakage. In certain cases, the source of severe leakage can be easily identified as a large fistula or massive intrinsic sphincter deficiency associated with a gaping (patulous) urethra. A local neurological examination, focusing on local sensations, pelvic floor muscle tone, and the presence of the bulbocavernosus reflex, provides clues to underlying neurological problems leading to voiding dysfunction.

A bladder log (a written record of the timing of urination, volume, timing of UI episodes, and fluid intake) is useful because it allows a semiquantitative analysis of the patterns of urinary elimination, UI, and associated symptoms. It can also be used to assess fluid intake or the patient's response to prompted voiding.[22] The patient is taught to record the time of voluntary urination, episodes of incontinence and associated factors (urgency, physical activity), and type and amount of fluids consumed. This record is used to determine voiding interval, frequency of UI episodes along with associated factors, and the total volume and types of fluids consumed. Recording fluid intake allows the nurse to calculate the cumulative volume of fluids consumed each day, as well as the proportion of fluids containing caffeine or alcohol, substances that exacerbate bothersome LUTS. A 3-day bladder log is strongly recommended, but valuable information can be obtained from a 1- or 2-day document if a 3-day record is not available.[23]

Urinalysis serves several useful purposes in the evaluation of the patient with UI. The presence of nitrites and leukocytes on dipstick analysis or bacteriuria and pyuria on microscopic analysis indicates a clinically relevant urinary tract infection. Blood in the urine may coexist with a urinary tract infection, or it may indicate significant hematuria demanding prompt management (see later discussion). In the patient receiving palliative care, glucosuria may indicate poorly controlled diabetes mellitus causing osmotic diuresis and subsequent UI. In contrast, a low specific gravity may indicate diabetes mellitus or excessive fluid intake from oral or parenteral sources.

Other diagnostic tests are completed when indicated. For example, a urine culture and sensitivity analysis is obtained if the urinalysis reveals bacteriuria and pyuria, and an endoscopy is indicated if significant hematuria is present without an obvious explanation. Urodynamic testing is indicated after acute UI is excluded and if simpler examinations have failed to establish an accurate diagnosis leading to an effective plan for management.

The management of UI is based on its type, the desires of the patient and family, and the presence of complicating factors. Acute UI is managed by addressing its underlying cause.[24] A urinary tract infection should be treated with sensitivity-driven antibiotics. Similarly, medication regimens are altered as feasible if they produce or exacerbate UI. Atrophic urethritis may be managed with topical hormone replacement if feasible. Alternatively, topical vitamin E preparations may offer some benefit if hormone replacement therapy is contraindicated. Fecal impaction must be relieved and constipation aggressively managed, using a combination of fluids and fiber. After disimpaction, a scheduled elimination program is frequently indicated. This program usually combines a peristaltic stimulant, such as a warm cup of coffee or tea or a suppository, and a scheduled elimination program. In addition, stool softeners or laxatives may be used if simpler programs fail to alleviate constipation. Refer to Chapter 11 for a detailed discussion of bowel elimination problems.

A number of techniques are used to manage chronic or established UI. Every patient should be counseled about lifestyle alterations that may alleviate or occasionally relieve UI and associated LUTS.[25,26] Patients are advised to avoid routinely restricting fluid intake to reduce UI, because this strategy only increases the risk of constipation and concentrates the urine, irritating the bladder wall. Instead, they should be counseled to obtain the recommended daily allowance for fluids (30 mL/kg or 0.5 oz/lb),[27] to sip fluids throughout the day, and to avoid intake of large volumes of fluids over a brief period. Patients may also be taught to reduce or avoid bladder irritants that increase urine production or stimulate detrusor muscle tone, including caffeine and alcohol, depending on the goals of care and the short-term prognosis.

Containment devices may be used to provide protection while treatments designed to address underlying UI are undertaken, or they may be used for added protection if these interventions improve but fail to eradicate urine loss.[28] Women and men should be counseled about the disadvantages of using home products and feminine hygiene pads when attempting to contain urine. Specifically, they should be counseled that home products, such as tissues or paper towels, are not designed to contain urine and feminine hygiene products are designed to contain menstrual flow. As an alternative, patients should be advised about products specifically designed for UI, including disposable and reusable products, inserted pads, and containment undergarments.

If the patient experiences primarily stress UI, the initial management is with behavioral methods. Pelvic floor muscle training is strongly recommended for mild to moderate stress UI.[29] Ideally, visual biofeedback is used to assist the patient to identify, isolate, and contract the pelvic floor muscles. If visual biofeedback is not available, vaginal palpation may be used to assist the patient to identify and contract the pelvic muscles. This task may be supplemented by asking the patient to occasionally interrupt the urinary stream during micturition, but this maneuver should not be routinely employed because it interferes with the efficiency of bladder evacuation. After the patient demonstrates mastery of muscle identification, isolation, and contraction, he or she is taught the "knack" of pelvic muscle contractions in response to physical exertion.[30] This maneuver increases urethral closure and resistance to UI and relieves or sometimes corrects stress UI.

Medications also may be used to treat stress UI in selected cases.[31] Pseudoephedrine, an α-adrenergic agonist, is available in over-the-counter preparations (e.g., Sudafed SA). Imipramine, a tricyclic antidepressant with both α-adrenergic effects that increase urethral resistance and anticholinergic actions, may be useful for patients who experience stress UI or mixed stress and urge UI symptoms.[32] Although these agents often alleviate stress UI, their potential benefits must be weighed carefully against their side effects. In addition to enhancing urethral sphincter closure, α-adrenergic agonists may cause tachycardia, restlessness, insomnia, and hypertension. Imipramine may produce these side effects as well as dysrhythmias and anticholinergic effects, including dry mouth, blurred vision, flushing, and heat intolerance. It also may affect the central nervous system and may be associated with short-term memory impairment, hallucinations, and nightmares. These side effects may be particularly significant in aged patients and in those with preexisting cognitive defects related to a primary tumor or disease.

An indwelling catheter may be indicated if intrinsic sphincter deficiency and subsequent stress UI are severe. Although not usually indicated, a larger catheter size may be required, to prevent urinary leakage (bypassing) around the catheter.[33] A detailed discussion of catheter management is provided later in this chapter.

Overactive bladder dysfunction, with or without urge UI, is also managed by behavioral or pharmacological modalities (or both) whenever possible.[34] In addition to the lifestyle and dietary factors discussed earlier, biofeedback methods are used to teach the patient to identify and contract the pelvic muscles. These skills are applied to a technique called *urge suppression,* which is used to inhibit specific episodes of urgency before UI occurs. When a sudden urge to urinate occurs, the patient is taught to stop, tighten the pelvic muscles in rapid succession using several "quick flick" contractions until the urge has subsided, and proceed to the bathroom at a normal pace. The patient also may be taught relaxation or other distraction techniques to cope with specific urge episodes. Behavioral methods are particularly helpful for the patient who is at risk for falling and related injuries.

Anticholinergic or antispasmodic medications also may be used to manage urge UI. A variety of agents are available, but three relatively new drugs, extended-release tolterodine (Detrol LA), extended-release oxybutynin (Ditropan XL), and transdermal oxybutynin (Oxytrol) are preferred because they are associated with fewer side effects when compared to other anticholinergic medications (Table 14–3).[35,36] Anticholinergic medications work by increasing the functional bladder capacity, inhibiting overactive detrusor contractions, and reducing voiding frequency. Their principal side effect is dry mouth, which can be severe and can interfere with appetite and mastication.[31] Other side effects include blurred vision, constipation, flushing, heat intolerance, and cognitive effects such as nightmares or altered short-term memory.

Although antispasmodic medications are often viewed as an alternative to behavioral therapies, they are better viewed as complementary modalities.[37] Specifically, all patients who wish to use anticholinergic medications for urge UI should be advised to void according to a timed schedule (usually every 2 to 3 hours, depending on the urinary frequency documented on a bladder log obtained during assessment) and taught urge-suppression skills. Similarly, patients whose urge UI is not managed adequately by behavioral methods should be counseled about anticholinergic medications before placement of an indwelling catheter is recommended.

Intermittent catheterization or an indwelling catheter may be used in selected cases if urge UI is severe and proves refractory to other treatments. It is also indicated if urge UI is complicated by clinically relevant urinary retention or if the patient is near death and immobile.

Because reflex UI is typically associated with diminished sensations of bladder filling, it is not usually responsive to behavioral treatments.[38] A minority of patients with reflex UI retain the ability to urinate spontaneously, but most cases must be managed with an alternative program. For men, a condom catheter may be used to contain urine. A condom that is latex free is typically selected. In some patients, an α-adrenergic blocking agent such as terazosin, doxazosin, tamsulosin, or alfuzosin is administered, to minimize obstruction caused by detrusor–sphincter dyssynergia.[39] Intermittent catheterization is encouraged whenever feasible. The patient and at least one significant other should be taught a clean intermittent catheterization technique. For the patient with reflex UI, an anticholinergic medication is usually required in addition to catheterization, to prevent UI. If intermittent catheterization is not feasible, an indwelling catheter is used to manage reflex UI. Although the indwelling catheter is associated with serious long-term complications and is avoided in patients with spinal cord injury and a significant life expectancy, it is a more attractive alternative for the patient receiving palliative care.

Functional UI is treated by minimizing barriers to toileting and the time required to prepare for urination.[40,41] Strategies designed to remove barriers to toileting are highly individualized and are best formulated with the use of a multidisciplinary team, combining nursing with physical and occupational therapy as indicated. Strategies used to maximize mobility and access to the toilet include using assistive devices such as a walker or wheelchair, widening bathroom doors, adding support bars, and providing a bedside toilet or urinal. The time required for toileting may be reduced by selected alterations in the patient's clothing, such as substituting tennis shoes with good traction for slippers or other footwear with slick soles and substituting Velcro- or elastic-banded clothing for articles with multiple buttons, zippers, or snaps.

If the patient has significant contributing cognitive disorders, functional UI is usually managed by a prompted voiding program.[42,43] Baseline evaluation includes a specialized bladder log, which is completed over a 48- to 72-hour period. The caregiver is taught to assist the patient to void on a fixed schedule, usually every 2 to 3 hours. The caregiver is taught to help the patient move to the toilet and prepare for urination; the caregiver also uses this opportunity to determine whether the pad incontinence brief reveals evidence of UI since the previous scheduled toileting. Patients who are successful, dry, and able

Table 14–3
Pharmacologic Management: Agents Used to Decrease Bladder Contractility

Drug	Action	Dosage	Adverse Effects	Nursing Considerations
Extended Release and Transdermal Agents				
Extended–release tolterodine (Detrol LA), 2 mg and 4 mg capsules	Antimuscarinic: inhibits overactive detrusor contractions, reduces frequency of urge UI episodes and voiding frequency, increases functional bladder capacity	Usual adult dosage: 4 mg capsule taken once daily	Dry mouth (usually mild to moderate), flushing, constipation, drowsiness, blurred vision	May administer at bedtime to minimize dry mouth; dry mouth is less prevalent and less severe when compared to classic anticholinergic agents; all antimuscarinic and anticholinergic agents are contraindicated in patients with narrow-angle glaucoma
Trospium chloride (Sanctura), 20 mg tablets	Antimuscarinic actions, similar to tolterodine	Usual adult dosage: 20 mg taken twice daily	Dry mouth (usually mild to moderate), constipation, headache	Similar to tolterodine
Extended-release oxybutynin (Ditropan XL), 5, 10, 15 mg tablets	Anticholinergic: inhibits overactive detrusor contractions, reduces frequency of urge UI episodes and voiding frequency, increases functional bladder capacity	Usual adult dosage: 10 mg tablet taken once daily, may titrate to 30 mg daily Child: 5 mg tablet once daily	Dry mouth (usually mild to moderate), flushing, constipation, drowsiness, blurred vision	Osmotic releasing system comprises skeleton, active drug, and small osmotic sponge; advise patient that skeleton is excreted in stool 1–2 days after swallowing; dry mouth less severe than that associated with immediate-release formulation of oxybutynin; tablets must be swallowed whole and cannot be chewed, divided, or crushed
Transdermal oxybutynin (Oxytrol) 3.9 mg matrix patch	Anticholinergic: same as above	Apply 1 patch twice weekly (every 3.5 days)	Dry mouth (usually), flushing, constipation, drowsiness, blurred vision; skin irritation (pruritus) at site of patch application	Teach patient to rotate patch placement to reduce risk of skin irritation; advise patient to apply patch to clean, dry skin and avoid applying lotions or oils before application; counsel patient to apply barrier cream if skin irritation occurs

(continued)

Table 14–3
Pharmacologic Management: Agents Used to Decrease Bladder Contractility *(continued)*

Drug	Action	Dosage	Adverse Effects	Nursing Considerations
Classic Anticholinergics				
Propantheline (Pro-Banthine)	Anticholinergic: same as above	Child: 0.5 mg/kg bid–qid Adult: 7.5 mg, up to 30 mg bid–qid	Dry mouth, flushing, diminished sweating, constipation, drowsiness, increased heart rate, behavioral changes, blurred vision	Dry mouth may be moderate to severe
Immediate release oxybutynin (Ditropan) 7.5–15 mg tablets	Anticholinergic: same as above	Child < 5 y: Age in years = mL/dose bid–tid Child > 5 y: 0.2 mg/kg bid–qid Adult: 2.5–5 mg bid–qid Geriatric: 2.5–5 mg daily to bid	Same as above	Dry mouth may be moderate to severe; available in liquid formulation for children unable to swallow pill
Hyoscyamine, oral tablets. (Levsin, Levbid), hyoscyamine sublingual (Levsin SL) 0.125–0.375 mg tablets	Anticholinergic: same as above	Child: 2–12 y: 1/2–1 tablet q4h Child: ≥12 y: 1–2 tablet q4h	Same as above	Available in elixir and extended–release formulation (administered bid)
Dicyclomine hydrochloride (Bentyl), 10 mg capsules 20 mg tablets, 10 mg/5 mL solution	Antimuscarinic, anticholinergic: same as above	Adult: 20–40 mg qid	Same as above	—
Flavoxate (Urispas), 100 mg tablets	Direct spasmolytic effect on smooth muscle	Adult (> 12 y): 100–200 mg tid–qid	Dry mouth, flushing, diminished sweating, constipation, drowsiness, increased heart rate, behavioral changes, blurred vision	—
Belladonna and opium suppository, 16.2 mg belladonna and 30 or 60 mg opium	Antimuscarinic, spasmolytic	Adult: 1 suppository q4–6h	Dry mouth, drowsiness, dizziness, constipation, blurred vision, sensitivity to light	Moisten suppository before insertion; advise patient to place suppository adjacent to rectal wall and not in fecal mass

Source: References 34–37, 39.

to urinate with prompting on more than 50% of attempts completed during this trial period are considered good candidates for an ongoing prompted voiding regimen; those who are unsuccessful are considered poor candidates and are managed by alternative methods, including indwelling catheterization in highly selected cases.

Because extraurethral UI is caused by a fistulous tract and produces continuous urinary leakage, it must be managed initially by containment devices and preventive skin care.[3] The type of containment device depends on the severity of the UI; an incontinent brief is frequently required. Preventive skin care consists of routine cleansing with water and an incontinence cleanser or mild soap, followed by thorough drying using a soft towel and hair dryer on the low (cool) setting. Additionally, a skin barrier may be applied if altered skin integrity is particularly likely.

In some cases, the fistula may be closed by conservative (nonsurgical) means. An indwelling catheter is inserted, and the fistula is allowed to heal spontaneously.[44] This intervention is most likely to work for a traumatic (postoperative) fistula. If the fistula is a result of an invasive tumor or radiation therapy, it is not as likely to heal spontaneously. In such cases, cauterization and fibrin glue may be used to promote closure.[45] Alternatively, a suspension containing tetracycline may be prepared and used as a sclerosing agent. The adjacent skin is prepared by applying a skin barrier (e.g., a petrolatum-based ointment) to protect it from the sclerosing agent. Approximately 5 to 10 mL of the tetracycline solution is injected into the fistula by a physician, and the lesion is monitored for signs of scarring and closure. If UI persists for 15 days or longer, the procedure may be repeated under the physician's direction. For larger fistulas or those that fail to respond to conservative measures, surgical repair is undertaken if feasible.

Assessment and Management of Bothersome LUTS: Urinary Stasis or Retention

A precipitous drop or sudden cessation of urinary outflow is a serious urinary system complication that may indicate oliguria or *anuria* (failure of the kidneys to filter the blood and produce urine), *urinary stasis* (blockage of urine transport from the upper to lower urinary tracts), or *urinary retention* (failure of the bladder to evacuate itself of urine). The following sections review the pathophysiology and management of urinary stasis or acute postrenal failure caused by bilateral ureteral obstruction and urinary retention.

Obstruction of the Upper Urinary Tract

Upper urinary tract stasis in the patient receiving palliative care is usually caused by obstruction of one or both ureters.[46] The obstruction is typically attributable to a primary or metastatic tumor, and most arise from the pelvic region. In men, prostatic cancer is the most common cause, whereas pelvic (cervical, uterine, and ovarian) malignancies produce most ureteral obstructions in women. In addition to malignancies, retroperitoneal fibrosis secondary to inflammation or radiation may obstruct one or both ureters. Unless promptly relieved, bilateral ureteral obstruction leads to acute renal failure with uremia and elevated serum potassium, which can cause life-threatening arrhythmias.

When a single ureter is obstructed, the bladder continues to fill with urine from the contralateral (unobstructed) kidney. In this case, urinary stasis produces symptoms of ureteral or renal colic. Left untreated, the affected kidney is prone to acute failure and infection, and it may produce systemic hypertension because of increased renin secretion.

Urinary Retention

Urinary retention is the inability to empty the urinary bladder despite micturition.[47] Acute urinary retention is an abrupt and complete inability to void. Patients are almost always aware of acute urinary retention because of the increasing suprapubic discomfort produced by bladder filling and distention and the associated anxiety. Chronic urinary retention occurs when the patient is partly able to empty the bladder by voiding but a significant volume of urine remains behind. Although no absolute cutoff point for chronic urinary retention can be defined, most clinicians agree that a residual volume of 200 mL or more deserves further evaluation.

Urinary retention is caused by two disorders, bladder outlet obstruction or deficient detrusor contraction strength. Bladder outlet obstruction occurs when intrinsic or extrinsic factors compress the urethral outflow tract. For the patient receiving palliative care, malignant tumors of the prostate, urethra, or bladder may produce anatomic obstruction of the urethra, whereas lesions affecting spinal segments below the brainstem micturition center but above the sacral spine cause functional obstruction associated with detrusor–sphincter dyssynergia.[48] In addition, brachytherapy may cause inflammation and congestion of the prostate, producing a combination of urinary retention and overactive bladder dysfunction.[49] In the patient receiving palliative care, deficient detrusor contraction strength usually occurs as a result of denervation or medication. Alternatively, it may result from histological damage to the detrusor muscle itself, usually caused by radiation therapy or by detrusor decompensation after prolonged obstruction. Neurological lesions commonly associated with deficient detrusor contraction strength include primary or metastatic tumors affecting the sacral spine or spinal column, multiple sclerosis lesions, tertiary syphilis, and diseases associated with peripheral polyneuropathies, such as advanced-stage diabetes mellitus or alcoholism. Poor detrusor contraction strength also may occur as a result of unavoidable denervation from large abdominopelvic surgeries, such as abdominoperineal resection or pelvic exenteration.

Assessment and Management of Upper Tract Obstruction and Urinary Retention

Accurate identification of the cause of a precipitous drop in urine output is essential, because the management of upper urinary tract obstruction and of urinary retention are different. Because both conditions cause a precipitous drop in urinary output, the LUTS reported by the patient may be similar. Both may cause difficulty initiating urination and a dribbling, intermittent flow, or both may produce few or no bothersome symptoms in some instances. However, upper urinary tract obstruction is more likely to produce flank pain, whereas acute urinary retention is more likely to produce discomfort localized to the suprapubic area. The flank pain associated with upper urinary tract obstruction is usually localized to one or both flanks, although it may radiate to the abdomen and even to the labia or testes if the lower ureter is obstructed. Its intensity varies from moderate to intense. It typically is not relieved by changes in position, and the patient is often restless. The discomfort associated with acute urinary retention is typically localized to the suprapubic area or the lower back. The patient with acute urinary retention also may feel restless, although this perception is usually attributable to the growing and unfulfilled desire to urinate.

A focused physical examination assists the nurse to differentiate urinary retention from upper urinary tract obstruction. The patient with bilateral ureteral obstruction and acute renal failure may have systemic evidence of uremia, including nausea, vomiting, and hypertension. In some cases, obstruction may by complicated by pyelonephritis, causing a fever and chills. An abdominal assessment also should be performed. Physical assessment of the patient with upper urinary tract obstruction reveals a nondistended bladder, whereas the bladder is grossly distended and may extend above the umbilicus in the patient with acute urinary retention. Blood analysis reveals an elevated serum creatinine, blood urea nitrogen, and potassium in the patient with bilateral ureteral obstruction, but these values are typically normal in the patient with urinary retention or unilateral ureteral obstruction.[46] Ultrasonography of the kidneys and bladder reveals ureterohydronephrosis above the level of the obstruction or bladder distention in the patient with acute urinary retention.

In contrast to the patient with ureteral obstruction or acute urinary retention, many patients with chronic retention remain unaware of any problem, despite large residual volumes of 500 mL or more.[47] When present, LUTS vary and may include feelings of incomplete bladder emptying, a poor force of stream, or an intermittent urinary stream. Patients are most likely to complain of diurnal voiding frequency and excessive nocturia (often arising four times or more each night), but these symptoms are not unique to incomplete bladder emptying. Although acute renal failure is uncommon in the patient with chronic urinary retention, the serum creatinine concentration may be elevated, indicating renal insufficiency attributable to lower urinary tract pathology.

Obstruction of the upper urinary tract is initially managed by reversal of fluid and electrolyte imbalances and prompt drainage.[46] Urinary outflow can be reestablished by insertion of a ureteral stent (drainage tube extending from the renal pelvis to the bladder) via cystoscopy. A ureteral stent is preferred because it avoids the need for a percutaneous puncture and drainage bag. In the case of bilateral obstruction, a stent is placed in each ureter under endoscopic guidance; a single stent is placed if unilateral obstruction is diagnosed. The patient is advised that the stents will drain urine into the bladder. However, because the stents often produce bothersome LUTS, the patient is counseled to ensure adequate fluid intake while avoiding bladder irritants, including caffeine and alcohol. In certain cases, an anticholinergic medication may be administered to reduce the irritative LUTS or bladder spasms that sometimes are associated with a ureteral stent.

If the ureter is significantly scarred because of radiation therapy or distorted because of a bulky tumor, placement of a ureteral stent may not be feasible and a percutaneous nephrostomy tube may be substituted. The procedure may be done in an endoscopy suite or an interventional radiographic suite under local and systemic sedation or anesthesia. Unlike the ureteral stent that drains into the bladder, the nephrostomy tube is drained via a collection bag. The patient and family are taught to monitor urinary output from the bag and to secure the bag to the lower abdomen or leg in a manner that avoids kinking. The success of placement of a ureteral stent or nephrostomy tube is measured by the reduction in pain and in serum creatinine and potassium concentrations, indicating reversal of acute renal insufficiency.

Acute urinary retention is managed by prompt placement of an indwelling urethral catheter.[47] The patient is closely monitored as the bladder is initially drained, because of the very small risk of brisk diuresis associated with transient hyperkalemia, hematuria, hypotension, and pallor.[50] This risk may be further reduced by draining 500 mL, interrupted by a brief period during which the catheter is clamped (approximately 5 minutes), and followed by further drainage until the retained urine is evacuated; or by draining the bladder slowly using a small-bore tube or intravenous set. The catheter is left in place for up to 1 month; this allows the bladder to rest and recover from the overdistension typical of acute urinary retention. After this period, the bladder may be slowly filled with saline, preferably heated to body temperature, and the catheter removed.[51] The patient is allowed to urinate, and the voided volume is measured. This volume is compared with the volume infused, to estimate the residual volume; or a bladder ultrasound study can be completed to assess the residual volume. If the patient is able to evacuate the bladder successfully, the catheter is left out and the patient is taught to recognize and promptly manage acute urinary retention. If the patient is unable to urinate effectively, the catheter may be replaced or an intermittent catheterization program may be initiated, depending on the cause of the retention and the patient's ability to perform self-catheterization.

The patient with chronic urinary retention may be managed by behavioral techniques, intermittent catheterization, or an indwelling catheter.[47] Behavioral methods are preferred because they are noninvasive and not associated with any risk of adverse side effects. Scheduled toileting with double voiding may be used in the patient with low urinary residual volumes (approximately 200 to 400 mL). The patient is taught to attempt voiding every 3 hours while awake and to double void (urinate, wait for 3 to 5 minutes, and urinate again before leaving the bathroom). Higher urinary residual volumes and clinically relevant complications caused by urinary retention, including urinary tract infection or renal insufficiency, are usually managed by intermittent catheterization or an indwelling catheter.

Many factors enter into the choice between intermittent and indwelling catheterization, including the desires of the patient and family, the presence of obstruction or low bladder wall compliance (e.g., a small or contracted bladder), and the prognosis. From a purely urological perspective, intermittent catheterization is preferable because it avoids long-term complications associated with an indwelling catheter, including chronic bacteriuria, calculi, urethral erosion, and catheter bypassing. However, an indwelling catheter may be preferable in a palliative care setting when the urethra is technically difficult to catheterize, the patient has a small capacity with low bladder wall compliance, the patient is experiencing significant pain or limited upper extremity dexterity that interferes with the ability to effectively evacuate the bladder via micturition, or UI is complicated by retention.

Managing the Indwelling Catheter

Although the decision to insert a catheter may be directed by a physician or nurse practitioner, decisions concerning catheter size, material of construction, and drainage bag are usually made by the nurse.[33,52,53] A relatively small catheter is typically sufficient to drain urine from the bladder. A 14- to 16-Fr catheter is adequate for men and a 12- to 14-Fr catheter is usually adequate for women. Larger catheters (18 to 20 Fr) are reserved for patients with significant intrinsic sphincter deficiency, hematuria, or sediment in the urine. Silastic, Teflon-coated tubes are avoided if the catheter is expected to remain in place more than 2 to 3 days. Instead, a silicone- or hydrophilic, low-friction catheter is selected because of its reduced affinity for bacterial adherence and increased comfort.

In men, water-soluble lubricating jelly should be injected into the urethra before catheterization, and in women such jelly should be liberally applied to the urethral meatus and adjacent mucosa before catheterization. A lubricant containing 2% Xylocaine may be used to reduce the discomfort associated with catheter insertion. The catheter is inserted to the bifurcation of the drainage port. A 5-mL balloon is filled with 10 mL to fill the dead space in the port while ensuring proper inflation, and the inflated balloon is gently withdrawn to near the bladder neck.

A drainage bag that provides adequate storage volume and reasonable concealment under clothing should be chosen. A bedside bag is preferred for bed-bound patients and for overnight use in ambulatory persons. The bedside bag should hold at least 2000 mL, should contain an antireflux valve to prevent retrograde movement of urine from bag to bladder, and should include a drainage port that is easily manipulated by the patient or care provider. In contrast, a leg bag is preferred for ambulatory patients. It should hold at least 500 mL, should be easily concealed under clothing, and should attach to the leg by elastic straps or a cloth pocket rather than latex straps, which are likely to irritate the underlying skin.

The patient is taught to keep the drainage bag level with or below the symphysis pubis and to secure the catheter so that unintentional traction against the thigh is avoided. Typically, the patient is encouraged to drink at least the recommended daily allowance of fluids, and to drink additional fluids if hematuria or sediment is present. However, these recommendations may be altered depending on the clinical setting and the patient's short-term prognosis. The catheter is routinely monitored for blockage caused by blood clots, sediment, or kinking of the drainage bag above the urinary bladder. The patient and family are also advised to monitor for signs and symptoms of clinically relevant infection, including fever, new hematuria, or urinary leakage around the catheter. They are also advised that bacteriuria is inevitable, even with the use of catheters containing a bacteriostatic coating, and that only clinically relevant (symptomatic) urinary tract infections should be treated.

CASE STUDY

DY, a Patient with an Indwelling Catheter, Hematuria, and Clot Retention

DY is a 69-year-old white woman with type 2 diabetes mellitus, hypertension, and idiopathic cirrhosis with a mild coagulopathy. She was diagnosed with endometrial cancer at age 65 years and treated with external beam radiation therapy and interstitial radium seed implants. She began noting LUTS, including frequency, urgency, and dysuria, and she developed gross hematuria with clots approximately 3 years after completing radiation therapy. She was initially treated with continuous bladder irrigation, intravesical alum, and prostaglandin instillations with minimal response. She underwent a cystoscopy for evacuation of blood clots. At that time, random bladder biopsies were obtained, which revealed chronic inflammation, hemorrhage, hemosiderin-laden macrophages, and vascular telangiectasia. There was no evidence of malignancy. Several areas of bleeding were cauterized. Hyperbaric oxygen therapy was attempted, but the patient did not tolerate the procedure well and refused further treatments. Over the next 3 months, she continued to have intermittent episodes of gross hematuria and progressive weakness.

DY again sought assistance when she experienced a particularly severe episode of hematuria with clot retention and a hematocrit of 12%. She was admitted to hospital for transfusions and management of recurring hemorrhagic cystitis. A voiding cystourethrogram (VCUG) was obtained on admission, and she was treated with transfusions and continuous bladder irrigations until her sixth hospital day, when she was taken to the operating room for a cystoscopy, performed under anesthesia. Before the cystoscopy, Vaseline gauze was placed on the perineal skin. Because left vesicoureteral reflux was noted on the VCUG, a Fogarty balloon was passed into the distal left ureter and inflated to occlude the ureter. The bladder was filled, and her capacity was determined to be 300 mL. A total of 150 mL of a 1% formalin solution was slowly infused into the bladder and retained for 20 minutes. The bladder was then drained and irrigated with saline. A three-way indwelling catheter was placed, and continuous bladder irrigation was restarted. Her hematuria partially resolved, and she returned to the operating room 3 days later for instillation of 150 mL of a 3% formalin solution. The hematuria resolved after this second instillation, and the continuous bladder irrigation was discontinued within 24 hours.

At the time of discharge the next day, she was voiding well and her urine remained free of hematuria. Postprocedure pain was managed by a combination of urinary analgesics, such as phenazopyridine (Pyridium), and an oral narcotic analgesic (oxycodone). Both medications were discontinued 1 week after the final instillation.

Four months later, DY presented with recurrent dysuria, hematuria, and clots requiring transfusion and repeated cystoscopy with instillation of a 1% formalin solution. She responded to this treatment and was discharged 2 days after treatment.

This case demonstrates the risk of recurrent hemorrhagic cystitis after treatment with a combination of external beam and interstitial radiotherapy. This patient's coagulopathy may have exacerbated the risk for significant hematuria. In this case, the initial episode of hematuria occurred 3 years after therapy, and it recurred over a period of 22 months despite treatment with continuous bladder irrigation, cystoscopy with electrocauterization, hyperbaric oxygen, intravesical alum, and prostaglandin. Ultimately, the condition failed to respond to intravesical instillation of a 1% formalin solution, but it did respond to a 3% solution. Nonetheless, the patient experienced a single recurrence within a period of 4 months, which responded to a single instillation of a 1% formalin solution. She remained symptom-free at 1 year.

Fortunately, life-threatening blood loss is a rare complication of hemorrhagic cystitis and bladder tumors. Treatment usually begins with bladder irrigation, evacuation of clots, and intravesical instillations such as alum or silver nitrate and progresses to therapy with intravesical prostaglandin and formalin. Because of the significant risk of toxicity if formalin is absorbed, a Fogarty catheter must be introduced to prevent reflux of formalin into the upper urinary tract and renal capillaries. Alternatives include cystoscopy with electrical cauterization or laser coagulation of individual bleeding sites. Selective embolization or ligation of the hypogastric artery, palliative cystectomy, or radical nephrectomy may be required as a last resort.

Assessment and Management of Bothersome LUTS: Bladder Spasm

Irritative LUTS, including a heightened sense of urgency and urethral discomfort, are common in patients with a long-term indwelling catheter or ureteral stent. In certain cases, these irritative symptoms are accompanied by painful bladder spasms. Bladder spasms are characterized by intermittent episodes of excruciating, painful cramping localized to the suprapubic region. They are caused by high-pressure, overactive detrusor contractions in response to a specific irritation.[46] Urine may bypass (leak around) the catheter or cause urge UI in the patient with a stent. Painful bladder spasms may be the direct result of catheter occlusion by blood clots, sediment, or kinking; or they may be associated with a needlessly large catheter, an improperly inflated retention balloon, or hypersensitivity to the presence of the catheter or stent or to principal constituents. Other risk factors include pelvic radiation therapy, chemotherapeutic agents (particularly cyclophosphamide), intravesical tumors, urinary tract infections, and bladder or lower ureteral calculus.

Bladder spasms are managed by altering modifiable factors or by administering anticholinergic medications if indicated (Table 14–4). Changing the urethral catheter may relieve bladder spasms. An indwelling catheter is usually changed every 4 weeks or more often because of the risk of blockage and encrustation with precipitated salts, hardened urethral secretions, and bacteria.

In addition to changing the catheter, the nurse should consider altering the type of catheter. For example, a catheter with a smaller French size may be inserted if the catheter is larger than 16 Fr, unless the patient is experiencing a buildup of sediment causing catheter blockage. Similarly, a catheter with a smaller retention balloon (5 mL) may be substituted for a catheter with a larger balloon (30 mL), to reduce irritation of the trigone and bladder neck. Use of a catheter that is constructed of hydrophilic polymers or latex-free silicone may relieve bladder spasms and diminish irritative LUTS because of their greater biocompatibility when compared with Teflon-coated catheters.

Instruction about the position of the catheter, drainage tubes, and bags is reinforced; and the drainage tubes and urine are assessed for the presence of sediment or clots likely to obstruct urinary drainage. In certain cases, such as when the urethral catheter produces significant urethritis with purulent discharge from the urethra, a suprapubic indwelling catheter may be substituted for the urethral catheter. A suprapubic catheter also may be placed in patients who have a urethra that is technically difficult to catheterize, or who tend to encrust the catheter despite adequate fluid intake. Once established, these catheters are changed monthly, usually in the outpatient, home care, or hospice setting.

Patients with indwelling catheters who are prone to rapid encrustation and blockage present a particular challenge for the palliative care nurse. Options for management include frequent catheter changes (sometimes as often as one or two times per week) and irrigation of the catheter with a mildly acidic solution such as Renacidin. Irrigation may be completed once or several times weekly, and a small volume of solution is used (approximately 15 mL) to provide adequate irrigation of the catheter while avoiding irritation of the bladder epithelium.[54]

Bladder spasms also may indicate a clinically relevant urinary tract infection. The catheter change provides the best opportunity to obtain a urine specimen. This specimen should be obtained from the catheter and never from the drainage bag. Although bacteriuria is inevitable with a long-term indwelling catheter, cystitis associated with painful bladder spasms should be managed with sensitivity-guided antibiotic therapy.

Table 14–4
Conditions Associated with Detrusor Overactivity in the Patient Receiving Palliative Care

Condition	Disorder
Neurological lesions above the brainstem micturition center	(Overactive bladder, with or without urge UI) Posterior fossa tumors causing intracranial pressure increased
Primary or metastatic tumors of the spinal segments	Cerebrovascular accident (stroke) Diseases affecting the brain, including multiple sclerosis, AIDS
Neurological lesions below the brainstem neicturition center but above sacral spinal segments	Reflex UI with vesicosphincter dyssynergia Primary or metastatic tumors of the spinal cord Tumors causing spinal cord compression because of their effects on the spinal column Systemic diseases directly affecting the spinal cord, including advanced-stage AIDS, transverse myelitis, Guillain-Barré syndrome
Inflammation of the bladder	(Overactive bladder, with or without urge UI) Primary bladder tumors, including papillary tumors or carcinoma in situ Bladder calculi (stones) Radiation cystitis, including brachytherapy Chemotherapy-induced cystitis
Bladder outlet obstruction	(Overactive bladder usually without urge UI) Prostatic carcinoma Urethral cancers Pelvic tumors causing urethral compression

AIDS, acquired immunodeficiency syndrome; UI, urinary incontinence.

The patient is taught to drink sufficient fluids to meet or exceed the recommended daily allowance of 30 mL/kg (0.5 oz/lb) whenever feasible. Reduced consumption of beverages or foods containing bladder irritants, such as caffeine or alcohol, also may alleviate bladder spasms in some cases.

If conservative measures or catheter modification fail to relieve bladder spasms, an anticholinergic medication may be administered. These medications work by inhibiting the overactive contractions that lead to painful bladder spasms. Table 14–4 summarizes the dosage, administration, and nursing considerations of common anticholinergic medications used to manage bladder spasms, as well as urge or reflex UI.

CASE STUDY

BA, a 76-Year-Old Man with Advanced Prostate Cancer

BA is a 76-year-old African-American man who presented with stage T4, Gleason grade 9, adenocarcinoma of the prostate gland at the time of initial evaluation. The initial management was by androgen deprivation therapy for 30 months, but BA then presented with a rising prostate-specific antigen (PSA) level and evidence of several metastatic lesions on follow-up imaging studies. His prostate cancer continued to progress despite maximal androgen ablation therapy, radiation therapy, and several courses of chemotherapy. Recently, he has experienced progressive difficulty urinating, recurring episodes of hematuria, and an episode of acute urinary retention that required placement of an indwelling catheter for 2 weeks. Attempts to discontinue the indwelling catheter were unsuccessful, and his postvoid residual urine volumes remained elevated at 500 to 670 mL. A number of bladder management options were discussed with the patient and his spouse, and both agreed that they wished to leave an indwelling catheter in place, to avoid the risk for recurring episodes of acute urinary retention and accompanying LUTS.

Initially, BA managed the catheter well, but he subsequently developed multiple painful bladder spasms, sometimes associated with catheter bypassing (leakage of urine around the catheter). A urine culture was obtained which revealed $>10^5$ colony-forming units of *Proteus mirabilis*, pyuria, and microscopic hematuria. He was treated with a 10-day course of levofloxacin based on sensitivity reports. Within 3 days, the frequency and severity of his bladder spasms had diminished to two to three episodes per day, and leakage around the catheter had stopped entirely. A regimen of Ditropan XL, 10 mg qd, was then started to alleviate residual bladder spasms. Telephone follow-up 2 weeks later revealed that his spasms had stopped altogether.

Hematuria

Hematuria is defined as the presence of blood in the urine. It results from a variety of renal, urological, and systemic processes. When gross hematuria was present as an initial complaint or finding in an adult, further evaluation in one study revealed that 23% of patients had an underlying malignancy.[53,55] In the palliative care setting, hematuria occurs more commonly after pelvic irradiation or chemotherapy or as the result of a major coagulation disorder or a newly diagnosed or recurring malignancy.

Hematuria is divided into two subtypes according to its clinical manifestations. Microscopic hematuria is characterized by hemoglobin or myoglobin on dipstick analysis and more than 3 to 5 red blood cells (RBCs) per high-power field (hpf) under microscopic urinalysis, but the presence of blood remains invisible to the unaided eye. Macroscopic (gross) hematuria is also characterized by dipstick and microscopic evidence of RBCs in the urine, as well as a bright red or brownish discoloration that is apparent to the unaided eye.

In the context of palliative care, hematuria can also be subdivided into three categories depending on its severity.[56] Mild hematuria is microscopic or gross blood in the urine that does not produce obstructing clots or cause a clinically relevant decline in hematocrit or hemoglobin. Moderate and severe hematuria are associated with more prolonged and high-volume blood losses; hematuria is classified as moderate if ≤6 units of blood is required to replace blood lost within the urine and as severe if ≥6 units is required. Both moderate and severe hematuria may produce obstructing clots that lead to acute urinary retention or obstruction of the upper urinary tract.

Pathophysiology

Hematuria originates as a disruption of the endothelial–epithelial barrier somewhere within the urinary tract.[57] Inflammation of this barrier may lead to the production of cytokines, with subsequent damage to the basement membrane and passage of RBCs into the urinary tract. Laceration of this barrier may be caused by an invasive tumor, iatrogenic or other trauma, vascular accident, or arteriovenous malformation. Hematuria that originates within the upper urinary tract is often associated with tubulointerstitial disease or an invasive tumor, whereas hematuria originating from the lower urinary tract is typically associated with trauma, an invasive tumor, or radiation- or chemotherapy-induced cystitis.

In the patient receiving palliative care, significant hematuria most commonly occurs as the result of a hemorrhagic cystitis related to cancer, infection (viral, bacterial, fungal, or parasitic), chemical toxins (primarily from oxazaphosphorine alkylating agents), radiation, anticoagulation therapy, or an idiopathic response to anabolic steroids or another agent.[56] Radiation and chemotherapeutic agents account for most cases of moderate to severe hematuria.

Radiation cystitis is typically associated with pelvic radiotherapy for cancer of the uterus, cervix, prostate, rectum, or lower urinary tract. Most of these patients (80% to 90%) experience bothersome LUTS (diurnal voiding frequency, urgency, and dysuria) that reach their maximum intensity near the end of treatment and subside within 6 to 12 weeks after cessation therapy. However, about 10% to 20% of patients experience clinically relevant cystitis that persists well beyond the end of treatment or occur months or even years after radiotherapy.[58,59] In addition to bothersome LUTS, these patients experience pain and hematuria caused by mucosal edema, vascular telangiectasia, and submucosal hemorrhage. They also may experience interstitial and smooth muscle fibrosis with low bladder compliance and markedly reduced bladder capacity.[56] Severe fibrosis associated with radiotherapy can lead to moderate to severe hematuria, as well as upper urinary tract distress (ureterohydronephrosis, vesicoureteral reflux, pyelonephritis, and renal insufficiency) caused by chronically elevated intravesical pressures.

Chemotherapy-induced cystitis usually occurs after treatment with an oxazaphosphorine alkylating agent, such as cyclophosphamide or isophosphamide.[56] A urinary metabolite produced by these drugs, acrolein, is believed to be responsible. Hemorrhage usually occurs during or immediately after treatment, but delayed hemorrhage may occur in patients undergoing long-term therapy. The effects on the bladder mucosa are similar to those described for radiation cystitis.

Assessment

Because bleeding can occur at any level in the urinary tract from the glomerulus to the meatus, a careful, detailed history is needed to identify the source of the bleeding and to initiate an appropriate treatment plan. The patient should be asked whether the hematuria represents a new, persistent, or recurrent problem. This distinction is often helpful, because recurrent or persistent hematuria may represent a benign predisposing condition, whereas hematuria of new or recent onset is more likely to result from conditions related to the need for palliative care. A review of prior urinalyses also may provide clues to the onset and history of microscopic hematuria in particular. The patient is queried about the relation of grossly visible hematuria to the urinary stream. Bleeding limited to initiation of the stream is often associated with a urethral source, bleeding during the entire act of voiding usually indicates a source in the bladder or upper urinary tract, and bleeding near the termination of the stream often indicates a source within the prostate or male reproductive system.

The patient with gross hematuria should also be asked about the color of the urine: a bright red hue indicates fresh blood, whereas a darker hue (often described as brownish, rust, or "Coke" colored) indicates older blood. Some patients with severe hematuria report the passage of blood clots. Clots that are particularly long and thin, resembling a shoestring or fishhook, suggest an upper urinary tract source; larger and bulkier clots suggest a lower urinary tract source.

The patient is asked about any pain related to the hematuria; this questioning should include the site and character of the pain and any radiation of pain to the flank, lower abdomen, or groin. Flank pain usually indicates upper urinary tract problems, abdominal pain radiating to the groin usually indicates lower ureteral obstruction and bleeding, and suprapubic pain suggests obstruction or infection causing hematuria.

In addition to questions about the hematuria, the nurse should ask about specific risk factors, including a history of urinary tract infections; systemic symptoms suggesting infection or renal insufficiency including fever, weight loss, rash, and recent systemic infection; any history of primary or metastatic tumors of the genitourinary system; and chemotherapy or radiation therapy of the pelvic or lower abdominal region. A focused review of medications includes all chemotherapeutic agents used currently or in the past and any current or recent administration of anticoagulant medications, including warfarin, heparin, aspirin, nonsteroidal antiinflammatory drugs, and other anticoagulant agents.

Physical Examination

Physical examination also provides valuable clues to the source of hematuria. When completing this assessment, the nurse should particularly note any abdominal masses or tenderness, skin rashes, bruising, purpura (suggesting vasculitis, bleeding, or coagulation disorders), or telangiectasia (suggesting von Hippel-Lindau disease). Blood pressure should be assessed, because a new onset or rapid exacerbation of hypertension may suggest a renal source for hematuria. The lower abdomen is examined for signs of bladder distention, and a rectal assessment is completed to evaluate apparent prostatic or rectal masses or induration.

Laboratory Testing

A dipstick and microscopic urinalysis is usually combined with microscopic examination when evaluating hematuria. This provides a semiquantitative assessment of the severity of hematuria (RBCs/hpf), and it excludes pseudohematuria (reddish urine caused by something other than RBCs, such as ingestion of certain drugs, vegetable dyes, or pigments).

Urinalysis provides further clues to the likely source of the bleeding.[60] Dysmorphic RBCs, cellular casts, renal tubular cells, and proteinuria indicate upper urinary tract bleeding. In contrast, hematuria from the lower urinary tract is usually associated with normal RBC morphology.

Additional evaluation is guided by clues from the history, physical examination, and urinalysis. For example, the presence of pyuria and bacteriuria suggests cystitis as the cause of hematuria and indicates the need for culture and sensitivity testing. The calcium/creatinine ratio should be assessed in a random urine sample for patients with painful macroscopic hematuria, to evaluate the risk for stone formation, particularly for individuals with hyperparathyroidism or prolonged immobility. A random urine protein/creatinine ratio and measurement of the C3 component of complement are obtained in all patients with proteinuria or casts, to evaluate for glomerulopathy or interstitial renal disease. Further studies also may be completed, to evaluate the specific cause of hematuria and implement a treatment plan.

In selecting those who should undergo a more extensive evaluation, one should also consider the presence of other risk factors for urological cancer, such as age >40 years, tobacco use, analgesic abuse, pelvic irradiation, cyclophosphamide use, and occupational exposure to rubber compounds or dyestuffs.[61]

Imaging Studies

Ultrasonography is almost always indicated in the evaluation of hematuria in the patient receiving palliative care.[56] It is used to identify the size and location of cystic or solid masses that may act as the source of hematuria and to assess for obstruction, most stones, larger blood clots, and bladder-filling defects. An intravenous pyelogram also may be used to image the upper and lower urinary tracts, but its clinical use is limited by the risk of contrast allergy or nephropathy. Cystoscopy is performed if a bladder lesion is suspected, and ureteroscopy with retrograde pyelography may be completed if an upper urinary tract source of bleeding is suspected.

Management

The management of hematuria is guided by its severity and its source or cause. Preventive management for chemotherapy-induced hematuria begins with administration of sodium 2-mercaptoethanesulfonate (mesna) to patients receiving an alkylating agent for cancer.[62] This is given parenterally, and it oxidizes to a stable, inactive form within minutes after administration. It becomes active when it is excreted into the urine, where it neutralizes acrolein (the metabolite postulated to cause chemotherapy-induced cystitis and hematuria) and slows degradation of the 4-hydroxy metabolites produced by administration of alkylating drugs. It is given with cyclophosphamide (20 mg/kg at time 0 and every 4 hours for 2 or 3 doses). When combined with vigorous hydration, it has been shown to protect the bladder from subsequent damage and hematuria.

Mild urinary retention is managed by identifying and treating its underlying cause. For example, sensitivity-guided antibiotics are used to treat a bacterial hemorrhagic cystitis, and extracorporeal lithotripsy may be used to treat hematuria associated with a urinary stone. While the hematuria persists, the patient is encouraged to drink more than the recommended daily allowance for fluids, to prevent clot formation and urinary retention. In addition, the patient is assisted in obtaining adequate nutritional intake to replace lost blood, and iron supplementation is provided if indicated.

In contrast to mild hematuria, moderate to severe cases often lead to the formation of blood clots, causing acute urinary retention and bladder pain. In these cases, complete evacuation of clots from the bladder is required before a definitive assessment and treatment strategy are implemented.[46] A large-bore urethral catheter (24 or 26 Fr in the adult) is placed, and manual irrigation is performed with a Toomey syringe. The bladder is irrigated with saline until no further clots are obtained and the backflow is relatively clear.[46] A 22- or 24-Fr three-way indwelling catheter is then placed, to allow continuous bladder irrigation using cold or iced saline. Percutaneous insertion of a suprapubic catheter is not recommended because of limitations of size and the potential to "seed" the tract if a bladder malignancy is present.

Unsuccessful attempts to place a urethral catheter or recurrent obstruction of the irrigation catheter provides a strong indication for endoscopic evaluation. Rigid cystoscopy is preferred because it allows optimal evacuation of bladder clots and further evaluation of sites of bleeding; retrograde pyelography or ureteroscopy may also be completed if upper urinary tract clots are suspected. Based on the findings of endoscopic evaluation, sites of particularly severe bleeding are cauterized or resected.

After the initial evacuation of obstructing clots, bladder irrigations or instillations may be completed if multiple sites of bleeding are observed or if the risk of recurrence is high, as in the case of radiation- or chemotherapy-induced hematuria. Table 14–5 summarizes agents used to stop moderate to severe hematuria and their route, administration, and principal nursing considerations.

Table 14–5
Treatment Options for Hemorrhagic Cystitis*

Agent	Action	Route of Administration/Dosage	Problems/Contraindications
ε-Aminocaproic Acid	Acts as an inhibitor of fibrinolysis by inhibiting plasminogen activation substances	5 g loading dose orally or parenterally, followed by 1–1.25 g hourly to max of 30 g in 24 h; Maximum response in 8–12 h	Potential thromboembolic complications Increased risk of clot retention Contraindicated in patients with upper urinary tract bleeding or vesicoureteral reflux Decreased blood pressure
Silver nitrate	Chemical cautery	Intravesical instillation: 0.5% to 1.0% solution in sterile water instilled for 10–20 min followed by no irrigation; multiple instillations may be required	Reported as 68% effective Case report of renal failure in patient who precipitated silver salts in renal collecting system, causing functional obstruction.
Alum (may use ammonium or potassium salt of aluminum)	Chemical cautery	Continuous bladder irrigation: 1% solution in sterile water, pH = 4.5 (salt precipitates at pH of 7)	Requires average of 21 h of treatment Thought to not be absorbed by bladder mucosa; however, case reports of aluminum toxicity in renal failure patients
Formalin (aqueous solution of formaldehyde)	Cross-links proteins; exists as monohydrate methylene glycol and as a mixture of polymeric hydrates and polyoxyethylene glycols; rapidly "fixes" the bladder mucosa	Available as 37–40%, aqueous formaldehyde (= 100% formalin) diluted in sterile water to desired concentration (1% formalin = 0.37% formaldehyde); instillation: 50 mL for 4–10 min or endoscopic placement of 5% formalin-soaked pledgets placed onto bleeding site for 15 min and then removed	Painful, requires anesthesia Vesicoureteral reflux (relative contraindication): patients placed in Trendelenburg position with low-grade reflux or ureteral occlusive balloons used with high-grade reflux Extravasation causes fibrosis, papillary necrosis, fistula, peritonitis

Source: References 62–70.

CASE STUDY

FH, a 21-Year-Old Man with Muscular Dystrophy

FH is a 21-year-old man with Duchenne's muscular dystrophy who was admitted to the hospital with tachypnea, respiratory distress, and increasing problems with handling his secretions or swallowing well. On examination, his weight was 28 kg, respiratory rate 36, pulse 144. In general, he was a very thin, frail-appearing man who could respond only by nodding his head or moving a few fingers. He had severe contractions of his extremities. His lips were dry and cracked, but his mucous membranes moist. On pulmonary examination, he had coarse breath sounds bilaterally with decreased sounds in the right base. His pulse rate was increased, but no murmurs were heard. Bowel sounds were present, but severe abdominal distention was noted. Genitourinary examination noted diaper containment. Erythema of the sacrum was present, but no skin breakdown was noted.

FH was admitted to the intensive care unit with a diagnosis of right lower lobe pneumonia. His course deteriorated, and he appeared septic with decreased cardiac output, requiring intubation and respiratory support. Because of decreased urine output, repeated attempts were made to place a Foley catheter without success, and eventually bleeding was noted from the urethra. At that time, both urology and surgery specialists were consulted. Plain abdominal radiographs were remarkable for profoundly distended bowel loops containing an enormous amount of fecal material. An attempt was made to manually disimpact without success. At the time of the urology consultation, blood was noted at the meatus and a decision was made to perform a bedside cystoscopic examination for direct visualization and catheter placement. A very dense stricture and a large false passage were noted at the bulbous urethra. The stricture would not accommodate the scope, so under direct vision the green wire was advanced through the correct lumen into the bladder. Dilators were passed sequentially up to 12 Fr, which was the largest size that could be accommodated. The 12-Fr dilator was then left in place overnight, and the decision was made to take FH to the operating room for suprapubic catheter placement and surgical bowel disimpaction. In the operating room, because of his body habitus and the fact that the bladder was displaced by bowel, ultrasound guidance was used and a 14-gauge Bonanno suprapubic tube was placed percutaneously, stitched into place and attached to a drainage bag.

Eventually, FH improved and was extubated, now with bilevel positive airway pressure with oxygen, and he was discharged home with Home Health nursing care in addition to in-home hospice care. FH had made himself a "Do Not Intubate" code status, and everyone anticipated imminent death.

FH was scheduled to return to clinic for a suprapubic catheter change 1 month after discharge. However, the family failed to keep this appointment. Six weeks after the 14-gauge Bonanno catheter had been placed, FH returned to the emergency room with an obstructed catheter, with the nurses and family reporting inability to flush the catheter on a regular basis. He had been voiding per urethra intermittently. The catheter would not flush, and a guide wire could not pass through it. Eventually, with ultrasound guidance, a new Bonanno SP tube catheter was placed, and instructions were given for flushing daily with normal saline. This catheter obstructed 21 days later and could not be irrigated. A guide wire was placed, and a new Bonanno catheter was inserted over the top of the wire. FH returned 10 days later to the angiography suite, where an Amplatz wire was placed down the indwelling catheter; the catheter was removed, and serial dilatation of the tract and fascia was then performed. Over the Amplatz wire, a 12-Fr Uresil nephrostomy tube was advanced into the bladder, and the distal coil was engaged. This was then connected to a drainage bag, and the patient was discharged home with a plan to return in 4 weeks for an upgrading in size and changing of the catheter. However, after 1 week the catheter became obstructed and was not flushed or drained. He was then taken to the operating room, where an open procedure was done to place an 18Fr Foley catheter through a 22-Fr sheath. The balloon was inflated to 10 cc, and then the Foley was stitched in place and attached to a drainage bag. His subsequent bladder management program comprised daily normal saline flushes and outpatient Foley catheter changes monthly.

This case was particularly difficult in that FH was critically ill and unstable, and everyone thought death was imminent. The initial placement of a small Bonanno catheter was done because of his severe abdominal distention and stool impaction. The Bonanno catheter is only 14 gauge diameter and is made of Teflon, both factors that increase the risk of obstruction and encrustation. Daily irrigations with normal saline were ordered on discharge, but because a variety of home health nurses, hospice workers, and family members were involved in his care, there was confusion and the flushes were only being done as needed.

For long-term catheterization, the Bonanno-type suprapubic catheter, which is a Teflon catheter of only 14-gauge size, should not be used. The large-bore silicon Foley catheter (18 Fr and greater) is much preferred. The balloon should be inflated to at least 10 cc. If there are problems with the catheter coming out, a catheter with a 30-cc balloon could be used. Once the tract is matured with a good-sized catheter, the monthly replacement procedure can be taught to the home health or hospice nurse and done in the home.

It is recommended that an extra Foley catheter be kept in the home, so that if, for some reason, the catheter falls out, the nurse can immediately prepare the site with Betadine, lubricate the catheter, and insert it into the tract and bladder; otherwise, the tract tends to contract fairly quickly. The urology team must always be notified if there are problems with uncontrolled urine leakage, skin erosion, obstruction, hematoma formation, or symptoms of urinary tract infection.

Summary

Patients receiving palliative care frequently experience urinary system disorders. A malignancy or systemic disease may affect voiding function and produce UI, urinary retention, or upper urinary tract obstruction. In addition, upper acute renal insufficiency or renal failure may occur if the upper urinary tract becomes obstructed. These disorders may be directly attributable to a malignancy or systemic disease, or they may be caused by a specific treatment such as radiation, chemotherapy, or a related medication. Nursing management of patients with urinary system disorders is affected by the nature of the urological condition, the patient's general condition, and the nearness to death.

REFERENCES

1. Gray M, Brown KC. Genitourinary system. In: Thompson JM, McFarland GK, Hirsh JE, Tucker SM, eds. Clinical Nursing, 5th ed. St. Louis: Mosby, 2002:917–999.
2. Gray ML. Physiology of voiding. In: Doughty DB, ed. Urinary and fecal incontinence: Nursing Management. St. Louis: Mosby, 2000:1–27.
3. Gray M. UI Pathophysiology. WOCN Continence Conference, January 1999, Austin, TX.
4. deGroat WC. Central nervous system control of micturition. In: O'Donnell PD, ed. Urinary Incontinence. St. Louis: Mosby, 1997:33–47.
5. Langworthy OR, Kolb LC. The encephalic control of tone in the musculature of the urinary bladder. Brain 1933;56:371–375.
6. Bruggermann J, Shi T, Apkarian AV. Squirrel monkey lateral thalamus: II. Viscerosomatic convergent representation of urinary bladder, colon and esophagus. J Neurosci 1994;14:6796–6814.
7. Sakakibara R, Hattori T, Yasuda K, Yamanishi T. Micturitional disturbance after hemispheric stroke: Analysis of the lesion site by CT and MRI. J Neurol Sci 1996;137:47–56.
8. Fowler CJ. Neurological disorders of micturition and their treatment. Brain 1999;122:1213–1231.
9. Kohama T. Neuroanatomical studies of pontine urine storage facilitatory areas in the cat brain. Jpn J Urol 1992;83:1478–1483.
10. De Groat WC. Innervation of the lower urinary tract: An overview. Presented at the 20th Annual Meeting of the Society for Urodynamics and Female Urology, Dallas, Texas, May 1, 1999.
11. Elbadawi A. Functional anatomy of the organs of micturition. Urol Clin North Am 1996;23:177–210.
12. Chai TC, Steers WD. Neurophysiology of voiding. Urol Clin North Am 1996;23:221–236.
13. Eglen RM, Choppin A, Dillon MP, Hegde S. Muscarinic receptor ligands and their therapeutic potential. Curr Opin Chem Biol 1999;3:426–432.
14. de Groat WC, Fraser MO, Yoshiyama M, Smerin S, Tai C, Chancellor MB, Yoshimura N, Roppolo JR. Neural control of the urethra. Scand J Urol Nephrol Suppl 2001; (207):35-43; discussion 106–125.
15. Thor KB. Serotonin and norepinephrine involvement in efferent pathways to the urethral rhabdosphincter: implications for treating stress urinary incontinence. Urology 2003;62(4 Suppl):3–9.
16. Urinary Incontinence Guideline Panel. Acute and Chronic Incontinence. Publication 96-0682. Rockville, Md.: Department of Health and Human Services, 1996.
17. Abrams P, Cardozo L, Fall M, Griffiths D, Rosier P, Ulmstem U, van Kerrebroeck P, Wein A. The standardization of terminology of lower urinary tract function: report for the standardization sub-committee of the International Continence Society. Neurourol Urodyn 2002;21:167–178.
18. McGuire EJ, English SF. Periurethral collagen injection and female sphincteric incontinence: ndications, techniques and result. World J Urol 1997;15:306–309.
19. Gray M. Reflex urinary incontinence. In: Doughty DB, ed. Urinary and Fecal Incontinence: Nursing Management, 2nd ed. St. Louis: Mosby, 2000:105–143.
20. Jirovec MM, Wells TJ. Urinary incontinence in nursing home residents with dementia: The mobility–cognition paradigm. Appl Nurs Res 1990;3:112–117.
21. Gray M, Marx RM, Peruggio M, Patrie J, Steers WD. A model for predicting motor urge urinary incontinence. Nurs Res 2001; 50:116–122.
22. Robinson D, McClish DK, Wyman JF, Bump RC, Fantl JA. Comparison between urinary diaries with and without intensive patient instructions. Neurourol Urodyn 1996;15:143–148.
23. Sampselle CM. Teaching women to use a voiding diary. Am J Nurs 2003;103:62–64.
24. Peggs JF. Urinary incontinence in the elderly: Pharmacologic therapies. Am Fam Physician 1992;46:1763–1769.
25. Tomlinson BU, Doughery MC, Pendergrast JF, Boyington AR, Coffman PA, Pickens SM. Dietary caffeine, fluid intake and urinary incontinence in older rural women. Int J Urogynecol Pelvic Floor Dysfunct 1999;10:22–28.
26. Gray ML. Altered patterns of urinary elimination. In: Ackley BJ, Ladwig GB, eds. Nursing Diagnosis Handbook. St. Louis: Mosby, 1999:643–646.
27. National Academy of Sciences, Food and Nutrition Board. Recommended Daily Allowances, 9th ed. Washington, DC: National Academy of Sciences, 1980.
28. Brink CA. The value of absorbent and containment devices in the management of urinary incontinence. J Wound Ostomy Cont Nurs 1996;23:2–4.
29. Gray M, Marx R. Results of behavioral treatment for urinary incontinence in women. Curr Opin Urol 1998;8:279–282.
30. Miller JM, Ashton-Miller JA, Delancey JO. A pelvic muscle precontraction can reduce cough-related urine loss in selected women with mild SUI. J Am Geriatr Soc 1998;46:870–874.
31. Ghoneim GM, Hassouna M. Alternative for the pharmacologic management of stress urinary incontinence in the elderly. J Wound Ostomy Cont Nurs 1997;24:311–318.
32. Hunsballe JM, Djurhuus JC. Clinical options for imipramine in the management of urinary incontinence. Urol Res 2001;29: 118–125.
33. Moore KN, Rayome RG. Problem solving and troubleshooting: The indwelling catheter. J Wound Ostomy Cont Nurs 1995; 22:242–247.
34. Burgio KL, Locher JL, Goode PS, Hardin JM, McDowell BJ, Dombrowski M, Candib D. Behavioral vs. drug treatment for urge urinary incontinence in older women: A randomized controlled trial. JAMA 1998;280:1995–2000.
35. Larsson G, Hallen B, Nilvebrant L. Tolterodine in the treatment of overactive bladder: Analysis of pooled phase II efficacy and safety data. Urology 1999;53:990–998.

36. Gelason DM, Susset J, White C, Munoz DR, Sand PK. Evaluation of a new once daily formulation of oxybutynin for the treatment of urge incontinence. Ditropan XL study group. Urology 1999; 54:420–423.
37. Burgio KL, Locher JL, Goode PS. Combined behavioral and drug therapy for urge incontinence in older women. J Am Geriatr Soc 2000;48:370–374.
38. Smith DA. Devices for continence. Nurse Pract Forum 1994; 5:186–189.
39. Nickel JC. The use of alpha1-adrenoceptor antagonists in lower urinary tract symptoms: Beyond benign prostatic hyperplasia. Urology 2003;62(3 Suppl 1):34–41.
40. Anson C, Gray M. Secondary urologic complications of spinal injury. Urol Nurs 1993;13:107–112.
41. Van Gool JD, Vijverberg MA, Messer AP, Elzinga-Plomp A, De Jong TP. Functional daytime incontinence: Non-pharmacologic treatment. Scand J Urol Nephrol 1992;141:93–105.
42. Colling J, Ouslander J, Hadley BJ, Eisch J, Campbell E. The effects of patterned urge response toileting (PURT) on urinary incontinence among nursing home residents. J Am Geriatr Soc 1992;40:135–141.
43. Schnelle JF, Keeler E, Hays RD, Simmons S, Ouslander JG, Siu AL. A cost and value analysis of two interventions with incontinent nursing home residents. J Am Geriatr Soc 1995;43:1112–1117.
44. Golomb J, Ben-Chaim J, Goldwasser B, Korach J, Mashiach S. Conservative treatment of a vesicocervical fistula resulting from Shirodkar cervical cerclage. J Urol 1993;149:833–834.
45. Tostain J. Conservative treatment of urogenital fistula following gynecological surgery: The value of fibrin glue. Acta Urol Belg 1992;60:27–33.
46. Norman RW. Genitourinary disorders. In: Oxford Textbook of Palliative Medicine. Oxford: Oxford University Press, 1998: 667–676.
47. Gray M. Urinary retention: Management in the acute care setting. Am J Nurs 2000;15:42–60.
48. Gray M. Functional alterations: Bladder. In: Gross J, Johnson BL, eds. Handbook of Oncology Nursing. Boston: Jones and Bartlett, 1998:557–583.
49. Stock RG, Stone NN, DeWyngaert JK, Lavagnini P, Undger PD. Prostate specific antigen findings and biopsy results following interactive ultrasound guided transperineal brachytherapy for early stage prostate carcinoma. Cancer 1996;77:2386–2392.
50. Perry A, Maharaj D, Ramdass MJ, Naraynsingh V. Slow decompression of the bladder using an intravenous giving set. Int J Clin Pract 2002;56:619.
51. Thees K, Dreblow L. Trial of voiding: What's the verdict? Urol Nurs 1999;19:20–24.
52. Fiers S. Management of the long-term indwelling catheter in the home setting. J Wound Ostomy Cont Nurs 1995;22:140–144.
53. Copley JB. Asymptomatic hematuria in the adult. Am J Med Sci 1986;29:101–111.
54. Getliffe K. Managing recurrent urinary catheter blockage: Problems, promises, and practicalities. J Wound Ostomy Cont Nurs 2003;30:146–151.
55. Openbrier D. Asymptomatic hematuria. Adv Nurse Pract 2003;11:81–88.
56. DeVries CB, Fuad SF. Hemorrhagic cystitis: A review. J Urol 1990;143:1–7.
57. Herrin JT. General urology: Workup of hematuria and tubular disorders. In: Gonzales ET, Bauer SB, eds. Pediatric Urology Practice. Philadelphia: Lippincott Williams & Wilkins, 1999:69–79.
58. Levenbach C, Eifel PJ, Burke TW, Morris M, Gershenson DM. Hemorrhagic cystitis following radio therapy for stage Ib cancer of the cervix. Gynecol Oncol 1994;55:206–210.
59. Dean RJ, Lytton B. Urologic complications of pelvic irradiation. J Urol 1978;119:64–67.
60. Stapleton FB. Morphology of urinary red blood cells: A simple guide in localizing the site of hematuria. Pediatr Clin North Am 1987;34:561–563.
61. Catalona WJ. Urothelial tumors of the urinary tract. In: Walsh PC, Retik AB, Stamey T, Vaughan ED, eds. Campbell's Urology, 6th ed. Philadelphia: WB Saunders, 1992:1094–1158.
62. Droller MJ, Saral R, Santos G. Prevention of cyclophosphamide-induced hemorrhagic cystitis. Urology 1982;20:256.
63. Lowe BA, Stamey TA. Endoscopic topical placement of formalin soaked pledgets to control localized hemorrhage due to radiation cystitis. J Urol 1997;158:528–529.
64. Praveen BV, Sankaranarayanam A, Vaibyanathan S. A comparative study of intravesical instillation of 15(s) 15 Me alpha and alum in the management of persistent hematuria of vesical origin. Int J Clin Pharmacol Ther Toxicol 1992;30:7–12.
65. Shoskes DA, Radzinski CA, Struthers NW, Honey RJ. Aluminum toxicity and death following intravesical alum irrigation in a patient with renal impairment. J Urol 1992;147:697–699.
66. Perazella M, Brown E. Acute aluminum toxicity and alum bladder irrigation in patients with renal failure. Am J Kidney Dis 1993;21:44–46.
67. Norkool DM. Hyperbaric oxygen therapy for radiation-induced hemorrhagic cystitis. J Urol 1993;150:332–334.
68. DelPizzo JJ, Chew BH, Jacobs SC. Treatment of radiation induced hemorrhagic cystitis with hyperbaric oxygen: long-term follow-up. J Urol 1998;160:731–733.
69. Singh I, Laungani Gobinl B. Intravesical epsilon aminocaproic acid in management of intractable bladder hemorrhage. Urology 1992;40:227–229.
70. Dewan AK, Mohan GM, Ravi R. Intravesical formalin for hemorrhagic cystitis following irradiation of cancer of the cervix. Int J Gynecol Obstet 1993;42:131–135.

15

Jean K. Smith

Lymphedema Management

Will the swelling just keep increasing and increasing?—A metastatic lymphoma patient

Finally someone is listening and knows how to help!—A primary lymphedema patient

- ***Key Points***
- *Lymphedema and edema are frequently neglected by health providers.*
- *Lymphedema is caused by irreversible lymphatic transport capacity failure.*
- *Edema indicates that the capillary filtration rate exceeds lymphatic transport capacity.*
- *Long-term lymphedema management, including external compression, is fundamental to successful management.*

Lymphedema and edema are seen regularly in palliative and acute care settings. Both are often neglected despite their capacity to cause pain, immobility, infection, skin problems, and significant patient distress. Long-term, neglected edemas, such as lower extremity venous insufficiency, can develop into chronic lymphedema. Discerning the difference between edema and lymphedema allows appropriate treatment. Because nurses have access to large, diverse patient populations, they constitute an ideal resource for improving patient care. This text prepares nurses to understand, assess, and manage both edema and lymphedema. Information is applicable to various clinical settings, including acute, outpatient, and palliative care.[1,2]

Definitions

Edema, a symptom, refers to excessive accumulation of fluid within interstitial tissues. One or several factors precipitate an imbalance in extracellular fluid volume. *Lymphedema* is edema that arises principally from failure of lymphatic function. Lymphedema, a chronic disorder, results in both extracellular and lymphatic stasis. Excess fluids, proteins, immunological cells, and debris in affected tissues can produce chronic inflammation and connective tissue proliferation, including hypertrophy of adipose tissue. Some degree of progression usually occurs and can produce subcutaneous and dermal thickening and hardening. Lymphedema and edema are contrasted in Table 15–1, which provides definitions, signs and symptoms, and basic pathophysiology.[2–4]

Prevalence

The world prevalence of edema is unknown,[2] and that of lymphedema is poorly documented. Campisi[5] estimated that the worldwide incidence of lymphedema, based on 1984 data, was some 150 million.

Table 15–1
Comparison of Edema and Lymphedema

	Edema	Lymphedema
Disorder	A symptom of various disorders	A chronic, currently incurable edema
Definition	Swelling caused by the excessive fluid in tissues (interstitially) due to imbalance between capillary filtration and lymph drainage over time	Swelling (edema) caused by accumulation of fluid within tissues as a result of lymphatic drainage failure, increased production of lymph over time, or both
Signs and Symptoms	Swelling, decreased skin mobility Tightness, tingling, or bursting Decreased strength and mobility Discomfort (aching to severe pain) Possible skin color change *Pitting scale is often used*: 1+ Edema barely detectable 2+ Slight indentation with depression 3+ Deep indentation for 5–30 sec with pressure 4+ Area 1.5–2 times greater than normal	Swelling, decreased skin mobility Tightness, tingling or bursting sensations Decreased strength and mobility Discomfort (none to severe pain) Progressive skin changes (color, texture, tone, temperature), integrity such as blisters, weeping (lymphorrhea), hyperkeratosis, warts, papillomatosis, and elephantiasis
Pathophysiology	Capillary filtration rate exceeds lymph transport capacity *Example:* Heart failure, fluid overload, and/or venous thrombosis are common causes of increased capillary pressure, leading to an increased capillary filtration rate that causes edema *Note:* Timely treatment of the underlying cause or causes usually reduces edema Prolonged, untreated edema can transition to lymphedema	Inadequate Lymph transport capacity *Primary*—Inadequately developed lymphatic pathways *Secondary*—Damage outside lymphatic pathways (obstruction/obliteration) *Initial sequelae of transport failure:* Lymphatic stasis → Increased tissue fluid → Accumulated protein and cellular metabolites → Further increased tissue water and pressure *Potential long-term sequelae:* Macrophages seek to decrease inflammation Increased fibroblasts and keratinocytes cause chronic inflammation Gradual increase in adipose tissue Lymphorrhea (leakage of lymph through skin) Gradual skin and tissue thickening and hardening progressing to hyperkeratosis, papillomatosis and other problems Ever-increasing risk of infection and other complications

Source: References 2, 3, 107–110.

Secondary (acquired) lymphedema results from obstruction or obliteration of lymphatic channels.[6] Cancer, trauma, surgery, severe infections, and immobilizing or paralyzing diseases are major causes of secondary lymphedema in developed nations.[6] In industrialized nations with sophisticated cancer treatment facilities, secondary lymphedema occurs most often in breast cancer survivors undergoing standard axillary node dissections or radiation therapy or both.[1,6] Prevalence has been reported as 20% to 28%.[7,8] Sentinel node biopsy has, at least initially, decreased the incidence to 2% to 3%.[9] Other cancers associated with lymphedema risk include breast, gynecological, and prostate cancers; sarcoma; melanoma; and lymphoma. Infection and thrombosis are known to precipitate lymphedema in patients treated for breast and other cancers.[2]

Filariasis, a tropical disease in underdeveloped nations, is the predominant worldwide cause of secondary lymphedema. Mosquitoes transmit filariasis nematodes, which embed in human lymphatics to cause progressive lymphatic damage. Mortimer[3,10] estimated the worldwide incidence of filariasis at 750 million. Sequelae are enormous from untreated lymphatic tissue destruction caused by this disease.[3,10]

Currently, primary lymphedema is attributed to embryonic developmental abnormalities, which may be sporadic or part of a syndrome caused by either chromosomal abnormalities (e.g., Turner's syndrome) or inherited single-gene defects. Prevalence documentation is poor but has been reported as 1 in every 6000 individuals, with a male-to-female ratio of 1:3.[11]

Impact

Without proper management, lymphedema generally becomes worse over time and triggers a number of complications.[12] Early diagnosis and long-term management are essential for complication avoidance and optimal outcomes.[12,13] Research has documented numerous detrimental effects of lymphedema associated with breast cancer treatment, including varying levels of pain,[14] fatigue,[15] activity and exercise restriction, arm function losses,[16] obvious disfigurement along with a sense of being different,[17] depression and anxiety, and decreased sexual health.[13] A sense of victory over cancer and full recovery are diminished by a visibly enlarged limb,[18] which can potentially represent cancer recurrence and not just lymphatic dysfunction.

Additional potential sequelae include overall functional limitations capable of causing loss of self-sufficiency and long-term disability, skin changes and pathologies, and weight gain.[19] Surgery or injury to the affected area increases the risk of both infection and progression.[20] Prolonged stasis can lead to severe skin and tissue symptoms, sometimes referred to as elephantiasis. Symptoms include hyperkeratosis (hard, reptile-like skin), warts, and papillomas (engorged and raised lymph vessels on the skin surface).[1] Chronic lymphedema, over a number of years, has also been associated with the development of the rare, usually fatal cancer, lymphangiosarcoma.[21]

Anatomy, Physiology, and Pathophysiology

Edema

Edema is a symptom that results from an imbalance between capillary filtration and lymph drainage. Edema requires treatment of the underlying disorder that is precipitating tissue

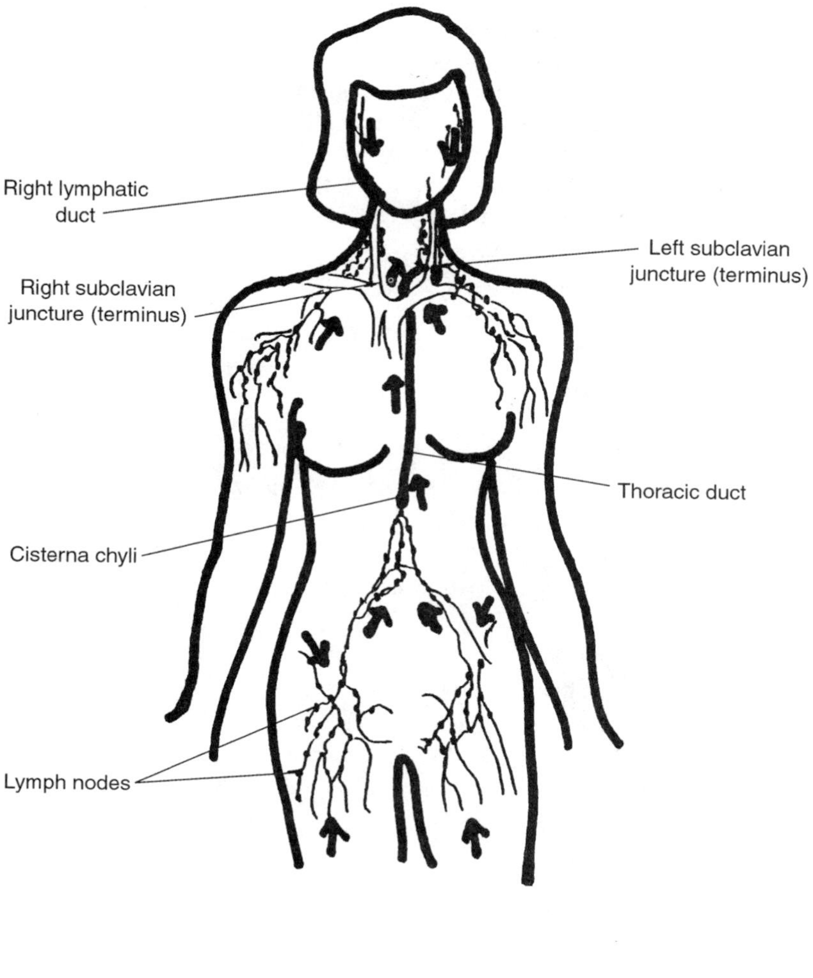

Figure 15–1. Major components of lymphatic circulation. Large lymph vessels and key concentrations of lymph nodes are displayed. One-way directional flow causes all lymph to move to the subclavian junctures via either the thoracic duct or the right lymphatic duct. The largest vessel, the thoracic duct, originates in the cisterna chyli. (Principles adapted from References 1–3, 25. Original drawing by Dale Matson, Penrose Cancer Center.)

fluid excess. Precipitators can include cardiac, hepatic, renal, allergic, or hypoproteinic disease; venous obstruction; and medication complications[22] (see Table 15–1). Edema can develop into secondary lymphedema after sufficient lymphatic damage, such as in venous insufficiency or fractures of the lower extremities.[3,23,24]

Lymphedema

A healthy lymphatic system helps regulate the tissue cellular environment, including collecting and returning plasma and proteins.[3] Daily, 20% to 50% of the total accumulating plasma proteins travel through 2 to 4 L of lymph fluid in a healthy lymphatic system.[25] Lymphatics also remove cellular waste products, mutants, and debris; eliminate nonself antigens, and regulate local immune defense in the process of maintaining homeostasis.[3] Unidirectional vessels traverse from superficial to deep lymphatics through 600 to 700 lymph nodes, carrying lymph fluid to the venous system at the right or left venous angle of the anterior chest on either side of the neck (Figure 15–1). Lymph nodes purify lymph fluid, eliminating defective cells, toxins, and bacteria, explaining the increased risk of infection for patients with compromised lymphatics.[3] Lymphedema pathology signifies malfunction in any part of the process of collecting, transporting, and depositing lymph into the venous system. Lymphedema pathophysiology signifies disruption of these processes and is described in Table 15–1.

Assessment

Physical assessment is the most common means of evaluating lymphedema.[8] Assessment allows optimal management and fosters the well-known medical goal, "Do no harm." Practitioner diagnostic tools are also available that provide insight and criteria for lymphedema assessment.[1] No validated nursing lymphedema assessment tool exists. "Best Practice"[26] components of lymphedema nursing assessment are displayed in Table 15–2.

The first assessment priority is proper diagnosis. For example, assessment revealed that early symptoms of congestive heart failure were responsible for a suspected lymphedema in one elderly, frail patient referred for lymphedema assistance. When the results of the physical assessment and patient history were combined with dialogue, the patient reported that she had replaced her cardiac medication with several natural supplements in order to save money and avoid "toxic drugs." Edema resolved within several days after she resumed her cardiac medications. Some patients, especially those who are elderly, chronically ill, or significantly distressed, are not able to accurately provide a medical history. Requesting physician (physician assistant or nurse practitioner) dictations can provide excellent assessment information.

A patient health history questionnaire facilitates assessment. Useful health categories include patient demographics; health history; etiology; signs and symptoms; complications; work and household responsibilities; support people; spiritual health[27]; and lymphedema goals. Completion of the questionnaire before the initial assessment is performed improves assessment accuracy and content and allows additional time for important nurse–patient dialogue.[28] Dialogue helps nurses gain essential patient knowledge: (1) view of lymphedema, (2) readiness for instruction and treatment, (3) pertinent work and lifestyle matters, (4) spiritual concerns, (5) illness and adjustment issues, and (6) desired goals. Often the patient's initial goal is cure, which is unattainable. In this situation, the patient needs time to adopt new goals. Nurse awareness of patient quality-of-life goals[29] fosters collaboration and management success. Instruction, support, multidisciplinary referrals, goal-setting, assistance with

Table 15–2
Sequential Components of Lymphedema Assessment

Rule out or address immediate complications (i.e., infection, thrombosis, severe pain, new or recurrent cancer, significant nonrelated disorders)
History and physical examination
Routine physical assessments: vital signs, blood pressure, height and weight, body mass index
Past and current health status, including medications and allergies (especially antibiotic allergies and history of infection, trauma, or surgery in affected area)
Current activities of daily living (job, home responsibilities, leisure activities, sleep position, activities that aggravate lymphedema)
Current psychological health, support people, view of lymphedema and health
History of lymphedema etiology, presentation, duration, and progression
Patient knowledge of and response to lymphedema, interest in assistance and goals
Third party payer status
Quantification of lymphedema status (lymphedema signs and symptoms, volume, pain and other neurological symptoms, tissue status, range of motion of nearby joints, site-specific and overall patient function)

self-care, complication avoidance, and long-term management are improved by this knowledge.[30,31]

For example, a 58-year-old woman presented with large lower extremity primary lymphedema. She expressed a positive, easy-going life view; had a boyfriend, children, and grandchildren; cared for an elderly mother; and worked full-time, 50 miles away from home. Her stated treatment goal was to "wear boots." If the nurse's goals were complete limb reduction and perfect compliance, both the nurse and the patient would be likely to experience frustration and failure. This failure *could* cause the nurse to conclude that the patient's poor outcome was caused by poor compliance. Alternatively, the nurse could incorporate the patient's life view, goals, and responsibilities into a workable treatment and self-care program.

A definitive lymphedema diagnosis is often determined solely from a history and physical examination,[8] especially if conservative management is planned and symptoms are not severe. Questionable clinical symptoms or etiology may require imaging evaluation. Lymphoscintigraphy (isotope lymphography) is currently the optimal lymphedema diagnostic test.[3] Lymphography (direct), formerly the only test available, is now rarely used in lymphedema patients[32] because of its potential to cause lymphatic injury and its inability to clarify function.[3]

Assessment for infection, thrombosis, or cancer metastasis (Figure 15–2) is required at every patient contact.[33,34] Although later signs of infection or thrombosis are well known, awareness and careful assessment allow early diagnosis and treatment. Lymphedema progression or treatment resistance may be the earliest sign of complication or may represent a lack of response to current treatment. Changes in pain or comfort, skin (color, temperature, condition), or mobility and range of motion are other possible early signs of these three major

Figure 15–2. Assessment of complications in lymphedema management. ADLs, activities of daily living; BMI, body mass index; BP, blood pressure; DO, doctor of osteopathy; F/U, follow-up; MD, doctor of medicine; NP, nurse practitioner; PA, physician assistant; PCP, primary care physician; TPR, temperature, pulse, and respirations; US, ultrasonography.

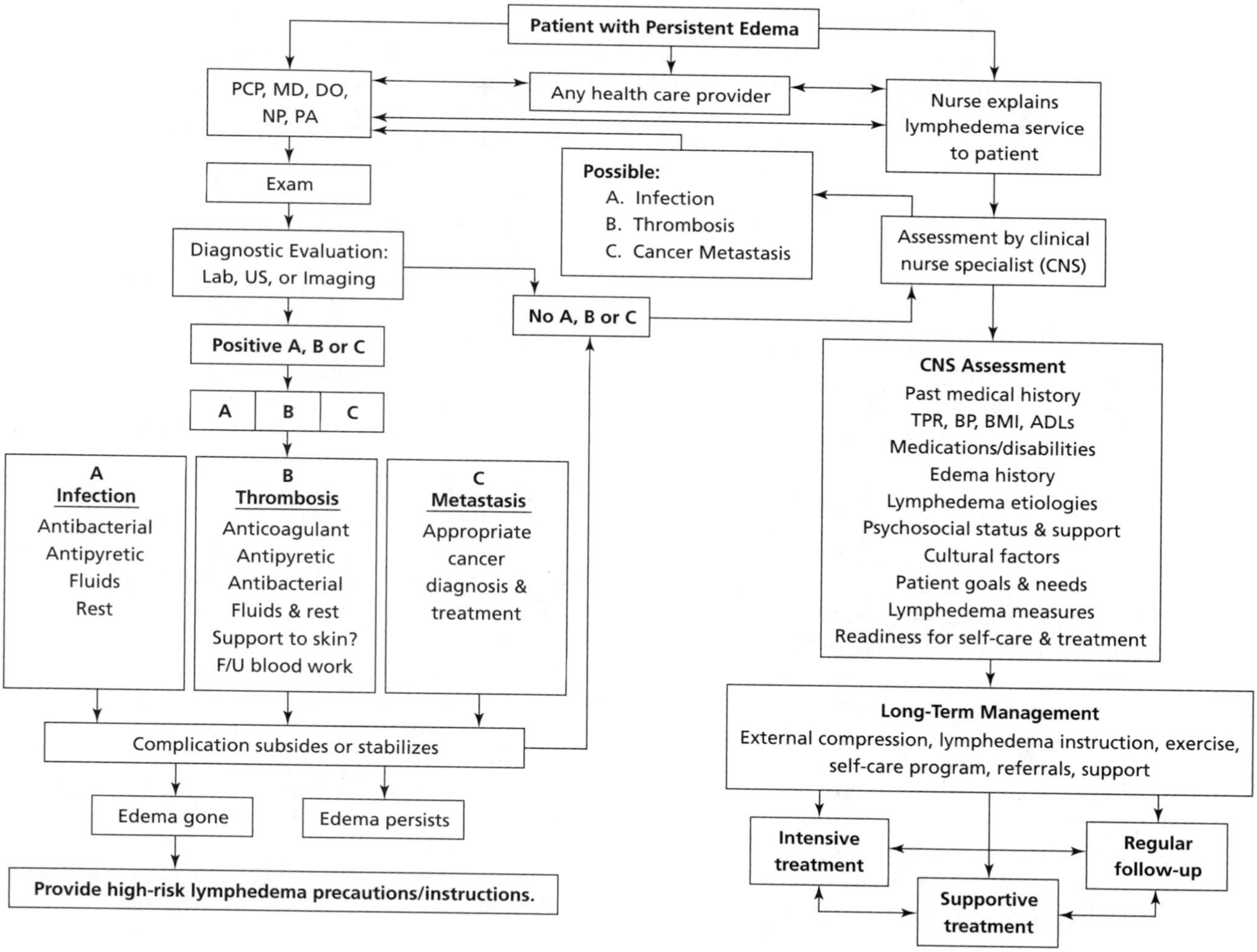

complications. Most infections develop subcutaneously, beneath intact skin. Cultures are not recommended, because they rarely document a bacterial source and can further increase the risk of infection.[35] Suspected thrombosis or new or recurring cancer requires appropriate diagnostic evaluation (e.g., Doppler ultrasonography, magnetic resonance imaging, positron emission tomography, computed tomographic scanning). Venous ultrasonography is reported to be safer than venography for evaluation of suspected thrombosis in a limb with, or at high risk for, lymphedema.[36]

Figure 15–2 depicts ongoing complication assessment and decision-making. Basic treatment of complications is also included. Signs and symptoms of metastasis can include pain, neuropathies, new masses or lesions, skin/tissue color and texture changes, and treatment-resistant rashes. For thrombosis, signs can include distended veins, venous telangiectasis, and rapid edema progression beyond the affected limb.[23,37] Thrombosis requires anticoagulation, pain control, rest, and avoidance of use of external compression. Currently, no research clarifies the appropriate timing for use of compression after thrombosis, and the traditional 6-month delay until use of compression should be assumed.[31] Discussion of this issue with the presiding physician is appropriate. Compression refers to the deliberate application of pressure to produce a desired clinical effect.[2] In contrast, some physicians recommend the use of limb support for several days or longer after painful thrombosis-related swelling, especially in the presence of metastatic cancer. Support signifies the retention and control of tissue without application of pressure.[2] Until research enables a practice standard, the presiding physician must determine the use and timing of support and compression.

A diagnosis of early thrombosis was achieved for a 67-year-old patient with advanced metastatic lymphoma and leukemia when left leg thrombosis developed rapidly while the patient was hospitalized for a cancer complication. Thrombosis encompassed the entire leg. During anticoagulation, leg edema, pain, and signs of venous insufficiency continued to progress. Several weeks later, the patient was referred to the clinical nurse specialist for assistance. Excess edema volume in the affected leg (compared with the nonaffected leg) was 94% (4816 mL). A Tensoshape product (BSN Medical Ltd., Brierfield, England) was provided (with physician approval) for 1 week, and 9% limb reduction was achieved. Good product tolerance was reported. A demonstration ContourSleeve (lower extremity, full-leg product that uses high-low foam and a spandex compression sleeve; Peninsula Medical, Inc., Scotts Valley, CA) was then provided with instructions to use it as tolerated, reverting to the Tensoshape product whenever the ContourSleeve was removed. One week later, follow-up assessment revealed edema reduction of 43%, compared with the initial volume. Excess volume had decreased from 94% to 54% (2730 mL). The patient also agreed to referral to a lymphedema therapist to obtain daytime compression stockings and to undergo several sessions of lymphatic drainage massage. Five weeks after the initial assessment, the patient returned for follow-up wearing her new stockings, her "tight-legged" slacks, her wig, and a large smile. Pain level, skin color and condition, gait, and range of motion of the ankle, knee, and hip were significantly improved (Figure 15–3A). Edema reduction in the lymphedema limb was 81%; excess volume was 18% (926 mL). By 4½ months following the initial assessment, edema reduction had continued. Treatment included daytime stockings and ContourSleeve usage several nights a week. Edema reduction at this time was 87%. Excess limb volume, compared to the contralateral leg, was 12% (634 mL). Figure 15–3B displays improvement from the initial assessment through the 4-month follow-up.

Lymphedema Precautions

No research has demonstrated that "prevention" of lymphedema is possible. Rigid prevention measures may promote fears and frustration. The term "precaution" appears more accurate.[38,39] One essential precaution is achieving and maintaining ideal body weight, because excess body weight is associated with decreased lymphatic function.[40–48]

Infection prevention is a vital lymphatic function[3]; infection is a significant risk factor and is the most frequent lymphedema complication. Risk increases with breaches in skin integrity. Blood withdrawal provides minimal risk because the skin puncture is small and no irritant is injected. Occasional drawing of blood, when no other reasonable option exists, is necessary for some patients. Patients can request an experienced phlebotomist and emphasize their increased infection risk. Subcutaneous, intramuscular, or intravenous injections can cause an allergic or inflammatory response and/or infection that compromises a weakened lymphatic system. These risks must be compared with the benefit and risk of use of a central venous catheter or suboptimal venipuncture site such as the lower extremity.[39,49] Diabetes potentially increases breast cancer patients' lymphedema risk when the affected limb is used for continual blood sticks or insulin injections. Patients with bilateral limb risk, especially of the upper extremities, face lifelong decisions regarding adherence to precautions.

Breast cancer disease and treatment factors are associated with increased lymphedema risk, including advanced cancer stage at diagnosis and radiation therapy to the axilla or supraclavicular area after a mastectomy. Box and associates[50] provided excellent evidence regarding the benefit of early nurse interventions in decreasing the occurrence and severity of secondary lymphedema in breast cancer survivors. Nurses can assist high-risk patients by presenting or reinforcing precaution information and encouraging use of a compression sleeve at the earliest sign of edema. Emphasis on self-protection rather than rigid rules fosters patient empowerment.[39] For example, an empowered patient assumes responsibility for reminding staff to avoid use of the affected arm rather than expecting medical personnel to remember to do so.

Exercise restrictions have long been recommended for breast cancer survivors. However, a growing body of evidence suggests that exercise does not necessarily increase lymphedema

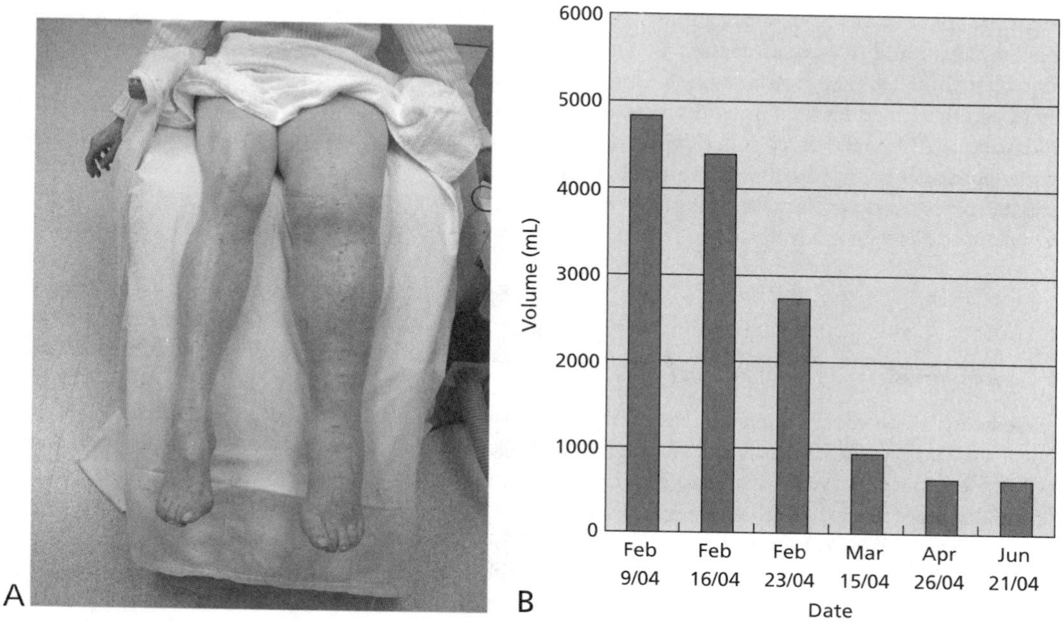

Figure 15–3. Metastatic lymphoma patient with severe deep venous thrombosis in the left leg, showing excess edema volume (mL) in the affected compared with the unaffected leg. The graph shows the improvement in the lymphedema over time.

risk.[41,51–54] Miller,[34] a physical therapist, emphasized the important role exercise plays in general health, weight control, and quality of life. She explored the use of exercise to foster lymphatic function for breast cancer survivors. In addition to surgical recovery exercises, Miller oversaw progressive patient flexibility, strengthening, and aerobic exercises. She also established a guideline for monitoring limb exercise tolerance: (1) decrease exercise activity if any adverse response occurs (e.g., pain, increased edema, neurological changes); (2) decrease exercise if skin and tissue texture becomes firm and/or limb size increases for more than a brief period after exercise; and (3) consider the use of a compression garment during exercise. Although additional research is needed, preliminary research suggests that breast cancer survivors should be encouraged to carry out all postoperative exercises, resume normal precancer activities and be as fit as possible, while regularly monitoring their high-risk or affected limb.[34,53–55]

Table 15–3
Components of Long-Term Lymphedema Management

History, physical examination, and ongoing assessment and support
Individualized and holistic care coordination
Multidisciplined referrals
Comprehensive initial and ongoing patient instruction
Ongoing psychosocial support
Promotion of ongoing optimal self-care management
Facilitation of appropriate evidence-based, individualized treatment
Patient and practice outcome measurement
Access and long-term follow-up and management
Communication and collaboration with related health care providers

Long-Term Management Versus Treatment

Edema usually subsides with proper treatment, whereas lymphedema requires long-term management.[31] Components of long-term lymphedema management are listed in Table 15–3 and described throughout the chapter. Long-term management is a process of fostering optimal physical, functional, psychosocial, and spiritual wellness. Spiritual care guidelines have been gradually evolving in nursing for several decades. Spiritual care supports patients' efforts to make meaning out of illness and to redefine themselves in their new state of being. Specific spiritual interventions can include (1) support during the struggle with and exploration of life's ambiguities, (2) acknowledgment of patients' real and potential losses and victories; and (3) guidance in patients' exploration of end-of-life issues and decisions.[27,56,57]

Long-term management requires quantification of ongoing patient, nurse, and program outcomes.[26,58] Limb size is commonly used in both research and practice to evaluate treatment effectiveness. Other important objective outcomes include pain level, skin condition, range of motion of nearby joints, affected area and overall patient function, body mass index (BMI), incidence of infection, and other complications.[14,44,54,59,60] Patient self-care compliance and overall satisfaction are subjective outcomes that contribute to management success. Outcome measurement has been mandated by the Joint Commission on Accreditation of Healthcare Organizations (JCAHO).[58] Collecting and reviewing outcomes with patients over time fosters ongoing instruction, complication avoidance, sustained lymphedema improvement, and patient empowerment.[19,31,61]

CASE STUDY

Mary, A Breast Cancer Survivor with Lymphedema

Mary was diagnosed with breast cancer at age 60 years. Five years earlier, a diagnosis of polyradiculopathy had required early retirement from a demanding career. Every aspect of Mary's life had been disrupted by this life-threatening muscle disorder. She had coped and adapted through adherence to a set schedule of daily activities, personal problem-solving, assertion of her locus of control, and her husband's loving support.

Lymphedema manifested during radiation therapy, 4 months after conservative breast surgery that included standard axillary node dissection. Lymphedema was accompanied by erythema and petechiae, which varied in intensity throughout each day. Antibiotic therapy did not provide benefit and was poorly tolerated. Edema volume in the surgical arm, compared with the nonaffected arm, was 29% (734 mL). No previous treatment had been available to Mary, who lived and received her breast cancer treatment 60 miles away from the lymphedema facility.

Mary was attentive and participatory during assessment and instruction. When a daytime compression garment was recommended, she emphatically rejected this treatment, convinced that the product would increase the symptoms of her muscle disorder. No data existed to support or refute this belief. Acceptance and support of Mary's viewpoint validated her coping activities and fostered future self-care decision-making.[57] Patient readiness for and acceptance of treatment is crucial to successful chronic disease management and warrants nurses' patience.[58] Mary agreed to use demonstration nighttime compression products (a ContourSleeve and Medi glove) for 6 to 8 hours at a time. Instruction was provided, including removal of the product (until she could speak with the clinical nurse specialist) if pain, numbness, tingling, infection, bleeding, or worrisome signs or symptoms occurred. One month later, she obtained her ContourSleeve and assumed full responsibility for regular replacement.

Over time, Mary gradually increased her product-wearing time. Eight months after assessment, she had achieved 45% limb reduction. Excess limb volume, compared with the nonaffected arm, had decreased from 29% to 16% (405 mL). She never experienced pain or other neurological symptoms. One year after assessment, Mary requested assistance in obtaining a compression sleeve and glove for daytime use. Over the next several months, daytime compression resulted in an 83% limb volume reduction compared with the initial pretreatment volume. Edema volume in the affected arm was reduced to 5% (124 mL). Patient self-reported satisfaction and compliance with management was consistently high, and no limb complications occurred. Asymptomatic mild erythema has continued. Follow-up is currently every 6 months.

Edema Treatment

Edema treatment focuses on detection and intervention related to the causative factor or factors. Effective treatment stabilizes the interstitial fluid volume.[3] Tissue support and/or gentle compression can be useful in relieving edema that might progress to lymphedema.

Lymphedema Treatment

Lymphedema treatment, evolving over the past 20 years, has lacked scientific rigor.[62,63] Sequelae to the evidence deficit included (1) ongoing unsubstantiated treatment fads,[64,65] (2) lack of practice and outcome standards, (3) lack of physician support and referrals,[66,67] (4) inadequate third party payer reimbursement,[38] and (5) reimbursement-driven rather than research-driven planning. For example, decongestive lymphatic therapy (DLT) is commonly recommended as the "gold standard" lymphedema treatment, and credentialing has been established.[38,69] However, recent research in patients with breast cancer–related lymphedema indicates that compression bandaging alone provides limb reduction equivalent to that attained through bandaging combined with lymph drainage massage (LDM).[69a,b] Clearly, gold standard lymphedema treatment must be re-evaluated. Additionally, since no outcome standards exist to quantify current treatment outcomes, any treatment strategy can be called "successful," and treatment results cannot be compared individually or in meta-analysis.[69] Controlled trials are needed to provide evidence that allows establishment of valid practice and outcome standards, which must address cost-effectiveness, third party payer limitations, patient satisfaction, quality of life, and long-term outcomes.[70]

Nevertheless, over the last few years, research has reported several treatment principles. Delay of lymphedema treatment and larger edema volumes are associated with poorer lymphedema treatment outcomes.[71–74] Barriers to lymphedema treatment are time, cost, and lifestyle disruption.[75] Thus, in conclusion, the research deficit has dramatically hindered lymphedema treatment efficacy, and this can only be addressed through appropriate scientific investigation.

Infection Treatment

Infection is the most common lymphedema complication.[3] Lymph stasis, decreased local immune response, tissue congestion, and accumulated proteins and other debris foster infection.[76] Traditional signs and symptoms (fever, malaise, lethargy, and nausea) are often present.[14] Decades of literature support prompt oral or intravenous antibiotic therapy.[3,35,77,78] Because streptococci and staphylococci are frequent precipitators, antibiotics must cover normal skin flora, as well as gram-positive cocci,[79] and have good skin penetration.[80] Early detection and treatment can help prevent the need for intravenous therapy and hospitalization.[35] Intravenous antibiotic therapy is recommended for systemic signs of infection or insufficient response to oral antibiotics.[80] Nursing activities include assisting patients in obtaining prompt antibiotic therapy, monitoring and reporting signs and symptoms, and providing instruction regarding high fluid intake, rest, elevation of the infected limb, and avoidance of strenuous activity. Garment-type compression is encouraged as soon as tolerable during infection.[81] Wound care or infectious disease specialists can be helpful in complicated cases. Infection prophylaxis has been highly effective for patients who experience repeated serious infections or inflammatory episodes.[77,82–84] Effective edema reduction and control may also help prevent lymphedema infection.[84]

The feet, which are especially susceptible to fungal infections in lower extremity lymphedema, can exhibit peeling, scaly skin, and toenail changes. Antifungal powders are recommended prophylactically. Antifungal creams should be used at the first sign of fungus. Diabetic-like skin care and use of cotton socks and well-fitted, breathable (leather or canvas), sturdy shoes are beneficial.[85]

Pain Treatment

Foldi[86] reported that pain is not associated with lymphedema and requires further investigation if present. Others have reported a 30% to 60% incidence of pain in breast cancer-related lymphedema. Causes of pain included infection, postoperative changes in the axilla, postmastectomy pain syndrome, brachial plexopathy, various arthritic conditions, peripheral entrapment neuropathies, vascular compromise, and cancer recurrence.[14,80] Sudden onset of pain requires careful assessment for complications (see Figure 15–2). Patient quantification of pain level at regular intervals is helpful.[14] Use of the 0-to-10 pain scale developed by Serlin and colleagues[87] is recommended for cancer pain assessment. Standard pain management principles are applicable for lymphedema-related pain.

Elevation and Self-Care

Because elevation is recommended for edema, it has often been emphasized for lymphedema patients. Elevation is impractical for lymphedema patients, and documentation of benefit has not been established.[80,88,89] Patient avoidance of limb dependency, as possible, appears to be a more appropriate lymphedema precaution. Optimal patient self-care typically includes adherence to precautions, use of compression products and other treatments, weight management, fitness and lymphedema exercises, optimal nutrition and hydration, healthy lifestyle practices, and seeking assistance for lymphedema-related problems. Patient empowerment for optimal self-care is a great impetus to long-term management success.[90]

For example, one female patient attended school, worked part-time, and was a single parent of two sons. She had experienced many lymphedema treatment failures after her initial presentation of lymphedema at age 5 years. Treatments had been painful, distressing, and unsuccessful. Emotional scars had resulted from having legs so different from those of her friends. Five years of intermittent support and encouragement were required to achieve patient treatment readiness. Achieving a successful treatment program required another year and included surgical repair of ingrown toenails. Use of outcomes provided concrete data that fostered excellent compression compliance (daytime garment and nighttime lower leg ContourSleeves). Ultimately, external compression reduced pain and fatigue sufficiently to allow 3 extra hours of activity per day. Long-term treatment success included sustained reduction of lymphedema and pain, elimination of recurrent infections, excellent compression compliance and self-care, high treatment satisfaction, and minimal need for lymphedema assistance.

Exercise

Exercise guidelines described earlier (see Lymphedema Precautions) are applicable for lymphedema management, including fitness exercise. Physician approval for exercise may be required. Cardiac or pulmonary disease and limb progression may require exercise restriction.[88]

Skin Care

Diabetic-like care fosters skin health and integrity as well as infection prevention.[85] Diligent care is especially important for patients with lower extremity, genital, breast, head, neck, or late-stage lymphedema, additional skin alterations, or unrelated debilitating conditions. Lymphedema can cause skin dryness and irritation, which is increased with long-term use of compression products. Bland, nonscented products are recommended for daily cleansing and moisturizing.[76] Low pH moisturizers (e.g., AmLactin), which discourage infection, are recommended for advanced lymphedema, because skin and tissue changes increase infection risk. Water-based moisturizers, which are absorbed more readily, are less likely to damage compression products but are not suitable for all patients. Cotton clothing allows ventilation and is absorbent.

Advanced lymphedema can cause several skin complications, including lymphorrhea, lymphoceles, papillomas, and hyperkeratosis. Lymphorrhea is leakage of lymph fluid through the skin that occurs when skin cannot accommodate accumulated fluid. Nonadherent dressings, good skin care, and compression are used to alleviate leakage. Compression and good skin care also reduce the occurrence of lymphoceles, papillomas, and hyperkeratosis; these complications reflect skin adaptation to excess subcutaneous lymph.

External Compression

Because human skin expands as needed to maintain integrity, it does not resist progressive edema. External compression provides resistant pressure and is currently the most essential part of all lymphedema treatment.[91] Physiological effects of compression include edema control or reduction, decreased accumulated protein, decreased arteriole outflow into the interstitium, improved muscle pump effect with movement and exercise of the affected area, and protection of skin. Gradient external pressure provides the greatest pressure distally and less pressure proximally; this is optimal for improved lymphatic transport.[92] Compression that is not uniform on a limb (e.g., blood pressure cuffs, tourniquets, watches, elastic sleeves) can be detrimental by decreasing peripheral lymphatic function.

Bandages

Multilayer, low-stretch bandages provide external compression. They may be used as a single treatment modality, as part of DLT, or as part of a compression regimen that uses daytime garments and nighttime bandages. This third strategy is especially important for patients with severe lymphedema, such as can occur with morbid obesity or neglected primary lymphedema. Foam or other padding is often used under bandages to improve edema reduction and foster limb uniformity. The time, effort, and dexterity required for bandaging can become burdensome or impossible for some patients, necessitating the use of an alternative compression method. Kelly[1] emphasized avoidance of bandaging because of arterial insufficiency in patients with an ankle/brachial index (ABI) of < 0.8.

Compression Garments

Compression garments are universally recommended for all patients with lymphedema of the extremities.[68,92,93] Some experts have recommended early compression to manage lymphedema without the need for DLT.[24,65,94] A national consensus meeting provided the following garment recommendations: (1) guidelines for selection and use of garments remain unclear; (2) cost and patient tolerance of the garments warrant consideration when prescribing; (3) hand swelling may develop or become problematic if an arm sleeve is used without hand protection, and patients should be made aware of this risk before obtaining a garment; (4) garments should be replaced after they lose elasticity; and (5) use of garments is recommended during physical activity and exercise.[88] Garment use recommendations vary from daytime only, after DLT,[1,95] to continual use as a first-line treatment.[94] Svensson[94] reported a 50% to 100% limb reduction through continual use of garments as a sole treatment. Bertelli and colleagues[96] reported a 17% reduction with 6 hours of daily use of compression alone.

Garment usage requires frequent laundering of products (daily to every other day), daily skin care and complication monitoring, and 2 replacements every 6 months. Various helpful products exist to assist patients in applying garments, an especially important task for elderly and disabled patients. Hand arthritis or neuropathy can hinder tolerance of garments. Garment removal is required if compression causes pain, neurological symptoms, or color or temperature changes. Readjustment and movement may remedy the problem; often product replacement is required. Because a variety of products exist, staff and patient persistence is likely to result in good patient tolerance. Rubber gloves (dish-washing gloves) facilitate application of garments and extend their longevity. Timely garment replacement (usually every 6 months) is essential for good edema control.[92]

Other Compression Products

A growing number of alternative commercial compression products have become available. Semirigid products (e.g., ReidSleeve [Peninsula Medical, Inc., Scotts Valley CA], CircAid [CircAid, San Diego, CA]) use foam and Velcro straps to provide nonelastic compression designed to simulate bandaging while saving time and energy. JoVi (Innovative Medical Solutions, Inc., Selah, WA) and ContourSleeve products use foam and an outer spandex compression sleeve. The ContourSleeve allows adjustment for limb size changes, which can be ideal for limb reduction or increase or for weight changes affecting limb size. Distinct advantages of these products include ease and speed of application, overall comfort and tolerance, and product longevity. Haslett and Aitken[97] reported that the Tribute Solaris (LymphaCare, New York, NY) appeared to contribute to maintenance of previously achieved DLT reduction. Lund[98] reported that use of CircAid provided an acceptable substitute for bandaging. Research is needed to provide insight and direction regarding the use of these promising products.[95] Use of CircAid products on the lower extremities is currently contraindicated with ABI < 0.8.[98]

Decongestive Lymphatic Therapy and Lymph Drainage Massage

DLT evolved in Europe when Michael Foldi[86] combined Vodder's Manual Lymph Drainage (MLD) technique with bandaging, exercises, and specialized skin care. Dr. Foldi described his four-modality lymphedema treatment as "Complete Decongestive Therapy" (CDT). Information has already been provided on skin care, exercise and compression. Vodder's MLD technique consisted of a specialized light touch (skin-stretching) massage that stimulates peripheral lymphatics and assists lymph transport across watersheds to allow alternative transport routes. The term "Lymphatic Drainage Massage" (LDM) is used in this text. The National Lymphedema Network has established DLT credentialing in the United States. Nevertheless, two randomized controlled clinical trials have demonstrated that compression bandaging (CB) alone is as effective at reducing arm volumes in breast cancer–related lymphedema as CB in combination with LDM/MLD. Thus, scientific research demonstrates that compression bandaging is the single most optimal lymphedema treatment.

Pneumatic (Mechanical) Pumps

Mechanical pumps use electricity to inflate a single-chamber or multichamber sleeve and produce external limb compression. A decreased tissue capillary filtration rate (documented by lymphoscintigraphy) produces tissue fluid reduction and, consequently, limb volume decrease.[99] Lymph formation decreases, but lymph transport, which would address lymphedema pathophysiology, is not affected. Badger and coworkers[62] initiated a Cochrane review of physical therapies used to treat lymphedema. Regarding pumps, she reported: (1) pumps are used as a way of both reducing lymphedema and controlling it; (2) opinion is divided on the use of pumps for lymphedema treatment; (3) pump use has reduced swelling, but concern exists regarding the way in which swelling is decreased as well as the rapid displacement of fluid elsewhere in the body; and (4) use of pumps does not eliminate the need for compression garments and may not provide more benefit than garments alone. Brennan and Miller[88] presented a consensus view of reservations related to tissue injury from improper pump prescription and use. Investigations have reported several pump complications, including lymphatic congestion and injury proximal to the pump sleeve, increased swelling adjacent to the pump cuff in up to 18% of patients,[100] lack of benefit in all but stage I (reversible) lymphedema, and development of genital lymphedema in up to 43% of patients with cancer-related lower extremity lymphedema.[100,101] After more than 50 years of pump use in lymphedema care[1] and long-established Medicare reimbursement, no guidelines exist, significant complications are reported, and research has not clarified benefit.

Surgical Treatments

For a number of decades, surgical intervention has been described as a last resort in the treatment of lymphedema.[102] Several surgical interventions have been reported, including microsurgical anastomoses, debulking, and liposuction. Surgery does not cure lymphedema, and follow-up use of compression is necessary.[94,91] Surgery has provided cosmetic improvement in eyelid or genital edema.[2]

Liposuction surgery has demonstrated greater than 100% reduction for patients with treatment-resistant lymphedema.[93,94] Lack of response to conventional treatment resulted from formation of excess subcutaneous adipose tissue secondary to slow or absent lymph flow.[103] Liposuction has increased skin capillary blood flow and does not further impair already decreased lymph transport capacity in breast cancer patients with lymphedema.[91,104] No surgical complications occurred in 81 patients over a period of 9 years (data collection is ongoing). The average percentage of limb reduction for all patients 1 or more years after surgery (including 78 breast cancer survivors) was 107%. Fifteen study patients who underwent liposuction 8 or more years previously had a mean limb reduction of 120%. Patients have maintained these excellent limb reductions with 24-hour use of Elvarex compression garments (BSN-JOBST, Inc., Emmerick, Germany) and regular follow-up.[103]

CASE STUDY

GR, a Breast Cancer Survivor with Resistant Lymphedema

GR, a California breast cancer survivor, developed lymphedema in 1977; she intermittently used garments and pumps for the next two decades. After relocating to Colorado in 1996, she was assisted by a Lymphedema Clinical Nurse Specialist. Over the next 3 years, GR was referred for two courses of intensive DLT. The second course was provided at a well-known Arizona treatment center. Lymphedema gradually and continually progressed, in spite of good compliance to the use of compression products. The patient met liposuction surgery criteria and obtained third party payer approval for liposuction surgery in Sweden. Preoperatively, excess limb volume was 2315 mL; no pitting was present. The patient had agreed to lifelong use of compression and underwent liposuction surgery in April of 2001. The surgical aspirate contained 90% adipose tissue. One month after surgery, she had achieved 125% edema reduction.

Patient follow-up takes place at least every 6 months, and garments are replaced at each of these follow-ups. Three years after surgery, edema reduction was 119%. Hand edema has returned. GR has continued 100% compliance with use of compression products. She has also regained significant quality of life. In late 2004, GR began using a ContourSleeve at nighttime along with her Elvarex glove. She continues daytime use of the Elvarex sleeve and glove. Greater than 100% edema reduction has been maintained. GR reported relief at the variation between her daytime and nighttime products. Figures 15–4 and 15–5 display the results of lymphedema treatment for this patient.

Pharmacological Interventions

Pharmacological treatment of lymphedema is supportive and includes antimicrobials, antifungals, and diuretics. Infection treatment has already been described. Physicians commonly use diuretics to treat edema and lymphedema. Diuretics generally provide little benefit in normal lymphedema management, because they limit capillary filtration by reducing the circulating systemic blood volume. Depleted systemic fluid volume can lead to hypotension and altered electrolyte status while achieving minimal to no lymphedema volume reduction.[3] Isotope lymphography has substantiated that removal of fluid from the blood of lymphedema patients decreases the rate of lymphatic drainage.[104]

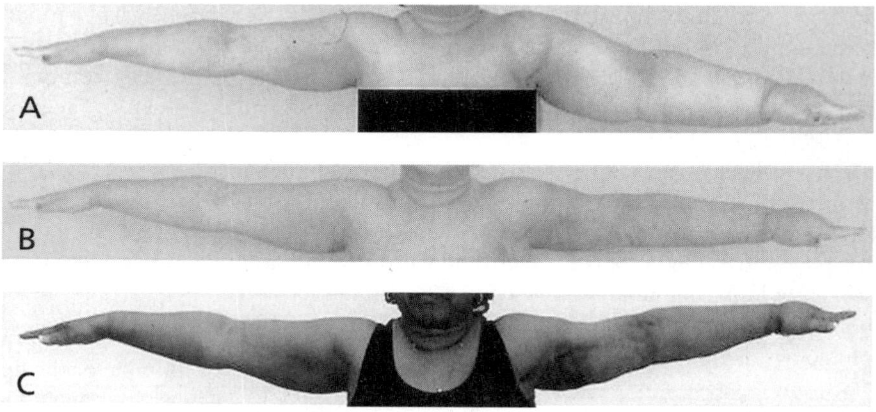

Figure 15–4. Photographs showing results of lymphedema treatment in GR, a breast cancer survivor (see Case Study). A. Preoperative—2315 ml. B. Four weeks postoperative—100 ml. C. Three years postoperative—210 ml.

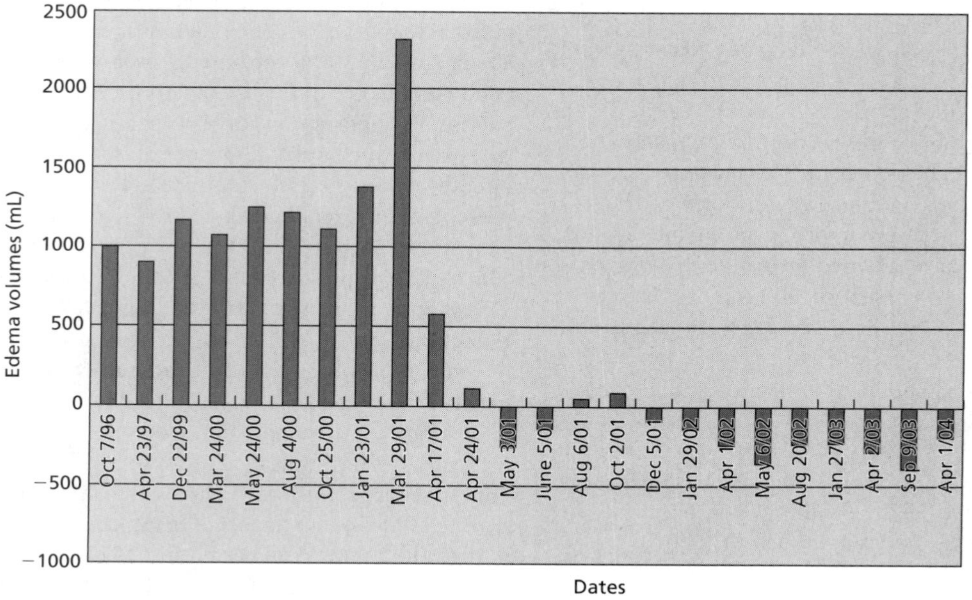

Figure 15–5. Affected arm excess edema volume, compared with nonaffected arm, over time. The patient, GR, underwent liposuction of the affected arm in April 2001.

Diuretics can be useful in some lymphedema-related conditions, including lymphedema of mixed origin; effusion of lymph into body cavities or organs (abdomen, thorax, genitals); lymphatic obstruction associated with malignancy, especially in hard-to-treat areas; and short-term use after infection, thrombosis, or trauma.[2,95]

Unusual Lymphedemas

Palliative care may require the management of unusual and challenging lymphedema sites, such as breast, head, neck, trunk, or genitals.[105] LDM, skin-softening techniques, foam chip pads, and external compression (if possible) are recommended.[2] External compression may be achieved with collars, vests, custom pants or tights, scrotal supports,[76] or spandex type exercise apparel. The assistance of occupational or physical therapists and a seamstress may be helpful. Nationally, instructional courses are available to provide guidance for managing these difficult lymphedemas.

Conclusion

Edema is a symptom usually relieved by addressing the causative factor. Lymphedema, often labeled as edema, is a chronic disorder that requires long-term management. Although external compression is essential to effective lymphedema management, third party payer reimbursement is inadequate and frustrating, patients are frequently fitted with products they cannot tolerate, and many patients have not been adequately prepared for compression products and therefore discontinue use when their product does not cure the lymphedema. Newer compression products, such as the CircAid,

Legacy, and ContourSleeve, offer exciting product alternatives but lack controlled research substantiation. Benefits of two commonly supported treatments, DLT and pneumatic compression pumps, have not been substantiated by randomized controlled clinical trials, according to several expert literature reviews. Controlled clinical trials are essential for establishing "gold standard" treatments and should be the basis for third party payer reimbursement. Research deficit has also precluded establishment of outcome and practice standards, allowing an "anything goes" treatment environment. Nevertheless, over the last 10 years, progress has been achieved in both lymphedema awareness and scientific research. Oncology nurses and other nurses have increasingly contributed to lymphedema management as they have improved cancer survivorship.[106] Nursing's unique focus and scope of practice is ideally suited to chronic illness management, both at entry and at the advanced practice levels. Combined with nurses' immense and diverse patient contact, enormous potential exists for nurses to dramatically improve both edema and lymphedema management.

REFERENCES

1. Kelly DG. A Primer on Lymphedema. Upper Saddle River, NJ: Prentice-Hall, 2002.
2. Mortimer PS, Badger C. Lymphoedema. In Doyle D, Hanks GW, Cherny N, Calman K, eds. Oxford Textbook of Palliative Medicine. New York: Oxford University Press, 2004:640–647.
3. Mortimer P. Lymphoedema. In: Warrell DA, Cox TM, Firth JD, eds. Oxford Textbook of Medicine, Vol 2, 2nd ed. Oxford: Oxford University Press, 2003:1202–1208.
4. Brorson H, Aberg M, Svensson H. Chronic lymphedema and adipocyte proliferation: Clinical therapeutic implications. The Lymphatic Continuum. National Institutes of Health, Bethesda, USA, 2002. Lymphatic Research and Biology 2003;1:88.
5. Campisi C. Global incidence of tropical and non-tropical lymphoedema. Int Angiol 1999;18:3–5.
6. Rockson S. Lymphedema [review]. Am J Med 2001;110:288–295.
7. Ozaslan C, Kuru B. Lymphedema after treatment of breast cancer. Am J Surg 2004;187;69–72.
8. Hull MM. Lymphedema in women treated for breast cancer. Semin Oncol Nurs 2000;16:226–237.
9. Golshan M, Martin WJ, Dowlatshahi K. Sentinel lymph node biopsy lowers the rate of lymphedema when compared with standard axillary lymph node dissection. Am Surg 2003;69: 209–211.
10. Cheville AL, McGarvey CL, Petrek JA, Russo SA, Tylor ME, Tiadens SR. Lymphedema management. Semin Radiat Oncol 2003;13:290–301.
11. Hafez H, Wolfe J. Lymphedema. Ann Vasc Surg 1996;10:88–95.
12. Casley-Smith J. Modern treatment of lymphedema. Mod Med 1992;35:70–83.
13. Passik SD, McDonald MV. Psychosocial aspects of upper extremity lymphedema in women treated for breast carcinoma. Cancer 1998;83(12 Suppl American):2817–2820.
14. Brennan M. The complexity of pain in post breast cancer lymphedema. NLN Newsletter 1999;11(1):1–8.
15. Armer JM, Porock D. Self-reported fatigue among women with post-breast cancer LE. Lymph Link 2001;13(3):1,2,4.
16. Bosompra K, Ashikaga T, O'Brien PJ, Nelson L, Skelly J. Swelling, numbness, pain and their relationship to arm function among breast cancer survivors: A disablement process model perspective. Breast J 2002;8:338–348.
17. Ryan T. Skin failure and lymphedema. NLN Newsletter 1996; 8:1,2,5.
18. Ryan M, Stainton MC, Jaconelli C, Watts S, MacKenie P, Mansberg T. The experience of lower limb lymphedema for women after treatment for gynecologic cancer. Oncol Nurs Forum 2003;30:417–423.
19. Smith JK, Zobec A. Lymphedema management. In: Ferrell B, Coyle N, eds. The Oxford Textbook of Palliative Nursing. New York: Oxford University Press, 2001:92–203.
20. Foldi M, Idiazabal G. The role of operative management of varicose veins in patients with lymphedema and/or lipedema of the legs. Lymphology 2000;33:67–71.
21. Budd G. Management of angiosarcoma. Curr Oncol Rep 2002; 4:515–519.
22. Firth J. Idiopathic oedema of women. In: Warrell DA, Cox TM, Firth JD, eds. Oxford Textbook of Medicine. Oxford: Oxford University Press, 2004:1209–1210.
23. Szuba A, Razavi M, Rockson SG. Diagnosis and treatment of concomitant venous obstruction in patients with secondary lymphedema. J Vasc Interv Radiol 2002;13:799–803.
24. Rockson S. Secondary lymphedema of the lower extremities. NLN Newsletter 1998;10(3):1,2,12,13.
25. Ganong WF. Dynamics of blood and lymph flow. In: Ganong WF. Review of Medical Physiology. Chicago: Lange Medical Books, McGraw-Hill Medical Publishing Division, 2001: 570–571.
26. Murphy-Ende K. Advanced practice nursing: Reflections on the past, issues for the future. Oncol Nurs Forum 2002;29:106–112.
27. Parran L. Spiritual care is elemental and fundamental to the heart. ONS News 2003;8(3):1,4,5.
28. Woods M. Using philosophy, knowledge and theory to assess a patient with lymphoedema. Int J Palliat Nurs 2002;8:176, 178–181.
29. Movsas B. Quality of life in oncology trials: A clinical guide. Semin Radiat Oncol 2003;13:235–247.
30. Johansson K, Holmstrom H, Nilsson I, Ingvar C, Albertsson M, Ekdahl C. Breast cancer patients' experiences of lymphoedema. Scand J Caring Sci 2003;17:35–42.
31. Rymal C. Comprehensive decongestive therapy for lymphedema in patients with a history of cerebral vascular accident. Clin J Oncol Nurs 2003;7:677–678.
32. Szuba A, Rockson SG. Lymphedema: Classification, diagnosis and therapy. Vasc Med 1998;3:145–156.
33. Caban ME. Trends in the evaluation of lymphedema. Lymphology 2002;35:28–38.
34. Smith JK, Miller L. Management of patients with cancer-related lymphedema. Oncol Nurs Updates 1985;5:1–12.
35. Simon M, Cody R. Cellulitis after axillary lymph node dissection for carcinoma of the breast. Am J Med 1992;93:543–548.
36. Balzarini A, Millela M, Civelli E, Sigari C, De Conno F. Ultrasonography of arm edema after axillary dissection for breast cancer: a preliminary study. Lymphology 2001;34:152–155.
37. Smith JK. Collaborative approach to treatment of lymphedema with breast cancer complications: A case study. NLN Newsletter 1997;9(1):1–3,6,7.
38. Rymal C. Teach your patients about lymphedema precautions. Lymphedema Management Special Interest Group Newsletter 2001;12(3):2.

39. Witte C, Witte M. Consensus and dogma. Lymphology 1998; 31:98–100.
40. Bertelli G, Venturini M, Forno G, Macciavello F, Dini D. An analysis of prognostic factors in response to conservative treatment of post-mastectomy lymphedema. Surg Gynecol Obstet 1992;175:455–460.
41. Kocak Z, Overgaard J. Risk factors of arm lymphedema in breast cancer patients. Acta Oncol 2000;39:389–392.
42. Martlew B. Seroma and other factors influencing the development of breast oedema following breast cancer treatment. Macmillan Lymphoedema Specialist Website, 2001. Available at: http://www.lymphoedema.org/bls/blsc0035.htm (accessed December 30, 2004).
43. Mason M. The influence of body mass index (BMI) on lymphoedema. Adelaide Lymphoedema Clinic 2001;5–7.
44. Meek A. Lymphedema prevention: a one-year survey. Lymph Link (National Lymphedema Network) 2001;13(3);1–3. Available at: http://www.lymphnet.org/newsletter.html (accessed June 9, 2005).
45. Petrak J, Senie RT, Peters M, Rosen PP. Lymphedema in a cohort of breast carcinoma survivors 20 years after diagnosis. Cancer 2001;92:1368–1377.
46. Werner R, McCormick B, Petrek J, Cox L, Cirrincione C, Gray JR, Yahalom J. Arm edema in conservatively managed breast cancer: Obesity is a major predictive factor. Radiology 1991; 180:177–184.
47. Pezner R. Arm lymphedema in patients treated conservatively for breast cancer: Relationship to patient age and axillary node dissection technique. Radiat Oncol 1986;12:2079–2083.
48. Treves N. An evaluation of the etiological factors of lymphedema following radical mastectomy: An analysis of 1,007 cases. Cancer 1957;10:444–449.
49. Venipuncture Policy. Penrose–St. Francis Health Services. Nursing Policy Committee, Colorado Springs, CO:2003.
50. Box RC, Reul-Hirche HM, Bullock-Saxton JE, Furnival CM. Physiotherapy after breast cancer surgery: Results of a randomised controlled study to minimise lymphedema. Breast Cancer Research Treatment 2002;75:51–64.
51. Kissin M, della Rovere GQ, Easton D, Westbury G. Risk of lymphoedema following the treatment of breast cancer. Br J Surg 1986;73:580–584.
52. Segerstrom K, Bjerle P, Graffman S, Nystrom A. Factors that influence the incidence of brachial oedema after treatment of breast cancer. Scand J Plast Reconstr Hand Surg 1992;26:223–227.
53. Harris SR, Niesen-Vertommen S. Challenging the myth of exercise-induced lymphedema following breast cancer: A series of case reports. J Surg Oncol 2000;74:95–98.
54. Johannson K, Ohlsson K, Ingvar C, Albertsson M, Ekdahl C. Factors associated with the development of arm lymphedema following breast cancer treatment: A match pair case-control study. Lymphology 2002;35:59–71.
55. Erickson VS, Pearson ML, Ganz PA, Adams J, Kahn KL. Arm edema in breast cancer patients. J Natl Cancer Inst 2001;93:96–111.
56. Highfield ME. Providing spiritual care to patients with cancer. Clin J Oncol Nurs 2000;4:115–120.
57. Taugher T. Helping patients search for meaning in their lives. CJON 2002;6:239–240.
58. Habel M. Patient education helping patients, families take charge of their health. Nurseweek (Mountainview) 2002;3:3–4, 29–30.
59. Stanton AWB, Badger C, Sitzia J. Non-invasive assessment of the lymphedematous limb. Lymphology 2000;33:122–135.
60. Gerber LH. A review of measures of lymphedema. Cancer (Suppl)1998;83:2803–2804.
61. Hoskins CL, Daugherty D. Disease management: Establishing standards of care for lymphedema treatment. Lymph Link 2003;15(4):5,26.
62. Badger C, Preston N, Seers K, Mortimer P. Physical therapies for reducing and controlling lymphoedema of the limbs. Cochrane Database Syst Rev 2004;(4):CD003141.
63. Sitzia J, Harlow W. Lymphoedema 4: Research priorities in lymphoedema care. Br J Nurs 2002;11:631–641.
64. Lerner R. Lymphedema: A 25 year perspective. NLN Newsletter 1997;9(4):1,2,11.
65. Harris SR, Hugi MR, Olivotto IA, Levine M; Steering Committee for Clinical Practice Guidelines for the Care and Treatment of Breast Cancer. Clinical practice guidelines for the care and treatment of breast cancer: 11. Lymphedema. CMAJ 2001;164: 191–199.
66. Susman E. Patients, doctors not on same page in recognizing lymphedema complications. Oncology Times 2000;(November):4.
67. Dotts T. Despite the risk, oncologists admit they know little about lymphedema. Hem Onc Today 2004;5(2):14.
68. Megens A, Harris SR. Physical therapist management of lymphedema following treatment for breast cancer: A critical review of its effectiveness. Phys Ther 1998;78:1302–1311.
69. Johnston RV, Anderson JN, Walker BL. Is physiotherapy an effective treatment for lymphedema secondary to cancer treatment? Med J Aust 2003;178:236–237.
69a. Anderson L, Horjis I, Erlanson M, Andersen J. Treatment of breast-cancer-related lymphedema with or without manual lymphatic drainage: a randomized study. Acta Oncol 2000;39(3): 399–405.
69b. McNeely M, Magee D, Lees AW, Bagnall KM, Haykowsky M, Hanson J. The addition of manual lymph drainage to compression therapy for breast cancer related lymphedema: a randomized controlled trial. Breast Cancer Res Treat, 2004;86(2): 95–106.
70. Lyman GH, Kuderer NM, Balducci L. Cancer care in the elderly: Cost and quality-of-life considerations. Cancer Control 1998;5: 347–354.
71. Erickson V. Arm edema in breast cancer patients. J Natl Cancer Inst 2001;93:96–111.
72. Woods M. Patients' perceptions of breast-cancer-related lymphoedema. Eur J Cancer Care 1993;2:125–128.
73. Dennis B. Acquired lymphedema: A chart review of nine women's responses to intervention [review]. Am J Occup Ther 1993;47:891–899.
74. Ramos SM, O'Donnell LS, Knight G. Edema volume, not timing, is the key to success in lymphedema treatment. Am J Surg 1999;178:311–315.
75. Carter BJ. Women's experiences of lymphedema. ONF 1997;24 (5):875–881.
76. Regnard C, Allport S, Stephenson L. ABC of palliative care: Mouth care, skin care, and lymphoedema. Br Med J 1997;315: 1004–1005.
77. Babb R, Spittell JA, Martin WJ, Schirger A. Prophylaxis of recurrent lymphangitis complicating lymphedema. JAMA 1966;195: 183–185.
78. Britton R, Nelson P. Causes and treatment of postmastectomy lymphedema of the arm. JAMA 1962;180:95–102.
79. Mallon E, Powell S, Mortimer P, Ryan T. Evidence for altered cell-mediated immunity in postmastectomy lymphoedema. Br J Dermatol 1997;137:928–933.
80. Cohen SR, Payne DK, Tunkel RS. Lymphedema: Strategies for management. Cancer 2001;92(4 Suppl):980–987.
81. Macdonald JM. Wound healing and lymphedema: A new look at an old problem. Ostomy Wound Manage 2001;47(4):52–57.

82. Mortimer P. Inflammation and infection in the lymphedema limb. Newsletter of the Lymphedema Association of Australia 1997;3–4.
83. Olszewski W. Inflammatory changes of skin in lymphedema of extremities and efficacy of benzathine penicillin administration. NLN Newsletter 1996;8(4):1–3.
84. Ko DS, Lerner R, Klose G, Cosimi AB. Effective treatment of lymphedema of the extremities. Arch Surg 1998;133:452–458.
85. Williams AE, Bergl S, Twycross RG. A 5-year review of a lymphoedema service. Eur J Cancer Care 1996;5:56–59.
86. Foldi E. The treatment of lymphedema. Cancer 1998;83(12 Suppl American):2833–2834.
87. Serlin R, Mendoza T, Nakamura Y, Edwards KR, Cleeland CS. When is cancer pain mild, moderate or severe? Grading pain severity by its interference with function. Pain 1995;61: 277–284.
88. Brennan MJ, Miller LT. Overview of treatment options and review of the current role and use of compression garments, intermittent pumps, and exercise in the management of lymphedema. Cancer 1998;83(12 Suppl American):2821–2827.
89. Petrak JA, Lerner R. Lymphedema. In: Harris JR, Lippman ME, Morrow M, Osborne CK. Diseases of the Breast, 2nd ed. Philadelphia: Lippincott Williams & Wilkins, 2000:1033–1040.
90. Mortimer PS. Managing lymphedema. Clin Exper Dermatol 1995;20:98–106.
91. Brorson H, Svensson H. Skin blood flow of the lymphedematous arm before and after liposuction. Lymphology 1997;30: 165–172.
92. Rymal C. Compression modalities in lymphedema therapy. Innovations in Breast Cancer Care 1998;3(4):88–92.
93. Brorson H, Svensson H. Complete reduction of lymphoedema of the arm by liposuction after breast cancer. Scand J Plast Reconstr Surg Hand Surg 1997;31:137–143.
94. Svensson H. Liposuction combined with controlled compression therapy reduces arm lymphedema more effectively than controlled compression therapy alone. Plast Reconstr Surg 1998;31:156–172.
95. Cheville AJ. Lymphedema and palliative care. Lymph Link 2002;14(1):1–4.
96. Bertelli G, Venturini M, Forno G, Macciavello F, Dini D. Conservative treatment of postmastectomy lymphedema: A controlled, randomized trial. Ann Oncol 1991;2:575–578.
97. Haslett ML, Aitken MJ. Evaluating the effectiveness of a compression sleeve in managing secondary lymphoedema. J Wound Care 2002;11:401–404.
98. Lund E. Exploring the use of the CircAid legging in the management of lymphoedema. Int J Palliat Nurs 2000;6:383–391.
99. Miranda F Jr, Perez MC, Castiglioni ML, Juliano Y, Amorim JE, Nakano LC, de Barros N Jr, Lustre WG, Burinah E. Effect of sequential intermittent pneumatic compression on both leg lymphedema volume and on lymph transport as semi-quantitatively evaluated by lymphoscintigraphy. Lymphology 2001;34:135–141.
100. Lynnworth M. Greater Boston lymphedema support group pump survey. NLN Newsletter 1998;10(1):6–7.
101. Boris M, Weindorf S, Lasinski B. The risk of genital edema after external pump compression for lower limb lymphedema. Lymphology 1998;31:15–20.
102. Brennan MJ, DePompolo RW, Garden FH. Focused review: Postmastectomy lymphedema. Arch Phys Med Rehabil 1996;77:S74–S80.
103. Brorson H, Aberg M, Svensson H. Liposuction of arm lymphedema: A well established method giving complete reduction with long-lasting result—9 years follow-up. Lymphology. In press.
104. Tiedjen K. Isotopenlymphographische Untrusting (Technetium-Zinn-II-Schwefelkolloid) oberer Extremitäten beg Zustand nach Mammaamputation und Bestrahlung. Phlebol Proktol 1983;12:196.
105. Cheville AJ. Lymphedema and palliative care. Lymph Link 2002;14(1):1–4.
106. Ferrell BR. The role of oncology nursing to ensure quality care for cancer survivors: A report commissioned by the National Cancer Policy Board and Institute of Medicine. Oncol Nurs Forum 2003;30(1):E1–E11.
107. Brorson H. How to treat chronic arm lymphedema. Congress Booklet 2001. ESPRAS, Rome.
108. Olszewski W. Lymph Stasis: Pathophysiology, Diagnosis and Treatment. Boca Raton, FL: CRC Press, 1991.
109. Barrett J. The assessment and treatment of patients with lymphoedema. Nursing Standard 1997;11(21):48–53.
110. Cho S, Atwood JE. Idiopathic oedema of women (Chapter 15.18). In: Warrell DA, Cox TM, Firth JD, eds. Oxford Textbook of Medicine (Vol 2) (2nd ed). New York: Oxford University Press, 2003:1209–1210.

16A

Barbara M. Bates-Jensen

Skin Disorders: Pressure Ulcers—Assessment and Management

I always thought that bedsores came from neglect. I feel so guilty that I let this happen.
—A patient's family member

- ***Key Points***
- *Pressure ulcer prevention includes repositioning at frequent intervals, with attention to adequate pain relief interventions before movement.*
- *Palliative care for pressure ulcers includes attention to prevention measures, obtaining and maintaining a clean wound, management of exudates and odor, and prevention of complications such as wound infection.*
- *It is essential to involve caregivers and family members in the plan of care.*

Palliative care for skin disorders is a broad area, encompassing prevention and care for pressure ulcers, management of malignant cutaneous wounds and fistulas, and management of stomas. The goals of treatment are often to reduce discomfort, manage odor and drainage, and provide for optimal functional capacity. In each area, involvement of the caregiver and family in the plan of care is important. Management of skin disorders involves significant physical care as well as attention to psychological and social care. To meet the needs of the patient and family, access to the multidisciplinary care team is crucial, and consultation by an Enterostomal Therapy nurse or a certified Wound, Ostomy, Continence nurse is highly desirable.

Because skin disorders are such an important issue in palliative nursing care, Chapter 16 has been divided into two distinct parts. Part 16A addresses pressure ulcers in depth, and Part 16B addresses tumor necrosis, fistulas, and stomas.

Definition

Pressure ulcers are areas of local tissue trauma that usually develop where soft tissues are compressed between bony prominences and external surfaces for prolonged periods. Mechanical injury to the skin and tissues causes hypoxia and ischemia, leading to tissue necrosis. Caring for the patient with a pressure ulcer can be frustrating for clinicians because of the chronic nature of the wound and because additional time and resources are often invested in the management of these wounds. Pressure ulcer care is costly, and treatment costs increase as the severity of the wound increases. Additionally, not all pressure ulcers heal, and many heal slowly, causing a continual drain on caregivers and on financial resources. The chronic nature of a pressure ulcer challenges the health care provider to design more effective treatment plans.

Once a pressure ulcer develops, the usual goals are to manage the wound and to support healing. However, some patients will benefit most from a palliative care approach. Palliative wound care means that the goals are comfort and limiting the extent or impact of the wound, but without the intent of healing. Palliative care for chronic wounds, such as pressure ulcers, is appropriate for a wide variety of patient populations. Palliative care is often indicated for terminally ill patients, such as those with terminal-stage cancer or other diseases. Institutionalized older adults with multiple comorbidities and older adults with severe functional decline may also benefit from palliative care. Sometimes individuals with long-standing wounds and other life expectations benefit from a palliative care approach for a specified duration of time. For example, a wheelchair-bound young adult with a sacral pressure ulcer may make an informed choice to continue to be up in a wheelchair to attend school even though this choice severely diminishes the expectation for wound healing. The health care professional may decide jointly with the patient to treat the wound palliatively during this time frame.

The foundation for designing a care plan for the patient with a pressure ulcer is a comprehensive assessment. This is true even if the goals of care are palliative. Comprehensive assessment includes assessment of wound severity, wound status, and the total patient. Generally, management of the wound is best accomplished within the context of the whole person, particularly if palliation is the outcome. Assessment is the first step in maintaining and evaluating a therapeutic plan of care. Without adequate baseline wound and patient assessment and valid interpretation of the assessment data, the plan of care for the wound may be inappropriate or ineffective—at the least, it may be disjointed and fragmented due to poor communication. An inadequate plan of care may lead to impaired or delayed healing, miscommunication regarding the goals of care (healing versus palliation), and complications such as infection.

Pathophysiology of Pressure Ulcer Development

Pressure ulcers are the result of mechanical injury to the skin and underlying tissues. The primary forces involved are pressure and shear.[1–5] Pressure is the perpendicular force or load exerted on a specific area; it causes ischemia and hypoxia of the tissues. High-pressure areas in the supine position are the occiput, sacrum, and heels. In the sitting position, the ischial tuberosities exert the highest pressure, and the trochanters are affected in the side-lying position.[2,6]

As the amount of soft tissue available for compression decreases, the pressure gradient increases. Likewise, as the tissue available for compression increases, the pressure gradient decreases. For this reason, most pressure ulcers occur over bony prominences, where there is less tissue for compression.[6] This relationship is important to understand for palliative care, because most of the likely candidates for palliative care will have experienced significant changes in nutritional status and body weight, with diminished soft tissue available for compression and a more prominent bony structure. This more prominent bony structure is more susceptible to skin breakdown from external forces, because the soft tissue that is normally used to deflect physical forces (e.g., pressure, shear) is absent. Therefore, the tissues are less tolerant of external forces, and the pressure gradient within the vascular network is altered.[6]

Alterations in the vascular network allow an increase in the interstitial fluid pressure, which exceeds the venous flow. This results in an additional increase in the pressure and impedes arteriolar circulation. The capillary vessels collapse, and thrombosis occurs. Increased capillary arteriolar pressure leads to fluid loss through the capillaries, tissue edema, and subsequent autolysis. Lymphatic flow is decreased, allowing further tissue edema and contributing to the tissue necrosis.[3,5,7–9]

Pressure, over time, occludes blood and lymphatic circulation, causing deficient tissue nutrition and buildup of waste products due to ischemia. If pressure is relieved before a critical time period is reached, a normal compensatory mechanism, reactive hyperemia, restores tissue nutrition and compensates for compromised circulation. If pressure is not relieved before the critical time period, the blood vessels collapse and thrombose, causing tissue deprivation of oxygen, nutrients, and waste removal. In the absence of oxygen, cells utilize anaerobic pathways for metabolism and produce toxic byproducts. The toxic byproducts lead to tissue acidosis, increased cell membrane permeability, edema, and, eventually, cell death.[3,7]

Tissue damage may also be caused by reperfusion and reoxygenation of the ischemic tissues or by postischemic injury.[10] Oxygen is reintroduced into tissues during reperfusion after ischemia. This triggers oxygen free radicals, known as superoxide anion, hydroxyl radicals, and hydrogen peroxide, which induce endothelial damage and decrease microvascular integrity. Ischemia and hypoxia of body tissues are produced when capillary blood flow is obstructed by localized pressure. The degree of pressure and the amount of time necessary for ulceration to occur have been a subject of study for many years. In 1930, Landis,[11] using single-capillary microinjection techniques, determined normal hydrostatic pressure to be 32 mm Hg at the arteriolar end and 15 mm Hg at the venular end. His work has served as a criterion for measuring occlusion of capillary blood flow. Generally, a range from 25 to 32 mm Hg is considered normal and is used as the marker for adequate relief of pressure on the tissues. In severely compromised patients, even this level of pressure may be too high.

Pressure is greatest at the bony prominence and soft tissue interface and gradually lessens in a cone-shaped gradient to the periphery.[2,12,13] Therefore, although tissue damage apparent on the skin surface may be minimal, the damage to deeper structures can be severe. In addition, subcutaneous fat and muscle are more sensitive than the skin to ischemia. Muscle and fat tissues are more metabolically active and, therefore, more vulnerable to hypoxia with increased susceptibility to pressure damage. The vulnerability of muscle and fat tissues to pressure forces explains pressure ulcers, in which large areas of muscle and fat tissue are damaged yet the skin opening is relatively small.[8] In patients with severe malnutrition and weight loss, there is less tissue between the bony prominence and the surface of the skin, so the potential for large ulcers with extensive undermining or pocketing is much higher.

There is a relationship between intensity and duration of pressure in pressure ulcer development. Low pressures over a long period of time are as capable of producing tissue damage as high pressures for a shorter period.[2] Tissues can tolerate higher cyclic pressures compared with constant pressure.[14] Pressures differ in various body positions. They are highest (70 mm Hg) on the buttocks in the lying position and in the sitting position can be as high as 300 mm Hg over the ischial tuberosities.[2,6] These levels are well above the normal capillary closing pressures and are capable of causing tissue ischemia. If tissues have been compressed for prolonged periods, tissue damage will continue to occur even after the pressure is relieved.[12] This continued tissue damage relates to changes at the cellular level that lead to difficulties with restoration of perfusion. Initial skin breakdown can occur in 6 to 12 hours in healthy individuals and more quickly (less than 2 hours) in those who are debilitated.

More than 95% of all pressure ulcers develop over five classic locations: sacral/coccygeal area, greater trochanter, ischial tuberosity, heel, and lateral malleolus.[4] Correct anatomical terminology is important when identifying the true location of the pressure ulcer. For example, many clinicians often document pressure ulcers as being located on the patient's hip. The hip, or iliac crest, is actually an uncommon location for pressure ulceration. The iliac crest, located on the front of the body, is rarely subject to pressure forces. The area most clinicians are referring to is correctly termed the greater trochanter. The greater trochanter is the bony prominence located on the side of the body, just above the proximal, lateral aspect of the thigh, or "saddlebag" area. The majority of pressure ulcers occur on the lower half of the body. The location of the pressure ulcer may affect clinical interventions. For example, the patient with a pressure ulcer on the sacral/coccygeal area with concomitant urinary incontinence requires treatments that addresses the incontinence problem. Ulcers in the sacral/coccygeal area are also more at risk for friction and shearing damage due to the location of the wound. Figure 16–1 shows the correct anatomical terminology for pressure ulcer locations. Typical pressure ulcer locations for palliative care patients are the sacral/coccygeal area, trochanters, and heels. Patients with contractures are at special risk for pressure ulcer development due to the internal pressure of the bony prominence and the abnormal alignment of the body and its extremities. Institutionalized older adults with severe functional decline are particularly susceptible to contractures due to immobilization for extended periods of time in conjunction with limited efforts for maintenance of range of motion.

Risk Factors for Pressure Ulcers

Pressure ulcers are physical evidence of multiple causative influences. Factors that contribute to pressure ulcer development can be thought of as those that affect the pressure force over the bony prominence and those that affect the tolerance of the tissues to pressure.

Mobility, sensory loss, and activity level are related to the concept of increasing pressure. Extrinsic factors including shear, friction, and moisture, as well as intrinsic factors such as nutrition, age, and arteriolar pressure, relate to the concept of tissue tolerance.[15] Several additional areas may influence pressure ulcer development, including emotional stress, temperature, smoking, and interstitial fluid flow.[16]

Immobility

Immobility, inactivity, and decreased sensory perception affect the duration and intensity of the pressure over the bony prominence. Immobility or severely restricted mobility is the most important risk factor for all populations and a necessary condition for the development of pressure ulcers. Mobility is the state of being movable. The immobile patient cannot move, or facility or ease of movement is impaired. Closely related to immobility is limited activity.

Inactivity

Activity is the production of energy or motion and implies an action. Activity is often clinically described by the ability of the individual to ambulate and move about. Those persons who are bed- or chair-bound, and thus inactive, are more at risk for pressure ulcer development.[17,18] A sudden change in activity level may signal significant change in health status and increased potential for pressure ulcer development.

Sensory Loss

Sensory loss places patients at risk for compression of tissues and pressure ulcer development, because the normal mechanism for translating pain messages from the tissues is dysfunctional.[19] Patients with intact nervous system pathways feel continuous local pressure, become uncomfortable, and change their position before tissue ischemia occurs. Spinal cord–injured patients have a higher incidence and prevalence of pressure ulcers.[20,21] Patients with paraplegia or quadriplegia are unable to sense increased pressure; if their body weight is not shifted, pressure ulceration develops. Likewise, patients with changes in mental status or functioning are at increased risk for pressure ulcer formation. They may not feel the discomfort from pressure, may not be alert enough to move spontaneously, may not remember to move, may be too confused to respond to commands to move, or may be physically unable to move.[19] This risk factor is particularly evident in the palliative care population, in which individuals may be at the end of life, may not be alert enough to move spontaneously, or may be physically unable to move.

Shear

Extrinsic risk factors are those forces that make the tissues less tolerant of pressure. Extrinsic forces include shear, friction, and moisture. Whereas pressure acts perpendicularly to

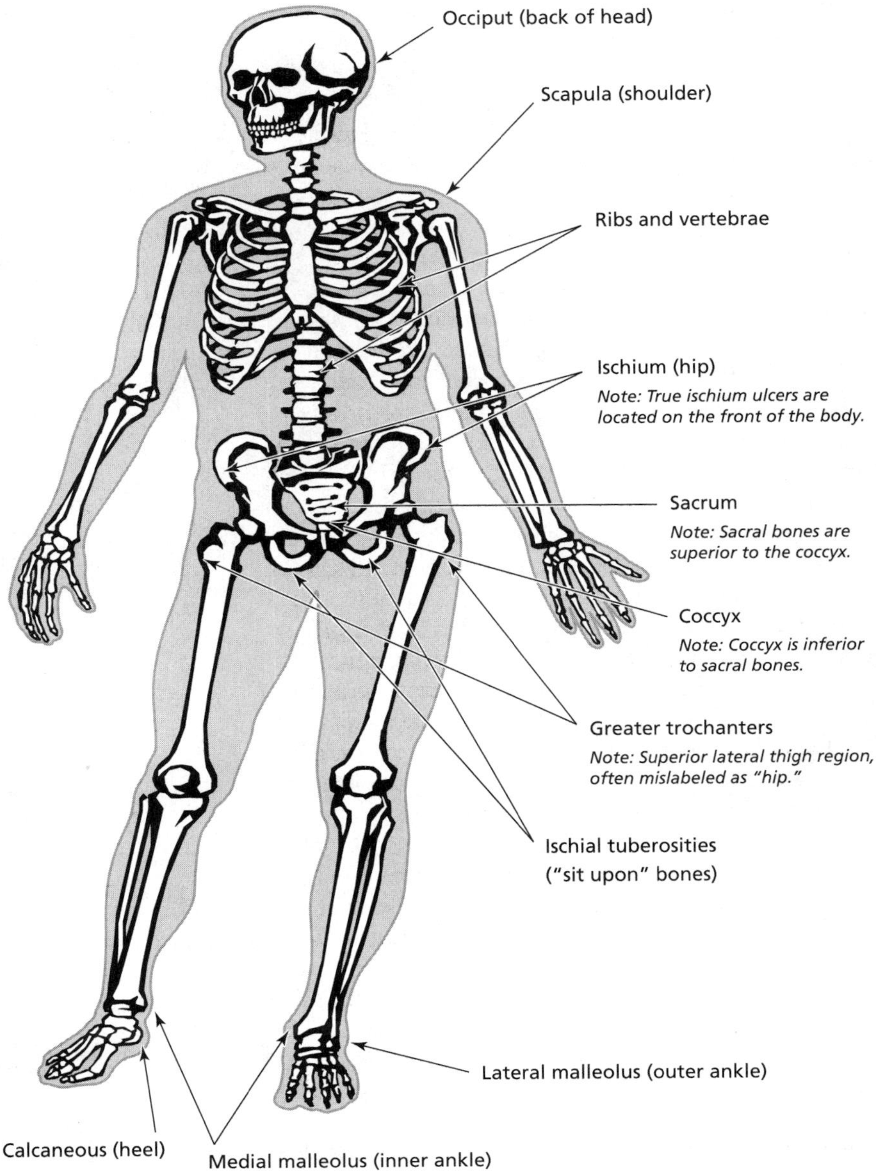

Figure 16A-1. Common anatomical locations of pressure ulcers.

cause ischemia, shear causes ischemia by displacing blood vessels laterally and thereby impeding blood flow to tissues.[22–24] Shear is caused by the interplay of gravity and friction. Shear is a parallel force that stretches and twists tissues and blood vessels at the bony tissue interface; as such, it affects the deep blood vessels and deeper tissue structures. The most common example of shear is seen in the bed patient who is in a semisitting position with knees flexed and supported by pillows on the bed or by head-of-bed elevation. If the patient's skeleton slides down toward the foot of the bed, the sacral skin may stay in place (with the help of friction against the bed linen). This produces stretching, pinching, and occlusion of the underlying vessels, resulting in ulcers with large areas of internal tissue damage and less damage at the skin surface.

Friction

Friction and moisture are not direct factors in pressure ulcer development, but they have been identified as contributing to the problem by reducing tolerance of tissues to pressure.[24] Friction occurs when two surfaces move across one another. Friction acts on tissue tolerance to pressure by abrading and damaging the epidermal and upper dermal layers of the skin. Additionally, friction acts with gravity to cause shear. Friction abrades the epidermis, which may lead to pressure ulcer development by increasing the skin's susceptibility to pressure injury. Pressure combined with friction produces ulcerations at lower pressures than does pressure alone.[24] Friction acts in conjunction with shear to contribute to the development of sacral/coccygeal pressure ulcers on patients in the semi-Fowler position.

Moisture

Moisture contributes to pressure ulcer development by removing oils on the skin, making it more friable, as well as interacting with body support surface friction. Constant moisture on the skin leads to maceration of the tissues. Waterlogging leads to softening of the skin's connective tissues. Macerated tissues are more prone to erosion, and once the epidermis is eroded, there is increased likelihood of further tissue breakdown.[25] Moisture alters the resiliency of the epidermis to external forces. Both shearing force and friction increase in the presence of mild to moderate moisture. Excess moisture may be caused by wound drainage, diaphoresis, or fecal or urinary incontinence.

Incontinence

Urinary and fecal incontinence are common risk factors associated with pressure ulcer development. Incontinence contributes to pressure ulcer formation by creating excess moisture on the skin and by chemical damage to the skin. Fecal incontinence has the added detrimental effect of bacteria in the stool, which can contribute to infection as well as skin breakdown. Fecal incontinence is more significant as a risk factor for pressure ulceration because of the bacteria and enzymes in stool and their effects on the skin.[19,26] Inadequately managed incontinence poses a significant risk factor for pressure ulcer development, and fecal incontinence is highly correlated with pressure ulcer development.[17,27]

Nutritional Risk Factors

There is some disagreement concerning the major intrinsic risk factors affecting tissue tolerance to pressure. However, most studies identify nutritional status as playing a role in pressure ulcer development. Hypoalbuminemia, weight loss, cachexia, and malnutrition are commonly identified as risk factors predisposing patients to pressure ulcer development.[28–31] Low serum albumin levels are associated both with having a pressure ulcer and with developing a pressure ulcer.

Age

Age itself may be a risk factor for pressure ulcer development, with age-related changes in the skin and in wound healing increasing the risk of pressure ulcer development.[32] The skin and support structures undergo changes in the aging process. There is a loss of muscle, a decrease in serum albumin levels, diminished inflammatory response, decreased elasticity, and reduced cohesion between dermis and epidermis.[32,33] These changes combine with other changes related to aging to make the skin less tolerant of pressure forces, shear, and friction.

Medical Conditions and Psychological Factors

Certain medical conditions or disease states are also associated with pressure ulcer development. Orthopedic injuries, altered mental status, and spinal cord injury are such conditions.[20,21,31,34,35] Other psychological factors may affect risk for pressure ulcer development.[36–38] Self-concept, depression, and chronic emotional stress have been cited as factors in pressure ulcer development; and the emerging role of cortisol levels in pressure ulcer development bears monitoring.

Environmental Resources

Environmental resources include socioeconomic, psychosocial, health care system, and therapy resources. These factors are less understood than other risk factors; however, several of them play important roles in determining risk for pressure ulcer development and course of pressure ulcer care in patients receiving palliative care. Socioeconomic resources that may influence pressure ulcer development and healing are cost of therapy, type of payor (insurance type), and access to health care. In palliative care, cost of therapy becomes an important issue, particularly in long-term care facilities, where financial resources are limited and cost of therapy may hinder access to treatment.

Health care system resources are the type of health care setting and the experience, education level, and discipline of health care professionals. Patients receiving palliative care are often in long-term care facilities and dependent on the direct care practices of nurse aides with minimal education in health care, nursing, and, especially, the needs of the palliative care patient. Therapy resources include topical treatments for wounds and systemic treatments. Palliative care patients often receive concomitant therapy that impairs mobility or sensory perception (e.g., pain medication) or normal healing mechanisms (e.g., steroids).

Psychosocial resources include adherence to the therapy plan, cultural values and beliefs, social support network (family and caregiver support), spiritual support, and alternative medicine use. The social support network is a key factor for palliative care. Patients receiving palliative care are often cared for in the home or in a long-term care facility. Home caregivers may be family members of the patient, often the spouse or significant other. If the patient is older and frail, it is typical to find that the caregiver is also older and frail, yet responsible for providing direct care 24 hours a day with minimal respite or support. Many times the nurse is dealing with two patients, the patient receiving palliative care and the patient's caregiver, who may also be frail and in need of services. The family member may be physically unable to reposition the patient or to provide other care services. In long-term care facilities, the problem may not be physical inability to perform the tasks but lack of time or motivation. The availability of nurse attendants in the long-term care facility may be such that turning and repositioning of palliative care patients are not high-priority tasks.

In summary, environmental resources are not all well defined and typically are not included in formal risk-assessment tools for development of pressure ulcers. However, the importance of environmental resources in both the development and healing of pressure ulcers is clinically relevant in palliative care.

Use of Risk-Assessment Scales

For practitioners to intervene in a cost-effective way, a method of screening for risk factors is necessary. Several risk-assessment instruments are available to clinicians. Screening tools assist in prevention by distinguishing those persons who are at risk for pressure ulcer development from those who are not. The only purpose in identifying patients who are at risk for pressure ulcer development is to allow for appropriate use of resources for prevention. The use of a risk-assessment tool allows for targeting of interventions to specific risk factors for individual patients. The risk-assessment instrument selected is based on its reliability for the intended raters, its predictive validity for the population, its sensitivity and specificity under consideration, and its ease of use including the time required for completion. The most common risk-assessment tools are Braden's Scale for Predicting Pressure Sore Risk and Norton's Scale. There is minimal information on the use of either instrument in palliative care patients, but both tools have been used in long-term care facilities, where many patients are assumed to be receiving palliative care. This is an area in which further study is warranted.

Norton's Scale. The Norton tool is the oldest risk-assessment instrument. Developed in 1961, it consists of five subscales: physical condition, mental state, activity, mobility, and incontinence.[39] Each parameter is rated on a scale of 1 to 4, with the sum of the ratings for all five parameters yielding a total score ranging from 5 to 20. Lower scores indicate increased risk, with scores of 16 or lower indicating "onset of risk" and scores of 12 or lower indicating high risk for pressure ulcer formation.[40]

Braden Scale for Predicting Pressure Sores. The Braden Scale was developed in 1987 and is composed of six subscales that conceptually reflect degrees of sensory perception, moisture, activity, nutrition, friction and shear, and mobility.[15,16] All subscales are rated from 1 to 4, except for friction and shear, which is rated from 1 to 3. The subscales may be summed for a total score ranging from 6 to 23.

Lower scores indicate lower function and higher risk for development of a pressure ulcer. The cutoff score for hospitalized adults is considered to be 16, with scores of 16 and lower indicating at-risk status.[16] In older patients, some have found cutoff scores of 17 or 18 to be better predictors of risk status.[15,30] Levels of risk are based on the predictive value of a positive test. Scores of 15 to 16 indicate mild risk, with a 50% to 60% chance of developing a stage I pressure ulcer; scores of 12 to 14 indicate moderate risk, with 65% to 90% chance of developing a stage I or II lesion; and scores lower than 12 indicate high risk, with a 90% to 100% chance of developing a stage II or deeper pressure ulcer.[30,34] The Braden Scale has been tested in acute care and long-term care with several levels of nurse raters and demonstrates high interrater reliability with registered nurses.

Validity has been established by expert opinion, and predictive validity has been studied in several acute care settings, with good sensitivity and specificity demonstrated.[16,30] The Braden Scale is the model used in this chapter for prevention of pressure ulcers in patients requiring palliative care.

Regardless of the instrument chosen to evaluate risk status, the clinical relevance is threefold. First, assessment for risk status must occur at frequent intervals. Assessment should be performed at admission to the health care organization (within 24 hours), at predetermined intervals (usually weekly), and whenever a significant change occurs in the patient's general health and status. The second clinical implication is the targeting of specific prevention strategies to identified risk factors. The final clinical implication is for those patients in whom prevention is not successful. For patients with an actual pressure ulcer, the continued monitoring of risk status may prevent further tissue trauma at the wound site and development of additional wound sites.

Prevention of Pressure Ulcers

Prevention strategies are targeted at reducing risk factors and can be focused on eliminating specific risk factors. Early intervention for pressure ulcers is risk factor specific and prophylactic in nature. The prevention strategies are presented here by risk factor, beginning with general information and ending with specific strategies to eliminate particular risk factors. Prevention is a key element for palliative care. If pressure ulcers can be prevented, the patient is spared tiresome, sometimes painful, and often overwhelming treatment. The Braden Scale is the basis for these prevention interventions. Prevention interventions that are appropriate to the patient's level of risk and specific to individual risk factors should be instituted.[18] For example, the risk factor of immobility is managed very differently for the comatose patient compared with the patient with severe pain on movement or the patient who is still mobile even if bed bound. The comatose patient requires caregiver education and caregiver-dependent repositioning. The patient with severe pain on movement requires special support surface intervention and minimal movement methods with a foam wedge. The patient who is still mobile but bed bound requires self-care education and may be able to perform self-repositioning. The interventions for the risk factor of immobility are very different for these patients.

Immobility, Inactivity, and Sensory Loss

Patients who have impaired ability to reposition and who cannot independently change body positions must have local pressure alleviated by any of the following: passive repositioning by caregivers, pillow bridging, or pressure relief or reduction support surfaces for bed and chair.[18,19,34] In addition, measures to increase mobility and activity and to decrease friction and shear should be instituted. This is true for persons receiving palliative care until the terminal stage of the disease process. The difference for those receiving palliative care is the emphasis on providing adequate pain management as part of prevention interventions related to movement and repositioning.

Overhead bed frames with trapeze bars are helpful for patients with upper body strength and may increase mobility and independence with body repositioning. Wheelchair-bound patients with upper body strength can be taught and encouraged to do wheelchair pushups to relieve pressure and allow for reperfusion of the tissues in the ischial tuberosity region. For patients who are weak from prolonged inactivity, providing support and assistance for reconditioning and increasing strength and endurance may help prevent further decline.[19] Mobility plans for each patient should be individualized, with the goal of attaining the highest level of mobility and activity possible in light of the goals of overall care. Caregivers in the home are often left to fend for themselves for prevention interventions and may be frail and have health problems themselves. A return demonstration of a repositioning procedure can be very informative to the nurse. The nurse may need to coach, improvise, and think of creative strategies for caregivers to use in the home setting to meet the patient's needs for movement and tissue reperfusion.

Passive Repositioning by Caregiver. Turning schedules and passive repositioning by caregivers is the normal intervention response for patients with immobility risk factors. Typically, turning schedules are based on time or event. If time-based, turning is usually done every 2 hours for full-body change of position and more often for small shifts in position. Event-based schedules relate to typical events during the day (e.g., turning the patient after each meal). Full-body change of position involves turning the patient to a new lying position, such as from the right side-lying position to the left side-lying position or the supine position. If the side-lying position is used in bed, avoidance of direct pressure on the trochanter is essential. To avoid placing pressure on the trochanter, the patient is placed in a 30-degree, laterally inclined position instead of the commonly used 90-degree side-lying position, which increases tissue compression over the trochanter. The 30-degree, laterally inclined position allows for distribution of pressure over a greater area. Small shifts in position involve moving the patient but keeping the same lying position, such as changing the angle of the right side-lying position or changing the position of the lower extremities in the right side-lying position. Both strategies are helpful in achieving reperfusion of compressed tissues, but only a full-body change of position completely relieves pressure.

A foam wedge is very useful in positioning for frail caregivers and for patients with severe pain on movement. The foam wedge should provide a 30-degree angle of lift when fully inserted behind the patient, usually extending from the shoulders to the hips/buttocks. Once it is in place, even the most frail of caregivers can easily pull the wedge out slightly every hour, providing for small shifts in position and tissue reperfusion. Even patients with pain on movement find the slight movement from the foam wedge tolerable. There are other techniques to make turning patients easier and less time-consuming. Turning sheets, draw sheets, and pillows are essential for passive movement of patients in bed. Turning sheets are useful in repositioning the patient to a side-lying position. Draw sheets are used for pulling patients up in bed; they help prevent dragging of the patient's skin over the bed surface.

The recommended time interval for a full change of position is every 2 hours, depending on the individual patient profile. Similar approaches to repositioning are useful for patients in chairs. Full-body change of position involves standing the patient and then re-sitting the patient in a chair. Small shifts in position for those in chairs might involve changing the position of the lower extremities or inserting a small foam pillow or wedge. For the chair-bound patient, it is also helpful to use a foot stool to help reduce the pressure on the ischial tuberosities and to distribute the pressure over a wider surface. Attention to proper alignment and posture is essential. Individuals at risk for pressure ulcer development should avoid uninterrupted sitting in chairs, and clinical practice guidelines suggest repositioning every hour. The rationale behind the shorter time frame is the extremely high pressures generated on the ischial tuberosities in the seated position.[42] Those patients with upper-body strength should be taught to shift weight every 15 minutes, to allow for tissue reperfusion. Again, pillows may be used to help position the patient in proper body alignment. Physical therapy and occupational therapy can assist in body-alignment strategies with even the most contracted patient.

In many instances, patients receiving palliative care at home spend much of their time up in recliner chairs. The ability of recliner chairs to provide a pressure-reduction support surface is not known, and individual recliner chairs probably have various levels of pressure-reducing capability. Therefore, it is still prudent to institute a repositioning schedule for those using recliner chairs. Repositioning of patients in recliner chairs is more difficult due to the physical properties of the chair and requires some creativity. The repositioning schedule should mimic the schedule for those in wheelchairs.

For patients with significant pain on movement, premedication 20 to 30 minutes before a scheduled large position change may make routine repositioning more acceptable for the patient and the family. In those close to death, repositioning schedules may be used solely for maintaining comfort, with few or no attempts to reposition as a strategy for preventing skin problems.

Pillow Bridging. Pillow bridging involves the use of pillows to position patients with minimal tissue compression. The use of pillows can help prevent pressure ulcers from occurring on the medial knees, the medial malleolus, and the heels. Pillows should be placed between the knees, between the ankles, and under the heels.

Pillow use is especially important for reducing the risk of development of heel ulcers regardless of the support surface in use.[18] The best prevention strategy for eliminating pressure ulcers on the heels is to keep the heels off the surface of the bed. Use of pillows under the lower extremities keeps the heel from making contact with the support surface of the bed. Pillows help to redistribute the pressure over a larger area, thus reducing high pressures in one specific area. The pillows should extend and support the leg from the groin or perineal area to the ankle. Use of donut-type or ring cushion devices is contraindicated. Donut ring cushions cause venous congestion and edema and actually increase pressure to the area of concern.[18]

Use of Pressure Relief and Pressure-Reduction Support Surfaces. There are specific guidelines for the use of support surfaces to prevent and manage pressure ulcers.[42–44] Regardless of the type of support surface in use, written repositioning and turning schedules remain essential. Support surfaces serve as adjuncts to strategies for positioning and careful monitoring of patients. The type of support surface chosen is based on a multitude of factors, including clinical condition of the patient, type of care setting, ease of use, maintenance, cost, and characteristics of the support surface. The primary concern should be the therapeutic benefit to the palliative care patient. Table 16A–1 categorizes the types of support surfaces available and their general performance characteristics.[42]

Pressure-Reducing Support Surfaces. Pressure-reduction devices lower tissue interface pressures but do not consistently maintain interface pressures below capillary closing pressures in all positions on all body locations. Pressure-reducing support surfaces are indicated for patients who are at risk for pressure ulcer development, who can be turned, and who have skin breakdown involving only one sleep surface.[18,19] Patients with an existing pressure ulcer who are at risk for development of further skin breakdown should be managed on a pressure-reducing support surface.

Pressure-reduction devices can be classified as static or dynamic. Static devices do not move; they reduce pressure by spreading the load over a larger area. A simple definition of a static support surface is one that does not require electricity to function, usually a mattress overlay (which is placed on top of the standard hospital mattress). Examples of static devices are foam, air, or gel mattress overlays and water-filled mattresses. The difficulties with foam devices include retaining moisture and heat and not reducing shear. Air and water static devices also have difficulties associated with retaining moisture and heat.

Dynamic support surfaces move. A simple definition of a dynamic support surface is one that requires a motor or pump and electricity to operate. One example is the alternating-pressure air mattress. Most of these devices use an electric pump to alternately inflate and deflate air cells or air columns, thus the term "alternating-pressure air mattress." The key to determining effectiveness is the length of time over which cycles of inflation and deflation occur. Dynamic support surfaces may also have difficulties with moisture retention and heat accumulation.[42] Dynamic devices may be preferable for palliative care patients, especially those with significant pain on movement, because they may help with tissue reperfusion when patients cannot be turned because of pain. When using pressure-reduction devices, the caregiver must ensure that the device is functioning properly and that the patient is receiving pressure reduction.

One concern when using mattress overlays, whether they are static or dynamic, is the "bottoming-out" phenomenon. Bottoming-out occurs when the patient's body sinks down, the support surface is compressed beyond function, and the patient's body lies directly on the hospital mattress. When bottoming-out occurs, there is no pressure reduction for the bony prominence of concern. Bottoming-out typically happens when the patient is placed on a static air mattress overlay that is not appropriately filled with air or when the patient has been on a foam mattress for extended periods. The nurse can monitor for bottoming-out by inserting a flat, outstretched hand between the overlay and the patient's body part at risk. If the caregiver feels less than an inch of support material, the patient has bottomed-out. It is important to check for bottoming-out when the patient is in various body positions

Table 16A–1
Selected Characteristics for Classes of Support Surface

Performance Characteristics	High Air Loss (Air Fluidized)	Low Air Loss	Alternating Air (Dynamic)	Static Flotation (Air or Water)	Foam	Standard Hospital Mattress
Increased support area	Yes	Yes	Yes	Yes	Yes	No
Low moisture retention	Yes	Yes	No	No	No	No
Reduced heat accumulation	Yes	Yes	No	No	No	No
Shear reduction	Yes	?	Yes	Yes	No	No
Pressure reduction	Yes	Yes	Yes	Yes	Yes	No
Dynamic	Yes	Yes	Yes	No	No	No
Cost per day	High	High	Moderate	Low	Low	Low

Source: Bergstrom et al. (1994), reference 42.

and to check at various body sites. For example, when the patient is lying supine, check the sacral/coccygeal area and the heels; and when the patient is side-lying, check the trochanter and lateral malleolus.[42]

Pressure-Relieving Support Surfaces. Pressure-relief devices consistently reduce tissue interface pressures to a level below capillary closing pressure in any position and in most body locations. Pressure-relief devices are indicated for patients who are at high risk for pressure ulcer development and who cannot turn independently or have skin breakdown involving more than one body surface. Most commonly, pressure-relief devices are grouped into low air loss, fluidized air or high air loss, and kinetic devices. These devices often assist with pain control as well as relieving pressure.

Low air loss therapy devices use a bed frame with a series of connected air-filled pillows with surface fabrics of low-friction material. The amount of pressure in each pillow can be controlled and calibrated to provide maximal pressure relief for the individual patient. These devices provide pressure relief in any position, and most models have built-in scales. Low air loss therapy devices that are placed on top of standard hospital mattresses may be of particular benefit for palliative care patients at home.

Fluidized air or high air loss therapy devices consist of bed frames containing silicone-coated glass beads and incorporate both air and fluid support. The beads become fluid when air is pumped through the device, making them behave like a liquid. High air loss therapy has bactericidal properties due to the alkalinity of the beads (pH 10), the temperature, and entrapment of microorganisms by the beads. High air loss therapy relieves pressure and reduces friction, shear, and moisture (due to the drying effect of the bed). These devices cause difficulties when transferring patients because of the bed frame. The increased airflow can increase evaporative fluid loss, leading to dehydration. Finally, if the patient is able to sit up, a foam wedge may be required, limiting the beneficial effects of the bed on the upper back. In palliative care cases, use of high air loss therapy is typically not indicated for pressure ulcers alone but may be indicated for patients with significant pain as well as pressure ulcers.

Support Surface Selection. Determining which support surface is best for a particular patient can be confusing. The primary concern must always be the effectiveness of the surface for the individual patient's needs. The Agency for Healthcare Research and Quality (AHRQ, formerly Agency for Health Care Policy and Research [AHCPR]) recommends the following criteria as guidelines for determining how to manage tissue loading and support surface selection.[18]

1. Assess all patients with existing pressure ulcers to determine their risk for developing additional pressure ulcers. If the patient remains at risk, use a pressure-reducing surface.
2. Use a static support surface if the patient can assume a variety of positions without bearing weight on an existing pressure ulcer and without "bottoming-out."
3. Use a dynamic support surface if the patient cannot assume a variety of positions without bearing weight on an existing pressure ulcer, if the patient fully compresses the static support surface, or if the pressure ulcer does not show evidence of healing.
4. If a patient has large stage III or stage IV pressure ulcers on multiple turning surfaces, a low air loss bed or a fluidized air (high air loss) bed may be indicated.
5. If excessive moisture on intact skin is a potential source of maceration and skin breakdown, a support surface that provides airflow can be important in drying the skin and preventing additional pressure ulcers.
6. Any individual who is at risk for developing pressure ulcers should be placed on a static or dynamic pressure-reducing support surface.

Seating Support Surfaces. Support surfaces for chairs and wheelchairs can be categorized similarly to support surfaces for beds. In general, providing adequate pressure relief for chair-bound or wheelchair-bound patients is critical. The patient at risk for pressure ulcer formation is at increased risk in the seated position because of the high pressures across the ischial tuberosities. Most pressure-reducing devices for chairs are static overlays, such as those made out of foam, gel, air, or some combination. Positioning of chair- or wheelchair-bound individuals must include consideration of individual anatomy and body contours, postural alignment, distribution of weight, balance, and stability in addition to pressure relief.

Reducing Friction and Shear

Measures to reduce friction and shear relate to passive or active movement of the patient. To reduce friction, several interventions are appropriate. Providing topical preparations to eliminate or reduce the surface tension between the skin and the bed linen or support surface assists in reducing friction-related injury. To lessen friction-induced skin breakdown, appropriate techniques must be used when moving patients so that skin is never dragged across the linens. Patients who exhibit voluntary or involuntary repetitive body movements (particularly movements of the heels or elbows) require stronger interventions. Use of a protective film such as a transparent film dressing or a skin sealant, a protective dressing such as a thin hydrocolloid, or protective padding helps to eliminate the surface contact of the area and decrease the friction between the skin and the linens.[19] Even though heel, ankle, and elbow protectors do nothing to reduce or relieve pressure, they can be effective aids against friction.

Most shear injury can be eliminated by proper positioning, such as avoidance of the semi-Fowler position and limited use of upright positions (i.e., positions more than 30 degrees inclined). Avoidance of upright positions may prevent sliding- and shear-related injuries. Use of foot boards and knee Gatch (or pillows under the lower leg) to prevent sliding and to maintain position is also helpful in reducing shear effects on the skin. Observation of the patient when sitting is also important, because the patient who slides out of the chair is at equally high risk for shear injury. Use of footstools and the foot pedals on wheelchairs, together with appropriate 90-degree flexion of the hip (which may be achieved with the use of pillows, special seat cushions, or orthotic devices) can help prevent chair sliding.

Nutrition

Nutrition is an important element in maintaining healthy skin and tissues. There is a strong relationship between nutrition and pressure ulcer development.[28] The severity of pressure ulceration is also correlated with severity of nutritional deficits, especially low protein intake and low serum albumin levels.[28,30,31] Nutritional assessment is key in determining the appropriate interventions for the patient. A short nutritional assessment should be performed at routine intervals on all patients who are determined to be at risk for pressure ulcer formation.

Malnutrition may be diagnosed if the serum albumin level is lower than 3.5 mg/dL, the total lymphocyte count is less than 1800 cells/mm^3, or body weight has decreased by more than 15%.[42] Malnutrition impairs the immune system, and total lymphocyte counts are a reflection of immune competence. If the patient is diagnosed as malnourished, nutritional supplementation should be instituted to help achieve a positive nitrogen balance. Examples of oral supplements are assisted oral feedings and dietary supplements. Tube feedings have not been effective for patients with pressure ulcers. The goal of care is to provide approximately 30 to 35 calories per kilogram of weight per day and 1.25 to 1.5 g of protein per kilogram of weight per day.[42] It may be difficult for a pressure ulcer patient or an at-risk patient to ingest enough protein and calories necessary to maintain skin and tissue health. Oral supplements can be very helpful in boosting calorie and protein intake, but they are designed only to be an adjunct to regular oral intake. Monitoring of nutritional indices is helpful to determine the effectiveness of the care plan. Serum albumin, protein markers, body weight, and nutritional assessment should be performed every 3 months to monitor for changes in nutritional status if appropriate.

In palliative care, nutrition can be a major risk factor for pressure ulcer development. Nutritional supplementation may not be possible in all cases; however, if the patient can tolerate it, supplementation should be encouraged if it is in keeping with the overall goals of care. Involvement of a dietitian during the early assessment of the patient is important to the overall success of the plan. Maintenance of adequate nutrition to prevent pressure ulcer development and to repair existing pressure ulcers in palliative care patients is fraught with differing opinions. The issue is how to balance nutritional needs for skin care without providing artificial nutrition to prolong life. One of the problems in this area is the limited research available. The inadequate evidence base leaves clinicians to rely on expert opinion and their own clinical experience. Perhaps the best advice is to look at the whole clinical picture rather than focusing only on the wound. Viewing the pressure ulcer as a part of the whole, within the contextual circumstances of the patient, should provide some assistance in determining how aggressive to be in providing nutrition. The overriding concern in palliative care is to provide for comfort and to minimize symptoms. If providing supplemental nutrition aids in providing comfort to the patient and is mutually agreed upon by the patient, family caregivers, and health care provider, then supplemental nutrition (in any form) is very appropriate for palliative wound care. If the patient's condition is such that to provide supplemental nutrition (in any form) increases discomfort and the prognosis is expected to be poor and rapid, then providing supplemental nutrition should not be a concern and is not appropriate for palliative wound care. It is important to remember that little evidence exists for either of these viewpoints, yet expert opinions on the topic abound.

Managing Moisture

The preventive interventions related to moisture include general skin care, accurate diagnosis of incontinence type, and appropriate incontinence management.

General Skin Care. General skin care involves routine skin assessment, incontinence assessment and management, skin hygiene interventions, and measures to maintain skin health. Routine skin assessment involves observation of the patient's skin, with particular attention to bony prominences. Reddened areas should not be massaged. Massage can further impair the perfusion to the tissues.

Incontinence Management. Volumes have been written about various incontinence management techniques. This discussion is meant to serve as a stepping stone to those resources available to clinicians concerning management of incontinence. It does not include all management strategies and only briefly mentions several strategies that are most pertinent to palliative care patients at high risk of development of pressure ulcers. Management of incontinence is dependent on assessment and diagnosis of the problem (see Chapter 14).

Incontinence Assessment. Assessment of incontinence should include history of the incontinence, including patterns of elimination, characteristics of the urinary stream or fecal mass, and sensation of bladder or rectal filling. The physical examination is designed to gather specific information related to bladder or rectal functioning and therefore is limited in scope. A limited neurological examination should provide data on the mental status and motivation of the patient and caregiver, specific motor skills, and condition of back and lower extremities. The genitalia and perineal skin are assessed for signs of perineal skin lesions and perineal sensation.

The environmental assessment should include inspection of the patient's home or nursing home facility to evaluate for the presence of environmental barriers to continence. A voiding/defecation diary is very helpful in planning the treatment and management of incontinence. In cognitively impaired patients, the caregiver may complete the diary, and management strategies can be identified from the baseline data.

Incontinence Management Strategies. Palliative care patients who are at risk for pressure ulcer development may be candidates for behavioral management strategies for incontinence. Incontinence in palliative care patients may be successfully managed with scheduled toileting. Scheduled toileting is caregiver dependent and requires a motivated caregiver to be successful. Adequate fluid intake is an important component of a scheduled toileting program.

Scheduled toileting, or habit training, is toileting at planned time intervals. The goal is to keep the patient dry by assisting him or her to void at regular intervals. There can be attempts to match the interval to the individual patient's natural voiding schedule. There is no systematic effort to motivate patients to delay voiding or to resist the urge to void. Scheduled toileting may be based on the clock (e.g., toileting every 2 hours) or on activities (e.g., toileting after meals and before transferring to bed).

Underpads and briefs may be used to protect the skin of patients who are incontinent of urine or stool. These products are designed to absorb moisture, wick the wetness away from the skin, and maintain a quick-drying interface with the skin. Studies in both infants and adults demonstrate that products that are designed to present a quick-drying surface to the skin and to absorb moisture do keep the skin drier and are associated with a lower incidence of dermatitis.[45] The critical feature is the ability to absorb moisture and present a quick-drying surface, not whether the product is disposable or reusable. Regardless of the product chosen, containment strategies imply the need for a check-and-change schedule for the incontinent patient, so that wet linens and pads may be removed in a timely manner. Underpads are not as tight or constricting as briefs. Kemp[25] suggested alternating use of underpads and briefs. This recommendation echoes the early work of Willis,[46] who studied warm-water immersion syndrome and found that the effects of water on the skin could be diminished by allowing the skin to dry out between wet periods. Use of briefs when the patient is up in a chair, ambulating, or visiting and use of underpads when the patient is in bed is one suggestion for combining the strengths of both products.[25]

External collection devices may be more effective with male patients. External catheters or condom catheters are devices applied to the shaft of the penis that direct the urine away from the body and into a collection device. Newer models of external catheters are self-adhesive and easy to apply. For patients with a retracted penis, a special pouching system, similar to an ostomy pouch, is available. A key concern with the use of external collection devices is routine removal of the product for inspection and hygiene of the skin.

There are special containment devices for fecal incontinence as well. Fecal incontinence collectors consist of a self-adhesive skin barrier attached to a drainable pouch. Application of the device is somewhat dependent on the skill of the clinician. To facilitate success, the patient should be put on a routine for changing the pouch before leakage occurs. The skin barrier provides a physical obstacle to keep the stool away from the skin and helps to prevent dermatitis and associated skin problems. Skin barrier wafers without an attached pouch can be useful in protecting the skin from feces or urine.

Use of moisturizers for dry skin and use of lubricants for reduction of friction injuries are also recommended skin care strategies.[18] Moisture barriers are used to protect the skin from the effects of moisture. Although products that provide a moisture barrier are recommended, the reader is cautioned that the recommendation is derived from usual practice and clinical practice guidelines and is not research based. The success of the particular product is linked to how it is formulated and the hydrophobic properties of the product.[25] Generally, pastes are thicker and more repellent of moisture than ointments. As a quick evaluation, one can observe the ease with which the product can be removed with water during routine cleansing: if the product comes off the skin with just routine cleansing, it probably is not an effective barrier to moisture. Mineral oil may be used for cleansing some of the heavier barrier products (e.g., zinc oxide paste) to ease removal from the skin.

Pressure Ulcer Assessment

The foundation for designing a palliative care plan for the patient with a pressure ulcer is a comprehensive assessment. Comprehensive assessment includes assessment of wound severity, wound status, and the total patient.

Wound Severity

Assessment of wound severity refers to the use of a classification system for diagnosing the severity of tissue trauma by determining the tissue layers involved in the wound. Classification systems such as staging pressure ulcers provide communication regarding wound severity and the tissue layers involved in the injury.

Pressure ulcers are commonly classified according to grading or staging systems based on the depth of tissue destruction. The National Pressure Ulcer Advisory Panel (NPUAP) recommended the use of a universal four-stage classification system to describe depth of tissue damage. Staging systems measure only one characteristic of the wound and should not be viewed as a complete assessment independent of other indicators. Staging systems are best used as a diagnostic tool for indicating wound severity. Table 16A–2 presents pressure ulcer staging criteria according to the NPUAP. Pressure-induced skin damage that manifests as purple, blue, or black areas of intact skin may represent deep tissue injury (DTI).

Table 16A–2
Pressure Ulcer Staging Criteria

Pressure Ulcer Stage	Definition
Stage I	An observable pressure-related alteration of intact skin whose indicators, as compared with the adjacent or opposite area on the body, may include changes in one or more of the following: • skin temperature (warmth or coolness) • tissue consistency (firm or boggy feel) • sensation (pain, itching) The ulcer appears as a defined area of persistent redness in lightly pigmented skin, whereas in darker skin tones, the ulcer may appear with persistent red, blue, or purple hues.
Stage II	Partial-thickness skin loss involving epidermis or dermis or both. The ulcer is superficial and presents clinically as an abrasion, blister, or shallow crater.
Stage III	Full-thickness skin loss involving damage or necrosis of subcutaneous tissue, which may extend down to, but not through, underlying fascia. The ulcer presents clinically as a deep crater with or without undermining of adjacent tissue.
Stage IV	Full-thickness skin loss with extensive destruction, tissue necrosis, or damage to muscle bone or supporting structures (such as tendon, joint capsule).

Source: National Pressure Ulcer Advisory Panel (1995), reference 47.

These lesions commonly occur on heels and the sacrum and signal more severe tissue damage below the skin surface. DTI lesions reflect tissue damage at the bony tissue interface and may progress rapidly to large tissue defects.

Wound Status

Pressure ulcer assessment is the base for maintaining and evaluating the therapeutic plan of care. Assessment of wound status involves evaluation of multiple wound characteristics. Initial assessment and follow-up assessments at regular intervals to monitor progress or deterioration of the sore are necessary to determine the effectiveness of the treatment plan. Adequate assessment is important even when the goal of care is comfort, not healing. The assessment data enable clinicians to communicate clearly about a patient's pressure ulcer, provide for continuity in the plan of care, and allow evaluation of treatment modalities. Assessment of wound status should be performed weekly and whenever a significant change is noted in the wound. Assessment should not be confused with monitoring of the wound at each dressing change. Monitoring of the wound can be performed by less skilled caregivers, but assessment should be performed on a routine basis by health care practitioners. Use of a systematic approach with a comprehensive assessment tool is helpful.

There are few tools available that encompass multiple wound characteristics to evaluate overall wound status and healing. Two available tools are the Pressure Ulcer Scale for Healing (PUSH)[48] and the Bates-Jensen Wound Assessment Tool (BWAT, revised Pressure Sore Status Tool).[49]

The PUSH tool incorporates surface area measurements, exudate amount, and surface appearance. These wound characteristics were chosen based on principal component analysis to define the best model of healing.[48] The clinician measures the size of the wound, calculates the surface area (length times width), and chooses the appropriate size category on the tool (0 to 10). Exudate is evaluated as none (0), light (1), moderate (2), or heavy (3). Tissue type choices include closed (0), epithelial tissue (1), granulation tissue (2), slough (3), and necrotic tissue (4). The three subscores are then summed for a total score.[48]

Reliability testing of the tool with a large sample is under way.[48] The PUSH tool may offer a quick assessment to predict healing outcomes. The PUSH tool is best used as a method of prediction of wound healing. Therefore, it may not be the best tool for palliative care patients, because healing is not an expected outcome of care. Assessment of additional wound characteristics may still be needed, to develop a treatment plan for the pressure ulcer. The BWAT includes additional wound characteristics that may be helpful in designing a plan of care for the wound.

The BWAT or Pressure Sore Status Tool (Figure 16A–2), developed in 1990 by Bates-Jensen[50] and revised in 2001, evaluates 13 wound characteristics with a numerical rating scale and rates them from best to worst possible. The BWAT is recommended as a method of assessment and monitoring of

BATES-JENSEN WOUND ASSESSMENT TOOL NAME ______________________

Complete the rating sheet to assess wound status. Evaluate each item by picking the response that best describes the wound and entering the score in the item score column for the appropriate date.

Location: Anatomic site. Circle, identify right (**R**) or left (**L**) and use "**X**" to mark site on body diagrams:

____ Sacrum & coccyx
____ Trochanter
____ Ischial tuberosity
____ Lateral ankle
____ Medial ankle
____ Heel
Other Site ____

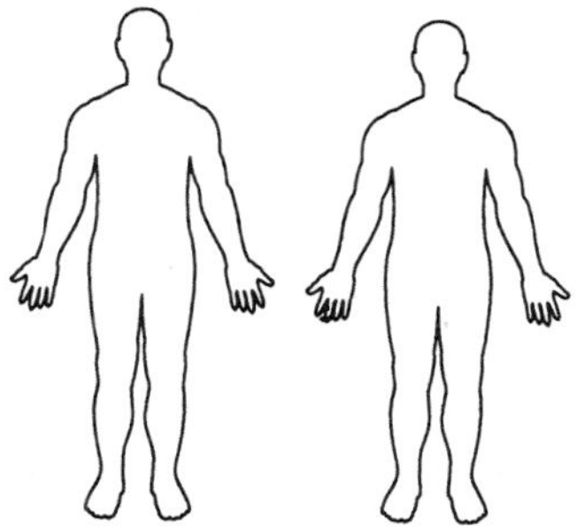

Shape: Overall wound pattern; assess by observing perimeter and depth.

Circle and date appropriate description:

____ Irregular
____ Round/oval
____ Square/rectangle
____ Linear or elongated
____ Bowl/boat
____ Butterfly
Other Shape ____

Item	Assessment	Date Score	Date Score	Date Score
1. Size	1 = Length x width <4 sq cm 2 = Length x width 4–<16 sq cm 3 = Length x width 16.1–<36 sq cm 4 = Length x width 36.1–<80 sq cm 5 = Length x width >80 sq cm			
2. Depth	1 = Non-blanchable erythema on intact skin 2 = Partial thickness skin loss involving epidermis &/or dermis 3 = Full thickness skin loss involving damage or necrosis of subcutaneous tissue; may extend down to but not through underlying fascia; &/or mixed partial & full thickness &/or tissue layers obscured by granulation tissue 4 = Obscured by necrosis 5 = Full thickness skin loss with extensive destruction, tissue necrosis or damage to muscle, bone or supporting structures			
3. Edges	1 = Indistinct, diffuse, none clearly visible 2 = Distinct, outline clearly visible, attached, even with wound base 3 = Well-defined, not attached to wound base 4 = Well-defined, not attached to base, rolled under, thickened 5 = Well-defined, fibrotic, scarred or hyperkeratotic			
4. Under-mining	1 = None present 2 =Undermining < 2 cm in any area 3 = Undermining 2–4 cm involving < 50% wound margins 4 = Undermining 2–4 cm involving > 50% wound margins 5 = Undermining > 4 cm or tunneling in any area			
5. Necrotic Tissue Type	1 = None visible 2 = White/grey non-viable tissue &/or non-adherent yellow slough 3 = Loosely adherent yellow slough 4 = Adherent, soft, black eschar 5 = Firmly adherent, hard, black eschar			
6. Necrotic Tissue Amount	1 = None visible 2 = < 25% of wound bed covered 3 = 25% to 50% of wound covered 4 = > 50% and < 75% of wound covered 5 = 75% to 100% of wound covered			

Figure 16A-2. The Bates-Jensen Wound Assessment Tool (BWAT) for measuring pressure sore status.

Item	Assessment	Date Score	Date Score	Date Score
7. Exudate Type	1 = None 2 = Bloody 3 = Serosanguineous: thin, watery, pale red/pink 4 = Serous: thin, watery, clear 5 = Purulent: thin or thick, opaque, tan/yellow, with or without odor			
8. Exudate Amount	1 = None, dry wound 2 = Scant, wound moist but no observable exudate 3 = Small 4 = Moderate 5 = Large			
9. Skin Color Surrounding Wound	1 = Pink or normal for ethnic group 2 = Bright red &/or blanches to touch 3 = White or grey pallor or hypopigmented 4 = Dark red or purple &/or non-blanchable 5 = Black or hyperpigmented			
10. Peripheral Tissue Edema	1 = No swelling or edema 2 = Non-pitting edema extends <4 cm around wound 3 = Non-pitting edema extends ≥4 cm around wound 4 = Pitting edema extends < 4 cm around wound 5 = Crepitus and/or pitting edema extends ≥4 cm around wound			
11. Peripheral Tissue Induration	1 = None present 2 = Induration < 2 cm around wound 3 = Induration 2–4 cm extending < 50% around wound 4 = Induration 2–4 cm extending ≥ 50% around wound 5 = Induration > 4 cm in any area around wound			
12. Granulation Tissue	1 = Skin intact or partial thickness wound 2 = Bright, beefy red; 75% to 100% of wound filled &/or tissue overgrowth 3 = Bright, beefy red; < 75% & > 25% of wound filled 4 = Pink &/or dull, dusky red &/or fills ≤ 25% of wound 5 = No granulation tissue present			
13. Epithelialization	1 = 100% wound covered, surface intact 2 = 75% to <100% wound covered &/or epithelial tissue extends >0.5cm into wound bed 3 = 50% to <75% wound covered &/or epithelial tissue extends to <0.5cm into wound bed 4 = 25% to < 50% wound covered 5 = < 25% wound covered			
	TOTAL SCORE			
	SIGNATURE			

WOUND STATUS CONTINUUM

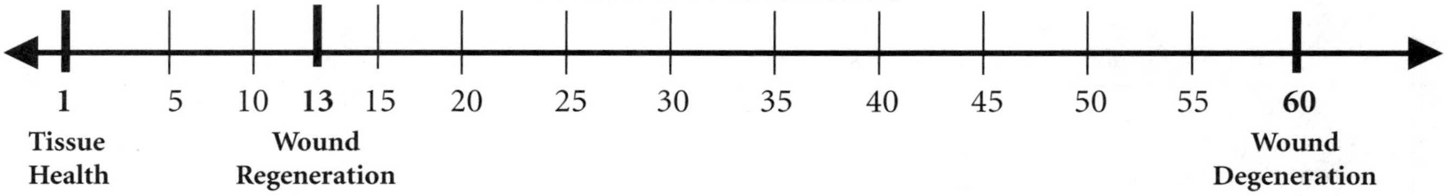

Plot the total score on the Wound Status Continuum by putting an "X" on the line and the date beneath the line. Plot multiple scores with their dates to see-at-a-glance regeneration or degeneration of the wound.

Figure 16A-2. *(continued)*

pressure ulcers and other wounds. It is a pencil-and-paper instrument comprising 15 items: location, shape, size, depth, edges, undermining or pockets, necrotic tissue type, necrotic tissue amount, exudate type, exudate amount, surrounding skin color, peripheral tissue edema, peripheral tissue induration, granulation tissue, and epithelialization. Two items, location and shape, are nonscored. The remaining 13 are scored items, and each appears with characteristic descriptors rated on a scale of 1 (best for that characteristic) to 5 (worst attribute of the characteristic). It is recommended that wounds be scored initially for a baseline assessment and at regular intervals to evaluate therapy. Once a lesion has been assessed for each item on the BWAT, the 13 item scores can be added to obtain a total score for the wound. The total score can then be monitored to determine "at a glance" the progress in healing or degeneration of the wound. Total scores range from 13 (skin intact but always at risk for further damage) to 65 (profound tissue degeneration). Appendix 16A–1 presents the instructions for use of the BWAT.

Reliability of the tool has been evaluated in an acute care setting with enterostomal therapy (ET) nurses (nurses with additional training in wound care)[51] and in long-term care with a variety of health care professionals and one ET nurse expert in wound assessment.[52] Interrater reliability ranged from $r = 0.915$ ($P = 0.0001$) for the ET nurses[51] to 0.78% agreement for the variety of health care professionals.[52] The BWAT or the Pressure Sore Status Tool is the most widely used of the instruments available.

Wound Characteristics

Adequate initial wound assessment should encompass a composite of wound characteristics, which forms a base for differential diagnosis, therapeutic intervention, and future reassessment comparisons.[53] The indices for wound assessment include all of the following: location, size of ulcer, depth of tissue involvement, stage or classification, condition of wound edges, presence of undermining or tunneling, necrotic tissue characteristics, exudate characteristics, surrounding tissue conditions, and wound healing characteristics of granulation tissue and epithelialization.[54–58] Wound characteristics of concern for the palliative care patient include wound edges, undermining and tunneling, necrotic tissue characteristics, exudate characteristics, and surrounding tissue conditions. These five characteristics, as well as healing attributes of granulation tissue and epithelialization, are discussed in the following sections.

Edges or Margins. Wound edge, or margin, includes characteristics of distinctness, degree of attachment to the wound base, color, and thickness. In pressure ulcers, as tissues degenerate, broad and indistinct areas, in which the wound edge is diffuse and difficult to observe, become shallow lesions with edges that are more distinct, thin, and separate. As tissue trauma from pressure progresses, the reaction intensifies with a thickening and rolling inward of the epidermis, so that the edge is well defined and sharply outlines the ulcer, with little or no evidence of new tissue growth. In long-standing pressure ulcers, fibrosis and scarring result from repeated injury and repair, with the edges hyperpigmented, indurated, and firm[59] and possible impairment in the migratory ability of epithelial cells.[60] Pressure ulcers in palliative care may show significant tissue damage, and the edges may indicate areas of full-thickness tissue loss with other areas of partial-thickness damage. In palliative care, pressure ulcers may be present for prolonged periods with no change in the wound; the wound edges often exhibit hemosiderin staining or hyperpigmentation in conjunction with their rolled-under and thickened appearance.

When assessing edges, the nurse should look at the clarity and distinctness of the wound outline. With edges that are indistinct and diffuse, there are areas in which the normal tissues blend into the wound bed and the edges are not clearly visible. Edges that are even with the skin surface and the wound base are attached to the base of the wound. This means that the wound is flat, with no appreciable depth. Well-defined edges, on the other hand, are clear and distinct and can be outlined easily on a transparent piece of plastic. Edges that are not attached to the base of the wound imply a wound with some depth of tissue involvement. A crater or bowl or boat shape indicates a wound with edges that are not attached to the wound base. The wound has walls or sides. There is depth to the wound.

As the wound ages, the edges become rolled under and thickened to palpation. The edge achieves a unique hyperpigmented coloring due to hemosiderin staining. The pigment turns a gray or brown color in both dark- and light-skinned persons. Long-standing wounds may continue to thicken, with scar tissue and fibrosis developing in the wound edge, causing the edge to feel hard, rigid, and indurated. The wound edges are evaluated by visual inspection and palpation.

Undermining and Tunneling. The terms *undermining* and *tunneling* refer to the loss of tissue underneath an intact skin surface. Undermining, or pocketing, usually involves a greater percentage of the wound margins and more shallow length, compared with tunneling. Undermining usually involves subcutaneous tissues and follows the fascial planes next to the wound.

Wounds with undermining have more aerobic and anaerobic bacteria than do wounds that are in the process of healing with no undermining.[61] The degree and amount of undermining indicate the severity of tissue necrosis. As subcutaneous fat degenerates, wound pockets develop. Initially, deep fascia limits the depth of pocketing, encouraging more superficial internal spread of undermining. Once the fascia is penetrated, undermining of deeper tissues may proceed rapidly.[59] Internal dimensions of wound undermining are commonly measured with the use of cotton-tipped applicators and gentle probing of the wound. There are also premeasured devices that can be inserted under the wound edge and advanced into the deeper tissues to aid in determination of the extent of undermining.

Undermining and wound pockets should be assessed by inserting a cotton-tipped applicator under the wound edge, advancing it as far as it will go without using undue force, raising the tip of the applicator so that it may be seen or felt on the surface of the skin, marking the surface with a pen, and measuring the distance from the mark on the skin to the edge of the wound. This process is continued all around the wound. Then the percentage of the wound involved is determined with the help of a transparent metric measuring guide with concentric circles divided into quadrants. Another noninvasive method of assessment of wound pockets is the use of ultrasound to evaluate the undermined tissues. Ultrasonography provides a visual picture of the impaired tissues and can be repeated to monitor for improvement.

Necrotic Tissue Type and Amount. Necrotic tissue characteristics of color, consistency, adherence, and amount present in the wound must be incorporated into wound assessment. As tissues die during wound development, they change in color, consistency, and adherence to the wound bed. The level and type of tissue death influence the clinical appearance of the necrotic tissue. For example, as subcutaneous fat tissues die, a collection of stringy, yellow slough is formed. As muscle tissues degenerate, the dead tissue may be more thick or tenacious.

The characteristic "necrotic tissue type" is a qualitative variable, with most clinicians using descriptions of clinical observations of a composite of factors as a method of assessment. The characteristics of color, consistency, and adherence are most often used to describe the type of necrosis. Color varies, as necrosis worsens, from white/gray nonviable tissue, to yellow slough, and finally to black eschar. Consistency refers to the cohesiveness of the debris (i.e., thin or thick, stringy or clumpy). Consistency also varies on a continuum as the necrotic area deepens and becomes more dehydrated.

The terms *slough* and *eschar* refer to different levels of necrosis and are described according to color and consistency. A slough is described as yellow (or tan) and as thin, mucinous, or stringy, whereas eschar is described as black, and as soft or hard; eschar represents full-thickness tissue destruction. *Adherence* refers to the adhesiveness of the debris to the wound bed and the ease with which the two may be separated. Necrotic tissue tends to become more adherent to the wound bed as the level of damage increases. Clinically, eschar is more firmly adherent than is yellow slough.

Necrotic tissue is assessed for color, consistency, and adherence to the wound bed. The predominant characteristic present in the wound should be chosen for assessment. Necrotic tissue type changes as it ages in the wound, as debridement occurs, and as further tissue trauma causes increased cellular death. Slough usually is nonadherent or loosely adherent to the healthy tissues of the wound bed. By definition, nonadherent tissue appears scattered throughout the wound; it appears as if the tissue could easily be removed with gauze. Loosely adherent tissue is attached to the wound bed; it is thick and stringy and may appear as clumps of debris attached to wound tissue.

Eschar Signifies Deeper Tissue Damage. Eschar may be black, gray, or brown in color. It is usually adherent or firmly adherent to the wound tissues and may be soggy, soft or hard, or leathery in texture. A soft, soggy eschar is usually strongly attached to the base of the wound but may be lifting from (and loose from) the edges of the wound. A hard, crusty eschar is strongly attached to the base and edges of the wound. Hard eschars are often mistaken for scabs. Sometimes nonviable tissue appears before a wound is apparent. This can be seen as a white or gray area on the surface of the skin. The area usually demarcates within a day or two, when the wound appears and interrupts the skin surface.

Necrotic tissue retards wound healing because it is a medium for bacterial growth and a physical obstacle to epidermal resurfacing, wound contraction, and granulation. The greater the amount of necrotic tissue present in the wound bed, the more severe the insult to the tissue and the longer the time required to heal the wound. The amount of necrotic tissue usually affects the amount of exudate from the wound and causes wound odor, both of which are distressing to the patient and to caregivers. Because of the amount of necrotic tissue present, modifications of treatment and debridement techniques may be made. The depth of the wound cannot be assessed in the presence of necrosis that blocks visualization of the total wound.

The amount of necrotic tissue present in the wound is one of the easier characteristics to assess. The nurse uses a transparent measuring guide with concentric circles divided into quadrants laying it over the wound. The percentage of necrosis present is judged by looking at each quadrant. The judgments from each quadrant are added to determine the total percentage of the wound involved. Alternatively, the length and width of the necrotic tissue may be measured to determine the surface area involved in the necrosis.

Exudate Type and Amount. Wound exudate (also known as wound fluid, wound drainage) is an important assessment feature, because the characteristics of the exudate help the clinician to diagnose signs of wound infection, to evaluate appropriateness of topical therapy, and to monitor wound healing. Wound infection retards wound healing and must be treated aggressively. Proper assessment of wound exudate is also important because it affirms the body's brief, normal inflammatory response to tissue injury. Accurate assessment and diagnosis of wound exudate and infection are critical components of effective wound management. One of the main goals of palliative wound care is to prevent infection and to control exudate, because these conditions lead to discomfort from the wound.

The healthy wound normally has some evidence of moisture on its surface. Healthy wound fluid contains enzymes and growth factors, which may play a role in promoting reepithelialization of the wound and provide needed growth factors for all phases of wound repair. The moist environment produced by wound exudate allows efficient migration of epidermal cells and prevents wound desiccation and further injury.[62,63]

In pressure ulcers, increased exudate is a response to the inflammatory process or infection. Increased capillary permeability causes leakage of fluids and substrates into the injured tissue. When a wound is present, tissue fluid leaks out of the open tissue. This fluid normally is serous or serosanguineous.

In the infected wound, the exudate may thicken, become purulent in nature, and continue to be present in moderate to large amounts. Examples of exudate character changes in infected wounds are the presence of *Pseudomonas,* which produces a thick, malodorously sweet-smelling, green drainage,[64] or *Proteus* infection, which may have an ammonia-like odor. Wounds with foul-smelling drainage are generally infected or filled with necrotic debris, and healing time is prolonged as tissue destruction progresses.[61] Wounds with significant amounts of necrotic debris often have a thick, tenacious, opaque, purulent, malodorous drainage in moderate to copious amounts. True wound exudate must be differentiated from necrotic tissue that sloughs off the wound as a result of debridement efforts. Exudate from sloughing necrotic tissue is commonly attached to or connected with the necrotic debris; frequently, the only method of differentiation is adequate debridement of necrotic tissue from the wound site. Liquefied necrotic tissue occurs most often as a result of enzymatic or autolytic debridement. Often, removal of the necrotic tissue reduces the amount and changes the character of wound exudate.

Exudate should be assessed for the amount and type of drainage that occurs. The type and color of wound exudate vary depending on the degree of moisture in the wound and the organisms present. Characteristics used to examine exudate are color, consistency, adherence, distribution in the wound, and presence of odor.

Estimating the amount of exudate in the wound is difficult due to wound size variability and topical dressing types. One problem with assessment of exudate amount is the size of the wound. What might be considered a large amount of drainage for a smaller wound may be considered a small amount for a larger wound, making clinically meaningful assessment of exudate difficult.

Certain dressing types interact with or trap wound fluid to create or mimic certain characteristics of exudate, such as color and consistency of purulent drainage. For example, both hydrocolloid and alginate dressings mimic a purulent drainage on removal of the dressing. Preparation of the wound site for appropriate assessment involves removal of the wound dressing and cleansing with normal saline to remove dressing debris in the wound bed, followed by evaluation of the wound for true exudate.

Although it is not a part of exudate assessment, evaluation of the wound dressing provides the clinician with valuable data about the effectiveness of treatment. Evaluation of the percentage of the wound dressing involved with wound drainage during a specific time frame is helpful for clinical management that includes dressings beyond traditional gauze. In estimating the percentage of the dressing involved with the wound exudate, clinical judgment must be quantified by putting a number to visual assessment of the dressing. For example, the clinician might determine that 50% percent of the hydrocolloid dressing was involved with wound drainage over a 4-day wearing period. Based on the data, the clinician might quantify the judgment for this type of dressing, length of dressing wear time, and wound cause as being a "minimal" amount of exudate. Clinical judgment of the amount of wound drainage requires some experience with expected wound exudate output in relation to phase of wound healing and type of wound, as well as knowledge of absorptive capacity and normal wear time of topical dressings.

Certain characteristics of exudate indicate wound degeneration and infection. If signs of cellulitis (erythema or skin discoloration, edema, pain, induration, purulent drainage) are present at the wound site, the exudate amount may be copious and seropurulent or purulent in character. The amount of exudate remains high or increases, and the character may change to frank purulence, with further wound degeneration. Wound infection must be considered in these cases.

Pressure ulcers manifest with a variety of wound exudate types and amounts. In partial-thickness pressure ulcers, the wound exudate is most likely to be serous or serosanguineous in nature and to be present in minimal to moderate amounts. In clean full-thickness pressure ulcers, the wound exudate is similar, with minimal to moderate amounts of serous to serosanguineous exudate. As healing progresses in the clean full-thickness pressure ulcer, the character of the exudate changes; it may become bloody if the fragile capillary bed is disrupted, and it lessens in amount.

For full-thickness pressure ulcers with necrotic debris, wound exudate is dependent on the presence or absence of infection and the type of therapy instituted. Exudate may appear moderate to large but, in fact, is related to the amount of necrotic tissue present and to liquefaction of the debris in the wound. Typically, the necrotic full-thickness pressure ulcer manifests with serous to seropurulent wound exudate in moderate to large amounts. With appropriate treatment, the wound exudate amount may temporarily increase, as the character gradually assumes a serous nature.

Surrounding Tissue Condition. The tissues surrounding the wound should be assessed for color, induration, and edema. The tissues surrounding the wound are often the first indication of impending further tissue damage and are a key gauge of successful prevention strategies. Color of the surrounding skin may indicate further injury from pressure, friction, or shearing. The tissues within 4 cm of the wound edge should be assessed. Dark-skinned persons show the colors "bright red" and "dark red" as a deepening of normal skin color or a purple or blacker hue. As healing occurs in dark-skinned persons, the new skin is pink and may never darken. In both light- and dark-skinned patients, new epithelium must be differentiated from tissues that are erythematous. To assess for blanchability in light-skinned patients, the nurse presses firmly on the skin with a finger, then lifts the finger and looks for "blanching," or sudden whitening, of the tissues followed by prompt return of color to the area. Nonblanchable erythema signals more severe tissue damage.

Edema in the surrounding tissues delays wound healing in the pressure ulcer. It is difficult for neoangiogenesis, or growth of new blood vessels into the wound, to occur in edematous tissues. Again, tissues within 4 cm of the wound edge are assessed. Nonpitting edema appears as skin that is shiny and taut, almost glistening. Pitting edema is identified by firmly pressing a finger down into the tissues and waiting for 5 seconds; on release of pressure, tissues fail to resume their previous position and an indentation appears. Crepitus is the accumulation of air or gas in tissues. The clinician should measure how far edema extends beyond the wound edges.

Induration is a sign of impending damage to the tissues. Along with skin-color changes, induration is an omen of further pressure-induced tissue trauma. Tissues within 4 cm of the wound edge are assessed. Induration is an abnormal firmness of tissues with margins. The nurse should palpate where the induration starts and where it ends by gently pinching the tissues. Induration results in an inability to pinch the tissues. Palpation proceeds from healthy tissue, moving toward the wound margins. It is usual to feel slight firmness at the wound edge itself. Normal tissues feel soft and spongy; induration feels hard and firm to the touch.

Granulation Tissue and Epithelialization. Granulation and epithelial tissues are markers of wound health. They signal the proliferative phase of wound healing and usually foretell wound closure. Granulation tissue is the growth of small blood vessels and connective tissue into the wound cavity. It is more observable in full-thickness wounds because of the tissue defect that occurs in such wounds. In partial-thickness wounds, granulation tissue may occur so quickly, and in concert with epithelialization, or skin resurfacing, that it is unobservable in most cases. The granulation tissue is healthy when it is bright, beefy-red; shiny; and granular with a velvety appearance. The tissue looks "bumpy" and may bleed easily. Unhealthy granulation tissue, resulting from poor vascular supply, appears pale pink or blanched to a dull, dusky red. Usually, the first layer of granulation tissue to be laid down in the wound is pale pink and, as the granulation tissue deepens and thickens, the color becomes bright, beefy red.

The percentage of the wound that is filled with granulation tissue and the color of the tissue are characteristics indicative of the health of the wound. The clinician makes a judgment as to what percent of the wound has been filled with granulation tissue. This is much easier if there is some past history with the wound. If the wound has been monitored by the same person over multiple observations, it is simple to judge the amount of granulation tissue present. If the initial observation was done by a different observer or if the data are not available, the clinician simply must use his or her best judgment to determine the amount of tissue present.

Partial-thickness wounds heal by epidermal resurfacing and regeneration. Epithelialization occurs via lateral migration at the wound edges and the base of hair follicles as epithelial cells proliferate and resurface the wound. Full-thickness wounds heal by scar formation: the tissue defect fills with granulation tissue, the edges contract, and the wound is resurfaced by epithelialization. Therefore, epithelialization may occur throughout the wound bed in partial-thickness wounds but only from the wound edges in full-thickness wounds.

Epithelialization can be assessed by evaluating the amount of the wound that is surrounded by new tissue and the distance to which new tissue extends into the wound base. Epithelialization appears as pink or red skin. Visualization of the new epithelium takes practice. A transparent measuring guide is used to help determine the percentage of wound involvement and the distance to which the epithelial tissue extends into the wound.

Monitoring the Wound. In palliative care, monitoring of the wound is important, to continue to meet the goals of comfort and reduction in wound pain and wound symptoms such as odor and exudate. Evaluation of wound characteristics at scheduled intervals allows the nurse to revise the treatment plan as appropriate and often provides an indication of the overall health of the patient. In many cases, the pressure ulcer worsens as death approaches and as the patient's condition worsens. The skin may be the first organ to actually "fail," with other systems following the downward trend. Progressive monitoring is also important to determine whether the treatment is effectively controlling odor, managing exudate, preventing infection, and minimizing pain—the goals of wound care during palliative care.

Total Patient Assessment

Comprehensive assessment includes assessment of the total patient as well as of wound severity and wound status. Generally, diagnosis and management of the wound are best accomplished within the context of the whole person. Comprehensive assessment includes a focused history and physical examination, attention to specific laboratory and diagnostic tests, and a pain assessment. Table 16A–3 presents an overview of assessment for the patient with a pressure ulcer.

It is important to obtain a focused history and physical examination as part of the initial assessment. The patient history determines which relevant systems reviews are needed in the physical examination. The goals for treatment and the direction of care (e.g., curative with a goal of wound closure, palliative with a goal of reduced wound pain) can be determined with, at a minimum, the following patient history information: reason for admission to care facility or agency; expectations and perceptions about wound healing; psychological, social, cultural, and economic history; presence of medical comorbidities; current wound status; and previous management strategies.

The systems review portion of the patient history and physical examination provides information on comorbidities that may impair wound healing. Specific comorbidities such as diabetes,[65–68] vascular disease,[69,70] and immunocompromise[71–73] have been related to impaired healing. The individual's capacity to heal may be limited by specific disease effects

Table 16A-3
Pressure Ulcer Assessment Overview

Assessment Parameter	Assessment Methods	Notes & Considerations	Frequency
Wound severity	Pressure ulcer staging classification Partial vs. full thickness classification	Provides diagnosis of severity of tissue insult	• Baseline, initial observation of wound • Reassess if wound deteriorates • Does not change over time
Wound status	Evaluate wound characteristics (location, size, shape, depth, edges, undermining, and tunneling), necrotic tissue characteristics, exudate characteristics, surrounding skin characteristics, granulation tissue and epithelialization	Use of standardized tool is easiest: Pressure Sore Status Tool (BWAT)	• Baseline or initially • Weekly • Whenever significant change in wound status is noted
Total patient:			
History	Interview or patient questionnaire. Include review of systems and specific questions: • Goals for care? • Reason for admission to facility? • Expectations about wound progress? • Psychosocial, cultural, economic history? • Presence of medical comorbidities? • Previous wound treatments?	Look for relevant systems to then include in physical examination	• Baseline data
Physical examination	Focus on items identified during patient history	Focus on areas that would affect wound healing, such as disease effects on tissue perfusion, tissue integrity, mobility, nutrition, and risk for infection	• Baseline data
Laboratory and diagnostic tests	Nutritional parameters: serum albumin Tissue perfusion: arterial blood gases, hemoglobin and hematocrit, blood glucose levels, glycosylated hemoglobin	Specific tests depend on individual patient	• Baseline or initially • Every 3 months for nutritional markers, tissue perfusion markers • If performing self-blood glucose monitoring, daily levels are helpful
Pain	Assess for wound pain before and during procedures and when no procedure is occurring	Use 0–10 point scale, with 0 = no pain and 10 = worst pain ever, and have patient state level of pain. For nonverbal patients, observe for grimacing, pulling away, crying out, or withdrawal	• Baseline or initially • Every day as needed • Before and during procedures such as dressing changes, debridement, or repositioning

on tissue integrity and perfusion, patient mobility, nutrition, and risk for wound infection. Therefore, throughout the patient history, systems review, and physical examination, the clinician considers host factors that affect wound healing.

Specific laboratory and diagnostic tests in a comprehensive assessment include data on nutrition, glucose management, and tissue oxygenation and perfusion. Nutritional parameters typically include evaluation of serum albumin. Serum albumin is a measure of protein available for healing; a normal level is greater than 3.5 mg/dL. Clinicians should evaluate laboratory values such as arterial blood gases to assess tissue perfusion and oxygenation abilities. Review of laboratory values is prudent to determine the level of diabetic control. Normal glucose levels are 80 mg/dL. Concentrations of 180 to 250 mg/dL or higher indicate that glucose levels are out of control. The nurse should look specifically for a fasting blood glucose concentration lower than 140 mg/dL and a glycosylated hemoglobin concentration (HgbA1C) lower than 7%. The HgbA1C helps to determine the level of glucose control the patient has had over the last 2 to 3 months.

The final aspect of the comprehensive assessment is pain assessment. Pain is thought to be an important factor in healing. Until recently, chronic wound pain was largely ignored as a cofactor in healing. Krasner[74] proposed a chronic wound pain experience model and described the typical pain experiences for persons with chronic wounds in four categories: noncyclic acute wound pain (e.g., sharp debridement), cyclic acute wound pain (e.g., with daily dressings or repositioning), and chronic wound pain (e.g., persistent pain with no wound manipulation). Krasner[74] suggested that the model is best used as a guide for assessment, intervention, and evaluation.

Wound pain is evaluated by having the patient rate the pain on a numerical scale from 0 to 10, with 0 equal to no pain and 10 equal to the worst pain ever felt, or by use of a visual analog scale. Patients who are nonverbal are observed for withdrawal, grimacing, crying out, or other nonverbal signs of pain. Pain assessments should be done before and during wound procedures, such as dressing changes or debridement, and also at times when the dressing is intact and no procedures are in progress. The patient or caregiver should be encouraged to keep a pain diary, because the data may be valuable in evaluating changes in wound pain over time. The focused history, physical examination, evaluation of laboratory and diagnostic data, and pain assessment provide the context for the wound itself and, along with wound severity and wound status assessment, the basis for pressure ulcer treatment. Total patient assessment should also encompass evaluation of treatment appropriateness in light of the overall condition of the patient and the goals of palliative care.

Pressure Ulcer Management

Pressure ulcer management can be based on clinical practice guidelines. Existing guidelines are helpful in developing a palliative care plan. The existing guidelines are broad based and general and, as such, form a good basis for wound care when the goal is comfort as well as when the goal is healing.

In the United States, most pressure ulcer care is based on the 1994 AHRQ algorithms for treatment.[42] The guidelines present a general approach to use in developing a care plan for the patient with a pressure ulcer. Although they were published in 1994, the general principles of ulcer management remain the same. Pressure ulcer care is focused on nutritional assessment and support, management of tissue loads, and ulcer care, including management of bacterial colonization and infection.[42] These general guidelines are also appropriate for palliative care.

Nutritional Support. Because many studies have linked malnutrition with pressure ulcers, adequate nutritional support is an important part of pressure ulcer management. Figure 16A–3 presents the nutritional assessment and support algorithm for pressure ulcer management from the AHRQ guidelines. The clinician must ensure that dietary intake is adequate in the patient with a pressure ulcer. Prevention of malnutrition reduces the patient's risk for further tissue trauma related to pressure or impaired wound healing. As noted in the discussion of prevention, maintenance of adequate nutrition in the palliative care patient may not be possible.

Management of Tissue Loads. Management of tissue loads refers to care related to those with pressure ulcers who are at risk for development of additional pressure ulcers. Figure 16A–4 presents an algorithm for management of tissue loads with support surfaces algorithm. This is an important part of pressure ulcer treatment, because many individuals with a pressure ulcer are at risk for further pressure-induced tissue trauma. More information on support surfaces and management of tissue loads was presented in the earlier discussion of prevention of pressure ulcers. It is important to understand that the goal of managing tissue loads in the palliative care patient is to ease suffering and discomfort from the wound. Use of pressure-reduction devices, such as alternating air mattresses, is particularly appropriate for palliative care.

Ulcer Care: Debridement. Direct pressure ulcer care involves adequate debridement of necrotic material, management of bacterial colonization and infection, wound cleansing, and selection of topical dressings. Figure 16A–5 presents an algorithm for ulcer care.

Adequate debridement of necrotic tissue is necessary for wound healing. Necrotic debris in the wound bed forms an obstacle to healing and provides a medium for bacterial growth. The patient's condition and the goals of care determine the method of debridement. Sharp, mechanical, enzymatic, or autolytic debridement techniques may be used if there is no urgent need for drainage or removal of devitalized material from the wound. In the presence of advancing cellulitis, sepsis, or large and adherent amounts of necrotic debris, sharp debridement should be performed. In palliative care, debridement is still important, because the removal of nonviable material decreases wound odor. In the case of the black eschar that forms on heels, debridement may not be necessary. Observation of the black heel with attention to the development of pathological signs such as erythema, drainage, odor, or bogginess of the tissues is necessary. If signs of erythema, drainage, odor, or bogginess appear, then the heel eschar must be debrided.

Mechanical debridement includes the use of wet-to-dry dressings at specific intervals, hydrotherapy, or wound irrigation. Of these three methods, wound irrigation is the most favorable for wound healing. Wet-to-dry dressings are not favorable because of the time and labor involved in performing the dressing technique correctly and the potential for pain. Wet-to-dry dressings are not recommended for palliative care

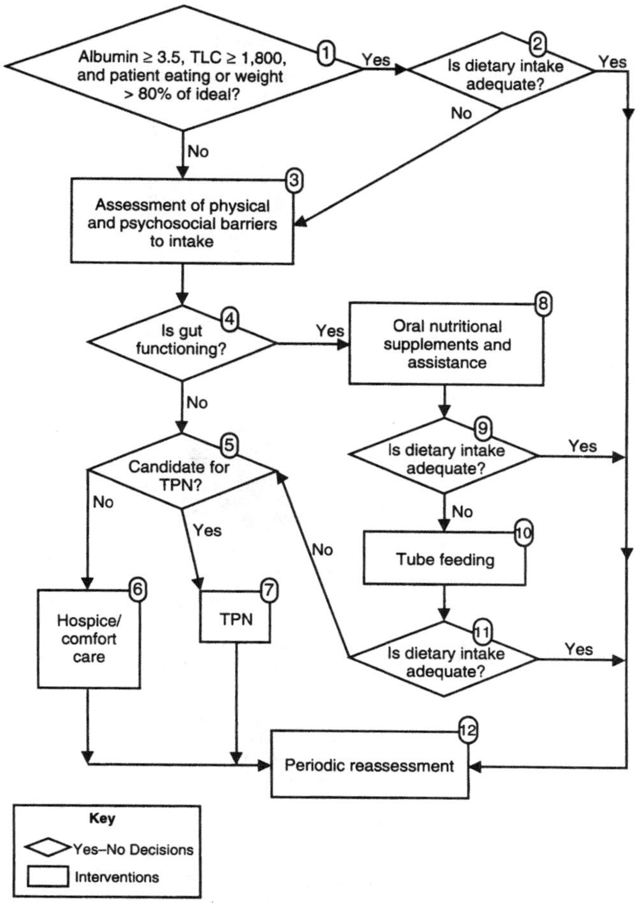

Figure 16A-3. Nutritional assessment and support algorithm from the United States Agency for Health Care Policy and Research (AHCPR). TLC, total lymphocyte count; TPN, total parenteral nutrition. *Source*: From Bergstrom et al. (1994), reference 42, with permission.

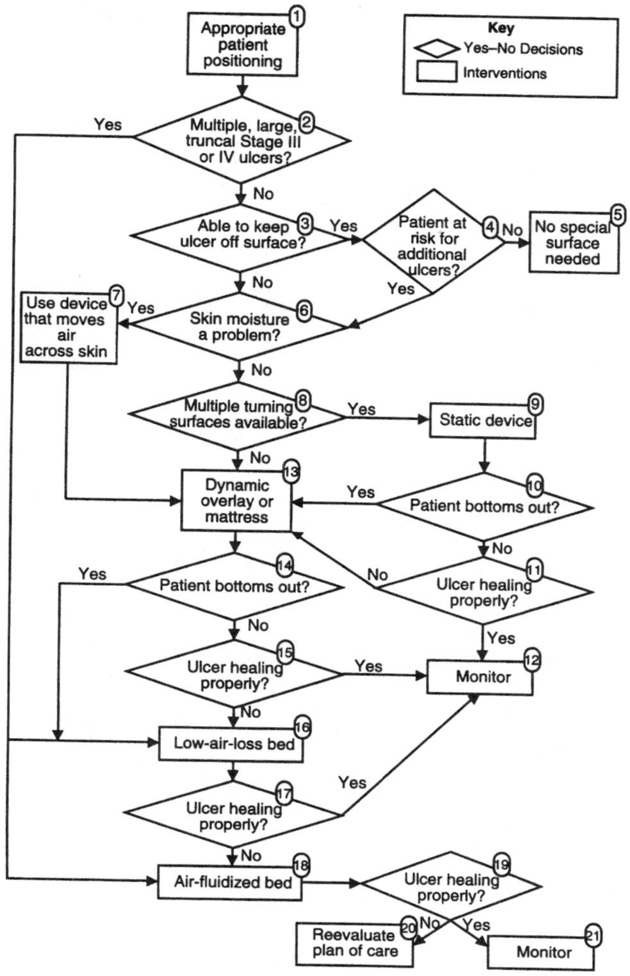

Figure 16A-4. Management of tissue loads algorithm from the United States Agency for Healthcare Research and Quality (AHRQ), formerly the Agency for Health Care Policy and Research (AHCPR). *Source*: From Bergstrom et al. (1994), reference 42, with permission.

because of the frequency of dressing changes and the increased potential for wound pain. Hydrotherapy or whirlpool treatments may be helpful for wounds with large amounts of necrotic debris adherent to healthy tissues. In these cases, hydrotherapy helps to loosen the material from the wound bed for easier removal with sharp debridement.

Enzymatic debridement is performed by applying a topical agent containing an enzyme that destroys necrotic tissue. Enzymatic debridement should be considered if the patient is not a candidate for sharp debridement or is in long-term care or home care. Enzymes may be used alone or in conjunction with other debridement techniques. Enzymatic debridement may be an appropriate method for palliative care, because the frequency of dressing changes is usually once a day and the method is easy to use in conjunction with periodic sharp debridement.

Autolytic debridement involves the use of moisture-retentive dressings to cover the wound and allow necrotic tissue to self-digest from enzymes normally found in wound fluid or exudate. Autolytic debridement may be used in conjunction with other debridement methods such as intermittent sharp debridement or wound irrigation. Again, autolytic debridement may be particularly effective for palliative care. Autolytic debridement has the added benefit of decreased frequency of dressing changes (typically every 3 to 5 days), so the suffering associated with dressing changes is diminished.

Ulcer Care: Bacterial Colonization and Infection. Open pressure ulcers are typically colonized with bacteria. In most cases, adequate debridement and wound cleansing prevent the bacterial colonization from proceeding to the point of clinical infection. Figure 16A–6 presents a preferred pathway for management of bacterial colonization and infection. Wound management can be enhanced in pressure ulcers by attention to debridement of necrotic debris and adequate wound cleansing. These two steps alone are often sufficient to prevent wound infection in pressure ulcers, because they remove the debris that supports bacterial growth.[42] Prevention of infection is an

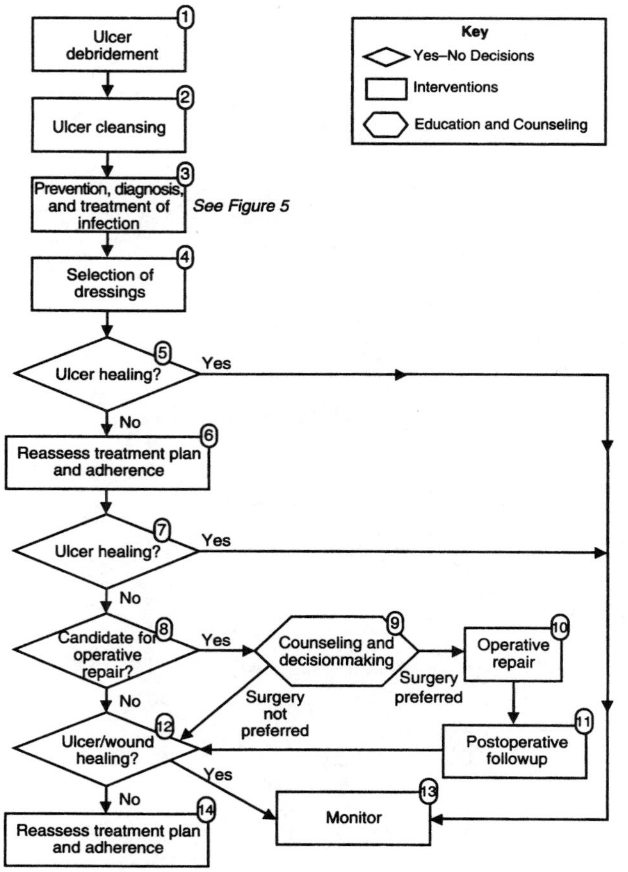

Figure 16A-5. Ulcer care algorithm from the United States Agency for Healthcare Research and Quality (AHRQ), formerly the Agency for Health Care Policy and Research (AHCPR). *Source*: From Bergstrom et al. (1994), reference 42, with permission.

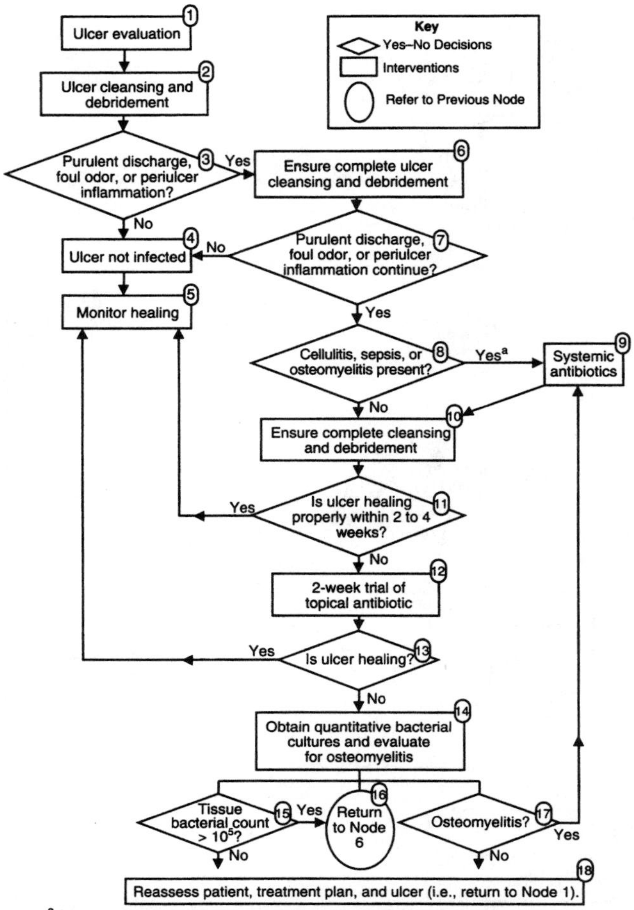

[a] Suspicion of sepsis requires urgent medical evaluation and treatment. Treatment of sepsis is not discussed in this guideline.

Figure 16A-6. Managing bacterial colonization and infection algorithm from the United States Agency for Healthcare Research and Quality (AHRQ), formerly the Agency for Health Care Policy and Research (AHCPR). *Source*: From Bergstrom et al. (1994), reference 42, with permission.

important goal for the palliative care patient. Use of prolonged silver-release topical dressings helps control wound surface bacteria and is effective against a broad range of pathogens, including methicillin-resistant *Staphylococcus aureus* (MRSA).

Identification of infection is best accomplished by clinical assessment. Routine swab cultures should not be used to identify infection in most pressure ulcers. Swab cultures simply reflect the bacterial contamination on the surface of the wound and may not truly identify the organisms causing tissue infection. The recommended technique for diagnosis of tissue infection in pressure ulcers is needle aspiration or tissue biopsy.[42] An alternative method involves use of surface swabs. After cleansing the wound with normal saline to remove any dressing debris, the nurse swabs a 1 cm^2 area of the wound bed with the surface swab for 5 seconds, until tissue fluid is apparent on the swab, and then sends the swab directly to the laboratory. This technique may better reflect actual bacterial invasion of the wound tissues than standard swab methods do.

Use of topical antimicrobial solutions is not indicated for clean pressure ulcers. Indeed, most topical antimicrobial solutions are toxic to the fibroblast, which is the cell responsible for wound healing and may cause a burning sensation, adding to the patient's discomfort. Topical antiseptics, such as povidone iodine, iodophor, sodium hypochlorite, hydrogen peroxide, and acetic acid, do not significantly reduce the number of bacteria in wound tissue; however, they do harm the healthy wound tissues.[42] As such, these substances usually have no place in the treatment of clean pressure ulcers. In wounds filled with necrotic debris, antiseptic/antimicrobial solutions may be used for a short course of therapy (typically 2 weeks), to assist with surface bacteria and odor reduction, and then evaluated for further use.

Ulcer Care: Wound Cleansing. Cleansing of a wound assists healing because it removes necrotic tissue, excess wound exudate, and metabolic wastes from the wound bed. Wound healing is optimized and the potential for wound infection is decreased when wound cleansing is a part of the treatment plan for pressure ulcers. Wound cleansing involves the selection of a solution for cleansing and a method of delivering the solution to the wound. Routine wound cleansing should be accomplished with minimal trauma to the wound bed. Wounds should be cleansed initially and at each dressing change. Minimal force should be applied when using gauze, sponges, or cloth to clean the wound bed. Skin cleansers and antimicrobial solutions are not indicated as solutions for cleaning pressure ulcers because they destroy the healthy wound tissues and are toxic to the fibroblast cell.[42] Normal saline is the preferred solution, because it is physiological and will not harm healing tissues.

When wound irrigation is used to cleanse wounds, the irrigation pressure should fall within the range of 4 to 15 pounds per square inch (psi). Higher pressures may drive bacteria deeper into wound tissues or cause additional wound trauma. A 35-mL syringe with a 19-gauge angiocatheter delivers saline at 8 psi and is an effective method for removing bacteria from the wound bed.

Ulcer Care: Dressings. In general, moisture-retentive wound dressings are the most appropriate type for pressure ulcers. For palliative care, they are the dressings of choice because of the decreased frequency of required changes (typically every 3 to 5 days). The goal of the wound dressing is to provide an environment that keeps the wound bed tissue moist and the surrounding intact skin dry. Use of moist wound healing dressings supports a better rate of healing than use of dry gauze dressings[42]; more importantly in palliative care, moist wound healing dressings contain odor, absorb exudate, and minimize dressing change discomfort. Clinical judgment is needed to determine the best dressing for the wound. The appropriate dressing should keep the surrounding intact skin dry while controlling wound exudate and should provide a minimal amount of pain during dressing changes.

The clinician must be aware of the absorptive capacity and pain reduction properties of the major dressing types. In general, thin film dressings have no absorptive capacity and minimize pain by covering exposed nerve endings. Thin film dressings are adherent to the skin surrounding the wound and sometimes to the wound itself, making dressing removal more likely to be painful. Hydrocolloids, hydrogels, and foam dressings typically have a minimal to moderate absorptive capacity. Hydrocolloid dressings are occlusive and reduce pain by preventing exposure of the wound to air. They have adhesive properties and can cause pain if removed improperly. Foam dressings are moderately absorptive and nonadherent, resulting in reduced pain during dressing changes. Hydrogel dressings are cool and soothing and are particularly effective in wounds that induce a burning sensation. Hydrogel dressings are nonadherent, reducing wound pain during dressing changes. Calcium alginates, alginate collagen dressings, and exudate absorbing beads, flakes, pastes, or powders absorb large amounts of drainage. Dressings with a large absorptive capacity reduce pain related to maceration of surrounding tissues and to pressure caused by the excess exudate. Calcium alginates and exudate-absorbing dressings are nonadherent and are easily removed from the wound during dressing changes. Soft silicone dressings absorb minimal amounts of drainage but are nonadherent and reduce pain associated with dressing changes.

Wounds with small or minimal amounts of exudate can benefit from a variety of dressings, including hydrocolloids, hydrogels, thin film dressings, and foam dressings. Wounds with moderate amounts of exudate may require dressings with a higher absorptive capacity, such as hydrocolloids, foam dressings, hydrogel sheet dressings, or composite dressings (those including a combination of products, such as a thin film with a foam island in the center). Wounds with a large amount of drainage require dressings that are capable of absorbing it, such as calcium alginates, alginate collagen combinations, or specific beads, pastes, or powders designed to handle large amounts of drainage. Wounds with significant odor benefit from dressings formulated with charcoal, such as charcoal foam and dressings with a charcoal filter overlay.

If a wound shows a significant loss of tissue or if undermining or pockets are present, the wound cavities should be loosely filled with dressing to eliminate the potential for abscess formation. Eliminating the dead space helps to prevent premature wound closure with resulting abscess formation. Dressings such as calcium alginates, impregnated hydrogel gauze strips, or wound cavity fillers are useful for eliminating the dead space. Loose filling of the undermined areas also assists with exudate management, because these wounds tend to have large amounts of exudate.

Wounds in the sacral area require additional protection from stool or urine contamination. Because dressings near the anus may be difficult to maintain, the clinician must monitor dressings in this area more frequently. Some hydrocolloid dressings have been designed with specific shapes to improve their ability to stay in place over sacral/coccygeal wounds.

Wound pain must be managed with the same attention given to choice of wound dressings. In general, pain that is moderate to severe should be managed pharmacologically (see Chapters 5 and 6). The pressure ulcer alone may not require continuous pharmacological analgesia, but medication before procedures is essential. Lower levels of pain may be manageable with appropriate wound dressing choice and topical wound analgesia. Techniques useful for noncyclic and cyclic wound pain associated with procedures (e.g., debridement, dressing changes) include use of distraction (e.g., talking to the patient while performing the procedure), allowing the patient to call a "time-out" during the procedure, allowing the patient to control and participate in the procedure, providing opioids and/or nonsteroidal anti-inflammatory drugs 30 minutes before the procedure and afterwards, and administering topical anesthetics or topical opioids using hydrogels as a transport media. The lidocaine patch 5% (Lidoderm) blocks sodium channels and has been approved for postherpetic neuralgia. It is effective for chronic neuropathic pain. Another option is EMLA cream (eutectic mixture of lidocaine 2.5% and prilocaine 2.5%), which reduces debridement pain scores and might have a vasoactive effect cutaneously.[75–78] Low-dose topical morphine was been used successfully in two small pilot studies to control pressure ulcer–related pain.[79,80]

As evidenced by this discussion, attention to multiple wound characteristics helps to determine the most appropriate wound dressing. Evaluation of wound characteristics in follow-along assessments provides the basis for changes in topical dressings. For example, a wound that is heavily exudative may be treated topically with a calcium alginate dressing for several weeks; as the amount of wound exudate decreases, the wound dressing may appear dry at dressing changes. This indicates that use of a dressing with high absorptive capacity may not be needed any longer, and the wound dressing can be changed to one with minimal to moderate absorptive capacity, such as a hydrocolloid dressing. As the wound continues to heal and wound exudate becomes minimal or nonexistent, a thin film dressing may be used to provide protection from the environment.

Patient and Caregiver Teaching Guidelines

Patient and caregiver instruction in self-care must be individualized according to specific pressure ulcer development risk factors, individual learning styles and coping mechanisms, and the ability of the patient or caregiver to perform procedures. In teaching prevention guidelines to caregivers, it is particularly important to use return demonstration to evaluate learning. Observing the caregiver perform turning maneuvers, repositioning, managing incontinence, and providing general skin care can be enlightening and provides a context in which the clinician supports and follows up education. In palliative care, it is important to include the reasons for specific actions, such as the continuation of some level of turning and repositioning to prevent further tissue damage and lessen discomfort from additional wounds.

Summary

Poorly managed pressure ulcers can increase pain and suffering in those with a chronic debilitating illness. Although preventive measure in patients identified as at risk for developing such pressure ulcers can be effective, some patients do develop pressure ulcers that require expert nursing management. Expert nursing management includes instituting preventive measure to preserve intact skin, obtaining and maintaining a clean wound, management of exudate and odor, and prevention of complications such as a superimposed wound infection. Because many dying and chronically ill debilitated patients are cared for at home, educating family members about the development of pressure ulcers and involving family caregivers in the plan of care is critical.

REFERENCES

1. Daniel RK, Priest DL, Wheatley DC. Etiologic factors in pressure sores: An experimental model. Arch Phys Med Rehabil 1981; 62:492–498.
2. Kosiak M. Etiology and pathology of ischemic ulcers. Arch Phys Med Rehabil 1959;40:62–69.
3. Reuler JB, Cooney TG. The pressure sore: pathophysiology and principles of management. Ann Intern Med 1981;94:661.
4. Seiler WD, Stahelin HB. Recent findings on decubitus ulcer pathology: implications for care. Geriatrics 1986;41:47–60.
5. Witkowski JA, Parish, LC. Histopathology of the decubitus ulcer. J Am Acad Dermatol 1982;6:1014–1021.
6. Lindan O, Greenway RM, Piazza JM. Pressure distributor on the surface of the human body. Arch Phys Med Rehabil 1965;46:378.
7. Scales JT. Pressure on the patient. In: Kenedi RM, Cowden JM, eds. Bedsore Biomechanics. London: University Park Press, 1976.
8. Parish LC, Witkowski JA, Crissey JT. The Decubitus Ulcer. New York: Masson, 1983.
9. Slater H. Pressure Ulcers in the Elderly. Pittsburgh, PA: Synapse, 1985.
10. Parish LC, Witkowski JA, Crissey JT. The Decubitus Ulcer in Clinical Practice. Berlin: Springer, 1997.
11. Landis EM. Micro-injection studies of capillary blood pressure in human skin. Heart 1930;15:209.
12. Husain T. An experimental study of some pressure effects on tissues, with reference to the bedsore problem. J Pathol Bacteriol 1953;66:347–358.
13. Salcido R, Donofrio JC, Fisher SB, LeGrand EK, Dickey K, Carney JM, Schosser R, Liang R. Histopathology of decubitus ulcers as a result of sequential pressure sessions in a computer-controlled fuzzy rat model. Adv Wound Care 1994;7(5):40.
14. Kosiak M, Kubicek WG, Olsen ME. Evaluation of pressure as a factor in the production of ischial ulcers. Arch Phys Med Rehabil 1958;39:623.
15. Braden BJ, Bergstrom N. A conceptual schema for the study of etiology of pressure sores. Rehabil Nurs 1987;12:8–12.
16. Bergstrom N, Demuth PJ, Braden BJ. A clinical trial of the Braden Scale for Predicting Pressure Sore Risk. Nurs Clin North Am 1987;22:417–428.
17. Allman RM, Goode PS, Patrick MM, Burst N, Bartolucci AA. Pressure ulcer risk factors among hospitalized patients with activity limitations. JAMA 1995;273:865–870.
18. Panel for the Prediction and Prevention of Pressure Ulcers in Adults. Pressure Ulcers in Adults: Prediction and Prevention. Clinical Practice Guideline Number 3. Publication AHCPR 92–0047. Rockville, MD: Agency for Health Care Policy and Research, U. S. Department of Health and Human Services, 1992.
19. Maklebust J, Sieggreen MY. Pressure Ulcers: Guidelines for Prevention and Nursing Management, 2nd ed. Springhouse, PA: Springhouse, 1996.
20. Curry K, Casady L. The relationship between extended periods of immobility and decubitus ulcer formation in the acutely spinal cord injured individual. J Neurosci Nurs 1992;24:185–189.
21. Hammond MC, Bozzacco VA, Stiens SA, Buhrer R, Lyman P. Pressure ulcer incidence on a spinal cord injury unit. Adv Wound Care 1994;7:57–60.
22. Reichel SM. Shearing force as a factor in decubitus ulcers in paraplegics. JAMA 1958;166:762–763.
23. Bennett L, Kavner D, Lee BY, Trainor FS, Lewis JM. Skin stress and blood flow in sitting paraplegic patients. Arch Phys Med Rehabil 1969;65:186–190.
24. Dinsdale SM. Decubitus ulcers: role of pressure and friction in causation. Arch Phys Med Rehabil 1974;55:147–152.
25. Kemp MG. Protecting the skin from moisture and associated irritants. J Gerontol Nurs 1994;20:8–14.

26. Bates-Jensen B. Incontinence management. In: Parish LC, Witkowski JA, Crissey JT, eds. The Decubitus Ulcer in Clinical Practice. Berlin: Springer, 1997:189–199.
27. Maklebust J, Magnan MA. Risk factors associated with having a pressure ulcer: A secondary analysis. Adv Wound Care 1994; 7:25–42.
28. Pinchcovsky-Devin G, Kaminsky MV Jr. Correlation of pressure sores and nutritional status. J Am Geriatr Soc 1986;34:435–440.
29. Bobel LM. Nutritional implications in the patient with pressure sores. Nurs Clin North Am 1987;22:379–390.
30. Bergstrom N, Braden B. A prospective study of pressure sore risk among institutionalized elderly. J Am Geriatr Soc 1992;40: 747–758.
31. Allman RM, Laprade CA, Noel LB, Walker JM, Moorer CA, Dear MR, Smith CR. Pressure sores among hospitalized patients. Ann Intern Med 1986;105:337–342.
32. Jones PL, Millman A. Wound healing and the aged patient. Nurs Clin North Am 1990;25:263–277.
33. Eaglestein WH. Wound healing and aging. Clin Geriatr Med 1989;5:183.
34. Bergstrom N, Braden BJ, Boynton P, Bruch S. Using a research-based assessment scale in clinical practice. Nurs Clin North Am 1995;30:539.
35. Versluysen M. Pressure sores in elderly patients: The epidemiology related to hip operations. J Bone Joint Surg Br 1985; 67:10–13.
36. Shannon ML. Pressure sores. In: Norris CM, ed. Concept Clarification in Nursing. Rockville, Md.: Aspen, 1982.
37. Anderson TP, Andberg MM. Psychosocial factors associated with pressure sores. Arch Phys Med Rehabil 1979;60:341–346.
38. Vidal J, Sarrias M. An analysis of the diverse factors concerned with the development of pressure sores in spinal cord patients. Paraplegia 1991;29:261–267.
39. Norton D, McLaren R, Exton-Smith NA. An Investigation of Geriatric Nursing Problems in Hospitals. London: National Corporation for the Care of Old People, 1962.
40. Norton D. Calculating the risk: Reflections on the Norton scale. Decubitus 1989;2:24–31.
41. Braden B, Bergstrom N. Clinical utility of the Braden scale for predicting pressure sore risk. Decubitus 1989;2:44–51.
42. Bergstrom N, Bennett MA, Carlson CE, et al. Treatment of Pressure Ulcers. Clinical Practice Guideline Number 15. Publication AHCPR 95-0652. Rockville, Md.: Agency for Health Care Policy and Research, U. S. Department of Health and Human Services, 1994.
43. McLean J. Pressure reduction or pressure relief: making the right choice. J ET Nurs 1993;20:211–215.
44. Krouskop TA, Garber SL, Cullen BB. Factors to consider in selecting a support surface. In: Krasner D, ed. Chronic Wound Care. King of Prussia, Pa.: Health Management Publications, 1990;135–141.
45. Zimmerer RE, Lawson KD, Calvert CJ. The effects of wearing diapers on skin. Pediatr Dermatol 1986;3:95–101.
46. Willis I. The effects of prolonged water exposure on human skin. J Invest Dermatol 1973;60:166–171.
47. National Pressure Ulcer Advisory Panel. Consensus statement. Adv Wound Care 1995;8:32–33.
48. Thomas DR, Rodeheaver GT, Bartolucci AA, Franz RA, Sussman C, Ferrell BA, Cuddigan J, Stotts N, Maklebust J. Pressure Ulcer Scale for Healing: Derivation and validation of the PUSH tool. Adv Wound Care 1997;10:96–101.
49. Bates-Jensen BM, Vredevoe DL, Brecht ML. Validity and reliability of the Pressure Sore Status Tool. Decubitus 1992;5:20–28.
50. Bates-Jensen B. New pressure ulcer status tool. Decubitus 1990; 3:14–15.
51. Bates-Jensen BM, Vredevoe DL, Brecht ML. Validity and reliability of the Pressure Sore Status Tool. Decubitus 1992;5:20–28.
52. Bates-Jensen BM, McNees P. Toward an intelligent wound assessment system. Ostomy Wound Manage 1995;41(Suppl 7A):80–87.
53. Bates-Jensen B. The Pressure Sore Status Tool: An outcome measure for pressure sores. Top Geriatr Rehabil 1994;9:17–34.
54. Bates-Jensen BM. The Pressure Sore Status Tool a few thousand assessments later. Adv Wound Care 1997;10:65–73.
55. Cooper DM. Indices to include in wound assessment. Adv Wound Care 1995;8:28-15–28-18.
56. Lazarus GS, Cooper DM, Knighton DR, Mrgolis DJ, Pecorar RE, Rodeheaver G, Robson MC. Definitions and guidelines for assessment of wounds and evaluation of healing. Arch Dermatol 1994;130:489–493.
57. Van Rijswijk L. Wound assessment and documentation. In: Kane DP, Krasner D, eds. Chronic Wound Care: A Clinical Sourcebook for Healthcare Professionals, 2nd ed. Wayne, PA: Health Management Publications, 1997:16–28.
58. Yarkony GM, Kirk PM, Carlson C, Roth EJ, Lovel L, Heinemann A, King R, Lee MY, Betts HB. Classification of pressure ulcers. Arch Dermatol 1990;126:1218–1219.
59. Shea JD. Pressure sores: Classification and management. Clin Orthop Rel Res 1975;112:89–100.
60. Seiler WD, Stahelin HB. Identification of factors that impair wound healing: A possible approach to wound healing research. Wounds 1995;6:101–106.
61. Sapico FL, Ginunas VJ, Thornhill-Hoynes M, Canawati HN, Capen DA, Klen NE, Khawa S, Montgomerie JZ. Quantitative microbiology of pressure sores in different stages of healing. Diagn Microbiol Infect Dis 1986;5:31–38.
62. Winter GD. Formation of the scab and the rate of reepithelialization of superficial wounds in the skin of the young domestic pig. Nature 1965;193:293–294.
63. Kerstein MD. Moist wound healing: the clinical perspective. Ostomy Wound Manage 1995;41(Suppl 7A):37S–44S.
64. Stotts NA. Impaired wound healing. In: Carrieri-Kohlman VK, Lindsay AM, West, CM, eds. Pathophysiological Phenomena in Nursing, 2nd ed. Philadelphia: WB Saunders, 1993:343–366.
65. Bagdade JD, Root RK, Bulger RJ. Impaired leukocyte function in patients with poorly controlled diabetes. Diabetes 1974;23:9–15.
66. Pecoraro RE, Ahroni JH, Boyko EJ, Stensel VL. Chronology and determinants of tissue repair in diabetic lower extremity ulcers. Diabetes 1991;40:1305–1313.
67. Goodson WH 3rd, Hunt TK. Studies of wound healing in experimental diabetes mellitus. J Surg Res 1977;22:221–227.
68. Yue DK, McLennan S, Marsh M, Mai YW, Spaliviero J, Delbridge L, Reeve T, Turtle JR. Effects of experimental diabetes, uremia, and malnutrition on wound healing. Diabetes 1987;36:295–299.
69. Coleridge Smith PD, Thomas P, Scurr JH, Dormandy JA. Causes of venous ulceration: A new hypothesis. BMJ 1998;296:1726–1727.
70. Falanga V. Growth factors and wound healing. Dermatol Clin 1993;11:667–674.
71. Barbul A, Lazarou SA, Efron DT, Wasserkrug HL, Efron G. Arginine enhances wound healing and lymphocyte immune responses in humans. Surgery 1990;108:331–336.
72. Kagan RJ, Bratescu A, Jonasson O, Matsuda T, Teodorescu M. The relationship between the percentage of circulating B cells,

corticosteroid levels, and other immunologic parameters in thermally injured patients. J Trauma 1989;29:208–213.
73. Mosiello GC, Tufaro A, Kerstein M. Wound healing and complications in the immunosuppressed patient. Wounds 1994;6: 83–87.
74. Krasner D. The chronic wound pain experience: A conceptual model. Ostomy Wound Manage 1995;41:20–27.
75. Argoff, CE, New Analgesics for neuropathic pain: the lidocaine patch. Clin J Pain, 2000;16(2 Suppl):S62–S66.
76. Briggs M, Nelson EA. Topical agents or dressings for pain in venous leg ulcers. Cochrane Database Syst Rev 2003;(1):CD001177.
77. Hafner HM, Thomma SR, Eichner M, Steins A., Junger M. The influence of EMLA cream on cutaneous microcirculation. Clin Hemorrheol Microcirc 2003;28:121–128.
78. Popescu A, Salcido R. Wound pain: A challenge for the patient and wound care specialist. Adv Skin Wound Care 2004;17:14–20.
79. Zeppetella G, Paul J, Ribeiro M. Analgesic efficacy of morphine applied topically to painful ulcers. J Pain Symptom Manage 2003;25:555–558.
80. Flock P. Pilot study to determine the effectiveness of diamorphine gel to control pressure ulcer pain. J Pain Symptom Manage 2003;25:547–554.

APPENDIX 16A-1

Bates-Jensen Wound Assessment Tool

General Guidelines:

Fill out the attached rating sheet to assess a wound's status after reading the definitions and methods of assessment described below. Evaluate once a week and whenever a change occurs in the wound. Rate according to each item by picking the response that best describes the wound and entering that score in the item score column for the appropriate date. When you have rated the wound on all items, determine the total score by adding together the 13-item scores. The HIGHER the total score, the more severe the wound status. Plot total score on the Wound Status Continuum to determine progress.

Specific Instructions:

1. **Size:** Use ruler to measure the longest and widest aspect of the wound surface in centimeters; multiply length x width.

2. **Depth:** Pick the depth, thickness, most appropriate to the wound using these additional descriptions:
   1 = tissues damaged but no break in skin surface.
   2 = superficial, abrasion, blister or shallow crater. Even with, &/or elevated above skin surface (e.g., hyperplasia).
   3 = deep crater with or without undermining of adjacent tissue.
   4 = visualization of tissue layers not possible due to necrosis.
   5 = supporting structures include tendon, joint capsule.

3. **Edges:** Use this guide:

Indistinct, diffuse	=	unable to clearly distinguish wound outline.
Attached	=	even or flush with wound base, no sides or walls present; flat.
Not attached	=	sides or walls are present; floor or base of wound is deeper than edge.
Rolled under, thickened	=	soft to firm and flexible to touch.
Hyperkeratosis	=	callous-like tissue formation around wound & at edges.
Fibrotic, scarred	=	hard, rigid to touch.

4. **Undermining:** Assess by inserting a cotton tipped applicator under the wound edge; advance it as far as it will go without using undue force; raise the tip of the applicator so it may be seen or felt on the surface of the skin; mark the surface with a pen; measure the distance from the mark on the skin to the edge of the wound. Continue process around the wound. Then use a transparent metric measuring guide with concentric circles divided into 4 (25%) pie-shaped quadrants to help determine percent of wound involved.

5. **Necrotic Tissue Type:** Pick the type of necrotic tissue that is predominant in the wound according to color, consistency and adherence using this guide:

White/gray non-viable tissue	=	may appear prior to wound opening; skin surface is white or gray.
Non-adherent, yellow slough	=	thin, mucinous substance; scattered throughout wound bed; easily separated from wound tissue.
Loosely adherent, yellow slough	=	thick, stringy, clumps of debris; attached to wound tissue.
Adherent, soft, black eschar	=	soggy tissue; strongly attached to tissue in center or base of wound.
Firmly adherent, hard/black eschar	=	firm, crusty tissue; strongly attached to wound base and edges (like a hard scab).

6. **Necrotic Tissue Amount:** Use a transparent metric measuring guide with concentric circles divided into 4 (25%) pie-shaped quadrants to help determine percent of wound involved.

7. **Exudate Type:** Some dressings interact with wound drainage to produce a gel or trap liquid. Before assessing exudate type, gently cleanse wound with normal saline or water. Pick the exudate type that is predominant in the wound according to color and consistency, using this guide:

Bloody	=	thin, bright red
Serosanguineous	=	thin, watery pale red to pink
Serous	=	thin, watery, clear
Purulent	=	thin or thick, opaque tan to yellow
Foul purulent	=	thick, opaque yellow to green with offensive odor

8. **Exudate Amount:** Use a transparent metric measuring guide with concentric circles divided into 4 (25%) pie-shaped quadrants to determine percent of dressing involved with exudate. Use this guide:

None	=	wound tissues dry.
Scant	=	wound tissues moist; no measurable exudate.
Small	=	wound tissues wet; moisture evenly distributed in wound; drainage involves $\leq$ 25% dressing.
Moderate	=	wound tissues saturated; drainage may or may not be evenly distributed in wound; drainage involves > 25% to $\leq$ 75% dressing.
Large	=	wound tissues bathed in fluid; drainage freely expressed; may or may not be evenly distributed in wound; drainage involves > 75% of dressing.

9. **Skin Color Surrounding Wound:** Assess tissues within 4 cm of wound edge. Dark-skinned persons show the colors "bright red" and "dark red" as a deepening of normal ethnic skin color or a purple hue. As healing occurs in dark-skinned persons, the new skin is pink and may never darken.

10. **Peripheral Tissue Edema & Induration:** Assess tissues within 4 cm of wound edge. Non-pitting edema appears as skin that is shiny and taut. Identify pitting edema by firmly pressing a finger down into the tissues and waiting for 5 seconds, on release of pressure, tissues fail to resume previous position and an indentation appears. Induration is abnormal firmness of tissues with margins. Assess by gently pinching the tissues. Induration results in an inability to pinch the tissues. Use a transparent metric measuring guide to determine how far edema or induration extends beyond wound.

11. **Granulation Tissue:** Granulation tissue is the growth of small blood vessels and connective tissue to fill in full thickness wounds. Tissue is healthy when bright, beefy red, shiny and granular with a velvety appearance. Poor vascular supply appears as pale pink or blanched to dull, dusky red color.

12. **Epithelialization:** Epithelialization is the process of epidermal resurfacing and appears as pink or red skin. In partial thickness wounds it can occur throughout the wound bed as well as from the wound edges. In full thickness wounds it occurs from the edges only. Use a transparent metric measuring guide with concentric circles divided into 4 (25%) pie-shaped quadrants to help determine percent of wound involved and to measure the distance the epithelial tissue extends into the wound.

16B

Barbara M. Bates-Jensen, Susie Seaman, and Lynne Early

Skin Disorders: Tumor Necrosis, Fistulas, and Stomas

This constant drainage smells so bad, and my skin is so sore, life isn't worth living—I don't belong among people.—A palliative care patient

- ***Key Points***
- *Management of drainage and odor are key components of palliative care for malignant cutaneous wounds or tumor necrosis.*
- *Palliative care for the person with an ostomy is focused on maintenance of an efficient management plan and provision for optimal functional capacity.*
- *It is essential to involve caregivers and family members in the plan of care.*

TUMOR NECROSIS

Definition

Tumor necrosis, also known in the literature as fungating tumors, ulcerative malignant wounds, or malignant cutaneous wounds, presents both a physical and an emotional challenge for the patient and even the most experienced clinician. These wounds are frequently associated with pain, odor, bleeding, and an unsightly appearance. They may be a blow to self-esteem and may cause social isolation just when the patient needs more time with loved ones. The goals in the care of patients with tumor necrosis include pain management; control of exudate, odor, and bleeding; and prevention of infection.

Malignant cutaneous lesions occur in up to 5% of patients with cancer and 10% of patients with metastatic disease. Lookingbill and colleagues[1] retrospectively reviewed data accumulated over a 10-year period from the tumor registry at Hershey Medical Center in Pennsylvania. Of 7316 patients, 367 (5.0%) had cutaneous malignancies. Of these, 38 patients had lesions as a result of direct local invasion, 337 had metastatic lesions, and 8 had both. A secondary analysis from the same registry found that 420 patients (10.4%) of 4020 with metastatic disease had cutaneous involvement.[2] In women, the most common origins of metastasis were breast carcinoma (70.7%) and melanoma (12.0%). In men, melanoma (32.3%), lung carcinoma (11.8%), and colorectal cancer (11.0%) accounted for the most common primary tumors. Although these types of cancer account for the majority of skin involvement, it is important to note that metastatic cutaneous lesions may arise from any type of malignant tumor.[3,4]

Pathophysiology of Tumor Necrosis

Tumor necrosis may occur from infiltration of the skin by local invasion of a primary tumor or by metastasis from a distant site.[5] Local invasion may initially manifest as inflammation with induration, redness, heat, tenderness, or some combination of these features. The skin may have a peau d'orange appearance and may be fixed to underlying tissue. As the tumor spreads and further tissue destruction occurs, the skin eventually ulcerates. The presentation differs in metastatic cutaneous infiltration. Tumor cells detach from the primary site and travel via blood or lymphatic vessels, or tissue planes, to distant organs, including the skin.[3,4] These lesions may initially manifest as well-demarcated, painless nodules ranging in size from a few millimeters to several centimeters. Their consistency may vary from firm to rubbery. Pigmentation changes may be noted over the lesions, from deep red to brown-black. Over time, these nodules may ulcerate, drain, and become very painful.

As both locally invasive and metastatic lesions extend, changes in vascular and lymphatic flow lead to edema, exudate, and tissue necrosis.[5,6] The resulting lesion may be fungating, in which the tumor mass extends above the skin surface with a fungus or cauliflower-like appearance, or it may be erosive and ulcerative.[7] The wound bed may be pale to pink with very friable tissue, completely necrotic, or a combination of both. The surrounding skin may be erythematous, fragile, and exceedingly tender to touch. The skin may also be macerated in the presence of excessive wound exudate. The presence of necrotic tissue is an ideal culture medium for bacterial colonization, which results in significant malodor.[8] The degree of pain experienced by the patient depends on wound location, depth of tissue invasion and damage, nerve involvement, and the patient's previous experience with pain and analgesia.[7]

Tumor Necrosis Assessment

Assessment of tumor necrosis provides the clinician with information to develop a treatment plan, adjust the treatment plan as assessment parameters change, and observe for wound complications. Specifically, wound location, size, appearance, exudate, odor, and condition of the surrounding skin guide local therapy. Associated symptoms should be noted so that appropriate measures can be taken to provide comfort. The potential for serious complications such as hemorrhage, vessel compression or obstruction, or airway obstruction should be noted so that the caregiver can be educated regarding their palliative management. Table 16B-1 presents highlights for the assessment of tumor necrosis and associated symptoms.

Haisfield-Wolfe and Baxendale-Cox[9] proposed a staging classification system for assessment of malignant cutaneous wounds. Use of wound classification may increase the effectiveness of communication among health care practitioners and make evaluation of treatment effectiveness consistent. In a pilot study with 13 wounds, they proposed a staging classification system that evaluates wound depth with clinical descriptors, predominant color of the wound, hydration status of the wound, drainage, pain, odor, and presence of tunneling or undermining. Use of this system provides a basis for a standard set of descriptors that nurses can use to both understand and assess tumor necrosis wounds.

Wounds secondary to tumor necrosis are expected to change over time based on the aggressiveness of the cancer and whether the patient is undergoing palliative surgery, chemotherapy, or radiation. Although palliative treatment may result in regression or even disappearance of the cutaneous lesion, it can be expected to recur eventually.[10] Ongoing assessment allows the clinician to tailor the local wound management based on the current needs of the patient and wound.

Tumor Necrosis Management

The goals of care for patients with tumor necrosis include control of infection and odor, management of exudate, prevention and control of bleeding, and management of pain. In determining the appropriate treatment regimen, the abilities of the caregiver must also be considered. The limited information on treatment effectiveness reflects the absence of evidence-based care in this area and the extreme need for further research and dissemination of findings. Many articles are based on expert opinion and the personal experience of practitioners knowledgeable in palliative and hospice care. Although research-based treatment is the gold standard of care, anecdotal reports on successful treatment of these challenging wounds is helpful to nurses striving to provide the best care.

Infection and Odor Control. Control of infection and odor is achieved by controlling local bacterial colonization with wound cleansing, wound debridement, and use of local antibiotic agents. Because malignant cutaneous lesions are frequently associated with necrotic tissue and odor, wound cleansing is essential to remove necrotic debris, decrease bacterial counts, and thus reduce odor. If the lesion is not very friable, the patient may be able to get in the shower. This not only provides for local cleansing but also gives the added psychological benefit of helping the patient to feel clean. The patient should be instructed to allow the shower water to hit the skin above the wound and then run over the wound. If there is friable tissue (i.e., tissue that bleeds easily with minimal trauma) or the patient is not able to shower, the nurse or caregiver should gently irrigate the wound with normal saline or a commercial wound cleanser. Skin cleansers, which contain mild soaps and antibacterial ingredients used in bathing, can be very helpful in controlling local colonization and odor. As long as they do not cause burning, they may be sprayed directly on the wound and can be quite effective at controlling odor. If pain and burning occur with use of skin cleansers in the wound, they should be used only on the surrounding skin. Topical antimicrobial agents such as hydrogen peroxide, Dakin's solution, and povidone iodine are recommended by some authors[10]; however, their use should be weighed against the potential negative effects of local pain, wound desiccation with subsequent pain and bleeding on dressing removal, and unpleasant odor associated with some agents (Dakin's and povidone iodine), which may be bothersome to patients. In the authors' experience, the skin cleansers described provide cleansing and odor reduction without many of the negative effects of the topical antimicrobial agents.

Table 16B–1
Assessment of Cutaneous Malignancy

Assessment	Rationale
Wound Location	
Is mobility impaired?	Consider occupational therapy referral to facilitate activities of daily living
Located near wrinkled or flat skin?	Affects dressing selection
	Affects dressing fixation
Wound Appearance	
Size: length, width, depth, undermining, deep structure exposure	Affects dressing selection, provides information on deterioration or response to palliative treatment
Fungating or ulcerative	Affects dressing selection and fixation
Percentage of viable vs. necrotic tissue	Need for cleansing/debridement
Tissue friability and bleeding	Need for nonadherent dressings and other measures to control bleeding
Presence of odor	Need for odor-reducing strategies
Presence of fistula	Possible need for pouching
Exudate amount	Affects dressing selection
Wound colonized or clinically infected	Need for local versus systemic care
Surrounding Skin	
Erythematous	Infection or tumor extension
Fragile or denuded	Impacts dressing type and fixation
Nodular	Tumor extension/metastasis
Macerated	Need for improved exudate management
Radiation-related skin damage	Need for topical care of skin, affects dressing fixation
Symptoms	
Deep pain: aching, stabbing, continuous	Need to adjust systemic analgesia
Superficial pain: burning, stinging, may be associated only with dressing changes	Need for topical analgesia and rapid-onset, short-acting analgesics
Pruritus	Related to dressings? If not, may need systemic antipruritic medications
Potential for Serious Complications	
Lesion is near major blood vessels: potential for hemorrhage	Need for education of patient/family about palliative management of severe bleeding
Lesion is near major blood vessels: potential for vessel compression/obstruction	Need for education of patient/family about palliative management of severe swelling and pain, possible tissue necrosis
Lesion is near airway: potential for obstruction	Need for education of patient/family about palliative management of airway obstruction

Necrotic tissue in tumor necrosis is typically moist yellow slough. Occasionally, in the absence of exudate, there may be dry black eschar, but this is uncommon. Debridement is best done with the use of autolytic and/or gentle mechanical methods, as opposed to wet-to-dry dressings, which are traumatic and can cause significant bleeding on removal. Autolytic debridement can be achieved with the use of dressings that support a moist wound environment,[11] but odor may be increased under occlusion and/or with the use of hydrogels. Local debridement may be performed by very gently scrubbing the necrotic areas with gauze saturated with skin or wound cleanser. Low-pressure irrigation with normal saline using a 35-mL syringe and a 19-gauge needle can be used to remove loose necrotic tissue and decrease bacterial counts. Care should be taken to avoid causing pain with either procedure. In addition, careful sharp debridement by clinicians trained in this procedure can be done to remove loose necrotic tissue. Care should be taken to avoid penetrating viable tissue, because bleeding may be difficult to control. If necrotic tissue on the tumor is extensive, surgical debridement may be indicated to allow for infection prevention, odor control, and exudate management, if compatible with the palliative goals of care for the patient.

Local colonization and odor can be reduced with the use of topical antibacterial preparations. Odor control is by far the most difficult management aspect of tumor necrosis. The literature supports use of topical metronidazole, which has a wide range of activity against anaerobic bacteria, to control wound odor.[12–17] Topical therapy is available by crushing metronidazole tablets in sterile water and creating either a 0.5% solution (5 mg/mL) or a 1% solution (10 mg/mL).[12,15,18] This may be used as a wound irrigant, or gauze may be saturated with the solution and packed into wound cavities. Care must be taken not to allow the gauze packing to desiccate, because dressing adherence may lead to bleeding and pain. Gomolin and Brandt[12] reported the use of a 1% metronidazole solution in the treatment of four geriatric patients with malodorous pressure ulcers. Odor was completely eradicated in three of the patients within 3 to 7 days, and it was dramatically decreased in the fourth patient within 2 days.

An easy, effective alternative to metronidazole solution is MetroGel Topical Gel (metronidazole 0.75%; Galderma Laboratories), which is applied to the wound in a layer one-eighth inch thick. Poteete[16] evaluated the use of metronidazole 0.75% gel in the treatment of 13 patients with malodorous wounds. Metronidazole gel was applied to the wounds daily and covered with either saline-moistened or hydrogel-saturated gauze. At the end of the 9-day observation period, no odor was detected in any wound after the dressings were removed. Finlay and associates[17] prospectively studied subjective odor and pain, appearance, and bacteriological response in 47 patients with malodorous wounds treated with daily application of metronidazole 0.75% gel. Patients were assessed at study entry, at 7 days, and at 14 days. Ninety-five percent of the patients reported decreased odor at 14 days. Anaerobic colonization was discovered in 53% of patients and eliminated in 84% of these cases after treatment. Patients reported decreased pain at day 7, and both discharge and cellulitis were significantly decreased by the end of the study. Because the cost of this product is significantly higher than that of metronidazole 1% solution, practitioners may want to use the gel product initially, to eradicate odor, and then switch to the irrigation solution for maintenance. Systemic metronidazole should not be used for local bacterial colonization, but should only be used if the wound is clinically infected.

Another topical antimicrobial agent is Iodosorb gel, an iodine complexed in a starch copolymer (cadexomer iodine). This product contains slow-release iodine and has been shown to decrease bacterial counts in wounds without cytotoxicity. Seaman[11] reported her clinical experience with this product for reduction of odor associated with venous ulcers. Cadexomer iodine is available in a 40-g tube and is applied to the wound in a one-eighth inch layer. An advantage of this product is exudate absorption: each gram absorbs 6 mL of fluid. Disadvantages include cost (comparable to metronidazole 0.75% gel) and possible burning on application.

Less conventional methods of odor management are also available. Topical use of yogurt or buttermilk has been reported to be successful at eliminating some tumor necrosis odors.[19,20] The yogurt or buttermilk is applied topically to the wound after cleansing. These substances may work by decreasing the wound pH, thus stunting bacterial proliferation and the resultant odor. It is theorized that the low pH of the lactobacilli present in the yogurt or buttermilk is responsible for the alteration in wound pH. There are limited studies supporting the use of yogurt or buttermilk, and none has addressed specific limitations or contraindications for use. Use of peppermint oil or other aromatherapy products, as well as cat litter, in the environment around the patient may also help to eliminate wound odor.

Use of charcoal dressings, which absorb and trap odor, may also be helpful in odor management. Charcoal dressings may be used as either primary or secondary dressings. Because these dressings vary in their application and performance, package inserts should be reviewed before use. A basket of charcoal under the bed or table may also help to rid the environment of wound odor in the home setting.[21]

Although local colonization is treated with topical cleansing, debridement, and antibacterial agents, clinical infection (as evidenced by erythema, induration, increased pain and exudate, leukocytosis, and fever) should be treated with systemic antibiotics. Cultures should be used to identify infecting organisms once the wound is diagnosed with an infection based on clinical signs; cultures should not be used routinely to diagnose infection. Because of the local inflammatory effects of the tumor, wounds may have many of the same signs as infection, so the clinician must be discriminating in differentiating between the two. A complete blood count, assessing the white cell count and differential, may be helpful in guiding assessment and therapy. It is crucial to avoid treating patients with oral antibiotics if they are only colonized and not infected, to prevent side effects and emergence of resistant organisms.

Management of Exudate. Because of the inflammation and edema commonly associated with these wounds, there tends to be significant exudate. Dressings should be chosen to conceal and collect exudate and odor. It is essential to use dressings that contain the exudate, because a patient who experiences unexpected drainage on clothing or bedding may suffer significant feelings of distress and loss of control. Specialty dressings, such as foams, alginates, or starch copolymers, are notably more expensive than gauze pads or cotton-based absorbent pads. However, if such dressings reduce the overall cost by reducing the need for frequent dressing changes, they may be cost-effective. Table 16B–2 summarizes tumor necrosis dressing considerations. Nonadherent dressings are best for the primary contact layer, because they minimize the trauma to the wound associated with dressing changes.

Seaman[11] suggested using nonadherent contact layers, such as Vaseline gauze, for the primary dressing on the wound bed,

Table 16B–2
Dressing Choices for Tumor Necrosis or Malignant Cutaneous Lesions

Type of Wound and Goals of Care	Dressing Choice
Low Exudate	
Maintain moist environment Prevent dressing adherence and bleeding	Nonadherent contact layers • Adaptic (Johnson & Johnson) • Dermanet (DeRoyal) • Mepitel (MöInlycke) • Petrolatum gauze (numerous manufacturers) • Tegapore (3M Health Care) Amorphous hydrogels Sheet hydrogels Hydrocolloids: contraindicated with fragile surrounding skin, may increase odor Semipermeable films: contraindicated with fragile surrounding skin
High Exudate	
Absorb and contain exudate Prevent dressing adherence in areas of lesion with decreased exudate	Alginates Foams Starch copolymers Gauze Soft cotton pads Menstrual pads (excessive exudate)
Malodorous Wounds	
Wound cleansing (see text) Reduce or eliminate odor	Charcoal dressings Topical metronidazole (see text) Iodosorb Gel (Healthpoint): iodine-based, may cause burning

and covering these with soft, absorbent dressings, such as gauze and ABD pads, for secondary dressings to contain drainage. The entire dressing is changed once a day; the secondary dressing should be changed twice a day if drainage strikes through to the outside of the bandage. Menstrual pads may be advantageous, not only because of their excellent absorption but also because the plastic backing blocks exudate and protects clothing. Protection of the surrounding skin is another goal of exudate management.

The skin around the tumor necrosis may be fragile secondary to previous radiation therapy, inflammation due to tumor extension, repeated use of adhesive dressings, or maceration. Although adhesive dressings may assist with drainage and odor control, their potential to strip the epidermis on removal may outweigh their benefit. Using ostomy skin barriers on the skin surrounding the wound and then taping the dressings to the skin barriers (changing them every 5 to 7 days) is one method of protecting surrounding skin from excess drainage and also from the skin stripping that results with dressing changes when tape is used. Another method of protecting the surrounding skin is to use a barrier ointment or skin sealant on the skin surrounding the ulcer. These barriers protect the fragile tissue from maceration and the irritating effects of the drainage on the skin. Dressings can then be held in place with Montgomery straps or tape affixed to a skin barrier placed on healthy skin, flexible netting, tube dressings, sports bras, panties, and the like.

Controlling Bleeding. The viable tissue in a malignant lesion may be very friable, bleeding with even minimal manipulation. Prevention is the best therapy for controlling bleeding. Prevention involves use of a gentle hand in dressing removal and thoughtful attention to the use of nonadherent dressings or moist wound dressings. On wounds with a low amount of exudate, the use of hydrogel sheets, or amorphous hydrogels under a nonadherent contact layer, may keep the wound moist and prevent dressing adherence. Even highly exudating wounds may require a nonadherent contact layer to allow for atraumatic dressing removal. If dressings adhere to the wound on attempted removal, they should be soaked away with normal saline to lessen the trauma to the wound bed. If bleeding does occur, the first intervention should be direct pressure applied for 10 to 15 minutes. Local ice packs may also assist in controlling bleeding. If pressure alone is ineffective, several other options exist. Haisfield-Wolfe and Rund[22] suggested the use of calcium alginate or collagen dressings, because both have hemostatic properties. Waller and Caroline[23] advised use of gauze soaked in 1:1000 epinephrine over the bleeding point or application of sucralfate paste (a 1-g sucralfate tablet crushed in 2 to 3 mL of water-soluble gel) over widespread oozing. As an alternative, use of a topical absorbable hemostatic sponge or foam (e.g., Gelfoam) may be appropriate. Small bleeding points can be controlled with silver nitrate sticks. More aggressive therapy may be necessary in cases of significant bleeding, including transcatheter embolization of the arteries feeding the tumor,[24] intraarterial infusion chemotherapy and radiotherapy,[25] or surgery if compatible with palliative care goals of the patient. Clinicians should not hesitate to consider these options if they will improve the quality of life in patients with tumor necrosis.

Pain Management. Several types of pain are associated with tumor necrosis: deep pain, neuropathic pain, and superficial pain related to procedures.[7] Deep pain should be managed by premedication before dressing changes. Opioids for preprocedural medication may be needed, and rapid-onset, short-acting analgesics may be especially useful for those already receiving other long-acting opioid medication. For management of superficial pain related to procedures, topical lidocaine or benzocaine may be helpful.[26] These local analgesics may be applied to the wound immediately after dressing removal, with wound care delayed until adequate local anesthesia is obtained. Ice packs used before or after wound care may also be helpful to reduce pain.

Another option for topical analgesia is the use of topical opioids, which bind to peripheral opioid receptors.[27–29] Back and Finlay[28] reported on the use of diamorphine 10 mg added to an amorphous hydrogel and applied to the wounds of three patients on a daily basis. Two of the patients had painful pressure ulcers, and the third had a painful malignant ulceration. All three were receiving systemic opioid therapy. The patients noted improved pain control on the first day of treatment. Krajnik and Zbigniew[29] reported the case of a 76-year-old woman with metastatic lesions on her scalp that caused her severe tension pain. Ibuprofen (400 mg three times daily) was ineffective. Because the pain was in a limited area, the authors applied morphine gel 0.08% (3.2 mg morphine in 4 g of amorphous hydrogel). The patient's pain decreased from 7 to 1 on a 10-point visual analog scale within 2 hours after gel application. Pain increased back to 6 at 25.5 hours after application. Therefore, the gel was reapplied daily and maintained pain control with no side effects. Similar results have been obtained by other authors in the care of patients with painful ulcers.[30,31] Additionally, Ballas[32] noted success in treating two patients with painful sickle cell ulcers using topical crushed oxycodone for one patient and topical crushed meperidine for the other one. Nurses should discuss this option for topical pain relief with individual patients and physicians. Because wound care is performed frequently in these patients, topical opioids may be an excellent adjunct to the pain management plan.

Patient and Caregiver Education

The same education provided to patients and caregivers about basic wound care should be provided to those dealing with tumor necrosis. Frequency and procedures for dressing changes, including time of premedication for pain management and alternatives for odor control, should be presented and reinforced. Patient and caregiver education must also focus on the psychosocial aspects of tumor necrosis. Patients are often unable to separate themselves from the wound and may feel as if their bodies are rotting away. Indeed, patients are often unable to view the wound, may become nauseous or retch when dressing changes are performed, or may exhibit other signs of low self-esteem related to the wound. The nurse can facilitate a trusting relationship with the patient by reviewing the goals of care and by openly discussing issues that the patient may not have talked about with other providers. For example, it is helpful to acknowledge odor openly and then discuss how it will be managed. Attention to the cosmetic appearance of the wound with the dressing in place can assist the patient in dealing with body image disturbances. Use of flexible dressings (e.g., foam dressings) and dressings that can fill a defect (e.g., calcium alginates, soft nonwoven gauze) may be appropriate to restore symmetry and provide adequate cosmesis for the patient.

Isolation may result from embarrassment, shame, or guilt. Caregivers may be overcome by the appearance of the wound or the other associated characteristics, such as odor. Assisting the patient and the caregiver to deal with the distressing symptoms of the tumor necrosis so that odor is managed, pain is alleviated, and exudate contained improves the quality of life for these patients and contributes to the goal of satisfactory psychological well-being. Education must include realistic goals for the wound. In cases of tumor necrosis, the goal of complete wound healing is seldom achievable, but through attention to exudate, odor, and pain, quality of life can be maintained even as the tumor necrosis wound degenerates. Determination of priority goals in palliation may be the first step in patient and caregiver education. For example, if the patient is most disturbed by odor, measures to address wound odor should be foremost in the treatment plan. Continual education and evaluation of the effectiveness of the treatment plan are essential to maintaining quality of life for those with tumor necrosis.

FISTULAS

Definition

A fistula is an abnormal passage or opening between two or more body organs or spaces. The most frequently involved organs are the skin and either the bladder or the digestive tract, although fistulas can occur between many other body organs and/or spaces. Often, the organs involved and the location of the fistula influence management methods and complicate care. For example, fistulas involving the small bowel and the vaginal vault and those involving the esophagus and skin create extreme challenges in care related to both the location and the organs involved in the fistula. Although spontaneous closure occurs in at least 50% of all enteric or small-bowel fistulas, the time required to achieve closure is 4 to 7 weeks, so long-term treatment plans are required for all patients with fistulas. Ninety percent of those fistulas that close spontaneously do so within the 4- to 7-week time frame.[33] Therefore, if the fistula has not spontaneously closed with adequate medical treatment within 7 weeks, the goal of care may change to palliation, particularly if chances of closure are limited by other factors. Factors that inhibit fistula closure include complete disruption of bowel continuity, distal obstruction, presence of a foreign body in the fistula tract, an epithelium-lined tract contiguous with the skin, presence of cancer, previous radiation, and Crohn's disease. The presence of any of these factors can be deleterious for spontaneous closure of a fistula. The goals of management for fistula care involve containment of effluent, management of odor, comfort, and protection of the surrounding skin and tissues.

Pathophysiology of Fistula Development

In cancer care, those with gastrointestinal cancers and those who have received irradiation to pelvic organs are at highest risk for fistula development. Fistula development occurs in 1% of patients with advanced malignancy.[33] In most cases of advanced malignancy, the fistula develops in relation to either obstruction from the malignancy or irradiation side effects. Radiation therapy damages the vasculature and underlying structures. In cancer-related fistula development, management is almost always palliative. However, fistula development is not limited to patients with cancer.

In addition to cancer and radiation therapy, postsurgical adhesions, inflammatory bowel disease (Crohn's disease), and small-bowel obstruction place an individual at high risk for fistula development. The number one cause of fistula development is postsurgical adhesions. Adhesions are scar tissues that cause fistula development by providing an obstructive process within the normal passageway. Those with inflammatory bowel disease, Crohn's disease in particular, are prone to fistula development by virtue of the effects of the disease process on the bowel itself. Crohn's disease often involves the perianal area, with fissures and fistulas being common findings. Because Crohn's disease is a transmural disease, involving all layers of the bowel wall, patients are prone to fistula development. Crohn's disease can occur anywhere along the entire gastrointestinal tract, and there is no known cure. Initially, the disease is managed medically with steroids, immunotherapy, and metronidazole for perianal disease. If medical management fails, the patient may be treated with surgical creation of a colostomy, to remove the portion of bowel affected by the disease. In later stages of disease, if medical and surgical management have failed, multiple fistulas may present clinically, and the goal for care becomes living with the fistulas and palliation of symptoms.

Other factors contributing to fistula development include the presence of a foreign body next to a suture line, tension on a suture line, improper suturing technique, distal obstruction, hematoma/abscess formation, tumor or additional disease in anastomotic sites, and inadequate blood supply. Each of these can contribute to fistula formation by promoting an abnormal passage between two body organs. Typically, the contributing factor provides a tract for easier evacuation of stool or urine along the tract rather than through the normal route. Such is the case with a foreign body next to the suture line and with hematoma or abscess formation. In some cases, the normal passageway is blocked, as with tumor growth or obstructive processes. Finally, in many cases, the pathology relates to inadequate tissue perfusion, as with tension on the suture line, improper suturing, and inadequate blood supply.

Fistula Assessment

Assessment of the fistula involves assessment of the source, surrounding skin, output, and fluid and electrolyte status. Evaluation of the fistula source may involve diagnostic tests such as radiographs to determine the exact structures involved in the fistula tract. Assessment of the fistula source involves evaluation of fistula output, or effluent, for odor, color, consistency, pH, and amount. These characteristics provide clues to the origin of the output. Fistulas with highly odorous output are likely to originate in the colon or may be related to cancerous lesions. Fistula output with less odor may have a small-bowel origin. The color of fistula output also provides clues to the source: clear or white output is typical of esophageal fistulas, green output is usual of fistulas originating from the gastric area, and light brown or tan output may indicate small-bowel sources. Small-bowel output is typically thin and watery to thick and pasty in consistency, whereas colonic fistulas have output with a pasty to a soft consistency. The volume of output is often an indication of the source. For small-bowel fistulas, output is typically high, with volumes ranging from 500 to 3000 mL over 24 hours, for low-output and high-output fistulas, respectively. Esophageal fistula output may be as high as 1000 mL over 24 hours. Fistulas can be classified according to output, with those producing less than 500 mL over 24 hours classified as low output and those producing greater volumes classified as high output.[32]

The anatomical orifice location, proximity of the orifice to bony prominences, the regularity and stability of the surrounding skin, the number of fistula openings, and the level at which the fistula orifice exits onto the skin influence treatment options. Fistulas may be classified according to the organs involved and the location of the opening of the fistula orifice. Fistulas with openings from one internal body organ to another (e.g., from small bowel to bladder, from bladder to vagina) are internal fistulas; those with cutaneous involvement (e.g., small bowel to skin) are external fistulas.[33]

The location of the fistula often impedes containment of output. Skin integrity should be assessed for erythema, ulceration, maceration, or denudation from fistula output. Typically, the more caustic the fistula output, the more impaired the surrounding skin integrity. Multiple fistula tracts may also impede containment efforts.

Assessment of fluid and electrolyte balance is essential because of the risk of imbalance in both. In particular, the patient with a small-bowel fistula is at high risk for fluid volume deficit or dehydration and metabolic acidosis due to the loss of large volumes of alkaline small-bowel contents. Significant losses of sodium and potassium are common with small-bowel fistulas. Laboratory values should be monitored frequently. Evaluation for signs of fluid volume deficit is also recommended.

Fistula Management

Wherever anatomically possible, the fistula should be managed with an ostomy pouching technique. The surrounding skin should be cleansed with warm water without soap or antiseptics; skin barrier paste should then be used to fill uneven skin surfaces, so that a flat surface is created to apply the pouch. Pediatric pouches are often smaller and more flexible and may be useful for hard-to-pouch areas where flexibility is needed, such as the neck for esophageal fistulas. The type of pouch should be chosen based on the output of the fistula. For example, if the fistula output is watery and thin, a pouch with a narrow spigot or tube for closure is chosen; in contrast, a fistula with a thick, pasty output would be better managed with a pouch with an open end and a closure clamp. Pouches must be emptied frequently, at least when one-third to one-half full. There are several wound drainage pouching systems on the market that allow for visualization and direct access to the fistula through a valve or door that can be opened and closed. These wound management pouches are available in large sizes and often work well for abdominal fistulas. Pouching of the fistula allows for odor control (many fistulas are quite malodorous), containment of output, and protection of the surrounding skin from damage. Gauze dressings with or without charcoal filters may be used if the output from the fistula is less than 250 mL over 24 hours and is not severely offensive in odor. Colostomy caps (small closed-end pouches) can be useful for low-output fistulas that continue to be odorous.

There are specific pouching techniques that are useful in complex fistula management, including troughing, saddlebagging, and bridging. These techniques are particularly helpful when dealing with fistulas that occur in wounds, most commonly the small-bowel fistula that develops in the open abdominal wound. Troughing is useful for fistulas that occur in the posterior aspect of large abdominal wounds.[34] The skin surrounding the wound and fistula should be lined with a skin barrier wafer and the edge nearest the wound sealed with skin barrier paste. Then, thin film dressings are applied over the top or anterior aspect of the wound, down to the fistula orifice and the posterior aspect of the wound. Finally, a cut-to-fit ostomy pouch is used to pouch the opening in the thin film dressing at the fistula orifice. Wound exudate drains from the anterior portion of the wound (under the thin film dressing) to the posterior portion of the wound and out into the ostomy pouch, along with fistula output. The trough technique does not prevent fistula output from contaminating the wound site.

The bridging technique prevents fistula output from contaminating the wound site and allows for a unique wound dressing to be applied to the wound site. Bridging is appropriate for fistulas that occur in the posterior aspect of large abdominal wounds, where it is important to contain fistula output away from the wound site. Using small pieces of skin barrier wafers, the clinician builds a "bridge" by consecutively layering the skin barriers together until the skin barrier has the appearance of a wedge or bridge and is the same height as the depth of the wound.[33] With the use of a skin barrier paste, the skin barrier wedge is adhered to the wound bed (it does not harm the healthy tissues of the wound bed), next to the fistula opening. An ostomy pouch is then cut to fit the fistula opening, using the wedge or bridge as a portion of intact surrounding skin to adhere the pouch.[33] The anterior aspect of the wound may then be dressed with the dressing of choice.

Saddlebagging is used for multiple fistulas, if it is important to keep the output from each fistula separated and the fistula orifices are close together. Two cut-to-fit ostomy pouches (or more for more fistulas) are used. The fistula openings are cut on the back of the pouch, off-center or as far to the side as possible, and the second pouch is cut to fit the next fistula, off-center as far to the other side as possible. The skin is cleansed with warm water, and skin barrier paste is applied around the orifices. Ostomy pouches are applied, and, where they contact each other (down the middle), they are affixed or adhered to each other in a "saddlebag" fashion. Multiple fistulas can also be managed with one ostomy pouching system that accommodates the multiple openings. Consultation with an enterostomal therapy (ET) nurse or ostomy nurse is extremely advantageous in these cases.

Another method of managing fistulas is by a closed suction wound drainage system. Jeter and colleagues[35] described the use of a Jackson-Pratt drain and continuous low suction in fistula management. After the wound is cleansed with normal saline, the fenestrated Jackson-Pratt drain is placed in the wound, on top of a moistened gauze that has been opened up to line the wound bed (primary contact layer); a second fluffed wet gauze is placed over the drain, and the surrounding skin is prepared with a skin sealant. Next, the entire site is covered with a thin film dressing, which is crimped around the tube of the drain where it exits the wound. The tube exit site is filled with skin barrier paste, and the drain is connected to low continuous wall suction; the connection site may need to be adjusted and may require use of a small "Christmas tree" connector or device and tape to secure it. Jeter and colleagues[35] advised changing the system every 3 to 5 days. Others have used a similar setup for pharyngocutaneous fistulas.[36] A wound closure device that provides intermittent or continuous subatmospheric pressure offers additional options for fistula management.

Pouches to contain the fistula output usually involve odor as well. If odor continues to be problematic with an intact pouching system, internal body deodorants such as bismuth subgallate, charcoal compositions, or peppermint oil may be helpful.[37] Taking care to change the pouch in a well-ventilated room also helps with odor. If odor is caused by anaerobic bacteria, use of 400 mg metronidazole orally three times a day may be helpful. Management of high-output fistulas may be improved with administration of octreotide 300 mcg subcutaneously over 24 hours.[33]

Nutrition management and fluid and electrolyte maintenance are essential for adequate fistula care. Fluid and nutritional requirements may be greatly increased with fistulas, and there are difficulties with fistulas that involve the gastrointestinal system. As a general guideline, the intestinal system should be used whenever possible for nutritional support. If nutrition can bypass the fistula site, absorption and tolerance are better with use of the intestinal tract. For small-bowel fistulas, bypass of the fistula orifice is not always feasible. If the small-bowel fistula is located distally, enough of the intestinal tract may be available to adequately absorb nutrients before the fistula orifice is reached. If the fistula is located more proximally, there may not be enough intestinal tract available for nutrient absorption ahead of the fistula orifice. Many of these patients must be given intravenous hyperalimentation during the early stages of fistula management. The specific goals of fluid and electrolyte and nutritional support for fistula management must be discussed with the patient and family in view of the palliative nature of the overall care plan.

Patient and Caregiver Education

Patient and caregiver teaching first involves adequate assessment of the self-care ability of the patient and of the caregiver's abilities. The patient and caregiver must be taught the management method for the fistula, including pouching techniques, how to empty the pouch, odor control methods, and strategies for increasing fluid and nutritional intake. Many of the pouching techniques used to manage fistulas are complicated and may require continual surveillance by an expert such as an ET nurse or ostomy nurse.

PALLIATIVE STOMA CARE

The significance of palliative care for an individual with a stoma is to improve well-being during this critical time and to attain the best quality of life possible. In regard to the stoma, palliative care is achieved by restoring the most efficient management plan and providing optimal functional capacity. It is essential to involve the family in the plan of care and to provide care to the extent of the patient's wishes.

Management of the ostomy includes physical care as well as psychological and social care. To meet the needs of the patient and family, access to the multidisciplinary care team is crucial. This team may include the ET nurse, physicians such as the surgeon and oncologist, a nutritionist, and social service personnel. The urinary or fecal stoma can be managed (by the ET nurse) to incorporate the needs and goals of both the patient and the caregiver and to provide the highest quality of life possible.

Pathophysiology

A stoma is an artificial opening in the abdominal wall that is surgically created to allow urine or stool to be eliminated by an alternative route. The most common indications for the creation of a stoma are as follows:

1. Cancers that interfere with the normal function of the urinary or gastrointestinal system
2. Inflammatory bowel diseases such as Crohn's or ulcerative colitis
3. Congenital diseases such as Hirschsprung's disease or familial adenomatous polyposis
4. Trauma

In planning the care of an individual with a stoma, it is necessary to understand the type of ostomy that was created, including the contents that will be eliminated.

Types of Diversion

The three types of diversion created with a stoma as the outlet for urine or stool are the ileoconduit (urinary output), the ileostomy (fecal output), and the colostomy (fecal output). Construction of any of these diversions requires the person to wear an external appliance to collect the output.

Ileoconduit. Since the early 1950s, the Bricker ileoconduit has been the primary method for diverting urinary flow in the absence of bladder function. This procedure involves isolation of a section of the terminal ileum. The proximal end is closed, and the distal end is brought out through an opening in the abdominal wall at a site selected before surgery. The ileal segment is sutured to the skin, creating a stoma. The ureters are implanted into the ileal segment, urine flows into the conduit, and peristalsis propels the urine out through the stoma. An external appliance is worn to collect the urine; it is emptied when the pouch is one-third to one-half full, or approximately every 4 hours.

Ileostomy. The ileostomy is created to divert stool away from the large intestine, typically using the terminal ileum. The stoma is created by bringing the distal end of the ileum through an opening surgically created in the abdominal wall and suturing it to the skin. The output is usually a soft, unformed to semiformed stool. Approximately 600 to 800 mL/day is eliminated. An external appliance is worn to collect the fecal material; it is emptied when the bag is one-third to one-half full, usually four to six times per day.

An ileostomy may be temporary or permanent. A temporary ileostomy usually is created when the colon needs time to heal or rest, such as after colon surgery or a colon obstruction. A permanent ileostomy is necessary if the entire colon, rectum, and anus has been surgically removed, such as in colorectal cancer or Crohn's disease.[38]

Colostomy. The colostomy is created proximal to the affected segment of the colon or rectum. A colostomy may be temporary or permanent. There are three sections of the colon: the ascending, transverse, and descending colon. The section of colon used to create the stoma determines in part the location and the consistency of output, which may affect the nutritional and hydration status of the individual at critical times. The ascending colon stoma usually is created on the right midquadrant of the abdomen, and the output is a semiformed stool. The transverse stoma is created in the upper quadrants and is the largest stoma created; the output is usually a semiformed to formed stool. The descending colon stoma most closely mirrors the activity of normal bowel function; it usually is located in the lower left quadrant.

The stoma is created by bringing the distal end of the colon through an opening surgically created in the abdominal wall and suturing it to the skin. An external appliance is worn to collect the fecal material; it is emptied when the bag is one-third to one-half full, usually one or two times per day. A second option for management is irrigation, to regulate the bowel. The patient is taught to instill 600 to 1000 mL of lukewarm tap water through the stoma, using a cone-shaped irrigation apparatus. This creates bowel distention, stimulating peristaltic activity and therefore elimination within 30 to 45 minutes. Repetition of this process over time induces bowel dependence on the stimulus, reducing the spillage of stool between irrigations. The elimination process after initial evacuation is suppressed for 24 to 48 hours.[39,40]

Assessment

Stoma Characteristics. Viability of the stoma is assessed by its color. This should be checked regularly, especially in the early postoperative period. Normal color of the stoma is deep pink to deep red. The intestinal stomal tissue can be compared with the mucosal lining of the mouth. The stoma may bleed when rubbed because of the capillaries at the surface. Bleeding that occurs spontaneously or excessively from stoma trauma can usually be managed by the application of pressure. Bleeding that persists or that originates from the bowel requires prompt investigation, with the management plan based on the cause of the bleeding and the overall status of the individual.[39,40]

A stoma with a dusky appearance ranging from purple to black, or a necrotic appearance, indicates impairment of circulation and should be reported to the surgeon. A necrotic stoma may develop from abdominal distention that causes tension on the mesentery, from twisting of the intestine at the time of surgery, or from arterial or venous insufficiency. Necrotic tissue below the level of the fascia indicates infarction and potential intraabdominal urine or stool leakage. Prompt recognition and surgical reexploration are necessary.

Stoma edema is normal in the early postoperative period as a result of surgical manipulation. This should not interfere with stoma functioning, but a larger opening will need to be cut in the appliance to prevent pressure or constriction of the stoma. Most stomas decrease by 4 to 6 weeks after surgery, with minor changes over 1 year. Teaching the individual to continue to measure the stoma with each change of appliance should alleviate the problem of wearing an appliance with an aperture too large for the stoma. The stoma needs only a space one-eighth of an inch in diameter to allow for expansion during peristalsis.

Stoma herniation occurs when the bowel moves through the muscle defect created at the time of stoma formation and into the subcutaneous tissue. The hernia usually reduces spontaneously when the patient lies in a supine position, as a result of decreased intraabdominal pressure. Problems associated with the formation of a peristomal hernia are increased difficulty with ostomy pouch adherence and possible bowel strangulation and obstruction. The peristomal hernia may be managed conservatively with the use of a peristomal hernia belt to maintain a reduction of the hernia. The belt is an abdominal binder with an opening to allow for the stoma and pouch. The belt is applied with the patient in a supine position, while the hernia is reduced, creating an external pressure that maintains the bowel in a reduced position. Aggressive treatment includes surgical intervention for correction of the peristomal hernia. However, this is usually reserved for emergency situations, such as obstruction or strangulation of the bowel. Colostomy patients who irrigate should be taught to irrigate with the hernia in a reduced position, to prevent perforation of the bowel.

Stoma prolapse occurs as a result of a weakened abdominal wall caused by abdominal distention, formation of a loop stoma, or a large aperture in the abdominal wall. The prolapse is a telescoping of the intestine through the stoma. Stoma prolapse may be managed by conservative or surgical intervention. Surgical intervention is required if there is bowel ischemia, bowel obstruction, or prolapse of excessive length and unreducible segment of bowel. Conservative management includes reducing the stoma while in a supine position to decrease the intraabdominal pressure, then applying continuous gentle pressure at the distal portion of the prolapse until the stoma returns to skin level. If the stoma is edematous, cold soaks or a hypertonic solution such as salt or sugar is applied to reduce the edema before stoma reduction is attempted. Once the stoma is reduced, a support binder is applied to prevent recurrence. In most cases, it is necessary to alter the pouching system by including a two-piece appliance and cutting the barrier size opening larger to accommodate changes in stoma size.

Retraction of the stoma below skin level can occur in the early postoperative period due to tension on the bowel or mesentery or related to breakdown at the mucocutaneous junction. Late retraction usually occurs as a result of tension on the bowel from abdominal distention, most likely as a result of intraperitoneal tumor growth or ascites. Stomal retraction is managed by modification of the pouching system—for example, by using a convex appliance to accommodate changes in skin contour. Stomas that retract below the fascia level require prompt surgical intervention.

Stenosis of the stoma can occur at the skin level or at the level of the fascia. Stenosis that interferes with normal bowel elimination requires intervention. Signs and symptoms of stenosis include change in bowel habits (e.g., decreased output, thin-caliber stools), abdominal cramping, abdominal distention, flank pain from urinary stomas, and nausea or vomiting. The stenotic area may be managed conservatively by dilatation or may require surgical intervention by local excision or laporatomy.[39,40] Many of the stoma problems discussed can occur from simple stretching and displacement of normal organs due to bulky tumors, as might occur in the end stages of some disease states.

Peristomal Skin Problems. Peristomal skin complications commonly include mechanical breakdown, chemical breakdown, rash, and allergic reaction. Mechanical breakdown is caused by trauma to the epidermal skin layer. This is most often related to frequent appliance changes that cause shearing or tearing to the epidermal skin. The result is denuded skin or erythematous, raw, moist, and painful skin. The use of pectin-based powder with or without a light coating of skin sealant aids in healing and protecting the skin from further damage while allowing appliance adherence.

Chemical breakdown is caused by prolonged contact of urine or fecal effluent with the peristomal skin. Inappropriate use of adhesive skin solvents may also result in skin breakdown. The result of chemical breakdown is denudation of the peristomal skin that has been exposed to the caustic effects of the stool, urine, or adhesive solvents. Prompt recognition and management are essential. Modification of the pouching system, such as using a convex wafer instead of a flat wafer or adding protective skin products such as a paste (or both) can be used to correct the underlying problem. Instructing patients and caregivers to thoroughly cleanse the skin with plain water after using the skin solvent can eliminate the problem of denuded skin. Treatment of denuded skin is the same as described previously.

A peristomal fungal rash can occur as a result of excessive moisture or antibiotic administration that results in overgrowth of yeast in the bowel or, at the skin level, due to perspiration under a pouch or leakage of urine or stool under the barrier. The rash is characterized as having a macular, red border with a moist, red to yellow center; it is usually pruritic. Application of antifungal powder, such as nystatin powder, to the affected areas usually produces a prompt response. Blotting the powder with skin preparation or sealant may allow the pouching system to adhere more effectively.

Allergic reactions are most often caused by the barrier and tape used for the pouching system. Erythematous vesicles and pruritus characterize the area involved. Management includes removal of the offending agent. The distribution of the reaction can usually aid in defining the allergen. It may be necessary to perform skin testing if the causative agent is not clear. Patients with sensitive skin and those who use multiple products may respond to simple pouching techniques such as using water to clean the skin, patting the skin dry, and applying the wafer and pouch without the use of skin preparations. Changing to products from a different manufacturer may also eliminate the allergen. A nonadhesive pouching system may be used temporarily for patients with severe blistering and hypersensitivity, to allow healing and prevent further peristomal skin damage. Patients with severe blistering and pruritus may also require temporary use of systemic or topical antihistamines or corticosteriods.[39,40]

Principles and Products for Pouching a Stoma. The continuous outflow of urine or stool from the stoma requires the individual to wear an external appliance at all times. Ideally, the stoma protrudes one-half to three-fourths of an inch above the skin surface, to allow the urine or stool to drain efficiently into a pouch.[40] The objective of stoma management is to protect the peristomal skin, contain output, and control odor.

The skin around the stoma should be cleaned and thoroughly dried before the appliance is positioned over the stoma. An effective pouch should adhere for at least 3 days, although this is not always possible. If no leakage occurs, the same pouch may remain adhered to the skin for up to 10 days. It should then be changed for hygienic reasons and to observe the peristomal area. Today, there is an ever-changing supply of new appliances. Materials and design are being updated rapidly to provide the consumer with the best protection and easiest care.[41] Factors to consider when choosing a pouch include the consistency and type of effluent, the contour of the abdomen, the size and shape of the stoma, and the extent of protrusion, as a well as patient preferences.

Pouching systems are available as one-piece or two-piece systems. The one-piece system is constructed with the odor-proof pouch joined to a barrier ring that adheres to the skin. The barrier can be precut to the size of the stoma, or it can be customized with a cut-to-fit barrier. A two-piece system usually consists of an individual barrier with a flange ring and an odor-proof pouch, which attach (snap) together by matching the ring size of the barrier and pouch. The pouch barrier may be flat or convex and is chosen based on the contour of the abdomen and the extent of stoma protrusion. The colostomy pouch may be closed-ended or open-ended with a clip for closure. Some individuals choose to clean the pouch daily. The pouch of the one-piece system can be cleaned by instilling water into the pouch (with a syringe or turkey baster) and rinsing while preventing the water from reaching the stoma area. The pouch of the two-piece system can be cleaned daily by detaching and washing it in the sink with soap and water and drying it before reattaching it to the barrier.

The urinary pouch has a spout opening to allow for controlled emptying of the pouch. This end may also be attached to a bedside bag or bottle to collect urine. It typically holds up to 2000 mL of urine. The urinary system can be easily disassembled and cleaned with soap and water. After cleaning, a vinegar-and-water solution should be rinsed through the tubing and bag/bottle to prevent urine crystallization.

Skin barriers, skin sealants, powders such as Stomahesive powder or karaya powder, and pastes such as Stomahesive paste

Table 16B–3
Pouch Options

Type	Barrier	Odor-Proof Pouch
1-piece	Flat	Open end with clip (ileostomy with colostomy)
2-piece	Convex	Closed end (colostomy)
	Cut-to-fit	Spout opening (urostomy)
	Precut	

or karaya paste are available to protect the peristomal skin from the caustic affects of urine or stool. These products may also be used to aid in the healing of peristomal skin problems.

Belts and binders are available to assist in maintaining pouch adherence and for management of certain stoma problems.[40] Table 16B-3 presents an overview of pouching options for patients with fecal or urinary diversions.

Interventions

Prevention of Complications. Stoma surgery performed as a palliative measure is not intended to provide a cure but rather to alleviate difficulties such as obstruction, pain, or severe incontinence. Unfortunately, at a difficult time in patients' and families' lives, the created stoma disrupts normal physical appearance, normal elimination of urine or stool, and control of elimination with in some cases loss of body parts and/or sexual function. The patient then has to learn to care for the stoma or allow someone else to care for them. Physically and psychologically, the patient has to come to terms with the presence of the stoma, its function, and care. This takes time and energy to cope emotionally, physically, and socially.[38,39]

Educating the patient and family regarding management issues related to ostomy care and palliation could assist in the physical and psychological adaptation to the ostomy. Additional therapies that may be required for treatment of the underlying disease or a new disease process, such as progressed or recurrent cancer, may affect the activity of the stoma or the peristomal skin. Additional therapies may include chemotherapy, radiation therapy, or analgesics for pain management.

Chemotherapy and radiation therapy may affect a fecal stoma by causing diarrhea. Associated symptoms include abdominal discomfort, larger quantities of loose or liquid stool produced per day, and potential dehydration and loss of appetite with prolonged diarrhea. The ostomy bag requires more frequent emptying, and the ostomy pouch seal needs to be monitored more closely for leakage. In addition, radiation therapy that includes the stoma in the radiation field can cause peristomal skin irritation, particularly redness and maceration. The effects on the peristomal skin may be exacerbated by leakage of urine or stool, as described earlier.[39]

Analgesic use may result in constipation and ultimately bowel obstruction. It is necessary to coadminister stool softeners or laxatives for the prevention of constipation. Irrigation of the colostomy may also assist in treating constipation. The patient and family need to be instructed regarding these measures so that they can be used to treat and prevent constipation. The patient and family need to be aware that adequate pain relief and prevention of constipation can be achieved.[38,39]

Patients may become very tired or may experience anxiety, nausea, or pain as a result of their condition and palliative management. Patients often want to remain as independent as possible but may allow assistance from family and staff. For example, the patient may want to perform the actual pouch change but allow someone else to gather and prepare the supplies. This allows for conservation of energy during part of the task to be accomplished. The patient may also choose the time of day to perform such tasks—when he or she has the most energy and maximal pain and nausea control.[42]

Nutrition and Hydration. Anorexia and dehydration can be major problems for the patient with advancing disease or disease-related treatments such as chemotherapy and radiation therapy. Compromised ingestion, digestion, and absorption can have major influences on nutritional and hydration status.

Anorexia is the loss of appetite resulting from changes in gastrointestinal function, including changes in taste, changes in metabolism, psychological behaviors, and the effects of disease and treatment. Decreased oral intake and changes in metabolism, including decreased protein and fat metabolism, increased energy expenditure, and increased carbohydrate consumption, result in loss of muscle mass, loss of fat stores, and fatigue, leading to weight loss and malnutrition.[43]

Managing the underlying cause of poor nutritional and hydration status, such as controlling the cancer or disease, treating an infection, or slowing down the high-volume ileostomy output, can improve the nutritional state. However, despite effective treatment, other assistance may be necessary, such as small and more frequent meals, nutritional liquid supplements, appetite stimulants (e.g., megestrol acetate), corticosteroids, and parenteral or enteral support.[44] Foods and drinks need to be appealing to the patient. Strong odors and large-portion meals may result in appetite suppression. Promoting comfort before meals may also increase appetite; this may include administering antiemetics or analgesics, oral care, or resting for 30 minutes before mealtime.[43]

Management Issues

Controlling odor, reducing gas, and preventing or managing diarrhea or constipation are management issues related to patients with a colostomy. Odor can be controlled by ensuring that the pouch seal is tight, that odor-proof pouches are used, and that a clean pouch opening is maintained. In addition, deodorants such as bismuth subgallate or chlorophyllin copper complex may be taken orally. Gas can be reduced by decreasing intake of gas-producing foods such as broccoli, cabbage, beans, and beer. Peppermint or chamomile tea may be effective in gas reduction.[38,39]

Diarrhea can be managed as in a patient with an intact rectum and anus. Diarrhea may be a result of viral illness or use of a chemotherapeutic agent. Management includes increased fluid intake, a low-fiber and low-fat diet, and administration of antidiarrhea medications such as loperamide (Imodium), bismuth subsalicylate (Pepto-Bismol), or diphenoxylate plus atropine (Lomotil) by prescription.[40,45] If the patient irrigates, it is necessary to hold irrigation until formed stools return. Constipation more commonly occurs in patients with advanced malignancies due to the affects of analgesic use, reduced activity level, and reduced dietary fiber intake. Management of constipation includes administration of laxatives such as milk of magnesia, mineral oil, or lactulose and initiation of a plan for prevention of constipation with use of stool softeners and laxatives as needed. Cleansing irrigation may be necessary for patients who normally do not irrigate. Cleansing irrigation is performed as described previously for individuals with a colostomy who irrigate for control of bowel movements.[40]

Skin protection, fluid and electrolyte maintenance, prevention of blockage, and modification of medications are management issues related to an ileostomy. Because of the high-volume liquid or loose stools, protecting the skin from this effluent is critical. Leakage of effluent can cause chemical skin breakdown and pain from the irritated skin. The ET nurse can work with the patient and family to determine the cause of the effluent leak. It may be necessary to modify the pouching system, to ensure a proper fit. The peristomal skin may need to be treated with a powder or skin sealant, or both, to aid in healing. The transit time of food and wastes through the gastrointestinal system and out through the ileostomy is rapid and potentially contributes to dehydration and fluid and electrolyte imbalance. Ensuring adequate fluid and electrolyte intake is essential and may be accomplished by ingestion of sports drinks or nutrition shakes. Patients with an ileostomy are instructed to include fiber in their diet, to bulk stools and promote absorption of nutrition and medications.

Food blockage occurs when undigested food particles or medications partially or completely obstruct the stoma outlet at the fascia level. It is necessary to instruct the patient and family about the signs of a blockage, including malodorous, high-volume liquid output or no output accompanied by abdominal cramping, distention, and/or nausea and vomiting. These symptoms should be reported as soon as they occur. Blockage is resolved by lavage or mini-irrigation performed by the physician or ET nurse. A catheter is gently inserted into the stoma until the blockage is reached, 30 to 60 mL of normal saline is instilled, and the catheter is removed to allow for the return. This process is repeated until the blockage has resolved. Patient teaching should be reinforced regarding the need to chew food well before swallowing, to prevent food blockage. Time-release tablets and enteric-coated medications should be avoided because of inadequate or unpredictable absorption. Medications often come in various forms, including liquid, noncoated, patch, rectal suppository, subcutaneous or intravenous administration. Choosing the most appropriate route that provides the greatest efficacy for the individual is essential. For example, a transdermal patch may be used for analgesia instead of a time-released pain tablet. For patients who have an intact rectum that is no longer in continuity with the proximal bowel, rectal administration of medications is effective.[45]

Management issues for an individual with an ileoconduit include prevention of a urinary tract infection, stone formation, peristomal skin protection, and odor control. Each of these issues is preventable by the maintenance of dilute and acidic urine through adequate fluid intake (1800 to 2400 mL/day). Vitamin C (500 to 1000 mg/day) and citrus fruits and drinks may assist in accomplishing acidic urine. Alkaline urine can cause encrustations on the stoma and peristomal skin damage with prolonged exposure. Acetic acid soaks may be applied three or four times per day to treat the encrustations until they dissolve. Adjustments in the pouching system may be necessary to prevent leakage of urine onto the skin, and the temporary addition of powder, paste, skin sealant, or some combination of these products may be needed to aid healing of the affected skin.[40]

CASE REPORT
Mrs. P, a Patient with Bladder Cancer

Mrs. P is a 75-year-old woman with bladder cancer. She was diagnosed 2 months ago. She presented with symptoms of difficulty passing urine, hematuria, and painful urination. She had a 15-pound weight loss, significant fatigue, and anorexia. Investigations demonstrated a large mass within the bladder with ureteral obstruction, intraabdominal mass, and liver lesions. Mrs. P's care was complicated by underlying medical conditions including sick sinus syndrome, chronic hyperkalemia, nutritional depletion, and fatigue. Her past medical history included treatment for ovarian cancer 38 years earlier with radiation therapy. She met with the urological surgeon, medical oncologist, and radiation oncologist. The plan of care was determined to be palliative care, with the goal to keep her as comfortable as possible and provide the best quality of life. Her son became her primary caregiver, with assistance from a daughter who lives out of town.

Mrs. P underwent placement of an ileoconduit and began chemotherapy. Radiation therapy was not an option because she had already received maximum radiation exposure. She required placement of a pacemaker at the initiation of chemotherapy. She developed a hypersensitivity reaction, erythema without desquamation, on her abdomen at the site of a prior radiation reaction. This resolved with a short course of oral steroids. Because of her limited activity, she developed a stage II partial-thickness pressure sore at the midlumbar vertebral body. The pressure sore was clean and the wound bed was pink, with granulation tissue present, minimal exudate, no necrotic tissue, and intact surrounding tissue.

Wound management included daily cleaning with soap and water when assisted with bathing. Mrs. P reported pain at the site as being a 1 or 2 on a pain scale of 0 to 10. She was able to empty and change the ileoconduit pouch with assistance from her son every 3 to 4 hours, including at night. She changed the barrier and pouch every 3 days to avoid leakage. She was able to eat orally without difficulty; however, she had little to no appetite. Her serum albumin concentration was 2.8 mg/dL. She also experienced nausea with the chemotherapy. Unfortunately, she experienced increasing pain in her lower abdomen and required increasing amounts of narcotics. The use of the narcotics caused constipation and bowel obstruction, which was complicated by radiation changes to the bowel resulting from prior treatment.

To assist this patient in the promotion of palliation and comfort, the following measures were advised. Mrs. P was given a large bag to be connected to the ileoconduit pouch at night, to allow for a full night's sleep for both patient and caregiver. The ileoconduit pouching system was changed to a convex barrier, which decreased the frequency of appliance change to every 5 to 7 days instead of every 3 days. In terms of the pressure sore, the patient and her son were taught pressure relief techniques including side-lying and use of pillows. The son was also taught placement of a hydrocolloid dressing over the wound site and to change this dressing every 3 days. The patient was given a bowel regimen to assist in prevention of bowel obstruction; this regimen included stool softeners, laxatives, and increased fluids. Mrs. P was encouraged to continue her pain medication regimen to maintain comfort. She was given antinausea medication to minimize nausea associated with the chemotherapy.

Summary

Skin disorders are both emotionally and physically challenging for patients and caregivers. Cutaneous symptoms may be the result of disease progression (e.g., tumor necrosis, fistula development), complications associated with end-stage disease or the end of life (e.g., pressure ulcers), or simple changes in function of urinary or fecal diversions. All cutaneous symptoms require attention to basic care issues, creativity in management strategies, and thoughtful attention to the psychosocial implications of cutaneous manifestations. Palliative care intervention strategies for skin disorders reflect an approach similar to those for nonpalliative care. Although the goals of care do not include curing the condition, they always include alleviating the distressing symptomology and improving quality of life. The most distressing symptoms associated with skin disorders are odor, exudate, and pain. The importance of attention to skin disorders for palliative care is related to the major effect of these conditions on the quality of life and general psychological well-being of the patient.

REFERENCES

1. Lookingbill DP, Spangler N, Sexton FM. Skin involvement as the presenting sign of internal carcinoma. J Am Acad Dermatol 1990;22:19–26.
2. Lookingbill DP, Spangler N, Helm KF. Cutaneous metastases in patients with metastatic carcinoma: A retrospective study of 4020 patients. J Am Acad Dermatol 1993;29:228–236.
3. Rosen T. Cutaneous metastasis. Med Clin North Am 1980;64:885–900.
4. Brodland DG, Zitelli JA. Mechanisms of metastasis. J Am Acad Dermatol 1992;27:1–8.
5. Ivetic O, Lyne PA. Fungating and ulcerating malignant lesions: a review of the literature. J Adv Nurs 1990;15:83–88.
6. Grocott P, Cowley S. The palliative management of fungating malignant wounds: Generalising from multiple-case study data using a system of reasoning. Int J Nurs Stud 2001;38:533–545.
7. Naylor W. Assessment and management of pain in fungating wounds. Br J Nurs 2001;10(22 Suppl):S33–S36,S38,S40.
8. Clark J. Metronidazole gel in managing malodorous fungating wounds. Br J Nurs 2002;11(6 Suppl):S54–S60.
9. Haisfield-Wolfe ME, Baxendale-Cox LM. Staging of malignant cutaneous wounds: A pilot study. Oncol Nurs Forum 1999;26:1055–1064.
10. Van Leeuwen BL, Houwerzijl M, Hoekstra HJ. Educational tips in the treatment of malignant ulcerating tumours of the skin. Eur J Surg Oncol 2000;26:506–508.
11. Seaman S. Dressing selection in chronic wound management. J Am Podiatr Med Assoc 2002;92:24–33.
12. Gomolin IH, Brandt JL. Topical metronidazole therapy for pressure sores of geriatric patients. J Am Geriatr Soc 1983;31:710–712.
13. Newman V, Allwood M, Oakes RA. The use of metronidazole gel to control the smell of malodorous lesions. Palliat Med 1989;3:303–305.
14. Bower M, Stein R, Evans TRJ, Hedley A, Pert P, Coombes RC. A double-blind study of the efficacy of metronidazole gel in the treatment of malodorous fungating tumours. Eur J Cancer 1992;28A:888–889.
15. Rice TT. Metronidazole use in malodorous skin lesions. Rehabil Nurs 1992;17:244–245,255.
16. Poteete V. Case study: Eliminating odors from wounds. Decubitus 1993;6(4):43–46.
17. Finlay IG, Bowszyc J, Ramlau C, Gwiezdzinski Z. The effect of topical 0.75% metronidazole gel on malodorous cutaneous ulcers. J Pain Symptom Manage 1996;11:158–162.
18. Whedon MA. Practice corner: What methods do you use to manage tumor-associated wounds? Oncol Nurs Forum 1995;22:987–990.
19. Welch LB. Simple new remedy for the odour of open lesions. RN 1981;44:42–43.
20. Schulte MJ. Yogurt helps to control wound odor. Oncol Nurs Forum 1993;20:1262.
21. Cormier AC, McCann E, McKeithan L. Reducing odor caused by metastatic breast cancer skin lesions. Oncol Nurs Forum 1995;22:988–999.
22. Haisfield-Wolfe ME, Rund C. Malignant cutaneous wounds: A management protocol. Ostomy Wound Manage 1997;43:56–66.
23. Waller A, Caroline NL. Smelly tumors. In: Waller A, Caroline NL, eds. Handbook of Palliative Care in Cancer. Boston: Butterworth-Heinemann, 1996:69–73.

24. Rankin EM, Rubens RD, Reidy JF. Transcatheter embolisation to control severe bleeding in fungating breast cancer. Eur J Surg Oncol 1988;14:27–32.
25. Murakami M, Kuroda Y, Sano A, Okamoto Y, Nishikawa T, Shimura S, Matsuue S. Validity of local treatment including intraarterial infusion chemotherapy and radiotherapy for fungating adenocarcinoma of the breast. Am J Clin Oncol 2001;24: 388–391.
26. Sawynok J. Topical and peripherally acting analgesics. Pharmacol Rev 2003;55:1–20.
27. Stein C. The control of pain in peripheral tissue by opioids. N Engl J Med 1995;332:1685–1690.
28. Back IN, Finlay I. Analgesic effect of topical opioids on painful skin ulcers. J Pain Symptom Manage 1995;10:493.
29. Krajnik M, Zbigniew Z. Topical morphine for cutaneous cancer pain. Palliat Med 1997;11:325.
30. Zeppetella G, Paul J, Ribeiro M. Analgesic efficacy morphine applied topically to painful ulcers. J Pain Symptom Manage 2003;25:555–558.
31. Flock P. Pilot study to determine the effectiveness of diamorphine gel to control pressure ulcer pain. J Pain Symptom Manage 2003;25:547–554.
32. Ballas SK. Treatment of painful sickle cell leg ulcers with topical opioids. Blood 2002;99:1096.
33. Bryant RA. Management of drain sites and fistula. In: Bryant RA, ed. Acute and Chronic Wounds: Nursing Management. St. Louis: Mosby Year Book, 1992:248–287.
34. Wiltshire BL. Challenging enterocutaneous fistula: A case presentation. J Wound Ostomy Cont Nurs 1996;23:297–301.
35. Jeter KF, Tintle TE, Chariker M. Managing draining wounds and fistula: New and established methods. In: Krasner D, ed. Chronic Wound Care. King of Prussia, PA: Health Management Publications, 1990:240–246.
36. Harris A, Komray RR. Cost-effective management of pharyngocutaneous fistulas following laryngectomy. Ostomy Wound Manage 1993;39:36–44.
37. McKenzie J, Gallacher M. A sweet smelling success. Nurs Times 1989;85:48–49.
38. Breckman B. Rehabilitation in palliative care: Stoma management. In: Doyle D, Hanks G, MacDonald N, eds. Oxford Textbook of Palliative Medicine. New York: Oxford University Press, 1998:543–549.
39. Doughty D. Principles of fistula and stoma management. In: Berger A, Portenoy R, Weissman D, eds. Principles and Practice of Supportive Oncology. New York: Lippincott-Raven, 1998: 285–294.
40. Erwin-Toth P, Doughty DB. Principles and procedures of stomal management. In: Hampton BG, Bryant RA, eds. Ostomies and Continent Diversions: Nursing Management. Philadelphia: Mosby Year Book, 1992:29–94.
41. Anonymous. The 1998 ostomy/wound management buyers guide. Ostomy/Wound Manage 1998;44:4.
42. Dodd M. Self-care and patient/ family teaching. In: Yarbro C, Frogge M, Goodman M, eds. Cancer Symptom Management. Boston: Jones and Bartlett, 1999:20–32.
43. Tait N. Anorexia–cachexia syndrome. In: Yarbro C, Frogge M, Goodman M, eds. Cancer Symptom Management. Boston: Jones and Bartlett, 1999:183–208.
44. Bruera E. ABC of palliative care: Anorexia, cachexia, and nutrition. BMJ 1997;315:1219–1222.
45. Martz C. Diarrhea. In: Yarbro C, Frogge M, Goodman M, eds. Cancer Symptom Management. Boston: Jones and Bartlett, 1999:522–545.

17

Michelle Rhiner and Neal E. Slatkin

Pruritus, Fever, and Sweats

The constant itching is worse than the pain. There is no rest; it continues day and night. It feels like a thousand ants are crawling all over my body.—A patient

- ***Key Points***
- *Pruritus is not a pain state, but it causes considerable distress that affects patients psychologically, physically, socially, and spiritually.*
- *Treatment choices for pruritus should be made based on the type of pruritus involved and should use both local and systemic measures.*
- *The management of fever and sweats in palliative care should be focused on comfort measures.*

PRURITUS

Pruritus, derived from the Latin word *prurire,* which means "to itch," is a common and poorly understood symptom of both localized and systemic disorders (Table 17-1). The difficulties of defining the clinical characteristics of pruritus are in part related to the ambiguities of the available terminology and difficulties in quantifying this subjective disorder. "Itch," while describing the actual experience of sensory discomfort, is sometimes confused with scratching, the response used to relieve the discomfort. The literature is also less than clear on the distinction between itching and pruritus.[1,2] "Itch" is probably best reserved to describe the actual sensory discomfort that may arise in response to a fleeting stimulus or a pathological disorder.[3] The term "pruritus," is generally used to refer to a pathological condition in which the sensations of itch are intense and often generalized and trigger repeated scratching in an attempt to relieve the discomfort. Quantification of itch intensity, which is necessary for both clinical management and intervention studies, usually relies on the same 0-to-10 scale used to rate pain and other subjective symptoms. An assessment can also be made of "itch behaviors," such as rubbing and scratching, or the physical manifestations of these behaviors, such as the severity and distribution of scratch-induced excoriation.

Although itching is not normally considered a pain state, its neurotransmission parallels that of pain, and the discomfort it causes can be just as distressing as conditions ordinarily considered painful. Words used to describe pruritus include "intense itch," "stinging," "burning," "pins and needles," "tickle," "a creeping or crawling sensation," and "pain." The particular descriptor used often depends on whether the cause of the itch is primarily cutaneous or neuropathic and, in the case of cutaneous conditions, which inflammatory mediators have been activated. Like persistent pain, persistent itch, especially when generalized, can cause considerable distress, including alterations in mood and

Table 17–1
Differential Diagnoses for Pruritus

Systemic Causes

Endocrine/metabolic

 Hyperthyroidism and hypothyroidism

 Hyperparathyroidism and hypoparathyroidism

 Diabetes mellitus

 Zinc deficiency

 Pyridoxine (vitamin B_6) and niacin deficiency

 Chronic renal insufficiency and failure

 Dialysis dermatosis

Hepatic

 Cholestasis (e.g., primary biliary cirrhosis, drug-induced)

 Extrahepatic biliary obstruction

 Hepatitis

Connective tissue disorders

 Sjögren syndrome

 Systemic lupus erythematosus

 Chronic graft versus host disease

Infectious

 Syphilis

 Human immunodeficiency virus

 Parasitic (e.g., onchocerciasis, filariasis)

Neurological disorders

 Stroke, brain tumor, brain injury (hemipruritus)

 Multiple sclerosis (hemipruritus or paroxsymal pruritus)

 Peripheral neuropathy (usually small-fiber neuropathy)

 Post-herpes zoster

 Tabes dorsalis

 Notalgia paresthetica

Other

 Sarcoid

 Pregnancy

Psychological/psychiatric

 Psychosis, psychogenic causes

Malignancies

 Polycythemia rubra vera

 Carcinoid syndrome

 Cutaneous T-cell lymphomas (mycosis fungoides, Sézary syndrome)

 Other lymphomas and Hodgkin's disease

 Plasma cell dyscrasias (e.g., multiple myeloma) with paraproteinemias

 Other solid tumors

Hematological

 Iron deficiency anemia

 Systemic mastocystosis

Drug-Induced Causes

Release of endogenous mediators

 Opioids

 Amphetamines

 Cocaine

Hypersensitivity

 Acetylsalicylic acid (aspirin)

 Quinidine

 Niacinamide

 Etretinate

Other medications

Dermatological Causes

Infections

 Dermatophytosis

 Folliculitis

Infestations

 Pediculosis (lice)

 Scabies

Inflammatory

 Atopic dermatitis

 Contact dermatitis

 Drug hypersensitivity

 Eczema

 Psoriasis

 Urticaria

Miscellaneous

 Insect bites

 Systemic mastocytosis

 Pregnancy-associated

 Xerosis (dry skin)

 Sunburn

Source: Lowitt and Bernhard (1992), reference 12.

loss of sleep. Moreover, persistent scratching can cause skin excoriations and cutaneous infection, which can also be painful and contribute to the vicious cycle of itching.[4]

Skin Anatomy

The skin is the body's first line of defense and its largest organ system. It consists of two layers, the *epidermis* (outer layer) and the *dermis* (inner layer), with a basement membrane zone dividing the two. Subcutaneous tissue, consisting primarily of fat and connective tissue, lends support to the neural and vascular systems that supply the skin and contains *eccrine* glands (ordinary sweat glands) and deep hair follicles.

The cells of the epidermis produce *keratin* (a fibrous protein), which imparts durability to the skin and protection against real-world frictions, and *melanin*, which protects against ultraviolet radiation. There are five layers of the epidermis: stratum corneum, stratum lucidum, stratum granulosum, stratum spinosum, and stratum germinativum (the single layer of basal cells attached to the basal membrane). Within these layers are found four major cell types: *keratinocytes* (which produce keratin), *melanocytes* (pigment-synthesizing cells), *Langerhans' cells* (derived from bone marrow cells, which assist in cutaneous immune responses and produce prostaglandins), and *Merkel's cells* (mechanoreceptors).[5]

The dermis separates the epidermis from the subcutaneous tissues and is well vascularized, providing nutrients to the more superficial layers of skin. The two layers of the dermis are the *papillary dermis* (which contains capillary venules, lymph vessels, and nerve fibers) and the *reticular dermis* (the thicker layer of the dermis, consisting of collagen bundles interlaced by elastic fibers and ground substance). The cell types found in the dermis include *fibroblasts* (which secrete enzymes necessary to remodel the connective tissue matrix), *macrophages* (which synthesize enzymes that enhance or suppress lymphocytic activity and express inflammatory mediators), *lymphocytes,* and *mast cells* (which contain among other substances the pruitogenic mediator histamine).

Pathophysiology

Neural innervation of the skin is complex. As the barrier that functionally separates the self from the nonself, the skin's sensory innervation must allow for all manner of touch, temperature, and pain sensitivity while at the same time responding to changes in environmental conditions. Receptors for pain, heat, cold, touch, pressure, and pleasure are distributed widely within the skin. These receptors are in turn innervated by a variety of afferent nerve types, including well-myelinated A fibers (which relay sharp pain, proprioception, direction of movement along the skin), myelinated D fibers, and unmyelinated C fibers. Afferent C fibers comprise 70% of all peripheral neurons transmitting to the central nervous system (CNS) and are of three types: C mechanoreceptors, cold thermoreceptors, and C polymodal nociceptors. Maintenance of the skin's function as a protective barrier and temperature-regulating organ also requires a motor, or efferent, nerve supply. The ongoing turnover and replacement of epidermal cells, which maintains the skin's function as a protective barrier, requires a rich vascular supply. This vascular supply is in part regulated by sympathetic efferent fibers. The skin's function as a temperature-regulating system also depends on changes in cutaneous vascularity as well as the function of sweat glands and erector pili muscles (pilomotor muscles are responsible for "goosebumps"). Thermoregulatory sympathetic nerves help to modulate body temperature by either vasodilatation or vasoconstriction and by controlling the function of the sweat glands.

The sensation of itch can arise from either exogenous or endogenous stimuli. Regardless of the origin, evidence suggests that the sensation is transmitted by otherwise inactive nonmyelinated C nerve fibers. Such cutaneous sensory nerves can be activated by a variety of chemical or physical stimuli and serve as the final common sensory pathway for transmission of the itch stimulus. The ultimate sensation of itch, therefore, often provides little information about the etiology or provoking factors of itch. Chemical stimuli include caustic and abrasive substances, which cause skin injury, as well as a variety of potential topical allergens, including additives in perfumes and cleaning products. Physical stimuli that can cause pruritus include sunburn, negative pressure, moving suddenly from cold to heat in the presence of moisture, low-voltage electrical stimulation, and the epicutaneous application of caustic substances. Through uncertain mechanisms, repeated scratching itself can promote itch. Scratching causes *lichenification,* or thickening of the epidermis, which may decrease the sensitivity of large nerve fibers that may "gate" the perception of itch.[6] The exact mechanisms by which chemical and physical stimuli cause itch are in some instances stimulus-dependent, generally acting either directly on the free nerve endings or indirectly through the release of histamine (from dermal mast cells) or other inflammatory mediators.

As discussed above, the neurotransmission of itch typically begins with activation of the free, or penicillate, nerve endings of unmyelinated polymodal C nociceptive fibers, which lie at the epidermal–dermal junction. The terminal ends of these fibers form a rich arborization throughout the granular layers of the epidermis and dermis. Why some signals carried by these fibers are interpreted as itch and others as burning pain appears to depend on the pattern of neural firing and/or of coactivation of other nerve fibers.[7,8] Activated C polymodal nociceptive fibers transmit their signals back to their nerve cells in the dorsal root ganglia and then to the spinal cord to synapse in the substantia gelatinosa of the dorsal horn. After interacting with interneurons within the dorsal horn, fibers ascend in the anterolateral pathways (including the spinothalamic tract) to terminate within the brain stem and thalamus. The role played by the cerebral cortex in the mediation of itch remains undetermined but, as will be indicated below, appears to at least in part inhibitory. In both the laboratory and the clinic, brain injury can result in clinical itching.[9–11]

The neurochemical mediation of itch begins with activation of the polymodal nociceptive C fibers. These contain neuropeptides such as substance P, neurokinin A, vasoactive intestinal peptide, and calcitonin gene–related peptide.[3,12] Of these, substance P is the best studied and most abundant; it acts as the major puritogenic peptide. Its local release in response to neural activation may secondarily activate release of histamine from dermal mast cells, as well as other inflammatory mediators. These mediators may include prostaglandins, interleukins, serotonin, and neuropeptides such as endogenous opiates.[1,3,4] Capsaicin, an alkaloid from the chili pepper plant, typically evokes pain when applied to the mucous membranes or skin, due to release of substance P. When applied at very low concentrations, however, the sensation of itch rather than pain may occur. When chronically applied, capsaicin depletes substance P and, therefore, can block transmission of both itch and pain. Prostaglandins can lower the threshold to chemically induced itch, though prostaglandin antagonists do not typically have antipruritic effects except in certain hematological disorders such as polycythemia vera.[13] Other mediators that produce itch are the endopeptidases. These include such enzymes as trypsin, chymotrypsin, bradykinin, kallikrein, and papain, which have been demonstrated to cause pruritus when injected into the skin even in the absence of dermal histamine. Itching powder, or cowhage, which is derived from the legume *Mucuna pruriens,* contains endopeptidases that cause the sensation of itch.[6] One mechanism by which microorganisms, such as bacteria, fungi, and parasites, may cause itching is the release of endopeptidases and other inflammatory mediators.

Serotonin is also an important mediator of pruritus, as revealed by the response of various pruritic states to antiserotonergic therapy. 5-hydroxytryptamine-3 (5-HT_3) antagonists (e.g., ondansetron, granisetron) have been used to palliate pruritus associated with uremia and cholestasis.[14,15] The temperature-dependent pruritus seen with polycythemia and lymphoreticular malignancies may also respond to antiserotonergic therapies.

Etiology

Pruritus, like pain, is multifactorial in origin and can be a symptom of diverse pathophysiologies. Like pain, pruritus can at times serve as a warning sign of external or internal threats to the organism or exist only as a discomforting and unwelcome symptom. Management of pruritus must begin with a thorough assessment of the various etiological causes. Several different classification systems for pruritus have been proposed and are useful in conceptualizing its causes. When no cause can be found, even after a meticulous evaluation, it is referred to as primary, or idiopathic, pruritus. When symptoms are severe and generalized, the patient should remain under continued surveillance for the development of a possible malignancy.[16–18] Secondary pruritus can arise from either dermatological or nondermatological causes, and the distribution can be localized or systemic. Acute localized onset of pruritus is less suggestive of systemic disease than is chronic generalized pruritus.

Secondary Pruritus. Secondary pruritus can be related to either exogenous agents, such as scabies, insect bites, and fungi, or endogenous factors, for example, atopic dermatitis, psoriasis, and biliary obstruction. Pruritus caused by a specific disease may require medical or surgical intervention. As noted above, itch can arise from a variety of exogenous physical and chemical stimuli, as well as from a large number of endogenous causes. Other endogenous causes for pruritus are not as well understood. In metabolic disorders, malignancies, and conditions of organ failure, pruritus may be due to hormonal imbalance, excessive production of cytokines, or build-up of metabolic by-products. Some of the most common causes of pruritus in the palliative care setting include senile pruritus, cholestasis, skin dermatoses, drugs, uremia, and psychogenic etiologies.[19]

Various Common Clinical Situations

Atopic Dermatitis. Pruritus in atopic dermatitis (AD) arises from the release of proinflammatory cytokines from mast cells and keratinocytes.[19] It is postulated that there is a dysfunction of bone marrow–derived cells migrating to the skin rather than an intrinsic cutaneous defect. Lymphocytic infiltrates of AD consist of T-helper cells. Both the Langerhans' cells and macrophages found in AD lesions have surface-bound immunoglobulin E (IgE). The patterns of cytokine production are also distinctive, due to the presence of interleukin-4 (IL-4) with the acute inflammatory phase and IL-5 and eosinophil infiltration with chronic inflammation.[20]

Cholestatic Jaundice. In cholestatic liver disease, the accumulation of bile salts is presumed to be a causative factor in pruritus, though an association with bile levels in the skin and blood has not been consistently demonstrated.[21,22] Moreover, the response of pruritus to a variety of agents, each with differing mechanisms of action (e.g., ondansetron, rifampin, opiate antagonists, propofol, cholestyramine, norethandrolone, etc.) renders the primary causative factor even more obscure.[23–27] More recent evidence points to the accumulation of pruritogenic endogenous opiates.[28–30]

Opioid-Induced Pruritus. Opioids can cause pruritus, whether administered by the systemic, intraspinal, or intracisternal route. Clinically, itching is most commonly seen after intrathecal administration; then, typically, it is initially localized and most severely experienced in and about the face. Epidural administration, due to the higher systemic levels of opiate achieved with this route, tends to cause more generalized itching. Among opioid-naive cesarean section patients, as many as 60% to 80% receiving epidural morphine report pruritus, with more than half of these requiring treatment.[31,32] The occurrence among palliative care patients, most of whom are not opiate-naive at the time of epidural placement, is considerably less, suggesting that tolerance to the pruritogenic effects of opiates develops with continued opioid exposure. The mechanisms for opioid-induced pruritus are several. Opioids are known to trigger mast-cell degranulation with histamine release, which probably accounts for the pruritus seen with systemic opioid administration. Opioid antagonists can attenuate histamine-induced itch unrelated to opioid administration, suggesting that endogenous opioids play an intermediary role in some forms of chemically induced pruritus.[33] Morphine, which appears to cause greater histamine release than fentanyl, meperidine, or oxymorphone, is most frequently implicated in opioid-induced pruritus. Changing to an alternative opioid (opioid rotation) may be a successful management strategy.[34–38] The fact that pruritus can be caused by either intrathecal or intracisternal opioid administration also speaks to a direct pruritogenic effect of opioids on the CNS.

Pruritus Associated with Lesions of the Central Nervous System. Pruritus may also arise from disorders of the CNS (e.g., cerebrovascular accident pruritus).[10] Cases of hemipruritus have been described following stroke and with multiple sclerosis (MS). Phantom itch can occur in the amputated limb.[39] Paroxysmal itching may also result from nerve root demyelination in MS.[40,41]

Anorectal Pruritus (Pruritus Ani). While sometimes mistakenly viewed as a discrete diagnosis, anorectal pruritus is a common symptom of a large number of disorders affecting the lower colorectal area. Common etiologies include hemorrhoids, pinworms and other parasites, fungal infection, rectal irritation and dryness from detergent soaps, rectal seepage, and cryptitis from undigested food particles. Premalignant conditions, such as Bowen's disease and Paget's disease, may also present with these symptoms. In one reported series, 16% of 109 patients evaluated for pruritus ani were found to have a neoplastic lesion in the anorectal area.[42,43]

Uremia. Pruritus can be a disabling symptom of end-stage renal disease and is not relieved by dialysis. Between 80% and 90% of patients undergoing hemodialysis suffer from this symptom.[44] As with many systemic causes of pruritus, the pathogenesis is poorly understood. Recent studies have shown affected patients to have high plasma histamine levels. These levels, as well as clinical pruritus, were significantly reduced by therapy with recombinant erythropoietin, the treatment reaching its maximal efficacy after 3 to 4 weeks.[45] Other potential causes of pruritus include secondary hyperparathyroidism, uremic and other forms of polyneuropathy, xerosis, and hypervitaminosis A.

Evaluation of the Patient with Pruritus

Evaluation of pruritus should be thorough and systematic, applying the same principles used when assessing pain. Quantify as much as possible any physical findings as well as subjective responses to the pruritus (e.g., distress associated with the itch based on a scale of 0–10, with 0 being "no distress" and 10 representing "severe distress").

Location. It is important to recognize whether the itch reported by the patient is generalized throughout the body, focal to a single region, or more widespread but in a particular pattern. Itching around skin creases of the wrists, axilla, and intertriginous areas, as well as the umbilicus and nipples, suggests scabies mite infestation. Anogenital itching may be due to contact dermatitis (e.g., from menstrual or continent pads, deodorants, washing products), *Candida* or other fungal infection, other infestations, or potentially psychogenic causes. Localized dermatitis, for instance, with a dermatomal distribution, may indicate prior herpes zoster infection or other segmental neurological abnormality. Generalized pruritus may arise from a large number of causes, including organ failure, endocrinopathy, or dry skin.

Presence or Absence of Rash. Pruritus resulting from systemic disease is seldom characterized by a rash, though with histamine and serotonin release, a mild flush may be present. It is important to distinguish between a true rash and the stigmata of frequent scratching, including excoriations and dermatographia. Focal rash may indicate contact sensitivity, evolving skin infection, or dryness of skin with associated flaking.

Quality of Symptoms. The common itch consists of an irresistible and persistent tickling sensation, which is usually, at least transiently, relieved with scratching. In addition to bearing the tickling sensation common to the itch experience, itch from irritant dermatitis and herpes zoster typically has a burning quality. Actual pain may coexist with itch in herpes zoster and other neuropathic lesions or arise from the trauma of repeated scratching.

Aggravating and Alleviating Factors. Topical application of heat often worsens itching, whereas cold diminishes the sensation. Worsening of pruritus after a hot shower is typical of Hodgkin's disease, myeloid metaplasia, and polycythemia vera. Consumption of alcohol may also induce itching in these conditions.

Laboratory Evaluations. Laboratory tests are used most commonly in cases where the manifestation of pruritus is of the generalized type. In such cases, the evaluation should be directed towards an underlying systemic cause. Laboratory tests should include a complete blood count (with differential leukocyte count), and liver, renal, and thyroid panels.[19]

Treatment/Management of Pruritus

Local Dermatological Measures

Topical Treatment. Dry skin (xerosis) is common in patients who have undergone chemotherapy or radiation therapy. Xerosis arises either as a direct effect of therapy or as a manifestation of anorexia, dehydration, impaired nutrition, or weight loss because the skin becomes more vulnerable under these conditions to everyday traumas.[46]

Xerosis is also a common cause of pruritus in the aged. Other causes are related to reduced activity of the sebaceous and sweat glands, thinning of the skin, decreased subcutaneous tissue padding, and alterations in skin elasticity. Hydration of the skin is essential and can be accomplished by soaking in a warm bath for 15 to 20 minutes. The area should be patted dry, followed by application of an occlusive or moisturizer (Table 17-2). This is referred to by Nicol and Boguniewicz[20] as the "soak and seal" method and can relieve dryness by trapping moisture in the skin. Vaseline is considered an occlusive but must be used after hydration because it does not contain moisture. Moisturizers can be classified as lotions, creams, or ointments. Lotions can potentially be more drying to the skin since they contain more water and evaporate more quickly. There are a number of moisturizers (among them Eucerin, Aquaphor, Vanicream, Moisturel, and Cetaphil) available in large containers that are alcohol- and fragrance-free. Among patients for whom cost is a treatment-limiting factor, a cooking shortening, such as Crisco, can be an inexpensive alternative moisturizer. Moisturizers and occlusives should be applied several times per day. Patients should also be advised to wear clothing that is loose fitting, less irritating, and minimizes retention of heat and sweating to help reduce the itch sensation. The best type of fabric to wear is cotton clothing.[47]

For patients with pruritus, skin cleansing is important, especially if there are skin excoriations due to scratching. Many patients additionally seek relief by bathing or skin washing. The skin cleansers used in these situations should have a neutral pH and minimal defatting activity. Examples of such products include Dove, Oil of Olay, Basis, and Aveeno. Oatmeal baths and cold packs can be used to dry vesicles and relieve itch. Other topical agents such as calamine and topical Benadryl contain an antihistamine, which soothes and dries vesicles and decreases scratching. Camphor, phenol, and pramoxine may have local anesthetic properties, and menthol, a counterirritant, gives the impression of a cooling effect to the skin.[48]

A morphine- and lidocaine-based cream has been used in our clinical practice for pruritus described as burning and painful. Topical applications have been used for bullous pemphigoid lesions associated with graft versus host disease, cutaneous skin lesions associated with chest-wall recurrence of breast cancer, and macerated rectal skin from persistent seepage. The preparation, when applied three times a day over affected areas, was highly effective at decreasing pain and pruritus. Creams compounded with antidepressants, such as doxepin (Zonalon), may decrease itch by local inhibition of H1 and H2 receptors, as well as through antiserotonergic effects.[4,20]

Topically applied corticosteroids can reduce inflammation and itching associated with urticaria and other acute conditions but are generally not indicated for chronic use. Key considerations when prescribing topical steroids are the potency of the product (high to low potency), the vehicle used (lotion, cream, ointment, solution, gel), and the area of application. Examples of high-potency steroids include betamethasone dipropionate (Diprolene 0.05%) ointment/cream and desoximetasone (Topicort 0.25%) ointment/cream; mid-range preparations include triamcinolone (Kenalog 0.1%) ointment/cream and betamethasone valerate (Valisone 0.1%) ointment; hydrocortisone (Hytone 2.5%) and 1% ointment/cream/lotion represent low-potency preparations.[20] The side effects from prolonged use may include thinning and hypopigmentation of the skin, secondary skin infections, acne, and striae. If high-potency topical steroids are used under occlusive dressings, greater skin and systemic absorption can occur, which increases the likelihood of localized atrophy and systemic side effects (e.g., Cushing's disease, cataracts, hyperglycemia, and avascular necrosis).[20,49,50] In the same manner, ointments are more occlusive than other vehicles and, therefore, may be associated with a higher skin penetration as well as a greater likelihood of side effects upon prolonged use. In hot, humid conditions, ointments may also cause folliculitis, thereby increasing pruritus. Under these conditions, creams may be a better option. Topical steroids should generally not be applied more often than twice a day. Hydration of the skin before each application will promote absorption through the stratum corneum, thereby improving local absorption and efficacy.[50] It is typical to start with a high-potency preparation and to move to a lower-potency agent as the dermatitis/pruritus improves.[49]

Antifungal Treatment. The most frequent superficial fungal infection of the skin is *Candida albicans.* Typical areas of infection involve the inframammary areas, inguinal folds, and vulvovaginal areas, with pruritus being a common manifestation. Patients predisposed to candidiasis include those who are obese and have overlapping skin folds, those who are immunosuppressed, are on broad-spectrum antibiotics, are receiving corticosteroids, or have diabetes. Skin involvement in the inframammary or inguinal folds often appears as a creamy white layer, but gentle removal of this layer may reveal an erythematous base, with areas of maceration and even papules and pustules. Vulvovaginal infections will have a cheesy vaginal discharge, with itching and excoriation of the vulva.

Topical antifungal agents in use fall into three classifications: the polyene group (nystatin), the azole group (ketoconazole, fluconazole, itraconazole), and the allylamine/benzylamine

Table 17–2
Occlusives and Moisturizers

Vaseline (Chesebrough Ponds, Greenwich, CT)
Aquaphor ointment (Allscrips, Vernon Hills, IL)
Eucerin cream (Allscrips)
Vanicream (Pharm Spec, Rochester, MN)
Cetaphil cream (Galderma, Fort Worth, TX)
Moisturel cream (Westwood/Squibb, Buffalo, NY)
Crisco (Procter & Gamble, Cincinnati, OH)

group (ciclopiroxolamine, terbinafine).[51] The allylamine/benzalamine group is the newest generation of antifungals. They have greater bioavailability and a high cure rate with a shorter duration of treatment. To prevent recurrence, antifungal treatment should continue for 5 to 7 days after signs of infection have resolved. Ketoconazole should not be used in individuals with sulfite sensitivity. Some antifungals are prepared with corticosteroids; however, these should be avoided to prevent side effects from the corticosteroids.

Fungal infections not responsive to topical therapy will require systemic treatment. Systemic antifungals include griseofulvin, the azoles, and the allylamines. Gastrointestinal distress, headaches, exanthema, and liver toxicity (griseofulvin and fluconazole) are common side effects.

Tar preparations may reduce inflammation and limit the use of topical steroids in chronic pruritus/dermatitis. They may be used at night and washed off in the morning. Tar products are less costly; however, the smell and staining that occur with these products make them less than desirable.

Phototherapy with ultraviolet A may be an option for some individuals. Initially, treatments are given three or four times per week and, after several weeks, may progress to weekly. An oral preparation of psoralen before phototherapy may also be used for a wide range of disorders from AD to renal disease.[4] Side effects include sunburn and an increased risk of skin cancer.[20]

Systemic Measures

Opioid Antagonists. Naloxone hydrochloride (Narcan) is effective for relieving pruritus related to systemic and intraspinal opiates.[33,52,53] Infusion of naloxone at an hourly dose of 0.25 mg/kg was successful at relieving pruritus in patients receiving a continuous morphine infusion and appeared to enhance rather than diminish postoperative analgesia.[52] Nalbuphine, an agonist–antagonist analgesic, has also shown efficacy under similar conditions.[54] Naltrexone and nalmephene are oral agents, with a longer half-life than naloxone, that have been used in the treatment of pruritus associated with cholestasis, uremia, AD, and urticaria.[29,55] It is not known whether all centrally acting opioid antagonists are equal in their antipruritic effects. When naltrexone was used for pruritus in a patient with mycosis fungoides after initial success with subcutaneous naloxone, it was found to actually exacerbate itching[56] (Table 17-3). Because of the potential of opiate antagonists to induce a withdrawal syndrome, neither pure antagonists nor agonist–antagonists should be prescribed for the treatment of pruritus except by those experienced in their use.

Systemic Corticosteroids. Systemic corticosteroids can be highly effective in patients with pruritus related to inflammatory conditions, neoplasms, and certain dysmetabolic states. The presumed mechanism of action is inhibition of inflammatory and pruritogenic factors. Long-term use of these agents is limited by the well-known sequelae of chronic steroid use, including increases in skin friability, hyperglycemia, and the risks of fungal and other opportunistic infections. All of these can worsen preexisting pruritus. Other side effects may include avascular necrosis, hypertension, proximal muscle weakness, fluid retention, and osteoporosis.[57]

Antihistamines. H1-specific antihistamines are useful primarily for histamine-mediated pruritus, such as that associated with hives; but these agents often fail to provide meaningful relief in other conditions. A trial of the more sedating histamines is often recommended in initial treatment, but many patients find that negative side effects outweigh the minimal benefit achieved. A trial of the nonsedating antihistamines (fexofenadine, cetirizine, and loratidine) may be a more reasonable first step in the treatment of nonspecific itch because these agents are well tolerated. The more sedating antihistamines, such as diphenhydramine, chlorpheniramine, clemastine, hydroxyzine, and cyproheptadine, can be useful at night when itch interferes with sleep. In addition to its antihistaminic effects, cyproheptadine has antiserotonergic activity, which may provide increased relief in some patients.

Local Anesthetics. Mexiletine (Mexitil) is similar in its chemical properties to lidocaine and has been used in patients with intractable pruritus. Other anesthetic agents given IV, intradermally, or intraarterially can block sensory transmission, including pruritus.[1,58] Side effects include lightheadedness, dizziness, tremors, and nervousness. Interferon-α has been reported to be effective in relieving pruritus refractory to antihistamines and steroids in B-cell chronic lymphocytic leukemia and in non-Hodgkin's lymphoma. It is thought to inhibit the proliferation of eosinophil differentiation.[59,60] Dermatomyositis induced pruritus has been treated with high-dose human immunoglobulin.[61]

Antidepressants. Doxepin, amitriptyline, nortriptyline, and imipramine have been used in the treatment of numerous neuropathic pain states. Pruritus is frequently a comorbid feature of neuropathic pain, and anecdotal reports suggest that the same tricyclic antidepressants that are efficacious in certain forms of neuropathic pain may also be beneficial in treating pruritus.[62–64] As the most antihistaminic of the group, doxepin may be the most effective. Mirtazapine also has potent H1 antagonism, as well as antiserotonergic effects at both the 5-HT_2 and 5-HT_3 receptors. Since antagonism at each of these individual receptor types has been associated with antipruritic effects, mirtazepine may possess a theoretical advantage in pruritus treatment. The SSRI Paroxetine (paxil) has been shown to be effective in patients with generalized pruritus during terminal illness. The addition of a 5-HT_3 agent such as ondansetron (Zofran) and mirtazapine may enhance the efficacy of paxil in this setting.[47,65]

Propofol. Subhypnotic doses of propofol have been successfully used in the treatment of pruritus resulting from neuraxial administration of opioids and cholestasis from pancreatic

Table 17–3
Medications Used to Treat Pruritus in Selected Conditions

Allergic/Autoimmune

- Drug rotation or discontinuation[1]
- Avoidance of offending allergen
- 5-HT_3 antagonists[13]
- Antihistamines (e.g., diphenhydramine, cyproheptadine)
- Corticosteroids
  - Topical
  - Systemic
- Other immunosuppressive therapy

Opioid-Induced Pruritus

- Opiate rotation (e.g., from morphine to alternative opiate, such as fentanyl)
- Low-dose naloxone infusion
- Low-dose nalbuphine infusion
- Propofol[24]

Cholestatic Disorders

Acute palliative effects

- Propofol
- Naloxone and other opioid antagonists or agonist–antagonists
- Ondansetron
- External biliary drainage

Chronic palliative effects

- Cholestyramine
- Androgenic steroids
- Phototherapy
- Plasmapheresis
- Rifampicin (enhances hepatic microsomal function)
- Ursodeoxycholic acid
- Barbiturates
- IV heparin
- Charcoal

Neuropathic Disorders

- Local anesthetics (e.g., lidocaine, mexiletine, topical EMLA cream, lidoderm patch)
- Anticonvulsant agents (e.g., for paroxysmal symptoms of multiple sclerosis)
- Capsaicin[13]

Dermatoses

- Skin cooling: increases the itch threshold, can break vicious cycle

Uremia

- 5-HT_3 antagonists[14,15]
- Ultraviolet ß phototherapy
- Erythropoietin
- Parathyroidectomy
- Thalidomide
- Lidocaine

Polycythemia vera

- Nonsteroidal antiinflammatory agents
- α-interferon

neoplasm, hepatic and bile duct metastasis, and primary biliary cirrhosis. Patients achieved rapid symptomatic control following both single injections and continuous low-dose infusion.[23,24,66] While the mechanism of action is unclear, the effect was unrelated to sedation.[23,24,66]

Anticonvulsants. In general, anticonvulsant agents have not been investigated for utility in the treatment of pruritus. Several anticonvulsant agents, such as carbamezepine and gabapentin, are of established clinical efficacy in the treatment of a variety of neuropathic pain syndromes. When pruritus complicates a known neuropathic disorder (e.g., postherpetic neuralgia), a therapeutic trial of one of these agents should be considered.

Other Agents. Ondansetron, a 5-HT_3 antagonist, has been used in cholestatic, uremic, and opioid-induced pruritus.[15,67,68] Benzodiazepines, such as lorazepam and alprazolam, may be helpful in relieving itch if anxiety is also present.[69] Benzodiazepines are not suggested for long-term use.

Sensory modulation can be accomplished through counterirritants, heat or cold, and transcutaneous electrical nerve stimulation (TENS). The Roman physician Scribonius Largus used the voltages of certain fish (electric rays and torpedo fish) in 47 A.D. for treatment of gout and headaches.[68] With the advent of the battery, TENS units that provided a more reliable source of current were developed. When applied directly over the pruritic area, surrounding area, or acupressure points, TENS may block transmission of polymodal nociceptive C fibers, thereby blocking pain and pruritus.[70,71,72]

Capsaicin depletes substance P when applied repeatedly to the mucous membrane or skin, decreasing both pain and itch sensations. When given in low concentrations, the stinging, burning itch may initially be exacerbated.[2]

The gate control theory of pain states that impulses carried by noxious stimuli to the spinal cord via thin myelinated and unmyelinated fibers are blocked at the dorsal horn by stimulation of larger-diameter myelinated nerve fibers by pressure, vibration, or a TENS unit.[71] Thick nerve fibers have a lower threshold than thin fibers and adapt more readily. No adaptation takes place in the large fibers when scratching or vibration occurs. This may explain why scratching or rubbing the affected part sometimes relieves mild to moderate pain.[71]

Nonpharmacological Measures. In a palliative care setting, most patients are in the terminal phase of their disease. Pruritus during this phase of illness is primarily a result of changing organ functions. For example, liver and kidney function may be deteriorating. Thus, systemic therapy might be more toxic to patients in the terminal phase of their illness. Hence, it is important to attempt nonpharmacological antipruritus measures to minimize further injury to organ functions and also to maintain quality of life (Table 17-4).

Table 17–4
General and Topical Antipruritic Measures in Palliative Care

Prevent dry skin, excessive heat.
Humidify ambient environment.
Lubricate frequently, especially after bathing.
Avoid contact irritants (e.g., wool, hairy pets, cleansers).
Apply cold application (ice, compress).
Wear loose-fitting, cotton clothing.
Apply appropriate topical antipruritic agents.

Sources: Adapted from Krajnik (2001), reference 104; Pittelkow (2004), reference 105; and Charlesworth (2002), reference 106.

CASE STUDY

Ms. S, a Patient with Pruritus

Ms. S is a 75-year-old woman with a history of non-Hodgkin's lymphoma, cervical cancer, breast cancer, chronic renal failure, hypothyroidism, hypertension, and seizure disorder. She was treated for a disseminated herpes zoster infection diagnosed 3 months earlier that involved several dermatomes (T2–L2). Ms. S was seen in clinic for complaints of pruritus in the right posterior chest that had been present for 3 months and thought to be a postherpetic neuralgia. The patient described the pruritus as a burning, unrelenting itch and stated she was "ready to give up." The following medications were prescribed and reported to be ineffective: amitriptyline (Elavil) 20 mg at bedtime (qhs), hydroxyzine (Atarax) 25 mg three times a day (tid), diphenhydramine (Benadryl) 25 mg tid po, and doxepin cream 5% to the affected area four times (qid) a day. Nondrug interventions included ice pack to the back for 20 min tid. Famotidine (Pepcid) 20 mg twice a day (bid), prednisone 20 mg bid, and triamcinolone acetonide (Kenalog) cream 0.025 topically applied tid were also used, again without relief. The patient was admitted to the hospital for cellulitus in the right arm, presumably a secondary bacterial infection resulting from the scratching, and was given cefazolin (Ancef) IV.

The patient denied any contact with pets, no new or changed soap/detergents, cosmetics, body lotions/creams, medications, and no exposure to scabies or to new foliage. She denied pruritus in any area other than her back.

Clinical evaluation: a frail, elderly woman who appeared uncomfortable and at times restrained herself from scratching. No vesicular eruptions were noted. Dry blood and numerous scratch marks are present over the posterior thorax. Three raised erythematous areas were noted, in the right scapular, lower thorax, and lumbar areas. Skin turgor was good. There was no allodynia, and no lymphadenopathy in the head/neck, supraclavicular area, or axilla. There was no evidence of a rash, infection, or tracks. Blood urea nitrogen and creatinine were stable, and thyroid function tests were within normal limits.

The impression was that this woman with a history of herpes zoster infection had developed postherpetic neuralgia.

Ms. S's pruritus was treated as a postherpetic neuralgia, and a prescription for mexiletine (Mexitil) 150 mg bid was given with instructions to take with food to minimize gastrointestinal side effects. Ms. S was asked to titrate by one pill (150 mg) every 5 days to a total of 300 mg tid. Amitriptyline (Elavil) 10 mg was prescribed with instructions to take every evening at 8:00. By taking this medication earlier in the evening, the patient was less likely to feel "hungover" in the morning.

The patient reported improvement in the "itchiness and discomfort" in her back once the mexiletine was started; however, she developed a tremor that she noted while in church. The patient became frightened and stopped the medication. Ms. S was evaluated in an urgent-care clinic by an on-call physician. Upon examination, an essential tremor was diagnosed and the patient was advised to restart the mexiletine at 150 mg tid for 24 hours and then to increase to 300 mg tid. Ms. S was reevaluated later that week and reported "dizziness" when taking mexiletine 300 mg tid. She stopped the amitriptyline at night and continued to report relief of the pruritus with the use of this drug. The patient was asked to decrease the mexiletine to 150 mg tid and to restart the amitriptyline 10 mg qhs. The patient called several days later to report that the pruritus was not controlled at this dose and that she was afraid to increase the dose because of side effects (i.e., tremor). The patient was seen in clinic, and it was decided that since the mexiletine was the only medication that provided any relief of her symptoms, the dose would be adjusted again to 150 mg in the morning and evening and 300 mg at hs; propranolol (Inderal) 10 mg tid was added to decrease the tremor.

Nursing Implications

Assessment

1. Describe and document the color, characteristics, and size of any lesions.
2. Obtain a thorough history of any new products (detergents, lotions, soap), exposure to new pets, recent travel and outdoor exposure, or any new medications.
3. Obtain a thorough patient and family history of allergies (e.g., food or seasonal), treatments previously used and their success, travel, hikes, and any exposure to known infectious agents/insect bites. Do other members of the family or others with whom the patient has had social contact have pruritus?
5. What has been the general health of the patient during the several weeks preceding the development of pruritus?
6. A skin biopsy may be required to determine the etiology of the pruritus.

Management

1. Teach safety measures with use of sedating antihistamines, such as not driving or operating potentially dangerous equipment until tolerance to the sedating effects of these medications has been established.
2. Psychological support is needed for any new diagnosis of malignancy.
3. Educate patients concerning the proper use of topical medications and the potential side effects.
4. Frequently assess the skin in pruritic areas for the presence of any secondary infections.

FEVER

Fever is defined as a rise in normal body temperature (above 37° ± 1°C), as a temperature ≥38°C for three consecutive readings performed 1 hour apart, or as one reading ≥38.5°C.[73] Fevers can be a result of inflammation (including malignancy), infection, immunological disorders, hypermetabolic states (e.g., thyrotoxicosis), hyperthermia, heat stroke, or, uncommonly, disorders of the CNS (e.g., cerebral stroke) (Table 17-5). Febrile illnesses have been recorded in the medical literature as far back as Hippocrates (5th century B.C.E.), though it was not possible to actually measure body temperature until the development of the thermometer in the mid-19th century.[74,75] Determining the etiology of a fever is often essential to providing the most appropriate treatment of this symptom as well as of its underlying causes. Deciding when to treat the actual symptom of fever depends to a great extent on the symptoms associated with it (e.g., tachypnea, tachycardia, hyperhydrosis, feeling of dissipation, fatigue), age, general medical condition, any comorbid conditions or diseases, and the goals of care relative to the patient's stage of illness. For example, the treatment of fever and associated tachycardia in an older patient with a known history of advanced coronary artery disease but few other comorbid illnesses may itself be life-saving. Treating fever usually provides improved patient comfort. However, treating fever may at times have the unintended effect of inhibiting immunological responses mounted as a means of defense against infectious pyrogens.[75] To what extent such inhibitory responses are of clinical significance is largely unknown.

In the setting of palliative care, decisions on treating an infectious etiology of fever can at times trigger controversy since the treatment may prolong the dying process. How aggressively infection should be treated at the end of life depends on the factors listed above and the plan of care agreed upon by the patient, family, and health care professionals.

Pathophysiology

The body's thermoregulatory system is controlled by the preoptic region of the anterior hypothalamus. Under ordinary circumstances, the hypothalamus maintains the core body temperature by establishing a thermal set-point. This set-point, analogous to a thermostatic control, may be affected by the presence of various *pyrogens,* or fever-causing substances. Pyrogens may be produced by and released directly from infectious pathogens (bacteria, viruses, or fungi). These are typically called "exogenous" pyrogens. Pathogenic agents may also stimulate the release of endogenous pyrogens from the immune system. The four best recognized endogenous pyrogens are IL-1, IL-6, tumor necrosis factor-α (TNF-α), and interferon (IFN). Systemic release of either exogenous or endogenous pyrogens can trigger the fever response by elevating the hypothalamic set-point so that compensatory temperate lowering mechanisms are not activated until higher-than-normal

Table 17–5
Common Causes of Fevers

Tumor
- Hodgkin's and non-Hodgkin's lymphoma (cell-mediated immune deficiency)
- Hypernephroma
- Carcinoma metastatic to the liver
- Leukemia
- Multiple myeloma (altered humoral immunity)
- Ewing's sarcoma
- Tumors that become necrotic, with secondary infections
- Adrenal carcinoma/pheochromocytoma
- Primary or metastatic tumors of the thermoregulatory areas of the brain
- Obstructive solid tumors of the GI, genitourinary, or respiratory system

Cancer and treatment
- Changes in the body's natural defenses
- Foreign bodies (catheters, venous access devices)
- Degree and duration of neutropenia
- Immunosuppression
- Chemotherapeutic agents (e.g., bleomycin)
- Blood products
- Splenectomy

Inflammatory processes
- Thrombophlebitis
- Radiation
- Heat
- Trauma
- Surgery
- Cell necrosis (ischemic)
- Pulmonary embolism
- Regional enteritis
- Granulomatous disease of the colon
- Ulcerative colitis

Autoimmune and allergic processes
- Connective tissue disorders (systemic lupus)
- Anaphylactoid reactions
- Rheumatoid arthritis
- Polymyalgia rheumatica
- Acquired immunodeficiency syndrome
- Medications. (e.g., antibiotics)

Infections
- Bacteria, fungi, viruses, and parasites
- Tuberculosis
- Infective endocarditis
- Liver abscess/subphrenic abscess
- Anicteric hepatitis
- Nosocomial infection

Environmental
- Microbial flora that colonize in the nasopharynx, small and large bowel, and skin
- Travel to third-world countries
- Exposure to microorganisms from farm animals
- Allergic response to environmental allergens

Foods (immunocompromised patients)
- Fresh fruits and vegetables
- Fresh flowers
- Spices
- Tobacco

Others
- Constipation
- Dehydration

temperatures are reached. At this time, it is not known if peripherally released cytokines cross the blood–brain barrier to directly influence the hypothalamic set point, or whether this process occurs through other cytokine mediators or even neural means. At the hypothalamic level, prostaglandins, especially prostaglandin E2, appear to play an important role in establishing the hypothalamic set-point. It is presumably through these inhibiting prostaglandin mediators that aspirin and certain other antipyretic agents work. Regardless of the actual mechanism, the hypothalamus continues to regulate body temperature, though this regulation is now around a higher set-point. When an antipyretic is given or the pyrogen level is decreased, the hypothalamic temperature is reset back to normal.[73,75,76] Temperatures above 41°C suggest that the source of fever may be either abnormal heat production (as in malignant hyperthermia) or problems with heat dissipation (as in heat stroke).

Phases of Fevers

There are often three stages of a fever. The "cold stage" occurs when there is a physiological discrepancy between the hypothalamic set-point, now at a higher level, and the existing body temperature. In response, hypothalamic mechanisms signal for peripheral vasoconstriction to occur, which diminishes cutaneous heat loss, and for shivering, which generates heat through increased muscle activity. The "hot stage," or febrile phase, occurs when body heat is maintained at a higher-than-normal level due to the higher set-point of hypothalamic thermoregulaton. During the febrile stage, symptoms often include flushing of the skin, increased sense of thirst, sensation of increased body warmth, lethargy, and restlessness or irritability. Less commonly seen CNS manifestations include hallucinations and seizures, though the latter are seen almost exclusively in young children. During febrile states, the basal metabolic rate is increased as tissue metabolism and oxygen requirements increase by 10% to 13% for each 1°C increase in body temperature. Associated physiological changes include tachycardia with an increase in cardiac output and workload.[76,77] Decreases in the level of pyrogen produced or administration of an antipyretic at least temporarily resets the hypothalamic set-point. During the defervescence stage, or stage 3, heat dissipation is increased due to vasodilatation and sweating, causing an increase in evaporative skin cooling.[77,78] Heat-generating mechanisms (e.g., shivering) are inhibited, and the body temperature falls back within the normal range.[79,80]

Etiology

Immunological Responses. Blood products and certain medications, as well as allergic reactions and connective tissue disorders, liberate substances which, in turn, activate release of endogenous pyrogens, the three best recognized being IL-1, IL-6, TNF, and IFN. A variety of secondary immune reactions may trigger the release of pyrogens, including anaphylactic reactions (e.g., asthma), cytotoxic reactions (e.g., blood-transfusion reactions), immune complex–mediated reactions (e.g., serum sickness), and delayed hypersensitivity reactions (e.g., contact dermatitis and allograft rejection). Primary immune disorders that may be associated with a fever include systemic lupus erythematosus, giant cell arteritis, and rheumatoid arthritis.

Infections. Infectious pathogens elaborate pyrogens, such as bacterial lipopolysaccharides, which, in turn, promote the release of endogenous pyrogenic cytokines by stimulating the body's immune and other defensive reactions. The principal origins of these cytokines are activated monocytes, macrophages, and lymphocytes, which are recruited to respond to the infection. Endogenous pyrogens can also be produced by endothelial cells and fibroblasts.

Of pathogens found in new fevers, 85% to 90% are of bacterial origin. Common origins of bacterial infections in cancer and immunosuppressed patients include the breakdown of skin integrity and mucosal barriers due to multiple venipunctures and lines or catheters, other invasive procedures, decubitus ulcers, cutaneous infections including herpes zoster, and mucositis. Bacteria, as well as other pathogens, induce the production of endogenous pyrogens in macrophages and monocytes. These pyrogens include TNF-α and IL-1β. Release of these substances into the inflammatory mix in turn stimulates the cascade of other cytokines, including IL-1, IL-6, and the prostaglandins.[73]

Increasing body temperature can itself increase phagocytic activity and affect the type and amount of pyrogenic cytokine released.[77] Although fever may contribute in this fashion to stimulation of the immune system, the tachycardia and hypermetabolism caused by the fever can prove fatal in an individual who is immunocompromised, in advanced cancer patients, and in those with acquired immunodeficiency syndrome (AIDS).[76,79,80]

Inflammation. Inflammation occurs with cellular damage due to cytotoxic agents, trauma (including surgery), radiation therapy, or exposure to heat. Fibroblasts and endothelial cells, as well as macrophages, release endogenous pyrogens, such as IL-1, IL-6, and TNF.[73,74,77] Postoperative fluid collections and large internal hematomas are therefore common causes of fever in the surgical patient. Although circumscribed superficial inflammation rarely causes significant fever, inflammation can predispose to secondary infection and a febrile state.[76,79,80] Radiation therapy, for example, can cause fevers through several mechanisms. First, immunocytes and endothelial cells damaged by radiation may release endogenous pyrogens. Second, radiation therapy may alter skin integrity (dry and moist desquamation) and damage mucosal barriers, thereby increasing the patient's predisposition to infection. Infection may also be associated with radiation-related myelosuppression when the radiation field includes the primary sites of blood cell production, such as the sternum, long bones, and iliac crests.[81–83] Finally, cranial radiation may cause temporary perturbations in the hypothalamic set-point.

Vascular causes of fever may include thrombophlebitis with or without pulmonary emboli, and regional or systemic tumor-associated vasculitis. The cause of fevers in these settings is thought to be release of pyrogens from phagocytic and endothelial cells. Several cancers, especially lymphomas and gastrointestinal malignancies, are associated with a higher-than-expected risk for developing deep-vein thrombosis. It is not uncommon, in fact, for fever to be the earliest sign of thrombophlebitis. In one study of pulmonary emboli, approximately 18% of the patients had malignancies, 54% had a fever >37.5°C, and 19.6% had a fever >38°C.[84]

Even in the absence of vascular inflammation, fever may be the presenting symptom of many malignancies, including Hodgkin's lymphoma, bronchogenic carcinoma, breast cancer, non-Hodgkin's lymphoma, and multiple myeloma. Fevers related to tumors may be associated with the release of pyrogens, such as TNF-α and IL-6, either directly from the tumor or from tumor-reactive hypersensitivity reactions.[73,76,77]

Pulsatile release of tumor pyrogens can cause a waxing and waning of fever, which correlates with disease activity.[73,76,85–87] The naproxen test has been used as a diagnostic tool to differentiate between a neoplastic fever and a fever associated with an infection. Chang and Gross[88] reported complete response of neoplastic fevers to naproxen within 24 hours of starting the drug, whereas no patient with an infectious fever showed any improvement.[73,81] It was postulated that the fever suppression was related to the interference/suppression or release of humoral factor(s).[88] The specificity of this test is uncertain, and the possibility of infection should not be dismissed on the basis of this test alone. Other noninfectious etiologies, such as allergic reaction, drug toxicity, and adrenal insufficiency, also need to be considered.[73]

Blood Transfusions. Allergic responses to white blood cells in blood products may be avoided by using irradiated blood products, removing white blood cells from blood (leukapheresis), or premedicating with antihistamines, hydrocortisone, and/or antipyretics.[78]

Medications Associated with Fevers. Certain medications may be antigenic; that is, they are interpreted by the body as a foreign substance, thereby initiating an allergic or immune response with accompanying fever. The categories of drug most often associated with a febrile response include antibiotics, cytotoxic agents, cardiovascular drugs, and biological therapies such as the interferons and interleukins.[80] The classes of antibiotics most commonly associated with fevers are the penicillins, cephalosporins, and certain antifungals, such as amphotericin.[73] Cytotoxic drugs such as bleomycin trigger a fever in 25% of individuals, and anaphylaxis results in 1% of cases.[73]

Hemorrhage. Gastrointestinal bleeding may result in fever within 24 hours, which may last a few days to a few weeks.[73,74] Although this has been mentioned in the literature, no clear explanation has been offered, but fever may be related to the release of IL-1 from the damaged gastrointestinal mucosa.[74]

Neutropenia. Neutropenia is defined as a polymorphonuclear neutrophil count of 500/mL or less, which may arise from decreased production of white blood cells (myelosuppression from chemotherapy or radiation therapy or tumor infiltration of bone marrow with inhibition of white blood cell production) or increased loss of white blood cells (usually through an autoimmune process). Of patients with neutropenia, 50% to 70% experiencing a fever will die within 48 hours if left untreated because of rapidly progressive sepsis.[78,80,89]

Miscellaneous Factors. Several general medical problems can be identified as contributing to fever (see Table 17-5). Dehydration limits the body's compensatory response of heat loss through sweating. Severe obstipation has been associated with fever, due possibly to associated dehydration or ischemia of the bowel, causing a local inflammatory response. Hospitalization itself is a frequent cause of infection and fever, probably because of the frequency of procedures, such as venipuncture and the placement of IV catheters, which violate the integrity of skin defense mechanisms. Nosocomial infections account for more than 80% of infections in cancer patients.[90]

Opioids. Opioids have been found to cause a flush (vasodilatation) and sweating, especially involving the face, but have not been associated with fever.[91] Meperidine hydrochloride (pethidine hydrochloride) in combination with a monoamine oxidase inhibitor can cause hyperpyrexia, muscle rigidity, CNS excitability, or depression that can be severe or fatal.[73,92] Abrupt opioid cessation results in withdrawal symptoms, including restlessness, rhinitis, abdominal pain, and fever. Withdrawal from benzodiazepines may also cause a fever.[73]

Clinical Evaluation

Patient History. A thorough history must be obtained to determine if there are coexisting symptoms suggestive of a urinary tract infection, upper respiratory infection, or any exposure to a person with infection or who has had a live-virus vaccination. A bowel history should be conducted to rule out constipation. If the patient has cancer, when was the last surgery? When was the last course of chemotherapy or immunotherapy? When was the last course of radiation therapy? Is there any history of blood transfusion within the preceding 6 months? It is important to determine the pattern of the patient's fevers, the time of day they occur, and the number of temperature peaks over 24 hours. In patients receiving end-of-life care, the focus of the treatment plan is palliation of symptoms. Determining the source of the fever will guide the clinician as to the appropriate intervention. If the patient is severely constipated, laxative-induced evacuation may not only reduce the fever but also improve nutritional status and eliminate or reduce nausea, if present. Treating a urinary infection may also improve comfort, promote rest, and improve cognition. Use of oral antibiotics to treat a urinary tract or upper respiratory infections may be appropriate to palliate symptoms, such as the distress that may accompany tachypnea, tachycardia, or shaking chills. Antibiotics are used in this manner to palliate symptoms due to infection rather than to eradicate the infection properly. If antibiotic therapy causes increased physical distress in the form of pruritus, drug-induced fevers, or nausea and vomiting, the role of antibiotic treatment needs to be reevaluated, to keep the focus of care on quality-of-life issues. As with all palliative treatments, it is important to routinely reassess goals with the patient and family to be certain that everyone is in agreement.

Physical Examination. Since common sites of infection include the skin, respiratory tract, urinary system, perianal region, oral cavity, and sinuses, a comprehensive evaluation for infection should not overlook any of these sites. In chronically ill and emaciated patients, special attention should be paid to the skin overlying bony prominences as well as the perineal and perianal regions, evaluating for decubitus lesions and other areas of skin breakdown, necrotic tumors, and/or infection. If the patient has an IV line, central catheter, or other central venous access device (e.g., Porta-Cath), these need to be carefully evaluated for signs of infection. Decisions on the appropriateness of blood and sputum cultures and radiographic tests need to be made on a case-by-case basis, depending on the patient's status and the likelihood that test results will lead to a meaningful therapeutic intervention. This said, performance of a urinalysis is noninvasive and inexpensive and can provide information leading to straightforward therapies offering symptom relief.

Management of Common Sources of Skin Infection in End-of-Life Care

There are several interventions nurses can initiate to manage skin infections based on the location, characteristics of the affected area, and organism(s) involved. Dakin's solution is composed of bleach, sodium bicarbonate, and sterile water. It can be prepared as a 0.25%, 0.5%, 0.75%, or full-strength solution, depending on the contamination of the wound, and may be used to irrigate or pack wounds contaminated with *Pseudomonas*. Clean, healthy skin should not come in contact with Dakin's solution because it is extremely irritating.

Hypertonic saline gels (Panafil) can debride thick, necrotic eschar on a decubitus without surgical intervention. Morphine (powder or concentrated solution) is added to commercially prepared ointments and substances used for wound healing, such as Silvadene and lidocaine, and to DuoDERM powder to pack inside wounds. These mixtures may be helpful in reducing secondary skin infections as well as promoting comfort, and can be used to pack a venous stasis ulcer, decubitus, or fungating lesion. Fungal infections, generally characterized by a foul odor, maceration of the skin, and occasionally superficial bleeding, are commonly seen in the intertriginous areas (inframammary and inguinal folds). Daily cleansing with soap and water, thorough drying of the affected area, and use of antifungal powder or lotion (nystatin, clotrimazole) can be applied twice or three times a day until healed.

Treatment of Fever

Comfort should be the primary goal for the dying patient with a fever. Treatment should be initiated with antipyretics, such as acetaminophen, aspirin, or ibuprofen, which are the only drugs approved by the Food and Drug Administration for this purpose.

Acetaminophen can be administered in tablet, liquid, or suppository form. For tumor-related fever, a nonsteroidal antiinflammatory drug (NSAID) may be especially beneficial. The presence of thrombocytopenia may be a limiting factor in the selection of NSAIDs. The specific cyclooxygenase-2 (COX-2)–inhibiting antiinflammatory agents, such as celecoxib (Celebrex), may in certain instances be preferred in this setting.

Cooling measures, such as a tepid cloth to the patient's forehead, may be comforting; otherwise, cooling measures (such as ice bags and cool cloths) should be avoided because they cause shivering, which is heat-generating. Oral fluids and/or ice chips should be encouraged, but the benefit of using parenteral or enteral fluids is highly debated, and it remains undetermined whether hydration improves cognition, especially in individuals using opioids.[93,94] Oral care with soft applicators should be offered frequently by the family caregiver; in addition to promoting the patient's comfort, this allows the caregiver to participate in the loved one's care. A salt-and-soda solution can be used instead of mouthwash. A solution can be made by boiling 1 quart of water and adding 1 teaspoon of salt and 1 teaspoon of baking soda. Chill the solution and use several times a day, as desired. Discard any unused solution after 1 week. Vaseline or other lubricants should be placed on the patient's lips to prevent dryness and cracking. Special attention to skin is essential, especially to skinfolds; clothing and linens should be changed frequently. Aquaphor, Eucerin, aloe vera, or Vaseline Intensive Care can be applied to maintain skin integrity. Lymphedema patients using a Jobst and Sigvarus compression garment should be instructed to avoid products that contain petroleum because they break down the rubber in the garment. Avoid skin products that contain alcohol because they may actually increase dryness and cause chemical irritation.

A bowel history should be obtained and a laxative or suppository given if constipation is present. An enema or disimpaction may be required. Corticosteroids are effective as antipyretics and can reduce inflammation and pain but are potentially dangerous insofar as immune function is hampered and an infectious process may be masked.[77] The risk:benefit ratio with respect to goals of care must always be considered. In a palliative care setting, neuroleptic agents can be used for centrally mediated fevers. Chlorpromazine (Thorazine) has been used primarily in this setting, probably because among the neuroleptics it is most likely to cause vasodilatation.[95]

Palliative radiation may be needed if the fever is tumor-related, as indicated by the tumor type and general condition of the patient.

CASE STUDY

Mr. D, a Patient with Fever

Mr. D was an 80-year-old retired pediatrician with a recent history of fever of unknown origin, leukocytosis, elevated erythrocyte sedimentation rate (ESR), anemia, and myalgias. The patient had been in good health until his return from Mexico 2 months earlier, when he developed chills, myalgias, nonproductive cough, and fevers. Antibiotics were prescribed when a chest x-ray showed a left lower-lobe infiltrate. Myalgias continued, especially in the triceps muscles and shoulder girdle muscles. The myalgias were partially relieved by NSAIDs. Throughout the 2 months, he had intermittent spikes of fever, with episodes of profuse diaphoresis, generalized malaise, anorexia, and a 15-lb. weight loss. He was admitted to a local hospital, where he underwent extensive testing.

The past medical history included Guillain-Barré syndrome in 1945, right bundle-branch block, transurethral prostatectomy in 1988, and prostate cancer without evidence of metastatic disease. There was no history of rheumatic fever or heart murmur.

Clinical evaluation revealed the patient as an alert, oriented man with intact cognitive functions. Funduscopic examination was impeded by cataract formation, but no Roth spots or areas of hemorrhage were visible. There was slight focal tenderness of the proximal superficial temporal artery, barely notable on the right and mild on the left. There was no nodularity or induration along the course of either of these arteries. Carotid bruits were absent and extracranial artery pulsations were normal. There was no nuchal rigidity. Motor examination was normal for age, without muscle masses or tenderness, except in the calves. He was, however, unable to rise from a chair without the use of his arms and was unsteady on his feet. Gait was wide-based and waddling, with some unsteadiness. Sensation was intact to all modalities, though Romberg's sign was positive for postural imbalance and tandem gait was slightly abnormal. Radial pulses were equal, and pedal pulses were present bilaterally. No cutaneous stigmata of infection or vasculitis was appreciated. Heart sounds were normal, without murmur. There was no hepatomegaly or abdominal tenderness. Areas of bone tenderness were absent.

The impressions were (1) fever of unknown origin, and (2) rule out temporal arteritis.

The diagnostic data were as follows: lumbar puncture was negative, carotid ultrasound showed moderate amount of plaque formation in both common carotid arteries with no significant stenosis, and temporal artery biopsy showed giant cell arteritis.

The patient was treated with prednisone 20 mg tid, with regular monitoring of ESR.

The patient enjoyed complete relief of fevers, night sweats, and myalgias. He was encouraged to exercise, and bone-density studies and blood-sugar levels were monitored during the time he was on prednisone. His ESR returned to normal, and prednisone was gradually tapered.

SWEATS

The sweat glands of the skin, the piloerector muscles, and the vascular skin blood vessels are controlled, at least in part, by the sympathetic nervous system and are intimately involved in temperature regulation. Vasodilatation and sweating allow for evaporative heat loss to lower body temperature in a hot environment, with fevers, or during exercise. Approximately 5% of cancer patients experience sweating as a direct result of malignant disease.[96–98]

Pathophysiology

The hypothalamus interprets signals from the central and peripheral thermoreceptors. There are two types of thermosensitive neurons, warm-sensitive and cold-sensitive, both of which are located in the preoptic anterior hypothalamus. The more abundant warm-sensitive neurons respond to a rise in temperature in the periphery, whereas the cold-sensitive neurons are triggered by a decrease in body temperature in the periphery.[1] Body temperature is read at various thermoreceptors in the skin, spinal cord, and brain stem. Hypercapnia, plasma osmolality, intravascular blood volume changes, and dehydration can affect body temperature and set-point.[1]

The autonomic nervous system both transmits the thermoregulatory adjustments to the CNS and has a measure of thermoregulatory control independent of the CNS. Postganglionic sympathetic axons innervate sweat glands, blood vessels, and piloerector muscles. Through adjustments in adrenergic vasoconstrictor nerve fibers, cutaneous blood flow is increased or decreased depending on the need to dissipate or conserve heat. Cholinergic fibers innervate the eccrine glands. Thermal sweating occurs when the hypothalamic set-point is exceeded. Signals are transmitted from the hypothalamus by the autonomic nervous system to the effector sweat glands and cutaneous vasculature. Generalized diaphoresis ensues, which lowers body temperature. Emotional sweating is controlled primarily by the limbic system rather than the hypothalamus, and may affect areas of the body differently. Whereas sweating may be either depressed or increased over the trunk and proximal limbs, sweating always increases in the palms of the hands and soles of the feet. Under given circumstances, the quantity of sweating in response either to temperature elevation or emotion is often dependent on age, gender, exercise, hydration, ambient temperature, and sweat gland blood flow. Disorders of sweating include *hyperhidrosis* (excessive sweating), *anhidrosis* (absent or decreased sweating), and *gustatory sweating* (primarily of the face, associated with diabetes). Each of these disorders can arise from dysfunction of either the neural innervation or the sweat glands themselves or both.

Etiology

Anhydrotic ectodermal hypoplasia is an inherited condition in which heat loss through perspiration may be inadequate to lower body temperature. Other cooling methods must be used for thermoregulation (e.g., submersion in cool water, exposure to cool ambient temperatures, cool cloths) to lower temperature.

Hyperhidrosis may be a compensatory mechanism for anhidrosis of other body areas. Thermoregulatory sweat testing can be conducted to assess the peripheral and central sympathetic pathways. Reduced or absent sweating patterns can be identified and the pathology identified as either pre- or postganglionic abnormalities or abnormalities of the sweat glands. Abnormalities of sweating, either excessively dry or wet skin, accompanied by trophic skin changes and thin shiny skin are signs of a peripheral neuropathic disorder. When seen in the setting of limb pain, they typically indicate that the pain is arising, at least in part, on a neuropathic basis.

Generalized hyperhydrosis can occur with various endocrine disorders, such as estrogen deficiency due to menopause (related either to the climacteric medical treatment), hyperthyroidism, or hypoglycemia, as well as with various neuroendocrine tumors, such as carcinoid and pheochromocytoma. Hyperhidrosis may also be a sign of chronic infection, such as tuberculosis, or of inflammatory illnesses (e.g., lupus, vasculitis, regional enteritis) even in the absence of fevers. Various malignancies, most notably lymphomas, cause drenching sweats, especially at night. Such night sweats may be an early sign of tumor recurrence. Hyperhidrosis may announce many abstinence syndromes, such as from barbiturates, opioids, or ethanol.[1] With opioids, both agonists, such as morphine and methadone, and mixed agonists–antagonists, such as butorphanol and pentazocine, have been associated with excessive sweating, probably due to cutaneous vasodilatation. An opioid rotation may be beneficial in reducing this symptom.[1]

It is important to evaluate all reported regional disturbances of sweating. Patients with an area of anhidrosis (e.g., related to a Pancoast tumor as a component of Horner's syndrome) may not notice a decrease in sweating on the affected area but, instead, report hyperhidrosis on the unaffected side.

Nocturnal hyperhidrosis, or night sweats, can be associated with decreased estrogen production such as from menopause, other endocrine disorders, and malignancies. Hormonal therapy for breast and prostate cancers is often associated with troublesome hot flashes, which interfere with sleep patterns. Seventy-five percent of men receiving hormonal therapy experience hot flashes, although the symptom is often overlooked.

Clinical Evaluation/Treatment Options for Hot Flashes

Hot flashes occur as a result of estrogen depletion related to surgery, adjuvant chemotherapy, and hormonal therapy (such as tamoxifen, leuprolide [Lupron], and flutamide [Eulexin]). In the United States, estrogen replacement therapy (ERT) generally is not given to women with a history of breast cancer. Such women are predisposed not only to hot flashes but also to other problems associated with estrogen deficiency, such as osteoporosis and heart disease. In the nonhormonal treatment of hot flashes, such agents as ergotamine tartrate plus phenobarbital (Bellergal), methyldopa, and clonidine have been tried, but often with limited success. Other purported remedies include moderate doses of vitamin E, certain antidepressant agents such as paroxetine (Paxil), venlafaxine Hcl (Effexor),[101] and anticholinergic agents such as oxybutynin chloride (Ditropan).[100] Oxybutynin is an antispasmodic, anticholinergic agent indicated for the treatment of urge incontinence and bladder hyperactivity disorders; it often effectively reduces sweating. It is now available in a sustained-release form, which minimizes the side effects of sleepiness and dry mouth. Patients living in hot climates must be cautioned against overactivity in the heat because diminished sweating can lead to heat stroke when taking anticholinergic agents. Adequate hydration is important to avoid confusion and hyperthermia. In clinical practice, propranolol hydrochloride (Inderal) has been found to decrease the sympathetic symptoms of hot flashes and night sweats in a variety of illnesses, such as Parkinson's disease. Thalidomide has been reported to decrease TNF-α production and sweating in patients with tuberculosis, leprosy, rheumatoid arthritis, graft versus host disease, and mesothelioma (where TNF-α levels were elevated).[96] There are numerous references in the professional and lay literature regarding use of evening primrose oil and phytoestrogens for menopausal symptoms. Phytoestrogens are found in more than 300 plants (coumestans: bean sprouts, red clover, and sunflower seeds; lignans: rye wheat, sesame seeds, linseed). Constituent isoflavones are reportedly similar in efficacy to endogenous estrogen at minimizing the symptoms of menopause (hot flashes) and premenstrual syndrome. A recent study evaluating soy phytoestrogens for treatment of hot flashes in breast cancer survivors concluded the soy product did not alleviate hot flashes.[99] Black cohosh (*Cimicifuga racemosa*) is a perennial herb that has emerged as a treatment for hot flashes, but there is no good evidence from controlled trials to support its use.[102,103]

CASE STUDY

Mrs. M, a Patient with Hot Flashes

Mrs. M is a 60-year-old woman with a prior history of oophorectomy, who was diagnosed in 1994 with breast cancer. Treatment included a lumpectomy, followed by a segmental resection with axillary node dissection and external radiation therapy. Since her diagnosis, she has taken tamoxifen 10 mg twice a day as a prophylactic measure. Hot flashes were reported as her most distressing symptom. The patient described these episodes as being "drenched," and they impacted negatively on her quality of life. Sleep was interrupted due to frequent linen changes (two or three per night), and frequent changes of nightwear were required. Past medical history included mitral valve prolapse, type II diabetes, hypertension, hypercholesterolemia, stress incontinence (status post bladder suspension), and oophorectomy.

Mrs. M is a very pleasant, well-developed, well-nourished woman in no distress. Vital signs: T: 35.9°C; P: 95; BP: 162/92; Wt: 84 kg. The physical examination was unremarkable except for the area of the right breast, where a well-healed surgical deficit was present. There was increased density in the tissue of the right breast. There was no erythema and no palpable mass. There was no lymphadenopathy in the supraclavicular region or axillae. There was no nipple discharge.

Diagnostic data included fasting blood sugar of 115. The impression is that the hot flashes are related to tamoxifen use.

The patient was given a prescription for a clonidine TTS-1 patch, to be worn weekly, to block the symptoms of excessive sympathetic outflow that caused her hot flashes and sweats, and to treat her hypertension. The clonidine was tried for 1 month, but after this, the patient discontinued the patch, feeling it was ineffective and reporting symptoms of orthostatic hypotension. Hyosphen (Bellergal), which contains phenobarbital, ergotamine, and belladonna, was prescribed, twice a day.

This agent was tried for several days, and while it had some efficacy, the patient found its sedating properties to be unacceptable. Oxybutynin chloride (Ditropan), an anticholinergic and antispasmodic agent, was prescribed. At the starting dose of 5 mg bid, the patient reported that the frequency and intensity of her hot flashes were considerably reduced and that her urinary urgency was also better controlled.

The patient's quality of life reportedly improved when she was able to sleep through the night without experiencing the hot flashes or nocturia. She was able to decrease the dose of oxybutynin to 5 mg once a day at bedtime.

Conclusion

Pruritus, fever, and sweats are frequently seen in end-of-life care but are still not well managed. New pharmacological therapies have evolved in the palliation of these symptoms, and the physiological processes are better understood. Symptoms of pruritus, fever, and sweats should be assessed and recognized as causing distress to the patient and negatively impacting on the patient's quality of life. In the palliative care setting, treatment of the underlying disease process may be limited but comfort should be a priority.

REFERENCES

1. Pittelkow MR, Loprinzi CL. Pruritus and sweating. In: Doyle D, Hanks G, Cherny N, Calman K, eds. Oxford Textbook of Palliative Medicine, 3rd ed. Oxford: Oxford University Press, 2004:573–587.
2. Fleischer AB Jr, Michaels JR. Pruritus. In: Berger A, Portenoy RK, Weissman DE, Principles and Practice of Supportive Oncology. Philadelphia: Lippincott Williams & Wilkins, 1998:245–250.
3. Denman ST. A review of pruritus. J Am Acad Dermatol 1986; 14:375–392.
4. Fleischer AB, Michaels JR. Pruritus. In: Berger A, Portenoy RK, Weissman DE, Principles and Practice of Supportive Oncology. Philadelphia: Lippincott Williams & Wilkins, 1998:245–250.
5. Simandl G. Alterations in skin function and integrity. In: Porth CM, ed. Pathophysiology Concepts of Altered Health States 3rd Ed. Philadelphia: JB Lippincott, 1990:106–143.
6. Herndon JH Jr. Itching: the pathophysiology of pruritus. Int J Dermatol 1975;14:465.
7. Tuckett RP, Denman ST, Chapman CR, et al. Pruritus, cutaneous pain, and eccrine gland and sweating disorders. J Am Acad Dermatol 1985; 5:1000–1006.
8. Handwerker HO, Forster HC, Kirchhoff C. Discharge patterns of human C-fibers induced by itching and burning stimuli. J Neurophysiol 1991;66:307–315.
9. Bradford FK. Ablations of frontal cortex in cats with special reference to enhancement of the scratch reflex. J Neurophysiol 1939;2:192–201.
10. King CA, Huff FJ, Jorizzo JL. Unilated neurogenic pruritus: paroxysmal itching associated with central nervous system lesions. Ann Intern Med 1982;97:222–223.
11. Massey EW. Unilateral neurogenic pruritus following stroke. Stroke 1984;15:901–903.
12. Lowitt MH, Bernhard JD. Quantitation of itch and scratch. Semin Neurol 1992;12:374–384.
13. Lovell CR, Burton PA, Duncan EHL, Burton JL. Prostaglandins and pruritus. Br J Dermatol 1976;94:273.
14. Schworer H, Ramadori G. Treatment of pruritus: a new indication for serotonin type 3 receptor antagonists. Clin Invest 1993;71:659–662.
15. Raderer M, Muller C, Scheithauer W. Ondansetron for pruritus due to cholestasis. N Engl J Med 1994;330:1540.
16. Radossi P, Tison T, Vianello F, Dazzi F. Intractable pruritus in non-Hodgkins lymphoma/CLL: rapid response to IFN α. Br J Haematol 1996;94:579–583.
17. Cooper DL, Gilliam AC, Perez MI. Hyperprolactinemic galactorrhea in a patient with Hodgkin's disease and intense pruritus. South Med J 1993;86:829–830.
18. Apel RL, Fernandes BJ. Malignant lymphoma presenting with an elevated serum CA-125 level. Arch Pathol Lab Med 1995;119: 373–376.
19. Krajnik, M., and Zylicz, Z. Understanding pruritus in systemic disease. J Pain Symptom Manage 2001;21:151–168.
20. Nicol NH, Boguniewicz M. Understanding and treating atopic dermatitis. Nurse Pract Forum 1999;10:48–55.
21. Malet KM. Pruritus associated with cholestasis. A review of pathogenesis and management. Dig Dis Sci 1994;39:1–8.
22. Losowsky T Jr. Opioid peptides and primary biliary cirrhosis. BMJ 1988;297:1501–1504.
23. Borgeat A, Savioz D, Mentha G, Giostra E, Suter PM. Intractable cholestatic pruritus after liver transplantation–management with propofol. Transplantation 1994;58:727–730.
24. Borgeat A, Wilder-Smith OHG, Saiah M, Rifat K. Subhypnotic doses of propofol relieve pruritus induced by epidural and intrathecal morphine. Anesthesiology 1992;76:510–512.
25. Bachs L. Rifampin more effectively relieves pruritus in patients with primary biliary cirrhosis, compared with phenobarbital. Lancet 1989;1:574–576.
26. Jones EA, Bergasa NV. The pruritus of cholestasis: from bile acids to opiate agonists. Hepatology 1990;11:884–887.
27. Abboud TK, Lee K, Zhu J, et al. Prophylactic oral naltrexone with intrathecal morphine for cesarean section: effects on adverse reactions and analgesias. Anesth Analg 1990;71:367–70.
28. Thornton JR, Losowsky MS. Opioid peptides and primary biliary cirrhosis. BMJ 1988;297:1501–1504.
29. Bergasa NV, Alling DW, Talbot TL, et al. Effects of naloxone infusions in patients with the pruritus of cholestasis. A double-blind, randomized, controlled trial. Ann Intern Med 1995;123:161–167.
30. Khandelwal M, Malet PF. Pruritus associated with cholestasis: a review of pathogenesis and management. Dig Dis Sci 1994;39: 1–7.
31. Fuller JG, McMorland GH, Douglas MJ. Epidural morphine for analgesis after caesarean section: a report of 4880 cases. Can J Anaesth 1990;37:636–640.
32. Cohen SE, Ratner EF, Kreitzman TR, et al. Nalbuphine is better than naloxone for treatment of side effects after epidural morphine. Anesth Analg 1992;75:747–752.
33. Bernstein JE, Swift RM, Soltani K, Lorincz A. Anti-pruritic effect of an opiate antagonist, naloxone hydrochloride. J Invest Dermatol 1982;78:82–83.
34. Ackerman W, Juneja M, Kaczorowski D, Colclough G. A comparison of the incidence of pruritus following epidural opioid administration in the patient. Can J Anaesth 1989;36:388–391.

35. Hermens JM, Ebertz JM, Hanifin JM, Hirshman CA. Comparison of histamine release in human skin mast cells induced by morphine, fentanyl, and oxymorphone. Anesthesiology 1985;62:124–129.
36. Sinatra RS, Lodge K, Sibert K, et al. A comparison of morphine, meperidine, and oxymorphone as utilized in patient-controlled analgesia following cesarean delivery. Anesthesiology 1989;70:585–590.
37. Woodhouse A, Hobbes AFT, Mather LE, Gibson M. A comparison of morphine, pethidine and fentanyl in the postsurgical patient-controlled analgesis environment. Pain 1996;64:115–121.
38. Bergasa NV, Talbot TL, Alling DW, et al. A controlled trial of naloxone infusions for the pruritus of chronic cholestasis. Gastroenterology 1992;102:544–549.
39. Bernhard JD. Phantom itch, pseudophantom itch and senile pruritus. Int J Dermatol 1992;33:856–857.
40. Yamamoto M, Yabuki S, Hayabara T, Otsuki S. Paroxysmal itching in multiple sclerosis: a report of three cases. J Neurol Neurosurg Psychiatry 1981;44:19–22.
41. Osterman PO. Paroxysmal itching in multiple sclerosis. Br J Dermatol 1976;95:555.
42. Daniel GL, Longa WE, Vernava AM III. Pruritus ani: causes and concerns. Dis Colon Rectum 1994;37:670–674.
43. Hejna M, Valencak J, Raderer M. Anal pruritus after cancer chemotherapy with gemcitabine. N Engl J Med 1999;340:655–656.
44. Gilchrest BA. Pruritus: pathogenesis, therapy and significance in systemic disease states. Arch Intern Med 1982;142:101–105.
45. De Marchi SD, Cecchin E, Villalta D, Sepiacci G, Santini G, Bartoli E. Relief of pruritus and decreases in plasma histamine concentrations during erythropoietin therapy in patients with uremia. N Engl J Med 1992;326:15.
46. Hunnuksela A, Kinnunen T. Moisturizers prevent irritant dermatitis. Acta Derm Venereol 1992;72:42–44.
47. Pittelknow MR, Loprinzi CL. Pruritus and sweating in palliative medicine. In: Doyle D, Hanks G, Cherny N, Calman K, eds. Oxford Textbook of Palliative Medicine, 3rd ed. New York: Oxford University Press, 2004: 573–587.
48. Gatti S, Serri F. Pruritus in Clinical Medicine. New York: McGraw Hill, 1991:90–105.
49. Nicol NH, Baumeister LL. Topical corticosteroid therapy: considerations for prescribing and use. Prim Care 1997;1:62–69.
50. Chaffman MO. Topical corticosteroids: a review of properties and principles in therapeutic use. Nurse Pract Forum 1999;10:95–105.
51. Rudy SJ. Superficial fungal infections in children and adolescents. Nurse Pract Forum 1999;10:56–66.
52. Gan TJ, Ginsberg B, Glass PSA, Fortney J, Jhaveri R, Perno R. Opioid-sparing effects of a low-dose infusion of naloxone in patient-administered morphine sulfate. Anesthesiology 1997;87:1075–1081.
53. Sullivan JR, Watson A. Naltrexone: a case report of pruritus from an antipruritic. Australas J Dermatol 1997;38:196–198.
54. Kendrick WD, Woods AM, Daly MY, Birch RF, DiFazio C. Naloxone versus nalbuphine infusion for prophylaxis of epidural morphine-induced pruritus. Anesth Analg 1996;82:641–647.
55. Monroe EW. Efficacy and safety of nalmefene in patients with severe pruritus caused by chronic urticaria and atopic dermatitis. J Am Acad Dermatol 1989;21:135–136.
56. Sullivan JR, Watson A. Naltrexone: a case report of pruritus from an antipruritic. Australas J Dermatol 1997;38:196–198.
57. Howser RL. What you need to know about corticosteroid therapy. Am J Nurs 1995:95;44–48.
58. Fishman S, Stojanovic MP, Borsook D. Intravenous lidocaine for treatment-resistant pruritus. Am J Med 1997;102:584–585.
59. Radossi P, Tison T, Vianello F, Dazzi F. Intractable pruritus in non-Hodgkin lymphoma/CLL: rapid response to IFN alpha. Br J Haematol 1996;94:579–583.
60. Neuber K, Berg-Drewniock B, Volkenandt M, Neumaier M, Gross G, Ring J. B cell chronic lymphocytic leukemia associated with high serum IGE levels and pruriginous skin lesions: successful therapy with IFN α after failure on IFN Γ. Dermatology 1996;192:110–115.
61. Kikuchi-Numagami K, Sato M, Tagami H. Successful treatment of a therapy resistant severely pruritic skin eruption of malignancy associated dermatomyositis with high dose intravenous immunoglobulin. J Dermatol 1996;23:340–343.
62. Freilich RJ, Seidman AD. Pruritus caused by 3-hour infusion of high-dose paclitaxel and improvement with tricyclic antidepressants. J Natl Cancer Inst 1995;87:933–934.
63. Liddell K. Post-herpetic pruritus. BMJ 1974;4:165.
64. Procacci P, Maresca M. Case report. Pain 1991;45:307–308.
65. Zylicz Z, Smits C, Krajnik M. Paroxetine for pruritus in advanced cancer. J Pain Symptom Manage 1998;16:121–124.
66. Saiah M, Borgeat A, Wilder-Smith HG, Rifat K, Suter PM. Epidural morphine-induced pruritus: propofol versus naloxone. Anesth Analg 1994;78:1110–1113.
67. Wilde MI, Markham A. Ondansetron: a review of its pharmacology and preliminary clinical findings in novel applications. Drugs 1996;52:773–794.
68. Larijani GE, Goldberg ME, Rogers KH. Treatment of opioid induced pruritus with ondansetron: report of four patients. Pharmacotherapy 1996;16:958–960.
69. Fried RG. Evaluation and treatment of psychogenic pruritus and self excoriation. J Am Acad Dermatol 1994;30:993–999.
70. Ostrowski MJ. Pain control in advanced malignant disease using transcutaneous nerve stimulation. Br J Clin Pract 1979;33:157–162.
71. Ostrowski MJ, Dodd A. Transcutaneous nerve stimulation for relief of pain in advanced malignant disease. Nurs Times 1977; 11:1233–1238.
72. Carlsson CA, Augustinsson LE, Lund S, Roupe G. Electrical transcutaneous nerve stimulation for relief of itch. Experientia 1975;31:191.
73. Cleary J. Fever and sweats: including the immunocompromised hosts. In: Berger A, Portenoy RK, Weissman DE, Principles and Practice of Supportive Oncology. Philadelphia: Lippincott Williams & Wilkins, 1998:119–131.
74. Porth CM, Curtis RL. Alteration in temperature regulation. In: Porth CM, ed. Pathophysiology Concepts of Altered Health States, 3rd ed. Philadelphia: JB Lippincott, 1990:95–105.
75. Styrt B, Sugarman B. Antipyresis and fever. Arch Intern Med 1990;150:1591–1597.
76. Carpenter R. Fever. In: Chernecky CC, Berger BJ, eds. Advanced and Critical Care Oncology Nursing: Managing Primary Complications. Philadelphia: WB Saunders, 1998:156–171.
77. Bruce JL, Grove SK. Fever: pathology and treatment. Crit Care Nurse 1992;12:40–49.
78. Chernecky CC, Berger BJ. Fever. In: Chernecky CC, Berger BJ, eds. Advanced and Critical Care Oncology Nursing: Managing Primary Complications. Philadelphia: WB Saunders 1998:156–171.
79. Pizzo PA. Management of fever in patients with cancer and treatment induced neutropenia. N Engl J Med 1993;328:1323–1332.
80. Pizzo PA. Fever in immunocompromised patients. N Engl J Med 1999;341:893–897.

81. Wujcik D. Infection control in oncology patients. Nurs Clin North Am 1993;20:639–650.
82. Lokkevik E, Skovlund E, Reitan JB, Hannidsdal E, Tanum G. Skin treatment with bepanthen cream versus no cream during radiotherapy. Acta Oncol 1996;35:8.
83. Omand M, Meredith C. A study of acute side-effects related to palliative radiotherapy treatment of lung cancer. Eur J Cancer Care 1994;3:149–152.
84. Manganelli D, Palla A, Donnamaria V, Giuntini C. Clinical features of pulmonary embolus. Doubts and certainties. Chest 1995;107:S25–S32.
85. Pitz CCM, Lokhorst HM, Hoekstra JBL. Fever as a presenting symptom of multiple myeloma. Neth J Med 1998;53:256–259.
86. Scully RE, Mark EJ, McNeely WF, Ebeling SH. Case presentation. N Engl J Med 1996;335:1514–1521.
87. Gucalp R. Management of the febrile neutropenic patient with cancer. Oncology 1991;5:137–144.
88. Chang JC, Gross HM. Neoplastic fever responds to adequate dose of naproxen. J Clin Oncol 1985;3:552–558.
89. Burke MB, Wilkes GM, Berg DB, Bean CK, Ingwersen K. Cancer Chemotherapy: A Nursing Process Approach. Boston: Jones and Bartlett, 1991:49–138.
90. Finkbiner KL, Ernst TF. Drug therapy management of the febrile neutropenic cancer patient. Cancer Pract 1993;1:295–304.
91. Rogers AG. Considering histamine release in prescribing opioid analgesics. J Pain Symptom Manage 1991;6:44.
92. Coyle N, Cherny N, Portenoy R. Pharmacologic management of cancer pain. In: McGuire DB, Henke Yarbro C, Ferrell B, eds. Cancer Pain Management, 2nd ed. Boston: Jones and Bartlett, 1995:89–130.
93. Waller A, Hershkowitz M, Adunsky A. The effect of intravenous fluid infusion on blood and urine parameters of hydration and on state of consciousness in terminal cancer patients. Am J Hospice Palliat Care 1994;11:22–37.
94. Fainsinger RL. Rehydration in palliative care. Palliat Med 1996; 10:165–166.
95. Takata Y, Kurihara J, Suzuki S, Okubo Y, Kato H. A rabbit model for evaluation of chlorpromazine-induced orthostatic hypotension. Biol Pharm Bull 1999;22:457–462.
96. Gates LK, Cameron AJ, Nagorney DM, Goellner JR, Farley DR. Primary leiomyosarcoma of the liver mimicking liver abscess. Am J Gastroenterol 1995;90:649–652.
97. Tuckett RP, Wei JY. Response to an itch-producing substance in CAT II cutaneous receptor populations with unmyelinated axons. Brain Res 1987;413:95–103.
98. Deaner P. Thalidomide for distressing night sweats in advanced malignant disease. Palliat Med 1998;12:208–209.
99. Quella SK, Loprinzi CL, Barton DL, Knost JA, Sloan JA, LaVasseur BI, Swan D, Krupp KR, Miller KD, Notovny PJ. Evaluation of soy phytoestrogens for the treatment of hot flashes in breast cancer survivors: A North Central Cancer Group Trial. J Clin Oncol 2000;18:1068–1074.
100. Stearns V, Isaacs C, Rowland J, Crawford J, Ellis MJ, Kramer R, Lawrence W, Hanfelt JJ, Haynes DF. A pilot trial assessing the efficacy of paroxetine hydrochloride (Paxil) in controlling hot flashes in breast cancer survivors. Ann Oncol 2000;11:17–22.
101. Loprinzi CL, Pisansky TM, Fonseca R, Sloan JA, et al. Pilot evaluation of venlafaxine hydrochloride for the therapy of hot flashes in cancer survivors. J Clin Oncol 1998;16:2377–2381.
102. Petit J. Alternative medicine. Black cohosh. Clin Rev 2000;10: 117–121.
103. Lisle E. Therapeutic efficacy and safety of Cimicifuga racemosa for gynecologic disorders. Adv Ther 1998;15:45–53.
104. Krajnik M, Zylicz, Z. Understanding pruritus in systemic disease. Journal of Pain and Symptom Management, 2001;21 (2):151–168.
105. Pittelkow MR, Loprinzi CL. Pruritus and sweating. In: Doyle D, Hanks G, Cherny, N, Calman, K, eds. Oxford Textbook of Palliative Medicine, 2nd Ed. Oxford University Press, 2004: 573–587.
106. Charlesworth E, Beltrani V. Pruritic dermatoses: overview of etiology and therapy. The American Journal of Medicine, 2002; 113(9A): 25S–33S.

18

Judith A. Paice

Neurological Disturbances

The seizures never stopped. It was awful to witness. We will never forget how he suffered.
—A mother

- ***Key Points***
- *Myoclonus, uncontrolled rhythmic jerking movements, often is due to accumulation of opioid metabolites, particularly in patients with renal dysfunction.*
- *Seizures may arise from central nervous system neoplasms, metabolic dysfunction, medications, stroke and other causes. Aggressive management is indicated to reduce pain and exhaustion.*
- *Spasms, involving uncontrolled movement, rigidity, and hyperreflexia, can impair mobility and cause pain. Palliative care includes pharmacological and nonpharmacological management, along with safety measures.*

Myoclonus is frequently seen in palliative care settings, particularly during the final days of life. If left untreated, this neurological disturbance may progress to seizures. Seizures also may occur due to central nervous system (CNS) lesions, metabolic disorders, or medications. A third neurological disturbance, spasticity, involves involuntary movements that may produce discomfort and fatigue. Astute palliative care clinicians can prevent some of these disorders and treat those that cannot be prevented. Patient and family involvement is mandatory since comfort and safety issues are prevalent with all three syndromes.

Myoclonus

Myoclonus consists of sudden, uncontrollable, nonrhythmic jerking, usually of the extremities.[1] Frequently seen in the palliative care setting, myoclonus can be exhausting and can progress to more severe neurological dysfunction, including seizures. Early identification and rapid treatment are critical.

Causes of Myoclonus

In the palliative care setting, myoclonus is most often associated with opioids. The prevalence of opioid-induced myoclonus ranges greatly, from 2.7% to 87%.[1] Nocturnal myoclonus is common and often precedes opioid-induced myoclonus.[2] The precise cause of opioid-induced myoclonus is unknown; however, several mechanisms have been proposed.[3,4] High doses of opioids result in the accumulation of neuroexcitatory metabolites. The best characterized are morphine-3-glucuronide and hydromorphone-3-glucouronide.[5,6] Serum and cerebrospinal fluid levels, as well as the ratios of these metabolites, are elevated in patients receiving morphine for cancer and nonmalignant pain.[7] This is particularly true for patients with renal dysfunction.[8] However, clinical evidence of myoclonus does not consistently correlate with serum levels of morphine-3-glucuronide.[9] Hyperalgesia is particularly associated with these metabolites, although other opioids with no known metabolites have also produced myoclonus.[10] A variety of other metabolites of opioids exist, including morphine-6-glucuronide and hydromorphone-6-glucuronide, but these have been implicated in nausea and vomiting, as well as sedation, rather than myoclonus.

Opioids given in high doses may result in myoclonus.[3] Bruera and Pereira[11] reported the development of acute confusion, restlessness, myoclonus, hallucinations, and hyperalgesia due to an inadvertant administration of 5000-mcg intravenous (IV) fentanyl (the patient had been receiving 1000 mcg/hour subcutaneously). These symptoms were successfully treated with several doses of 0.1 to 0.2 mg of IV naloxone, followed by a continuous IV naloxone infusion of 0.2 mg/hour. The patient did not demonstrate withdrawal symptoms initially, yet began to complain of return of pain after several hours (see Chapter 6 regarding the use of diluted naloxone to reverse adverse effects associated with opioids). Other opioids, including methadone,[12] meperidine,[13] and transdermal fentanyl[14] have been implicated in the development of myoclonus.

Other reported causes of myoclonus include surgery to the brain,[15] placement of an intrathecal catheter,[16] AIDS dementia,[17] hypoxia,[18] chlorambucil,[19] and a paraneoplastic syndrome.[20] This paraneoplastic syndrome is rare, occurring in fewer than 1% of people with cancer. The etiology of the paraneoplastic syndrome can also be viral and is believed to be immunologically mediated. Symptoms of this paraneoplastic (also called opsoclonus-myoclonus) syndrome include myoclonus, opsoclonus, ataxia, and encephalopathic features.[21] Treatment of the underlying tumor or infection and immunosuppression are possible treatments.[20,21]

Assessment

An accurate history from the patient and family is essential. An analogy to help patients describe the symptoms is to compare the jerking to the feeling that often happens when one is close to falling asleep (a common condition called nocturnal myoclonus). The difference is that myoclonus is usually continuous. Physical exam will reveal jerking of the extremities, which is uncontrolled by movement or other activities. Jerking can be induced by single or repeated tapping of a muscle group.

Treatment

Opioid rotation is the primary treatment of myoclonus, particularly if the patient is receiving higher doses of an opioid and has renal dysfunction.[1] There is great variation in individual response to opioids, thus, different agents may have a greater likelihood of producing myoclonus or other adverse effects. Presently, there are no tests that predict individual response, and trials are the only strategy for determining effectiveness as well as adverse effects. In addition, cross-tolerance is not complete, and thus, lower equianalgesic doses of an alternate opioid may provide analgesia. Methadone has been successfully used as an alternative agent,[7] although other opioids may be easier to titrate, and methadone also has been reported to cause myoclonus.[12] Strategies, such as adding adjuvant analgesics, that reduce the necessary amount of opioid could reduce or eliminate myoclonus.

Little research is available regarding agents used to reduce myoclonic jerking. Benzodiazepines, including clonazepam, diazepam, and midazolam, have been recommended.[1,22] The antispasmodic baclofen has been used to treat myoclonus due to intraspinal opioid administration.[23] Dantrolene has been used, yet it produces significant muscle weakness and hepatotoxicity.[24]

Patient and Family Education

Safety measures are essential, as are interventions designed to reduce fatigue during myoclonus. Use padding around bed rails and assistive devices if the patient is ambulatory. Provide a calm, relaxing environment. Pain assessment is critical as opioids are rotated since equianalgesic conversions are approximations and wide variability exists. Therefore, patients and family members are encouraged to track pain intensity as opioids are titrated to provide optimal relief.

Seizures

Of the many neurological disorders that occur in advanced disease, seizures are the most frightening. This fear exists for the patient and for their caregivers. Furthermore, seizures can be exhausting for the patient, eliminating the few energy reserves that might be better spent on quality activities. Therefore, seizures must be prevented whenever possible. When prevention is not feasible, all attempts should be made to limit the extent of the seizure and ensure safety measures to prevent trauma during these episodes.

Seizures occur when a large number of neurons discharge abnormally.[25] This abnormal discharge produces involuntary paroxysmal behavioral changes. There are two types of seizure, including primary (also called generalized) and focal (also called partial). Primary seizures involve large parts of the brain and include both grand mal and petit mal types. Focal seizures are isolated to specific regions of the brain, and symptoms reflect the area of disturbance.[25] For example, Jacksonian motor seizures result from abnormal discharge in the motor cortex. These patients may have involuntary twitching of muscle groups, usually on the contralateral side of the body. If the tumor is located in the left motor cortex (anterior to the central sulcus), the activity is seen on the right side of the body. Often, activity begins in one area and spreads throughout that side of the body as abnormal discharge spreads to nearby cortical neurons. Patients generally remain conscious, unless the abnormal cortical discharge spreads to the opposite hemisphere. In the palliative care setting, there are many potential causes of seizure activity.

Causes of Seizures

Careful consideration of the many causes of seizure activity must be included in the assessment of patients at the end of life, whether the patient has demonstrated seizure activity or not. This allows prevention whenever possible. Primary or metastatic neoplasms to the brain are common causes of seizures in palliative care, as are preexisting seizure disorders.[26] Medications, including phenothiazines, butyrophenones, and tricyclic antidepressants, can lower the seizure threshold. Other medication-related causes of seizures include metabolites (e.g., normeperidine), preservatives within these compounds (e.g., sodium bisulfite), or the abrupt discontinuation of certain drugs (e.g., benzodiazepines).[3,27] Additional causes of seizures at the end of life include metabolic disorders, infection, HIV, stroke, hemorrhage, oxygen deprivation, and some rare paraneoplastic syndromes (Table 18–1).[26,28,29]

Primary or Metastatic Brain Tumors. Brain tumors can result in either primary generalized or focal seizures. Seizures occur in approximately 25% of those with brain metastases.[30] Patients with malignancies known to metastasize to the brain, such as breast, lung, hypernephroma, and melanoma, should be considered at risk for seizures. Leukemias and lymphomas are also known to produce infiltrates in the brain. Multiple metastases or brain and leptomeningeal disease are more commonly associated with seizures.[30] The tumor location, size, and histology dictate whether seizures may result and the resulting symptoms associated with the seizure.

Medications. Medications can lead to seizures in the palliative care setting through several mechanisms. Medications such as the phenothiazines, butyrophenones, and tricyclic antidepressants can place patients at risk by lowering the seizure threshold. These agents should be used cautiously in patients with intracranial tumors or infection. There are reports of patients developing seizures due to fluoroquinolones, including ofloxacin and ifosfamide (more likely if serum creatinine is elevated and the patient has had prior treatment with cisplatin), as well as cephalosporins and monobactams.[31–35] In very high doses, any opioid can lead to seizures. Several opioids are associated with much higher risk due to their metabolites that cause seizures. Meperidine is converted to normeperidine during metabolism.[13] Individuals with renal dysfunction cannot excrete normeperidine efficiently; the metabolite then accumulates in the bloodstream and leads to seizures. Therefore, the clinical practice guidelines developed by the American Pain Society for cancer pain strongly discourage the use of meperidine in any patient, a practice long known to those in palliative care.[36] These guidelines also discourage the use of propoxyphene (the weak opioid in Darvon) in persons with cancer due to the metabolite norpropoxyphene.[36]

More recently, morphine and hydromorphone have been found to be metabolized by glucuronidation to morphine-3-glucuronide or hydromorphine-3-glucuronide, respectively. These metabolites may produce hyperalgesia (elevated pain intensity), myoclonus (see previous section), and seizure in patients unable to excrete these efficiently.[7,10] Clinically, patients respond acceptably to the opioid for the first day or two, then develop symptoms after the metabolite has accumulated. Alternately, the patient may have obtained good relief in the absence of opioid neurolotoxicity, until renal status diminishes, with concomitant difficulties in clearing the metabolite. Another opioid, tramadol, has been associated with seizure risk, especially when taken with other drugs that lower the seizure threshold.

Compounds added to medications to preserve the drug or prevent its breakdown (such as sodium bisulfite) are normally present in extremely small amounts. However, when high doses of a drug, usually opioids, are needed to treat severe pain, the concomitant dose of these additives increases. In this setting, there have been rare reports of seizures.[27] Using preservative-free solutions when administering high doses of any agent may prevent this activity. Hagen and Swanson[3] report a syndrome of opioid hyperexcitability that progressed to seizures in five patients with high-dose infusions. Parenteral midazolam infusion was used to treat the seizures, the patients were rotated to alternative opioids (including levorphanol and methadone), and aggressive supportive care was provided during the episodes.

Rapid cessation of various drugs can lead to seizure activity in the palliative care setting. Often, this occurs when staff are unaware that a patient uses certain medications and, as a result, these drugs are not provided when patients are hospitalized or unable to independently dispense their own drugs. Benzodiazepines, barbiturates, and baclofen are the most common drugs associated with seizures during abstinence.[25] This also can occur when the patient abuses these compounds or alcohol and the staff or family is unaware. Alcohol abuse often is underrecognized in the palliative care setting.[37]

Table 18–1
Causes of Seizures in Palliative Care

Primary or metastatic neoplasm to the brain
Preexisting seizure disorder
Medications
Lower seizure threshold
Metabolites
Preservatives, antioxidants, or other additives
Abstinence
Metabolic disorders
Infection
Trauma
Strokes and hemorrhage
Paraneoplastic syndromes

Other Causes of Seizures in Palliative Care. Infection within the brain, as may be seen in persons with human immunodeficiency virus (HIV) or acquired immunodeficiency syndrome (AIDS), can lead to seizure activity.[17,29] The syndrome of inappropriate antidiuretic hormone, associated with lung cancer and other malignancies, can result in increased water and sodium content within the cells.[38] The resultant swelling of neuronal cells within the brain causes increased intracranial pressure (ICP). Anoxia deprives the brain of needed nutrients, resulting in an inability to drive sodium out of neuronal tissue. Water follows into the cells, creating increased ICP. Hyponatremia (<130 mEq/L) can also lead to mental status changes and seizures, especially when of rapid onset.

Assessment

Conduct a thorough history from the patient and caregiver to ascertain any symptoms existing with the onset of the seizure, the specific type of seizure activity, and whether there was any aura immediately before the seizure.[25] Headache, nausea, and projectile vomiting are associated with increased ICP and can occur immediately before seizure activity.[30] The family may relate a staring-type behavior, where the patient does not respond to stimuli for a brief moment.

The past medical history might reveal a seizure disorder. Review all drugs recently added to the plan of care for agents that might lower the seizure threshold or produce metabolites. Question whether the patient recently discontinued a drug, including recreational drugs. If the patient is currently taking anticonvulsants or corticosteroids for seizures and increased ICP, determine if there could be reasons that the drugs were not ingested or absorbed. These might include compliance issues or nausea and vomiting.

Often, the clinician may not witness the seizure and must rely on the observation and memory of family members and caregivers. Assist family members in differentiating between seizures and myoclonus (see previous section) or altered level of consciousness due to other etiologies. A thorough examination is indicated, with attention to bruises and other signs of trauma. If these occur, additional teaching for family and caregivers regarding safety measures is warranted.

Measuring serum levels of anticonvulsants may be indicated to insure that the drug is adequately absorbed.[39] Dose adjustments may be done empirically based on the patient's condition. Electroencephalography may be used to identify the site of abnormal discharge. Brain lesions may be scanned using computed tomography (CT) or magnetic resonance imaging (MRI). These tests should only be considered if they will provide information that will guide therapy and if they are consistent with the patient's and family's goals of care.

Treatment

Anticonvulsants are used when patients have demonstrated seizures (Table 18–2). The prophylactic use of anticonvulsants in patients who have not had a seizure is controversial. Only in the case of brain metastases from melanoma has prophylactic anticonvulsant therapy demonstrated benefit. The potential benefits must be weighed against the side effects associated with these agents.

The most common anticonvulsants used in the United States to prevent seizures are phenytoin, carbamazepine, valproate, and phenobarbital (see Table 18–2).[39] Newer anticonvulsants, such as gabapentin, vigabatrin, and lamotrigine, have not been extensively studied in the palliative care setting.[39,40] Agents used during a seizure include diazepam, lorazepam, midazolam, phenytoin, and phenobarbital (Table 18–3).

A particular challenge in palliative care is the administration of these drugs when the patient is unable to take oral medications. The intramuscular route can be used for some (diazepam and phenobarbitol), but since this route is painful and absorption is unpredictable, its use should be reserved for situations when no other access is practical or possible. Diazepam is available in a rectal gel. Doses are 200 mcg/kg body weight, rounded down to the next available unit dose (10-mg, 15-mg, and 20-mg unit doses for adults) in debilitated patients. Phenobarbital is available in a solution for parenteral delivery, and pentobarbital (used more commonly in Canada and Europe) is available in rectal formulations. Intravenous phenytoin can lead to the purple-glove syndrome, a potentially serious local complication including edema, discoloration, and pain distal to the injection site.[41,42] Fosphenytoin, although more expensive, has an advantage in palliative care because it can be given subcutaneously (by either intermittent injection or infusion) for prevention or treatment of seizures. Dosing is based on phenytoin equivalents, generally 5- to 10-mg phenytoin equivalent/kg. Little research has compared the efficacy of these agents, particularly in the palliative care setting. The choice of agent is often based on the availability of the drug, comfort level of the practitioner, ability to use nonoral routes, and other factors. Because most medications are administered by nonprofessional caregivers in the home, often elderly spouses of aged patients, it is best to keep the drug regimen simple.

Many patients with seizure disorders will also be taking dexamethasone. Dexamethasone is technically not an anticonvulsant, yet this compound is critical when intracranial lesions that might increase ICP are present.[39] Although most texts suggest four-times-a-day (qid) dosing, the long half-life of dexamethasone allows daily dosing with adequate serum levels maintained throughout the 24-hour period. Of additional concern is the interaction between phenytoin and dexamethasone. Phenytoin can decrease the bioavailability of dexamethasone by as much as 20%. Additionally, dexamethasone inhibits the metabolism of phenytoin, reducing the anticonvulsant effect of this drug. Thus, extreme care must be exercised when adding or titrating either drug when using combinations. Phenytoin can alter plasma levels of several drugs (Table 18–4). In the palliative care setting, if a patient decides to stop all corticosteroids, the professional must evaluate the likelihood of developing seizures. Prophylactic therapy must be considered.

Table 18–2
Prophylactic Pharmacological Management of Seizures

Drug	Adult Dose	Adverse Effects	Comments
Phenytoin (Dilantin) Tablets Capsules Suspension Parenteral	Loading dose: 5 mg/kg PO q3h × 3 doses (loading dose not to be used in patients with renal or hepatic disease) Maintenance: 5 mg/kg PO	Nystagmus, ataxia, slurred speech, mental confusion, Stevens-Johnson syndrome Too rapid IV injection (>50 mg/min) can result in cardiac toxicity	Usual serum level 10–20 mcg/mL (or 10–20 mg/L or 40–80 µmol/L)
Carbamazepine (Tegretol) Tablets Suspension	400 mg/day: Tablet: 200 mg bid Suspension: 1 teaspoon qid Maximum dose: 1600 mg/24 h	Aplastic anemia, agranulocytosis Patients with known sensitivity to tricyclic antidepressants may be hypersensitive to carbamazepine.	Periodic blood counts and liver function tests indicated Therapeutic plasma levels 4–12 mcg/mL
Valproic acid (Depakene) Capsules Syrup	15 mg/kg daily, increasing weekly in 5–10 mg increments Syrup can be given rectally by a red rubber catheter 250–500 mg tid.	Hepatic failure, coagulopathies, nausea, vomiting, sedation	Therapeutic plasma levels 50–100 mcg/mL
Divalproex sodium (Depakote) Capsules Sprinkles Tablets	Same dosing for valproic acid and divalproex, although peaks and troughs may differ	Chewing may produce irritation of the mouth and throat.	
Phenobarbital Tablets Elixir Parenteral	Oral: 60–200 mg/day Parenteral: 3–4–mg/kg q24h continuous SQ infusion	Sedation, paradoxical excitation	
Midazolam (Versed) Parenteral	1–3 mg/h continuous SQ or IV Infusion	Sedation, respiratory depression if overdose	Antagonist, flumazenil, can result in seizures. Use same extreme caution as when giving naloxone for suspected opioid overdose.

SQ = subcutaneous; IV = intravenous.

Table 18–3
Acute Treatment of Seizures

Drug	Dose
Diazepam (Valium)	5–10 mg slow IV push (stop other infusions to prevent incompatibility problems) or 5–10 mg IM every 5–10 min if no IV access, can also use diazepam (Diastat) rectal gel, usually 10 mg per rectum
Fosphenytoin (Cerebyx)	15–20 mg phenytoin equivalents/kg IV loading dose
Lorazepam (Ativan)	1 mg/min up to 5 mg
Midazolam (Versed)	0.02–0.10 mg/kg continuous hourly infusion
Phenobarbital	20 mg/kg IV at a rate of 100 mg/min
Phenytoin (Dilantin)	Acute treatment: 20 mg/kg IV infusion over 20–30 min. An additional 5–10 mg/kg can be given if seizures persist. However, IV injections can cause severe local reactions, including edema, pain, and discoloration.

Table 18–4
Drugs that Interact with Phenytoin

Drugs that may increase phenytoin serum levels
Alcohol, amiodarone, choramphenicol, chlordiazepoxide, diazepam, dicumarol, disulfiram, estrongens, H_2 antagonists, halothane, isoniazide, methylphenidate, phenothiazines, phenylbutazone, salicylates, succinimides, sulfonamides, tolbutamide, trazodone
Drugs that may decrease phenytoin serum levels
Carbamazepine, chronic alcohol abuse, reserpine, sucralfate, antacids with calcium (should not be taken with phenytoin but at a different time)
Drugs that may have reduced efficacy due to phenytoin
Corticosteroids (including dexamethasone), coumarin anticoagulants, digitoxin, doxycycline, estrogens, furosemide, oral contraceptives, quinidine, rifampin, theophylline, vitamin D

Status epilepticus is a seizure that persists longer than 5 minutes or repeated seizures without a return to consciousness between each episode.[43] This is considered a neuro-oncological emergency. Clear the airway, ensure adequate perfusion, give glucose (usually 50 mL of a 50% solution), evaluate electrolytes, and administer IV benzodiazepine (such as diazepam or lorazepam), followed by a loading dose of IV phenytoin. The Veterans Administration Cooperative Trial of Status Epilepticus revealed response rates during first-line treatment as follows: lorazepam 64.9%, phenobarbitol 58.2%, diazepam plus phenytoin 55.8%, and phenytoin alone 43.6%.[44] These results suggest that lorazepam should be the first drug of choice. If the seizure is not relieved in 5 to 7 minutes, add phenytoin or fosphenytoin. If recurrent, continuous infusion of phenobarbital or diazepam is indicated. In extreme cases, barbiturate anesthesia, neuromuscular blockade, and propofol may be indicated.[45]

Patient and Family Education

Witnessing a seizure can be extremely frightening for family members and caregivers. Preparation is critical. Explain that restraining the patient or attempting to place objects in the mouth can lead to significant harm. Educate family members to move items that might cause trauma out of the way and to get the patient to lay on one side if possible. Caregivers may be given information regarding the jaw-lift technique if the airway is compromised. Pillows placed around the bed, between the patient and the siderails (if a hospital-style bed is in use), and around the room can be quickly positioned to prevent trauma. Caution family members to refrain from feeding or providing fluids until the patient is fully alert and able to swallow. However, if the patient has grossly unstable blood sugar levels and is prone to developing hypoglycemia, candy, glucose, juice, or other sources of glucose can be given only if the patient is able to swallow. Glucagon can also be given subcutaneously. Inform family members that loss of continence is common during a seizure and does not imply that the patient is not able to control these functions at other times. Encourage them to assist the patient while being considerate of the patient's ability and dignity.

To help recovery after a seizure, the patient may benefit from reduced stimulation. Lower the lights, reduce the sound of televisions or radios, and speak softly and reassuringly. Assess for pain and treat accordingly. Relaxation exercises also may be helpful. Often, patients will sleep for several hours after the seizure.

CASE STUDY

A 31-Year-Old Man with Intractable Nausea and Vomiting

A 31-year-old man was admitted to the oncology unit with intractable nausea and vomiting, presumably due to appendiceal cancer with omental and peritoneal metastases. He previously had been treated with a right hemicolectomy and diverting ileostomy, systemic chemotherapy, and a venting gastrostomy tube with total parenteral nutrition when obstruction occurred. Abdominal pain was treated with IV hydromorphone 26 mg/hour, with 26 mg every 15 minutes as needed. Several hours after admission to the unit he developed myoclonus, hyperreflexia, agitation, delirium, and eventually, tonic–clonic seizures. Evaluation revealed acute obstructive renal failure (BUN 37 mg/dL, creatinine 4.2 mg/dL) secondary to diffuse carcinomatosis.

Because the opioid metabolite hydromorphone-3-glucuronide was suspected as the likely cause of these neurological disturbances, the hydromorphone dose was reduced by 50% and the bolus dose was discontinued. Phenytoin (Dilantin) 1 gram followed by a 200-mg IV bolus every 12 hours did not stop the seizures; neither did valproate sodium (Depakon) 500-mg IV infusion every 12 hours, chlorpromazine (Thorazine) 25-mg slow IV push every 6 hours, lorazepam 2-mg IV every 2 hours, or diazepam 5 mg every 5 to 10 minutes. Despite these efforts, the generalized tonic-clonic movements increased in intensity and frequency (every 8 to 10 minutes) to status epilepticus. The patient was disoriented, yet remained arousable,

able to follow simple commands, and appeared to be in pain during these seizures.

Because the family's goals were to keep the patient comfortable, a midazolam infusion was begun at 1 mg/hour and rapidly titrated upward to 96 mg/hour, without change in frequency or intensity of seizures unfortunately. A nationwide shortage of phenobarbital prompted the use of pentobarbital 1 gram over 1 hour, followed with a 40-mg/hour infusion, with no change in seizure activity. A propofol (Diprivan) infusion was started, with a bolus of 80 mg given over 1 hour, and an infusion of 160 mg/hour. The patient experienced three more seizures, and then they stopped; he died approximately 6 hours later in apparent comfort.[45]

Spasticity

Spasticity is a movement disorder that results in a partial or complete loss of supraspinal control of spinal cord function. Patients may exhibit involuntary movement, abnormal posture, rigidity, and exaggerated reflexes. Spasticity may interfere with all aspects of life by limiting mobility, disturbing sleep, and causing pain.[46] Spasticity is often associated with advanced multiple sclerosis (MS), spinal cord trauma, tumors of the spinal cord, stroke meningitis, and other infections.[47–49] In a study of 2104 patients with nontraumatic spasticity seen in a regional neuroscience center in the United Kingdom, 17.8% had MS, 16.4% had neoplasm, and 4.1% had motor neuron disease.[50]

Assessment

Patients will describe a gradual onset of loss of muscle tone, followed by resistance and jerking when muscles are flexed. A recent history of urinary tract infection, decubitus ulcer, constipation, or pain may immediately predate the onset, or increased episodes, of spasticity.

Physical exam will yield resistance and spasticity when doing passive limb movement. The faster the passive movement, the more pronounced the effect. Reflexes may be hyperactive, particularly in the affected area. Bruises are common as patients inadvertently and uncontrollably move their limbs, resulting in trauma.

Management

The standard therapies for reducing spasticity include oral baclofen, a gamma-aminobutyric acid-B agonist. Baclofen is generally started with lower doses, 5 to 10 mg/day, and titrated upward gradually, using three- or four-times-a-day dosing. Although effective for some patients, higher doses are often necessary, frequently resulting in cognitive changes and dizziness. For this reason, intrathecal baclofen has been administered with good results.[51] Those in palliative care must weigh the benefits of intrathecal baclofen therapy given the patient's prognosis, the availability of skilled clinicians to administer the therapy, cost, and other factors.

Muscle relaxants, such as dantrolene 50 to 100 mg/day, diminish the force of the contraction.[47] Start at 25 mg daily and increase by 25-mg increments in divided doses every 4 to 7 days. The contents can be mixed with liquids if the patient is unable to swallow capsules. Although this reduces spasticity, significant impairment in muscle strength can occur. Therefore, dantrolene is not recommended in ambulatory patients. Furthermore, dantrolene can cause hepatotoxicity. Marijuana, and its active ingredient delta-9-tetrahydrocannabinol (THC), has been described by patients as useful in the relief of spinal cord spasticity.[52] Although not approved for this purpose, there is general agreement within the medical community that the treatment of spasticity is a legitimate use of THC. However, despite data supporting its safety and the availability of a commercially prepared product (Marinol), some patients, family members, and health care professionals continue to feel uneasy regarding the use of this compound.

Patient and Family Education

Patients and their caregivers should be educated about factors that may worsen spasticity, including constipation, urinary tract infection, pressure ulcers, fatigue, and psychosocial concerns. Strategies to prevent and relieve these conditions should be clearly communicated, and early communication regarding their onset should be encouraged. When spasticity occurs, the patient and family members must understand the rationale for drug therapy. Nonpharmacological therapy also may be helpful. Family members may be encouraged to gently massage the affected extremities, although this may produce increased spasticity in some patients. Repositioning, heat, and range-of-motion exercises have been described by patients as being helpful. As with other neurological disorders, safety measures are imperative. Padding wheelchairs, bed rails, and any other furniture that might come in contact with spastic extremities will reduce trauma.

Conclusion

Neurological disorders, including myoclonus, seizures, and spasticity, create fear, reduce energy levels, increase pain, and can complicate the course of a patient's illness. The goal in palliative care is prevention whenever possible. When not possible, early diagnosis and treatment are critical. Knowledge of pharmacotherapy is essential, including agents that might precipitate these disorders, drugs that are used to treat these syndromes, and drug interactions that might occur in the palliative care setting. As with all aspects of palliative care, the patient and family are the center of care. Nurses skilled in palliative care can empower them through education and support. The interdisciplinary approach exemplified by palliative care is key.

REFERENCES

1. Mercadante S. Pathophysiology and treatment of opioid-related myoclonus in cancer patients. Pain 1998;74:5–9.
2. Nunez-Olarte J. Opioid-induced myoclonus. Euro J Palliat Care 1995;2:146–150.
3. Hagen N, Swanson R. Strychnine-like multifocal myoclonus and seizures in extremely high-dose opioid administration: treatment strategies. J Pain Symptom Manage 1997; 14:51–58.
4. Hemstapat K, Monteith GR, Smith D, Smith MT. Morphine-3-glucuronide's neuro-excitatory effects are mediated via indirect activation of N-methyl-D-aspartic acid receptors: mechanistic studies in embryonic cultured hippocampal neurones. Anesth Analg 2003;97:494–505, table of contents.
5. Smith MT. Neuroexcitatory effects of morphine and hydromorphone: evidence implicating the 3-glucuronide metabolites. Clin Exp Pharmacol Physiol 2000;27:524–528.
6. Wright AW, Mather LE, Smith MT. Hydromorphone-3-glucuronide: a more potent neuro-excitant than its structural analogue, morphine-3-glucuronide. Life Sci 2001;69:409–420.
7. Sjogren P, Thunedborg LP, Christrup L, Hansen SH, Franks J. Is development of hyperalgesia, allodynia and myoclonus related to morphine metabolism during long-term administration? Six case histories. Acta Anaesthesiol Scand 1998;42:1070–1075.
8. Lee MA, Leng ME, Tiernan EJ. Retrospective study of the use of hydromorphone in palliative care patients with normal and abnormal urea and creatinine. Palliat Med 2001;15:26–34.
9. Klepstad P, Borchgrevink PC, Dale O, Zahlsen K, Aamo T, Fayers P, et al. Routine drug monitoring of serum concentrations of morphine, morphine-3-glucuronide and morphine-6-glucuronide do not predict clinical observations in cancer patients. Palliat Med 2003;17:679–687.
10. Gong QL, Hedner J, Bjorkman R, Hedner T. Morphine-3-glucuronide may functionally antagonize morphine-6-glucuronide induced antinociception and ventilatory depression in the rat. Pain 1992;48:249–255.
11. Bruera E, Pereira J. Acute neuropsychiatric findings in a patient receiving fentanyl for cancer pain. Pain 1997;69:199–201.
12. Sarhill N, Davis MP, Walsh D, Nouneh C. Methadone-induced myoclonus in advanced cancer. Am J Hosp Palliat Care 2001; 18:51–53.
13. Kaiko RF, Foley KM, Grabinski PY, Heidrich G, Rogers AG, Inturrisi CE, et al. Central nervous system excitatory effects of meperidine in cancer patients. Ann Neurol 1983;13:180–185.
14. Han PK, Arnold R, Bond G, Janson D, Abu-Elmagd K. Myoclonus secondary to withdrawal from transdermal fentanyl: case report and literature review. J Pain Symptom Manage 2002;23: 66–72.
15. Nishigaya K, Kaneko M, Nagaseki Y, Nukui H. Palatal myoclonus induced by extirpation of a cerebellar astrocytoma. Case report. J Neurosurg 1998;88:1107–1110.
16. Ford B, Pullman SL, Khandji A, Goodman R. Spinal myoclonus induced by an intrathecal catheter. Mov Disord 1997;12: 1042–1045.
17. Maher J, Choudhri S, Halliday W, Power C, Nath A. AIDS dementia complex with generalized myoclonus. Mov Disord 1997;12:593–597.
18. Werhahn KJ, Brown P, Thompson PD, Marsden CD. The clinical features and prognosis of chronic posthypoxic myoclonus. Mov Disord 1997;12:216–220.
19. Wyllie AR, Bayliff CD, Kovacs MJ. Myoclonus due to chlorambucil in two adults with lymphoma. Ann Pharmacother 1997; 31:171–174.
20. Pranzatelli MR, Tate ED, Kinsbourne M, Caviness VS, Jr., Mishra B. Forty-one year follow-up of childhood-onset opsoclonus-myoclonus-ataxia: cerebellar atrophy, multiphasic relapses, and response to IVIG. Mov Disord 2002;17:1387–1390.
21. Batchelor TT, Platten M, Hochberg FH. Immunoadsorption therapy for paraneoplastic syndromes. J Neurooncol 1998;40:131–136.
22. Eisele JH, Jr., Grigsby EJ, Dea G. Clonazepam treatment of myoclonic contractions associated with high-dose opioids: case report. Pain 1992;49:231–232.
23. Stayer C, Tronnier V, Dressnandt J, Mauch E, Marquardt G, Rieke K, et al. Intrathecal baclofen therapy for stiff-man syndrome and progressive encephalomyelopathy with rigidity and myoclonus. Neurology 1997;49:1591–1597.
24. Mercadante S. Dantrolene treatment of opioid-induced myoclonus. Anesth Analg 1995;81:1307–1308.
25. Sirven JI. Classifying seizures and epilepsy: a synopsis. Semin Neurol 2002;22:237–246.
26. Lassman AB, DeAngelis LM. Brain metastases. Neurol Clin 2003;21:1–23, vii.
27. Gregory RE, Grossman S, Sheidler VR. Grand mal seizures associated with high-dose intravenous morphine infusions: incidence and possible etiology. Pain 1992;51:255–258.
28. Steeghs N, de Jongh FE, Sillevis Smitt PA, van den Bent MJ. Cisplatin-induced encephalopathy and seizures. Anticancer Drugs 2003;14:443–446.
29. Romanelli F, Ryan M. Seizures in HIV-seropositive individuals: epidemiology and treatment. CNS Drugs 2002;16:91–98.
30. Schaller B, Ruegg SJ. Brain tumor and seizures: pathophysiology and its implications for treatment revisited. Epilepsia 2003;44: 1223–1232.
31. Walton GD, Hon JK, Mulpur TG. Ofloxacin-induced seizure. Ann Pharmacother 1997;31:1475–1477.
32. Kushner JM, Peckman HJ, Snyder CR. Seizures associated with fluoroquinolones. Ann Pharmacother 2001;35:1194–1198.
33. Steinmann RA, Rickel MK. A 23-year-old with refractory seizures following an isoniazid overdose. J Emerg Nurs 2002; 28:7–10.
34. Bassilios N, Restoux A, Vincent F, Rondeau E, Sraer JD. Piperacillin/Tazobactam inducing seizures in a hemodialysed patient. Clin Nephrol 2002;58:327–328.
35. Sugimoto M, Uchida I, Mashimo T, Yamazaki S, Hatano K, Ikeda F, et al. Evidence for the involvement of GABA(A) receptor blockade in convulsions induced by cephalosporins. Neuropharmacology 2003;45:304–314.
36. Miaskowski C, Cleary J, Burney R, Coyne P, Finley R, Foster R, et al. Guideline for the Management of Cancer Pain in Adults and Children. APS Clinical Practice Guidelines Series, No. 3. Glenview, IL: American Pain Society, 2005.
37. Bruera E, Moyano J, Seifert L, Fainsinger RL, Hanson J, Suarez-Almazor M. The frequency of alcoholism among patients with pain due to terminal cancer. J Pain Symptom Manage 1995; 10:599–603.
38. Daniels AC, Chokroverty S, Barron KD. Thalamic degeneration, dementia, and seizures. Inappropriate ADH secretion associated with bronchogenic carcinoma. Arch Neurol 1969; 21:15–24.
39. Beydoun A, Passaro EA. Appropriate use of medications for seizures. Guiding principles on the path of efficacy. Postgrad Med 2002;111:69–70,73–68, 81–62.

40. Kasteleijn-Nolst Trenite DG, Hirsch E. Levetiracetam: preliminary efficacy in generalized seizures. Epileptic Disord 2003; 5:S39-S44.
41. O'Brien TJ, Cascino GD, So EL, Hanna DR. Incidence and clinical consequence of the purple glove syndrome in patients receiving intravenous phenytoin. Neurology 1998;51: 1034–1039.
42. O'Brien TJ, Meara FM, Matthews H, Vajda FJ. Prospective study of local cutaneous reactions in patients receiving IV phenytoin. Neurology 2001;57:1508–1510.
43. Rosenow F, Arzimanoglou A, Baulac M. Recent developments in treatment of status epilepticus: a review. Epileptic Disord 2002; 4:S41–51.
44. Bleck TP. Management approaches to prolonged seizures and status epilepticus. Epilepsia 1999;40:S59-S63.
45. Golf M, Paice JA, Feulner E, O'Leary C, Marcotte S, Mulcahy M. Refractory status epilepticus. J Palliat Med 2004;7:85–88.
46. Gianino J, York M, Paice J. Intrathecal Drug Therapy for Spasticity and Pain. New York: Springer-Verlag, 1996:67-76.
47. Ben-Zacharia AB, Lublin FD. Palliative care in patients with multiple sclerosis. Neurol Clin 2001;19:801–827.
48. Lorenz R. A causistic rationale for the treatment of spastic and myocloni in a childhood neurodegenerative disease: neuronal ceroid lipofuscinosis of the type Jansky-Bielschowsky. Neuroendocrinol Lett 2002;23:387–390.
49. Watkins CL, Leathley MJ, Gregson JM, Moore AP, Smith TL, Sharma AK. Prevalence of spasticity post stroke. Clin Rehabil 2002;16:515–522.
50. Moore AP, Blumhardt LD. A prospective survey of the causes of non-traumatic spastic paraparesis and tetraparesis in 585 patients. Spinal Cord 1997;35:361–367.
51. Thompson E, Hicks F. Intrathecal baclofen and homeopathy for the treatment of painful muscle spasms associated with malignant spinal cord compression. Palliat Med 1998;12:119–121.
52. Fox SH, Kellett M, Moore AP, Crossman AR, Brotchie JM. Randomised, double-blind, placebo-controlled trial to assess the potential of cannabinoid receptor stimulation in the treatment of dystonia. Mov Disord 2002;17:145–149.

19

Jeannie V. Pasacreta, Pamela A. Minarik, and Leslie Nield-Anderson

Anxiety and Depression

I am not complete because my body does not function now. Before I was almost a normal person. Everything functioned even though I had pain for many years. I'm impotent now—I can't do what I want to. Yesterday my grandchild fell on a broom. I felt so bad I couldn't run to save her. I feel so inadequate in this world. This dependency is driving me crazy.—A patient

- ***Key Points***
- *The psychosocial issues in persons facing life-threatening illness are influenced by individual, sociocultural, medical, and family factors.*
- *Emotional turmoil may occur at times of transition in the disease course.*
- *Anxiety and depression are common symptoms in individuals facing chronic or life-threatening illness but should not be regarded as an inevitable consequence of advanced disease.*
- *These symptoms warrant evaluation and appropriate use of pharmacological and psychosocial interventions.*

This chapter provides information regarding the assessment and treatment of anxiety and depression among individuals who are faced with chronic or life-threatening illness and delineates psychosocial interventions that are effective at minimizing these troubling symptoms. Practical guidelines regarding patient management and identifying patients who may require formal psychiatric consultation are offered.

CASE STUDY

Mrs. Brady, a Patient with Depression

Mrs. Brady, a 42-year-old housewife and mother of two small children, was referred for consultation following segmental resection for probable stage IV breast cancer, with 15 positive nodes and one small area of questionable bone metastasis noted on her left hip. On being told that she required chemotherapy, she refused, saying "It is hopeless—why bother?" Both her husband and oncologist persuaded her to discuss her decision with a psychiatric consultation-liaison nurse, and she reluctantly agreed. She was depressed and withdrawn, although moderately anxious. She wrung her hands throughout the interview, reporting intrusive thoughts of death that kept her from sleeping at night, and stated that she preferred that her children remembered her as she was. An early death would be preferable to the lingering debilitation she believed would be associated with chemotherapy. On further review, she described being 13 years old when her mother was diagnosed with breast cancer and that she had always feared that it would happen to her too. Her mother's mastectomy had been followed by painful bone metastasis despite chemotherapy. Mrs. Brady had distressing memories of her mother's suffering and had taken lengthy steps with her physicians to assure that mammograms and frequent breast exams would allow her to be diagnosed early should breast cancer develop. Several areas of calcification had been monitored for more than a year. She now had anger toward her physician that her life was needlessly compromised by late diagnosis of something she had attempted to avoid for so long. The anger and hopelessness together were overwhelming, and she could not focus on anything else.

Changes in Health Care that have Accentuated Psychiatric Symptoms

Changes in health care delivery and rapid scientific gains are simultaneously increasing the number of individuals receiving or in need of palliative care at any given time, the longevity and course of chronic diseases, and the prevalence and intensity of the psychological symptoms that accompany them.[1,2] Furthermore, psychological distress is experienced within an increasingly complex, fragmented, and impersonal health care system that intensifies symptoms. Despite these realities, psychological symptoms receive minimal attention, and health care providers often lack the education and support regarding assessment, treatment, and referral of these common problems.

Advances in science and technology have moved the crisis of a life-threatening medical diagnosis to the prediagnostic period, extending life expectancy and the number of treatment courses delivered over a lifetime. Individuals are being diagnosed earlier and living longer, with increasing opportunities to experience simultaneous, interrelated psychosocial and medical comorbidity. The human genome project has theoretically and, in some cases, practically moved the psychosocial implications of chronic disease into the prediagnostic period. Concurrent treatment discoveries have increased quantity of life, albeit with ill-defined consequences to quality of life.[2,3] For example, an individual who learns of an inherited predisposition to cancer at age 25 is diagnosed at age 50, and receives intermittent treatment until death at age 79 incurs innumerable insults to her mental health and psychological well-being.

Soaring medical costs, managed-care arrangements, and the stigma associated with mental illness have simultaneously placed a low priority on the recognition and treatment of psychosocial distress within our health care system. There is abundant documentation that psychiatric morbidity, particularly depression, and anxiety enhance vulnerability and create formidable barriers to integrated health care.[3] Psychological factors have long been implicated as barriers to disease prevention, early diagnosis, and comprehensive treatment.[3,4] Lack of assessment and treatment of the common psychiatric sequelae to chronic disease have been linked to such problems as treatment-resistant depression and anxiety, family dysfunction, lack of compliance with prevention and treatment recommendations, potentiation of physical symptoms, and suicide, to name just a few.[3–6] These issues create long-term problems that drive up health care expenses and diminish access, quality, and efficiency of care. In health care settings, physical problems assume priority in the growing competition for scarce resources. Clinicians confronted with ambiguous symptoms are likely to interpret them within diagnostic paradigms most consistent to their specialty and theoretical orientation. As a consequence, the psychological symptoms that accompany life-threatening conditions are often interpreted and treated inappropriately, rendering care that is not comprehensive or cost effective.

We are at a critical juncture in the evolution of health care in this country. Systems are being overwhelmed by serious, often preventable, diseases that are not being treated comprehensively after diagnosis. Furthermore, in spite of cutting-edge therapies, a significant number of individuals experience unfavorable outcomes. As budget constraints limit the use of psychiatric specialists, these issues have intensified, and the importance of educating "front line" health providers to recognize and address psychiatric morbidity is clear and compelling. In a health care system focused largely on pathogenesis, cure, and cost, psychological symptoms are all too often unrecognized and untreated in clinical settings, despite their insidious harm to patients, caregivers, and the health professionals who feel ill prepared to manage them. As psychiatric-consultation liaison nurses who work primarily in nonpsychiatric settings, the authors have been consistently impressed by the lack of knowledge of nursing and medical staff regarding key signs and symptoms that characterize depression and anxiety in the medically ill. Often, young patients with particularly poor prognoses, who elicit anxiety and sadness from staff, rather than their objectively depressed or anxious counterparts, are referred for psychiatric evaluation. Among depressed and/or anxious patients who are referred for evaluation, the decision to intervene with psychotherapy or pharmacological agents is often based largely on the philosophy, educational background, and past experience of individual clinicians. Often, a diagnosis of clinical anxiety or depression is ruled out if the symptoms seem reactive and appropriate to the situation or are viewed as organic in nature. Patients who exhibit depressive or anxious symptoms not considered severe enough to classify for "psychiatric" status are often not offered psychotherapeutic services, and the natural history of their symptoms is rarely monitored over time. The lack of attention to assessment and treatment of depression and anxiety among the medically ill may lead to ongoing dysphoria, family conflict, noncompliance with treatment, increased length of hospitalization, persistent worry, and suicidal ideation, to name just a few risks. Because depression and anxiety are common among individuals with chronic illness, and particularly because they are often responsive to treatment, recognition of those afflicted is of unquestionable clinical relevance. Patients, family, and professional caregivers need to be informed of the factors that affect psychological adjustment, the wide range of psychological responses that accompany chronic and progressive disease, and the efficacy of various modes of intervention at minimizing psychological distress and thus promoting adaptation.

The Clinical Course of Chronic Illness

Acute stress is a common response to the diagnosis of a life-threatening chronic illness that occurs at transitional points in the disease process (beginning treatment, recurrence, treatment failure, disease progression).[7] The response is characterized by shock, disbelief, anxiety, depression, sleep and appetite disturbance, and difficulty performing activities of daily living. Under favorable circumstances, these psychological symptoms should resolve within a short period.[7,8] The time period is variable, but the general consensus is that once the crisis has passed and individuals know what to expect in terms of a treatment plan, psychological symptoms diminish.[7,9] The stage of disease at the time of diagnosis and its clinical course, including medical treatments, recurrence, and prominent symptoms, impact the psychosocial profiles of individuals. To a large extent, these factors will determine the emotional issues that are most pressing at any given point. Patients who are diagnosed with late-stage disease or have aggressive illnesses with no hope for cure are often most vulnerable to psychological distress, particularly anxiety, depression, family problems, and physical discomfort.

Diagnostic Phase

The period from time of diagnosis through initiation of a treatment plan is characterized by medical evaluation, the development of new relationships with unfamiliar medical personnel, and the need to integrate a barrage of information that, at best, is frightening and confusing. Patients and families experience heightened responsibility, concern, and isolation during this period. They are particularly anxious and fearful when receiving initial information regarding diagnosis and treatment. Consequently, care should be taken by professionals to repeat information over several sessions and to inquire about patients' and families' understanding of facts and options. Weissman and colleagues described the first 100 days following a cancer diagnosis as the period of "existential plight."[8] Psychological distress varied according to patient diagnosis. Individuals with lung cancer who had predominantly late-stage disease were more distressed than individuals with early-stage disease, supporting the need for palliative care services directed toward psychological symptoms. During the diagnostic period, patient concerns focus on existential issues of life and death more than on concerns related to health, work, finances, religion, self, or relationships with family and friends. While it is unusual to observe extreme and sustained emotional reactions as the first response to diagnosis, it is important to assess the nature of early reactions because they are often predictive of later adaptation.[10,11] Early assessment by clinicians can help to identify individuals at risk for later adjustment problems or psychiatric disorders and are in the greatest need of ongoing psychosocial support.[7,12] The initial response to diagnosis may be profoundly influenced by a person's prior association with a particular disease.[13] Those with memories of close relatives with the same illness often demonstrate heightened distress, particularly if the relative died or had negative treatment experiences. During the diagnostic period, patients may search for explanations or causes for their disease and may struggle to give personal meaning to their experience. Since many clinicians are guarded about disclosing information until a firm diagnosis is established, patients may develop highly personal explanations that can be inaccurate and provoke intensely negative emotions. Ongoing involvement and accurate information will minimize uncertainty and the development of maladaptive coping strategies based on erroneous beliefs. While the literature substantiates the devastating emotional impact of a life-threatening chronic illness, it also well documents that many individuals cope effectively. Positive coping strategies, such as taking action and finding favorable characteristics in the situation, have been reported to be effective.[14] Contrary to the beliefs of many clinicians, denial also has been found to assist patients in coping effectively,[15] unless sustained and used excessively to a point that it interferes with appropriate treatment. Health care practitioners play an important role in monitoring and supporting psychosocial adjustment. With an awareness of the unique meaning the individual associates with the diagnosis, it is vital that practitioners keep patients informed and involved in their care. Even though patients may not be offered hope for cure, assisting them in maintaining comfort and control promotes adaptation and improved quality of life.

Recurrence and Progressive Disease

Development of a recurrence after a disease-free interval can be especially devastating for patients and those close to them. The point of recurrence often signals a shift into a period of disease progression and is clearly a time when palliative care services aimed at alleviating psychological symptoms are indicated. The medical workup is often difficult and anxiety-provoking;[16] psychosocial problems experienced at the time of diagnosis frequently resurface, often with greater intensity.[17,18] Shock and depression often accompany relapse and require individuals and their families to reevaluate the future. This period is a difficult one, during which patients may also experience pessimism, renewed preoccupation with death and dying, and feelings of helplessness and disenchantment with the medical system. Patients tend to be more guarded and cautious at this time and feel as if they are in limbo.[18] Silverfarb and colleagues[18] examined emotional distress in a cross-sectional study of 146 women with breast cancer at three points in the clinical course (diagnosis, recurrence, stage-of-disease progression). The point of recurrence was found to be the most distressing time, with an increase in depression, anxiety, and suicidal ideation. As a disease progresses, the person often reports an upsetting scenario that includes frequent pain, disability, increased dependence on others, and diminished functional ability, which often potentiates psychological symptoms.[19] Investigators studying quality of life in cancer patients have demonstrated a clear relationship between an individual's perception of quality of life and the presence of discomfort.[20] As uncomfortable symptoms increase, perceived quality of life diminishes. Thus, an important goal in the psychosocial treatment of patients with advanced chronic illness focuses on symptom control.

An issue that repeatedly surfaces among patients, family members, and professional care providers deals with the use of aggressive treatment protocols in the presence of progressive disease. Often, patients and families request to participate in experimental protocols even when there is little likelihood of extending survival. Controversy continues about the efficacy of such therapies and the role health professionals can play in facilitating patients' choices about participating. These issues become even more important because changes in the health care system may limit payment for costly and highly technical treatments, such as bone marrow transplants. It is essential for health care professionals to establish structured dialogue with patients, family members, and care providers regarding treatment goals and expectations. Despite the existence of progressive illness, certain individuals may respond to investigational treatment with increased hope. Efforts to separate and clarify values, thoughts, and emotional reactions of care providers, patients, and families to these delicate issues is important if individualized care with attention to psychological symptoms is to be provided. Use of resources such as psychiatric consultation-liaison nurses, psychiatrists, social workers, and chaplains can be invaluable in assisting patients, family members, and staff to grapple with these issues in a meaningful and productive manner.

Terminal Disease and Dying

Once the terminal period has begun, it is usually not the fact of dying but the quality of dying that seems to be the overwhelming issue confronting the patient and family.[21,22] Continued palliative care into the terminal stage of cancer relieves physical and psychological symptoms, promotes comfort, and increases well-being. Often, patients and families who have received such services along the illness trajectory will be more open and accepting of palliative efforts in the final stage of life. In addition, it is important that nurses caring for the terminally ill recognize the emotional impact on themselves and attend to self-care. Patients living in the final phase of any advanced chronic illness experience fears and anxiety related to uncertain future events, such as unrelieved pain, separation from loved ones, burden on family, and loss of control. Psychological maladjustment is more likely in persons confronting diminished life span, physical debilitation associated with functional limitation, and/or symptoms associated with toxic therapies for which there are no effective interventions.[20,23] Therapeutic interventions should be directed toward increasing patients' sense of control and self-efficacy within the context of functional decline and increased dependence. In addition, if patients so desire, it is often therapeutic to let them know that there is help available to discuss the existential concerns that often accompany terminal illness. Personal values and beliefs, socioeconomic and cultural background, and religious belief systems influence patients' expectations about quality of life and palliative care. Cultural affiliation has a significant influence on perception of pain; for example, the findings of Bates and colleagues[24] indicate that the best predictors of pain intensity are ethnic group affiliation and locus of control style. For example, an individual's stoic attitude, which serves to minimize or negate discomfort, may be related to a cultural value learned and reinforced through years of family experiences. Similarly, an individual's highly emotional response to routine events may become exaggerated during the terminal phase of illness and not necessarily signal maladjustment but, rather, a cultural norm. Awareness of the family system's cultural, religious, ethnic, and socioeconomic background is important to the understanding of their beliefs, attitudes, practices, and behaviors related to illness and death. Cultural patterns play a significant role in determining how individuals and families cope with illness and death.[25,26] Delirium, depression, suicidal ideation, and severe anxiety are among the most common psychiatric complications encountered in terminally ill cancer patients.[27] When severe, these problems require urgent and aggressive assessment and treatment by psychiatric personnel, who can initiate pharmacological and psychotherapeutic treatment strategies. Psychiatric emergencies require the same rapid intervention as distressing physical symptoms and medical crises. In spite of the seemingly overwhelming nature of psychosocial responses along the chronic illness trajectory, most patients do indeed cope effectively. Periods of intense emotions, such as anxiety and depression, are not necessarily the same as maladaptive coping.

Factors That Affect Psychological Adjustment

Psychological responses to chronic illness vary widely and are influenced by many individual factors. A review of the literature points to key factors that may impact psychological adjustment and the occurrence and expression of anxiety and depression. Three of the most important factors are previous coping strategies and emotional stability, social support, and symptom distress. In addition, there are common medical conditions, treatments, and substances that may cause or intensify symptoms of anxiety and depression (Table 19–1, Table 19–2).

Previous Coping Strategies and Emotional Stability

One of the most important predictors of psychological adjustment to chronic illness is the emotional stability and coping strategies used by the person prior to diagnosis.[28] Individuals with a history of poor psychological adjustment and of clinically significant anxiety or depression are at highest risk for emotional decompensation[29] and should be monitored closely throughout all phases of treatment. This is particularly true for people with a history of major psychiatric syndromes and/or psychiatric hospitalization.[30]

Table 19–1
Common Medical Conditions Associated with Anxiety and Depression

Anxiety	Depression
• Endocrine disorders: hyperthyroidism and hypothyroidism, hyperglycemia and hypoglycemia, Cushing's disease, carcinoid syndrome, pheochromocytoma • Cardiovascular conditions: myocardial infarction, paroxysmal atrial tachycardia, angina pectoris, congestive heart failure, mitral valve prolapse, hypovolemia • Metabolic conditions: hyperkalemia, hypertemia, hypoglycemia, hyperthermia, anemia, hyponatremia • Respiratory conditions: asthma, chronic obstructive pulmonary disease, pneumonia, pulmonary edema, pulmonary embolus, respiratory dependence, hypoxia • Neoplasms: islet cell adenomas, pheochromocytoma • Neurological conditions: akathisia, encephalopathy, seizure disorder, vertigo, mass lesion, postconcussion syndrome	• Cardiovascular: cardiovascular disease, congestive heart failure, myocardial infarct, cardiac arrhythmias • Central nervous system: cerebrovascular accident, cerebral anoxia, Huntington's disease, subdural hematoma, Alzheimer's disease, human immunodeficiency virus (HIV) infection, dementia, carotid stenosis, temporal lobe epilepsy, multiple sclerosis, postconcussion syndrome, myasthenia gravis, narcolepsy, subarachnoid hemorrhage • Autoimmune: rheumatoid arthritis, polyarteritis nodosa • Endocrine: hyperparathyroidism, hypothyroidism, diabetes mellitus, Cushing's disease, Addison's disease • Other: alcoholism, anemia, systemic lupus erythematosus, Epstein-Barr virus, hepatitis, malignancies, pulmonary insufficiency, pancreatic or liver disease, syphilis, encephalitis, malnutrition

Sources: Stoudemire (1996), reference 77; Fernandez et al. (1995), reference 45; Kurlowicz (1994), reference 98; Wise & Taylor (1990), reference 19.

Table 19–2
Common Medications and Substances Associated with Anxiety and Depression

Anxiety	Depression
Alcohol and nicotine withdrawal	Antihypertensives
Stimulants including caffeine	Analgesics
Thyroid replacement	Antiparkinsonian agents
Neuroleptics	Hypoglycemic agents
Corticosteroids	Steroids
Sedative–hypnotic withdrawal or paradoxical reaction	Chemotherapeutic agents
Bronchodilators and decongestants	Estrogen and progesterone
Cocaine	Antimicrobials
Epinephrine	L-dopa
Benzodiazepines and their withdrawal	Benzodiazepines
Digitalis toxicity	Barbiturates
Cannabis	Alcohol
Antihypertensives	Phenothiazines
Antihistamines	Amphetamines
Antiparkinsonian medications	Lithium carbonate
Oral contraceptives	Heavy metals
Anticholinergics	Cimetidine
Anesthetics and analgesics	
Toxins	

Sources: Stoudemire (1996), reference 77; Fernandez et al. (1995), reference 45; Kurlowicz (1994), reference 98; Wise & Taylor (1990), reference 19.

Social Support

Social support consistently has been found to influence a person's psychosocial adjustment to chronic illness.[31] The ability and availability of significant others in dealing with diagnosis and treatment can significantly affect the patient's view of him- or herself and potentially the patient's survival.[32] Individuals diagnosed with all types of life-threatening chronic disorders experience a heightened need for interpersonal support. Individuals who are able to maintain close connections with family and friends during the course of illness are more likely to cope effectively with the disease than those who are not able to maintain such relationships.[33] This is especially true during the palliative care period.

Symptom Distress

The effects of treatment for a variety of chronic diseases as well as the impact of progressive illness can inflict transient and/or permanent physical changes, physical symptom distress, and functional impairments in patients. It is a well-known clinical fact supported by research[34] that excessive psychological distress can exacerbate the side effects of cancer-treatment agents. Conversely, treatment side effects can have a dramatic impact on the psychological profiles of patients.[35] The potential for psychological distress, particularly anxiety and depression, appears to increase in patients with advanced illness,[36–39] especially when cure is not viable and palliation of symptoms is the issue. In a study that elicited information from oncology nurses regarding psychiatric symptoms present in their patients, almost twice as many patients with metastatic disease were reported to be depressed in contrast to those with localized cancers.[40] Investigators studying quality of life in cancer patients have demonstrated a clear relationship between an individual's perception of quality of life and the presence of discomfort.[20] As uncomfortable symptoms increase, perceived quality of life diminishes and psychiatric symptoms often worsen. The presence of increased physical discomfort combined with a lack of control and predictability regarding the occurrence of symptoms often amplifies anxiety, depression, and organic mental symptoms in patients with advanced disease.

Differentiating Psychiatric Complications from Expected Psychological Responses

Differentiating between symptoms related to a medical illness and symptoms related to an underlying psychiatric disorder is particularly challenging to health care practitioners. Anxiety and depression are normal responses to life events and illness and occur throughout the palliative care trajectory. It is the intensity, duration, and extent to which symptomatology affects functioning that distinguishes an anxiety or depressive disorder from symptoms that individuals generally experience in the progression of an illness. Symptoms following stressful events (employment difficulties, retirement, death of a family member, loss of a job, diagnosis of a medical illness/life-threatening illness) in a person's life are expected to dissipate as an individual copes, with reassurance and validation from family and friends, and adapts to the situation. When responses predominantly include excessive nervousness, worry, and fear, diagnosis of an adjustment disorder with anxiety is applied. If an individual responds with tearfulness and feelings of hopelessness, he or she is characterized as experiencing an adjustment disorder with depressed mood. An adjustment disorder with mixed anxiety and depressed mood is characterized by a combination of both anxiety and depression.[41]

Referrals from primary care providers for psychiatric assistance with psychopharmacological treatment are indicated when symptoms continue, intensify, or disrupt an individual's life beyond a 6-month period, or when symptoms do not respond to conventional reassurance and validation by the primary care provider and support from an individual's social network. Most patients develop transient psychological symptoms that are responsive to support, reassurance, and information about what to expect regarding a disease course and its treatment. There are some individuals, however, who require more aggressive psychotherapeutic intervention, such as pharmacotherapy and ongoing psychotherapy. Following are guidelines to help clinicians identify patients who exhibit behavior that suggests the presence of a psychiatric syndrome.

If the patient's problems become so severe that supportive measures are insufficient to control emotional distress, referral to a psychiatric clinician is indicated. Factors that may predict major psychiatric problems along the chronic illness trajectory include past psychiatric hospitalization; history of significant depression, manic-depressive illness, schizophrenia, organic mental conditions, or personality disorders; lack of social support; inadequate control of physical discomfort; history of or current alcohol and/or drug abuse; and currently prescribed psychotropic medication. The need for psychiatric referral among patients receiving psychotropic medication deserves specific mention because it is often overlooked in clinical practice. Standard therapies used to treat major chronic diseases, such as surgery and chemotherapy, and/or disease progression itself can significantly change dosage requirements for medications used to treat major psychiatric syndromes such as anxiety, depression, and bipolar disorder. For example, dosage requirements for lithium carbonate, commonly used to treat the manic episodes associated with bipolar disorder and the depressive episodes associated with recurrent depressive disorder, can change significantly over the course of treatment for a number of chronic diseases. Therapeutic blood levels of lithium are closely tied to sodium and water balance. Additionally, lithium has a narrow therapeutic window, and life-threatening toxicity can develop rapidly. Treatment side effects such as diarrhea, fever, vomiting, and resulting dehydration warrant scrupulous monitoring of dosage and side effects. Careful monitoring is also indicated during pre- and postoperative periods. Another common problem among patients treated with psychotropic medication is that medications may be discontinued at specific points in the treatment process, such as the time of surgery, and not restarted. This may produce an avoidable recurrence of emotionally disabling psychiatric symptoms when the stress of a life-threatening chronic disease and its treatment is burden enough. For some patients, psychological distress does not subside with the usual supportive interventions. Unfortunately, clinically relevant and severe psychiatric syndromes are often unrecognized by nonpsychiatric care providers.[41,42] Particularly, as a chronic illness progresses, anxiety and depression may occur in greater numbers of patients and with greater intensity.[43] One of the reasons that it may be difficult to detect serious anxiety and depression in patients is that several of the diagnostic criteria used to evaluate their presence, such as lack of appetite, insomnia, decreased sexual interest, psychomotor agitation, and diminished energy, may overlap with usual disease and treatment effects.[44]

Additionally, health care providers may confuse their own fears about chronic illness with the emotional reactions of their patients (e.g., "I too would be extremely depressed if I were in a similar situation").

The Coexisting Nature of Psychiatric and Medical Symptoms

Depression and anxiety are appropriate to the stress of having a serious illness, and the boundary between normal and abnormal symptoms is often unclear. Even when diagnostic criteria are met for a major depressive episode or anxiety disorder, there is disagreement regarding the need for psychiatric treatment as psychiatric symptoms may improve upon initiation of medical treatment. A major source of diagnostic confusion is the overlap of somatic symptoms associated with several chronic illnesses and their treatments and those pathognomic to depression and anxiety themselves (e.g., fatigue, loss of appetite, weakness, weight loss, restlessness, agitation). Separating out whether a symptom is due to depression, anxiety, the medical illness and its treatment, or a combination of factors is often exceedingly difficult.

Figure 19–1 diagrams the overlap between the symptoms of a chronic medical condition and/or its treatment effects and the clinical manifestations of anxiety or depression. The symptoms of anxiety or depression may be intrinsic to the medical disorder or induced by certain treatment agents. Symptoms may cease when the medical disorder is treated or the medication is discontinued or decreased. Whether the psychiatric symptoms have a primary psychiatric etiology, occur following the medical diagnosis or receive equal causal contributions from medical, and psychiatric sources, neurovegetative symptoms are not reliable assessment parameters and treatment may be delayed or never treated.

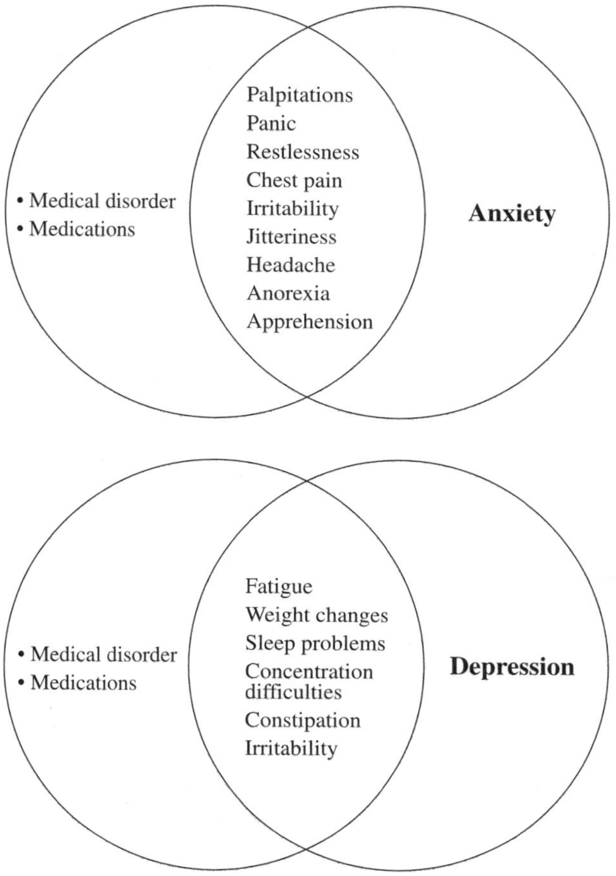

Figure 19–1. Symptoms of depression and anxiety with medical etiologies. *Source:* Leslie Nield-Anderson, unpublished, adapted from Derogatis & Wise (1989), reference 102.

Anxiety or Depression with a Medical or Pharmacological Etiology

During progressive or active treatment phases of a chronic disease, symptoms of anxiety or depression may recur at various intervals relative to a specific causative agent, the stress associated with the illness or a combination of those as well as other factors. Diagnostic data from earlier points, both before the onset of the current illness and at various points along the illness course, are vital and should routinely be incorporated into the plan of care. As psychiatric symptoms become more prevalent within the context of the lengthening chronic illness trajectory, attention to the collection of this diagnostic information is a vital and intrinsic aspect of quality comprehensive care. History and physical, medication history, mental status, psychosocial and psychiatric histories (see Table 19–3 for screening instruments), electrocardiogram, comprehensive laboratory tests including toxicology screening, and relevant family information regarding available support systems, changes in lifestyle and functioning will promote accurate assessment and close monitoring throughout the palliative

Table 19–3
Brief Screening Measures Used in Nonpsychiatric Settings for Cognitive Functioning, Anxiety, and Depression

Folstein Mini-Mental Exam
Beck Depression Inventory
Center for Epidemiological Studies of Depression Scale
Geriatric Depression Scale
Hamilton Depression Scale
Hamilton Rating Scale for Anxiety
Hospital Anxiety and Depression Scale
Zung Self-Rating Depression Scale
Zung Self-Rating Anxiety Scale
Speilberger State-Trait Anxiety Inventory

care trajectory. This information will assist the health care team in determining the etiology of anxiety and depressive symptoms and, as such, treat and monitor them appropriately.

Some patients may have a primary psychiatric disorder that precedes the diagnosis of their chronic medical condition. This situation is increasingly encountered in primary care and chronic illness treatment settings. During the diagnostic phase, fear and anxiety are expected reactions to the diagnosis of a life-threatening or potentially life-threatening disease. Heightened apprehension coincides with the anticipated course of treatment, uncertainty, and concerns about the potential impact on lifestyle. These initial responses usually resolve in a few weeks with the support of family and friends, use of personal resources, provision of professional care, and hope.[45,46] Lingering reports of feeling weak, dizzy, worried, or tense and of difficulty concentrating are often confusing to providers and may suggest an anxiety disorder. When anxiety is accurately diagnosed and treated, somatic complaints often diminish. However, if symptoms are not correctly identified and treated, clinicians must rule out a worsening medical condition, and the course of illness, treatment and suffering can become needlessly prolonged.[39,41]

Depression occurs frequently during the recurrence and progressive disease phase. An illness course marked with recurrences engenders anxiety and fear with each relapse, as well as feelings of desperation. Individuals experiencing depression do not always present with a dysphoric effect or report distressing feelings of hopelessness and helplessness.[47] Instead, they may present with somatic complaints such as dizziness, headaches, excessive fatigue, sleep disturbances, or irritability. Accurate diagnosis and treatment, including pharmacological and psychotherapeutic management and education, can expedite somatic complaints and, importantly, the underlying depressive disorder that often causes or exaggerates them.

Disturbances in appetite, sleep, energy, and concentration are hallmark symptoms of depression. However, in the medically ill, these symptoms are frequently caused by the medical illness.[48] Symptoms such as fearfulness, depressed appearance, social withdrawal, brooding, self-pity, pessimism, a sense of punishment, and mood that cannot be changed (e.g., cannot be cheered up, not smiling, does not respond to good news) are considered to be more reliable. It has been recommended that assessment of these affective symptoms provides more accurate diagnostic information for depression in medically ill patients than neurovegetative symptoms commonly used in healthy individuals.[48–51] Tables 19–4 and 19–5 list

Table 19–4
Symptoms Indicating an Anxiety Disorder in the Medically Ill

Chronic apprehension, worry, inability to relax not related to illness or treatment
Difficulty concentrating
Irritability or outbursts of anger
Difficulty falling asleep or staying asleep not explained by illness or treatment
Trembling or shaking not explained by illness or treatment
Exaggerated startle response
Perspiring for no apparent reason
Chest pain or tightness in the chest
Fear of places, events, certain activities
Unrealistic fear of dying
Fear of "going crazy"
Recurrent and persistent ideas, thoughts, or impulses
Repetitive behaviors to prevent discomfort

Sources: Barraclough (1997), reference 46; Fernandez et al. (1995), reference 45; American Psychiatric Association (2000), reference 99.

Table 19–5
Symptoms Indicating a Depressive Disorder in the Medically Ill

Enduring depressed or sad mood, tearful
Marked disinterest or lack of pleasure in social activities, family, and friends
Feelings of worthlessness and hopelessness
Excessive enduring guilt that illness is a punishment
Significant weight loss or gain not explained by dieting, illness, or treatments
Hopelessness about the future
Enduring fatigue
Increase or decrease in sleep not explained by illness or treatment
Recurring thoughts of death or suicidal thoughts or acts
Diminished ability to think and make decisions

Sources: American Psychiatric Association (2000), reference 99; Cassem (1995), reference 43; Cavanaugh (1995), reference 44; Kurlowicz (1994), reference 98.

general criteria to diagnosis an anxiety and depressive disorder in the medically ill.[41,50,51] Whenever symptoms are unremitting or intensify and do not respond to conventional professional and family support, psychiatric evaluations for psychopharmacological and psychotherapeutic interventions are essential.

Untreated or undertreated psychiatric disorders can be profoundly disabling and, as such, can precipitate or exacerbate the physical manifestations of chronic disease. The degree of anxiety and depression experienced by an individual at any given point depends on the degree to which individuals and their families have been prepared for what to expect. These considerations include: the physical and psychological manifestations, the speed and extent of physical devastation expected, including the likelihood of pain and other potential discomforts and available treatment options, and the individual's history of psychiatric illness and the impact that those symptoms and treatments may have on the clinical picture and treatment options.[40]

Anxiety and depression typically accompany difficult decisions regarding both the addition of comfort measures and the withdrawal of diagnostic procedures and aggressive medical treatments. Despair regarding separation from family and friends, worries about burdening caregivers, overwhelming self and others with end-of-life decisions, and living in existential uncertainty are just a few of the issues that individuals and families must confront during terminal phases of illness. Severe distress, thoughts of suicide, panic, and/or questions about assisted suicide may occur, despite the supportive interventions provided by professional and family caregivers. Such responses require immediate attention and intervention. Suicide and assisted suicide are discussed at a later point in this chapter.

Anxiety or Depression Precipitated by a Medical Disorder

In many cases, an anxiety or depressive disorder occurs secondary to the diagnosis of a chronic medical condition. The stress of the medical illness itself typically induces anxiety or depression. Often these symptoms diminish when treatment is explained and initiated and hope is offered. When a patient with a chronic illness experiences increasing physical dependence on others, prolonged pain, progressive loss of function and/or immobility, anxiety and depression can become severe and prolonged. Disease progression may affect body image, self-esteem, social relationships, employment, and family roles. The extent and speed at which disabling aspects of a chronic illness occur will impact an individual's ability to react and to integrate the upsetting changes and, subsequently, to develop adjustment skills. The development of adaptive coping strategies is influenced by many factors, particularly the patient's premorbid coping strategies and the availability of outside support.

Within the context of a chronic medical condition, anxiety and depression often occur simultaneously. In general, anxiety precedes depression, and depression is more likely to persevere in individuals who also have an anxiety disorder. When anxiety and depression coexist, assessment and treatment may be more challenging, underscoring an aggressive, ongoing approach to assessment and treatment.

A common but erroneous assumption by clinicians is that the psychological distress that accompanies a medical condition, even when it is severe and unremitting, is natural and expected and, therefore, does not require or respond to treatment. This is particularly true when hope for a cure is unavailable or the prognosis is grave, leading to underrecognition and undertreatment of disabling symptoms and needlessly promoting suffering.[52] Receiving a life-threatening medical diagnosis and undergoing invasive treatment are potent catalysts for an acute stress response that is not typically expected, planned for, or routinely addressed in health care settings. Providers' dominant concerns are usually centered around treatment options, the pursuit of a cure, improving prognosis, and relieving physical discomfort. Often, providers are desensitized to the intrusiveness of medical protocols and treatment environments. Most patients are not comfortable and are not encouraged to address feelings of helplessness, dependency, or fear with professional or family care providers. In fact, they often avoid such discussions to decrease burden on others, and untreated psychological symptoms may lead to a diagnosis of posttraumatic stress disorder. Posttraumatic stress disorders (PTSD), typically induced by exposure to extreme stress and/or trauma, increasingly are being linked in the literature to medical treatment situations. Providers are apt to confuse PTSD symptoms such as avoidance and withdrawal as nonpathological responses, e.g., acceptance adjustment. It is common for providers to hear "I do not remember anything about the hospitalization; it is a blur. I feel like I was in a daze . . . ask my wife/husband . . . my memory isn't so great." In the treatment of PTSD, psychopharmacological agents alone are inadequate and must be accompanied by aggressive psychotherapeutic interventions, education and support. PTSD is best treated by a professional with skill treating this disorder. Routine psychiatric assessment and the availability of prompt treatment across the palliative care trajectory is critical to reduce the prevalence and morbidity of posttraumatic stress disorders that occur in response to medical diagnosis and treatment.[35]

Assessment and Screening Considerations

Assessment of Anxiety

The experience of anxiety is universal, especially when a person has a serious chronic illness. Anxiety is a vague, subjective feeling of apprehension, tension, insecurity, and uneasiness, usually without a known specific cause. Normally, anxiety serves as an alerting response resulting from a real or perceived threat to a person's biological, psychological, or social integrity, as well as to self-esteem, identity, or status. This alert occurs in response to actual happenings or to thoughts about happenings, in the past, present, or future. The greater the perceived threat, the greater the anxiety response.[26] A wide variety of signs and symptoms accompany anxiety along the continuum of mild, moderate, severe, and panic levels. Table 19–6 illustrates how anxiety affects attention, learning, and adaptation, all of which are essential to coping during the palliative care trajectory.[53] Anxiety responses can be adaptive, and anxiety can be a powerful motivating force for productive problem-solving. Talking, crying, sleeping, exercising, deep breathing, imagery, and relaxation techniques are adaptive anxiety-relief strategies. Responses to anxiety also can be maladaptive and may indicate psychiatric disorder, but not all distressing symptoms of anxiety indicate a psychiatric disorder. Table 19–4 lists anxiety symptoms that indicate a psychiatric disorder and call for psychiatric assessment and treatment. Skill in early recognition of anxiety is crucial so that care providers can intervene immediately to alleviate symptoms, to prevent escalation and loss of control, and to enable adjustment and coping. Anxiety is interpersonally contagious. As a result, therapeutic effectiveness can be severely compromised when care providers fail to recognize and manage their own anxiety.

Table 19–6
Symptoms of Anxiety and Effects on Attention, Learning, and Adaptation

Mild
Awareness, alert attention, skill in seeing relationships or connections available for use
Notices more than previously, ability to observe improved
If the person has well-developed learning and adaptive skills, will be able to use all steps in the learning process, from observing and describing to analyzing, testing, and using what is learned
Moderate
Perceptual field is narrowed, ability to observe decreased, does not notice peripheral stimuli but can notice more if directed to do so (selective inattention)
If the person has well-developed learning and adaptive skills, will be able to use all steps in the learning process, from observing and describing to analyzing, testing, and using what is learned
Severe
Perceptual field is greatly reduced, focus on one detail or scattered details
May be able to notice what is pointed out by another person, but as anxiety escalates will be unable to attend
May dissociate to prevent panic (i.e., fail to notice what is happening in reference to self)
Even with well-developed learning and adaptive skills, behavior will orient toward getting immediate relief
Automatic (not requiring thought) behaviors used to reduce anxiety
Panic
Feelings of panic, awe, dread
Previous foci of attention "blown up" or scattering of details increased
Tendency to dissociate to prevent panic
Inability to focus attention even when directed by another person
Even with well-developed learning and adaptive skills, behavior will orient toward getting immediate relief
Automatic (not requiring thought) behaviors used to reduce anxiety

Source: Peplau (1963), reference 52.

Assessment of Depression

Often underrecognized and undertreated, depression has the potential to decrease immune response, decrease survival time, impair ability to adhere to treatment, and impair quality of life.[54] The assessment of depression in any setting depends on the provider's awareness of its potential to occur. In addition, providers must be cognizant of the risk factors associated with depression and its key signs, symptoms, and historical aspects. In addition to medical comorbidity, risk factors that favor the development of a depressive disorder include prior episodes of depression, family history of depression, prior suicide attempts, female gender, age under 40 years, postpartum period, lack of social support, stressful life events, personal history of sexual abuse, and current substance abuse.[55] The experience of chronic and progressive disease may increase dependence, helplessness, and uncertainty and generate a negative, self-critical view. Cognitive distortions can easily develop, leading to interpretation of benign events as negative or catastrophic. Motivation to participate in care may be diminished, leading to withdrawal. Patients may see themselves as worthless and burdensome to family and friends. Family members may find themselves immobilized, impatient, or angry with the patient's lack of communication, cooperation, or motivation.[55]

Cultural Considerations

Culture can be a powerful influence on the occurrence and presentation of psychiatric morbidity. In some cultures, anxiety and depression may be expressed through somatic symptoms rather than affective/behavioral symptoms such as guilt or sadness. Complaints of "nerves" and headaches (in Latino and Mediterranean cultures); of weakness, tiredness, or "imbalance" (in Chinese or Asian cultures); of problems of the "heart" (in Middle Eastern cultures); or of being "heartbroken" (among the Hopi) may be depressive equivalents. Cultures may differ in judgments about the seriousness of dysphoria; for example, irritability may be a greater concern than sadness or withdrawal. Experiences distinctive to certain cultures, such as fear of being hexed or vivid feelings of being visited by those who have died, must be differentiated from actual hallucinations or delusions that may be part of a major depressive episode with psychotic features. However, a symptom should not be dismissed because it is seen as characteristic of a particular culture (see Table 19–5).[41,48,49,51]

Conceptual and Diagnostic Considerations

The conceptualization of psychological distress is varied. Depression in particular, has a variety of meanings and has been used to describe a broad spectrum of human emotions and behaviors, ranging from expected, transient, and nonclinical sadness following upsetting life events to the clinically relevant extremes of suicidality and major depressive disorder. Depression is common among people with chronic illness. The term "depressive syndromes" refers to a specific constellation of symptoms that comprise a discrete psychiatric disorder, such as major depression, dysthymia, organic affective disorder, and adjustment disorder with depressed features. Depressive symptoms describe varying degrees of depressed feelings not necessarily associated with psychiatric illness. Five major theoretical viewpoints have been used to understand and treat depression. In the psychoanalytic view, depression represents the introjection of hostility subsequent to the loss of an ambivalently loved object.[56] Cognitive views emphasize the mediating role that distorted and negative thinking plays in determining mood and behavior.[57] In the sociological view, depression is a social phenomenon in which a breakdown of self-esteem involves the loss of possessions such as status, roles and relationships, and life meaning.[58] Cultural and societal factors, including illness, increase vulnerability to depression. The biological view of depression emphasizes genetic vulnerability and biochemical alterations in neurotransmitters.[59] In studies of medically ill patients, depression is often equated with a crisis response, in which demands on the individual exceed the ability to respond.[60]

Conceptual viewpoints are important to the extent that they influence the understanding and subsequent treatment of the psychiatric symptoms experienced by patients with chronic physical illness. Diverse conceptualizations do not diminish the ability to plan and deliver effective care and most often simply offer complementary ideas concerning the etiological significance of symptoms. In many health care settings, nurses have the most patient contact and are likely to talk with individuals about their physical and emotional problems and thus to detect psychiatric symptoms and syndromes. Specific screening instruments, such as those listed in Table 19–3, may be used for assessment. In addition, direct questioning and clinical observation of mood, behavior, and thinking can be carried out concomitant with physical care. Questions related to mood may include the following: How have your spirits been lately? How would you describe your mood now? Have you felt sad or blue? Questions about behavior relate to sleeping patterns, appetite, activity level, and changes in energy: How are you sleeping lately? How much energy do you have now compared with 1 month or 6 months ago? Have you experienced recent changes in your appetite? Have you lost or gained weight? What do you usually do to cope with stress (talk to someone? go to a movie? work? exercise? drugs? alcohol?)? Questions related to cognition are as follows: What do you see in your future? What are the biggest problems facing you now? Are you as interested as usual in your family and friends, work, hobbies, etc.? Have you felt satisfied with yourself and with your life? Can you concentrate as well as you usually can? Do you have family or close friends readily available to help you? Do you feel able to call on them? As noted previously, disturbances in appetite, sleep, energy, and concentration may be caused by the illness and not necessarily indicative of depression.

Screening for Anxiety and Depression

In chronic illness settings, the need for routine psychiatric screening has been well documented for identifying patients at high risk for psychiatric morbidity, as well as to identify those who can benefit from early-intervention programs. Patients may require different interventions based on their placement on the distress continuum. Researchers[61] concluded that newly diagnosed patients who are highly distressed can benefit from evaluation and treatment for psychiatric consequences of illness and that adaptation to the disease can be improved through the use of psychosocial interventions and close monitoring. A number of tools have been developed to screen for psychological distress but have not been consistently incorporated into clinical care.[62–63] One tool that is easy to administer, reliable, and palatable to patients is the Distress Thermometer. This tool, developed by a team led by Dr. Jimmie Holland at Memorial Sloan Kettering Cancer Center, is similar to pain measurement scales that ask patients to rate their pain on a scale from 0 to 10, and consists of two cards. The first card is a picture of a thermometer, and the patient is asked to mark his or her level of distress. A rating of 5 or above indicates that a patient has symptoms indicating a need to be evaluated by a mental health professional and potential referral for services. The patient is then handed a second card and asked to identify which items from a six-item problem list relate to the patient's distress, that is, illness-related, family, emotional, practical, financial, or spiritual. This tool is part of the National Comprehensive Cancer Network (NCCN) distress-management practice guidelines in oncology. This interdisciplinary workgroup chose the term "distress management" because it was "more acceptable and less stigmatizing than psychiatric, psychosocial or emotional," and could be defined and measured by self report.[64]

Again, striving for simplicity and clinical utility, Harvey Chochinov and colleagues compared the performance of four brief screening measures for depression in the terminally ill.[50] They found that asking the question "Are you depressed?" was reliable and valid for diagnosing depression and was extraordinarily useful in care of the terminally ill. Both the NCCN Practice Guidelines for distress management and the simple three-word screening sentence for depression can easily be incorporated into daily clinical practice.

Addressing Deficits in Case-finding Strategies

Individuals are living longer with chronic illnesses within the context of aggressive physically and psychologically debilitating treatments. These trends promise to continue, and further study is needed to identify effective approaches to treatment. Available data clearly support a policy of routine psychological assessment in chronic-illness settings. Additional studies are needed to support intervention development that, at a minimum, will likely lead to improved quality of life for patients and cost savings at the systems level. In clinical settings, detection and case identification are particularly difficult. As mentioned, this is due to several factors including: the high prevalence of clinically significant "subsyndromal" psychiatric symptoms in medically ill samples (symptoms not severe enough or of sufficient duration to be classified as a psychiatric disorder), and the overlapping nature of physical and neurovegetative symptoms, such as fatigue, changes in appetite, sleep, and sex drive. Different clinical sites have their own unique limitations, including lack of knowledge, comfort, or time by health professionals to assess patients for these symptoms. Consequently, recognition of significant psychological distress (psychiatric morbidity) is seriously impeded in clinical settings. Clinicians need to be trained to recognize the prognostic importance of comorbid medical illness and psychiatric symptoms and to understand how the subtleties of case identification can affect treatment planning. The range in severity of psychiatric symptoms and the often rapid change in both psychiatric and physical symptoms across the treatment trajectory create both a great variance and the need to observe and record the dynamic interchange between physical and psychological phenomena over a small time span. The difficulties in case identification discussed may be highlighted by the severity of physical symptoms and the low prevalence of prior mood disorder. The presence of acute physical illnesses places the individuals under severe physiological as well as psychological and psychosocial stress. In addition, patients are often removed from their usual social support systems to receive treatment and are exposed to psychosocial stressors unique to the treatment setting (e.g., dependency on hospital staff, unfamiliar and sometimes painful diagnostic and therapeutic procedures, altered eating, bathing, and sleep routines, and uncertain prognosis). Symptom assessments must strike a balance between overly inclusive (e.g., mistakenly treating the fatigue of cancer treatment as depression) and overly exclusive (e.g., erroneously dismissing the patient's mood symptoms as "understandable"). Case identification is a crucial first step. The approach to identifying psychiatric symptoms potentially confounded by medical illnesses must be defined explicitly. Choice of an inclusive approach avoids premature exclusion of relevant phenomena. The use of similar screening instruments across clinical sites would greatly facilitate comparisons of information and standardization of assessment and case-finding guidelines.

Suicide

Suicide is the ninth leading cause of death in the United States. Five percent of suicides occur in patients with chronic medical illnesses, with spinal cord injuries, multiple sclerosis, cancer, and human immunodeficiency virus disease.[65] Because of underreporting, statistics underestimate the magnitude of suicide; intentional overdoses by the terminally ill and intentional car accidents are rarely labeled as suicides. The strongest suicide predictor is the presence of a psychiatric illness, especially depression and alcohol abuse, although a chronic deteriorating medical illness with perceived poor health, recent diagnosis of a life-threatening illness, and recent conflict or loss of a significant relationship also are considered to be predictive.[65] Males, over age 45 years, and living alone and lacking a social support system are risk factors.[66] In one study, hopelessness was found to be more important than depression as a clinical marker of suicidal ideation in the terminally ill.[67] Individuals with progressive chronic illness, particularly during the terminal stages, are at increased risk for suicide.[68] Other cancer-related risk factors include oral, pharyngeal, or lung cancer; poor prognosis; confusion and delirium; inadequately controlled pain; and the presence of deficits, such as loss of mobility, loss of bowel or bladder control, amputation, sensory loss, inability to eat or swallow, and exhaustion.[69] The highest-risk patients are those with severe and rapidly progressive disease producing rapid functional decline, intractable pain, and/or history of depression, suicide attempts, or substance abuse.[70]

Physician-Assisted Suicide

Whereas suicide is the intentional ending of one's own life, physician-assisted suicide (PAS) refers to a physician acting to aid a person in the ending of his or her life.[71] Public demand for PAS has been fueled by burdensome, exhausting, and expensive dying in acute care settings.[72] It is highly controversial; the American Medical Association, the American Nurses Association, and the National Hospice and Palliative Care Organization have taken strong positions against it.[73,74] Implications for health care providers include the following: to be knowledgeable about the legal and moral/ethical aspects of PAS; to do a personal evaluation and prepare responses for situations with patients where the topic may arise; to improve education about pain management, symptom control, and related issues in the care of dying and seriously ill patients; to conduct rigorous research on the attitudes and practices of health care professionals with respect to assisted suicide; and to develop effective mechanisms to address conflicts.[72,74] There is an ongoing debate about the legalization of PAS. Only in Oregon have the voters approved legalization of PAS.[75] The controversy potentially affects pain management in palliative care. Current efforts to create a federal ban on PAS may have a "chilling" effect on the widely supported approach to pain management in terminal care of high doses of opiates, regardless of secondary effects on respiration and length of life. Some fear that providing adequate pain relief might be seen as assisting the patient to die.[76] Although the Oregon law remains in dispute, the public dialogue in that state led to palliative care reform that significantly improved end-of-life care in Oregon.[75] Events in Oregon highlight care as a priority and increase the understanding about the distinction between assisting suicide and honoring patient preferences for limiting life-sustaining treatment.[75] Patient concerns most often related to desire to suicide are unrelieved pain, poorly managed symptoms, depression, worries about loss of control, being a burden, being dependent on others for personal care, and loss of dignity.[76] Valente and Trainor[66] identified poor quality of life, failed requests for treatment withdrawal, and distressing treatments as typical reasons for suicide in the critically ill. Further, patient requests for PAS are not rare, and physicians do provide such services, even though they are not legal.[77] Requests to physicians may also be indirect, as in the reported case of a patient asking for pain relief with the unspoken intent to cause death.[78] To further complicate the issue for health care providers, requests for suicide may be rational and not simply a symptom of depression.[76] Rationality has been defined as the capacity to deliberate, to communicate in relationships, and to reflect on and to examine one's own values and purposes.[76] The accepted criteria for rational suicide among adults with terminal illness include the following: rational considerations, understandable motives, careful planning, review of alternatives, absence of coercion, and recognition of consequences.[76] The patient's decisional capacity may be impaired by agitation, disorientation, major depression, poor reality orientation, grief and loss, medications, effects of illness, and ambivalence. Particularly in these circumstances, a formal psychiatric evaluation is warranted. See Chapter 59, Palliative Care and Requests for Assistance in Dying, for a more in-depth review.

Assessment of Suicide Risk

Assessment and treatment of depression, often overlooked in chronic-illness treatment settings, is a key suicide-prevention strategy. In addition, managing symptoms, communicating, and helping patients to maintain a sense of control are vitally important prevention strategies. An assessment of depression should always include direct questions about suicidal thinking, plans or attempts, despair or hopelessness, distress from poorly managed symptoms, and personal or family history of suicidal ideation, plans, or attempts.[76] When any indicator of suicide risk is recognized, risk factors, clues, suicidal ideation, level of depression, hopelessness and despair, and symptom distress should be thoroughly evaluated to estimate individual lethality. The rationality of the suicidal request or intent must also be evaluated. The nurse should interview the patient and family members to find out why the patient is thinking about suicide now.[76] Find out what method the patient is considering and whether the means are available. Ask the patient what has prevented suicide before and if he or she wants help or hopes someone else will decide.[76] Most people are relieved to be asked about suicidal thoughts because it opens communication. Initial and periodic evaluation of suicidal potential is necessary for patients with a history, thoughts, or risk factors of suicide.

Recognition of Clues

Suicidal persons usually give verbal and/or behavioral clues, such as isolated or withdrawn behavior or death wishes or death themes in art, writing, play, or conversation. Clues may be subtle or obvious, for example, joking about suicide, asking questions concerning death (e.g., "How many of these pills would it take to kill someone?"), comments with a theme of giving up, or statements that indicate hopelessness or helplessness. Resistance or refusal of treatments, food, or fluids may indicate suicidal ideation or intent and require further assessment.[74,76] Keys to determining lethality are suicide plan, method, intended outcome (e.g., death or rescue), and availability of resources and ability to communicate.[74,76] Lethal means include guns, knives, jumping from heights, drowning, or carbon monoxide poisoning. Other potentially lethal means include hanging or strangulation (using strong pieces of twine, rope, electric cords, sheets), taking high doses of aspirin or Tylenol, being in a car crash, or undergoing exposure to extreme cold. Low to moderately lethal methods are wrist cutting and mild aspirin overdose.

Suicide Interventions

Severely depressed and/or potentially suicidal patients must be identified as soon as possible to ensure a safe environment and appropriate treatment. Prompt action should be taken including provision of safety, supervision, and initiation of psychiatric evaluation. A patient with an immediate, lethal, and precise suicide plan needs strict safety precautions such as hospitalization and continuous or close supervision. The low-risk patient should not be underestimated. If circumstances change, risk could change. In all cases, notify the primary provider, and document the patient's behavior and verbatim statements, suicide assessment, and rationale for decisions, as well as the time and date the provider was notified.[76] If the provider is not responsive to the report of the patient's suicidal ideation, it is important to maintain observation and to pursue psychiatric consultation. The motivation for suicide can be reduced through palliative care interventions such as improved pain and symptom management; referral and treatment for depression or other psychiatric disorders; discussion of alternative interventions to improve quality of life; referral to spiritual, social, and psychiatric resources; and education and accurate facts about options for terminal care or end-of-life decision-making. Openness to talking about suffering, distress, death preferences, and decision-making in a sensitive and understanding manner and advocacy to aid communication with others is helpful for patients and their families.[76,77]

Management of Anxiety and Depression

Psychosocial interventions can exert an important effect on the overall adjustment of patients and their families to chronic illness and treatment.[78] Several studies document the beneficial effect of counseling on anxiety, feelings of personal control,[79] depression, and generalized psychological distress.[80] Increased length of survival from time of diagnosis has highlighted the need for psychopharmacological, psychotherapeutic, and behaviorally oriented interventions to reduce anxiety and depression and to improve quality of life for patients diagnosed with a chronic illness.

Pharmacological Interventions

Pharmacotherapy, as an adjunct to one or more of the psychotherapies, can be an important aid in bringing psychological symptoms under control.

Pharmacological Management of Anxiety. The prevalence of anxiety in medical illness is relatively high. As described in Figure 19–1, a variety of disorders have anxiety as a prominent symptom of the clinical presentation (see Tables 19–1 and 19–2), and many commonly used medications are associated with anxiety as a side effect. Studies have shown a high prevalence in cardiovascular, pulmonary, cerebrovascular, and gastrointestinal diseases, as well as cancer and diabetes. In addition, patients with a history of anxiety disorders have increased rates of diabetes, heart disease, arthritis, and physical handicaps compared to the general population. Pain, metabolic abnormalities, hypoxia, and drug withdrawal states can present as anxiety. Before instituting pharmacological treatment, any patient with acute or chronic symptoms of anxiety should be thoroughly evaluated, including a review of medications to assess the contribution of medical condition and/or medication-related etiologies for their complaints.

The following brief review of pharmacological treatment must be supplemented with other references concerning assessment, intervention, evaluation, and patient education (Table 19–7). Benzodiazepines are the most frequently used medications for anxiety in both medical and psychiatric settings. When longer-acting benzodiazepines, such as diazepam, are used in the elderly or in the presence of liver disease, dosages should be decreased and dosing intervals increased. They may suppress respiratory drive. Consultation-liaison services often use lorazepam in medically ill patients because its elimination half-life is relatively unaffected by liver disease, age, or concurrent use of selective serotonin reuptake inhibitors (SSRIs) or nefazodone. Drawbacks include amnestic episodes and interdose anxiety caused by its short half-life. The latter can be remedied by more frequent dosing. If medically ill patients need a longer-acting benzodiazepine for panic disorder or generalized anxiety disorder, clonazepam is often used because it is not affected by concurrent use of SSRIs. Clonazepam may accumulate and result in oversedation and ataxia

Table 19–7
Medications Appropriate for the Treatment of Anxiety in the Medically Ill

Benzodiazepines
Diazepam (Valium and others)
Flurazepam (Dalmane and others)
Halazepam (Paxipam)
Chlordiazepoxide (Librium and others)
Alprazolam (Xanax)
Triazolam (Halcion)
Clorazepate (Tranxene)
Prazepam (Centrax)
Midazolam (Versed, IM, IV, and S/C only)
Quazepam (Doral)
Estazolam (ProSom)
Clonazepam (Klonopin)
Lorazepam (Ativan and others)
Temazepam (Restoril and others)
Oxazepam (Serax and others)
Azapirones
Buspirone (Buspar)
Cyclic Antidepressants
Amitriptyline (Elavil and others)
Imipramine (Tofranil and others)
Nortriptyline (Pamelor and others)
Protriptyline (Vivactil)
Trazodone (Desyrel and others)
Desipramine (Norpramin and others)
Amoxapine (Asendin)
Maprotiline (Ludiomil)
Doxepin (Sinequan and others)
Trimipramine (Surmontil)
Other Antidepressants
Fluoxetine (Prozac), an SSRI
Sertraline (Zoloft), an SSRI
Paroxetine (Paxil), an SSRI
Bupropion (Wellbutrin), a dopaamine reuptake blocker
Nefazodone (Serzone), 5-HT2 receptor antagonist
Venlafaxine (Effexor), a serotonin/norepinephrine reuptake inhibitor
Other Medications Selectively Used for Their Anxiolytic Effects
β-Adrenergic blocking agents, such as propranolol
Monoamine oxidase inhibitors
Neuroleptics (antipsychotics), such as haloperidol

Source: Stoudemire (1996), reference 77

in the elderly; therefore, low doses are used. Temazepam is useful as a sedative-hypnotic.[35] Buspirone, used primarily for generalized anxiety disorder, is preferable for anxiety in the medically ill because of its lack of sedation, lack of negative effects on cognition, insignificant effect of age on elimination half-life, and limited effect of liver disease on half-life. Buspirone has almost no clinically significant interactions with drugs commonly used in general medicine. It may stimulate the respiratory drive, which makes it useful in patients with pulmonary disease or sleep apnea.[35] Cyclic antidepressants are well established as anxiolytic agents, which are particularly effective in the treatment of panic disorder and in generalized anxiety disorder. If these drugs are used for anxiety in depressed medically ill patients or used because of their sedating properties in patients with major depression or panic disorder, the side effects must be carefully considered. Potentially deleterious side effects in the medically ill are sedative, anticholinergic, orthostatic hypotensive, and quinidine-like. Liver disease and renal disease may affect metabolism and excretion of the drug and, therefore, require careful dosage titration.[34] Other drugs that may be used for anxiety include the β-adrenergic blocking agents, antihistamines, monoamine oxidase inhibitors, and neuroleptics. Beta-adrenergic blocking agents may be used for milder forms of generalized anxiety, but there are cautions and contraindications in the presence of pulmonary disease, diabetes, and congestive heart failure. Antihistamines are sometimes used, although the effects are largely nonspecific and sedative. Side effects, such as sedation and dizziness, can be significant for medically ill patients. Monoamine oxidase inhibitors are rarely used in the medically ill because of the precautions that must be taken to prevent drug interactions. Neuroleptics, such as haloperidol in low doses, are used for anxiety associated with severe behavioral agitation or psychotic symptoms.[34] When anxiety develops in the context of the terminal stages of cancer, it is often secondary to hypoxia and/or an untreated pain syndrome. Intravenous opiates and oxygen if hypoxia is present are usually an effective palliative treatment.[81] Anxiolytics are most effective when doses are scheduled; if given on an as-needed basis, anxiety may increase in patients already frightened and anxious. Anxiolytic medications help patients gain control over agonizing anxiety. Use of these medications may also assist the patient in psychotherapy, which can help control symptoms. All pharmacological treatments must be monitored for effectiveness and side effects. The effects of benzodiazepines are felt within hours, with a full response in days. Buspirone has no immediate effect, with a full response after 2 to 4 weeks. The sedating effects of benzodiazepines are associated with impaired motor performance and cognition. Benzodiazepines have dependence and abuse potential and the possibility of withdrawal symptoms when discontinued. Buspirone has no association with dependence or abuse.

Pharmacological Management of Depression. Patients with chronic illness commonly exhibit transient depressive symptoms at various points in the disease trajectory, particularly during the palliative care period when a hope for cure is no longer possible. As explained previously, depressive symptoms can be caused by the medical disorder itself, associated with medications used for treatment or symptom management, or caused or worsened by the stress related to coping with illness. Depression can also predate and recur with the medical illness. To further complicate matters, individuals with medical illness are often older, with potentially greater risk of adverse effects from both psychotropic and nonpsychotropic medications. Medical illnesses and the medications required to treat or manage symptoms may impose significantly modified prescribing regimens on the use of antidepressants. Therefore, it is necessary to evaluate the possible role of existing medical conditions and medications that could cause the depressive symptoms. Other general guidelines include: (1) use the medication with the least potential for drug–drug interactions and for adverse effects based on the patient's drug regimen and physiological vulnerabilities, and the greatest potential for improving the primary symptoms of the depression; (2) begin with low dosage, increase slowly, and establish the lowest effective dosage; and (3) reassess dosage requirements regularly.[81]

In the past, antidepressant drug selection was limited by the nearly sole availability of tricyclic antidepressants, but new drugs, such as the SSRIs, bupropion, and venlafaxine, have vastly simplified pharmacological treatment of depression in the medically ill.[82] No one medication is clearly more effective than another. The SSRIs have fewer long-term side effects than the tricyclic antidepressants and, in general, are the first line of pharmacological antidepressant treatment unless specific side effect profiles associated with other classes of drugs are desired.

Psychostimulants such as dextroamphetamine and methylphenidate have been useful in the treatment of depression in medically ill patients.[83–85] Advantages include rapid onset of action and rapid clearance if side effects occur.[86] They can also counteract opioid-induced sedation and improve pain control through a positive action on mood.[87] Common side effects of psychostimulants include insomnia, anorexia, tachycardia, and hypertension,[83] although incremental dosage increases allow adequate monitoring of therapeutic versus side effects. In patients with cardiac conduction problems, stimulants may be the treatment of choice. In medically ill patients, a 1- to 2-month trial can provide remission from depression even after discontinuation of the drug. Different studies have shown a 48% to 80% improvement in depressive symptoms,[87] and this class of medication is often quite effective but underutilized in medical settings (Table 19–8).

Certain medications and treatment agents can produce severe depressive states. As reiterated throughout this chapter, a diagnosis of major depression in medically ill patients relies heavily on the presence of affective symptoms such as hopelessness, crying spells, guilt, preoccupation with death and/or suicide, diminished self-worth, and loss of pleasure in most activities, for example, being with friends and loved ones. The

Table 19–8
Medications Appropriate for the Treatment of Depression in the Medically Ill

For Patients with Cardiovascular Disease	
Selective serotonin reuptake inhibitors (SSRIs)	**Dopamine reuptake blocking compounds**
Sertraline (Zoloft)	Bupropion (Wellbutrin, Zyban)
Paroxetine (Paxil)	**Serotonin/norepinephrine reuptake inhibitors**
Fluoxetine (Prozac)	Venlafaxine (Effexor)
Fluvoxamine (Luvox)	**5-HT_2 receptor antagonist properties**
Citalopram (Celexa)	Nefazodone (Serzone)
	Trazodone (Desyrel)
For Patients with Gastrointestinal Disease	
Tricyclic antidepressants	**5-HT_2 receptor antagonist properties**
Amitriptyline (Elavil)	Nefazodone (Serzone)
Amoxapine (Asendin)	Trazodone (Desyrel)
Clomipramine (Anafranil)	**Dopamine reuptake blocking compounds**
Desipramine (Norpramin)	Bupropion (Wellbutrin, Zyban)
Doxepin (Sinequan)	
Imipramine (Tofranil)	
Maprotiline (Ludiomil)	
Nortriptyline (Aventyl, Pamelor)	
Protriptyline (Vivactil)	
Trimipramine (Surmontil)	
For Patients with Renal Disease	
Tricyclic antidepressants	**Selective serotonin reuptake inhibitors**
Amitriptyline (Elavil)	Sertraline (Zoloft)
Amoxapine (Asendin)	Paroxetine (Paxil)
Clomipramine (Anafranil)	Fluoxetine (Prozac)
Desipramine (Norpramin)	Fluvoxamine (Luvox)
Doxepin (Sinequan)	Citalopram (Celexa)
Imipramine (Tofranil)	**Serotonin/norepinephrine reuptake inhibitors**
Maprotiline (Ludiomil)	Venlafaxine (Effexor)
Nortriptyline (Aventyl, Pamelor)	**Noradrenergic agonist**
Protriptyline (Vivactil)	Mirtazapine (Remeron)
Trimipramine (Surmontil)	
For Patients with Hepatic Disease	
Tricyclic antidepressants	
Amitriptyline (Elavil)	Imipramine (Tofranil)
Amoxapine (Asendin)	Maprotiline (Ludiomil)
Clomipramine (Anafranil)	Nortriptyline (Aventyl, Pamelor)
Desipramine (Norpramin)	Protriptyline (Vivactil)
Doxepin (Sinequan)	Trimipramine (Surmontil)

(*continued*)

Table 19–8
Medications Appropriate for the Treatment of Depression in the Medically Ill (*continued*)

Selective serotonin reuptake inhibitors	**5-HT$_2$ receptor antagonist properties**
Sertraline (Zoloft)	Nefazodone (Serzone)
Paroxetine (Paxil)	Trazodone (Desyrel)
Fluoxetine (Prozac)	**Noradrenergic agonist**
Fluvoxamine (Luvox)	Mirtazapine (Remeron)
Citalopram (Celexa)	
Serotonin/norepinephrine reuptake inhibitors	
Venlafaxine (Effexor)	
For Medically Ill Patients with Anergic Depression	
Psychostimulants	**Dopamine reuptake blocking compounds**
Dextroamphetamine (Dexedrine)	Bupropion (Wellbutrin, Zyban)
Methylphenidate	

Source: Beliles & Stoudemire (1998), reference 100.

neurovegetative symptoms that usually characterize depression in physically healthy individuals are not good predictors of depression in the medically ill because disease and treatment can also produce these symptoms. A combination of psychotherapy and antidepressant medication will often prove useful in treating major depression in medically ill patients.[88] Peak dosages of antidepressants, regardless of drug class, are usually substantially lower than those tolerated by physically healthy individuals. Antidepressant medications may take 2 to 6 weeks to produce their desired effects. Patients may need ongoing support, reassurance, and monitoring before experiencing the antidepressant effects of medication. It is essential that patients are monitored closely by a consistent provider during the initiation and modification of psychopharmacological regimens. Patient education is essential in this area to decrease the possibility of nonadherence to the medication regimen.

Psychotherapeutic Modalities

Psychosocial interventions are defined as systematic efforts applied to influence coping behavior through educational or psychotherapeutic means.[18] The goals of such interventions are to improve morale, self-esteem, coping ability, sense of control, and problem-solving abilities, and to decrease emotional distress. The educational approach is directive, using problem-solving and cognitive methods. It is important that the educational approach both clarify medical information that may be missed due to fear and anxiety or misconceptions and/or misinformation regarding illness and treatment, and normalize emotional reactions throughout the illness trajectory. The psychotherapeutic approach uses psychodynamic and exploratory methods to help the individual understand aspects of the medical condition such as emotional responses and personal meaning of the disease. Psychotherapeutic interventions, as opposed to educational interventions, should be delivered by professionals with special training in both mental health and specific interventional modalities as applied to patients with chronic medical illnesses and palliative care needs. Psychotherapy with a patient who has cancer should maintain a primary focus on the illness and its implications, using a brief therapy and crisis-intervention model.[78] Expression of fears and concerns that may be too painful to reveal to family and friends is encouraged. Normalizing emotional distress, providing realistic reassurance and support, and bolstering existing strengths and coping skills are essential components of the therapeutic process. Gathering information about previous associations with the medical condition experienced through close relationships can also be instrumental in clarifying patients' fears and concerns and establishing boundaries for and differences from the current situation.

Depending on the nature of the problem, the treatment modality may take the form of individual psychotherapy, support groups, family and marital therapy, or behaviorally oriented therapy such as progressive muscle relaxation and guided imagery. A primary role for clinicians is to facilitate a positive adjustment in patients under their care. Periodic emotional distress and coping problems can be expected during the palliative-care trajectory and monitored routinely. Emotional display is not the same as maladaptive coping. Understanding an individual's unique circumstances can assist nurses in supporting the constructive coping abilities that seem to work best for a particular patient.[78]

Psychotherapeutic Interventions Targeted to Symptoms of Anxiety

Anxiety responses can be thought of as occurring along a continuum, from mild to moderate to severe to panic. Lazarus and Folkman's[92] differentiation of problem-focused coping and emotion-focused coping provides a framework for intervention strategies matched to the continuum of responses (Table 19–9). As a person moves along the continuum to moderate, severe, and panic levels of anxiety, the problem-causing distress is lost sight of and distress itself becomes the focus of attention. Both preventive and treatment strategies can be used with patients and family members in a variety of settings. Before assuming that anxiety has a psychological basis, consider the models of interaction and review the patient's history for recent changes in medical condition and/or medications. Asking whether the

Table 19–9
Hierarchy of Anxiety Interventions

Anxiety Level	Interventions
Level 1 Mild to moderate	*Prevention Strategies*
	Provide concrete objective information.
	Ensure stressful-event warning.
	Increase opportunities for control.
	Increase patient and family participation in care activities.
	Acknowledge fears.
	Explore near-miss events, past and/or present.
	Control symptoms.
	Structure uncertainty.
	Limit sensory deprivation and isolation.
	Encourage hope.
Level 2 Moderate to severe	*Treatment Strategies*
	Use presence of support person as "emotional anchor."
	Support expression of feelings, doubts, and fears.
	Explore near-miss events, past and/or present.
	Provide accurate information for realistic restructuring of fearful ideas.
	Teach anxiety-reduction strategies, such as focusing, breathing, relaxation, and imagery techniques.
	Use massage, touch, and physical exercise.
	Control symptoms.
	Use antianxiety medications.
	Delay procedures to promote patient control and readiness.
	Consult psychiatric experts.
Level 3 Panic	*Treatment Strategies*
	Stay with the patient.
	Maintain calm environment and reduce stimulation.
	Use antianxiety medications and monitor carefully.
	Control symptoms.
	Use focusing and breathing techniques.
	Use demonstration in addition to verbal direction.
	Repeat realistic reassurances.
	Communicate with repetition and simplicity.
	Consult psychiatric experts.

Sources: Minarik (1996), reference 17; Leavitt & Minarik (1989), reference 101.

patient was taking medications for "nerves," depression, or insomnia will help to determine whether drugs were inappropriately discontinued or whether anxiety symptoms predated the current illness. In addition, ask about over-the-counter medications, illegal drugs, alcohol intake, and smoking history. Documentation and communication of findings are essential to enhance teamwork among providers.

Frequently, patients can identify the factors causing their anxiety, as well as coping skills effective in the past, and when they do, their discomfort decreases. Anxiety may be greatly reduced by initiating a discussion of concerns that are painful, frightening, or shameful, such as being dependent or accepting help. Use open-ended questions, reflection, clarification, and/or empathic remarks, such as "You're afraid of being a burden?" to help the patient to identify previously effective coping strategies and to integrate them with new ones. Use statements such as "What has helped you get through difficult times like this before?" "How can we help you use those strategies now?" or "How about talking about some new strategies that may work now?" Encourage the patient to identify supportive individuals who can either help emotionally or with tasks.

Preventive Strategies. Preventive strategies can help to maintain a useful level of anxiety, one that enhances rather than interferes with problem-solving (see Table 19–9). Effective preventive strategies that can be used by all providers involved with the patient follow[26,90]:

1. Provide concrete objective information. Fear of the unknown, lack of recent prior experience, or misinterpretations about an illness, procedure, test, or medication, especially when coupled with a tendency to focus on emotional aspects of experiences, may be a source of anxiety. Help patients and families know what to expect, and focus attention by realistically describing the potentially threatening experience with concrete objective information.[91] Describe both the typical subjective (e.g., sensations and temporal features) and objective (e.g., timing, nature of environment) features of stressful health care events using concrete terminology. Avoid qualitative adjectives, such as "terrible." Also known as mental rehearsal and stress inoculation, concrete information increases the patient's understanding of the situation, allows for preparation under less emergent and more supportive conditions, and facilitates coping. Encourage the patient to ask questions, and then match the detail of the preparatory information to the request. Since anxiety hinders retention, use of understandable terms and repetition is helpful. Too much information at once may increase anxiety.
2. Ensure stressful event warning before the event. For example, a person may experience magnetic resonance imaging as entrapping or traumatic or the placement of a central line as painful and threatening. Giving time to anticipate and mentally rehearse coping with the experience helps the person to maintain a sense of control and endure the procedure.
3. Increase opportunities for control. Illness can seriously disrupt a person's sense of control and increase anxiety. Help the patient to make distinctions between what is controllable, partially controllable, or not controllable. Focus on what is controllable or partially controllable and create decision-making and choice opportunities that fit the patient's knowledge. Ask patients to make choices about scheduling the day of the visit and the readiness for and timing of procedures and interventions.
4. Increase patient and family participation in care. Participation in care helps directly in coping and can be taught to both the patient and family members. Participation may reduce helplessness and increase a sense of control. Patients and family members may vary in their interest in participating and in their ability to do so. Often, female family members are more likely to be caregivers. Other factors influencing the ability to participate include family roles such as spouse, parent, and sibling; quality of relationships; presence or absence of conflicts; and other commitments, such as work or other family roles. Cultures also vary in expectations and the duty or obligation about caregiving based on gender or family position. Participation may also help with the resolution of ineffective denial when a person's condition is deteriorating. Family members who are caring for a person may recognize and adjust to the deterioration.
5. Encourage self-monitoring and the use of a stress diary. Self-monitoring of stress is a cognitive-behavioral intervention. Ask the patient to record the situations, thoughts, and feelings that elicit stress and anxiety. The patient may record incidences of treatment-related stress, illness-related stress, or other unrelated anxiety-provoking situations. Not only does this intervention provide assessment information, it also enhances collaboration with the patient and helps the patient understand the relationship between situations, thoughts, and feelings.
6. Acknowledge fears. Encourage and listen to the expression of feelings. Avoid denying the existence of problems or reassuring anxious people that "everything will be fine." Structure your availability. Refrain from avoiding anxious persons or their fears. Avoidance is likely to increase vulnerability, isolation, helplessness, and anxiety. Early structured intervention is more economical of time and more effective.
7. Explore near-miss events. Past or current exposure to a near-miss event is a potent generator of extreme stress and anxiety, with heightened vigilance. A near-miss is a harrowing experience that overwhelms the ability to cope. It may be a one-time experience, such as a person's own near-death experience, the cardiac arrest of another person in similar circumstances, or

something faced repeatedly, such as daily painful skin and wound care. Near-misses should be explored, fears acknowledged and realistically evaluated in view of the person's situation, and help given in developing coping strategies.

8. Manage symptoms. Managing symptoms such as pain, dyspnea, and fatigue is an essential part of promoting self-control. Symptoms such as pain signal threat and may lead to worries about the meaning of the symptom and whether necessary treatments will be worse or more frightening. Ensure pain control, especially before painful or frightening procedures. Severe anxiety may increase the perception of pain and increase the requirement for analgesia. Symptom management reduces distress and allows for rest.
9. Structure uncertainty. Even when there are many unknowns, the period of uncertainty can be framed with expected events, procedures, updates, and meetings with providers.
10. Reduce sensory deprivation. Sensory deprivation and isolation can heighten attention to various signals in the environment. Without the means for the patient to accurately interpret the signals, to be reassured, and to feel in control, the signals take on frightening meanings, such as abandonment and helplessness. Feeling isolated and helpless increases the sense of vulnerability and danger.
11. Build hope. Provide information about possible satisfactory outcomes and means to achieve them. Hope also may be built around coping ability, sustaining relationships, revising goals such as pain-free or peaceful death, and determination to endure.[92] Many additional suggestions are provided in this text.

Treatment Strategies. When it is evident that the person's anxiety level has escalated to the point of interfering with problem solving or comfort, the following strategies may be helpful.[26,90]

1. Presence of supportive persons. Familiar and supportive people, a family member, friend, or staff member can act as an "emotional anchor." Family and friends may need coaching to enable them to help in the situation without their own anxiety increasing.
2. Expression of feelings, doubts, and fears. Verbalizing feelings provides the opportunity to correct or restructure unrealistic misconceptions and automatic anxiety-provoking thoughts. Accurate information allows restructuring of perceptions and lends predictability to the situation. Aggressive confrontation of unrealistic perceptions may reinforce them and is to be avoided.
3. Use of antianxiety medications. If medications are used, they should be given concurrently with other interventions and monitored. Use caution to avoid delirium from toxicity, especially in the aged person.
4. Promoting patient control and readiness. If a patient is very frightened of a particular procedure, allow time for the patient to regain enough composure to make the decision to proceed. Forging ahead when a patient is panicked may appear to save time in the immediate situation, but it will increase the patient's sense of vulnerability and helplessness, possibly adding time over the long term.
5. Management of panic. When anxiety reaches panic, use presence and acknowledgment: "I know you are frightened. I'll stay with you." Communicate with repetition and simplicity. Guide the person to a smaller, quieter area away from other people and use quiet reassurance. Maintain a calm manner and reduce all environmental stimulation. Help the patient to focus on a single object (see below), and guide the patient in recognizing the physical features of the object while breathing rhythmically. Consider using prescribed anxiolytic medication.
6. Massage, touch, and physical exercise. For those who respond well to touch, massage releases muscle tension and may elicit emotional release. Physical exercise is a constructive way of releasing energy when direct problem-solving is impossible or ineffective because it reduces muscle tension and other physiological effects of anxiety.
7. Relaxation techniques. Relaxation techniques are likely to be effective for patients with mild to moderate anxiety who are able to concentrate and who desire to use them. Some techniques require learning and/or regular practice for effectiveness. Environmental awareness is reduced by focusing inward, with deliberate concentration on breathing, a sound, or an image, and suggestions of muscle relaxation. Progressive relaxation and autogenic relaxation are commonly used techniques, which require approximately 15 minutes. Relaxation and guided imagery scripts are readily available for use by clinicians.[26,93]
8. Breathing techniques. Simple and easy to learn, breathing exercises emphasize slow, rhythmic, controlled breathing patterns that relax and distract the patient while slowing the heart rate, thus decreasing anxiety. Ask the patient to notice his or her normal breathing. Then ask the patient to take a few slow, deep abdominal breaths and to think "relax" or "I am calm" with each exhalation. Encourage practice during the day. Some patients are helped by seeing photographs and drawings of lungs and breathing to visualize their actions.[94]
9. Focusing techniques. Useful for patients with episodes of severe-to-panic levels of anxiety, focusing repeatedly on one person or object in the room helps the patient to disengage from all other stimuli and promotes control. A combination of focusing with demonstration and coaching of slow, rhythmic breathing with a calm, low-pitched voice is helpful.

These techniques enhance the patient's self-control, which is desirable when the stress reaction is excessive and the stressful event cannot be changed or avoided. Both focusing and deep-breathing techniques can be used without prior practice and during extreme stress.

10. Music therapy. Soothing music or environmental sounds reduce anxiety by providing a tranquil environment and prompting recall of pleasant memories, which interrupt the stress response through distraction or direct sympathetic nervous system action.[95,96] Music most helpful for relaxation is primarily of string composition, low-pitched, with a simple and direct musical rhythm and a tempo of approximately 60 beats per minute,[95] although music with flute, a cappella voice, and synthesizer is also effective.
11. Imagery and visualization techniques. Imagery inhibits anxiety by invoking a calm, peaceful mental image, including memories, dreams, fantasies, and visions. Guided imagery is the deliberate, goal-directed use of the natural capacities of the imagination. Using all the senses, imagery serves as a bridge for connecting body, mind, and spirit.[76] Imagery, especially when combined with relaxation, promotes coping with illness by anxiety reduction, enhanced self-control, feeling expression, symptom relief, healing promotion, and dealing with role changes. Regular practice of imagery enhances success. Guided imagery for pain or anxiety reduction should not be attempted the first time in periods of extreme stress. Imagery in conversation is subtle and spontaneous. Often without awareness, health care providers' questions and statements to patients include imagery. Easily combined with routine activities, the deliberate use of conversational imagery involves listening to and positive use of the language, beliefs, and metaphors of the patient. Be aware of descriptors used for the effects of medications or treatments because they affect the patient's attitude and response. Health care providers can enhance hope and self-control if they give empowering, healing messages that emphasize how the treatment will help.

Psychotherapeutic Interventions Targeted to Symptoms of Depression

Depression is inadequately treated in palliative care, although many patients experience depressive symptoms. Goals for the depressed patient are (1) to ensure a safe environment, (2) to assist the patient in reducing depressive symptoms and maladaptive coping responses, (3) to restore or increase the patient's functional level, (4) to improve quality of life if possible, and (5) to prevent future relapse and recurrence of depression.

Crisis Intervention. Crisis intervention is appropriate treatment for a grief-and-loss reaction and when a patient feels overwhelmed. Effective strategies also include providing guidance on current problems, reinforcing coping resources and strengths, and enhancing social supports.[26]

Cognitive Interventions. Cognitive interventions (Table 19–10) are based on a view of depression as the result of faulty thinking. A person's reaction depends on how that person perceives and interprets the situation of chronic illness. Patterns of thinking associated with depression include self-condemnation, leading to feelings of inadequacy and guilt; hopelessness, which is often combined with helplessness; and self-pity, which comes from magnification or catastrophizing about one's problems. Cognitive approaches involve clarification of misconceptions and modification of faulty assumptions by identifying and correcting distorted, negative, and catastrophic thinking. Cognitive approaches are effective in treating forms of depression.[69] Therapy is usually brief, with the primary goal of reversing and decreasing the likelihood of recurrence of the symptoms of depression by modifying cognitions. It requires effort on the part of the patient. The effect is more powerful if homework and practice are included. Cognitive restructuring is one of the strategies used in cognitive therapy. In this strategy, patients are aided in identifying and evaluating maladaptive attitudes, thoughts, and beliefs by self-monitoring and recording their automatic thoughts when they feel depressed. The patient is then helped to replace self-defeating patterns of thinking with more constructive patterns. For example, "The treatment is not working. I can't cope; nothing works for me," could be replaced with a rational response such as "I can cope. I have learned how to help myself and I can do it." New self-statements and their associated feeling responses can also be written on the self-monitoring form. Over time, the patient learns to modify thinking and learns a method for combating other automatic thoughts.[67]

Imagery rehearsal is a useful strategy for helping patients to cope with situations in which they usually become depressed. The first step is to anticipate events that could be problematic, such as a magnetic resonance procedure. The patient is helped to develop constructive self-statements; then, imagery is used to provide an opportunity for the patient to mentally rehearse how to think, act, and feel in the situation. The combination of imagery with cognitive restructuring increases the effectiveness.[67]

Interpersonal Interventions. Interpersonal interventions (see Table 19–10) focus on improved self-esteem, the development of effective social skills, and dealing with interpersonal and relationship difficulties. Interpersonal difficulties that could be a focus include role disruptions or transitions, social isolation, delayed grief reaction, family conflict, or role enactment. Psychotherapies include individual, group, and support groups led by a trained professional. Patient-led support groups or self-help groups are effective for the general chronic illness population but less able to address the needs of depressed persons.[68]

Table 19–10
Nonpharmacological Interventions for Treatment of Depression

Cognitive Interventions

Review and reinforce realistic ideas and expectations.

Help the patient test the accuracy of self-defeating assumptions.

Help the patient identify and test negative automatic thoughts.

Review and reinforce patient's strengths.

Set realistic, achievable goals.

Explain all actions and plans, seek feedback and participation in decision-making.

Provide choices (e.g., about the timing of an activity).

Teach thought stopping or thought interruption to halt negative or self-defeating thoughts.

Encourage exploration of feelings only for a specific purpose and only if the patient is not ruminating (e.g., constant repeating of failures or problems).

Direct the patient to activities with gentle reminders to focus as a way to discourage rumination.

Listen and take appropriate action on physical complaints, then redirect and assist the patient to accomplish activities.

Avoid denying the patient's sadness or depressed feelings or reason to feel that way.

Avoid chastising the patient for feeling sad.

Interpersonal Interventions

Educate the patient about the physical and biochemical causes of depression and the good prognosis.

Enhance social skills through modeling, role playing, rehearsal, feedback, and reinforcement.

Build rapport with frequent, short visits.

Engage in normal social conversation with the patient as often as possible.

Give consistent attention, even when the patient is uncommunicative, to show that the patient is worthwhile.

Direct comments and questions to the patient rather than to significant others.

Allow adequate time for the patient to prepare a response.

Mobilize family and social support systems.

Encourage the patient to maintain open communication and share feelings with significant others.

Supportively involve family and friends and teach them how to help.

Avoid sharing with the patient your personal reactions to the patient's dependent behavior.

Avoid medical jargon, advice giving, sharing personal experiences, or making value judgments.

Avoid false reassurance.

Behavioral Interventions

Provide directed activities.

Develop a hierarchy of behaviors with the patient and use a graded task assignment.

Develop structured daily activity schedules.

Encourage the at-home use of a diary or journal to monitor automatic thoughts, behaviors, and emotions; review this with the patient.

Use systematic application of reinforcement.

Encourage self-monitoring of predetermined behaviors, such as sleep pattern, diet, and physical exercise.

Focus on goal attainment and preparation for future adaptive coping.

Specific Behavioral Strategies

Observe the patient's self-care patterns, then negotiate with the patient to develop a structured, daily schedule.

Develop realistic daily self-care goals with the patient to increase sense of control.

Upgrade the goals gradually to provide increased opportunity for positive reinforcement and goal attainment.

Use a chart for monitoring daily progress; gold stars may be used as reinforcement; a visible chart facilitates communication, consistency among caregivers, and meaningful reinforcement (i.e., praise and positive attention from others).

Provide sufficient time and repetitive reassurance ("You can do it") to encourage patients to accomplish self-care actions.

Positively reinforce even small achievements.

Provide physical assistance with self-care activities, especially those related to appearance and hygiene, that the patient is unable to do.

Adjust physical assistance, verbal direction, reminders, and teaching to the actual needs and abilities of the patient; and avoid, increasing unnecessary dependence by overdoing.

Teach deep breathing or relaxation techniques for anxiety management.

Complementary Therapies

Guided imagery and visualization

Art and music therapies

Humor

Aerobic exercise

Phototherapy

Aromatherapy and massage

Sources: Minarik (1996), reference 17; Leavitt & Minarik (1989), reference 101.

Behavioral Interventions. Behavioral interventions (see Table 19–10) are based on a functional analysis of behavior and on social learning theory. These interventions are often used in combination with cognitive interventions, such as self-monitoring and imagery rehearsal. The key to the behavioral approach is to avoid reinforcement of dependent or negative behaviors. Instead, provide a contingency relationship between positive reinforcement and independent behavior and positive interactions with the environment. This approach suggests that, by altering behavior, subsequent thoughts and feelings are positively influenced. It is helpful to structure this approach using the following self-care functional areas: behavior related to breathing, eating, and drinking; elimination patterns; personal hygiene behavior; rest and activity patterns; and patterns of solitude and social interaction. The aim is to maintain involvement in activities associated with positive moods and, if possible, to avoid situations that trigger depression.[97] This approach has been effective at helping family members of terminally ill patients see and accept functional decline.

Alternative and Complementary Therapies. Complementary therapies may help reduce mild depressive symptoms, or they may be used as an adjunct to other therapies for more severe depressive symptoms.[68] Strategies described for anxiety, such as guided imagery and visualization, the use of drawings or photographs, and music therapy, also may be used for depression. Art therapy for creative self-expression, use of humor and laughter, aerobic exercise, and aromatherapy massage have been helpful for mild depressive symptoms.[68] Phototherapy, which is exposure to bright, wide-spectrum light, has shown promise in patients with cancer.[68] See Chapter 25, Complementary and Alternative Therapies in Palliative Care, for a more in-depth review.

Conclusion

The psychosocial issues in persons facing life-threatening illness are influenced by individual, sociocultural, medical, and family factors. Most patients receiving palliative treatment and their families experience expected periods of emotional turmoil that occur at transition points, as is seen, for example, along the clinical course of cancer. Some patients experience anxiety and depressive disorders. This chapter has described the spectrum of anxiety and depressive symptoms during the palliative care trajectory; models of interaction useful for understanding the interaction of psychiatric and medical symptoms and for designing appropriate treatments; guidelines for referral to trained psychiatric clinicians; and a range of treatments for anxiety and depression. Supportive psychotherapeutic measures, such as those described in this chapter, should be used routinely because they minimize distress and enhance feelings of control and mastery over self and environment. Assessment and treatment of psychosocial problems, including physical symptoms, psychological distress, caregiver burden, and psychiatric disorders, can enhance quality of life throughout the palliative care trajectory.

This was reflected in Mrs. Brady's outcome. Following clarification that she would be receiving chemotherapy to halt disease progression plus awareness that her reason for refusing was based on memories of her mother and, thus, assumptions about her own outcome, led the patient to reconsider and accept treatment recommendations. A low-dose anxiolytic was suggested for use at bedtime, which the patient received on a short-term basis. Mrs. Brady was still well at the 1-year follow-up.

REFERENCES

1. Zabora J, Brintzenhofeszoc K, Curbow B, Hooker C, Piantadosi S. The prevalence of psychological distress by cancer site. Psychooncology 2001;10:19.
2. Richardson JL, Zamegar Z, Bisno B, Levine A. Psychosocial status at initiation of cancer treatment and survival. J Psychosom Res 1990;34:189.
3. Wellisch DK, Centeno J, Guzman J, Belin T, Schiller GJ. Bone marrow transplantation vs high-dose cytorabine-based consolidation chemotherapy for acute myelogenous leukemia: a long-term follow-up study of quality-of-life measures of survivors. Psychosomatics 1996;37:144.
4. Syrjala KL, Chapko MK, Vitaliano PP, et al. Recovery after allogenic marrow transplantation: a prospective study of predictors of long-term physical and psychosocial functioning. Bone Marrow Transplant 1993;11:319.
5. Tschuschke V, Hertenstein B, Arnold R, et al. Associations between coping and survival time of adult leukemia patients receiving allogeneic bone marrow transplantation: results of a prospective study. J Psychosom Res 2001;50:277.
6. Steinhauser KE, Christakis NA, Clipp EC, et al. Factors considered important at the end of life by patients, family, physicians, and other care providers. JAMA 2000;284:2476.
7. Holland J. Clinical course of cancer. In: Holland JC, Rowland JH, eds. Handbook of Psychooncology: Psychological Care of the Patient with Cancer. New York: Oxford University Press, 1989:75–110.
8. Weissman A, Worden JW. The existential plight in cancer: significance of the first 100 days. Int J Psychiatry Med 1976;7:1.
9. Endicott J. Measurement of depression in patients with cancer. In: Proceedings of the Working Conference on Methodology in Behavioral and Psychosocial Cancer Research. American Cancer Society, St. Petersburg Beach, FL, April 21–23, 1983;2243–2247.
10. Graydon JE. Factors that predict patients' functioning following treatment for cancer. Int J Nurs Stud 1988;25:117–124.
11. Richardson JL, Zamegar Z, Bisno B, Levine A. Psychosocial status at initiation of cancer treatment and survival. J Psychosom Res 1990;34:189.
12. Vickberg SMJ, Duhamel KN, Smith MY, et al. Global meaning and psychological adjustment among survivors of bone marrow transplant. Psychooncology 2001;10:29.
13. Pasacreta JV, Pickett M. Psychosocial aspects of palliative care. Semin Oncol Nurs 1998;26:77–92.
14. Watson M, Greer S, Blake S, Sharpnell K. Reaction to a diagnosis of breast cancer: relationship between denial, delay, and rates of psychological morbidity. Cancer 1984;53:2008–2012.

15. Molassiotis A, Van Den Akker OBA, Milligan DW, Goldman JM. Symptom distress, coping style and biological variables as predictors of survival after bone marrow transplantation. J Psychosomatic Res 1997;42:275.
16. Bope E. Follow-up of the cancer patient: surveillance for metastasis. Prim Care 1987;14:391–401.
17. Minarik P. Psychosocial intervention with ineffective coping responses to physical illness: anxiety-related. In: Barry PD, ed. Psychosocial Nursing: Care of Physically Ill Patients and Their Families. New York: Lippincott-Raven, 1996:301–322.
18. Silverfarb PM, Maurer LH, Crouthamel CS. Psychosocial aspects of neoplastic disease: I. Functional status of breast cancer patients during different treatment regimens. Am J Psychiatry 1980; 137:450–455.
19. Wise MG, Taylor SE. Anxiety and mood disorders in medically ill patients. J Clin Psychiatry 1990;51 (Suppl 1):27–32.
20. Breitbart W. Identifying patients at risk for and treatment of major psychiatric complications of cancer. Support Care Cancer 1995;3:45–60.
21. McGrath P. End-of-life care for hematological malignancies: the "technological imperative" and palliative care. J Palliat Care 2002;18:39.
22. Steinhauser KE, Christakis NA, Clipp EC, et al. Factors considered important at the end of life by patients, family, physicians, and other care providers. JAMA 2000;284:2476.
23. Emanuel EJ, Emanuel LL. The promise of a good death. Lancet 1998;351:21.
24. Bates MS, Edwards WT, Anderson KO. Ethnocultural influences on variation in chronic pain perception. Pain 1993;;52:101–112.
25. Pickett M. Cultural awareness in the context of terminal illness. Cancer Nurs 1993;16:102–106.
26. Tang ST, McCorkle R. Determinants of place of death for terminal cancer patients. Cancer Invest 2001;19:165.
27. Roth AJ, Breitbart W. Psychiatric emergencies in terminally ill cancer patients. Hematol Oncol Clin North Am 1996;10: 235–259.
28. Minarik P. Psychosocial intervention with ineffective coping responses to physical illness: depression-related. In: Barry PD, ed. Psychosocial Nursing: Care of Physically Ill Patients and Their Families. New York: Lippincott-Raven, 1996;323–339.
29. Levenson J, Lesko LM. Psychiatric aspects of adult leukemia. Semin Oncol Nurs 1990;6:76–83.
30. Pasacreta JV, Pickett M. Psychosocial aspects of palliative care. Semin Oncol Nurs 1998;14:110–20.
31. Bloom JR. Social support, accommodation to stress and adjustment to breast cancer. Soc Sci Med 1982;16:1329–1338.
32. Molassiotis A, Van Den Akker OBA, Boughton BJ. Perceived social support, family environment and psychosocial recovery in bone marrow transplant long-term survivors. Soc Sci Med 1997;44:317.
33. Andrykowski MA, Brady MJ, Henslee-Downey PJ. Psychosocial factors predictive of survival after allogenic bone marrow transplantation for leukemia. Psychosom Med 1994;56:432.
34. Molassiotis A, Van Den Akker OBA, Milligan DW, Goldman JM. Symptom distress, coping style and biological variables as predictors of survival after bone marrow transplantation. J Psychosom Res 1997;42: 275.
35. Burish TG, Lyles JN. Effectiveness of relaxation training in reducing adverse reactions to cancer chemotherapy. J Behav Med 1981;4:65–78.
36. Worden JW. Psychosocial screening of cancer patients. J Psychosoc Oncol 1983;1:1–10.
37. Derogatis LR, Morrow GR, Fetting J, et al. The prevalence of psychiatric disorders among cancer patients. JAMA 1983;249:751–757.
38. Massie MJ, Gagnon P, Holland JC. Depression and suicide in patients with cancer. J Pain Symptom Manage 1994;9:325–340.
39. Pasacreta JV, Massie MJ. Psychiatric complications in patients with cancer. Oncol Nurs Forum 1990;17:19–24.
41. Pasacreta JV, McCorkle R. Psychosocial aspects of cancer. In: McCorkle R, Grant M, Stromborg MF, Baird S, eds. Cancer Nursing: A Comprehensive Textbook 2nd ed. Philadelphia: WB Saunders, 1991:1074–1090.
42. McDaniel JS, Messelman DL, Porter MR, Reed DA, Nemeroff CB. Depression in patients with cancer. Diagnosis, biology and treatment. Arch Gen Psychiatry 1995;52:89–99.
43. Cassem EH. Depressive disorders in the medically ill. Psychosomatics 1995;36:S2–S10.
44. Cavanaugh S. Depression in the medically ill. Psychosomatics 1995;36:48–59.
45. Fernandez R, Levy JK, Lachar BL, Small GW. The management of depression and anxiety in the elderly. J Clin Psychiatry 1995;56(Suppl 2):20–29.
46. Barraclough J. ABC of palliative care: depression, anxiety, and confusion. BMJ 1997;315:1365–1368.
47. Morse JM, Doberneck B. Delineating the concept of hope. Image: J Nurs Scholarsh 1995;27:277–285.
48. Loge JH, Abrahamsen AF, Ekeberg O, Kaasa S. Fatigue and psychiatric morbidity among Hodgkin's disease survivors. J Pain Symptom Manage 2000;19:91.
49. McCoy, D.M. Treatment considerations for depression in patients with significant medical comorbidity. J Fam Pract 1996; 43(Suppl):S35–44.
50. Chochinov HM, Wilson KG, Enns M, Lander S. Depression, hopelessness, and suicidal ideation in the terminally ill. Psychosomatics 1998;39:366–370.
51. Wettergren L, Langius A, Bjorkholm M, Bjorvell H. Posttraumatic stress symptoms in patients undergoing autologous stem cell transplantation. Acta Oncol 1999;38:475.
52. Peplau H. A working definition of anxiety. In: Burd SF, Marshall MA, eds. Some Clinical Approaches to Psychiatric Nursing. New York: Macmillan, 1963:323–327.
53. Sarna L, McCorkle R. Living with lung cancer: a prototype to describe the burden of care for patient, family and caregivers. Cancer Pract 1996;4:245–251.
54. McCorkle R, Yost LS, Jespon C, et al. A cancer experience: relationship of patient psychosocial responses to caregiver burden over time. Psychooncology 1993;2:21.
55. Robinson LA, Berman JS, Neimeyer RA. Psychotherapy for the treatment of depression: a comprehensive review of controlled outcome research. Psychol Bull 1990;108:30–49.
56. Beck AT, Rush AJ, Shaw BF, et al. Cognitive Therapy of Depression. A Treatment Manual. New York: Guilford Press, 1979.
57. Beck AT. Cognitive therapy: a 30-year retrospective. Am Psychol 1991;46:368–375.
58. Johnson J, Weissman MM, Klerman GL. Service utilization and social morbidity associated with depressive symptoms in the community. JAMA 1992; 267: 1478–1483.
59. Koenig HG, George LK, Peterson BL, Pieper CF. Depression in medically ill hospitalized older adults: prevalence characteristics, and course of symptoms according to six diagnostic schemes. Am J Psychiatry 1997;154:1376-1383.
60. Holland J, Massie MJ, Straker N. Psychotherapeutic interventions. In: Holland JC, Rowland JH, eds. Handbook of Psychooncology:

Psychological Care of the Patient with Cancer. New York: Oxford University Press, 1989:455–469.
61. DiMatteo MR, Lepper HS, Croghan TW. Depression is a risk factor for noncompliance with medical treatment: meta-analysis of the effects of anxiety and depression on patient adherence. Arch Intern Med 2000;160:2101-2107.
62. Barg F, Cooley M, Pasacreta JV, Senay B, McCorkle R. Development of a self-administered psychosocial cancer screening tool. Cancer Pract 1994;2:288–296.
63. Roth AJ, Kornblith AB, Batel-Copel L, Holland J. Rapid screening for psychologic distress in men with prostate carcinoma. Cancer 1998;82:1904–1908.
64. Pasacreta JV, McCorkle R, Jacobsen P, Lundberg J, Holland JC. Distress management training for oncology nurses: description of an innovative and timely new program. Cancer Nurs. In Press.
65. Hall RCW, Platt DE. Suicide risk assessment: a review of risk factors for suicide in 100 patients who made severe suicide attempts: evaluation of suicide risk in a time of managed care. Psychosomatics 1990;40:18–27.
66. Valente SM, Trainor D. Rational suicide among patients who are terminally ill. AORN J 1998;68:252–264.
67. Eisendrath SJ. Psychiatric Problems. In: FS Bongard, DY Sue, eds. Current Critical Care Diagnosis and Treatment. Norwalk, CT: Appleton and Lange, 1994:233–244.
68. Back AL, Wallace JI, Starks HE, Pearlman RA. Physician-assisted suicide and euthanasia in Washington State. Patient requests and physician responses. JAMA 1996;275:919–925.
69. Scanlon C. Euthanasia and nursing practice—right question, wrong answer. N Engl J Med 1996;344:1401–1402.
70. Daley BJ, Berry D, Fitzpatrick JJ, Drew B, Montgomery K. Assisted suicide: implications for nurses and nursing. Nurs Outlook 1997;45:209–214.
71. St John PD, Man-Son-Hing M. Physician-assisted suicide: the physician as an unwitting accomplice. J Palliat Care 1999;15:56–58.
72. Tilden VP, Tolle SW, Lee MA, Nelson CA.Oregon's physician-assisted suicide vote: its effect on palliative care. Nurs Outlook 1996;44:80–83.
73. Fawzy FL, Fawzy NW, Arndt LA, Pasnau RO. Critical review of psychosocial interventions in cancer care. Arch Gen Psychiatry 1995;52:100.
74. Thomas C Jr., Petry T, Goldman JR. Comparison of cognitive and behavioral self-control treatments of depression. Psychol Rep 1987;60:975-982.
75. Robinson LA, Berman, JS Neimeyer RA. Psychotherapy for the treatment of depression: a comprehensive review of controlled outcome research. Psychol Bull 1990;108:30–49.
76. Eisenberg L. Treating depression and anxiety in primary care: closing the gap between knowledge and practice (1992). N Engl J Med 1992; 326:1080-1084.
77. Stoudemire A. Epidemiology and psychopharmacology of anxiety in medical patients. J Clin Psychiatry 1996;57(Suppl 7):977–986.
78. Bailey K. Lippincott's Need-to-Know Psychotropic Drug Facts. Philadelphia: Lippincott Williams & Wilkins, 1998.
79. Stuber ML, Reed GM: "Never been done before": consultative issues in innovative therapies. Gen Hosp Psychiatry 1991; 13:337.
80. Koenig HG, Breitner JCS. Use of antidepressants in medically ill older patients. Psychosomatics 1990;31:22–32.
81. Frank L, Revicki DA, Sorensen SV, Shih YC. The economics of selective serotonin reuptake inhibitors in depression: a critical review. CNS Drugs 2001;15:59–83.
82. Katzelnick DJ, Kobak KA, Jefferson JW. Prescribing pattern of antidepressant medications for depression in a HMO. Formulary 1996;31:374–388.
83. Shuster JL, Stern TA, Greenberg DB. Pros and cons of fluoxitine for the depressed cancer patient. Oncology 2002;11:45–55.
84. Reich MG, Razavi D. Role of amphetamines in cancerology: a review of the literature. Bull Cancer 1996;83:891–900.
85. Hyma SE, Arana GW. Other agents: psychostimulants, beta adrenergic blockers and clonidine. In: SE Hyman, GW Arana, eds. Handbook of Psychiatric Drug Therapy. Boston: Little, Brown and Co., 1997:134–152.
86. Vigano A, Watanabe S, Bruera E. Methylphenidate for the management of somatization in terminal cancer patients. J Pain Symptom Manage 1995;10:167–170.
87. Woods SW, Tesar GE, Murray GB. (1996). Psychostimulant treatment of depressive disorders secondary to medical illness. J Clin Psychiatry 1996;47:12–15.
88. American Psychiatric Association. Practice guidelines for major depressive disorder in adults. Am J Psychiatry 1993;150:1–21.
89. Anderson CM, Griffin S, Rossi A. A comparative study of the impact of education vs process groups for families of patients with affective disorders. Fam Process 1986;25:185–204.
90. Gallagher DE, Thompson LW. Treatment of major depressive disorder in older adult outpatients with brief psychotherapies. Psychotherapy: Theory, Research and Practice 1982;19:482–490.
91. Persons JB, Burns DD, Perloff JM. Predictors of dropout and outcome in cognitive therapy for depression in a private practice setting. Cognitive Therapy Research 1998;12;557–574.
92. Lazarus RS, Folkman S. Stress, Appraisal and Coping. New York: Springer, 1984.
92a. Leavitt M, Minarik PA. The agitated, hypervigilant response. In: Riegel B, Ehrenreich D, eds. Psychological Aspects of Critical Care Nursing. Rockville, MD: Aspen, 1989:49–65.
93. Christman NJ, Kirchhoff KT, Oakley MG. Concrete objective information. In: Bulechek GM, McCloskey JC, eds. Nursing Interventions: Essential Nursing Treatments, 2nd ed. Philadelphia: WB Saunders, 1992.
94. Morse JM, Doberneck B. Delineating the concept of hope. Image: J Nurs Scholarsh 1995;27:277–285.
95. Dossey BM. Imagery: awakening the inner healer. In: Dossey BM, Keegan L, Guzzetta CE, Kolkmeier LG, eds. Holistic Nursing: A Handbook for Practice. Rockville, MD: Aspen, 1988.
96. White JM. Music therapy: an intervention to reduce anxiety in the myocardial infarction patient. Clin Nurse Spec 1992;6:58.
97. Tommassini N. The client with a mood disorder (depression). In: Antai-Otong D, ed. Psychiatric Nursing: Biological and Behavioral Concepts. Philadelphia, PA: WB Saunders, 1995: 178–189.
98. Kurlowicz LH. Depression in hospitalized medically ill edlers; evoluation of the concept. Arch Psychiatric Nurs 1994;7:124–136.
99. American Psychiatric Association. Diagnostic and Statistical Manual of Mental Disorders, Text Revision (DSM-IV-TR), 4th ed. Washington DC: APA, 2000.
100. Beliles K, Stoudemire A. Psychopharmacologic treatment of depression in the medically ill. Psychosomatics 1998;39:S2–S19.
101. Leavitt M, Minarik PA. The agitated, hypervigilant response. In: Rigel B, Ehrenreich D, eds. Psychological Aspects of Critical Care Nursing. Rockville, MD: Aspen, 1989:49–65.
102. Derogatis LR, Wise TN. Anxiety and Depressive Disorders in the Medical Patient. Washington, DC: American Psychiatric Press, 1989.

20

Kim K. Kuebler, Debra E. Heidrich, Catherine Vena, and Nancy English

Delirium, Confusion, and Agitation

Herein lies a paradox [delirium], a condition that is often reversible, yet is the hallmark of dying in most patients. The challenge for the clinician is to identify and treat the reversible underlying causes in a manner that is consistent with the overall goals of care.—P. Lawlor[1]

- ***Key Points***
- *Delirium, confusion, and agitation are common symptoms at the end of life and are extremely distressing to both patient and family.*
- *Identifying patients at risk of developing these symptoms can lead to early recognition and prompt treatment.*
- *The etiology of these symptoms is frequently multi-factorial; some causes are reversible and others not.*
- *Patient and family education regarding the reasons for these mental changes and how they will be managed is essential.*

The human "living" experience will eventually tread the path toward the inevitable physical decline that accompanies age, disease, and death. Yet each individual's dying experience is as unique as the life that he or she has lived. Many of the common threads that often create fear in the dying process are similar and include the fear of pain, the fear of loss, and the fear of losing control over one's physical, emotional, and mental capacities. As nurses caring for those that are facing the end of their lives and their families, it is important that we understand how to empower both patients and families and how to reassure them that they will receive the care and support necessary to control symptoms at life's end.

Unmanaged physical and psychiatric symptoms impact negatively upon the quality of life for each person and his or her family.[2] To ensure optimal quality of life, prompt recognition, assessment, and intervention of all symptoms become crucial for the well-being of the patient living and dying from advanced disease. The patient is often faced with many stressors throughout the course of his or her illness, and the accompanying psychological distress experienced is as varied and individualized as the patient's personality, coping ability, social support, and medical factors.[2] Cognitive disorders are frequently seen in dying patients. For example, in the advanced cancer patient, delirium has been found to be the main reason for cognitive failure.[2–4] This chapter specifically discusses the symptoms of delirium, confusion, agitation, and dementia and provides nurses with a framework for approaching patients with cognitive disorders in the palliative care setting.

Prevalence

The elderly, postoperative patients, critical care patients, and those facing the last days and hours of life are subject to alterations in cognition. Many patients develop psychiatric symptoms during the terminal phase of illness, either alone or in combination with other physical symptoms. The varied psychiatric complications include anxiety, depression, and cognitive disorders.[2,4,5] Cognitive disorders have a negative impact upon patient functional capacity and often lead to a poor prognosis.[2,4,5] Losing one's sense of "self" is one of the most feared aspects of dying, and maintaining intellectual activity has been highlighted as an important area within the "good death" literature.[6–8] A recent survey revealed that 92% of the seriously ill respondents identified mental awareness as an important aspect for a good death, while only 65% of their physicians viewed this as a priority.[8] Maintaining a mental capacity facilitates the patient's ability to strengthen his or her relationships with loved ones, and achieves a sense of control and the ability to complete life by resolving past issues and contributing to others.[6–8] Clinically, observations focusing on global consciousness within several palliative care settings have identified that the percentages of "alert" patients often ranged from 25% to 82% during the final week of life. This decreased dramatically to 10% to 45% in the last 3 days of life, therefore, concluding that only 34% of these patients were able to "speak lucidly" before death.[9]

Delirium is considered the most common cognitive disorder in the palliative care setting and is found in as many as 80% of patients with advanced cancer.[3] Elderly and terminally ill cancer patients with pain are twice as likely to develop cognitive disorders, often a result of opioid use, than those without pain.[2] Delirium has been reported in 24% to 40% of hospitalized patients evaluated by a psychiatric consultation.[10] About 30% percent of patients in the intensive care unit (ICU) and 40% to 50% of elderly patients after hip replacement surgery have delirium.[11,12] Up to 60% of elderly hospitalized patients develop delirium as a complication during their hospitalized course.[11] A recent report indicated that 66% to 84% of elderly hospitalized patients with delirium are misdiagnosed.[13] Many studies have reported the lack of detection and identification of delirium. These studies include many reasons for the lack of reporting delirious patients:[14–17]

- Differing diagnostic terms or descriptors from clinician to clinician (vague descriptors such as confusion, agitation, acute brain syndrome, or metabolic encephalopathy)
- Varying presentations of delirium or fluctuations (hypoactive, hyperactive, etc.)
- Attributing cognitive changes to dementia, depression, or senescence
- Lack of baseline assessment using validated assessment tools
- Inexperienced clinicians

Some clinicians may consider delirium to be the "hallmark" of dying, or a metaphor for what is termed "terminal drop," which distinguishes delirium for those who are actively dying.[18] Its relevance to palliative care is evident. Delirium is also one of the most commonly encountered mental disorders in general hospital practice[19] and has been referred to as "everyman's psychosis," which accounts for the fact that everybody is potentially susceptible. For patients who are actively dying, the metaphor of delirium might be used as an aid to diagnosis and to management, while keeping it distinct from the delirium encountered among those not recognized at the outskirts of dying.[18] While delirium can occur at any age, the high incidence in elderly patients is often overlooked. Delirium has also been referred to as the "reversible madness," which no clinician should overlook. Studies have indicated that approximately 30% to 67% of delirium episodes are reversible.[3] Delirium is often unrecognized early in its onset, when manifestations are mild and easily treated. Failure to recognize this symptom and provide early management contributes not only to significant morbidity and mortality but also to an underestimation of its prevalence. Therefore, early detection and assessment are likely to improve patient quality of life. Objective monitoring and a high level of clinical awareness and skill are necessary to detect and treat cognitive symptoms within the palliative setting.

Definition (Terminology of Cognitive Changes)

Understanding the many symptoms, syndromes, and diagnoses associated with cognitive changes in persons with an advanced illness can be difficult at best, and the use of these definitions is often inconsistent in both clinical practice and the nursing and medical literature. "Confusion," for example, may at times be used to describe a symptom; at other times, "confusion" may be used to describe a syndrome. Terms such as "encephalopathy" and "acute confusional state" are often used to describe changes in mental status instead of using a psychiatric classification based upon set criteria from the DSM-IV.[20] Delirium, for example, may also be referred to as an acute confusional state, acute brain syndrome, and/or an acute organic reaction.[21] In addition, many of these are complex disorders having overlapping yet distinct etiologies and clinical characteristics. Cognitive disorders in the medically ill interface between medicine and psychiatry and all too often owned by neither.[21] The use of imprecise terminology can lead to mislabeling of behaviors, miscommunication among health care professionals, and misdiagnoses of cognitive changes. Therefore, the potential for the mismanagement of any cognitive change is extremely high.

Symptoms Associated with Cognitive Changes

The various labels used to categorize cognitive changes are based on the observation and evaluation of symptoms and behaviors. A common language regarding these symptoms is essential for accurate communication among health care professionals, which can decrease the variabilities often seen in caring for patients with reversible symptoms (i.e., delirium).

Anxiety

Abrupt changes in cognition can lead to anxiety. Cognitive impairment, regardless of the underlying cause, can disrupt both the receiving and the processing of sensory information. This results in a diminished ability to handle stressful situations and can contribute to the sensation of anxiety.[22] Anxiety may be described as a fear of the unknown (not knowing what is expected) or fear of the known (knowing what to expect), and is considered a universal human experience. Factors contributing to anxiety may include previous or underlying anxiety disorders, unmanaged pain, and associated medical factors (metabolic abnormalities, medication side effects, and withdrawal states).[3]

Anxious patients may complain of tension, restlessness, jitteriness, autonomic hyperactivity, vigilance, insomnia, distractibility, shortness of breath, numbness, apprehension, and worry or rumination.[2] However, the patient will most often present with a chief complaint identifying the somatization of anxiety that, therefore, is often overshadowed with a physical complaint.[2] The assumption that anxiety is a normal companion to the terminal phase is not considered helpful to both the assessment and the interventions associated with this symptom.[2]

There are multiple factors that can contribute to anxiety in the terminal setting. Many studies have identified a higher prevalence of anxiety when combined with depression.[2,23] Patients with anxiety often have multiple etiologies, and the clinician should not exclude psychological and existential issues as contributory factors, particularly in the alert and oriented patient.[2,23,24]

Confusion

Confusion is common among terminally ill patients and has broad consequences for their care and well-being.[25] A recent study that highlighted nurse-identified confusion in 299 hospice patients compared confused patients with nonconfused patients. The median age of patients studied was 78 years, and there was an incidence of malignancy in 54%. The data identified 50% of the patients as confused the week before assessment, and of those patients, 36% were severely confused or disabled by confusion. Compared with the nonconfused patients, the confused patients were more likely to have cancer (64% vs. 43%) and to live in the long-term care setting (21% vs. 33%).[25] Of these patients, common manifestations included disorientation to time and place, impaired short-term memory, drowsiness, and easy distractibility. From this data, inappropriate mood, a cancer diagnosis, agitation, and age were considered variables that predicted problematic confusion.[25]

Acute confusion or delirium is a manifestation of compromised brain function and has been identified as the most frequently occurring cognitive disorder in the elderly.[26–28] The American Psychiatric Association (APA) (2000) defines acute confusion as a syndrome that is characterized by a disturbance of consciousness and changes in cognition that develop abruptly (over a short period of time).[20] If untreated, acute confusion in the elderly patient can contribute to excessive disability, morbidity, and mortality.[29,30]

Incidence rates of acute confusion in the elderly hospitalized patient range from 33% to 80%, with an estimated mean at 40%.[26,31] However, the assessment and effective management for confused elderly hospitalized patients is problematic, and it is predicted that as many as 7 of 10 older patients who experience acute confusion will not receive an accurate diagnosis, thereby contributing to poor management.[26,32]

Several older studies have laid the groundwork to help clinicians understand the various etiologies and risk factors associated with the diagnosis of confusion, which include the following work and associated factors:

- Foreman (1992): low potassium, elevated glucose, elevated sodium, elevated blood urea nitrogen/creatinine ratio[33]
- Inouye, Viscoli, Horwitz, Hurse, & Tinetti (1993): vision impairment, severity of illness, cognitive impairment, high blood urea nitrogen, and creatinine ratios[34]
- Pompei, Foreman, Rudberg, Inouye, Brand, & Cassell (1994): cognitive impairment, burden of comorbidity, depression, and alcoholism[35]
- Inouye & Charpentier (1996): malnutrition, three new medications, internal bladder catheter, an iatrogenic event, use of physical restraints[36]

Other contributing factors associated with the onset of acute confusion identified in long-term care residents include a diagnosis of dementia, polypharmacy, fluid and electrolyte imbalances, metabolic disturbances, sensory impairment, and multiple disease processes.[37]

Agitation

Agitation has been used to describe specific behaviors, syndromes, and outcomes of multiple psychiatric or medical etiologies.[38] Allen[22] has described agitation as being better understood as a group of symptoms that might characterize an underlying disorder. Agitation can include many different behaviors or manifestations including anxiety, aimless wandering, pacing, cursing, screaming, calling out to a passerby, and arguing. In a factor analysis of agitated behaviors, Cohen-Mansfield and Billing[39] identified four types of agitation:

1. Physically aggressive behaviors: hitting, kicking, tearing, pushing, and cursing
2. Physically nonaggressive behaviors: pacing, inappropriate robing or disrobing, repetitious mannerism, and handling things inappropriately
3. Verbally agitated behaviors: constant request for attention, screaming, complaining, and negativism
4. Hiding/hoarding behaviors

These researchers further identified correlations between medical diagnoses and types of agitated behavior. They noted that nursing home residents who typically manifest agitation through physical behaviors usually suffer from dementia but are not otherwise generally ill. Verbal agitation was found to be prevalent in persons with a generally ill condition and in persons with unrelieved pain. However, verbal agitation was not associated with dementia. The researchers believed that the correlation of verbal agitation with disease and pain might be explained by the possibility that agitation is a form of expression of suffering from a medical disorder. This study illustrates the importance of describing the agitated behaviors and not necessarily describing the patient as being agitated.[39]

Other researchers have also noted a relationship between disease progression and specific agitated behaviors. Persons with dementia, for example, often exhibit agitation.[38,40] This is most likely a direct result of brain alterations that contribute to impairments in memory, judgment, and impulse control. Agitation may be a person's attempt to express feelings and needs that cannot be verbalized, either physical or emotional (pain, dyspnea, or frustration).[39]

Delirium

Delirium is a complex psychiatric syndrome and has attracted growing attention in the medical and nursing literature. Descriptions of delirium can be found in medical writings from 2500 years ago to the present.[40] In spite of this history, the terms used to describe the syndrome have been inconsistent, overlapping, poorly defined, and often related to the discipline or specialty observing the condition. Historically, terms such as organic brain syndrome, acute secondary psychosis, exogenous psychosis, and sundown syndrome have been used to describe delirium.[41] A review of the recent literature reveals a continuing use of a variety of terms to characterize delirium, including acute brain failure, acute confusional state, terminal restlessness/agitation, and ICU psychosis.[29,42–45] The APA first used the term "delirium" to describe the syndrome, and established diagnostic criteria in the third edition of the Diagnostic and Statistical Manual of Mental Disorders (DSM-III), published in 1980.[46] These criteria were revised in the DSM-III-R and DSM-IV. While diagnostic criteria in the earlier editions were developed from the opinions of committees of experts, the latest edition (DSM-IV) published in 1994, relied on comprehensive review of the literature and data from prospective studies of delirium.[47]

Based on the DSM-IV criteria, delirium may be defined as an acute and fluctuating organic brain syndrome characterized by global cerebral dysfunction that includes disturbances in attention, the level of consciousness, and basic cognitive functions (thinking, perception, and memory).[20] Other features commonly associated with delirium include increased or decreased psychomotor activity, disturbances in the sleep-wake cycle, and emotional lability.[41]

The diagnosis of delirium is primarily clinical, based upon careful observation and awareness of key features.[40,47] Because the signs and symptoms are nonspecific, the clinician must look for a constellation of findings (subtle change or disturbance in consciousness and/or a change in cognition), identify the rapidity of onset, and assess for associated medical and environmental risks that lead to a definitive diagnosis. Delirium is frequently unrecognized and misdiagnosed by clinicians.[48] The fact that demented, depressed, and anxious patients may develop delirium additionally makes the diagnosis difficult.[49] However, because of delirium's prevalence in the hospitalized elderly, the ICU, cancer patients, and the terminally ill, any patient with deterioration in mental status is best presumed to be delirious until it is proved otherwise.[13,32,50,51] The distinguishing characteristics of delirium and dementia are outlined in Table 20-1.

An understanding of delirium, both its clinical course and its assessment, is particularly important for the palliative care nurse. The palliative care patient population has a high prevalence of commonly identified risk factors for delirium that include advanced age, dementia/cognitive impairment, severe medical illness and the use of multiple medications (sedative/hypnotics, anticholinergics, corticosteroids, and opioids).[34,52–54] Furthermore, the consequences of delirium can be severe for both patients and caregivers. The presence of delirium is associated with increased mortality and morbidity, including prolonged hospital stays, functional decline, long-term care placement, and, in the case of the imminently dying, a distressing and uncomfortable death.[30,55–58] In addition to medical morbidity, there is evidence that psychosocial morbidity is also significant. A significant number of patients who recover from delirium remember the episode and report distress from the experience that includes anxiety, helplessness, and fear.[59–62] Caring for patients with hyperactive delirium has obvious stressors for both families and nurses; however, hypoactive delirium is also stressful, especially for families who regret premature separation from a patient who can no longer communicate.[47] Delirium robs patients and families of valuable time.

Because of the subtle presentation of symptoms and fluctuating course associated with delirium, nurses, who have more frequent and continuous contact with patients, are key to the early recognition of delirium.[28] However, research during the past decade continues to show that nurses fail to recognize delirium when it is present, especially in its hypoactive forms.[62] This is partly due to assessments of cognitive status that rely primarily on orientation, to the exclusion of other aspects such as memory, attention, and perception.[28,63,64] Useful tools have been developed to evaluate cognitive status and screen for delirium in patients in a variety of settings (hospital, home, long-term care, ICU). These tools are reviewed later in this chapter. Consistent use could improve early recognition of delirium by nurses.[65,66] However, to better understand the manifestations of delirium, it may be helpful to discuss each diagnostic criterion in more detail.

Disturbance of Consciousness. The term "disturbance of consciousness," while inherently vague, is a critical feature in delirium.[67] Disturbance of consciousness refers to impairments in attention and the ability to be aware of and sustain attention to the environment. Attention is typically fluctuating and may present as a change in the level of consciousness, slowed or inadequate reactions to stimuli or the environment, and easy distractibility. Due to this distractibility, individuals may be

Table 20–1
Differentiating Delirium and Dementia

	Delirium	Dementia
Onset	Acute or subacute, occurs over a short period of time (hours–days).	Insidious, often slow and progressive.
Course	Fluctuates over the course of the day, worsens at night. Resolves over days to weeks.	Stable over the course of the day; is progressive.
Duration	If reversible, short term.	Chronic and nonreversible.
Consciousness	Impaired and can fluctuate rapidly. Clouded, with a reduced awareness of the environment.	Clear and alert until the later stages. May become delirious, which will interfere.
Cognitive Defects	Impaired short-term memory, poor attention span.	Poor short-term memory; attention span less affected until later stage.
Attention	Reduced ability to focus, sustain, or shift attention.	Relatively unaffected in the earlier stages.
Orientation	Disoriented to time and place.	Intact until months or years with the later stages. May have anomia (difficulty recognizing common objects) or agnosia (difficulty recognizing familiar people).
Delusions	Common, fleeting, usually transient and poorly organized.	Often absent.
Hallucinations	Common and usually visual, tactile, and olfactory.	Often absent.
Speech	Often uncharacteristic, loud, rapid, or slow (hypoactive).	Difficulty in finding words and articulating thoughts; aphasia.
Affect	Mood lability.	Mood lability.
Sleep–Wake Cycle	Disturbed; may be reversed.	Can be fragmented.
Psychomotor activity	Increased, reduced, or unpredictable; variable depending on hyper/hypo delirium.	Can be normal; may exhibit apraxia.

Sources: Adapted from Ely et al. (2001), reference 12; Morrison (2003), reference 19; Brown & Boyle (2002), reference 21.

unable to follow conversations or complete simple tasks.[68] For example, patients may be slow to respond, unable to maintain eye contact, or may fall asleep between stimuli. Increasing stimuli (touch, sound) may be needed to elicit a response. Conversely, patients may be hyperalert and over-attentive to cues or objects in the environment.[69] The ability to focus can be assessed by the patient's inability to complete a particular task such as spelling "world" backwards, or subtracting serial 7s.[67]

Change in Cognition. Many aspects of cognitive function are impaired in delirium, including orientation, memory, language, thinking, and perception.[67,68] Disorientation usually manifests as disorientation to time or place, with time disorientation being the first to be affected. Disorientation to other people commonly occurs, but disorientation to self is very rare.[68] Short-term memory deficits are the most evident memory impairments. Patients may not remember conversations, television shows, or verbal instructions. They may have no recollection of the conversation or remember only bits and pieces. For example, the person experiencing cognitive changes may remember the nurse visiting but not anything the nurse said or did. Language disturbances associated with delirium range from a lack of fluency and spontaneity to rambling discourse that switches from topic to topic. The content of language may be rich in imagery or extremely simple. There may be long pauses in the conversation or use of repetitious phrases by the patient. The person experiencing delirium may also have difficulty finding the correct word to use in conversation or naming objects (anomia). Thinking is usually disorganized, as evidenced by incoherent speech, deficits in logic, and responses that are irrelevant to questions asked.[67,69] Perceptual disturbances may include misinterpretations, illusions, or hallucinations. Visual misperceptions and hallucinations are most common, but auditory, tactile, gustatory, and olfactory misperceptions or hallucinations can also occur. The individual with delirium may have the delusional conviction that the hallucination is real and exhibit emotional and behavioral responses consistent with the hallucination's content.[68]

Additional Features of Delirium. Although not required for the diagnosis of delirium, other features, including sleep–wake disturbances, psychomotor activity changes, and emotional lability, often accompany delirium. It is helpful to assess for these symptoms and monitor for any changes in these over time. Disturbance in sleep patterns is frequently observed in persons with delirium and was one of the criteria for delirium in the DSM-IIIR (3rd ed., revised) definition. However, this criterion was excluded from the DSM-IV definition of delirium because it lacked specificity.[47] It is common to observe daytime sleepiness, nighttime agitation, and disturbances in sleep continuity in addition to other features of delirium.[68]

Persons with delirium may also exhibit disturbed psychomotor activity. Continuing research has indicated that there are several subtypes based on motor activity of delirium. These include a hyperactive/hyperalert subtype, a hypoactive/hypoalert subtype, and a mixed subtype that features components of the other two (Table 20–2).[69–72] According to this description, hyperactive/hyperalert patients are restless, agitated, with overactivity of the sympathetic nervous system. Clinicians expect delirium to present with agitation, hallucinations, and inappropriate behavior. Indeed, the hyperalert–hyperactive variant of delirium is most commonly recognized.[28] Characteristics of hyperactive–hyperalert delirium include plucking at bedclothes, wandering, verbal or physical aggression, and increased alertness to stimuli, psychosis, and mood lability.

Hypoactive/hypoalert patients appear lethargic and drowsy, respond slowly to questions, and do not initiate movement. This type of delirium is characterized by withdrawal from people and usual activities and decreased responsiveness to stimuli. Because these patients are quiet and withdrawn, the delirium is often overlooked or attributed to dementia, depression, or senescence.[28,47] Differentiating delirium from the normal aging process, dementia, or depression requires careful and repeated assessment.[73]

A patient with a mixed subtype shows alternating periods of both types of behavior. Clinicians are likely to recognize the delirium only during periods of agitation, combativeness, or perceptual disturbance. Periods of lethargy may be seen as clinical improvements, when, in fact, the delirium may be continuing and increasing in severity.[41,69] A complete assessment of all symptoms of delirium is required before a change in behavior can be labeled as an improvement.

Persons with delirium may exhibit emotional disturbances. Anxiety, fear, depression, irritability, anger, euphoria, and apathy are common, with anxiety being the prevailing emotion. The delirious patient may be emotionally labile, rapidly and unpredictably shifting from one emotional state to another.[68]

Prodromal and Subsyndromal Signs of Delirium. Some patients manifest prodromal symptoms such as restlessness, anxiety, irritability, distractibility, or sleep disturbance in the days before the onset of delirium. These may progress to overt delirium over 1 to 3 days.[67] Recently, Cole and colleagues described a condition known as subsyndromal delirium (SSD).[74] The symptoms of subsyndromal delirium were similar to prodromal symptoms but never progressed to overt delirium. Patients with SSD had the same risk factors and similar outcomes as those with delirium. These findings may support the notion that delirium is a spectrum disorder in which increasing numbers of symptoms are associated with increasingly adverse consequences. Patients noted to be exhibiting one or more prodromal symptoms or who report feeling "mixed up," having difficulty judging the passing of time, and having difficulty thinking or concentrating should be assessed for potentially reversible causes of delirium (such as dehydration, medications, and hypercalcemia), and appropriate interventions should be initiated.

Differentiation of Delirium and Dementia. Dementia, in contrast to delirium, occurs in patients who are relatively alert and with little or no clouding of consciousness. Dementia differs

Table 20–2
Subtypes of Delirium: Frequency of Occurrence and Manifestations

Occurrence	Manifestations
Hyperactive	
Occurs in approximately 15% of patients with delirium	Agitation Anxiety Insomnia Hallucinations Nightmares Combative/violent behaviors Loud abnormal speech patterns
Hypoactive	
Occurs in 19% of patients diagnosed with delirium	Decrease in physical activity Lethargy Somnolence Apathy Depression Withdrawn Mental clouding
Mixed Subtypes	
Most common form and diagnosed in 52% of patients with delirium	Combined features of both hyperactive and hypoactive delirium

Sources: Adapted from Morrison (2003), reference 19, Brown & Boyle (2002), reference 21.

in its presence by occurring gradually and progressively over time and is not associated with an acute onset as noted in delirium.[19,21] The sleep–wake cycle is not disrupted in dementia but significantly interferes with short-term memory loss, while long-term memory remains intact.[19,21] Dementia has a pronounced impact upon judgment and abstract thinking and is associated with disturbances in higher cortical functions (apraxia, aphasia).[21]

Dementia is a strong risk factor for the development of delirium.[75] It has been noted in the elderly that up to two thirds of cases of delirium are superimposed on dementia. It has also been postulated that delirium may lead to chronic cognitive impairment. Many patients who have experienced delirium are slow to recover to their previous level of function and are at greater risk for developing dementia.[57,76] The symptom profile of delirium is very similar in patients with and without dementia. Patients with dementia, however, tend to have more symptoms of delirium, especially psychomotor agitation/retardation, disorganized thinking, and disorientation.[77] While some have postulated that hypoactive delirium is more prevalent in dementia, both subtypes have been identified.[75,77]

Differentiating dementia from delirium is a challenge for clinicians. In one study, presence of dementia was found to be a significant risk factor for nurses' nonrecognition of delirium.[28] Careful observation and comprehensive history taking is essential to identify acute mental status changes in demented patients that may indicate a superimposed delirium. While both conditions share the features of impaired memory, thinking, and judgment, the features of acute onset, altered level of consciousness, and fluctuating course are specific for delirium.[40] Likewise, psychotic symptoms and agitation are also common in both disorders. However, in dementia, the symptoms are consistent and generally do not wax and wane (See Table 20-2).

Assessment

As discussed above, delirium is often unrecognized and misdiagnosed by clinicians. Factors contributing to under-diagnosis of acute confusion in the elderly include lack of formal training in gerontology, knowledge deficits about acute confusion, and lack of knowledge about the availability and use of established, standardized instruments to assess changes in cognition.[78] It is likely similar factors contribute to inadequate recognition of delirium in the palliative care setting. A number of delirium assessment instruments have been developed for use in various populations. These tools vary in the goals, type of data collected, qualifications required of rater, number of items, and time required to complete.[79] Some are burdensome and difficult to use in daily clinical practice.[80] Palliative care nurses must identify persons at greatest risk for delirium and use standardized, reliable tools to assist in the diagnosis of delirium in daily practice.

Predicting Delirium. Knowledge of the risk factors associated with delirium is required to identify the population at greatest risk and to assist in early diagnosis. One model used in hospitalized elderly patients is the Risk Assessment Model for Delirium.[81] Factors present on admission that are associated with the development of delirium during hospitalization are visual impairment, severe illness, dehydration, and previous cognitive impairment. Events associated with the onset of delirium during hospitalization (precipitating factors) include use of physical restraints, malnutrition, more than three medications added to the medication profile, and insertion of an indwelling catheter.[81] Using this information, nurses can identify those elderly at greatest risk for delirium, intervene to prevent delirium, and initiate early treatment if delirium does occur.

Based on multiple studies on delirium, Sarhill and colleagues[82] identified the following as predisposing factors for delirium in persons with advanced cancer: medications (opioids, steroids, metoclopramide, and phenothiazine), age 65 and older, brain metastasis, infection, hypoxia, dehydration, hypercalcemia, anemia, and renal failure. Persons were more likely to develop delirium if five or more of these predisposing were present, with each medication considered a separate factor. Identification of these risk factors alerts the palliative care nurse to those patients who require a more detailed assessment for early identification of delirium.

Delirium Assessment Instruments. The Mini-Mental State Examination (MMSE) provides a systematic, scored method for evaluating cognitive function.[83–85] This scored examination can indicate early changes in cognition as it relates to the cortical function of the brain.[3] Orientation, attention, recall, and language are evaluated. Scores below 24 (out of a maximum of 30) are indicative of cognitive changes.[84] The MMSE is intended to measure cognitive change over time, but does not differentiate among delirium, dementia, anxiety, and depression.[3,86,87] Thus, the MMSE may best be used as a predictive instrument that directs the clinician to use a delirium assessment instrument for additional information.

Table 20-3 provides an overview of instruments used to assess delirium. These instruments are reviewed because they distinguish delirium from dementia and assess at least several of the multiple features of delirium. While all of these instruments require further study to determine application across varied settings and among different patient populations, the following have shown good reliability and validity in identifying delirium in selected populations.[79]

- The Memorial Delirium Assessment Scale (MDAS) (Figure 20-1) is based on the DSM-IV criteria[3,88,89] and is psychometrically valid and reliable in palliative care settings.[81,90] The MDAS requires minimal training for use and is appropriate for both clinical practice and research.
- The Delirium Rating Scale (DRS) is the most widely used assessment instrument based on the DSM-III criteria[86,91] and is useful in the assessment of delirium in the terminally ill.[88] It also has the best results for screening symptom severity. However, it lacks administrative ease for the clinician, and no publications are available on the use of the DRS by nurses.[79]

Table 20–3
Overview of Delirium Assessment Scales

	MDAS	DRS	CAM	NCS	BCS
DSM-IV Criterion					
Acute Onset		✓	✓		
Fluctuating Nature		✓	✓		
Physical Disorder		✓	✓		
Consciousness	✓		✓		✓
Attention/Concentration	✓		✓	✓	✓
Thinking	✓	✓	✓	✓	✓
Disorientation	✓		✓	✓	
Memory	✓	✓	✓	✓	✓
Perception		✓	✓		
Purpose					
Screening/diagnosis		✓	✓	✓	✓
Symptom severity	✓	✓			
Number of Items	10	10	9	9	2
Time to Complete (minutes)	10	**Not specified**	<5	10	<2

MDAS, Memorial Delirium Assessment Scale; DRS, Delirium Rating Scale; CAM, Confusion Assessment Method; NCS, NEECHAM Confusion Scale; BCS, Bedside Confusion Scale

- The Confusion Assessment Method (CAM) is designed for use by a trained interviewer to assess cognitive functioning in elderly patients on a daily scheduled basis.[92,93] Despite its attempt to streamline a diagnosis, the CAM is a complex instrument that requires extensive instruction for the rater due to its subtleties.
- Nurses designed the NEECHAM Confusion Scale (NCS) to use in routine assessments of hospitalized elderly.[94] No published studies in the palliative care setting are found.
- The Bedside Confusion Scale (BCS) (Table 20-4) correlates with the CAM and is designed for use in the palliative care setting.[80,82] It requires minimal training and only about 2 minutes to complete.

Delirium assessment protocols in hospitalized elderly and palliative care patients may include daily or even every-shift evaluations for delirium. Given the prevalence of delirium in these settings, this frequency makes sense. There are no published recommendations on the frequency with which delirium assessment tools should be used in outpatient and home care settings, although some of these patients may be at as great a risk as those in inpatient settings. Too frequent evaluation for delirium in persons at low risk for delirium is burdensome to both the patient and the clinician. It does make sense to complete a baseline evaluation on all patients and then base the frequency of follow-up assessments on the number of risk factors for delirium present.

Factors Contributing to Delirium

There are numerous factors that can contribute to cognitive changes in the palliative setting. Multiple medications and more predominantly, the use of polypharmacy (using more than one drug from the same class) can contribute to delirium. Accumulation of specific medications and their metabolites can be seen especially from drugs coming from the benzodiazepines, anticholinergics, opioid analgesics, etc. Other contributing causes include organ failure, for example patients who have end-stage liver failure are unable to effectively manage the metabolism of medications that undergo hepatic oxidation (e.g. benzodiazepines). Therefore, to summarize, common underlying medical conditions that contribute to delirium include:

- Medication toxicities, especially noted in the use of anticholinergic agents, anticonvulsants, anti-parkinsonism agents, corticosteroids, cimetidine, opioids, sedatives, alcohol, and illicit drugs
- Withdrawal from alcohol, sedatives, benzodiazepines, and barbiturates

INSTRUCTIONS: Rate the severity of the following symptoms of delirium based on current interaction with subject or assessment of his/her behavior or experience over past several hours (as indicated in each time.)

ITEM 1—REDUCED LEVEL OF CONSCIOUSNESS (AWARENESS): Rate the patient's current awareness of and interaction with the environment (interviewer, other people/objects in the room; for example, ask patients to describe their surroundings).
- ☐ 0: none (patient spontaneously fully aware of environment and interacts appropriately)
- ☐ 1: mild (patient is unaware of some elements in the environment, or not spontaneously interacting appropriately with the interviewer; becomes fully aware and appropriately interactive when prodded strongly; interview is prolonged but not seriously disrupted)
- ☐ 2: moderate (patient is unaware of some or all elements in the environment, or not spontaneously interacting with the interviewer; becomes incompletely aware and inappropriately interactive when prodded strongly; interview is prolonged but not seriously disrupted)
- ☐ 3: severe (patient is unaware of all elements in the environment with no spontaneous interaction or awareness of the interviewer, so that the interview is difficult-to-impossible, even with maximal prodding

ITEM 2—DISORIENTATION: Rate current state by asking the following 10 orientation items: date, month, day, year, season, floor, name of hospital, city state, and country.
- ☐ 0: none (patient knows 9–10 items)
- ☐ 1: mild (patient knows 7–8 items)
- ☐ 2: moderate (patient knows 5–6 items)
- ☐ 3: severe (patient knows no more than 4 items)

ITEM 3—SHORT-TERM MEMORY IMPAIRMENT: Rate current state by using repetition and delayed recall of 3 words [patient must immediately repeat and recall words 5 min later after an intervening task. Use alternate sets of 3 words for successive evaluations (for example, apple, table, tomorrow; sky, cigar, justice)].
- ☐ 0: none (all 3 words repeated and recalled)
- ☐ 1: mild (all 3 repeated, patient fails to recall 1)
- ☐ 2: moderate (all 3 repeated, patient fails to recall 2, 3)
- ☐ 3: severe (patient fails to repeat 1 or more words)

ITEM 4—IMPAIRED DIGIT SPAN: Rate current performance by asking subjects to repeat first 3, 4, then 5 digits forward and then 3, then 4 backwards; continue to the next step only if patient succeeds at the previous one.
- ☐ 0: none (patient can do at least 5 numbers forward and 4 backward)
- ☐ 1: mild (patient can do at least 5 numbers forward, 3 backward)
- ☐ 2: moderate (patient can do 4–5 numbers forward, cannot do 3 backward)
- ☐ 3: severe (patient can do no more than 3 numbers forward)

ITEM 5—REDUCED ABILITY TO MAINTAIN AND SHIFT ATTENTION: As indicated during the interview by questions needing to be rephrased and/or repeated because patient's attention wanders, patient loses track, patient is distracted by outside stimuli or over-absorbed in a task.
- ☐ 0: none (none of the above; patient maintains and shifts attention normally)
- ☐ 1: mild (above attentional problems occur once or twice without prolonging the interview)
- ☐ 2: moderate (above attentional problems occur often, prolonging the interview without seriously disrupting it)
- ☐ 3: severe (above attentional problems occur constantly, disrupting and making the interview difficult-to-impossible)

ITEM 6—DISORGANIZED THINKING: As indicated during the interview by rambling, irrelevant, or incoherent speech, or by tangential, circumstantial, or faulty reasoning. Ask patient a somewhat complex question (for example, "Describe your current medical condition.").
- ☐ 0: none (patient's speech is coherent and goal-directed)
- ☐ 1: mild (patient's speech is slightly difficult to follow; responses to questions are slightly off target but not so much as to prolong the interview)
- ☐ 2: moderate (disorganized thoughts or speech are clearly present, such that interview is prolonged but not disrupted)
- ☐ 3: severe (examination is very difficult or impossible due to disorganized thinking or speech)

(*continued*)

Figure 20–1. Memorial Delirium Assessment Scale (MDAS). (Copyright © 1996 Memorial Sloan-Kettering Cancer Center. Reproduced with permission.)

ITEM 7—PERCEPTUAL DISTURBANCE: Misperceptions, illusions, hallucinations inferred from inappropriate behavior during the interview or admitted by subject, as well as those elicited from nurse/family/chart accounts of the past several hours or of the time since last examination:

☐ 0: none (no misperceptions, illusions, or hallucinations)
☐ 1: mild (misperceptions or illusions related to sleep, fleeting hallucinations on 1–2 occasions without inappropriate behavior)
☐ 2: moderate (hallucinations or frequent illusions on several occasions with minimal inappropriate behavior that does not disrupt the interview)
☐ 3: severe (frequent or intense illusions or hallucinations with persistent inappropriate behavior that disrupts the interview or interferes with medical care)

ITEM 8—DELUSIONS: Rate delusions inferred from inappropriate behavior during the interview or admitted by the patient, as well as delusions elicited from nurse/family/chart accounts of the past several hours or of the time since the previous examination.

☐ 0: none (no evidence of misinterpretations or delusions)
☐ 1: mild (misinterpretations or suspiciousness without clear delusional ideas or inappropriate behavior)
☐ 2: moderate (delusions admitted by the patient or evidenced by his/her behavior that do not or only marginally disrupt the interview or interfere with medical care)
☐ 3: severe (persistent and/or intense delusions resulting in inappropriate behavior, disrupting the interview or seriously interfering with medical care)

ITEM 9—DECREASED OR INCREASED PSYCHOMOTOR ACTIVITY: Rate activity over past several hours, as well as activity during interview, by circling (a) hypoactive, (b) hyperactive, or (c) elements of both present.

☐ 0: none (normal psychomotor activity)
☐ a b c 1: mild (Hypoactivity is barely noticeable, expressed as slightly slowing of movement. Hyperactivity is barely noticeable or appears as simple restlessness.)
☐ a b c 2: moderate (Hypoactivity is undeniable, with marked reduction in the number of movements or marked slowness of movement; subject rarely spontaneously moves or speaks. Hyperactivity is undeniable, subject moves almost constantly; in both cases, exam is prolonged as a consequence.)
☐ a b c 3: severe (Hypoactivity is severe; patient does not move or speak without prodding or is catatonic. Hyperactivity is severe; patient is constantly moving, overreacts to stimuli, requires surveillance and/or restraint; getting through the exam is difficult or impossible.)

ITEM 10—SLEEP-WAKE CYCLE DISTURBANCE (DISORDER OF AROUSAL): Rate patient's ability to either sleep or stay awake at the appropriate times. Utilize direct observation during the interview, as well as reports from nurses, family, patient, or charts describing sleep-wake cycle disturbance over the past several hours or since last examination. Use observations of the previous night for morning evaluations only.

☐ 0: none (at night, sleeps well; during the day, has no trouble staying awake)
☐ 1: mild (mild deviation from appropriate sleepfulness and wakefulness states: at night, difficulty falling asleep or transient night awakenings, needs medication to sleep well; during the day, reports periods of drowsiness or, during the interview, is drowsy but can easily fully awaken him/herself)
☐ 2: moderate (moderate deviations from appropriate sleepfulness and wakefulness states: at night, repeated and prolonged night awakening; during the day, reports of frequent and prolonged napping or, during the interview, can only be roused to complete wakefulness by strong stimuli)
☐ 3: severe (severe deviations from appropriate sleepfulness and wakefulness states: at night, sleeplessness; during the day, patient spends most of the time sleeping or, during the interview, cannot be roused to full wakefulness by any stimuli)

Figure 20–1. *(Continued)*

- Metabolic abnormalities that include hypoglycemia, organ failure (hepatic, renal, pulmonary), fluid and electrolyte imbalances, and endocrinopathies (hypothyroidism, hyperparathyroidism)
- Systemic infections
- Head trauma
- Neoplastic disease
- Vascular disorders (transient ischemic attack, thrombosis, myocardial infarction, cardiac failure)[19,21]

Dehydration

People with chronic illness and the elderly are at risk for fluid deficits due to a number of causes, including use of medications (diuretics), infections/fever, and inadequate fluid intake.[95] Fluid deficits, whether they are volume depletion (intravascular water and electrolytes) or dehydration (total body water deficit), place patients at risk for numerous adverse consequences, including changes in behavior, cognition, and energy level.[82] Dehydration can cause confusion,

Table 20–4
The Bedside Confusion Scale

Parameter	Scoring
Level of Alertness	Normal = 0 Hyperactive = 1 Hypoactive = 1
Test of Attention: timed recitation of the months of the year in reverse order	Delay of >30 seconds = 1 1 omission = 1 2 omissions = 2 ≥ 3 omissions, reversal of task, termination of task = 3 Inability to perform = 4

Total BCS score is point score of Level of Alertness plus score of Test of Attention; range is 0–5.

0 = normal

1 = borderline

2-5 = diagnostic of confusion

Source: Adapted from Stillman & Rybicki (2000), reference 80.

restlessness, and neuromuscular irritability.[96] On the other hand, reduced intravascular volume and glomerular filtration are known to precipitate prerenal failure. The subsequent accumulation of drugs normally excreted by the kidneys may precipitate further adverse effects.[1] Fluid deficits can also increase the risk of pressure sores, precipitate fatigue, fever, constipation, and postural hypotension.[97,98] Furthermore, dehydration has been identified as a risk factor for delirium.[32,53]

In patients whose death is not imminent, correction of fluid deficits is imperative. However, fluid replacement for patients approaching death is controversial. In most care settings, aggressive maintenance of fluid and electrolyte balance is common practice. Yet some palliative care practitioners argue against the appropriateness of fluid replacement in the last days of life. Common arguments concerning the benefits of not correcting fluid deficits include: (a) decreased stress on the pulmonary system; (b) decreased brain swelling and discomfort related to headaches and confusion; (c) reduction in cardiopulmonary problems (congestive heart failure, pulmonary edema); (d) decreased airway secretions; (e) reduction in urinary incontinence with decreased urine output; and (f) decrease in pain from the potential release of endorphins.[100–102] On the other hand, some palliative care providers have challenged the idea that dehydration is universally beneficial in dying patients.[97,103] The potential burdens of fluid deficit include: (a) precipitation of confusion, restlessness, or neuromuscular irritability from buildup of toxins and metabolites; (b) confusion and syncope when dehydration is rapid (diarrhea, paracentesis); (c) discomforting symptoms such as thirst, dry mouth, cracked, parched or painful oral mucosa; and (d) the lay perspective of dehydration as contributing to an uncomfortable death.[96,99]

There is no evidence from randomized controlled trials to support approaches to fluid deficits in terminally ill patients. Thus, we do not know the benefits and risks of fluid deficit or whether hydration really can improve symptoms, quality of life, or quantity of life when used in a situation in which the patient likely has a life expectancy that might be measured in days as opposed to months. In their absence, current opinion on the benefits and risks of terminal dehydration rests primarily on clinical observation and descriptive studies conducted in the last decade. These studies primarily involved patients with late stage, terminal cancer and, therefore, findings may not be pertinent to other populations. They do, however, provide beginning insight into the experience of fluid deficit. For example, the distress experienced by dehydrated patients appears to be minimal.[100–102] Other studies have shown that patients who are clinically dehydrated may have normal laboratory parameters.[102,103] While experience of thirst and dry mouth has been found to be related to dehydration and hyperosmolality,[6] others have found little relationship between fluid status and fluid therapy.[102–105] On the other hand, dehydration may contribute to neurotoxicity (restlessness, delirium, myoclonus) when it leads to renal failure and accumulation of metabolites and toxins.[51,106] Since dehydration most likely has an interactive effect on development of delirium, rehydration may or may not affect the course of delirium in the terminal phase.[107,108]

It is possible that clinicians may provide comfort for dying patients by either avoiding or providing artificial hydration in the dying days. Decisions of hydration should be based on careful patient assessment and the goals of the individual patient and family. The decision to avoid artificial hydration in favor of oral fluids and meticulous oral hygiene may avoid problems such as pulmonary edema and intrusive technology. For patients in distress from neurotoxicity or thirst, a time-limited trial of hydration via carefully monitored intravenous (IV) or subcutaneous fluid administration may provide relief and promote comfort.[96,98]

Pharmacological Interventions for the Management of Delirium

The APA has developed a practice guideline to support the management of patients diagnosed with delirium.[109] After a complete history and physical examination and discerning reversible contributing factors to delirium, a prompt psychiatric consultation should always be considered in the primary management for this patient population. Psychiatry may be able to point out important environmental factors that the primary care team has not considered, such as an increase or decrease in sensory input or opportunities that would improve orientation.[110] Despite the conciseness and comprehensiveness of these guidelines, there is little information on the safety and efficacy of the newer antipsychotic that will be briefly described below.

Understanding that the use of sedative hypnotics (e.g., benzodiazepines) can actually contribute to the symptom of delirium, a recent physician survey identified the lack of knowledge and skills in successfully treating delirium. The impetus for this survey was based upon the concerns that benzodiazepines were too commonly prescribed for the management of general delirium in older hospitalized patients.[111] There is a substantial body of literature that can guide clinicians in the management of delirious medically ill older patients, who constitute the highest risk of developing this symptom.[111] The APA clearly articulates that there is substantial clinical confidence and available data suggesting that the use of benzodiazepines as monotherapy may be ineffective in the treatment of delirium, with the exception, however, of those patients who are experiencing delirium as a result of withdrawal from alcohol or benzodiazepines.[109] The physician survey was mailed to physicians thought to have experience caring for older patients who would at some point experience delirium in the course of their illness. A total of 286 surveys were collected to discern the clinical management of delirium.[111]

In the setting of severe delirium, 4% of those queried chose no treatment with drugs; 180 of the respondents, however, considered haloperidol as a single agent (64%). Seven considered risperidone, one thioridazine, and one loxapine. Therefore, 66% of the respondents chose an antipsychotic agent.[111] Lorazepam as monotherapy was the choice in 20% of the survey respondents, and lorazepam in combination with haloperidol was selected as an intervention by 8%. Seven of the respondents who chose haloperidol for severe delirium would prescribe lorazepam for mild delirium. Thirty percent of the respondents chose lorazepam alone or in combination with haloperidol for the treatment of choice in patients with mild or severe delirium.[111] The respondents who did choose haloperidol as an intervention for the management of delirium in their patient population chose low-dosing schedules. From this data, 20% of the respondents selected lorazepam as monotherapy to treat severe delirium. The investigators of this study identified concern, given the ability of benzodiazepines themselves to cause cognitive impairment and create

Table 20–5
Pharmaceutical Management

Anxiety/Agitation			
Alprazolam	0.25–1 mg	tid/qid	8 mg
Amitriptyline	10–25 mg	qhs	150 mg
Chlorpromazine	10–25 mg	tid/qid	600 mg
Citalopram	10–20 mg	qd	60 mg
Diazepam	2–5 mg	q 8–12	60 mg
Haloperidol	0.5–2 mg	bid/q4	20 mg
Mirtazapine	7.5–1.5 mg	qhs	45 mg
Olanzapine	2.5 mg	bid	20 mg
Delirium			
Chlorpromazine	12.5–50 mg	q4–12	600 mg
Haloperidol*	0.5–5 mg	q4–12	20 mg
Lorazepam*	0.5–2 mg	q1–4 hr	10 mg
Midazolam	1–5 mg load	c/i	60 mg
Phenobarbital	1–3 mg/kg load	c/i	600 mg
*Combination is recommended as first line in patients with an anxiolytic component to their restlessness			
Terminal Sedation			
Similar medications as in treating delirium.			
Midazolam	2–6 mg/hr	sq/IV drip	
Triazolam	0.25 mg	all day (sl/pr)	
Chlorpromazine	100–200 mg	titrate up to 800 mg (sl, pr, sq, IM)	
Droperidol	1.25–2.5 mg	q2–4 hr (IM IV)	
Clonazepam	0.5–2 mg	bid/tid (sl, pr, IV)	
Phenobarbital	10–20 mg	bid/qid (sl, pr, sq)	

Sources: Adapted from Smith & Kuebler (2002), reference 37; Schwartz & Masand (2002), reference 110; Caraceni & Grassi (2003), reference 114; Passik & Cooper (1999), reference 116.

delirium.[112] The APA's consensus is that benzodiazepines have proven ineffective in the treatment of delirium. The APA further suggests that the use of benzodiazepines used in combination with haloperidol should only be considered for patients who cannot tolerate low doses of antipsychotic medications or for those with problematic anxiety or agitation.[109]

The adverse effects of benzodiazepines are well documented in the delirium literature and include profound sedation, respiratory depression, and hypoxia.[113] Benzodiazepines have been shown to contribute to troubling behavioral side effects such as anger, agitation, restlessness, hostility, and violent and aggressive behaviors.[113,114] The rationale for choosing to use a benzodiazepine for the delirious patient outside of alcohol or benzodiazepine withdrawal should be clearly defined.[114] Since benzodiazepines contribute to and worsen the symptom of delirium, they may be considered for use in patients who are extremely agitated or anxious and require sedation.[114] (Table 20-5)

Haloperidol is most often considered as the drug of choice in the management of delirium with the exception of alcohol or benzodiazepine withdrawal.[3,110,114] Haloperidol has very few anticholinergic side effects, has limited active metabolites, and is not as sedating as benzodiazepines. It is readily available for oral, intramuscular, subcutaneous, and IV administration (the latter two are not FDA approved in the United States and United Kingdom).[110,114]

Haloperidol should be dosed at 1 to 2 mg every 2 to 4 hours as needed, with dose increases for agitated patients. Haloperidol can, however, prolong the QT interval and may require that patients be monitored if receiving IV dosing.[110] Because most dopamine antagonist's antipsychotics are effective in the treatment of delirium, using the newer atypical antipsychotics may be considered. However, there are currently few randomized and controlled studies to promote strong evidence, but there is a need to investigate this area further.

Risperidone is widely accepted for use in elderly agitated and aggressive demented patients, with doses ranging from 0.5 mg to 1.5 to 2 mg/day for dementia patients and lower doses in delirious patients.[115] In the literature, there have been a few case reviews that demonstrate the effectiveness of risperidone on delirium. Though the evidence is limited, it appears that risperidone could be used to effectively manage the psychotic symptoms often associated in the setting of delirium.[110,114]

Olanzapine has been useful in a series of anecdotal case reports.[116,117] It does not create extrapyramidal effects and is often considered as a second-line agent in patients who cannot tolerate the extrapyramidal effects of haloperidol. Olanzapine is initiated at 5 mg at bedtime and may be increased to 10 mg, with 2.5 mg as needed throughout the day.[116]

Clinicians prescribing antipsychotics for delirium should have a basic knowledge of the drug interactions with other concomitant medications that the patient may encounter. For example, haloperidol, which is metabolized through the P450 enzyme system, inhibits the specific isoenzyme CYP 2D6 when combined with analgesics such as codeine or oxycodone.[118] Haloperidol when combined with SSRIs (serotonin reuptake inhibitors) and TCAs (tricyclic antidepressants) can interfere with the metabolism of haloperidol.[119]

Nonpharmacological Nursing Interventions

Delirium Risk Reduction. Given the correlation between the number of predisposing factors and the incidence of delirium, it makes sense to intervene promptly to reduce the number of risk factors. Inouye and colleagues[87] demonstrated that the rate of delirium in elderly patients receiving multicomponent, targeted interventions to reduce risk factors was significantly lower than in those receiving usual care. The protocol included providing orientation communication tools, engaging patients in cognitively stimulating activities, promoting ambulation or active range of motion, administering a nonpharmacological sleep protocol if patient has difficulty falling asleep, using or repairing visual and hearing aids as needed, and instituting volume repletion in the presence of hydration. These interventions were most effective in patients who were at intermediate risk for delirium. The interventions had no significant effect on the severity of delirium once an episode had occurred, demonstrating that primary prevention is the most effective strategy. Although no similar studies are found in the palliative care setting, these should be part of basic nursing care for all patients, and most can be taught to patients' caregivers.

Restful Environment. In the presence of delirium, the interventions such as orientation and ambulation may no longer be as helpful. A quiet, restful environment is a means of reducing the internal and external sensory stimuli that often insult the delirious patient's cortical brain.[10,120,121] Familiar sounds, smells, and textures convey warmth and caring for the agitated and restless patient. Patients who experience confusion as a result of a delirious episode may have a greater need to relate to the familiar voice of a significant caregiver or to the soft touch of a favorite pet. Since the visual field may present distorted images, sound, smell, and touch are avenues that nurses and caregivers can use to communicate understanding and reassurance for the cognitively impaired patient. Reorienting to time is of minimal value as time has little meaning to the patient. Television and extraneous noise should be avoided. By reducing the excess stimuli, pertinent relaxing sounds of music or a familiar voice can be received.[121]

The sound of familiar music can also quiet the restless mind. Learning from the family or caregiver what the patient's favorite music has been in the past and encouraging its use not only includes the family but also promotes a soothing environment. When deemed appropriate by the professional support team, integrating the use of psalms and prayer may be of value to the family whose background is influenced by the Judeo-Christian religions. Knowledge of rituals used in various cultures, along with individual/family belief systems, is essential.

Supportive Care for Terminal Agitation. The importance of supportive interventions for patients in the final hours of life and their family members should not be underestimated.[10,121,122] It is important for the nurse to distinguish between acute confusion, signaling a possibly treatable and reversible delirium, and "nearing death awareness." Callahan and Kelly[123] define nearing death awareness as a special knowledge about the process of dying; it may reveal what dying is like and what is needed to die peacefully. Nurses have a unique role in helping caregivers understand this symbolic communication. Themes of nearing death awareness include describing a place, talking to or being in the presence of someone who is not alive, knowledge of when death will occur, choosing the time of death, needing reconciliation, preparing for travel or change, being held back, and symbolic dreams. When nurses understand these themes, what may sound like confused words to others may be understood as symbolic expressions of the patient's own awareness that he or she is dying. For example, a plea of "I want to go home" may be answered with "I know, it's time and you can go when you are ready," rather than with the more literal "You are home."[123]

When the caregiver and nurse communicate compassionate understanding, the patient's restlessness is often subdued.[114,123,124] Caregivers can offer insight into the patient's restlessness if queried on issues that may remain unresolved for the patient.[120] Byock,[125] identifies five requirements for relationship completion, by saying: "I forgive you"; "Forgive me"; "Thank you"; "I love you"; and "Goodbye." Pain and resentment within the family that has been kept hidden during the patient's illness may emerge when death is on the threshold. A counselor, chaplain, or other spiritual caregiver in the palliative care setting can offer families solace and support.

Use of Smell. The faint scent of freshly baked bread often conveys a sense of safety in one's remote memory. A pleasant scent is remembered as a time of joy, a safe and secure moment of love and caring. The sense of smell travels by way of the olfactory nerve to the central part of the brain, known as the limbic system. The limbic system is known as the "seat of emotion," where anxiety and fear are labeled as threatening to the self.[14]

In palliative care settings throughout England and Ireland, scents are used as an intervention in the form of essential oils. Essential oils are aromatic substances extracted from plants.[126,127] A minute drop of oil can be added to massage oil and applied to the skin in the form of a massage. Clinical studies have indicated a positive and prolonged effect in reducing anxiety when using scented oils in conjunction with massage.[14,127] A review of clinical studies of patients in the palliative care setting concluded that providing massage with essential oil is of therapeutic benefit.[127]

When patients experience the anxiety and fear associated with a delirious episode, a simple hand massage with lavender oil can help provide a calming and relaxing effect. The essential oil of lavender (*Lavandula angustifolia*) acts primarily on the central nervous system, resulting in a sedative effect. The relaxation effect is believed to be a direct result of the biochemical properties of lavender due to its high content of linalyl acetate (ester). In the home setting, scented candles can be placed in the room. The use of candles can also symbolize a sacred space of solitude and peace.

Use of Touch. Touch with intent offered by the caregiver, nurse, or volunteer, may express caring and safety to the confused mind of the patient. The clinical experience of nurses using therapeutic touch has value in calming the patient who has reached the end of life's journey. Therapeutic touch, a gentle and noninvasive expression by a nurse or caregiver, will relax the physical body, an effect that may be observed in the patient's facial expression and relaxation of muscles as the breath ceases. Cathleen Fanslow-Brunjes,[128] a nurse clinician who worked with Elisabeth Kübler-Ross and later at Calvary Hospital in the Bronx, pioneered the use of therapeutic touch while caring for the dying. The hand–heart connection developed by Fanslow-Brunjes[128] is a relevant intervention for use in terminal restlessness and terminal anguish. Based on the principles of therapeutic touch, in conjunction with the ancient healing system of Tibetan Buddhism and Ayurvedic medicine, it encourages "letting go."

Patient and Family Teaching

Patient and family education is the cornerstone of comprehensive end-of-life care. Through proper education and support, cognitive disorders may be avoided, recognized early, or shortened. When a cognitive disorder leads to distress, appropriate education and support can decrease the severity of symptoms by providing open and adequate communication to lessen the stimuli that exacerbate symptoms.[126] Teaching activities associated with cognitive disorders at the end of life involve prevention, identification, intervention, and supportive care issues.

Preventing Terminal Anguish. As terminal anguish is related to unresolved issues, often involving guilt,[120] it is important to encourage the patient and family to identify and to address unresolved issues. This sensitive topic can be introduced by telling the patient that many times people hold old grudges and hurts inside because they seem too painful or difficult to talk about. However, the common experience is that not talking about these concerns makes treating somatic symptoms even more emotional and difficult.

Preventing Delirium in the Dying. As medications are the most common reversible and preventable cause of delirium,[129] patients and families require education on the proper dosing and scheduling of all medications. Delirium can be caused by both taking too much medication (leading to toxicity) or too little (causing discomfort or potential withdrawal). It is important for nurses who care for patients in home care and clinic settings to review all medications with the patient and primary caregiver. Ideally, patients or family caregivers will recognize both the generic and trade names of their medications. Patients and family caregivers need to know the schedule for each medication, the side effects of each to report to their clinicians, and what to do if they should lose or run out of a medication. Medication charts, pillboxes, and medication information cards or sheets may be useful tools.

Patients and family also need to understand that any discomfort that is not adequately addressed can lead to complications, such as feeling nervous, confused, or worse. Thus, education for managing symptoms such as pain, nausea, constipation, and insomnia is an important component of the teaching plan to prevent delirium.[19,21]

Knowing that sensory deprivation, sensory overload, and unfamiliar or threatening surroundings may contribute to the development of delirium, it becomes evident that patient and family education should include evaluating the patient's sensory environment and developing strategies to provide appropriate levels of sensory stimulation. For some patients, this may mean encouraging interactions with caregivers and others (e.g., hospice volunteers), having the television or radio at a level pleasing to the patient, being sure the patient can see out a window to sense day and night clues, encouraging touch (e.g., massage or range-of-motion exercises), and assuring that the patient uses any needed sensory aides, such as eyeglasses or hearing aides.

Conversely, the patient who is in an environment where sensory overload is a potential requires education on decreasing sensory stimuli. Acute care settings are well known for the potential for sensory overload. However, many times, the potential for sensory overload in the home is not assessed. The combination of noises from vacuums, mixers, dishwashers, televisions, radios, conversations, and patient equipment (e.g., oxygen concentrators) can be overwhelming. In the susceptible patient, it may be helpful to close room doors, to run dishwashers or other equipment at different times of the day, to turn off or turn down televisions and radios when conversing, or to unplug the telephone at certain times of the day.

Being in a strange or threatening environment can contribute to delirium. Should a patient need to be admitted to an acute care or extended care setting, it is important to make that environment as familiar as possible. Encourage the patient and family to bring in familiar photographs or objects, establish a plan for familiar persons to visit regularly, teach family to greet their loved one at eye level, and encourage the use of touch, since this is very reassuring to the patient.

Early Identification of the Symptoms of Delirium. The prodromal symptoms of delirium may be easily overlooked. It is not uncommon for persons with advanced diseases to feel restless, anxious, depressed, irritable, angry, or emotionally labile. These symptoms may go unnoticed, only to be recalled later in family interviews.[10,109] Therefore, it is important to teach the patient and family to report any new feelings of uneasiness, anxiety, restlessness, or mood changes.

Lessening the Severity of the Symptoms of Delirium. The individual experiencing delirium may be very frightened regarding what is happening. Clinicians need to provide reassurance that delirium is usually temporary and that the symptoms are part of a medical condition.[109] This intervention may significantly decrease fear and anxiety. The purpose of all supportive measures needs to be explained to both the patient and the family. For example, discuss the purpose of any hydration ordered, the importance of adequate rest, and the rationale for orienting interactions on the part of nursing staff and family.[130]

The family should be informed regarding the fluctuating nature of delirium[19,21] to prepare them for the changes in behavior and to prevent them from misinterpreting these frequent changes. Reorienting the patient to time, place, and persons in the environment may assist him or her to stay oriented. Repetition is important to compensate for memory impairment.[120] Thus, the family should be taught to correct the patient's orientation errors gently and regularly. If, however, correcting orientation errors leads to increased distress in the patient, this strategy should be discontinued.[19,21]

The delirious patient is at risk for misinterpreting the environment. The family should be encouraged to evaluate the patient's environment for over- or undersensory stimulation. Interventions to correct the potential for sensory deprivation or overload, as mentioned above, may be appropriate.

Behaviors associated with delirium can be distressing for family caregivers to observe and may lead to fears that their loved one has "gone crazy."[109,120] The family needs to hear that delirium is the result of a biological disorder and that the symptoms are generally temporary. The family should also be included in discussions of current, predicted, or resolving delirium in the patient. In addition, the family should be encouraged not to take behavior personally.[22]

Teaching Following an Episode of Delirium. Follow-up teaching will include a discussion with the patient about the apparent cause of delirium so that both the patient and family are aware of risk factors. The individual may or may not recall events during delirious episodes. Some individuals have frightening recollections of the delirious episode. Thus, it is important to assess the presence of any distressing memories. Extra psychotherapeutic support to work through the experience may be appropriate.[2,109]

CASE STUDY

M.H., a Patient with Metastatic Breast Cancer

M.H. is a 54-year-old Caucasian woman who has self treated her metastatic breast cancer in the belief that herbs and vitamins would help her disease better than what the traditional medical community could provide her. She had been living with her illness for more than 5 years and had allowed her right breast to ulcerate on several occasions, leaving a huge scar and disfigured chest wall, with no resemblance of breast tissue. M.H. was the owner of a natural herbs-and-vitamins business with her husband, who had died 5 months before from a metastatic malignancy of unknown etiology. M.H. had two young adult daughters who both lived out of town.

M.H. was enrolled in a local hospice program and was receiving opioids for treatment of severe pain. Her primary caregiver (her best friend, and a registered nurse) contacted a local palliative care nurse practitioner (NP) to evaluate her status, believing that she was receiving too many opioids, which were contributing to significant side effects such as sedation, cognitive clouding, constipation, nausea, vomiting, and anorexia. The NP made a home visit to evaluate M.H. and quickly identified her reluctance to use and embrace the practices offered by Western medicine. Therefore, after a long discussion with the patient and her caregiver, the NP was allowed to perform a limited physical examination. M.H. would not allow the NP to evaluate her affected breast or palpate for associated lymphadenopathy; the NP was allowed to obtain vital signs and listen to both heart and lung sounds. Because of her distrust of the medical community, M.H. had limited diagnostics performed to a bone scan, which she received from an alternative therapy clinic, and which revealed extensive bone metastasis. The NP focused her attention on the medications that the patient had been prescribed and noted 100 mcg of transdermal fentanyl, 80 mg of sustained-release morphine every 8 hours, and 30 mg of immediate-release morphine for incident pain. She was prescribed lorazepam 1 mg every 4 to 6 hours for nausea and vomiting and was using her own preparation of cascara for constipation as needed. M.H. also had promethazine 50-mg suppositories in her refrigerator and was using them every 6 hours for her nausea and vomiting.

The NP noted that M.H. required direct control of her medical management and, despite the inappropriate use of medications, noted that it would require deliberate time and energy to gain trust and confidence in the NP to better control her symptoms. It was also clear to the NP that M.H. was extremely nervous and agitated about her illness, and during the home visit, she learned that M.H. was planning to travel to a clinic in Mexico, where she believed she would be cured of her disease. The NP focused on the immediate needs and identified the following problems that could promptly be managed: dehydration, constipation, unmanaged pain, anorexia, anxiety, agitation, sedation, and cognitive clouding, and, despite the patient's insistence that she was not depressed. The NP initiated hydration of 1000 mL of NACL 0.9% IV over 2 hours, discontinued lorazepam and fentanyl, changed her sustained-release opioid schedule to a 12-hour schedule (not changing the total daily dose), and discouraged the use of promethazine. The NP, in conversation with her collaborative physician, then prescribed dexamethasone 16 mg every day (to support her complaints of somatic pain, assist with nausea and vomiting, and help with anorexia and depression), haloperidol 2 to 5 mg every 4 to 6 hours for complaints of nausea and vomiting and agitation, and encouraged routine use of her cascara (every 8 hours) to aid her constipation. The NP planned a return home visit the next day to evaluate her symptoms. During the next visit, the patient and caregiver were both ecstatic about the benefit and changes in her condition, and by the following Sunday the patient attended religious services, which she had been unable to attend for many weeks.

M.H. continued to do extremely well and began to plan her trip to Mexico seeking cure. Because of her physical improvement, she did travel to Mexico and returned home only to become very ill from the treatment she had received. The NP was consulted and upon arrival to her home realized that M.H. was actively dying and that she was extremely agitated, since she was convinced that it would have been the "miracle." Her two daughters had been called from out of town and were present during the home visit, along with the caregiver and hospice nurse. M.H. was having episodes of insomnia, calling out inappropriately at night, and refusing to stay in bed. Because M.H. had done so well before her travel, many of the medications that she had been taking previously were discontinued. While in the Mexican clinic, she had discontinued all medications except her opioids. The NP noted the apparent changes in the patient's cognition and considered hypercalcemia and dehydration, but M.H. refused laboratory analysis. She did, however, accept hydration through hypodermoclysis. The NP also prescribed haloperidol 5 mg every 6 hours, discussing its benefits with the family, caregiver, and hospice nurse.

The NP was frantically contacted the next day because M.H., despite her weakness, was extremely agitated and on her hands and knees in her hospital bed, rocking back and forth and yelling out at her family. The NP made an emergency home visit and inquired about the use and amount of haloperidol. She promptly discovered that the hospice nurse did not feel comfortable using haloperidol and had discouraged the family from its use, instead encouraging the use of lorazepam 2-mg every 4 hours. The NP was faced with a challenging patient and family situation—they apparently had gone online to learn more about haloperidol because the hospice nurse was not in favor of this intervention, and were reluctant to use it. After a prolonged discussion of the benefits associated with this intervention, haloperidol was initiated subcutaneously at 10 mg until the patient became less agitated (lorazepam was titrated to a low dose 0.5 mg sublingual every 12 hours). M.H. was then able to relax and be placed back in her bed. She kept her eyes closed yet was able to respond appropriately to questions regarding her comfort. The NP suggested that the caregiver continue with haloperidol 5-mg subcutaneous injections every 6 hours. This intervention was successful and M.H. died early the next morning, peaceful and surrounded by her family.

Summary

This case illustrates many issues related to a dying patient who experiences agitation and confusion. M.H. required individualized assessment and respect for her beliefs regarding her disease and treatment. The NP's skilled assessment of her multiple and changing symptoms was also essential. This case also illustrates the necessity of distinguishing related symptoms and modifying drug regimens as symptoms progress, particularly at the end of life, and including the participation of the family in the plan of care, especially when the patient is dying at home.

Conclusion

The nurse is the bedside advocate in discerning changes in the patient's cognition. Early and prompt recognition of cognitive changes can help to initiate appropriate interventions and discourage the progressive nature of delirium. Delirium is a broad category for many alterations in the cognitive realm of the person experiencing advanced disease and can be reversible. Becoming better acquainted with the assessment, etiology, and interventions to promote an improved quality of life is essential when providing optimal symptom management to ease the transition for the dying patient.

REFERENCES

1. Lawlor P, Delirium and dehydration: some fluid for thought. Support Cancer Care 2002;10:445–454.
2. Breitbart W, Chochinov HM, Passik S. Psychiatric symptoms in palliative care. In: Doyle D, Hanks G, Cherny N, Calman K, eds. Oxford Textbook of Palliative Medicine, 3rd ed. Oxford: Oxford University Press, 2004:746–771.
3. Elsayem A, Driver L, Bruera E. The M.D. Anderson Symptom Control and Palliative Care Handbook, 2nd ed. Houston: The University of Texas Health Science Center at Houston, 2003:61–68.
4. Portenoy R, Brietbart W. Foreword. In: Caraceni A, Grassi L, eds. Delirium: Acute Confusional States in Palliative Medicine, Oxford: Oxford University Press, 2004:vii-ix.
5. Marcantonio E, Simon S, Bergmann M, Jones R, Murphy K. Delirium symptom in post-acute care: prevalent, persistent and associated with poor functional recovery. J Am Geriatrics Soc 2003;51:4–9.
6. Mortia T, Tei Y, Inoue S. Impaired communication capacity and agitated delirium in the final week of terminally ill cancer patients: prevalence and identification of research focus. J Pain Symptom Manage 2003;26:827–833.
7. Singer P, Martin D, Kelner M. Quality end of life care. Patient's perspectives. JAMA 1999;281:163–168.
8. Steinhauser K, Christakis N, Clipp E, et al. In search of a good earth: observations of patients, families and providers. Ann Intern Med 200;132:825–832.
9. Turner K, Chye R, Aggarwal G, et al. Dignity in dying: a preliminary study of patients in the last three days of life. J. Palliat Care 1996;12:7–13.
10. Ingham J, Caraceni A. Delirium. In: Berger A, Portenoy R, Weissman D, eds. Principles and Practice of Palliative Care and Supportive Oncology, 2nd ed. Philadelphia: Lippincott Williams & Wilkins; 2002:555–576.
11. Marshall M, Soucy M. Delirium in the intensive care unit. Crit Care Nurse 2003;26:172–178.
12. Antai-Otong D. Managing geriatric psychiatric emergencies: delirium and dementia. Nurs Clin North Am 2003;38:123–135.
13. Ely E, Margolin R, Francis J. Evaluation of delirium in critically ill patients: validation of the confusion assessment method of the intensive care unit (CAM-ICU). Crit Care Med 2001;29: 1370–1379.
14. Kales H, Kamholz B, Visnic S, et al. Recorded delirium in a national sample of elderly inpatients: potential implications for recognition. J Geriatr Psychiatry Neurol 2003;16:32–38.
15. Inouye S, Schlesinger M, Lydon T. Delirium: a symptom of how hospital care is failing older persons and a window to improve quality of hospital care. Am J Med 1999;106:565–573.
16. Johnson J, Identifying and recognizing delirium. Dement Geriatr Cogn Disord 1999;10:353–358.
17. McNicoll L, Pisani M, Zhang Y, et al. Delirium in the intensive care unit: occurrence and clinical course in older patients. J Am Geriatrics Soc 2003;51:591–598.
18. Rockwood K, Lindesay J. Delirium and dying. Int Psychogeriatr 2002;14:235–238.
19. Morrison C. Identification and management of delirium in the critically ill patient with cancer. AACN Critical Issues 2003; 14:92–111.
20. American Psychiatric Association. Diagnostic and Statistical Manual of Mental Disorders, 4th ed. Washington DC: American Psychiatric Association, 2000.
21. Brown T, Boyle M. ABC of psychological medicine: delirium. BMJ 2002;325:644–647.
22. Allen L. Treating agitation without drugs. Am J Nurs 1999;99:36–41.
23. Massie M, Payne D. Anxiety in palliative care. In: Chochinov H, Brietbart W, eds. Handbook of Psychiatry in Palliative Medicine. New York: Oxford University Press, 2000:63–74.
24. Holland J. Anxiety and cancer: the patient and family. J Clin Psychiatry 1989;50:20–25.
25. Nowels D, Bublitz C, Kassner C, Kutner J. Estimation of confusion prevalence in hospice patients. J Palliat Med 2002;5:687–695.
26. McCarthy M. Detecting acute confusion in older adults: comparing clinical reasoning of nurses working in acute, long-term, and community health care environments. Res Nurs Health 2003;26:203–212.
27. Inouye S. Delirium: a barometer for quality of hospital care. Hosp Practice 2001;36:37–39.
28. Inouye S, Foreman M, Mion L, et al. Nurses' recognition of delirium and its symptoms: comparison of nurse and researcher ratings. Arch Intern Med 2001;161:2467–2473.
29. Cacchione P, Culp K, Laing J, Tripp-Reimer T. Clinical profile of acute confusion in the long-term care setting. Clin Nurse Res 2003;12:145–158.
30. Inouye S, Rusing J, Foreman M, et al, Does delirium contribute to poor hospital outcomes? A three site epidemiologic study. J Gen Med 1998;13:234–242.
31. Dolan M, Hawkes W, Zimmerman S. Delirium on hospital admission in aged hip fracture patients: prediction of mortality and 2-year functional outcomes. J Gerontol 2000;55:M527-M534.

32. Inouye S, Delirium in older hospitalized patients. Clin Geriat Med 1998;14:745–764.
33. Foreman M, Wakefield B, Culp K, Milisen K. Delirium in elderly patients: an overview of the state of science. J Gerontol Nurs 2001;27:12–20.
34. Inouye S, Charpentier P. Precipitating factors for delirium in hospitalized elderly persons: predictive model and interrelationships with baseline vulnerability. JAMA 1996;275: 852–857.
35. Pompei P, Foreman M, Rudberg M, et al. Delirium in hospitalized older persons: outcomes and predictors. J Am Geriatr Soc 1994;42:809–815.
36. Matteson M, Linton B, Cleary S, Barnes J, Lichtenstein L. Management of problematic behavioral symptoms associated with dementia: A cognitive developmental approach. In: Funk S, Tornquist M, Leeman J, Miles M, Harrell J, eds. Key Aspects of Preventing and Managing Chronic Illness. New York: Springer Publishing, 2000:323–341.
37. Smith H, Kuebler, K, Agitation. In: Kuebler K, Esper P, eds. Palliative Practices from A-Z for the Bedside Clinician. Pittsburgh: Oncology Nursing Society, 2002:5–8.
38. Cohen-Mansfield J, Billing N. Agitated behaviors in the elderly. I. A conceptual review. J Am Geriatr Soc 1986;34:711–721.
39. Haskell R, Frankel H, Rotondo M. Agitation. AACN Clin Issues 1997;8:335–350.
40. Clary GL, Krishnan KR. Delirium: diagnosis, neuropathogenesis, and treatment. J Psychiatr Pract 2001;7:310–323.
41. Lipowski AJ. Delirium: Acute Confusional States. New York: Oxford University Press, 1990:132–137.
42. Barber JM. Pharmacologic management of integrative brain failure. Crit Care Nurs Quarterly 2003;26:192–207.
43. Maluso-Bolton T. Terminal agitation. J Hospice Palliative Nurs 2000;2:9–20.
44. McGuire BE, Basten CJ, Ryan CJ, Gallagher J. Intensive care unit syndrome: a dangerous misnomer. Arch Intern Med 2000;160: 906–909.
45. Travis SS, Conway J, Daly M, Larsen P. Terminal restlessness in the nursing facility: assessment, palliation, and symptom management. Geriatr Nurs 2001;22:308–312.
46. American Psychiatric Association. Diagnostic and statistical manual of mental disorders. Washington, DC: American Psychiatric Association, 1980:133–179.
47. Liptzin B. What criteria should be used for the diagnosis of delirium? Dement Geriatr Cogn Disord 1999;10:364–367.
48. Casarett DJ, Inouye SK. American College of Physicians—American Society of Internal Medicine End-of-Life Care Consensus Panel. Diagnosis and management of delirium near the end of life. Ann Intern Med 2001; 135:32–40.
49. Armstrong SC, Cozza KL, Watanabe KS. The misdiagnosis of delirium. Psychosomatics 1997;38:433–439.
50. Insel KC, Badger TA. Deciphering the 4 D's: cognitive decline, delirium, depression and dementia—a review. J Adv Nurs 2002; 38:360–368.
51. Lawlor PG, Gagnon B, Mancini IL, et al. Occurrence, causes, and outcome of delirium in patients with advanced cancer: a prospective study. Arch Intern Med 2000;160:786–794.
52. Massie MJ, Holland J, Glass E. Delirium in terminally ill cancer patients. Am J Psychiatry 1983; 140:1048–1050.
53. Eden BM, Foreman MD, Sisk R. Delirium: comparison of four predictive models in hospitalized critically ill elderly patients. Appl Nurs Res 1998; 11:27–35.
54. Elie M, Cole MG, Primeau FJ, Bellavance F. Delirium risk factors in elderly hospitalized patients. J Gen Intern Med 1998;13:204–212.
55. Martin NJ, Stones MJ, Young JE, Bedard M. Development of delirium: a prospective cohort study in a community hospital. Int Psychogeriatr 2000;12:117–127.
56. Breitbart W, Strout D. Delirium in the terminally ill. Clin Geriatr Med 2000;16:357–372.
57. Ely EW, Gautam S, Margolin R, et al. The impact of delirium in the intensive care unit on hospital length of stay. Intensive Care Med 2001; 27:1892–1900.
58. Marcantonio ER, Simon SE, Bergmann MA, Jones RN, Murphy KM, Morris JN. Delirium symptoms in post-acute care: prevalent, persistent, and associated with poor functional recovery. J Am Geriatr Soc 2003;51:4–9.
59. McCusker J, Cole M, Abrahamowicz M, Primeau F, Belzile E. Delirium predicts 12-month mortality. Arch Intern Med 2002; 162:457–463.
60. Breitbart W, Gibson C, Tremblay A. The delirium experience: delirium recall and delirium-related distress in hospitalized patients with cancer, their spouses/caregivers, and their nurses. Psychosomatics 2002;43:183–194.
61. Laitinen H. Patients' experience of confusion in the intensive care unit following cardiac surgery. Intensive Crit Care Nurs 1996;12:79–83.
62. Schofield I. A small exploratory study of the reaction of older people to an episode of delirium. J Adv Nurs 1997;25:942–952.
63. Schuurmans MJ, Duursma SA, Shortridge-Baggett LM. Early recognition of delirium: review of the literature. J Clin Nurs 2001;10:721–729.
64. Morency CR, Levkoff SE, Dick KL. Research considerations: delirium in hospitalized elders. J Gerontological Nurs 1994;20:24–30.
65. Souder E, O'Sullivan PS. Nursing documentation versus standardized assessment of cognitive status in hospitalized medical patients. Appl Nurs Res 2000;13:29–36.
66. Lacko L, Bryan Y, Dellasega C, Salerno F. Changing clinical practice through research: the case of delirium. Clin Nurs Res 1999; 8:235–250.
67. Tune LE. Delirium. In: Coffey CE, Cummings JL, eds. Textbook of Geriatric Neuropsychiatry. Washington, DC: American Psychiatric Press, Inc., 2000:441–452.
68. Anonymous. Practice guideline for the treatment of patients with delirium. Am J Psychiatry 1999;156:1–20.
69. Miller J, Neelon V, Champagne M, et al. The assessment of acute confusion as part of nursing care. Appl Nurs Res 1997;10:143–151.
70. Camus V, Burtin B, Simeone I, Schwed P, Gonthier R, Dubos G. Factor analysis supports the evidence of existing hyperactive and hypoactive subtypes of delirium. Int J Geriatric Psychiatry 2000; 15:313–316.
71. Meagher DJ, Trzepacz PT. Motoric subtypes of delirium. Semin Clin Neuropsychiatry 2000;5:75–85.
72. Ross CA, Peyser CE, Shapiro I, Folstein MF. Delirium: phenomenologic and etiologic subtypes. Int Psychogeriatr 1991;3:135–147.
73. Milisen K, Foreman MD, Godderis J, Abraham IL, Broos PL. Delirium in the hospitalized elderly: nursing assessment and management. Nurs Clin North Am 1998;33:417–439.
74. Cole M, McCusker J, Dendukuri N, Han L. The prognostic significance of subsyndromal delirium in elderly medical inpatients. J Ame Geriatrics Soc 2003; 51:754–760.
75. Fick DM, Agostini JV, Inouye SK. Delirium superimposed on dementia: a systematic review. J Am Geriatrics Soc 2002;50: 1723–1732.

76. Rockwood K, Cosway S, Carver D, Jarrett P, Stadnyk K, Fisk J. The risk of dementia and death after delirium. Age Ageing 1999; 28:551–556.
77. Cole MG, McCusker J, Dendukuri N, Han L. Symptoms of delirium among elderly medical inpatients with or without dementia. J Neuropsychiatry Clin Neurosciences 2002;14:167–175.
78. Rapp C, Wakefield B, Kundrat M, Mentes J, Tripp-Reimer T, et al. Acute confusion assessment instruments: clinical versus research usability. Appl Nurs Res200;13:37–45.
79. Schuurmans M, Deschamps P, Markham S, Shortridge-Baggett L, et al. Measurement of delirium: review of scales. Res Theory Nurs Pract 2003;17:207–224.
80. Stillman M, Rybicki L. The bedside confusion scale: development of a portable bedside test for confusion and its application to the palliative medicine population. J Palliat Med 2000; 3:449–456.
81. Caraceni A. Delirium in palliative medicine. Eur J Palliat Care 1995;2:62–67.
82. Sarhill N, Walsh D, Nelson K, LeGrand S, Davis M. Assessment of delirium in advanced cancer: the use of the bedside confusion scale. Am J Hospice Palliative Care 2001;18:335–341.
83. Kuebler KK. Hospice and Palliative Care Clinical Practice Protocol: Terminal Restlessness. Pittsburgh: Hospice and Palliative Nurses Association, 1997.
84. de Stoutz N, Tapper M, Fainsinger R. Reversible delirium in terminally ill patients. J Pain Symptom Manage 1995;10:249–253.
85. Folestein M, Folstein S, McHugh P. Mini-mental state: a practical method for grading the cognitive status of patients for the clinician. J Psychiatr Res 1975;12:189–193.
86. Armstrong-Esther C, Browne K. The influence of elderly patients' mental impairment on nurse–patient interactions. J Adv Nurs 1986;11:379–387.
87. Inouye SK, Bogardus S, Charpentier P, et al. A multicomponent intervention to prevent delirium in hospitalized older patients. N Engl J Med 1999;340:669–676.
88. de Stoutz N, Stiefel F. Assessment and management of reversible delirium. In: Portenoy R, Bruera E, eds. Topics in Palliative Care. New York: Oxford University Press, 1997:21–43.
89. Smith M, Brietbart W, Platt W. A critique of instruments and methods to detect, diagnose and rate delirium. J Pain Symptom Manage 1995;10:35–70.
90. Kemp C. Neurological problems and interventions. In: Terminal Illness Guide to Nursing Care. Philadelphia: JB Lippincott, 1995; 149–153.
91. Kaasa T, Loomis J, Gills K, Bruera E, Hanson J. The Edmonton functional assessment tool: preliminary development and evaluation for use in palliative care. J Pain Symptom Manage 1997; 13:10–17.
92. Trzepacz P. Cognitive Disturbances Basic Perspectives: Symptoms in Terminal Illness: A Research Workshop. Rockville, MD: National Institutes of Health, September 22–23,1997, http://ninr.nih.gov/ninr/wnew/symptoms_in_terminal_illness.html (accessed March 8, 2005).
93. Inouye S, Viscoli C, Horwitz R, Hurst L, Tinetti M. A predictive model for delirium in hospitalized elderly medical patients and evaluation for use in palliative care. Ann Intern Med 1993;119: 474–481.
94. Csokasy J. Assessment of acute confusion: use of the NEECHAM Confusion Scale. Appl Nurs Res 1999;12:51–55.
95. Bennett JA. Dehydration: hazards and benefits. Geriatr Nurs 2000;21:84–88.
96. Fainsinger RL, Bruera E. When to treat dehydration in a terminally ill patient? Support Care Cancer 1997;5:205–211.
97. Bruera E, MacDonald N. To hydrate or not to hydrate: how should it be? J Clin Oncolog 2000; 18:1156–1158.
98. Sharill N, Walsh D, Nelson K, Davis M. Evaluation and treatment of cancer-related fluid deficits: volume depletion and dehydration. Supp Care Cancer 2001;9:408–419.
99. Huffman JL, Dunn GP. The paradox of hydration in advanced terminal illness. J Am Coll Surgeons 2002;194:835–839.
100. Zerwekh JV. Do dying patients really need IV fluids? Am J Nurs 1997;97:Nurse Pract Extra Ed:26–31.
101. Steiner N, Bruera E. Methods of hydration in palliative care patients. J Palliat Care 1998;14:6–13.
102. Ellershaw JE, Sutcliffe JM, Saunders CM. Dehydration and the dying patient. J Pain Symptom Manage 1995;10:192–197.
103. McCann RM, Hall WJ, Groth-Juncker A. Comfort care for terminally ill patients. The appropriate use of nutrition and hydration. JAMA 1994;272:1263–1266.
104. Vullo-Navich K, Smith S, Andrews M, Levine AM, Tischler JF, Veglia JM. Comfort and incidence of abnormal serum sodium, BUN, creatinine and osmolality in dehydration of terminal illness. Am J Hospice Palliative Care 1998;15:77–84.
105. Burge FI. Dehydration symptoms of palliative care cancer patients. J Pain Symptom Manag 1993;8:454–464.
106. Morita T, You T, Tsunoda J, Inoue S, Chihara S. Underlying pathologies and their associations with clinical features in terminal delirium of cancer patients. J Pain Symptom Manage 2001;22: 997–1006.
107. Cerchietti L, Navigante A, Sauri A, Palazzo F. Clinical trial. Hypodermoclyisis for control of dehydration in terminal-stage cancer. Int J Palliative Nurs 2000;6:370–374.
108. Viola RA, Wells GA, Peterson J. The effects of fluid status and fluid therapy on the dying: a systematic review, J Palliative Care 1997;13:41–52.
109. American Psychiatric Association. Practice guideline for the treatment of patients with delirium. Am J Psychiatry 1999;156(Suppl 5):1–20.
110. Schwartz T, Masand P. The role of atypical antipsychotics in the treatment of delirium. Psychsomatics 2002;43:171–173.
111. Carnes M, Howell T, Rosenberg M, Francis J, et al. Physicians vary in approaches to the clinical management of delirium. J Am Geriatr Soc 2003;51:234–239.
112. Gray S, Lai K, Larson E. Drug-induced cognitive disorders in the elderly: incidence, prevention and management. Drug Safety 1999;21:101–122.
113. Olshaker J, Flanigan J. Flumazenil reversal of lorazepam-induced acute delirium. J Emerg Med 2003; 24:181–183.
114. Caraceni A, Grassi L. (eds). Acute confusional states in palliative medicine. Oxford: Oxford University Press, 2003:172–179.
115. Ravona-Springer R, Dolberg O, Hirschmann S, Grunhaus L. Delirium in elderly patients treated with risperidone: a report of three cases. J Clin Psycopharmacol 1998;18:171–172.
116. Passik S, Cooper M. Complicated delirium in a cancer patient successfully treated with olanzapine. J Pain Symptom Manage 1999;17:219–223.
117. Sipahimalani A, Massand P. Olanzapine in the treatment of delirium. Psychosomatics 1998;39:422–430.
118. Gagnon B, Bielech M, Watanabe S, Walker P. et al. The use of intermittent subcutaneous injections of oxycodone for opioid rotation in patients with cancer pain. Support Cancer Care 1999;7:265–270.

119. Bernard S, Bruera E. Drug interactions in palliative care. J Clin Oncol 2000;18:1780–1799.
120. Furst C, Doyle D. The terminal phase. In: Doyle D, Hanks G, Cherny N, Calman K, eds. Oxford Textbook of Palliative Medicine, 3rd ed. Oxford: Oxford University Press, 2004:1117–1134.
121. Boyle-McCaffery D, Abernathy G, Baker L, Wall A. End-of-life confusion in patients with cancer. Oncol Nurs Forum 1998; 25:1335–1343.
122. Shuster J. Delirium. Confusion and agitation at the end-of-life. J Palliat Med 1998;1:177–185.
123. Callahan C, Kelly P. Final Gifts. New York: Poseidon Press, 1992:67–71.
124. Macleod A. The management of delirium in hospice practice. Eur J Palliat Care 1997;4:116–120.
125. Byock I. Dying well: the prospect for growth at the end of life. New York: Riverhead Books, 1997: 43–45.
126. Fox M, Sheldrake R. The Physics of Angels: Exploring the Realm Where Science and Spirit Meet. San Francisco: Harper Collins, 1996:184 .
127. Vickers A. Complementary therapies in palliative care. Eur J Palliat Care 1996;3:150–153.
128. Fanslow-Brunjes C. Therapeutic touch: compassion for dying persons and their families. Lecture Presentation, Annual Conference of Nurse Healers–Professional Associates Annual Conference, Wichita, KS, October 15, 1988.
129. Inoute SK. The dilemma of delirium: clinical and research controversies regarding controversies regarding diagnosis and evaluation of delirium in hospitalized elderly medical patients. Am J Med 1994; 97:278–288.
130. Stiefel F, Fainsinger R, Bruera E. Acute confusional states in patients with advanced cancer. J Pain Symptom Manage 1992; 7:94–98.

21

Margaret Anne Lamb

Sexuality

My husband and I have been married for over 50 years. When I was diagnosed with ovarian cancer 9 months ago, it was devastating for both of us. The nights I spent in the hospital after my exploratory surgery were some of the roughest times in my life. Before then, I could count on one hand how many nights since our marriage we had not spent together in the same bed. Now it seems that number is growing exponentially. I wish we could have some time alone together. Now that the doctors have said the chemotherapy isn't working, there seems to be a steady stream of people through our house, both night and day. Our three grown children live in the area and often drop by to see us. Along with them come their spouses and grandchildren. Hospice has started paying daily visits, and friends and neighbors come by often. I long for just a little privacy with my husband. Just to hold each other, maybe snuggle and kiss or even just fall asleep in each other's arms would mean the world to me.—A patient with end-stage ovarian cancer

- ***Key Points***
- *Sexuality is an integral part of the human experience. It can relieve suffering and diminish the threat to identity that facing a terminal illness often causes.*
- *Health care providers often overlook the sexual needs of those receiving palliative care.*
- *Communication, privacy, and practical solutions to physical impediments to sexual functioning can foster sexual health within the realm of terminal illness.*

Sexuality is a basic aspect of human life, seen by many as fundamental to "being human." It is a complex phenomenon that basically comprises the greatest intimacy between two humans. The ability to give and to receive physical love is very important for many individuals, even through the trajectory of an incurable illness.[1,2] The ability to maintain close sexual relations can be viewed as maintaining an essential part of one's "self." Sexuality can affirm love, relieve stress and anxiety, and distract one from the emotional and physical sequelae of an eventually terminal chronic illness. Sexual expression can foster hope and accentuate spirituality. Health care providers in all clinical settings where palliative care is provided can be pivotal in facilitating the expression of sexuality in the terminal stages of life. Holistic palliative care throughout the trajectory of an incurable illness should include the promotion of sexual expression and assistance in preventing or minimizing the negative effects of an illness's progression on a couple's intimacy. Sexual partners' caring can comfortably include sexual expression if both parties are interested and able.

Importance of Physical Intimacy

The patient and family are at the center of palliative care. A patient's desire for and interest in maintaining sexual relations is highly variable. Some may find expression of physical love an important aspect of their life right up to death, while others may relinquish their "sexual being" early in their end-of-life trajectory. Each individual's identity is influenced, in part, by his or her sexual identity. Roles between spouses or sexual partners are additionally defined by the sexual intimacy between them.

Sexual integrity can be both altered and compromised during the course of an incurable disease, deleteriously affecting both the identity and the role fulfillment of the affected persons. Health care providers should not make assumptions about the level of interest or capacity a couple has for physical intimacy.

Sexuality goes far beyond "sexual intercourse." Sexuality may encompass physical touch of any kind, as well as experiences of warmth, tenderness, and the expression of love. The importance of physical intimacy vacillates throughout a relationship and may be diminished or rekindled by a superimposed illness. Long-term palliative care providers may see sexual desire and expression ebb and flow between a couple throughout the course of care. The patient may view sexual expression as an affirmation of life, a part of being human, a means to maintain role relationships, or the expression of passion in and for life itself. Some patients may view sexual expression as an essential aspect of their being, while others may see it as ancillary or unimportant. Some patients may enter palliative care with an established sexual partner; some may lose a partner during this period through separation, divorce, or widowhood; and others may begin a relationship during this time. Some patients may have several sexual partners; some couples may be gay or lesbian; while others, without a sexual partner, may gain pleasure by erotic thoughts and masturbation. All of these scenarios are within the realm of the palliative care provider's patient base. Understanding the various forms of sexual expression and pleasure is paramount in providing comprehensive care.

A sexual partner's interest and ability to maintain sexual relations throughout the palliative care trajectory can also be affected by many variables. Sexual expression may be impeded by the partner's mood state (anxiety, depression, grief, or guilt), exhaustion from caregiving and assuming multiple family roles, and misconceptions about sexual appropriateness during palliative care. Anxiety and depression have profound effects on sexual functioning. Decreases in libido and sexual activity result from depressive and anxious states.[3] A partner may feel that the patient is "too ill" to engage in sexual activity. In turn, the partner may feel remorse or guilt for even thinking about their loved one in a sexual capacity during this time. Partners may fear that they may injure their loved one during sexual activity due to their perceived or actual weakened state or appearance. Furthermore, a partner may have difficulty adjusting to the altered physical appearance of the patient (cachexia, alopecia, stomatitis, pallor, amputation, etc.). The role of caregiver may seem incompatible with that of sexual partner. As the ill partner's health deteriorates, the well partner may assume caretaking roles that may seem incompatible with those of a lover. Furthermore, the myriad of responsibilities sequentially assumed by the well partner may leave him or her exhausted. This can impede sexual interest and performance. Finally, the partner may harbor misconceptions about sexual relations with a terminally ill partner, including diminishing the patient's waning energy reserves or causing the illness to progress more rapidly.

Cultural issues may also play a part in the couple's willingness or interest in maintaining sexual intimacy during palliative care. In Part IX of this book, the international perspective of palliative care is addressed. There exists tremendous diversity among cultural, religious, and spiritual beliefs in relation to sexual intimacy and death.[4] Culture often guides interactions between people, even the mores within sexual interactions. Culturally competent health care providers should take into consideration the effect of culture on sexual expression between a couple during palliative care. For example, does the couple possess the same cultural identity? If not, are their identities similar in respect to beliefs about intimacy? What are the couple's health, illness, and sexual beliefs and practices? What are their customs and beliefs about intimacy, illness, and death? Issues such as personal space, eye contact, touch, and permissible topics to discuss with health care providers and/or members of the opposite sex may influence one's ability to intercede within the realm of intimate relations. A cultural assessment is key to determining if these factors are an issue. Variations in sexual orientation must also be considered within the area of cultural competence. The beliefs, actions, and normative actions of homosexual and bisexual couples are important considerations when providing palliative care to a couple with alternate sexual expression.[5–7] Gay and lesbian couples may be offended by the assumption that they are heterosexual. An example demonstrating the need for acknowledging and respecting individual sexuality follows:

CASE STUDY

A 67-Year-Old Man with Prostate Cancer

A 67-year-old man dying of prostate cancer once stated, "I am gay but I was married years ago and have three grown children. I have maintained a close supportive relationship with my ex-wife and children. However, for the past 17 years I've been in a homosexual relationship with Todd. We are very close emotionally, spiritually, and physically. We have been very forthright about our sexual orientation with our family and friends, but it is difficult when I'm admitted to the hospital. Both my ex-wife and my partner visit me regularly. The staff acknowledge my ex-wife but seem to think Todd is my business partner because I first introduced him as 'my partner.' From the onset, this was an embarassing assumption on their part, and one I felt awkward in correcting. I have Todd accompany me more often than my ex-wife, but they see him as a friend who gives me rides. I know I should just come right out and explain the nature of my relationship; the problem is, I see so many different providers. I feel like I would have to keep going over this again and again. I don't want to be put in this position repeatedly. Todd is very frustrated by this misunderstanding, and I hate to see him upset. It is difficult enough to be going through the terminal cancer experience without adding another layer of embarrassment and confusion."

Developmental issues also play a part in the patient's ability to maintain intimacy during palliative care. Often, health care providers assume sexual abstinence in the elderly and, to some degree, in adolescents and unmarried young adults. However, intimacy may be a vital part of these individuals' lives.[8] Chronological age may or may not be a determination of sexual activity. For underage patients, parental influence may interfere with the ability to express physical love. Likewise, the elderly may be inhibited by perceived societal values and judgments about their sexuality. Maintaining an open, nonjudgmental approach to patients of all ages, sexual orientations, and marital status when inquiring about intimacy aspects will foster trust and communication.

Privacy

One of the main external obstacles to maintaining intimate relations during palliative care is the lack of privacy. In Part VI of this book, the various settings in which end-of-life care may take place and the concomitant issues raised within each setting are addressed. In the acute care setting, privacy is often difficult to achieve. However, this obstacle can be removed or minimized by recognizing the need for intimacy and making arrangements to ensure quiet, uninterrupted time for couples. Private rooms are, of course, ideal. However, if this is not possible, arranging for roommates and visitors to leave for periods of time is necessary. Furthermore, a sign should be posted on the door that alerts health care providers, staff, and visitors that privacy is required. Finally, many rooms in the acute care setting have windows as opposed to walls, requiring the use of blinds and/or curtains to assure privacy. The nurse should offer such strategies rather than expecting patients to suggest privacy measures.

Similar issues may arise in the long-term care environment. If privacy is a scarce commodity, assisting couples to maintain intimate relations as desired is crucial in providing holistic care. Nurses in long-term care can initiate strategies similar to those enumerated for the acute care setting. Furthermore, this issue may be even more paramount to the patient because often the stay in long-term care is quite extended. In both the acute care and long-term care settings, nurses can play a vital role in setting policy to allow for the expression of intimacy.

Home care may present an array of different obstacles for maintaining intimate relations. The ongoing presence of a health care provider other than the sexual partner is such an obstacle. Furthermore, the home setting is often interrupted by professional visits as well as visits from family, friends, and clergy. These visits may be unplanned or unannounced. The telephone itself may be an unwelcome interruption. Furthermore, the patient may have been moved from a more private, bedroom setting to a more convenient central location, such as a den or family room, to aid care giving and to maintain an integral role in family life. However, this move does not foster the privacy usually sought for intimate activity. There may not be a door to close. Alternately, proximity of the patient's bed to the main rooms of the house may inhibit a couple's intimate activities. Negotiating for private time is often necessary. Necessary steps to maintaining sexual relations include scheduling "rest periods" when one will not be disturbed; turning the ringer on the phone off; asking health care providers, friends, and clergy to call before visiting; and having family members allow periods of uninterrupted time.

CASE STUDY

A 26-Year-Old Woman with Hodgkin's Disease

"I am a single woman but have been in a serious relationship for the past 2 years. My boyfriend has been very understanding and supportive during my diagnosis and treatment for Hodgkin's disease. Sex is a very important part of our relationship. We have lived together for the past year. I was admitted to the hospital several days ago. The nurses, doctors, and others come and go all day long. I wanted a private room but really couldn't afford the extra expense. One night, just before visiting hours were over, we decided to try to have a 'quickie.' We thought my roommate was asleep and tried to be very quiet. We pulled the curtains around the bed and turned off the lights. All of a sudden, the light went on and the curtain was pulled back. Come to find out my roommate heard the noise I was making and thought I was having difficulty breathing. She had put on her call light for the nurse. We were so embarrassed. My boyfriend left quickly and I'm afraid I won't see him again. I think this is just too much for a 28-year-old guy."

Sexual Assessment

The promotion or restoration of sexual health begins with a sexual assessment. The assessment should include the patient as well as his or her partner. Securing permission to include the sexual partner is necessary. For the nurse to perform this assessment, she or he must be comfortable with the topic of sexuality. Comfort with one's sexuality conveys comfort to others. Additionally, the nurse's values, beliefs, and attitudes regarding sexuality greatly influence the capacity to discuss these issues in a nonjudgmental way. Perceived insufficient knowledge on the part of the health care provider is often an obstacle to frank sexual discussions. Additional sexual education and consistent assessment and counseling approaches will allay this discomfort. Education can be gained informally via discussions with colleagues and through consultation with experts in the area of human sexuality. Formal training is gained through in-service education offerings, workshops, and sexual-attitude reassessment programs. Knowledge can also be fostered by keeping abreast of new developments within the field by attending conferences and reviewing journals and professional information via the Internet.

Assessment of sexuality begins with a sexual history and is then supplemented by data regarding the patient and partner's physical health as it influences intimacy, psychological sequelae of the chronic illness, sociocultural influences, and possible environmental issues. Since sexual health is viewed as a relative matter, it is essential to determine if the couple is satisfied with their current level of sexual functioning. Celibacy, for example, may have been present in the relationship for years. However, the trajectory of palliative care may have forced celibacy on an otherwise sexually active couple. Determining the couple's need for interventions and assistance in this area is key. The health care provider has many interventions available to prevent or minimize the untoward effects that palliative care may impose on intimacy.

Obtaining a sexual history and performing a subsequent sexual assessment can be augmented using several communication techniques—assuring privacy and confidentiality; allowing for ample, uninterrupted time; and maintaining a nonjudgmental attitude. Addressing the topic of sexuality early in the relationship with a palliative care patient legitimizes the issue of intimacy. It delivers the message that this is an appropriate topic for concern within the professional relationship, and is often met with relief on the part of the patient and couple. Often, sexuality concerns are present but unvoiced.

Incorporating several techniques of therapeutic communication enhances the interview. These techniques include asking open-ended questions ("Some people who have an incurable illness are frustrated by their lack of private time with their spouse/sexual partner. How is this experience for you?"); using questions that refer to frequency as opposed to occurrence ("How often do you have intimate relations with your wife/husband/partner?" as opposed to "Do you have intimate relations with your wife/husband/partner?"); and "unloading" the question ("Some couples enjoy oral sex on a regular basis, while others seldom or never have oral sex. How often do you engage in oral sex?"). This last technique legitimizes the activity and allows the patient to feel safe in responding to the question in a variety of ways.

Gender and age may also play a part in the patient's comfort with sexual discussions. An adolescent boy may feel more comfortable discussing sexual concerns with a male health care provider, whereas an elderly woman may prefer to discuss sexual issues with a woman closer to her own age. Assessment of these factors may include statements like the following: "Many young men have questions about sexuality and the effect their illness may have on sexual functioning. This is something we can discuss or, if you'd be more comfortable, I could have one of the male nurses talk to you about this. Which would you prefer?"

If the sexual history reveals a specific sexual problem, a more in-depth assessment is warranted. This would include the onset and course of the problem, the patient's or couple's thoughts about what caused the problem, any solutions that have been attempted, and potential solutions and their acceptability to the patient/couple. For example, use of a vibrator in the case of male impotence may be entirely acceptable to some couples but abhorrent to others. Determining what is and is not acceptable regarding potential solutions is part of the logical next step in sexual assessment.

Finally, documentation in the patient's chart should reflect the findings of the sexual assessment. Many institutions have a section for sexual assessment embedded within their intake form. This can be completed and more thorough notes added to the narrative section on the chart. Findings, suggestions for remediation, and desired outcomes should be documented. This will prevent duplication of efforts, communication within the health care team, and continuity of care within the realm of sexual health.

Interventions to Augment Sexual Health in End-of-Life Care

The specific sexual needs and concerns of the patient and couple determine the approach and type of intervention. The intervention can address current needs or focus on potential future needs in the form of anticipatory guidance. Although dated, the P-LI-SS-IT model developed by Annon[9] remains a cornerstone in sexual rehabilitation. The assessment phase, previously outlined, comprises the "P," or permission, phase of this intervention model. Permission simply refers to the openness about discussing sexual concerns. In assessing sexual health, the health care provider has begun intervening in the realm of sexuality. By initiating a discussion about the effects that palliative care may have on an individual's or couple's intimate relations, one legitimizes these concerns.

Limited information regarding actual or potential problems is addressed once the assessment phase of the intervention is complete. This is the "LI" of the acronym. Specific information and suggestions can then be given to assist the patient or couple with adapting to changes in intimacy brought on by incurable illness or end-of-life care. Questions can be answered, what is normal can be acknowledged, and myths and misconceptions can be dispelled. False assumptions about intimacy during palliative care can be addressed, and anticipatory guidance regarding what to expect as a result of advancing disease and palliative treatment is included in this discussion.

Specific suggestions (SS) go beyond limited information, and counseling is employed to rectify specific problems or to attain a mutually stated goal. A stated goal is key to this phase because the resultant plan will aim at attaining that outcome. Specific suggestions usually pertain to communication, symptom management, and alternate physical expression. Fostering open communication between the couple about sexuality in end-of-life care is essential. Candid discussions regarding their emotional response to this phase of their relationship, their fears and concerns, and their hopes and desires are included in these interactions. Symptom management is essential to optimizing sexual expression. The following section of this chapter addresses specific symptoms, their effect on the expression of intimacy, and strategies to effectively manage them while not compounding sexual problems. Alternate expressions of physical intimacy may be necessary if sexual disruption is due to organic changes. If intercourse is difficult, painful, or impossible, the couple may have to expand their sexual repertoire. A thorough discussion of the couple's values, attitudes, and preferences should be done before suggesting alternatives. Using language that is understandable to the patient/partner is essential. However, the use of slang or street language may be unacceptable to the health care provider. Therefore, defining terms early in the discussion will alleviate this potential problem.

There are many ways of giving and receiving sexual pleasure—genital intercourse is only one way of expressing physical love. Other suggestions include hugging, massage, fondling, caressing, cuddling, kissing, hand-holding, and masturbation, either mutually or singularly. Sexual gratification may be derived from manual, oral, and digital stimulation. Intrathigh, anal, and intramammary intercourse are also options if the female partner is unable to continue vaginal penetration.

Intensive therapy (IT), the last stage of this model, is not usually suggested in end-of-life care. This therapy is generally for couples who have long-standing sexual or marital problems. The feasibility of this type of therapy during palliative care for a terminal illness is questionable.

Management of Alterations in Sexual Functioning During End-of-Life Care

Terminal illness and end-of-life care can interfere with sexual functioning in many ways. All of the following can impact sexual functioning: physiological changes; tissue damage; other organic manifestations of the disease; attempts to palliate the symptoms of advancing disease, such as fatigue, pain, nausea and vomiting; and psychological sequelae such as anxiety, depression, and body-image changes. Environmental issues that may affect sexual expression were addressed in the previous section. Management of the patient's biological and psychological sequelae is addressed below.

Fatigue

Fatigue may be due to an array of factors. In Chapter 7, the etiology and management of fatigue were thoroughly addressed. Fatigue may render a patient unable to perform sexually. If fatigue is identified as a factor in the patient's ability to initiate or maintain sexual arousal, several strategies may be suggested to diminish these untoward effects. Minimizing exertion during intimate relations may be necessary. Providing time for rest before and after sexual relations is often a sufficient strategy to overcome the detrimental effects of fatigue. Likewise, avoiding the stress of a heavy meal, alcohol consumption, or extremes in temperature may be helpful. Experimenting with positions that require minimal patient exertion (male-patient, female astride; female-patient, male astride) is often helpful. Finally, timing should be taken into consideration. Sexual activity in the morning upon awakening may be preferable over relations at the end of a long day. Planning for intimate time rather than spontaneity can be a beneficial strategy.

Pain

Sexual arousal and performance are often impaired by the presence of pain. Additionally, the use of pain medication (especially opiates) can interfere with sexual arousal.[10] In Chapters 5 and 6, the issues of pain assessment and management are discussed in a comprehensive manner. The goal of pain therapy is to alleviate or minimize discomfort. However, in attaining that goal, sexual responsiveness (i.e., libido or erectile function) may be hindered. Temporarily adjusting pain medications or experimenting with complementary methods of pain management should be explored. For example, using relaxation techniques before intimacy may be helpful. Romantic music may decrease discomfort through distraction and relaxation, while enhancing sexual interest. Sexual activity itself can be viewed as a form of distraction and subsequent relaxation. The couple should be encouraged to explore positions that offer the most comfort. Traditional positions may be abandoned for more comfortable ones, such as sitting in a chair or a side-lying position. Pillows can be used to support painful limbs or to maintain certain positions. A warm bath or shower before sexual activity may help pain relief and be seen as preparatory to intimate relations. Massage can be used as both an arousal technique and a therapeutic strategy for minimizing discomfort. Finally, suggesting the exploration of alternate ways of expressing tenderness and sexual gratification may be necessary if the couple's traditional intimacy repertoire is not feasible due to discomfort.

Nausea and Vomiting

Nausea and vomiting are common during the palliative care trajectory and negatively impact sexual functioning. Chapter 9 discusses the etiology and treatment of these symptoms. There are many medications that suppress nausea; however, they may interfere with sexual functioning due to their sedative effects.[10] If the patient complains of sexual difficulties secondary to treatment for nausea and vomiting, an assessment of the prescribed antiemetics may shed light on a pharmacological culprit. Using alternate nonpharmacological methods to control nausea and vomiting or changing to another antiemetic may be warranted. Such strategies include eating small and frequent meals, serving foods at room temperature, avoiding spicy foods, assuring a well-ventilated dining area, and using relaxation and distraction techniques. Providing fresh air through an open window in the bedroom, for example, may decrease noxious olfactory stimuli. As with fatigue, timing may be an important consideration for intimate relations. If the patient/couple notes that nausea is more prevalent during a certain time of the day, planning for intimacy at alternate times may circumvent this problem.

Neutropenia and Thrombocytopenia

Neutropenia and thrombocytopenia, per se, do not necessarily interfere with intimacy, but they do pose some potential problems. Sexual intimacy during neutropenic phases may jeopardize the compromised patient. Severe neutropenia predisposes a patient to infection. Close physical contact may be inadvisable if the sexual partner has a communicable disease, such as an upper respiratory infection or influenza. Specific sexual practices, such as anal intercourse, are prohibited during neutropenic states due to the likelihood of subsequent infection. The absolute neutrophil count, if available, is a good indicator of neutropenic status and associated risk for infection. Patient and partner education about the risks associated with neutropenia is essential.

Thrombocytopenia and the associated risk of bleeding, bruising, or hemorrhage should be considered when counseling a couple about intimacy issues. Again, anal intercourse is contraindicated due to risk for bleeding. Likewise, vigorous genital intercourse may cause vaginal bleeding. Indeed, even forceful or energetic hugging, massage, or kissing may cause bruising or bleeding. Preventative suggestions might include such strategies as gentle lovemaking, with minimal pressure on the thrombocytopenic patient, or having the patient assume the dominant position to control force and pressure.

Dyspnea

Dyspnea is an extremely distressing occurrence in the end-of-life trajectory. In Chapter 13, the management of this symptom is reviewed. Dyspnea, or even the fear of initiating dyspnea, can impair sexual functioning. General strategies can be employed to minimize dyspnea during sexual play. These can include using a waterbed to accentuate physical movements, raising the dyspneic patient's head and shoulders to facilitate oxygenation, using supplementary oxygen and/or inhalers before and during sexual activity, performing pulmonary hygiene measures before intimacy, encouraging slower movements to conserve energy, and modifying sexual activity to allow for enjoyment and respiratory comfort.

Neuropathies

Neuropathies can be a result of disease progression or complication of prior aggressive treatment. Neuromuscular disturbances are discussed in depth in Chapter 18. Neuropathies can manifest as pain, paresthesia, and/or weakness. Depending on the location and severity of the neuropathy, sexual functioning can be altered or completely suppressed. Management or diminution of the neuropathy may or may not be feasible. If not, creative ways to evade the negative sequelae of this occurrence are necessary. Such strategies might include creative positioning, use of pillows to support affected body parts, or alternate ways of expressing physical love. The distraction of intimacy may temporarily minimize the perception of the neuropathy.

Mobility and Range of Motion

Mobility issues and compromised range of motion may interfere with sexual expression. Similar to issues related to fatigue, a decrease in mobility can inhibit a couple's customary means of expressing physical love. A compromise in range of motion can result in a similar dilemma. For example, a female patient may no longer be able to position herself in such a way as to allow penile penetration from above due to hip or back restrictions. Likewise, a male patient may have knee or back restrictions that make it impossible for him to be astride his partner. Regardless of the exact nature of the range-of-motion/mobility concern, several suggestions can be offered. Experimenting with alternate positions, employing relaxation techniques before sexual play, massage, warm baths, and exploring acceptable alternative methods of expressing physical intimacy should be encouraged.

Erectile Dysfunction

Erectile dysfunction can be caused by physiological, psychological, and emotional factors. These factors include vascular, endocrine, and neurological causes; chronic diseases, such as renal failure and diabetes; and iatrogenic factors, such as surgery and medications. Surgical severing of the small nerve branches essential for erection is often the untoward effect of radical pelvic surgery, radical prostatectomy, and aortoiliac surgery.[11–13] Vascular and neurological causes may not be reversible; however, endocrine causes may be minimized. For example, the use of estrogen in advanced prostate cancer may be terminated in palliative care, thus allowing for the return of erectile function. Many medications decrease desire and erectile capacity in men. The most common offenders are antihypertensives, antidepressants, antihistamines, antispasmodics, sedatives or tranquilizers, barbiturates, sex hormone preparations, narcotics, and psychoactive drugs.[10–12] Often, these medications cannot be discontinued to permit the return of erectile function. For those patients, penile implants may be possible. The use of sildenafil (Viagra), vardenafil HCl (Levitra), tadalafil (Cialis), and yohimbine (Yohimbine) have not been researched in the area of terminal care. These medications are classified as selective enzyme inhibitors. They relax smooth muscle, increase blood flow, and facilitate erection.[10] If a vascular component is part of the underlying erectile dysfunction, the use of one of these medications may correct the problem. Certainly, contraindications such as underlying heart disease and other current medications should be taken into consideration. Otherwise, digital or oral stimulation of the female partner may be suggested as well as use of a vibrator, if that is acceptable.

Dyspareunia

Dyspareunia, like erectile dysfunction, can be caused by physiological, psychological, and emotional factors. These factors include vascular, endocrine, and neurological causes as well as iatrogenic factors such as surgery and medications.[11,12,14,15] Again, while vascular and neurological causes may not be reversible, endocrine causes may be minimized. For example, the use of estrogen replacement therapy (ERT), vaginal estrogen creams, or water-soluble lubricants may be helpful in diminishing vaginal dryness, which can cause painful intercourse. Gynecological surgery and pelvic irradiation may result in physiological changes that prevent comfortable intercourse. Postirradiation changes, such as vaginal shortening, thickening, and narrowing, may result in severe dyspareunia. For women, as with male patients, many medications decrease desire and function. These drugs include antihypertensives, antidepressants, antihistamines, antispasmodics, sedatives or tranquilizers, barbiturates, sex hormone preparations, narcotics, and psychoactive drugs.[10–13] Often, these medications cannot be discontinued to permit the return of sexual function. For those patients, digital or oral stimulation of the male partner may be suggested, if acceptable. Additionally, intrathigh and intramammary penetration may be suggested to women who find vaginal intercourse too painful.

Body Image Disturbances

Sexuality is closely related to how one views oneself in the physical sense. An incurable illness and concomitant end-of-life care can alter one's physical appearance. Additionally, past treatments for disease often irrevocably alter body appearance and function. Issues such as alopecia, weight loss, cachexia, the presence of a stoma, or amputation of a body part, to name a few, can result in feelings of sexual inadequacy and/or disinterest. End-of-life care can focus on the identification and remediation of issues related to body image changes. Although an altered appearance may be permanent, counseling and behavior modification, as well as specific suggestions to minimize or mask these appearances, can improve body image to a level compatible with feelings of sexual adequacy and empowerment.

The use of a wig, scarf, or headbands can mask alopecia. Some patients, rather than try to conceal hair loss, choose to emphasize it by shaving their heads. Weight loss and cachexia can be masked through clothing and the creative use of padding. The presence of an ostomy can significantly alter body image and negatively affect sexual functioning. Specific interventions for minimizing the effect that the presence of an ostomy has on sexual functioning depend, in part, on the particular type of ostomy. Some patients are continent, while others need an appliance attached at all times. If the patient has a continent ostomy, timing sexual activity can allow for removal of the appliance and covering the stoma. If the ostomy appliance cannot be safely removed, the patient should be taught to empty the appliance before intimate relations and to use a cover or body stocking to conceal the appliance. Alternate positions may also be considered, and in the event of a leak, sexual activity can continue in the shower. The United Ostomy Association (http://www.uoa.org) publishes four patient information booklets on sexuality and the ostomate: *Sex, Courtship, and the Single Ostomate* by D.P. Binder, *Sex and the Female Ostomate* by G.L. Dickman and C.A. Livingston, *Sex and the Male Ostomate* by E. Gambrell, and *Gay and Lesbian Ostomates and Their Caregiver* by the Gay Lesbian Organization.

Anxiety and Depression

Anxiety and depression related to the incurable and terminal aspects of the disease may interfere with sexual desire and response. As two of the most common affective disorders during end-of-life care, they are thoroughly discussed in Chapter 19. Both anxiety and depression have profound effects on sexual functioning.[3] Decreases in sexual desire, libido, and activity are common sequelae of these affective disorders. However, some interventions, especially pharmacological management, can further compromise sexual functioning. A thorough assessment of the patient's psychological state and an evaluation of the medications currently prescribed for this condition may reveal the source of the problem. Anxiolytics such as lorazepam and alprazolam are commonly prescribed. Antidepressants, such as tricyclic antidepressants, selective serotonin reuptake inhibitors (SSRIs), and monoamine oxidase inhibitors, are often prescribed. All of these have the potential for interfering with sexual functioning.[10] Unfortunately, one may end up having to choose psychological comfort and compromised intimacy. Alternately, the health care provider may suggest a nonpharmacological approach to the management of these affective disorders, especially if the disorder is mild. Relaxation techniques, imagery, and biofeedback may lower anxiety to a tolerable level. Additionally, the release of sexual tension may itself resolve anxiety. If desire is maintained and function alone is compromised for male patients, the couple may explore alternate ways of pleasing each other. For female patients, use of water-soluble lubricants can offset the interference with arousal if interest remains intact. Once again, open communication between both the couple and the health care provider allows for frank discussions and the presentation of possible alternatives to expressing physical affection during palliative care.

Summary

Incurable illness and end-of-life care may result in compromising a couple's intimacy. To prevent or minimize this, health care providers should assume a leading role in the assessment and remediation of potential or identified alterations in sexual functioning. Clearly, not all couples will find intimacy a concern at this point of their life together. However, if intimacy is desired, all attempts should be made to facilitate this important aspect of life. Many find being physically close to the one they love life-affirming and comforting. As patients draw close to the end of life, they remain human and holistic. Their needs, hopes, and concerns remain as intact as all others. If those needs and hopes include maintaining intimacy with a partner, this should be included in the assessment and provision of care. The health care provider's offer of information and support can make a significant difference in a couple's ability to adjust to the changes in intimacy related to end-of-life care.

The realm of sexual functioning and intimacy during end-of-life care remains an area in which further research is warranted. Much of the information presented in this chapter resulted from clinical practice and inferences made from other, tangentially related research. Incorporating intimacy research into end-of-life care research is a natural and much-needed marriage.

REFERENCES

1. Hordern AJ, Currow DC. A patient-centered approach to sexuality in the face of life-limiting illness. Med J Aust 2003;179(Suppl 6):S8–S11.
2. Rice A. Sexuality in cancer and palliative care: effects of disease and treatment. Int J Palliative Nurs 2000;6:392–397.
3. Varcarolis E. Foundations of Psychiatric Mental Health Nursing, 4th ed. Philadelphia: WB Saunders, 2002.
4. Laqueur T. Making Sex: Body and Gender from the Greeks to Freud. Cambridge, MA: Harvard University Press, 2000.
5. Lipson JG, Dibble SL, Minarik PA. Culture and Nursing Care. San Francisco: UCSF Nursing Press, 1996.
6. Stein GL, Bonuck KA. Attitudes on end-of-life care and advance care planning in the lesbian and gay community. J Palliative Med 2001;4:173–190.
7. Saulnier CF. Deciding who to see: lesbians discuss their preferences in health and mental health care providers. Soc Work 2002;47:355–365.
8. Hajjar RR, Kamel HK. Sexuality in the nursing home: attitudes and barriers to sexual expression. J Am Med Dir Assoc 2003;3:152–156.
9. Annon JS. The Behavioral Treatment of Sexual Problems. Honolulu: Mercantile Printing, 1974.
10. Skidmore-Roth L. Mosby's 2004 Nursing Drug Reference. Philadelphia: Mosby, 2004.
11. LeMome P, Burke KM. Medical Surgical Nursing: Critical Thinking in Patient Care, 2nd ed. Menlo Park, CA: Addison-Wesley, 2000.
12. Lewis SM, Heitkemper MM, Dirksen SF (eds). Medical Surgical Nursing: Assessment and Management of Clinical Problems, 6th ed. Philadelphia: Mosby, 2003.
13. Rondorf-Klym LM. Quality of life after radical prostatectomy. Oncol Nurs Forum 2003;30:24–32.
14. Sormanti M, Kayser K. Partner support and changes in relationships during life-threatening illness: women's perspectives. J Psychosoc Oncol 2000; 18:45–66.
15. Ekwall E, Ternestedt B, Sorbe B. Important aspects of health care for women with gynecologic cancer. Oncol Nurs Forum 2003; 30:313–319.

22

Patrick J. Coyne, Laurie Lyckholm, and Thomas J. Smith

Clinical Interventions, Economic Outcomes, and Palliative Care

"Would you tell me please which way I have to go from here?"
"That depends a good deal on where you want to get to."
—Lewis Carroll, Alice's Adventures in Wonderland.

- ***Key Points***
- *The scope of nursing and nursing education has expanded to include multiple domains, many of which overlap other disciplines such as wellness, disease prevention, and health services administration.*
- *Economic outcome is an area in which nursing plays an essential role in providing efficient, cost-effective, and appropriate palliative care.*
- *Health services research regarding economic outcomes, while limited, may help create a framework for addressing how to make palliative care available to everyone in an ethical, economic, and effective manner.*

Why Are Economic Outcomes Important?

Health care spending and health care quality are major problems in the United States, with health care spending reaching $1.6 trillion, a number expected to triple in the next 10 years. In 2002, there was an annual increase of 9.3%. Drug costs and rising hospital expenses fueled much of this spending.[1] The financial costs of cancer are great both for the individual and for society as a whole. The economic burden is likely to increase as the population ages, the absolute number of people treated for cancer increases, and newer technologies and expensive treatments are adopted as standards of care.[2] Already in the year 2004, the National Institutes of Health estimated overall annual costs for cancer to be $189.8 billion, with direct medical costs totaling $69.4 million, and indirect costs from lost productivity to be $16.9 billion due to illness and $103.5 billion due to premature death.[3] Lack of health insurance and other barriers to health care prevent many Americans from receiving optimal medical care. According to the 2003 National Health Interview Survey data, nearly 27% of Americans between the ages of 18 and 24 and 20% of Americans between the ages of 25 and 44 reported not having a regular source of health care.[4] Additionally, 17% of Americans under age 65 have no health insurance, and about one third of older individuals only have Medicare coverage.[4] Nearly one third of all Medicare spending is on patients in their last year of life[5,6]; we are spending a significant amount on high-technology care for the elderly, and those funds cannot be spent on preventive services or chronic disease conditions for the same population.[7] The pressure on health care funds will increase due to heightened demands for care from an educated elderly population, more elderly long-term survivors, new and expensive technologies, new diseases, and demands for cost cutting. All health care interventions, regardless of intention, active therapy, or palliative care, are delivered at a price. Cost effectiveness of interventions must

Table 22–1
Types of Needed Health and Service Research Studies

Type of Study	Question Posed
Policy analysis	What outcomes justify treatment? Who should make those decisions?
Type of care: chemotherapy vs. best or other types of supportive care	Does chemotherapy save money compared to best supportive care when all costs are considered?
Site of service	Is home site more effective and less costly compared to hospital?
Structural and process changes in care	Can costs be reduced by changing how care is delivered, e.g., by inpatient hospice or at home?
Hospice vs. nonhospice	Does hospice improve quality of life and/or reduce costs of care?
Advance directives and do-not-resuscitate orders	Do advance directives influence medical treatment decisions and/or change costs?
Nursing ability to impact cost at end of life	Can skilled palliative care nurses effectively palliate patients and effect a savings of resources?

be continually assessed; less is not necessarily better, but whatever is spent must maximize the resources available.[8] The question of when, where, and why to use high-tech interventions falls into the middle of this debate and must be carefully explored.

Care is not optimal for all patients, and quality of palliative care must improve. The Study to Understand Prognoses and Preferences for Outcomes and Risks of Treatment (SUPPORT) showed that half of all dying patients had unnecessary pain and suffering in their final days of life while in the hospital.[9] Cleeland and colleagues found that nearly half of all patients suffer unnecessary pain, even when cared for by oncologists.[10]

The whole neglected issue of cancer care quality is now under discussion, with active efforts to improve it.[11] The relationship of volume to quality is striking[12]: (1) a significant (5% to 10%) overall survival advantage at a breast cancer specialty center versus community hospitals[13,14]; (2) better survival for testicular cancer patients treated at specialist centers[15]; (3) better survival and fewer complications for ovarian cancer surgery performed by specialist gynecological oncologists rather than general surgeons or gynecologists[16]; and (4) better survival for prostate cancer patients at high-volume centers.[17] Until the science of palliative care becomes better known, one can reasonably speculate that palliative care will improve in high-volume or specialized centers.[18]

Clearly, there is a need for additional research to address these questions of quality care. We have identified some important questions about economic outcomes and palliative care, which are listed in Tables 22–1 and 22–2.

Table 22–2
Outcomes that Justify a Medical Intervention

Justify	Do Not Justify
Improved overall survival	False hope that survival will be improved
Improved disease-free survival	
Improved quality of life	
Less toxicity	
Improved cost effectiveness	Cost alone

The Ethics of Adding Economic Outcomes

In the modern arena of health care, nonmedical concerns, such as cost control, oversight and audit, utilization review, and decreasing liability risk, have assumed a significant role. Some authorities have argued that such management tools are not inherently unethical.[19] Cost control is certainly not so, but should be considered secondary to the goal of quality care. The goals of nursing and medicine are grounded in a tradition of promoting health and providing comfort and relief of suffering in a just manner. Cost control through aggressive disease management, or "critical paths," may actually promote these goals by making more and/or better care available if we avoid the current systems that reward/pay for hi-tech interventions but fail to reimburse effective low-tech treatments.[20] An example of this discrepancy is that insurance will reimburse a patient-controlled analgesia pump but will not reimburse oral analgesics.

Cost control must be differentiated from profit motivation and entrepreneurship, which have not traditionally been considered the goals of medicine. These activities in the context of health care are unethical in that they may make medical care more expensive and difficult to access, especially for those who are socially disadvantaged. They may also create further conflicts of interest in already precarious fiduciary relationships between clinicians and their patients. A code of ethics that covers all professionals, rather than medicine alone, might be useful.[21]

Tolerance of suboptimal care is an equally important ethical issue and one that is rarely mentioned in either ethical or management studies. Studies such as SUPPORT have revealed that many aspects of end-of-life care are still suboptimal. The national dialogue about physician-assisted suicide might also indicate that end-of-life care has not been optimized, thus resulting in despair and frustration so significant as to urge dying persons to consider suicide to end their suffering. If palliative care can be improved and/or made less costly without sacrificing quality, it must be done in the service of promoting the values of beneficence, compassion, and respect for autonomy. Palliative care has emerged as a national movement, with the advent of several important initiatives (e.g., Project on Death in America, Oncology Nursing Society efforts, Education for Physicians on End-of-Life Care by the American Medical Association, established programs such as the Center to Improve Care of the Dying at George Washington University), plus the development of palliative care programs all over the world. The Healthcare Finance Administration's approval of an International Classification of Diseases-9 code for palliative care was hoped by some to indicate its significance in the health care system.[21] The economic outcomes are not known and may be difficult to measure, but regardless, the ethical impetus to correct the deficiency is critical.

Another serious ethical question is the ownership of disease-management models. Should management tools that improve care be protected or available to the general public? If a tool that improved care at a markedly lower cost were developed, one could argue that it should be made available for widespread distribution, much like polio vaccine. Another example would be an algorithm that eased dyspnea rapidly in end-stage disease, with minimal economic impact and no requirement for technology.

Some have argued that budgets should not be balanced with penalty to one group, such as the elderly or those on Medicare.[22,23] Many health care goods are rationed justly (benefit versus risk) according to age, such as transplants, coronary bypass, and hemodialysis, based on the theory of equality of opportunity according to ability to benefit from such procedures.[24] However, palliative care is different in that age does not determine whether a person stands to benefit. In this circumstance, the ethic of distributive justice supports the concept that medical and social needs dictate who stands to benefit most from palliative care.

Daniels[25] reported that "it does not seem reasonable to postulate that the medical needs of the elderly terminally ill are any less than those of younger patients, and indeed they may be greater because of multiple additional pathologies associated with aging." Sidgwick's[26] argument that each moment of life is equally valuable no matter when it occurs is most poignant in the instance of palliative care. This would also apply to extending palliative care to neonates expected to live only a short time after birth.

Patients may view benefit and toxicity in ways very different from their health care providers and from those who are well. According to a recent study, dying patients would undergo almost any treatment toxicity for a 1% chance of short-term survival, while their doctors and nurses would not; and these decisions were not changed after patients experienced the toxicity of treatment.[27] A study of palliative radiotherapy for brain tumor patients showed little survival, modest functional benefit, and a substantial decrease in intellectual function; but most patients and families would still want it.[28,29] This is a complex appraisal that needs further study.

What Is the Right Amount to Spend on Health Care?

How much to spend on health care cannot be determined without knowing the economic and cultural particulars of a country or even a health system. Blanket statements about a percentage of the gross national product (GNP) may be misleading if a comparison country spends a higher percentage on social net programs but less on direct medical care costs. Comments about health care spending as a percent of the GNP may also reflect opinions about alternative uses; for example, "We should stop spending money on defense and spend it on health care." In the United States, the amount spent on education has declined from 6% to 5% of the GNP, while the amount spent on health care (especially for the elderly) has risen from 6% to about 14%.[30] Clearly, in all countries, the entire system of health

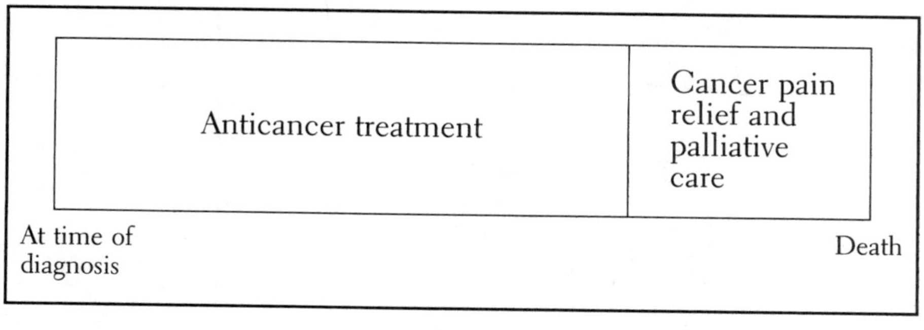

Figure 22–1. Present allocation worldwide of cancer resources. Palliative care must receive more of these resources. *Source:* World Health Organization (1990), reference 91. Reproduced by permission of WHO.

care needs to be explored with policies designed to ensure that palliative care is a component of the overall health care system (Figure 22-1).[31]

Should There Be Special Economic or Policy Considerations for Palliative Care?

We believe that, in general, there should be no special considerations for palliative care. Most health care policy analysts and economists would argue that all care should be evaluated equally. For example, a therapy that gains 1 week for 52 patients should be valued as much as a therapy of equivalent cost that gains 52 weeks for 1 patient.[32] Recently, some health economists have argued that time given to those who are most at risk should be valued more (e.g., time added in the last 6 months of life should be given triple value).[33] The analogy was made to food and hunger: a sandwich given to a starving person would be of more intrinsic value than one given to a person who already had many sandwiches. Such discussions, while interesting, are outside the scope of this chapter, but many of the ethical concepts applied to these global discussions have relevance to decisions about palliative care.

The World Health Organization (WHO) has listed priorities for health care. In cancer, palliative care has always been included in the same category as curative therapy. In part, this was done because most palliative care is relatively inexpensive. Current allocation of resources greatly favors curative care with less support for palliative care. As Figures 22–2 and 22–3 illustrate, WHO advocates a more equal distribution of resources in developed countries and an even greater support of palliative care in developing countries, where most of the population will experience advanced disease rather than cure or long-term survival.

One approach to funding treatments has been based on cost-effectiveness ratios.[34] Laupacis and colleagues[34] in Canada proposed explicit funding criteria: (1) treatments that work better and are less expensive should be adopted; (2) treatments with cost-effectiveness ratios of less than C$20,000 per additional life year (LY) gained should be accepted, with the recognition that they cost additional resources; (3) treatments with cost-effectiveness ratios of $20,000 to C$100,000/LY should be examined on a case-by-case basis with caution; (4) and treatments with cost-effectiveness ratios of greater than C$100,000/LY should be rejected. These criteria are valid in a system where all resources are shared equally; it is not clear how they apply to other health care systems, where resources may not be shared.[35] Alternatively, patients might be allowed to purchase additional insurance for expensive treatments or pay for them out of pocket. In the United States, there has been no accepted answer, but most authorities have agreed on an implicitly defined benchmark of $35,000 to $50,000/LY saved.[32] For example, an individual with a pathological fracture of a femur is sent to the operating room for pinning. This surgery will

Figure 22–2. Proposed allocation of cancer resources in developed countries. Curative and palliative care are not mutually exclusive. Resources should be dispensed to allow the greatest benefits for the majority of individuals. *Source:* World Health Organization (1990), reference 91. Reproduced by permission of WHO.

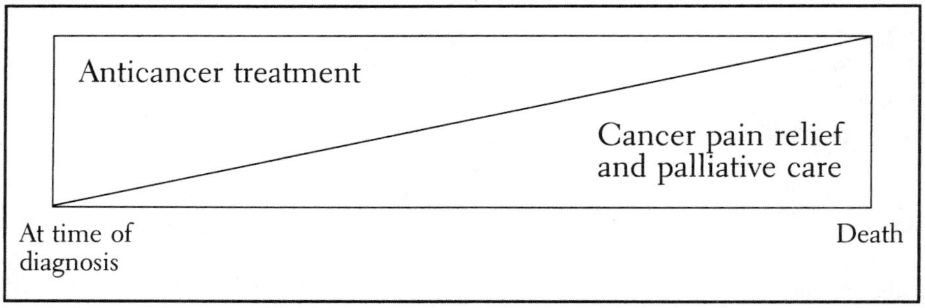

Figure 23–3. Proposed allocation of cancer resources in developing countries. As developing countries are the least likely to prevent, detect, and cure cancers, the distribution of resources should be further tailored to best meet the needs of their population. (It is a great ethical dilemma: do you cure one to allow 1000 more to suffer?) *Source:* World Health Organization (1990), reference 91. Reproduced by permission of WHO.

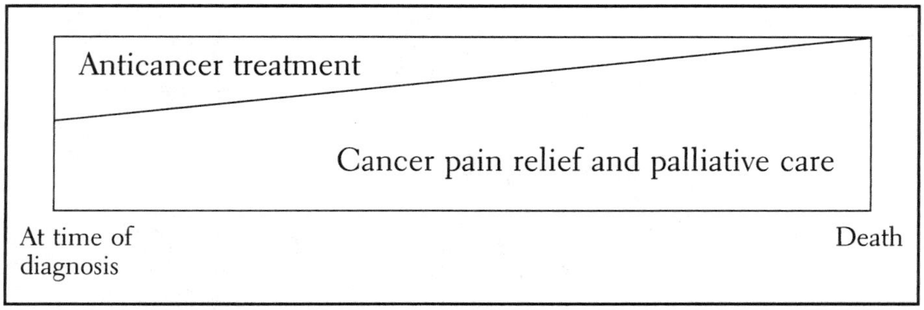

aid in relieving pain, improving function, and probably decreasing other potential complications, such as decubitus ulcer and deep venous thrombosis.

What Are Important Economic Outcomes?

Economic outcomes are not different from clinical outcomes, and cost must be considered along with clinical benefit. Only one medical group, the American Society of Clinical Oncology (ASCO), has published recommendations on what benefit is justified to recommend a medical intervention, as listed in Table 22–2.[35] Of note, ASCO could not define the lowest amount of benefit that justified an intervention, for example, 2 weeks of quality survival, but recommended that the benefit be weighed against the toxicity and costs. If cost-effectiveness data are not available, then cost consciousness with attention to lowest costs for comparable results would be appropriate; cost alone is not sufficient since more expensive treatments, such as bone marrow transplantation for relapsed leukemia, may give better survival at reasonable cost effectiveness.[32]

The economic data necessary to make decisions about treatment may be collected in much the same way as clinical information, and standard formats for collection and analysis are now available.[36] Some standard definitions are listed in Table 22–3.

It is important to organize data in a way that balances clinical and cost information side by side, as shown in Table 22–4. Cost effectiveness is the amount of money someone must pay to gain additional months or years of life. The usual benchmark is "life years gained" or LYs. The standard cost-effectiveness question is $\Delta C/\Delta E = (C_2 - C_1)/(E_2 - E_1)$ where C = costs and E = effectiveness of treatment measured in time. To adjust for quality of life, when the quantity does not change, the concept of utility is used. Utility is the value placed on time in a particular state of health. Perfect health would be assigned a utility value of 1.0 and death a value of 0.0. When utility, or the time × the utility value, is added, the equation becomes $\Delta C/\Delta U$ where $\Delta U = U_2 - U_1$. For example, a therapy that does not improve survival but increases utility by 10% will increase U by (1 year) × (0.10) = 0.1 year. If this treatment costs an additional $10,000/year, then the cost-utility ratio is:

$$\Delta C = C_2 - C_1 = \$10{,}000 = \$100{,}000/\text{QALY}.$$

$$\Delta U = U_2 - U_1 = 0.10$$

Table 22–3
Standard Definitions for Economic Outcome Analysis

Term	Definition	Comment
Resource utilization	Number of units used (e.g., 9 hospital days)	Best collected prospectively, using a combination of clinical research forms, hospital bills, and patient diaries for outpatient or off-site events.
Charge	What is billed to the patient	May be fair representation of the cost of service. Can be accurately converted to costs using ratio of charges to cost.[92]
Cost	What it costs society to provide the service	This is different from the charge because many services cost more or less than what is billed.
Direct medical cost	Costs of standard medical interventions	Usual "cost-drivers" include hospital days, professional fees, diagnostic tests, pharmacy fees, other (e.g., blood products, operating room, emergency services)
Direct nonmedical cost	Costs of medical interventions not usually captured but directly caused	Includes transportation, time lost from work, caregiver costs, etc. Most are not covered by insurance and may be "out-of-pocket" costs.
Perspective	The viewpoint of the analysis	Should be explicitly stated. Most analyses are done from the perspective of society (valuing this intervention vs. other uses of the same money) or a health care system (valuing this intervention against other local health care needs). The perspective of the individual patient or provider may give less attention to the needs of others.[36]
Discounting	Adjusts value of intervention for future benefit to present-time amount	Health effects and costs should normally be discounted at 3% per year. Health benefits in the present are worth more than those in the future.

Source: Smith (1993), reference 35.

Table 22–4
Ways to Balance Clinical Evaluation and Cost Studies

Type of Study	Advantages and Disadvantages
Clinical outcomes only	Ignore costs. Easy to choose among clearly superior therapies such as cisplatin for testicular cancer; harder among all others that give lesser benefits at high costs.
Cost only (e.g., cost of treating febrile neutropenia)	Ignores clinical outcomes. Does not help choose among clinical strategies. The cost of colony-stimulating factor (CSF) mobilization of stem cells may be higher than that of bone marrow collection, but it saves money later by reducing hospital stay.[35]
Costs and clinical outcomes together	
Cost minimization	Assumes that two strategies are equal; lowest cost strategy is preferred.
Cost effectiveness	Compares two strategies; assigns dollar amount per additional year of life (life year [LY]) saved by strategy. Example: at present, CSFs have not improved survival, so cost must be lower for therapy to be cost-effective.
Cost utility	Compares two strategies; assigns dollar amount per additional LY saved by strategy, then estimates the quality of that benefit in cost per quality adjusted LY. No data show significant improvement in quality of life or utilities in patients who have received CSFs, so they are unlikely to have major impact.
Cost benefit	Compares two strategies but converts the clinical benefits to money (e.g., a year of life is worth $100,000). This is possible but is rarely done due to difficulty in assigning monetary value to benefit; requires assigning a monetary value to human life.

Such values can be compared to other medical interventions, as shown in Table 22-5. Many authorities use a cost effectiveness ratio of $50,000/life year as an informal benchmark to decide about payment for care. To an economist, 1 week of additional life for 52 people is equal to 52 weeks of life for one person, so a therapy that gains 8 weeks, with an improvement in utility from 0.50 to 0.70 could still be valued as long as the $/LY is acceptable.

Chemotherapy is often thought of as a curative treatment, but it is often palliative in nature, with a goal of symptom relief or prolonging survival. Chemotherapy may be a good treatment decision in palliative care as long as the switch to palliative care is made while resources and quality time are still available.[37,38]

It is possible to give chemotherapy and either save money or have a cost effectiveness within accepted limits, as shown in Table 22-5. Patients treated with chemotherapy for non-small-cell lung cancer have a small benefit, estimated at 2 to 4 months in most cases,[39,40] and symptom relief in up to 60% of cases.[41] Both the ASCO[42] and the Ontario government[43] recommend consideration of chemotherapy for suitable patients. Jaakimainen and coworkers[44] found that chemotherapy actually saved disease-management costs compared to best supportive care by preventing hospitalizations late in the disease course. The cost-effectiveness ratios ranged from C$8000 (cost saving) to C$20,000 (costs more than supportive care) for each additional year of life.[44] Chemotherapy with cisplatin and vinorelbine compared to vinorelbine alone or cisplatin and vindesine added substantial clinical benefit[45] at a reasonable cost effectiveness of C$15,000 to C$17,000/LY.[46] Given the benefit and low cost of the drugs, vinorelbine and cisplatin compared to best supportive care would give results similar to those of Jaakimainen and colleagues.[44] Evans and colleagues[47] used decision analysis to show that chemotherapy in combination with radiation and/or surgery for stage IIIA or IIIB disease in comparison to treatment without chemotherapy would improve survival at a cost of C$3348 to C$14,958 per year of life saved. The model showed benefit at a reasonable cost under all situations of reasonable clinical efficacy. The chemotherapy treatments fit existing monetary guidelines for use.[48,49]

A trial of fluorouracil-based chemotherapy for gastrointestinal cancer patients randomized to first-line chemotherapy versus best supportive care, which could include later chemotherapy for symptom control, showed benefit at acceptable cost-effectiveness ratios.[50] For the whole group, chemotherapy enhanced survival by about 5 months at a cost of about $20,000/LY gained, within accepted bounds.[32] For subsets of types of cancer, such as gastric cancer, the treatment was effective at a reasonable cost. For most other subsets, the patient numbers were too small to draw meaningful conclusions about either clinical effect or cost effectiveness.

In a metastatic prostate cancer study, mitoxantrone added a clinical benefit in terms of pain relief and symptom control in

Table 22–5
Chemotherapy vs. Best Palliative Care or Alternative Treatments

Topic	Conclusion
Lung cancer Chemotherapy vs. best supportive care in non-small-cell lung cancer.[44, 46]	Chemotherapy gained 8–13 weeks compared to best supportive care.[44] Chemotherapy generally saved money for the province of Ontario, from a savings of $8000 to an additional cost of $20,000 depending on assumptions. Similar results were found for vinorelbine and cisplatin.[46]
Combined modality including chemotherapy vs. radiation or surgery for stage III non-small-cell lung cancer.[47–49]	Chemotherapy in combination with radiation or surgery adds clinical benefit; for chemotherapy plus radiation, 1- and 5-year survival rates are increased from 40% to 54% and from 6% to 17%, respectively. The addition of chemotherapy to IIIB patients added cost of $15, 866, and addition of chemotherapy to IIIB patients added $8912. The cost per year of life gained was well within accepted bounds at $3348 to $14,958 CAN.
Alternating chemotherapy for small-cell lung cancer[84]	The alternating chemotherapy arm cost more, but because it was more effective, the marginal cost effectiveness was only $4560/year of life.
Gastrointestinal cancer Chemotherapy vs. best supportive care followed by chemotherapy for gastrointestinal cancer patients[50]	Chemotherapy added 5 months median survival if given early rather than late, with symptom palliation for 4 months. The additional cost of about $20,000 per life year was within accepted bounds.
Prostate cancer Palliative chemotherapy with mitoxantrone plus prednisone vs. prednisone[51, 52]	Mitoxantrone did not improve survival but did improve quality of life as measured by several indices, and the mitoxantrone strategy cost less than prednisone supportive care.
Breast cancer High-dose chemotherapy for limited metastatic disease vs. standard chemotherapy[56]	High-dose chemotherapy added 6 months at a cost of $58,000, or $116,000 per life year; this is palliative care because this treatment has not been shown to be curative.
Other Acute myelogenous leukemia[58]	Chemotherapy, compared to supportive care, added additional cost, but the cost effectiveness was $18,000/life year, within acceptable limits.

23 of 80 patients, lasting for 6 months more than prednisone alone, but did not alter survival when compared to prednisone alone.[51] Although initial drug costs were higher, total disease costs were lower in the group that received mitoxantrone as initial treatment,[52] so good chemotherapy palliation could be accomplished at no additional cost to society. Total androgen blockade produced small clinical benefit at an acceptable cost to society compared to single androgen blockade.[53]

There have been no studies on the effectiveness or cost effectiveness of chemotherapy for metastatic breast cancer compared to best supportive care. Hospitalization accounts for the majority of costs, while chemotherapy has been a relatively trivial cost in the United Kingdom.[54] High-dose chemotherapy is commonly used for incurable metastatic disease, and in the one randomized controlled trial, it doubled overall survival from 10.4 to 20.8 months but did not produce a long-term survival plateau.[55] In the only available study of comparative treatment, Hillner and associates[56] compared best standard chemotherapy to high-dose chemotherapy with a stem-cell transplant. High-dose chemotherapy added about 6 months at a cost-effectiveness ratio of $116,000/LY gained, outside the bounds of accepted treatments. Of interest, drug costs for most breast cancer patients amount to less than 10% of the total cost.[57]

Sometimes, highly expensive chemotherapy can be a "good value" for society if it gains substantial amounts of time, or if the comparative treatment is also expensive. Chemotherapy for acute myelogenous leukemia costs more than supportive care, but was effective enough to gain months or years compared to certain death, so the cost-effectiveness ratio was acceptable. Allogenic transplant was even more expensive than usual second-line chemotherapy, but the transplant survival benefit of 48% versus 21% at 5 years was sufficient to offset higher costs of treatment and make the cost-effectiveness ratio about $18,000/LY.[58]

The less expensive the setting, the less costly the intervention, as shown in Table 22–6. Home opioid infusions had lower total costs due to lower hospital costs despite higher drug equipment and nursing costs.[59] Outpatient administration of chemotherapy was less expensive than inpatient administration.[60] Home chemotherapy compared to outpatient chemotherapy was accepted well, with only two of 424 patients electing to discontinue home treatment; it was safe and no more costly, with an average cost of $50 as compared to $116 in the hospital and equal total costs.[61]

Disease-management strategies have shown some modest improvements, with better quality of care, less cost, and high patient satisfaction. The available studies are shown in Table 22–7.

Coordinated care may be one of the most successful disease-management strategies. The Medicare Hospice Benefit requires nurse coordination, team management, easy access to low per diem hospital beds for respite or temporary care, and expanded drug coverage.[62,63] Adding a nurse coordinator for terminally ill patients in England did not change any disease outcomes: patients still died, and most still had some unrelieved symptoms; however, patient and family satisfaction was helped slightly.[64] Total costs were reduced from £8814 to £4414 due to decreased hospital days, for a cost savings of 41% in almost all conditions. Home nursing care was associated with more patients dying at home.[65]

One center did a pain-management intervention with enhanced institutional education programs, a highly visible respected consultative team, and a pain-resource center for nurses and families. This was associated with a decrease in admissions and readmissions for pain control and marked cost savings.[66] The study was not randomized and could not account for other significant changes, such as the growth of managed care with restricted admission policies. However, the conclusion must be that this is better pain management and better medical care and probably saves money.[67]

Teaching staff about choices for intensive care unit (ICU) use can improve economic outcomes. In one setting, an ethicist in the surgical ICU addressed the issues of patient choice about dying and the ethics of futile care. This was associated with a decrease in length of stay from 28 to 16 days, and a decrease in surgical intensive care days from 2028 to 1003, far greater than observed in other parts of the hospital. Cost savings were estimated at $1.8 million.[68] In a similar project, Dowdy and colleagues[69] did proactive ethics consultations for all mechanically ventilated patients beyond 4 days and showed improved length of stay (less use of the ICU, either by discontinuing futile care or transferring the patient to lesser-intensity units) and a decrease in costs.

Clinical practice guidelines for supportive care may decrease costs, but formal data have not been published.[63] While there have been significant anecdotal data and clinical opinion that hospice provides improved quality and decreased cost, the available data do not show that hospice improves care or saves money, as shown in Table 22–8.[63,70,71] A

Table 22–6
Site of Service

Topic	Conclusion
Opioids in home infusion	Per diem costs were higher for home patients, but total costs were lower, with equivalent palliation.[59]
Inpatient or outpatient	Outpatient administration was less expensive, $184 vs. $223US.[60]
Home or inpatient/ clinic chemotherapy	Home chemotherapy was safe, well accepted, and cost less per treatment.[61]

Table 22–7
Process or Structural Changes in Care

Topic	Conclusion
Reducing uncontrolled pain admissions	A system-wide intervention of focus on pain management, a supportive-care consultation team, and a pain resource center. This was associated with a reduction in admissions from 255/5772 (4.4%) to 121/4076 (3.0%), at a project cost savings of $2,719,245.[66]
Presence of nursing care for end of life	Nursing care availability allowed more patients to die at home, consistent with the wishes of most patients.[65]
Clinical practice guidelines for supportive care: antiemetics, treatment of febrile neutropenia, treatment of pain	A division changed practice to standardized oral antiemetics and once-daily ceftriaxone and gentamicin. Cost savings were estimated at $250,000 for each intervention, yearly.[63,85,86]

Table 22–8
Hospice vs. Nonhospice Care

Topic	Conclusion
Randomized controlled trial of hospice vs. nonhospice care in Veterans Hospital	Hospice did not improve or worsen quality of care by any measured benchmark (pain, ability to perform activities of daily living). There was no difference in diagnostic procedures. Total costs were $15,000 per patient, with no difference in the arms.[87]
Hospice election vs. standard care, Medicare beneficiaries, 1992	Medicare saved $1.65 for each $1 spent on hospice programs; most of the savings occurred during the last month of life.[72]
Hospice election vs. standard care, Medicare beneficiaries, 1988	Medicare saved $1.26 for each $1 spent on hospice programs; most of the savings occurred during the last month of life.[74]
Total costs from databases	No significant difference in total costs from diagnosis to death, but significant cost savings of 39% for hospice patients who were in hospice more than 2 weeks.[88]
Total disease-management costs comparing those who elected hospice to those who did not	No different or slightly higher costs among Medicare beneficiaries who elected hospice. Within the hospice period, average 27 days, costs were slightly lower for those who elected hospice.[63]
Home care	Home care provided by relatives is not much different ($4563 for each 3-month period) from costs in a nursing home or similar setting. The sicker the patient became, the more the cost to the family regardless of diagnosis. Costs were lowest when the patient and caregiver lived in the same household.[89,90]
Matching resource use to the dying patient	Hospice patients were likely to receive more home nursing and to spend less time in the hospital than conventional care patients. Conventional care was the least expensive when overall disease management costs were calculated, but hospital-based hospice ($2270) and home care hospice ($2657) were less.

large, randomized controlled trial of hospice versus standard care showed that hospice did not improve quality of care by any measured benchmark (pain, ability to perform activities of daily living). Patients still used many hospital days (48 for controls, and 51 for hospice), but more of the hospice patients were hospitalized on the hospice unit. There was no difference in diagnostic procedures or total costs (about $15,000 per patient).

More recent data suggest that hospice care can be cost saving.[18,72,73] Smith and colleagues and Brumley and colleagues demonstrated that integrating palliative care into a curative practice model earlier in a disease trajectory improved patient satisfaction while decreasing needs of acute care and lowering health care costs. In the 1992 Medicare files, those cancer patients who elected hospice cost less than those who did not elect hospice. For those who enrolled in hospice in the last month of life, typically over half of Medicare hospice patients, Medicare saved $1.65 for each $1 spent. However, those who elected hospice tended to use more resources in the months from diagnosis until about 3 months before death, so the total disease-management savings were close to zero. Similar findings were reported previously.[74]

Hospice may actually not save total disease-management costs but just shift them to costs not captured by our current accounting systems. In our own study of Medicare hospice use in Virginia, total disease-management costs were actually higher for those who eventually elected hospice. Those who elect hospice tend to have resources to absorb more home care costs, more out-of-pocket drug costs, etc. The data are consistent with an affluent group of patients using all of the resources needed for treatment, then using hospice resources in addition. There are no published data on whether the medically underserved use hospice, whether they will accept its philosophy, or how much they will cost the system.[63]

Database studies have shown similar results. In a retrospective study of 12,000 patients at 40 centers, Aiken[75] found that hospice patients were more likely to receive home nursing care and to spend less time in the hospital than conventional care patients. Of the three models of care evaluated, conventional care was the least expensive when overall disease-management costs were calculated, but hospital-based hospice ($2270) and home care hospice ($2657) were less expensive than conventional care ($6100) in the last month of life.

Table 22–9
Use of Advanced Directives, Do-Not-Resuscitate (DNR) Orders

Study	Conclusion
California durable power of attorney for health care placed on chart[78]	No effect on treatment charges, types of treatment, or health status.
DNR[93]	Average of $57,334 for those without DNR orders, compared to $62,594 for those with DNR orders.
Advance directives in SUPPORT hospitals[77]	No cost savings with advance directives. Before the SUPPORT intervention, there was a 23% reduction in cost associated with presence of advance directives ($21,284 versus $26,127).
	Intervention patients were more likely to have advance directives documented.
	Average cost was $24,178 for those without advance directives, $28,017 for those with advance directives on the intervention arm.

Advanced directives, such as "do-not-resuscitate" (DNR) orders, have been advocated to allow patients to make autonomous choices about their care at the end of life and possibly to reduce costs by preventing futile care. However, as reviewed by Emanuel and Emanuel,[70,76] there has been no cost saving associated with the use of either advanced directives or DNR orders (Table 22–9). These findings have been confirmed in the more recent SUPPORT study.[77]

End-of-life or advanced planning is clearly a part of palliative care and care of the dying. Levinsky[22] has questioned whether end-of-life planning has become an economic strategy as much as a way to respect a patient's wishes: "Confusion between advance planning as a method to find out what the patient wants and advance planning as a mechanism to reduce medical care and thereby contain costs represents a clear danger to the goals of informed consent and autonomy for patients." In a randomized study of 204 patients with life-threatening diseases, it was found that in those who executed an advance directive, there was no significant positive or negative effect on well-being, health status, medical treatments, or medical treatment charges.[78]

Nursing Issues

Clearly, many issues related to nursing impact need to be explored. Role utilization and its potential impact will vary within each setting. For example, an entire multidisciplinary palliative care team may be necessary to meet the needs of the population in a large university-based hospital, yet a specially trained nurse may be adequate in a small community hospital. Such impact of services needs to be evaluated in many fields to examine quality of care and cost effectiveness.[79] The role of the advance practice nurse may be a powerful tool in identifying and coordinating the needs of patients/families requiring palliation. Advance practice nurses may fill a void within the hospital, hospice, and nursing home for this population.[80,81]

A cost not truly examined is the out-of-pocket cost that the patient's significant others bear in caring for them, specifically in terms of lost work hours, expended resources, and simple care hours not reimbursed through the health care system. Also to be determined is the increased health care costs of the caregivers due to the stressful, often exhausting requirements.[82]

Nursing needs to continue to advocate for this population while supporting effective quality care, and fair utilization of resources must be frequently assessed. For example, the use of advanced technology, especially expensive diagnostic tests, may be accepted as routine in an acute care hospital, even though it is costly, unnecessary, and not consistent with the goals of palliative care. Consider the following examples.

1. An 82-year-old man with end-stage chronic obstructive pulmonary disease requests removal from a respirator and comfort measures only. He is deemed competent, yet it is questionable if he will be able to survive off the respirator. His wishes are followed, and he is extubated. While adamantly refusing any discussion regarding reintubation, he continues to have arterial blood gases sampled every 2 to 3 hours around the clock. Clearly, use of such sampling is academic because the patient refuses reintubation. Sampling of arterial blood gases is costly and painful and does not contribute to the goals of comfort.

2. A 32-year-old man with widely metastatic colon cancer arrives in your facility with a bowel obstruction related to his disease. He has been in the local hospice program. After evaluation, his prognosis is confirmed as approximately 6 weeks. He has a nasogastric tube placed to relieve persistent nausea, vomiting, and abdominal discomfort. After 4 days of decompression, the surgeon offers to place a gastrostomy tube for drainage and decompression. While the surgery will be costly, placement of the gastrostomy tube meets the goals of both comfort and providing the patient with the ability to return home.
3. A 29-year-old woman with acquired immunodeficiency syndrome is admitted for severe debilitating neuropathic pain, unresponsive to typical adjunctive analgesic agents. The patient is losing her ability to ambulate due to the pain. She is given a trial of epidural opioids with local anesthetics, which offer almost complete pain relief. An intrathecally implanted pump, at a cost of several thousand dollars, is placed. While the initial cost is staggering, the long-term benefits are considerable, including measurable improved functional status, decreased occurrence of depression, decrease in required skilled and nonskilled nursing care hours, decreased opportunistic infection, and improved quality of life for both the patient and her significant others.
4. A 60-year-old woman with multiple myeloma is admitted with an adjusted serum calcium level of 179 mg/dL. The myeloma is now progressing and refractory to therapy. Intravenous fluids, diuretics, biphosphates, and calcitonin are administered, and serum calcium is drawn every 12 hours. The patient's disease is irreversible. The present interventions will perhaps delay an inevitable outcome, but they will cost thousands of dollars, while not improving the patient's quality of life, and may potentially cause discomfort.

   This process of reassessment and recognition should be fostered through education and role modeling and should begin in the very basic nursing courses. It must be integrated throughout the longitudinal nursing curriculum, as patients dealing with end-of-life disease processes exist in almost all health care settings. It is imperative that outcomes research accompanies education to ensure the best and most cost-efficient palliative care available.
5. A 36-year-old man with a self-inflicted gunshot wound arrives in your emergency room. The neurosurgical team determines the injury to the brain is devastating and that the prognosis is grave. The family requests all measures to keep him alive "no matter what." They demand ongoing ventilator and nutritional support. What role should the nurse take in this situation? What options might the health care team have, should the family be unwilling to understand the illness trajectory of their relative? What role should the hospital take in this matter? How will you advocate?
6. A 68-year-old previously healthy woman has suffered a traumatic subdural hematoma, with significant brain damage. She only opens her eyes to verbal stimuli and does not follow commands 2 weeks after her injury. She has been receiving NG feedings. The patient has a living will that clearly states no artificial nutrition if her condition becomes irreversible. The social worker informs the medical team that she cannot place this patient in a nursing home unless she becomes "skilled," which a PEG feeding tube would accomplish. What is your role? The hospital could lose considerable revenue if the patient is not placed in a nursing home? What presently happens in your facility? What role would your ethics and risk management play in this case?

Summary

Economic outcomes are increasingly important for all types of health care, including palliative care. The few studies show substantial opportunities for improvement by using disease-management strategies. Chemotherapy for some cancers (non-small-cell lung cancer, prostate cancer, and gastrointestinal cancer) is reasonably effective and has acceptable cost-effectiveness ratios; this does not apply to any regimen that has not been formally evaluated. Coordination of palliative care shows no major clinical benefit but does show major cost savings. Directed, ethically motivated interventions about futile care appear to produce significant cost savings. The use of advance directives or hospice care may be good medical care but has not been shown to produce major economic benefit.

The cost of care is rising due to the increasing age of the population, more cancer cases and chronic diseases, increased demand for treatment, and new and expensive technologies. Our limited resources must be rationed wisely so that we can provide both curative and palliative care. The ethical implications of using economic and management outcomes rather than traditional health outcomes include shifting emphasis from helping at all cost to helping at a cost society can afford, as well as how much society is willing to pay; the value of care to the dying versus those with curable illnesses; and tolerance of suboptimal care.

The outcomes of palliative care do not differ from those of other cancer treatment, from the perspective of economics or health service research. For treatment to be justified, there must be some demonstrable improvement in disease-free or overall survival, toxicity, quality of life, or cost effectiveness. Palliative care usually does not change survival, and it does not have a measurable cost-effectiveness ratio since it does not gain years of life. There may be little change in quality-adjusted life years because the improvements in health state are too small to measure with current instruments or are lost in the impact of the disease.

Only a few studies have assessed the economic outcomes of palliative therapy. The major areas of interest include the following: (1) palliative chemotherapy versus best supportive care; (2) supportive care for cancer symptoms; (3) the process and structure of care; (4) follow up; and (5) hospice care. Palliative first-line chemotherapy for stage III and IV non-small-cell lung cancer, mitoxantrone for prostate cancer, and fluorouracil-based chemotherapy for gastrointestinal cancer have acceptable cost-effectiveness ratios. Supportive care effectiveness and cost for infections, nausea, and pain can be improved. Research outside of cancer is scant. Hospice care saves at best 3% of total care cost but gives care equal to nonhospice care. Coordination of palliative care will save 40% of costs but will not improve the clinical outcomes of dying patients.[83] Nursing clearly has the ability to impact the care and cost for this population and should be in the forefront of these issues. [81]

ACKNOWLEDGEMENTS

This work is based on a chapter published in Topics in Palliative Care, Vol. 5, edited by R.K. Portenoy and E. Bruera: Economic outcomes and palliative care, by Thomas J. Smith and Laurie Lyckholm. New York: Oxford University Press, 2001: 157–175.

REFERENCES

1. Centers for Medicare and Medicaid Services. National Health Expenditures and selected economic indicators, levels and average annual percent change: selected calendar years 1990–2013, http://www.cms.hhs.gov/statistics/nhe/projections-2003/t1.asp (accessed April 2, 2005).
2. National Cancer Institute. Cancer Progress Report: 2003 Update, http://progressreport.cancer.gov (accessed January 9, 2005).
3. American Cancer Society. Cancer Facts & Figures 2005. Atlanta: Author, 2005.
4. National Heart, Lung and Blood Institute. Fact Book Fiscal Year 2003, http://www.nhlbi.nih.gov/about/03factbk.pdf (accessed January 10, 2005).
5. Lubitz JD, Riley GF. Trends in Medicare payments in the last year of life. N Engl J Med 1993;328:1092–1096.
6. Lubitz J, Beebe J, Baker C. Longevity and Medicare expenditures. N Engl J Med 1995;332:999–1003.
7. Welch HG, Wennberg DE, Welch WP. The use of Medicare home health care services. N Engl J Med 1996;335:324–329.
8. Brunner D. Cost effectiveness of palliative care. Semin Oncol Nurs 1998;14:164–167.
9. SUPPORT Principal Investigators. A controlled trial to improve care for seriously ill hospitalized patients. The Study to Understand Prognoses and Preferences for Outcomes and Risks of Treatments (SUPPORT). JAMA 1995;274:1591–1598.
10. Cleeland CS, Gonin R, Hatfield AK, et al. Pain and its treatment in outpatients with metastatic cancer. N Engl J Med 1994;330: 592–596.
11. Bevan, G. Taking equity seriously: a dilemma for government from allocating resources to primary care groups. BMJ 1998;316:39–43.
12. Hillner BE, Smith TJ. Hospital volume and patient outcomes in major cancer surgery: a catalyst for quality assessment and concentration of cancer services. JAMA 1998;280:1784.
13. Gillis CR, Hole DJ. Survival outcome of care by specialist surgeons in breast cancer: a study of 3786 patients in the west of Scotland. BMJ 1996;312:145–148.
14. Sainsbury R, Haward R, Rider L, Johnstone C, Round C. Influence of clinician workload and patterns of treatment on survival from breast cancer. Lancet 1995;345:1265–1270.
15. Feuer EJ, Frey CM, Brawley OW, et al. After a treatment breakthrough: a comparison of trial and population-based data for advanced testicular cancer. J Clin Oncol 1994;12:368–377.
16. Nguyen HN, Averette HE, Hoskins W, Penalver M, Sevin B, Steren A. National survey of ovarian carcinoma, Part V. The impact of physician's specialty on patient's survival. Cancer 1993;72:3663–3670.
17. Desch CE, Penberthy L, Newschaffer C, et al. Factors that determine the treatment of local and regional prostate cancer. Med Care 1996;34:152–162.
18. Smith T, Coyne P, Cassel B, Penberthy L, Hopson A, Hager M. A high-volume specialist palliative care unit and team may reduce in-hospital end-of-life care costs. J Palliative Med 2003;6: 699–705.
19. Berger JT, Rosner F. The ethics of practice guidelines. Arch Intern Med 1996;156:2051–2056.
20. Olson V, Coyne P, Smith V, Hudson C. Critical pathway improves outcomes for patients with sickle-cell disease. Oncol Nurs Forum 1997;24:1682.
21. Smith R. An ethical code for everybody in health care: a code that covered all rather than single groups might be useful. BMJ 1997;315:1633–1634.
22. Levinsky NG. The purpose of advance medical planning—autonomy for patients or limitation of care? N Engl J Med 1996; 335:741–743.
23. Callahan D. Controlling the costs of health care for the elderly—fair means and foul. N Engl J Med 1996;335:744–746.
24. Randall F. Palliative Care Ethics: A Good Companion. New York: Oxford University Press, 1996.
25. Daniels N. Just Health Care. New York: Cambridge University Press, 1985.
26. Sidgwick H. The Methods of Ethics. London: McMillan, 1907.
27. Slevin ML, Stubbs L, Plant HJ, et al. Attitudes to chemotherapy: comparing views of patients with cancer with those of doctors, nurses, and general public. BMJ 1990;300:1458–1460.
28. Davies E, Clarke C, Hopkins A. Malignant cerebral glioma—I: survival, disability, and morbidity after radiotherapy. BMJ 1996; 313:1507–1512.
29. Davies E, Clarke C, Hopkins A. Malignant cerebral glioma—II: perspectives of patients and relatives on the value of radiotherapy. BMJ 1996;313:1512–1516.
30. Lamm RD. The ghost of health care future. Inquiry 1994;31 :365–367.
31. Coyne P. International efforts in cancer pain relief. Semin Oncol Nurs 1997;13:57–62.
32. Smith TJ, Hillner BE, Desch CE. Efficacy and cost-effectiveness of cancer treatment: rational allocation of resources based on decision analysis. J Natl Cancer Inst 1993;85:1460–1474.
33. Waugh N, Scott D. How should different life expectancies be valued? BMJ 1998;316:1316.

34. Laupacis A, Feeny D, Detsky AS, Tugwell PX. How attractive does a new technology have to be to warrant adoption and utilization? Tentative guidelines for using clinical and economic evaluation. Can Med Assoc J 1992;146:473–481.
35. Smith TJ. Which hat do I wear? JAMA 1993;270:1657–1659.
36. Brown M, Glick H, Harrell F, et al. Integrating economic analysis into cancer clinical trials: The National Cancer Institute--American Society of Clinical Oncology Economics Workbook, 1998:1.
37. Smith TJ, Hillner BE, Schmitz N, et al. Economic analysis of a randomized clinical trial to compare filgrastim-mobilized peripheral blood progenitor cell transplantation and autologous bone marrow transplantation in patients with Hodgkin and non-Hodgkin lymphoma. J Clin Oncol 1997;15:5–10.
38. Smith TJ, Desch CE, Hillner BE. Ways to reduce the cost of oncology care without compromising the quality. Cancer Invest 1994;12:257–265.
39. Blair SN, Kohl HWI, Barlow CE, Paffenbarger RS Jr, Gibbons LW, Macera CA. Changes in physical fitness and all-cause mortality. A prospective study of healthy and unhealthy men. JAMA 1995; 273:1093–1098.
40. Souquet PJ, Chauvin F, Boissel JP, et al. Polychemotherapy in advanced non-small cell lung cancer: a meta-analysis. Lancet 1993;342:19–21.
41. Adelstein DJ. Palliative chemotherapy for non-small cell lung cancer. Semin Oncol 1995;22:35–39.
42. American Society of Clinical Oncology. Clinical practice guidelines for the treatment of unresectable non-small-cell lung cancer. J Clin Oncol 1997;15:2996–3018.
43. Evans WK, Newman T, Graham I, et al. Lung cancer practice guidelines: lessons learned and issues addressed by the Ontario Lung Cancer Disease Site Group. J Clin Oncol 1997;15: 3049–3059.
44. Jaakimainen L, Goodwin PJ, Pater J, Warde P, Murray N, Rapp E. Counting the costs of chemotherapy in a National Cancer Institute of Canada randomized trial in non-small cell lung cancer. J Clin Oncol 1990;8:1301–1309.
45. Le Chevalier T, Brisgand D, Douillard JY, et al. Randomized study of vinorelbine and cisplatin versus vindesine and cisplatin versus vinorelbine alone in advanced non-small cell lung cancer: results of a European multicenter trial including 612 patients. J Clin Oncol 1994;12:360–367.
46. Smith TJ, Hillner BE, Neighbors DM, McSorley PA, Le Chevalier T. An economic evaluation of a randomized clinical trial comparing vinorelbine, vinorelbine plus cisplatin and vindesine plus cisplatin for non-small cell lung cancer. J Clin Oncol 1995;13: 2166–2173.
47. Evans WK, Will BP, Berthelot JM, Earle CC. Cost of combined modality interventions for stage III non-small-cell lung cancer. J Clin Oncol 1997;15:3038–3048.
48. Evans WK, Will BP. The cost of managing lung cancer in Canada. Oncology (Huntingt) 1995;9(Suppl 11):147–153.
49. Evans WK, Will BP, Berthelot JM, Wolfson MC. The economics of lung cancer management in Canada. Lung Cancer 1996;14:13–17.
50. Glimelius B, Hoffman K, Graf W, et al. Cost-effectiveness of palliative chemotherapy in advanced gastrointestinal cancer. Ann Oncol 1995;6:267–274.
51. Tannock IF, Osoba D, Stockler MR, et al. Chemotherapy with mitoxantrone plus prednisone or prednisone alone for symptomatic hormone-resistant prostate cancer: a Canadian randomized trial with palliative end points. J Clin Oncol 1996;14:1756–1764.
52. Bloomfield DJ, Krahn MD, Tannock IF, Smith TJ. Economic evaluation of chemotherapy with mitoxantrone plus prednisone for symptomatic hormone resistant prostate cancer (HRPC) based on a Canadian randomized trial (RCT) with palliative endpoints. Proc Am Soc Clin Oncol 1997;17:2272–2279.
53. Hillner BE, McLeod DG, Crawford E, Bennett CL. Estimating the cost effectiveness of total androgen blockade with flutamide in M1 prostate cancer. Urology 1995;45:633–640.
54. Richards MA, Braysher S, Gregory WM, Rubens RD. Advanced breast cancer: use of resources and cost implications. Br J Cancer 1993;67:856–860.
55. Bezwoda WR, Seymour L, Dansey RD. High-dose chemotherapy with hematopoietic rescue as primary treatment for metastatic breast cancer: a randomized trial. J Clin Oncol 1995;13:2483–2489.
56. Hillner BE, Smith TJ, Desch CE. Efficacy and cost-effectiveness of autologous bone marrow transplantation in metastatic breast cancer. Estimates using decision-analysis while awaiting clinical trial results. JAMA 1992;267:2055–2061.
57. Holli K, Hakama M. Treatment of the terminal stages of breast cancer. BMJ 1989;298:13–14.
58. Welch HG, Larson EB. Cost-effectiveness of bone marrow transplantation in acute nonlymphocytic leukemia. N Engl J Med 1989;321:807–812.
59. Ferris FD, Wodinsky HB, Kerr IG, Sone M, Hume S, Coons C. A cost-minimization study of cancer patients requiring a narcotic infusion in hospital and at home. J Clin Epidemiol 1991;44:313–327.
60. Wodinsky HB, DeAngelis C, Rusthoven JJ, et al. Re-evaluating the cost of outpatient cancer chemotherapy. Can Med Assoc J 1987;137:903–906.
61. Lowenthal RM, Piaszczyk A, Arthur GE, O'Malley S. Home chemotherapy for cancer patients: cost analysis and safety. Med J Aust 1996;165:184–187.
62. Harris NJ, Dunmore R, Tscheu MJ. The Medicare hospice benefit: fiscal implications for hospice program management. Cancer Manage 1996;May/June:6–11.
63. Smith TJ. End of Life Care: Preserving Quality and Quantity of Life in Managed Care. Alexandria, VA. ASCO: Education Book 33rd Annual Meeting, 1997;303–307.
64. Raftery JP, Addington-Hall JM, MacDonald LD, et al. A randomized controlled trial of the cost-effectiveness of a district coordinating service for terminally ill cancer patients. Palliat Med 1996;10:151–161.
65. McWhinney IR, Bass MJ, Orr V. Factors associated with location of death (home or hospital) or patients referred to a palliative care team. Can Med Assoc J 1995;152:361–370.
66. Grant M, Ferrell BR, Rivera LM, Lee J. Unscheduled readmissions for uncontrolled symptoms. Nurs Clin North Am 1995;30:673–682.
67. Chandler S, Payne R. Economics of unrelieved cancer pain. Am J Hospice Palliat Care 1998;15:223–225.
68. Holloran SD, Starkey GW, Burke PA, Steele G, Jr, Forse RA. An educational intervention in the surgical intensive care unit to improve ethical decisions. Surgery 1995;118:294–298.
69. Dowdy MD, Robertson C, Bander JA. A study of proactive ethics consultation for critically and terminally ill patients with extended lengths of stay. Crit Care Med 1998;26:252–259.
70. Emanuel EJ. Cost savings at the end of life. What do the data show? JAMA 1996;275:1907–1914.
71. Emanuel EJ, Emanuel LL. The economics of dying. The illusion of cost savings at the end of life. N Engl J Med 1994;330:540–544.
72. National Hospice Organization. An Analysis of the Cost Savings of the Medicare Hospice Benefit. Miami: Lewin-VHI, 1997.

73. Brumley R, Enguidanos S, Cherin D. Effectiveness of a home-based palliative care program for end-of-life. J Palliat Med 2004;6:715–724.
74. Kidder D. The effects of hospice coverage on Medicare expenditures. Health Serv Res 1992;27:195–217.
75. Aiken LH. Evaluation and research and public policy: lessons learned from the National Hospice study. J Chronic Dis 1986; 39:1–4.
76. Emanuel EJ, Emanuel LL. The economics of dying: the illusion of cost savings at the end of life. N Engl J Med 1994;330:540–544.
77. Teno J, Lynn J, Connors AF, Jr, et al. The illusion of end-of-life resource savings with advance directives. SUPPORT Investigators: Study to Understand Prognoses and Preferences for Outcomes and Risks of Treatment. J Am Geriatr Soc 1997; 45:513–518.
78. Schneiderman LJ, Kronick R, Kaplan RM, Anderson JP, Langer RD. Effects of offering advance directives on medical treatments and costs. Ann Intern Med 1992;117:599–606.
79. Kassirer JP. Rationing by any other name. N Engl J Med 1997; 336:1668–1669.
80. Coyne PJ. Evolution of the advanced practice nurse within palliative care. J Palliat Med 2003;6: 767–768.
81. Reb A. Palliative and end of life care: policy analysis. Oncol Nurs Forum 2003;30:35–50.
82. Levine C. The loneliness of the long-term care giver. N Engl J Med 1999;340:1587–1590.
83. Payne P, Coyne P, Smith T. The health economics of palliative care. Oncology 2002;16:801–808.
84. Goodwin PJ, Feld R, Evans WK, Pater J. Cost-effectiveness of cancer chemotherapy: an economic evaluation of a randomized trial in small-cell lung cancer. J Clin Oncol 1995;13:248.
85. Smith, TJ. Reducing the cost of supportive care. I: Antibiotics for febrile neutropenia. Clin Oncol Alert 1996;11:49–47.
86. Smith, TJ. Reducing the cost of supportive care. II: Anti-emetics. Clin Oncol Alert 1996;11:62–64.
87. Kane RL, Berstein L, Whales J, Leibowitz A, Kaplan S. A randomized control trial of hospice care. Lancet 1984;1:890–894.
88. Brooks CH, Smyth-Staruch K. Hospice home care cost savings to third party insurers. Med Care 1984;22:691–703.
89. Stommel M, Given CW, Given BA. The cost of cancer home care to families. Cancer 1993;71:1867–1874.
90. Given BA, Given CW, Stommel M. Family and out-of-pocket costs for women with breast cancer. Cancer Pract 1994;2: 187–193.
91. World Health Organization. Cancer Pain Relief and Palliative Care. Technical Report Series 304. Geneva: Author, 1990.
92. Schwartz M, Young DW, Siegrist R. The ratio of costs to charges: How good a basis for estimating costs? Inquiry 1995; 32:476–481.
93. Maksoud A, Jahnigen DW, Skibinski CI. Do not resuscitate orders and the cost of death. Arch Intern Med 1993;153: 1249–1253.

23

Ashby C. Watson

Urgent Syndromes at the End of Life

He not busy being born is busy dying.—Bob Dylan

- ***Syndromes Covered in This Chapter Include:***
- *Superior vena caval obstruction*
- *Pleural effusion*
- *Pericardial effusion*
- *Hemoptysis*
- *Spinal cord compression*
- *Hypercalcemia*
- *See individual topics for Key Points*

Hallmarks of palliative care are skilled assessment and rapid evaluation and management of symptoms that impact negatively on patient and family quality of life. This chapter addresses select syndromes that unless recognized and treated promptly will cause unnecessary suffering for the patient and family.

SUPERIOR VENA CAVAL OBSTRUCTION

CASE STUDY 1

Mr. W, a Patient with Small-Cell Lung Cancer

Mr. W, a 72-year-old retired Army colonel, recently had a central-venous access device placed in preparation for chemotherapy for small-cell lung cancer. He is also receiving concurrent radiation therapy. You meet Mr. W and his wife for the first time in the outpatient oncology clinic. They are nervous about chemotherapy, but he says "I'll do anything to beat this thing." His wife tells you in his presence, "I think his arm has swelled some since they put that catheter in. His face seems 'fuller' in the morning when he wakes up and he looks different. Is that normal?" Mr. W says, "Oh honey, you worry about everything," and turns to you, winks, and says, "There's nothing wrong, right?" He then asks his wife to leave the room so he can talk to you privately. He says "I want to know what I'm facing, but I don't want my wife to worry."

- ***Key Points***
- *Superior vena caval obstruction can cause distressing symptoms that are amenable to palliation.*
- *The common presenting symptoms are dyspnea, facial swelling, and feeling of fullness in the head.*

- *The patient's swollen and distorted facial features can be highly upsetting to the patient and family.*
- *The diagnosis of vena caval syndrome can usually be made on clinical grounds.*

Definition

Superior vena caval obstruction (SVCO) is a disorder produced by obstruction of blood flow in the superior vena cava, which results in impairment of blood flow through the superior vena cava into the right atrium. Severity of the syndrome depends on rapidity of onset, location of the obstruction, and whether or not the obstruction is partial or complete. Obstruction may occur acutely or gradually, and symptoms may be severe and debilitating.[1,2]

Epidemiology

The patient most likely to experience SVCO is a 50- to 70-year-old man with a primary or metastatic tumor of the mediastinum. More than 90% of SVCO cases are due to cancer, most commonly, endobronchial tumors.[3,4] In the majority of patients, the presence of SVCO is not a poor prognostic indicator of survival.[5] The prognosis of patients with SVCO strongly correlates with the prognosis of underlying disease.

Two types of obstruction[1] may cause SVCO: (1) intrinsic obstruction, and (2) extrinsic obstruction. Intrinsic obstruction is usually caused by primary tracheal malignancies that invade the airway epithelium, that is, squamous cell carcinoma and adenoid cystic carcinoma, as well as other benign and malignant tumors. Extrinsic obstruction occurs when airways are surrounded and compressed by external tumors or enlarged lymph nodes, that is, lymphoma, and locally advanced thyroid, lung, or esophageal cancers. Obstruction may be caused by a tumor arising in the right main or upper-lobe bronchus or by large-volume lymphadenopathy in the right paratracheal or precarinal lymph node chains.[6]

Thrombosis of the superior vena cava (SVC) is also associated with insertion of indwelling intracaval catheters and central-venous access devices, which are thought to damage the intima of vessels. Both adults and children may experience thrombosis of the SVC. More than compression or tumor, thrombosis is likely to cause acute and complete obstruction of the SVC.[7] Cancer patients are also at greater risk of experiencing hypercoagulopathies, which increase the risk of experiencing thrombosis and SVCO. Other less common nonmalignant causes associated with SVCO are mediastinal fibrosis from histoplasmosis and iatrogenic complications from cardiovascular surgery.[7,8]

Pathophysiology

The superior vena cava is located in the rigid thoracic cavity and is surrounded by a number of structures, including the sternum, trachea, right bronchus, aorta, pulmonary artery, and several lymph node chains. There is little room for structures to move or expand within this cavity, thus the superior vena cava is vulnerable to any space-occupying lesion in its vicinity. Venous drainage from the head, neck, upper extremities, and upper thorax collects in the SVC on its way to the right atrium. The SVC has a thin wall, and normally, blood flows through the vessel under low pressure. When the vessel is compressed, blood flow is slowed, fluid pressure is increased, and occlusion may occur.[9]

When venous collateral circulation has time to develop, the symptoms of SVCO are likely to develop insidiously.[10] The presence of collateral circulation, tumor growth rate, and extent and location of the blockage are factors in determining how rapidly SVCO develops.[11]

Signs and Symptoms

The onset of symptoms is often insidious. Patients may report subtle signs that include venous engorgement in the morning hours after awakening from sleep, difficulty removing rings from fingers, and an increase in symptoms when bending forward or stooping, all of which may not be noticed initially.[1,9,12,13] The most common symptom of the syndrome is dyspnea.[12,14,15] Swelling of the neck and face is seen in 50% of patients. Other common symptoms are cough (54%), arm swelling (18%), chest pain (15%), and dysphagia (9%).[7] Physical findings include venous distention of the neck (66%), venous distention of the chest wall (54%), facial edema (46%), plethora, a very ruddy facial complexion (19%), and cyanosis (19%). Patients may experience tachypnea, hoarseness, nasal stuffiness, periorbital edema, redness and edema of the conjunctivae, and, rarely, paralyzed vocal cord.[16]

In severe or rapid cases, where collateral circulation has not yet made accommodation for increased blood flow, symptoms may be immediately life-threatening. Patients may experience orthopnea, stridor, respiratory distress, headache, visual disturbances, dizziness, syncope, lethargy, and irritability. As the condition further progresses, significant mental status changes occur, including stupor, coma, seizures, and, ultimately, death.[17]

Diagnostic Procedures

Plain chest x-ray films are the least invasive diagnostic modality.[7] Computed tomography (CT) is the most widely available and used modality to elucidate the location, extent of obstruction or stenosis, presence and extent of thrombus formation, and status of collateral circulation,[18–20] and can be performed unless the patient is so debilitated that no further treatment is indicated or desired by the patient.[21] Magnetic resonance imaging (MRI) is another diagnostic tool that can confirm the diagnosis of SVC[21] and distinguish between tumor mass or thrombosis.

Palliation of Symptoms

The effectiveness of palliation of symptoms of SVCO in patients who have persistent or recurrent small-cell lung cancer

(SCLC) has been reviewed.[5] Chemotherapy or mediastinal radiation therapy were found to be very effective as initial treatment for patients who have SCLC and SVCO at first presentation, as well as in those with recurrent or persistent disease. It was recommended that radiation therapy should be used in those patients who have been previously treated with chemotherapy. However, due to side effects, large fractions should be avoided.[5] When comparing the treatment modalities used to treat SVCO, including chemotherapy alone, chemotherapy and radiation therapy, and radiation therapy alone, none has proved superior.[6] Adverse prognostic indicators are dysphagia, hoarseness, and stridor.

SVC Stenting

Current American College of Chest Physicians (ACCP) guidelines state that lung cancer patients with symptomatic SVCO can be treated with radiation therapy, insertion of an SVC stent, or both. [22] More recent evidence indicates that symptomatic patients may possibly be better treated initially by SVC stenting. Although there are no controlled studies comparing radiation therapy with SVC stenting, several reviews and nonrandomized studies indicate that this procedure can relieve edema, promote improved superficial collateral vein drainage, and improve neurological impairment. It can also relieve dyspnea, provide greater relief of obstruction, create few or minor complications,[6,17,23–26] and allow for the full use of chemotherapy and radiation therapy,[17] thus providing more rapid relief in a higher proportion of patients.[6] Complications associated with SVC stenting procedures include bleeding due to anticoagulation, arrhythmia, septic episodes, thrombosis, fibrosis, and migration of the stent.

Thrombolytic Therapies

Thrombolytic therapy has often been successful in the lysing of SVC thrombi.[27] Another alternative, percutaneous angioplasty with or without thrombolytics, may open SVC obstructions. Documented thrombi may be treated with tissue plasminogen activators (TPS).

Drug Therapy

Steroids have been one of the standard therapies for treatment of SVCO in spite of the lack of evidence to support their use. Prednisone and methylprednisolone have both been used to reduce inflammation in the treatment of SVCO. Prednisone dosages range from 5 to 60 mg orally once a day or are given in a divided dosage schedule of either twice daily or four times daily. The drug is then tapered over 2 weeks as symptoms resolve. Methylprednisolone may be given in an initial IV dosage of 125 to 250 mg. The maintenance dose is 0.5–1 mg/kg/dose every 6 hours for up to 5 days.[28]

Diuretics, such as furosemide, may be given to promote diuresis, thus decreasing venous return to the heart, which reduces pressure in the SVC. In general, a 20- to 80-mg dose is given once, then repeated every 6 to 8 hours as necessary, and may be increased by 20 to 40 mg per dose if necessary. The dose should be individualized to the requirements of each patient.[28]

Nursing Management

The primary nursing goals are to identify patients at risk for developing SVC syndrome, to recognize the syndrome if it does occur, and to relieve dyspnea and other symptoms. Reduction of anxiety is an important nursing goal. The patient and family may experience significant distress not only because of physical symptoms experienced but also because of an altered physical appearance, including a ruddy, swollen, distorted face and neck.

The nurse monitors the patient for side effects of treatment and provides symptom management. For example, if the patient is receiving radiation therapy, be alert for signs of dyspnea (which may indicate presence of tracheal edema), pneumonitis, dysphagia, pharyngitis, esophagitis, leukopenia, anemia, skin changes, and fatigue. If the patient is receiving chemotherapy, be alert for signs of stomatitis, nausea and vomiting, fatigue, leukopenia, anemia, and thrombocytopenia. If the patient is receiving steroid therapy, educate the patient and family about the potential for developing proximal muscle weakness, mood swings, insomnia, oral candida, and hyperglycemia. Aspects of palliative nursing care always of primary importance are early recognition and management of symptoms, educating the patient and family about these symptoms and what to report, and providing reassurance that these symptoms, if they occur, will be controlled.

PLEURAL EFFUSION

CASE STUDY 2

Ms. B, a Patient with Breast Cancer

Ms. B, a 42-year-old divorced woman, has been living with breast cancer for the last 5 years. She has received numerous therapies, none of which has halted the progression of her disease, but she wants to continue with chemotherapy. She now has widely metastatic disease in her bone, liver, and both lungs. In the clinic, you are preparing her chemotherapy as she tells you that over the past several weeks she has been feeling more fatigued and has no appetite. She has also been feeling more short of breath, which first occurred when she was walking but now is present all the time. She complains of feeling pressure and pain in her chest and especially when taking in a deep breath. "I . . . know . . . it's the . . . cancer taking . . . over. I'm losing . . . the battle," she tells you breathlessly. Her pulse is rapid and her respirations are 24 a minute. You notice that she is using her accessory breathing muscles to breathe. You listen to her lungs and she has decreased breath sounds on the left side; she also has decreased diaphragmatic excursion on her left side. When you percuss the lungs, you also notice dullness on the left side.

- ***Key Points***
- *The treatment of pleural effusion is palliative and symptomatic.*
- *The treatment approach depends on clinical circumstances, the patient's general condition, and nearness to death.*
- *Preemptive pain management is a critical nursing function when patients undergo invasive procedures.*

Definition

Pleural effusion is defined as a disparity between secretion and absorption of fluid in the pleural space secondary to increased secretion, impaired absorption, or both, resulting in excessive fluid collection.[29–32]

Epidemiology

More than 150,000 pleural effusions (PE) are diagnosed each year in the United States.[33] Parapneumonic disease is the most common cause of pleural effusions, followed by malignant disease. Bronchogenic, breast, and lymphoma malignancies account for 75% of all malignant pleural effusions (MPE),[34] followed by ovarian cancer and gastric cancer, in order of descending frequency.[35] Almost half of patients with metastatic disease will experience a pleural effusion sometime during the course of their disease.[36–40]

Pleural effusions occur in 7% to 27% of hospitalized human immunodeficiency virus (HIV) patients.[41] The three leading causes of PE in those with HIV disease are parapneumonic infection, pulmonary Kaposi's sarcoma (KS), and tuberculosis.[42–44] The overall mortality rate associated with pleural effusion in HIV patients is 10% to 40%.[44] Unfortunately, the presence of malignant pleural effusion is usually associated with widespread disease and poor clinical prognosis, particularly in those with malignancy or AIDS. The overall mean survival for cancer patients who have MPE is 4 to 12 months.[45,46] Lung cancer patients usually die within 2 to 3 months, breast cancer patients within 7 to 15 months, and ovarian cancer patients within 9 months.[47–49] The mean survival period of those with pulmonary KS and MPE is 2 to 10 months; for those who have lymphoma and MPE, it is about 9 months.[50–52] Nearly all patients who have malignant pleural effusion are appropriate candidates for hospice care.[47]

Pathophysiology

Each lung is covered with a serous membrane called the pleura. A closed cavity is located between the pleura and the surface of each lung, called the pleural cavity. Under normal circumstances, it is bathed with 10 to 120 mL of almost protein-free fluid that continuously flows across the pleural membrane. The fluid moves from the systemic circulation into the pleural cavity and then into the pulmonary circulation.[53] Osmotic and hydrostatic pressure act to ensure that equilibrium is maintained between absorption and production of fluid in the pleural space. When this equilibrium is disturbed, fluid can accumulate in the pleural cavity.[54–56]

A number of factors may disturb this equilibrium: (1) metastatic implants or inflammation that cause increased hydrostatic pressure in pulmonary circulation; (2) inflammatory processes that increase capillary permeability and increase oncotic fluid pressure in the pleural space; (3) hypoalbuminemia that decreases systemic oncotic pressure; (4) tumor obstruction or lung damage that creates increased negative intrapleural pressure; (5) impaired absorption of lymph when channels are blocked by tumor; and (6) increased vascular permeability caused by growth factors expressed by tumor cells. [29–31,57,58] Patients with large pleural effusions have demonstrated left-ventricular diastolic collapse and cardiac tamponade, which resolved with thoracentesis. [59,60]

Diagnostic Procedures

A chest x-ray will usually establish the presence of the pleural effusion and should also differentiate the presence of free versus loculated pleural fluid.[61] CT can show pleural or lung masses, adenopathy, pulmonary abnormalities, such as infiltrates or atelectasis, or distant disease.[62–64] Chest ultrasound may differentiate between pleural fluid and pleural-thickening disease.[65,66]

In some cases, once evidence of the effusion has been established and obvious nonmalignant causes have been ruled out, a diagnostic thoracentesis may be helpful in establishing the diagnosis. Sonographic guidance can avoid problems associated with performing "blind" thoracentesis.[64]

Signs and Symptoms

Dyspnea is the most common symptom of pleural effusion and occurs in about 75% of patients.[29,33,35–37,67] Its onset may be insidious or abrupt and depends on how rapidly the fluid accumulates.[47] It is almost always related to collapse of the lung from the increase of pleural fluid pressure on the lung.[57]

The patient's inability to expand the lung leads initially to complaints of exertional dyspnea. As the effusion increases in volume, resting dyspnea, orthopnea, and tachypnea develop. The patient may complain of a dry, nonproductive cough, and an aching pain or heaviness in the chest. Pain is often described as dull or pleuritic in character.[68] Generalized systemic symptoms associated with advanced disease may also be present: malaise, anorexia, and fatigue.[30,34,66]

Physical examination reveals the presence of dullness to percussion of the affected hemithorax, decreased breath sounds, egophony, decreased vocal fremitus, whispered pectoriloquy, and decreased or no diaphragmatic excursion.[30,69,70] A large effusion may cause mediastinal shift to the side of the effusion; tracheal deviation may be present. Cyanosis and plethora, a ruddy facial complexion that occurs with partial caval obstruction, may also be present.[30,70]

Medical and Nursing Management

Overall medical management of malignant pleural effusion depends on multiple factors. The history of the primary tumor, prior patient history and response to therapy, extent of disease and overall medical condition, goals of care, and severity of symptom distress. In some cases, systemic therapy, hormonal therapy, or mediastinal radiation therapy may provide control of pleural effusions.[64] Symptomatic management of symptoms with pharmacotherapy includes the use of opioids to manage both pain and dyspnea, as well as anxiolytics to control concomitant anxiety.[34]

If the patient is to have a chest tube placed or other invasive procedures to drain the fluid or to prevent fluid reaccumulation, the nurse must aggressively manage the patient's pain and anxiety. Educating the patient about what to expect, staying with them during the procedure and medicating them preemptively are important aspects of palliative nursing care. Use of patient-controlled analgesia (PCA) for pain management is appropriate. Unfortunately, pain assessment and management is frequently not recognized as a priority when patients undergo these procedures.

Thoracentesis Alone

Thoracentesis has been shown to relieve dyspnea associated with large pleural effusions.[64] When thoracentesis is undertaken, relief of symptoms may rapidly occur, but fluid reaccumulates quickly, usually within 3 to 4 days, and in 97% of patients, within 30 days.[71] The decision to perform repeated thoracenteses should be tempered by the knowledge that risks include empyema, pneumothorax, trapped lung from inadequate drainage and/or loculated fluid, and the possibility of increasing malnutrition as a result of the removal of large amounts of protein-rich effusion fluid.[57]

Repeated thoracenteses rarely provide lasting control of malignant effusions.[72–74] There are no studies that compare repeated thoracenteses to other management approaches.[2] Instead of a second thoracentesis, a thoracostomy with pleurodesis should be considered.[47] It can be used to reduce adhesions, draw off fluid, and initiate drainage, all at the same time.

Tube Thoracostomy and Pleurodesis

Palliative treatment, especially for those with a life expectancy of months rather than weeks, is best accomplished by performing closed-tube thoracoscopy, using imaging guidance with smaller bore tubes.[47] The goal of this therapy is to drain the pleural cavity completely, expand the lung fully, and then to instill the chemical agent into the pleural cavity. However, if there is a large effusion, only 1000 mL to 1500 mL should be drained initially.[47] Too-rapid drainage of a large volume of fluid can cause reexpansion pulmonary edema, and some patients have developed large hydropneumothoraces following rapid evacuation of fluid.[47] The thoracoscopy tube should then be clamped for 30 to 60 minutes. Approximately 1000 mL can be drained every hour until the chest is completely empty, but a slow rate of drainage is recommended.[64,75] The chest tube is then connected to a closed-drainage device. To prevent reexpansion pulmonary edema, water-seal drainage alone and intermittent tube clamping should be used to allow fluid to drain slowly.

Complications of chest tube placement include bleeding and development of pneumothorax, which occurs when fluid is rapidly removed in patients who have an underlying noncompliant lung. Patients who have chest tubes inserted should receive intrapleural bupivacaine or epidural and intravenous (IV) conscious sedation, as the procedure can be moderately to severely painful.[34,74,76–81]

Pleurodesis

Chest radiography is used to monitor the position of the thoracostomy tube after thoracostomy is completed. It is thought that tube irritation of the pleural cavity may encourage loculations, which can lessen the effectiveness of potential sclerosing agents.[57] Current evidence indicates that it is not necessary to wait for drainage to fall below a certain level, and that the sclerosing agent can be injected as soon as the lung is fully reexpanded.[76] If the lung fails to expand and there is no evidence of obstruction or noncompliant lung, additional chest tube placement may be considered. Fibrinolysis with urokinase or streptokinase may improve drainage in those cases where fluid is still present or is thick or gelatinous.[82] Intrapleural instillation of urokinase 100,000 units in 100-mL 0.9% saline can be attempted, and the chest tube clamped for 6 hours, with suction then being resumed for 24 hours. Once the pleural fluid has been drained and the lung is fully expanded, pleurodesis may be initiated. This can usually take place the day after chest tube insertion.[36,74,83–85]

The purpose of pleurodesis is to administer agents that cause inflammation and subsequent fibrosis into the pleural cavity to produce long-term adhesion of the visceral and parietal pleural surfaces. The goal of this procedure is to prevent reaccumulation of pleural fluid.[35,72,86] Various sclerosing agents are used to treat MPE. They include bleomycin, doxycycline, and sterilized asbestos-free talc.[76] The overall response rate to chemical pleurodesis is 64%.[76]

Pleuroperitoneal Shunt

This procedure is useful for patients who have refractory MPE despite sclerotherapy.[29,72,73,87–89] Two catheters are connected by a pump to a chamber between the pleural cavity and the peritoneal cavity. Manually pushing the pumping chamber moves fluid from the pleural cavity to the peritoneal cavity. Releasing the compression moves the fluid from the pleural cavity into the chamber.

The major advantage of this device is that it can be used on an outpatient basis and allows the patient to remain at home. Its disadvantages include obstruction risk, infection, tumor seeding, general anesthesia is needed for placement, and the device requires motivation and ability on the part of the patient to operate it. Most patients with advanced disease are unable to physically overcome the positive peritoneal pressure required to pump the device. Pumping is required hundreds of times a day, and therefore this device is not likely to be useful in those who are close to death.[90]

Pleurectomy

Surgical stripping of the parietal pleura, with or without lung decortication (if the underlying lung is trapped), is more than 90% effective, but it has a high complication rate[67,72] and should be reserved for only those who have a reasonable life expectancy and physical reserve to withstand surgery.[29,32] Video-assisted thoracoscopy (VATS) and pleurectomy have been performed successfully in small selected groups of patients.[91] However, it is likely to be an inappropriate choice in the palliative care patient at end of life.

Indwelling Pleural Catheters

Indwelling pleural catheters can be placed under local anesthesia.[34] Those who meet criteria for ambulatory therapy, that is, those with symptomatic, unilateral effusions, and who have a reasonable performance status may benefit from this therapy. It has been suggested that tunneled pleural catheters may permit long-term drainage and control of MPE in more than 80 to 90% of patients.[36,92,93] These catheters can be used to treat trapped lungs and large locules. Spontaneous pleurodesis may occur in up to 40% of patients.

Small-bore tubes attached to gravity drainage bags or vacuum drainage have been reported to be successful on an outpatient basis.[47] Rare complications include tumor seeding, obstruction, infection, cellulitis of tract site, and pain during drainage. If spontaneous pleurodesis does not occur, then continuing drainage may present management challenges. This treatment offers the potential for better quality of life and reduction in overall health care costs.

Subcutaneous Access Ports

In this procedure a fenestrated catheter is placed in the pleural cavity. It can be accessed for repeated drainage without risk of pneumothorax or hemothorax.[47] Complications include occlusion, kinking, and wound infection.

Nursing Management

Dyspnea and anxiety are primary symptoms experienced by the patient who has a pleural effusion. When invasive diagnostic procedures are being considered, these choices should be guided by the stage of disease, prognosis, the risk/benefit ratio of tests or interventions, pain-management considerations, and the desires of the patient and family.[94] The nurse can educate the patient and family about each procedure, including its purpose, how it is carried out, how pain will be addressed, and possible side effects or complications that may occur. This not only allows for informed consent but also may help to reduce anxiety and thus decrease dyspnea.[94]

A variety of nonpharmacological techniques can relieve the patient's dyspnea and pain and can be used in combination with opioids and anxiolytics, as well as concurrently with medical treatment. These approaches include positioning the patient to comfort, using relaxation techniques, and providing oxygenation as appropriate.[94] Aggressive pain assessment and monitoring are particularly important for patients who receive invasive procedures.

PERICARDIAL EFFUSION

CASE STUDY 3
Mr. S, a Patient with Leukemia in Remission

Mr. S, a 28-year-old married man with a diagnosis of leukemia, has been in remission following a second induction therapy. His sperm had been banked before starting therapy, and he and his wife have a baby girl. He is now rehospitalized in blast crisis. When you ask his oncologist if end-of-life discussions have been held with the family, he tells you, "I'm pulling out all the stops on this one. He's going on another clinical trial." His wife draws you aside and says, "Don't tell him that I told you this, but he's been coughing a lot more at home lately, and I've noticed that he can't seem to catch his breath. He won't let me tell the doctor. I'm afraid and I don't know what to do." You begin your nursing assessment and notice that the patient is tachycardic and anxious. You try to listen to his heart but the sounds are very faint. You are concerned, but he says, "Let's get this chemo going. I've got a daughter to get home to."

- ***Key Points***
- *Malignant pericardial effusions occur in less that 5% of patients with cancer, but the incidence may be nearer to 20% in patients with lung cancer.*
- *Effusions usually develop in patients with advanced disease and are usually a poor prognostic sign.*
- *The clinical features depend on the volume of pericardial fluid, the rate of accumulation of fluid, and the underlying cardiac function.*
- *Dyspnea is the most common presenting symptom.*

Definition

A pericardial effusion is defined as an abnormal accumulation of fluid or tumor in the pericardial sac.[95] Pericardial effusions can lead to life-threatening sequelae. They can be caused by malignancies and their treatment, and by nonmalignant conditions. Pericardial effusions can lead to cardiac tamponade, which, if not treated, will cause cardiovascular collapse and death.[95]

Epidemiology

Malignant disease is the most common cause of pericardial effusions.[96] Pericardial effusion is most commonly associated with lung and breast cancer, leukemia, and lymphoma.[96] Twenty-five percent to 50% of all patients who require surgical pericardial drainage have malignant pericardial involvement.[96] Metastatic spread or local extension from esophageal tumors and from sarcomas, melanomas, and liver, gastric, and pancreatic cancers can also occur.[97–100] Many pericardial effusions are asymptomatic and are discovered only on autopsy.[101] Up to 40% of cancer patients who have a symptomatic pericardial effusion will have a benign cause of the effusion.[57] Nonmalignant causes of pericardial effusions include pericarditis, congestive heart failure, uremia, myocardial infarction, and autoimmune disease, such as systemic lupus erythematosus. Other causes are infections, fungi, virus, tuberculosis, hypothyroidism, renal and hepatic failure, hypoalbuminemia, chest trauma, aneurysm, and complications of angiographic and central venous catheter procedures.[102,103]

A treatment-related cause of pericardial effusion is radiation therapy to the mediastinal area of more than 4000 cGy, which can lead to pericarditis and possible cardiac tamponade.[99,104,105] The anthracycline-based chemotherapies, such as doxorubicin, can also cause pericardial effusions.[106]

Pathophysiology

The heart is covered by a thin sac called the pericardium. There are usually 15 to 50 mL of fluid between the pericardium and the heart itself.[57] Pericardial fluid originates in lymphatic channels surrounding the heart and is reabsorbed and drained by the lymph system into the mediastinum and into the right side of the heart.[10,11] This fluid minimizes friction, provides a barrier against inflammation, supports the chambers of the heart, and maintains the heart's position in the chest against accelerational and gravitational forces.[107–110] A pericardial effusion occurs when there is excessive fluid in this space. This fluid causes increased pressure to build in the pericardial sac, and the heart cannot fill or pump adequately. A pericardial effusion refers to the increased fluid or tumor in the pericardial sac. Cardiac tamponade is the physiological hemodynamic response of the heart to the effusion.[9]

Malignancies can cause effusions in the pericardial space by: (1) blocking lymph and blood drainage and preventing their resorption, (2) producing excess fluid in the space, (3) bleeding into the space, and (4) growing tumor into the space. The pericardial sac can hold up to 1800 mL of fluid before the heart begins to decompensate.[111,112] Thus, volume of fluid and distensibility will affect the impact of effusion on intrapericardial pressure.

Cardiac tamponade occurs when the heart cannot beat effectively because of excess pressure being exerted on its muscle.[99,102] As the pressure of fluid in the pericardial sac increases, the heart chambers are compressed. First, the right side of the heart, including the right atrium and right ventricle, is compressed. Less blood volume returns to the right side of the heart, thus increasing venous pressure. As the ventricles are further compressed, the heart cannot fill adequately, which leads to decreased stroke volume and cardiac output, and poor perfusion throughout the body. The body attempts to compensate by activating the adrenergic nervous system to keep the heart stimulated and its chambers filled with circulating blood volume. Heart rate increases, veins constrict, and the kidneys increase sodium and fluid retention. The heart ultimately is overwhelmed due to increased fluid, decreased filling, and decreased cardiac output, which leads to hypotension and circulatory collapse.[10,110,111]

Pericardial effusion can develop gradually over a period of weeks or months. The pericardium becomes more compliant, stretching to accommodate as much as 2 liters or more of fluid, with minimal effect on pericardial pressure. This is known as the "stress relaxation" phenomenon. Unfortunately, patients with chronic pericardial effusions may not exhibit physical signs of cardiac tamponade until compression of the heart and surrounding structures occurs, leading to sudden, life-threatening cardiac decompensation.[113–115]

Signs and Symptoms

Pericardial tamponade that results from metastatic disease has a gradual onset that may be chronic and insidious.[9,107,114] Vague symptoms may be reported. Early in the decompensation process it may be difficult to differentiate symptoms of cardiac dysfunction from the effects seen in advancing cancer. The severity of symptoms is related to volume of the effusion, rate of accumulation, and the patient's underlying cardiac function.[10,99,111,116] Generally, rapid accumulation of fluid is associated with more severe cardiac tamponade. The most powerful predictor of the development of cardiac tamponade is the size of the pericardial effusion.[117]

Dyspnea is the most common presenting symptom.[118,119] The patient may complain of the inability to catch his or her breath, which progresses from dyspnea on exertion to dyspnea at rest. In advanced stages, the individual may be able to speak only one word at a time. Chest heaviness, cough, and weakness are also symptoms.[57] Pressure on adjacent structures, that is, the esophagus, trachea, and lung may increase.[120]

Tachycardia occurs as a response to decrease in cardiac output. A narrowing pulse pressure (difference between systolic and diastolic blood pressure) may be seen when blood backs up in the venous system, causing the systolic blood pressure to decrease and the diastolic blood pressure to increase.[9,120] Compression of the mediastinal nerves may lead to cough, dysphagia, hoarseness, or hiccups.[11] Increased venous pressure in the chest may lead to gastrointestinal (GI) complaints, such as nausea.[121,122] Retrosternal chest pain that increases when the patient is supine and decreases when he is leaning forward may occur but is often not present.[110,120] Engorged neck veins, hepatomegaly, edema, and increased diastolic blood pressure are late signs of effusion. Anxiety, confusion, restlessness, dizziness, lightheadedness, and agitation related to hypoxemia may be present as the process progresses.[10,13,99,110,118,123] Poor cardiac output will lead to complaints of fatigue and weakness.

As the effusion increases and the heart begins to fail, symptoms worsen and dyspnea and orthopnea progress. Increasing venous congestion leads to peripheral edema. As cerebral perfusion worsens and hypoxemia increases, confusion increases. Ultimately, there is cardiovascular collapse, anuria, and decreased tissue perfusion, which causes obtundation, coma, and death.[10] Patients with chronic symptomatic pericardial effusions will often exhibit tachycardia, jugular venous distension, hepatomegaly, and peripheral edema.[120]

When examining the patient, one should listen for early signs of cardiac tamponade: (1) muffled heart sounds and perhaps a positional pericardial friction rub, and weak apical pulse; (2) presence of a compensatory tachycardia; (3) abdominal venous congestion and possible peripheral edema; and (4) a fever.[13,110,118,120,124] The signs and symptoms of pericardial effusion and cardiac tamponade may be mistaken for those of other pulmonary complications or pleural effusions. Many cancer patients have both pleural and pericardial effusions.[110,118] Unfortunately, symptoms of cardiac tamponade may be the first indication of the presence of pericardial effusion.

The triad of hypotension, increased jugular venous pressure, and quiet heart sounds that are diagnostic for pericardial effusion occurs in less than a third of patients.[125] If clear lung fields are present, this can help the clinician differentiate between pericardial effusion and congestive heart failure.[125] Pulsus paradoxus is a cardinal sign of cardiac tamponade. It occurs in 77% of those with acute tamponade and in only about 30% of those with chronic pericardial effusion.[114,125] However, its absence does not rule out pericardial effusion. Pulsus paradoxus is a fall in systolic blood pressure of greater than 10 mmHg with inspiration. Normally, blood pressure lowers on inspiration, but when the heart is compressed it receives even less blood flow. The resulting lowered volume and output result in a greater decrease in blood pressure.[110,121,126] Hepatojugular reflux is a late sign of cardiac tamponade.[10,123]

Late in the process of deterioration, diaphoresis and cyanosis are also present. The patient develops increasing ascites, hepatomegaly, peripheral edema, and central venous pressure. Decreased renal flow progresses to anuria. Further impairment in tissue perfusion leads to loss of consciousness, obtundation, coma, and death.[9,10,13,99,110,118]

Diagnostic Procedures

Initially, a standard chest x-ray is likely to show a change in the size or contour of the heart and clear lung fields.[57] A pleural effusion may be evident in up to 70% of patients. Chest x-ray can also demonstrate mediastinal widening or hilar adenopathy. This diagnostic tool is cost-effective, minimally invasive, readily available, and may detect tamponade before the patient becomes symptomatic. However, when used alone, it is not specific enough to diagnose pericardial effusions and does not indicate the level of heart decompensation.[10,121] 2-D echocardiogram (2-D echo) is the most sensitive and precise test to determine if pericardial effusion or cardiac tamponade is present.[22,118] It can be used at the bedside and is noninvasive.

Some cancer patients may have both pericardial effusions and pleural effusions.[110,118] Pleural effusions can mimic the signs and symptoms of pericardial tamponade, causing symptoms of dyspnea and respiratory distress. Chest x-ray may hide or mimic the presence of pericardial tamponade, so depending on the goals of care, a 2D-echo should be performed to differentiate between these phenomena and to detect decompensation of the heart.

Other tests, including MRI and CT, can be used to detect effusions, pericardial masses and thickening, and cardiac tamponade. However, these tests do not indicate how well the heart is functioning, and they have limited use due to safety and comfort concerns in very ill patients.[118,120] If echocardiography is not available, a cardiac catheterization, which will detect depressed cardiac output and pressure levels in all four chambers of the heart, may be considered on a case-by-case basis.[120]

Medical and Nursing Management

Options for medical management include pericardiocentesis with or without catheter drainage, pericardial sclerosis, percutaneous balloon pericardiotomy, pericardiectomy, pericardio-peritoneal shunt, tunneled pericardial catheters, and radiation therapy and chemotherapy, and aggressive symptom management without invasive procedures.

Pericardiocentesis

The most simple, safe, and effective (97%) treatment is echocardiography-guided pericardiocentesis, with a procedural morbidity of 2% to 4% and mortality of 0%.[127–130] Since more than 50% of pericardial effusions reoccur, it is recommended that a 60-cm pigtail catheter (6 to 8 French) be threaded over the needle to allow for drainage of fluid over time.[120,127,131] The procedure can be performed emergently at the bedside, blindly, or with ECG guidance, but it should not be attempted in this manner except in extreme emergencies.[132] Adverse complications of the blind procedure include myocardial laceration, myocardial "stunning," arrhythmias, pneumothorax, abscess, and infection.[95,133,134] The failure rate of this procedure is 10% to 20% because of posterior pericardial loculation or catheter obstruction.

Pericardial Sclerosis

Patients who experience pericardial tamponade face a 50% rate of recurrence when the underlying disease is not effectively treatable.[120] Pericardial sclerosis should be considered in those patients whose disease is not being actively or effectively treated. Pericardial sclerosis is defined as the instilling of chemicals through an indwelling catheter into the pericardial sac for the purpose of causing inflammation and fibrosis, to prevent further fluid reaccumulation. Doxycycline and bleomycin are the most common drugs instilled into the pericardial space.[126] A common side effect of sclerosing therapy is severe retrosternal chest pain, especially with talc administration, and sometimes with bleomycin therapy.[126] A preemptive pain management plan is essential for the well-being of the patient. Arrhythmias, catheter occlusion, and transient fever of up to 38°C without associated bacteremia are also associated complications, primarily of talc and bleomycin therapy.[114,135,136] While sclerosing therapy may initially be "successful," that is, evidence of disappearance of effusion or absence of tamponade symptoms for more than 30 days, multiple instillations may be necessary for true success.[120] The use of thiotepa has been recommended for pericardial instillation because it can be instilled into the drained space, is not associated with severe pain, and is reasonably effective.[126] A major complication is pericardial constriction. A serious discussion of risks, benefits, side effects of the therapy, and its impact on quality of life should take place in the context of end-of-life decision-making.

Percutaneous Balloon Pericardiotomy

This is a safe, nonsurgical method that can be used to relieve the symptoms of chronic recurrent pericardial effusions.[120] It is performed in a cardiac catheterization lab under fluoroscopic guidance using IV conscious sedation and local anesthesia. A guidewire is inserted into the pericardial space, and a small pigtail catheter is inserted over the wire. The wire is removed and some pericardial fluid is withdrawn. Next, the pigtail catheter is removed and replaced with a balloon-dilating catheter that is advanced into the pericardial space and inflated. A pericardial drainage catheter is left in place and is removed when there is less than 100 mL of drainage daily.[137] Patients have reported experiencing severe pain during and after this procedure. A plan for aggressive pain management must be in place before this procedure and rapidly implemented if pain occurs.

Fever and pneumothorax are the most common complications.[137] Pleural effusion has also been associated with the procedure. It is suggested that percutaneous balloon pericardiotomy can be used in place of surgical drainage in patients with malignancy and a short life expectancy.[138]

Surgical Pericardiectomy

Another option is to surgically create a pericardial "window" (partial pericardiectomy), a small opening in the pericardium and suture it to the lung. This allows pericardial fluid to drain out of the pericardial cavity, especially loculated effusions.[126] When other procedures fail and the patient is expected to have long-term survival and good quality of life, partial or complete pericardiectomy may be considered.[120]

Video-Assisted Thoracoscopic Surgery

Video-assisted thoracoscopic surgery (VATS), a minimally invasive procedure, can be used to manage chronic pericardial effusions. In this case, a thoracoscope is introduced into the left or right chest and a pericardial window is performed under thoracoscopic vision.[139,140] The pleura and pericardium can be visualized, tissue diagnosis can be obtained, and loculated effusions can be drained.[141] It has a 100% long-term success rate, and there is no significant morbidity or mortality associated with its use.[120]

Radiation Therapy and Chemotherapy

In some cases, radiation therapy can be used to treat chronic effusions after the pericardial effusion has been drained,[120] and when tamponade is not present. It can be effective in radiosensitive tumors such as leukemias and lymphomas, but is less so in solid tumors.[114] Systemic chemotherapy can be considered if the malignancy is chemotherapy sensitive.[119]

Chronic pericardial effusions and their management can be challenging. Treatment of symptomatic chronic pericardial effusions will depend on patient prognosis, extent of symptoms, presence of concurrent medical conditions, and general condition. In many cases, treatment may be planned and carried out in a less urgent manner, keeping in mind the long-term benefits and side effects of interventions. Optimal treatment should focus on relieving symptoms caused by pressure on adjacent structures and, in the case of underlying malignancy, the first priority should be the promotion of comfort. When choosing a plan, the ability to treat the underlying cause, the long-term prognosis, and patient comfort should be of greatest importance.[120]

Nursing Management

The priority goals in managing this condition are to provide comfort, to promote pain relief, and to reduce anxiety. The nurse should know both early and late signs of cardiac tamponade. Early recognition of these signs and their implications is most important because early intervention may prevent life-threatening sequelae.[9]

Aggressive symptom management includes the administration of opioids and anxiolytics to reduce pain and anxiety. If invasive cardiac procedures are carried out in an emergency at the bedside, the nurse should be present to provide support to the patient and family, to control pain and anxiety, and to monitor vital signs as indicated.[9]

HEMOPTYSIS

CASE STUDY 4

Mr. J, a Patient with Bronchogenic Lung Cancer

Mr. J, a 56-year-old married man, has a long history of cigarette smoking. He recently has been diagnosed with bronchogenic lung cancer. Last week he had one brief episode of moderate hemoptysis at home that was stopped with laser treatment in the emergency room. He has now been admitted to your unit for uncontrollable cough, dyspnea, and chest pain. His wife of 30 years and their two grown children are at his bedside. The oncologist has just told them that any further treatment will be futile. During your initial nursing assessment, Mr. J tells you, "I'm not afraid of dying. If you can just keep me comfortable and help my family, I'll be happy." The family agrees with his desire not to be resuscitated, and plans are being made for him to return home under hospice care. His wife asks you, "The oncologist told me that there might be more bleeding from his lungs. What do we need to be prepared for at home?"

- ***Key Points***
- *Hemoptysis occurs commonly in patients with advanced cancer and is most commonly due to malignant infiltration or infection.*
- *Hemoptysis should be distinguished from gastrointestinal and nasopharyngeal bleeding.*
- *Hemoptysis frequently provokes considerable anxiety.*
- *Massive hemoptysis, while rare, is a life-threatening crisis for patient, family, and staff. Massive hemoptysis occurs in fewer than 5% of cases, but the mortality rate is 85% if surgery is not feasible.*
- *Skilled palliative nursing intervention includes provision of 24-hour psychological support and guidance.*

Definition

Hemoptysis is defined as blood that is expectorated from the lower respiratory tract. Hemoptysis can be classified according to the amount of blood expectorated: (1) mild—less than 15 to 20 mL in a 24-hour period, (2) moderate—greater than 15 to 20 mL but less than 200 mL in a 24-hour period, and (3) massive—greater than 200 mL to 600 mL in a 24-hour period.[142] The primary risk to the patient is asphyxiation from blood-clot formation obstructing the airway rather than from exsanguination. Massive hemoptysis carries a high mortality rate if not treated.

Epidemiology

Tuberculosis is the most common worldwide cause of hemoptysis.[143] The most common causes of hemoptysis in the United States are bronchitis, bronchiectasis, and bronchogenic carcinoma.[143] Other nonmalignant causes of hemoptysis are lung abscess, sarcoidosis, mycobacterium invasion, emphysema, fungal diseases, and AIDS. There is no underlying cause found in 15% to 30% of hemoptic episodes.[143-145]

Metastatic lung disease caused by other primary tumors is associated with nonfatal hemoptysis.[146] Tumors in the trachea usually cause obstructive symptoms rather than massive bleeding.[147] Massive hemoptysis occurs in fewer than 5% of cases, but the mortality rate is 85% if surgery is not feasible.[148,149] Bleeding occurs most often from proximal endobronchial tumors that are not amenable to surgical intervention. Prognosis is usually grim in the case of end-stage lung disease and in the setting of massive hemoptysis.

Pathophysiology

Each lung is supplied with blood by way of two circulatory systems. Pulmonary circulation delivers blood under low pressure from the right ventricle to the alveolar capillaries, where oxygen and carbon dioxide are exchanged. Bronchial circulation arises from the systemic circulation that branches off the aorta, which delivers blood to the lungs under high pressure. These systems anastomose in precapillary pulmonary arterioles and pulmonary veins.[146]

The bronchial venous system returns blood to the heart by two pathways: (1) blood is returned to the right atrium by way of the azygous, hemiazygous, or intercostal veins, and (2) blood is returned to the left ventricle by way of the pulmonary veins. The second pathway carries the bulk of bronchial venous return to the heart.[146]

In the setting of inflammation, tumor, or infection, the bronchial vasculature develops new vascularization pathways. Bronchial blood flow increases as the result of increases in both size and number of these collateral vessels. When these vessels are damaged by inflammation, malignancy, or other injury, blood flow is increased and this raises pulmonary vascular pressure. Hemoptysis occurs in the setting of multiple collateral vessels, high vascular pressure, and damaged, enlarged, and diseased airways.[146,150,151]

In patients who have HIV disease, bacterial pneumonia and infections cause 63% of episodes of hemoptysis. Kaposi's sarcoma causes 10% of episodes, and pulmonary embolism causes 4% of episodes.[152] Patients on anticoagulant or thrombolytic therapy may also experience hemoptysis.[149,153]

Diagnostic Procedures

Flexible fiberoptic bronchoscopy is initially the quickest and surest way to visualize the source of bleeding in the upper lung lobes and to localize it in the lower respiratory tract.[143] This procedure can be done at the bedside without putting the patient under general anesthesia, and it can also visualize distal airways.[146] If there is brisk bleeding, the rigid bronchoscope can suction more efficiently, remove clots and foreign bodies, allow for better airway control, and can be used to obtain material for diagnostic purposes.[154] In some cases, bronchoscopy may locate the area of bleeding but not the direct source of bleeding. In this case, the segment of affected tissue may be purposely suctioned until it collapses.[43] Bronchoscopy should not be undertaken if there is evidence of pulmonary embolism, pneumonia, or bronchitis, or when the patient's condition is so poor or unstable that no further intervention would be undertaken no matter what the results.[151]

If treatment is to be initiated, the combination of bronchoscopy and high-resolution CT can identify the cause of hemoptysis in 81% of patients. It is also quick, noninvasive, and less costly than other modalities.[143] If pulmonary embolism is suspected and therapy is to be initiated, a ventilation-perfusion scan may be warranted.[155]

Signs and Symptoms

Respiratory complaints that raise suspicion of bleeding into the lungs may include cough, dyspnea, wheezing, chest pain, sputum expectoration, and systemic clues, such as fever, night sweats, and weight loss. Clues to nasopharyngeal bleeding as the possible source include frequent nosebleeds, throat pain, tongue or mouth lesions, dysphonia, and hoarseness.[156] Clues to GI bleeding as the possible source include the presence of dyspepsia, heartburn, dysphagia. Coffee grounds-colored vomitus and blood in vomitus does not rule out hemoptysis because blood from respiratory sources can be swallowed. Patients and family members should be asked to describe the color of blood, and should be asked about any changes in color and pattern of bleeding in vomitus and stool.[156]

During an active bleeding episode, a focused examination should be performed as quickly as possible. If possible, the nasopharynx, larynx, and upper airways should be thoroughly visually examined to rule out an upper airway source of bleeding.[143,154,156] If bleeding is brisk and views are obstructed, examination may best be accomplished with bronchoscopy. The patient may be coughing or vomiting blood, and may be short of breath. If possible, sputum, blood and vomitus should be examined. [143,151] Some patients may not yet have a diagnosis of malignancy. In these cases one should note clubbing of fingernails and presence of cervical or supraclavicular adenopathy. This may indicate the presence of a malignancy.[156]

Massive bleeding may take place in the lung without the presence of hemoptysis, so listening to lung sounds is very important. Auscultation of the lungs may reveal localized wheezing, an indication of possible airway obstruction.[156] Fine diffuse rales and asymmetric chest excursion may indicate the presence of an infectious or consolidative process.[156] If petechiae and ecchymosis are present, then there should be strong suspicion that a bleeding diathesis is present.[156]

Medical and Nursing Management

If the episode of bleeding is severe and the goal is active treatment or prolongation of life, then the primary focus is to maintain an adequate airway. This will usually require endotracheal intubation, which may have to be performed immediately at the bedside, and oxygenation. If bleeding can be localized and controlled quickly, a short period of intubation may be considered if it will allow for improved quality of life.[146]

Specific methods of treatment include radiation therapy, laser coagulation therapy, bronchial arterial embolization, endobronchial balloon tamponade, epinephrine injection, and iced saline lavage, and, in very rare cases, surgical resection.

Radiation Therapy

External-beam radiation therapy can stop hemoptysis in more than 80% of cases, especially in those patients who have unresectable lung cancers.[157] The goal is to provide therapy in the shortest time period possible, at the lowest dose to achieve symptom control while minimizing side effects. Complications of therapy are radiation fibrosis, and, unfortunately, massive hemoptysis.[158]

Endobronchial brachytherapy has been effective in some patients who have failed previous external-beam radiation attempts.[159,160] Brachytherapy and bronchoscopy laser therapy have also resulted in resolution of hemoptysis. Results have not been as favorable in patients who have failed previous external-beam radiation therapy or when combined with laser therapy.[161] Side effects associated with brachytherapy, particularly high-dose brachytherapy, include mucositis, fistula formation, and fatal hemoptysis.[162-164] The benefits of this treatment should be carefully weighed against potential side effects and their impact on quality of life, particularly in those patients who have short-term prognoses.

Endobronchial Tamponade

In this procedure, flexible bronchoscopy is used to find the bleeding site after the site has been lavaged with iced saline. A balloon catheter attached to the tip of the bronchoscope is placed on the site and is then inflated and left on the bleeding site for 24 to 48 hours.[165] In the case of life-threatening hemoptysis, a rigid bronchoscope should be used. This is not a uniformly successful procedure, and should be considered a temporizing measure only.[143]

Laser Coagulation Therapy

In the case of obstructing tracheal tumors, Nd-YAG photocoagulation may control bleeding from endobronchial lesions, and it has a response rate of 60%.[164,166] Anecdotal reports of the effectiveness of electrocautery to control hemoptysis have been reported; argon plasma coagulation has led to resolution of hemoptysis for at least a 3-month followup. However, highly vascular tumors are at risk for bleeding when exposed to laser therapy.[165]

Bronchial Arterial Embolization

When an endoscopically visualized lung cancer is the source of bleeding, bronchial artery embolization is effective as a palliative intervention. It stops bleeding in 77% to 93% of cases.[154,167] Bronchial artery embolization, preceded by bronchoscopy, involves injecting a variety of agents angiographically into the bronchial artery to stop blood flow.[151,168] Thirty percent of patients will rebleed within the first or later months, and repeated embolizations may be required.[168,169]

There are major risks of this procedure, including transverse myelitis, paraplegia, ischemic colitis, severe pneumonia, esophagobronchial fistula formation, and temporary severe retrosternal pain.[170] Superselective catheterization now reduces the chance of inadvertently catheterizing the spinal cord branch of the bronchial artery, which has led to spinal cord paraplegia in the past.[171] The risks of rebleeding and the prospect of having repeated embolizations should be carefully reviewed and discussed with the patient and family before carrying out this therapy.

Endobronchial Epinephrine Injections

A 1:10,0000 epinephrine solution may be instilled on visualized lesions to constrict veins and reduce bleeding. Vasopressin and chlorpromazine have also been used in this procedure, which is performed in patients who are not candidates for surgery and when bronchial artery embolization is not available.[143,154]

Iced Saline Lavage

Iced saline solution lavage has been used as a temporary nonstandard measure to provide improved visualization and localization of the bleeding site. It does not appear to improve outcomes.[143,154]

Surgery

In rare cases, some patients who continue to have life-threatening hemorrhage after receiving other therapies may be considered as candidates for surgical intervention. Only those whose life expectancy, condition, ability to tolerate major surgery, and ability to maintain an airway make them suitable candidates, should be considered. It is important to remember that most lung cancers are well advanced at diagnosis and that undertaking this procedure may not meet quality-of-life goals for those with short-term prognoses.[143]

Palliative Care

When a decision has been made to forgo aggressive treatment measures, then promotion of comfort for the patient is the primary goal. Death from massive hemoptysis is usually rapid, occurring within minutes. However, even when the family has been carefully "prepared" for this possibility and coached in a step-by-step manner in what to do, family members inevitably remain unprepared and distraught if a massive hemorrhage does occur, especially in the home, without medical personnel around. Preemptive planning includes anxiolytic and opioids readily available in the home, a 24-hour palliative care number to call for immediate guidance and support, and dark-colored towels to make the viability of blood less overwhelming.

SPINAL CORD COMPRESSION

CASE STUDY 5
Mr. L, a Patient with Prostate Cancer

Mr. L, a 79-year-old widowed ex-postal worker, has been treated with hormone therapy for his prostate cancer for the past 2 years. You've seen him once since he was discharged from the hospital 6 months ago. "I told them I didn't want any of that chemotherapy stuff, and I didn't want to go under the knife either." He lives with his 44-year-old divorced daughter, who works two jobs and is home only at night. Mr. L has done well until the last few weeks, when he began to complain of increasing low-back pain, especially at night. He's been taking Tylox for the pain and says "it helps some." You receive a call from Mr. L, who tells you "I took a bit of a fall last night, but I'm OK now. Could you come out and check me over?" When you arrive at his house, you notice that Mr. L has a bruise under his right eye but no other visible injuries. He tells you "I just got weak and slid to the floor. I feel fine now." On further questioning, you learn that his back pain has markedly increased in severity at night, although it decreases when he stands. In addition, Mr. L complains of more difficulty in moving his bowels and some difficulty in urinating. He attributes the pain to "just an old disk problem I had some years back." He finally admits that he's been having more difficulty walking lately, but doesn't want to worry his daughter—"She's got enough on her mind as it is." Before you can make any recommendations, Mr. L says, "I don't want to go back to the hospital for any tests. I don't want them to do anything else to me."

- ***Key Points***
- *Pain is the primary presenting symptom of spinal cord compression. It may be present long before neurological dysfunction occurs.*
- *The pain is classically worse when lying flat and improved when upright.*
- *In a patient with cancer, increasing back pain that is worse when lying flat and improved when standing is presumed to be cord compression until proven otherwise.*
- *Early detection and treatment may prevent permanent loss of function. It is therefore considered a medical emergency.*
- *The use of steroids and radiation therapy in patients with far advanced cancer can decrease the pain and usually preserve function. Steroids alone can usually decrease pain and preserve function in those who are close to death and do not want to undergo radiation therapy, even in truncated form.*

Definition

Spinal cord compression (SCC) is compression of the thecal sac at the level of the spinal cord or cauda equina. Spinal cord injury may cause progressive and irreversible neurological damage and requires immediate intervention to prevent disability. SCC in the presence of malignancy often carries a poor prognosis, with a life expectancy of 3 months or less.[172]

Epidemiology

Compression of the spinal cord and cauda equina is a major cause of morbidity in patients with cancer. It occurs in approximately 5% to 10% of patients with malignant disease,[173,174] and is most commonly associated with metastatic disease from tumors of the breast, lung, and prostate. Less than 50% of patients will regain functional losses due to SCC.[10,174–176]

Compression of the spine in 85% to 90% of cases is caused by direct hematological extension of solid tumor cells into a vertebral body.[150,177–180] A less common pathway is by direct extension of tumor from adjacent tissue through the intervertebral foramina. Tumor cells can also enter the epidural space directly by circulating in the cerebral spinal fluid (CSF). Paraneoplastic syndromes, leptomeningeal disease, and toxicity of chemotherapy drugs can cause spinal cord syndromes.[181]

Nonmalignant causes of SCC include benign tumors, degenerative, inflammatory, and infectious diseases that affect the spinal column, and from trauma, herniated disks, osteoporosis, or other structural diseases.[22,181]

Pathophysiology

There are 26 vertebrae in the vertebral column: 7 cervical, 12 thoracic, 5 lumbar, 1 sacral, and 1 coccygeal. Inside this flexible protective vertebral column is the spinal cord, which is an elongated mass of nervous tissue covered and protected by membranes called meninges. The outermost layer is the dura mater, the middle layer is the arachnoid membrane, and the innermost layer closest to the spinal cord is the pia mater. The epidural space is located between the outer layer of the dura mater and the vertebral column.[10]

The spinal cord begins where it is attached to the medulla oblongata in the brain and descends through the foramen magnum of the skull until it ends at the level of the first lumbar vertebra. Lumbar and sacral nerve roots then descend below the distal tip of the vertebral column and spread to the lumbar and sacral areas. These long nerve roots resemble a horse's tail that is called the cauda equina. Thirty-one pairs of spinal nerves exit from the spinal cord. [176,182,183] Transmission of nerve impulses travels the length of the spinal cord to and from the brain in ascending and descending tracts. Impulses from the spinal cord to the brain travel through the anterior spinothalamic tracts, and impulses from the brain to the spinal cord travel through the lateral corticospinal tracts. Injury to these nerves or to the cord itself can result in sensory-motor and autonomic impairment.[176]

Eighty-five percent of SCCs are extradural in nature.[9,10,174,184] That is, they originate outside the cord itself. Extradural metastatic tumors may be osteolytic, where lesions invade the marrow of the vertebrae and cause absorption of bone tissue, which leads to bone destruction. They may also be osteoblastic, where lesions invade the bone marrow and cause bone development, tumor invasion, and collapse of the vertebral body, which then pushes tumor or bone fragments into the spinal cord.[10,182,184] Neurological deficits caused by SCC include direct compression on the cord or cauda equina, vascular supply interruption, or pathological fracture, causing vertebral collapse. When nerve tissue dies, neurological regeneration is not always possible. Function may be quickly and irreversibly lost.

Diagnostic Procedures

Plain spinal x-rays are an excellent screening tool and can determine the presence of tumor and the stability of spine.[181] They can identify lytic or blastic lesions in up to 85% of vertebral lesions. However, false negatives can occur due to poor visualization, mild pathology, or poor interpretation.[177] More than 50% collapse, and pedicle erosion must be present before x-ray can detect SCC.[185,186] Epidural spread of tumor through the foramina may not always be visualized using plain x-rays. A bone scan may detect vertebral abnormalities when plain films are negative.[187–189]

MRI is the imaging choice for emergent SCC.[186] It is noninvasive and does not require injection with contrast material. It has an advantage over CT because it can image the entire spine, thus detecting multiple areas of compression.[173,181,190] Decisions about diagnostic testing will be tempered by a number of factors, including the potential for treatment, prognosis, patient's condition, and the family's wishes for treatment.

Signs and Symptoms

The presence of increasing back pain, worse on lying flat and improved on standing, with or without signs of bowel and bladder impairment, in a patient with a history of cancer, should presumed to be SCC until proven otherwise. Neurological function before initiation of therapy is the single most important prognostic factor in SCC.[16] Misdiagnosis of SCC has been attributed to poor history, inadequate examination, and insufficient diagnostic evaluation.[191] Patients who have only localized back pain and a normal neurological examination may have more than 75% of the spinal cord compressed. Upper motor neuron weakness may occur above the L1 vertebral body in 75% of patients with SCC at diagnosis. Sensory changes occur in about half of patients at presentation. Sensory change without pain complaint is extremely rare.

A thorough history should pay special attention to the onset of pain, its location, its intensity, duration, quality, and what activities increase or decrease the pain.[180,184,192] A history of sensory or motor weakness and autonomic dysfunction should be evaluated and should include onset and degree of weakness; heaviness or stiffness of limbs; difficulty walking; numbness in arms, hands, fingers, toes, and trunk; and change in temperature or touch. Specific questions about bowel, bladder, and sexual function should be asked directly, because patients may not volunteer these symptoms, such as difficulty in passing urine or stool, incontinence of bowel or bladder, loss of sphincter control, and ability to obtain and maintain an erection. Constipation usually precedes urinary retention or incontinence.[184]

Physical examination includes observation of the spine, muscles, extremities and skin, and palpation and gentle percussion of vertebrae. Spinal manipulation to elicit pain responses should be carried out cautiously because it may cause muscle spasm or further injury.[181] Mental status, cranial nerve, motor function, reflexes, sensation, coordination, strength, and gait should be evaluated (where appropriate to the patient's status and closeness to death). Focused examination may include performing straight leg raises until the patient feels pain, then dorsiflex the foot. If this action increases pain down the back of the leg, this suggests that nerve root compression is present. Testing of reflexes will indicate the presence and impact of nerve root compression on motor ability. Cord compression may cause hyperactive deep-tendon reflexes while nerve-root compression may cause decreased deep-tendon reflexes. A positive Babinski sign and sustained ankle clonus indicate motor involvement.[184]

Sensory function should be tested by assessing pain (sharp, dull), temperature (hot, cold), touch (light), vibration (tuning fork test), and position senses (fingers and toes). Examination may reveal a demarcated area of sensory loss and brisk or absent reflexes.[184] The mapping of positive sensation can be used to pinpoint the level of SCC, usually one or two levels below the site of compression.[184] Bladder percussion and digital rectal examination will elicit retention and laxity of sphincter control, a late sign of SCC.

Pain may be reported for weeks to months before any obvious neurological dysfunction.[173] Pain may be local initially (in the central back, for example), then progress to a radicular pattern that follows a particular dermatome.[175,181] Local pain may be caused by stretching of bone periosteum by tumor or vertebral collapse, and is usually described by the patient as constant, dull, aching, and progressive in nature. Radicular pain is caused by pressure of tumor along the length of the nerve root.[10,123,176] The patient who reports radicular pain will describe it as shooting, burning, or shocklike in nature and will state that it is worsened by movement, sneezing, straining, neck flexion, or by lying down.

A classic sign of cord compression is if pain is relieved by sitting up or standing and is worsened by lying flat. Also, if pain increases at night when the patient is lying down to sleep, one should be suspicious of SCC rather than degenerative or disk disease.[173] Radicular pain is present in 90% of lumbosacral SCC, 79% in cervical SCC, and in 55% of thoracic SCC.[193] Radicular pain is typically bilateral in thoracic lesions, and is often described as a tight band around the chest or abdomen, but it may also be experienced in only part of one dermatome.[173,177] Nonradicular referred pain may also be associated with vague paresthesias and point tenderness.[173,177,181] Vigilance is called for when these radicular symptoms occur: (1) shoulder tip pain from C7/T1 metastases; (2) anterior or abdominal, flank, or hip pain from T12-L2 metastases; or (3) lateral or anterior rib pain from thoracic metastases.[181]

The sequence of neurological symptoms usually progresses in the following manner—first there is pain, then motor weakness that progresses to sensory loss, then motor loss, and finally, autonomic dysfunction.[9] The patient will initially complain of heaviness or stiffness in the extremities, loss of coordination, and ataxia.[194,195] Sensory complaints include paresthesias and numbness, and loss of heat sensation. Dysfunction begins in the toes and ascends in a stocking-like pattern to the level of the lesion.[173] Loss of proprioception, deep pressure and vibration are late signs of sensory loss.[10,22,123,176] When the cauda equina is affected, sensory loss is bilateral; the dermatome that follows the perianal area, posterior thigh, and lateral aspect of the leg is involved. Late signs of SCC are motor loss and paralysis. Loss of sphincter control is associated with poor return to functionality.[10,22,176]

Medical and Nursing Management

The focus of management of SCC should be the relief of pain and preservation or restoration of neurological function. Rapid intervention is required to prevent permanent loss of function and concomitant quality of life. The patient status (e.g., goals of care and closeness to death), rate of neurological impairment, and prior radiation therapy experience are other factors to consider.[184] Corticosteroids, surgical decompression, radiation therapy, and adjuvant chemotherapy or hormonal therapy are the standard treatments for SCC.[13,184,196]

Corticosteroids

Corticosteroids decrease vasogenic edema and inflammation and thus relieve pain and neurological symptoms, and may have some oncolytic effect on tumor.[192] Dexamethasone is the preferred corticosteroid because it is less likely to promote systemic edema caused by other steroids or to cause cognitive and behavioral dysfunction, and it improves overall outcomes after specific therapy.[173]

There has been controversy about dosage and scheduling of dexamethasone therapy in the management of SCC.[173,185] There is good evidence to support the use of high-dose therapy because substantially more patients are ambulatory after this treatment. It reverses edema and relieves back pain more rapidly. In animal studies, neurological status has improved more rapidly with high-dose therapy. [2,177,178,197–200] High-dose dexamethasone is recommended in ambulatory patients with subclinical SCC.[201]

Currently, high-dose therapy regimens recommend administering a 100-mg IV bolus of dexamethasone, followed by 24-mg dexamethasone orally QID for 3 days, then tapering the dose over 10 days. High-dose therapy may increase analgesia but can also increase side effects that are significant. These include GI bleeding, hyperglycemia, depression and psychosis, myopathy, osteoporosis, and acute adrenal insufficiency with abrupt withdrawal.[182] Low-dose dexamethasone therapy is better tolerated but does not improve the chance of remaining ambulatory. This regimen recommends administering a 10-mg IV bolus of dexamethasone, followed by 4-mg IV QID for 3 days, then tapering the dose over 14 days.[173,172] Rapid IV push of corticosteroids causes severe burning pain in the perineum, and the patient needs to be warned that this will occur but does not signify that anything is wrong. Corticosteroids are metabolized by the cytochrome P-450 system, and there are implications for interactions with other medications, particularly anticonvulsants.

Decompressive Surgery

The goals of surgery are to decompress neural structures, resect tumor if possible, establish local disease control, achieve spinal stability, restore the ability to ambulate, treat pain, and improve quality of life. Surgery for SCC has been used to (1) establish a diagnosis when tissue is required for histologic analysis; (2) halt rapidly deteriorating function; (3) achieve cure for primary malignancy; (4) treat those with previously irradiated radio-resistant tumor and who have continuing symptomatic progressive loss of function; (5) rule out infection or hematoma; (6) alleviate respiratory paralysis caused by high cervical spinal cord lesions; and (7) decompress and stabilize spine structure.[10,13,22,184] Benefits and burden of surgery to the patient in a palliative care setting must be carefully weighed so that the patient and family can make an informed decision.

Radiation Therapy

Fractionated external-beam radiation therapy (XRT) to the spine is given to inhibit tumor growth, restore and preserve neurological function, treat pain, and improve quality of life.[9,202] It has been the primary treatment for SCC.[173] Only symptomatic sections of the spine are treated. Seventy percent of patients who are ambulatory at the start of treatment will retain their ability to walk. Thirty-five percent of paraparetic patients will regain their ability to walk, while only 5% of completely paraplegic patients will do so.[16,203] Primary side effects of radiation therapy include skin alterations of erythema, dry or moist desquamation, pigmentation changes, as well as generalized fatigue.

Nursing Management

The goal of nursing management is to identify patients at high risk for cord compression, to educate the patient and family regarding signs and symptoms to report, to detect early signs of SCC, and to work as a member of the palliative care team in managing symptoms during management of SCC. In those patients who have far advanced disease, palliative care efforts focus on promoting comfort, relieving pain and family support.

HYPERCALCEMIA

CASE STUDY 6

Mrs. H, a Patient with Multiple Myeloma

Mrs. H, a 65-year-old retired LPN, has been receiving outpatient chemotherapy for multiple myeloma. This most recent treatment is under the auspices of an NCI clinical trial, and the patient knows that her cancer is incurable. "I'm a tough ol' bird. I've been around the block a few times, and I know what's what. They can sugarcoat it all they want. I know this is just buying time, but if it helps somebody else, I'm doin' it." Mrs. H lives in a nearby inner-city assisted-living facility. Her children live out of state. She was brought to the hospital when her friends at the facility noticed that she has become more fatigued and lethargic over the past few days, complained of nausea and frequent need to urinate, and seemed a little more confused than usual. You review her lab panels and notice that her ionized calcium is 11.

- ***Key Points***
- *Hypercalcemia occurs in 8% to 10% of patients with cancer, with an incidence of 40% in patients with breast cancer and multiple myeloma.*
- *Common presenting signs are fatigue, lethargy, nausea, polyuria, and confusion.*
- *The combination of nausea and polyuria can lead to dehydration and worsening of hypercalcemia.*
- *Severity of symptoms depends on the level of free ionized calcium and the speed with which the level rises.*
- *The serum calcium level is adjusted according to the serum albumin in patients with significant hypoalbuminemia.*
- *All patients with hypercalcemia who are symptomatic warrant a trial of therapy.*
- *Control of hypercalcemia will not affect prognosis but may greatly improve symptoms and quality of life in these patients.*

Definition

Hypercalcemia is an excessive amount of ionized calcium in the blood.[204,205] If hypercalcemia is left untreated, the patient may experience irreversible renal damage, coma, or death. Mortality from untreated hypercalcemia approaches 50%.

Epidemiology

About 10% to 20% of cancer patients will develop hypercalcemia at some time during their illness.[204,206–208,210] Carcinomas of the breast and lung, multiple myeloma, and squamous cell carcinomas of the head, neck, and esophagus are the most common malignancies associated with hypercalcemia. Incidence ranges from 30% to 40% for breast cancer with bone metastases, 20% to 40% for multiple myeloma, 12.5% to 35% for the squamous cell lung carcinomas, and 2.9% to 25% for head and neck malignancies.[204] Hypercalcemia is rare in prostate cancer, GI cancers, and cancers of the biliary tract.[204]

Primary hyperparathyroidism as a cause of hypercalcemia is more common in the ambulatory and asymptomatic population.[209,211,216] Other conditions associated with hypercalcemia include lithium therapy, Addison's disease, Paget's disease, granulomatous disease, vitamin D intoxication, hyperthyroidism, vitamin A intoxication, and aluminum intoxication.[205,212]

Pathophysiology

Calcium helps the body to maintain its acid-base balance, maintain permeability of cell membranes, promote coagulation, and maintain proper nerve and muscle function.[213] Under normal circumstances, bone resorption and bone formation are in a steady state and are regulated by three hormones—parathyroid hormone (PTH), calcitriol (1,25 dihydroxyvitamin D, a metabolite of vitamin D), and calcitonin.[205] These hormones act at bone sites, in the intestine, and in the kidney. PTH directly increases resorption of calcium from the bone and calcium resorption in the renal tubule. Calcitriol stimulates absorption of calcium in the intestine. It enhances bone resorption and increases renal resorption. Calcitonin is excreted by the thyroid gland and inhibits bone resorption and increases excretion of calcium.

Bone undergoes constant remodeling in the human body. Osteoblasts form bone and osteoclasts resorb bone. About 99% of the body's calcium is found in bone. The remaining 1% circulates in the blood or is found inside cells. Half of plasma calcium is bound to either protein (albumin) or to other ions, such as phosphate, carbonate, or citrate. The remaining calcium circulates as free ions. Since free calcium is biologically active, its level is maintained in a narrow range in the normally physiological state.

Hypercalcemia in malignant disease is primarily due to increased mobilization of calcium from bone. Increased renal tubular calcium resorption is also a factor in hypercalcemia of malignancy. There are three major mechanisms that contribute to the development of malignant hypercalcemia.[206] First, higher levels of PTHrP (parathyroid hormone-related protein) are found in hypercalcemic patients who have solid tumors, particularly squamous cell carcinomas. The presence of elevated PTHrP levels is associated with more advanced cancer, a worse prognosis, and a poor response to bisphosphonate therapy. Approximately 80% of cases of malignant hypercalcemia are related to the presence of this protein.

Second, osteolysis of bone is caused by the release of tumor and other cell mediators. When this mechanism is operating, hypercalcemia occurs late in disease and is usually associated with extensive osteolytic bone metastases. Third, the increased production of calcitriol by lymphoma tumor cells, for example, leads to increased resorption of calcium in the gut. Hypercalcemia induced by calcitriol usually responds to corticosteroid therapy.

The kidney normally adapts to disturbances in calcium homeostasis. However, in the presence of malignancy, patients may experience treatment or disease-related side effects including vomiting, mucositis, anorexia, dysphagia, and fever, all of which can lead to volume depletion.[204] This imbalance signals the kidney to reabsorb sodium to correct extracellular volume depletion. Calcium and sodium resorption are closely linked in the body; when sodium is resorbed, calcium is also resorbed. As calcium ions are resorbed in the kidney, the tubules lose their ability to concentrate urine, leading to high-output polyuria and further dehydration. Poor renal perfusion, reduced glomerular filtration and compromised excretion of calcium lead to a further increase of calcium in the blood. Ultimately, renal failure will occur.

A high calcium level can alter the patient's mental status significantly, which, in turn, can greatly affect the patient's ability to drink fluids. Cellular dehydration and resulting hypotension are exacerbated by decreased proximal renal tubule reabsorption of sodium, magnesium, and potassium. Bone loss due to immobilization, lack of physical exercise, inappropriate use of thiazide diuretics, poor diet, and general physiological wasting will also increase the amount of free calcium ions in the circulation, further increasing calcium levels.

Diagnostic Tests and Procedures

The ionized calcium concentration is the most important laboratory test to use in the diagnostic workup for hypercalcemia. It is the most accurate indicator of the level of calcium in the blood. (There is only a fair correlation between the total serum calcium level and ionized calcium.) When ionized calcium cannot be used as a diagnostic tool, the total serum calcium value may be used, but it must be corrected for serum albumin. A rule of thumb is to add 0.8 for each 1 g/dL the albumin has dropped below the normal range (3.7 to 5 g/dL).[204,205]

Signs and Symptoms

Symptoms of hypercalcemia, their severity, and how quickly they appear will vary from patient to patient. The extent of metastatic bone disease is not associated with hypercalcemia levels.[208,209,210,214] It is important to remember that patients, especially the elderly and the debilitated,[204,209,212,215] may experience severe symptoms when serum calcium is not extremely elevated.[204] Symptoms of hypercalcemia, such as vomiting, nausea, anorexia, weakness, constipation, and impaired mental status, may be mistakenly attributed to the disease or effects of treatment. Factors that will influence patients' response to hypercalcemia include age, performance status, renal or hepatic failure, and sites of metastatic disease.

Patients with a corrected serum calcium level less than 12 mg/dL who are asymptomatic can be considered to have mild hypercalcemia. Patients who have a serum calcium level between 12 and 14 mg/dL should be closely monitored and may require urgent intervention, depending on goals of care in the palliative setting. Those patients with a calcium level greater than 14 mg/dL will require urgent treatment, again depending on goals of care in the palliative setting.[206]

The patient may complain of numerous symptoms that can mimic symptoms of advanced malignancy.[204] These include GI symptoms of nausea, vomiting, anorexia, constipation, obstipation and even complete ileus. Polydipsia and polyuria may also be present. Muscle weakness, fatigue, and difficulty climbing stairs or getting out of a car, are musculoskeletal symptoms that can progress to profound weakness, hypotonia, and fracture. Neuropsychological symptoms can begin with confusion, personality change, restlessness, and mood alterations and progress to slurred speech, psychotic behavior, stupor, and coma. These are also symptoms that must be evaluated. The patient may also complain of bone pain, although the precise mechanism of bone-pain hypercalcemia is unknown.

Early signs of delirium in the hypercalcemic patient are associated with multiple factors that include electrolyte imbalance, metabolic disturbance, and renal failure, among others. If recognized early, treatment of the condition can alleviate and possibly reverse the symptoms.[216] Management of confusion includes both pharmacotherapy and a reassuring and calm environment.

Medical and Nursing Management

Regardless of the goals of care, active treatment goals are to promote alleviation of distressing symptoms. All patients with hypercalcemia who are symptomatic warrant a trial of therapy. When the goal is to reverse the hypercalcemia, this is accomplished by replenishing depleted intravascular volume, promoting diuresis of calcium, shutting down osteoclast activity in the bone, inhibiting renal tubular reabsorption of calcium, and promoting patient mobilization to the extent it is possible.[205,206]

Hydration is the first step in treatment. The purpose of hydration is to increase urinary calcium excretion, which improves renal function.[207] One to 2 liters of isotonic saline is administered over 1 to 4 hours, and the patient's fluid intake and urinary output are closely monitored. The rate of fluid administration depends on the clinical estimate of the extent of hydration, patient cardiovascular function, and renal excretion capacity.[206]

Electrolytes and other laboratory values are closely monitored in appropriate patients. These include serum calcium (ionized or corrected), potassium, magnesium, as well as other electrolytes, and albumin and bicarbonate levels. Renal function tests, including BUN and creatinine, are monitored. In rare cases, dialysis may be considered. In most patients, cardiac effects of hypercalcemia are minimal and outcomes are not usually affected, so cardiac monitoring is not usually necessary.

Bisphosphonate Therapy

Most hypercalcemic patients are treated with bisphosphonate therapy. It is an effective therapy for a number of cancers.[218-221] Bisphosphonate therapy inhibits bone resorption by osteoclasts, thus reducing the amount of calcium released into the bloodstream. Several IV bisphosphonates and aminobisphosphonates are available for use in patients.[222,223] Pamidronate and etidronate are available in the United States.[208,217,224,225] Newer agents include risedronate sodium, ibandronate, and zoledronic acid.[226]

Pamidronate has been the most frequently used bisphosphonate. It is more potent and produces a longer response that often begins within 24 hours of IV administration and lasts for 15 days.[211,217,225,227] Pamidronate appears to be safe in the usual dose of 60 mg to 90 mg IV given approximately every 3 to 4 weeks. In general, there is a 60% response to a 60-mg dose and a 100% response to a 90-mg dose.[211]

Since hypercalcemia tends to recur, pamidronate must be given approximately every 2 to 3 weeks. Side effects of pamidronate therapy include low-grade fever appearing within 48 hours of treatment, redness, induration, and swelling at the site of catheter. Hypomagnesia and hypocalcemia may also occur. Rapid administration of IV bisphosphonates can cause significant pain and this practice should be avoided. Subcutaneous administration of clodronate has been found to be an efficient treatment for malignant hypercalcemia.[228] This route may be particularly useful in hospital, home, and hospice settings and spares the patient discomfort and the costs associated with transportation and IV administration in the hospital environment.

Calcitonin

Calcitonin inhibits resorption of calcium and can rapidly restore normocalcemia, often within 2 to 4 hours of administration. It is much less effective than pamidronate. Its role in managing hypercalcemia is limited to short-term use, usually of only 2 to 3 days' duration. Side effects are usually mild and include nausea and vomiting, skin rashes, and flushing.

Gallium Nitrate and Plicamycin

Gallium nitrate is an effective bone resorptive agent. Its mechanism of action is unknown.[229] Its main disadvantages are that it has potential to cause nephrotoxicity, and it must be given as a continuous IV infusion over 5 days.[205,217] Plicamycin is an antitumor antibiotic.[230,231] Its mechanism is unknown. It has a hypocalcemic effect that occurs within 48 hours of administration and that lasts for 3 to 7 days, but it exhibits marrow, hepatic, and renal toxicities.[205] Individual response variations make this drug unpredictable, and it must be administered repeatedly.

Corticosteroids

Corticosteroids have a limited role in the treatment of hypercalcemia.[206]

Dialysis

The use of dialysis has been reserved for those patients who have severe hypercalcemia, renal failure, congestive heart failure, and cannot be given saline hydration.[232,233] The decision to offer this therapy is made on a case-by-case basis, but, in general, dialysis is not offered in the palliative care arena.

Palliative Nursing Care

Hypercalcemia can cause significantly painful and distressing symptoms, including bone pain, agitation and confusion, severe constipation, and delirium. Treatment of hypercalcemia can reduce pain and other symptoms, improve quality of life, and reduce hospitalizations. At end of life, the promotion of comfort and management of symptoms are the primary goals of the palliative nursing care. If hypercalcemia cannot be reversed or the patient decides that the burden of interventions is greater than the benefit, the patient should be given the option of discontinuing such treatment. Ongoing management of symptoms, including sedation if desired, must be guaranteed to the patient and their family.

CONCLUSION

This chapter addressed a group of syndromes, which, unless recognized and treated promptly, will cause unnecessary suffering for the patient and family. Emphasis has been given to the epidemiology and basic pathophysiology of each syndrome as well as diagnostic assessment. Providing this information, although by necessity limited in detail, enables the palliative care nurse to explain to the patient and/or family why particular symptoms are occurring and why a particular management approach is being suggested. Treatment advice and decisions are always couched within the framework of "Is the underlying cause reversible or not?," "What is the benefit/burden ratio of the treatment and how does that fit in with the patient's values and goals?," "What is the likely outcome if the syndrome is not treated?," "How will resultant symptoms be managed?," "Is palliative sedation available to a patient at end of life if desired?," and "Will the site of care impact on treatment decisions?"

REFERENCES

1. Haapoja I, Blendowski C. Superior vena cava syndrome. Sem Oncol Nurs 1999;15:183–189.
2. Kvale PA, Simoff M, Prakash UBS. Palliative care. Chest 2003; 123(Suppl):284S-311S.
3. Ostler PJ, Clarke DP, Watkinson AF. Superior vena cava obstruction: a modern management strategy. Clin Oncol 1997; 9:83–89.
4. Woolard WL, Hogan DK. Oncologic emergencies: implications for nurses. J IV Nurs 1996;19:256–263.
5. Chan RH, Dar AR, Yu E, et al. Superior vena cava obstruction in small-cell lung cancer. Internat J Rad Onc Biol Phys 1997;38: 513–520.
6. Rowell NP, Gleeson FV. Steroids, radiotherapy, chemotherapy and stents for superior vena caval obstruction in carcinoma of the bronchus: a systematic review. Clin Oncol 2002;14:338–351.
7. Yaholom J. Superior vena cava syndrome. In: Devita VT, Hellman S, Rosenberg SA, eds. Cancer Principles and Practice of Oncology, 6th ed. Philadelphia: Lippincott Williams & Wilkins, 2001:2609–2616.
8. Beeson, M.S. Superior Vena Cava Syndrome. Available at Http://www.emedicine.com/EMERG/topic561.htm (accessed December 6, 2004).
9. Flounders JA. Oncology emergency modules: spinal cord compression. Oncol Nurs Forum 2003;30:E17–23.
10. Schafer S. Oncologic complications. In: Otto S, ed. Oncology Nursing, 3rd ed. St. Louis: Mosby, 1997:406–476.
11. Uaje C, Kathsen K, Parish L. Oncology emergencies. Crit Care Nurs Quarterly 1996;18:26–34.
12. Armstrong BA, Perez CA, Simpson JR. Role of irradiation in the management of superior vena cava syndrome. Int J Rad Onc Biol Physics 1987;13:531–539.
13. Hunter J. Structural emergencies. In: Itano J, Taoka K, eds. Core Curriculum for Oncology Nursing, 3rd ed. Philadelphia: W.B. Saunders, 1998:340–354.
14. Parish JM, Marschke RF, Dines DE. Etiologic considerations in superior vena cava syndrome. Mayo Clinic Proceed 1981;56: 407–413.
15. Bell DR, Woods RL, Levi JA. Superior vena caval obstruction: a 10–year experience. Med J Aust 1986;145:566–568.
16. Falk S, Fallon M. ABC of palliative care: emergencies. BMJ 1997;315:1525–1528.
17. Urruticoechea A, Mesia R, Dominquez J, et al. Treatment of malignant superior vena cava syndrome by endovascular stent insertion: experience on 52 patients with lung cancer. Lung Cancer 2004;43:209–214.
18. Yedlicka JW, Schultz K, Moncada R. CT findings in superior vena cava obstruction. Sem Roentgenol 1989;24:84–90.
19. Quinadli SD, El Heajjam M, Bruckert F. Helical CT phlebography of the superior vena cava: diagnosis and evaluation of venous obstruction. Am J Roentgen 1999;172:1327–1333.
20. Moncada R, Cardella R, Demos TC. Evaluation of superior vena cava syndrome by axial CT and CT phlebography. Am J Roentgen 1984;143:731–736.
21. Silvestri GA, Tanoue LT, Margolis ML. The noninvasive staging of non-small cell lung cancer: the guidelines. Chest 2003;123: 147S–156S.
22. DeMichele A, Glick J. Cancer-related emergencies. In: Lenhard R, Osteen R, Gansler T, eds. Clinical Oncology. Atlanta, GA: American Cancer Society, 2001:733–764.
23. Sasano S, Onuki T, Mae M. Wallstent endovascular prosthesis for the treatment of superior vena cava syndrome. Japan Thoracic Cardiovasc Surg 2001;49:165–170.
24. Tanigawa N, Sawada S, Mishima K. Clinical outcome of stenting in superior vena cava syndrome associated with malignant tumors: comparison with conventional treatment. Acta Radiologica 1998;39:669–674.
25. Nicholson AA, Ettles DF, Arnold A. Treatment of malignant superior vena cava obstruction: metal stents or radiation therapy. J Vasc Intervent Radiol 1997;8: 781–788.
26. Irving JD, Dondelinger RF, Reidy JF. Gianturco self-expanding stents: clinical experience in the vena cava and large veins. Cardiovasc Intervent Radiol 1992;15:328–333.

27. Gauden SJ. Superior vena cava syndrome induced by bronchogenic carcinoma: is this an oncological emergency? Australas Radiol 1993;37:363–366.
28. National Cancer Institute (NCI). Cancer Information Service: Physicians Desk Query Supportive Care Guideline: Superior Vena Cava Syndrome. http://www.nci.nih.gov/cancertopics/pdq/supportivecare/superior-vena-cava (accessed February 15, 2004).
29. Fiocco M, Krasna, MJ. The management of malignant pleural and pericardial effusions. Hem Onc Clinics N America 1997;11:253–265.
30. Hausheer FH, Yarbro JW. Diagnosis and management of malignant pleural effusions. Sem Oncol 1985;12: 54–75.
31. Andrews CO, Gora ML. Pleural effusions: pathophysiology and management. Ann Pharmacother 1994; 28:894–903.
32. Woodruff R. Palliative Medicine, 2nd ed. Melbourne: Asperula Pty Ltd., 1996:143.
33. American Thoracic Society. Management of malignant pleural effusions. Am J Resp Crit Care Med 2000;162:1987–2001.
34. Erasmus JJ, Patz EF. Treatment of malignant pleural effusions. Curr Opinion Pulm Med 1999;5:250.
35. Sahn SA. Malignancy metastatic to the pleura. Clin Chest Med 1998;19:351–361.
36. Pollak JS. Malignant pleural effusions: treatment with tunneled long-term drainage catheters. Curr Opin Pulm Med 2002; 8:302–307.
37. Grossi F, Pennucci MC, Tixi L, et al. Management of malignant pleural effusions. Drugs 1998;55:47–58.
38. Tattersall DJ. Management of malignant pleural effusion. Aust N Z J Med 1998;28:394–396.
39. Baker GL, Barnes HJ. Superior vena cava syndrome: etiology, diagnosis, and treatment. Am J Crit Care 1992;1:54–64.
40. Kreamer K. Superior vena cava syndrome. In: Gross J, Johnson BL, eds. Handbook of Oncology Nursing, 2nd ed. Boston: Jones and Bartlett, 1994:628–638.
41. Afessa B. Pleural effusions and pneumothoraces in AIDS. Curr Opin Pulm Med 2001;7: 202–209.
42. Armbruster C, Schalleschak J, Vetter N, et al. Pleural effusions in human immunodeficiency virus-infected patients: correlation with concomitant pulmonary diseases. Acta Cytol 1995;39: 698–700.
43. Joseph J, Strange C, Sahn SA. Pleural effusions in hospitalized patients with AIDS. Ann Intern Med 1993;118:856–859.
44. Soubani AO, Michelson MK, Karnik A. Pleural fluid findings in patients with the acquired immunodeficiency syndrome: correlation with concomitant pulmonary disease. South Med J 1999;92: 400–403.
45. Burrows CM, Mathews WC, Colt HG. Predicting survival in patients with recurrent symptomatic malignant pleural effusions: an assessment of the prognostic values of physiologic, morphologic, and quality of life measures of extent of disease. Chest 2000;117:73–78.
46. Heffner J, Nietert P, Barbieri C. Pleural fluid pH as a predictor of survival for patients with malignant pleural effusions. Chest 2000;117:79–86.
47. American Society of Clinical Oncology (ASCO). Optimizing cancer care—the importance of symptom management (Vol II): Malignant pleural effusions. ASCO Curriculum 2001. Dubuque, IA: Kendall/Hunt Publishing Company, 2001:1–27.
48. Chernow B, Sahn SA. Carcinomatous involvement of the pleura. Am J Med 1977;63:695–702.
49. Yano S, Herbst RS, Shinohara H, et al. Production of experimental malignant pleural effusion of human lung adenocarcinoma by inhibition of vascular endothelial growth factor receptor tyrosine kinase phosphorylation. Clin CA Research 2000;6:957–965.
50. Light RW, MacGregor MI, Luchsinger PC, et al. Pleural effusions: the diagnostic separation of transudates and exudates. Ann Intern Med 1972;77:507–513.
51. Gill PS, Akil B, Colletti P, Rarick M, Loweiro C, Bernstein-Singer M. Pulmonary Kaposi's sarcoma: clinical findings and results of therapy. Am J Med 1989;87:57–61.
52. Levine AM. Acquired immunodeficiency syndrome-related lymphoma: clinical aspects. Semin Oncol 2000;27:442–453.
53. Milne ENC, Pistolesi M. Pleural effusions: normal physiology, pathophysiology, and diagnosis. In: Reading the Chest Radiograph: A Physiologic Approach. Patterson S., ed. St. Louis: Mosby-Year Book, 1993:120–163.
54. Black LF. The pleural space and pleural fluid. Mayo Clin Proceed 1972;47:493–506.
55. Meyer PC. Metastatic carcinoma of the pleura. Thorax 1966; 21:437–443.
56. Leff A, Hopewell PC, Costello J. Pleural effusion from malignancy. Ann Intern Med 1978;88:532–537.
57. Ruckdeschel JC, Robinson LA. Management of pleural and pericardial effusions. In: In Berger AM, Portenoy RK, Weissman DE, eds. Principles and Practice of Palliative Care and Supportive Oncology, 2nd ed. Philadelphia: Lippincott Williams & Wilkins, 2002: 389–412.
58. Wailer A. Caroline NL. Handbook of Palliative Care in Cancer. Boston: Butterworth-Heineman, 1996: 217.
59. Vaska K, Wann LS, Sagar KK, et al. Pleural effusion as a cause of right ventricular collapse. Circulation 1992;86:609–617.
60. Kaplan LM, Epstein SK, Schwartz SL, et al. Clinical, echocardiographic, and hemodynamic evidence of cardiac tamponade caused by large pleural effusions. Am J Resp Crit Care Med 1995; 151:904–908.
61. Woodring JH, Loh FK, Kryscio RJ. Mediastinal hemorrhage: an evaluation of radiographic manifestations. Radiology 1984: 23:393–397.
62. Doust BD, Baum JK, Maklad NF. Ultrasonic evaluation of pleural opacities. Radiol 1975;114:135–140.
63. Ravin CE, Chotas HC. Chest radiography. Radiology 1997;204: 593–600.
64. Nemchek AA. Management of malignant pleural effusions. J Vasc Interv Radiol 1998;9:115–120.
65. Gryminski J, Krakowka P, Lypacewicz G. The diagnosis of pleural effusion by ultrasonic and radiologic techniques. Chest 1976;70:83–87.
66. Bartter T, Santarelli R, Akers S, et al. The evaluation of pleural effusion. Chest 1994;106:1209–1214.
67. Martini N, Eisenberg B, Baisden CE. Indications for pleurectomy in malignant effusion. Cancer 1975;35:734–738.
68. Nally AT. Critical care of the patient with lung cancer. AACN Clin Issues: Adv Practice Acute Crit Care 1996;7:79–94.
69. Chernecky C, Shelton B. Pulmonary complications in patients with cancer: diagnostic and treatment information for the noncritical care nurse. AJN 2001;101:24A,24E,24G–24H.
70. Ruckdeschel JC. Management of malignant pleural effusion: an overview. Semin Oncol 1988;15:24–28.
71. Anderson CB, Philpott GW, Ferguson TB. The treatment of malignant pleural effusions. Cancer 1974;33:916–922.

72. Light RW. Malignant pleural effusions. In: Light RW, ed. Pleural Diseases, 3rd ed. Baltimore: Williams and Wilkins, 1995:94–116.
73. Belani CP, Patz EF. Malignant pleural effusion: advances in management. Pittsburgh: University of Pittsburgh Medical Center, 1995, monograph.
74. Antunes G, Neville E. Management of malignant pleural effusions. Thorax 2000;55:981–983.
75. Ratliff JL, Chavez CM, Majchuk A. Re-expansion pulmonary edema. Chest 1973;64:654–656.
76. DeCamp MM, Mentzer SJ, Swanson SJ. Malignant effusive disease of the pleura and pericardium. Chest 1997;112 (Suppl):291S–295S.
77. Clarke K. Effective pain relief with intrapleural analgesia. Nurs Times 1999;95:49–50.
78. Short K, Scheeres D, Mlakar J, et al. Evaluation of intrapleural analgesia in the management of blunt traumatic chest wall pain: a clinical trial. Am Surg 1996;62:488–493.
79. Reigler FX. Pro: Intrapleural anesthesia is useful for thoracic analgesia. Con: Unreliable benefit after thoracotomy—epidural is a better choice. J Cardiothorac Vasc Anesth 1996;10:429–431.
80. McIlvaine WB. Intrapleural anesthesia is useful for thoracic analgesia. Pro: Intrapleural anesthesia is useful for thoracic analgesia. J Cardiothorac Vasc Anesth 1996;10:425–428.
81. Gaeta RR, Marcario A, Brodsky JB, et al. Pain outcomes after thoracotomy: lumbar epidural hydromorphone versus intrapleural bupivacaine. J Cardiothorac Vasc Anesth 1995;9:534–537.
82. Robinson LA, Mouton AL, Fleming WH, et al. Intrapleural doxycycline control of malignant pleural effusions. Am Thorac Surg 1993;55:1115–1122.
83. Piehler JM, Pluth JR, Schaff HV, et al. Surgical management of effusive pericardial disease: influence of extent of pericardial resection on clinical course. J Thoracic Cardiovasc Surg 1985;90: 506–516.
84. Gilkeson RC, Silverman P, Haaga JR. Using urokinase to treat malignant pleural effusions. Am J Roent 1999;173:781–783.
85. Lee KA, Harvey JC, Reich H, et al. Management of malignant pleural effusions with pleuroperitoneal shunting. J Am College of Surg 1994;178:586–588.
86. Holt JW. Malignant pleural effusions. Semin Resp Crit Care Med 1995;16:333–339.
87. Petrou M, Kaplan D, Goldstraw P. Management of recurrent malignant pleural effusions: the complementary role of talc pleurodesis and pleuroperitoneal shunting. Chest 1995;75:801–805.
88. Woodruff R. Palliative Medicine, 2nd ed. Melbourne: Asperula Pty Ltd., 1996:143.
89. Sherman S, Raviskrishnan KP, Patel AS. Optimum anesthesia with intrapleural lidocaine during chemical pleurodesis with tetracycline. Chest 1988;94:533–536.
90. Leslie WK, Kinasewitz GT. Clinical characteristics of the patient with nonspecific pleuritis. Chest 1988;94:603–608.
91. Harvey JC, Erdman CB, Beattie EJ. Early experience with videothorascopic hydrodissection pleurectomy in the treatment of malignant pleural effusion. J Surg Onc 1995;59:243–245.
92. Pollak JS, Burdge CM, Rosenblatt M, et al. Treatment of malignant pleural effusions with tunneled long-term drainage catheters. J Vasc Interventional Radiol 2001;12:201–208.
93. Patz EF Jr, McAdams HP, Goodman PC, et al. Ambulatory sclerotherapy for malignant pleural effusions. Radiol 1996;99: 133–135.
94. Dudgeon DJ, Lertzman M, Askew GR. Physiological changes and clinical correlates of dyspnea in cancer outpatients. J Pain Symptom Manage 2001;21:373–379.
95. Braunwald E. Cardiac tampanade. In: Braunwald E, ed. Heart Disease: A Textbook of Cardiovascular Medicine. Philadelphia: W.B. Saunders, 1997:1446–1496.
96. Weinberg BA, Conces DJ Jr, Waller BF. Cardiac manifestations of noncardiac tumors. Part 1: Direct effects. Clin Cardiol 1989;12: 289–296.
97. Palatianos GM, Thurer RJ, Pompeo MQ, Kaiser GA. Clinical experience with subxiphoid drainage of pericardial effusions. Ann Thorac Surg 1989;48:381–385.
98. Mills SA, Graeber GM, Nelson MG. Therapy of malignant tumors involving the pericardium. In: Roth J, Ruckdeschel JC, Weisenburger T, eds. Thoracic Oncology, 2nd ed. Philadelphia: W.B. Saunders, 1995:492–513.
99. Knoop T, Willenberg K. Cardiac tamponade. Semin Oncol Nurs 1999;15:168–175.
100. McAllister H, Hall R, Cooley D. Tumors of the heart and pericardium. Curr Prob Cardiol 1999;24: 57–116.
101. National Hospital Discharge Summary: Annual Survey 1993. U.S. Department of Health and Human Services, Public Health Service. Centers for Disease Control and Prevention, National Center for Health Statistics. Hyattsville, MD, 1993, DHHS Publication No. (PHS) 93–1775.
102. Bullock B. Altered cardiac function. In: Bullock B, Henze R, eds. Focus on Pathophysiology. Philadelphia: Lippincott Williams & Wilkins, 2000: 455–502.
103. Lawler P. Effusions. In: Yarbro C, Frogge M, Goodman M, eds. Cancer Symptom Management, 2nd ed. Boston: Jones and Bartlett, 1999:419–433.
104. Chabner B, Myers C. Antitumor antibiotics. In: DeVita V, Hellman S, Rosenberg S, eds. Cancer Principles and Practice of Oncology, 4th ed. Philadelphia: J. B. Lippincott, 1993.
105. Harken A, Hammond G, Edmunds L. Pericardial diseases. In: Edmunds L, ed. Cardiac Surgery in the Adult. New York: McGraw Hill, 1997:1303–1317.
106. Smeltzer S, Bare B. Oncology: Nursing the patient with cancer. In: Smeltzer S, Bare B, eds. Brunner and Suddarth's Textbook of Medical-Surgical Nursing, 8th ed. Philadelphia: Lippincott-Raven, 1996: 309–316.
107. Spodick DH. Effective management of congestive cardiomyopathy: relation to ventricular structure and function. Arch Intern Med 1982;4:689–692.
108. Miller RR, McGregor DH. Hemorrhage from carcinoma of the lung. Cancer 1980;46:200–205.
109. Pories WJ, Gaudiani VA. Cardiac tamponade. Surg Clin N Am 1975;55:573–589.
110. Beauchamp K. Pericardial tamponade: an oncologic emergency. Clin J Oncol Nurs 1998;2:85–95.
111. Spodick DH. Pericardial windows are suboptimal. Am J Cardiol 1983;51:607.
112. Ruckdeschel JC. Preoperative paclitaxel plus carboplatin for patients with intermediate-risk non-small cell lung cancer. Semin Oncol 1996;23:62–67.
113. Freeman GL, LeWinter MM. Pericardial adaptations during chronic cardiac dilation in dogs. Circ Res 1984;54:294–300.
114. Press OW, Livingston R. Management of malignant pericardial effusion and tamponade. JAMA 1987;8:1088–1092.
115. Fowler NO, Gabel M. The hemodynamic effects of cardiac tamponade: mainly the result of atrial, not ventricular, compression. Circulation 1985;71:154–157.
116. Posner J. Neurologic Complications of Cancer. Philadelphia: F.A. Davis, 1995.

117. Buck M, Ingle JN, Giulani ER, Gordon JR, Therneau TM. Pericardial effusion in women with breast cancer. Cancer 1987;60:263–269.
118. Shepherd F. Malignant pericardial effusion. Curr Opin Oncol 1997;9:170–174.
119. Vaitkus PT, Herrmann HC, LeWinter MM. Treatment of malignant pericardial effusion. JAMA 1994;272:59–64.
120. Stouffer GA, Sheahan RG, Lenihan DJ, et al. Diagnosis and management of chronic pericardial effusions. Am J Med Sciences 2001:322:79–87.
121. Mangan C. Malignant pericardial effusions: pathophysiology and clinical correlates. Oncol Nurs Forum 1992;19:1215–1223.
122. Nguyen DM, Schrump DS. Malignant pleural and pericardial effusions. In: DeVita V, Hellman S, Rosenberg S, eds. Cancer Principles and Practice of Oncology, 7th ed. Philadelphia: Lippincott Williams & Wilkins, 2005: 2381–2392.
123. Dietz K, Flaherty A. Oncologic emergencies. In: Groenwald S, Frogge M, Goodman M, Yarbro C, eds. Cancer Nursing, 3rd ed. Boston: Jones and Bartlett, 1993:800–839.
124. Bickley L. Bates' Guide to Physical Examination and History Taking, 7th ed. Philadelphia: Lippincott Williams & Wilkins, 1999.
125. Gueberman B, Fowler N, Engel P. Cardiac tamponade in medical patients. Circulation 1987;64:633–640.
126. Keefe D. Cardiovascular emergencies in the cancer patient. Semin Oncol 2000;27:244–255.
127. Kopecky SL, Callahan JA, Tajik AJ, Seward JB. Percutaneous pericardial catheter drainage: report of 42 consecutive cases. Am J. Cardiol 1986:7:633–635.
128. Tsang TS, Freeman, WK, Sinah LJ, Seward JB. Echocardiographically guided pericardiocentesis: evolution and state-of-the-art technique. Mayo Clin Proc 1998;73:647–652.
129. Callahan JA, Seward JB, Tajik AJ. Cardiac tamponade: pericardiocentesis directed by two-dimensional echocardiography. Mayo Clin Proc 1985;60:344–347.
130. Tsang TS, Barnes ME, Hayes SN, Freeman WK, Dearani JA, Butler SL. Clinical and echocardiographic characteristics of significant pericardial effusions following cardiothoracic surgery and outcomes of echo-guided pericardiocentesis for management: Mayo Clinic experience, 1979–1998. Chest 1999;116:322–331.
131. Tsang TS, Seward JB, Barnes ME, Bailey KR, Sinah LJ, Urban LH. Outcomes of primary and secondary treatment of pericardial effusion in patients with malignancy. Mayo Clin Proc 2000; 73:248–253.
132. Chong HH, Plotnick GD. Pericardial effusion and tamponade: evaluation, imaging, modalities, and management. Compr Ther 1995;21:378–385.
133. Shepherd F. Malignant pericardial effusion. Curr Opin Onc 1997;9:170–174.
134. Davis S, Ramboti P, Grigani F. Intrapericardial tetracycline sclerosis in the treatment of malignant pericardial effusion: an analysis of thirty-three cases. J Clin Oncol 1984;2:631–636.
135. Lissoni P, Barni S, Ardiozzoia A. Intracavitary administration of interleukin-2 as palliative therapy for neoplastic effusion. Tumori 1992;78:118–120.
136. Maher EA, Shepherd FA, Todd T Jr. Pericardial sclerosis as the primary management of malignant pericardial effusion and cardiac tamponade. J Thorac Cardiovasc Surg 1996;112:637–643.
137. Ziskind AA, Pearce AC, Lemmon CC, et al. Percutaneous balloon pericardiotomy for the treatment of cardiac tamponade and large pericardial effusions: descriptions of technique and report of the first 50 cases. J Am Coll Cardiol 1993;21:1–5.
138. Jackson G, Keane D, Mishra B. Percutaneous balloon pericardiotomy in the management of recurrent malignant of recurrent malignant pericardial effusions. Br Heart J 1992;68:613–615.
139. Shapira OM, Aldea GS, Fonger, JD, Shemin RJ. Video-assisted thoracic surgical techniques in the diagnosis and management of pericardial effusion in patients with advanced lung cancer. Chest 1993;104:1262–1263.
140. Hurley JP, McCarthy J, Wood AE. Retrospective analysis of the utility of video-assisted thoracic surgery in 100 consecutive procedures. Eur J Cardiothorac Surg 1994;8:589–592.
141. Liu H, Chang C, Lin P, et al. Thoracoscopic management of effusive pericardial disease: indication and technique. Ann Thorac Surg 1994;58:1695–1697.
142. Lewis MM, Read CA. Hemoptysis, part 1: identifying the cause. J Resp Dis 2000;21:335–341.
143. Corder R. Hemoptysis. Emerg Med Clinics N Am 2003;21: 421–435.
144. Harries ML, Morrison M. Management of unilateral vocal cord paralysis by injection medialization with Teflon paste—quantitative results. Ann Otol Rhinol Laryngol 1998;107: 332–336.
145. Schwartz AR, Smith PL, Kashima HK, et al. Respiratory function of the upper airways. In: Murray JF, Nadel JA, eds. Respiratory Medicine. Philadelphia: W.B. Saunders, 1994:1451–1470.
146. Lipchik RJ. Hemoptysis. In: Berger AM, Portenoy RK, Weissman DE, eds. Principles and Practice of Palliative Care and Supportive Oncology, 2nd ed. Philadelphia: Lippincott Williams & Wilkins, 2002: 372–377.
147. Rizzi A, Rocco G, Robustellini M, et al. Results of surgical management of tuberculosis: experience in 206 patients undergoing operation. Ann Thoracic Surg 1995;59:896–900.
148. Chan C, Elazar-Popovic E, Farver C, et al. Endobronchial involvement in uncommon diseases. J Bronch 1996;3:53–63.
149. Levine MN, Raskob G, Landefeld S, et al. Hemorrhagic complications of anticoagulant treatment. Chest 1995;108:276–290S.
150. Levine MN, Goldhaber SZ, Gore JM, et al. Hemorrhagic complications of thrombolytic therapy in the treatment of myocardial infarction and venous thromboembolism. Chest 1995;108: 291–301S.
151. Corey R, Hla KM. Major and massive hemoptysis: reassessment of conservative management. Am J Med Sci 1987;294:301–309.
152. Luce K, O'Donnell EE, Morton AR. A combination of calcitonin and bisphosphonate for the emergency treatment of severe tumor-induced hypercalcemia. Calcif Tissue Int 1993;52:70–71.
153. Boyars M. Current strategies for diagnosing and managing hemoptysis. J Crit Ill 1999;14:148–156.
154. Lewis MM, Read CA. Hemoptysis, part 2: treatment options. J Resp Dis 2000;21:392–394.
155. Saltzman HA, Alavi A, Greespan RH. Value of the ventilation/perfusion scan in acute pulmonary embolism: results of the prospective investigation of pulmonary embolism diagnosis. JAMA 1990;263:2753–2759.
156. Colice GL. Hemoptysis: three questions that can direct management. Postgrad Med 1996;100:227–236.
157. Awan AM, Weichselbarum RR. Palliative radiotherapy. Hem Onc Clinics N Am 1990;4:1169–1181.
158. Makker HK, Barnes PC. Fatal hemoptysis from the pulmonary artery as a late complication of pulmonary irradiation. Thorax 1991;46:609–610.
159. Villaneuva AG, Lo TCM, Beamis JF. Endobronchial brachytherapy. Clin Chest Med 1995;16: 445–454.

160. Gollins SW, Burt PA, Barber PV, et al. High dose rate intraluminal radiotherapy for carcinoma of the bronchus: outcome of treatment of 406 patients. Radiother Oncol 1994;33:31–40.
161. Sutedgja G, Baris G, Schaake-Koning C, et al. High dose rates brachytherapy in patients with local recurrences after radiotherapy of non-small cell lung cancer. Int J Radiation Oncol Biol Phys 1992;24: 551–553.
162. Hatlevoll R, Karlsen KO, Skovlund E. Endobronchial radiotherapy for malignant bronchial obstruction or recurrence. Acta Oncologica 1999;38: 999–1004.
163. Khanavkar B, Stern P, Alberti W, et al. Complications associated with brachytherapy alone or with laser in lung cancer. Chest 1991;99:1062–1065.
164. Langendijk JA, Tjwa MKT, de Jong JMA, et al. Massive hemoptysis after radiotherapy in inoperable non-small cell lung carcinoma: is endobronchial brachytherapy really a risk factor? Radiother Oncol 1998;49:175–183.
165. Aurora R, Milite F, Vander Els N. Respiratory emergencies, Semin Oncol 2000;27:256–269.
166. Schray MF, McDougall JC, Martinez A, et al. Management of malignant airway compromise with laser and low dose brachytherapy: the Mayo Clinic experience. Chest 1988;93: 264–269.
167. Hayakawa K, Tanaka F, Torizuka T, et al. Bronchial artery embolization for hemoptysis: immediate and long-term results. Cardiovasc Intervent Rad 1992;15:154–158.
168. Adelman M, Haponik E, Bleeker E, et al. Cryptogenic hemoptysis. Ann Intern Med 1985;102:829–834.
169. Mal H, Rullon I, Mellot F, et al. Immediate and long-term results of bronchial artery embolization for life-threatening hemoptysis. J Crit Ill 1999;14: 148–156.
170. Brinson G, Noone P, Mauro M, et al. Bronchial artery embolization for the treatment of hemoptysis in patients with cystic fibrosis. Am J Resp Crit Care Med 1998;157:1951–1958.
171. Hirscherg B, Biran I, Glazer M, et al. Hemoptysis: etiology, evaluation, and outcome in a tertiary referral hospital. Chest 1997; 112:440–444.
172. Tan SJ. Recognition and treatment of oncologic emergencies. J Infusion Nurs 2002;25:182–188.
173. Quinn J, DeAngelis L. Neurologic emergencies in the cancer patient. Semin Oncol 2000;27:311–321.
174. Byrne TN. Metastatic epidural spinal cord compression. In: Black P, Loeffler J, eds. Cancer of the Nervous System. London: Blackwell Scientific, 1997:664–673.
175. Byrne TN. Spinal cord compression from epidural metastases. N Engl J Med 1992;327:614–619.
176. Wilkes G. Neurological disturbances. In: Yarbro C, Frogge M, Goodman M, eds. Cancer Symptom Management, 2nd ed. Boston: Jones and Bartlett, 1999: 344–381.
177. Posner J. Neurologic Complications of Cancer. Philadelphia: F.A. Davis, 1995:111–142.
178. Portenoy RK.Chronic nociceptive pain syndromes: cancer pain. In: North RB, Levy RM, eds. Neurosurgical Management of Pain. New York: Springer-Verlag, 1997:62–74.
179. Perrin RG, Janjan NA, Langford LA. Spinal axis metastases. In: Levin VA, ed. Cancer in the Nervous System. New York: Churchill Livingstone, 1996:259.
180. Caraceni A, Martini C, Simonetti F. Neurological disturbances in advanced cancer. In: Doyle D, Hanks G, Cherny N, Calman K, eds. Oxford Textbook of Palliative Medicine. Oxford: Oxford University Press, 2004:702–726.
181. Weinstein SM. Management of spinal cord and cauda equina compression. In: Berger AM, Portenoy RK, Weissman DE, eds. Principles and Practice of Palliative Care and Supportive Oncology, 2nd ed. Philadelphia: Lippincott Williams & Wilkins, 2002: 532–543.
182. Belford K. Central nervous system cancers. In: Groenwald S, Frogge M, Goodman M, Yarbro C, eds. Cancer Nursing, 4th ed. Boston: Jones and Bartlett, 1997:721–741.
183. Henze R. Traumatic and vascular injuries of the central nervous system. In: Bullock B, Henze R, eds. Focus on Pathophysiology. Philadelphia: Lippincott Williams & Wilkins, 2000: 938–978.
184. Bucholtz J. Metastatic epidural spinal cord compression. Semin Oncol Nurs 1999;15:150–159.
185. Fuller BG, Heiss JD, Oldfield EH. Spinal cord compression. In: Devita VT, Hellman S, Rosenberg SA, eds. Cancer Principles and Practice of Oncology, 6th ed. Philadelphia: Lippincott Williams & Wilkins, 2001:2617–2632.
186. Hewitt DJ, Foley KM. Neuroimaging of pain. In: Greenberg JO, ed. Neuroimaging. New York: McGraw-Hill, 1995:41.
187. Frank JA, Ling A, Patronas NJ. Detection of malignant bone tumors: MRI imaging vs. scintigraphy. Am J Roentgenol 1990; 155:1043–1048.
188. Algra PR, Bloem JL, Tissing H. Detection of vertebral body metastases: comparison between MR imaging and bone scintigraphy. Radiograph 1991;11: 219–232.
189. St. Amour TE, Hodges SC, Laakman RW, et al. MRI of the Spine. New York: Raven, 1994:435.
190. Sze G. Magnetic resonance imaging in the evaluation of spinal tumors. Cancer 1991;67:1229–1241.
191. Burger EL, Lindeque BG. Sacral and non-spinal tumors presenting as a backache: a retrospective study of 17 patients. Acta Orthoped Scand 1994;65: 344–346.
192. Abrahm JL. Management of pain and spinal cord compression in patients with advanced cancer. Ann Intern Med 1999;131:37–46.
193. Gilbert RW, Kim JH, Posner JB. Epidural spinal cord compression from metastatic tumor: diagnosis and treatment. Ann Neurol 1978;3:40–51.
194. Hainline B, Tuzynski MH, Posner JB. Ataxia in epidural spinal cord compression. Neurol 1992;42:2193–2195.
195. Gudesblatt M, Cohen JA, Gerber O. Truncal ataxia presumably due to malignant spinal cord compression. Ann Neurol 1987;21:511–512.
196. Patchell R, Tibbs PA, Regine WF, et al. A randomized trial of direct decompressive surgical resection in the treatment of spinal cord compression caused by metastasis. Proceed Am Society Clin Oncol 2003;22(abstract 2):1.
197. Greenberg HS, Kim JH, Posner JB. Epidural spinal cord compression from metastatic tumor: results from a new treatment protocol. Ann Neurol 1980;8:1–366.
198. Delattre JY, Arbit E, Thaler HT. A dose response study of dexamethasone in a model of spinal cord compression caused by epidural tumor. J Neurosurg 1989;70:920–925.
199. Loblaw D, Laperriere N. Emergency treatment of malignant extradural spinal cord compression: an evidence-based guideline. J Clin Oncol 1998;16:1613–1624.
200. Grant R, Papadopoulos SM, Greenberg HS. Metastatic epidural spinal cord compression. Neurol Clin 1991;9:825–841.
201. Jenis LG, Dunn EJ, An HS. Metastatic disease of the cervical spine. A review. Clin Orthoped 1999;359:89–103.

202. Flower CDR, Jackson JE. The role of radiology in the investigation and management of patients with hemoptysis. Clin Radiol 1996;51:391–400.
203. Sitton E. Nursing implications of radiation therapy. In: Itano J, Toaka K, eds. Core Curriculum for Oncology Nursing, 3rd ed. Philadelphia: W.B. Saunders, 1998:616–629.
204. Clayton, K. Cancer-related hypercalcemia: how to spot it, how to manage it. AJN 1997;97:42–48.
205. Morton AR, Ritch PS. Hypercalcemia. In: Berger AM, Portenoy RK, Weissman DE, eds. Principles and Practice of Palliative Care and Supportive Oncology, 2nd ed. Philadelphia: Lippincott Williams & Wilkins, 2002:493–507.
206. Warrell RP. Metabolic emergencies. In: Devita VT, Hellman S, Rosenberg SA, eds. Cancer Principles and Practice of Oncology, 6th ed. Philadelphia: Lippincott Williams & Wilkins, 2001: 2633–2645.
207. Bajorunas D. Clinical manifestations of cancer-related hypecalcemia. Semin Oncol 1990;17:16–24.
208. Mundy GR. Pathophysiology of cancer-associated hypercalcemia. Semin Oncol 1990;17:10–15.
209. Ralston SH. Pathogenesis and management of cancer-associated hypercalcemia. In: Rubens RD, Fogelman I, eds. Bone Metastases: Diagnosis and Treatment. New York: Springer Verlag, 1991:149–169.
210. Gaich G, Burtis WJ. The diagnosis and treatment of malignancy-associated hypercalcemia. New Eng J Med 1992;326:1196–1203.
211. Nussbaum SR. Pathophysiology and management of severe hypercalcemia. Endocrinol Metabol Clin North Am 1993; 2:343–362.
212. Kovacs CS, MacDonald SM, Chik CL, et al. Hypercalcemia of malignancy in the palliative care patient: a treatment strategy. J Pain Symptom Manage 1995;10:224–232.
212a. Lange B, D'Angio G, Ross AJ, et al. Oncologic emergencies. In: Pizzo PA, Poplack DG, eds. Principles and Practice of Pediatric Oncology. Philadelphia: J.B. Lippincott, 1989:799–819.
213. King PA. Oncologic emergencies: assessment, identification, and interventions in the emergency department. J Emerg Nurs 1995;21:213–218.
214. Burtis WJ. Parathyroid hormone-related protein: structure, function, and measurement. Clin Chem 1992;38:2171–2183.
215. Mercadante S. Malignant bone pain: pathophysiology and treatment. Pain 1997;69:1–18.
216. Kuebler KK. Palliative nursing care for the patient experiencing end-stage renal failure. Urol Nurs 2001:21:167–168,171–178.
217. Flombaum CD. Oncologic emergencies: metabolic emergencies. Semin Oncol 2000;27:322–334.
218. Djulbvegovic B, Wheatley K, Ross J, Clark O, Bos G, et al. Bisphosphonates in multiple myeloma. Cochrane Database Syst Rev 2002;3:CD0031188.
219. Pavlakis N, Stockler PN. Bisphosphonates for breast cancer. Cochrane Library Database Rev, 2003, 2: http://80–www.cochranelibrary.com.proxy.library.vcu.edu/Abs/ab0003474.htm, (accessed October 23, 2003).
220. American Society of Clinical Oncology (ASCO). Optimizing cancer care—the importance of symptom management: malignant pleural effusions. ASCO Curriculum. Dubuque, IA: Kendall/Hunt Publishing Company, 2001:1–27.
221. Wong R, Wiffen PJ. Bisphosphonates for the relief of pain secondary to bone metastases. Cochrane Library, 2003, 2, http://80cochranelibrary.com.proxy.library.vcu.edu/Abs/ab002068.htm, (accessed October 23, 2003).
222. Ralston SH, Gallacher SJ, Patel U, et al. Comparison of three intravenous bisphosphonates in cancer-associated hypercalcemia. Lancet 1989;2:1180–1182.
223. Gallacher SJ, Ralston SH, Fraser WD. A comparison of low versus high dose pamidronate in cancer-associated hypercalcemia. Bone Mineral 1991; 15:249–256.
224. Gucalp R, Theriault R, Gill I, et al. Comparative study of pamidronate disodium and etidronate disodium in the treatment of cancer-related hypercalcemia. J Clin Oncol 1992;10:134–142.
225. Purohit OP, Radstone CR, Anthony C, et al. A randomized double-blind comparison of intravenous pamidronate and clodronate in the hypercalcemia of malignancy. Br J Cancer 1995;72:1289–1293.
226. Major P, Lortholary A, Hon J, et al. Zoledronic acid is more effective than pamidronate for hypercalcemia of malignancy. Evid based Oncol 2001;2: 159–162.
227. Thurlimann B, Waldburger R, Senn HF, et al. Plicamycin and pamidronate in symptomatic tumor-related hypercalcemia: a prospective randomized crossover trial. Ann Oncol 1992;3:619–623.
228. Roemer-Becuwe C, Vigano A, Romano F, et al. Safety of subcutaneous clodronate and efficacy in hypercalcemia of malignancy: a novel route of administration. J Pain Symptom Manage 2003;26:843–848.
229. Warrell RP Jr, Bockman RS, Coonley CJ, et al. Gallium nitrate inhibits calcium resorption from bone and is effective treatment for cancer-related hypercalcemia. J Clin Invest 1984; 73:1487–1490.
230. Smith IE, Powles T.J. Mithramycin for hypercalcemia associated with myeloma and other malignancies. BMJ 1975;1:268–269.
231. Mundy GR. Mechanisms of bone metastasis. Cancer 1997;80: 1546–1556.
232. Koo WS, Jeon DS, Ahn SJ, et al. Calcium-free dialysis for the management of hypercalcemia. Nephron 1996;72:424–428.
233. Leehey DJ, Ing TS. Correction of hypercalcemia and hypophosphatemia by hemodialysis using a conventional, calcium-containing dialysis solution enriched with phosphorus. Am J Kidney Dis 1997;29:288–290.

24

Patti Knight, Laura A. Espinosa, and Eduardo Bruera

Sedation for Refractory Symptoms and Terminal Weaning

You wouldn't let a dog suffer like this!—Wife of terminal cancer patient with severe dyspnea from obstructive terminal lung cancer before palliative sedation

I wish everyone could see all the tubes and the equipment that it took to sustain my husband in a lifeless state of nonexistence, only then to die of cancer. He looked so peaceful after we removed all the tubes and equipment that sustained him.—Wife of dying patient in intensive care unit

- ***Key Points***
- *Palliative sedation is sedation used to control refractory and unendurable symptoms at the end of life when control of these symptoms is not possible with less aggressive measures.*
- *Determining refractoriness of symptoms and prognosis of hours to days to live is difficult and requires assessment and management by skilled practitioners with advanced palliative training.*
- *Patient/family/proxy involvement is critical in decision-making concerning use of palliative sedation or terminal weaning. Clear communication with significant others, clear documentation of the meeting, and informed consent are necessary.*
- *Withholding or withdrawing life support has increased dramatically, from 51% of all intensive cae unit (IXU) deaths in 1987 to 90% in 1993.*[24,25]
- *Nursing professionals in the acute units and the ICU should train new nurses in the skills required to withdraw and withhold treatment. These skills do not come easily; a concerted effort should be made to provide proper training to ensure patients a painless, dignified, peaceful death.*
- *The principle of double effect holds that an act with more than one potential effect (at least one good and one bad) is ethical if certain conditions are met. For example, medications administered in the process of terminal weaning from a ventilator or palliative sedation for refractory dyspnea are intended to provide comfort rather than hasten death.*

In the United States, approximately 2.5 million people die each year, with >60% of those deaths occurring in hospitals.[1] These statistics are alarming and support the public's concern for the dying. The results of a survey by the Last Acts Coalition, funded by the Robert Wood Johnson Foundation, suggested that the public feels that deaths in hospital settings are not well managed; 93% of respondents stated that it was "very important" or "somewhat important" to improve how the health care system cares for dying Americans.[2] This survey also stated that patients and their family members clearly want to be involved in decision-making (42%) and to be comfortable at the end of life, with well-managed symptoms (39%) and with care that does not exhaust their life savings (73%).

Palliative care providers are faced with the challenge of managing a multitude of complex symptoms in terminally ill patients. Although many of these symptoms respond to skilled palliative management, others may remain refractory to treatment.[3–7] Suffering at the end of life involves physical, psychological, social, and spiritual distress. In most situations, multidisciplinary palliative interventions provide effective comfort.[6,7] However, in some instances, suffering becomes refractory and unbearable.[8] Information about end-of-life decision-making is scarce and usually is obtained after the death by retrospective research methods. Therefore, decisions about starting or forgoing potentially life-prolonging or life-shortening therapy are not well understood.[9]

Research and experience suggest that much work must be done in palliative care in the areas of sedation and advanced therapy decision-making, both before and at the end of life. This chapter explores the use of palliative sedation and terminal weaning in the hospital setting. Specifically, it presents case studies involving palliative sedation and withholding or withdrawing life support, definitions of palliative sedation, incidence of sedation use, reasons for sedation, sedative medications, treatment locations, guidelines for use of sedation, nursing care, ethical issues, informed consent, time to death, and the role of the nurse caregiver.

The following cases provide examples of clinical situations in which decision-making regarding sedation and terminal weaning was required.

CASE STUDY I

Mr. M, a 35-Year-Old Man with Metastatic Lung Cancer

Mr. M, a 35-year-old Asian patient with widely metastatic lung cancer, was transferred to the acute palliative inpatient unit for management of severe delirium. His mother and his life partner, a nurse, accompanied the patient to the unit. He was also under psychiatric care for bipolar disorder and was taking six psychotropic mediations. Although Mr. M. had uncontrolled large muscle movements, he was arousable and could follow simple commands. Both his mother and his significant other were very distressed. This is a fairly typical patient presentation to an acute palliative unit. Approximately 25% to 35% of this type of delirium is reversible.[10]

CASE STUDY II

Mr. Z, a 52-Year-Old Man with Mesothelioma

Mr. Z, a 52-year-old man was admitted to the intensive care unit (ICU) status post left pneumonectomy with mesothelioma in his remaining lung. He had been married for 30 years and had two adult children: a 23-year-old daughter and 26-year-old son. He was awake and alert but ventilator dependent, with a tracheostomy, and in renal failure. Renal dialysis was being discussed by the physicians. The patient was surrounded by his wife, daughter, and family friends. When the patient was informed that his lung cancer was metastatic, he expressed his desire to go home and discontinue mechanical ventilation. The patient's request to discontinue mechanical ventilation was unrealistic but began the dialogue for terminal weaning.

Definitions

There is no standardized or consistent search term for palliative sedation across databases. The phrase "terminal sedation" was first used by Enck,[11] who employed the term after a review of patient cases in which physical symptoms were treated with sedation at the end of life. Since that time, numerous efforts have been made to define terminal sedation clearly and to separate it from sedation used in other medical settings.[4–7,12–14] Terminology for palliative sedation varies and includes palliative sedation,[4,6,7,13] terminal sedation,[8] total sedation,[15] sedation for intractable symptoms,[16] and sedation for distress in the imminently dying.[4] Palliative sedation has also been termed "slow euthanasia,"[17] but terms such as this should not be used, because the intent of palliative sedation should be comfort rather than hastening death. Currently, most authors have elected to use the term "palliative sedation."[6,7]

At the authors' institution, the term "palliative sedation" is used. It is defined as the monitored use of medications (midazolam or propofol) that induce sedation to control refractory and unendurable symptoms near the end of life when control of these symptoms is not possible with less aggressive measures. The purpose is to control symptoms, not to hasten death. The acceptance of the term "palliative sedation" over "terminal sedation" has evolved to emphasize the difference between management of refractory symptoms and euthanasia. Table 24–1

Table 24–1
Palliative Sedation Definitions

Euthanasia: the "deliberate termination of life of a patient by active intervention at the request of the patient in the setting of uncontrolled suffering" (Cherny [2000], reference 63).

Existential suffering (sometimes referred to as terminal anguish): refractory psychological symptoms (Lanuke et al. [2003], reference 35).

Imminent death: death that is expected to occur within hours to days based on the person's condition, disease progression, and symptom constellation.

Intent: the purpose or state of mind at the time of an action. Intent of the patient/proxy and health care provider is a critical issue in ethical decision-making regarding palliative sedation. Relief of suffering, not hastening or causing death, is the intent of palliative sedation.

Palliative sedation: the monitored use of medications intended to provide relief of refractory symptoms by inducing varying degrees of unconsciousness, but not death, in terminally ill patients (Hospice and Palliative Nurses Association [2003], reference 55).

Double effect: in terminal sedation, an act with more than one potential effect (one good and one bad) is ethical if (1) the intended end (relief of distressing symptoms) is a good one, (2) the bad effect (death) is foreseen but not intended, (3) the bad effect is not the means of bringing about the good effect (death is not what relieves the distress), and (4) the good effect outweighs the bad effect (in a dying patient, the risk of hastening death for the benefit of comfort is appropriate) (Thorns [2002], reference 84).

Refractory symptom: a symptom that cannot be adequately controlled in a tolerable time frame despite the aggressive use of usual therapies and that seems unlikely to be adequately controlled by further invasive or noninvasive therapies without excessive or intolerable acute or chronic side effects.

Terminal weaning (slow withdrawal): removal of mechanical ventilation, which is performed by gradually reducing the fraction of inspired oxygen (F_{IO_2}) and/or mandatory ventilator rate, leading to the development of hypoxemia and hypercarbia, when the patient is not expected to survive.[18,20]

Terminal extubation (abrupt withdrawal): removal of an endotracheal tube.[19]

lists common terms used in relation to palliative sedation and terminal weaning.

The term "terminal wean" is used when mechanical ventilation is withdrawn and the patient is not expected to survive.[18] In 1983, Grenvik was the first to describe a systematic approach to ventilator withdrawal, suggesting a gradual reduction in the ventilator setting over several hours.[19] Many strong opinions exist regarding slow withdrawal versus abrupt withdrawal. A commonly used expression is "terminal extubation," which is removal of the endotracheal tube. This technique usually occurs after administration of boluses of sedatives or analgesics, or both. Another term used to describe this technique is "terminal wean," which is performed by gradually reducing the fraction of inspired oxygen (FIO_2) and/or mandatory ventilator rate, which may lead to the development of hypoxemia or hypercarbia or both.[20] The decision to remove the endotracheal tube during or after a terminal weaning process is practitioner dependent at this time. Perhaps best practices could be decided by further research.

Incidence of Use

It is difficult to determine how often palliative sedation occurs in practice. The exact frequency of palliative sedation is unknown, but is reported to be used in 5% to 52% of dying patients. The wide variation results in part from inconsistencies in definition and reporting and from cultural differences.[4–7,21] Because patients with refractory symptoms are often hospitalized, 81% of the reported cases of palliative sedation occur in inpatient settings such as a hospital or hospice.[13]

Approximately half of those who die in a hospital have been cared for in an ICU within the previous 3 days, and one third of them spend at least 10 days in the ICU during their final hospitalization.[22] In 1995, 20% of all deaths in the United States occurred in an ICU.[20,22] Many studies in the United States have shown that the majority of ICU deaths involve withholding or withdrawing life-sustaining treatments.[23] Withholding or withdrawing life support has increased dramatically, from 51% of all ICU deaths in 1987 to 90% in 1993.[24,25]

A 1997 survey of the Critical Care section of the American Thoracic Society revealed that 96% of the physician respondents had withheld or withdrawn some form of life support.[26] A survey by Luce and Pendergast demonstrated wide geographical variation in the proportion of deaths in ICUs that are preceded by withdrawal of life support (0% to 79%) and the proportion that are preceded by a do-not-resuscitate (DNR) order (0% to 83%).[27] Other studies have shown that 70% to 90% of ICU patients who die do so as a consequence of a decision to withhold or withdraw life support.[25]

In a 1992 survey of Society of Critical Care Medicine physicians about general ICU patients in need of extubation, 33% preferred terminal weaning, 13% preferred extubation, and the remainder used both.[28] Surgeons and anesthesiologists were more likely to use terminal weaning, and internists and pediatricians were more likely to use extubation. The primary advantage of terminal weaning, including administration of sedatives and analgesics, is that patients do not develop any signs of upper airway obstruction during the withdrawal process. Terminal weaning can be viewed as less disruptive than extubation, reducing the anxiety of family and caregivers. On the other hand, it has been argued that the principal advantages of extubation are that the dying process is not prolonged and the patient is returned to a more natural appearance.[25]

Reasons for Sedation

Although sedation has been used to control noxious symptoms and for surgical anesthesia, its use at the end of life has not been so generally accepted.[13,17,29–31] Common symptoms at the end of life include pain, dyspnea, delirium, and nausea and vomiting, as well as hopelessness, remorse, anxiety, and loss of meaning for the patient.[4,5] Palliative sedation is most commonly used for physical symptoms that are not responding to aggressive symptom management and are causing life to become unbearable. Table 24–2 outlines common symptoms for which palliative sedation is used. Fainsinger and associates,[32] in a multicenter international study, found that 1% to 4% of terminally ill patients needed sedation for pain, 0% to 6% for nausea and vomiting, 0% to 13% for dyspnea, and 9% to 23% for delirium. In a review of 27 reports, 342 patients had more than one symptom.[13] Chater's survey of palliative care experts found that more than half of patients had more than one symptom and that 34% received sedation for nonphysical symptoms such as anguish, fear, panic, anxiety, terror, and emotional, spiritual or psychological distress.[8]

The concept of refractoriness of nonphysical symptoms or existential suffering is not as clear.[7,8,32,33] Although there is no clear consensus on palliative sedation for existential suffering, the Oregon experience with physician-assisted suicide indicates that patients want assisted suicide to avoid dependence on others and to control the timing and manner of their death.[34] Psychological suffering is a more nebulous symptom for sedation, but it can be just as distressful and refractory as physical

Table 24–2
Symptoms Requiring Palliative Sedation

Symptom	Frequency (%)
Agitation/restlessness	26
Pain	21
Confusion	14
Shortness of breath	12
Muscle twitching	11
Anguish	9
Other	7

Source: Cowen and Palmer (2002), reference 6.

Table 24–3
Refractory Physical Symptoms

Symptom	Considerations Before Defining a Symptom As Refractory
Agitation and confusion	Discontinue all nonessential medications
	Change required medications to ones less likely to cause delirium
	Check for bladder distention and rectal impaction
	Evaluate for undiagnosed or undertreated pain
	Review role of hydration therapy
	Consider evaluation and therapy for potentially reversible processes, such as hypoxia, hyponatremia, and hypercalcemia
Pain	Maximize opioid, nonopioid, and adjuvant analgesics including agent, route, and schedule
	Consider other therapies, including invasive/neurosurgical procedures, environmental changes, wound care, physical therapy, and psychotherapy
	Anticipate and aggressively manage analgesic side effects
Shortness of breath	Provide oxygen therapy
	Maximize opioid and anxiolytic therapy
	Review the role of temporizing therapy, including thoracentesis, stents, and respiratory therapy
Muscle twitching	Differentiate from seizure activity
	Remember the use of opioid rotation, clonidine, and benzodiazepines if muscle twitching is caused by high-dose opioids

Source: Cowen and Palmer (2002), reference 6.

suffering.[34,35] Table 24–3 identifies interventions that should be made before defining a physical symptom as refractory.

In the ICU setting, reasons for terminal sedation are related to both refractory symptom management and terminal weaning from a ventilator. The decision for terminal weaning may occur if the patient's condition is terminal, attempts to wean from the ventilator have failed, and the family or patient concurs with futility. "Futility" is defined as the perception that the patient has a poor prognosis and is not likely to survive.[25] Singer and colleagues[36] described five domains that indicate good end-of-life care: good symptom management, avoiding inappropriate prolongation of the dying process, achieving a sense of control, relieving burden, and strengthening the patient's relationship with loved ones.

Medications

Drugs used in palliative sedation outside the ICU are benzodiazepines, neuroleptics, barbiturates, and anesthetics.[6,7,13,16] Midazolam is the most commonly used of these drugs.[6,37] The drug and route chosen vary based on the route available, location of the patient, and cost, as well as the preference of the provider.[6] Usually in inpatient settings the medications are given intravenously or subcutaneously and continuously. In palliative sedation, in general, the chosen medication is started at a low dose and titrated upward until the symptom is controlled. Before palliative sedation is started, administration of all previous comfort medications should be continued.[7] Types and routes are presented in Table 24–4. The type of medication used may be influenced by state regulatory agencies for nursing, medicine, and pharmacy. For example, the Texas Board of Nurse Examiners expresses concern regarding the administration of anesthetics by nurses not certified as nurse anesthetists in nonmonitored settings.

The drugs of choice for refractory symptoms and terminal weaning in the ICU are opiates and benzodiazepines.[18,20,38,39] These drugs can be continually infused and titrated until the patient appears comfortable. Morphine is a drug of choice because it provides analgesia, sedation, and reduction of dyspnea.[18] In some instances, barbiturates, haloperidol, and propofol are used.[40,41] Neuromuscular blocking agents have no therapeutic effect; they should not be started, or should be

Table 24–4
Medications Used for Palliative Sedation

Medication	Dose and route	Comments
Benzodiazepines/midazolam	Loading dose of 0.5–5.0 mg, followed by 0.5–10 mg/h continuously infused IV or SQ	Monitor for paradoxical agitation with all benzodiazepines
Lorazepam	0.5–5.0 mg every 1–2 h PO, SL, or IV	—
Neuroleptics/haloperidol	Loading dose of 0.5–5.0 mg PO, SL, SC, or IV, followed by an IV bolus of 1–5 mg every 4 h or 1–5 mg/h continuously infused IV or SQ	Monitor for extrapyramidal side effects
Chlorpromazine	12.5–25.0 mg every 2–4 h PO, PR, or IV	More sedating than haloperidol
Barbiturates/pentobarbital	60–200 mg PR every 4–8 h; loading dose of 2–3 mg/kg bolus IV, followed by 1–2 mg/kg/h continuously infused IV	Do not mix with other drugs when given IV
Phenobarbital	Loading dose of 200 mg, followed by 0.5 mg/kg/h continuously injected SQ or IV	—
Anesthetics/ propofol	Begin with 2.5–5.0 μg/kg/ min and titrate to desired effect every 10 min by increments of 10–20 mg/h	—

IV, intravenously; SQ, subcutaneously; PO, per os; SL, sublingually, PR, per rectum.
Source: Lynch (2003), reference 7.

stopped if already prescribed, before life-sustaining therapies are withdrawn.[38,42] Neuromuscular blockades make it difficult to assess a patient's comfort level because their use makes movement impossible. Patients may be experiencing pain, respiratory distress, and anxiety but unable to communicate their symptoms.[43]

If the skilled clinician is available and the patient's family agrees, the withdrawal of life support can ethically occur in the presence of neuromuscular blockade.[42,44] This is useful in cases in which death is expected to be rapid and certain after removal of the ventilator and if the burden to the patient and family of waiting for the neuromuscular blockade to clear the system (up to several days), is inappropriate.

Treatment Locations

Many hospitals do not have palliative care units. Although the number of fellowship programs for Palliative Medicine in the United States has grown to 20,[39] most hospitals and communities do not have access to these specialists. Because palliative sedation should be a last resort for intractable symptoms, expertise in symptom management and end-of-life care to verify refractoriness is needed.[6,45] The drugs of choice are classified as anesthesia medications, but institutional polices may limit the choice of agents used. Unfortunately, inappropriate use of benzodiazepines for palliative sedation occurs, and sedation may be implemented by professionals not trained in palliative care.

Unfortunately, palliative sedation seems at cross-purposes with the goals of intensive care. The original intent of admission to an ICU is to aggressively stabilize the patient faced with life-threatening events. The ICU environment allows rapid identification and treatment of life-threatening changes to avoid death.[46] Patients and families come to the ICU expecting miracles, and they often are familiar with stories of those who have survived similar experiences, whether real cases or from television. The challenge for health care practitioners in the ICU is to know when to transition from curative to palliative care and then to communicate with the family regarding the patient's prognosis and decisions about sedation. Once

Table 24–5
Palliative Sedation Checklist

Part A. Background

____ Confirm patient has

- Irreversible advanced disease.
- Apparent imminent death within hours, days, or weeks.
- A "do not attempt resuscitation" order.

____ Confirm that symptoms are refractory to other therapies that are acceptable to the patient and have a reasonable/practical potential to achieve comfort goals.

____ Consider obtaining a peer consultation to confirm that the patient is near death with refractory symptoms.

____ Complete informed consent process for palliative sedation (PS).

____ Discontinue interventions not focused on comfort.

- Discontinue routine laboratory and imaging studies.
- Review medications, limit to those for comfort, and adjust for ease of administration (timing and route).
- Discontinue unnecessary cardiopulmonary and vital sign monitoring.
- Review the role of cardiac support devices (e.g., pacemaker) and disable functioning implanted defibrillators.
- Integrate a plan to discontinue ventilator support with PS.

____ Develop a plan for the use or withdrawal of nutrition and hydration during PS.

____ Identify a location and an environment acceptable for providing PS.

____ Use providers familiar with PS and the use of sedatives.

Part B. Treatment/Care of the Patient

____ Institute and maintain aspiration precautions.

____ Provide mouth care and eye protection.

____ Use oxygen only for comfort, not to maintain a specific blood oxygen saturation.

____ Provide medications primarily by IV or SQ route.

____ Maintain bowel, bladder, and pressure point care.

____ Continue, do not taper, routine opioids.

____ Provide sedating medication:

- Around the clock.
- Titrate to symptom control not level of consciousness, using frequent re-evaluation.
- Limit vital sign monitoring to temperature and respiratory rate for dyspnea.

____ Choose sedating medication based on provider experience, route available, and patient location.

Home initial dosing (choose one):

- Chlorpromazine, 25 mg suppository or 12.5 mg IV infusion every 4–6 h.
- Midazolam, 0.4 mg/h by continuous IV or SQ infusion.
- Lorazepam, 0.5–2.0 mg IV sublingually every 4–6 h.

Hospital initial dosing (choose one):

- Chlorpromazine, 12.5–25.0 mg every 4–6 h.
- Midazolam, 0.4 mg/h by continuous IV or SQ infusion.
- Amobarbital or thiopental, 20 mg/h by continuous IV infusion.
- Propofol, 2.5 mg/kg/min by continuous IV infusion.

Source: Lynch, (2003), reference 7.

there is a consensus, the challenge is then to transform the high-tech, fast-paced, often loud ICU setting into a peaceful, serene environment conducive for dying. Even in ideal settings, where palliative care and ICUs coexist, there are still challenges in transferring patients to a less restrictive environment in a safe, timely manner due to the patient's critical, fragile state. Copies of protocols from the authors' institution are include in Appendices 24-1 through 24-3 at the end of this chapter.

Guidelines for Use

The use of sedation for refractory symptoms varies. Therefore, the use of clinical pathways or checklists is recommended to ensure optimal and consistent standards of care.[6,21] Table 24–5 is a sample checklist for palliative sedation. Table 24–6 is a sample checklist used in an ICU setting for terminal weaning. Although evidence is often anecdotal, there has been concern that palliative sedation could be used inappropriately.[6,21,45] Four factors need to be present for a patient to be considered for sedation. First, the patient should have a terminal diagnosis. Second, the patient should have symptoms that are unbearable and refractory. Consultation with an expert to confirm that the patient is near death with refractory symptoms is recommended. Third, a DNR order must be in effect. Fourth, death must be imminent (within hours to days), although this can be challenging to determine.[6,7,45] In the presence of the first three conditions, sedation may be appropriate for a patient with severe distress that has been unresponsive to skilled palliative interventions. Ethics committees or patient advocate services may be useful if there appear to be irresolvable family or staff conflicts. Studies have shown that ethics consultations are useful in resolving conflicts that may otherwise prolong futile and unwanted treatments in the ICU.[47]

A major function for palliative care is to assist families to make the transition in goals of treatment from cure to comfort. Refractory symptoms and the distress they cause create a very difficult and abrupt need for this transition phase. Use of the interdisciplinary team to both plan for treatment options and participate in family meetings is critical to the success of the team. The social worker plays a vital role in assessing caregiver stress and family dynamics and coordinating family meetings. The chaplain and other psychosocial professionals provide spiritual assistance and counseling in redefining hope and supporting the decision-makers through anticipatory and actual grief.

Nursing Care: Back to Basics

Communication

An important role of the nurse in the end-of-life process is to facilitate communication and establish trust between the patient, family, and health care providers.[48] Communication is vital to developing a relationship of trust and avoiding conflict during any illness, but it becomes more important at the end of life. The team has to build a trusting relationship with patients and families as they make difficult decisions. If a patient or family members do not trust the health care team, conflict is likely to result.[49] Communication includes (1) being honest and truthful, (2) letting patients and families know they will not be abandoned, (3) including them in care decisions, (4) helping the patients and families explore all options, (5) asking clearly what they need from the team, (6) working to ensure that the entire team knows and understands the plan, and (7) most important, active listening.[48,50]

When the decision is made to use either terminal sedation or terminal weaning, caring and thoughtful communication make a tremendous difference in the family's experience with the death. The concept of "presence" with the patient and family during the death vigil is difficult to quantify but critical during periods of extreme distress.[51–53] Untreated symptoms cause families and staff to be traumatized by a "horrible death." For example, 77% to 85% of all cancer patients experience delirium before death.[54] Some delirium, 25% to 35%, is reversible,[10] and all patients should be treated for delirium and other distressing symptoms. Loss of inhibition is the hallmark of delirium as global brain function diminishes. Symptoms of moaning, groaning, and restlessness are often interpreted by the family as physical pain. An explanation of the delirium and aggressive treatment is important to comfort the family, who also need support for anxiety, grief, and sadness as they prepare for the death of their loved one. They need continual explanations of and reassurance about what to expect and the opportunity to express their feelings of grief.[6]

Physical Care

Nurses play an essential role at the bedside to administer sedation and monitor symptom response to sedation. It is also important to continually reinforce with the family that the intent of sedation is symptom control and not hastening of death.[6] In collaboration with the physician, evaluation of symptom response and possible need for titration of medication should be done at least every 24 hours once the symptoms are stable.

As the patient becomes more sedated, protective reflexes decrease. The ability to clear secretions decreases, necessitating suctioning and/or medications. Make sure the family understands that the patient can no longer safely swallow. The blink reflex decreases and eyes can become very dry, requiring frequent eye drops (artificial tears). Bowel and bladder management needs to be carefully monitored to maintain comfort. A urinary catheter is often appropriate to minimize the need for frequent changing and cleaning and to prevent skin breakdown. General nursing care for immobilized patients is vital; mattress pads that decrease pressure, excellent skin care, and attention to positioning are all important.[50,55]

Table 24–6
Checklist for Intensive Care Unit Personnel End-of-Life Criterion Checklist

Assessment	MET	NOT MET
1. Determine that primary physician, critical care physician, family and possibly patient are in agreement with discontinuation of life sustaining treatment.	——	——
2. Assist family in preparation or fulfillment of familial or religious predeath rituals.	——	——
3. Place, "do not resuscitate" orders on chart.	——	——
4. Turn off neuromuscular blockade agents (e.g., paralytics).	——	——
5. Provide a calm, quiet, restful atmosphere free of medical devices and technology for the patient and family, including dimming the lights in the room.	——	——
6. Turn off arrhythmia detection and turn off or decrease all auditory alarms at bedside and central station.	——	——
7. Remove all monitoring equipment from patient and patient's room except for the electrocardiograph (ECG).	——	——
8. Remove all devices unless the removal of the device would create discomfort for the patient (e.g., sequential compression device, nasogastric tube).	——	——
9. Remove or discontinue treatments that do not provide comfort to the patient.	——	——
10. Obtain orders to discontinue test and laboratory studies.	——	——
11. Liberalize visitation.	——	——
12. Notify respiratory therapist of end-of-life care.	——	——
13. Notify chaplain and social worker of end-of-life care; obtain grief packet from chaplain.	——	——
14. Determine that family participants in the end-of-life process are present, if appropriate; place sufficient chairs in the patient's room for family members.	——	——
15. Maintain the patient's personal comfort and dignity with attention to hygiene, hairstyle, and providing moisturizers for lips and eyes.	——	——
16. Gather ordered sedation and analgesics. Frequent assessment of the patient's condition assists in titrating medications per end-of-life protocol and level of patient discomfort.	——	——
17. Document the patient's signs and symptoms that indicate discomfort, including but not limited to the following: Agitated behavior Altered cognition Anxiety Autonomic hyperactivity Confusion Coughing Dyspnea Grimacing Increased work of breathing Irritation Moaning Pain Perspiration	——	——

(*continued*)

Table 24–6
Checklist for Intensive Care Unit Personnel End-of-Life Criterion Checklist *(continued)*

Assessment	MET	NOT MET
Restlessness; Self-report of symptoms; Splinting; Stiffness; Tachycardia; Tachypnea; Tension; Trembling		
18. Remain at bedside to a. assess patient for comfort/discomfort. b. promptly administer sedation, analgesics. c. provide emotional support to patient and family. d. ask patient/family if additional comfort measures are needed.	____	____
19. Obtain physician orders for additional or alterations in pain and sedation medications if the end-of-life protocol medications are ineffective in controlling the patient's discomfort.	____	____
20. Respiratory therapist should remain in room until ventilator is function at minimal capacity or patient is extubated and the ventilator is removed from the room.	____	____
21. Support and educate the patient's family regarding interpretation of the clinical signs and symptoms the patient may experience during the end of life.	____	____
22. Assess the family's need to be alone with the patient during and after the death process.	____	____
23. Assess the family to determine the amount of support they require during the end-of-life process.	____	____
24. Assist the family in meeting its needs and the patient's needs for communication, final expressions of love and concern (e.g., holding a hand, talking with the patient, remembering past events).	____	____
25. Discuss signs of death and how the physician will pronounce the patient; the family will be asked to leave the room while the physician examines the patient.	____	____
26. If the patient is transferred to the general care floors during end-of-life care, provide the accepting nurse a verbal report and discuss the dosage of IV medications and the signs and symptoms for medication titration. Suggest to the critical care physician or attending physician a patient referral to or consultation with palliative care services.	____	____
27. Notify intensive care unit physician to pronounce patient. An ECG strip of a straight line or asystole is not needed to document patient death.	____	____
28. Notify primary care physician.	____	____
29. Assist family with decisions regarding need for autopsy.	____	____
30. Notify clinical nurse specialist Monday through Friday before 3 P.M. to complete death paperwork.	____	____
31. Notify in-house administrator after 3 P.M. and on weekends to complete death paperwork.	____	____

(continued)

Table 24–6
Checklist for Intensive Care Unit Personnel End-of-Life Criterion Checklist *(continued)*

Assessment	MET	NOT MET
32. Notify chaplain, if chaplain not present.	____	____
33. If the patient is to have an autopsy, leave all tubes in place; if no autopsy, remove all tubes (IV lines may be clamped instead of removed).	____	____
34. Permit family visitation after the patient has been cleaned and tubes removed.	____	____
35. Prepare patient for the morgue, shroud etc.	____	____

MET, Indicates that the individual is prepared, follows suggested steps in appropriate sequence, and demonstrates minimal safe practice; NOT MET, Indicates that the individual is unprepared, needs repeated assistance or suggestions in order to proceed, and or omits necessary steps.

Source: M.D. Anderson Cancer Center, Houston, Texas. Reprinted with permission.

Special Considerations in the Intensive Care Unit

Immediately before terminal weaning, the physician should briefly review the procedure and be available to answer any questions family members may have. Nurses should ask family members whether they have any last-minute questions or concerns. Nurses can reassure the family that comfort is the primary goal and that pain medication is available. If appropriate, nurses should also explain that the patient may need to be asleep to be comfortable. Nurses should also make clear that sometimes the patient may experience involuntary movements but that they do not indicate pain.

Before beginning the weaning process, the nurse should turn off the physiological monitoring alarms and remove any unnecessary tubes or equipment (e.g., restraints, nasogastric tubes). Any unnecessary medications (e.g., vasoactive drips, antibiotics) should be stopped. Before extubation, medications should be administered to establish adequate symptom control as ordered by the physician. Opioids are the most effective agents for relieving the sense of breathlessness, and benzodiazepines are most effective for relieving anxiety. Any additional medications should be readily available. Oxygen should be set at 21% or as ordered by the physician.

The need for additional medications should be continually assessed and readjusted. Once the patient appears to be comfortable, the physician or respiratory therapist removes the endotracheal tube. Throughout this process the nurse should allow space for the patient's family at the bedside. The decision to stay at the bedside or not is a personal decision and nurses can validate and support whatever decision is made by the family. The family also should be encouraged to assist by wiping the patient's forehead, holding the patient's hand, or talking to the patient.[56] The patient and family should be offered chaplaincy or other psychosocial services support throughout the process. After the patient dies, the family should be allowed adequate time to begin the grieving process.

Time to Death

One of the concerns many have with palliative sedation is that it might hasten death. Part of this concern stems from the difficulty in predicting the time of death.[57,58] Several studies using different methodologies have examined effects of sedation on survival rates.[13,29] The mean time to death in a large four-country study ranged from 1.9 to 3.2 days,[32] and the median time to death in a Taiwanese study was 5 days.[58a] A study of patients in Japanese hospices indicated that sedating medications did not shorten the lifespan.[59] However, because of ethical considerations, none of these studies were controlled trials, so it is not possible to determine whether sedation may or may not result in hastening the death. In situations of unbearable distress, sedation remains an appropriate option to relieve suffering.

Ethical Considerations

This section describes ethical principles applicable to palliative sedation, which includes "slow euthanasia" and terminal weaning. The ethical and legal principles that apply to palliative sedation are patient autonomy (patient's choice), beneficence (do good), nonmaleficence (do no harm), futility, and the principle of double effect.[6,16,29,60,61] Patient autonomy is defined as freedom to make and act on decisions.[6] This requires informed consent with adequate decision-making capacity. Conflicts can occur if patient, family, and staff beliefs about the goal of therapy are in conflict. Autonomy conflicts with beneficence and nonmaleficence if the roles of the medical and nursing caregivers as healers conflict. The issue of medical futility creates great distress for the physician who is accountable for medical care of a patient or family requesting further treatment that is deemed by the medical team to be futile. Refusal to treat does not mean ignoring patient or family wishes but reflects a concern about doing harm instead of good.

This issue becomes more complicated for nurses at the bedside. Nurses are required to care for the patient based on the physician's orders with varying ability to express personal beliefs.[53] With skilled palliative management, nurses are included in the entire process. Resolution of dilemmas is difficult but is facilitated by ensuring that the nurse understands the goals and is allowed the option to decline assignment to a patient if uncomfortable with the treatment plan. Nursing leaders across the country are working diligently to create systems that support patients and their families as well as the nurses at the bedside during end-of-life care.

The principle of double effect holds that an act with more than one potential effect is ethical if certain conditions are met. The doctrine of double effect emphasizes four basic conditions: (1) the nature of the act is morally good and is not in a category that is absolutely prohibited or intrinsically wrong; (2) the intent of the act is good, even in the presence of a foreseen bad effect; (3) the means of attaining the good effect (relief of suffering) is not bad; (4) the intended good effects balance or are greater than the bad effects (rule of proportionality).[61] Cowan and Palmer[6] added a fifth condition: that there are no other means to achieve the intended good effect. However, Quill and coworkers[62] argued that clinical justification of palliative sedation is ambiguous, making double effect inappropriate, because palliative sedation causes death and the intentions are not always clear. Cherny[63] suggested that relieving a symptom and proportionality are more appropriate than double effect.

Some authors have suggested that palliative sedation and slow euthanasia are morally equivalent.[17,64] Billings and Block[17] defined slow euthanasia as the clinical practice of treating a terminally ill patient in a fashion that will assuredly lead to a comfortable death, but not too quickly. Mount[65] argued that Billings and Block's definition is more a definition of palliative care. Whereas euthanasia is the deliberate termination of life by active intervention of a medical provider for a patient with uncontrolled suffering, palliative sedation is not euthanasia because it is not intended to end life primarily but rather to relieve the distressing symptoms.

The U.S. Supreme Court in 1997 ruled unanimously that "there is no constitutional right to physician-assisted suicide" but "terminal sedation is intended for symptom relief and not assisted suicide . . . .and is appropriate in the aggressive practice of palliative care."[66,67] The American Nurses Association (ANA) and the Oncology Nursing Society (ONS) have position papers opposed to physician-assisted suicide.[68,69] Although neither addresses the exact issue of palliative sedation or terminal weaning, both support the risk of hastening death through treatments aimed at alleviating suffering or controlling symptoms as ethically and legally acceptable. The Hospice and Palliative Nurses Association has issued a position paper in support of palliative sedation.[55] Hospitals are being encouraged to develop policies for terminal sedation and against euthanasia and to understand that aggressive and readily available palliative care (included sedation) might actually reduce the demand for euthanasia or assisted suicide.[70] The issue of palliative sedation for existential suffering remains controversial.[4]

In Case Study I, cited earlier, before the transfer to the palliative unit, the primary physician felt uncomfortable with the high level of sedation required for this young and otherwise healthy man to stay sedated. This physician did not object to the patient's being sedated, but she was concerned with the amount of medication required to appropriately sedate him. The physician initially refused to transfer the patient to the palliative service or to accept the palliative's team orders for sedation. Although the primary physician never used the term "slow euthanasia," her actions suggested this concern. The nurses on this medical oncology floor were concerned about "killing the patient with medicine" but also expressed concern that the patient might die of suffocation while awake. The palliative physician requested a medical ethics consultation, but it was not needed because the patient was transferred to the palliative care unit.

The ethical principles that apply to withdrawal of mechanical ventilation are patient autonomy, nonmaleficence, and beneficence. Patient autonomy is the process that allows the patient to make an informed and voluntary decision regarding his or her care. The basis for the ethical dilemma in withholding or withdrawing life support is the balance between patient autonomy and physician autonomy or professional and institutional integrity.[71] A conflict may arise if the patient or family insist that "everything be done" and the health care team believes that continued aggressive support would be inappropriate or futile. In Case Study II, the family could have argued that the patient was not in a condition to make end-of-life decisions and insisted that everything be done or, at the very least, that mechanical ventilation be continued. The patient or family also could have requested further treatment (e.g., chemotherapy, dialysis).

Withdrawal of life-sustaining therapy may be justified if the therapy in question is deemed futile. Medical futility refers to interventions that are unlikely to produce a significant benefit. Practitioners should carefully consider each intervention and whether there would be benefit or harm for the patient. Terminal weaning can be disturbing for those who do not understand the principles that guide caregivers' actions. The administration of opioids in this setting is justified ethically by the principle of double effect. The double effect principle draws a distinction between the intended effects of a person's action and the unintended, though anticipated, effects of that action.[40] During the terminal weaning process, the caregiver's first responsibility is to relieve pain and suffering, whereas the potential for hastening death is tolerated as a necessary evil. The clinican's primary intent is to relieve the patient's suffering and not to cause death.[40] The terminal weaning process can be more difficult for the caregiver if the patient is awake and alert enough to participate in the decision to withdraw life support, but the guiding principles remain the same.

In Case Study II, another ethical principle that should be considered is nonmaleficence, or duty not to inflict harm. The patient's nurse might have viewed the withdrawal of ventilation and corresponding sedation requirements as inflicting harm. In the case presented, does the patient's physician have the right to withhold dialysis? Medical futility refers to interventions that are unlikely to produce a significant benefit to the patient. Practitioners should carefully consider each intervention and whether there would be any benefit for the patient. In the case presented, continuing ventilation would only prolong death. There is no reasonable likelihood that the patient could ever have been weaned off the ventilator, because his cancer had spread to his remaining lung. Use of life-sustaining or invasive interventions in a patient who is terminally ill may only prolong the dying process.[38] Also, the intervention of dialysis for the patient would only have prolonged the dying process.

Ethical issues are not clearcut. Although respect for patient autonomy is important, it does not mean that health care workers are obligated to provide requested sedation in all circumstances. Principles of intent provide safeguards for palliative sedation and terminal weaning. Closeness to imminent death needs to be assessed, as well as refractoriness of distressing symptoms. With careful application of criteria, palliative sedation cannot be equated with slow euthanasia.[16,31,59]

Informed Consent

Palliative sedation is a joint decision and not an arbitrary medical decision. In the palliative care setting, a consent for sedation should be obtained as soon as a symptom is identified as possibly refractory. Sedation can then be quickly arranged if needed. Informed consent regarding palliative sedation or terminal weaning should be more than simply a signature on a form. There is a tendency to discuss the plan of care for the patient at the convenience of the physician and not that of the patient or family. A well planned, compassionate, and clear discussion at the end of life should occur with the family and the patient. The bedside nurse should attend these meetings to provide insight into the care and support needed by the family. It is vital to plan these meetings carefully to ensure that the appropriate family members are present. Allowing the designated decision-maker to invite important people to the planned meeting allows key participants to hear the information at the same time. A religious or spiritual representative may be helpful at these meetings if desired.

Family meetings work well for cohesive and connected family units. In families with more disparity, family members may appear to agree in the group but individually continue to have conflicts about agreed-upon decisions. Nurses and staff need to respond to all questions and be prepared to repeat information and provide support.[72]

The primary physician should begin the family meeting with a brief, clear report on the current condition of the patient. Any supporting documentation of the current condition, such as recent laboratory data or other diagnostic test results, may be helpful in certain cases. Either at the end of the family meeting or the next day in nonemergency cases, an informed consent document needs to be signed by the patient, family, or medical proxy. The family should be provided time to raise all concerns and clarify information.

Next, the treatment options should be discussed. When discussing terminal sedation options, it is important to assess the patient's and family's cultural and religious beliefs and concerns. Documentation of the informed consent should include the patient's name and diagnosis, the parties present, the reason for sedation (symptom distress), and the primary goal (patient comfort), as well as patient terminal status, notation of any professional consultations, documentation that the patient is near death and has refractory symptoms, planned discontinuance of treatments not focused on comfort, plan for hydration and nutrition, and anticipated risks or burdens of sedation.[6] Because it usually is not possible to communicate with the sedated patient, it is important to make sure that the patient and family are ready to proceed with sedation.[73] A well-planned family meeting decreases miscommunication and supports the family during a difficult decision-making time by allowing all pertinent parties to hear the same information at the same time.

In the ICU setting, there should also be a succinct description of the terminal weaning process. One of the most common reasons for withholding or withdrawing life support is the perception that the patient has a poor prognosis.[74] Although there are many published guidelines for withholding and withdrawing life support, the actual implementation of such measures is often difficult for the health care team members as well as the patient and family. Physicians may have a difficult time discussing such interventions with patients and families, and this often leads to the continuation of treatments that are medically inappropriate or futile. The patient and family members should also be allowed sufficient time to reach a consensus about whether to discontinue life support. All members of the multidisciplinary team should understand and be able to discuss the plan of care. The nurse and physician should also carefully document the plan. Because withholding and withdrawing life support and administering palliative sedation can involve health care practitioners other than the attending physician, the health care team should participate in the planning phase.[75] A team approach is vital during this phase of care delivery, because disagreement among professional caregivers about the goal of care can increase liability.[76]

Withholding and withdrawing life support are legally justified primarily by the principles of informed consent and informed refusal.[75] These principles were applied in the Karen Ann Quinlan and Nancy Cruzan cases. In the Quinlan case, the New Jersey Supreme Court upheld a patient's right to refuse medical treatment.[77] The patient Quinlan was in a persistent vegetative state, and her parents, acting as her surrogate, were granted the right to refuse mechanical ventilation. In the Cruzan case, the Missouri Court held that sufficient evidence of the patient's wishes had been offered and made the ruling to permit tube withdrawal.[78] These cases were milestones because they allowed the families, not the physicians, to determine which treatments were appropriate and which were futile. The Patient Self-Determination Act of 1990 further opposed the culture against the traditional medical paternalism and fostered patients' rights.[78]

The Nurse Caregiver

In most settings, the nursing staff is involved in the terminal sedation or weaning process. Nurses must be provided with the proper educational training to rectify knowledge and skill deficits and to provide nurses the opportunity to seek alternative employment in another setting if they do not feel comfortable with palliative sedation or the terminal weaning process.[79,80] Nurses involved in caring for these patients should be allowed to abstain from doing so until they feel comfortable with the process.

It may also be helpful for the nurse to have education and support regarding personal death awareness. Personal death awareness is defined as one's comfort with death and can be affected by personality, cultural, social, and spiritual belief systems. The nurse must be allowed to adapt to caring for dying patients, which may require the nurse to explore, experience, and express his or her feelings regarding death. If the nurse is not allowed to explore his or her personal beliefs, this may result in inappropriate defense mechanisms, such as emotional distancing or avoidance and withdrawal from dying patients and families.

Cumulative loss is experienced by nurses working with patients with life-threatening illnesses. Cumulative loss can be described as a succession of losses experienced by nurses who care for dying patients. Systems of support must be in place to help the nurse deal with loss. Palliative care recognizes that no one can do this work alone. Nurses at the bedside can be supported by professionals from many other disciplines, including social workers, chaplains, counselors, advanced practice nurses, and physicians. Nurses who work with patients requiring palliative sedation and terminal weaning are at increased risk of burnout if not intimately involved with the team decision-making process. It is vital that these nurses be involved in the decision-making process, because they have high responsibility but often low autonomy. Bedside nurses are intimately involved in palliative sedation and the terminal weaning process, but, if left out of decision-making processes such as the team planning and family conferences, they are denied the information needed for effective counseling at the bedside.[81] There must be a formal and informal support system as well as education in end-of-life care, spiritual support, and individual support as needed.

An interdisciplinary team meeting after death in these cases can function as both a learning experience and a debriefing process. Working in an environment that recognizes the need for support and education for staff, and one that recognizes the importance of mentors and advance practice nurses, allows nurses to face these challenges as they arise.[81]

Case Study Conclusions

CASE STUDY I

Mr. M—Conclusion

After 5 days of aggressive attempts to reverse the delirium, a family meeting was held with all significant people present. The decision was made to provide palliative sedation for a trial of psychotropic drug discontinuation with the hope that the hyperactive delirium might reverse. The mother and significant other understood that sedation could be terminal but clearly agreed that Mr. M's distress was unbearable. The family opted for continued hydration, no parenteral nutrition, chaplain and counseling support, and a course of midazolam. Attempts to decrease the midazolam dose 2 days later resulted in renewed agitation, so the dose was returned to maintenance level and the patient died the next day with his loved ones at his side. The family was referred to bereavement services in the state where they live.

CASE STUDY II

Mr. Z—Conclusion

The ethics team reviewed the case to determine the patient's capacity and understanding of terminal weaning. The nurse was also concerned that withdrawing life support from this awake, alert patient would appear "Kevorkian-like" or give the impression of euthanasia. The ethics team believed that the patient had made his wishes clear. He did not want to continue his life if it meant being dependent on mechanical ventilation. The patient's wife was supportive of his wishes, as were his two adult children. The team's conclusion and recommendation was to support the patient's wishes and the physician's decision to withhold further treatment, dialysis, and to withdraw ventilator support. The ethics team also felt the patient was making an informed decision.

A decision was reached between the ICU attending physician and the patient that the ventilator would be withdrawn the next morning. The following day the patient had his family at his bedside while the ventilator adjustments were made. He was sedated, and comfort measures were taken. The patient was made comfortable and within 10 minutes after weaning from the ventilator he died peacefully with his family, physician, and nurse at the bedside.

Conclusion

In today's ICU environment, advances in technology that are designed to prolong life have outpaced those designed to return patients to a reasonable quality of life.[82] This disparity has caused ICU nurses to view death as an acceptable outcome, maintaining palliative care and symptom management, and ensuring a dignified, tolerable death with the more traditional goals of curing disease, restoring health and function, and promoting life and survival. Nursing professionals in the ICU should train new nurses in the skills required to withdraw and withhold care. These skills do not come easily; a concerted effort should be made to provide proper training to ensure patients a painless, dignified, peaceful death.

Although many may disagree about what a "good death" is, there is general agreement about what is a "bad death." Palliative sedation and terminal weaning are ethical and realistic interventions in a percentage of dying patients whose symptoms remain unbearable despite aggressive palliative interventions. The concerns and challenges appear to be related to the lack of consistency in providing care skillfully across all settings. The confusion between slow euthanasia and sedation remains, as does a lack of agreement on palliative sedation for existential suffering. The ability to determine refractoriness of symptoms is complicated by the lack of palliative care experts in all settings as well as the continued challenge of accurately predicting time to death. When all patients have access to nurses and physicians with specialized training in palliative sedation and terminal weaning, the dying process will improve significantly.

REFERENCES

1. Miller PA, Forbes S, Boyle DK. End-of-life care in the intensive care unit: A challenge for nurses. Am J Crit Care 2001;10:230–237.
2. Robert Wood Johnson Foundation. Survey Results: What Americans Think About the American Way of Death. 2002, http://www.rwjf.org (accessed April 14, 2004). http://ww2.rwjf.org/news/special/meansSummary.jhtml.
3. Ventafridda V, Ripamonte C, De Conno F, Tamburini M, Cassileth BR. Symptom prevalence and control during cancer patients' last days of life. J Palliat Care 1990;6:7–11.
4. Wein S. Sedation in the imminently dying patient. Oncology 2000;14:585–601.
5. Beel A, McClement S, Harlos M. Palliative sedation therapy: A review of definitions and usage. Int J Palliat Nurs 2002;8:190–199.
6. Cowan JD, Palmer TW. Practical guide to palliative sedation. Curr Oncol Rep 2002;4:242–249.
7. Lynch M. Palliative sedation. Clin J Oncol Nurs 2003;7:653–667.
8. Chater S, Viola R, Paterson J, Jarvis V. Sedation for intractable distress in the dying: A survey of experts. Palliat Med 1998;12:255–269.
9. Volker DL. Assisted dying and end of life symptom management. Cancer Nurs 2003;26:392–399.
10. Bruera E, Franco J, Maltoni M, Wantanabe S, Suarez-Almazor M. Changing pattern of agitated impaired mental status in patients with advanced cancer: Association with cognitive monitoring, hydration and opioid rotation. J Pain Symptom Manage 1995;10:287–291.
11. Enck RE. Drug induced terminal sedation for symptom control. Am Hospice Palliat Care 1991;84:332–337.
12. Cherny NI, Portenoy RK. Sedation in the management of refractory symptoms: Guidelines for evaluation and treatment. J Palliat Care 1994;10:31–38.
13. Cowan JD, Walsh D. Terminal sedation in palliative medicine: Definition and review of literature. Support Cancer Care 2001; 9:403–407.
14. Morita T, Tsuneto S, Shima Y. Proposed definitions of sedation for symptom relief: A systematic literature review and a proposal of operation criteria. J Pain Symptom Manage 2002;24:447–453.
15. Peruselli C, Di Giulio P, Toscani F, Gallucci M, Brunelli C, Costantini M, Tamburini M, Paci E, Miccinesi G, Addington-Hall JM, Higginson U. Home palliative care for terminal cancer patients: A survey on the final week of life. Palliat Med 1999;13:233–241.
16. Krakauer EL, Penson RT, Troug RD, King LA, Chabner BA, Lynch TJ Jr. Sedation for intractable distress of a dying patient: Acute palliative care and the principle of double effect. Oncologist 2000;5:53–62.
17. Billings JA, Block SD. Slow euthanasia. J Palliat Care 1996;12:21–30.
18. Campbell ML, Carlson RW. Terminal weaning from mechanical ventilation: Ethical and practical considerations for patient management. Am J Crit Care 1992:1:52–56.
19. Grenvik A. "Terminal weaning": Discontinuance of life-support therapy in the terminally ill patient. Crit Care Med 1983;11:394–395.
20. Truog RD, Cist AF, Brackett SF, Burns JP, Curley MAQ, Danis M, DeVita MA, Rosenbaum SH, Rothenberg DM, Sprung CL, Webb SA, Wlody GS, Hurford WE. Recommendations for end-of-life care in the intensive care unit: The Ethics Committee of the Society of Critical Care Medicine. Crit Care Med 2001;29:2332–2348.
21. Rousseau P. Existential suffering and palliative sedation: A brief commentary with a proposal for clinical guidelines. Am J Hospice Palliat Care 2001;18:151–153.
22. Curtis JR, Patrick DL. How to discuss death and dying in the ICU. In: Curtis JR, Rubenfeld GD, eds. Managing Death in the ICU. New York: Oxford University Press, 2001:85–102.
23. Rocker GM, Curtis JR. Caring for the dying in the intensive care unit: In search of clarity. JAMA 2003;290:820–822.
24. Prendergast TJ, Luce JM. Increasing incidence of withholding and withdrawal of life support from the critically ill. Am J Respir Crit Care Med 1997;155:15–20.
25. Ardagh M. Futility has no utility in resuscitation medicine. J Med Ethics 2000:26;396–399.
26. Asch DA, Hansen-Flaschen J, Lanken PN. Decisions to limit or continue life-sustaining treatment by critical care physicians in the United States: Conflicts between practices and patients' wishes. Am J Respir Crit Care Med 1995;151:288–292.
27. Luce JM, Prendergast TJ. The changing nature of death in the ICU. In: Curtis JR, Rubenfeld GD, eds. Managing Death in the Intensive Care Unit. New York: Oxford University Press, 2001:19–29.
28. Faber-Langendoen K. The clinical management of dying patients receiving mechanical ventilation: Survey of physician practice. Chest 1994;106:880–888.
29. Sykes N, Thorns A. Sedative use in the last week of life and the implications for end of life decision making. Arch Intern Med 2003;163:341–344.
30. Jansen LA, Sulmasy DP. Sedation, alimentation, hydration, and equivocation: Careful conversation about care at the end of life. Ann Intern Med 2002;136:845– 849.
31. Hallenbeck JL. Terminal sedation: Ethical implications in different situations. J Palliat Med 2000;3:313–320.
32. Fainsinger RL, Waller A, Bercovici M, Bengtson K, Landman W, Hosking M, Nunez-Olarte JM, deMoissac D. A multicentre international study of sedation for uncontrolled symptoms in terminally ill patients. Palliat Med 2000;14:257–265.

33. Ferris FD, vonGunten CF, Emanuel LA. Competency in end of life care: Last hours of life. J Palliat Med 2003;6:605–613.
34. Ganzini L, Dobscha SK, Heintz RT, Press N. Oregon physicians' perceptions of patients who request assisted suicide and their families. J Palliat Med 2003:6:381–390.
35. Lanuke K, Fainsinger RL, Demoissac D, Archibald J. Two remarkable dyspneic men: When should terminal sedation by administered? J Palliat Med 2003;6:277–281.
36. Singer PA. Martin DK, Kelner M. Quality end of life care: Patients' perspectives. JAMA 1999;281:163–168.
37. Cheng C, Roemer-Becuwe C, Pereira J. When midazolam fails. J Pain Symptom Manage 2002;23:256–265.
38. Rubenfield GD, Curtis JR. Improving care for patients dying in the intensive care unit. Clin Chest Med 2003;24:763–773.
39. Abraham JL. Update in palliative medicine and end-of-life care. Annu Rev Med 2003;54:53–72.
40. Truog RD, Berde CB, Mitchell C, Grier HE. Barbiturates in the care of the terminally ill. N Engl J Med 1992;327:1678–1681.
41. Casarett DJ, Inouye SK. Diagnosis and management of delirium near the end of life. Ann Intern Med 2001:135:32–40.
42. Truog, RD, Burns JP, Mitchell C, Johnson J, Robinson, W. Sounding board: Pharmacological paralysis and withdrawal of mechanical ventilation at the end of life. N Engl J Med 2000;342:508–511.
43. Rushton CH, Terry PB. Neuromuscular blockade and ventilator withdrawal: Ethical controversies. Am J Crit Care 1995;4:112–115.
44. Nelson RM. Extubation or euthanasia: Getting the facts clear. Crit Care Med 2000;28:3120–3121.
45. Braun TC, Hagen NA, Clark T. Development of a clinical practice guideline for palliative sedation. J Palliat Med 2003;6:345–350.
46. Ahrens T, Yancey V, Kollef M. Improving family communications at the end of life: Implications for length of stay in the intensive care unit and resource use. Am J Crit Care 2003;12:317–323.
47. Schneiderman LJ, Gilmer T, Teetzel HD, Dugan DO, Blustein J, Cranford R, Briggs KB, Komatsu GI, Goodman-Crew P, Cohn F, Young EWD. Effects of ethics consultations on nonbeneficial life-sustaining treatments in the intensive care setting. JAMA 2003;209:1166–1172.
48. Matzo ML, Sherman DW, Sheehan DC, Ferrell BR, Penn B. Communication skills for end of life nursing care. Nurs Educ Perspect 2003;24:176–183.
49. Caplan AL. Odds and ends: Trust and the debate over medical futility. Ann Intern Med 1996:125:688–689.
50. End of Life Nursing Education Consortium (ELNEC) Project. Funded by the Robert Wood Johnson Foundation to the American Association of Colleges of Nursing and City of Hope National Medical Center 2003, http://www.aacn.nche.edu/elnec (accessed January 6, 2005).
51. Walsh SM, Hogan NS. Oncology nursing education: Nursing students' commitment of "presence" with the dying patient and the family. Nurs Educ Perspect 2003;24:86–90.
52. Pitorak EF. Care at the time of death: How nurses can make the last hours of life a richer, more comfortable experience. Am J Nurs 2003;103:42–53.
53. Hayes C. Ethics in end of life care. J Hospice Palliat Nurs 2004;6:36–43.
54. Pereira J, Hanson J, Bruera E. The frequency and clinical course of cognitive impairment in patients with terminal cancer. Cancer 1997;79:835–842.
55. Hospice and Palliative Nurses Association. Position paper: Palliative sedation at the end of life. J Hospice Palliat Nurs 2003;5: 235–237.
56. American Medical Association. Education for Physicians on End-of-Life Care: Participant's Handbook. Module 11: Withholding, Withdrawing Therapy. Available at: http://www.amaassn.org/ethic/epec/download/module_11.pdf (accessed January 6, 2005).
57. The SUPPORT Principal Investigators. A controlled trial to improve care for seriously ill hospitalized patients: The Study to Understand Prognosis and Preferences for Outcomes and Risks of Treatments (SUPPORT). JAMA 1995;274:1591–1598.
58. Lo B. Improving care near the end of life: Why is it so hard? JAMA 1995;274:1634–1636.
58a. Chiu TY, Hu WY, Lue BH, Cheng SY, Chen CY. Sedation for refractory symptoms of terminal cancer patients in Taiwan. J Pain Symptom Manage 2001;21:467–472.
59. Morita T, Tsunoda J, Inoue S, Chihara S. Effects of high dose opioids and sedatives on survival in terminally ill cancer patients. J Pain Symptom Manage 2001;21:282–289.
60. Quill TE, Byock IR. Responding to intractable terminal suffering: The role of sedation and voluntary refusal of food and fluids. Ann Intern Med 2000;132:408–414.
61. Rousseau P. The ethical validity and clinical experience of palliative sedation. Mayo Clin Proc 2000;75:1064–1069.
62. Quill TE, Dresser R, Brock DW. The rule of double effect: A critique of its role in end of life decision making. N Engl J Med 1997;337:1768–1771.
63. Cherny NI. The use of sedation in the management of refractory pain. Principles and Practice of Supportive Oncology Updates 2000;3:1–11.
64. Fondras J. Sedation and ethical contradictions. Eur J Palliat Care 1996;3:17–20.
65. Mount B. Morphine drips, terminal sedation, and slow euthanasia: Definitions and fact, not anecdotes. J Palliat Care 1996; 12:31–37.
66. Orentlicher D. The Supreme Court and physician-assisted suicide: Rejecting assisted suicide but embracing euthanasia. N Engl J Med 1997;337:1236–1239.
67. Burt RA. The Supreme Court speaks: Not assisted suicide but a constitutional right to palliative care. N Engl J Med 1997;337: 1234–1236.
68. American Nurses Association. Code of Ethics for Nurses with Interpretive Statements. Washington, DC: Author, 2001.
69. Oncology Nursing Society. Position statement on the nurse's responsibility to the patient requesting assisted suicide, 2001. Available at: http//www.ons.org/publications/positions/AssistedSuicide.shtml (accessed January 6, 2005).
70. Cranford RE, Gensinger RG. Hospital policy on terminal sedation and euthanasia. HEC Forum 2002;14:259–264.
71. Halevy A, Brody BA. Policy perspectives: A multi-institution collaborative policy on medical futility. JAMA 1996;276: 571–574.
72. Davies R. Supporting families in palliative care. In: Ferrell B, Coyle N, eds.. Textbook of Palliative Care. Oxford: Oxford University Press, 2001:363–373.
74. Keenan SB, Busche KD, Chen LM, McCarthy L, Inman KJ, Sibbald WJ. A retrospective review of a large cohort of patients undergoing the process of withholding or withdrawal of life support. Crit Care Med 1997;25:1324–1321.
75. Luce JM, Alpers A. Legal aspects of withholding and withdrawing life support from critically ill patients in the United States and providing palliative care to them. Am J Respir Crit Care Med 2000;162:2029–2032.
76. Alpers A. Criminal act or palliative care? Prosecutions involving the care of the dying. J Law Med Ethics 1998;26:308–331.

77. Angell M. The legacy of Karen Ann Quinlan. Trends in Health Care Law and Ethics 1993:8;17–19.
78. Cogliano JF. The medical futility controversy: Bioethical implications for the critical care nurse. Crit Care Nurse Q 1999; 22:81–88.
79. Frederich ME, Strong R, von Gunten CF. Physician-nurse conflict: Can nurses refuse to carry out doctor's orders? J Palliat Med 2002;5:155–158.
80. King P, Jordan-Welch M. Nurse assisted suicide: Not an answer in end of life care. Issues Ment Health Nurs 2003;24:45–57.
81. Vachon M. The nurses role: The world of palliative nursing. In: Ferrell B, Coyle N. Textbook of Palliative Nursing. Oxford: Oxford University Press, 2001:647–662.
82. McGee DC, Weinacker AB, Raffin TA. Withdrawing life support from the critically ill. Chest 2000;118:1238–1239.
83. Curtis JR, Rubenfeld GD. Managing Death in the Intensive Care Unit: The Transition from Cure to Care. New York: Oxford University Press, 2001.
84. Thorns A. Sedation, the doctrine of double effect and the End of Life commentary. Int J Palliat Nurs 2000;341–343.

APPENDIX 24-1

End-of-Life Protocol

Introduction

The Intensive Care Unit (ICU) healthcare team provides complex medical and nursing interventions to stabilize and improve the physical status of critically ill patients. However, there are frequent situations in which the patient cannot be stabilized, their status cannot be improved or continued life-sustaining interventions would be medically inappropriate.

The End-of-life Protocol is a guide and educational tool for the ICU healthcare team. Consequently the patient will benefit from expert, competent, compassionate, consistent end-of-life care.

The End-of-Life Protocol should be initiated subsequent to a patient care conference and a written DNR order.

Definitions

ICU healthcare team—The ICU healthcare team is multidisciplinary and the participants vary according to the needs of the patient or family. Members may include: physicians, nurses, social worker, respiratory therapist, ethicist, dietician, physical therapy, pharmacist, chaplain, and others depending on the patient's physical and mental status.

Intensive care physician—The Intensive Care Physician supervising the initiation of the End-of-Life Protocol will sign the End-of Life Orders and will be readily available to consult with the nurse and family during the patient's end-of-life care.

Contact alternate physician—If the Intensive Care Physician is unavailable during the patient's end-of-life care, the Intensive Care Physician will indicate a physician that will assume supervision of the patient's care. This physician will be known as the Alternate Physician Contact and will be identified on the End-of-Life Orders by name and pager number.

Comfort measures—Comfort measures are interventions that ease the patient's discomfort. Comfort measures may include: regulation of hypothermia or hyperthermia, oral care, basic hygiene, music therapy, control of pain and sedation.

Family—Family includes spouse, mother, father, sibling, guardian, or any significant other to the patient.

Patient care conference—The family and or patient meets with the Intensive Care Physician, Attending Physician, nurse, social worker and other appropriate members from the ICU healthcare team to discuss the patient's medical status. The goal for the Patient Care Conference is to develop a plan of care that may include the End-of-Life Protocol.

Plan of care—The plan of care gives direction and prioritizes the care the patient receives.

Signs and symptoms of discomfort—Signs and symptoms of discomfort include, but are not limited to: agitated behavior, altered cognition, anxiety, autonomic hyperactivity, confusion, coughing, dyspnea, grimacing, increased work of breathing, irritation, moaning, pain, restlessness, tachycardia, splinting, tenseness, self-report of discomfort, perspiration, stiffness, trembling and tachypnea.

When appropriate—The terms "when appropriate" or "appropriate" in reference to the End-of-Life Protocol defines a time when the patient, family and ICU healthcare team are present and prepared to initiate the steps outlined in the Protocol. The timing for Protocol initiation will accommodate the needs of the patient and family.

Purpose

The purpose for the End-of-Life Protocol is to guide the ICU healthcare team, promote consistency of care, and improve the quality of care provided during the patient's end-of-life.

Goal

The goal for the End-of-Life Protocol is to maximize patient comfort and dignity without prolongation of life, extension of the dying process or hastening the dying process.

Objectives

The End-of-Life Protocol and care may include the following actions:

- Create a quiet, calm, restful atmosphere with minimal medical devices and technology in the patient's room.
- Remove or discontinue treatments that do not provide comfort for the patient.
- Provide controlled and comfortable end-of-life care for the patient.
- Promote patient comfort with a variety of approaches including medications.
- Provide physical, psychological, social, emotional, and spiritual resources for the patient and family.
- Educate and support the patient's family regarding the progression of end-of-life care and the interpretation of the clinical signs and symptoms the patient may experience.
- Assist the family in meeting their needs and the patient's needs for communication, final expressions of love, and concern.
- Assist the family in fulfilling familial, cultural or religious death rituals.

APPENDIX 24-2

Sample Institutional Policy on Palliative Sedation

Institutional Policies

Volume XI
Book J Division of Nursing Procedures
Chapter 24 Palliative Care
Policy XI.J.24.01

NURSING ADMINISTRATION OF MIDAZOLAM AND PROPOFOL TO NON-INTUBATED PATIENTS FOR PALLIATION OF SEVERE INTRACTABLE SYMPTOMS FOR TERMINALLY ILL CANCER PATIENTS ON THE PALLIATIVE CARE UNIT

PURPOSE

To establish an institutional standard for administering and monitoring sedation using midazolam and/or propofol for palliation of severe intractable symptoms for terminally ill cancer patients on the Palliative Care unit (PCU). This protocol does not address the use of midazolam or propofol or other benzodiazepines for conscious sedation or anesthesia.

GENERAL INFORMATION

Administration of anesthetic agents by RNs to non-intubated patients be practiced in accordance with the following guidelines. These are systematically developed recommendations that will provide nurses with criteria for making decisions about the administration of anesthetic agents that are consistent with evidence-based practice guidelines and the position statement of the Texas Board of Nurse Examiners on Anesthesia by RNs.

SCOPE

The Texas Board of Nurse Examiners states: "The clinical effects for patients receiving anesthetic agents may vary widely within a negligible dose range. Because of the danger of unintended deep sedation and/or general anesthesia with pharmacologic agents classified as "anesthetic" agents, the Board advises caution for registered nurses who are not qualified anesthesia providers in administering such agents in non-intubated patients. Both nurses and facilities should consider evidence-based practice guidelines put forth by the respective specialty group(s) for a given practice area in developing the appropriate guidance for the RN in the specific practice setting."

The procedure covers the administration of midazolam or propofol continuous infusion for the purposes of palliation of severe and unendurable symptoms, such as agitated delirium, severe dyspnea, or active severe bleeding. This procedure applies to terminally ill cancer patients under the care of the Palliative Care service. These symptoms can be a source of great distress to the patient and family. Sedation is a widely used intervention by Palliative Care providers, in the U.S. and internationally, to control symptoms in these rare circumstances. The practice is widely supported by the Palliative Care Literature. Midazolam is the most frequently reported agent in use. Propofol is also an agent of choice due to its speed of onset, easy titration and easy reversibility. See also "Palliative Sedation Policy for the Symptom Control and Palliative Care Service".

DEFINITIONS

Palliative sedation (previously known as terminal sedation) is defined as the monitored use of medications (midazolam or propofol) that induce sedation to control refractory and unendurable symptoms near the end of life when the control of these symptoms is not possible using less aggressive measures.
The purpose is to control symptoms and not to hasten death.

Refractory Symptoms are defined as those symptoms that cannot be adequately relieved or controlled despite aggressive use of usually effective therapies (e.g. medications, other interventions), and seem unlikely to respond to further invasive or non-invasive therapies in a timely way without excessive or intolerable side effects/complications.

Continuous infusion administration is defined as the administration of medication directly into an intravenous or subcutaneous site continuously by measured and metered dosage using an infusion pump.

Midazolam is a very short acting benzodiazepine (onset of action within 3-5 minutes after intravenous injection with peak effect seen in 20-60 minutes), used most frequently as an induction agent for general anesthesia or to provide conscious sedation during brief invasive diagnostic procedures. The drug is given by IV/SQ infusion with starting dose of 0.5-1mg/Hr.

Propofol is an intravenous sedative hypnotic agent useful in the induction and maintenance of general anesthesia, and in sedation of mechanically ventilated patients. The onset of action is given by continuous infusion with a staring dose of 0.15mg/kg/Hr.

ORDERING/ADMINISTERING PROCEDURES

PRIVILEGES

1. The Department of Palliative Care and Rehabilitation Medicine will recommend the award of privileges for Palliative Care Staff physicians for palliative sedation on the PCU using midazolam and propofol. This privilege covers evaluation of terminally ill patients for the need for the procedure, and the issuance of orders for palliative sedation.

2. Nurses who have successfully completed the Palliative Sedation Competency may administer palliative sedation as described by the Palliative care physician.

3. If ordered for palliative sedation, each of the following criteria must be met in order for midazolam or propofol to be administered.

   Irreversible advanced disease with death appearing imminent (within days to weeks).

   Severe unendurable symptoms.

   Refractory symptoms to conventional interventions.

   Anti cancer therapies have been discontinued and all interventions are tailored to patient comfort.

   DNR order in place.

   Meets medical necessity criteria based on medical judgment of a palliative care physician.

CONSENT

4. If ordered for palliative sedation, the patient and/or family receive education about the goal of palliative sedation, which is to control intractable symptoms rather than hasten death. Efforts are made to develop consensus among family members concerning the goal of this intervention. Informed consent is obtained prior to the procedure and documented in the patient medical records. If the patient is disoriented or comatose, the consent may be obtained from the individual having Medical Power of Attorney. A final review by members of the Clinical Ethics Service may be offered to the patient and/or family prior to implementation,

   These medications have the potential to induce conscious sedation and/or general anesthesia, and must be monitored accordingly. "Palliative Sedation Policy for the Symptom Control and Palliative Care Service".

PROTOCOL

5. a. Midazolam or propofol continuous infusions, administered by subcutaneous or intravenous routes, may be used for the control of refractory symptoms in the PCU (Palliative Care Unit) using Palliative Sedation Physician Orders.

   b. If midazolam or propofol continuous infusion is being considered for the management of refractory symptoms, a palliative care consultation should be established and if considered appropriate the patient will be moved to the palliative care unit where less aggressive symptom management trials may be attempted by the palliative care team. The decision to institute sedation using continuous IV midazolam or propofol should be made by the palliative care attending and documented in the patient medical records.

   c. An intravenous (IV) or subcutaneous (SQ) line is established prior to the administration of midazolam continuous infusion. An intravenous line is established before starting propofol.

   d. Assess and document vital signs prior to administration of drug.

e. Maintain aspiration precaution, provide mouth and eye care, maintain bowel and bladder care and avoid pressure sores by turning the patient regularly from side to side.

f. Continue opioids, oxygen and other medications as needed for comfort measures.

g. A patient receiving a midazloam or propofol by continuous infusion is monitored for respiratory depression and sedation. Patient monitoring requires assessment of level of consciousness and respiratory rate as medically appropriate using the Palliative Sedation record

h. Midazolam or propofol is never pushed or bolused. Administer at a continuous rate only in the Palliative Care Unit, with titration (increases or decreases in dose) no more frequently than q1h.

STARTING ANALGESIA

6. a. For Midazolam start at a dose of 0.5-1mg/hr by continuous IV or subcutaneous infusion

b. Use propofol at a starting dose of 0.15mg/kg/hr by continuous IV infusion.

c. Keep flumazenil 0.2 mg IV handy for immediate reversal of respiratory depression from infusion.

MONITORING

7. a. The registered nurse managing the care of the patient receiving IV or SQ palliative sedation shall have no other responsibilities that would leave the patient unattended until the medication is titrated to adequate symptom control. The RN will check respiratory rate as medically appropriate.

b. Use the smallest effective dose to control symptoms.

c. The order for palliative sedation should be reviewed daily by a Palliative Care physician and renewed if necessary.

REFERENCES

1. Fainsinger RL, Waller A, Bercovici M, Bengtson K, Landman W, Hosking M, Nunez-Olarte JM, deMoissac D. A multicentre international study of sedation for uncontrolled symptoms in terminally ill patients. Palliative Med 2000; 14:257–265.
2. Cowan JD, Walsh D. Terminal sedation in palliative medicine—definition and review of the literature. Support Care Cancer, 2001; 9:403–407.
3. Gremaud G, Zulian GB. Letter, Indications and limitations of intravenous and subcutaneous Midazolam in a palliative care center. J Pain Symptom Manag 1998; 15:331–333.
4. Chater S, Viola R, Paterson J, Jarvis V. Sedation for intractable distress in the dying—a survey of experts. Palliative Med 1998; 12:255–269.
5. Cherny NI, Coyle N, Foley KM. The treatment of suffering when patients request elective death. J Palliat Care 1994; 10:71–79.

6. Fainsinger RL. Use of sedation by a hospital palliative care support team. J Palliat Med 1998; 14:51–54.
7. Glover ML, Kodish E, Reed MD. Continuous propofol infusion for relief of treatment-resistant discomfort in a terminally ill pediatric patient with cancer. J Pediatr Hematol+ Oncol 1996; 18:377–380.
8. Mercadante S, De Conno F, Ripamonti C. Propofol in terminal care. J Pain Symptom Manag 1995; 10:639–642.
9. Moyle J. The use of propofol in palliative medicine. J Pain Symptom Manag 1995; 10:643–646.
10. Ramani S, Karnad AB. Long-term subcutaneous infusion of midazolam for refractory delirium in terminal breast cancer. South Med J 1996; 89:1101–1103.
11. Stone P, Phillips C, Spruyt O, Waight C. A comparison of the use of sedatives in a hospital support team and in a hospice. Palliat Med 1997; 11:140–144.
12. Vainio A, Auvinen A. and members of the Symptom Prevalence Group. Prevalence of symptoms among patients with advanced cancer: an international collaborative study. J Pain Symptom Manag 1996; 12:3–10.

APPENDIX 24-3

Sample ICU End-of-Life Orders

Date Printed:
09/24/2004

THE UNIVERSITY OF TEXAS MD ANDERSON CANCER CENTER

Inpatient Physician Orders

MRN:

Pt Name:

DOB: Sex:

ICU End of Life Orders

Attending Physician: ______________________

Height: _________**cm** **Weight:** ___________**Kg**

Primary Diagnosis: ______________________ **Admitting Diagnosis** ________________

Allergies: ______________________

Provider's signature indicates all orders with boxes checked are activated.

☐ Verify that physician determination of resuscitation status is consistent with a plan to optimize patient comfort.
☐ Titrate medications to alleviate the patient's signs and symptoms of discomfort.
☐ Contact Chaplain of family's choice for spiritual support.

Transitional Care:

☐ Discontinue neuromuscular blockade agents prior to weaning ventilator.
☐ Discontinue all tests and laboratory studies.
☐ Remove all monitoring equipment from the patient and patient's bedside except for the ECG.
☐ Suspend arrhythmia detection at bedside and central station.
☐ Suspend or decrease all auditory alarms at bedside and central station.
☐ Discontinue medications and fluids when appropriate:
 ☐ Hydration ☐ Vasoactive medication ☐ other ____________
☐ Discontinue mechanical support devices:
 ☐ Dialysis ☐ IABP ☐ other ____________
☐ Assess and monitor the patient for signs and symptoms of discomfort.
☐ Liberalize visitation

Medications:

☐ Morphine drip at ________ mg/hr **or** ☐ Fentanyl drip at ________ mcg/hr.
☐ Lorazepam drip at ________ mg/hr **or** ☐ Midazolam drip at ________ mg/hr.
☐ Other medication drips (i.e. benzodiazepine, barbiturate, propofol):
 ☐ ____________ mg/mcg/kg/hr ☐ ____________ mg/mcg/Kg/hr
 ☐ ____________ mg/mcg/kg/hr ☐ ____________ mg/mcg/Kg/hr
☐ For signs of patient discomfort give IV bolus of medication equal to drip rate every 3 minutes until patient is comfortable.
☐ To **maintain** patient comfort, increase drip rate up to 50 % of prior rate.
☐ Contact physician and charge nurse regarding patient status.

Ventilator:

☐ Initiate ventilator wean once patient appears comfortable.
☐ Oscillatory Ventilation converted to conventional ventilator.
☐ Initial Ventilator setting: F_iO_2 ________ Bilevel – High PEEP ______ Low PEEP ________
 PS ______ IMV ________ PEEP ________
☐ Reduce all ventilator alarms to minimum settings.
☐ Transition F_iO_2 to 0.21 and PEEP to zero.
☐ Assess for signs and symptoms of patient discomfort while decreasing the tidal volume and rate.
☐ When the patient is comfortable on minimal ventilator support, select one:
 ☐ extubate to room air ☐ T-piece ☐ remain on ventilator

Signature / Credentials / ID Code: ______________________________

Pager: ________________ **Date:** ________ **Time:** ________

FAX COMPLETED ORDERS TO PHARMACY
File under: Physician Order

Page 1 of 1

POS ICU 00032 V2 10/25/04

25

Susan Berenson

Complementary and Alternative Therapies in Palliative Care

I was in so much distress that I wanted to let go. You gave me the reflexology and now I feel like I want to go on living.—A patient

- ***Key Points***
- *Complementary therapies improve quality of life in patients with advanced cancer.*
- *Complementary therapies reduce physical, psychosocial, and spiritual symptoms and provide comfort.*
- *Nurses bring hope and power to patients and families through education and guidance to safe complementary therapies.*

CASE STUDY

Mary, a 64-Year-Old Woman with Stage IV Lung Cancer

Mary was a 64-year-old vivacious, beautiful woman with a zest for life, a wonderful sense of humor, and a terrific Welsh accent. She appeared much younger than her stated age. She was born in Wales and immigrated to the United States at the age of 23. She was happily married for 29 years and had a 23-year-old son, whom she adored. Mary was a strong woman who had managed to stay sober in Alcoholics Anonymous one day at a time for 10 years, and who was able to stop smoking after 35 to 40 years of smoking. She had numerous friends and was cherished by many.

Mary was in good health until a tumor was discovered in 1998 on a routine chest radiograph. She had a right upper lobectomy and was diagnosed with non–small cell lung cancer. No follow-up treatment was done. She was devastated by the diagnosis, but once she recovered from the surgery, she seemed to be back to her old self. In the fall of 1999, Mary suffered from several bouts of pneumonia, shortness of breath, sore throat, and fatigue. In summer of 2000, some cervical lymphadenopathy was noticed; positron emission tomography (PET) scanning showed multiple lymph node involvement, including right supraclavicular, right adrenal, right paraspinal, right diaphragmatic, and mediastinal spread. She sought out a second opinion and transferred her care to a major cancer center, where biopsy of the right supraclavicular lymph node confirmed metastatic non–small cell lung cancer.

The nurses at the cancer center informed Mary about the Integrative Medicine Service (IMS). Mary came to IMS several weeks after her biopsy. She had a consultation with the clinical nurse specialist (CNS), who also administered several of the therapies to inpatients and outpatients. The CNS explained that all of the therapies and classes were focused on stress management, symptom control, and improving quality of life. The verbal assessment of the patient by the CNS revealed the following symptoms: tenderness in the right lower neck, anxiety, fatigue, nausea, and depression. The CNS discussed the various therapies and asked the patient what she thought she might like. It was decided to begin with acupuncture to help reduce the neck pain and the nausea. Mary had a few sessions of acupuncture and was pleased to see a reduction in neck pain and nausea. A few weeks later, Mary came in and talked about how worried she was about the tumor and her symptoms. She was asked to rate her symptoms on a scale of 1 to 10. She reported nausea 7/10, fatigue 9/10, anxiety 9/10, and depression 5/10. It was decided to give reflexology as an attempt to reduce her symptoms. After the 60-minute reflexology session, Mary was smiling and excited to see the rather rapid reduction of her symptoms as she rated nausea 1/10, fatigue 1/10, anxiety 0/10, and depression 0/10.

The following week, Mary reported that her treatment of chemotherapy was to be given the following week and she was experiencing a great deal of anxiety and muscle tension. A light to moderate medical massage was given, with reported relief of anxiety and muscular tension. The following week, Mary came to IMS the day after her first chemotherapy. She reported fatigue 7/10, anxiety 8/10, depression 6/10, and some pain 5/10 in her upper back. She was given again a light to moderate massage with the resulting reduction of fatigue 1/10, anxiety 0/10, depression 3/10, and pain 2/10. She left smiling and said, "This was a great way to end my day."

Mary continued to come weekly to IMS as she received her chemotherapy. She reported more fatigue and cried at times about her son, her thinning hair, wondering if there would be a future, and being less able "to do life." Because she was weaker and had very low platelet counts, reflexology was more the therapy of choice, with the resulting relief of anxiety and some of the fatigue. She reported, "I feel like I could go out dancing." Mary's disease course was complicated by shortness of breath, chest pain from a pulmonary embolus, a deep vein thrombosis (DVT) in the right neck, and a DVT of the left lower leg. She required hospitalization and was very frightened. Reflexology and massage were contraindicated, but Reiki was offered. Mary responded beautifully to Reiki; as her anxiety decreased, she reported, "You are my angels that help me get through these tough times."

Mary was discharged after the placement of a Greenfield filter to prevent further movement of emboli and was started on the anticoagulant Fragmin. She returned to IMS to learn meditation and attended the chair aerobics class to learn exercises to help decrease breathlessness and fatigue and to increase her endurance for everyday activities.

Mary did well for another month but then it became clear that her disease was progressing with the development of pleural effusions, chest pain, and increasing shortness of breath. She required constant nasal oxygen and wore a Fentanyl patch for her chest pain. Mary eventually needed to be admitted again, and this time it was for the last time. IMS saw her frequently and was able to offer her the soothing benefits of light touch Reiki and music therapy. Often, both were offered at the same time. The nursing staff was grateful that the IMS team came and could always offer Mary something that made her feel better. Mary never declined the offer of these services, always had a smile when IMS appeared at her hospital door, always nodded yes, and raised her weakened hand, beckoning us to approach her bedside. Her husband and son, often in attendance, were taught some of the Reiki touch techniques and were encouraged to join in the singing and gentle drumming of the music. The last words that IMS staff heard from Mary's lips were, "My angels."

After reading this chapter, the reader should begin to understand the rationale for the choices that Mary and her caregivers made as she moved through the last stages of her life.

Introduction to Complementary and Alternative Therapies

There is worldwide use of complementary and alternative medicine (CAM) by cancer patients for many reasons (Table 25–1), but many of the oncologists and nurses that provide care for cancer patients have limited or no knowledge of these therapies or their benefits versus risks. Complementary medicine has become an important aspect of palliative and supportive cancer care.[1] The management of debilitating physical

Table 25–1
Reasons for Use of Complementary and Alternative Medicine

Poor prognosis
Focus of care is comfort not cure
Desire to be more active in one's own health care
Reduce side effects of treatment
Reduce side effects of the disease
Desire to cover all the options
Suggestions by family/friends/society to try it
Philosophical or cultural orientation
Less expensive than conventional medicine
Easier access to health food store than physician
Dissatisfaction with or loss of trust in conventional medicine
Desire to treat the disease in a "natural" way
Hope of altering the disease progression
Decrease the feelings of helplessness and hopelessness
Improve the immune system
Improve overall health
Improve the quality of one's life

symptoms, particularly in terminally ill patients, is integral to good palliative care. When curative treatment is no longer an option, the emphasis of care shifts to palliation and symptom management. Comfort measures become the main focus.[2]

Many patients in the advanced stages of cancer seek treatments outside conventional medicine in hopes of a cure and better management of the debilitating physical symptoms. Some CAM therapies can improve quality of life, such as management of pain, dyspnea, nausea and vomiting, fatigue, anxiety, depression, insomnia, and peripheral neuropathy, whereas others may be potentially harmful or useless. It is difficult, if not impossible, for most readers to distinguish between reputable treatments and promotions of unproven alternatives pushed by vested interests. CAM is complicated because of its unfamiliar terminology, large numbers of available therapies, and the controversial anecdotal stories versus good research studies. It is confusing for patients, families, doctors and nurses to find their way through to the most effective and safest choices.

In this chapter, the focus is on the most helpful complementary therapies. Cancer is used as a model of chronic progressive disease. Most of the literature and research on CAM is related to cancer but can be expanded to cardiac, liver, and lung disease, diabetes, and other illnesses. Evidence-based complementary therapies are shown to affect in safe ways patients' physical, emotional, and spiritual well-being. Individuals who can participate in their care in the last stages of their illnesses are often more hopeful and positive than those who are passive participants. Patients in the advanced stages of their disease can participate in their care by knowing that they have options to promote comfort and quality of life. It is the role of nurses to educate themselves, their patients, and families to assist in the critical decision-making of CAM.

The goals of this chapter are (1) to define terms related to CAM; (2) to list, define, and describe the benefits and risks of the most common CAM therapies; (3) to emphasize the most beneficial evidenced-based complementary therapies along with the supportive research; and (4) to describe the role of the nurse as an educator, researcher, and clinical practitioner in the setting of CAM. Patients look to their nurses to guide them to make informed and safe complementary therapy choices. Nurses can bring hope and power to their patients and families by teaching, supporting, and encouraging the use of safe complementary therapies when indicated.

Definitions

CAM can include anything that is not conventional Western medicine or found in hospitals.[3,4] CAM is a group of diverse medical and health care systems, practices, therapies, and products that are not presently considered to be part of conventional medicine. "They range from adjunctive modalities that effectively enhance quality of life and promising antitumor herbal remedies now under investigation to bogus therapies that claim to cure cancer and that harm not only directly, but also indirectly by encouraging patients to avoid or postpone effective cancer care."[5] The list of what is considered to be CAM changes continually, as therapies that are proven to be safe and effective become adopted into conventional health care.

Although they are grouped together, complementary and alternative therapies are very different. Complementary therapies are used together with conventional care. They are not promoted as cancer cures but are used as soothing, noninvasive therapies to provide comfort and increase the quality of life to patients (Table 25–2). The goals of complementary cancer care are to promote relaxation, reduce stress and anxiety, relieve pain and other symptoms, reduce adverse effects of conventional therapies, and improve sleep.[1] An example of a complementary therapy is the use of reflexology to help to lessen patients' anxiety as they await a painful procedure.

In contrast, alternative therapies are used in place of surgery, chemotherapy, and radiation therapies. They are invasive, biologically active, and unproven and are promoted as viable cures and alternatives to be used in place of mainstream cancer treatments.[6] Some examples of alternative therapies are Laetrile, dietary cancer cures, oxygen therapy, and biomagnetics. There is not a single alternative intervention (as opposed to mainstream therapies) that has been demonstrated to constitute an effective cure for cancer.[1] Alternative therapies can misguide, raise false hopes, and financially exploit patients and may be associated with significant risks. They may prevent patients from seeking known, helpful medical oncological interventions.[7]

Integrative oncology medicine promotes the use of evidence-based complementary therapies along with mainstream cancer treatments. At a major comprehensive cancer center, Memorial Sloan-Kettering Cancer Center (MSKCC) in New York

Table 25–2
Evidence-based Complementary Medicine Therapies for Symptom Control and Quality of Life

Physical	Cognitive
Acupuncture	Art therapy
Acupressure	Biofeedback
Aromatherapy	Creative visualization
Chiropractic medicine	Focused breathing
Exercise	Guided imagery
Massage	Hypnosis
Nutrition	Meditation
Polarity	Music therapy
Qi gong	Progressive muscle relaxation
Reflexology	
Reiki	
Shiatsu	
Therapeutic touch	
Yoga	

City, Integrative Medicine practitioners of massage, reflexology, Reiki, meditation, acupuncture, art therapy, and music therapy work with inpatients who have been self-referred or referred by doctors, nurses, or other hospital professionals. Outpatients are offered these same therapies along with nutritional counseling, yoga, Tai chi, Qi gong, and other exercise classes.

History

The history of medicine is filled with descriptions of persons using herbs, potions, and physical and spiritual manipulations to heal the sick. Traditional medicine came into being in the United States in the late 1890s when physicians began to develop the science of medicine, with a focus on cure. Anything other than the allopathic physician using science-based diagnosis and prescribing tested medicines began to be considered quackery.[8] The healer became passé. Recently, however, there has been a resurgence of interest in the use of herbal and other CAM therapies that fall outside mainstream medicine. People are living longer with chronic diseases, cancer being one of them. Patients look to CAM therapies to help with quality of life, to allow them to participate in their own self-care, and to provide a glimmer of hope and maybe a cure. Physicians and nurses are voicing concerns that patients are being misled about CAM therapies, are wasting their time and money, are putting themselves in harm's way, and are not reporting the use of these therapies to the medical team.

The increasing use of CAM by the American people prompted the United States Congress to establish in 1992 the Office of Alternative Medicine (OAM) as part of the National Institutes of Health (NIH). In 1998, the name was changed to the National Center for Complementary and Alternative Medicine (NCCAM), and a larger budget was assigned. NCCAM's mission is to explore complementary and alternative healing practices in the context of rigorous science, to train CAM researchers, and to inform the public and health professionals about the results of CAM research studies.

Prevalence

General Population

The use of CAM by the general population in the United States is common, widespread, and on the rise. In a national health interview survey conducted by the Centers for Disease Control and Prevention (CDC) in 2002, use of CAM therapies among U.S. adults was 36% when prayer was excluded and 62% when prayer for health reasons was included.[9] Some publications cite prayer as a CAM therapy. Prayer has been with us for a long time and is not considered to be a CAM in the strict sense of the term; it is excluded from further discussion as a CAM therapy in this chapter. Other findings of the CDC study were that women are more likely than men, black adults more likely than white or Asian adults, persons with higher educations more likely than those with lower education, and those who have been hospitalized in the past year more likely than those who have not been hospitalized to use CAM.

Cancer Population

Among cancer patients, rates of CAM use are usually higher than in the general population. But Ernst and Cassileth,[10] in 1998, found that the average use in 26 surveys from 13 countries was 31.4%, ranging from 7% to 64%. They believed that lack of specificity and inconsistent definitions of CAM to have contributed to this variability. For example, some studies included counseling, group therapy, prayer, wellness regimens, and self-help efforts as CAM, whereas others counted these as mainstream therapies. Another study reported 63% use of CAM therapies by adult cancer patients enrolled in an National Cancer Institute (NCI) clinical trial.[11] Higher use among women and among patients with higher education was also observed. Sixty-two percent of the patients in this study reported that they would have liked to talk to their physicians about the use of these therapies, but 57% said that their physicians did not ask them about CAM therapies.

Rural Cancer Population

One study looked at the use of only complementary therapies in a rural cancer population.[12] Eighty-seven percent of the patients were using at least one complementary therapy, most commonly prayer, humor, support group, and relaxing music and visualization. Again, women were found to be more interested in CAM, but education and income did not seem to make a difference in this population.

Comprehensive Cancer Center

In an outpatient clinic in a comprehensive cancer center, 83% of the patients had used at least one CAM therapy.[13] When psychotherapy and spiritual practices were eliminated, 68.7% had used at least one other CAM therapy. Use of multiple CAM therapies with conventional treatment was widespread, disclosure of CAM to the physician was low, and seeking information about CAM was high.

Breast Cancer Patients

The prevalence of CAM among breast cancer patients varies but is higher than in the general population. New use of CAM after surgery in patients with early-stage breast cancer (28.1%) was thought to be a marker for greater psychosocial distress and worse quality of life.[14] It was suggested that physicians take note of such usage and evaluate patients for anxiety, depression, and physical symptoms. The prevalence of CAM use among breast cancer survivors in Ontario, Canada, was 66.7% and was mostly associated with the hope of boosting the immune system.[8,15] Women with breast cancer tended to use more CAM, compared with patients with other malignancies

(63% versus 83%, respectively).[8,16] In the largest patient cohort to date (500 women with breast and gynecological cancers), 48% of the breast cancer patients used CAM therapies, and the number increased to 58% after patients who had recurrent disease were included.[17] These higher percentages may be indicative of the patients' high level of distress, but they may also indicate the seeking of hope and attempts to control their situations.

Pediatric Population

CAM therapies are infrequently studied in pediatric populations. Parents of patients were surveyed in British Columbia between 1989 and 1995. CAM was found to be used by 42% of the patients.[18] Relaxation techniques and imagery were used to reduce chemotherapy side effects in children and adolescents.[19] At MSKCC, reflexology, imagery, and music therapy are successful used in the pediatric population for the symptoms of pain and anxiety. There is some evidence from letters published in the New England Journal of Medicine[20] that some parents choose alternative approaches, where evidence of efficiency is lacking, rather than conventional evidence-based therapies. Use of conventional and alternative therapies simultaneously is also of concern, because there could be a harmful reaction between the two. The possibility of simultaneous use calls for education and discussion with the parents and families about known risks and the recognition that "doing everything" may be harmful.[21]

Ethnic Differences

There appears to be a relation between ethnicity and CAM use. In a diverse population in Hawaii, CAM use was highest among Filipino and Caucasian patients, intermediate among the Native Hawaiians and Chinese, and significantly lower among Japanese patients.[22] The preferences were as follows: Filipinos, religious healing or prayer; Japanese, vitamins and supplements; Chinese, herbal therapies; Native Hawaiians, religious healing, prayer, vitamins, supplements, massage, and bodywork; and Caucasians, vitamins and supplements along with support groups and homeopathy. A study by Lee and associates[23] on the use and choices of CAM by women with breast cancer in four ethnic populations revealed that Blacks most often chose spiritual healing, Chinese chose herbal remedies, Latinas chose dietary therapies and spiritual healing, and Whites chose dietary methods and physical methods such as massage and acupuncture. Another study of Navajo patients revealed that 62% used Native healers but did not see a conflict between the use of a native healer and use of conventional medicine.[24] These studies suggest that culture can influence CAM choices and should be considered when caring for patients.

Elderly

Another study[25] found CAM use in older adults (65 years of age and older) to be 64%. This study also revealed that only 35% of all self-reported supplements actually were documented in the patient's chart by the physician. This created potential risks, because some patients were found to be taking CAM with anticoagulant properties along with prescribed anticoagulants.

Cost

Most insurance companies do not reimburse for CAM. The cost of CAM may prevent many patients from receiving these therapies. There is a movement before the U.S. Congress to begin to acknowledge the value of these therapies and to reimburse for them. It is suggested that patients check with their insurance companies to see whether use of CAM can be reimbursed. There is hope that reimbursement will be soon forthcoming.

Overview of Complementary and Alternative Therapies

CAM therapies have been grouped into five major domains by the NCCAM: (1) alternative medical systems (traditional Chinese medicine, ayurvedic medicine, homeopathic medicine, naturopathic medicine, Native American medicine, and Tibetan medicine); (2) mind–body interventions (meditation, focused breathing, progressive muscle relaxation, guided imagery, creative visualization, hypnosis, biofeedback, music therapy, and art therapy); (3) biologically based therapies, nutrition, and special diets (e.g., macrobiotics, megavitamin and orthomolecular therapies, metabolic therapies, individual biological therapies such as shark cartilage) and herbal medicine; (4) manipulative and body-based methods (massage, aromatherapy, reflexology, acupressure, Shiatsu, polarity, chiropractic medicine, yoga, and exercise); and (5) energy therapies (Reiki, Qi gong, and therapeutic touch). The currently popular therapies are discussed in the following sections. Many of these methods are not proven, whereas others have been documented as helpful complementary therapies.

Counseling, group therapy, prayer, and spirituality, which we already know to be very helpful to cancer patients, are not included in this CAM chapter, because many view them as part of mainstream therapies.

Alternative Medical Systems

Instead of disease-oriented therapies, ancient systems of healing were based on attributing health, illness, and death to an invisible energy or life force and the suggestion of an interaction between the human body, human kind, the spirit world, and the universe. In the earliest of times, there seemed to be a link between religion, magic, and medicine. This is in contrast to modern Western medicine, which is focused on the cause and curing of the disease. These alternative medicine systems are briefly discussed in this chapter because they are followed by many people today. The best known examples of alternative medical systems are traditional Chinese medicine (TCM), India's Ayurvedic medicine, homeopathic medicine, naturopathic medicine, Native American medicine, and Tibetan medicine. Ancient healing systems tend to remain unchanged, unlike modern medicine, which keeps growing and expanding on a regular basis. A common feature across alternative medical systems is an emphasis on working with internal natural forces to achieve a harmonic state of mind and body, which can promote a sense of well-being and comfort. This idea, although outmoded and unscientific, has great appeal for many in the general public and especially for cancer patients dealing with advanced disease.

Traditional Chinese Medicine

The cornerstone concept in Chinese medicine is qi (life force), which is energy that flows through the body along pathways known as meridians. TCM views people as ecosystems in miniature.[26] Any imbalance or disruption in the circulation of Chi or qi (pronounced "chee") is thought to result in illness. Restoration of one's health is therefore dependent on returning the balance and flow of the life force. A TCM diagnosis is based on examination of the person's complexion, tongue, radial pulse, and detection of scents in bodily materials. Treatment is geared toward correcting imbalances or disruptions of the qi, primarily with herbal formulas and acupuncture.[26]

Acupuncture is one of the best known forms of CAM. It is one component of TCM. It is based on the belief that qi, the life force, flows through the human body in vertical energy channels known as meridians. There are 12 main meridians, which are believed to be dotted with acupoints that correspond to every body part and organ. To restore the balance and flow of qi, very fine disposable needles are inserted into the acupoints just under the skin. Other stimuli can be used along with acupuncture, such as heat (moxibustion), suction (cupping), external pressure (acupressure), and electrical currents (electroacupuncture). The biological basis of qi or meridians has not been found, but is thought that acupuncture needling releases endorphins and other neurotransmitters in the brain.[27] There is good evidence in the oncology literature that acupuncture helps control pain and nausea and vomiting. There is current research on its possible effectiveness for fatigue and dyspnea. Risks associated with acupuncture include mild discomfort or occasionally a drop of blood and or a small bruise at the site of the insertion, but they can include more serious problems, such as an infection or (in the most extreme case) a pneumothorax, which is rare and depends on the training and experience of the acupuncturist.

Ayurvedic Medicine

The term Ayurveda comes from Sanskrit words ayur (life) and veda (knowledge) and is about 5000 years old. Ayurvedic medicine is based on the idea that illness is the absence of physical, emotional, and spiritual harmony.[28] Many of the basic principles are similar to those of Chinese medicine. Ayurveda is a natural system of medicine that uses diet, herbs, cleansing and purification practices, meditation, yoga, astrology, and gemstones to bring about healing. It sees causation of disease as an accumulation of toxins in the body and an imbalance of emotions. It prescribes individualized diets, regular detoxification, cleansing from all orifices, meditation, and yoga as some of the therapies. There is no scientific evidence that Ayurvedic medicine healing techniques cure illness.

Homeopathic Medicine

Homeopathy is a medical system that was devised by Samuel Hahnemann 200 years ago, when the causes of diseases, bacteria and viruses, were unknown and little was understood about the workings of the bodily organs. The thinking was that symptoms of ill health represent expressions of disharmony within the person and attempts of the body to heal itself and to return to a state of balance. It is the person, not the disease, that needs treatment. The treatment of disease is based on the principle, "Like cures like." Homeopathic medicines are made by taking original substances from plants, animals, and minerals and highly diluting them. It is believed that the body's own healing ability is stimulated by these medicines. Homeopathic medicines are sold over the counter without prescription. They are so dilute that they are thought to have no side effects and at the same time to be ineffectual for medical conditions, including cancer-related conditions.

Naturopathic Medicine

Naturopathy is more of a philosophical approach to health than a particular form of therapy. It is an alternative medical system that attempts to cure disease by harnessing the body's own natural healing powers, and restoring good health and preventing disease. Rejecting synthetic drugs and invasive procedures, it stresses the restorative powers of nature, the search for the underlying causes of disease, and the treatment of the whole person. It takes very seriously the motto, "First, do no harm." Naturopathic medicine began as a quasispiritual "back to nature" movement in the 19th century. European founders advocated exposure to air, water, and sunlight as the best therapy for all ailments and recommended spa treatments such as hot mineral baths as virtual cure-alls. This system relies on natural healing approaches such as herbs, nutrition, and movement or manipulation of the body. Most naturopathic remedies are considered harmless by conventional practitioners, but using naturopathy instead of conventional medicine is not wise.[28]

American Indian Medicine

Native American medicine is a system of healing that is used as the primary source of medical care or in combination with

Western medicine. Physical illness is attributed to spiritual causes or evil spirits. Healing involves activities that appease the spirits, rid the individuals of impurities, and restore them to a healthful, spiritually pure state.[28] The central figure in American Indian healing is the medicine man (healer, sorcerer, seer, educator, and priest), often called shaman. Shamans are trained spiritual healers who seek to drive the evil spirits out. Four healing techniques are practiced by Native Americans: purifying and purging the body through the sweat lodge, the use of herbs, involvement of shamanic healers, and symbolic rituals. Shamanistic methods included incantations, charms, prayers, dances, shaking of rattles, beating of drums, and sucking to remove disease. Native American healing is more spiritual and magical than scientific. There are anecdotal reports of healers curing diseases, but these have not been formally investigated.[28] The most important evidence of Native American influence on traditional American medicine is the fact that >200 indigenous medicines that were used by one or more tribes have been listed in the Pharmacopeia of the United States of America.[29]

Tibetan Medicine

Tibetan medicine views the human body as an ecological system, a microcosm directly related to the macrocosm of the world. It attempts to investigate the root causes of illness. The belief is that all of the material that makes up our universe is based on the qualities of five basic elements (earth, water, fire, wind, and space). It is understood through experience that natural environmental forces can influence the functioning of the human organism. The Tibetan doctor bases his practice of diagnosis on his own spiritual practice, intellectual training, and intuition. The Tibetan medical diagnosis is a result of the patient interview, observation of the urine, taking of the 12 pulses, looking at the sclera and surface of the tongue, and feeling for sensitivity on certain parts of the body. The treatment is similar to that used in Chinese medicine, especially herbs.

Mind–Body Interventions

Mind–body medicine uses a variety of techniques designed to enhance the mind's capacity to effect change in bodily functions and symptoms. The ability to influence health with the mind is an extremely appealing concept, especially for patients who feel out of control. These are distraction techniques. To affirm the power of the individual, when a person can feel so powerless, is very attractive. Some good documentation supports the effectiveness of meditation, guided imagery, biofeedback, and yoga in stress reduction and the control of symptoms. The ability to control stress or other symptoms was expanded to the notion of controlling or curing the disease. There is no evidence that patients can control their disease through mental work. Furthermore, this approach can backfire on patients; they may feel guilty, responsible, and a failure as disease progresses despite their best mental efforts.

Meditation

Meditation is the intentional self-regulation of attention. It enhances concentration and awareness as the individual focuses systematically and intentionally on particular aspects of inner or outer experience. It allows one to stay present in the moment and without judgment.[30] Historically, most meditation practices were developed within a spiritual or religious context with the goal of spiritual growth, personal transformation, or transcendental experience.[31]

There are two categories of meditation: concentration and mindfulness. Concentrative methods cultivate one-pointedness of attention and start with mantras (sounds, words, or phrases repeated), as in Transcendental Meditation (TM). Mindfulness-based stress reduction (MBSR) practices start with the observation of thoughts, emotions, and sensations without judgment as they arise in the field of awareness.[30] "Meditation can help individuals connect with what is deepest and most nourishing in themselves, and to mobilize the full range of inner and outer resources available to them."[30] Meditation has been helpful for terminally ill cancer patients. It has shown to be helpful in the relief of physical and emotional pain when integrated into a palliative care program. Many dying cancer patients discover that the calmness and quiet of meditation promotes a profound feeling of acceptance, well-being, and inner peace.[30]

Walking meditation is appealing to those that cannot sit still. The focus might be on taking one step at a time, smelling the fresh air, taking in one breath at a time, or listening to the birds as one walks along.

Relaxation Techniques

Relaxation techniques are those simple techniques that, when learned by the patient, can promote relaxation. They include progressive muscle relaxation (contracting and relaxing muscle groups one at a time from head to toe), passive progressive muscle relaxation (no contraction of muscles, but focusing in the mind on sequentially relaxing groups of muscles),[32] focused breathing (counting of breaths as one exhales, which can be used by itself or as an introduction to guided imagery).

Guided Imagery

"Imagery is the thought process that invokes and uses the senses: vision, audition, smell, taste, sense of movement, position, and touch. It is the communication mechanism between perception, emotion, and bodily change."[33] Imagery is a natural phenomenon in our lives that occurs all day long. For example, when we wake in the morning, we might imagine our day, where we will be going, what we will wear, what we will eat. Imagery is used as a distraction technique that allows the patient to shift the focus from distress (e.g., pain, anxiety, nausea) to the sensory details of a past pleasant experience. This usually distracts the patient enough so that some of the physical and emotional symptoms decrease. Guided imagery allows a practitioner to help the cancer patient through his or her own past positive experiences or to create a positive image of the future along with the patient. It is a very effective therapy for symptom control. Guided imagery can be taught to nurses and family members so that they can affect the quality of the patient's life.[32] Guided imagery is contraindicated in a patient with cognitive impairment.

Creative Visualization

Creative visualization is the technique of using the imagination to create what one wants in life physically, emotionally, mentally, or spiritually. It is using the imagination to create a clear image of something one wishes to manifest. For the patient in the end stage of disease, visualization might take the form of imagining being at home again, feeling calm or more comfortable, visiting with a loved one, or going to that quiet still place within. The patient continues to focus on the idea or image regularly, giving it positive energy, until what is being visualized is achieved. It is preceded by relaxing into a deep meditative state. It is based on the following principles: the physical universe is energy (including individuals and their thoughts); energy is magnetic (energy of a certain quality attracts energy of a similar quality); form follows idea (the idea has energy that attracts and creates that form on the material plane; it magnetizes and guides the physical energy to flow into that form and eventually manifest on the physical plane); and the law of radiation and attraction (we attract into our lives what we think about).[34] The point is that each individual is the constant creator of his or her life and has the means to bring himself or herself to a more comfortable place physically, emotionally, mentally, and spiritually. There is no evidence that creative visualization is curing cancer, but it can be very effective for symptom management.

Hypnosis

Relaxation and imagery techniques are often used to induce an altered state of consciousness or a hypnotic trance state. All hypnosis is self-hypnosis. A trained professional can teach a patient to enter a hypnotic trance state. It is important, clinically, to recognize and this state, because in it the individual is typically more suggestible, or more receptive to new ideas and initiation of new behaviors. According to Milton Erikson, in hypnosis the "limits of one's usual frame of reference and beliefs are temporarily altered so that one can be receptive to other patterns of association and modes of mental functioning that are more conducive to problem solving."[35] Hypnosis has been shown to be helpful in the management of pain, dyspnea, anxiety, and phobias. It is contraindicated in patients with cognitive impairment.

Biofeedback

Biofeedback involves the use of devices that amplify physiological processes (e.g., blood pressure, muscle activity, skin temperature, perspiration, pulse, respiratory rate, and electroencephalography) that ordinarily cannot be perceived without amplification. Patients are guided through relaxation and imagery exercises and are instructed to alter their physiological processes using as a guide the provided biofeedback (typically visual or auditory data). The primary objective of biofeedback is to promote relaxation. It is a noninvasive procedure. It has been shown to be effective for anxiety and tension headaches.

Music Therapy

Music therapy in the palliative care setting is essential. Music can break the cyclic nature of pain, alter mood, promote relaxation, and improve communication.[36] Music can facilitate the participation of the patient with family and hospital staff. Music therapists apply psychotherapeutic skills in the setting of music as they care for patients with advanced cancer. Music therapy interventions consist of use of precomposed songs (reflecting messages or feelings that are foremost in the patient's thoughts), improvisation (offering opportunities for spontaneous expression and discovery), chanting and toning (use of vocalization to promote attentiveness and relaxation), imagery (exploration of images and feelings that arise in the music), music listening techniques (which facilitate reminiscence and build self-esteem through reflection on accomplishments), and taping of the music session as a gift for the family.[36] Music therapy may help to facilitate a life review for the patient. It can also help in management of the most common symptoms of advanced cancer: pain,[37] anxiety and depression,[38] nausea and vomiting,[39] shortness of breath,[40] and sleeplessness.[39] Live music has been shown to be more effective than taped music.[41]

Art Therapy

Art therapy is a form of psychotherapy. Art therapists are trained professionals. Art therapy focuses on assisting patients to express, explore, and transform sensations, emotions, and thoughts connected with physical and psychological suffering.[36] In art therapy, the art therapist and the art materials (e.g., paper, colored markers, oil pastels, cut-up images from magazines) help patients get in touch with their feelings, their fears, and their hopes and put them out onto the paper, thus helping patients process their experience of illness. It can easily be accommodated to hospitalized inpatients as well as to outpatient art groups or individuals. Art therapy can assist patients with advanced-stage cancer in the management of pain, fatigue, and stress.[42] Art images can serve to help the dying patient with issues of anger, bereavement, and loss. The art therapist may help dying patients find "personal symbols" to express something so powerful and so mysterious as the end of life.[42]

Biologically Based Therapies

Alternative diets have an ancient history, both medical and cultural, of plants and herbs as the first medicines. The example of vitamin C curing scurvy reinforces the idea of foods being medicines and curing illness. Some of the ancient medicine systems are still being practiced today; for example, Ayurvedic medicine uses special diets, herbs, and cleansings to treat illness and promote health.

Today's food pyramid recommends fiber, grains, fruits and vegetables, and less protein, meat, and dairy products than was emphasized in earlier U.S. Department of Agriculture government guidelines. It emphasizes balance. Changes in guidelines are based on carefully controlled scientific studies. Many alternative and fad diets, herbs, and supplements are either not scientifically validated or are marketed despite having been found worthless or harmful.

Nutrition

Some alternative practitioners believe that dietary treatments can prevent cancer or even go a step further to believe that foods or vitamins can cure cancer. The American Cancer Society Guidelines on Nutrition form the basis for a healthful diet that emphasizes vegetables, fruits, legumes, and whole grains; low-fat or nonfat dairy products; and limited amounts of red meat (lean preferred). Special dietary problems should be discussed with the doctor and an oncology registered dietitian. It should be emphasized to the patient and family that the doctor should be informed before the patient takes any vitamin, mineral, or herb.

Special Diets

Macrobiotics. The philosophy of the microbiotic diet is curing through diet. It was developed in the 1930s by a Japanese philosopher, George Ohsawa. Originally, the diet consisted of brown rice with very little liquid. It was nutritionally deficient. Today it consists of 50% to 60% whole grains, 25% to 30% vegetables, and the remainder beans, seaweeds, and soups. Soybean foods are encouraged, and a small amount of fish is allowed. In-season foods are preferred. Proponents of this diet believe that it cures cancer. There is no evidence that the macrobiotic diet is beneficial for cancer patients.

Megavitamin and Orthomolecular Therapy. Some alternative practitioners believe that huge doses of vitamins can cure cancer. Linus Pauling coined the term orthomolecular, meaning large quantities of minerals and other nutrients. His claim that large doses of vitamin C could cure cancer was disproved. There was no evidence in 1979 that megavitamin or orthomolecular therapy was effective in treating any disease.[43] In 1985, Moertel and colleagues[44] showed that vitamin C was ineffective against advanced malignant cancer. There are side effects to the overdosing of vitamins and minerals.[28] A nutritionally healthy diet is recommended for overall good health. Some people have special needs and may require supplements. Patients should not attempt to treat themselves with megadoses of vitamins or minerals, but should seek professional attention for nutritional advice.

Metabolic Therapies. Metabolic therapies are based on the theory that disease is caused by the accumulations of toxic substances in the body. The goal of treatment is to eliminate the toxins. Metabolic therapies usually include a special diet; high-dose vitamins, minerals, or other dietary supplements; and detoxification with coffee enemas or irrigation of the colon. Colon detoxification is not used in mainstream medicine, and there are no data to support the claims that dried food and toxins remain stuck in the walls of the colon. The development of metabolic therapy is attributed to Max Gerson, a physician who emigrated from Germany in 1936. Today, cancer is the most common illness treated with metabolic therapies. Research does not substantiate the beliefs and practices of metabolic therapies, and patients may lose valuable time during which they could be receiving treatments with proven benefits.

Individual Biological Therapy. Advocates of shark and bovine cartilage therapy claim that it can reduce tumor size, slow or stop the growth of cancer, and help reverse bone diseases such as osteoporosis. More importantly, shark and bovine cartilage are thought to play a role in angiogenesis, which involves halting the blood supply to cancer cells. There is no firm evidence that cartilage treatment is effective against cancer.

Herbal Medicine

Herbs have been used as medicines going back to ancient times. Belief in the magic of herbs for the treatment of cancer exists today, especially in the face of advanced cancer and few or no options. There is a romance about herbs in that they are natural and come from the earth and therefore must be pure, safe, and harmless. A major concern exists that patients are using herbs indiscriminately on a routine basis without knowledge that they interact with drugs, can interfere with the efficacy of anticancer drugs, and can cause death.[45] There is a lack of knowledge that most herbal remedies have not been tested in carefully designed clinical studies.[46] Currently, some herbal remedies are being studied for their ability to induce or extend a cancer remission. We must remember and teach our patients that herbs have potency comparable to that of pharmaceuticals.[47] They can cause medical problems such as allergic reactions, toxic reactions, adverse effects, drug interactions, and drug contamination.[26]

An important aspect of cancer care is to recognize that herbs can be toxic to cancer patients and should be discussed with the doctor and other qualified practitioners. MSKCC advises patients to avoid taking any herbs for 2 weeks before any cancer therapy and to refrain from using supplements while in the hospital. Some herbs, such as St. John's wort,[48] may interfere with the effectiveness of chemotherapy. Garlic may alter clotting times in a surgical candidate. Dong qui may make the skin more sensitive to burns during radiation. The active ingredients in many herbs are not known. In the United States, herbal and other dietary supplements are not regulated by the U.S. Food and Drug Administration (FDA) as drugs.

This means that they do not have to meet the same standards as drugs and over-the-counter medications for proof of safety and effectiveness. Identifying the active ingredients and understanding how they affect the body are important areas of research being done by NCCAM. Differences have been found in some cases between what is listed on the label and what is in the bottle, and some contaminants have been identified as heavy metals, microorganisms, or unspecified prescription drugs and adulterants. Standardization and authentication of herbs is important. An excellent resource to obtain information about herbs can be found on MSKCC's website for Integrative Medicine[49] and in a resource book on herb-drug interactions.[50] The website has a consumer version as well as a professional version; both are available to all at no cost. Neither the author, the hospital, nor the publisher makes any medical recommendations about herbs; the website is specifically for information.

Mikail and colleagues[51] found in a study of medical residents that they had a knowledge deficit concerning herbal medicines. Ninety percent of them wanted to learn more about herbal medicine, including uses of herbs, contraindications, and drug interactions, as well as talking to patients about their use. As the prevalence of herbal remedy use grows, equipping nurses and doctors with information and vocabulary will help them discuss with and offer their patients proper precautions. Patients should be encouraged to talk to their doctors and nurses about the herbs they are taking. It is important to listen with patience, and then to respond without judgment. This approach promotes open, ongoing communication between the patient and the doctor and nurse.

Manipulative and Body-Based Methods

Touch is the first sense to develop, and it is the primary way of experiencing the world, starting with infancy up until the moment of our last breath.[52] It is critical to growth and development. Infants, the elderly, the ill, and animals that do not receive regular touch fail to thrive and eventually die. In ancient times, the "laying on of hands" was the early practice of healing by touch. Medicine consisted of touch before the advent of pharmaceutical therapies. Today drugs, technology, paperwork, and heavy patient loads keep the doctor and nurse from the bedside. Patients comment, "I don't get touched very much any more. If I do it is a medical touch, and it can hurt. My family and friends don't seem to touch either, maybe out of fear." Touch is a healing agent, but is underutilized by healing practitioners. Touch is our most social sense and implies a communication between two people. Cultural differences in touching are essential to keep in mind so as to always be respectful.

Massage

Massage therapy is one of the oldest health care practices in use. Chinese medical texts referred to it more than 4000 years ago. It is one of the most widely accepted forms of complementary therapies today. Massage employs the manual techniques of rubbing, stroking, tapping, or kneading the body's soft tissues to influence the whole person. Simms[2] suggested that touch is a fundamental element in patient care that can encourage better communication and promote comfort and well-being. The concern of the medical profession and patients has been that massage would spread cancer cells. There is no evidence that this is the case, because the stimulation caused by massage is no more than everyday exercise.[53] The benefits of massage are many and include improving circulation, relaxing muscles and nerve tissue, releasing tension, reducing pain, decreasing anxiety and depression, energizing, and promoting an overall sense of well-being. Massage is contraindicated under some circumstances: over metastatic bones (for risk of bone fracture or breakage), if the platelet count is <35,000 to 40,000/mm^3 (for risk of bruising), over sites of blood clots (for risk of promoting movement of a thrombus in the circulation), and over surgical sites or rashes. Medical massage for the cancer patient, and especially for the end-stage cancer patient, uses light pressure. Deep tissue massage is not appropriate and is potentially harmful.

Aromatherapy

Aromatherapy is the controlled use of plant essences for therapeutic purposes. Essential oils are the aromatic essences of plants in the form of oil or resin, which has been extracted in a highly concentrated solution.[54] The history of medicinal use of plant oils goes back to ancient Egypt, China, and Renaissance Europe. Essential oils are thought to have different mechanisms of action: antiviral, antiseptic, antibacterial, anti-inflammatory, fungicidal, sedative, and easing congestion. Aromatherapy is often practiced with massage and has been found to destress, empower, and promote communication and a sense of security.[55] Aromatherapy is a delightful tool in enhancing yoga.[56] Aromatherapy should be administered only by a certified practitioner. Essential oils should not be administered orally or applied undiluted to the skin. Possible contraindications to the use of essential oils are contagious disease, venous thrombosis, open wounds, and recent surgery. Possible adverse events are photosensitivity, allergic reactions, nausea, and headache. Many essential oils have the potential to enhance or reduce the effects of prescribed medications.[57]

Reflexology

Reflexology is touch therapy that goes back 5000 years to ancient Egypt. It is based on the assumption that the body contains energy flowing through it. Reflexology is an art and a science that is based on the principle that there are reflex points and areas in the ears, hands, and especially the feet that correspond to every gland, organ, and part of the body. By skillful stimulation of these areas and points with hand, finger, and thumb techniques, the body systems are facilitated to greater balance.[58] Reflexology should be done to the tolerance of the patient; it should not hurt. Reflexology is generally used to reduce stress, to promote relaxation and sleep, to improve circulation, to energize, to diminish symptoms of pain, anxiety, nausea, and peripheral neuropathy, and to promote an overall sense of well-being. It can be made special and pleasant when preceded by an aroma foot bath. It is contraindicated if blood clots, infection, skin rash, bruising, or wounds are present on the extremities. Reflexology can be performed anywhere, requires no special equipment, is noninvasive, and does not interfere with the patient's privacy. It can easily be taught to the family to empower them to provide comfort to their loved one.

Acupressure

Acupressure is the pressing of a single point or specific acupuncture point to relieve pain and stress in a particular area or part of the body. It is acupuncture without the needles. It involves placing the finger firmly on an acupoint. More than 300 acupoints dot the lengths of the hypothesized meridians (channels) that run vertically head to toe. The acupoint to be pressed is determined by the energy channel that is blocked and is causing the problem.[28] Acupressure promotes relaxation and comfort. It should be done to the tolerance of the patient. It need not be painful. It should not be applied near areas of fractures or broken bones, or near blood clots, wounds, sores, or bruises.

Shiatsu

Shiatsu is a modern outgrowth of ancient acupressure. It is a Japanese body therapy that works on the energetic pathways (meridians) and points of access to acupuncture points in order to harmonize the energy flow (qi). The philosophy is rooted in TCM, which views illness as being caused by energy imbalances. Shiatsu, a touch therapy, was developed from an ancient form of Japanese massage into the use of pressure with thumbs, palms, elbows, and knees and stretching, applied to these meridians and to the specific acupoints that are located on these pathways. The focus is on prevention and healing. Shiatsu is contraindicated with widespread bone metastases, pulmonary emboli, and deep vein thromboses. The benefits are relaxation, higher energy levels, improved physical capability, and enhanced symptom control. Light touch is suggested for the palliative care patient.[59]

Polarity

Polarity views good health as a balance among internal energies, such as earth, air, fire, water, and space. When these energies are blocked due to stress or other factors, physical and emotional problems follow. The therapist provides a series of gentle stretching, light rocking, and holding of pressure points until the body's energy is brought into balance. Most often patients report a deep sense of relaxation.

Chiropractic

The hands-on joint manipulation known as chiropractic is particularly helpful for lower back pain. Chiropractic medicine is a system of therapy based on the premise that the relationship between structure (primarily the spine) and function (as coordinated by the nervous system) in the human body is a significant health factor. Disease is considered to be the result of irregular or misaligned vertebrae and abnormal functioning of the nervous system. Back pain is one of the most frequent health problems, although neck, shoulder, head, and carpal tunnel syndrome are frequently treated by chiropractors. The normal transmission and expression of nerve energy are essential to the restoration and maintenance of health. Chiropractic medicine emphasizes the inherent recuperative power of the body to heal itself without the use of drugs or surgery. The method of treatment usually involves manipulation of the spinal column and other body structures to realign or readjust joints. Research evidence does not support chiropractic claims that cancer can be cured with spinal manipulation. Chiropractic is not recommended for patients with advanced cancer.

Yoga

Yoga is the Sanskrit word for union or oneness. It is a centuries-old Eastern philosophy, science, and art form that can be used as a tool to achieve inner peace and freedom. Through mental (meditation) and physical (movement and simple poses with deep breathing) techniques, pathways lead into the yoga state of oneness.[56] Yoga helps align the body, promotes relaxation, and reduces fatigue. There are different types of yoga: hatha yoga (physical posturing), pranayama (yoga breathing), mantra yoga (sacred sound symbols in the sound of a chant designed to awaken the left hemisphere of the brain to rational thinking and clarity), and yantra yoga (visualizing symbols and energy patterns). Yoga can be accommodated to any patient, in any position, at any stage of their cancer. It should be guided by an accredited yoga teacher and done to the tolerance of the patient, starting out very slowly and simply.

Exercise

Patients with cancer often experience lack of energy and loss of physical performance and strength.[60] Researchers have found that exercise can alleviate patients' fatigue and improve their physical performance and psychological outlook.[61] A pilot study demonstrated that myeloma patients with bone lesions were able to do a home-based exercise program, once taught, without supervision and without injury.[60] Another pilot study supported the suitability of exercise for the palliative care population who were given an exercise program, which included 5-minute walks, arm exercises with a resisted rubber band in a chair, marching on a spot, or dancing to their favorite music.[62] All patients expressed a sense of satisfaction in attaining their activity levels. Individuals who knowingly and actively participate in their care have a more positive outlook than those who are passive participants.[63] Patients with advanced cancer should be assessed first by a medical professional and then given an individualized exercise program that they can gradually work into.

Energy Therapies

NCCAM has classified Reiki, Qi gong, and Therapeutic Touch (TT) as biofield therapies. Biofield therapies are defined as those therapies intended to affect energies that purportedly surround and interpenetrate the human body. They are thought to be able to rebalance the biofield. Some believe that these therapies can remove the subtle causes of illness and enhance overall resilience. The existence of such fields has not yet been scientifically proven.

Reiki

Reiki is a vibrational or subtle energy most commonly facilitated by light touch. Rei means universal or highest energy, and ki means subtle energy. Reiki therapy is thought to balance the biofield and to strengthen the body to heal itself. Reiki is offered to a fully clothed individual and involves placement of hands on the head and front and back; it may include placement of hands on the site of discomfort, if desired. The gentle touch is soothing to patients and promotes deep relaxation.

Qi gong

Qi gong is a component of traditional Chinese medicine that combines movement, meditation, and regulation of breathing to enhance the flow of qi (vital energy) in the body, to improve circulation, and to enhance immune function. With practice, qi gong can lower stress levels, reduce anxiety, and provide an increased well-being and peace of mind. It is important to note that there is no evidence that qi gong exercises can increase resistance to illness or cure existing disease.[28]

Therapeutic Touch

TT, as described by Dolores Krieger,[64] is "the conscious, intentional act of directing universal energy with the intent to help and heal." It is defined by Nurse Healers Professional Associates[65] as an intentionally directed process of energy exchange during which the practitioner uses the hands as a focus to facilitate the healing process. TT was developed by Kreiger and Dora Kunz in the 1970s from studying techniques of ancient healing practices. It is believed that healing is promoted when the body's energies are in balance. The hands are usually passed over the patient so that the practitioner can detect energy imbalances and facilitate rebalancing. It is believed to affect a profound relaxation response and to help with pain.[66] The effectiveness of TT was evaluated in a meta-analytic review.[67] The results seemed to indicate that TT has a positive and medium effect on physiological and psychological variables, although the studies had significant methodological issues. More research needs to be done. Until then, TT is safe to use and seems to provide comfort to patients, even without scientific evidence.

Pre-therapy Nursing Assessment

The nurse needs to assess the patient first, before any therapy is given or ordered.

Current Medical History

The practitioner should determine the diagnosis, extent of disease, location of tumors, sites of metastatic disease, medications, CAM therapies (including vitamins, supplements, and herbs), site of blood clots, surgical site, site of radiation, and blood counts. He or she should determine which positions are most comfortable for the patient. All information must be obtained from the chart, doctor, or patient before doing a touch therapy.

Remember:

- Do not massage on bones where there is metastatic disease, because bones are at risk for fracture or breakage; if the platelet count is <35,000 to 40,000/mm,[3] because there is risk for bruising; on a site of current radiation, due to increased fragility of the skin; or where there are blood clots, due to the risk of setting a clot free to travel.
- There is no deep tissue massage given especially in a patient with advanced disease. Gentle light massage is most appropriate.

Symptoms

Ask patients what symptoms they are currently experiencing. Ask patients to rate their symptoms on a scale of 0 to 10 as an estimate of their level of distress. This is necessary to select the most appropriate and the most effective CAM therapy. If the patient has pain, medicate first, before therapy is provided; the patient is much more likely to enjoy it. Have patients rate their individual symptoms after the chosen therapy, to make clear to the patient and medical staff the benefit of the therapy.

Religious/Cultural Background

What culture is the patient from? What therapies were used at home? Are there any cultural taboos? For example, it is not acceptable for a Hasidic Jewish man to be touched by a woman.

Previous Use

What do the patients know about these therapies? Have they had previous experiences? Were they positive or negative experiences? Do they have any fears or reticence?

Patient's Requests

Who is asking for these therapies? Is it the patient or the family? What would the patient like to try?

Symptom Management with Evidence-Based Complementary Therapies

Dying patients experience a heavy symptom burden, including pain, nausea and vomiting, anxiety, depression, fatigue, dyspnea, insomnia, and peripheral neuropathy. When some of these symptoms are treated with medicines such as opioids, additional problematic side effects, such as sedation, delirium, and constipation, can occur. Complementary therapies have fewer, if any, side effects and may be more consistent to the patient's and family's culture and health care beliefs.[68]

Complementary Therapies for Control of Pain

A multicenter trial of seriously ill hospitalized patients with diverse diagnoses documented that 50% of patients who died in the hospital had moderate to severe pain during the last few days before death.[69] Pain is highly prevalent for the patient with advanced-stage cancer. Cancer pain can be very difficult to control; analgesic drugs do not always completely relieve it. Pain can isolate the patient from everything and everyone as it completely takes over, preventing communication between the patient and family. It can prevent a peaceful good-bye. The following adjuvant complementary therapies can provide much-needed extra help for pain control: acupuncture, massage, reflexology, hypnosis, music, Reiki, and art therapy. They can be chosen based on the nurse's assessment and the patient's wishes.

Control of pain is the best known use of acupuncture. Randomized trials support the use of acupuncture for acute pain, in dental surgery,[70] and for chronic pain such as migraine headaches.[71] In one study, pain control was achieved for at least 1 month in all of the patients with mild to moderate pain and in 72% of those with severe pain[72]; 48% of the patients in another study reported pain relief for 3 days and an increase in mobility.[73] Auricular acupuncture has demonstrated analgesic effects for cancer pain.[74] One very interesting study with pediatric patients, ages 6 to 18 years, successfully used acupuncture and hypnosis for chronic pain.[75] Acupuncture was also easily integrated into an outpatient clinic, where it provided 71% relief of pain.[76]

Massage therapy and aromatherapy provide pain relief and a sense of well-being in cancer patients experiencing pain.[77–79] Ferrell-Torry and Glick[80] reported that massage reduced pain perception by an average of 60%. Of note is a study by Walach and colleagues,[81] which found that pain improvement lasted until the 3-month follow-up visit. NCCAM recommends massage for treatment of refractory cancer pain. Reflexology has a significant effect on the symptom of pain.[78,80,82,83] It is a relatively simple nursing intervention and can be quite effective in <10 minutes. Relaxation and imagery can provide some pain relief.[84,85] Marcus and associates[86] suggested numbing parts of the body where there is pain through the use of hypnosis. These therapies require that the patient be alert and not in too much pain to concentrate.

In palliative care, music therapists provide services to treat pain.[40] Music increases the patient's comfort, is soothing, and creates a safe environment to ease the dying process. Reiki, which is safe and noninvasive, facilitates relaxation and decreases pain. Hartford Hospital, which has a hospital Reiki program, reports that Reiki provides significant pain relief for surgery patients.[87] Reiki, because it is a light holding touch, can be given to any patient. MSKCC uses art therapy to help patients communicate the painful side of their illness in such a way that they can feel understood and respected.[88] This intervention, with the guidance of a trained art therapist, uses a "body outline" that allows the patient to draw the location and type of physical pain and express the feelings around it without guilt or shame. This may be the starting point for some patients who seem to be verbally unreachable and might benefit from communicating their physical and emotional pain with the result of lessening the distress.

Complementary Therapies for Control of Nausea and Vomiting

Nausea and vomiting can greatly compromise patients' quality of life. The causes may be multiple, including a reaction to medications (chemotherapy, antibiotics, opiates), bad taste in the mouth, or bowel obstruction. Nausea and vomiting can be so severe that patients would rather discontinue their chemotherapy, or wish to die. Acupuncture, relaxation techniques, acupressure, reflexology, massage, music, imagery art therapy and meditation are effective therapies for nausea and vomiting.

Acupuncture can be used along with antiemetics. There is clear evidence that needle acupuncture is efficacious for adult postoperative and chemotherapy-related nausea and vomiting.[89] There is often an element of anxiety with nausea and vomiting. Progressive muscle relaxation has been shown to be very effective in decreasing nausea and vomiting as well as anxiety.[90] In a small pilot study, finger acupressure decreased nausea in women undergoing chemotherapy for breast cancer.[91] They were taught to apply pressure to the anterior surface of the forearm (P6) and the back of the knee (ST36), an intervention that is easy to learn and use. Reflexology was effective in promoting relaxation, which improved nausea.[82] Music therapy distracts patients by having them pick their own music, listen to live music, sing, or play an instrument, resulting in decreased nausea.[92] Music therapy is easy to implement. Guided imagery encourages patients to focus on past pleasant images to distract from the negative experience of nausea.[93,94] Art therapy can be used as a distraction intervention to reduce nausea and vomiting.[95] Meditation can also distract from the unpleasant sensation of nausea.

Complementary Therapies for Control of Anxiety

People with advanced stages of cancer may live with chronic anxiety and pain. The most common causes of anxiety in cancer patients with advanced disease are situational anxiety, previous history of anxiety, poorly controlled pain, abnormal metabolic states (e.g., hypoxia, sepsis, delirium), and side effects of medications (e.g., corticosteroids, neuroleptics).[96] The complementary therapies that are effective for the control of anxiety are massage, reflexology, meditation, relaxation, guided imagery, Reiki, music therapy, and exercise.

Massage promoted relaxation and significantly reduced the perception of pain and anxiety.[80] Meek[97] reported that her hospice patients, who were in the terminal stage of illness, received a slow stroke back massage and were provided comfort and induced relaxation. Cassileth and Vickers[98] have demonstrated a 52.2% reduction in anxiety with massage. In bone marrow transplant patients, the strongest effects were seen immediately after massage, with a reduction in diastolic blood pressure, anxiety, and nausea.[99] A significant reduction in anxiety was seen 3 months after massage by Walach and colleagues.[81] Family members can be taught to provide slow massage strokes to soothe the patient. Reflexology reduced anxiety in a randomized trial of patients with breast or lung cancer.[83] Gambles and associates[100] found that hospice patients reported 91% relief from tension and anxiety after a course of six reflexology sessions.

"Many dying patients find that the calmness and silence of meditation bring profound feelings of acceptance, well-being and inner peace."[30] Cancer patients frequently experience anxiety as they anticipate entering the final stages of life. Hypnotic relaxation has been found to significantly reduce terminal anxiety.[86] Relaxation training reduced treatment-related anxiety.[101] Imagery work can be a distraction that removes the patient from the stressor of the present. Reiki, which is a light touch therapy, promotes stress reduction and relaxation.[87] Music therapy reduced mood disturbance in cancer patients during hospitalization for autologous bone marrow transplantation.[38] Live music was found to be more effective than taped recorded music.[41] Music therapy was found to be more effective in decreasing anxiety in ventilator-dependent patients than quiet time.[102] Exercise is an intervention that may assist in the reduction of anxiety.[103]

Complementary Therapies for Control of Depression

The National Comprehensive Cancer Network (NCCN) in their guidelines of 2003, chose to focus on the patient's distress management. They recognized that distress extends along a continuum, ranging from feelings of vulnerability, sadness, and fear to disabling conditions such as clinical depression, anxiety, panic, isolation, and existential or spiritual crisis.[104] An estimated 20% to 25% of cancer patients experience depression at some time during their illness. In the advanced stages of cancer, the incidence of major depressive syndromes increases to 58%.[105] Factors that place patients at greater risk for depression are history of depression, advanced stage of cancer, poorly controlled pain, and medications. The following complementary therapies are effective for the relief of depression: mind–body therapies, massage, and music.

Depression was significantly reduced with the use of progressive muscle relaxation together with guided imagery in patients with advanced cancer.[106] MBSR was effective in reducing anxiety and depression in cancer outpatients.[107] Massage therapy achieved major reduction in pain, fatigue, nausea, anxiety, and depression at a major cancer center.[98] Music therapy reduced mood disturbance in patients hospitalized for autologous stem cell transplantation.[38] "Music therapy is an invaluable resource for diminishing suffering in advanced cancer"; and can help the patient link to inner strengths, restore a sense of identity, and open doorways during times of pain and loss.[37] Music can help the patient begin a life review and facilitate finding meaning and purpose in life.[39]

Complementary Therapies for Control of Fatigue

Fatigue is a common symptom among patients with advanced cancer. A multivariate analysis found that fatigue severity in advanced cancer was significantly associated with pain and dyspnea.[108] Portenoy and Itri[109] reported that fatigue can profoundly undermine the quality of life of patients with cancer. There are some nonpharmacological interventions for cancer-related fatigue. The following complementary therapies are recommended for cancer-related fatigue: acupuncture, exercise, massage, reflexology, mind–body therapies, and music.

MSKCC reported a 31.1% reduction in fatigue with acupuncture in a population of cancer patients with postchemotherapy fatigue.[110] Decreased physical activity, regardless of the reason, leads to decreased energetic capacity. A pilot study provided an exercise program for advanced cancer patients, resulting in increased energy and decreased fatigue.[62] There is a Chair Aerobics exercise class in the Integrative Medicine department at MSKCC that is run by an oncology clinical nurse specialist and personal trainer. This class is a fitness program targeted to help breathlessness and fatigue and to improve physical and psychological well-being of cancer patients. There are currently several stage IV patients in this class, who report that it is hard to get to class because of fatigue, but that after class they feel energized and proud to have accomplished something. Nail[111] summarized a number of nonpharmacological interventions for fatigue, including aerobic exercises and attention-restoring exercises. Coleman and colleagues[60] suggested tailoring exercise to the patients' capabilities as they move through the disease continuum, so that they do not get discouraged. Massage and reflexology can be very stimulating as well as relaxing. Imagery can include visualization of oneself as being very active. Patients can be very stimulated by listening to energetic music or by playing an instrument, especially the drums.

Complementary Therapies for Control of Dyspnea

Breathlessness is an extremely distressing and frightening symptom that can completely dominate a patient's life. It can cause physical disability, high anxiety, dependence, and loss of self-esteem. The following complementary therapies are recommended for dyspnea: relaxation techniques, Reiki, reflexology, gentle massage, music, specific exercise, acupuncture, and hypnosis.

Lung cancer patients using breathing retraining, simple relaxation techniques, activity pacing, and psychosocial support were able to reduce breathlessness from 73% to 27%.[112] Reiki has been shown to reduce anxiety,[113] as have reflexology, gentle massage, and music. Reduction of anxiety aids in the reduction of perceived breathlessness. Chair aerobics exercise helps decrease breathlessness, control panic, and improve muscle tone. Acupuncture was shown to promote quality of life in patients with chronic obstructive asthma.[114] For patients with active, progressive, or far advanced disease, and for those with a short life expectancy, hypnosis can provide reduction of dyspnea and enhance coping.[86]

Complementary Therapies for Control of Insomnia

Insomnia is a prevalent problem in cancer. Studies conducted among heterogeneous samples of cancer patients suggest that between 30% and 50% of cancer patients have sleep difficulties.[115] The contributing factors, especially for advanced cancer, are hypoxia, pain, anxiety, delirium, medications, or withdrawal from medications. The causes need to be treated, but, in addition, therapies that promote stress reduction and relaxation can be considered. The following complementary therapies can be helpful in the management of insomnia: mind–body therapies (relaxation and imagery), massage, reflexology, Reiki, exercise, and music.

Mind–body therapies such as relaxation, imagery, meditation, and biofeedback may be chosen to reduce body tension and anxiety and promote sleep.[31] Massage, reflexology, and Reiki, being touch therapies, can promote relaxation. Exercise is an intervention that can help reduce anxiety and improve quality of life in cancer patients.[63,116] Music can promote relaxation for sleep.

Complementary Therapies for Control of Peripheral Neuropathy

Peripheral neuropathy is a common problem for cancer patients receiving certain chemotherapies and for those with diabetes. It is a difficult problem to treat, and its severity and recovery can vary with each patient. It can be so severe that the oncologist may have to stop the chemotherapy. It may be described by patients as numbness, tingling, or burning. Cisplatin is known to induce sensory peripheral neuropathy, and paclitaxel causes sensory and motor neuropathy. Neurological toxicity eventually decreases the patient's ability to perform physical functions necessary for activities of daily living and thus can interfere with quality of life.[117]

One study looked at the prevalence and patterns of use of CAM therapies in a group of outpatients with peripheral neuropathy.[118] Reportedly, 43% of the patients used CAM for peripheral neuropathy. The following complementary therapies can be helpful in the management of peripheral neuropathy: reflexology and acupuncture.

Support for the Family

Caregivers of patients with cancer experience stress. They must learn to participate in complicated medical regimens, assist patients in daily activities of living, drive or accompany them to clinics or treatments, and perhaps at the same time be responsible for finances, running of the household, and preparing for the death.[119,120] Perception of discomfort in the dying patient may be another stress factor for the relatives.[121] Family members have difficulty dealing with patients' pain, dyspnea, appetite loss,[122] and delirium.[123] Caregivers of cancer patients undergoing autologous hematopoietic stem cell transplantation were enrolled in a study to receive massage therapy. Massage significantly reduced anxiety, depression, and fatigue; it reduced motivation fatigue and emotional fatigue.[119]

A program of care for family members is offered at MSKCC. Family members are offered massage, reflexology, meditation, yoga, and other evidence-based complementary therapies for stress reduction. "Touch Therapy for the Caregiver" is a monthly program offered to family members, who are taught how to give light upper back and neck massage to provide comfort to the patient. They are instructed to check with the patient's doctor to determine where it will be safe to do gentle massage.

Complementary and Alternative Therapies for the Nurse

Stress and burnout in oncology is well documented.[124–128] Stress and burnout are particularly relevant in oncology nursing, where nurses work closely with patients and families and bear witness to suffering and dying on a daily basis.

MSKCC's Integrative Medicine Service offers massage to the nursing staff as well as reflexology, meditation, and yoga classes to provide a program of care for nurses. MSKCC is invested in their nurses and knows the great benefit these therapies can offer them. Programs are offered in which nurses are taught Reiki, as well as very simplified versions of gentle upper body massage and reflexology, which they can integrate into their nursing practice after reviewing the indications and contraindications. These skills are a necessary part of any palliative care program.

Summary

It is a privilege to work with cancer patients, but especially to care for those approaching their last days of life. Gone are the days when a patient or a family might be told, "There is nothing more we can do." There remain many treatment options, including complementary therapies, that patients can choose and receive as a part of palliative care.

Nurses can educate patients and families about the safe choices of evidence-based complementary therapies that can affect their quality of life. But first, they need to educate themselves about CAM:—what these therapies are, what are their specific benefits and risks, and which ones are safe—before guiding patients. Nurses want to be respectful of the patient's desire to seek out CAM in the setting of advanced disease. Nurses must listen to the patient and then give suggestions of effective complementary therapies for comfort. Palliative care nurses are exposed to an abnormal amount of suffering and death and need to take care of themselves in order to give to others. Use of complementary therapies for themselves will benefit all.

Nurses can help patients live their lives to the last with hope. One patient said, "I didn't mind returning to the hospital, because I knew Integrative Medicine would be there for me." Another inpatient reported, after her reflexology session, "You have made me want to stay alive longer, I feel so good." And yes, there is Mary, our case history, who always looked for us in her hospital doorway and called us her angels. We cannot change the course of patients' terminal illnesses, but we can accompany them on the last days of their journey with gentle touch.

REFERENCES

1. Ernst E. Complementary therapies in palliative cancer care. Cancer 2001;91:2181–2185.
2. Sims S. The significance of touch in palliative care. Palliat Med 1998;2:58–61.
3. Ernst E, Resch KL, Mills S, Hill R, Mitchell A, Willoughby M, White A. Complementary medicine: A definition. Br J Gen Pract 1995;45:506.
4. Zollman C, Vickers A. What is complementary medicine? BMJ 1999;319:693–696.
5. Cassileth BR. Evaluating complementary and alternative therapies for cancer patients [review]. CA Cancer J Clin 1999;49:362–375.
6. Schraub S. Unproven methods in cancer: a worldwide problem. Support Care Cancer 2000;8:10–15.
7. Vickers A, Cassileth BR. Unconventional therapies for cancer and cancer-related symptoms. Lancet Oncol 2001;2:226–232.
8. Morris T, Johnson N, Homer L, Walts D. A comparison of complementary therapy use between breast cancer patients and patients with other primary tumor sites. Am J Surg 2000;179: 407–411.
9. Barnes P, Powell-Griner E, McFann K, Nahin R. Complementary and alternative medicine use among adults: United States, 2002. U.S. Department of Health and Human Services, Centers for Disease Control and Prevention, National Center for Health Statistics. CDC Advance Data Reprt No. 343. May 27, 2004.
10. Ernst E, Cassileth BR. The prevalence of complementary/alternative medicine in cancer. Cancer 1998;83:777–782.
11. Sparber A, Bauer L, Curt G, Eisenberg D, Levin T, Parks S, Steinberg SM, Wootton J. Use of complementary medicine by adult patients participating in cancer clinical trials. Oncol Nurs Forum 2000;27:623–630.
12. Bennet M, Lengacher C. Use of complementary therapies in a rural cancer population. Oncol Nurs Forum 1999;26:1287–1294.
13. Richardson MA, Sanders S, Palmer J, et.al. Complementary/alternative medicine use in a comprehensive cancer center and the implications for oncology. J Clin Oncol 2000;18:2505–2514.
14. Burstein H, Gelber S, Guadagnoli E, Weeks J. Use of alternative medicine by women with early-stage breast cancer. N Engl J Med 1999;340:1733–1739.
15. Boon H, Stewart M, Kennard MA, Gray R, Sawka C, Brown JB, McWilliam C, Gavin A, Baron RA, Aaron D, Haines-Kamka T. Use of complementary/alternative medicine by breast cancer survivors in Ontario: Prevalence and perceptions. J Clin Oncol 2000;18:2515–2521.
16. DiGianni L, Garber J, Winer E. Complementary and alternative medicine use among women with breast cancer. J Clin Oncol 2002;20;34s–38s.
17. Navo M, Phan P, Vaughan C, Palmer J, Michaud L, Jones K, Bodurka D, Basen-Engquist K, Hortobagyi G, Kavanagh J, Smith J. An assessment of the utilization of complementary and alternative medication in women with gynecologic or breast malignancies. J Clin Oncol 2004;22:671–677.
18. Fernandez CV, Stutzer CA, MacWilliam L, Fryer C. Alternative and complementary use in pediatric oncology patients in British Columbia:prevalence and reasons for use and nonuse. J Clin Oncol 1998;16:1279–1286.
19. McQuaid E, Nassau J. Empirically supported treatments of disease-related symptoms in pediatric psychology: Asthma, diabetes, and cancer. J Pediatr Psychol 1999;24:333–334.
20. Coppes M, Anderson R, Egeler R, Wolff J. Alternative therapies for the treatment of childhood cancer. N Engl J Med 1998; 339:846–847.
21. Fernandez C, Pyesmany A, Stutzer C. Alternative therapies in childhood cancer. N Engl J Med 1999;340:569–570.
22. Maskarinec G, Shumay D, Kakai H, Gotay C. Ethnic differences in complementary and alternative medicine use among cancer patients. J Altern Complement Med 2000;6:531–538.
23. Lee M, Lin S, Wrensch M, Adler S, Eisenberg D. Alternative therapies used by women with breast cancer in four ethnic populations. J Natl Cancer Inst 2000;92:42–47.
24. Kim C, Kwok Y. Navajo use of native healers. Arch Intern Med 1998;158:2245–2249.
25. Cohen R, Ek K, Pan C. Complementary and alternative medicine (CAM) use by older adults. J Gerontol 2002;57:223–227.
26. Cassileth BR, Deng G. Complementary and alternative therapies for cancer. Oncologist 2004;9:80–89.
27. Kaptchuk T. Acupuncture: Theory, efficacy, and practice. Ann Intern Med 2002;136:374–383.
28. Cassileth BR. The Alternative Medicine Handbook: The Complete Reference Guide to Alternative and Complementary Therapies. New York: WW Norton, 1998.
29. Vogel V. American Indian Medicine. Norman, OK: The Civilization of the American Indian Series, University of Oklahoma Press, 1970.

30. Kabat Zinn J, Massion A, Hebert J, Rosenbaum E. Meditation. In: Holland J, ed. Psycho-oncology. Oxford: Oxford University Press, 1998.
31. Astin J, Shapiro S, Eisenberg D, Forys K. Mind-body medicine: State of the science, implications for practice. J Am Board Fam Pract 2003;16:131–147.
32. Berenson S. The cancer patient. In: Zhourek R, ed. Relaxation and Imagery: Tools for Therapeutic Communication and Intervention. Philadelphia: WB Saunders, 1988.
33. Achterberg J. Imagery in Healing: Shamanism and Modern Medicine. Boston, New Science Library/Shambhala, 1985.
34. Gawain S. Creative Visualization. New York: Bantam New Age Book, 1979.
35. Erikson M. Hypnotherapy: An Exploratory Casebook. New York: Irvington, 1979.
36. Magill L, Luzzatto P. Music therapy and art therapy. In: Berger A, Portenoy R, Weissman D, eds. Principles and Practice of Palliative Care and Supportive Oncology, 2nd ed. Philadelphia: Lippincott Williams & Wilkins, 2002.
37. Magill L. The use of music therapy to address the suffering in advanced cancer pain. J Palliat Care 2001;17:167–172.
38. Cassileth BR, Vickers A, Magill L. Music therapy for mood disturbance during hospitalization for autologous stem cell transplantation. Cancer 2003;98:2723–2729.
39. Halstead M, Roscoe S. Restoring the spirit at the end of life: Music as an intervention for oncology nurses. Clin J Oncol Nurs 2002;6:332–336.
40. Hilliard R. Music therapy in pediatric care: Complementing the interdisciplinary approach. J Palliat Care 2003;19:127–132.
41. Bailey L. The effects of live music versus tape-recorded music on hospitalized cancer patients. Music Ther 1983;3:17–28.
42. Luzzatto P, Gabriel B. Art therapy. In: Holland, J, ed. Psycho-oncology. Oxford: Oxford University Press, 1998.
43. Creagan ET, Moertel CG, O'Fallon JR, Schutt A, O'Connell M, Rubin J, Frytak S. Failure of high-dose vitamin C (ascorbic acid) therapy to benefit patients with advanced cancer: A controlled study. N Engl J Med 1979;301:687–690.
44. Moertel CG, Fleming TR, Creagan ET, Rubin J, O'Connell M, Ames M. High-dose vitamin C versus placebo in the treatment of patients with advanced cancer who have had no prior chemotherapy: A randomized double-blind comparison. N Engl J Med 1985;312:137–141.
45. Sparreboom A, Cox M, Acharya M, Figg W. Herbal remedies in the United States: Potential adverse interactions with anticancer agents. J Clin Oncol 2004;22:2489–2503.
46. Cassidy A. Are herbal remedies and dietary supplements safe and effective for breast cancer patients? Breast Cancer Res 2003; 5:300–302.
47. Cassileth BR, Vickers A. Complementary and alternative cancer therapies. In: Holland J, Frei E, eds. Cancer Medicine, Vol 1. Hamilton, Ontario: BC Decker, 2003.
48. Barone G, Gurley B, Ketel B, Lightfoot M, Abul-Ezz S. Drug interaction between St John's wort and cyclosporine. Ann Pharmacother 2000;34:1013–1016.
49. Integrative Medicine Service at Memorial Sloan-Kettering Cancer Center, New York. Available at: http://www.mskcc.org/integrativemedicine (accessed January 6, 2005).
50. Cassileth BR, Lucarelli C. Herb-Drug Interactions in Oncology. Hamilton, Ontario: BC Decker, 2003.
51. Mikail C, Hearney E, Nemesure B. Increasing physician awareness of the common uses and contraindications of herbal medicines: Utility of a case-based tutorial for residents. J Altern Complement Med 2003;9:571–576.
52. Field T. Touch. Cambridge, MA: MIT Press, 2001.
53. Kassab S, Stevensen C. Common misunderstandings about complementary therapies for patients with cancer. Complement Ther Nurs Midwifery 1996;2:62–65.
54. Betty P, Andrusia D. Essential Beauty: Using Nature's Essential Oils to Rejuvenate, Replenish, and Revitalize. Los Angeles: Keats Publishing, 2000.
55. Dunwoody L, Smyth A, Davidson R. Cancer patients' experiences and evaluations of aromatherapy massage in palliative care. Int J Palliat Nurs 2002;8:497–504.
56. Cummins S. Peaceful Journey: A Yogi's Travel Kit. Hauppauge, NY: Barrons, 2001.
57. Perez C. Clinical aromatherapy. Part I: An introduction into nursing practice. Clin J Oncol Nurs 2003;7:595–598.
58. Norman L. Feet First: A Guide to Foot Reflexology. New York: Simon & Schuster, 1988.
59. Cheesman S, Christian R, Cresswell J. Exploring the value of shiatsu in palliative care day services. Int J Palliat Nurs 2001; 7:234–239.
60. Coleman E, Hall-Barrow J, Coon S, Stewart C. Facilitating exercise adherence for patients with multiple myeloma. Clin J Oncol Nurs 2003;7:529–534.
61. Dimeo F. Effects of exercise on cancer-related fatigue. Cancer 2001;92:1689–1693.
62. Porock D, Kristjanson L, Tinnelly K, Duke T, Blight J. An exercise intervention for advanced cancer patients experiencing fatigue: A pilot study. J Palliat Care 2000;16:30–36.
63. Wall L. Changes in hope and power in lung cancer patients who exercise. Nurs Sci Q 2000;13:234–242.
64. Kreiger D. The Therapeutic Touch: How to Use Your Hands to Help or to Heal. Englewood Cliffs, NJ: Prentice-Hall, 1979.
65. Nurse Healers Professional Associates International. Available at: http://www.therapeutic-touch.org (accessed January 6, 2005).
66. Samarel N, Fawcett J, Davis M, Ryan F. Effects of dialogue and therapeutic touch on preoperative and postoperative experiences of breast cancer surgery: An exploratory study. Oncol Nurs Forum 1998;25:1369–1376.
67. Peters R. The effectiveness of therapeutic touch: A meta-analytic review. Nurs Sci Q 1999;12:52–61.
68. Pan C, Morrison S, Ness J, Fugh-Berman A, Leipzig R. Complementary and alternative medicine in the management of pain, dyspnea, and nausea and vomiting near the end of life: A systematic review. J Pain Symptom Manage 2000;20:374–387.
69. SUPPORT Principal Investigators. A controlled trial to improve care for seriously ill hospitalized patients: The Study to Understand Prognoses and Preferences for Outcomes and Risks of Treatments (SUPPORT). JAMA 1995;274:1591–1598.
70. Lao L, Bergman S, Langenberg P, Wong R, Berman B. Efficacy of Chinese acupuncture on postoperative oral surgery pain. Oral Surg Oral Med Oral Pathol 1995;79:423–428.
71. Melchart D, Linde K, Fisher P, White A, Allais G, Vickers A, Berman B. Acupuncture for recurrent headaches: A systematic review of randomized controlled trials. Cephalalgia 1999;19:779–786.
72. Xu S, Liu Z, Li Y. Treatment of cancerous abdominal pain by acupuncture on Zusanli (ST36): A report of 92 cases. J Tradit Chin Med 1995;15:189–191.
73. Filshie J, Redman D. Acupuncture and malignant pain problems. Eur J Surg Oncol 1985;11:389–394.

74. Alimi D, Rubino C, Leandri E, Brule S. Analgesic effects of auricular acupuncture for cancer care. J Pain Symptom Manage 2000;19:81–82.
75. Zeltzer L, Tsao J, Stelling C, Powers M, Levy S, Waterhouse M. A phase I study on the feasibility and acceptability of an acupuncture/hypnosis intervention for chronic pediatric pain. J Pain Symptom Manage 2002;24:437–446.
76. Johnstone P, Polston G, Niemtzow R, Martin P. Integration of acupuncture into the oncology clinic. Palliat Med 2002;16:235–239.
77. Gray R. The use of massage therapy in palliative care. Complement Ther Nurs Midwifery 2000;6:77–82.
78. Weinrich S, Weinrich M. The effect of massage on pain in cancer patients. Appl Nurs Res 1990;3:140–145.
79. Wilkinson S, Aldridge J, Salmon I, Cain E, Wilson B. An evaluation of aromatherapy massage in palliative care. Palliat Med 1999;13:409–417.
80. Ferrell-Torry A, Glick O. The use of therapeutic massage as a nursing intervention to modify anxiety and the perception of cancer pain. Cancer Nurs 1993;16:93–101.
81. Walach H, Guthlin C, Konig M. Efficacy of massage therapy in chronic pain: A pragmatic randomized trial. J Altern Complement Med 2003;9:837–846.
82. Grealish L, Lomasney A, Whiteman B. Foot massage: A nursing intervention to modify the distressing symptoms of pain and nausea in patients hospitalized with cancer. Cancer Nurs 2000; 23:237–43.
83. Stephenson N, Weinrich S, Tavakoli A. The effects of foot reflexology on anxiety and pain in patients with breast and lung cancer. Oncol Nurs Forum 2000;27:67–72.
84. Fleming U. Relaxation therapy for far–advanced cancer. Practitioner 1985;229:471–475.
85. Syrjala K, Donaldson G, Davis M, Kippes M, Carr J. Relaxation and imagery and cognitive-behavioral training reduce pain during cancer treatment: A controlled clinical trial. Pain 1995; 63:189–198.
86. Marcus J, Elkins G, Mott F. The integration of hypnosis into a model of palliative care. Integr Cancer Ther 2003;2:365–370.
87. Miles P, True G. Reiki—Review of a biofield therapy: History, theory, practice, and research. Altern Ther 2003;9:62–72.
88. Luzzatto P, Sereno V, Capps R. A communication tool for cancer patients with pain: The art therapy technique of the Body Outline. 2003;1:135–142.
89. Shen J, Wenger N, Glaspy J, Hays R, Albert P, Choi C, Shekelle P. Electroacupuncture for control of myeloablative chemotherapy-induced emesis. JAMA 2000;284:2755–2761.
90. Arakawa S. Relaxation to reduce nausea, vomiting, and anxiety induced by chemotherapy in Japanese patients. Cancer Nurs 1997;20:342–349.
91. Dibble S, Chapman J, Mack K, Shih A. Acupressure for nausea: Results of a pilot study. Oncol Nurs Forum 2000;27:41–47.
92. Bender C, McDaniel R, Murphy-Ende K, Pickett M, Rittenberg C, Rogers M, Schneider S, Schwartz R. Chemotherapy-induced nausea and vomiting. Clin J Oncol Nurs 2002;6:94–102.
93. King C. Nonpharmacologic management of chemotherapy-induced nausea and vomiting. Oncol Nurs Forum 1997;24:41–48.
94. Van Fleet S. Relaxation and imagery for symptom management: Improving patient assessment and individualizing treatment. Oncol Nurs Forum 2000;27:501–510.
95. Gabriel B, Bromberg E, Vandenbovenkamp J, Walka P, Komblith A, Luzzatto P. Art therapy with adult bone marrow transplant patients in isolation: A pilot study. Psycho-oncology 2001; 10:114–123.
96. Massie MJ. Anxiety, panic, and phobias. In: Holland JC, Rowland JH, eds. Handbook of Psychooncology: Psychological Care of the Patient with Cancer. Oxford: Oxford University Press, 1990.
97. Meek S. Effects of slow stroke back massage on relaxation in hospice clients. IMAGE: J Nurs Schol 1993;25:17–21.
98. Cassileth BR, Vickers A. Massage therapy for symptom control: Outcome study at a major cancer center. J Pain Symptom Manag, 2004. In press.
99. Ahles T, Tope D, Pinkson B, Walch S, Hann D, Whedon M, Dain B, Weiss J, Mills L, Silberfarb P. Massage therapy for patients undergoing autologous bone marrow transplantation. J Pain Symptom Manage 1999;18:157–163.
100. Gambles M, Crooke M, Wilkinson S. Evaluation of a hospice based reflexology service: A qualitative audit of patient perceptions. Eur J Oncol Nurs 2002;6:37–44.
101. Luebbert K, Dahme B, Hasenbring M. The effectiveness of relaxation training in reducing treatment related symptoms and improving emotional adjustment in acute non-surgical cancer treatment: A meta-analytical review. Psycho-oncology 2001;10: 490–502.
102. Wong H, Lopez–Nahas V, Molassiotis A. Effects of music therapy on anxiety in ventilator-dependent patients. Heart Lung 2001;30: 376–387.
103. Blanchard C, Courynea K, Laing D. Effects of acute exercise on state anxiety in breast cancer survivors. Oncol Nurs Forum 2001;28:1617–1621.
104. National Comprehensive Cancer Network. Distress management: Clinical practice guidelines. J Compr Cancer Network 2003; 1:344–374.
105. Breitbart W. Identifying patients at risk for, and treatment of major psychiatric complications of cancer. Supportive Cancer Care 95;3:45–60.
106. Sloman R. Relaxation and imagery for anxiety and depression control in community patients with advanced cancer. Cancer Nurs 2002;25:432–435.
107. Speca M, Carlson L, Goodey E, Angen M. A randomized, wait-list controlled clinical trial: The effect of a mindfulness meditation-based stress reduction program on mood and symptoms of stress in cancer outpatients. Psychosom Med 2000; 62:613–622.
108. Stone P, Hardy J, Broadley K, Tookman A, Kurowska A, A'Hern R. Fatigue in advanced cancer: A prospective controlled cross-sectional study. Br J Cancer 1999;79:1479–1486.
109. Portenoy R, Itri L. Cancer-related fatigue: Guidelines for evaluation and management. Oncologist 1999;4:1–10.
110. Vickers A, Straus D, Fearon B, Cassileth BR. Acupuncture for post-chemotherapy fatigue: A phase II study. J Clin Oncol 2004; 22:1731–1735.
111. Nail L. CLIR: Center for Leadership, Information, and Research/ Continuing Education: Fatigue in patients with cancer. Oncol Nurs Forum 2002;29;537–546.
112. Hately J, Laurence V, Scott A, Baker R, Thomas P. Breathlessness clinics within specialist palliative care settings can improve the quality of life and functional capacity of patients with lung cancer. Palliat Med 2003;17:410–417.
113. Wardell D, Engebretson J. Biological correlates of Reiki touch healing. J Adv Nurs 2001;33:439–445.
114. Maa SH, Sun MF, Hsu KH, Hung TJ, Chen HC, Yu CT, Wang CH, Lin HC. Effect of acupuncture or acupressure on quality of life of patients with chronic obstructive asthma: A pilot study. J Altern Complement Med 2003;9:659–670.

115. Savard J, Morin C. Insomnia in the context of cancer: A review of a neglected problem. J Clin Oncol 2001;19:895–908.
116. Courneya K. Exercise in cancer survivors: An overview of research. Med Sci Sports Exerc 2003;35:1846–1852.
117. Almadrones L, McGuire D, Walczak J, Florio C, Tian C. Psychometric evaluation of two scales assessing functional status and peripheral neuropathy associated with chemotherapy for ovarian cancer: A gynecologic oncology group study. Oncol Nurs Forum 2004;31:615–623.
118. Brunelli B, Gorson K., The use of complementary and alternative medicines by patients with peripheral neuropathy. J Neurol Sci 2004;218:59–66.
119. Rexilius S, Mundt C, Megel M, Agrawal S. Therapeutic effects of massage therapy and healing touch on caregivers of patients undergoing autologous hematopoietic stem cell transplant. Oncol Nurs Forum 2002;29:E35–E34.
120. Mok E, Chan F, Chan V, Yeung E. Family experience caring for terminally ill patients with cancer in Hong Kong. Cancer Nurs 2003;26:267–275.
121. Bruera E, Sweeney C, Willey J, Palmer J, Strasser F, Strauch E. Perception of discomfort by relatives and nurses in unresponsive terminally ill patients with cancer: A prospective study. J Pain Symptom Manage 2003;26:818–826.
122. Ogasawara C, Kume Y, Andou M. Family satisfaction with perception of and barriers to terminal care in Japan. Oncol Nurs Forum 2003;30:763–766.
123. Brajtman S. The impact on the family of terminal restlessness and its management. Palliat Med 2003;17:454–460.
124. Kushnir T, Rabin S, Azulai S. A descriptive study of stress management in a group of pediatric oncology nurses. Cancer Nurs 1997;20:414–421.
125. Kash K, Holland JJ, Breitbart B, Berenson S, Dougherty J, Ouellette-Kobasa S, Lesko L. Stress and burnout in oncology. Oncology (Huntingt) 2000;14:1621–1633.
126. Penson R, Dignan F, Canellos G, Picard C, Lynch TJ Jr. Burnout: Caring for the caregivers. Oncologist 2000;5:425–434.
127. Grunfeld E, Whelan T, Zitzelsberger L, Willan AR, Montesanto B, Evans WK. Cancer care workers in Ontario: Prevalence of burnout, job stress and job satisfaction. CMAJ 2000;163:166–169.
128. Medland J, Howard-Ruben J, Whitaker E. Fostering psychosocial wellness in oncology nurses: Addressing burnout and social support in the workplace. Oncol Nurs Forum 2004;31:47–54.

III

Psychosocial Support

26

Mary Ersek

The Meaning of Hope in the Dying

I have these three gremlins in my head. One of them is on one side saying, "Jack, you're going to lick this—don't worry." Another gremlin is on the other side saying, "Jack, you dope, you know you aren't going to make it." And on the middle of this is this third little guy who has to make sense of both of them and help me to keep going on with my life day after day. Sometimes, they get so loud I can't think, but most of the time I keep them locked up, and when I'm busy they don't bother me.
—37-year-old-man with malignant melanoma[1]*

Every time life asks us to give up a desire, to change our direction or redefine our goals; every time we lose a friend, break a relationship, or start a new plan, we are invited to widen our perspectives and to touch, under the superficial waves of our daily lives, the deeper currents of hope.
—Henri Nouwen[2]

- ***Key Points***
- *Hope is a key factor in coping with and finding meaning in the experience of life-threatening illness.*
- *People facing life-threatening illness and their families do not invariably lose hope; in fact, hope can increase at the end of life.*
- *Nurses can implement evidence-based practices to foster and sustain hope for patients and families at the end of life.*
- *Nurses need to understand and respect individual variations in hope processes to provide sensitive, effective care to patients and their families at the end of life.*

Hope has long been recognized as fundamental to the human experience. Many authors have contemplated hope, extolling it as a virtue and an energy that brings life and joy.[2–5] Fromm[5] called hope "a psychic commitment to life and growth." (p. 12). Some authors assert that life without hope is impossible.[3,6]

Despite its positive connotations, hope is intimately bound with loss and suffering.[4,7] As the French philosopher Gabriel Marcel[4] observed, "Hope is situated within the framework of the trial" (p. 30). It is this paradox that manifests itself so fully at the end of life.

Indeed, the critical role that hope plays in human life takes on special meaning as death nears. The ability to hope often is challenged, and it can elude patients and families during terminal illness. Hope for a cure is almost certainly destroyed, and even a prolonged reprieve from death is unlikely. Many patients and families experience multiple losses as they continue an illness trajectory that is marked by increasing disability and pain.

Even when hope appears to be strong within the dying person or the family, it can be problematic if hopefulness is perceived to be based on unrealistic ideas about the future.[8,9] Tension grows within relationships as people become absorbed in a struggle between competing versions of reality. Important issues may be left unresolved as individuals continue to deny the reality of impending death.

Despite these somber realities and the inevitable suffering, many people do maintain hope as they die, and families recover and find hope even within the experience of loss. How can this be? Part of the reason lies in the nature of hope itself—its resiliency and capacity to coexist with suffering. As witnesses to suffering and hope, palliative care nurses must understand these complexities and be confident and sensitive in their efforts to address hope and hopelessness in the people for whom they care.

*From *The Human Side of Cancer: Living with Hope, Coping with Uncertainty* by Jimmie Holland, M.D., and Sheldon Lewis.[1] (Reprinted with permission from HarperCollins Publishers, Inc.)

To assist palliative care nurses, this chapter explores the many dimensions of hope and identifies its possible influence on health and quality of life. Nursing assessment and strategies to foster hope are described. In addition, specific issues such as "unrealistic hopefulness" and cultural considerations in the expression and maintenance of hope are discussed. The goals of the chapter are to provide the reader with an understanding about this complex but vital phenomenon; to offer guidance in the clinical application of this concept to palliative nursing care; and to explore some of the controversies about hope that challenge clinicians.

Definitions and Dimensions of Hope

Hope is an important concept for many disciplines, including philosophy, theology, psychology, nursing, and medicine. Many authors have attempted to define hope and describe its attributes.[10–13] Some authors are more successful than others in capturing its complexity. A classic nursing theory of hope, developed by Karin Dufault[12,14] and based on qualitative research involving elderly people with cancer, is particularly notable in its comprehensiveness and expansion of previous psychological models of hope.[15] Dufault[14] described hope as "a multidimensional, dynamic life force characterized by a confident yet uncertain expectation of achieving a future good which, to the hoping person, is realistically possible and personally significant" (p. 380). Dufault also theorized that hope has two interrelated spheres: particularized and generalized. *Particularized hope* is centered and dependent on specific, valued goals or hope objects. An example is the hope of a terminally ill patient to live long enough to celebrate a particular holiday or event. In contrast, *generalized hope* is a broader, nonspecific sense of a more positive future that is not directly related to a particular goal or desire. Dufault likened this sphere to an umbrella that creates a diffuse, positive glow on life.

Dufault postulated several dimensions of hope that were incorporated into later research and theories.[10,11,16–18] These dimensions include affective, spiritual, relational, cognitive, behavioral, and contextual aspects of hope. The *affective* dimension of hope encompasses a myriad of emotions. Of course, hope is accompanied by many positive feelings, including joy, confidence, strength, and excitement. The full experience of hope, however, also includes uncertainty, fear, anger, suffering, and, sometimes, despair.[4,19–24] The philosopher Gabriel Marcel, for example, argued that in its fullest sense hope could only follow an experience of suffering or trial.[4] Marcel's thesis is corroborated by the experiences described by people with cancer who see their disease as "a wake-up call" that has opened their eyes to a greater appreciation for life and an opportunity for self-growth—in other words, an event that has forced them to confront their mortality while also inspiring hope.[25,26]

The *spiritual* dimension is a central component of hope.[27–33] Hopefulness is associated with spiritual well-being,[32,34,35] and qualitative studies have shown that spirituality and spiritual practices provide a context in which to define hope and articulate hope-fostering activities.[11,14,16,23,29,36] These activities include religious beliefs and rituals but extend to broader conceptualizations of spirituality that encompass meaning and purpose in life, self-transcendence, and connectedness with a deity or other life-force.[33,37] Although spirituality is almost always viewed as a hope-fostering influence, serious illness and suffering can challenge one's belief and trust in a benevolent deity or be viewed as punishment from God; either interpretation of suffering can result in hopelessness.[38]

Relationships with significant others are another important dimension of hope. Interconnectedness with others is cited as a source of hope in virtually every study, and physical and psychological isolation from others is a frequent threat to hope.[11,31,39] Hope levels are positively associated with social support.[39–41] In addition to family members and friends, patients also have identified nurses as having a significant influence on hope.[42,43] Despite being vital sources of hope, other people can threaten a patient's hope by distancing themselves from the patient, showing disrespect, discounting the patient's experiences, disclosing negative information, or withholding information.[12,36,44]

The *cognitive* dimension of hope encompasses many intellectual strategies, particularly those involving specific goals that require planning and effort to attain. Identifying goals can motivate and energize people, thereby increasing hope.[10,45] When identifying goals, people assess what they desire and value within a context of what is realistically possible. They appraise the resources necessary to accomplish their goals against the resources that are available to them. They then take action to secure the resources or meet the goals, and they decide on a reasonable time frame in which to accomplish the goals.[10,12,45] Active involvement in one's situation and attainment of goals increases the sense of personal control and self-efficacy, which, in turn, increases hope.[10,46] If a person repeatedly fails to attain valued goals, hopelessness and passivity can result.[10,45]

The *behavioral,* goal-focused thoughts and activities that foster hope are similar to the problem-focused coping strategies originally described by Lazarus and Folkman.[47] This similarity is not surprising, because hope is strongly associated with coping.[20,39] The exact relationship between the two concepts, however, is unclear. Hope has been identified as a foundation or mediator for successful coping,[20,48] a method of coping,[49] and an outcome of successful coping.[39] Many strategies that people use to maintain hope have been previously identified as coping methods, and models of maintaining hope overlap substantially with models of coping.[8,10,11,45] Strategies to maintain hope include problem-focused coping methods (e.g., setting goals, actively managing symptoms, getting one's affairs in order) and emotion-focused strategies (e.g., using distraction techniques, appraising the illness in nonthreatening ways).[8,10,11]

Contextual dimensions of hope are the life circumstances and abilities that influence hope—for example, physical health, financial stability, and functional and cognitive abilities.[30,48,50–52] Common threats to hope include acute, chronic, and terminal illness; cognitive decline; fatigue; and impaired functional status. These factors, particularly physical illness and impairment, do not inevitably decrease hope, if people are able to overcome the threat through cognitive, spiritual, relational, or other strategies.

Influence of Hope and Hopelessness on Adaptation to Illness

Hope influences health and adaptation to illness. Empirical evidence indicates that diminished hope is associated with poorer quality of life,[53,54] increased severity of suicidal intent,[50,54] and higher incidence of suicide.[50,54–56] Hopelessness also increases the likelihood that people will consider physician-assisted suicide as an option for themselves.[57–59] If hopelessness occurs, anxiety and depression can result.[51,53,60] Lower levels of hope also are associated with lower self-esteem.[40,41,61]

In addition to its influence on psychological states and behaviors, there is some evidence to suggest that hope affects physical states as well. Researchers have found an association between hope and immune function.[62,63] Moreover, decreased hope is associated with a worse prognosis in several patient populations.[64–66]

Variations in Hope Among Different Populations

The preceding description of hope is derived from studies involving diverse populations, including children, adolescents, adults, and the elderly. In addition, research has been conducted in inpatient, outpatient, and community settings with well persons and those with a variety of chronic and life-threatening illnesses. The experiences of families also have been described. Over these diverse populations and settings, many core concepts have been identified that transcend specific groups. However, some subtle but important differences exist. For this reason, hopefulness in selected populations is addressed in the following sections.

Hope in Children and Adolescents

A few investigators have examined hope in pediatric populations. In an early study, Wright and Shontz[67] studied hope in children with chronic disabilities and significant adults in their lives (e.g., parents, teachers, physical therapists). Both the children and the adults were interviewed, allowing for the identification of differences between the two samples. The investigators found that hope for the children in their study was two-dimensional. Hoping involved (1) an awareness of the positive and (2) a sense of time orientation. For younger children, hope was present-focused, whereas older children had a future orientation to hope. Younger children also saw adults as being in control of a situation and were less concerned about assessing how realistic their particular hopes were. In contrast, adults actively assessed the realities of the present and possibilities for the future.

Artinian[68] explored hope in older children, aged 10 to 20 years, who underwent bone marrow transplantation. The findings suggested that ways to reduce stress and instill hope among younger patients and their parents include managing physical discomforts, making children and parents feel cared for, being nonjudgmental when children and parents vent anger, preventing boredom, and assisting with making and altering plans.

A program of research by Hinds and colleagues elucidated the experience of hoping in adolescents.[13,42,44,69,70] These investigators conducted studies in well adolescents, adolescents undergoing inpatient treatment for substance abuse, and adolescents with cancer. Based on qualitative studies, Hinds defined adolescent hopefulness as "the degree to which an adolescent possesses a comforting or life-sustaining, reality-based belief that a positive future exists for self and others"[13] (p. 85). Interestingly, inclusion of the phrase "and others" arose from the sample of adolescent cancer patients. Hinds found that only in this sample did adolescents express a concern and articulate their hopes for others. Examples of this attribute included such hopes as "My parents will be O.K. if I die," and "There will be a cure soon so patient 'X' will not die"[13] (p. 85). This ability to go beyond oneself and hope for others may be influenced by the adolescents' sense of mortality that accompanies the cancer diagnosis.[13]

Despite the stress of life-threatening illness, many adolescents are able to remain hopeful. Ritchie[61] examined hopefulness and self-esteem in 45 adolescents with cancer. She found that the average hopefulness and self-esteem scores for her sample were as high as those for healthy adolescents. Moreover, high self-esteem was an important predictor of hopefulness. These results suggest that teens are able to respond to serious illness with intact self-esteem and hope.

Hope and Older Adults

Numerous studies have examined hope in ill and healthy older adults.[12,17,30,35,66,71,72] Findings from these studies suggest that certain hope-related themes and factors take on special significance for this age group. For example, religious beliefs and spiritual well-being are strongly associated with hope in elders;[35] these factors also were prominent themes in qualitative studies.[12,30,71] Common health-related factors, such as impaired physical functioning, poor physical health, decreased mobility, fatigue, and cognitive impairment, are negatively associated with hope in older adults.[30,52,71,73] Although chronic illness that impairs physical functioning is linked with decreased hope, diagnosis of a life-threatening disease, such as cancer, is not associated with low levels of hope.[74] This finding may reflect an attitude among older adults that the quality of life that remains matters more than the quantity.

Among younger European American adults, hope tends to be tied to being productive; personal and professional achievements figure prominently in one's ability to nurture and maintain hope. In contrast, older adults are more likely to focus on spirituality, relationships, and other factors that are not linked with accomplishment.[71,75] Hope-fostering activities include reminiscing, participating in purposeful volunteer activities, religious activities, and connecting with others.

Hope from the Family Caregiver's Perspective

Family caregivers are an integral component in palliative care. Patients and families influence each other's hope, and nursing interventions must focus on both groups. Often, the physical and psychological demands placed on family caregivers are great, as are threats to hope.[76–78] Threats to hope in caregivers include isolation from support networks and from God; concurrent losses, including loss of significant others, health, and income; and inability to control the patient's symptoms. Caregivers with poor health status, high fatigue, multiple losses, and sleep disturbances were significantly less hopeful than caregivers without these problems.[78]

Yates and Stetz[76] found that as awareness of dying increased, caregivers hoped for relief from suffering rather than for a cure. Herth[78] reported that as death became imminent, the need "to do" for the patient was replaced by a wanting simply "to be" with the patient. In addition, little emphasis was placed on the "future" in caregivers' descriptions of hope.[78]

Strategies to maintain hope in family caregivers are similar to those found in patients, with a few differences. Spending time with others in the support network was very important for caregivers. In addition, being able to reprioritize demands helped caregivers conserve much-needed energy. Caregivers also maintained hope through engaging in relaxing activities, such as listening to or playing music, gardening, or watching a sunset.[78]

Hope in Terminally Ill Patients: Is Hope Compatible with Death?

Research demonstrates that many people are able to maintain hope during acute and chronic illness. Hope also can thrive during the terminal phase of an illness, despite the realization that no cure is possible. In one study, the hope in terminally ill patients and their caregivers actually increased over time as death neared.[36,78]

Although hope levels may not decrease, the nature of hope often is altered through the dying process. Hope tends to be defined more in terms of "being" rather than "doing."[43,79] Other changes in hope at the end of life include an increased focus on relationships and trusting in others, as well as a desire to leave a legacy and to be well remembered.[12,80,81] Spirituality also increases in importance during the terminal phases of illness. In a study of 160 terminally ill patients, decreased spiritual well-being was significantly associated with hopelessness.[82] People also adopt specific strategies to foster hope at the end of life.[36,45,80,83] Many of these approaches are summarized in Table 26–1.

Table 26–1
Sources of Hope/Hope-Fostering Strategies in Terminally Ill Adults

- Having one or more meaningful, shared relationships in which one feels a sense of "being needed" or "being a part of something"
- Maintaining a feeling of lightheartedness; feeling delight, joy, or playfulness and communicating that feeling; using humor
- Recalling joyous, meaningful events
- Having one's individuality acknowledged, accepted, and honored; having one's worth affirmed by others
- Identifying positive personal attributes such as courage, determination, serenity
- Having spiritual beliefs and engaging in spiritual practices that provide a sense of meaning for their suffering
- Focusing attention and effort on the short-term future
- Thinking about and directing efforts at specific, short-term attainable aims (earlier in terminal illness)
- Thinking about global, positive aims that are focused on others (e.g., support for the bereaved, happiness for their children) (later in terminal illness)
- Desiring serenity, inner peace, eternal rest (last days and weeks of life)

Source: Adapted from Herth (1990), reference 36.

Although hope tends to change in people with terminal illness, maintaining a delicate balance between acceptance of death and hope for a cure often remains an important task up until the time of death, even when people acknowledge that cure is virtually impossible.[45,80] The dying person also needs to envision future moments of happiness, fulfillment, and connection. For example, Benzein and colleagues[80] reported that people with life-threatening illness needed to dream about possibilities and situations even if the imagined events and goals were unlikely to occur. As one of their participants related,[80]

> Sometimes I let myself imagine that I'll live until Christmas and sometimes in the night I lie and think about where to put the tree. I know it's silly but it feels good to think about myself sitting there by the tree with everyone . . . a lovely picture (p. 122).

The first quotation that appears at the beginning of this chapter also captures the ways in which dying patients and their families must walk the tightrope between hope and despair. As Wilkinson[84] stated, people confronting the end of their lives must change their perspectives "from dying from a terminal illness to living with a life-threatening illness" (p. 661) in order to maintain hope.

Multicultural Views of Hope

Over the past three decades, understanding of the clinical phenomenon of hope has increased dramatically through theoretical discourse and empirical investigation. Although knowledge regarding the components, processes, and outcomes of hope has grown dramatically, progress in multicultural research on hope has been limited. The samples in many studies that examine hope or hopelessness are ethnically homogeneous,[16,39] or their ethnic composition is unknown.[10,80] The studies that do include ethnically diverse samples are small,[85–87] precluding any comparisons or generalization of findings.

Several excellent European studies have contributed greatly to the general understanding of hope.[21,24,80,88–92] However, many of these investigations use frameworks and instruments developed by U.S. researchers whose work is founded on homogeneous samples. Moreover, it may be that hopefulness for Europeans is more similar to that of middle-class Americans than it is different.

Some descriptive research using translations of instruments developed by American investigators has been conducted in Korean and Taiwanese cancer patients.[19,51,90,93,94] Although findings from these studies generally are consistent with those conducted in the United States and Canada, discrete differences may reflect cultural dissimilarities. For example, Lin and associates[93] hypothesized that cultural differences in physicians' willingness to disclose a cancer diagnosis may have contributed to changes in hope levels in Taiwanese cancer patients.

Despite the growing body of research in diverse samples, existing research may not adequately reflect the experience of hope for people from non-European cultures. Several known cultural differences could certainly limit the applicability of current conceptualizations of hope, especially within the palliative care context. Three issues that theoretically could have a major impact on multicultural views of hope are time orientation, truth-telling, and one's beliefs about control.

Time orientation is identified as a cultural phenomenon that varies among cultural groups. Some cultural groups, particularly those within the Euro-American culture, tend to be future oriented. Within these groups, people prefer to look ahead, make short- and long-term plans, and organize their schedules to meet goals.[95] Because hope is defined as being future-oriented, with hopeful people more likely to identify and take action to meet goals, members of these future-oriented cultures may possibly appear more hopeful than people who are predominantly present-focused. On the other hand, people who are more focused on the present may be better able to sustain hope at the end of life, when the ability to make long-range goals is hindered by the uncertainty surrounding a terminal diagnosis. Additional research is needed to clarify these relationships.

The value for truth-telling in Western health care systems also may affect hope. Current ethical and legal standards require full disclosure of all relevant health care information to patients.[96] Informed consent and patient autonomy in medical decision-making, two eminent values in American health care, are impossible without this disclosure.[96] Although few would advocate lying to patients, truth-telling is not universally viewed as helpful or desirable. In some cultures, it is believed that patients should be protected from burdensome information that could threaten hope.[97,98] Truthful, but blunt, communication may also be seen as rude and disrespectful in some cultures, and the feeling of being devalued and disrespected has a negative impact on hope.[97,98] In addition to the threats to hope that frank discussion is believed to engender, people who prefer nondisclosure of threatening information may be seen as attempting to cling to unrealistic hopes by refusing to listen to discouraging facts about their condition.

A third cultural concept that may affect hope is one's feeling of being in control. As described earlier, control is a core attribute in many conceptualizations of hope. Although hope can be relinquished to others, including health care providers or a transcendent power, personal control often is central to the hoping process. In Euro-American cultures, applying one's will and energy to alter the course of an illness or to direct the dying process seems natural and desirable. Advance directives are one culturally sanctioned way in which members of these societies exert control over the dying process.[99] However, this desire for and belief in personal control is not a common feature in many other cultures. In cultures where death is viewed as part of the inherent harmony of living and dying, attempts to exert any influence over the dying process may seem unnatural or inappropriate.[100] People from diverse cultures who take a more passive role in their health care or who do not espouse a desire to control their illness or the dying process may be viewed as less hopeful than people who manifest a "fighting spirit" and active stance.

More research needs to be conducted to test theories of hope in multicultural groups, to ensure the appropriate application of current conceptualizations to diverse cultural groups and to develop new theories that are relevant for these groups. Until this work is done, palliative care clinicians must be cautious in applying current hope theories and sensitive to the possible variations in diverse populations.

Models of Maintaining Hope for People with Life-Threatening Illnesses

Several investigators have identified factors that foster hope and strategies that enable people to sustain hope despite life-threatening or chronic illness.[12,16,23,30,36,78,80,101–103] Although there is considerable concordance across these studies regarding many of the major themes, various models emphasize different styles and strategies that demonstrate the diversity in hope-fostering strategies.

As described previously, many people with terminal illness turn to activities and coping strategies that cultivate generalized hope rather then an emphasis on achievement and control. These strategies reflect a sense of peace and acceptance of

Table 26–2
Structure of "Keeping It In Its Place": Hope-Maintaining Strategies In People with Life-Threatening Illness

I. Appraising the illness in a nonthreatening manner
- A. Seeing the disease/treatment as a challenge or a test
- B. Seeing the disease/treatment as a positive influence
  - 1. Reprioritizing one's life
  - 2. Becoming altruistic
  - 3. Looking at the bright side

II. Managing the cognitions related to the illness experience
- A. Joking about it
- B. Avoiding thinking or talking about the negative
- C. Keeping distracted
- D. Forgetting about it
- E. Not dwelling on it
- F. Focusing on loved ones

III. Managing the emotional response to the illness experience
- A. Limiting the emotional response
- B. Severing the cognitive from the emotional response
- C. Shifting from one emotion to another
- D. Translating emotional pain into physical pain

IV. Managing the sense of control
- A. Maintaining control
  - 1. Getting information/staying informed
  - 2. Restraining the disease through exercise, diet, and stress management
  - 3. Decisional control—making decisions about treatment or other aspects of life to exert control
- B. Relinquishing control
  - 1. To a deity
  - 2. To the medical and nursing staffs
  - 3. To medical science

V. Taking a stance toward the illness and treatment
- A. Fighting the illness
  - 1. "Go down fighting"
  - 2. Imagining the illness as the enemy or an evil being
- B. Accepting the illness
  - 1. "It's God's will"
  - 2. "It's just part of the process"
  - 3. Expecting the disease/death

VI. Managing uncertainty
- A. Minimizing the uncertainty
  - 1. "Knowing" the future
  - 2. "Having to believe"
- B. Maximizing the uncertainty
  - 1. "They (the physicians) could always be wrong"
  - 2. "I'm not a statistic!"—beating the odds

VII. Managing the focus on the future
- A. Living day to day
- B. Focusing on long-term goals
  - 1. Making mutable goals
  - 2. Establishing interim goals
  - 3. Using previously met goals as a source of hope
  - 4. Using unmet goals as a source of hope

VIII. Managing the view of the self in relation to the illness
- A. Minimizing the illness and the treatment
  - 1. "It (the disease) is just a flaw in my system"
  - 2. "It (the therapy) is just a temporary inconvenience"
- B. Maximizing personal strength
  - 1. Identifying personal attributes of strength
  - 2. Making downward comparisons with others (e.g., "At least I don't have AIDS")
  - 3. Focusing on successful others
  - 4. Identifying a history of personal strength

Source: Adapted from Ersek (1991), reference 25, and Ersek (1992), reference 16, with permission.

death and center on "being" rather than "doing." These strategies are described in Table 26–1.

In contrast, some models focus more on active, goal-oriented or problem-solving strategies.[16,25,45] This author[16,25] found that adults with leukemia undergoing bone marrow transplantation maintained hope by using many active, cognitive strategies to minimize the psychological distress of life-threatening disease. The resulting model emphasizes that maintaining hope requires a dynamic interplay, or dialectic, between two categories of hope-sustaining strategies: "Dealing with It" and "Keeping It in Its Place." "Dealing with It" is defined as the process of confronting the negative possibilities inherent in the illness experience, including death, and allowing the full range of thoughts, behaviors, and emotions resulting from the recognition. "Keeping It in Its Place" is defined as the process of managing the impact of the disease and its treatment by controlling one's response to the disease, prognosis, and therapy (Table 26–2). This model underscores the complex and sometimes contradictory nature of sustaining hope through serious illness. People use multiple strategies that allow them to confront and to avoid the negative aspects of illness and death. Although the strategies used to manage the threat of death often seem to predominate, these activities occur within a background of recognition and acknowledgment of the possibility of death. This process of negotiating between acknowledgment and management of these fears has been identified in other studies of people with life-threatening illnesses.[21,46,104]

Gum and Snyder[45] elaborated a model of hoping that emphasizes the need for people to set goals and take action to achieve them. Although some people continue to search for a cure after receiving a terminal diagnosis, most people eventually accept their prognosis and mourn the loss of their original goals. At this point, they need to develop and pursue alternative goals that are possible in light of their diminished physical function, end-of-life symptoms, and loss of energy.

These different approaches for maintaining hope are important to describe and understand because they assist the palliative care nurse in designing effective strategies to foster hope. They increase clinicians' awareness regarding the various ways that people respond to chronic and terminal illness and guide clinicians in their interactions with patients and families to sustain hope. They also help palliative care providers understand difficult or troubling responses, such as unrealistic hopefulness.

The Issue of Unrealistic Hopefulness

Reality surveillance is a feature of many conceptualizations of hope. Often, clinicians, researchers, and theorists believe that mentally healthy people should choose and work toward realistic goals. In these frameworks, adhering to unrealistic hopes or denying reality is a sign of maladaptive cognitions that could lead to negative health outcomes. Therefore, denial and unrealistic hopes and ideas are discouraged and treated as pathological.[8,9]

Clinical examples of unrealistic hopes that cause consternation are numerous and diverse. For instance, one patient with advanced cancer might hope that his persistent, severe sciatica is from exercise and overuse rather than spinal metastases. The nurse working with this patient may continually contradict his theory, asserting that his denial of the probable, malignant cause of the pain will delay effective treatment. Another patient might insist that a new cure for her illness is imminent, causing distress for the nurse who knows that it is unlikely that a cure will be found and who believes that the patient's unrealistic hopes will hinder acceptance of and preparation for death.

Despite these concerns, however, some investigators argue that the nurses' fears may be unfounded. This perspective is based on findings from studies, conducted over the past few decades, which have led social psychologists to question the view that denial and unrealistic hopes are always maladaptive. Instead, these researchers argue that human interpretation of information from the environment is inherently biased and inaccurate.[9,45,46]

Shelley Taylor and colleagues developed this idea further in their theory of positive illusions, which is based on an extensive program of research spanning more than two decades.[105–108] They describe positive illusions as general, enduring cognitive patterns, involving error and/or bias, that provide a foundation for successful adaptation to many threatening events, including serious illness. Especially important are unrealistically positive evaluations of the self, exaggerated perceptions of control, and unrealistic optimism about the future.[109] They support their theory with empirical evidence that denial and positive illusions often are associated with positive outcomes, such as better psychological adjustment to illness, less physical and emotional distress, and even decreased mortality.[46,107,108,110,111]

In addition to promoting positive outcomes, unrealistic hopes need to be assessed within the context of uncertainty. No one really does know exactly what the future will bring. So, if a person hopes for something in the future that appears highly unlikely, can it be known for certain that it will not occur? Sometimes, patients and families need to focus on this uncertainty to sustain hope.

Another frequent cause of concern is the way in which people exploit uncertainty to maximize hope. For instance, people frequently respond to dire prognostic news with observation that they can always "beat the odds." Given the fact that no one can predict the future with absolute certainty, it is impossible to predict which individuals with a 2% chance of remission or recovery will actually be cured. Also, consider the case of a person with life-threatening disease who believes that God can provide a cure. Spontaneous "miracle" cures, however rare, have been documented. No one can predict with complete confidence that there is no possibility of a cure. These observations raise the question: do all people who hope against poor odds need help to become more "realistic"?

A third argument against aggressive "reality orientation" for all patients and families is the evidence that unrealistic hopes and illusions often are abandoned over time and without intensive intervention from professionals.[12,107,109] In other words, most people acknowledge and accept distressing information, but need to do so on their own schedules.

The preceding discussion may seem to imply that clinicians should not be concerned about unrealistic hopefulness. Of course, that is not the case. Despite their adaptive potential, illusions and denial may result in adverse outcomes. For example, unrealistic hopes may lead parents to insist on aggressive, futile therapy that increases their child's suffering without curing or controlling the disease. Similarly, a person who denies that his illness is terminal may isolate himself from his family to protect his beliefs and avoid contradictory opinions. Unfortunately, in these cases and others, there is insufficient research to inform clinicians fully regarding situations that are potentially maladaptive, and even less guidance about appropriate therapeutic strategies. However, evidence exists that some situations should be viewed with caution and may indicate a need for gentle interventions, such as offering alternative hopes or providing skillful counseling. Table 26–3

Table 26–3
Assessing Unrealistic Hopes

1. Is the focus of the unrealistic hope broad or severe (e.g., complete denial of a disease that has been documented)?
2. Is the persistence of the unrealistic hope severe, i.e., does it persist despite multiple pieces of information from multiple sources (e.g., family, physicians, nurses) that the hope is unlikely to be realized?
3. Is the person's adherence to the unrealistic hope *complete,* or does the person admit at times that there are limitations and acknowledge negative possibilities? Does the person continually use words such as "knowing" what will happen, rather than acknowledging that what he or she hopes for might *not* occur?
4. Does the hope cause the person to engage in reckless behaviors?
5. Does the hope cause the person to ignore warning signs (e.g., angina, increased pain) that should be treated promptly?
6. Does the hope cause great distress for family members and significant others?
7. Has the person become isolated from others, either to avoid their challenges to the unrealistic hope or because others are uncomfortable in responding to the person?
8. Does it appear that adhering to the hope actually is causing distress and anxiety for the person (who may tacitly doubt or disbelieve in the illusion or hope, but is afraid to discuss that possibility with others)?
9. Is death imminent, and the unrealistic hopefulness is hindering efforts to get affairs in order, say good-bye, or receive emotional support?

lists several questions regarding unrealistic hopes. If the answer to any of these question is "Yes," then further assessment and possible intervention may be necessary.

Assessing Hope

As in all nursing care, thorough assessment of physical and psychosocial factors must precede thoughtful planning and implementation of therapeutic strategies. Therefore, consistent and comprehensive evaluations of hope should be included in the palliative nursing assessment. Some conceptual elements of hope, such as those focusing on meaning and purpose in life, are included in a spiritual assessment. Rarely, however, are comprehensive guides to assessing hope included in standardized nursing assessment forms.

The guidelines produced by Farran, Wilken, and Popovich[131] for the clinical assessment of hope appropriately use the acronym *HOPE* to designate the major areas of evaluation: The areas are **H**ealth, **O**thers, **P**urpose in Life, and **E**ngaging Process. The term "engaging process" refers to identifying goals, taking actions to achieve goals, sense of control over one's situation, and identifying hope-inspiring factors in one's past, present, and future. In Table 26–4, this framework has been adapted and applied to terminally ill patients. It includes examples of questions and probes that can be used to assess hope.

Like pain, hope is a subjective experience and assessment should focus on self-report. However, behavioral cues can also provide information regarding a person's state of hope or hopelessness. Hopelessness is a central feature of depression; therefore, behaviors such as social withdrawal, flat affect, alcohol and substance abuse, insomnia, and passivity may indicate hopelessness.

As discussed earlier, the patient's terminal illness affects the hope of family caregivers, who, in turn, influence the hope of the patients. Therefore, the hope of the patients' family caregivers and other significant support people also should be assessed.

Over the past decades, researchers from several disciplines have developed instruments to measure hope and hopelessness. The theoretical and empirical literature documents the comprehensiveness and face validity of these tools. Advances in psychometric theory and methods have allowed the evaluation of multiple dimensions of validity and reliability. The development and use of well-designed and well-tested tools has contributed greatly to the science of hope. Although a thorough discussion of these measures is beyond the scope of this chapter, Table 26–5 provides a brief description of several widely used and tested instruments. More complete descriptions and evaluations of these scales can be found elsewhere.[11,112]

Nursing Interventions to Maintain Hope at End of Life

Clinicians, theorists, and researchers recognize that nurses play an important role in instilling, maintaining, and restoring hope in people for whom they care. Researchers have identified many ways in which nurses assist patients and families to sustain hope in the face of life-threatening illness,[44,87,102,113,114]

Table 26–6 provides a summary of nursing approaches to instill hope. A brief perusal of this table reveals an important point about these strategies: For the most part, nursing care to maintain patients' and families' hope fundamentally is about providing excellent physical, psychosocial, and spiritual palliative care. There are few unique interventions to maintain hope, and yet there is much nurses can do. Because hope is inextricably connected to virtually all facets of the illness experience—including physical pain, coping, anxiety, and spirituality—improvement or deterioration in one area has repercussions in other areas. Attending to these relationships reminds clinicians that virtually every action they take can influence hope, negatively or positively.

Another vital observation about hope-inspiring strategies is that many approaches begin with the patient and family. The experience of hope is a personal one, defined and determined

Table 26–4
Guidelines for the Clinical Assessment of Hope in Palliative Care

Interview Question/Probe	Rationale
Health (and Symptom Management)	
1. Tell me about your illness. What is your understanding of the probable course of your illness?	Explore the person's perceptions of the seriousness of the illness and possible trajectories.
2. How hopeful are you right now, and how does your illness affect your sense of hope?	Determine the person's general sense of hope and the effect of the terminal illness on hope.
3. How well are you able to control the symptoms of your illness? How do these symptoms affect your hope?	Uncontrolled end-of-life symptoms have been found to negatively influence hope.[36, 78]
Others	
1. Who provides you with emotional, physical, and spiritual support?	Identify people in the environment who provide support and enhance hope.
2. Who are you most likely to confide in when you have a problem or a concern?	Identify others in whom the person has trust.
3. What kinds of difficult experiences have you and your family/partner/support network had to deal with in the past? How did you manage those experiences?	Explore experiences of coping with stressful situations.
4. What kinds of things do family, support people, health care providers do that make you more hopeful? Less hopeful?	Identify specific behaviors that affect hope. Recognize that other people can also *decrease* hope.
Purpose in Life	
1. What gives you hope?	Identify relationships, beliefs, and activities that provide a sense of purpose and contribute positively to hope.
2. What helps you make sense of your situation right now?	Identify the ways in which the person makes meaning of difficult situations.
3. Do you have spiritual or religious practices or support people that help you? If "yes," what are these practices / people?	Identify if and how spirituality acts as a source of hope.
4. Has your illness caused you to question your spiritual beliefs? If "yes," how?	Terminal illness can threaten one's basic beliefs, and test one's faith.
5. How can we help you maintain these practices and personal connections with spiritual support people?	Identify ways in which clinicians and others can support spiritual practices that enhance hope.
Goals	
1. Right now, what are your major goals?	Identify major goals and priorities. Examine whether these goals are congruent with the views of others.
2. What do you see are the chances that you will meet these goals?	Explore how realistic the person thinks the goals are; if the goals are not perceived as being attainable, assess the impact on hope.

(*continued*)

Table 26–4
Guidelines for the Clinical Assessment of Hope in Palliative Care *(continued)*

Interview Question/Probe	Rationale
3. What actions can you take to meet these goals?	Identify specific actions the person can take to meet the goals.
4. What actions have you already taken to meet these goals?	Identify how active the person has been in attaining the goals.
5. What resources do you have for meeting these goals?	Determine other resources to which the person has access for the purpose of attaining goals.
Sense of Control	
1. Do you feel that you have much control over your current situation?	Determine whether the person feels any ability to control or change the situation. Explore whether the person *wants* to have more control.
2. Are there others who you feel have some control over your current situation? If "yes," who are they and in what ways do they have control?	Determine whether the person feels as though trusted others (e.g., health care providers, family, deity) can control or change the situation.
Sources of Hope over Time	
1. In the past, what or who has made you hopeful?	Identify sources of hope from the person's past that may continue to provide hope during the terminal phase.
2. Right now who and what provides you with hope?	Identify current sources of hope.
3. What do you hope for in the future?	Assess generalized and specific hopes for the future.

Source: Adapted from Farran et al. (1992), reference 131, and Farran et al. (1995), reference 11.

by the hoping person. Although others greatly influence that experience, ultimately the meanings and effects of words and actions are determined by the person experiencing hope or hopelessness. Many approaches used by people with life-threatening illness to maintain hope are strategies initiated with little influence from others. For example, some people pray; others distract themselves with television watching, conversation, or other activities; and many patients use cognitive strategies, such as minimizing negative thoughts, identifying personal strengths, and focusing on the positive.[16] For many patients and families, careful observation and active support of an individual's established strategies to maintain hope will be most successful.

A final point is to remind the reader that family caregivers and other support people should be included in these approaches. Ample evidence exists that patients and people within their support systems reciprocally influence one another's hope. In addition, family and significant others are always incorporated into the palliative care plan and considered part of the unit of care. Maintenance of hope also is a goal after death, in that hope-restoring and -maintaining strategies must be an integral part of bereavement counseling.[115]

Specific Interventions

The framework for the following discussion is adapted from Farran, Herth, and Popovich,[11] who articulated four central attributes of hope: experiential, spiritual/transcendent, relational, and rational thought. These areas encompass the major themes found in the literature, and although they are not mutually exclusive, they provide a useful organizing device. This section also includes a brief discussion of ways in which nurses need to explore and understand their own hopes and values in order to provide palliative care that fosters hope in others.

Experiential Process Interventions

The experiential process of hope involves the acknowledgment and acceptance of suffering, while at the same time using

Table 26–5
Descriptions of Selected Instruments to Measure Hope and Hopelessness

Instrument Name	Brief Description	Selected References
Beck Hopelessness Scale	20-item, true-false format Based on Stotland's definition of hopelessness: system of negative expectancies concerning oneself and one's future Developed to assess psychopathological levels of hopelessness; correlates highly with attempted and actual suicide	50, 55, 56, 82, 121,122
Herth Hope Index	12-item, 4-point Likert scale; total score is sum of all items; range of scores 12–48 Designed for well and ill populations Assesses three overlapping dimensions: (1) cognitive–temporal, (2) affective–behavioral, (3) affiliative–behavioral Spanish, Thai, Chinese, Swedish translations available	18, 19, 28, 36, 39, 51, 53, 78, 88, 123, 124
Hopefulness Scale for Adolescents (Hinds)	24-item visual analog scale Assesses the degree of the adolescent's positive future orientation Assesses only the relational and rational thoughts processes of hope Tested in several populations of adolescents: well, substance abusers, adolescents with emotional and mental problems, cancer patients	61, 70, 125, 126
Miller Hope Scale	40-item scale, 5-point Likert scale Assesses 10 elements: (a) mutuality/affiliation, (b) avoidance of absolutizing, (c) sense of the possible, (d) psychological well-being and coping, (e) achieving goals, (f) purpose and meaning in life, (g) reality surveillance–optimism, (h) mental and physical activation, (i) anticipation, (j) freedom Chinese and Swedish versions	35, 127, 128
Snyder Hope Scale	12-item, 4-point Likert scale Based on Stotland's definition of hope; focus is on goals identification and achievement Tested in healthy adults and adults with psychiatric illness Also has developed tool to measure hope in children	129, 130

the imagination to move beyond the suffering and find hope.[87] Included in these types of strategies are methods to decrease physical suffering and cognitive strategies aimed at managing the threat of the terminal illness.

Uncontrolled symptoms, such as pain, fatigue, dyspnea, and anxiety, cause suffering and challenge the hopefulness of patients and caregivers. Timely and adept symptom prevention and management is central to maintaining hope. In home care settings, teaching patients and families the knowledge and skills to manage symptoms confidently and competently also is essential.

Other ways to help people find hope in suffering is to provide them a cognitive reprieve from their situation. One powerful strategy to achieve this temporary suspension is through humor. Several studies and lay publications have identified the central place of humor and lightheartedness in promoting hope.[16,44,83,116] According to patients' views, humor helps put things in perspective and frees the self, at least momentarily, from the onerous burden of illness and suffering. Making light of a grim situation brings a sense of control over one's response to the situation, even when one has little influence over it. In one study, a respondent noted, "I may not have much control over the nearness of death, but I do have the power to joke about it"[36] (p. 1255). Of course, the use of humor with patients and families requires sensitivity as well as a sense of timing. Otherwise, humor becomes a belittling and hope-destroying

Table 26–6
Interventions to Foster Hope

Experiential Processes

- Prevent and manage end-of-life symptoms
- Use lightheartedness and humor appropriately
- Encourage the patient and family to transcend their current situation
- Encourage aesthetic experiences
- Encourage engagement in creative and joyous endeavors
- Suggest literature, movies, and art that are uplifting and highlight the joy in life
- Encourage reminiscing
- Assist patient and family to focus on present and past joys
- Share positive, hope-inspiring stories
- Support patient and family in positive self-talk

Spiritual/Transcendent Processes

- Facilitate participation in religious rituals and spiritual practices
- Make necessary referrals to clergy and other spiritual support people
- Assist the patient and family in finding meaning in the current situation
- Assist the patient/family to keep a journal
- Suggest literature, movies, and art that explore the meaning of suffering

Relational Processes

- Minimize patient and family isolation
- Establish and maintain an open relationship
- Affirm patients' and families' sense of self-worth
- Recognize and reinforce the reciprocal nature of hopefulness between patient and support system
- Provide time for relationships (especially important in institutional settings)
- Foster attachment ideation by assisting the patient to identify significant others and then to reflect on personal characteristics and experiences that endear the significant other to the patient.[118]
- Communicate one's own sense of hopefulness

Rational Thought Processes

- Assist patient and family to establish, obtain, and revise goals without imposing one's own agenda
- Assist in identifying available and needed resources to meet goals
- Assist in procuring needed resources; assist with breaking larger goals into smaller steps to increase feelings of success
- Provide accurate information regarding patient's condition and treatment
- Facilitate reality surveillance as appropriate
- Help patient and family identify past successes
- Increase patients' and families' sense of control when possible

mistake. The nurse should take cues from the patient and family, observe how they use humor to dispel stress, and let them take the lead in joking about threatening information and events. In general, humor should be focused on oneself or on events outside the immediate concerns of the patient and family.

Other ways to move people cognitively beyond their suffering is to assist them in identifying and enjoying that which is joyful in life. Engagement in aesthetic experiences, such as watching movies or listening to music that is uplifting, can enable people to transcend their suffering. Sharing one's own hope-inspiring stories also can help.

Another strategy is to support people in their own positive self-talk. As noted earlier, many people naturally cope with stress by comparing themselves with people they perceive to be less fortunate or by identifying attributes of personal strength that help them find hope.[16,117] For example, an elderly, married woman with advanced breast cancer may comment that, despite the seriousness of her disease, she feels luckier than another woman with the same disease who is younger or without social support. By comparing herself with less fortunate others, she can take solace in recognizing that "things could be worse." Similarly, a person can maintain hope by focusing on particular talents or previous accomplishments that indicate an ability to cope with illness. In one study on hope, a woman asserted that her ability to survive an abusive marriage provided evidence that she could also cope with and manage her illness and treatment.[25] People may also cite their high level of motivation as a reason to feel hopeful about the future. Acknowledgment and validation of these attributes supports hope and affirms self-worth for patients and families.

Spiritual Process Interventions

Several specific strategies can foster hope while incorporating spirituality. These strategies include providing opportunities for the expression of spiritual beliefs and arranging for involvement in religious rituals and spiritual practices.

Assisting patients and families to explore and make meaning of their trials and suffering is another useful approach. Encouraging patients and families to keep a journal of thoughts and feelings can help people in this process. Suggesting books, films, or art that focuses on religious or existential understanding and transcendence of suffering is another effective way to help people make sense of illness and death.

Palliative care nurses also should assess for signs of spiritual distress and make appropriate referrals to clergy and other professionals with expertise in counseling during spiritual and existential crises. Other spiritual and existential strategies are described in chapters 30, 31 and 32 of this text.

Relational Process Interventions

To maximize hope, nurses should establish and maintain an open relationship with patients and members of their support network, taking the time to learn what their priorities and needs are and then addressing those needs in timely, effective ways. Demonstrating respect and interest, and being available to listen and be with people—that is, affirming each person's worth—are essential.

Fostering and sustaining connectedness among the patient, family, and friends can be accomplished by providing time for uninterrupted interactions, which is especially important in institutional settings. Nurses can increase hope by enlisting help from others to help achieve goals. For example, recruiting friends or arranging for a volunteer to transport an ill person to purchase a gift for a grandchild can cultivate hope for everyone involved. It is important to help others realize how vital they are in sustaining a person's hope.

Miller[118] recommended that another method of instilling hope is to foster attachment ideation. Attachment ideation is the preoccupation with significant others, such as a child or spouse. To encourage this attachment, a nurse assists a person in identifying and reviewing characteristics that endear and attract the person to the significant other. In this way, the person can focus on the loved one during times of distress or pain, thereby maintaining hope.

Rational Thought Process Interventions

The rational thought process is the dimension of hope that specifically focuses on goals, resources, personal control and self-efficacy, and action. Interventions related to this dimension include assisting patients and families in devising and attaining goals. Providing accurate and timely information about the patient's condition and treatment helps patients and families decide which goals are achievable. At times, gentle assistance with monitoring and acknowledging negative possibilities helps the patient and family to choose realistic goals. Helping to identify and procure the resources necessary to meet goals also is important.

Often, major goals need to be broken into smaller, shorter-term achievements. For example, a patient with painful, metastatic lung cancer might want to attend a family event that is 2 weeks away. The successful achievement of this goal depends on many factors, including adequate pain control, transportation, and ability to transfer to and from a wheelchair. By breaking the larger goal into several smaller ones, the person is able to identify all the necessary steps and resources. Attainment of a subgoal, such as being able to transfer with minimal assistance, can empower patients and families and help energize them to reach more difficult and complex goals.

Supporting patients and families to identify those areas of life and death in which they do have real influence can increase self-esteem and self-efficacy, thereby instilling hope. It also helps to review their previous successes in attaining important goals.

Programs to Enhance Hopefulness

In addition to discrete actions that individual nurses take to foster hope, several investigators have developed and tested programs to enhance hope in people with life-threatening illness. Rustøen and colleagues[91] designed a theoretically based group intervention to increase hope in people with cancer. The eight weekly meetings each lasted 2 hours. After an initial introductory session, the subsequent seven sessions focused on a major topic such as believing in oneself, relationships, active involvement, and spiritual beliefs and values. In a randomized trial, Rustøen and coworkers[92] compared the effects of their hope intervention with those of a group self-help/education intervention and a control group. They reported that, 1 to 2 weeks after the interventions, participants in the hope group showed significantly increased hope scores compared with the other two groups. At the 6-month follow-up, however, these differences were no longer significant.

Herth[87,102] also designed and tested a Hope Intervention Program, which she evaluated in a group of people with recurrent cancer. Based on her empirically derived theory of hope, the intervention consists of eight sessions delivered in a nurse-facilitated group setting. Six sessions focus on strategies that specifically address the four hope processes: experiential, relational, spiritual/transcendent, and rational thought. During the final session, participants develop an individual plan with strategies to maintain and foster hope. When Herth tested this intervention, she found significantly increased hope levels in the treatment group compared with two control groups. These significant differences persisted at the 3-, 6-, and 9-month follow-up measurements.[102]

Hinds and colleagues developed a Psychosocial Research–Translation Team to integrate evidence-based hope intervention guidelines into the cancer care department at St. Jude Children's Hospital.[119] Using this innovative approach, the multidisciplinary team reviewed the literature on hope and interviewed experts on the topic. The team used this information to develop its own definition of hope and to identify potential projects aimed at translating the evidence-based guidelines on hope into practice. These projects included (1) adding information about hope to the parent handbook; (2) developing patient, parent, and staff educational sheets about hope; (3) developing a telephone hotline that allows for the efficient and personal delivery of messages of hope to callers; and (4) designing and launching websites about hope. This program demonstrates the creative and diverse approaches that health care providers can use to support and promote hope among patients and families facing life-threatening illnesses.

Ensuring the Self-Knowledge Necessary to Provide Palliative Care

Providing holistic palliative care requires a broad range of skills. Astute management of physical symptoms and a solid command of technical skills must be matched with an ability to provide psychosocial and spiritual care for patients and families at a time of great vulnerability. To nurture these latter skills, nurses should continually reflect on and evaluate their own hopes, beliefs, and biases[6,120] and identify how these factors influence their care. Within particular clinical situations, they should evaluate how patients' and families' responses and strategies to maintain hope affect them. For example, does it anger or frustrate the nurse that the patient seems to refuse to acknowledge that his or her disease is incurable? Is this anger communicated nonverbally or verbally to the patient or family? In addition to self-reflection, it is important for palliative care nurses to maintain hopefulness while working with dying patients by engaging in self-care activities.

Summary

Hope is central to the human experience of living and dying, and it is integrally entwined with spiritual and psychosocial well-being. Although terminal illness can challenge and even temporarily diminish hope, the dying process does not inevitably bring despair. The human spirit, manifesting its creativity and resiliency, can forge new and deeper hopes at the end of life. Palliative care nurses play important roles in supporting patients and families with this process by providing expert physical, psychosocial, and spiritual care. Sensitive, skillful attention to maintaining hope can enhance quality of life and contribute significantly to a "good death" as defined by the patient and family. Fostering hope is a primary means by which palliative care nurses accompany patients and families on the journey through terminal illness.

REFERENCES

1. Holland J, Lewis S. The human side of cancer: Living with hope, coping with uncertainty. New York: Quill, 2000.
2. Nouwen H, Gaffney W. Aging. New York: Image Books, 1990.
3. Menninger K. Hope. Bull Menninger Clin 1987;51:447–462.
4. Marcel G. Homo Viator: Introduction to a Metaphysic of Hope. New York: Harper and Row, 1962.
5. Fromm E. The Revolution of Hope. New York: Bantam Books, 1968.
6. Scanlon C. Creating a vision of hope: The challenge of palliative care. Oncol Nurs Forum 1989;16:491–496.
7. Lynch W. Images of Hope: Imagination as Healer of the Hopeless. New York: New American Library, 1965.
8. Ersek M. Examining the process and dilemmas of reality negotiation. Image: J Nurs Scholarship 1992;24:19–25.
9. Snyder CR, Rand KL. The case against false hope. Am Psychol 2003;58:820–822; authors' reply 823–824.
10. Nekolaichuk CL, Jevne RF, Maguire TO. Structuring the meaning of hope in health and illness. Soc Sci Med 1999;48:591–605.
11. Farran CJ, Herth KA, Popovich JM. Hope and Hopelessness: Critical Clinical Constructs. Thousand Oaks, CA: Sage Publications, 1995.
12. Dufault K. Hope of Elderly Persons with Cancer. Unpublished dissertation. Cleveland: Case Western Reserve University, 1981.
13. Hinds PS. Adolescent hopefulness in illness and health. Adv Nurs Sci 1988;10:79–88.
14. Dufault K, Martocchio B. Hope: Its spheres and dimensions. Nurs Clin North Am 1985;20:379–391.
15. Stotland E. The Psychology of Hope. San Francisco: Jossey-Bass, 1969.
16. Ersek M. The process of maintaining hope in adults undergoing bone marrow transplantation for leukemia. Oncol Nurs Forum 1992;19:883–889.
17. Cutcliffe JR, Grant G. What are the principles and processes of inspiring hope in cognitively impaired older adults within a continuing care environment? J Psychiatr Ment Health Nurs 2001;8: 427–436.

18. Herth K. Development and refinement of an instrument to measure hope. Sch Inq Nurs Pract 1991;5:39–51.
19. Hsu TH, Lu MS, Tsou TS, Lin CC. The relationship of pain, uncertainty, and hope in Taiwanese lung cancer patients. J Pain Symptom Manage 2003;26:835–842.
20. Wineman NM, Schwetz KM, Zeller R, Cyphert J. Longitudinal analysis of illness uncertainty, coping, hopefulness, and mood during participation in a clinical drug trial. J Neurosci Nurs 2003; 35:100–106.
21. Kylma J, Vehvilainen-Julkunen K, Lahdevirta J. Hope, despair and hopelessness in living with HIV/AIDS: A grounded theory study. J Adv Nurs 2001;33:764–775.
22. Morse JM, Penrod J. Linking concepts of enduring, uncertainty, suffering, and hope. Image: J Nurs Scholarship 1999; 31:145–150.
23. Hall BA. Ways of maintaining hope in HIV disease. Res Nurs Health 1994;17:283–293.
24. Kylma J, Vehvilainen-Julkunen K, Lahdevirta J. Dynamically fluctuating hope, despair and hopelessness along the HIV/AIDS continuum as described by caregivers in voluntary organizations in Finland. Issues Ment Health Nurs 2001;22:353–377.
25. Ersek M. The Process of Maintaining Hope in Adults with Leukemia Undergoing Bone Marrow Transplantation. Doctoral dissertation. Seattle: University of Washington, 1991.
26. Taylor EJ. Whys and wherefores: Adult patient perspectives of the meaning of cancer. Semin Oncol Nurs 1995;11:32–40.
27. Mickley JR, Soeken K, Belcher A. Spiritual well-being, religiousness and hope among women with breast cancer. Image: J Nurs Scholarship 1992;24:267–272.
28. Herth KA. The relationship between level of hope and level of coping response and other variables in patients with cancer. Oncol Nurs Forum 1989;16:67–72.
29. Holt J, Reeves JS. The meaning of hope and generic caring practices to nurture hope in a rural village in the Dominican Republic. J Transcult Nurs 2001;12:123–131.
30. Bays CL. Older adults' descriptions of hope after a stroke. Rehabil Nurs 2001;26:18–20.
31. Cutcliffe JR, Herth K. The concept of hope in nursing 1: Its origins, background and nature. Br J Nurs. 2002;11:832–840.
32. Gibson LM. Inter-relationships among sense of coherence, hope, and spiritual perspective (inner resources) of African-American and European-American breast cancer survivors. Appl Nurs Res 2003;16:236–244.
33. Haase JE, Britt T, Coward DD, Leidy NK, Penn PE. Simultaneous concept analysis of spiritual perspective, hope, acceptance and self-transcendence. Image: J Nurs Scholarship 1992;24: 141–147.
34. Carson V, Soeken KL, Shanty J, Terry L. Hope and spiritual well-being: essentials for living with AIDS. Perspect Psychiatr Care 1990;26:28–34.
35. Fehring RJ, Miller JF, Shaw C. Spiritual well-being, religiosity, hope, depression, and other mood states in elderly people coping with cancer. Oncol Nurs Forum 1997;24:663–671.
36. Herth K. Fostering hope in terminally-ill people. J Adv Nurs 1990;15:1250–1259.
37. Yates P. Towards a reconceptualization of hope for patients with a diagnosis of cancer. J Adv Nurs 1993;18:701–706.
38. Borneman T, Brown-Saltzman K. Meaning in illness. In: Ferrell B, Coyle N, eds. Textbook of Palliative Nursing. New York: Oxford University Press, 2001:415–424.
39. Ebright PR, Lyon B. Understanding hope and factors that enhance hope in women with breast cancer. Oncol Nurs Forum 2002;29:561–568.
40. Foote AW, Piazza D, Holcombe J, Paul P, Daffin P. Hope, self-esteem and social support in persons with multiple sclerosis. J Neurosci Nurs 1990;22:155–159.
41. Piazza D, Holcombe J, Foote A, Paul P, Love S, Daffin P. Hope, social support and self-esteem of patients with spinal cord injuries. J Neurosci Nurs 1991;23:224–230.
42. Hinds PS. Fostering coping by adolescents with newly diagnosed cancer. Semin Oncol Nurs 2000;16:317–327.
43. Herth KA, Cutcliffe JR. The concept of hope in nursing 3: Hope and palliative care nursing. Br J Nurs 2002;11:977–983.
44. Hinds PS, Martin J, Vogel RJ. Nursing strategies to influence adolescent hopefulness during oncologic illness. J Assoc Pediatr Oncol Nurses 1987;4:14–22.
45. Gum A, Snyder CR. Coping with terminal illness: The role of hopeful thinking. J Palliat Med 2002;5:883–894.
46. Taylor SE, Kemeny ME, Reed GM, Bower JE, Gruenewald TL. Psychological resources, positive illusions, and health. Am Psychol 2000;55:99–109.
47. Lazarus RS, Folkman S. Stress, Appraisal, and Coping. New York: Springer Publishing, 1984.
48. Popovich JM, Fox PG, Burns KR. "Hope" in the recovery from stroke in the U.S. Int J Psych Nurs Res 2003;8:905–920.
49. Kim TS. Hope as a mode of coping in amyotrophic lateral sclerosis. J Neurosci Nurs 1989;21:342–347.
50. Patten SB, Metz LM. Hopelessness ratings in relapsing-remitting and secondary progressive multiple sclerosis. Int J Psychiatry Med 2002;32:155–165.
51. Lin CC, Lai YL, Ward SE. Effect of cancer pain on performance status, mood states, and level of hope among Taiwanese cancer patients. J Pain Symptom Manage 2003;25:29–37.
52. Harwood DG, Sultzer DL. "Life is not worth living": Hopelessness in Alzheimer's disease. J Geriatr Psychiatry Neurol 2002;15:38–43.
53. Evangelista LS, Doering LV, Dracup K, Vassilakis ME, Kobashigawa J. Hope, mood states and quality of life in female heart transplant recipients. J Heart Lung Transplant 2003;22:681–686.
54. Sullivan MD. Hope and hopelessness at the end of life. Am J Geriatr Psychiatry 2003;11:393–405.
55. Beck AT, Brown G, Steer RA. Prediction of eventual suicide in psychiatric inpatients by clinical ratings of hopelessness. J Consult Clin Psychol 1989;57:309–310.
56. Beck AT, Steer RA, Kovacs M, Garrison B. Hopelessness and eventual suicide: A 10-year prospective study of patients hospitalized with suicidal ideation. Am J Psychiatry 1985;142:559–563.
57. Ganzini L, Johnston WS, McFarland BH, Tolle SW, Lee MA. Attitudes of patients with amyotrophic lateral sclerosis and their care givers toward assisted suicide. N Engl J Med 1998;339:967–973.
58. Wilson KG, Scott JF, Graham ID, Kozak JF, Chater S, Viola RA, de Faye BJ, Weaver LA, Curran D. Attitudes of terminally ill patients toward euthanasia and physician-assisted suicide. Arch Intern Med 2000;160:2454–2460.
59. Breitbart W, Rosenfeld B, Pessin H, Kaim M, Funesti-Esch J, Galietta M, Nelson CJ, Brescia R. Depression, hopelessness, and desire for hastened death in terminally ill patients with cancer. JAMA 2000;284:2907–2911.
60. Johnson JG, Alloy LB, Panzarella C, Metalsky GI, Rabkin JG, Williams JB, Abramson LY. Hopelessness as a mediator of the association between social support and depressive

symptoms: Findings of a study of men with HIV. J Consult Clin Psychol 2001;69:1056–1060.
61. Ritchie MA. Self-esteem and hopefulness in adolescents with cancer. J Pediatr Nurs 2001;16:35–42.
62. Segerstrom SC, Taylor SE, Kemeny ME, Fahey JL. Optimism is associated with mood, coping, and immune change in response to stress. J Pers Soc Psychol 1998;74:1646–1655.
63. Bower JE, Kemeny ME, Taylor SE, Fahey JL. Cognitive processing, discovery of meaning, CD4 decline, and AIDS-related mortality among bereaved HIV-seropositive men. J Consult Clin Psychol. 1998;66:979–986.
64. Watson M, Haviland JS, Greer S, Davidson J, Bliss JM. Influence of psychological response on survival in breast cancer: A population-based cohort study. Lancet 1999;354:1331–1336.
65. Barefoot JC, Brummett BH, Helms MJ, Mark DB, Siegler IC, Williams RB. Depressive symptoms and survival of patients with coronary artery disease. Psychosom Med 2000;62:790–795.
66. Stern SL, Dhanda R, Hazuda HP. Hopelessness predicts mortality in older Mexican and European Americans. Psychosom Med 2001;63:344–351.
67. Wright BA, Shontz FC. Process and tasks in hoping. Rehabil Lit 1968;29:322–331.
68. Artinian BM. Fostering hope in the bone marrow transplant child. Matern Child Nurs J 1984;13:57–71.
69. Hinds PS, Martin J. Hopefulness and the self-sustaining process in adolescents with cancer. Nurs Res 1988;37:336–340.
70. Hinds PS, Quargnenti A, Fairclough D, Bush AJ, Betcher D, Rissmiller G, Pratt CB, Gilchrist GS. Hopefulness and its characteristics in adolescents with cancer. West J Nurs Res 1999; 21:600–616.
71. Herth K. Hope in older adults in community and institutional settings. Issues Ment Health Nurs 1993;14:139–156.
72. Farran CJ. A survey of community-based older adults: stressful life events, mediating variables, hope, and health. Dissertation Abstracts International 1985;46:113B.
73. Farran CJ, McCann J. Longitudinal analysis of hope in community-based older adults. Arch Psychiatr Nurs 1989;3: 272–276.
74. McGill JS, Paul PB. Functional status and hope in elderly people with and without cancer. Oncol Nurs Forum 1993;20:1207–1213.
75. Herth KA, Cutcliffe JR. The concept of hope in nursing 4: Hope and gerontological nursing. Br J Nurs 2002;11:1148–1156.
76. Yates P, Stetz KM. Families' awareness of and response to dying. Oncol Nurs Forum 1999;26:113–120.
77. Parker-Oliver D. Redefining hope for the terminally ill. Am J Hosp Palliat Care 2002;19:115–120.
78. Herth K. Hope in the family caregiver of terminally ill people. J Adv Nurs 1993;18:538–548.
79. Nekolaichuk CL, Bruera E. On the nature of hope in palliative care. J Palliat Care 1998;14:36–42.
80. Benzein E, Norberg A, Saveman BI. The meaning of the lived experience of hope in patients with cancer in palliative home care. Palliat Med 2001;15:117–126.
81. Tulsky JA. Hope and hubris. J Palliat Med 2002;5:339–341.
82. McClain CS, Rosenfeld B, Breitbart W. Effect of spiritual well-being on end-of-life despair in terminally-ill cancer patients. Lancet 2003;361:1603–1607.
83. Herth K. Contributions of humor as perceived by the terminally ill. Am J Hosp Care 1990;7:36–40.
84. Wilkinson K. The concept of hope in life-threatening illness. Prof Nurse 1996;11:659–661.
85. Herth K. Hope from the perspective of homeless families. J Adv Nurs 1996;24:743–753.
86. Herth K. Hope as seen through the eyes of homeless children. J Adv Nurs 1998;28:1053–1062.
87. Herth KA. Development and implementation of a hope intervention program. Oncol Nurs Forum 2001;28:1009–1016.
88. Benzein E, Berg A. The Swedish version of Herth Hope Index: An instrument for palliative care. Scand J Caring Sci 2003;17:409–415.
89. Kylma J, Vehvilainen-Julkunen K, Lahdevirta J. Dynamics of hope in HIV/AIDS affected people: An exploration of significant others' experiences. Res Theor Nurs Pract 2003;17:191–205.
90. Lee EH. Fatigue and hope: Relationships to psychosocial adjustment in Korean women with breast cancer. Appl Nurs Res 2001;14:87–93.
91. Rustøen T, Hanestad BR. Nursing intervention to increase hope in cancer patients. J Clin Nurs 1998;7:19–27.
92. Rustøen T, Wiklund I, Hanestad BR, Moum T. Nursing intervention to increase hope and quality of life in newly diagnosed cancer patients. Cancer Nurs 1998;21:235–245.
93. Lin CC, Tsai HF, Chiou JF, Lai YH, Kao CC, Tsou TS. Changes in levels of hope after diagnostic disclosure among Taiwanese patients with cancer. Cancer Nurs 2003;26:155–160.
94. Chen ML. Pain and hope in patients with cancer: A role for cognition. Cancer Nurs 2003;26:61–67.
95. Purnell L, Paulanka B. The Purnell Model for cultural competence. In: Purnell L, Paulanka B, eds. Transcultural Health Care: A Culturally Competent Approach, 2nd ed. Philadelphia: F.A. Davis, 2003:8–39.
96. Beauchamp TL, Childress JF. Principles of Biomedical Ethics, 5th ed. New York: Oxford University Press, 2001.
97. Blackhall LJ, Frank G, Murphy S, Michel V. Bioethics in a different tongue: The case of truth-telling. J Urban Health 2001;78:59–71.
98. Kagawa-Singer M, Blackhall LJ. Negotiating cross-cultural issues at the end of life: "You got to go where he lives." JAMA 2001; 286:2993–3001.
99. Ersek M, Kagawa-Singer M, Barnes D, Blackhall L, Koenig BA. Multicultural considerations in the use of advance directives. Oncol Nurs Forum 1998;25:1683–1690.
100. Hepburn K, Reed R. Ethical and clinical issues with Native-American elders: End-of-life decision making Clin Geriatr Med. 1995;11:97–111.
101. Hall BA. The struggle of the diagnosed terminally ill person to maintain hope. Nurs Sci Q 1990;3:177–184.
102. Herth K. Enhancing hope in people with a first recurrence of cancer. J Adv Nurs 2000;32:1431–1441.
103. Snyder CR, Rand KL, King EA, Feldman DB, Woodward JT. "False" hope. J Clin Psychol 2002;58:1003–1022.
104. Taylor SE, Armor DA. Positive illusions and coping with adversity. J Pers 1996;64:873–898.
105. Taylor SE. Adjustment to threatening events: A theory of cognitive adaptation. Am Psychol 1983;38:1164–1171.
106. Taylor SE, Lichtman RR, Wood JV. Attributions, beliefs about cancer, and adjustment to breast cancer. J Pers Soc Psychol 1984;46:489–502.
107. Taylor SE. Positive Illusions: Creative Self-Deception and the Healthy Mind. New York: Basic Books, 1989.
108. Taylor SE, Lerner JS, Sherman DK, Sage RM, McDowell NK. Are self-enhancing cognitions associated with healthy or unhealthy biological profiles? J Pers Soc Psychol 2003;85:605–615.
109. Taylor SE, Brown JD. Illusion and well-being: A social psychological perspective on mental health. Psychol Bull 1988;103:193–210.

110. Taylor SE, Brown JD. Positive illusions and well-being revisited: Separating fact from fiction. Psychol Bull 1994;116:21–27.
111. Taylor SE. Positive and negative beliefs and the course of AIDS: Taylor et al. (2000). Adv Mind Body Med 2001;17:47–49.
112. Stoner M. Measuring hope. In: Frank-Stromborg M, Olsen S, eds. Instruments for Clinical Health-Care Research, 3rd ed. Boston: Jones and Bartlett, 2004:215–228.
113. Miller JF. Developing and maintaining hope in families of the critically ill. AACN Clin Issues Crit Care Nurs 1991;2:307–315.
114. Herth K. Engendering hope in the chronically and terminally ill: Nursing interventions. Am J Hosp Palliat Care 1995;12:31–39.
115. Cutliffe JR. Hope, counselling and complicated bereavement reactions. J Adv Nurs 1998;28:754–761.
116. Cousins N. Head First: The Biology of Hope and the Healing Power of the Human Spirit. New York: Peguin, 1989.
117. Taylor SE, Lobel M. Social comparison under threat: Downward comparisons and upward contacts. Psychol Rev 1989;96:569–575.
118. Miller JF. Coping with Chronic Illness: Overcoming Powerlessness, 2 ed. Philadelphia: FA Davis, 1992.
119. Hinds PS, Gattuso JS, Barnwell E, Cofer M, Kellum LK, Mattox S, Norman G, Powell B, Randall E, Sanders C. Translating psychosocial research findings into practice guidelines. J Nurs Adm 2003;33:397–403.
120. Cutliffe JR. How do nurses inspire and instill hope in terminally ill HIV patients? J Adv Nurs 1995;22:888–895.
121. Minkoff K, Bergman E, Beck AT, Beck R. Hopelessness, depression, and attempted suicide. Am J Psychiatry 1973;130:455–459.
122. Beck AT, Weissman A, Lester D, Trexler L. The measurement of pessimism: The hopelessness scale. J Consult Clin Psychol 1974; 42:861–865.
123. Herth K. Relationship of hope, coping styles, concurrent losses, and setting to grief resolution in the elderly widow(er). Res Nurs Health 1990;13:109–117.
124. Herth K. Abbreviated instrument to measure hope: Development and psychometric evaluation. J Adv Nurs 1992;17:1251–1259.
125. Hinds PS, Gattuso JS. Measuring hopefulness in adolescents. J Pediatr Oncol Nurs 1991;8:92–94.
126. Hinds PS, Stoker HW. Adolescents' preferences for a scaling format: A validity issue. J Pediatr Nurs 1988;3:408–411.
127. Miller JF. Development of an instrument to measure hope. Dissertation Abstracts International, 47,1B. (University Microforms No. 8705572.), 1986.
128. Miller JF, Powers MJ. Development of an instrument to measure hope. Nurs Res 1988;37:6–10.
129. Snyder CR, Harris C, Anderson JR, Holleran SA, Irving LM, Sigmon ST, Yoshinobu L, Gibb J, Langelle C, Harney P. The will and the ways: Development and validation of an individual-differences measure of hope. J Pers Soc Psychol 1991;60:570–585.
130. Snyder CR, Hoza B, Pelham WE, Rapoff M, Ware L, Danovsky M, Highberger L, Rubinstein H, Stahl KJ. The development and validation of the Children's Hope Scale. J Pediatr Psychol 1997; 22:399–421.
131. Farran CJ, Wilken C, Popovich JM. Clinical assessment of hope. Issues Ment Health Nurs 1992;13:129–138.

27 Bereavement

Inge B. Corless

What is it like to know you are dying? I will tell you. I just want to go—just to go out in a flash like a light. This knowing that the end is coming and of all I will leave behind is killing me. How do you say goodbye, let go?—A patient

- ***Key Points***
- *Bereavement is the state of having lost a significant other.*
- *Loss is a generic term indicating the absence of a current or future possession or relationship.*
- *Grief is the emotional response to loss.*
- *Mourning encompasses the death rituals engaged in by the bereaved.*

On June 9, 2004, a faculty member died after a valiant battle to live. She had been afflicted with a type of cancer for which she received a bone marrow transplant. The transplant failed, and this gifted academician died leaving a bereft husband and five children, three of whom were triplets. On the same day, a young girl died. She was the daughter of a faculty member at the same academic program. The faculty member chose not to divulge the slow decline of her lovely 19-year-old daughter, thereby encapsulating the group to which she needed to reveal her sad news. The faculty was devastated to have encountered death in the first person among their ranks, wanting to offer support and condolences to the immediate family—which they did—and also confronting their own grief. Faculty members walked around their school in a daze grieving for their losses. They were the walking wounded.

Bereavement takes many forms. It is influenced first and foremost by culture. In Victorian times, bereaved women in the northeastern United States wore black for a year and used black-edged stationery, while men wore a black armband for a matter of days before resuming their regular activities. Bereavement is also influenced by religious practice, the nature of the relationship with the deceased, the age of the deceased, and the manner of death. In this chapter, the impacts of social and cultural forces on the form of bereavement are examined.

Changes have occurred in what is considered appropriate to the expression of grief. The wearing of black by a widow ("widow's weeds") for the remainder of her life and the presumption that grief will be "resolved" within a year are no longer societal expectations. There are other expectations, however, that color the expressions of bereavement, loss, mourning, and grief. Given that greater emphasis is given to the discussion of bereavement and grief, it behooves us to define these terms and examine their related elements.

A Matter of Definition

Bereavement

With the pronouncement of death, those who have the closest blood or legal connections to the deceased are considered bereaved. Stated simply, "bereavement is defined as the state of having experienced the death of a significant other."[1] Bereavement confers a special status on the individual, entailing both obligations and special rights. The obligations concern disposition of the body and any attendant ceremonies, as well as disposal of the worldly goods of the deceased, unless indicated otherwise in a legal document such as a last will and testament. The rights include dispensation from worldly activities such as work and, to a lesser degree, family roles for a variable period of time. Before an expanded discussion of bereavement is undertaken, it is important to distinguish the concept of bereavement from related terms as loss, mourning, and grief.

Loss

Loss is a generic term that signifies absence of an object, position, ability, or attribute. More recently it also has been applied to the death of an animal or person. Absence or loss of the same phenomenon has different implications, depending on the strength of the relationship to the owner. For example, loss of a dog with which there was an indifferent relationship results in less emotional disruption for the owner than the loss of a dog that was cherished. The term is often applied to the death of an individual, and it is the bereaved person who is considered to have experienced a loss. Robinson and McKenna[2] noted three critical attributes of loss:

1. Loss signifies that someone or something one has had, or ought to have had in the future, has been taken away.
2. That which is taken away must have been valued by the person experiencing the loss.
3. The meaning of loss is determined individually, subjectively, and contextually by the person experiencing it.

As is evident from the example of the loss of a dog, the individual determination of meaning indicates that the second attribute suggested by Robinson and McKenna, namely that what was lost was valued, is not necessarily congruent with the third attribute, which indicates individual evaluation, and is in fact superfluous. A loss occurs and its meaning is determined by the person who sustained the loss. The attributes of loss can be reformulated as follows:

1. Loss signifies the absence of a possession or future possession.
2. Each loss is valued differently and ranges from no or little value to great value.
3. The meaning of the loss is determined primarily by the individual sustaining it.

This suggests that it is wiser not to make assumptions about loss but to query further as to its meaning to the individual.

Mourning

Mourning has been described in various ways. Kagawa-Singer[3] described mourning as "the social customs and cultural practices that follow a death." This definition highlights the external manifestations of the process of separation from the deceased and the ultimate reintegration of the bereaved into the family and, to varying degrees, society. Durkheim,[4] one of the founders of sociology, stated that "mourning is not a natural movement of private feelings wounded by a cruel loss; it is a duty imposed by the group" (p. 443). This duty is participation in the customary rituals appropriate to membership in a given group. Participation in such rituals has meaning for the mourner and group.[5] These rituals and behaviors acknowledge that a loss has occurred for the individual and the group, and that the individual and the group are adjusting their relationships so as to move forward without the presence of the deceased individual.

DeSpelder and Strickland[6] highlighted two important aspects of mourning. They stated that mourning is "the process of incorporating the experience of loss into our ongoing lives" and also "the outward acknowledgment of loss" (p. 207). That outward acknowledgment consists of participation in various death and bereavement rituals. As noted, these vary by religious and cultural traditions as well as by personal preferences. Martinson[7] described the variation in practices in eastern Asia due to the influences of folk practices, Confucianism, Buddhism, and Christianity.

Whereas ancestor worship is important to varying degrees in Asia, Latin cultures believe in "the interdependence between life and death," a belief that reflects "the value that is placed on the continuity of relationships between the living and the dead.[8] This relationship is considered sacred and is expressed openly in some of the ritual practices dedicated to the dead."[8,9] These practices have many functions, including signifying respect for the deceased and providing a mechanism for the expression of feelings by the bereaved.

Grief

Grief has been defined as "a person's emotional response to the event of loss,"[5] as the "state of mental and physical pain that is experienced when the loss of a significant object, person, or part of the self is realized,"[6] and as "the highly personal and subjective set of responses that an individual makes to a real, perceived, or anticipated loss."[10] There are numerous definitions of grief, and these are only illustrative of variations on a theme. The process of grief has been studied and reformulated, phases identified, types proposed (anticipatory, complicated, disenfranchised), and expressions of grief described.

Given that nurses work largely with individuals and families but in some cases also with communities, several sections of this chapter focus on grief as it relates to these different entities. However, even in those sections that putatively deal with associated topics, the subject of grief is related and may be interwoven. With these preliminary definitions as a basis, bereavement, grief, and mourning can now be addressed in greater depth.

The Process of Bereavement

The process and meaning of bereavement vary depending on a number of factors, including age, gender, ethnicity, cultural background, education, and socioeconomic status. For African American widows, story-telling was the means by which the bereavement experience was described.[11] The themes identified in a study of these widows included awareness of death, caregiving, getting through, moving on, changing feelings, and financial security. These themes describe well the concerns of bereavement.

To measure core bereavement phenomena, Burnett and colleagues[12] identified 17 items that they considered central to the process of bereavement. They categorized these items under three subscales, namely images and thoughts (e.g., "Do you think about 'X'?"), acute separation (e.g., "Do you find yourself missing 'X'?"), and grief (e.g., "Do reminders of 'X,' such as photos, situations, music, or places, cause you to cry about 'X'?").[12] Although the purpose of this scale is to "assess the intensities of the bereavement reaction in different community samples of bereaved subjects," the bereavement reaction that is being addressed is grief.

The distinction between grief and depression in the bereaved is an important one. As Middleton and associates[13] concluded, "The bereaved can experience considerable pain and yet be coping adaptively, and they can fulfill many depressive criteria yet at the same time be experiencing phenomena that are not depressive in nature." Even in individuals with a history of "sadness or irritability" before bereavement, although they may have more intense expressions of grief, the rate of recovery is the same as for those without such a history.[14] Other authors are not as sanguine and caution that subsyndromal symptomatic depressions are "frequently seen complications of bereavement that may be chronic and often are associated with substantial morbidity."[15] Nortriptyline and psychotherapy have been found efficacious in the treatment of bereavement-related major depressive episodes.[16]

Boelen and coworkers[17] pointed out that traumatic grief is distinct from bereavement-related depression and anxiety. Identifying these differences clinically is essential for appropriate treatment. A Bereavement Risk Questionnaire with 19 possible factors for identifying complicated bereavement was distributed to 508 hospice bereavement coordinators. Of these, 262 (52%) responded. Significant risk factors for caregivers included lack of social support, caregiver history of drug or alcohol abuse, poor coping skills, history of mental illness, and "patient is a child."[18]

Bereavement-related grief was conceptualized by Rubin and Schecter[19] into two pathways: "a dimension concerned with how the bereaved individual functions following loss" and "a dimension concerned with the nature of that individual's relational bond to the deceased." They observed further that loss involves disruption of multiple spheres of the individual's life. The two-track model of bereavement was developed as a means of understanding and addressing the bereavement process and its outcome: "Track I focuses on the physiological, somatic, affective, cognitive, social and behavioral factors that are affected by loss—and Track II examines ways of transforming the bereaved's attachment to the deceased and establishing new forms of ongoing relationship to the memories of that person."[19,20] In essence, bereavement involves adjusting to a world without the physical, psychological, and social presence of the deceased.

Although Bernard and Guarnaccia[21] found differences between husbands and daughters of breast cancer patients, ultimately the family role relationship affected bereavement adjustment. The quality of the family relationship, with greater expression of family affect and cohesion, was found to be predictive of the expression of fewer grief symptoms over time.[22]

Bereavement becomes complicated (in the literature and in life) when adjustment is impeded, as in posttraumatic stress disorder.[23] Whether such bereavement occurs as a result of vehicular accident, war, or natural disaster, the suddenness or overwhelming nature of the event dislodges the sense that all is well with the world. Even in instances in which an elective medical procedure such as abortion occurs, the emotional response may not become evident until many years later.

Death before its time, as in children and young and middle-aged adults, not only affects the bereaved directly but also affects the social roles of the survivors, which require readjustment. The idea that parental outcomes are worse when a child's death is by suicide was not confirmed empirically.[24] Another myth is that divorce is more common among bereaved couples than in the general population. The empirical evidence is insufficient either to substantiate or disconfirm this myth.[24]

Hutton and Bradley,[25] in their study of the bereaved siblings of babies who were casualties of sudden infant death, were uncertain as to whether these siblings actually exhibited more behavioral problems or were thought to be doing so by mothers whose perceptions were distorted. The need for greater attention to children who are bereaved was underscored by Mahon,[26] who observed that most of the literature in this area concerns "parental impressions of children's grief and studies of adolescent bereavement." The hesitancy of children to exhibit their own sadness so as not to upset their parents requires that professionals encourage parents to give their children permission to be sad when that is how they feel. By taking care of their parents, children may not receive the attention they require. In a study that sought to identify those factors that helped or hindered adolescent sibling bereavement, a youngster stated: "What helped me the most was my mother who was totally honest with me from the time Sarah got sick through her death. My mother took the time to listen to how I felt as well as understand and hug me."[27]

Formal programs of bereavement for children's support include peer support programs and art therapy programs. Institutions with bereavement programs, whether for children or adults, often send cards at the time of a patient's death, on the birthday of the deceased, and at 3, 6, 12, and 24 months after the death.[28] Pamphlets with information about grief, a bibliography of appropriate readings, and contact numbers of support groups are also helpful.[28] Lev and McCorkle[29] cited Potocky's[30] finding that short-term programs of two to seven sessions or meeting as needed were the most effective. Maddocks[31] observed that routine bereavement care can be helpful in identifying people at risk for complicated grieving. Family bereavement programs also have been found to lead to improved parenting, coping, and caregiver mental health.[32] Given that the best therapy is prevention, palliative care teams who identify caregivers at risk for bereavement maladjustment can intervene early to prevent long term difficulties.[33]

Attention to bereavement support has also been given by institutional trauma programs, in emergency departments, and in critical care departments.[1,34–36] All of these programs maintain contact with the bereaved so as to provide support and make referrals to pastoral care personnel and other professionals as needed. Indeed, the combination of "religious psychotherapy" and a cognitive-behavioral approach was observed to be helpful to highly religious bereaved persons.[37] Religious psychotherapy for a group of Malays who adhered to the religion of Islam consisted of discussion and reading of verses of the Koran and Hadith, the encouragement of prayers, and a total of 12 to 16 psychotherapy sessions.[37] Targeting of the follow-up approach to the characteristics of the population eschews the notion that "one size fits all."

A bereavement support group intervention was demonstrated to have a significant impact on the grief of homosexual men who were or were not seropositive for the human immunodeficiency virus (HIV-1).[38] The need for support was found to be all the more necessary for bereaved women living with HIV, who "may be at increased risk for bereavement complicated with psychiatric morbidity and thoughts of suicide" (Summers et al., p.225).[39,40] Cognitive processing and finding meaning were found to have immunologic and health benefits independent of the baseline health status of bereaved HIV-positive homosexual men.[41] This outcome has implications for the approaches nurses use with other bereaved clients.

Cognitive processing and finding meaning can be helpful to a variety of clients. However, older persons have been noted to be more reluctant to express their feelings.[42] Nurses can be helpful to these clients by encouraging them to express their feelings and being available when needed.

Aside from such proactive approaches for all bereaved persons, Sheldon[43] reported the following predisposing factors for a poor bereavement outcome: ambivalent or dependent relationship; multiple prior bereavements; previous mental illness, especially depression; and low self-esteem. Billings[44] added prior physical health problems to these predisposing factors. Sheldon[43] identified the following factors at the time of death: sudden and unexpected death, untimely death of a young person, preparation for the death, stigmatized deaths (e.g., AIDS, suicide, culpable death), sex of the bereaved person (e.g., elderly male widower), caring for the deceased person for >6 months, and inability to carry out valued religious rituals. The impact of trauma characterized by violence on bereavement was found by Kaltman and Bonanno to lead to posttraumatic stress disorder symptoms beyond those of normal grief.[45]

Finally, after the death, such factors as level of perceived social support, lack of opportunities for new interests, and stress from other life crises, as well as dysfunctional behaviors and attitudes appearing early in the bereavement period, consumption of alcohol and drugs, smoking, morbid guilt, and the professional caregiver's gut feeling that this patient will not do well are predictive of poor outcomes.[43,44] Knowledge of and alertness to such predisposing factors are useful for the provision of help, both lay and professional, early in the course of the bereavement so as to prevent further debilitating events.

The Nature of Grief

Rando[46] observed that, although Freud was not the first person to examine the effects of bereavement, he nonetheless is taken as an important point of departure. The observation that grief is a normal process and that "a lost love object is never totally relinquished" are congruent with current thinking.[46] The notion that one needs to totally "let go" of the beloved, ascribed to Freud on the basis of some of his work, has influenced professionals to the current day.

The initiation of the modern study of death and dying, however, especially in America, is often attributed to Erich Lindemann, a physician at Massachusetts General Hospital, who responded to the survivors of a fire in Boston's Coconut Grove nightclub. Five hundred persons died as a result of the fire, which took place on Thanksgiving eve, 1942. Lindemann, a psychiatrist, was interested at the time in the emotional reaction of patients to body disfigurement and plastic surgery.[47] With this background, "Lindemann was struck by the similarity of responses between his patients' reactions to facial disfigurement or loss of a body part and the reactions of the survivors of the fire" (p. 105).[47]

Lindemann's study of 101 patients included (1) psychoneurotic patients who lost a relative during the course of treatment, (2) relatives of patients who died in the hospital, (3) bereaved disaster victims (Coconut Grove fire) and their close relatives, and (4) relatives of members of the armed forces.[48] Based on these patients, he determined the five indicators that are "pathognomonic for grief"[48]: (1) sensations of somatic distress, such as tightness in the throat, choking and shortness of breath; (2) intense preoccupation with the image of the deceased; (3) strong feelings of guilt; (4) a loss of warmth toward others with a tendency to respond with irritability and anger; and (5) disoriented behavior patterns.

Lindemann coined the term "grief work" to describe the process by which individuals attempt to adjust to their loss.[47]

Various theorists have developed a series of stages and phases of grief work.[49–52] The best known of these to the general public are the stages formulated by Elizabeth Kübler-Ross. Proposed for those facing a death, these stages have also been applied to those experiencing a loss. Kübler-Ross[53] identified five stages: denial and isolation, anger, bargaining, depression, and acceptance. The commonality among all theorists of the stages of grief is that the individual moves through (1) notification and shock, (2) experience of the loss emotionally and cognitively, and (3) reintegration. Rando,[54] for example, used the terms avoidance, confrontation, and reestablishment for these three phases. Building on the work of Worden,[55] Corr and Doka[56] propose the following tasks:

1. To share acknowledgment of the reality of death
2. To share in the process of working through to the pain of grief
3. To reorganize the family system
4. To restructure the family's relationship with the deceased and to reinvest in other relationships and life pursuits

In regard to the last task, some dispute has arisen concerning the degree to which separation from the deceased must occur. Klass and associates[57] made the compelling argument that such bonds continue. They advocated that "survivors hold the deceased in loving memory for long periods, often forever," and that maintaining an inner representation of the deceased is normal rather than abnormal. Winston's study of African-American grandmothers demonstrated that they maintained strong bonds with the deceased.[58]

The second area of dissension and new consensus is the expectation that grief must be resolved within a year, which is not to say that the expected trajectory of grieving is one in which grief continues at an intense pitch for years. The question of continuing bonds and the length of the grief process are addressed again at the close of the chapter. In this next section, types of grief are examined.

Types of Grief

The types of grief examined in this section are not exhaustive of all types of grief but rather encompass the major categories.

Anticipatory Grief

Anticipatory grief shares similarities with other forms of grief. It is also different. The onset may be associated with the receipt of bad news.[5] Anticipatory grief must be distinguished from the concept of forewarning. An example of forewarning is learning of a terminal diagnosis. Anticipatory grief is an unconscious process, whereas forewarning is a conscious process. With forewarning of a terminal diagnosis the question is, "What if we do?" With a death that question becomes, "What if we had done?" With the former question, there is the potential for hope; with the latter query, there may be guilt.

Stephenson[5] described a roller-coaster experience of hope followed by negative experience countered by hope. Even with forewarning, preparation for loss may not occur, given that this may be perceived to be a betrayal of the terminally ill person. There have also been instances of family members unconsciously preparing for the death of an individual and going through the grieving process, only to have that person recover to find no place in the lives of his or her loved ones. This is an example of anticipatory grief.

The question of the utility of forewarning is one of how this time is used. If it is used to make some preparation for role change, such as becoming familiar with the intricacies of the role the terminally ill person plays in the family (e.g., mastering a checking account or other financial aspects of the family), such time may be used to the benefit of all concerned. On the other hand, anticipatory grieving that results in reinvestment of emotional energy before the death of the terminally ill person is detrimental to the relationship.

Byrne and Raphael[59] found that "widowers who were unable to anticipate their wife's death, even when their wife had suffered a long final illness, had a more severe bereavement reaction." (The term "anticipate" is being used by Byrne and Raphael in the sense of forewarning.) Family members and friends are "warned" when their loved one is diagnosed with certain disease entities such as cancer with metastases. If the primary problem is Alzheimer's disease, there may be a long decline in which, ultimately, familiar figures are no longer recognized. In either situation, the death of the ill person may be experienced both with sadness and with a sense of relief that the caregiving burden is no more. The price of that relief is that the patient is no more.

The sense of relief experienced by caregivers is often a source of guilt feelings about wishing the patient dead. It is important to clarify for the family member or significant other that feelings of relief from being freed of the caregiver burden are not equivalent to wishing someone dead. A woman who experienced relief from not having to care for her large husband was assisted to examine this distinction and consequentially was able to grieve uncomplicated by feelings of guilt. Further, persons who have cared for a dying person may experience a sense of accomplishment knowing that they have done everything they could for their loved one.[60] Schultz and associates[61] pointed out that bereavement is "not only a phenomenon that affects caregivers after the death but also . . . one that affects many caregivers before the death occurs" (p. 8).

Duke,[62] in a qualitative study of anticipatory grief, enlarged the understanding not so much of anticipatory grief but of the status changes of widowhood. She interviewed five spouses in the second year of their bereavement. Although the findings may have been biased by the distortion of hindsight, they provide much food for thought. The research identified four areas of change[62]: role change from spouse to caregiver during the illness, followed by loss of those roles in bereavement and needing to be cared for; relationship changes from being with spouse to being alone; coping changes from being in suspense to being in turmoil; and the change from experiencing and gathering memories to remembering and constructing memories. It is interesting that these findings reflect the general changes that occur over a terminal illness and not the experience of anticipatory grief. Anticipatory grief, as noted previously, is unconscious preparation for status change and not a conscious, deliberative process. Anticipatory grief is contrasted with what is termed uncomplicated grief.

Uncomplicated Grief

Uncomplicated grief, or normal grief, was described by Cowles[63] as dynamic, pervasive, highly individualized, and a process. Worthington[64] depicted a linear model of grief based on adjustment. In this model, an individual in a normal emotional state experiences a loss that causes a reaction and an emotional low; subsequently, the individual begins a recovery to his or her former state. This process of recovery is occasioned by brief periods of relapse, but not to the depths experienced previously. Ultimately the individual moves to adjustment to the loss. Although this description simplifies the turmoil that may be experienced, discussion of expressions of grief later in this chapter capture the physical, psychological, behavioral, and social upset that characterizes even uncomplicated grief.

Niemeyer[65] offered a vital new perspective by focusing on meaning reconstruction. He developed a set of propositions to capture adaptation to loss:

1. Death as an event can validate or invalidate the constructions that form the basis on which we live, or it may stand as a novel experience for which we have no constructions.
2. Grief is a personal process, one that is idiosyncratic, intimate, and inextricable from our sense of who we are.
3. Grieving is something we do, not something that is done to us.
4. Grieving is the act of affirming or reconstructing a personal world of meaning that has been challenged by loss.
5. Feelings have functions and should be understood as signals of the state of our meaning-making efforts.
6. We construct and reconstruct our identities as survivors of loss in negotiations with others.

Niemeyer[65] viewed meaning reconstruction as the central process of grief. The inability to make meaning may lead to complications.

Complicated Grief

In her discussion of complicated mourning, Rando[46] made observations applicable to complicated grief. She observed that, after a suitable length of time, the mourner is attempting to "deny, repress, or avoid aspects of the loss, its pain, and its implications and . . . to hold onto, and avoid relinquishing, the lost loved one." These attempts, or some variants thereof, cause the complications in mourning."

Researchers have identified the diagnostic criteria for complicated grief disorder.[66] These criteria include "the current experience (>1 year after a loss) of intensive intrusive thoughts, pangs of severe emotion, distressing yearnings, feeling excessively alone and empty, excessively avoiding tasks reminiscent of the deceased, unusual sleep disturbances, and maladaptive levels of loss of interest in personal activities." Other researchers have underscored the need for the specification of complicated grief as a unique disorder and have developed an inventory of complicated grief to measure maladaptive symptoms of loss.[67–69] The Inventory of Complicated Grief is composed of 19 items with responses ranging from "Never" to "Rarely," "Sometimes," Often," and "Always." Examples of items include, "I think about this person so much that it's hard for me to do the things I usually do"; "Ever since she (or he) died it is hard for me to trust people"; "I feel that it is unfair that I should live when this person died"; and "I feel lonely a great deal of the time ever since she (or he) died."[69] This inventory may be helpful to health care practitioners because it differentiates between complicated grief and depression.[70] Finally, it is the severity of symptomatology and the duration that distinguishes abnormal and complicated responses to bereavement.[71]

The Inventory of Complicated Grief was used by Ott with 112 bereaved participants in a study in which those identified as experiencing complicated grief were compared with those who were not.[72] Those with complicated grief both identified more additional life stressors and felt they had less social support than the other bereaved individuals in the study.

It should be noted that there is some concern among professionals that what is a normal process is being medicalized by health care practitioners. Complicated grief, however, may require professional intervention.[72] More is said about this later in the chapter. Bearing this in mind, disenfranchised grief poses different but potentially related problems.

Disenfranchised Grief

Doka[73] defined disenfranchised grief as "the grief that persons experience when they incur a loss that is not or cannot be openly acknowledged, publicly mourned, or socially supported." Doka continued, "The concept of disenfranchised grief recognizes that societies have sets of norms—in effect, grieving rules—that attempt to specify who, when, where, how, how long, and for whom people should grieve" (p. 272).[73] In addition, these norms suggest who may grieve publicly and expect to receive support.

Those who are grieving the loss of relationships that may not be publicly acknowledged—for example, with a mistress or with a family conceived outside a legally recognized union, or in some cases with stepfamilies, colleagues, or friends—are not accorded the deference and support usually afforded the bereaved. Further nonsanctioned relationships, either heterosexual or homosexual, may result in the exclusion of individuals not legitimated by blood or legal union. Individuals in homosexual relationships of long standing who care for their partners throughout their last illness, may find themselves barred both from the funeral and from the home that was shared.[74]

For some time, infection with HIV was hidden from the community, thereby depriving both the infected and their caregivers of support. The AIDS quilt has done much to provide a public mourning ritual but has not alleviated the disenfranchised status of homosexual or lesbian partners. The result is what has been termed "modulated mourning."[74] This response to stigmatization constrains the public display of mourning by the griever. In this situation, the griever is not recognized.

There are other instances in which a loss has not been legitimized. Loss resulting from miscarriage or abortion has only recently been recognized. In Japan, a "cemetery" is devoted to letters written by families each year telling miscarried or aborted children about the important events that occurred in the family that year and also expressing continued grief at their loss. Grieving in secret is a burden that makes the process more difficult to complete. Disenfranchised grief may also be a harbinger of unresolved grief.

Unresolved Grief

Unresolved grief is a failure to accomplish the necessary grief work. According to Rando,[54] a variety of factors may give rise to unresolved grief, including guilt, loss of an extension of the self, reawakening of an old loss, multiple loss, inadequate ego development, and idiosyncratic resistance to mourning (pp. 64–65). In addition to these psychological factors, such social factors as social negation of a loss, socially unspeakable loss, social isolation and/or geographic distance from social support, assumption of the role of the strong one, and uncertainty over the loss (e.g., a disappearance at sea) may be implicated in unresolved grief (pp. 66–67). By helping significant others express their feelings and complete their business before the death of a loved one, unresolved grief and the accompanying manifestations can be prevented to some extent.

Eakes and coworkers[75] questioned whether closure is a necessary outcome. They explored the concept of "chronic sorrow" in bereaved individuals who experienced episodic bouts of sadness related to specific incidents or significant dates. These authors suggested the fruitfulness of maintaining an open-ended model of grief. With this in mind, grief is always unresolved to some degree; this is not considered pathological but rather an acknowledgment of a death.

Expressions of Grief

Symptoms of Grief

In some of the earlier sections of this chapter, various manifestations of grief were mentioned. In this section, expressions of grief that are within the range considered normal in this society are described. It is important to note that what is considered appropriate in one group may be considered deviant or even pathological in another.

In Table 27–1, physical, cognitive, emotional, and behavioral symptoms of grief are presented. Table 27–1 is not exhaustive of all of the potential symptoms but rather is illustrative of the expressions and manifestations of grief. What distinguishes so-called normal grief is that it is usually self-limited. Manifestations of grief at 1, 3, and 15 months after the death are not the same in intensity, nor are the outward manifestations that are the expressions of mourning.

Mourning

O'Gorman[76] contrasted death rituals in England with those in Ireland. She recalled the "Protestant hushed respectfulness which had somehow infiltrated and taken over a Catholic community."[76] The body was taken from the home by the funeral director. Children continued with school and stayed with relatives; they were shielded from the death. By way of contrast, in an Irish wake, "The body, laid out by a member of the family, in order to receive a 'special blessing,' would be in the parlour of a country house surrounded by flowers from the garden and lighted candles." The children, along with the adult members of the family, viewed the corpse. "When visitors had paid their last respects they would join the crowd in the kitchen who would then spend all night recounting stories associated with the dead person."[76] O'Gorman noted the plentiful availability of alcohol and stated, "By the end of the night to the uninitiated the event would appear to be more like a party than a melancholy event." Although O'Gorman initially found this distasteful, she "now believes that rituals like the Irish wake celebrate death as a happy occasion and bestow grace upon those leaving life and upon a community of those who mourn them."[76]

The Irish wake, like the reception held in a church basement, hall, restaurant, or private home, serves not only for the expression of condolences but also as an opportunity to reinforce the connections of the community. Anyone familiar with such events knows that a variety of social and business arrangements are made by mourners both within and outside the immediate family. And although some gatherings are more reserved and others lustier, giving the deceased a good send-off ("good" being defined by the group) is central to each. The good send-off is part of the function of the funeral as a piacular rite—that is, as a means of atoning for the sins of the mortal being and as preparation for life in the afterworld.[77] Fulton[77] noted two other functions of funerals, namely integration and separation. The former concerns the living; the latter refers to separation from the loved one as a mortal person. The value of the Irish wake, which in the United States may look more like the Protestant burial O'Gorman describes, is the time spent together sharing stories and feelings. In the Irish wake as practiced in Ireland, one is not alone with one's feelings but in the company of others who are devoting the time to mourning (integration).

Table 27–1
Manifestations of Grief

Physical	Cognitive	Emotional	Behavioral
Headaches	Sense of depersonalization	Anger	Impaired work performance
Dizziness	Inability to concentrate	Guilt	Crying
Exhaustion	Sense of disbelief and confusion	Anxiety	Withdrawal
Muscular aches	Idealization of the deceased	Sense of helplessness	Avoiding reminders of the deceased
Sexual impotency	Search for meaning of life and death	Sadness	Seeking or carrying reminders of the deceased
Loss of appetite	Dreams of the deceased	Shock	Overreactivity
Insomnia	Preoccupation with image of deceased	Yearning	Changed relationships
Feelings of tightness or hollowness	Fleeting visual, tactile, olfactory, auditory hallucinatory experiences	Numbness	
Breathlessness		Self-blame	
Tremors		Relief	
Shakes			
Oversensitivity to noise			

Source: Adapted from Doka, (1989), reference 10.

This devotion of time to mourning is also found in the Jewish religion, where the bereaved sit "shiva," usually for 7 days.[78] In Judaism, the assumption is that the bereaved are to focus on their loss and the grieving of that loss. They are to pay no attention to worldly considerations. This period of time of exemption from customary roles may facilitate the process. Certainly having a "minion," in which 10 men and women (10 men for Orthodox Jews) say prayers each evening, reinforces the reality of the death and the separation. For the Orthodox, the mourning period is 1 year.

A very different pattern is practiced by the Hopi in Arizona. The Hopi have a brief ceremony with the purpose of completing the funeral as quickly as possible so as to get back to customary activities.[78] The fear of death and the dead and of spirits induces distancing by the Hopi from nonliving phenomena.

Stroebe and Stroebe[78] contrasted Shinto and Buddhist mourners in Japan with the Hopi. Both Shinto and Buddhist mourners practice ancestor worship. As a result, the bereaved can keep contact with the deceased, who become ancestors. Speaking to ancestors as well as offering food is accepted practice.

In contrast to this Japanese practice, what occurs in the United States is that those bereaved who speak with a deceased person do so quietly, hiding the fact from others, believing others will consider it suspect or pathological. It is, however, a common occurrence. Bringing food to the ancestor or (e.g., to celebrate the Day of the Dead) to the cemetery, is part of the mourning practice in Hispanic and many other societies.

Practices, however, change with time, although one can often find the imprint of earlier rituals. The practice of saving a lock of hair or the footprint of a deceased newborn may have evolved from the practice in Victorian times of using hair for mourning brooches and lockets. As a salesperson of these items commented, "They liked to be reminded of their dead in those days. Now it's out of sight, out of mind."[79]

These mourning practices provide continuing bonds with the deceased and offer a clue to the answer to the question posed for the last section of this chapter: When is it over? Before addressing this question, another needs to be raised, and that is the question of support.

A Question of Support

Formal Support

Many of the mourning practices noted previously provide support by the community to the bereaved (Table 27–2). Formal support in the Jewish tradition is exemplified by the practice of attending a minion for the deceased person. The minion expresses support for the living. It is formal in that it is prescribed behavior on the part of observant Jews and incorporates a prayer service.

Other examples of formal support include support groups such as the widow-to-widow program and the Compassionate Friends, Inc. for families of deceased children. The assumption underlying the widow-to-widow program is that grief and mourning are not in and of themselves pathological and that lay persons can be helpful to one another. The widow-to-widow program provides a formal mechanism for sharing one's

Table 27–2
Bereavement Practices

Lay	Professional
1. Friendly visiting	1. Clergy visiting
2. Provision of meals	2. Clergy counseling
3. Informal support by previously bereaved	3. Nurse, M.D., psychologist, social worker, psychiatrist counseling
4. Lay support groups	4. Professionally led support groups
5. Participation in cultural and religious	5. Organization of memorial services by rituals hospice and palliative care organizations
6. A friendly listener	6. A thoughtful listener
7. Involvement in a cause-related group	7. Referral to individuals with similar cause-related concerns
8. Exercise	8. Referral to a health club
9. Joining a new group	9. Referral to a bereavement program

emotions and experience with individuals who have had a similar experience. The Widowed Persons Service offers support for men and women via self-help support groups and a variety of educational and social activities. The Compassionate Friends, Inc., also a self-help organization, seeks to help parents and siblings after the death of a child. Other support groups may or may not have the input of a professional to run the group.

Support groups may be open-ended (i.e., without a set number of sessions), or they may be closed and limited to a particular set of individuals. Support groups with a set number of sessions have a beginning and end and are therefore more likely to be closed to new members until a new set of sessions begins. Open-ended groups have members who stay for varying lengths of time and may or may not have a topic for each session.

Other formal support entails working with a therapist or other health care provider (bereavement counseling). Arnold[80] suggested that the nurse should follow a process to assess the meaning of loss, the nature of the relationship, expressions and manifestations of grief, previous experience with grief, support systems, ability to maintain attachments, and progression of grief. Further, Arnold underscored the importance of viewing grief as a healing process (Table 27–3). She gave the following example of a patient situation and two different approaches to diagnosis:[80]

> A newly widowed woman feels awkward about maintaining social relationships with a group of married couples with whom she had participated with her husband.
>
> - Grief as a pathological diagnosis: social isolation.
> - Grief as a healthy diagnosis: redefinition of social supports.

Table 27–3
Assessment of Grief

The bereaved often are weary from caring for the deceased. During this period they may not have looked after themselves. An assessment should include

1. A general health checkup and assessment of somatic symptoms
2. A dental visit
3. An eye checkup as appropriate
4. Nutritional evaluation
5. Sleep assessment
6. Examination of ability to maintain work and family roles
7. Determination of whether there are major changes in presentation of self
8. Assessment of changes resulting from the death and the difficulties with these changes
9. Assessment of social networks

The health care worker needs to bear in mind that there is no magic formula for grieving. The key question is whether the bereaved is able to function effectively. Cues to the need for assistance include

1. Clinical depression
2. Prolonged deep grief
3. Extreme grief reaction
4. Self-destructive behavior
5. Increased use of alcohol and/or drugs
6. Preoccupation with the deceased to the exclusion of others
7. Previous mental illness
8. Perceived lack of social support

In addition to conventional talking therapy, such techniques as letter writing, empty chair, guided imagery, and journal writing can be used (Table 27–4).[81] In letter writing, the empty chair technique, and guided imagery, the bereaved is encouraged to express feelings about the past or what life is like without the deceased. These techniques can be helpful as the "wish I had said" becomes said. A journal is also a vehicle for recording ongoing feelings of the lived experience of bereavement.

Another part of bereavement counseling is the instillation or reemergence of hope. As Cutcliffe[82] concluded, "There are many theories of bereavement counseling, with commonalities between these theories. Whilst the theories indicate implicitly the re-emergence of hope in the bereft individual as a result of the counseling, they do not make specific reference to how this inspiration occurs." Cutcliffe saw the clear need to understand this process.

In her exposition of the concept "hope," Stephenson[83] noted the association made by Frankl[84] between hope and meaning. Stephenson stated, "Frankl equated hope with having found meaning in life, and lack of hope as [having] no meaning in life."[83] Meaning-making appears key to the emergence of hope, and hope has been associated with coping.[85]

In hospice programs, health care providers encourage dying persons and their families to have hope for each day. This compression of one's vision to the here and now may also be useful for the person who is grieving the loss of a loved one. Hope for the future and a personal future is the process that Cutcliffe[82] wished to elucidate. It may be a process that is predicated on hope for each day and having found meaning for the past. Sikkema and colleagues[40] compared the effectiveness of individual and group approaches by evaluating individual psychotherapy and psychiatric services on demand with a support group format. The strategies employed in dealing with grief included establishing a sense of control and predictability, anger expression and management, resolution of guilt, promotion of self-mastery through empowerment, and development of new relationships. Those assigned to individual therapy may or may not have taken advantage of the option. Future research should examine three groups: those receiving individual counseling, those receiving group therapy, and those assigned no specific intervention but given information about various options for counseling and support in a pamphlet.

A therapist provides a vehicle for ongoing discussion of the loss that informal caregivers may be unable to provide. A support group of bereaved individuals or periodic contact by an institutional bereavement service may also prove useful. What is helpful depends on the individual and his or her needs and also on the informal support that is available.

Informal Support

Informal support that is perceived as supportive and helpful can assist the bereaved to come to terms with life after the death of the beloved. Whether the bereaved is isolated or is part of a family or social group is of tremendous import to the physical, psychological, and social welfare of the individual. Community in a psychosocial sense and a continuing role in the group are key factors in adjustment.

In societies where the widow has no role without her husband, she is figuratively if not literally disposed of in one way or another. It is for this reason that the woman who is the first in her group to experience widowhood has a much more difficult social experience than a woman who is in a social group where several women have become widows. In the former there is no reference group; in the latter there is.

The presence of family and friends takes on added significance after the initial weeks after the funeral. In those initial weeks, friendly visiting occurs with provision of a variety of types of foods considered appropriate in the group. After the initial period, friendly visiting is likely to decrease, and the bereaved individuals may find themselves alone or the objects of financial predators. The counsel by the health care provider or by family and friends, not to make life-altering decisions (e.g., moving) at this time unless absolutely necessary, continues to be valuable advice. On the other hand, the comment that "time makes it easier" is a half-truth that is not perceived as helpful by the bereaved.[86,87]

What is helpful is being listened to by an interested person. Quinton[87] disliked the term "counseling" in that is implies the availability of a person with good counsel to confer. What Quinton considered important was "lots of listening to what the victim wants to off-load." She observed, "The turning point for me was realizing that I had a right to feel sad, and to grieve and to feel miserable for as long as I felt the need."[87] By owning the grieving process, Quinton provided herself with the most important support for her recovery from a devastating experience—her mother's murder in a massacre by the Irish Republican Army in 1987. The lesson is applicable, however, to any bereaved person regardless of whether the death was traumatic or anticipated. Quinton's turning point is another clue to answering the question of the last section of this chapter: When is it over?

When Is It Over?

To use the colloquial phrase, it's not over until it's over. What does this mean? As long as life and memory persist, the deceased individual remains part of the consciousness of family and friends. When is the grieving over? Unfortunately, there is no easy answer and the only reasonable response, is "It depends." Lindemann's concept of grief work,[47,48] mentioned earlier in this chapter, is applicable. Sooner or later that work needs to be accomplished. Delay protracts the time when accommodation is made. And grief work is never over, in the sense that there will be moments in years to come when an occasion or an object revives feelings of loss. The difference is that the pain is not the same acute pain as that experienced when the loss initially occurred. How one

Table 27–4
Counseling Interventions

It must be emphasized that grief is not a pathology. It is a normal process that is expressed in individual ways. The following techniques may prove helpful to the individual who is experiencing guilt about things not said or done. This list is not exhaustive, merely illustrative.

1. Letter writing	The bereaved writes a letter to the deceased expressing the thoughts and feelings that may or may not have been expressed.
2. Empty chair	The bereaved sits across from an empty chair on which the deceased is imagined to be sitting. The bereaved is encouraged to express his or her feelings.
3. Empty chair with picture	A picture of the deceased is placed on the chair to facilitate the expressions of feelings by the bereaved.
4. Therapist assumes role of the deceased	In this intervention, the therapist helps the bereaved to explore his or her feelings toward the deceased by participating in a role play.
5. Guided imagery	This intervention demands a higher level of skill than, for example, letter writing. Guided imagery can be used to explore situations that require verbalization by the bereaved to achieve completion. Imagery can also be used to recreate situations of dissension with the goal of achieving greater understanding for the bereaved.
6. Journal writing	This technique provides an ongoing vehicle for exploring past situations and current feelings. It is a helpful intervention to many.
7. Drawing pictures	For the artistically and not so artistically inclined, drawing pictures and explaining their content is another vehicle for discussing feelings and concerns.
8. Analysis of role changes	Helping the bereaved obtain help with the changes secondary to the death, such as with balancing a checkbook or securing reliable help with various home needs; assists with some of the secondary losses with the death of a loved one.
9. Listening	The bereaved has the need to tell his or her story. Respectful listening and concern for the bereaved is a powerful intervention that is much appreciated.
10. Venting anger	The professional can suggest the following: • Banging a pillow on the mattress. If combined with screaming, it is the best to do with the windows closed and no one in the home. • Screaming—at home or parked in a car in an isolated spot with the windows closed. • Crying—at home, followed by a warm bath and cup of tea or warm milk.
11. Normality barometer	Assuring the bereaved that the distress experienced is normal is very helpful to the bereaved.

arrives at the point of accommodation is a process termed "letting go."

Letting Go

The term "letting go" refers to acknowledgment of the loss of future togetherness—physical, psychological, and social. There is no longer a "we," only an "I" or a "we" without the deceased. Family members speak of events such as the first time a flower or bush blooms, major holidays, birthdays, anniversaries, and special shared times. Corless[88] quoted Jacqueline Kennedy, who spoke about "last year" (meaning 1962–1963) as the last time that her husband, John Kennedy, experienced a specific occasion:

> On so many days—his birthday, an anniversary, watching his children running to the sea—I have thought, "but this day last year was his last to see that." He was so full of love and life on all those days. He seems so vulnerable now, when you think that each one was a last time.

Mrs. Kennedy also wrote about the process of letting go, although she didn't call it that[88]:

> Soon the final day will come around again—as inexorably as it did last year. But expected this time. It will find some of us different people than we were a year ago. Learning to accept what was unthinkable when he was alive changes you.

Finally, she addressed an essential truth of bereavement[88]:

> I don't think there is any consolation. What was lost cannot be replaced.

Letting go encompasses recognizing the uniqueness of the individual. It also entails finding meaning in the relationship and experience. It does not mean cutting oneself off from memories of the deceased.

Continuing Bonds

Klass and associates[57] contributed to the reformulation of thinking on the nature of accommodating to loss. Although theorists postulated that the grief process should be completed in 1 year, with one's emotional energies once again invested in the living, the experience of the bereaved suggested otherwise. Bereaved persons visit the grave for periodic discussions with the deceased. They gaze at a picture and seek advice on various matters. Such behavior is not pathological. The provocative thesis that those with higher scores on the Continuing Bonds Scale experience elevated grief suggests not only an additional tool for assessment but that grief is the price that is exacted in the dissolution of close relationships.[89]

It is a common expectation that teachers in the educational system will have an influence on their students. The students progress and may or may not have continuing contact with those educators. Given that assumption about education, how could we not expect to feel the continuing influence and memory of those informal teachers in our lives, our deceased family members and friends? Integration of those influences strengthens the individual at any point in his or her life.

A Turkish expression in the presence of death is, "May you live."[90] That indeed is the challenge of bereavement.

REFERENCES

1. Warren NA. Bereavement care in the critical care setting. Crit Care Nurs Q 1997;20:42.
2. Robinson DS, McKenna HP. Loss: An analysis of a concept of particular interest to nursing. J Adv Nurs 1998;27:782.
3. Kagawa-Singer M. The cultural context of death rituals and mourning practices. ONF 1998;25:1752.
4. Durkheim E. The Elementary Forms of Religious Life. New York: Collier, 1961.
5. Stephenson JS. Grief and mourning. In: Fulton R, Bendikson R, eds. Death and Identity, 3rd ed. Philadelphia: Charles Press, 1994: 136–176.
6. DeSpelder LA, Strickland AL. The Last Dance, 2nd ed. Mountain View, CA: Mayfield Publishing, 1987:207.
7. Martinson IM. Funeral rituals in Taiwan and Korea. ONF 1998; 25:1756–1760.
8. Chidester D. Patterns of Transcendence: Religion, Death and Dying. Belmont, CA: Wadsworth, 1990.
9. Munet-Vilaro F. Grieving and death rituals of Latinos. ONF 1998;25:1761.
10. Doka K. Grief. In: Kastenbaum R, Kastenbaum B, eds. Encyclopedia of Death. Phoenix, AZ: Oryx Press, 1989:127.
11. Rodgers L. Meaning of bereavement among older African-American widows. Geriatr Nurs 2004;25:10–16.
12. Burnett P, Middleton W, Raphael B, Martinek N. Measuring core bereavement phenomena. Psychol Med 1997;27:49–57.
13. Middleton W, Franzp MD, Raphael B, Franzp MD, Burnett P, Martinek N. Psychological distress and bereavement. J Nerv Ment Dis 1997;185:452.
14. Hays JC, Kasl S, Jacobs S. Past personal history of dysphoria, social support, and psychological distress following conjugal bereavement. J Am Geriatr Soc 1994;42:712–718.
15. Zisook S, Shuchter SR, Sledge PA, Paulus M, Judd LL. The spectrum of depressive phenomena after spousal bereavement. J Clin Psychiatry 1994;55(Suppl):35.
16. Reynolds CF, Miller MD, Pasternak RE, Frank E, Perel JM, Cornes C, Houck PR, Mazumdar S, Dew MA, Kupfer DJ. Treatment of bereavement-related major depressive episodes in later life: A controlled study of acute and continuation treatment with nortriptyline and interpersonal psychotherapy Am J Psychiatry 1999;156:202–208.
17. Boelen PA, van den Bout J, de Keijser J. Traumatic grief as a disorder distinct from bereavement-related depression and anxiety: A replication study with bereaved mental health care patients. Am J Psychiatry 2003;160:1339–1341.
18. Ellifritt J, Nelson, KA, Walsh D. Complicated bereavement: A national survey of potential risk factors. Am J Hosp Palliat Care 2003;20:114–120.
19. Rubin SS, Schecter N. Exploring the social construction of bereavement: Perceptions of adjustment and recovery in bereaved men. Am J Orthopsychiatry 1997;67:280.
20. Rubin SS, Malkinson R, Witzum E. Trauma and bereavement: Conceptual and clinical issues revolving around relationships. Death Studies 2003;27:667–690.
21. Bernard LL, Guarnaccia CA. Two models of caregiver strain and bereavement adjustment: A comparison of husband and daughter caregivers of breast cancer hospice patients. Gerontologist 2003;43:808–816.
22. Traylor ES, Hayslip B Jr., Kaminski PL, York C. Relationships between grief and family system characteristics: A cross-lagged longitudinal analysis. Death Studies 2003;27:575–601.
23. Stewart AE. Complicated bereavement and posttraumatic stress disorder following fatal car crashes: Recommendations for death notification practice. Death Studies 1997;23:289–321.
24. Murphy SA, Johnson JL, Lohan J. Challenging the myths about parents' adjustment after the sudden violent death of a child. J Nurs Schol 2003;35:359–364.
25. Hutton CJ, Bradley BS. Effects of sudden infant death on bereaved siblings: A comparative study. J Child Psychol Psychiat 1994;55:723–732.
26. Mahon MM. Childhood bereavement after the death of a sibling. Holistic Nurs Pract 1995;9:16.
27. Hogan NS, DeSantis L. Things that help and hinder adolescent sibling bereavement. West J Nurs Res 1994;16:137.
28. Coolican MB. Families facing the sudden death of a loved one. Crit Care Nurs Clin North Am 1994;6:607–612.
29. Lev EL, McCorkle R. Loss, grief and bereavement in family members of cancer patients. Semin Oncol Nurs 1998;4: 145–151.
30. Potocky M. Effective services for bereaved spouses: A content analysis of the empirical literature. Health Soc Work 1993;18: 288–301.
31. Maddocks I. Grief and bereavement. Med J Aust 2003;179 (6Suppl):S6–S7.
32. Sandler IN, Ayers TS, Wolchik SA, Tein JY, Kwok OM, Twohey-Jacobs J, Suter J, Lin K, Padgett-Jones S, Weyer JL, Cole E, Kriege G, Griffin WA. The family bereavement program: Efficacy evaluation of a theory-based prevention program for parentally bereaved children and adolescents. J Consult Clin Psychol 2003; 71:587–600.
33. Rossi Ferrario S, Cardillo V, Vicarfio F, Balzarini E, Zotti AM. Advanced cancer at home: Caregiving and bereavement. Palliat Med 2004;18:129–136.

34. Coolican MB, Pearce T. After care bereavement program. Crit Care Nurs Prog North Am 1995;7:519–527.
35. Snyder J. Bereavement protocols. J Emerg Nurs 1996;22:39–42.
36. LeBrocq P, Charles A, Chan T, Buchanan M. Establishing a bereavement program: Caring for bereaved families and staff in the emergency department. Accid Emerg Nurs. 2003;11:85–90.
37. Azhar MZ, Varma SL. Religious psychotherapy as management of bereavement. Acta Psychiatry Scand 1995;91:233–235.
38. Goodkin K, Blaney NT, Feaster DJ, Baldewicz T, Burkhalter JE, Leeds B. A randomized controlled clinical trial of a bereavement support group intervention in human immunodeficiency virus type 1–seropositive and –seronegative homosexual men. Arch Gen Psychiatry 1999;56:52–59.
39. Summers J, Zisook S, Sciolla AD, Patterson T, Atkinson JH, San Diego HIV Neurobehavioral Research Center (HNRC) Group. Gender, AIDS, and bereavement: A comparison of women and men living with HIV. Death Studies 2004;28:225–241.
40. Sikkema KJ, Hansen NB, Kochman A, Tate DC, Difranceisco W. Outcomes from a randomized controlled trial of a group intervention for HIV positive men and women coping with AIDS-related loss and bereavement. Death Studies 2004;28:187–209.
41. Bower JE, Kemeny ME, Taylor SE, Fahy JL. Cognitive processing, discovery of meaning, CD4 decline, and AIDS-related mortality among bereaved HIV-seropositive men. J Consulting Clin Pscyhol 1998;66:979–986.
42. Anderson KL, Dimond MF. The experience of bereavement in older adults. J Adv Nurs 1995;22:308–315.
43. Sheldon F. ABC of palliative care—Bereavement. BMJ 1998; 316:456.
44. Billings JA. Useful predictors of poor outcomes in bereavement. In: JA Billings, coordinator. Palliative Care Role Model Course. Boston, MA: Massachusetts General Hospital, 1999.
45. Kaltman S, Bonanno GA. Trauma and bereavement: Examining the impact of sudden and violent deaths. J Anxiety Disord 2003; 17:131–147.
46. Rando TA. Grief and mourning: Accommodating to loss. In: Wass H, Neimeyer RA, eds. Dying—Facing the Facts. Philadelphia: Taylor and Francis, 1995:211–241.
47. Fulton R, Bendikson R. Introduction—Grief and the Process of Mourning. In: Fulton R, Bendicksen R, eds. Death and Identity, 3rd ed. Philadelphia: Charles Press Publishers, 1994:105–109.
48. Lindemann E. Symptomatology and management of acute grief. Am J Psychiatry (Sesquicentennial Suppl) 1994;151(6):156.
49. Gorer G. Death, Grief and Mourning. London: Cresset Press, 1965.
50. Kavanaugh R. Facing Death. Baltimore: Penguin Books, 1974.
51. Raphael B. The Anatomy of Bereavement. New York: Basic Books, 1983.
52. Weizman SG, Kamm P. About Mourning: Support and Guidance for the Bereaved. New York: Human Sciences Press, 1985.
53. Kübler-Ross E. On Death and Dying. New York: Macmillan, 1969.
54. Rando TA. Grief, Dying and Death—Clinical Interventions for Caregivers. Champaign, IL: Research Press Company, 1984.
55. Worden JW. Grief Counseling and Grief Therapy: A Handbook for the Mental Health Practitioner, 2nd ed. New York: Springer, 1991.
56. Corr CA, Doka KJ. Current models of death, dying and bereavement. Crit Care Nurs Clin North Am 1994;6:545–552.
57. Klass D, Silverman P, Nickman S. Continuing Bonds. Philadelphia: Taylor and Francis Publishing, 1996.
58. Winston CA. African American grandmothers parenting AIDS orphans: Concomitant grief and loss. Am J Orthopsychiatry 2003;73:91–100.
59. Byrne GJA, Raphael B. A longitudinal study of bereavement phenomena in recently widowed elderly men. Psychol Med 1994; 23:411–421.
60. Koop PM, Strang V. Predictors of bereavement outcomes in families of patients with cancer: A literature review. Can J Nurs Res 1997;29:33–50.
61. Schultz R, Mendelsohn AB, Haley WE, Mahoney D, Allen RS, Zhang S, Thompson L, Belle SH. End-of-Life care and the effects of bereavement on family caregivers of persons with dementia. N Engl J Med 2003;349:1936–1942.
62. Duke S. An exploration of anticipatory grief: The lived experience of people during their spouses' terminal illness and in bereavement. J Adv Nurs 1998;28:829–839.
63. Cowles KV. Cultural perspectives of grief: An expanded concept analysis. J Adv Nurs 1996;23:287–294.
64. Worthington RC. Models of linear and cyclical grief—Different approaches to differenct experiences. Clin Pediatr 1994;33:297–300.
65. Neimeyer RA. Meaning reconstruction and the experience of chronic loss. In: Doka KJ, Davidson J, eds. Living with Grief: When Illness Is Prolonged. Philadelphia: Taylor and Francis, 1997:159–176.
66. Horowitz MJ, Siegel B, Holen A, Bonanno GA, Milbrath C, Stinson CH. Diagnostic criteria for complicated grief disorder. Am J Psychiatry 1997;154:904–910.
67. Prigerson HG, Frank E, Kasl SV, Reynolds CF, Anderson B, Zubenko GS, Houck PR, George CJ, Kupfer DJ. Complicated grief and bereavement-related depression as distinct disorders: Preliminary empirical validation in elderly bereaved spouses. Am J Psychiatry 1995;152:22–30.
68. Prigerson HG, Bierhals AJ, Kasl SV, Reynolds CF, Shear MK, Newsom JT, Jacobs S. Complicated grief as a disorder distinct from bereavement-related depression and anxiety: A replication study. Am J Psychiatry 1996;153:1484–1486.
69. Prigerson HG, Maciejewski PK, Reynolds CF III, Bierhals AJ, Newsom JT, Fasiczka A, Frank E, Doman J, Miller M. Inventory of Complicated Grief: A scale to measure maladaptive symptoms of loss. Psychiatry Res 1995;59:65–79.
70. Ogrodniczuk JS. Differentiating symptoms of complicated grief and depression among psychiatric outpatients. Can J Psychiatry 2003;48:87–93.
71. Krigger KW, McNeely JD, Lippmann SB. Dying, death and grief: Helping patients and their families through the process. Postgrad Med 1997;101:263–270.
72. Ott CH. The impact of complicated grief on mental and physical health at various points in the bereavement process. Death Studies 2003;27:249–272.
73. Doka KJ. Disenfranchised grief. In: DeSpelderf LA, Strickland AL, eds. The Path Ahead. Mountain View, CA: Mayfield, 1995: 271–275.
74. Corless IB. Modulated mourning: The grief and mourning of those infected and affected by HIV/AIDS. In: Doka KJ, Davidson J, eds. Living with Grief: When Illness Is Prolonged. Philadelphia: Taylor and Francis, 1997:108–118.
75. Eakes GG, Burke ML, Hainsworth MA. Chronic sorrow: The experiences of bereaved individuals. Illness Crisis Loss 1999;7:172–182.
76. O'Gorman SM. Death and dying in contemporary society: An evaluation of current attitudes and the rituals associated with death and dying and their relevance to recent understandings of health and healing. J Adv Nurs 1998;2:1127–1135.

77. Fulton R. The funeral in contemporary society. In Fulton R, Bendiksen R, eds. Death and Identity, 3rd ed. Philadelphia: Charles Press, 1994:288–312.
78. Stroebe W, Stroebe MS. Is grief universal? Cultural variations in the emotional reaction to loss. In Fulton R, Bendiksen R, eds. Death and Identity, 3rd ed. Philadelphia: Charles Press, 1994:177–207.
79. Byatt AS. Possession—A Romance. New York: Vintage Books, 1990:6.
80. Arnold J. Rethinking—Nursing implications for health promotion. Home Healthcare Nurse 1996;14:779–780.
81. Rancour P. Recognizing and treating dysfunctional grief. ONF 1998;25:1310–1311.
82. Cutcliffe JR. Hope, counselling, and complicated bereavement reactions. J Adv Nurs 1998;28:760.
83. Stephenson C. The concept of hope revisited for nursing. J Adv Nurs 1991;16:1456–1461.
84. Frankl V. Man's Search for Meaning: An Introduction to Logotherapy. New York: Simon and Schuster, 1959.
85. Herth KA. The relationship between level of hope and level of coping and other variables in patients with cancer. ONF 1989; 16:62–72.
86. Watson MA. Bereavement in the elderly. AORN J 1994;59:1084.
87. Quinton A. Permission to mourn. Nurs Times 1994;90:31–32.
88. Corless IB. And when famous people die. In: Corless IB, Germino BA, Pittman MA, eds. A Challenge for Living—Dying, Death, and Bereavement. Boston: Jones & Bartlett Publishers, 1995:398.
89. Field NP, Gal-Oz E, Bonanno GA. Continuing bonds and adjustment at 5 years after the death of a spouse. J Consult Clin Psychol 2003;71:110–117.
90. [Commentary by newscaster on Turkish earthquake.] ABC News, 1999.

28

Betty Davies

Supporting Families in Palliative Care

I hope someday you'll find a way for families to understand how they should act in order to help a patient. The best help you can get from your family is understanding, for them to listen to you and understand you. . . . To help the family understand the illness, to be a support for the person who is ill: That is the greatest treasure to the person with cancer.—Daughter of 73-year-old man with extensive colon cancer

- ***Key Points***
- *Family-centered care is a basic tenet of palliative care philosophy, which recognizes that terminally ill patients exist within the family system. The patient's illness affects the whole family, and, in turn, the family's responses affect the patient. Supporting families in palliative care means that nurses must plan their care with an understanding not only of the individual patient's needs but also of the family system within which the patient functions.*
- *Families with a member who requires palliative care are in transition. Families have described this as a "transition of fading away," characterized by seven dimensions that help nurses to understand families' experiences and to support them.*
- *Level of family functioning also plays a role in family experience and serves to guide nursing interventions for families with varying levels of functioning.*

Family-Centered Palliative Care

Recognizing the importance of a family focus necessitates clearly defining what is meant by "family." Most often, families in palliative care do consist of patients, their spouses, and their children.[1] But in today's world of divorce and remarriage, steprelatives must also enter into the family portrait. In other instances, people unrelated by blood or marriage may function as family. Therefore, the definition of family must be expanded. The family is a group of individuals inextricably linked in ways that are constantly interactive and mutually reinforcing. Family can mean direct blood relatives, relationships through an emotional commitment, or the group or person with which an individual feels most connected.[2] Moreover, family in its fullest sense embraces all generations—past, present, future; those living, those dead, and those yet to be born. Shadows of the past and dreams of the future also contribute to the understanding of families.

Palliative care programs are based on the principle that the family is the unit of care. In practice, however, the family is often viewed as a group of individuals who can either prove helpful or resist efforts to deliver care. Nurses and other health professionals must strive to understand the meaning of the palliative experience to the family. If quality care is to be provided, nurses need to understand how all family members perceive their experience, how the relationships fit together, and that a multitude of factors combine to make families what they are. However, only recently has research gone beyond focusing on the needs of dying patients for comfort and palliation to addressing issues relevant to other family members. Much of this research has focused on the family's perspective of their needs[3]; experiences and challenges faced[4–7]; adaptation and coping skills required for home care[3,8–11]; the supportiveness of nursing behaviors[12] or physician behaviors[13]; and satisfaction with care.[14,15] Most research has focused on families of patients with cancer, though recent reports extend to end-of-life care for other diagnostic populations, such as Parkinson's disease,[4] cardiac disease,[5] and dementia.[16] Findings make it clear that family members look to health professionals to provide quality care to the patient. Family members also expect health professionals to meet their own needs for information, emotional support, and assistance with care.[14]

Much of the research that purports to address the impact of cancer on the family is based on the perceptions of individuals—either the patient or adult family members (usually the spouse). As well, many of the studies were conducted retrospectively, that is, after the patient's death. But even studies conducted during the palliative period frequently exclude the patient—the one who is at the center of the palliative care situation. Examining the palliative experience of the family unit has been rare.

As a basis for offering optimal support to families in palliative care, this chapter focuses on describing the findings of a research program that prospectively examined the experiences of such families.[17] The research evolved from nurses' concerns about how to provide family-centered palliative care. Nurses in a regional cancer center constantly had to attend to the needs of not only patients but also patients' families, particularly as they moved back and forth between hospital and home. In searching the literature for guidelines about family-centered care, they found that many articles were about the needs of patients and family members, about levels of family members' satisfaction with care, and about family members' perceptions of nurses, but nothing really described the families' experiences as they coped with the terminal illness of a beloved family member. Research involving families included patients with advanced cancer, their spouses, and at least one of their adult children (>18 years of age). Since the completion of the original research, families with AIDS, Alzheimer's disease, and cardiac disease have provided anecdotal validation of the findings for their experiences. In addition, families of children with progressive, life-threatening illness have provided similar validation. Therefore, it seems that the conceptualization has relevance for a wide range of families in palliative care. The findings from this research program form the basis for the description that follows; references to additional research studies are also included to supplement and emphasize the ongoing development of knowledge in the field of family-centered end-of-life care.

The Transition of Fading Away

The common view is that transitions are initiated by changes, by the start of something new. However, as Bridges[18] suggests, most transitions actually begin with endings. This is true for families living with serious illness in a loved one. The nurses' research findings generated a theoretical scheme that conceptualized families' experiences as a transition—a transition that families themselves labeled as "fading away." The transition of fading away for families facing terminal illness began with the ending of life as they knew it. They came to realize that the ill family member was no longer living with cancer but was now dying from cancer.

Despite the fact that family members had been told about the seriousness of the prognosis, often since the time of diagnosis, and had experienced the usual ups and downs associated with the illness trajectory, for many the "gut" realization that the patient's death was inevitable occurred suddenly: "It struck me hard-it hit me like a bolt. Dad is not going to get better!" The awareness was triggered when family members saw, with "new eyes," a change in the patient's body or physical capacity, such as the patient's weight loss, extreme weakness, lack of mobility, or diminished mental capacity. Realizing that the patient would not recover, family members began the transition of fading away. As one patient commented, "My body has shrunk so much—the other day, I tried on my favorite old blue dress and I could see then how much weight I have lost. I feel like a skeleton with skin! I am getting weaker. . . . I just can't eat much now, I don't want to. I can see that I am fading. . . . I am definitely fading away."

The transition of fading away is characterized by seven dimensions: redefining, burdening, struggling with paradox, contending with change, searching for meaning, living day by day, and preparing for death. The dimensions do not occur in linear fashion; rather, they are interrelated and inextricably linked to one another. Redefining, however, plays a central role. All family members experience these dimensions, although patients, spouses, and children experience each dimension somewhat differently.

Redefining

Redefining involves a shift from "what used to be" to "what is now." It demands adjustment in how individuals see themselves and each other. Patients maintained their usual patterns for as long as possible and then began to implement feasible alternatives once they realized that their capacities were seriously changing. Joe, a truck driver, altered his identity over time: "I just can't do what I used to. I finally had to accept the fact that the seizures made it unsafe for me to drive." Joe requested to help out at his company's distribution desk. When he could no longer concentrate on keeping the orders straight, Joe offered to assist with supervising the light loading. One day, Joe was acutely aware he didn't have the energy to even sit and watch the others: "I couldn't do it anymore," Joe sighed. "I had reached the end of my work life and the beginning of the end of my life." Another patient, Cora, lamented that she used to drive to her son's home to baby-sit her toddler-aged grandchildren; then her son dropped the children off at her house to preserve the energy it took for her to travel; and now, her son has made other child care arrangements. He brings the children for only short visits because of her extreme fatigue.

Both Joe and Cora, like the other patients, accepted their limitations with much sadness and a sense of great loss. Their focus narrowed, and they began to pay attention to details of everyday life that they had previously ignored or overlooked. Joe commented, "When I first was at home, I wanted to keep in touch with the guys at the depot; I wanted to know what was going on. Now, I get a lot of good just watching the grandkids out there playing in the yard."

Patients were eager to reinforce that they were still the same on the inside, although they acknowledged the drastic changes in their physical appearance. They often became more spiritual in their orientation to life and nature. As Joe said, "I always liked being outside—was never much of an office-type person. But, now, it seems I like it even more. That part of me hasn't changed even though it's hard for some of the fellas (at work) to recognize me now." When patients were able to redefine themselves as Joe did, they made the best of their situation, differentiating what parts of them were still intact. Joe continued, "Yeah, I like just being outside, or watching the kids. And, you know, they still come to their Grandpa when their toy trucks break down—I can pretty much always fix 'em." Similarly, Cora commented: "At least, I can still make cookies for when my family comes, although I don't make them from scratch anymore." Patients shared their changing perceptions with family members and others, who then were able to offer understanding and support.

Patients who were unable to redefine themselves in this way attempted to maintain their regular patterns despite the obvious changes in their capacity to do so. They ended up frustrated, angry, and feeling worthless. These reactions distanced them from others, resulting in the patients' feeling alone and, sometimes, abandoned. Ralph, for example, was an educational administrator. Despite his deteriorating health, he insisted that he was managing without difficulty. "Nothing's wrong with me, really. . . . We are being accredited this year. There's a lot to do to get ready for that." Ralph insisted on going into the office each day to prepare the necessary reports. His increasing confusion and inability to concentrate made his reports inaccurate and inadequate, but Ralph refused to acknowledge his limitations or delegate the work. Instead, his colleagues had to work overtime to correct Ralph's work after he left the office. According to Ralph's wife, anger and frustration were commonplace among his colleagues, but they were reluctant to discuss the issue with Ralph. Instead, they avoided conversations with Ralph, and he complained to his wife about his colleagues' lack of interest in the project.

For the most part, spouses took the patient's physical changes in stride. They attributed the changes to the disease, not to the patient personally, and as a result, they were able to empathize with the patient. Patients' redefining focused on themselves, the changes in their physical status and intrapersonal aspects; spouses' redefining centered on their relationship with the patient. Spouses did their best to "continue on as normal," primarily for the sake of the patient. In doing so, they considered alternatives and reorganized their priorities.

Sherman[19] described the "reciprocity of suffering" that family members experience, which results from the physical and emotional distress that is rooted in their anguish of dealing with the impending death of the loved one and in their attempt to fill new roles as caregivers. The degree to which family members experienced this phenomenon varied according to patients' redefining. When patients were able to redefine themselves, spouses had an easier time. Such patients accepted spouses' offers of support; patients and spouses were able to talk about the changes that were occurring. Spouses felt satisfied in the care that they provided. But when patients were less able to redefine, then spouses' offers of support were rejected or unappreciated. For example, Ralph's wife worried about his work pattern and its impact on his colleagues. She encouraged him to cut back, but Ralph only ignored her pleas and implied that she didn't understand how important this accreditation was to the future of his school. Even when Ralph was no longer able to go to the office, he continued to work from home, frequently phoning his colleagues to supervise their progress on the report. His wife lamented, "For an educated man, he doesn't know much. I guess it's too late to teach an old dog new tricks."

In such situations, spouses avoided talking about or doing anything that reminded the patient of the changes he or she was experiencing but not acknowledging. The relationship between the spouse and patient suffered. Rather than feeling satisfied with their care, spouses were frustrated and angry, although often they remained silent and simply "endured" the situation. The ill person contributed significantly to the caregiver's ability to cope. Indeed, the ill person was not simply a passive recipient of care but had an impact on the experience of the caregiving spouse. Similarly, in their study of factors that influence family caregiving of persons with advanced cancer, Strang and Koop[20] found that the ill person contributed significantly to the capacity of the spouse to continue to provide care despite their experience of overwhelming emotional and physical strain. Caregivers drew strength from the dying person when the ill person accepted the impending death, had an understanding of the caregivers' needs, and had attitudes, values, and beliefs that sustained their caregivers.

Adult children also redefined the ill family member; they redefined their ill parent from someone who was strong and competent to someone who was increasingly frail. Children felt vulnerable in ways they had not previously experienced. Most often, children perceived that the changes in their ill parent were the result of disease and not intentional: "It's not my father doing this consciously." Younger adult children were particularly sensitive to keeping the situation private, claiming they wanted to protect the dignity of the patient, but seemed to want to protect their own sense of propriety. For example, one young woman in her early twenties was "devastated" when her father's urinary bag dragged behind him as he left the living room where she and her friends were visiting. It was difficult for some young adults to accept such manifestations of their parent's illness. Adolescents in particular had a difficult time redefining the situation. They preferred to continue on as if nothing was wrong and to shield themselves against any information that would force them to see the situation realistically.

When the ill parent was able to redefine to a greater degree, then children were better able to appreciate that death is part of life. They recognized their own susceptibility and vowed to take better care of their own health; older children with families of their own committed to spending more quality time with their children. Joe talked, although indirectly, with his son about the situation: "I won't be here forever to fix the kids' toys." Together, Joe and his son reminisced about how Joe had always been available to his son and grandchildren as "Mr. Fix-it." Joe valued his dad's active participation in his life and promised to be the same kind of father to his own sons. In contrast, when the ill parent was unable to redefine, then children tended to ignore the present. They attempted to recreate the past to construct happy memories they never had. In doing so, they often neglected their own families. Ralph's daughter described her dad as a "workaholic." Feeling as if she had never had enough time with her dad, she began visiting her parents daily, with suggestions of places she could take him. He only became annoyed with her unfamiliar, constant presence: "It's okay she comes over every day, but enough is enough."

The extent to which spouses and adult children commented on the important contribution made by the dying family member is a provocative finding that underscores the importance of relationships among and between family members in facilitating their coping with the situation of terminal illness.

Burdening

Feeling as if they are a burden for their family is common among patients. If patients see themselves as purposeless, dependent, and immobile, they have a greater sense of burdening their loved ones. The more realistically patients redefined themselves as their capacities diminished, the more accurate they were in their perceptions of burdening. They acknowledged other family members' efforts, appreciated those efforts, and encouraged family members to rest and take time to care for themselves. Patients who were less able to redefine themselves did not see that they were burdening other family members in any way. They denied or minimized the strain on others. As Ralph said during the last week of his life, "I can't do much, but I am fine really. Not much has changed. It's a burden on my wife, but not much. It might be some extra work. . . . She was a nursing aide, so she is used to this kind of work."

Most spouses acknowledged the "extra load" of caring for their dying partner, but indicated that they did not regard the situation as a "burden." They agreed that it's "just something you do for the one you love." Spouses did not focus on their own difficulties; they managed to put aside their own distress so that it would not have a negative impact on their loved one. They sometimes shared stories of loneliness and helplessness, but also stories of deepening respect and love for their partner. Again, spouses of patients who were able to redefine were energized by the patient's acknowledgment of their efforts and were inspired to continue on. Spouses of patients who were not able to redefine felt unappreciated, exhausted, and confessed to "waiting for the patient to die."

The literature provides a comprehensive description of the multidimensional nature of the burden experienced by family caregivers, but no attention has been given to the burdening felt by patients or adult children specifically. Caregiver burden, usually by spouses, has been described in terms of physical burden, which includes fatigue and physical exhaustion,[21] sleeplessness,[22] and deterioration of health.[23] Social burden encompasses limited time for self[24] and social stress related to isolation.[25] Regardless of the type of burden, however, most caregivers, including the ones in the fading away studies, expressed much satisfaction with their caregiving.[26] Despite feeling burdened, most caregivers would repeat the experience: "Yes, it was difficult and exhausting, and there were days I didn't think I could manage one more minute. But, if I had to do it over again, I would. I have no regrets for what I am doing."

Children, too, experienced burdening, but the source stemmed from the extra responsibilities involved in helping to care for a dying parent superimposed on their work responsibilities, career development, and their own families. As a result, adult children of all ages felt a mixture of satisfaction and exhaustion. Their sense of burdening was also influenced by the ill parent's redefining—if the ill parent acknowledged their efforts, they were more likely to feel satisfaction. However, children's sense of burdening was also influenced by the state of health of the well parent. If that parent also was ill or debilitated, the burden on children was compounded. If children were able to prioritize their responsibilities so that they could pay attention to their own needs as well as helping both their parents, they felt less burdened. Children seemed less likely than their well parents to perceive caregiving as something they themselves would do. Of course, they did not have the life experience of a long-term relationship that motivated the spouses to care for their partners.

Finding effective ways to support family caregivers is critical, because an increase in the proportion of elderly people in the population means growing numbers of people with chronic, life-threatening, or serious illness require care. The responsibility for the care of such individuals is increasingly being placed on families. Respite care is often suggested as a strategy for relieving burden in family caregivers.[3,4,9] One review[8] was conducted of studies examining the effect of respite provision on caregivers. Surprisingly, the researchers found little evidence that respite provision had either a consistent or an enduring beneficial effect on caregivers' well being. The authors offered two explanations: the studies were methodologically poor and respite care often failed to facilitate the development of socially supportive relationships to provide a moderating influence.

However, another potential factor influencing the success of respite care may be the dynamics within the family, in particular between the patient and family caregivers. Respite must be assessed in conjunction with the role of redefining in burdening. Support for this suggestion comes from a study,[10] based in the Netherlands, of the experiences of caregivers, which showed that support from informal and professional caregivers was not sufficient to balance the stresses of caregiving and the missing element may be internal to the family. These findings encourage greater exploration into respite care and its meaning to caregivers. In one study of home-based family caregiving, caregivers differentiated between cognitive and physical breaks.[11] They valued cognitive breaks during which they remained within the caregiving environment, but physical separation from the caregiving environment was valuable only if it contributed in some meaningful way to the caregiving.

Struggling with Paradox

Struggling with paradox stems from the fact that the patient is both living and dying. For patients, the struggle focuses on wanting to believe they will survive and knowing that they will not. On "good days," patients felt optimistic about the outcome; on other days, they succumbed to the inevitability of their approaching demise. Often, patients did not want to "give up" but at the same time were "tired of fighting." They wanted to "continue on" for the sake of their families but also wanted "it to end soon" so their families could "get on with their lives." Patients coped by hoping for miracles, fighting for the sake of their families, and focusing on the good days. As Joe said, "I like to think about the times when things are pretty good. I enjoy those days. But, on the bad days, when I'm tired, or when the pain gets the best of me, then I just wonder if it wouldn't be best to just quit. But you never know—maybe I'll be the one in a million who makes it at the last minute." He then added wryly, "Hmmm, big chance of that."

Spouses struggled with a paradox of their own: they wanted to care for and spend time with the patient, and they also wanted a "normal" life. They coped by juggling their time as best they could, and usually put their own life on hold. Spouses who managed to find ways of tending to their own needs usually were less exhausted and reported fewer health problems than spouses who neglected their own needs. For years, Joe and his wife had been square dancers. They hadn't been dancing together for many months when his wife resumed going to "dance night as a sub" or to prepare the evening's refreshments. "Sometimes, I feel guilty for going and leaving Joe at home, but I know I need a break. When I did miss dance night, I could see I was getting really bitchy—I need to get out for a breather so I don't suffocate Joe."

Children struggled with hanging on and letting go to a greater extent than their parents. They wanted to spend time with their ill parent and also to "get on with their own lives." Feeling the pressure of dual loyalties (to their parents and to their own young families), the demands of both compounded the struggle that children faced.

Contending with Change

Those facing terminal illness in a family member experience changes in every realm of daily life—relationships, roles, socialization, work patterns. The focus of the changes differed among family members. Patients faced changes in their relationships with everyone they knew. They realized that the greatest change of their life was underway and that life as they knew it would soon be gone. They tended to break down tasks into manageable pieces, and increasingly they focused inward. The greatest change that spouses faced was in their relationship with the patient. They coped by attempting to keep everything as normal as possible. Children contended with changes that were more all-encompassing. They could not withdraw as their ill parent did, nor could they prioritize their lives to the degree that their well parent could. They easily become exhausted. As Joe's son explained, "It's a real challenge coming by this often—I try to come twice a week and then bring the kids on the weekends. But I just got a promotion at work this year so that's extra work too. Seems like I don't see my wife much—but she's a real trooper. Her dad died last year so she knows what it's like."

Searching for Meaning

Searching for meaning has to do with seeking answers to help in understanding the situation. Patients tended to journey inward, reflect on spiritual aspects, deepen their most important connections, and become closer to nature: "The spiritual thing has always been at the back of my mind, but it's developing more. . . . When you're sick like that, your attitude changes toward life. You come not to be afraid of death."

Spouses concentrated on their relationship with the patient. Some searched for meaning through personal growth, whereas others searched for meaning by simply tolerating the situation. Some focused on spiritual growth, and others adhere rigidly to their religion with little, if any, sense of inner growth or insight. Joe's wife commented, "Joe and I are closer than ever now. We don't like this business, but we have learned to love each other even more than when we were younger—sickness is a hard lesson that way." In contrast, Ralph's wife said with resignation, "He's so stubborn—always has been. I sometimes wonder why I stayed. But, here I am." Spouses and patients may attribute different meanings to other aspects of their experience as well. For example, when seeing their loved one in pain, many spouses felt helpless and fearful. Once the pain was controlled, they felt peaceful and relaxed and interpreted this as an indication that the couple would return to their old routines. The patient's meaning of the experience, however, often focused on future consequences of the pain.[6] The meaning attributed to the patient's experience also influenced spousal bereavement. For example, spouses who witnessed the patient die a painful death and who believed that physician negligence was the cause of the pain experience elevated anger and much distress after the death.[27]

Children tended to reflect on and reevaluate all aspects of their lives: "It puts in perspective how important some of our goals are. . . . Having financial independence and being able to retire at a decent age. . . . Those things are important, but not at the expense of sacrificing today."

Living Day to Day

Not all families reached the point of living day to day. If patients were able to find some meaning in their experience, then they were better able to adopt an attitude of living each day. Their attitude was characterized by "making the most of it." As one patient described it, "There's not much point in going over things in the past; not much point in projecting yourself too far into the future either. It's the current time that counts." Patients who were unable to find much meaning in their experience, or who didn't search for meaning, focused more on "getting through it." As Ralph said with determination, "Sure, I am getting weaker. I know I am sick. . . . But I will get through this!"

Spouses who searched for meaning focused on "making the best of it" while making every effort to enjoy the time they had left with their partner. Other spouses simply endured the situation without paying much attention to philosophizing about the experience. Children often had difficulty concentrating on living day to day, because they were unable to defer their obligations and therefore were constantly worrying about what else needed to be done. However, some children were still able to convey an attitude of "Live for today, today—worry about tomorrow, tomorrow."

Preparing for Death

Preparing for death involved concrete actions that would have benefit in the future, after the patient died. Patients had their family's needs uppermost in their minds and worked hard to teach or guide family members with regard to various tasks and activities that the patient would no longer be around to do. Patients were committed to leaving legacies for their loved ones, not only as a means of being remembered, but also as a way of comforting loved ones in their grief. Joe spent time "jotting down a few Mr. Fix-it pointers" for his wife and son. Ralph's energy was consumed by focusing on the work he still had to do, so he was unable to consider what he might do for his wife and daughter.

Spouses concentrated on meeting the patient's wishes. Whatever the patient wanted, spouses would try to do. They attended to practical details and anticipated their future in practical ways. Children offered considerable help to their parents with legal and financial matters. They also prepared their own children for what was to come. A central aspect was reassuring the dying parent that they would take care of the surviving parent. Children also prepared for the death by envisioning their future without their parent: "I think about it sometimes, . . . about how my children will never have a grandfather. It makes me so sad. That's why the photos we have been taking are so important to me. . . . They will show our children who their grandfather was."

Palliative Care for Diagnoses Other Than Cancer

Traditionally, palliative care practice and discussions have focused on families of cancer patients. At the same time, care of the patient with cardiac disease, for example, has traditionally focused on restoring health and enabling a return to normal life. So, the idea of providing a patient with aggressive versus palliative treatment has, until recently, not been a well-discussed issue in the treatment of the patient with heart disease. For most patients with heart disease, and particularly for those with heart failure, the decline in functional status is slower than for patients diagnosed with cancer.[5] However, if palliative care is considered only after disease-related care fails or becomes too burdensome, the opportunity for patients to achieve symptom relief and for patients and family members to engage in the process of fading away may be lost. Consequently, following a model of care wherein issues of treatment and end-of-life care are discussed early and throughout the illness trajectory facilitates patient and family coping and enables nurses to optimally support families.

Varying disease trajectories for other conditions, such as dementia, also influence the nature of support that nurses provide patients and families. For example, in a comparative study of staff's assessment of support needed by families of dementia and cancer patients, staff in dementia care stressed significantly more the need for forming support groups for families, offering respite care, educating families, and trying to relieve families' feeling of guilt. In the cancer care group, staff assigned greater importance to being available to listen, creating a sense of security, and supporting the family after death.[16]

Family Involvement According to Location of Care

Over the past century, nursing homes and hospitals increasingly have become the site of death. A recent national study evaluated the U.S. dying experience at home and in institutional settings.[28] Family members of 1578 deceased individuals were asked via telephone survey about the patient's experience at the last place of care at which the patient spent >48 hours. Results showed that two thirds (67.2%) of patients were last cared for in an institution. Family members reported greater satisfaction with patient's symptom management and with emotional support for both the patient and family if they received care at home with hospice services. Families have greater opportunities for involvement in the care if home care is possible. Family involvement in hospital care also makes for better outcomes. Among geriatric patients receiving end-of-life care in a hospital setting, family involvement before death reduces the use of technology and increases the use of comfort care as patients die.[29] Nurses, therefore, must consider how best to include families in the care of their dying loved ones, regardless of the location of care.

Large variations exist in the provision of home-based palliative and terminal care across the United States, although the development of hospice home services has enabled increasing numbers of seriously ill patients to experience care at home. However, dying at home can present special challenges for family members. Lack of support and lack of confidence have been found to be determinants contributing to hospital admissions and the breakdown of informal caregiving for people with a life-threatening illness.[25] A lack of support from the health care system is given as the reason many caregivers have to admit their loved one to the hospital.[30] They also report that fragmentation of services and lack of forward planning jeopardizes the success of home care.[31–33]

Moreover, the decision for home care has a profound effect on family members.[34,35] In an ethnographic study investigating palliative care at home,[36,37] caregiver decisions for home care were characterized in three ways. Some caregivers made uninformed decisions, giving little consideration to the implications of their decision: "I made the decision just like that. . . . There wasn't much thought that went into it." Such decisions were made early in the patient's disease trajectory or when the patient was imminently dying, and they were often influenced by the unrealistic portrayal in the media about dying at home. Indifferent decisions occurred if caregivers felt they had little choice. The patient's needs and wishes often drove decisions, with caregivers paying little attention to their own needs. Negotiated decisions for home care typically occurred if caregivers and patients were able to talk openly about dying and had done so throughout the disease trajectory.

Family members' decisions were influenced by three major factors: making promises to care for the loved one at home, the desire to maintain as much as possible a "normal" life for the patient and themselves, and negative experiences with institutional care. Of interest, family members did not think of themselves as the target of professional interventions. They were reluctant to ask for help or to let their needs be known. Consequently, when working with caregiving families, health care providers could mediate discussions with the aim of coming to a mutually acceptable decision about home care. Such discussions could allow the sharing of perspectives to allow for decisions that would work well for all concerned. Ideally, such discussions should begin early in the disease trajectory.

Importantly, ongoing attention should be paid to improving hospital end-of-life care so that families feel they have a meaningful alternative to home care. A small scale study to develop and evaluate care pathways for the last days of life in a community setting was developed and tested in the United Kingdom, based on the pioneering work of Ellershaw.[38] The plan outlines the expected course of a patient's trajectory; brings together all the anticipated aspects of care, particularly with regard to symptom management and caregiver support; and encourages forward planning to avoid crisis admission to the hospital.[39] It serves as a model for how home care can be optimally delivered to those with terminal illness, echoing Doyle's[40] observation that good palliative care is an exercise in anticipation.

Clinicians must recognize the emotional impact of providing palliative care at home and must be sensitive to the sometimes overwhelming task that caregiving imposes on family caregivers. Acknowledging that availability and access to service is important, Stajduhar and Davies[41] specified that care must be provided within a team context so that families can benefit from a whole set of services needed to support death at home. Clinicians must work with the dying patients, with family caregivers, and with each other as equal partners in the caregiving process.

Clinicians must be available to families, offering anticipatory guidance and support throughout the caregiving experience. Health care professionals must assist family members as they traverse the maze of treatment and care decisions, ranging from whether to give particular "as needed" medications, or what food to make for the patient to eat, to whether or not to seek hospice care, to sign "do-not-resuscitate" documents, or to terminate treatment. It is critical that palliative care professionals continually engage with caregivers in forward planning, interpretation, and monitoring of the inevitable decline and dying process of the ill person, so as to facilitate the feeling in caregivers that they are secure and supported in their physically and emotionally exhausting work. Families need to know whom to call and when, and how to reach them.

Some simple guidelines for families can serve to encourage their coping. For example, caregivers should be told to keep a small notebook handy for jotting down questions and answers. The pages may be divided in half lengthwise, using the column on the left for questions and the other column for answers. Or, the left-sided page may be used for questions and the opposite page for the answers. They should be advised to have the notebook with them whenever they talk with a member of the palliative care team. Family members should be reassured that nothing is trivial. All questions are important, and all observations are valuable. They should be encouraged to say when they do not understand something, and to ask for information to be repeated as necessary. Palliative care professionals can help by spelling words that family members do not understand or by jotting down explanations. They should reassure family members that asking for help is not a sign of failure, but rather a sign of good common sense. Following such simple guidelines helps keep families from feeling overwhelmed. And, if they do feel "out of control," such guidelines, simple as they may seem, give family members some concrete action they can take to help with whatever the situation may be.

Clinicians must also remember that their own attitudes are critical; if families feel they are a "nuisance" to health care providers, they tend to be more anxious and to shy away from asking for help. Furthermore, clinicians are in ideal positions to advocate with politicians and policy makers to expand resources for home-based palliative care programs so that families can adequately and humanely be supported in their caregiving work.

Guidelines for Nursing Interventions

Much of the nursing literature, which provides guidelines for nursing care, addresses the importance of four major interventions that have relevance for all members of the palliative care team:

1. *Maintain hope* in patients and their family members. As families pass through the illness trajectory, the

nature of their hope changes from hope for cure, to hope for remission, to hope for comfort, to hope for a good death. Offering hope during fading away can be as simple as reassuring families that everything will be done to ensure the patient's comfort. Talking about the past also can help some families by reaffirming the good times spent together and the ongoing connections that will continue among family members. Referring to the future beyond the immediate suffering and emotional pain can also sustain hope. For example, when adult children reassure the ill parent that they will care for the other parent, the patient is hopeful that the surviving spouse will be all right.

2. *Involve families* in all aspects of care. Include them in decision-making, and encourage active participation in the physical care of the patient. This is their life—they have the right to control it as they will. Involvement is especially important for children when a family member is very ill. The more children are involved in care during the terminal phase, and in the activities that follow the death, the better able they are to cope with bereavement.[42]
3. *Offer information.* Tell families about what is happening in straightforward terms and about what they can expect to happen, particularly about the patient's condition and the process their loved one is to undergo. Doing so also provides families with a sense of control. Initiate the discussion of relevant issues that family members themselves may hesitate to mention. For example, the nurse might say, "Many family members feel as if they are being pulled in two or more directions when a loved one is very ill. They want to spend as much time as possible with the patient, but they also feel the pull of their own daily lives, careers, or families. How does this fit with your experience?"
4. *Communicate openly.* Open and honest communication with nurses and other health professionals is frequently the most important need of families. They need to be informed; they need opportunities to ask questions and to have their questions answered in terms that they can comprehend. Open communication among team members is basic to open communication with the families.

It is not an easy task for families to give up their comfortable and established views of themselves as death approaches. The challenge for members of the health care team is to help family members anticipate what lies ahead without violating their need to relinquish old orientations and hopes at a pace they can handle. These four broad interventions assist health care providers in providing good palliative care; the following guidelines offer further direction. They are derived from the direct accounts of patients, spouses, and children about the strategies they used to cope with the dimensions of fading away.

Redefining

Supporting patients and other family members with redefining requires that health care providers appreciate how difficult it is for family members to relinquish familiar perceptions of themselves and adopt unfamiliar, unwelcome, and unasked for changes into their self-perceptions. Disengagement from former perceptions and the adoption of new orientations occur over time. Nurses and other care providers are challenged to help family members anticipate and prepare for what lies ahead, while not pushing them at a pace that threatens their sense of integrity. Each family member redefines at his or her own pace; interventions must be tailored according to the individual needs of each. At the same time, health care providers must support the family as a unit by reassuring family members that their varying coping responses and strategies are to be expected.

Provide opportunities for patients to talk about the losses incurred due to the illness, the enforced changes, the adaptations they have made, and their feelings associated with these changes. Reinforce their normal patterns of living as long as possible and as appropriate. When they can no longer function as they once did, focus on what patients still can do, reinforcing those aspects of self that remain intact. Acknowledge that roles and responsibilities may be expressed in new and different ways and suggest new activities appropriate to the patient's interest and current capabilities.

The focus with spouses and children centers on explaining how the disease or treatment contributes to changes in the patient physically, psychologically, and socially. Provide opportunities for spouses to talk about how changes in the patient affect their marital relationship. Help children appreciate their parent from another perspective, such as in recalling favorite memories or identifying the legacies left. Discuss how they can face their own vulnerability by channeling concerns into positive steps for self-care. Reinforce the spouses' and children's usual patterns of living for as long as possible and as appropriate; when former patterns are no longer feasible, consider adjustments or alternatives.

Provide opportunities for spouses to discuss how they may reorganize priorities in order to be with and care for the patient to the degree they desire. Consider resources that enable the spouse to do this, such as the assistance of volunteers, home support services, or additional nursing services. Teach caregiving techniques if the spouse shows interest. With the children, discuss the degree to which they want to be open or private about the patient's illness with those outside the family. Acknowledge that family members will vary in their ability to assimilate changes in the patient and in their family life.

Burdening

Palliative care professionals can help patients find ways to relieve their sense of burden and can provide patients with opportunities to talk about their fears and concerns and to consider with whom they want to share their worries. In this way, patients may alleviate their concern for putting excessive demands on family members. Explain the importance of a break for family members and suggest that patients accept assistance from a volunteer or home support services at those times to relieve family members from worry. Explain that when patients affirm family members for their efforts, this contributes to family members' feeling appreciated and reduces their sense of burden.

Nurses and all members of the interdisciplinary team can assist spouses with burdening by supporting the spouse's reassurances to the patient that he or she is not a burden. Acknowledge spouses' efforts when they put their own needs on hold to care for the patient; help them to appreciate the importance of taking care of themselves as a legitimate way of sustaining the energy they need for the patient. Talk with spouses about how they might take time out, and consider the various resources they might use. Acknowledge the negative feelings spouses may have about how long they can continue; do not negate their positive desire to help.

For children, acknowledge the reorganization and the considerable adjustment in their daily routines. Explain that ambivalent feelings are common—the positive feelings associated with helping and the negative feelings associated with less time spent on careers and their own families. Acknowledge that communicating regularly with their parents by telephoning or visiting often is part of the "work" of caring; the extra effort involved should not be underestimated. Encourage children to take time out for themselves, and support them in their desire to maintain involvement in their typical lives.

Struggling with Paradox

Facing the usual business of living and directly dealing with dying is a considerable challenge for all members of the family. The care provider's challenge is to appreciate that it is not possible to alleviate completely the family's psychosocial and spiritual pain. Team members must face their own comfort level in working with families who are facing paradoxical situations and the associated ambivalent feelings. Like family members, nurses, social workers, physicians, and all team members may also sometimes want to avoid the distress of struggling with paradox. They may feel unprepared to handle conversations in which no simple solution exists and strong feelings abound.

Care providers can support patients and other family members by providing opportunities for all family members to ventilate their frustrations and not minimizing their pain and anguish. On the good days, rejoice with them. Listen to their expressions of ambivalence, and be prepared for the ups and downs and changes of opinion that are sure to occur. Reassure them that their ambivalence is a common response. Encourage "time out" as a way to replenish depleted energy.

Contending with Change

Palliative care team members must realize that not all families communicate openly or work easily together in solving problems. Nurses in particular can support patients and family members to contend with change by creating an environment in which families explore and manage their own concerns and feelings according to their particular coping style. Providing information so that families can explore various alternatives helps them to determine what adjustments they can make. Make information available not only verbally but also in writing. Or, tape-record informative discussions so that families can revisit what they have been told.

Rituals can be helpful during periods of terminal illness. A family ritual is a behavior or action that reflects some symbolic meaning for all members of the family and is part of their collective experience. A ritual does not have to be religious in nature. Rituals may already exist, or they can be newly created to assist the family in contending with change. For example, the writing of an "ethical will," whereby one passes on wisdom to others or elaborates on his or her hopes for their loved ones' future, can help ill family members communicate what they might not be able to verbalize to their loved ones. Developing new rituals can help with the changes in everyday life; for example, one woman had always been the sounding board for her children on their return from school. It was a pattern that continued as her children entered the work force. Cancer of the trachea prevented her participation in the same way. Instead, she requested her young adult children to sit by her side, hold her hand, and recount their days. Instead of words, the mother responded with varying hand squeezes to let them know she was listening. The altered daily ritual served both mother and children in adapting to the changes in their lives.

Searching for Meaning

Palliative care professionals help families search for meaning by enabling them to tell their personal story and make sense of it. It is essential that team members appreciate the value of storytelling—when families talk about their current situation and recollections of the past, it is not just idle chatter. It is a vital part of making sense of the situation and coping with it. Professional team members must appreciate that much of searching for meaning involves examining spiritual dimensions, belief systems, values, and relationships within and outside the family. Nurses can be supportive by suggesting approaches for personal reflection, such as journal writing or writing letters.

Living Day to Day

In living day to day, families make subtle shifts in their orientation to living with a dying family member. They move from thinking that there is no future to making the most of the time they have left. This is a good time to review the resources available to the family, to ensure that they are using all possible sources of assistance so that their time together is optimally spent.

Preparing for Death

In helping families prepare for death, nurses in particular must be comfortable talking about the inevitability of death, describing the dying process, and helping families make plans for wills and funerals. It is important not to push or force such issues; it is equally important not to avoid them because of the nurse's personal discomfort with dying and death. Encourage such discussions among family members while acknowledging how difficult they can be. Affirm them for their courage to face these difficult issues. Encourage patients to attend to practical details, such as finalizing a will and distributing possessions. Encourage them to do "last things," such as participating in a special holiday celebration.

Provide information to spouses and children about the dying process. If the plan is for death at home, provide information about what procedures will need to be followed and the resources that are available. Provide opportunities for family members to express their concerns and ask questions. Encourage them to reminisce with the patient as a way of saying "good-bye" and acknowledge the bittersweet quality of such remembrances. Provide information to the adult children about how they can help their own children with the impending death.

The foregoing guidelines are intended to assist nurses and all members of the palliative care team in their care of individual family members. The guidelines are summarized in Table 28–1. In addition, family-centered care also means focusing on

Table 28–1
Dimensions of Fading Away: Nursing Interventions for Family Members

Redefining

Appreciate that relinquishing old and comfortable views of themselves occurs over time and does not necessarily occur simultaneously with physical changes in the patient

Tailor interventions according to the various abilities of family members to assimilate the changes

Reassure family members that a range of responses and coping strategies is to be expected within and among family members

Provide opportunities for patients to talk about the illness, the enforced changes in their lives, and the ways in which they have adapted; for spouses to talk about how changes in the patient affect their marital relationship; and for children to talk about their own feelings of vulnerability and the degree to which they want to be open or private about the situation

Reinforce normal patterns of living for as long as possible and as appropriate. When patterns are no longer viable, consider adjustments or alternatives

Focus on the patient's attributes that remain intact, and acknowledge that roles and responsibilities may be expressed differently. Consider adjustments or alternatives when former patterns are no longer feasible

Help spouses consider how they might reorganize priorities and consider resources to help them do this

Help children appreciate their parent from another perspective, such as in recalling favorite stories or identifying legacies left

Burdening

Provide opportunities for patients to talk about fears and anxieties about dying and death, and to consider with whom to share their concerns

Help patients stay involved for as long as possible as a way of sustaining self-esteem and a sense of control

Assist family members to take on tasks appropriate to their comfort level and skill and share tasks among themselves

Support family members' reassurances to patient that he or she is not a burden. Explain that when patients reaffirm family members for their efforts, this contributes to their feeling appreciated and lessens the potential for feeling burdened

Explain the importance of breaks for family members. Encourage others to take over for patients on a regular basis so family members can take a break

Acknowledge the reorganization of priorities and the considerable adjustment in family routines and extra demands placed on family members. Acknowledge the "work" of caring for all family members

Realize that family members will vary in their ability to assimilate the changes and that a range of reactions and coping strategies is normal

Struggling with Paradox

Appreciate that you, as a nurse, cannot completely alleviate the psychosocial-spiritual pain inherent in the family's struggle

Assess your own comfort level in working with people facing paradoxical situations and ambivalent feelings

Provide opportunities for family members to mourn the loss of their hopes and plans. Do not minimize these losses; help them modify their previous hopes and plans and consider new ones

Listen to their expressions of ambivalence, and be prepared for the ups and downs of opinions

Ensure effective symptom management, because this allows patients and family members to focus outside the illness

Explain the importance of respite as a strategy for renewing energy for dealing with the situation

(continued)

Table 28–1
Dimensions of Fading Away: Nursing Interventions for Family Members *(continued)*

Contending with Change

- Create an environment in which family members can explore and manage their own concerns and feelings. Encourage dialogue about family members' beliefs, feelings, hopes, fears, and dilemmas so they can determine their own course of action
- Recognize that families communicate in well-entrenched patterns and their ability to communicate openly and honestly differs
- Normalize the experience of family members and explain that such feelings do not negate the positive feelings of concern and affection
- Provide information so families can explore the available resources, their options, and the pros and cons of the various options. Provide information in writing as well as verbally
- Explain the wide-ranging nature of the changes that occur within the patient's immediate and extended family

Searching for Meaning

- Appreciate that the search for meaning involves examination of the self, of relationships with other family members, and of spiritual aspects.
- Realize that talking about the current situation and their recollections of past illness and losses is part of making sense of the situation
- Encourage life reviews and reminiscing. Listen to the life stories that family members tell
- Suggest approaches for self-examination such as journal writing, and approaches for facilitating interactions between family members such as writing letters

Living Day to Day

- Listen carefully for the subtle shifts in orientation to living with a dying relative and gauge family members' readiness for a new orientation
- Ensure effective control of symptoms so that the patient can make the most of the time available. Assess the need for aids
- Without minimizing their losses and concerns, affirm their ability to appreciate and make the most of the time left
- Review resources that would free family members to spend more time with the patient

Preparing for Death

- Assess your own comfort level in talking about the inevitability of death, describing the dying process, and helping families make plans for wills and funerals
- Provide information about the dying process
- Discuss patients' preferences about the circumstances of their death. Encourage patients to discuss these issues with their family. Acknowledge how difficult such discussions can be
- Encourage patients to do important "last things," such as completing a project as a legacy for their family
- Provide opportunities for spouses and children to express their concerns about their future without the patient. Provide them with opportunities to reminisce about their life together. Acknowledge such remembrances will have a bittersweet quality

Source: Davies et al. (1995), reference 17.

the family as a unit. Health care providers must appreciate that the family as a whole has a life of its own that is distinct but always connected to the individuals who are part of it. Both levels of care are important.[17] The families in the "fading away" study also provided insights about how family functioning plays a role in coping with terminal illness in a family member.

Family Functioning and Fading Away

Families experienced the transition of fading away with greater or lesser difficulty, depending on their level of functioning according to eight dimensions: integrating the past, dealing with feelings, solving problems, utilizing resources, considering others, portraying family identity, fulfilling roles, and tolerating differences. These dimensions occurred along a continuum of functionality; family interactions tended to vary along this continuum rather than being positive or negative, good or bad.

Some families acknowledged the pain of past experience with illness, loss, and other adversity and integrated previous learning into how they were managing their current situation. These families expressed a range of feelings, from happiness and satisfaction, through uncertainty and dread, to sadness and sorrow. Family members acknowledged their vulnerabilities and their ambivalent feelings. All topics were open for discussion. There were no clearcut rights and wrongs, and no absolute answers to the family's problems. They applied a flexible approach to problem-solving and openly exchanged all information. They engaged in mutual decision-making, considering each member's point of view and feelings. Each family member was permitted to voice both positive and negative opinions in the process of making decisions. They agreed on the characteristics of their family and allowed individual variation within the family. They allocated household and patient care responsibilities in a flexible way. These families were often

Table 28–2
Dimensions of Family Functioning: Examples of the Range of Behaviors

More Helpful	Less Helpful
Integrating the Past	
Describe the painful experiences as they relate to present experience	Describe past experiences repeatedly
Describe positive and negative feelings concerning the past	Dwell on painful feeling associated with past experiences
Incorporate learning from the past into subsequent experiences	Do not integrate learning from the past to the current situation
Reminisce about pleasurable experiences in the past	Focus on trying to "fix" the past to create happy memories which are absent from their family life
Dealing with Feelings	
Express a range of feelings including vulnerability, fear, and uncertainty	Express predominantly negative feelings, such as anger, hurt, bitterness, and fear
Acknowledge paradoxical feelings	Acknowledge little uncertainty or few paradoxical feelings
Solving Problems	
Identify problems as they occur	Focus more on fault finding than on finding solutions
Reach consensus about a problem and possible courses of action	Dwell on the emotions associated with the problem
Consider multiple options	Unable to clearly communicate needs and expectations
Open to suggestions	Feel powerless about influencing the care they are receiving
Approach problems as a team rather than as individuals	Display exaggerated response to unexpected events
	Withhold or inaccurately share information with other family members
Utilizing Resources	
Utilize a wide range of resources	Utilize few resources
Open to accepting support	Reluctant to seek help or accept offers of help
Open to suggestions regarding resources	Receive help mostly from formal sources rather than from informal support networks
Take the initiative in procuring additional resources	
Express satisfaction with results obtained	Express dissatisfaction with help received
Describe the involvement of many friends, acquaintances, and support persons	Describe fewer friends and acquaintances who offer help
Considering Others	
Acknowledge multidimensional effects of situation on other family members	Focus concern on own emotional needs
Express concern for well-being of other family members	Fail to acknowledge or minimize extra tasks taken on by others
Focus concern on patient's well-being	
Appreciate individualized attention from health care professionals, but do not express strong need for such attention	Display inordinate need for individualized attention
Direct concerns about how other family members are managing rather than with themselves	
Identify characteristic coping styles of family unit and of individual members	Describe own characteristic coping styles rather than the characteristic way the family as a unit coped
Demonstrate warmth and caring toward other family members	Allow one member to dominate group interaction
Consider present situation as potential opportunity for family's growth and development	Lack comfort with expressing true feelings in the family group
Value contributions of all family members	Feign group consensus where none exists
Describe a history of closeness among family members	Describe few family interactions prior to illness

(continued)

Table 28–2
Dimensions of Family Functioning: Examples of the Range of Behaviors *(continued)*

More Helpful	Less Helpful
Fulfilling Roles	
Demonstrate flexibility in adapting to role changes	Demonstrate rigidity in adapting to role changes and responsibilities
Share extra responsibilities willingly	Demonstrate less sharing of responsibilities created by extra demands of patient care
Adjust priorities to incorporate extra demands of patient care and express satisfaction with this decision	Refer to caregiving as a duty or obligation
	Criticize or mistrust caregiving provided by others
Tolerating Differences	
Allow differing opinions and beliefs within the family	Display intolerance for differing opinions or approaches of caregiving
Tolerate different views from people outside the family	Demonstrate critical views of friends who fail to respond as expected
Willing to examine own belief and value systems	Adhere rigidly to belief and value systems

Source: Davies, et al. (1994), reference 46. Reprinted with permission.

amenable to outside intervention and were comfortable in seeking and using external resources. Such families were often appealing to palliative care nurses and other personnel, because they openly discussed their situation, shared their concerns, and accepted help willingly.

Other families were more challenging for palliative care professionals. These were families who hung on to negative past experiences and continued to dwell on the painful feelings associated with past events. They appeared to avoid the feelings of turmoil and ambivalence, shielding themselves from the pain, often indicating that they did not usually express their feelings. These families approached problems by focusing more on why the problem occurred and who was at fault rather than generating potential solutions. They often were unable to communicate their needs or expectations to each other or to health care professionals and were angry when their wishes were not fulfilled. They expressed discrepant views only in individual interviews, not when all members were present, and tended not to tolerate differences. Varying approaches by health care workers were not generally well tolerated either. These families did not adapt easily to new roles, nor did they welcome outside assistance. Such families showed little concern for others. They used few resources, because family members were often unable or reluctant to seek help from others. Such families often presented a challenge for nursing care. Nurses must realize expecting such families to "pull together" to cope with the stresses of palliative care is unrealistic. It is essential not to judge these families, but rather to appreciate that the family is coping as best it can under very difficult circumstances. These families need support and affirmation of their existing coping strategies, not judgmental criticisms.

Palliative care clinicians are encouraged to complete assessments of level of family system functioning early in their encounters with families.[43,44] This is the best time to begin to develop an understanding of the family as a whole, as a basis for the services to be offered. In fact, the value of focusing on patterns of family functioning has been demonstrated by a clinical approach that screens for families, rather than individuals, at high risk.[45] Assessment of family functioning provides a basis for effective interactions to ensure a family-focused approach in palliative care. The eight dimensions of family functioning provide a guideline for assessment. Table 28–2 summarizes these dimensions and gives examples of the range of behaviors evident in each dimension. The table summarizes those behaviors that on one end of the continuum are more helpful, and on the other end are less helpful to families facing the transition of fading away.

Understanding the concept of family functioning enhances the nurse's ability to assess the unique characteristics of each family. An assessment of family functioning enables the nurse to interact appropriately with the family and help them solve problems more effectively (Table 28–3). For example, in families where communication is open and shared among all members, the nurse can be confident that communication with one family member will be accurately passed on to other members. In families where communication is not as open, the nurse must take extra time to share the information with all members. Or, in families who dwell on their negative past experiences with the health care system, nurses must realize that the establishing trust is likely to require extra effort and time. Families who are open to outside intervention are more likely to benefit from resource referrals; other families may need more encouragement and time to open their doors to external assistance.

Table 28–3
Family Functioning: Guidelines for Interventions in Palliative Care

Assessing Family Functioning	Solving Problems
Use dimensions of family functioning to assess families. For example: Do members focus their concern on the patient's well-being and recognize the effect of the situation on other family members, or do family members focus their concerns on their own individual needs and minimize how others might be affected? Putting your assessment of all the dimensions together will help you determine to what degree you are dealing with a more cohesive family unit or a more loosely coupled group of individuals, and hence what approaches are most appropriate. *Be prepared to collect information over time and from different family members.* Some family members may not be willing to reveal their true feelings until they have developed trust. Others may be reluctant to share differing viewpoints in the presence of one another. In some families, certain individuals take on the role of spokesperson for the family. Assessing whether everyone in the family shares the viewpoints of the spokesperson, or whether different family members have divergent opinions but are reluctant to share them, is a critical part of the assessment. *Listen to the family's story and use clinical judgment to determine where intervention is required.* Part of understanding a family is listening to their story. In some families, the stories tend to be repeated and the feelings associated with them resurface. Talking about the past is a way of being for some families. It is important that the nurse determine whether family members are repeatedly telling their story because they want to be better understood or because they want help to change the way their family deals with the situation. Most often the stories are retold simply because family members want the nurse to understand them and their situation better, not because they are looking for help to change the way their family functions.	*Use your assessment of family functioning to guide your approaches.* For example, in families where there is little consensus about the problems, rigidity in beliefs, and inflexibility in roles and relationships, the common rule of thumb—offering families various options so they may choose those that suit them best—tends to be less successful. For these families, carefully consider which resource provides the best possible fit for that particular family. Offer resources slowly, perhaps one at a time. Focus considerable attention on the degree of disruption associated with the introduction of the resource, and prepare the family for the change that ensues. Otherwise, the family may reject the resource as unsuitable and perceive the experience as yet another example of failure of the health care system to meet their needs. *Be aware of the limitations of family conferences and be prepared to follow up.* Family conferences work well for more cohesive family units. However, where more disparity exists among the members, they may not follow through with the decisions made, even though consensus was apparently achieved. Though not voicing their disagreement, some family members may not be committed to the solution put forward and may disregard the agreed-upon plan. The nurse needs to follow up to ensure that any trouble spots are addressed. *Be prepared to repeat information.* In less-cohesive families, do not assume that information will be accurately and openly shared with other family members. You may have to repeat information several times to different family members and repeat answers to the same questions from various family members. *Evaluate the appropriateness of support groups.* Support groups can be a valuable resource. They help by providing people with the opportunity to hear the perspectives of others in similar situations. However, some family members need more individualized attention than a support group provides. They do not benefit from hearing how others have experienced the situation and dealt with the problems. They need one-to-one interaction focused on themselves with someone with whom they have developed trust. *Adjust care to the level of family functioning.* Some families are more overwhelmed by the palliative care experience than others. Understanding family functioning can help nurses appreciate that expectations for some families to "pull together" to cope with the stress of palliative care may be unrealistic. Nurses need to adjust their care according to the family's way of functioning and be prepared for the fact that working with some families is more demanding and the outcomes achieved are less optimal.

Source: Davies et al. (1995), reference 17.

Nurses, and all palliative care providers, must remember that each family is unique and comes with its own life story and circumstances; listening to their story is central to understanding the family. There may be threads of commonality, but there will not be duplicate experiences. Nurses must assist family members to recognize the essential role they are playing in the experience and to acknowledge their contributions. Most importantly, nurses must realize that each family is doing the best it can. Nurses must sensitively, creatively, and patiently support families as they encounter one of the greatest challenges families must face—the transition of fading away.

REFERENCES

1. Ferrell BR. The family. In Oxford Textbook of Palliative Medicine (D. Doyle, G. Hanks, and N. MacDonald, eds.). Oxford: Oxford University Press, 1998:909–91.
2. Field MJ, Cassell CK, eds. Approaching death: Improving care at the end of life. Washington, DC: National Academy Press, 1997.
3. Harrington V, Lackey NR, Gates MF. Needs of caregivers of clinic and hospice cancer patients. Cancer Nursing, 1996;19: 118–125.
4. O'Reilly F, Finnan F, Allwright S, Davey Smith G, Ben-Shlomo Y. The effects of caring for a spouse with Parkinson's disease on social, psychological and physical well-being. Br J Gen Pract 1996; 46:507–512.
5. Jaarsma T. End-of-life issues in cardiac patients and their families. Eur J Cardiovasc Nurs 2002;1:223–225.
6. Mehta A, Ezer H. My love is hurting: The meaning spouses attribute to their loved ones' pain during palliative care. J Palliat Care 2003;19:87–94.
7. Stajduhar K, Davies B. Palliative care at home: Reflections on HIV/AIDS family caregiving experiences. J Palliat Care 1998; 14:14–22.
8. McNally S, Ben-Shlomo Y, Newman S. The effects respite care on informal carers' well-being: A systematic review. Disab Rehab 1999;21:1–14.
9. Payne S, Smith P, Dean S. Identifying the concerns of informal carers in palliative care. Palliat Med 1999;13:37–44.
10. Proot IM, Abu-Saad HH, Crebolder HF, Goldsteen M, Luker KA, Widdershoven GA. Vulnerability of family caregivers in terminal palliative care at home: Balancing between burden and capacity. Scand J Caring 2003;17:113–121.
11. Strang V, Koop P, Peden J. The experience of respite during home-based family caregiving for persons with advanced cancer. J Palliat Care 2003;18:97–104.
12. Raudonis B, Kirschling M. Family caregivers' perspectives on hospice nursing care. J Palliat Care 1996;12:14–19.
13. Cantor J, Blustein J, Carlson MJ, Gould D. Next-of-kin perceptions in physician responsiveness to symptoms of hospitalized patients near death. J Palliat Med 2003;6:531–539.
14. Kristjanson LJ, Leis A, Koop P, Carriere KC, Mueller B. Family members' care expectations, care perceptions, and satisfaction with advanced cancer care: Results of a multi-site pilot study. J Palliat Care 1997;13:5–13.
15. Baker R, Wu AW, Teno JM, Kreling B, Daminano AM, Rubin HR, Roach MJ, Wenger NS, Phillips RS, Desbiens NA, Connors AF Jr, Knause W, Lynn J. Family satisfaction with end-of-life care in seriously ill hospitalized patients: Findings of the SUPPORT program. J Am Geriatr Soc 2000;48:S61–S69.
16. Albinsson L, Strang P. Differences in supporting families of dementia patients and cancer patients: A palliative perspective. Palliat Med 2003;17:359–367.
17. Davies B, Chekryn Reimer J, Brown P, Martens N. Fading Away: The Experience of Transition in Families with Terminal Illness. Amityville, NY: Baywood, 1995.
18. Bridges W. Transitions: Making Sense of Life's Changes. Reading, MA: Addison-Wesley, 1980.
19. Sherman DW. Reciprocal suffering: The need to improve family caregivers' quality of life through palliative care. J Palliat Care 1998;1:357–366.
20. Koop P, Strang V. The bereavement experience following home-based family caregiving for persons with advanced cancer. Clin Nurs Res 2003;12:127–144.
21. Yang C, Kirschling JM. Exploration of factors related to direct care and outcomes of caregiving. Cancer Nurs 1992;15: 173–181.
22. Carter PA. Caregivers' descriptions of sleep changes and depressive symptoms. Oncol Nurs Forum 2002;29:1277–1283.
23. Davies BD, Cowley SA, Ryland RK. The effects of terminal illness on patients and their caregivers. J Adv Nurs 1996;23: 512–520.
24. Steele R, Fitch M. Needs of family caregivers of patients receiving home hospice care for cancer. Oncol Nurs Forum 1996; 23:823–828.
25. Scott G, Whyler N, Grant G. A study of family carers of people with a life-threatening illness 1: The carers' needs analysis. Int Palliat Nurs 2001;7:290–297.
26. Emanuel EJ, Fairclough L, Slutsman J, Alpert H., Baldwin D, Emanuel LL. Assistance from family members, friends, paid care givers, and volunteers in the care of terminally ill patients. N Engl J Med 1999;341:956–963.
27. Carr D. A "good death" for whom? Quality of spouse's death and psychological distress among older widowed persons. J Health Social Behav 2003;44:215–232.
28. Teno JM, Clarridge BR, Casey V, Welch LC, Wetle T, Shield R, Mor V. Family perspectives on end-of-life care at the last place of death. JAMA 2004;291:88–93.
29. Tschann JM, Kaufman SR, Micco GP. Family involvement in end-of-life hospital care. J Am Geriatr Soc 2003;51:835–840.
30. Perreault A, Fothergill-Bourbonnais F, Fiset V. The experience of family members caring for a dying loved one. Int J Palliat Nurs 2004;10:133–143.
31. Jarrett N, Payne S, Wilkes RA. Terminally ill patients and lay carers perceptions of and experiences of community health services. J Adv Nurs 1999;29:476–483.
32. Beaver K, Luker K, Woods S. Primary care services received curing terminal illness. Int J Palliat Nurs 2000;6:220–227.
33. Thomas K. Out-of-hours palliative care: Bridging the gap. Eur J Palliat Care 2000;7:22–25.
34. Addington-Hall J, Karlsen S. Do home deaths increase distress in bereavement? Palliat Med 2000;14:161–162.
35. Aranda SK, Hayman-White K. Home caregivers of the person with advanced cancer: An Australian perspective. Cancer Nurs 2001;24:300–307.
36. Stajduhar KI. Examining the perspectives of family members involved in the delivery of palliative care at home. J Palliat Care 2003;19:27–35.
37. Stajduhar KI, Davies B. Variations in and factors influencing family members' decisions for palliative home care. Palliat Med. In press.
38. Ellershaw J, Foster A, Murphy D, Shea T, Overill S. Developing an integrated care pathway for the dying patients. Eur J Palliat Care 1997;4:203–207.
39. Pooler J, McCrory F, Steadman Y, Westwell H, Peers S. Dying at home: A care pathway for the last days of life in a community setting. Int J Palliat Nurs 2003;9:258–264.
40. Doyle D. Palliative medicine in the home: An overview. In: Doyle D, Hanks G, MacDonald N, eds. Oxford Textbook of Palliative Care, 2nd ed. Oxford: Oxford University Press, 2004: 1097–1114.
41. Stajduhar K, Davies B. Death at home: Challenges for families and directions for the future. J Palliat Care 1996;14:8–14.

42. Davies B. Environmental factors affecting sibling bereavement. In: Davies B. Shadows in the Sun: Experiences of Sibling Bereavement in Childhood. Philadelphia: Brunner/Mazel. 1999: 123–148.
43. Jassak P. Families: An essential element in the care of the patient with cancer. Oncol Nurs Forum 1992;19:871–986.
44. Gulla J. Family assessment and its relation to hospice care. Am J Hospice Palliat Care 1992(July/August):30–34.
45. Kissane DW, McKenzie M, McKenzie DP, Forbes A, O'Neill I, Block S. Psychosocial morbidity associated with patterns of family functioning in palliative care: Baseline data from the Family Focused Grief Therapy controlled trial. Palliat Med 2003;17: 527–537.
46. Davies B, Reimer J, Maartens N. Family functioning and its implications for palliative care. J Palliat Care 1994;10:35–36.

29

Patricia Berry and Julie Griffie

Planning for the Actual Death

There is a sweetness to being there when someone dies, as I was with my father. I held his hand as he died and will never forget how warm his hand was, even after he was gone. The veil between this life and the next, I believe, is thin. I sensed his spirit leave his body but it remained in the room long after he had died, as if he was trying to say to me, "Marsha, it was my time and I am now in a better place." As an obstetrics nurse, I have witnessed many births but few deaths, but am struck by the similarities between them. Birth and death—the beginnings and endings we all experience as humans—are indeed sacred events.—A daughter

- ***Key Points***
- *The care of patients and families near to death and afterward is an important nursing function—arguably one of the most important. There are often no dress rehearsals; nurses and other health care professionals often only have one chance to "get it right."*
- *Aggressive management of symptoms remains a priority as death approaches.*
- *As the dying person nears death, the goals of care often change with patient and family needs, desires, and perspectives, providing a different experience for everyone.*
- *Care of the body after death, including honoring rituals and individual requests, can clearly communicate to the family that the person who died was indeed important and valued.*

Issues and needs at the time of death are exceedingly important and, at the same time, exceedingly personal. Although the physiology of dying may be the same for most expected deaths, the psychological, spiritual, cultural, and family issues are as unique and varied as the patients and families themselves. As death nears, the goals of care must be discussed and appropriately redefined. Some treatments may be discontinued, and symptoms may intensify, subside, or even appear anew. Physiological changes as death approaches must also be defined, explained, and interpreted to the patient, whenever possible, as well as to the patient's family, close others, and caregivers. The nurse occupies a key position in assisting patients' family members at the time of death by supporting or suggesting death rituals, caring for the body after death, and facilitating early grief work. Most of the focus on death and dying in the past has been on dying in general, making the need for a chapter focused specifically on the actual death even more important.

Terminally ill persons are cared for in a variety of settings, including home settings with hospice care or traditional home care, hospice residential facilities, nursing homes, assisted living facilities, hospitals, intensive care units, prisons, and group homes. Deaths in intensive care settings may present special challenges, such as restrictive visiting hours and lack of space and less privacy for families—shortcomings that may be addressed by thoughtful and creative nursing care. Likewise, death in a nursing home setting may also offer unique challenges. Regardless of the setting, good management can minimize distressing symptoms and maximize quality of life. Families can be supported in a way that optimizes use of valuable time and lessens distress during the bereavement period. Like it or not, health professionals only have one chance to "get it right" when caring for dying persons and their families as death nears. In other words, there is no dress rehearsal for the time surrounding death; extensive planning ensures the least stressful and best possible outcome for all involved.

The patient's family is especially important as death nears. Family members may become full- or part-time caregivers;

daughters and sons may find themselves in a position to "parent" their parents; and family issues, long forgotten or ignored, may surface. Although "family" is often thought of in traditional terms, a family may take on several forms and configurations. For purposes of this chapter, the definition of family recognizes that many patients have nontraditional families and may be cared for by a large extended entity, such as a church community, a group of supportive friends, or the staff of a health care facility. Family is defined broadly to include not only persons bound by biology or legal ties but also those whom the patient defines or who define themselves as "close others" or who function for the patient in "familistic" ways. These functions can include nurturance; intimacy; economic, social, and psychological support in times of need; support in illness (including dealing with those outside the family); and companionship.[1,2]

The research regarding uncontrolled symptoms at the end of life is misleading. It is most often performed in palliative care units or other settings dedicated to end-of-life care, in which the goals of care are focused on ensuring maximal symptom management. However, most studies demonstrate that the majority of people do not have a death in which symptoms are well managed.[3,4] Up to 52% of persons have refractory symptoms at the very end of life that, at times, require terminal sedation.[5] Dyspnea may worsen as death approaches. The notion of a final crescendo of pain is supported in some studies and not in others. Many patients experience a higher frequency of noisy and moist breathing, urinary incontinence and retention, restlessness, agitation, delirium, and nausea and vomiting.[6,7] Less frequently, symptoms such as sweating, myoclonus, and confusion have been reported.[8]

Ventafridda and colleagues[8] reported that, although most patients (91.5%) die peacefully, 8.5% experience symptoms requiring additional intervention in the final 24 hours, such as hemorrhage or hemoptysis (2%), respiratory distress (2%), restlessness (1.5%), pain (1%), myocardial infarction (1%), and regurgitation (1%). The wide variation in frequency of symptoms and reported "good deaths" may result from differing populations and sites of care (e.g., home, specialized palliative care unit, inpatient hospice), differing measurement protocols or instruments, and the participants' cultural variations in reporting symptoms and approaching death. In most studies, symptoms requiring maximum diligence in assessment, prevention, and aggressive treatment during the final day or two before death were respiratory tract secretions, pain, dyspnea, restlessness, and agitation.[7,9] Some authors emphasized that persons with cognitive impairment require specific attention to symptoms, especially as death nears.[9] The nurse plays a key role in educating family members and other caregivers about the assessment, treatment, and continual evaluation of these symptoms.

Regardless of individual patient and family needs, attitudes, and "unfinished business," the nurse's professional approach and demeanor at the time near death is crucial and worthy of close attention. Patients experience total and profound dependency at this stage of their illness. Families are often called upon to assume total caregiving duties, often disrupting their own responsibilities for home, children, and career. Although there may be similarities, patients and families experience this time through the lens of their own perspective and form their own unique meaning.

Some authors suggest theories and guidelines as the basis for establishing and maintaining meaningful, helpful, and therapeutic relationships with patients or clients and their families. One example is Carl Rogers' theory of helping relationships, in which he proposed that the characteristics of a helping relationship are empathy, unconditional positive regard, and genuineness.[10] These characteristics, defined later as part of the nurse's approach to patients and families, are essential in facilitating care at the end of life. To this may be added "attention to detail," because this additional characteristic is essential for quality palliative care.[11,12] Readers are urged to consider the following characteristics in the context of their own practices, as a basis for facilitating and providing supportive relationships:

- *Empathy:* the ability to put oneself in the other person's place, trying to understand the patient or client from his or her own frame of reference; it also requires the deliberate setting aside of one's own frame of reference and bias.
- *Unconditional positive regard:* a warm feeling toward others, with a nonjudgmental acceptance of all they reveal themselves to be; the ability to convey a sense of respect and esteem at a time and place in which it is particularly important to do so.
- *Genuineness:* the ability to convey trustworthiness and openness that is real rather than a professional facade; also the ability to admit that one has limitations, makes mistakes, and does not have all the answers.
- *Attention to detail:* the learned and practiced ability to think critically about a situation and not make assumptions. The nurse, for example, discusses challenging patient and family concerns with colleagues and other members of the interdisciplinary team. The nurse considers every "what if " before making a decision and, in particular, before making any judgment. Finally, the nurse is constantly aware of how his or her actions, attitudes, and words may be interpreted—or misinterpreted—by others.[11]

The events and interactions—positive as well as negative—at the bedside of a dying person set the tone for the patient's care and form lasting memories for family members. The time of death and the care received by both the individual who has died and the family members who are present are predominant aspects of the survivors' memories of this momentous event.[13] Approaching patients and families with a genuine openness characterized by empathy and positive regard eases the way in making this difficult time meaningful, individualized, and deeply profound.

This chapter discusses some key issues surrounding the death itself, including advanced planning, the changing focus of care as death nears, common signs and symptoms of death and their management, and care of the patient and family at time of death. It concludes with two case examples illustrating the chapter's content.

Advanced Planning: Evolving Choices and Goals of Care

Health care choices related to wellness are generally viewed as clearcut or easy. We have an infection, we seek treatment, and the problem resolves. Throughout most of the lifespan, medical treatment choices are obvious. As wellness moves along the health care continuum to illness, choices become less clear and consequences of choices have a significantly greater impact.

Many end-of-life illnesses manifest with well-known and well-documented natural courses. Providing the patient and family with information on the natural course of the disease at appropriate intervals is a critical function of health care providers such as nurses. Providing an opening for discussion, such as, "Would you like to talk about the future?" "Do you have any concerns that I can help you address?" or "It seems you are not as active as you were before," may allow a much-needed discussion of fears and concerns about impending death. Family members may request information that patients do not wish to know at certain points in time. With the patient's permission, discussions with the family may occur in the patient's absence. Family members may also need coaching to initiate end-of-life discussions with the patient. End-of-life goal setting is greatly enhanced when the patient is aware of the support of family.

End-of-life care issues should always be discussed with patients and family members. The competent patient is always the acknowledged decision-maker. The involvement of family ensures maximal consensus for patient support as decisions are actually implemented. Decisions for patients who lack decision-making capacity should be made by a consensus approach, using family conference methodology. If documents such as a durable power of attorney for health care or a living will are available, they can be used as a guide for examining wishes that influence decision-making and goal-setting. The decision-maker, usually the person named as health care power of attorney (HCPOA) or the patient's primary family members, should be clearly identified. This approach may also be used with patients who are able to make their own decisions.

To facilitate decision-making, a family conference involving the decision makers (decisional patient, family members, and the HCPOA), the patient's physician, nurse, chaplain, and social worker is initiated. A history of how the patient's health care status evolved from diagnosis to the present is reviewed. The family is presented with the natural course of the disease. Choices on how care may proceed in the future are reviewed. Guidance or support for those choices is provided based on existing data and clinical experience with the particular disease in relation to the current status of the patient. If no consensus for the needed decisions occurs, decision-making is postponed. Third-party support by a trusted individual or consultant may then be enlisted. Personal fundamental values of the patient, family, and physician should be recognized and protected throughout this process.[14]

Decisions by patients and families cross the spectrum of care. They range from continuing treatment for the actual disease, such as undergoing chemotherapy or renal dialysis or utilization of medications, to initiating cardiopulmonary resuscitation (CPR). The health care provider may work with the patient and family, making care decisions for specific treatments and timing treatment discontinuance within a clear and logical framework. A goal-setting discussion may determine a patient's personal framework for care, such as

- Treatment and enrollment in any clinical studies for which I am eligible
- Treatment as long as statistically there is a greater than 50% chance of response
- Full treatment as long as I am ambulatory and able to come to the clinic or office
- Treatment only of "fixable" conditions such as infections or blood glucose levels
- Treatment only for controlling symptomatic aspects of disease

Once a goal framework has been established with the patient, the appropriateness of interventions such as CPR, renal dialysis, or intravenous antibiotics is clear. For instance, if the patient states a desire for renal dialysis as long as transportation to the clinic is possible without the use of an ambulance, the endpoint of dialysis treatment is quite clear. At this point, the futility of CPR would also be apparent. Allowing a patient to determine when the treatment is a burden that is unjustified by his or her value system, and communicating this determination to family and caregivers, is perhaps the most pivotal point in management of the patient's care. Table 29–1 suggests a format for an effective and comprehensive family conference.

Changing the Focus of Care as Death Nears

Vital Signs

As nurses, we derive a good deal of security in performing the ritual of measurement of vital signs, one of the hallmarks of

Table 29–1
Family Conference

I. Why: Clarify goals in your own mind.

II. Where: Provide comfort, privacy, circular seating.

III. Who: Include legal decision maker/health care power of attorney; family members; social support; key health care professionals.

IV. How:

- A. Introduction
  1. Introduce self and others.
  2. Review meeting goals: State meeting goals and specific decisions.
  3. Establish ground rules: Each person will have a chance to ask questions and express views; no interruptions; identify legal decision-maker, and describe importance of supportive decision-making.
- B. Review medical status
  1. Review current status, plan, and prognosis.
  2. Ask each family member in turn for any questions about current status, plan, and prognosis.
  3. Defer discussion of decision until the next step.
- C. Family discussion with decisional patient
  1. Ask patient, "What decision(s) are you considering?"
  2. Ask each family member, "Do you have questions or concerns about the treatment plan? How can you support the patient?"
- D. Family discussion with nondecisional patient
  1. Ask each family member in turn, "What do you believe the patient would choose if he (or she) could speak for himself (or herself)?"
  2. Ask each family member, "What do you think should be done?"
  3. Leave room to let family discuss alone.
  4. If there is consensus, go to V; if no consensus, go to E.
- E. When there is no consensus:
  1. Restate goal: "What would the patient say if he or she could speak?"
  2. Use time as ally: Schedule a follow-up conference the next day.
  3. Try further discussion: "What values is your decision based on? How will the decision affect you and other family members?"
  4. Identify legal decision-maker.
  5. Identify resources: minister/priest; other physicians; ethics committee.

V. Wrap-up

1. Summarize consensus, decisions, and plan.
2. Caution against unexpected outcomes.
3. Identify family spokesperson for ongoing communication.
4. Document in the chart who was present, what decisions were made, follow-up plan.
5. Approach discontinuation of treatment as an interdisciplinary team, not just as a nursing function.
6. Continuity: Maintain contact with family and medical team; schedule follow-up meetings as needed.

VI. Family dynamics and decisions

1. Family structure: Respect the family hierarchy whenever possible.
2. Established patterns of family interaction will continue.
3. Unresolved conflicts between family members may be evident.
4. Past problems with authority figures, doctors, and hospitals affect the process; ask specifically about bad experiences in the past.
5. Family grieving and decision-making may include
   - Denial: False hopes.
   - Guilt: Fear of letting go.
   - Depression: Passivity and inability to decide; or anger and irritability.

Source: Adapted from Ambuel & Weissman (2001), reference 50. Copyright © 2001, Medical College of Wisconsin, Inc.

nursing care. When death is approaching, we need to question the rationale for measuring vital signs. Are interventions going to change if it is discovered that the patient has experienced a drop in blood pressure? If the plan of care no longer involves intervening in changes in blood pressure and pulse rate, the measurements should cease. The time spent taking vital signs can then be channeled to assessment of patient comfort and provision of family support. Changes in respiratory rate are visually noted and do not require routine monitoring of rates, unless symptom management issues develop that could be more accurately assessed by measurement of vital signs. The measurement of body temperature using a noninvasive route should continue on a regular basis until death, allowing for the detection and management of fever, a frequent symptom that can cause distress and may require management.

Fever often suggests infection. As death approaches, goal setting should include a discussion of the nontreatment of infection. Indications for treatment of infection are based on the degree of distress and patient discomfort.[15] Pharmacological management of fever should be available with antipyretics, including acetaminophen, and nonsteroidal antiinflammatory drugs for all patients. Ice packs, alcohol baths, and cooling blankets should be used cautiously, because they often cause more distress than the fever itself.[16]

Fever may also suggest dehydration. As with the management of fever, interventions are guided by the degree of distress and patient discomfort. The appropriateness of beginning artificial hydration for the treatment of fever is based on individual patient assessment.

Cardiopulmonary Resuscitation

Patients and family members may need to discuss the issue of the futility of CPR when death is expected from a terminal illness. Developed in the 1960s as a method of restarting the heart in the event of sudden, unexpected clinical death, CPR was originally intended for circumstances in which death was unexpected or accidental. It is not indicated in certain situations, such as cases of terminal irreversible illness where death is not unexpected; resuscitation in these circumstances may represent an active violation of a person's right to die with dignity.[17,18]

Over the years, predictors of the success of CPR have become apparent, along with the predictors of the burden of CPR. In general, a poor outcome of CPR is predicted in patients with advanced terminal illnesses, patients with dementia, and patients with poor functional status who depend on others for meeting their basic care needs. Poor outcomes or physical problems resulting from CPR include fractured ribs, punctured lung, brain damage if anoxia has occurred for too long, and permanent unconsciousness or persistent vegetative state.[19] Most importantly, the use of CPR negates the possibility of a peaceful death. This is considered the gravest of poor outcomes.

Artificial Fluids

The issue of artificial hydration is emotional for many patients and families because of the role that giving and consuming fluids plays in our culture. When patients are not able to take fluids, concern surfaces among caregivers. A decision must be reached regarding the appropriate use of fluids within the context of the patient's framework of goals. Beginning artificial hydration is a relatively easy task, but the decision to stop is generally much more problematic given the emotional implications. Ethical, moral, and most religious viewpoints state that there is no difference between withholding and withdrawing a treatment such as artificial hydration. However, the emotional response attached to withdrawing a treatment adds a world of difference to the decision to suspend. It is therefore much less burdensome to not begin treatment, if this decision is acceptable in light of the specific patient circumstances.[20]

Most patients and families are aware that, without fluids, death will occur quickly. The literature suggests that fluids should not be routinely administered to dying patients, nor automatically withheld from them. Instead, the decision should be based on careful, individual assessment. Zerwekh[21] suggested consideration of the following questions when the choice to initiate or continue hydration is evaluated:

- Is the patient's well-being enhanced by the overall effect of hydration?
- Which current symptoms are being relieved by artificial hydration?
- Are other end-of-life symptoms being aggravated by the fluids?
- Does hydration improve the patient's level of consciousness? If so, is this within the patient's goals and wishes for end-of-life care?
- Does hydration appear to prolong the patient's survival? If so, is this within the patient's goals and wishes for end-of-life care?
- What is the effect of the infusion technology on the patient's well-being, mobility, and ability to interact and be with family?
- What is the burden of the infusion technology on the family in terms of caregiver stress, finance? Is it justified by benefit to the patient?

A study by Fainsinger and Bruera[22] suggested that, although some dying patients may actually benefit from dehydration, others may manifest symptoms such as confusion or opioid toxicity that can be corrected or prevented by parenteral hydration. In any case, the uniqueness of the individual situation, the goals of care, and the comfort of the patient must always be considered when this issue is addressed.[23]

Terminal dehydration refers to the process in which the dying patient's condition naturally results in a decrease in fluid intake. A gradual withdrawal from activities of daily living may occur as symptoms such as dysphagia, nausea, and fatigue become more obvious. Families commonly ask whether the patient will be thirsty as fluid intake decreases. In a study at St. Christopher's Hospice in Sydenham, England, although patients reported thirst, there was no correlation between thirst and hydration, resulting in the assumption that artificial hydration to relieve symptoms may be futile.[24] Artificial hydration has the potential to result in fluid accumulation, resulting in distressful symptoms such as edema, ascites, nausea and vomiting, and pulmonary congestion.

Does artificial hydration prolong life? Smith[25] cited two studies that reported longer survival times with no artificial hydration. Health care providers need to assist patients and family members to refocus on the natural course of the disease and the notion that the patient's death will be caused by the disease, not by dehydration, a natural occurrence in advanced illness and dying. Nurses may then assist families in dealing with symptoms caused by dehydration.

Dry mouth, a consistently reported distressing symptom of dehydration, can be relieved with sips of beverages, ice chips, or hard candies.[26] Another simple comfort measure for dry mouth is spraying normal saline into the mouth with a spray bottle or atomizer. (Normal saline is made by mixing one teaspoon of table salt in a quart of water.) Meticulous mouth care must be administered to keep the patient's mouth clean. Family members can be instructed to anticipate this need. The nurse can facilitate this care by ensuring that the necessary provisions are on hand to assist the patient.

Medications

Medications unrelated to the terminal diagnosis are generally continued as long as their administration is not burdensome. When swallowing pills becomes too difficult, the medication may be offered in a liquid or other form if available, considering patient and family comfort. Continuing medications, however, may be seen by some patients and families as a way of normalizing daily activities and therefore should be supported. Considerable tact, kindness, and knowledge of the patient and family are needed in assisting them to make decisions about discontinuing medications.

Medications that do not contribute to daily comfort should be evaluated on an individual basis for possible discontinuance. Medications such as antihypertensives, replacement hormones, vitamin supplements, iron preparations, hypoglycemics, long-term antibiotics, antiarrhythmics, laxatives, and diuretics, unless they are essential to patient comfort, can and should be discontinued unless doing so would cause symptoms or discomfort.[27] Customarily, the only drugs necessary in the final days of life are analgesics, anticonvulsants, antiemetics, antipyretics, anticholenergic medications, and sedatives.[27]

Implantable Cardioverter Defibrillator

Implantable cardioverter defibrillators (ICDs) are used to prevent cardiac arrest due to ventricular tachycardia or ventricular fibrillation. Patients with ICDs who are dying of another terminal condition may choose to have the defibrillator deactivated, or turned off, so that there will be no interference from the device at the time of death. Patients with ICDs who enter a hospice or palliative care program with diagnoses such as advanced terminal cancer or end-stage renal disease and have decided to stop dialysis are candidates for such consideration.

Patients with ICDs have been instructed to carry a wallet identification card at all times that provides the model and serial number of the implanted device.[28] The identification card will also have the name of the physician to contact for assistance. Deactivating the ICD is a simple, noninvasive procedure. Standard practice calls for the patient to sign a consent form. The device is tested after it is turned off to ensure that it is no longer operational, and the test result is placed in the patient record. Patients who are at peace with their impending death find this procedure important to provide assurance that death indeed will be quiet and easy, when it does occur.

Corticosteroids in Patients with Intracranial Malignancy

In most cases, the patient with an intracranial malignancy will be receiving a corticosteroid such as dexamethasone to control headaches and seizures caused by intracranial swelling. When the patient is nearing death and is no longer able to swallow, the corticosteroids may be discontinued with minimal or no tapering.[29] Discontinuation of the corticosteroid may lead to increased cerebral edema, and, consequently, headache and progressive neurological dysfunction.[29] Addition or adjustment of analgesics and anticonvulsant medications may be needed for the patient's continued comfort.

A patient who is still able to swallow medications may also request that treatment with corticosteroids be stopped because of continued deterioration and poor quality of life. Should this occur, the drug can be tapered, and at the same time an oral anticonvulsant medication can be increased. Careful assessment and control of headache and discomfort should be done twice a day, preferably by the same person. Resumption of the drug at any point is always an option that should be offered to the patient and family if the need becomes apparent.[27,29]

Renal Dialysis

Renal dialysis is a life-sustaining treatment, and as death approaches, it is important to recognize and agree on its limitations. Discontinuation of dialysis should be considered in the following cases[30]:

- Patients with acute, concurrent illness, who, if they survive, will be burdened with a great deal of disability as defined by the patient and family
- Patients with progressive and untreatable disease or disability
- Patients with dementia or severe neurological deficit

There is general agreement that dialysis should not be used to prolong the dying process.[31] The time between discontinuing dialysis and death varies widely, from a matter of hours or days (for patients with acute illnesses, such as those described earlier) to days, weeks, or even longer if some residual renal function remains.[30,31] Opening a discussion about the burden of treatment, however, is a delicate task. There may be competing opinions among the patient, family, and even staff about the tolerability or intolerability of continuing treatment. The nurse who sees the patient and family on a regular basis may be the most logical person to recognize the discrete changes in status. Gently validating these observations may open a much-needed discussion regarding the goals of care.

The discussions and decisions surrounding discontinuation or modification of treatment are never easy. Phrases such as, "There is nothing more that can be done" or "We have tried everything" have no place in end-of-life discussions with patients and families. Always reassure the patient and family members—and be prepared to follow through—that you will stand by them and do all you can to provide help and comfort.[32] This is essential to ensure that palliative care is not interpreted as abandonment.

Common Signs and Symptoms of Imminent Death and Their Management

There usually are predictable sets of processes that occur during the final stages of a terminal illness due to gradual hypoxia, respiratory acidosis, metabolic consequences of renal failure, and the signs and symptoms of hypoxic brain function.[5,33,34] These processes account for the signs and symptoms of imminent death and can assist the nurse in helping the family plan for the actual death.

The following signs and symptoms provide cues that death is only days away[4,5,33]:

- Profound weakness (patient is usually bedbound and requires assistance with all or most care)
- Gaunt and pale physical appearance (most common in persons with cancer if corticosteroids have not been used as treatment)
- Drowsiness and/or a reduction in awareness, insight, and perception (often with extended periods of drowsiness, extreme difficulty in concentrating, severely limited attention span, inability to cooperate with caregivers, disorientation to time and place, or semicomatose state)
- Increasing lack of interest in food and fluid with diminished intake (only able to take sips of fluids)
- Increasing difficulty in swallowing oral medications

During the final days, these signs and symptoms become more pronounced, and, as oxygen concentrations drop, new symptoms also appear. Measurement of oxygen concentration in the dying person is not advocated, because it adds discomfort and does not alter the course of care. However, knowledge of the signs and symptoms associated with decreasing oxygen concentrations can assist the nurse in guiding the family as death nears.[35] As oxygen saturation drops below 80%, signs and symptoms related to hypoxia appear. As the dying process proceeds, special issues related to normalizing the dying process for the family, symptom control, and patient and family support present themselves. Table 29–2 summarizes the physiological process of dying and suggests interventions for both patients and families.

As the imminently dying person takes in less fluid, third-spaced fluids, clinically manifested as peripheral edema, acites, or pleural effusions, may be reabsorbed. Breathing may become easier, and there may be less discomfort from tissue distention. Accordingly, as the person experiences dehydration, swelling is often reduced around tumor masses. Patients may experience transient improvements in comfort, including increased mental status and decreased pain. The family needs a careful and compassionate explanation regarding these temporary improvements and encouragement to make the most of this short but potentially meaningful time.

There are multiple patient and family educational tools available to assist families in interpreting the signs and symptoms of approaching death (Figure 29–1). However, as with all aspects of palliative care, consideration of the individual perspective and associated relationships of the patient or family member, the underlying disease course trajectory, anticipated symptoms, and the setting of care is essential for optimal care at all stages of illness, but especially during the final days and hours.

Care at the Time of Death, Death Rituals, and Facilitating Early Grieving

At the time of death, the nurse has a unique opportunity to provide information helpful in making decisions about organ and body donation and autopsy. In addition, the nurse can support the family's choice of death rituals, gently care for the body, assist in funeral planning, and facilitate the early process of grieving.

Family members' needs around the time of death change, just as the goals of care change. During this important time, plans are reviewed and perhaps refined. Special issues affecting the time of death, such as cultural influences, decisions regarding organ or body donation, and the need for autopsy, are also reviewed.

Under U.S. federal law, if death occurs in a hospital setting, staff must approach the family decision-maker regarding the possibility of organ donation.[37] Although approaching family at this time may seem onerous, the opportunity to assist another is often comforting. Some hospital-based palliative care programs include information about organ donation in their admission or bereavement information. Readers are urged to review their own organizations' policies and procedures.

Table 29–2
Symptoms in the Normal Progression of Dying and Suggested Interventions

Symptoms	Suggested Interventions
Early Stage	
Sensation/Perception	
• Impairment in the ability to grasp ideas and reason; periods of alertness along with periods of disorientation and restlessness are also noted	• Interpret the signs and symptoms to the patient (when appropriate) and family as part of the normal dying process; for example, assure them the patient's "seeing" and even talking to persons who have died is normal and often expected • Urge family members to look for metaphors for death in speech and conversation (e.g., talk of a long journey, needing maps or tickets, or in preparing for a trip in other ways)[36] and using these metaphors as a departure point for conversation with the patient • Urge family to take advantage of the patient's periods of lucidity to talk with patient and ensure nothing is left unsaid • Encourage family members to touch and speak slowly and gently to the patient without being patronizing • Maximize safety; for example, use bedrails and schedule people to sit with the patient
• Some loss of visual acuity	• Keep sensory stimulation to a minimum, including light, sounds, and visual stimulation; reading to a patient who has enjoyed reading in the past may provide comfort
• Increased sensitivity to bright lights while other senses, except hearing, are dulled	• Urge the family to be mindful of what they say "over" the patient, because hearing remains present; also continue to urge family to say what they wish not to be left unsaid
Cardiorespiratory	
• Increased pulse and respiratory rate • Agonal respirations or sounds of gasping for air without apparent discomfort • Apnea, periodic, or Cheyne-Stokes respirations • Inability to cough or clear secretions efficiently, resulting in gurgling or congested breathing (sometimes referred to as the "death rattle")	• Normalize the observed changes by interpreting the signs and symptoms as part of the normal dying process and ensuring the patient's comfort • Assess and treat respiratory distress as appropriate • Assess use and need for parenteral fluids, tube feedings, or hydration. (It is generally appropriate to either discontinue or greatly decrease these at this point in time.) • Reposition the patient in a side-lying position with the head of the bed elevated • Suctioning is rarely needed, but when appropriate, suction should be gentle and only at the level of the mouth, throat, and nasal pharynx • Administer anticholinergic drugs (transdermal scopolamine, hyoscyamine) as appropriate, recognizing and discussing with the family that they will not decrease already existing secretions.
Renal/Urinary	
• *Decreasing urinary output, sometimes urinary incontinence or retention*	• Insert catheter and/or use absorbent padding • Carefully assess for urinary retention, because restlessness can be a related symptom
Musculoskeletal	
• Gradual loss of the ability to move, beginning with the legs, then progressing	• Reposition every few hours as appropriate • Anticipate needs such as sips of fluids, oral care, changing of bed pads and linens, and so on

(continued)

Table 29–2
Symptoms in the Normal Progression of Dying and Suggested Interventions *(continued)*

Symptoms	Suggested Interventions
Late Stage	
Sensation/Perception	
• Unconsciousness • Eyes remain half open, blink reflex is absent; sense of hearing remains intact and may slowly decrease	• Interpret the patient's unconsciousness to the family as part of the normal dying process • Provide for total care, including incontinence of urine and stool • Encourage family members to speak slowly and gently to the patient, with the assurance that hearing remains intact
Cardiorespiratory	
• Heart rate may double, strength of contractions decrease; rhythm becomes irregular • Patient feels cool to the touch and becomes diaphoretic • Cyanosis is noted in the tip of the nose, nail beds, and knees; extremities may become mottled (progressive mottling indicates death within a few days); absence of a palpable radial pulse may indicate death within hours	• Interpret these changes to family members as part of the normal dying process • Frequent linen changes and sponge baths may enhance comfort
Renal/Urinary	
• A precipitous drop in urinary output	• Interpret to the family the drop in urinary output as a normal sign that death is near • Carefully assess for urinary retention; restlessness can be a related symptom

In any case, it is important to clarify specifically with family members what their desires and needs are at the time of death. Do they wish to be present? Do they know of others who wish to now say a final goodbye? Have they said everything they wish to say to the person who is dying? Do they have any regrets? Are they concerned about anything? Do they wish something could be different? Every person in a family has different and unique needs that, unless explored, can go unmet. Family members recall the time before the death and immediately afterward with great acuity and detail. As mentioned earlier, there is no chance for a dress rehearsal—we only have the one chance to "get it right" and make the experience an individual and memorable one.

Although an expected death can be anticipated with some degree of certainty, the exact time of death is often not predictable. Death often occurs when no health care professionals are present. Frequently, dying people seem to determine the time of their own death—for example, waiting for someone to arrive, for a date or event to pass, or even for family members to leave—even if the leave-taking is brief. For this reason, it is crucial to ask family members who wish to be present at the time of death whether they have thought about the possibility they will not be there. This opens an essential discussion regarding the time of death and its unpredictability. Gently reminding family members of that possibility can assist them in preparing for any eventuality.

Determining That Death Has Occurred

Death often occurs when health professionals are not present at the bedside or in the home. Regardless of the site of death, a plan must be in place for who will be contacted, how the death pronouncement will be handled, and how the body will be removed. This is especially crucial for deaths that occur outside a health care institution.

Death pronouncement procedures vary from state to state, and sometimes from county to county within a state. In some states, nurses can pronounce death; in others, they cannot. In inpatient settings, the organization's policy and procedures are followed. In hospice home care, generally the nurse makes a home visit, assesses the lack of vital signs, contacts the physician who verbally agrees to sign the death certificate, and then contacts the funeral home or mortuary. Local customs, the ability of a health care agency to ensure the safety of a nurse during the home visit, and provision for "do-not-resuscitate" orders outside a hospital setting, among other factors, account for wide variability in the practices and procedures surrounding pronouncement of death in the home. Although practices vary widely, the police or coroner may need to be called if the circumstances of the death were unusual, were associated with trauma (regardless of the cause of the death), or occurred within 24 hours of a hospital admission.[38]

HospiceCare
of Boulder and Broomfield Counties

SIGNS AND SYMPTOMS OF APPROACHING DEATH

This list of symptoms and what to do about them may appear frightening, but knowing what to expect may reduce some of your anxiety about the approaching death.

Each person approaches death in their own way, bringing to this last experience their own uniqueness. Our list of "Symptoms and What To Do" is a map to the goal of a peaceful death. Like all maps, there are many different routes to the same destination.

You may see all of these symptoms or none. Death will come in its own time, and its own way to each of us. It is important to remember that **dying is a natural process**.

1.	Withdrawal - Physical and emotional, and increased sleep.	Natural process of withdrawing from everything outside of one's self, looking inward, reviewing one's self and one's life. Your loved one may turn inward, withdraw physically and emotionally. This occurs in an attempt to cope with the many changes that are occurring.
2.	Reduced food and fluid intake.	Decreased need because body will naturally begin to conserve energy. Dehydration is a natural comfort measure, since the body systems can't process fluids effectively. At no time should food/fluids be forced.
3.	Confusion/Agitation can vary from mild to end stage agitation which may include trying to get out of bed, picking at covers, seeing things that are not apparent to us.	Talk calmly and assuredly. Keep lights on, use times when patient is alert for meaningful conversation. Music can be very calming. Medication often used to control this symptom.

Figure 29–1. Sample handout for families responsible for end-of-life care. (Courtesy of Hospice Care of Boulder and Broomfield Counties, Colorado, June 2004.)

4.	Change in breathing patterns.	This is common. You may see irregular breathing: very rapid, very slow, and/or 10 to 30 seconds of no breathing at all (called apnea). These symptoms are very common and indicative of a decrease in circulation. It does not mean that your loved one is uncomfortable or struggling.
5.	Oral secretions collect in back of throat causing noisy respiration.	Swallowing reflex may be absent. Patient may be breathing through the secretions. • This may be more uncomfortable for us as observers than patient experiencing it. • Elevate head of bed or turn patient on side.
6.	Incontinence of urine and stool.	Reduced intake results in reduced output with darker color. Bedpads and diapers can be used to protect bed linens. Cleanse patient and change linens frequently to maintain comfort and protect skin.
7.	Changes in skin temperature and color.	Decreased circulation can cause coolness and discoloration of skin. Use light covers, turn side to side frequently to maintain comfort and prevent skin breakdown (bedsores). Heating pads and electric blankets NOT recommended.

Hearing is the last sense to be lost, so the patient can hear all that is being said. This is a good time to say good-bye, reassure them that you will be all right even though you will miss them greatly. (You may tell them it's OK to "let go".) This permission is often helpful for a peaceful death.

How would you know death has occurred?

1. No breathing
2. No heartbeat or pulse

If you believe that death has occurred, call Hospice at 449-7740. **Do not call 911 or the physician.** We will come to your home to help you. (You may want to use the time until we arrive to say your last good-byes.)

signs & symptoms death: 7/04

Figure 29–1. *(continued)*

The practice of actual death pronouncement varies widely and is not often taught in medical school or residencies.[38] The customary procedure is to, first, identify the patient, then note the following[39]:

- General appearance of the body
- Lack of reaction to verbal or tactile stimuli
- Lack of pupillary light reflex (pupils will be fixed and dilated)
- Absent breathing and lung sounds
- Absent carotid and apical pulses (in some situations, listening for an apical pulse for a full minute is advisable)

Documentation of the death is equally important and should be thorough and clear. The following guidelines are suggested[38,39]:

- Patient's name and time of call
- Who was present at the time of death and at the time of the pronouncement
- Detailed findings of the physical examination
- Date and time of death pronouncement (either pronouncement by the nurse or the time at which the physician either assessed the patient or was notified)
- Who else was notified and when—for example, additional family members, attending physician, or other staff members
- Whether the coroner was notified, rationale, and outcome, if known
- Special plans for disposition and outcome (e.g., organ or body donation, autopsy, special care related to cultural or religious traditions)

Care of the Body After Death

Regardless of the site of death, care of the body is an important nursing function. In gently caring for the body, the nurse can continue to communicate care and concern for the patient and family members and model behaviors that may be helpful as the family members continue their important grief work. Caring for the body after death also calls for an understanding of the physiological changes that occur. By understanding these changes, the nurse can interpret and dispel any myths and explain these changes to the family members, thereby assisting the family in making their own personal decisions about the time immediately following death and funeral plans.

A time-honored and classic article regarding postmortem care, emphasized that, although postmortem care may be a ritualized nursing procedure, the scientific rationale for the procedure rests on the basics of the physiological changes that occur after death.[40] These changes occur at a regular rate depending on the temperature of the body at the time of death, the size of the body, the extent of infection (if any), and the temperature of the air. The three important physiological changes—rigor mortis, algor mortis, and postmortem decomposition—are discussed along with the relevant nursing implications in Table 29–3.

Care of and respect for the body after death by nursing staff should clearly communicate to the family that the person who died was indeed important and valued. Often, caring for the body after death provides the needed link between family members and the reality of the death, recognizing that everyone present at the time of death and soon after will have a different experience and a different sense of loss. Many institutions no longer require nursing staff to care for patients after death or perform postmortem care.[42] Further, the only published resources related to postmortem care are a series of three articles describing the procedure of "last offices" published in a British journal in 1998.[43–45] In a 1999 review of nursing textbooks, only 26% covered this important aspect of nursing care.[46] Family members will long remember the actions of the nurse after the death. A kind, gentle approach and meticulous attention to detail are imperative.

Rituals that family members and others present find comforting should be encouraged. Rituals are practices within a social context that facilitate and provide ways to understand and cope with the contradictory and complex nature of human existence. They provide a means to express and contain strong emotions, ease feelings of anxiety and impotence, and provide structure in times of chaos and disorder.[47] Rituals can take many forms—a brief service at the time of death, a special preparation of the body as in the Orthodox Jewish tradition, or an Irish wake, where, after paying respect to the person who has died, family and friends gather to share stories, food, and drink.[48] Of utmost importance, however, is to ensure that family members see the ritual as comforting and meaningful. It is the family's needs and desires that direct this activity—not the nurse's. There are, again, no rules that govern the appropriateness of rituals; rituals are comforting and serve to begin the process of healing and acceptance.

To facilitate the grieving process, it is often helpful to create a pleasant, peaceful, and comfortable environment for family members who wish to spend time with the body, according to their desires and cultural or religious traditions. The nurse should consider engaging family members in after-death care and ritual by inviting them to either comb the hair or wash the person's hands and face, or more, if they are comfortable. Parents can be encouraged to hold and cuddle their baby or child. Including siblings or other involved children in rituals, traditions, and other end-of-life care activities according to their developmental level is also essential. During this time, family members should be invited to talk about their loved one and encouraged to reminisce—valuable rituals that can help them begin to work through their grief.[49]

The family should be encouraged to touch, hold, and kiss the person's body, as they feel comfortable. Parents may wish to clip and save a lock of hair as a keepsake. The nurse may offer to dress the person's body in something other than a hospital gown or other nightclothes. Babies may be wrapped snugly in a blanket. Many families choose to dress the body in a favorite article of clothing before removal by the funeral home. It should be noted that, at times, when a body is being turned, air escapes from the lungs, producing a "sighing" sound. Informing family members of this possibility is wise. Again, modeling gentle and careful handling of the body can communicate care and concern on the part of the nurse and facilitate grieving and the creation of positive and long-lasting memories.

Postmortem care also includes, unless an autopsy or the coroner is involved, removal of any tubes, drains, and other devices. In home care settings, these can be placed in a plastic bag and given to the funeral home for disposal as medical waste or simply double-bagged and placed in the family's regular trash. Placing a waterproof pad, diaper, or adult incontinence brief on the patient often prevents soiling and odor as the patient's body is moved and the rectal and urinary bladder sphincters relax. Packing of the rectum and vagina is considered unnecessary, because not allowing these areas to drain increases the rate of bacterial proliferation that naturally occurs.[41]

Table 29–3
Normal Postmortem Physiological Changes and Their Implications for Nursing

Change	Underlying Mechanisms	Nursing Implications
Rigor mortis	Approximately 2 to 4 hours after death, adenosine phosphate (ATP) ceases to be synthesized due to the depletion of glycogen stores. ATP is necessary for muscle fiber relaxation, so the lack of ATP results in an exaggerated contraction of the muscle fibers that eventually immobilizes the joints. Rigor begins in the involuntary muscles (heart, gastrointestinal tract, bladder, arteries) and progresses to the muscles of the head and neck, trunk and lower limbs. After approximately 96 hours, however, muscle chemical activity totally ceases, and rigor passes. Persons with large muscle mass (e.g., body builders) are prone to more pronounced rigor mortis. Conversely, frail elderly persons and persons who have been bed bound for long periods are less subject to rigor mortis.[41]	In many cultures, the body is viewed within 24–48 hours after death. Therefore, post-death positioning becomes of utmost importance. In many cases, it is important to be sure the eyelids and jaw are closed and den tures are in place in the mouth. (Rolling a towel and placing it under the jaw often helps to keep it closed.) The position of the hands is also important. Position all limbs in proper body alignment. If rigor mortis does occur, it can often be "massaged out" by the funeral director.[41] Finally, by understanding this physiology, the nurse can also reassure the family about the myth that due to rigor mortis, muscles can suddenly contract and the body can appear to move.
Algor mortis	After the circulaton ceases and the hypothalamus stops functioning, internal body temperature drops by approximately 1° C or 1.8° F per hour until it reaches room temperature. As the body cools, skin loses its natural elasticity. If a high fever was present at death, the changes in body temperature are more pronounced and the person may appear to "sweat" after death. Body cooling may also take several more hours.[41]	The nurse can prepare family members for the coolness of the skin to touch or the increased moisture by explaining the changes that happen after death. The nurse may also suggest kissing the person on their hair instead of their skin. The skin, due to loss of elasticity, becomes fragile and easily torn. If dressings are to be applied, it is best to apply them with either a circular bandage or paper tape. Handle the body gently as well, being sure to not place traction on the skin.
Postmortem decomposition or "liver mortis"	Discoloration and softening of the body are caused largely by the breakdown of red blood cells and the resultant release of hemoglobin that stains the vessel walls and surrounding tissue. This staining appears as a mottling, bruising, or both in the dependent parts of the body as well as parts of the body where the skin has been punctured (e.g., intravenous or chest tube sites).[41] Often this discoloration becomes extensive in a very short time. The remainder of the body has a gray hue. In cardiac-related deaths, the face often appears purple in color regardless of the positioning at or after death.[41]	As the body is handled (e.g., while bathing and dressing), the nurse informs the family member about this normal change that occurs after death.

Occasionally families, especially in the home care setting, wish to keep the person's body at home, perhaps to wait for another family member to come from a distance and to ensure that everyone has adequate time with the deceased. If the family wishes the body to be embalmed, this is best done within 12 hours. If embalming is not desired, the body can remain in the home for approximately 24 hours before further decomposition and odor production occur. The nurse should suggest to the family that they make the immediate area cooler to slow down natural decomposition, either by turning down the furnace or by turning up the air conditioning.[41] Be sure, however, to inform the funeral director that the family has chosen to keep the body at home a little longer. Finally, funeral directors are a reliable source of information regarding postdeath changes, local customs, and cultural issues.

The care of patients and families near the time of death and afterward is an important nursing function—arguably one of the most important. As the following case studies are reviewed, consider how the nurse interceded in a positive manner, mindful of the changing tempo of care and the changing patient and family needs, desires, and perspectives.

CASE STUDY

James, a 45-Year-Old Man with Amyotrophic Lateral Sclerosis

James was a 45-year-old, self-employed investment banker with a 2-year history of rapidly progressive amyotrophic lateral sclerosis (ALS). After unsuccessful treatment, including participation in clinical trials, James, with the blessing of his wife, Ruth, and their adult children, decided to focus on symptom management and ensuring the quality of his remaining life. However, when his physician suggested hospice, he resisted, claiming that "hospice" was synonymous with death, and, although he knew he was dying, he did not feel the need to talk about it outside of his immediate family. He also stated that he wanted time to sell his business and ensure that his long-time clients had continuity. His physician consulted the palliative care team at the hospital where James had received care, and James and Ruth agreed to meet with the palliative care clinical nurse specialist that day.

> *Goals and framework of care:* Gentle and respectful explanation of the available options and their meaning for care, first understanding and then incorporating James' and his family's goals and needs.

After meeting with the clinical nurse specialist, James and Ruth agreed they would think about a referral to the local hospice program. The following week, they enrolled and became acquainted with the hospice staff members who would be overseeing their care. James also decided to update his durable power of attorney for health care and to formalize his wish to not be resuscitated by wearing a bracelet communicating his wishes to the area emergency medical services. James's symptoms were well controlled and he was able to get out of the house with his wheelchair. Sometimes, a hospice volunteer would come and take him out to his favorite park. Although rapidly losing strength, he expressed a wish to go on a cruise with Ruth and his children.

> *Goals and framework of care:* Although they believed it to be inadvisable, the hospice staff chose to facilitate and honor James's wish despite his progressive illness. They advocated for him and his family with the cruise line and remained in communication with the physician and nurse on the cruise ship.

James and his family had an incredible "trip of a lifetime," according to James, but soon after their return he became increasingly weak, unable to swallow, and unable to breathe without continuous positive airway pressure (CPAP).

> *Goals and framework of care:* The hospice staff revisited James' goals in the context of his declining strength, understanding that there might indeed be things James wanted to accomplish before he died. They held a family meeting with James, Ruth, and the children to answer questions and discuss how his illness might progress. James made the decision to not use the CPAP any longer, and the hospice staff assured him that his symptoms would be well controlled.

The hospice provided volunteers who assisted James in transitioning his clients to the new owner of his business. As his illness worsened, his parents and siblings took turns coming and staying with James and Ruth. This gave Ruth needed respite from caregiving and James time alone with his parents—which had rarely happened in the past—as well as time alone with each of his siblings. The nurse was able to inform the family when his death neared, so all of the family members were present, as James had wished, when he died. During the visit at the time of James' death, Ruth helped the nurse prepare James' body for transportation to the mortuary, even choosing to dress James in his favorite flannel shirt. The nurse and James' wife, children, parents, and siblings reflected on how they had worked together and had empowered each other so that they could make this difficult experience James' very own.

> *Goals and framework of care:* The goals of care changed again to assisting James with accomplishing his final wishes and ensuring that his continued care needs were addressed. At the same time, James family began to prepare for his death by participating in early grief work.

Critical Points

- Coming to grips with death is a process and cannot be rushed. It is different for everyone.
- The needs of James and his family were listened to, honored, and not questioned or challenged.

He and his family remained in charge and in control.
- Time-of-death rituals—i.e., bathing and dressing the body—can often be comforting and memorable for family members.
- The care of a patient and family at end of life includes all family members, not just the immediate family. By supporting James' entire family, comforting memories were ensured.

CASE STUDY

Mrs. H, a 40-Year-Old Woman with Cancer of Unknown Origin

Mrs. H first presented to her primary care physician after noticing a new mass under her arm. The mass was biopsied and was determined to be an adenocarcinoma of unknown origin. Subsequent workup showed no evidence of disease elsewhere. Mammography, computed tomography, magnetic resonance imaging (MRI), chest radiography, and colonoscopy were negative. The biopsy slides were sent to another institution for review. After extensive review, it was determined that her cancer most closely mimicked the breast in origin, and treatment was begun based on that knowledge. The workup took approximately 3 weeks, a time of great anxiety for the patient and her family.

Mrs. H settled into chemotherapy on a weekly basis; her husband and sister accompanied her to her treatment sessions. She was employed by a local company who had pledged their full support to her in terms of job security and support by their staff for any needs. She was the mother of two children in college. Mrs. H reported that "life was full and good!"

Mrs. H asked for information on support programs. It was difficult for her to find appropriate group support, so she opted for individual counseling. She shared that she did not believe the situation was going to have a positive outcome. She desperately wanted to have a "kitchen table" conversation with her family but never felt successful in doing so. With the support of the nursing staff and social services staff, she settled for completing her advanced directive and putting her wishes in writing.

Goals and framework of care: "Treat and See"

Treatment continued for 6 months. No evidence of disease was noted after 4 months. It was determined that after 1 more month, treatments would be stopped and surveillance would begin. A feeling of relief and joy surrounded Mrs. H during her clinic visits. During her the last month of treatment, antiemetic treatment was noted to be more difficult, and dexamethasone was added to the treatment regimen.

A month after her last treatment, Mrs. H presented to clinic with a severe headache. An immediate MRI was ordered. Before it could be completed, Mrs. H became unconscious and was admitted to the intensive care unit (ICU). The results showed a brain mass compounded by a massive intracranial bleed.

Goals and framework of care: "Understanding the New Findings"

Comprehending the dramatic shift in the patient's condition, the extent of the disease, and the implications of the new findings was overwhelming to the family. Treating staff also struggled with the new findings. Time was needed. How much, though? How quickly could the family be moved to decision-making concerning life support for Mrs. H?

Clearly, a good deal of support would be needed for the family and staff. The family was asked to gather and to bring other supportive individuals who could assist them. Thirty-six hours after the MRI was done, the family gathered to hear the status of Mrs. H's condition and her prognosis. They were asked to consider what her wishes would be under the circumstances. Mrs. H's advance directive was reviewed; it clearly stated that she wished no advanced life support if meaningful recovery was not believed possible. The family was immobilized by the situation. They were asked to appoint a family spokesperson who could meet the next morning with the attending physician.

Goals and framework of care: "Continuing the Dialogue—Allowing for Time"

The next morning, the family spokesperson did not arrive to meet with the attending physician as planned. There were no phone calls from the family, and no communication from them for 24 hours. At this point, the family spokesperson was contacted by Mrs. H's nurse simply for the purpose of providing an update on Mrs. H's condition and asking if there were further questions. The reply was simply, "Thank you, no." The spokesperson shared with the nurse that the family simply did not know what to do and were not ready to come back to the hospital. They asked for more time. The ICU team agreed that, if there was no contact from the family by noon of the next day, Mrs. H's oncologist, who had been present at the family meeting, would make the next contact.

The next morning, the entire family arrived at the hospital and asked to plan with the team the most dignified way to remove Mrs. H from life support. They brought personal items, pictures of the family, their minister, and a special prayer to be read. The staff employed aggressive dyspnea management for Mrs. H and removed her from life support in the presence of her family. She died peacefully within 30 minutes after removal from the ventilator. Surrounded by the love of her family, who gave each other the support, Mrs. H died, much in the way the nursing staff in the oncology unit had heard her describe.

Critical Points

- Sudden changes in trajectories of care require time for the family to adjust, particularly if the patient is no longer able to speak or make decisions. Allowing realistic time frames for this process is critical.
- Frameworks of care must be clear to the patient, family, and all staff members involved in the patient's care throughout the process of treatment.

Summary

Assisting and walking alongside dying patients and their families, especially near and after death, is an honor and privilege. Nowhere else in the practice of nursing are we invited to be companions on such a remarkable journey as that of a dying patient and family. Likewise, nowhere else in the practice of nursing are our words, actions, and guidance more remembered and cherished. Caring for dying patients and families is indeed the essence of nursing. Take this responsibility seriously, understanding that, although it may be stressful and difficult at times, it comes with personal and professional satisfaction beyond measure. Listen to your patients and their families. They are the guides to this remarkable and momentous journey. Listen to them with a positive regard, empathy, and genuineness, and approach their care with an acute attention to every detail. They—in fact, all of us—are counting on you.

REFERENCES

1. Settles BH. A perspective on tomorrow's families. In: Sussman MB, Steinmetz SK, eds. Handbook of Marriage and the Family. New York: Plenum, 1987:157–180.
2. Matocha LK. Case study interviews: Caring for a person with AIDS. In: Gilgun JF, Daly K, Handel G, eds. Qualitative Methods in Family Research. Newbury Park, CA: Sage, 1992:66–84.
3. SUPPORT Study Principal Investigators. A controlled trial to improve care for seriously ill hospitalized patients: A Study to Understand Prognoses and Preferences for Outcomes and Risks of Treatments (SUPPORT). JAMA 1995;274:1591–1598.
4. Ellershaw J, Ward C. Care of the dying patient: The last hours or days of life. BMJ 2003;326:30–34.
5. Fürst CJ, Doyle D. The terminal phase. In: Doyle D, Hanks G, Cherny NI, Calman K, eds. Oxford Textbook of Palliative Medicine, 3rd ed. Oxford: Oxford University Press, 2004:1119–1133.
6. Wildiers H, Menten J. Death rattle: Prevalence, prevention and treatment. J Pain Symptom Manage 2002;23:310–317.
7. Klinkenberg M, Willems DL, van der Wal G, Deeg DJ. Symptom burden in the last week of life. J Pain Symptom Manage 2004; 27:5–13.
8. Ventafridda V, Ripamonti C, De Conno F, Tamburini M, Cassileth BR. Symptom prevalence and control during cancer patients' last days of life. J Palliat Care 1990;6:7–11.
9. Hall P, Schroder C, Weaver L. The last 48 hours of life in long-term care: A focused chart audit. J Am Geriatr Soc 2002;50:501–506.
10. Rogers C. On Becoming a Person: A Therapist's View of Psychology. Boston: Houghton Mifflin, 1961.
11. Twycross R. Symptom Management in Advanced Cancer, 2nd ed. Oxan, UK: Radcliffe Medical Press, 1997.
12. Du Boulay S. Cicely Saunders: Founder of the Modern Hospice Movement. London: Hodder and Stoughton, 1984.
13. Berns R, Colvin ER. The final story: Events at the bedside of dying patients as told by survivors. ANNA J 1998;25:583–587.
14. Karlawish HT, Quill T, Meier D (for the ACP-ASIM End of Life Care Consensus Panel). A consensus-based approach to providing palliative care to patients who lack decision making capacity. Ann Intern Med 1999;130:835–840.
15. Cleary JF. Fever and sweats. In: Berger AM, Portenoy RK, Weissman DE. Principles and Practice of Palliative Care and Supportive Oncology, 2nd ed. New York: Lippincott Williams & Wilkins, 2002:154–167.
16. Brody H, Campbell ML, Faber-Langendoen K, Ogle KS. Withdrawing intensive life-sustaining treatment: Recommendations for compassionate clinical management. N Engl J Med 1997;336: 652–657.
17. National Conference for Cardiopulmonary Resuscitation (CPR) and Emergency Cardiac Care (ECC). Standards of CPR and ECC. JAMA 1974;227:864–866.
18. Tomlinson T, Brody H. Sounding board: Ethics and communication in do-not-resuscitate orders. N Engl J Med 1988;318: 43–46.
19. McIntyre KM. Failure of predictors of CPR outcomes to predict CPR outcomes [editorial]. Arch Intern Med 1993;153:1293–1296.
20. Dunn H. Hard Choices for Loving People, 4th ed. Herndon, VA: A & A Publishers, 2001.
21. Zerwekh J. Do dying patients really need IV fluids? Am J Nurs 1997;97:26–31.
22. Fainsinger RL, Bruera E. When to treat dehydration in a terminally ill patient? Support Care Cancer 1997;5:205–211.
23. Hospice and Palliative Nurses Association. HPNA Position Statement: Artificial Nutrition and Hydration in End-of-Life Care. Pittsburgh: Hospice and Palliative Nurses Association, 2003.
24. Ellershaw JE, Sutcliffe JM, Saunders CM. Dehydration and the dying patient. J Pain Symptom Manage 1995;10:192–197.
25. Smith SA. Patient induced dehydration: Can it ever be therapeutic? Oncol Nurs Forum 1995;22:1487–1491.
26. McCann RM, Hall WJ, Groth-Juncker A. Comfort care for terminally ill patients: The appropriate use of nutrition and hydration. JAMA 1994;272:1263–1266.
27. Working Party on Clinical Guidelines in Palliative Care. Changing Gear—Guidelines for Managing the Last Days of Life. London: National Council for Hospice and Specialist Palliative Care Services, 1997.
28. Medtronic Inc. Restoring the Rhythms of Life: Your Implantable Defibrillator. St. Paul: Medtronic, Inc., 1994.
29. Weissman D. Glucocorticoid treatment for brain metastases and epidural spinal cord compression: A review. J Clin Oncol 1988;6: 543–551.
30. DeVelasco R, Dinwiddie LC. Management of the patient with ESRD after withdrawal from dialysis. ANNA J 1998;25:611–614.
31. Moss A. Ethics in ESRD patient care. To use dialysis appropriately: The emerging consensus on patient election guidelines. Adv Renal Replace Ther 1998;2:175–183.

32. Campbell ML. Forgoing Life-Sustaining Therapy. Aliso Viejo, CA: AACN Critical Care Publications, 1998.
33. Kelly C, Yetman L. At the end of life. Can Nurse 1987;83:33–34.
34. Smith JL. The process of dying and managing the death event. In: Schoenwetter RS, Hawke W, Knight CF. Hospice and Palliative Medicine Core Curriculum and Review Syllabus. Dubuque, IA: Kendall/Hunt, 1999.
35. Kelly C, Yetman L. At the end of life. Can Nurse 1987;83:33–34.
36. Callahan M, Kelley P. Final Gifts: Understanding the Special Awareness, Needs, and Communications of the Dying. New York: Bantam Books, 1993.
37. Department of Health and Human Services, Health Care Financing Administration. Medicare and Medicaid Programs; Hospital Conditions of Participation; Identification of Potential Organ, Tissue, and Eye Donors and Transplant Hospitals' Provision of Transplant-Related Data. Final rule. 63 Federal Register 119 (1998) (codified at 42 CFR §482.45).
38. Marchand LR, Siewert L. Death pronouncement: Survival tips for residents. Am Fam Physician 1998;58:284–285.
39. Heidenreich C, Assistant Professor of Medicine, Medical College of Wisconsin, Milwaukee, WI. Personal communication.
40. Pennington EA. Postmortem care: More than ritual. Am J Nurs 1978;75:846–847.
41. Hron J, Funeral Director, Gunderson Funeral Home, Madison, WI. Personal communication.
42. Speck P. Care after death. Nursing Times 1992; 88:20.
43. Nearny L. Practical procedures for nurses: Last offices—1. Nursing Times 1998;94(26): insert.
44. Nearny L. Practical procedures for nurses: Last offices—2. Nursing Times 1998;94(27): insert.
45. Nearny L. Practical procedures for nurses: Last offices—2. Nursing Times 1998; 94(28): insert.
46. Ferrell B, Virani R, Grant M. Analysis of end of life content in nursing textbooks. Oncol Nurs Forum 1999;26:869–876.
47. Romanoff BD, Terenzio M. Rituals and the grieving process. Death Studies 1998;22:697–711.
48. O'Gorman SM. Death and dying in contemporaty society: An evaluation of current attitudes and the rituals associated with death and dying and their relevance to recent understanding of health and healing. J Adv Nurs 1998;27:1127–1135.
49. Passagno RA. Postmortem care: Healing's first step. Nursing 97 1997;24:32a–32b.
50. Ambuel B, Weissman D. Fast Fact and Concept #016: Conducting a Family Conference. 2000, http://www.eperc.mcw.edu/FastFact/ff_016.htm (accessed February 2, 2005).

IV
Spiritual Care

30 Spiritual Assessment

Elizabeth Johnston Taylor

I agree that spiritual support is very important during a serious illness, but I also believe that it is a choice for the patients to make for themselves whether it be interactive with a professional caregiver. Some people prefer an intimate, personal relationship with God and may not feel comfortable revealing themselves. Others may welcome the genuine love and concern of others. It would have to be approached with utmost sensitivity and knowledge of people and their relationship with God.
—Spouse responding to a written survey

- ***Key Points***
- *Spiritual assessment precedes effective spiritual caregiving. Because palliative care patients and their family members use spiritual coping strategies, and spiritual well-being can buffer the distress of dying, spiritual care is integral to palliative care.*
- *Numerous typologies identifying the dimensions of spirituality exist and provide guidance for what to address in a spiritual assessment.*
- *A two-tiered approach to spiritual assessment allows the nurse to first conduct a superficial assessment to screen for spiritual problems or needs.*
- *The most streamlined assessment strategy suggests asking "How does your spirituality help you to live with your illness?" and "What can I/we do to support your spiritual beliefs and practices?"*
- *Spiritual assessment data allow diagnosis of a spiritual problem or need and should be documented.*

To solve any problem, one must first assess what the problem is. Consequently, the nursing process dictates that the nurse begin care with an assessment of the patient's health needs. Although palliative nurses are accustomed to assessing patients' pain experiences, hydration status, and so forth, they less frequently participate in assessing patients' and family members' spirituality.

Because spirituality is an inherent and integrating, and often extremely valued, dimension for those who receive palliative nursing care, it is essential that palliative care nurses know to some degree how to conduct a spiritual assessment. This chapter reviews models for spiritual assessment, presents general guidelines on how to conduct a spiritual assessment, and discusses what the nurse ought to do with data from a spiritual assessment. These topics are prefaced by arguments supporting the need for spiritual assessments, descriptions of what spirituality "looks like" among the terminally ill, and risk factors for those who are likely to experience spiritual distress. But first, a description of spirituality is in order.

What Is Spirituality?

A number of recent analyses of the concept of spirituality have identified key aspects of this ethereal and intangible phenomenon.[1] Conceptualizations of spirituality often include the following as aspects of spirituality: the need for purpose and meaning, forgiveness, love and relatedness, hope, creativity, and religious faith and its expression. A well-accepted definition for spirituality authored by Reed[2] proposed that spirituality involves meaning-making through intrapersonal, interpersonal, and transpersonal connection. A more recent definition that incorporates themes found in nursing literature is Dossey and Guzzetta's[3] description of "a unifying force of a person; the essence of being that permeates all of life and is manifested in one's being, knowing, and doing; the interconnectedness with self, others, nature, and God/Life Force/Absolute/Transcendent" (p. 7).

Usually, spirituality is differentiated from religion—the organized, codified, and often institutionalized beliefs and practices that express one's spirituality.[1] As Dossey and Guzzetta's[3] definition illustrates, care is often taken to allow for an open interpretation of what a person considers to be divine, or a transcendent Other. Although health care literature frequently uses phrases such as "higher power" in addition to "God," demographers of religion find that more than 90% of Americans believe in God.[4]

The spiritual assessment methods introduced in this chapter are all influenced inherently by some conceptualization of spirituality. Some, however, have questioned whether spiritual assessment is possible, given the broad, encompassing definition typically espoused by nurses.[5–6] Bash contended that spirituality is an "elastic" term that cannot be universally defined. Because a patient's definition of spirituality may differ from the nurse's assumptions about it, Bash argued that widely applicable tools for spiritual assessment are impossible to design. It is important to note, therefore, that the literature and methods for spiritual assessment presented in this chapter are primarily from the United States and United Kingdom, influenced most by Western Judeo-Christian traditions and peoples. Hence, they are most applicable to these peoples.

Why Is It Important for a Palliative Care Nurse to Conduct a Spiritual Assessment?

Spiritual awareness increases as one faces an imminent death.[7] While some may experience spiritual distress or "soul pain," others may have a spiritual transformation or experience spiritual growth and health.[8–10] There is mounting empirical evidence to suggest that persons with terminal illnesses consider spirituality to be one of the most important contributors to quality of life.[11] For example, two studies measuring various domains of quality of life found spiritual well-being to rank highest in samples of hospice patients.[12–13] McClain and colleagues[14] observed that spiritual well-being functioned to protect terminal cancer patients against end-of-life despair. They found spiritual well-being to have moderately strong inverse relationships with the desire for a hastened death, hopelessness, and suicidal ideations. Religious beliefs and practices (e.g., prayer, beliefs that explain suffering or death) are also known to be valued and frequently used as helpful coping strategies among those who suffer and die from physical illness.[15–17] Family caregivers of seriously ill patients also find comfort and strength from their spirituality that assists them to cope.[18–20] A national telephone survey of 1200 adults also confirmed that Americans project that their spiritual beliefs (e.g., beliefs in an afterlife, beliefs about life belonging to God, and being "born again") will be important sources of comfort when they are dying.[21]

The above themes from research imply that attention to the spirituality of terminally ill patients and their caregivers is of utmost importance. That is, if patients' spiritual resources assist them to cope, and if imminent death precipitates heightened spiritual awareness and concerns, and if patients view their spiritual health as most important to their quality of life, then spiritual assessment that initiates a process promoting spiritual health is vital to effective palliative care.

Underscoring these theoretical reasons for spiritual assessment is a very pragmatic one: the mandate of the Joint Commission on Accreditation of Healthcare Organizations (JCAHO) to conduct a spiritual assessment for clients entering an approved facility.[22] The Joint Commission states that a spiritual assessment, at least, should "determine the patients denomination, beliefs, and what spiritual practices are important." They do not stipulate how this assessment should be conducted, allowing the institution to develop its own process.

But why should palliative care nurses be conducting spiritual assessments? Hunt and colleagues[23] recognized that although chaplains are the spiritual care experts, all members of a hospice team participate in spiritual caregiving. In surveying hospice team members, Millison and Dudley[24] found nurses are often the ones responsible for completing spiritual assessments. Other nurse authors imply that nurses are pivotal in the process of spiritual assessment.[1,25–28] Considering nurses' frontline position, coordination role, and intimacy with the concerns of patients, the holistic perspective on care, and even their lack of religious cloaking, nurses are ideal professionals for completing a spiritual assessment.

However, nurses must recognize that they are not specialists in spiritual assessment and caregiving; they are generalists. Most oncology and hospice nurses perceive that they do not receive adequate training in spiritual assessment and care.[29–30] In fact, it is this lack of training, accompanied by role confusion, lack of time, and other factors that nurses often cite as barriers to completing spiritual assessments.[31–32] When a nurse's assessment indicates need for further sensitive assessment and specialized care, a referral to a specialist (e.g., chaplain, clergy, patient's spiritual director) is in order.

How Does Spirituality Manifest Itself?

To understand how to assess spirituality, the palliative care nurse must know what to look for. What subjective and objective observations would indicate spiritual disease or health? To approach an answer, it is helpful to consider two research studies exploring qualitatively what are clients' perceptions of spiritual need. Hermann[33] interviewed 19 hospice patients to determine what specifically their spiritual needs were. The 29 resulting spiritual needs were categorized under the following themes: need for involvement and control, need for companionship, need to finish business, need to experience nature, need for a positive outlook, as well as need for religion. Taylor[20] interviewed 28 cancer patients and family caregivers, some for whom death was imminent, and identified eight categories of spiritual need. These spiritual needs included the need to:

- Relate to God or an Ultimate Other (e.g., the need to believe God will or has healed, the need to remember God's providence, the need to remember that "there is Someone out there looking out for me")
- Have gratitude and optimism (e.g., the need to keep a positive outlook, to count one's blessings, or just enjoy life)
- Love others (e.g., to forgive or "get right" with others, to return others' kindnesses, to make the world a better place, to protect family members from witnessing the suffering from cancer)
- Receive love from others (e.g., the need to feel valued and appreciated by family, to know others are praying for you, or just being with others considered to be family)
- Review spiritual beliefs (e.g., wondering if religious beliefs are correct, thinking about the unfairness of personal circumstances, or asking "why?" questions)
- Create meaning, find purpose for cancer and for life (e.g., the need to "get past" asking "why me?" and becoming aware of positive outcomes from illness, lessening the frustration of not being able to do meaningful work, or sensing that there is a reason for being alive)
- Sustain religious experience (e.g., reading spirit-nurturing material, having quiet time to reflect, or receiving a sacrament from a religious leader)
- Prepare for death (e.g., balancing thoughts about dying with hoping for health, cognitively creating a purpose for death, or making sure personal business is in order).

Dudley and colleagues[34] found hospice spiritual assessment forms often include more specific spiritual problems, such as fear of death or abandonment, spiritual emptiness, unresolved grief, unresolved past experiences, confusion or doubts about beliefs, and the need for reconciliation, comfort, or peace.

Although the terminology "spiritual need" may suggest a problem, spiritual needs can also be of a positive nature. For example, patients can have a need to express their joy about sensing closeness to others, or have a need to pursue activities that allow expression of creative impulses (e.g., artwork, music making, writing). Although the following models for conducting a spiritual assessment will provide more understanding of how spirituality manifests, the reader is referred to Taylor[1] or Carpenito,[35] or Highfield and Cason's[36] seminal article for further concrete indicators of spiritual need.

Spiritual Assessment Models

Health care professionals from multiple disciplines offer models for spiritual assessment. Selected models from chaplaincy and pastoral counseling, medicine (including psychiatry), and nursing will be presented here. Although some assessment models have been published during the past few years, most were developed in the 1990s, when the research about spiritual care began to proliferate.

Chaplaincy/Pastoral Counseling

During the past several decades, as the field of chaplaincy and pastoral counseling has advanced, there have been several models for spiritual assessment published. However, most discussions of spiritual assessment in this field reflect the ideas of the Christian psychologist Pruyser.[37]

Pruyser proposed seven dimensions or traits to spirituality. Each dimension can be considered a continuum, with negative and unhealthy versus positive and healthy ends. These dimensions are presented in Table 30–1 with statements that terminally ill patients or their loved ones might make to illustrate each end of the continuum. Where a patient is on these continuums can change over time. Malony[38] asserted that one more dimension needs to be added to Pruyser's seven, a trait Malony labels "openness in faith." That is, a positive, healthy sense of openness in faith allows an individual to not be rigid or resistant to new ideas in his or her spiritual beliefs. Although Pruyser and Malony acknowledge this model as being molded by Christian perspectives, much of the model still offers non-Christians insight into what spiritual dimensions can encompass.

Fitchett[39] developed the "7 by 7" model for spiritual assessment. In addition to reviewing seven dimensions of a person (medical, psychological, psychosocial, family system, ethnic and cultural, societal issues, and spiritual dimensions), Fitchett advances seven spiritual dimensions to include in an assessment: beliefs and meaning (i.e., mission, purpose, religious and nonreligious meaning in life), vocation and consequences (what persons believe they should do, what their calling is), experience (of the divine or demonic) and emotion (the tone emerging from one's spiritual experience), courage and growth (the ability to encounter doubt and inner change), ritual and practice (activities that make life meaningful), community (involvement in any formal or informal community that shares spiritual beliefs and practices), and authority and guidance (exploring where or with whom one places trusts, seeks guidance).

Using an approach less complex than Fitchett's, van der Poel[40] offers five general questions for organizing the assessment of an incurably ill patient: What is the place of God in the patient's life? What is the patient's attitude toward self? How is the patient's relationship with family and friends? What is the patient's understanding of and interest in prayer? What is the patient's attitude toward his or her religion? Van

Table 30–1
Pruyser's Spiritual Dimensions

Spiritual Dimension	Negative, Less Healthy	Positive, More Healthy
Awareness of the Holy or God (sense of awe, reverence for that which is divine)	"When I hear the birds sing, they mock me; I see nothing sacred in nature—or anything else."	"I feel very close to God now and am dependent on God's help to face my death."
Acceptance of God's grace and steadfast love (experience of God as benevolent and unconditional in loving)	"I don't need or deserve any help or kindness; I'll handle things alone."	"Thank you for caring for me so tenderly; you mirror God for me."
Being repentant and responsible (openness to change, acceptance of responsibility for own feelings and behaviors)	"It's not my fault I feel bitter."	"How can I deal with my situation better?"
Faith (open, committed, and positive attitude toward life)	"There are some things in life I'd be afraid to do."	"I've enjoyed every minute of life! I try anything new."
Sense of providence (experience of God's leadership and direction)	"Where has God been for me? He left me when I got sick."	"I trust that God's will will be done in my life and dying."
Involvement in spiritual/religious community, and experience of communion	"Why should I have to ask for help from my church? They don't bother to even call me!"	"I still feel connected to my church because I know that they are praying for me."
Flexibility and commitment to living an ethical life	"There is no reason for me to still live. Let's pull the plug here."	"How I am choosing to die reflects my respect for the sacredness of my life; I have much to offer even while I'm in the process of dying."

Sources: Malony (1993), reference 38 and Kloss (1988), reference 62.

der Poel does specify substatements for each of these questions, but offers them in a tool that quantifies (using five-point response options) patient responses.

Hospice chaplain Muncy[41] assesses three dimensions of patients' spirituality. First, patient's self-understanding and attitudes about others are explored, since, in Muncy's view, how patients view self and others frequently portrays their view of God. Second, religious and spiritual history, including sense of purpose, are assessed. Last, patients are asked about their spiritual goals; this allows the clinician to discuss with the patient a plan for spiritual care.

Medicine

A number of physicians have offered approaches to spiritual assessment.[42–43] Most of these approaches befit the work of a physician or other health care professional who is needing to screen for spiritual need in an efficient way. These approaches generally involve asking about specified aspects of spirituality during a history taking. To remember these aspects of spirituality, many are organized to reflect a mnemonic. Several of these are summarized and illustrated in Table 30–2.

The Royal Free Interview Schedule developed in the United Kingdom by King, Speck, and Thomas[44] is a 2½-page self-report questionnaire. The tool showed acceptable reliability and various forms of validity when it was tested among 297 persons, who were primarily hospital employees and church members. Questionnaire items assess both spiritual and religious "understanding in life" (1 item), religious/spiritual beliefs (8 items), religious/spiritual practices (3 items), and "intense" spiritual or "near death" experiences (6 items). Response options for items include Likert scales, categorical options, and space for answering open-ended questions.

Family physician T.A. Maugens[45] offers the mnemonic SPIRIT for remembering six components to cover during a spiritual assessment, or "history" (to use Maugens's physician terminology). "**S**piritual belief system" refers to religious affiliation and theology. "**P**ersonal spirituality" refers to the spiritual views shaped by life experiences that are unique to the individual and not necessarily related to one's religion. "**I**ntegration and involvement with a spiritual community" reminds the clinician to assess for a patient's membership and role in a religious organization or other group that provides spiritual support. "**R**itualized practices and restrictions" are the behaviors and

Table 30–2
Spiritual Assessment: Mnemonics for Interviewing

Author	Components (Mnemonic)	Illustrative Questions
Maugens[45]	**S** (spiritual belief system)	What is your formal religious affiliation?
	P (personal spirituality)	Describe the beliefs and practices of your religion or spiritual system that you personally accept. What is the importance of your spirituality/religion in daily life?
	I (integration with a spiritual community)	Do you belong to any spiritual or religious group or community? What importance does this group have to you? Does or could this group provide help in dealing with health issues?
	R (ritualized practices and restrictions)	Are there specific elements of medical care that you forbid on the basis of religious/spiritual grounds?
	I (implications for medical care)	What aspects of your religion/spirituality would you like me to keep in mind as I care for you? Are there any barriers to our relationship based on religious or spiritual issues?
	T (terminal events planning)	As we plan for your care near the end of life, how does your faith impact on your decisions?
Anandarajah & Hight[46]	**H** (sources of hope)	What or who is it that gives you hope?
	O (organized religion)	Are you a part of an organized faith group? What does this group do for you as a person?
	P (personal spirituality or spiritual practices)	What personal spiritual practices, like prayer or meditation, help you?
	E (effects on medical care and/or end-of-life issues)	Do you have any beliefs that may affect how the health care team cares for you?
Puchalski	**F** (faith)	Do you have a faith belief? What is it that gives your life meaning?
	I (import or influence)	What importance does your faith have in your life? How does your faith belief influence your life?
	C (community)	Are you a member of a faith community? How does this support you?
	A (address)	How would you like for me to integrate or address these issues in your care?

lifestyle activities that influence one's health. "**I**mplications for medical care" reminds the nurse to assess how spiritual beliefs and practices influence the patient's desire and participation in health care. "**T**erminal events planning" reminds the clinician to assess end-of-life concerns. These components of a spiritual assessment are most appropriate for use in palliative care settings; the mnemonic may be helpful for remembering them.

Anandarajah and Hight[46] developed a simpler mnemonic for remembering aspects of a spiritual assessment: HOPE. "H" reminds the clinician to assess for sources of **h**ope, strength, comfort, meaning, peace, love, and connection. "O" refers to the patient's **o**rganized religion, while "P" stands for **p**ersonal spirituality and **p**ractices. "E" prompts the clinician to assess for spirituality **e**ffects on medical care and **e**nd-of-life decisions. Again, the mnemonic may be stretched, but the parsimony of the assessment strategy is appreciated.

Similarly, Puchalski[47] proposed the mnemonic of FICA as a strategy for spiritual assessment. FICA prompts the clinician to assess to what *faith* and beliefs the patient has (F), how *important* or *influential* this faith is (I), what faith *community* or spiritual support group they participate in (C), and how the client would like the health/hospice care team to *address* their spiritual needs (A). This mnemonic may be easier to recall, and is appropriate for the initial or standard spiritual assessments.

Two other screening approaches that are very concise have been proposed by physicians Lo and colleagues,[48] who suggested the following questions for use in palliative care settings:

- Is faith/religion/spirituality important to you in this illness?
- Has faith been important to you at other times in your life?
- Do you have someone to talk to about religious matters?
- Would you like to explore religious matters with someone?

Striving to have an even more streamlined spiritual assessment, Matthews and colleagues'[49] proposed initial spiritual assessments could be limited to asking "Is your religion (or faith) helpful to you in handling your illness?" and "What can I do to support your faith or religious commitment?"

CASE STUDY
Ms. B, a Patient With "Bone" Cancer

Ms. B, a 63-year-old African-American Pentecostal woman dying with "bone" cancer. Excerpts from an interview conducted by this author provide a partial picture of Ms. B's spirituality:

> If I ever wanted to be loved and appreciated, it is now! I just need to be with my grandkids, my kids all the time. I want to cook for them. I want to go places with them. I want to take some pictures. I just want to do it until that time comes . . . just the need to be wanted, not wanted because you this or you got that . . . a lot of love and laughter . . . just be needed, you know, for once, not because *I am your momma*, not because you have to, just be appreciative that we have each other . . .
>
> I believe that there is a God, that Jesus died for you. I have hope, because a Man is up there. But I can't go to church Sundays. With the pain, the pews are too hard, and I can't get to the restrooms quick enough.
>
> You never go 'til the Lord take you . . . and He says He "will never leave you or forsake you." God allows this to be a testimony to other people about Jesus, how he died for us. There are things you can be doing. Say, we could be helping someone else. I speak with someone else about it and give God all the praise. I could sit here and say "Oh, I'm ready for the Lord to take me whenever He ready" and I can die. 'Cause every time I get ready—and at first I did. But right now I wanna express so much what He has done that I'm not ready to go until I've expressed it.
>
> Nobody wants to go to Hell! Excuse me for sayin' it like that. So, the first thing you want to do is get life right and go to Heaven. Even though I am in the Word and you say, "Lord, Lord, Lord," maybe not to say you are going, but sometime, you feel like, "Am I already going to Hell?" or whatever! But you want to be as right as you can.
>
> I wish the nurses would just stay for a few minutes and say "you gonna be okay, it's in God's hands." That's just in an instant, nursing spirituality! Or, having a nurse say, "Okay, I'm gonna put you on my prayer list." But if the nurse is not a believer like me, it doesn't help. You gotta have to have a certain feelin' or vibe.

Assessment Using FICA

F (faith)—Pentecostal beliefs in God and Jesus. More specific beliefs include good behavior in present life means reward of Heaven in the after-life. God controls when she will die. In the meantime, she is to live her life as a "testimony" in praise of God.

I (import or influence)—This faith pervades her thinking and feeling, gives her hope, and allows joyfulness.

C (community)—Although she is used to attending Sunday services regularly at a local church, her terminal illness prevents it now. Her greatest desire is to receive and give love to her immediate family, including grandchildren (her spiritual community now).

A (address)—Would appreciate religiously like-minded nurses verbally reminding her of God's providence and praying for her.

Nursing

Recent years have brought a number of spiritual care texts for nurses.[1,26–28,50] These books generally include chapters on spiritual assessment. The nurse authors who have written about spiritual assessment are influenced by the writings of chaplains and pastoral counselors. However, they often go beyond a discussion of what dimensions to include in an assessment, to concrete suggestions about how to incorporate spiritual assessment into nursing care. Following is a review of what some nurse authors have suggested as spiritual dimensions for which to assess.

In a groundbreaking article, Stoll[51] suggests four areas for spiritual assessment:

- The patient's concept or God or deity
- Sources of hope and strength
- Religious practices
- The relationship between spiritual beliefs and health

Shelly[27] posited that there are three fundamental or underlying spiritual needs that should guide how a nurse completes a spiritual assessment. These needs are: "(1) to be loved and to love in return, (2) to experience forgiveness and extend it to others, (3) to find meaning and purpose in life and hope for the future" (p. 30).

Carpenito's[35] questions for collecting data to make a nursing diagnoses of "spiritual distress" or "potential for enhanced spiritual well-being" reflect Stoll's[51] approach. In addition to questions that simply ascertain a patient's religious affiliation, supportive clergy and helpful religious books as a source of strength and meaning, and questions that explore the link between spirituality and health are given (e.g., "What effect do you expect your illness (hospitalization) to have on your spiritual practices or beliefs?" "How can I help you maintain your spiritual strength during this illness?"). Furthermore, the North American Nursing Diagnosis Association (NANDA) criteria for spiritual distress can be used as indicators on an checklist-type assessment tool. Figure 30-1 provides an example of a spiritual self-assessment form.

Spiritual Self-Assessment

Often when people confront health challenges, they become more aware of their spirituality. For some, spiritual ways of thinking or living are especially helpful when health concerns emerge. For others, spiritual questions or doubts arise.

This form will guide you to think about spiritual issues. After completing it, you may choose to keep it or give it to your nurse, who may want to share it with other health care professionals who will be caring for you.

NAME: ______________________________

ROOM NUMBER: __________

Place an "X" on the lines to show the answer that comes closest to describing your feelings.

Recently, my spirits have been. . .

___ **awful** ___ **low** ___ **okay** ___ **good** ___ **great**

In general, I see myself as. . .

___ **not at all spiritual** ___ **a little spiritual** ___ **somewhat spiritual** ___ **fairly spiritual** ___ **very spiritual**

In general, I see myself as. . .

___ **not at all religious** ___ **a little religious** ___ **somewhat religious** ___ **fairly religious** ___ **very religious**

What can a nurse do that would help to nurture or boost your spirits? (check all that apply)

___ spend quiet time with you
___ have prayer with you
___ help you meditate
___ allow time and space for your private prayer or meditation
___ let you know nurse(s) are praying privately for you
___ read spiritually helpful literature to you
___ bring art or music to you that nurtures your spirit
___ bring you literature that you feel is spiritually helpful
___ help you to stay connected to your spiritual community
___ help you to observe religious practices
___ listen to your thoughts about certain spiritual matters
___ help you to remember how you have grown from previous difficult life experiences
___ help you to tell your life story
___ help you to face painful questions, doubts, or suffering
___ just be with you, not necessarily talking with you
___ just show a genuine and personal interest in you

I would also like help in boosting my spirits from:

___ my friends and family
___ other health care professionals
___ my own clergy or spiritual mentor
___ other clergy or spiritual leader
___ a chaplain at this institution

What would you like your nurse to know about your prayer or meditation beliefs and practices?

____
____

What literature, art, or music nurtures your spirit?

____
____

How can the nurse assist you with religious practices or fellowship?

____
____

What spiritual matters would you like to talk about most?

____
____

In what other ways can the nurse help to boost your spirits?

____
____

If there is anyone in particular you would like to meet with for spiritual fellowship, please so state. Or if there is someone you would like us to contact for you, please share what contact information you know:

____
____

Figure 30–1. Spiritual self-assessment form. *Source:* Taylor, Elizabeth Johnston. Spiritual Care: Nursing Theory, Research, and Practice. Upper Saddle River, NJ: Pearson Education, Inc., 2002. Copyright 2002 by Pearson Education, Inc. Reproduced with permission.

Dossey's[52] spiritual-assessment tool uses language that is less traditional (i.e., less overtly religious). This tool includes questions designed to assess meaning and purpose ("a person's ability to seek meaning and fulfillment in life, manifest hope, and accept ambiguity and uncertainty") and inner strength ("a person's ability to manifest joy and recognize strengths, choices, goals, and faith"). The tool also contains questions that assess interconnections, or what Dossey describes as "a person's positive self-concept, self-esteem, and sense of self; sense of belonging in the world with others; capacity to pursue personal interests; and ability to demonstrate love of self and self-forgiveness." Selected questions from Dossey's tool are found in Table 30–3, many in an adapted form.

While some spiritual care texts focus on how to conduct spiritual assessment interviews, some focus on paper-and-pencil type instruments for collecting information about spirituality.[1,26] These instruments include some that are psychometrically tested and can be used for research purposes and some that were developed specifically for nurse or client spiritual self-assessment. An example of a nurse-developed

Table 30–3
Selected Questions Adapted from Dossey's Spiritual-Assessment Tool

Meaning and Purpose

What gives your life meaning?

How does your illness interfere with your life goals?

How eager are you to get well—or to die?

What is the most important or powerful thing in your life?

Inner Strengths

What brings you joy and/or peace in your life?

What makes you feel alive and full of spirit?

What traits do you like about yourself? And how have these traits helped you to cope with your current situation?

Although physical healing may not be possible, what would help you to heal emotionally or spiritually?

How does your faith play a role in your health? In your preparation for death?

Interconnections

With Self

How do you feel about yourself right now?

What do you do to love yourself, or forgive yourself?

What do you do to heal your spirit?

With Others

Who are the people to whom you are closest? How can they help you now? How can you help them now?

How able are you to ask for help? To receive that help graciously?

How able are you to forgive others?

With Transcendent Other, Divinity

How important is it to you to worship a higher power or God? What forms of worship are most helpful to you now?

Does prayer, meditation, relaxation, or guided imagery, or anything like these, help you? How do they help you? For example, how are your prayers answered?

With the Environment, Nature

How connected to the earth do you feel?

Do you have spiritual insights when you enjoy nature's beauty?

How does your environment stress you, or contribute to your illness?

Source: Questions selected and adapted from Dossey (1998), reference 52.

self-assessment form for use with patients is presented in Figure 30-1.

Summary of Spiritual Assessment Models

The above summaries of various models for spiritual assessment identify spiritual dimensions that may be included in a spiritual assessment. Many of the dimensions identified in one model are observed (often using different language) in other models. The method necessary for completing the assessment generally requires the professional to make observations while asking questions, and listening for the patient's response. The vast majority of questions recommended for use in following such a model are open-ended. Several of the questions—indeed, the dimensions of spirituality—identified in this literature use "God language" or assume a patient will have belief in some transcendent divinity. The medical and nursing models that explicitly suggest assessment questions should address the linkage between spirituality and health, while the pastoral counseling models do not. All the models are developed by professionals who are influenced predominantly by Western, Judeo-Christian ways of thinking.

General Observations and Suggestions For Conducting a Spiritual Assessment

What Approach to Use

Whereas researchers often assess individuals' spirituality quantitatively with "paper and pencil" questionnaires, health care professionals generally assess spirituality using qualitative methods (e.g., participant observations, semistructured interviews). However, it is possible to use questionnaires during the clinical spiritual-assessment process.[1,26,28,40,53] This approach to conducting a spiritual assessment allows for identification, and possibly, measurement, of what one believes and how one behaves. This type of tool, however, should not "stand alone" in the process of spiritual assessment; rather, it can be the springboard for a more thorough assessment and deeper encounter with a patient, as appropriate. A quantitative tool should never replace human contact, instead, it should facilitate it. Although a quantitative spiritual self-assessment form provides an opportunity for health care teams to glean substantial information when screening for spiritual beliefs and practices, without spending any professional's time, it also is limited by its mechanistic, rigid, and nonindividualized nature.[6]

Other approaches to spiritual assessment have been described in addition to the interview and questionnaire techniques. LeFavi and Wessels[54] described how life reviews can become, in essence, spiritual assessments. Life reviews are especially valuable for persons who are dying, as they allow patients to make sense of and reconcile their life story. By doing a life review with a terminally ill patient, the nurse can assess many dimensions of spirituality (e.g., world views, commitments, missions, values) in a natural, noncontrived manner. Life reviews can be prompted by questions about the significant events, people, and challenges during the lifespan. A life review can also occur when inquiring about personal objects, pictures, or other memorabilia the patient wants to share.

Hodge[55] identified several creative approaches to collecting information about client spirituality. Diagrammatic tools such as a spiritual genogram, spiritual family tree, or spiritual map could be drawn by the patient to describe and organize their spirituality. Having clients draw a spiritual timeline that includes significant books, experiences, events, and so forth, will also yield rich information. Another unusual approach involves sentence completion. For example, a client may fill in the blank of sentences like "My relation to God . . ." or "What I would really like to be . . ." or "When I feel overwhelmed. . . ."

When to Assess

Dudley and colleagues[34] found that 100 of 117 hospices surveyed acknowledged that they did spiritual assessments routinely. In practice, if spiritual assessment is a routine, it generally occurs during the initial intake assessment. However, some experts agree that spiritual assessment should be an ongoing process.[1,45,57] The nurse does not complete a spiritual assessment simply by asking some questions about religion or spirituality during an intake interview. Instead, spiritual assessment should be ongoing throughout the nurse–patient relationship.

Stoll,[51] recognizing the significance of timing when asking patients questions about spirituality, suggested that spiritual assessment be separated from a sexual assessment because both topics are so sensitive and intimate. However, both spiritual and sexual assessment should occur during the general assessment for the purposes of screening for problems. Several authors remind their readers that spiritual assessments can only be effectively completed if the health care professional has first established trust and rapport with the patient.[6,51,57]

Levels of Assessment

Many advocate a two-tiered approach to spiritual assessment.[1,6,23,50] That is, a brief assessment for screening purposes is conducted when a patient enters a health care institution for palliative care. Matthews'[49] or Puchalski's[47] FICA guidelines work especially well for this screening. Ideally, what spiritual needs exist and how the palliative care team can care for these needs should be determined. Spiritual needs, however, are complex and often difficult to acknowledge, and more so, to describe with words. Furthermore, the patient may not yet feel comfortable divulging such intimate information to a nurse with whom rapport has not been established. General open-ended questions eliciting information about their faith, religiousness, or spiritual beliefs and practices are less upsetting than asking about "spiritual *need*" and can indirectly provide clues about needs. Kub and colleagues,[58] in their research with 114 terminally ill persons, found that a single question about the importance of religion to be more discriminating than a question about frequency of attendance at religious services.

If the screening assessment generates an impression that there are spiritual needs, then spiritual care can only be planned if further information is collected. The second tier of assessment allows for focused, in-depth assessment. For example, if a nurse observes a terminally ill patient's spouse crying and stating, "Why does God have to take my sweetheart?," then the nurse would want to understand further what factors are contributing to or may relieve this spiritual pain. To focus the assessment on the pertinent topic, the nurse would then ask questions that explore the spouse's "why" questions, beliefs about misfortune, perceptions of God, and spiritual coping strategies.

Prefacing the Spiritual Assessment

Because spirituality and religiosity are sensitive and personal topics (as are most other topics nurses assess), it is polite for a nurse to preface a spiritual assessment with an acknowledgment of the sensitivity of the questions and an explanation for why such an assessment is necessary.[1,45] For example, Maugens[45] suggested this preface:

> Many people have strong spiritual or religious beliefs that shape their lives, including their health and experiences with illness. If you are comfortable talking about this topic, would you please share any of your beliefs and practices that you might want me to know as your physician (p. 12).

Such a preface undoubtedly will help both the patient and the clinician to feel at ease during the assessment.

Assessing Nonverbal Indicators of Spirituality

Although this discussion of spiritual assessment has thus far focused on how to frame a verbal question and allow a patient to verbalize a response, the nurse must remember that most communication occurs nonverbally. Hence, the nurse must assess the nonverbal communication and the environment of the patient. A chaplain mentor instructed the author to observe the ABCs of spiritual assessment (personal communication, John Pumphries, October 1986). The observer must assess the **A**ffect, **B**ehaviors, and **C**ommunication of the patient and think, "Are these elements congruent?" An incongruency between affect and words indicates an area requiring care and further assessment. To illustrate, a patient who responds to "How are you?" with "Fine"—but with an angry tone of voice and demeanor and avoidance of eye contact, is sending incongruent messages. Such a patient is likely angry.

Assessment of the patient's environment can also provide clues about spiritual state.[1,27] Are there religious objects on the bedside table? Are there religious paintings or crucifixes on the walls? Get-well cards or books with spiritual themes? Are there indicators that the patient has many friends and family providing love and a sense of community? Are the curtains closed and the bedspread pulled over the face? Does the patient appear agitated or angry? Many of the factors a palliative care nurse usually assesses will provide data for a spiritual assessment as well as the psychosocial assessment.

Language: Religious or Spiritual Words?

One barrier to spiritual assessment is the nurse's fear of offending a nonreligious patient by using religious language. However, when one remembers the nonreligious nature of spirituality, this barrier disappears. Patients' spirituality can be discussed without God language or reference to religion.

To know what language will not be offensive during a spiritual assessment, the nurse must remember two guidelines. First, the nurse can begin the assessment with questions that are general and unrelated to religious assumptions. For example, "What is giving you the strength to cope with your illness now?" or "What spiritual beliefs and practices are important to you as you cope with your illness?" Second, the nurse must listen for the language of the patient, and use the patient's language when formulating more specific follow-up questions. If a patient responds to a question with "My faith and prayers help me," then the nurse knows "faith" and "prayer" are words that will not offend this patient. If a patient states that the "Great Spirit guides," then the sensitive nurse will not respond with, "Tell me how Jesus is your guide."

Asking Questions

Because asking a patient questions is an integral part of most spiritual assessments, it is good to remember some of the basics of formulating good questions. Asking close-ended questions that allow for short factual or yes/no responses is helpful when a nurse truly has no time or ability for further assessment. Otherwise, to appreciate the uniqueness and complexity of an individual's spirituality, the nurse must focus on asking open-ended questions. The best open-ended questions begin with how, what, when, who, or phrases like "Tell me about . . ." Generally, questions beginning with "why" are not helpful; they are often mixed with a sense of threat or challenge (e.g., "Why do you believe that?").

Listening to the Answers

Although it is easy to focus on and to worry about what to say during an assessment, the palliative care nurse must remember the importance of listening to the patient's responses. Discussion of active listening is beyond the scope of this chapter, yet a few comments are in order. Remember that silence is appropriate when listening to a patient's spiritual and sacred story. Listen for more than words; listen for symbols, listen for where the patient places energy, listen for emotion in addition to cognitions. The nurse will do well to listen to his or her own inner response. This response will mirror the feelings of the patient.

Overcoming the Time Barrier

Health care professionals may believe that they do not have enough time to conduct a spiritual assessment. Indeed, Maugens[45] observed that completing his spiritual history with patients took about 10 to 15 minutes. Although this is much less time than Maugen and his colleagues expected it to take, it is still a considerable amount of time in today's health care context. One response to this time barrier is to remember that spiritual assessment is a process that develops as the nurse gains the trust of a patient. It is ongoing.[56] The nurse can accomplish the assessment during "clinical chatterings." [45] Furthermore, data for a spiritual assessment can be simultaneously collected with other assessments or during interventions (e.g., while bathing or completing bedtime care). And finally, it can be argued that nurses do not have time to not conduct a spiritual assessment, considering the fundamental and powerful nature of spirituality.

Overcoming Personal Barriers

Nurses can encounter personal barriers to conducting a spiritual assessment. These barriers can include feelings of embarrassment or insecurity about the topic, or can result from projection of unresolved and painful personal spiritual doubts or struggles. Every nurse has a personal philosophy or world view that influences his or her spiritual beliefs. These beliefs can color or blind the nurse's assessment techniques and interpretation. Hence, an accurate and sensitive spiritual assessment requires that the nurse be spiritually self-aware. Nurses can increase their comfort with the topic and their awareness of their spiritual self if they ask themselves variations of the questions they anticipate asking patients. For example, "What gives my life meaning and purpose?" "How do my spiritual beliefs influence the way I relate to my own death?" "How do I love myself and forgive myself?"

Assessing Impaired Patients

Although verbal conversation is integral to a typical spiritual assessment, some terminally ill patients may not be able to speak, hear, or understand a verbal assessment. Patients who are unable to communicate verbally may feel unheard. In such situations, the nurse again must remember alternative sources of information. The nurse can consult with the family members and observe the patient's environment and nonverbal communications. Alternative methods for "conversing" can also be used. For patients who can write, paper-and-pencil questionnaires can be very helpful. Always be patient and be unafraid of the tears that can follow. Questions that demonstrate concern for their innermost well-being may release their floodgates for tears.

Assessing Children

Several strategies can be employed to assess the spirituality of children. The clinician must remember, however, that building trust and rapport with children is essential to completing a helpful spiritual assessment. Children are especially capable of ascertaining an adult's degree of authenticity. Children also are less likely to be offended by a question about religion. If a nurse creates a comfortable and nonjudgmental atmosphere in which a child can discuss spiritual topics, then the child will talk. Never underestimate the profoundness of a child's spiritual experience, especially a dying child's.

In addition to asking assessment questions verbally, the nurse can use play interviews, picture drawings, observations, and informal interviews.[59-60] The nurse may need to be more creative in formulating questions if the child's vocabulary is limited. For example, instead of asking the child about helpful religious rituals, the nurse may need to ask questions about what they do to get ready to sleep or what they do on weekends. When asking, "Does your mommy pray with you before you go to sleep?" or "What do you do on Sunday or Sabbath mornings?" the nurse can learn whether prayer or religious service attendance are a part of this child's life. An assessment question that Sexson's[60] colleague Patricia Fosarelli found to be particularly helpful with 6- to 18-year-olds was: "If you could get God to answer one question, what one question would you ask God?"

Understanding the family's spirituality is pivotal to understanding the child's. Structured interviews or unstructured conversations with parents and even older siblings will inform the health care team about the child's spirituality.[60] Barnes and colleagues[61] suggested the following questions as guides for assessing how a family's spirituality affects illness experience:

- How does the family understand life's purpose and meaning?
- How do they explain illness and suffering?
- How do they view the person in the context of the body, mind, soul, spirit, and so forth?
- How is the specific illness of the child explained?
- What treatments are necessary for the child?
- Who is the qualified person to address these various treatments for the various parts of the child's healing?
- What is the outcome measurement that the family is using to measure successful treatment (good death)?

While assessing children, it is vital to consider their stage of cognitive and faith development.[59,60] Questions must be framed in age-appropriate language (a 4-year-old will likely not understand what "spiritual belief" means!). Toddlers and preschoolers talk about their spirituality in very concrete terms, with an egocentric manner. School-aged and adolescent children should be addressed straightforwardly about how they see their illness. Inquiring about the cause of their illness is especially important, as many children view their illness and impending death as punishment.[60]

Assessing Diverse Spiritualities

Spiritual assessment methods must be flexible enough to obtain valid data from persons with diverse spiritual and religious backgrounds. Although the questions and assumptions presented in this chapter will be helpful for assessing most patients living in Western, Euro-American cultures, they may not be for some patients who do not share these presuppositions. For example, some may believe it is wrong to discuss their inner spiritual turmoil as they face death and will refuse to fully engage in the process of spiritual assessment. (While some Buddhists and Hindus may believe they must be in a peaceful state to be reincarnated to a better state, African-American Christians may think it is sinful to express doubts or anger towards God.) Framing spiritual assessment in a positive tone may overcome this type of barrier (e.g., "Tell me about how you are at peace now.") Others may assume they are void of spirituality and therefore decline any questions regarding their "spirituality." This barrier to assessment can be overcome with questions that are void of such language (e.g., "What gives your life meaning?" or "How is your courage?").

For patients who are religious, it is important to remember that no two members of a religious community or family are exactly alike. For example, one orthodoxly religious person may believe he should never consume any mind-altering drugs, such as morphine, while a less conservative member of the same denomination may understand that such drugs are a gracious Godly gift. Although having a cursory understanding of the world's major religious traditions provides nurses with some framework for inquiry, remaining open to the variation of religious experience and expression is essential.

The Next Step: What To Do with a Spiritual Assessment

Making a Diagnosis

The North American Nursing Diagnosis Association (NANDA) includes "spiritual distress," "risk for spiritual distress," and "potential for enhanced spiritual well-being" as validated diagnoses.[1,34] However, other language can be used to label a spiritual problem. For example, the NANDA diagnoses of "anxiety," "impaired adjustment," "ineffective family coping," "dysfunctional grieving," "fear," "hopelessness," "loneliness," "social isolation," "ineffective coping," and "defensive coping" can also refer to what may be essentially spiritual problems. O'Brien[28] offered a more complete taxonomy for spiritual problems that were identified during research on spirituality during life-threatening illness. O'Brien's labels for spiritual problems include spiritual pain, spiritual alienation, spiritual anxiety, spiritual guilt, spiritual anger, spiritual loss, and spiritual despair.

O'Brien's[28] list of potential spiritual problems begins to show the variety of diagnoses one patient could be given. Indeed, the NANDA primary diagnoses offer only a vague description; it is essential that the secondary or "related to" element of the NANDA diagnosis be determined.[1,35] Without specific identification of a spiritual problem and its etiology, appropriate and effective interventions cannot be implemented.

Documentation

Although assessments of physiological phenomenon are readily documented in patient charts, assessments and diagnoses of spiritual problems are less frequently documented. However, for many reasons, spiritual assessments and care should be documented. These reasons include: (1) to facilitate the continuity of patient care among palliative care team members, and (2) to document for the monitoring purposes of accrediting bodies, researchers, quality management teams, and so forth.

Formats for documenting spiritual assessments and diagnoses can vary. Some institutions encourage staff to use SOAP (**S**ubjective, **O**bjective, **A**ssessment, **P**lan) or similar formatting in progress notes shared by the multidisciplinary team. Others have developed quick and easy checklists for documenting spiritual and religious issues. Perhaps an assessment format that allows for both rapid documentation and optional narrative data is best. However, merely documenting one's religious affiliation and whether one desires a referral to a spiritual care specialist certainly does not adequately indicate a patient's spiritual status and need.

A summary of assessment forms created by professionals at hospices is reported by Dudley, Smith, and Millison.[34] These researchers synthesized the spiritual assessment forms from 53 hospices, finding questions about religious affiliation and rituals, religious problems or barriers, and questions about spiritual (nonreligious) topics, that is, questions void of overtly religious language. While Dudley and colleagues summarize the content of these forms, they do not review the format for documentation on these forms.

Conclusion

Spirituality is an elemental and pervading dimension for persons, especially those for whom death is imminent. Spiritual assessment is essential to effective and sensitive spiritual care. Indeed, spiritual assessment is the beginning of spiritual care. While the nurse questions a patient about spirituality, the nurse is simultaneously assisting the patient to reflect on the innermost and most important aspects of being human. The nurse is also indicating to the patient that grappling with spiritual issues is normal and valuable. The nurse also provides spiritual care during an assessment by being present and witnessing what is sacred for the patient.

REFERENCES

1. Taylor EJ. Spiritual Care: Nursing Theory, Research, and Practice. Upper Saddle River, NJ: Prentice Hall, 2002.
2. Reed PG. An emerging paradigm for the investigation of spirituality in nursing. Res Nurs Health 1992;15:349–357.
3. Dossey BM, Guzzetta CE. Holistic nursing practice. In: Dossey BM, Keegan L, Guzzetta CE (eds.). Holistic Nursing: A Handbook for Practice, 3rd ed. Rockville, MD: Aspen, 2000:5–26.
4. Gallup G, Jr. Religion in America. Harrisburg, PA: Morehouse Publishing, 1999.
5. Bash A. Spirituality: The emperor's new clothes? J Clin Nurs 2004;13:11–16.
6. McSherry W, Ross L. Dilemmas of spiritual assessment: considerations for nursing practice. J Adv Nurs 2002;38:479–488.
7. Taylor EJ. Spiritual and ethical end-of-life concerns. In: Groenwald SL, Frogge MH, Goodman M, Yarbro CH, eds. Cancer nursing: Principles and practice, 4th ed. Boston: Jones & Bartlett, 1997:1421–1434.
8. McGrath P. Spiritual pain: a comparison of findings from survivors and hospice patients. Am J Hosp Palliat Care 2003;20(1):23–33.
9. Thomas J, Retsas A. Transacting self-preservation: a grounded theory of the spiritual dimensions of people with terminal cancer. Internat J Nurs Stud 1999;36:19–201.
10. Greisinger AJ, Lorimor RJ, Aday L, Winn RJ, Baile WF. Terminally ill cancer patients: their most important concerns. Cancer Pract 1997;5:147–154.
11. Taylor EJ. Spiritual quality of life. In: King CR, Hinds PS, eds. Quality of Life: From Nursing and Patient Perspectives, 2nd ed. Sudbury, MA: Jones and Bartlett, 2000:93–116.
12. Thomson JE. The place of spiritual well-being in hospice patient's overall quality of life. Hospice J 2000;15:13–27.
13. McMillan SC, Weitzner M. How problematic are various aspects of quality of life in patients with cancer at the end of life? Oncol Nurs Forum 2000;27:817–823.
14. McClain CS, Rosenfeld B, Brietbart W. Effect of spiritual well-being on end-of-life despair in terminally ill cancer patients. Lancet 2003;361:1603–1607.
15. Feher S, Maly RC. Coping with breast cancer in later life: the role of religious faith. Psycho-Oncol 1999;8:408–406.
16. Taylor EJ, Outlaw FH. Use of prayer among persons with cancer. Holist Nurs Pract 2002;16:46–60.
17. Tatsumura Y, Maskarinec G, Shumay DM, Kakai H. Religious and spiritual resources, CAM, and conventional treatment in the lives of cancer patients. Altern Ther Health Med 2003;9:64–71.
18. Mickley JR, Pargament KI, Brant CR, Hipp M. God and the search for meaning among hospice caregivers. Hospice J 1998;13:1–17.
19. Abernethy AD, Chang HT, Seidlitz L, Evinger JS, Duberstine PR. Religious coping and depression among spouses of people with lung cancer. Psychosomat 2002;43:456–463.
20. Taylor EJ. Spiritual needs of cancer patients and family caregivers. Cancer Nurs 2003;26:260–266.
21. Spiritual Beliefs and the Dying Process: Key Findings. New York: Nathan Cummings Foundation and Fetzer Institute, October 1997.
22. Joint Commission on Accreditation of Healthcare Organizations. Spiritual assessment, http://www.jcaho.org/accredited+organizations/hospitals/standards/hospital+faqs/provision+of+care/assessment/spiritual+assessment.htm (accessed January 27, 2005).
23. Hunt J, Cobb M, Keeley VL, and Ahmedzai SH. The quality of spiritual care—developing a standard. Int J Palliat Nurs 2003; 9:208–215.
24. Millison M, Dudley JR. Providing spiritual support: a job for all hospice professionals. Hospice J 1992;8:49–65.
25. Maddox M. Teaching spirituality to nurse practitioner students: the importance of the interconnection of mind, body, and spirit. J Am Acad Nurse Pract 2001;13:134–139.
26. Burkhardt MA, Nagai-Jacobson MG. Spirituality: Living Our Connectedness. Albany, NY: Delmar, 2002.
27. Shelly JA. Spiritual Care: A Guide for Caregivers. Downers Grove, IL: Intervarsity Press, 2000.
28. O'Brien ME. Spirituality in Nursing: Standing on Holy Ground, 2nd ed. Sudbury, MA: Jones and Bartlett, 2003.
29. Taylor EJ, Highfield MF, Amenta MO. Predictors of oncology and hospice nurses' spiritual care perspectives and practices. Appl Nurs Res 1999;12:30–37.
30. Highfield MEF, Taylor EJ, Amenta MO. Preparation to care: the spiritual care education of oncology and hospice nurses. J Hosp Palliat Nurs 2000;2:53–63.
31. Kuuppelomaki M. Spiritual support for families of patients with cancer: a pilot study of nursing staff assessments. Cancer Nurs 2002;25:209–218.
32. Kristeller JL, Zumbrun CS, Schilling RF. "I would if I could": how oncology nurses address spiritual distress in cancer patients. Psycho-Oncol 1999;8:451–458.
33. Hermann CP. Spiritual needs of dying patients: a qualitative study. Oncol Nurs Forum 2001;28:67–72.
34. Dudley JR, Smith C, Millison MB. Unfinished business: assessing the spiritual needs of hospice clients. Am J Hospice Palliat Care 1995;12:30–37.
35. Carpenito LJ. Nursing diagnosis: Applications to clinical practice, 7th ed. Philadelphia: Lippincott Williams & Wilkins, 2000.
36. Highfield MF, Cason C. Spiritual needs of patients: are they recognized? Cancer Nurs 1983; 6:187–192.
37. Pruyser PW. The Minister as Diagnostician. Philadelphia: Westminster Press, 1976.
38. Malony HN. Making a religious diagnosis: the use of religious assessment in pastoral care and counseling. Pastoral Psychol 1993;41:237–246.
39. Fitchett G. Assessing Spiritual Needs: A Guide for Caregivers. Minneapolis: Fortress Press, 1993.
40. van der Poel CJ. (1998). Sharing the Journey: Spiritual Assessment and Pastoral Response to Persons with Incurable Illnesses. Collegeville, MN: Liturgical Press, 1998.
41. Muncy JF. Muncy comprehensive spiritual assessment. Am J Hosp Palliat Care 1996;13:44–45.
42. Koenig HG. Spirituality in Patient Care: Why, How, When, and What. Philadelphia: Templeton Foundation Press, 2002.
43. Massey K, Fitchett G, Roberts P. Assessment and diagnosis in spiritual care. In: Mauk KL, Schmidt NK, eds. Spiritual Care in Nursing Practice. Philadelphia: Lippincott Williams & Wilkins, 2004.
44. King M, Speck P, Thomas A. The royal free interview for spiritual and religious beliefs: development and validation of a self-report version. Psychol Med 2001;31:1015–1023.
45. Maugens TA. The SPIRITual history. Arch Fam Med 1996;5:11–16.
46. Anandarajah G, Hight E. Spirituality and medical practice: using the HOPE questions as a practical tool for spiritual assessment. Am Fam Physician 2001;63:81–89.

47. Puchalski CM. Taking a spiritual history: FICA. Spirituality and Medicine Connection 1999;3:1.
48. Lo B, Quill T, Tulsky J. Discussing palliative care with patients. Ann Intern Med 1999;130:744–749.
49. Matthews DA, McCullough ME, Larson DB, Koenig HG, Swyers JP, Milano MG. Religious commitment and health status: a review of the research and implications for family medicine. Arch Fam Med 1998;7:118–124.
50. Mauk CL, Schmidt NK. Spiritual care in nursing practice. Philadelphia: Lippincott Williams & Wilkins, 2004.
51. Stoll RI. Guidelines for spiritual assessment. Am J Nurs 1979; 79:1574–1577.
52. Dossey BM. Holistic modalities and healing moments. Am J Nurs 1998;98:44–47.
53. Salisbury SR, Ciulla MR, McSherry E. Clinical management reporting and objective diagnostic instruments for spiritual assessment in spinal cord injury patients. J Health Care Chaplaincy 1989;2:35–64.
54. LeFavi RG, Wessels MH. Life review in pastoral care counseling: background and efficacy for the terminally Ill. J Pastoral Care Council 2003;57:281–292.
55. Hodge DR. Spiritual assessment: a review of major qualitative methods and a new framework for assessing spirituality. Social Work 2001;46:203–214.
56. Brush BL, Daly PR. Assessing spirituality in primary care practice: is there time? Clin Excell Nurse Pract 2000;4:67–71.
57. Taylor EJ. Nurses caring for the spirit: patients with cancer and family caregiver expectations. Oncol Nurs Forum 2003;30: 585–590.
58. Kub JE, Nolan MT, Hughes MT, Terry PB, Sulmasy DP, Astrow A, Forman JH. Religious importance and practices of patients with a life-threatening illness: implications for screening protocols. Appl Nurs Res 2003;16:196–200.
59. Hart D, Schneider D. Spiritual care for children with cancer. Semin Oncol Nurs 1997;13:263–270.
60. Sexson SB. Religious and spiritual assessment of the child and adolescent. Child Adolesc Psychiatr Clin N Am 2004;13:35–47.
61. Barnes LP, Plotnikoff GA, Fox K, Pendleton S. Spirituality, religion, and pediatrics: Intersecting worlds of healing. Pediatrics 2000;104:899–908.
62. Kloss WE. Spirituality: the will to wellness. Harding J Relig Psychiatry 1988;7:3–8.

31 Spiritual Care Interventions

Charles Kemp

The purpose of life is reconciliation with God, self, and others.—Charles Kemp[1]
Management of physical symptoms is the first step in spiritual care.—William Breitbart[2]

- ***Key Points***
- *Hospice and palliative care emerged, in part, as a response to the increasing medicalization of death and dying.*
- *Terminal illness tends to bring into sharp focus man's search for meaning or sense of loss of meaning.*
- *The nursing challenge is to ensure that the sacred and the spiritual needs of the patient and family, so great at this time, are an integral part of their care.*

This chapter addresses the challenges of providing effective spiritual care to patients with terminal illness. The chapter is structured around the basic spiritual needs and is based on the certainty that there often is no one in a better position to provide spiritual care than the informed and committed nurse.

Definitions

There are many definitions of spirituality, religion, faith, and spiritual needs. For the purposes of this chapter, these terms are defined as follows:[1,3–6]

- *Religion:* An organized effort, usually involving ritual, dogma, and/or devotion, to manifest spirituality.
- *Faith:* The acceptance, without objective proof, of something, e.g., God.
- *Spirituality:* The incorporation of a transcendent dimension in life, usually, but not always, involving faith and religion.
- *Spiritual needs:* Human needs for transcendence that are addressed by most religions. The basic spiritual needs are meaning or purpose, hope, relatedness, forgiveness or acceptance, and transcendence.

Popular psychology or postmodern standards of political correctness often focus on spirituality without religion, faith, or God. However, in the real world of suffering, dying, and death, it is religion, faith, and God to which the majority of people turn.

Preparation

Providing spiritual care at the end of life can (and perhaps should) be a daunting task. Even the most academically and clinically prepared chaplain or counselor sometimes feels her or his own inadequacy to intervene effectively with a person facing the end of life. While there is an increase in education on spiritual issues and care in health professions education, there often is a lack of practical content or practice in actually providing spiritual care. This lack of preparation, coupled with the enormity of death and the nurse's personal doubts and uncertainties, may result in a reluctance to attempt to provide spiritual care—even when the need is apparent.[6-8]

Preparation to provide spiritual care includes clarification of goals, knowledge of spiritual needs, personal exploration, and willingness to apply knowledge of some basic interventions. Spiritual assessment and care should be introduced early in the course of care and reevaluated continuously. To facilitate a foundation of spiritual care, it is often essential for the nurse to first establish both a trusting relationship with the patient and good communication.

Clarification of Goals

The primary goal of spiritual care is to increase the opportunity for reconciliation with God (or a higher power) and self. This goal is based on the ideas that (1) life does indeed come from God, and (2) for many people, the process of living includes some degree of felt separation from God and faith. In the Western world, approximately 95% of people claim to believe in God, and worldwide about 85% of people claim to be religious,[9–11] so this goal would logically be as basic to persons with terminal illness as would relieving pain, dyspnea, and other symptoms. More specific goals of palliative care are clearly related to the spiritual needs, such as decreasing the sense of meaninglessness, purposelessness, or hopelessness or increasing a sense of relatedness, forgiveness, or acceptance. In terms of nursing diagnoses, the goal would likely be relieving spiritual distress, but the previously stated goals are more specific and function as etiologies (e.g., "spiritual distress related to hopelessness"). Note that the goal in spiritual care is not to provide one's own answers to ultimate questions or for the patient to achieve a particular belief. Most of the interventions and goals given here can apply to persons of any faith, or even to persons of no faith.

Knowledge of Spiritual Needs

Each of the spiritual needs is discussed below. Hope is also discussed more extensively in Chapter 26.

Meaning includes the reason for an event or events, the purpose of life, and the belief in a primary force in life. Meaning may be sought in a review of life achievements, in a review of relationships, in a moral or spiritual search, especially of life as it was lived, and in an effort to discern the meaning of dying, of human existence, of suffering, and of the remaining days of life.[3,4]

Hope is for the "expectation of a good that is yet to be."[12] There often is hope to not die, and, failing that, hope to live and die in a way perceived to be good.[8] In the struggle of terminal illness, spiritual hope may be distilled into achieving the purpose of life: reconciliation with God, with self, and with others.[1]

Relatedness for Christians, Jews, and Muslims is to God; for Hindus and Buddhists, relatedness may also be to (1) God or a god or (2) a system of spiritual faith or belief. Here, God is defined as supreme or ultimate reality, infinite, eternal, universal, all-knowing, and Being Itself. Relatedness for persons of any faith may also include relatedness to a religion or faith community.

Forgiveness by God is often seen in the West as a concept of Christianity, Judaism, or Islam. However, the Buddhist and Hindu concepts of karma and transmigration of souls also directly address forgiveness or at least another chance to rectify mistakes. Acceptance is related to forgiveness and meets the underlying need to deal with mistakes or misfortune in life.[1]

Transcendence is that which takes one beyond self and suffering—or attachment to self and suffering—beyond death. Transcendence can occur as a result of meeting other spiritual needs or as grace or manifestation of the divine, and thus may be seen as the outcome of spiritual needs or as the ultimate spiritual need.[1,13]

Understanding or working toward understanding these needs provides a framework for understanding and intervening in spiritual distress. Not every person fits neatly into spiritual distress related to one or more of these (unmet) needs, but at a minimum, these needs give nurses and others a place to start looking in a mindful manner at the spiritual dimension in terminal illness.

Personal Exploration

Working in palliative care is emotionally and spiritually challenging. Regardless of one's profession or role, those who work in palliative care operate, at least some of the time, at the edge of human existence and are often confronted by deep human suffering in all spheres of being (physical, psychological, social, and spiritual). To work gracefully and effectively in these circumstances, it is essential to explore one's own losses, grief, and fears. Such an exploration brings the practitioner face-to-face with existential challenges, such as the inevitability and finality of death, the isolation and separateness that are part of every life, and, if the truth be known, the inability to truly "deal with it." Sooner or later, personal exploration may then evolve into a spiritual search. Here again, though, the searcher may be found wanting. One may then look to the refuge intrinsic in every major faith. For here is the truth: Few of us in palliative care would presume to think "I can do the whole of the physical care"—in terms of the care for a particular patient, much less in terms of developing and putting into practice the theory and principles of palliative care! Few of us (clergy included) should then presume to think "I can do the whole of the spiritual care"—either in terms of the care for a particular patient, much less in terms of confronting and understanding the enormity of human existence, including death.

Personal spiritual exploration may lead to exploration of spiritual and religious resources such as church, synagogue, mosque, or temple. Of course, there are those who are spiritually well-grounded and able to provide quality spiritual care even though they do not participate in religious activities. However, a greater number do find that participation in spiritually based activities, specifically in religious activities where "universal values" are served by tradition, increases the capacity to provide spiritual care.[3,14]

In their seminal study of the spiritual practices of oncology nurses, Taylor, Amenta, and Highfield[15] found that 65% of oncology nurses surveyed attended religious services "frequently," ranging from one to three times per month (21%) to weekly or more often (44%). Both nurses and their patients benefit from the strongest possible spiritual foundation.

Basic Spiritual Care Interventions: "Watching With" and Prayer

Interventions related to basic spiritual needs are presented below; however, it is vital to keep in mind that the critical and most fundamental intervention is to remain present (to "watch through the night") in the face of suffering, fear, despair, and all the physical/emotional/social/spiritual trials of dying. [16] Being present on a consistent basis through the process of dying is primary spiritual care and addresses the most fundamental spiritual need—the need for transcendence. Granted, neither the patient nor the nurse may necessarily feel transcendent. Still, there is an undeniable element of transcendence in the willingness to go beyond self and suffering, and there is an undeniable need for this presence. The Bible presents the need for this presence in stark and universal terms: "My soul is very sorrowful, even to death; remain here, and watch with me" (Matthew 26:38).[17] And so the nurse and others working in palliative and hospice care have this opportunity to provide primary spiritual care that does not require understanding, answers, acceptance, or conquering—all that is required is to "watch with me."

A second, fundamental intervention is prayer. While many authors note prayer as an intervention, few are able to say how one implements this basic aspect of care (except as an expression of [usually Christian] spiritual practice). Here then are some of the author's thoughts and experiences in prayer.

For many, prayer is a deeply personal issue. For a nonclergyperson, moving into the dimension of prayer may be a difficult step. Knowing that somehow prayer would help, there still may be reluctance to (1) take the risk of spiritual rejection or (2) be put on the spot as a provider of frank spiritual care when there is certain knowledge of one's personal spiritual inadequacies. Yet we know prayer can be comforting, cleansing, and transcendent. The first one is the hardest.

A 17-Year-Old Girl with Bronchitis

I work mostly in primary care with medically indigent refugees and immigrants. Not long ago I walked into an exam room where a 17-year-old Mexican girl sat, ravaged by a 5-year history of central nervous system tumor, seizures, strokes, surgeries, and radiation. Her mother sat a few feet away, silent, dignified, very tired, and full of pain. The girl had bronchitis, and I prescribed the appropriate treatment. My anxiety about prayer fell away (Why was I ever concerned about *myself*?) and I asked the Mom if we could pray. She said yes, and we all held hands and I led the girl, Mom, translator, and nursing student in prayer. I thanked God for the Mom, the girl, for the doctors and nurses treating the girl, and for them coming to our clinic; I prayed for healing of body and spirit and for the strength to accept God's will.

So the first step is to see what is in front of one's eyes and forget about oneself. Invitations to prayer come from the heart. The words might include, "Could I say a prayer with you or for you?" or "Are you a praying person, because this feels like a time for a prayer." A noted physician and ethicist suggests that prayer may be gently introduced into a patient-care encounter by asking, "Would it be okay if we have a prayer? Even if it won't help you, it will help me."[18] Readers will readily see that such a request also is likely to have a salutary effect on the relationship between the patient and provider. Other interventions are discussed below.

Interventions: Spiritual Needs, Problems, and Practices

Each of the spiritual needs is examined below, including a discussion of the need, manifestations of the unmet need, and interventions to help in meeting the need. In actual practice, there often is overlap among problems resulting from the unmet needs. This may include needs that are never assessed and needs that are met or neglected to varying degrees. As with other frameworks for practice, patients and families do not always fit neatly into certain categories. In general, unmet spiritual needs may be expressed by direct statements of hopelessness, meaninglessness, despair, guilt, and so on. Indirect expressions of unmet spiritual needs may include anxiety, sadness/depression, fear, irritation, loneliness, and anger.[6] (See Chapter 30, Spiritual Assessment, for discussion of these signs.)

Meaning

For many people, serious questions about the meaning of life typically arise in the late teen years and into the early 20s. After that, these questions may be set aside or put into the background, as work, relationships, raising children, and other life demands take precedence over philosophical pursuits. Often, decisions are made and paths taken without regard to any component of meaning or other such concerns. In life, one does what one must do. Later, as the end of life approaches, questions of meaning may again arise.

Few people go through the process of terminal illness without experiencing some form of life review. It is important to note that those whose physical symptoms are unmanaged without remission are often unable to address meaning and other spiritual issues because they are more likely to focus only on physical needs and suffering.[2] That life review, whether conscious or unconscious, brings forth the question of, "What did my life mean and how well did I live it?" If the answer is, "My life was full of meaning and I lived it well," then meaning is more likely to be found in the last days, and those days are more likely to be lived well. If, on the other hand, the answer is, "My life had little meaning and I did not live it well," then meaning is less likely to be found in the last days, and those days are less likely to be lived well. The old adage of palliative care is again illustrated: without skilled intervention, most people die in a manner very similar to that of the rest of their lives.

However, there are those whose lives are characterized by spiritual emptiness and pain who then find meaning in life even as it draws to an end. For these, terminal illness may serve as a motivation to reach beyond self and suffering. To participate in such a process of spiritual growth is a privilege. Much of this chapter is focused on promoting this growth. A sense of meaninglessness in life as a whole may be first addressed by assisting the patient through a mindful life review.[19]

Previously it was noted that unless physical problems are overwhelming, almost everyone who is dying goes through some sort of life review. The problem with such life reviews is that many times they are undertaken in a time of despair, and/or they tend to focus on the negative. More importantly, these reviews are unproductive. This author is probably not alone in a tendency to wake during the night obsessing about a problem or personal deficit (in the midst of a life of plenty) and spend an hour or more going over and over and over that problem or deficit with little or no progress or insight achieved. The result is a sleepless night with nothing to show for the distress.

"Mindful life review" means that the nurse or other staff suggests to the patient a deliberate and thoughtful verbal or written review of the patient's life, including relationships, achievements, failures, high points, low points, and so on. It is essential to understand that such a review is not a one-time activity, or something that occurs early in the relationship, but, rather, is one valued aspect of an ongoing nurse–patient relationship. For example, in a home care setting, the nurse might ask the patient to think about one important relationship that was or is positive and one that was or is less positive and to talk about those during the next home visit. At that visit, the nurse listens to what the patient says about the relationships, helps the patient explore them in greater depth, and helps identify ways in which the relationships might be redefined or viewed in a more realistic manner. Specific to spiritual matters and meaning, the nurse might ask the patient to think about something that has been full of meaning in the patient's life and, conversely, to think of something important that seemed meaningless or possessed negative meaning. The interventions are contained (1) in the patient's explanation of the issue or issues and (2) in the nurse's help to the patient in breaking out of repetitious thinking about the issue(s).

The search for meaning in life as it has been lived is facilitated by asking the patient the very serious question, "If you had your life to live over again, what would you like to be different and what would you like to be the same?" In certain close and therapeutic relationships, this question can serve as a framework for the therapeutic aspect of the relationship. In a home care setting, for example, the question can be rephrased to address the various dimensions of a person's life (e.g., "In terms of your spiritual life, what would you . . ." or "In terms of relationships . . .").

This "If you had your life to live over" question is often painful for the patient. Who among us does not have painful memories and regrets? But the pain is not caused by the question. Most likely the pain was already there, perhaps suppressed or perhaps just hidden from others. This question serves not only to look at the past and the meaning of a person's life, but also to present circumstances, the future, and what meaning might emerge.

The meaning of dying, suffering, and death are difficult, if not impossible to understand in terms of psychological explanation. These meanings can be addressed by questions such as, "What does it mean to you that this (dying or suffering) is happening?" This is a very serious question, and often gets serious answers. The suffering of the dying is not in any way an academic issue. The questions of, "Why me; why am I suffering; why am I dying?" are not ones for the nurse or others to answer. Rather, they are questions to which the response is to stay with the patient in her or his time of questioning and doubt. Many times, providing an answer only stifles the patient's exploration of the suffering and its meaning.

Every religion acknowledges and deals with the problem of suffering and death, and every religion is rich in examples of compassionate reaction to human suffering and death.

> On Him let man meditate
> Always, for then at the last hour
> Of going hence from his body he will be strong
> In the strength of this yoga, faithfully followed:
> The mind is firm, and the heart
> So full, it hardly knows its love.
> —The Way to Eternal Brahman (Bhagavad-Gita)[20]

> Buddha's compassion is equal toward all people; but it
> is expressed with special care toward those, who,
> because of their ignorance, have heavier burdens of evil
> and suffering to bear.
> —Buddha's Relief and Salvation for Us[21]

I lift up my eyes to the hills.
From whence does my help come?
My help comes from the Lord, who made heaven and earth.
He will not let your foot be moved, he who keeps you will not slumber.
Behold, he who keeps Israel will neither slumber nor sleep.
The Lord is your keeper; the Lord is your shade on your right hand.
The sun shall not smite you by day, nor the moon by night.
The Lord will keep you from all evil; he will keep your life,
The Lord will keep your going out and your coming in from this time forth and for evermore.
—Psalm 121[17]

Let not your hearts be troubled; believe in God, believe also in me. In my Father's house are many rooms; if it were not so, would I have told you that I go to prepare a place for you? And when I go and prepare a place for you, I will come again and take you to myself, that where I am you may be also. And you know the way where I am going.
—John 14:1–4[17]

We heard his prayer and relieved his affliction. We restored to him his family and as many more with them: a blessing from Ourself and an admonition to worshipers.
—The Prophets[22]

For many patients, help in finding and discussing passages from the sacred books of their own faiths may provide the best kind of answer to the question of the meaning of suffering and death. Of course, worship, ritual, prayer, and meditation are, or should be, part of the spiritual care milieu. Encouraging these is important, both for the patient's and family's life, and for promoting their presence in the life of the institution or organization in which one practices.

Most people confront the questions of meaning in life, suffering, and death from the point of view of their own existence. The human condition and its tendency to isolation leads to the idea that the feelings of meaningless, emptiness, and brokenness are unique to the one who is experiencing them. Of course these feelings are not unique! Exploration of how and why a person feels this way, coupled with a gentle reminder that the person is not alone in these feelings may be helpful. Here again, the questions and responses lead to the realms of spirituality and religion. For Christian and Jewish patients, certain Psalms (e.g., 6, 32, 38, 39, 41, 51, 61, 69, 88, 91, 102, 103, 130, and 143) are especially appropriate to read and discuss with respect to the meaning of suffering. Better yet, find out from the patient what scripture is most meaningful to her or him.

Contemplating and exploring the questions of meaning in life, suffering, and death noted above is likely to lead to other questions about forgiveness, acceptance, punishment, and even transcendence. Once again the questions and responses lead to the realms of spirituality and religion. These questions may lead also to questions and exploration of the meaning or purpose of the remaining days of life and to the question of what might be done to make the most of that time, both in the present and in the future. As noted earlier, the primary goal of spiritual care is to increase the opportunity for reconciliation with God (or a higher power) and self. It is not overly directive to suggest that a person looking at a very limited future on earth might consider whether one or all three of these reconciliations are worth serious contemplation for at least part of future direction.

Finding meaning in the process of dying is largely dependent upon the degree to which the patient finds some meaning in his or her life when reviewing it. Looking at the question of what one would like to have done differently in life is critical to a fulsome review of life—the good and the bad. Bringing the whole of one's life into consciousness and applying sacred literature, worship, and prayer to the process of dying may lead directly to increased meaning in the present and future (Table 31–1). "What our patients need is unconditional faith in unconditional meaning."[15]

Table 31–1
Notes on the Search for Meaning: The Patient, Family, and Nurse

- Mindfully review life: the good and the bad.
- Integrate the sacred into the process of dying: prayer, reading, worship, and ritual.
- Set realistic goals for the remaining days: improving a relationship, reading portions of a sacred book, or praying regularly.
- The nurse and others consistently dispense loving and competent care, regardless of the extent to which the patient does or does not find meaning in the process.

Hope

Although Chapter 26 is devoted to hope, hope in a solely spiritual sense is also discussed here. Themes or "universal components of hope" include finding meaning through faith or spirituality, having affirming relationships, relying on inner resources, living everyday life, and anticipating survival.[23] Not all these may be achieved in the context of terminal illness—at least in a physical sense—but all are applicable to many people going through a terminal illness. Despite the realities and challenges of terminal illness, there may be much to hope for: to live another day, for relief from suffering, for a greater understanding of life, for a good death with dignity, for a healed relationship, to see a loved one, to not die at all, or simply to be able to go through the ordeal of dying.

Hope in terminal illness can be addressed directly by asking, "What do you hope for . . . in this illness (or situation)? . . . from others? . . . at this point in your life? . . . in just this day? . . . in or for yourself? . . . in your faith (or religion or spiritual life)? What would you like to hope for?" These questions are powerful at a time like this and can facilitate expression of deep feelings and issues. What a question to ask and issue to raise—hope in terminal illness! The answers to the questions are often a mix of hope and resignation. The critical point is to directly bring up the concept of hope for exploration and discussion.

Hope in this context includes hope for reconciliation with God and self. This does not, in any way, diminish the importance of hope in relation to other matters, especially hope to heal relationships with other people. Hearkening back to the earlier discussion of meaning and reconciliation, one quickly sees that making progress toward reconciliation will have a direct impact on the presence or absence of hope, whether spiritual or otherwise—or more commonly, on the waxing and waning of hope.

CASE STUDY

Mrs. P, a Patient with Cervical Cancer

Mrs P had a terribly difficult life. She grew up poor, and in her middle years survived war, torture, forced labor, and being a refugee several times over. When first admitted to hospice, she was an alcoholic and abusive to her children. She lived in a run-down one-bedroom apartment with her husband (also an alcoholic), a son who was a gangster, another son with Down syndrome, and a 12-year-old daughter, who was the primary caregiver. Mrs. P spent most of her days and nights lying on a small couch in the apartment's living room.

She had cervical cancer, with many complications. Symptom and disease management were complicated by her alcoholism, poverty, and limited English proficiency. Overall, and considering the circumstances, her symptoms were relatively well managed.

It was clear to all concerned that Mrs. P was spiritually bereft and without hope. Using both Buddhist and Christian translators, the hospice team tried counseling to address hope and other spiritual issues in several different ways. Although she was nominally Buddhist, she refused offers of transportation to the temple. On several occasions, she accepted gifts of objects sacred to Buddhists, but after a few days would put them away. Several Christian missionaries visited on a regular basis and, although she did not resist these visits, neither did she respond to them. Everything tried seemed to fail. She did, however, show appreciation for efforts to care for her and her family.

The only thing that seemed to affect her was when one day a nursing student knelt unbidden beside Mrs. P's couch and prayed. Although Mrs. P understood little of the prayer, tears began to run down her cheeks as the young woman prayed. Afterward, Mrs. P whispered, "Thank you."

As far as I know, this patient's spiritual needs were never met, and I never saw any evidence of hope or reconciliation. So what is the point of this case study? Where are the effective interventions and the insights? Unfortunately they are not to be found—except that those of us who tried to be effective and insightful never gave up. Though none of the caregivers, the patient, or the family ever experienced much in the way of transcendence, in retrospect, there were 2 years of transcending the desire to quit.

The week before she died, I went out of town for a conference. I returned late Sunday. On Monday, I left for work early so I could see Mrs. P first. I walked into her apartment and at that moment, she died.

There are two great hopes offered to the dying and to all others by faith and religion:

1. The hope to live more fully and deeply—after all these years, in so many cases, of superficiality. All the major faiths provide clear guidelines for living in connection to faith and God or whatever one calls ultimate reality. All the major faiths say without equivocation that living in this manner brings the greatest possible fulfillment.[2]
2. The hope for a life beyond this one. All the major world religions have definitive and hopeful beliefs in outcome, that is, in what happens or can happen after death. In fact, it is only religious belief that offers any possibilities about the future after death—other than the recyclable nature of our basic molecule, carbon.

Increasing or reaching these two great hopes begins with exploration of hope and hopelessness, and thence to sources of knowledge and insight into hope and truth. After looking at what hope and hopelessness exists, one may then in partnership with the patient begin looking at the patient's faith tradition for hope that may be found there (Table 31–2).

> Die, and you win heaven. Conquer and you enjoy the earth. Stand up now, son of Kunti, and resolve to fight.

Table 31–2
Notes on Hope: The Patient, Family, and Nurse

- Understand common hopes in the process of dying.
- Understand that two great hopes are offered by faith and religion: (1) to live fully and deeply, and (2) to expect life after death.
- Ask direct questions about hope, and explicate the presence or absence of hope.
- Integrate the sacred into the process of dying: prayer, reading, worship, and ritual.
- The nurse and others faithfully "watch through the night," whether the patient or others have or do not have hope.

> Realize that pleasure and pain, gain and loss, victory and defeat, are all one and the same: then go into battle. Do this and you cannot commit any sin.
> —The Yoga of Knowledge (Bhagavad-Gita)[20]

Relatedness

Relatedness in the spiritual sense is to faith, religion, and especially to God (or with whatever represents God), or to all three. Existentially, of course, many people feel very much alone in life and in the universe. The same holds true in terms of faith and/or religion.[4] Just as the quest for meaning in life may have been put into the background, so may a quest for spiritual growth or for a deep connection with faith been put away. In some people, there is a deep feeling of having been failed by their faith and the faith community. The result of any or all of these is a sense of isolation from faith and from God or anything greater than this—this life, this inadequacy, this suffering, this transience. It is possible, and even not unusual to spend an entire lifetime trying to avoid dealing with existential and spiritual isolation.

Terminal illness tends to bring everything into sharper focus, and loneliness or meaninglessness that once seemed a bearable part of life may come to the forefront after years of suppression. The need for reconciliation or reconnection then becomes a driving force in the remaining days of life.

For most people of most faiths, the reconnection is to God. Whether referred to as Yahweh, God, Lord, or Allah, the God of Judaism, Christianity, and Islam is clearly explicated. Contrary to some conceptions of Hinduism, Hindus also believe in "One God, who can be understood and worshipped in many different forms."[24] In the Buddhist canon, relatedness is to the faith and philosophy. However, in practice, many Buddhists believe in a divine "force" or "being," as expressed by the Buddha or existing as mystery and never explicated, but never denied in the teachings of the Buddha. From a psychological perspective, Carl Jung[25] wrote with deep insight that the presence or acknowledgment of God among virtually all peoples of all religions through all times is evidence of God as a universal archetype or "living psychic force" and that the imprint of God in this manner "presupposes an imprinter."

Given the incomplete and unenlightened nature of most of us, the primary way then to relatedness to or reconciliation with God is through religion and religious practice, including prayer, ritual, and worship. Ritual and worship are sometimes constrained, not so much by patient circumstances, but more by a lack of imagination on the part of regular sources of spiritual care. Thus, a church may not think to bring communion to the patient's home, nor a temple to offer an opportunity to give alms to monks. The nurse or other provider can then act as an advocate for the patient by giving direct suggestions to the source of spiritual care. The nurse may also in some cases provide/participate in ritual. Of course, the presence of chaplains in palliative care and hospice services is of great benefit to many patients in need of spiritual support, including ritual and worship.

Another form of relatedness is to a belief system and/or religion, which, paradoxically, may not necessarily mean a strong sense of relatedness to God.[26] In some cases, God seems too much to comprehend or relate to: If God is indeed "ultimate reality," then how are we to comprehend? In other cases, there may simply be an inability to take the leap to belief. Nevertheless, relatedness to a religion or a faith community may be a step toward relatedness to God, or if not relatedness to God, then toward spiritual comfort to the patient and family.

Ideally, the patient's source of help in finding or increasing a sense of relatedness is the patient's own faith and clergy. For a variety of reasons, such help is not always available, which tends to further increase a sense of separation. The nurse or others can explore with the patient her or his faith history, especially times when faith and relatedness were strong and when they were weak, and what influenced those changes (Table 31–3). As in other aspects of palliative care, it often is the nurse's willingness to bring up and explore difficult issues that is the most therapeutic measure taken. One cannot confer relatedness to God. But what can be conferred is the possibility that there is, indeed, something beyond this suffering and isolation. Here again, the ancient and priestly act of watching through the night of fear, suffering, and isolation may be the only spiritual care possible—not to mention, the best spiritual care available. Prayer with the patient, for the patient, or for the nurse or other caregivers is an important part of spiritual care in this and other issues. For Christians and Jews, the Psalms are especially appropriate and helpful readings.

> Oh God, thou hast rejected us, broken our defenses;
> thou hast been angry; oh, restore us . . .
> —Psalm 60[17]

Table 31–3
Notes on Relatedness: The Patient, Family, and Nurse

- Understand the common problem of existential and/or spiritual isolation.
- Relatedness may be to God or to religion or the faith community.
- Explore the patient's faith history to help rekindle a sense of relatedness—or uncover reasons for a lack of relatedness.
- When relatedness does not seem possible, the primary spiritual care is to watch with the patient through the night.
- Prayer with or for the patient, and for the caregivers is important.

Forgiveness or Acceptance

Every religion has rules and sanctions related to how one lives in the world and how one practices the religion and its precepts. Every religion also acknowledges that humans fail to fully follow its rules and has provisions for such failures. In Hinduism and Buddhism, there are cycles of birth and rebirth based on actions in life (we are born to be healed). Although sin and attendant suffering are issues in these faiths, the focus of practicing the faiths is more on acceptance of self and suffering than on forgiveness. In Judaism, Christianity, and Islam there is the concept of forgiveness of sins.

> To those who avoid the grossest sins and indecencies and commit only small offenses, your Lord will show abundant mercy. He knew you well when He created you of earth and when you were hidden in your mother's wombs. Do not pretend to purity; He knows best those who guard themselves against evil.
> —The Star[22]

Psychologically, there may also be a need for forgiveness or acceptance of self. While routinely considered psychological issues, the need for self-forgiveness or self-acceptance may be tied to spiritual issues. In most cases, a sense of forgiveness or acceptance from either source (self or God) promotes the same from the other source.

Earlier, it was suggested that persons who are dying (and others) benefit from a mindful life review that includes both the "good" and the "bad" of the person's life. Such a review inevitably leads to consideration of mistakes and/or unfortunate aspects of life. In many cases, there is at least some crumbling of defenses that functioned to hide certain painful aspects of life. Guilt is often the result, and it does not seem to matter whether the issue is something one did, such as a pattern of dishonesty, or if the issue is something that was experienced, such as growing up in an alcoholic family.

In the discussion of meaning, it was strongly suggested that the nurse employ the question, "If you had your life to live over again, what would you like to be different?" Clearly this question has direct application to the issue of forgiveness or acceptance. In the sort of deep and open relationship for which we strive in hospice and palliative care, this question often brings a strong response that may include a deep sense of regret or guilt. The question is really less of an assessment question than a starting point in a search for understanding and ultimately, forgiveness or acceptance (Table 31–4).

Table 31–4
Notes on Forgiveness or Acceptance: The Patient, Family, and Nurse

- Understand the universality of sin, regret, and guilt.
- Not all guilt is related to the patient's own doing.
- A life review almost always includes elements of the need for forgiveness or acceptance.
- Forgiveness and/or acceptance cannot be conferred by another, but the practice of mercy is a manifestation of forgiveness and acceptance.
- Integrate the sacred into the process of dying: prayer, reading, worship, and ritual.

CASE STUDY
Mrs. K., a Patient with Lung Cancer (the author's mother)

Mrs. K. was dying from small cell carcinoma of the lung, with metastases to brain and bone. Treatment of the primary tumor and metastases included several courses of chemotherapy and radiation, both initiated and discontinued at appropriate times. Her primary symptoms were pain, fatigue, and nausea, all of which were well managed. She lived in a cottage behind the house where her son, daughter-in-law, and grandson lived. She enjoyed warm, supportive relationships with her family and others. She had no financial worries.

However, there was an element of low-level unhappiness and vague suffering through much of her illness. In a series of difficult interactions in which she and her son struggled to share their deepest feelings about her life and their relationship, she was finally able to say truthfully how she saw herself: "I'm naked and ugly and skinny. I'm lying in the bottom of a pit and it's dirty and there are cigarette butts all around me." Her son responded, "That's not you—it's what you feel like, but it's not you." She replied by begging for forgiveness for the mistakes she had made. Her son told her not to beg, that he forgave her and hoped that she forgave him, but more importantly, God forgave her.

She felt a great sense of peace afterward and began making detailed plans for her funeral. Her choices of scripture and hymns were a lovely expression of her past and her future. She spent many hours talking about what these passages and hymns meant to her.

The role of the nurse or chaplain or other caregivers is not to try to confer forgiveness or acceptance or to convince a patient that her or his faith offers forgiveness. It is possible, however, to manifest forgiveness and acceptance through providing consistent loving care, and thereby hold out to the patient the possibility that forgiveness and acceptance are possible. This practice of mercy is a high ethical demand in nursing and related fields and may be seen in terms of beneficence, fidelity, and justice.[1] Similarly to the care in other spiritual issues, the nurse may help connect the patient to the sacred and the practice of faith: prayer (in this case for forgiveness or acceptance), reading (especially passages that acknowledge the reality of sin and forgiveness), and worship and ritual (especially ritual related to purification).

Transcendence

Transcendence is a quality of faith or spirituality that allows one to move beyond, to "transcend" what is given or presented in experience—in this case, the suffering and despair so often inherent in dying.[1]

> Beyond, beyond
> Beyond that beyond
> Beyond the Beyond.
> —Buddhist mantra

Transcendence is certainly more than resignation and is also more than what many think of as acceptance in the process of dying. At its highest level, there is an element of beauty or spiritual elevation in transcendence. At its most basic level, transcendence is the means by which one finds meaning "retroactively . . . even in a wasted life."[14] Even more than the need for forgiveness or acceptance, transcendence resists being conferred by others or problem-solving approaches. "Man is never helped in his suffering by what he thinks of for himself; only suprahuman, revealed truth lifts him out of his distress."[25]

Transcendence can occur in at least one of two ways:

1. The other spiritual needs are met and transcendence then is an outcome.
2. Transcendence occurs through grace, or as Jung would state it, through "suprahuman, revealed truth," and thus may exist independently of other spiritual needs; or of work, actions, or human interventions. In this latter case, we see that through transcendence, all other spiritual needs are met.

Transcendence is a profound issue that cannot be approached from a problem-solving perspective, and there are no specific interventions that lead to transcendence. One "watches" with the patient and practices mercy and is grateful when transcendence occurs.

It is well worth considering that there may be elements of transcendence in the practice of hospice and palliative care. Those who practice in this field operate at the edge of human existence. Sometimes we see that the practice also has elements of our own denial and fear of death, but sometimes, in the deep heart of the night, we transcend our own denials and fears and become—if only for a moment—a manifestation of the transcendent beauty seen when there is reconciliation with God, with self, and with others (Table 31–5).

Table 31–5
Notes on Transcendence: The Patient, Family, and Nurse

- Integration of the sacred into the process of dying may lead to transcendence.
- Transcendence is beyond human intervention.
- Take note of the times when transcendence occurs in the practice of hospice and palliative care.

General Notes on Providing Spiritual Care

The following are general suggestions for providing spiritual care. Not all are applicable in every case, and some may never be applicable to a particular patient or in a particular person's practice. They are offered here as ideas or suggestions that readers may add to in the effort to provide quality spiritual care.

- Remember that there often is nobody better placed or better qualified than the nurse to provide spiritual care.
- Patients and families often are reluctant to raise spiritual issues, but many respond positively to health professionals, who are "able to step beyond rigid professional boundaries."[6]
- Integration of the sacred into the process of dying should probably always be attempted, even if only in the nurse's life and the institution's milieu.
- There are situations in which the patient cannot physically tolerate going to a place of worship for a complete service, but can stay for a limited time. When this is the case, the patient may need help to choose which part of the service to attend, and the place of worship may need help in accommodating the patient's participation in the service. In some cases, the patient may need additional medication or portable equipment to make it through even part of the service.
- When, because of physical or other limitations, it becomes difficult for the patient to visit a place of worship, home or hospital visits from clergy should be considered. It is sometimes necessary for the nurse or other staff to make repeated appeals to the patient's clergy for such visits.
- Other religious activities that can take place at home or hospital include prayer, ritual, reading, and other spiritually oriented activities, including music. Music can be helpful to the patient and others, and might be provided by a few choir members coming to the home or by tapes or CDs of religious music.
- The presence of a religious book in the patient's home or room provides the opportunity for the nurse to pick up the book and discuss it with the patient. It is helpful for the nurse to actually take the book in hand when initiating discussion. It also is helpful to ask the patient to read aloud passages that are most important to her or him. If the patient is unable to read, the nurse or other caregiver can do the reading. (If the book is the Koran, the nurse should wash his or her hands before taking it in hand.)

- There is an understandable tendency for people to want to do things for the person who is dying. It is important to encourage the person who is dying to also do things for others. Creating or affirming memories and leaving a legacy is suggested by Lynn and Harrold.[27] This might include the patient giving a copy of the holy book of her or his faith to a loved one (e.g., a grandchild), planning the funeral service, making a point of reconciling with others, spending time to consider a mindful good-bye, and other means of making connection with others, including teaching the nurse what matters spiritually.
- Everyone dies, and while it is of no help to trivialize an individual's experience by pointing this out in a heedless manner, it may be helpful to carefully introduce the universality of the experience—especially the fact that many others have struggled with pain, fear, guilt, and other core issues in dying and death. All the major religions address the universality of death and suffering.
- Recall that hospice and palliative care emerged, in part, as humane responses to the increasingly technological nature of dying and death in the modern world. The serious question, "How can the spiritual and sacred become more a part of the process," arises both in terms of a particular patient and in terms of institutions.
- It is also important to always remember that key concepts in palliative care are respect for the person and protection of individual differences. Some patients and families may not want spiritual care, and these preferences should be respected.
- Prayer, invited and offered from the heart, is a powerful means of caring for the patient, family, and nurse.

And finally, the practice of mercy—of watching through the night—is central to hospice and palliative care and to the practice of every faith.

REFERENCES

1. Kemp CE. Terminal Illness: A Guide to Nursing Care, 2nd ed. Lippincott Williams & Wilkins, Philadelphia, 1999.
2. Breitbart W. Spirituality and meaning in supportive care: spirituality and meaning-centered group psychotherapy interventions in advanced cancer. Support Care Cancer 2002;10: 272–280.
3. Baylor University School of Nursing Report of Self-Study. Dallas, TX: Baylor University School of Nursing, 1991.
4. Kennedy C, Cheston SE. Spiritual distress at life's end: finding meaning in the maelstrom. J Pastoral Care & Counseling 2003; 57:131–141.
5. McClain CS, Rosenfeld B, Breitbart W. Effects of spiritual well-being on end-of-life despair in terminally ill cancer patients. Lancet 2003;361:1603–1607.
6. Murray SA, Kendall M, Boyd K, Worth A, Benton TF. Exploring the spiritual needs of people dying of lung cancer or heart failure: a prospective qualitative interview study of patients and their carers. Palliat Med 2004;18:39–45.
7. Musgrave CF, McFarlane EA. Oncology and nononcology nurses' spiritual well-being and attitudes toward spiritual care: a literature review. Oncol Nurs Forum 2003;30:523–527.
8. Volker DL. Assisted dying and end-of-life symptom management. Cancer Nurs 2003;26:392–399.
9. Johnstone P, Mandryk J. Operation World: 21st Century Edition. Waynesboro, GA: Paternoster USA, 2001.
10. Burton LA. The spiritual dimension of palliative care. Semin Oncol Nurs 1998;14:121–128.
11. Gallup International Institute. Spiritual Beliefs and the Dying Process. Princeton, NJ: Gallup International Institute, 1997:.
12. Nuland S. How We Die. New York: Alfred A. Knopf, 1994.
13. Taylor EJ. Nurses caring for the spirit: patients with cancer and family caregiver expectations. Oncol Nurs Forum 2003; 30: 585–590.
14. Frankl V. The Will to Meaning. New York: New American Library, 1969.
15. Taylor EJ, Amenta M, Highfield M. Spiritual care practices of oncology nurses. Oncol Nurs Forum 1995;22:31–39.
16. Saunders CM. Appropriate treatment, appropriate death. In: The Management of Terminal Disease, Saunders CM, ed. London: Edward Arnold, 1978:1–18.
17. The Bible: Revised Standard Version. New York: Thomas Nelson & Sons, 1952.
18. Foster D. (1999). Personal communication.
19. LeFavi RG, Wessels MH. Life review in pastoral counseling: background and efficacy for use with the terminally ill. J Pastoral Care & Counseling 2003;57:281–292.
20. Bhagavad-Gita. Translated by Swami Prabhavananda and C. Isherwood., New York: Mentor Religious Classics, 1991.
21. The Teaching of Buddha. Tokyo: Bukkyo Dendo Kyokai, 1981.
22. The Koran. Translated by N.J. Dawood. New York: Penguin Books, 1990.
23. Post-White J, Ceronsky C, Kreitzer MJ, Nickelson K, Drew D, Mackey KW, Koopmeiners L, Gutknecht S. Hope, spirituality, sense of coherence, and quality of life in patients with cancer. Oncol Nurs Forum 1996;23:1571–1579.
24. Green J. Death with dignity: Hinduism. Nurs Times 1989;85:50–51.
25. Jung CG. (1953). Psychology and alchemy. In: C.G. Jung: Psychological Reflection, Jacobi J, Hull RFC, eds. Princeton: Princeton University Press, 1953:338–339.
26. Nelson CJ, Rosenfeld B, Breitbart W, Galietta M. Spirituality, religion, and depression in the terminally ill. Psychosomatics 2002;43:213–220.
27. Lynn J, Harrold J, The Center to Improve Care of the Dying. Handbook for Mortals. New York: Oxford University Press, 1999.

32

Tami Borneman and Katherine Brown-Saltzman

Meaning in Illness

I cannot understand God's timing . . . . there's so much left for me to do. I've tried asking for more time . . . it seems that's not going to be granted, but I have great faith that God knows more than I do and that He's watching over me.—Cancer patient

In the driest whitest stretch
Of pain's infinite desert
I lost my sanity
And found this rose

—Galal al-Din Rumi; Persia, 1207–1273

- ***Key Points***
- *Finding meaning in illness is an important issue when facing the end of life.*
- *The process of finding meaning in illness involves a journey through sometimes very difficult transitions.*
- *A terminal illness can greatly impact the patient–caregiver relationship.*
- *It is essential for nurses to experience their own journey regarding the dying process and bring with them a willingness to be transformed by it.*

Is it possible to adequately articulate and give definition to meaning in illness? Or is meaning in illness better described and understood through using symbolism and metaphors such as the above poem? To try to define that which is enigmatic and bordering on the ineffable seems almost sacrilegious. The unique individual journey of finding meaning in illness experienced by each patient facing the end of life and their family caregiver would seem to be diminished by the very process that seeks to understand through the use of language.

Is it that we seek to find meaning in illness or is it that we seek to find meaning in the life that is now left and in those relationships and things we value? Do we seek to find meaning in illness itself as an isolated event or that which is beyond the illness, such as how to live out this newly imposed way of life? Terminal illness forces us to look at and possibly to reappraise the meaning in and of our life.[1] If we allow space in our lives for the process of meaning in illness to unfold, we then move from the superficial to the profound.

Terminal illness also forces us at some point to look directly at death, yet we resist getting in touch with the feelings that arise. Everything in us seeks life. Everything in us hopes for life. Everything in us denies death. There is something very cold, very unmoving, and very disturbing about it all. Does the end of one's human existence on earth need to be the sole metaphor for death?

Even though end-of-life issues have progressed nearer to the forefront of health care, the dying patient is still the recipient of an impersonal, detached, and cure-focused system, thereby exacerbating an already catastrophic situation. As necessary as it is for nurses to use the nursing process, it is not enough. The patient's illness odyssey beckons us to go beyond assessment, diagnosis, intervention, and evaluation to a place of vulnerability, not in an unprofessional manner but, rather, in a way that allows for a shared connectedness unique to each patient-nurse relationship. We need to be willing to use feelings appropriately as part of the therapeutic process. Separating ourselves from touching and feeling to protect ourselves only serves to make us more vulnerable, because we have then placed our emotions in isolation. Nurses can be a catalyst for helping the patient and family find meaning in the illness, and, in the process, help themselves define or redefine their own meaning in life, illness, and death.

Meaning Defined

Johnston-Taylor[2] presents several definitions for meaning (Table 32–1). In the dictionary,[3] one finds meaning defined simply as "something that is conveyed or signified" or as "an interpreted goal, intent, or end." But it is the etymology of the word "mean" that helps nursing come to understand our potential for supporting patients in the process of finding meaning in their lives, even as they face death. Mean comes from the Old English *maenan*, "to tell of." One does not find meaning in a vacuum; it has everything to do with relationships, spirituality, and connectedness. While the process of finding meaning depends greatly on an inward journey, it also relies on the telling of that journey. The telling may use language, but it may also be conveyed by the eyes, through the hands, or just in the way the body is held. Frankl[4] reminds us that the "will to meaning" is a basic drive for all of humanity and is unique to each individual. A life-threatening illness begs the question of meaning with a new urgency and necessity.

Cassell[5] tells us that "all events are assigned meaning," which entails judging their significance and value. Meaning cannot be separated from the person's past; it requires the thought of future and ultimately influences perception of that future (p. 67). Finding meaning is not a stagnant process; it changes as each day unfolds and the occurrences are interpreted. As one patient reflected upon her diagnosis, "Cancer changes your perception of your world and life."[6] Coming face to face with one's mortality not only defines what is important but also the poignancy of the loss of much that has been meaningful.

One's spirituality is often the key to transcending those losses and finding ways to maintain those connections, whether it is the belief that one's love, work, or creativity will remain after the physical separation or the belief that one's spirit goes on to an afterlife or through reincarnation. Meaning in life concerns the individual's realm of life on earth. It has to do with one's humanness, the temporal, and the composites of what one has done in life to give it meaning. Meaning of life has more to do with the existential. It is looking beyond one's earthly physical existence to an eternal, secure, and indelible God or spiritual plane. The existential realm of life provides a sense of security whereby one can integrate experiences.[7]

Spirituality has been defined as a search for meaning.[8] One of the Hebrew words for meaning is *biynah* (bee-naw), which is understanding, knowledge, meaning, and wisdom. It comes from the root word *biyn* (bene), to separate mentally or to distinguish.[9] How is it that one can come to knowledge and understanding? Patients receiving palliative care often describe a sense of isolation and loneliness. They frequently have endless hours available, while at the same time experiencing a shortening of their life. It is here that nursing has a pivotal role as the listener, for when the ruminations of the dying are given voice, there is an opportunity for meaning. Important life themes are shared, and the unanswerable questions are at least

Table 32–1
Definitions of Meaning

Meaning	". . . refers to sense, or coherence . . . A search for meaning implies a search for coherence. 'Purpose' refers to intention, aim, function . . . However, 'purpose' of life and 'meaning' of life are used interchangeably."[39]
	". . . a structure which relates purposes to expectations so as to organize actions . . . Meaning . . . makes sense of actions by providing reasons for it."[40]
Search for meaning	". . . is an effort to understand the event: why it happened and what impact it has had . . . [and] attempts to answer the questions(s), What is the significance of the event? . . . What caused the event to happen? . . . [and] What does my life mean now."[41]
	". . . is an attempt to restore the sense that one's life is orderly and purposeful."[42]
Personal search for meaning	". . . the process by which a person seeks to interpret a life circumstance. The search involves questioning the personal significance of a life circumstance, in order to give the experience purpose and to place it in the context of a person's total life pattern. The basis of the process is the interaction between meaning in and of life and involves the reworking and redefining of past meaning while looking for meaning in a current life circumstance."[1]

asked. As the stranger develops intimacy and trust, meaning takes hold.

Suffering creates one of the greatest challenges to uncovering meaning. For the dying patient, suffering comes in many packages: physical pain, unrelenting symptoms (nausea, pruritus, dyspnea, etc.), spiritual distress, dependency, multiple losses, and anticipatory grieving. Even the benefits of medical treatments given to provide hope or palliation can sometimes be outweighed by side effects (e.g., sedation and constipation from pain medication), inducing yet further suffering. The dictionary[3] defines suffering in this way: "To feel pain or distress; sustain loss, injury, harm, or punishment." But once again, it is the root word that moves us to a more primitive understanding, the Latin sufferer, which comprises *sub*, "below" and *ferre* "to carry." The weight and isolation of that suffering now becomes more real at the visceral level. Cassell[5] reminds us that pain itself does not foreordain suffering; it is, in fact, the meaning that is attributed to that pain that determines the suffering. In his clinical definition, "Suffering is a state of severe distress induced by the loss of the intactness of person, or by a threat that the person believes will result in the loss of his or her intactness" (p. 63). Suffering is an individual and private experience and will be greatly influenced by the personality and character of the person; for example, the patient who has needed control during times of wellness will find the out-of-control experience of illness as suffering.[5] In writing about cancer pain and its meaning, Ersek and Ferrell[10] provide a summary of hypotheses and theses from the literature (Table 32–2).

Although not always recognized, it is the duty of all who care for patients to alleviate suffering and not just treat the physical dimensions of the illness. This is no small task, for first, professionals must be free from denial and the need to self-protect to see the suffering of another. Then, they must be able to attend to it without trying to fix it or simplify it. The suffering needs to be witnessed; in the midst of suffering, presence and compassion become the balm and hope for its relief.

Table 32–2
Summary of Hypotheses and Theses from the Literature on Meaning

The search for meaning is a basic human need.	Frankl 1959[4]
Meaning is necessary for human fulfillment.	Steeves and Kahn 1987[43]
Finding meaning fosters positive coping and increased hopefulness.	Ersek 1991[44]
One type of meaning-making activity in response to threatening events is to develop causal attributions.	Gotay 1985[45]; Haberman 1987[46]; Steeves and Kahn 1987[43]; Taylor 1983[41]; Chrisman 1977[47]
Meaning-making can involve the search for a higher order.	Ersek 1991[44]; Ferrell et al. 1993[48]; Steeves and Kahn 1987[43]
Making meaning often involves the use of social comparisons.	Ferrell et al. 1993[48]; Taylor 1983[41]; Ersek 1991[44]; Haberman 1987[46]
Meaning can be derived through construing benefits from a negative experience.	Ersek 1991[44]; Haberman 1987[46]; Taylor 1983[41]
Meaning sometimes focuses on illness as challenge, enemy, or punishment.	Barkwell 1991[49]; Ersek 1991[44]; Lipowski 1970[50]
Pain and suffering often prompt a search for meaning.	Frankl 1959[4]; Steeves and Kahn 1987[43]; Taylor 1983[41]
Uncontrolled pain or overwhelming suffering hinder the experience of meaning.	Steeves and Kahn 1987[43]
One goal of care is to promote patients' and caregivers' search for and experiences of meaning.	Ersek 1991[44]; Ferrell et al. 1993[48]; Steeves and Kahn 1987[43]; Haberman 1988[51]

The Process of Finding Meaning in Illness

From years of working with terminally ill patients and their families, the authors have found that the process of finding meaning in illness invokes many themes. The title given to each theme is an attempt to represent observed transitions that many terminally ill patients seem to experience. Not all patients experience the transitions in order, and not all transitions are experienced. However, we have observed that these transitions are experienced by the majority of patients. Issues faced by family caregivers and health care professionals are discussed in later sections. The themes shared in this section are the imposed transition, loss and confusion, dark night of the soul, randomness and absence of God, brokenness, and reappraisal. In experiencing some or all of these transitions, one can perhaps find meaning in this difficult time of life.

The Imposed Transition

Being told that you have a terminal illness can be like hearing the sound of prison doors slam shut. Life will never be the same. The sentence has been handed down and there is no reversing the verdict. Terminal illness is a loss, and there is nothing we can do to change the prognosis even though we may be able to temporarily delay the final outcome. The essence of our being is shaken, and our souls are stricken with a panic unlike any other we have ever felt. For the first time, we are faced with an "existential awareness of nonbeing."[11] For a brief moment, the silence is deafening, as if suspended between two worlds, the known and the unknown. As one "regains consciousness," so to speak, the pain and pandemonium of thoughts and emotions begin to storm the floodgates of our faith, our coping abilities, and our internal fortitude, while simultaneously the word "terminal" reverberates in our heads. There is no easy or quick transition into the acceptance of a terminal diagnosis.

Facing the end of life provokes questions. Not only is the question "why me?" asked, but questions regarding the meaning *in* one's life as well as the meaning *of* one's life.[1] Whether we embrace with greater fervor the people and things that collectively give us meaning in life or we view it all as now lost, the loss and pain are real. Nothing can be done to prevent the inevitable. There is a sense of separation or disconnectedness in that while I am the same person, I have also become permanently different from you. Unless you become like me, diagnosed with a terminal illness, we are in this sense, separated. In a rhetorical sense, the meanings we gain in life from relationships and the material world serve to affirm us as participants in these meanings.[11] When these meanings are threatened by a terminal diagnosis, we fear the loss of who we are as functioning productive human beings. The affirmations we received from our meanings in life are now at a standstill.

A 50-year-old contractor, determined to fight for his life despite his terminal prognosis, was not only combating cancer but also trying to hold onto who he was. If word got out that he had cancer, he feared that no one would hire him. He felt that his wife depended on him to bring home a salary, so they kept the news of his illness even from close friends. He exhausted himself trying to keep up with work and the image that he was all right. When this was explored with him, he began to understand that he saw himself in limited functional ways, the contractor and the husband as a provider, and he feared losing what had defined his life. Having him define his life in terms of meaning, expanding his past limited view gave him new insight and gradually allowed him to open up and share his prognosis with close friends.

In addition to questioning meaning *in* life, those facing the end of life also question the meaning *of* life. A life-threatening illness makes it difficult to maintain an illusion of immortality.[12] What happens when we die? Is there really a God? Is it too late for reconciliation? For those believing in life after death, the questions may focus on uncertainty of eternal life, fear of what eternal life will be like, or the possibility of this being a test of faith. No matter what the belief system, the existential questions are asked. We reach out for a connection with God or something beyond one's self to obtain some sense of security and stability. Then, in this ability to transcend the situation, ironically, we somehow feel a sense of groundedness. Frankl[4] states, "It denotes the fact that being human always points, and is directed, to something or someone, other than oneself—be it a meaning to fulfill or another human being to encounter." There is an incredibly strong spiritual need to find meaning in this new senseless and chaotic world.

Loss and Confusion

One cancer patient stated, "Our lives are like big run-on sentences and when cancer occurs, it's like a period was placed at the end of the sentence. In reality, we all have a period at the end of the sentence, but we don't really pay attention to it."[13] With a terminal diagnosis, life is changed forever, for however long that life may be. Each day life seems to change as one is forced to experience a new aspect of the loss. There is a sense of immortality that pervades our lust for life, and when we are made to look at our mortality, it is staggering. With all of the many losses, coupled with the fear of dying, one can be left feeling confused from the infinite possibilities of the unknown. The panorama of suffering seems to be limitless.

The pain of loss is as great as the pleasure we derived from life.[14] The pain is pure and somewhat holy. The confusion comes not only from one's world having been turned upside down, but also from those who love us and care about us. It is not intentional; nevertheless, its impact is greatly felt. In trying to bring encouragement or trying to help one find meaning, the loss and pain are sometimes minimized by comparing losses, attempting to save God's reputation by denying the one hurting the freedom to be angry at God, or, by immediately focusing on the time left to live. The hurting soul needs to feel the depth of the loss by whatever means it can. The pain from loss is relentless, like waves from a dark storm at sea crashing repeatedly against rocks on the shoreline.

A 65-year-old woman with terminal lung cancer experienced further physical decline each day. She was surrounded by a family who lovingly doted on her. She was one who loved life and loved people. Many losses were experienced due to her condition. What added to these losses was the fact that her family wanted her to focus on life and not her disease or death. They knew she was going to die but felt that her quality of life would be better if these issues were not discussed. The patient had many thoughts and feelings to sort through and wanted to talk, but no one was listening. Her loss was not just physical; it also was an imposed emotional loss caused by a loving family trying to do the right thing. The communications with her family were different, constantly reminding her that nothing was the same, and, in turn, reminded her of her losses and impending death.

Dark Night of the Soul

The descent of darkness pervades every crack and crevice of one's being. One now exists in the place of Nowhere surrounded by nothingness that is void of texture and contour. One's signature is seemingly wiped away, taking with it the identification of a living soul.[14] Job states, "And now my soul is poured out within me; days of affliction have seized me. At night it pierces my bones within me, and my gnawing pains take no rest . . . My days are swifter than a weaver's shuttle, and come to an end without hope."[15] "One enters the abyss of emptiness—with the perverse twist that one is not empty of the tortured feeling of emptiness."[16] This is pain's infinite desert.

Darkness looms as one thinks about the past, full of people and things that provided meaning in life, and will soon have to be given up. Darkness looms as one thinks about the future, because death precludes holding on to all that is loved and valued. Darkness consumes one's mind and heart like fire consumes wood. It makes its way to the center with great fury, where it proceeds to take possession, leaving nothing but a smoldering heap of ashes and no hope of recovering any essence of life.[17]

A woman with young children relapsed after a bone marrow transplant and spent months in the hospital trying an experimental protocol. She suffered greatly, not only from the effects of the chemotherapy, but also from the long separations from her children. When it became clear that her leukemia had once again returned, she became tortured by the thought of abandoning her children at a time when they so greatly needed a mother, and the fact that she had gambled with the little time she had left and had lost. Now too ill to return home, in her mind, her children had the double loss of weeks of quality time she could have had with them and now her imminent death. She became inconsolable because of this darkness. Time to intervene was very limited. Allowing her the room for suffering, and being "present" to this suffering as a nurse, was essential. In addition, helping her to move back into her mothering role and providing for her children by helping to prepare them for her death became the pathway through the darkness and into meaning.

Though one might try, there are no answers theological or otherwise to the "whys" that engulf one's existence. Death moves from an "existential phenomenon to a personal reality."[18] All our presuppositions about life fall away and we are left emotionally naked. There is neither the physical, the emotional, nor the spiritual strength to help our own fragility. The world becomes too big for us and our inner worlds are overwhelming.[14] The enigma of facing death strips order from one's life, creating fragmentation and leaving one with the awareness that life is no longer tenable.

Randomness and the Absence of God

The pronouncement of a terminal diagnosis provokes inner turmoil and ruminating thoughts from dawn to dusk. Even in one's chaotic life, there was order. But order does not always prevail. A young athlete being recruited for a professional sport is suddenly killed in a tragic car accident. A mother of three small children is diagnosed with a chronic debilitating disease that will end in death. An earthquake levels a brand new home that a husband and wife had spent years saving for. A playful young toddler drowns in a pool. There seems to be no reason. It would be different if negligence were involved. For example, if the young athlete were speeding, or driving drunk, although still quite devastating, a "logical" reason could be assigned to the loss. But randomness leaves us with no "logical" explanation.[16]

The word "random" comes from the Middle English word *radon*, which is derived from the Old French word *randon*, meaning violence and speed. The word connotes an impetuous and haphazard movement, lacking careful choice, aim, or purpose.[3] The feeling of vulnerability is overwhelming. In an effort to find shelter from this randomness, meaning and comfort is sought from God or from something beyond one's self, but how do we know that God or something beyond ourselves is not the cause of our loss? Our trust is shaken. Can we reconcile God's sovereignty with our loss?[16] Can we stay connected to and continue to pull or gain strength and security from something beyond ourselves that may be the originator of our pain? There is a sense of abandonment by that which has been our stronghold in life. Yet to cut ourselves off from that stronghold out of anger would leave us in a state of total disconnection. A sense of connection is a vital emotion necessary for existence, no matter how short that existence may be. But facing death forbids us to keep our existential questions and desires at a distance. Rather, it seems to propel us into a deeper search for meaning as the questions continue to echo in our minds.

Brokenness

Does one come to a place of acceptance within brokenness? Is acceptance even attainable? Sometimes. Sometimes not. Coming to a place of acceptance is an individual experience for each person. Kearney,[19] in a wonderful analogy of acceptance, states, "Acceptance is not something an individual can choose at will. It is not like some light switch that can at will be flicked on or off. Deep emotional acceptance is like the settling of a cloud of silt in a troubled pool. With time the silt rests on the bottom and the water is clear"(p. 98). Brokenness does, however, open the door to relinquishing the illusion of immortality. Brokenness allows the soul to cry and to shed tears of anguish. It elicits the existential question "why?" once again, only this time not to gain answers but to find meaning.

A woman in her mid-60s, dying of lung cancer, shared how she came to a place of acceptance. When she was first diagnosed, the cancer was already well advanced. Her health rapidly declined, and she was more or less confined to bed or sitting. Out of her frustration, anger at God, sadness, and tears, came the desire to paint again. It was her way of coping, but it became more than that. It brought her to a place of peace in her heart. She had gotten away from painting due to busyness and was now learning to be blessed by quietness. She was very good at replicating Thomas Kinkade paintings, and her final picture, which was to be a gift, included many beautiful flowers. She was always surrounded by flowers.

If we go back to the poem at the beginning of this chapter, it wasn't until "sanity" was lost that the rose was found. A gradual perception takes place whereby we realize that the way out is by no longer struggling.[19] When we come to the end of ourselves and the need to fight the inevitable that is death, we give space for meaning to unfold. It isn't that we give up the desire, but we relinquish the need to emotionally turn the situation around and to have all our questions answered. Sittser,[16] a minister who experienced a sudden loss of several immediate family members, states, "My experience taught me that loss reduces people to a state of almost total brokenness and vulnerability. I did not simply feel raw pain; I was raw pain"(p. 164). Pain and loss are still profound, but in the midst of these heavy emotions there begins to be a glimmer of light. Like the flame of a candle, the light may wax and wane. It is enough to begin to silhouette those people and things that still can provide meaning.

Reappraisal

It is here where one begins to realize that something positive can come from even a terminal diagnosis and the losses it imposes. The good that is gained does not mitigate the pain of loss, but, rather, fosters hope. Hope that is not contingent on healing but on reconciliation, on creating memories with loved ones, on making the most of every day, on loving and being loved.[20] It's a hope that transcends science and explanations, and changes with the situation. It is not based on a particular outcome but, rather, focuses on the future, however long that may be. Despair undermines hope, but hope robs death of despair.[21]

A male patient in his late 30s, facing the end of life after battling leukemia and having gone through a bone marrow transplant, shared that he knew he was going to die. It took him a long time to be able to admit it to himself. The patient recalled recently visiting a young man who had basically given up and did not want his last dose of chemotherapy. He talked a while with this young man and encouraged him to "go for it." He told him that there's nothing like watching the last drop of chemo go down the tube and into his body, and the sense of it finally being all over. The patient shared with the young man that when he received his own last dose of chemotherapy, he stayed up until 3 in the morning to watch the last drop go down the tube. While the chemotherapy did not help him to the extent that he wanted, he wanted to encourage the young man to hope and not give up. Life was not yet over. He had tears in his eyes when he finished the story.

Facing end of life with a terminal diagnosis will never be a happy event. It will always be tragic because it causes pain and loss to everyone involved. But at a time unique to each person facing death, a choice can be made as to whether one wants to become bitter and devalue the remaining time, or value as much as possible the time that is left.

An important choice to be made during this time is whether to forgive or to be unforgiving—toward oneself, others, God, or one's stronghold of security in life. Being unforgiving breeds bitterness and superficiality. As we face the end of life, we need both an existential connection and a connection with others. Being unforgiving separates us from those connections, and it is only through forgiveness that the breech is healed. Forgiveness neither condones another's actions nor does it mean that this terminal diagnosis is fair. Rather, forgiveness is letting go of expectations that one somehow will be vindicated for the pain and loss. Whether by overt anger or by emotional withdrawal, in seeking to avoid being vulnerable to further pain and loss, we only succeed in making ourselves more vulnerable. Now we have chosen a deeper separation that goes beyond facing the death of the physical body—that of the soul.[16] Positive vulnerability through forgiveness provides a means of healing, and, when possible, reconciliation with others. It always provides healing and reconciliation with one's God or one's stronghold of security. Forgiveness allows both physical and emotional energy to be used for creating and enjoying the time left for living.

A 30-year-old woman was admitted to the hospital with advanced metastatic breast cancer. She was unknown to the hospital staff but had a good relationship with her oncologist. During the admissions assessment, the young woman could not give the name of anyone to contact in the event of an emergency. When pressed, she stated that she was alienated from her family and chose not to be in touch. She agreed that after her death her mother could be called, but not before. A social worker was summoned in the hope that something could be done to help with some unification. However, the social worker came out of the room devastated by the woman's resolve. The chaplain also found no way to reconnect this woman's family. The nursing staff experienced moral distress as they watched this woman die, all alone in the world. One of the authors worked with the staff to help them realize that they had become trusted and in a sense were her substitute family. One may not always be able to fix the pain of life's fractures or bring people to a place of forgiveness, but it is important not to underestimate what is happening in the moment. Healing for this patient came through the relationship with her doctors and nurses, and she died not alone, but cared for.

There are many emotions and issues with which those facing death must contend. It is not an easy journey and the process is wearing; nevertheless, the rose can be found.

Impact of the Terminal Illness on the Patient–Caregiver Relationship

Each of us comes to new situations with our life's experiences and the meanings we have gained from them. It is no different when being confronted with illness and the end of life. However, in this special episode of life, there are often no personal "reruns" from which to glean insight. Patient and family come together as novices, each helping the other through this unknown passage. Because different roles and relationships exist, the impending loss will create different meanings for each person involved.

Facing the loss of someone you love is extremely difficult. For the family caregiver, the process of finding meaning can either be facilitated or hindered by the meaning held by the one facing death.[22] One example experienced by one of the authors of this chapter involved a wife's short discussion with her terminally ill husband on the subject of heaven. She asked him if he thought he was going to heaven and if he was, would she be able to be with him even though she was from a different religion. He assured her that they would someday be together in heaven, and an immediate sense of peace came over his wife. He was not looking forward to dying, but for him, his death was not the end. He would see her again. His own meaning of death helped create a whole new meaning for his wife. He imparted to her a sense of eternal connection that allayed her fears of eternal separation from the most important person in her life. She could now face his death, with sorrow, but without fear.

In another example, a woman helped her family create meaning for themselves from the picture she had painted of herself sitting on the beach as a little girl next to a little boy. She explained that the little boy had his arm around her as they stared out at the sea. Each time the waves covered the surface of the beach and then retreated, the sea would carry with it bits and pieces of her fears and disease. The birds circling overhead would then swoop down to pick up and carry off any pieces not taken by the sea. The little boy's arm around her signified all the loving support she had received from others. When the time would come for her to die, she would be ready because she had been able to let go of life as she knew it. She had let the waves slowly carry that which was of life out to sea and yet had learned to hold on to the meaning that that life had represented. In doing so, she enabled her family to hold on to the meaning of their relationship with her and to realize that they would never be separated from that meaning.[23]

A final poignant story offers a different perspective. A 53-year-old woman with stage IV ovarian cancer was very angry at everyone and everything and could not seem to find any positive meaning. She was angry that her life would be cut short, and she would not live to see her grandchildren grow. She and her husband had made plans to travel and now she was too ill to make even one of the trips. She made life difficult for those who loved her. She made loving her and caring for her difficult. No one could seem to do anything right. She was bothered by company yet wanted someone with her all the time, and she did not like the intrusion of health care professionals in her home. She felt that her physician and family had given up on her and she resented it. She died a very angry and unhappy woman. This was extremely difficult for her family. The family was left feeling rather fragmented. What exactly did all of this mean? They had spent so much time trying to please the patient, which was almost impossible, that they never had time to synthesize the events and their feelings regarding the whole terminal illness trajectory. Not only did the family have their own pain from loss, they were left with final memories that created negative meanings. For example, various family members had begun to withdraw emotionally from the patient out of hurt and frustration, yet felt guilty for "abandoning" her. After her death, those family members still felt guilty because they had really wanted to be with her.

These actual patient stories were given to exemplify how the patient's meaning in illness affects the meaning held or created by family members. Differing or divergent meanings can be detrimental in a relationship, or they can be used to strengthen it, thereby increasing the quality of time left together. That is not to imply that the patient is responsible for the meaning created by family members, but how one affects the other. Germino, Fife, and Funk[22] suggest that the goal is not merely converging meanings within the patient-family dyad, but, rather, encouraging a sharing of individual meanings so that all can learn, and relationships can be deepened and strengthened.

There are many issues that family caregivers face in caring for a loved one nearing the end of life. They are discussed at length in the literature. There is one issue, however, that warrants more attention—the loss of dreams. The loss of dreams for a future with the person is in addition to the loss of the person. It is the loss of the way one used to imagine life, and how it would have been with that person. It is the loss of an emotional image of oneself and the abandonment of chosen plans for the future and what might have been.[24]

For a child and the surviving parent, those losses of dreams will be played out each time Mother or Father's Day arrives and important life-cycle events, such as graduations, weddings, or the birth of the first grandchild. As her mother lay dying, one child expressed that loss in the simple statement, "Mommy, you won't be here for my birthday!" The mother and child wept, holding and comforting each other. Nothing could change the loss, but the comforting would remain forever.

The loss of dreams is an internal process, spiritual for some, seldom recognized by others as needing processing.[24–27] Nurses have a wonderful opportunity at this point to verbally recognize the family caregivers' loss of dreams and to encourage them in their search to find meaning in the loss. The ability to transcend and connect to God or something greater than one's self helps the healing process.

Transcendence: Strength for the Journey That Lies Ahead

Transcendence is defined as lying beyond the ordinary range of perception; being above and independent of the material universe. The Latin root is *trans-*, "from or beyond," plus *scandere*, "to climb."[3] The images are many: the man in a pit climbing his way out one handhold at a time; the story of Job as he endured one defeat after another and yet found meaning; the climber who reaches the mountaintop, becoming closer to the heavens while still having the connection to the earth; or the dying patient who, in peace, is already seeing into another reality. The ability to transcend truly is a gift of the human spirit and often comes after a long struggle and out of suffering. It is often unclear which comes first—does meaning open the door for transcendence or, quite the opposite, does the act of transcendence bring the meaning? More than likely, it is an intimate dance between the two, one fueling the other. In the Buddhist tradition, suffering and being are a totality, and integrating suffering in this light becomes an act of transcendence.[28]

Transcendence of suffering can also be accomplished by viewing it as reparation for sins while still living, preparing the way for eternity, as in the Islamic tradition. In other traditions, transcendence is often relationship based, the connection to others, and sometimes to a higher power.[4] For example, the Christian seeing Christ on the cross connects one to the relationship and endurance of God and the reality that suffering is a part of life. For others, it is finding meaning in relating to others, even the act of caring for others. And for some, that relationship may be with the earth, a sense of stewardship and leaving the environment a better place. It is rare that patients reach a state of transcendence and remain there through their dying. Instead, for most it is a process in which there are moments when they reach a sense of expansion that supports them in facing death. The existential crisis does not rule, because one can frame the relationship beyond death; for example, "I will remain in their hearts and memories forever, I will live on through my children, or my spirit will live beyond my limited physical state."

Nursing Interventions

If one returns to the root word of meaning, *maenan*, "to tell of," this concept can be the guide that directs the nurse toward interventions. Given the nature of this work, interventions may not be the true representation of what is needed. For intervention implies action that the nurse has an answer and she can direct the course of care by intervening. It is defined as "To come, appear, or lie between two things. To come in or between so as to hinder or alter an action."[3] But finding meaning is process oriented; while finely honed psychosocial skills and knowledge can be immensely helpful, there is no bag of tricks. One example would be of a chaplain who walks in the room and relies only on offering prayer to the patient, preventing any real discourse or relationship building. The patient's personhood has been diminished and, potentially, more harm than good has been done.

So let us revisit "to tell of." What is required of the professional who enters into the healing dimension of a patient's suffering and search for meaning? It would seem that respect may be the starting point, respect for that individual's way of experiencing suffering and attempts of making sense of the illness. Secondly, allow for an environment and time for the telling. Even as this is written, the sighs of frustration are heard, "We have no time!" If nursing fails at this, if nurses turn their backs on their intrinsic promise to alleviate suffering, then nursing can no longer exist. Instead, the nurse becomes simply the technician and the scheduler—the nurse becomes a part of the problem. She has violated the Code for Nurses that states, "Nursing care is directed toward the prevention and relief of the suffering commonly associated with the dying process . . . and emphasizes human contact."[29]

If patients in the midst of suffering receive the message, nonverbal or directly, that there is no time, energy, or compassion, they will, in their vulnerability, withdraw or become more needy. Their alienation becomes complete. On the other hand, if privacy and a moment of honor and focused attention are provided, this allows for the tears to spill or the anguish to be spoken. Then the alienation is broken, and the opportunity for healing one dimension is begun. The terminally ill are a vulnerable population. They die and do not complete patient satisfaction surveys; their grievances, and their stories die with them. But the violation does not, for each nurse now holds that violation, as does society as a whole. The wound begets wounds, and the nurse sinks further into the protected and unavailable approach, alienated herself. The work holds no rewards, only endless days and demands. She has nothing left to give. The patient and family are ultimately abandoned. In the work of Kahn and Steeves,[30] one finds a model for the nurse's role in psychosocial processes and suffering. It represents the dynamic relationship of caring, acted out in caregiving as well as in the patient's coping, which transform each other.

For the nurse to provide this level of caregiving, she must understand the obstructions that may interfere. It is essential that the nurse undergo her own journey, visiting the intense emotions around the dying process and the act of witnessing suffering. We can serve the suffering person best if we ourselves are willing to be transformed through the process of our own grief as well as by the grief of others.[31] Presence may, in fact, be our greatest gift to these patients and their families. Still, imagine charting or accounting for presence on an acuity system! Presence "transcends role obligations and acknowledges the vulnerable humanness of us all . . . to be present means to unconceal, to be aware of tone of voice, eye contact, affect, and body language, to be in tune with the patient's messages."[31] Presence provides confirmation, nurturing, and compassion and is an essential transcendent act.

Touch becomes one of the tools of presence. Used with sensitivity, it can be as simple as the holding of the hand, or as powerful as the holding of the whole person. Sometimes, because of agitation or pain, direct touch becomes intrusive; even then touch can be invoked, by the touching of a pillow, the sheet, or the offering of a cold cloth. Healing touch takes on another level of intention through the directing energy of prayer.

If a key aspect of meaning is to tell, then one might be led to believe that the spoken word would be imperative. Yet over and over, it is silence that conveys the meaning of suffering, "a primitive form of existence that is without an effective voice and imprisoned in silence." Compassionate listeners in respect and presence become mute themselves.[31] They use the most intuitive of skills to carry the message. This may also be why other approaches that use symbols, metaphors, and the arts are the most potent in helping the patient to communicate and make sense of meaning. The arts, whether writing, music, or visual arts, often help the patient not only gain new insight, but convey that meaning to others. There are many levels on which this is accomplished. Whether it is done passively, through reading poetry, listening to music, or viewing paintings, or actively through creation, thoughts can be inspired, feelings moved, and the sense of connectedness and being understood can evolve. What once was ubiquitous can now be seen outside of one's soul, as feelings become tangible. It can be relational, because the act of creation can link one to the creator, or it can downplay the role of dependency, as the ill one now cares for others with a legacy of creational gifts.[32]

Meditation is another act of transcendence that can be extremely powerful for the dying.[33,34] Even those who have never experienced a meditational state can find that this new world in many ways links them to living and dying. The relaxation response that allows the anxious patient to escape into a meditative state, experiencing an element of control while relinquishing control. Many patients describe it as a floating state, a time of great peace and calm. Some, who have never had such an experience, can find the first time frightening, as the existential crisis, quelled so well by boundaries, is no longer confined. Most, given a trusting and safe teacher, will find that meditation will serve them well. The meditation can be in the form of prayer, guided imagery, breathing techniques, or mantras.

Prayer is well documented in the literature[35,36] as having meaning for patients and families; not only does it connect one to God, but it also again becomes a relational connection to others. Knowing that one is prayed for not only by those close at hand, but by strangers, communities, and those at a great distance can be deeply nurturing. Often forgotten is the role the patient can be empowered in, that of praying for others. One of the authors experienced her patient's prayers for her as the tables were turned, and the patient became the healer. The patient suddenly lost the sense of worthlessness and glowed with joy.

Leaving a legacy may be one of the most concrete ways for patients to find meaning in this last stage of their lives.[37] It most often requires the mastering of the existential challenges, in which patients know that death is at hand and choose to direct their course and what they leave behind. For some patients, that will mean going out as warriors, fighting till the end; for others, it will mean end-of-life planning that focuses on quality of life. Some patients will design their funerals, using rituals and readings that reveal their values and messages for others. Others will create videos, write letters, or distribute their wealth in meaningful ways. Parents who are leaving young children sometimes have the greatest difficulty with this aspect. On one hand, the feelings of horror at "abandoning" their children are so strong that they have great difficulty facing their death. Still, there is often a part of them that has this need to leave a legacy. The tug-of-war between these two willful emotions tends to leave only short windows of opportunity to prepare. The extreme can be the young father who began to push his toddler away, using excuses for the distancing. It was only after a trusting relationship had been established with one of the authors that she could help him to see how this protective maneuver was, in fact, harming the child. The father needed not only to see what he was doing, but to see how his love would help the child and how others would be there for the child and wife in their pain and grief. With relief, the father reconnected to his young son, creating living memories and a lifetime protection of love.

Another courageous parent anticipating the missed birthdays, bought cards and wrote a note in each one, so that the child would be touched not only by the individual messages, but the knowledge that the parent found a way to be there for him with each new year. A mother wrote a note for her young daughter, so that if she should ever marry, she would have a gift to be opened on her wedding day. The note described the mother's love, wisdom about marriage, and her daughter's specialness, already known through a mother's eyes. An elderly person may write or tape an autobiography or even record the family tree lest it be lost with the passing of a generation. The nurse can often be the one who inspires these acts, but always it must be done with great care so as not to instill a sense of "should" or "must," which would add yet another burden.

Helping patients to reframe hope is another important intervention. Recently, Dr. William Brietbart, Chief of the Psychiatry Services at Memorial Sloan-Kettering Cancer Center in New York City, designed and conducted research on a meaning-centered psychotherapeutic intervention to help terminally ill patients with cancer maintain hope and meaning as they face the end of their lives.[38] This research was inspired by the works of Dr. Victor Frankl, a psychiatrist and Holocaust survivor. Cancer patients attended an 8-week, group-focused, standardized course of experiential exercises that addressed constructs of despair at the end of life such as hopelessness, depression, loss of meaning, suicidal ideation, and desire for a hastened death. What was discovered during the study was that the patient's spiritual well-being, loss of meaning in part, was more highly correlated to the components that made up despair at the end of life than either depression or hopelessness alone. As a result, if the patient could manipulate or reframe his/her sense of meaning and spiritual well-being, this would positively affect the foundational elements of despair at the end of life. When patients are able to do this, their hope is sustained because they have been able to reframe the focus of their hope.

The Health Care Professional

While the health care professional can be educated about death and grieving, like the patient and family, it is in living out the experience that understanding is reached. It is a developmental process and, given the demands of the work, the nurse is at great risk for turning away from her feelings. There is often little mentoring that accompanies the first deaths, let alone formal debriefing or counseling. How can it be that we leave such important learning to chance? And what about cumulative losses and the years of witnessing suffering? Health care needs healing rituals for all of its health care professionals to support and guide them in this work. Individual institutions can develop programs that address these needs.

At one institution, "Teas for the Soul," sponsored by the Pastoral Care Department, provide respite in the workplace on a regular basis, as well as after difficult deaths or traumas. A cart with cookies and tea, plus soft music, are provided as physical nurturance, as well as nurturing the emotions of the staff and legitimizing the need to come together in support. Another support is a renewal program, the "Circle of Caring." This retreat supports health care professionals from a variety of institutions in a weekend of self care, integrating spirituality, the arts, and community building. The element of suffering is a focal point for a small group process that unburdens cumulative effects of the work and teaches skills and rituals for coping with the ongoing demands.

Clearly, there is much that can be done in this area to support nurses individually and to support organizations. There are many opportunities for assisting nurses in their own search for meaning and enhancing the care of patients and families. When the nurse takes the time to find meaning in this work, he or she is finding a health restorative practice that will protect her personally and professionally. Like the patient, he or she will need to choose this journey and find pathways that foster and challenge her.

> As long as we can love each other,
> And remember the feeling of love we had,
> We can die without ever really going away.
> All the love you created is still there.
> All the memories are still there.
> You live on – in the hearts of everyone you have
> Touched and nurtured while you were here.
> —Morrie Schwartz[52]

REFERENCES

1. O'Connor AP, Wicker CA, Germino BB. Understanding the cancer patient's search for meaning. Cancer Nurs 1990;13:167–175.
2. Taylor EJ. Whys and wherefores: adult patient perspectives of the meaning of cancer. Semin Oncol Nurs 1995;11:32–40.
3. The American Heritage Dictionary, 4th ed. Boston: Houghton Mifflin Co., 2000.
4. Frankl VE. Man's Search for Meaning: An Introduction to Logotherapy. Boston: Beacon, 1959.
5. Cassell EJ. The relationship between pain and suffering. Adv Pain Res Ther 1989;11:61–70.
6. Eick-Swigart J. What cancer means to me. Semin Oncol Nurs 1995;11:41–2.
7. Koestenbaum P. Is There an Answer to Death? Englewood Cliffs, NJ: Prentice-Hall, 1976.
8. Taylor EJ. Spiritual needs of patients with cancer and family caregivers. Cancer Nurs 2003;26:260–266.
9. Strong's Exhaustive Concordance. Nashville: Thomas Nelson Publishers, 1995.
10. Ersek M, Ferrell BR. Providing relief from cancer pain by assisting in the search for meaning. J Palliat Care 1994;10:15–22.
11. Tillich P. The Courage To Be. New Haven, CT: Yale University Press, 1952.
12. Benson H. Timeless Healing. New York: Simon and Schuster, 1997.
13. Putnam C. Verbal communication, 1999.
14. O'Donohue J. Eternal Echoes. New York: HarperCollins Publishers, 1999.
15. New American Standard Bible. Grand Rapids, MI: World Publishing, 1995.
16. Sittser G. A Grace Disguised. Grand Rapids, MI: Zondervan Publishing House, 1995.
17. Dark Night of the Soul. Kila, MT: Kessinger Publishing Company, 1942.
18. Kritek P. Reflections on Healing. Boston: Jones and Bartlett Publishers, 2003.
19. Kearney M. Mortally Wounded. New York: Simon and Schuster, 1996.
20. Martins L. The silence of God: the absence of healing. In: Cox RJ, Fundis RJ, eds. Spiritual, Ethical and Pastoral Aspects of Death and Bereavement. Amityville, NY: Baywood Publishing Company, 1992:25–31.
21. Pellegrino E, Thomasma D. The Christian Virtues in Medical Practice. Washington, DC: Georgetown University Press, 1996.
22. Germino BB, Fife BL, Funk SG. Cancer and the partner relationship: what is its meaning? Semin Oncol Nurs 1995;11:43–50.
23. Smith ED. Addressing the psychospiritual distress of death as reality: a transpersonal approach. Soc Work 1995;40:402–413.
24. Bowman T. Facing loss of dreams: a special kind of grief. Int J Palliat Nurs 1997;3:76–80.
25. Verbal communication. 1999.
26. Rando TA. Treatment of Complicated Mourning. Champaign, IL: Research Press 1993.
27. Garbarino J. The spiritual challenge of violent trauma. Am J Orthopsychiatry 1996;66:162–163.
28. Kallenberg K. Is there meaning in suffering? An external question in a new context. In: Cancer Nursing Changing Frontiers. Vienna: Blackwell Scientific, 1992: 21–24.
29. American Nurses Association Code for Nurses with Interpretive Statements. Washington, DC: American Nurses Publishing; 2001.
30. Kahn DL, Steeves RH. The significance of suffering in cancer care. Semin Oncol Nurs 1995;11:9–16.
31. Byock I. When suffering persists. J Pall Care 1994;10:8–13.

32. Bailey SS. The arts in spiritual care. Semin Oncol Nurs 1997;13: 242–247.
33. Sellers SC. The spiritual care meanings of adults residing in the midwest. Nurs Sci Q 2001;14:239–248.
34. Baldacchino D, Draper P. Spiritual coping strategies: a review of the nursing research literature. J Adv Nurs 2001;34:833–841.
35. Taylor EJ. Nurses caring for the spirit: patients with cancer and family caregiver expectations. Oncol Nurs Forum 2003;30:585–590.
36. Albaugh JA. Spirituality and life-threatening illness: a phenomenologic study. Oncol Nurs Forum 2003;30:593–598.
37. Kaut K. Religion, spirituality, and existentialism near the end of life. Am Behavioral Scientist 2002;46:220–234.
38. Breitbart W. Reframing hope: meaning-centered care for patients near the end of life. Interview by Karen S. Heller. J Palliat Med 2003;6:979–988.
39. Yalom ID. Existential Psychotherapy. New York: Basic Books, 1980.
40. Marris P. Loss and Change, 2nd ed. London: Routledge and Kegan Paul, 1986.
41. Taylor SE. Adjustment to threatening events: a theory of cognitive adaptation. Am Psychology 1983;38:1161–1173.
42. Thompson SC, Janigian AS. Life schemes: a framework for understanding the search for meaning. J Soc Clin Psychol 1988; 7:260–280.
43. Steeves RH, Kahn DL. Experience of meaning in suffering. Image: J Nurs Scholarship 1987;19:114–116.
44. Ersek M. The process of maintaining hope in adults with leukemia undergoing bone marrow transplantation [Unpublished doctoral dissertation]. Seattle: University of Washington, 1991.
45. Gotay CC. Why me? Attributions and adjustment by cancer patients and their mates at two stages in the disease process. Soc Sci Med 1985;20:825–831.
46. Haberman MR. Living with leukemia: the personal meaning attributed to illness and treatment by adults undergoing bone marrow transplantation [Unpublished doctoral dissertation]. Seattle: University of Washington, 1987.
47. Chrisman H. The health seeking process: an approach to the natural history of illness. Culture, Med Psychiatry 1977;1:351–377.
48. Ferrell BR, Taylor EJ, Sattler GR, Fowler M, Cheyney BL. Searching for the meaning of pain: cancer patients', caregivers', and nurses' perspectives. Cancer Pract 1993;1:185–194.
49. Barkwell DP. Ascribing meaning: a critical factor in coping and pain attenuation in patients with cancer-related pain. J Palliat Care 1991;7:5–10.
50. Lipowski Z. Physical illness, the individual and their coping processes. Int J Psychiatry Med 1970;1:101.
51. Haberman MR. Psychosocial aspects of bone marrow transplantation. Semin Oncol Nurs 1988;4:55–59.
52. Albom M. Tuesdays with Morrie. New York: Doubleday, 1997: 174.

33 Ruth Yorkin Drazen

Reflecting on the Journey: A Family Caregiver's Personal Perspective

We are all precious members of this universe and are here to make it a bit better through our resolve as honest, sincere partners in every moment.

I first met Ruth and Jerry in the summer of 1987. Jerry had advanced prostate cancer, and both he and Ruth were working hard to maintain a quality of life that gave continued meaning and purpose to their existence. After Jerry's death, Ruth continued to be part of our Pain and Palliative Care Service, always vocal with suggestions and always eager to come up with ways to help patients and families live to their fullest potential in the face of advancing disease as she and Jerry had strived to do. Communication was a constant theme—communication between patients and their doctors.

Out of this urge to improve communication, four films were born. The first was an outgrowth of Ruth's experience with the staff. She wondered what happened when a member of the staff or a member of their family got cancer—what happened to them as a person. The documentary When Doctors Get Cancer *was an outgrowth of that question and Ruth's first venture into the world of filmmaker as a producer and director. Her second film,* Cancer: A Personal Voyage, *grew out of the first film. Ruth had become friends with Peter Morgan, the youngest physician who participated in her film. After Peter's death, his family, having seen Ruth's first film, shared with her his diary, which detailed his journey with cancer.* Cancer: A Personal Voyage, *tells of his moving and courageous journey. Her third documentary,* Less Pain More Love, *depicts the struggle of children with cancer.*

In the meantime, Ruth's life was bound up in the life and work of Viktor Frankl. She found that no philosophy worked better for her than that of Frankl. She wanted people to recognize that the "greatest thing we have is the other," and she works to enable people to improve their lives through developing a meaningful mindset. Her fourth documentary, Frankl's Choice, *also known as* The Choice is Yours, *was born out of wanting to share with others what she had learned from Frankl. Ruth reflects on her own journey in the following piece.—Nessa Coyle*

It is 18 years since that fatal Monday morning when Jerry went into his final sleep. As I sat on his bed in the hospital with a nurse, sharing that unbelievable moment in our lives, she quietly kept on encouraging me—"Let him fly away and be free." I would touch his body that contained all the warmth of life and felt my unreality.

How could this be all over, I asked myself. Jerry never gave up. We had a "game" through all this. He would ask "If I make it to 85, is that good enough?" I always responded in the negative. "If the number is in the 90s?" I always said it was still not good enough. Our marriage of 28 years was like 28 days. As I recall it 18 years later, it was a shared journey.

Fortunately, the nurse was there to accompany me in those painful moments. When the funeral director asked me whether any family members wanted to say their goodbyes, I remained alone and asked the nurse to go with me. I had the first reality shock when I kissed Jerry's face and experienced his cold, stone-like body shouting in my ear, "I am no longer of your world." The burial was a blur of in-and-out detachment. I only recall covering Jerry with nature's blanket and asking him to wait for me to meet him again.

The months following Jerry's death were complicated. I felt a sense of abandonment. Yet, at the same time, I realized that I had the devotion of a few precious professionals who had been Jerry's caregivers both in New York and California. Even though we lived in New York City, Jerry chose to receive part of his care at a hospital in California because of their expertise in treating prostate cancer with radiation when surgery was not an option. He traveled to California every 4 months for 9 years.

The constancy of caring that I received from my friends at the cancer center was sacred to me. They understood my grief in countless loving ways. One particular time stands out in my memory. One Saturday morning, our Sabbath and our most holy day, Yom Kippur, I was sitting at my husband's bedside reading my prayer book when the door opened slightly. A hand motioned for me to come out into the hall. Here stood the neurologist who was treating Jerry for his severe pain. She stated that she had come to be with me on this day. We spent the day together in silence until sundown. I was overwhelmed.

The nurse, two of our physicians, and the hospital rabbi became "family" in ways that strengthened me and prepared me to live in my "new world." Grieving for each person is unpredictable. Jerry died on December 7, 1987. Our resident at the California Medical Center had grown very attached to us. We loved him. He phoned me regularly after Jerry's death, always checking on me. One dismal Friday February afternoon, the resident phoned to say that his chief had arranged for him to have a radiation rotation in New York. He was coming to stay with me. This was a miracle. I realized he wanted to help me in my grief. In spite of the disparity in age, we did things together. We exercised together, took walks together, cooked together, and most of all, laughed together. It was truly heaven until he had to return to California. On reflection, though many years ago, I still feel the capacity of this young man to empathize with the loneliness of another human being in those difficult days. He saw the need to rescue me. The capacity to find a new routine requires a good friend when family is unavailable.

As I ruminated on the future, I decided to go to Fordham University, which was a 10-minute walk from my apartment. During Jerry's illness, he had gone to Fordham and had thrived in that setting. In fact, I am certain that he tolerated his illness in remarkable ways because he had an environment that enabled him to realize the joy of learning was there for him. In 1989, I enrolled as a student at Fordham University— Jerry had been gone for 2 years. My 2½ years there stimulated me beyond belief. Life began to resonate again. Rediscovering the gift of learning energized my soul. It was then I became conscious of how I wanted to use whatever time would be allotted me on this earth. It was blatantly clear that my life with Jerry would enable me to give to others as we had totally given to each other. I started dreaming of how I might use my time to influence others who needed to discover ways of developing a meaningful mind-set. My passion to "reach for the moon" might seem bizarre, but I decided to go for it.

One afternoon I visited the New York neurologist who had cared for Jerry over the years, feeling comfortable to share my wild ideas with her. I explained how lucky Jerry had been to have me as his advocate. I told her that I had observed time and time again that most patients and families seemed unable to have an honest exchange with their physicians because neither party seemed to understand the value of true dialogue. To overcome this situation, I told her that I wanted to make a documentary involving physicians who had cancer. Her response was that Hollywood had made one recently; further, did I have the funds for this idea? When it was clear that I was a novice in filmmaking, the neurologist said to come back when I had the money. It took me 2 years to find the funds, but, with them, I found my life. I was now 75 years old.

In the 10 years that have followed, my life has been an adventure. I have produced four documentaries, each of which has enabled me to uncover a part of myself, continuously unlocking the mystery of living. I am convinced that my psychic suffering has been my "learning field." Experiencing the pain of Jerry's death, yet having the staying power to remain constant to my feelings in some indescribable way, opened up a creative universe for me. Producing my films enabled me to express my longings and my vision for those I may never meet but treasure in my being.

During Jerry's bout with cancer, he uncovered the wisdom of Viktor Frankl in *Man's Search for Meaning*. Frankl became my "companion" after Jerry was gone. His philosophy guided me through my darkest moments, teaching me that each of us has the capacity to transcend pain and disappointment. My creative journey has brought me into the lives of such remarkable people, and even though several of them are no longer here, they remain "alive" in different ways. I believe their contributions seen on film will continue to benefit those who view them. Each documentary has its own particular message. My film devoted to Frankl incorporates his concepts. I apply them to my daily life, inspiring me to give the best of myself to whatever task I undertake.

Living in the moment, every moment, has offered me rewards that are sometimes overwhelming. My responsibility is to be the best I can be in my daily tasks, from which I must not run. I find it helps me to acknowledge life's hurts, bruises, and disappointments, yet enables me to move on to a better space. Bringing something of beauty into each day is a continuing aspect of my agenda. Regardless of life's pressures, the ability to "feed" myself is essential. I awaken daily to Frankl's exercise of quickly naming the 10 best things in my life. I have found that they are always changing, which opens my mind to look, see, and be part of this glorious world. I reach for a favorite CD (Gustav Mahler), a poem, my memory bank, or some experience that I treasure. I have tested this system recently under a time of great personal stress and pain and can confirm its effectiveness. I believe caregivers in our society face constant challenges that surely require them to nurture themselves. It is only then that they can have the capacity to enter into and fully participate in the struggle of another.

The philosophy of Martin Buber explains the significance of the moment when we are called on to dialogue with another. It takes discipline and constant emotional energy to be able to feel the "Thou" of the other under powerful conditions. We all need to be understood and to be treated with respect—I did and do. Buber demonstrates the hurtfulness when one is perceived psychologically as an "It." A part of the divine is within each of us and requires us to honor the other.

In retrospect, witnessing Jerry's suffering was my real challenge. Over the 10 years he had cancer, we worked at our respective professions, always striving to live in a better space. One of my greatest pleasures was to read to him. In those last months at the Cancer Center in New York, Jerry and I meditated twice daily. We visualized the cancer cells being washed away. Many times it was like magic. He would announce "I feel terrific! Let's walk on the Champs Elysées" (the corridor around the nursing station). The corridors were filled with prints of great painters, many of which were impressionists. He would walk with his aluminum canes, viewing the pictures as we had done in the museums. There was a Monet, *The Beach At St. Addresse*, which was his favorite. One night he awakened at 2 AM as I slept on a cot in his room, asking me to take the print from our room and exchange it for the Monet. As you can imagine, I quickly slipped into my robe, took our "masterpiece" under my arm, secretly and softly removing the Monet and hanging the other in its place. Suddenly, the night nurse appeared. "What are you doing at this hour of the night, Ruth?" she questioned. I pleadingly explained that Jerry loved the Monet as she insisted that I had no right to move the picture from that wall. Since I already had it in hand, I told her Jerry had such a limited time to enjoy it and, therefore, it should be on "loan" for the duration of his stay. I marched back with it, and at that hour he was able to express his delight.

One memorable dialogue with me took place after the surgeon informed him that he was "coming down to the wire," and it appeared that there was nothing of benefit that could be offered. Jerry asked that I close the door. Alone with him, he insisted that I take an oath (this he had discovered to be a comforting and reassuring way to share his deepest concerns). Before his last hospital admission, Jerry determined he wanted to go to my analyst. The doctor gave him an appointment right after mine. I took him in his wheelchair, and he waited in the waiting room during my session, as I did during his session. Jerry elucidated his wishes that had probably been in his mind for many weeks. He had the analyst take an oath that he would never abandon me—that would enable him to die in peace. The oath asked of me was powerful—Jerry said, "I have had my care at two hospitals. I have thought of mistakes in both of them. But, as a lawyer, I can tell you, we all make mistakes, though most of us won't admit it. I have made plenty of mistakes in my life. So, I want you to swear that when I am gone, you will never fault them. They did the best they could and I love them." I agreed as we both reflected on that memorable day. Then I lit the incense and we held hands.

My struggle was bound up in separation. I wanted to have Jerry "inside of me" when we were not together and this I accomplished. I was able to recall him at any moment—during a meeting or alone on a bus, he could be present in my psyche. By giving Jerry my best, I never betrayed myself. As an octogenarian, life glistens for me in countless ways. Blessings abound: good health . . . my son . . . family, though far away . . . my work . . . and a few precious friends. With each day, I hope I can return the infinite goodness life has given me. We are all precious members of this universe and are here to make it a bit better through our resolve as honest, sincere partners in every moment.

V

Special Patient Populations

34

Polly Mazanec and Joan T. Panke

Cultural Considerations in Palliative Care

My mother went to the doctors like they said. But it was prayer and her healer that got her here this long. She is a cancer patient now, this year. But she has been a proud Indian woman all her life.—A daughter

- ***Key Points***
- *A multidimensional assessment of culture is essential to planning palliative care for patients and families.*
- *An individual's culture includes ethnicity, sexuality, family history, religion, and many other aspects.*
- *Issues of culture are important throughout any aspects. experience but are crucial in life-threatening disease.*

This chapter defines culture and its components as they relates to palliative care. It addresses cultural competence and the importance of recognizing how one's own values, practices, and beliefs impact care. Finally, selected palliative care issues influenced by culture are discussed. This chapter is not intended to be a "cookbook" approach to describing behaviors and practices of different cultures as they relate to palliative care, but, rather, a guide to raising awareness of the significance of cultural considerations in palliative care.

Culture and Palliative Care Nursing

The essence of palliative nursing is to provide holistic supportive care for the patient and the family living with a life-limiting illness. Palliative nursing strives to meet the physical, emotional, social, and spiritual needs of the patient and family across the disease trajectory.[1] In an effort to meet these needs, nurses must recognize the vital role that culture has on one's experience of living and dying. The beliefs, norms, and practices of an individual's cultural heritage guide one's behavioral responses, decision-making, and actions.[2] Culture shapes how an individual makes meaning out of illness, suffering, and death.[2,3] Nurses, along with other members of the interdisciplinary team, partner with the patient and family to ensure that patient and family values, beliefs, and practices guide the plan of care.

The following case illustrates the distress experienced by the patient, family, and health care team when cultural implications of care are not considered.

CASE STUDY

Mrs. Wu, a Patient with Lung Cancer

Mrs. Wu, a 78-year-old Chinese American woman, was diagnosed 7 months ago with non–small cell lung cancer.

Table 34–1
Panethnic Groups: Nations of Origin

Panethnic Groups	Nations of Origin
American Indian / Alaskan native	200 American Indian nations indigenous to North American Aleuts, and Eskimos in Alaska
Asian/ Pacific Islander	China, Japan, Hawaii, the Philippines, Vietnam, Asian India, Korea, Samoa, Guam, and the Remaining Asian/Pacific islands
Black	West coast of Africa; many African countries; West Indian islands, Dominican Republic; Haiti; Jamaica
Hispanic	Hispanic countries, Spain, Cuba, Mexico, Central and South America, Puerto Rico
White	Germany, England, Italy, Ireland, Former Soviet Union, and all other European countries

Source: Spector, Rachael E. Cultural care: Guides to heritage assessment and health traditions, 5th edition. © 2000. Reprinted by permission of Pearson Education, Inc., Upper Saddle River, NJ. (Reference 52)

She is admitted to the oncology unit of the hospital with severe dyspnea and weakness. Her husband died several years ago, and she has been living with her eldest unmarried son, who has taken a leave of absence from work to care for her. When asked how she is feeling, she states she is "fine" and reports no symptoms. The nurses note that she appears to be in severe pain, wincing with a furrowed brow and moaning with any movement. The son does not want his mother "sedated with pain medication" and tells the nurses "No one is to tell my mother that she has cancer. We have not told her and do not want her to know because she would give up hope." Mrs. Wu's only other child, a married son who lives 500 miles away, has come to visit and speaks privately with the nurse. He tells the nurse that he understands his mother is very ill and dying, but he must respect his brother's decisions about his mother's care. The nursing staff believes Mrs. Wu is suffering needlessly and should be fully informed of her diagnosis and prognosis. The nurses have struggled with the son's beliefs, trying to convince him to allow his mother to be medicated for pain. The nurses are upset at the son's request not to tell his mother her diagnosis. In addition, they are concerned that Mrs. Wu appears very depressed, never making eye contact with them and rarely talking.

On the second evening of the hospital stay, the nurse caring for Mrs. Wu asks the covering physician to consider ordering an antidepressant. While assessing Mrs. Wu, the physician tells her that she is dying from lung cancer. The family returns in the morning to find their mother quite distraught, and they are so angry that Mrs. Wu has been told her diagnosis that the eldest son threatens to sign his mother out of the hospital against medical advice. The patient, family, and staff are experiencing a great deal of distress as a result of the cultural conflict that has taken place.

Increasing Diversity in the United States Population

As the United States becomes increasingly diverse, the range of treasured beliefs, shared teachings, norms, customs, and languages challenge the nurse to understand and respond to a wide variety of perspectives. In 2000, the population in the United States exceeded 280 million people.[4] Population statistics illustrate that cultural diversity is increasing among the five most common pan-ethnic groups, which are federally defined as American Indian/Alaskan native, Asian/Pacific Islander, black, Hispanic, and white (Table 34–1). By 2030, the population of Hispanic and Asian/Pacific Islander will nearly double that of 1998. Immigrants and their children will account for nearly one half of the growth of the U.S. population.[4] Trends suggest that by 2050, one out of every two Americans will claim membership from what is currently an ethnic minority.[4]

Culture Defined

Culture is the "learned, shared and transmitted values, beliefs, norms and life ways of a particular group that guide their thinking, decision, actions in patterned ways—a patterned behavioral response."[5] Culture is shaped over time and is constantly changing.[6] It is a dynamic system in which the beliefs, values, and lifestyle patterns pass from one generation to another.[7] While culture is often thought of as race and ethnicity, the definition of culture expands far beyond, encompassing such dimensions as gender, age, differing abilities, sexual orientation, religion, financial status, residency, employment, and educational level.[2] Each dimension plays a role in shaping patient and family responses to life-threatening illness.

A broad definition of culture recognizes various subcultures an individual may associate with that shape experiences and responses in any given situation. The nurse must also be constantly aware that the culture of the health care system and the culture of the nursing profession shape how he or she responds to interactions with patients, families, and colleagues.

Components of Culture

Race

The commonly held misconception that "race" refers to biological and genetic differences and "ethnicity" refers to cultural variation is outmoded.[8] Race does not exist as a natural category, but as a social construct.[7,8] Any discussion of race must include the harsh reality of racism issues and disparities that have plagued society and continue to exist even today. Recent studies have demonstrated the discrimination of persons of certain races regarding health care practices and treatment options.[9–12] When viewed in relation to specific races, morbidity and mortality statistics point to serious gaps in access to quality care. Racial disparities are still evident even after adjustments for socioeconomic status and other access-related factors are taken into account.[13]

There is often an underlying mistrust of the health care system. Memories of the Tuskegee syphilis study and segregated hospitals remain with older African Americans.[3] The combination of mistrust, along with numerous other complex variables, influence issues such as medical decision-making and advance care planning.[3,14] Compounding the situation is the fact that health care providers often do not recognize existing biases within systems or themselves.

Ethnicity

Ethnicity refers to individuals with a common ancestry who share a similar sense of historical continuity.[7] The values, practices, and beliefs shared by members of the same ethnic group may influence behavior or response.[6] It is important to note, however, that although an individual may belong to a particular ethnic group, he or she may not identify strongly with that group.[15] Consider intergenerational differences and levels of acculturation. It is not unusual for members of the same family to have very different perspectives on certain issues. Assess each individual's beliefs and practices rather than assuming that he or she holds the beliefs of a particular group.[16] The tendency to assume that an individual will respond in a certain way contributes to stereotyping and can lead to inappropriate interventions.

Gender

Cultural norms dictate specific roles for men and women. The significance of gender is evident in areas such as decision-making, caregiving, and pain and symptom management. It is important to have an awareness of family dominance patterns, and determine which family member or members hold that dominant role. In some families, decision-making may be the responsibility of the male head of the family or eldest son; in others, it may be the eldest female. Discussing prognosis and treatment with an inappropriate member may create significant clashes with the health care team.[17]

Age

Age has its own identity and culture.[1] Age cohorts are characterized by consumer behaviors, leisure activities, religious activities, education, and labor force participation.[18] Each group has its own beliefs, attitudes and practices, which are influenced by their developmental stage and by the society in which they live. The impact of a life-limiting illness on persons of differing age groups is often influenced by the loss of developmental tasks associated with that age group. Consider also the cultural impact of age on decision-making, caregiving issues, and barriers to effective pain management.[10]

Differing Abilities

Individuals with physical disabilities or mental illness are at risk of receiving poorer quality health care. Those with differing abilities constitute a cultural group in themselves and often feel stigmatized. This discrimination is evident in cultures where the healthy are more valued than the physically, emotionally, or intellectually challenged. If patients are unable to communicate their needs, pain and symptom management and end-of-life wishes are not likely to be addressed. Taking time to determine an individual's goals of care, regardless of differing abilities, and identifying resources and support to improve quality of life is essential.

Sexual Orientation

Sexual orientation may carry a stigma when the patient is gay, lesbian, or transgendered. In palliative care, these patients have unique needs, due to the legal and ethical issues of domestic partnerships, multiple losses that may have been experienced as a result of one's sexual orientation, and unresolved family issues. Domestic partnerships, sanctioned by many cities and states in the United States, grant some of the rights of traditional married couples to unmarried homosexual couples who share the traditional bond of the family.[19] However, many cities and states do not legally recognize the relationship. If legal documents have not been drafted prior to death of a partner, survivorship issues, financial concerns, and lack of acknowledgment of bereavement needs may complicate grief.[2]

Religion and Spirituality

Religion is the belief and practice of a faith tradition, a means of expressing spirituality. Spirituality, a much broader concept, is the life force that transcends our physical being and gives meaning and purpose.[1,20] These terms are often mistakenly used interchangeably. It should be noted that an individual may be very spiritual, but not practice a formal religion. In addition, those who identify themselves as belonging to a religion do not necessarily adhere to all the practices of that religion. As with ethnicity, it is important to determine how strongly the individual aligns with his or her identified faith and the significance of its practice rituals.

Chaplains, clergy from a patient or family member's religious group, and ideally their own community clergy are key members of the interdisciplinary team. Often, individuals have misconceptions of the tenets of their own faith, and clergy can help ease spiritual distress.

Socioeconomic Status

One's socioeconomic status, place of residence, workplace, and level of education are important components of one's cultural identity and play a role in palliative care. For example, those who are socioeconomically disadvantaged face unique challenges when seeking health care and when receiving treatment. Patients and families in a supportive community have increased access to resources at end of life than other more vulnerable populations, such as those in prison and the homeless.[21]

However, regardless of financial status, an estimated 25% of families are financially devastated by a serious terminal illness.[2] Patients experiencing disease progression, or in whom treatment side effects preclude the ability to work, are forced to confront profound losses: loss of work and income, loss of identity, and loss of a network of colleagues. Those who are educationally disadvantaged struggle to navigate the health care system and to access information and support.

In addition to assessing the components of culture previously mentioned, when doing a thorough cultural assessment, it is important to determine communication styles, the meaning of food and food preferences and prohibitions, and death and dying rituals.

Cultural Considerations Related to Communication

Awareness of verbal and nonverbal communication styles assists the nurse in establishing trusting relationships, showing respect for variations, and identifying potential communication barriers early to avoid potential conflicts. Communication is an interactive, multidimensional process, often dictated by cultural norms, and provides the mechanism for human interaction and connection.

In any patient, family, or professional encounter, understanding communication styles and norms will help enhance that encounter. Factors to consider include clarifying who the decision-maker in the family is and with whom information should be shared (patient, family, or both). This is a key factor to address early on, as it establishes trust in the patient–provider and family–provider relationships. It is also important to determine the dominant language and dialect spoken and the literacy level of both patient and primary family caregiver(s). Additionally, find out if there are norms related to greetings (e.g., formal/informal; appropriateness of touch, handshake, smile). Attention to acceptable forms of nonverbal communication is as important as knowledge of verbal communication customs; for example, certain gestures, eye contact and silence that may be acceptable in some cultures yet unacceptable in others.[22,23]

If there is a language barrier, a professionally trained interpreter of the appropriate gender should be contacted. Family members should not be asked to serve as interpreters because this may force them into an uncomfortable role should sensitive issues arise. When using an interpreter, direct all verbal communication to the patient/family, not to the interpreter. Ongoing clarification that information is understood is critical.

Touch can be a powerful communication tool in palliative care; however, although intended to communicate reassurance and caring, touch may invade personal space and privacy, resulting in considerable distress. Norms regarding appropriateness of touching members of the opposite sex are important to note.[6] How close you should be to another, or the concept of personal space is closely related to communication styles. Sitting too close to a patient may be considered intrusive or disrespectful.[22] On the other hand, sitting or standing far away from the patient may communicate disinterest and lack of caring.[15] Asking the individual for guidance on these issues will avoid a great deal of unintended discomfort and avoid misunderstandings.

Meaning of Food and Nutrition

Across cultures, there is agreement that food is essential for life, to maintain body function and to produce energy.[6] Food serves another purpose in the building and maintaining of human relationships. It is used in rituals, celebrations, and rites of passage to establish and maintain social and cultural relationships with families, friends, and others. Because of food's importance for life and life events, a loss of desire for food and subsequent weight loss and wasting can cause suffering for both the patient and family. Culturally appropriate or favorite foods may be encouraged. However, families often need explanations when a patient is no longer able to enjoy favorite foods or family mealtime rituals. It is imperative that the health care team understands the meaning attached to food in a palliative care setting, when decisions regarding the potential burden of providing artificial nutrition and hydration for an imminently dying patient are being discussed.

Death Rituals and Mourning Practices

The loss of a loved one brings sadness and upheaval in the family structure across all cultures.[24] Each culture responds to these losses through specific rituals that assist the dying and the bereaved through the final transition from life. Respecting these rituals and customs will have tremendous impact on the healing process for family members following the death.

The tasks of grieving are universal: to accept the reality of the loss, to experience pain of grief, to begin the adjustment to new social and family roles, and to withdraw emotional energy from the dead individual and turn it over to those who are alive.[25] The expressions of grief, however, may vary significantly among cultures. What is acceptable in one culture may seem unacceptable, or even maladaptive, in another. Recognizing normal grief behavior (versus complicated grief) within a cultural context therefore demands knowledge about culturally acceptable expressions of grief. Important to note is that rituals may begin before death and may last for months or even years after death. Some may value being present at the time of death. Insure that any required spiritual, religious, or cultural practices are performed and that appropriate care of the body after death is carried out.

Cultural Competence

Cultural competence refers to a dynamic, fluid, continuous process of awareness, knowledge, skill, interaction, and sensitivity.[5] Cultural competence is an ongoing process, not an end point. It is more comprehensive than cultural sensitivity, implying not only the ability to recognize and respect cultural differences, but also to intervene appropriately and effectively.[6,26,27] Five components essential in pursuing cultural competence are cultural awareness, cultural knowledge, cultural skill, cultural encounter, and cultural desire.[28]

Integrating cultural considerations into palliative care requires first and foremost that the nurse becomes aware of how one's own values, practices, and beliefs influence care.[26,28,29] Cultural awareness begins with an examination of one's own heritage, family's practices, experiences, and religious or spiritual beliefs.[29,30] Each nurse brings his or her own cultural and philosophical views, education, religion, spirituality, and life experiences to the care of the patient and family. Cultural awareness challenges the nurse to look beyond his or her ethnocentric view of the world, asking the question "How are my values, beliefs, and practices different from the patient and family?" rather than "How is this patient and family different from me?"[31] Exploring one's own beliefs will raise an awareness of differences that have the potential to foster prejudice and discrimination and limit the effectiveness of care.[29] Often this exploration identifies more similarities than differences (Figure 34–1). The universal aspects of life, family, trust, love, hope, understanding, and caring unite us all.[32]

Acquiring knowledge about different cultural groups is the second component to gaining cultural competence, but knowledge alone is insufficient in providing culturally appropriate care. Yet, how does one attempt to gain knowledge and understanding of so many diverse cultures? No one can expect to have in-depth knowledge of all cultural variations of health and illness beliefs, values, and norms. A suggested strategy is to identify the most common ethnic group/cultures living in the nurse's community, and to integrate a basic understanding of norms and practices impacting issues likely to arise in palliative and end-of-life situations. Involve community members, organizations, faith communities, and leaders in a shared understanding of needs and concerns. Knowledge gained of a particular group should serve only as a guide to understanding the unique cultural needs of the patient and family that comes through individualized assessments. Other resources, such as cultural guides, literature and web-based resources are available to assist the nurse in acquiring knowledge about specific groups. Table 34–2 lists several useful web-based resources.

Cultural skill is the third component of cultural competency. Skills in cultural assessment, cross-cultural communication, cultural interpretation, and appropriate intervention can be learned. Multiple tools are available to assess cultural behavior and beliefs. Key assessment questions, applicable in the palliative care setting, will help the nurse address the patient's and family's needs in a culturally sensitive manner.[23]

Cultural Assessment

Cultural assessments involve questions that necessitate the development of a trusting relationship. When meeting the patient and family early in the disease trajectory, the palliative care clinician is able to establish trust. Often, though, the palliative care nurse may not have the luxury of time. Ideally, the patient's primary care team would have completed the assessment and communicated information gleaned from the assessment across settings.

When the timing of the assessment cannot be planned, inquiries of the patient or family can be helpful in assisting the nurse to gain the most helpful information for the situation at hand. Checklists do not necessarily build trust. Instead, asking the patient, or the family member to tell you about him or herself or the family, and then listening to those narratives can reveal many of their beliefs, values, and concerns. The speaker may give you clues that trigger important questions to ask so that you are able to clarify patient and family needs and goals. Examples of trigger questions are provided in Table 34–3.

Selected Palliative Care Issues Influenced by Culture

Cultural considerations impact all aspects of palliative care: assessment, planning, and implementation of care. This section focuses on cultural considerations regarding decision-making, pain, and symptom management.

Medical Decision-Making

Over the past 35 years in the United States, ethical and legal considerations of decision-making have focused on patient

CULTURAL KNOWLEDGE AND BELIEFS

1. List two cultural groups to which you belong (e.g. ethnicity, religion/spirituality).

   ____

   ____

   a. List three values that you attribute to each group listed above.

      ____

      ____

      ____

   b. List three rituals that you practice that have been learned from each cultural group.

      ____

      ____

      ____

2. Write down the first names of the 10 people with whom you spend the most time on a weekly basis. In the blank spaces below write down how many of them (0-10) differ from you in terms of:

Socioeconomic status	________	Health	________
Ethnicity	________	Race	________
Gender	________	Spirituality	________
Nationality	________	Sexual orientation	________
Cognitive abilities	________	Physical abilities	________
Age (5+/– years)	________	Mental abilities	________

3. Rank 1 to 5 the most common resources you use to learn about people from other cultural groups (1 = most frequent; 5 = least frequent).

   ______ Television shows
   ______ Ongoing personal relationships
   ______ Classroom presentations
   ______ Radio shows
   ______ Textbooks
   ______ Clients in clinical area
   ______ Research articles
   ______ Movies
   ______ Work relationships
   ______ Cultural events
   ______ Newspapers
   ______ Other (list)

4. Rank from 1 to 5 the most common reasons you are reluctant to or do not interact with people from other cultural groups (1 = most common; 5 = least common).

   ______ Don't know where to meet people
   ______ Family or peer pressure
   ______ Fear of rejection
   ______ Not interested
   ______ Fear of offending them
   ______ Fear of bodily harm
   ______ Past experiences
   ______ Language barriers
   ______ Nothing in common
   ______ Other (list)

Figure 34–1. Cultural knowledge and beliefs: a self-assessment questionnaire. (*Source:* JoAnne Banks-Wallace, PhD, RN, The University of Missouri, Sinclair School of Nursing, Columbia, MO. ONS Multicultural Tool Kit.)

Table 34–2
Web Resources for Acquiring Knowledge About Cultural Issues Affecting Health Care

This list offers suggestions of several useful resources. The list is not intended to be exhaustive, but serves as a starting point for gaining more information.

ACCESS—www.access2eolcare.org

ACCESS to End-of-Life Care: A Community Initiative is dedicated to improving end-of-life care services to culturally and ethnically diverse populations. The website offers in-depth information and an exceptional bibliography. Great links to other resources.

Cross Cultural Health Care Program (CCHPC)—http://www.xculture.org/

CCHCP addresses broad cultural issues that impact the health of individuals and families in ethnic minority communities.

Diversity Rx—http://DiversityRx.org

Models and practices, policy, legal issues, networking and links to other resources

EthnoMed—http://ethnomed.org/

The EthnoMed site contains information about cultural beliefs, medical issues and other related issues pertinent to the health care of recent immigrants to the US.

University of Michigan Cultural Competency Program—www.med.umich.edu/multicultural/ccp

Excellent source of information, tools, and resources.

Transcultural Nursing Society—www.tcns.org

The society, founded in 1974, serves as a forum to promote, advance, and disseminate transcultural nursing knowledge worldwide.

Audio Resource

Heart to Heart: Improving Care for the Dying through Public Policy—Part IV: Cultural Diversity and Discrimination. Perspectives on how death and dying are influenced by cultural and religious values. Ordering info: $12 per tape. By phone: 1-800-989-9455; E-mail: pfc@partnershipforcaring.org.

Video Resource

One Journey—Many Voices: Conversations About Serious Illness and Dying. Available at http://www.aarp.org/lce/video.

Other

Last Acts Diversity and End-of-Life Care Literature Review. Annotated bibliography. Washington, DC : Last Acts National Program Office, 2001; 13 p. MH04D6133. Free copies are available from Last Acts National Program Office, 1620 Eye Street, NW, Suite 202, Washington, DC 20006-4017; (phone) 202-296-8071; (fax) 202-296-8352.

autonomy.[33] This focus replaced the more paternalistic approach of decision-making as solely the physician's responsibility, with an approach that emphasizes a model of shared responsibility with the patient's active involvement. The Patient Self-Determination Act of 1991 sought to further clarify and to protect an individual's health care preferences with advance directives.[34,35] The principle of respect for patient autonomy points to a patient's right to participate in decisions about the care he or she receives. Associated with this is the right to be informed of diagnosis, prognosis, and the risks and benefits of treatment in order to make informed decisions.[17] Inherent in the movement for patient autonomy is the underlying assumption that all patients want control over their health care decisions. Yet, in fact, for some individuals, patient autonomy may violate the very principles of dignity and integrity it proposes to uphold.

This European-American model of patient autonomy has its origin in the dominant culture, a predominantly white middle-class perspective that does not take into consideration diverse cultural perspectives.[36] Emphasis on autonomy as the guiding principle assumes that the individual, rather than the family or other social group, is the appropriate decision-maker.[37]

Table 34–3
Key Cultural Assessment Questions

Formal cultural assessments are available for the nurse to use (see resources in Table 34–2). Remember that a checklist does not always instill trust. Below are some suggestions for ascertaining key cultural preferences from both patients and family caregivers.

- Tell me a little bit about yourself (for families, e.g., your mother, father, sister, brother, etc.) Where were you born and raised? (If an immigrant: How long have you lived in this country?)
- What language would you prefer to speak?
- Is it easier to write things down, or do you have difficulty with reading or writing?
- Whom do you go to for support (family, friends, community, religious or community leaders)?
- Is there anyone we should contact to come to be with you?
- I want to be sure I'm giving you all the information you need. What do you want to know about your condition? Whom should I speak to about your care?
- Whom do you want to know about your condition?
- How are decisions about health care made in your family? Should I speak directly with you, or is there someone else I should be discussing decisions with?
- *(Address to patient or designated decision maker.)* Tell me about your understanding of what has been happening up to this point? What does the illness mean to you?
- We want to work with you to be sure you are getting the best care possible, and that we are meeting all your needs. Is there anything we should know about any customs or practices that are important to include in your care?
- Many people have shared that it is very important to include spirituality or religion in their care. Is this something that is important for you? Our chaplain can help contact anyone that you would like to be involved with your care.
- We want to make sure we respect how you prefer to be addressed, including how we should act. Is there anything we should avoid? Is it appropriate for you to have male and female caregivers?
- Are there any foods you would like or that you should avoid?
- Do you have any concerns about how to pay for care, medications or other services?

Death Rituals and Practices

- Is there anything we should know about care of the body, about rituals, practices, or ceremonies that should be performed?
- What is your belief about what happens after death?
- Is there a way for us to plan for anything you might need both at the time of death and afterward?
- Is there anything we should know about whether or not a man or a woman should be caring for the body after death?
- Should the family be involved in the care?

However, in many non-European American cultures, the concept of interdependence among family and community members is more valued than individual autonomy.[33,37] Cultures that practice family-centered decision-making, such as Asian and Hispanic cultures, may prefer that the family, or perhaps a particular family member rather than the patient, receive and process information.[17] Patient autonomy may not be seen as empowering, but, rather, may seem burdensome for patients who are too sick to have to make difficult decisions.[31] The label of "truth-telling" itself is misleading. While full disclosure may not be appropriate, it is never appropriate to lie to the patient. If the patient does not wish to receive information and/or telling the patient violates the patient's and family's cultural norms, the health care provider may, in fact, not be respecting the patient's right to autonomously decide not to receive the information. Some cultures believe that telling the patient he has a terminal illness strips away any and all hope and causes needless suffering, and may indeed hasten death.[3,12,38,39]

The nurse must consider the harm that may occur when the health system or providers violate cultural beliefs and practices.[17] Assessing and clarifying the patient and family's perspectives, values, and practices may prevent a cultural conflict.[33] The nurse is in a key position to advocate these critical patient and family issues (see Table 34–3 for examples of questions to ask). By asking how decision are made, and whether or not the patient wishes to be involved in both being told information or participating in the decision-making process, patient autonomy is respected, and individual beliefs and values are honored.[14]

Withholding and Withdrawing

Another issue with the potential for cultural conflict is decision-making regarding withholding and withdrawing of life-sustaining treatments. Deciding to withhold or withdraw life-sustaining treatment is difficult because inherent in the decision is that the patient will most likely die.[34] Attitude surveys looking at initiating and terminating life support have demonstrated differences among several ethnic groups. When making difficult decisions, family members often feel that by agreeing to withdrawal of life support, they are, in fact, responsible for the death of their loved one. Recognize also that the words used in these decisions, including "do not resuscitate," all have negative connotations and involve the removing of something or the withholding of a particular intervention. Research suggests that groups including African Americans, Chinese Americans, Filipino Americans, Iranian Americans, Korean Americans, and Mexican Americans were more likely to start and to continue life support when such measures were felt by the health care team to be futile than were European Americans.[40] Because many ethical conflicts arise from differences in patients', families', and providers' values, beliefs, and practices, it is critical that individual members of the health care team be aware of their own cultural beliefs, understand their own reactions to the issue, and be knowledgeable about the patients' and families' beliefs to address the conflict.[33]

The Experience of Pain

Pain is a highly personal and subjective experience. Pain is whatever the person says it is, and exists whenever the person says it does.[41] Culture plays a role in the experience of pain, the meaning of pain, and the response to pain. A biocultural model of pain suggests that social learning from family and group membership can influence the psychological and physiological processing of pain, which then affects the perception and modulation of pain.[42]

Strong beliefs about expressing pain and expected pain behaviors exist in every culture.[43] Pain tolerance varies from person to person and is influenced by factors such as past experiences with pain, coping skills, motivation to endure pain, and energy level. Western society appears to value individuals that exhibit a high pain threshold.[44] As a result, those with a lower threshold, who report pain often, may be labeled as "difficult patients."

Pain assessment should be culturally appropriate, using terms that describe pain intensity across most cultural groups. "Pain," "hurt," and "ache" are words commonly used across cultures. These words may reflect the severity of the pain, with "pain" being the most severe, "hurt" being moderate pain, and "ache" being the least severe.[44] Focus on the words the patient uses to describe pain. To help facilitate an understanding of the severity of the pain experienced by someone who does not speak English, use pain rating scales that have been translated into numerous languages.[44] While it is important to base the assessment on the patient's self-report of pain intensity, it may be necessary to rely on nonverbal pain indicators such as facial expression, body movement, and vocalization to assess pain in the nonverbal, cognitively impaired patient, the older adult, or the infant, who are all at risk for inaccurate assessment and undertreatment of pain.[45–47]

Both cultural bias in pain reports and gender biases have been identified and documented.[13] Studies of gender variations in pain response have identified differences in sensitivity and tolerance to pain, and willingness to report pain.[48-51] Studies reveal that Hispanics, African Americans, and females are less likely to be prescribed opioids for pain.[47,51]

Incorporating culturally appropriate nondrug therapies may improve the ability to alleviate pain. Healing practices specific to cultures should be offered to the patient and family.[51] Herbal remedies, acupuncture, and folk medicines should be incorporated into the plan of care if desired. Keep in mind that certain nondrug approaches, such as hypnosis and massage, may be inappropriate in some cultures.[44]

Symptom Management

Similar to pain management, symptoms have cultural meanings associated with them that reflect cultural values, beliefs, and practices. Assessment and management of such commonly occurring symptoms in palliative care as fatigue, dyspnea, depression, nausea and vomiting, and anorexia/cachexia should be implemented within a cultural framework.

As noted earlier, it is important to understand the health and illness beliefs of the cultural groups living in your community. Table 34–4 lists cultural considerations for pain and symptom management for selected groups. Of note, there is a dearth of information in the literature regarding health and illness beliefs in the Caucasian, or what is often referred to as the European-American population. This group, as with other ethnic groups, migrated from numerous countries of origin. The reader is reminded that the groups listed in Table 34–4 also immigrated from various geographic areas. Therefore, the list serves as a guide only and does not replace individual assessment. The nurse recognizes guides as offering information based on generalizations, and that making assumptions without validating their significance to the individual and family may lead to harmful stereotyping.[27,32]

Summary

Given the changing population of the United States, we as nurses must advocate for the integration of cultural considerations in providing comprehensive palliative care. It is imperative that

Table 34–4
Cultural Considerations for Pain and Symptom Management

	American Indian/ Alaskan Native	Asian/Pacific Islander	Black	Hispanic
Pain	Rarely demonstrate pain behaviors or request medication; view pain as something that has to be endured; often under-treated	May not complain of pain May use nondrug therapies, e.g., acupuncture to relieve pain	Open expression of pain; avoids medications due to fears of addiction; believes pain must be endured	Ability to endure pain and suffering stoically is valued; males who express pain considered weak; type and amount of pain divinely predetermined
Dyspnea	May report "the air's heavy"	Caused by too much "yin"—may treat with hot soups/warm clothing	May report "difficulty catching breath"	Feels something is very wrong if oxygen is needed
Nausea and vomiting	Maybe embarrassed to report	Caused by too much "yin"—will treat with hot soups/broths	Prefers non-drug management	Willing to disclose symptom
Constipation/ diarrhea	Patient may be modest, but will report; may use elderberry flowers as remedy for diarrhea	Caused by too much "yang"; may treat with "yin" foods	May report "being blocked up"	Will disclose if asked; believe diarrhea is beneficial; may not want drug therapy
Fatigue	Tries to maintain a high level of activity despite poor health or impairment	Caused by too much "yin"—ginseng may be used for relief	Willing to disclose symptom	
Depression	Often psychiatric prob lems present as physical symptoms; vague generally recognized as "having a heart problem"	Family important in the care of mentally ill; tremendous stigma attached todiagnosis; readily not discussed	Seldom report depression—call it a "tired state"; will accept drug therapy	Not easily disclosed; considered a sign of weakness; family embarrassed

Source: Moller DW. Dancing with Broken Bones: Portraits of Death and Dying Among Inner-City Poor, © 2004 by Oxford University Press, Inc. Used by permission of Oxford University Press, Inc.

each of us moves beyond our own ethnocentric view of the world to appreciate and respect the similarities and differences in each other. We are challenged to embrace a better understanding of various perspectives. Becoming culturally competent first requires an awareness of how one's own cultural background impacts care. In addition, acquiring knowledge about cultures and developing skill in cultural assessment are essential to improving care to patients with life-limiting illnesses and their families.

This chapter encourages nurses to integrate cultural assessment and culturally appropriate interventions into palliative care. It is the hope of the authors that readers will enrich their practice by seeking new knowledge about different cultures through available resources and, most importantly, by using the most valuable resources on cultural considerations we have—our patients and their families.

REFERENCES

1. Sherman D. Cultural and spiritual backgrounds of older adults. In: Matzo M, Sherman D, eds. Gerontologic Palliative Care Nursing. St. Louis: Mosby, 2004:3–47.
2. End-of-Life Nursing Education Consortium (ELNEC), http://www.aacn.nche.edu/elnec/ (accessed December 16, 2004).
3. Kagawa-Singer M, Blackhall L. Negotating cross-cultural issues at the end of life. JAMA 2001;286:2993–3001.
4. U.S. Bureau of the Census (2000). Current Population Reports, http://www.census.gov/ipc/www/usinterimproj (internet release date March 18, 2004; accessed February 9, 2005).
5. Leininger M. Quality of life from a transcultural nursing perspective. Nursing Science Quarterly 1994:7:22–28.
6. Andrews M, Boyle J, eds. Transcultural Concepts of Nursing Care, 4th ed. Philadelphia: Lippincott Williams & Wilkins, 2003.

7. Kagawa-Singer M. Improving the validity and generalizability of studies with underserved U.S. populations: expanding the research paradigm. Ann Epidermiol 2000;10(Suppl 8): S92–103.
8. Koenig B, Gates-Williams J. Understanding cultural differences in caring for dying patients. West J Med 1995;163:244–249.
9. Doescher M, Saver B, Franks P, Fiscella K. Racial and ethnic disparities in perception of physician style and trust. Arch Fam Med 2000;9:1156–1167.
10. Cleeland C, Gonin R, Hatfield A, et al. Pain and its treatment in outpatients with metastatic cancer. NEJM 1994;330:592–596.
11. Gamble V. Under the shadow of Tuskegee: African Americans and healthcare. Am J Public Health 1997;87:1773–1778.
12. Gamble V. A legacy of distrust: African Americans and medical research. Am J Prev Med 1993;9:35–38.
13. Smedly B, Stith A, Nelson A. Unequal treatment: confronting racial and ethnic disparities in health care (Report of the Institute of Medicine). Washington, D.C.: National Academy Press, 2003.
14. Lapine A, Wang-Cheng R, Goldstein M, Nooney A, Lamb G, Derse A. When cultures clash: physician, patient, and family wishes in truth disclosure for dying patients. J Palliat Care 2001;4:475–480.
15. Giger J, Davidhizar R, eds. Transcultural Nursing: Assessment and Intervention, 3rd ed. New York: Mosby, 1999.
16. Crawley L, Marshall P, Lo B, Koenig B. Strategies for culturally effective end-of-life care. Ann Inter Med 2002;136:673–679.
17. Blackhall L, Murphy S, Frank G, Michel V, Azen S. Ethnicity and attitudes toward patient autonomy. JAMA 1995;274:820–825.
18. Matteson M, McConnell E, Linton A. Gerontological Nursing: Concepts & Practice, Philadelphia: W.B. Saunders, 1997.
19. Purnell L, Paulanka B. Transcultural Health Care: A Culturally Competent Approach. Philadelphia: F.A. Davis, 1998.
20. Conrad N. Spiritual support for the dying. Nurs Clin North Am 1985;20:415–425.
21. Flaskerud J, Winslow B. Conceptualizing vulnerable population's health-related research. Nurs Res 1998;47:69–78.
22. Wright F, Cohen S, Caroselli C. How culture affects ethical decision making. Crit Care Nurs Clin North Am 1997;9:63–74.
23. Lipson J, Meleis A. Culturally appropriate care: the case of immigrants. Top Clin Nurs 1985;7:48–56.
24. Kagawa-Singer M, Martinson I, Munet-Vilaro F. A multicultural perspective on death and dying. ONS 1998;25:1751–1756.
25. Worden J. Grief Counseling and Grief Therapy, 2nd ed., New York: Springer, 1991.
26. Zoucha R. The keys to culturally sensitive care. Am J Nurs 2000;100:24GG-24II.
27. Lipson J, Dibble S, Minarik P. Culture & Nursing Care: A Pocket Guide. San Francisco: UCSF Nursing Press, 1996.
28. Campinha-Bacote J. A model and instrument for addressing cultural competence in health care. J Nurs Educ 1999; 38: 203–207.
29. DeSpelder L. Developing cultural competence. In: Doka K, Davidson J, eds. Living with Grief. Washington, D.C.: Hospice Foundation of America, 1998.
30. Oncology Nursing Society, Multicultural Outcomes: Guidelines/or Cultural Competencies, Pittsburgh: Oncology Nursing Press, Inc., 1999.
31. Mazanec P, Kitzes J. Cultural competence in hospice and palliative care. In: Forman W, Kitzes J, Anderson R, Sheehan D, eds. Hospice and Palliative Care: Concepts and Practice. Boston: Jones & Bartlett, 2003:177–194.
32. Showalter S. Looking through different eyes: beyond cultural diversity. In: Living with Grief, Doka K, Davidson J, eds. Washington, DC: Hospice Foundation of American, 1998.
33. Ersek M, Kagawa-Singer M, Barnes D, Blackhall L, Koenig B. Multicultural considerations in the use of advance directives. Oncol Nurs Forum 1998;25:1683–1701.
34. Scanlon C. Ethical concerns in end-of-life care. AJN 2003; 103:48–55.
35. Pub L. No. 101–508: Omnibus Budget Reconciliation Act of 1990, Stat 4206, 751.
36. Pacquiao D. Addressing cultural incongruities of advance directives. Bioethics Forum 2001;17:27–31.
37. Hern H, Koenig B, Moore L, Marshall P. The differences culture can make in end-of-life decision-making. Camb Q Healthc Ethics 1998;7:27–40.
38. Kemp C, Chang BJ. Culture and the end of life: Chinese. J Hospice Palliat Nurs 2002;4:173–179.
39. Gostin L. Informed consent, cultural sensitivity, and respect for persons. JAMA 1995;274:844–845.
40. Klessig J. The effects of values and culture on life-support decisions. West J Med 1992;157:316–322.
41. McCaffrey M. Nursing Practice Theories Related to Cognition, Bodily Pain, and Man–Environment Interactions. Los Angeles: UCLA Student Store, 1968.
42. Bates MS, Edwards WT, Anderson KO. Ethnocultural influences on variation in chronic pain perception. Pain 1993;52:101–112.
43. Zborowski M. People in Pain. San Francisco: Jossey-Bass, 1969.
44. McCaffery M, Pasero C. Pain: Clinical Manual, 2nd ed. St. Louis: Mosby, 1999.
45. Pitorak E, Montana B. Pain assessment and management. In: Matzo M, Sherman D, eds. Gerontologic Palliative Care Nursing. Mosby, 2004.
46. Bernabei R, Gambassi G, Lapane K, et al. Management of pain in elderly patients with cancer. JAMA 1998;279:1877–1882.
47. Cleeland C. Undertreatment of cancer pain in elderly patients. JAMA 1998;279:1914–1915.
48. Miaskowski C. Women and pain. Crit Care Nurs Clin North Am 1997;9:453–458.
49. Robin O, Vinard H, Varnet-Maury E, Saumet J. Influence of sex and anxiety on pain threshold and tolerance. Funct Neurol 1987;2:173–179.
50. Vallerand A. Gender differences in pain. IMAGE: J Nurs Scholarsh 1995;27:235–237.
51. Lasch K. Culture, pain, and culturally sensitive pain care. Pain Manage Nurs 2000;1(Suppl 3):16–22.
52. Spector R. Cultural Care: Guides to Heritage Assessment and Health Traditions, 5th ed. Upper Saddle River, NJ: Pearson Education, 2000:9.

35 Elderly Patients

Susan Derby and Sean O'Mahony

Being elderly and sick is very frightening . . . your children have moved far away and many of your friends have died. Making decisions without support is scary and lonely.—An elderly woman, dying of cancer

- ***Key Points***
- *The majority of people who suffer from chronic disease are elderly.*
- *The trajectory of illness for the elderly is usually one of progressive loss of independence, with the development of multiple comorbid problems and symptoms.*
- *The last years of a frail elderly person's life are often spent at home in the care of family, with approximately 50% to 60% of the elderly dying in a hospital or long-term care facility.*
- *Evidence suggests that the end of life for many elderly is characterized by poor symptom control, inadequate advanced care planning, and increased burden on caregivers.*
- *Clinicians caring for the elderly often lack skills in providing palliative and end-of-life care.*

Aging is a normal process of life, not a disease, and infirmity and frailty do not always have to accompany being old. It is expected that most of us will live well into our 70s or 80s, and the aging of the population is projected to continue well into the 21st century. Projected growth for the elderly population is staggering. During the next 20 years, the fastest-growing segment of the population will be in the group aged 85 years and older. During the past decades, this increase in life expectancy has been mainly due to improvements in sanitation and infectious-disease control through vaccinations and antibiotics. Presently, the older population is growing older because of positive trends in the treatment of chronic diseases—cardiovascular and neurological, as well as cancer. This "swelling" of the older segment of the population reinforces the need for nurses, physicians, and all health care professionals to understand the special palliative care needs of the elderly. In our society, the majority of people who have chronic disease are elderly. One of the major differences from younger groups in treating illness in the elderly population is the need for extensive family support and care during the last weeks and months of life.

Comorbidity and Disability

The elderly have many comorbid medical conditions that contribute an added symptom burden to this palliative care population. The presence of existing comorbidities and disabilities renders them more susceptible to the complications of new illnesses and their treatments. The presence of chronic medical conditions is associated with disability and increased health care use, including institutionalization and hospitalization in the elderly (Table 35–1). Forty percent of community-dwelling adults older than 65 report impairment in their daily activities secondary to chronic medical conditions.[1] Sixteen percent of adults older than 65 report impairment in walking, increasing

Table 35–1
Age-Specific Prevalence of Chronic Medical Conditions in Noninstitutionalized U.S. Adults (per 1000)

	18–44 Years	45–64 Years	65–74 Years	>75 Years
Arthritis	52.1	268.5	459.3	494.7
Hypertension	64.1	258.9	426.8	394.6
Heart disease	40.1	129.0	276.8	349.1
Hearing impairment	49.8	159.0	261.9	346.9
Deformity/orthopedic impairment	125.3	160.6	167.9	175.5
Chronic sinusitis	164.4	184.8	151.2	160.0
Visual impairment	32.8	43.7	76.4	128.8
Diabetes	9.1	51.9	108.9	95.5
Cerebrovascular disease	1.9	17.9	54.0	72.6
Emphysema	1.6	15.2	50.0	38.9

Source: Seeman et al. (1989), reference 153.

to more than 32% in those older than 85. Comorbidity is highly prevalent in people over 65 years. In the United States, 49% of noninstitutionalized people over 60 have two or more chronic conditions. Much higher percentages are seen in adults older than 65 who are living in a nursing home or who are hospitalized.[1–11]

Sites of Residence and Place of Death

Sixty-six percent of older noninstitutionalized persons live in a family setting; this decreases with increasing age. Three out of every five women older than 85 live outside of a family arrangement. Rates of institutionalization are estimated to be 4% to 5% in the United States; this increases to 23% in the over-85 population. The wide range of care settings for the elderly is reflected in the sites of death of the elderly.[8,12–15]

Over the past 100 years, the site of death has shifted from the home to institutions. Data from the National Institute on Aging's *Survey of the Last Days of Life* (SLDOL) indicate that 45% of the elderly who died spent the night prior to death in a hospital and 24% in a nursing home, and 30% died at home.[15a] There was a significant drop in the proportion of patients in the older age group for both men and women who died in hospitals and an increase in proportions dying at home or nursing homes. Almost one third of older women died in nursing homes. Interestingly, the National Mortality Follow-Back Survey reported that only 8.7% of decedents were receiving home hospice, and less than 0.5% were receiving inpatient hospice care.[8–9]

In several studies, cancer and dementia are predictive of death at home rather than in institutions. Death in hospice appears to correlate with the local availability of hospice beds, as well as a diagnosis of cancer. For patients with a preference for death at home, the availability of home visits by physicians correlates with a higher rate of death at home. In patients expressing an initial wish to die at home, caregiver burnout and unrelieved symptoms are predictive of death in hospitals and hospice.[12–15] The available data suggest that with limited increase in the allocation of nursing support, dying patients' wishes to die at home can be met. Elderly women are more than twice as likely to be living alone than are elderly men. More than half of women 75 and older live alone.[12–15] Those living alone rely more heavily on the presence of social supports and assistance for the provision of health care.[12–15]

Palliative Care in Nursing Homes

End-of-life care in long-term care settings is described in greater detail in Chapter 40. It is estimated that of those who turned 65 years old in 1990, 43% will enter a nursing home before they die.[16] Because the fastest-growing segment of the population is those over 85 years, it is likely that these individuals will require long-term care in these settings. Pain management and end-of-life care in nursing homes represent management of the frailest individuals, often with minimal physician involvement. As many as 45% to 80% of nursing home residents have pain that contributes significantly to impaired quality of life.[17] Most mild pain in nursing homes is related to degenerative arthritis, low-back disorders, and diabetic and postherpetic neuropathy. Cancer pain accounts for the majority of severe pain.[18]

Barriers to palliative care in the nursing home include institutional, patient, and staff-related barriers (Table 35–2). Data from nursing homes suggest that as many as 30% to 80% of nursing home residents receive inadequate pain management.[19–25]

Table 35–2
Barriers to Palliative Care in Nursing Homes

Institution-Related
Low priority given to palliative care management by administration
Limited physician involvement in care, weekly or monthly assessments
Limited pharmacy involvement, no on-site pharmacy
Limited R.N. involvement in care; inadequate nurse–patient staff ratios
Primary care being administered by nonprofessional nursing staff
Limited radiological and diagnostic services, which impair determination of a pain diagnosis
Patient-Related
Physiological changes of aging, which affect distribution, metabolism, and elimination of medications
Multiple chronic diseases
Polypharmacy
Impaired cognitive status and Alzheimer's-type dementia
Underreporting of pain due to fear of addiction, lack of knowledge, fear of being transferred
Sensory losses that impede assessment
Increased incidence of depression, which may mask reporting and assessment of pain
Staff-Related
Lack of knowledge of symptom management at the end of life
Lack of knowledge in the assessment and management of chronic cancer pain
Lack of knowledge in use of opioid drugs, titration, and side-effect management
Fear of using opioids in elderly residents
Misconceptions about use of opioids in elderly patients (e.g., fear of addiction, "elderly feel less pain")
Lack of knowledge in use of nonpharmacological techniques
Lack of experience with other routes of administration including patient-controlled analgesia, transdermal, rectal, subcutaneous, and intravenous routes

Source: Adapted from Stein (1996), reference 154.

In one study comparing analgesic management of dying patients in a nursing home enrolled and not enrolled in Medicare Hospice program, 15% percent of hospice residents and 23% of nonhospice residents in daily pain received no analgesics; 51% of hospice residents and 33% of nonhospice residents received regular treatment for pain. These findings suggest that for nursing home residents in pain, analgesic management is better for hospice patients, but for many residents, pain management is sporadic and often inconsistent with American Medical Directors Association Guidelines.[26]

Many other obstacles to palliative care have been identified, including lack of communication among decision-makers, lack of agreement on a course for end-of-life care, failure to implement a timely end-of-life care plan, and failure to recognize treatment futility.[27] Only about half of nursing home residents have do-not-resuscitate (DNR) orders, fewer than one in five have advance directives, and fewer (14%) have living wills and do-not-hospitalize directives (4%).[28–30] One of the most troublesome concerns expressed by staff who care for nursing home residents is the difficulty in assessing pain in the cognitively impaired elderly resident.

Approximately 90% of the 4 million Americans with dementia will be institutionalized before death.[31] One of the barriers to end-of-life care in this population is that advanced dementia is often not viewed as a terminal condition. Because of this, palliative care often is not initiated until the final stages of life. In one retrospective study using the data from the Minimum Data Set,[32–33] 1784 residents with advanced dementia and 918 residents with terminal cancer were compared. Residents with advanced dementia were older, lived longer, and had higher activity of living scores than the terminal cancer residents. Six months after admission to the nursing home, only 20% of the residents with advanced dementia were perceived as having a life expectancy of less than 6 months. At the last assessment before death, only 4.1% were recognized as having a prognosis under 6 months; 55% had a DNR order, compared with 86.1% of the cancer patients.[34] With respect to nonpalliative interventions, residents dying with advanced dementia experienced more frequent uncomfortable or aggressive interventions at the end of life; 25% died with a feeding tube, 11% with restraints, and 10.1% with intravenous (IV) therapy. These findings suggest that palliative care for nursing home residents with advanced dementia is suboptimal, and encourages use of educational strategies to promote palliative care to these patients.

Economic Considerations in Caring for the Elderly

The higher rates of disability and comorbidity in the elderly, requiring the provision of long-term residential care as well as home care, result in considerable costs to the health care.

Health Care Financing Administration data indicate that 6% to 8% of Medicare enrollees die annually and account for 27% to 30% of annual Medicare expenses.[35] However, spending on aggressive interventions is not a major component of the hospital costs incurred in the dying elderly. Only 3% of Medicare beneficiaries who die sustain high costs associated with aggressive interventions such as surgery, chemotherapy, or dialysis.

While hospital costs in the last days of life are lower for the oldest old, the percentage of Medicare and Medicaid expenditure for nursing home care rises from 24% for the young-old

(65 to 74 years), to 62% for the oldest old (over 85 years).[36–38] Most required residential care occurs in the last days of life.

Determination of Prognosis and the Provision of Palliative Care

Providing palliative care to elderly patients is limited by the uncertain prognoses of many chronic illnesses in this population (congestive heart failure, chronic obstructive pulmonary disease [COPD], cerebrovascular disease, dementia). Because of the difficulty to accurately prognosticate and many other factors, most patients who have fatal illnesses do not use the Medicare hospice benefit until shortly before death.[38] Even the most complex prognostic scoring systems, such as the APACHE (Acute Physiology Age Chronic Health Evaluation), provide little information for the likelihood of an individual patient's death.[39]

The uncertain prognoses of chronic nonmalignant medical conditions can affect clinical decision-making. It may also lead to overuse of health care resources in acute care settings, even when death is imminent. An analysis of Medicare claim data for 6451 elderly hospice patients demonstrated that median survival after enrollment was only 36 days, with 15.6% dying within 7 days.[40–42]

Advance Directives and Decision-Making

Advance directives are especially important in elderly patients who are at high risk of morbidity and mortality. The presence, stability, and willingness to discuss advance care planning appears to be dependent upon several factors, including communication issues, value differences, cultural issues, ethnicity, and mental capacity.[43,44] In one study of advance care planning among nursing home residents, two variables were associated with the reduced likelihood of having DNR and do-not-hospitalize orders or restricting feeding, medication or other treatment: African-American ethnicity and less time in the facility.[44]

Many references in the literature support the notion that a patient's prior decision regarding treatment choices accurately reflects future choices,[45–48] however, not all studies support that. One prospective longitudinal study of 65 nursing home residents assessed stability of residents' preferences for life-sustaining interventions and evaluated factors that potentially affect these decisions.[49] Resident preferences changed over a 2-year period. Overall, a majority of participants consistently desired cardiopulmonary resuscitation, whereas somewhat fewer than half desired medical hydration and nutrition. As time progressed, a greater proportion of individuals favored medical hydration and nutrition. Because this study was of institutionalized residents who routinely witness the administration of hydration and nutrition to fellow residents, the authors concluded that such interventions become commonplace and are easily accepted by other residents. This practice, they believe, has an influence on the resident's decision to accept hydration.

Family/Caregiver Issues

Who Are the Caregivers for the Elderly?

The term *caregiver* refers to anyone who provides assistance to someone else who needs it. "Informal caregiver" is a term used to refer to unpaid individuals, such as family members and friends, who provide care. These persons can be primary or secondary caregivers, full or part time, and can live with the person being cared for or live separately. "Formal caregivers" are volunteers or paid care providers associated with a service system. Estimates vary on the numbers of caregivers in the United States.

According to the most recent *National Long Term Care Study* (NLTCS), more than 7 million people are informal caregivers, defined here as spouses, adult children, other relatives, and friends who provide unpaid help to older people with at least one limitation in their activities of daily living. An estimated 15% of American adults are providing care for seriously ill or disabled adults.[50] Of these, an estimated 12.8 million Americans need assistance to carry out activities such as eating, dressing, and bathing. About 57% are aged 65 or older (7.3 million). Spouses accounted for about 62% of primary caregivers. Approximately 72% of caregivers are female.[51] The majority of caregivers provide unpaid assistance for 1 to 4 years, 20% provide care for 5 years or longer.[51]

According to the 2000 *National Hospice Care Survey* (NHCS), 42% of patients enrolled in hospice programs were women and 33% were men. The majority (81%) were 65 years or older, and a significantly larger proportion of women than men were 85 years of age or older. Men were more likely to have a spouse as their primary caregiver, while women were more likely to be cared for by a child or child-in-law. The most common diagnosis for most of the hospice care patients included neoplasm, heart disease, and COPD.[52]

Involving Family in Caregiving for the Elderly: What Is the Burden?

The burden of caregiving has been well documented in the literature and includes a greater number of depressive symptoms, anxiety, diminished physical health, financial problems, and disruption in work. The amount of concrete needs the patient has strongly relates to family and caregiver psychological distress and burden of care.[53] Elderly patients who are dying require varying levels of assistance with personal care, meal preparation, shopping, transportation, paying bills, and submitting forms related to health care. The level of physical care may be tremendous and include bathing, turning and positioning, wound care, colostomy care, suctioning, medication administration, and managing incontinence. If the patient is confused or agitated, the strain is even greater, as 24-hour care may be necessary. In the palliative care setting, where the treatment goals are supportive and often include management of symptoms such as pain, respiratory distress, and delirium, the patient is frequently confined to home, with a greater burden placed on the live-in spouse or child.

In one study comparing the impact of caregiving in curative and palliative care settings, two study groups were evaluated—267 patients received active, curative treatment, and 134 patients received palliative care through a local hospice. Patients in the palliative care group were more physically debilitated and had poorer performance status. The mean age was 59.7 for the curative group and 57.9 for the palliative care group. Caregiver quality-of-life measures demonstrated that family caregivers of patients receiving palliative care had lower quality-of-life scores and worse overall physical health than family caregivers of patients receiving curative care.[54] Families with low socioeconomic status and those with less education were more distressed by the patient's illness.

Transitions in spousal caregiving have been investigated in respect to the level/intensity of caregiving and its impact on the overall health of the caregiver. In 428 subjects who were assessed at four intervals over a 5-year period, those who transitioned to heavy caregiving had more depressive symptoms than those who transitioned into moderate caregiving. Heavy caregivers scored higher in the number of health-risk behaviors between the second and third observations, concluding that these outcomes become worse over time.[55]

Family caregivers of people with dementia face particularly stressful demands because of the exhaustive phase of prolonged dependence. In one study, two goals of the caregiving to patients with dementia experience were looked at: the description of the caregiving experience, and the short- and long-term responses to bereavement. Two hundred sixty five in-home caregivers were assessed at 6-, 12-, and 18-month intervals. The mean length of caregiving was 3 years. More than one half of the caregivers reported that they felt they were on duty 24 hours a day, 48% had to reduce their work load, and 18% had to stop work entirely.

In another study of 231 caregivers of cancer patients who were at home, the goals were to evaluate family caregiver's quality of life, financial burden, and experience of managing cancer pain in the home.[57] Family caregivers scored worse in areas of coping difficulty, anxiety, depression, happiness, and feeling in control. In areas of physical well-being, the greatest problems were sleep changes and fatigue. Other quality-of-life disruptions included interference with employment, lack of support from others, isolation, and financial burden. The estimated average time spent caregiving was more than 12 hours per day; the estimated time for pain management was more than 3 hours per day. Family caregivers reported worse outcomes than patients did in their perception of the pain intensity, pain distress to themselves, feeling able to control the pain, and family concern about pain in the future. Caregivers reported fear of future pain, fear of tolerance, and concern about addiction and harmful effects of analgesics. The authors concluded that educational programs in pain management are needed and that further educational efforts should also address the emotional aspects of managing cancer pain in the home. Interventions directed toward improving the quality of life of direct caregivers include educational programs, improvement in home care supports, psychoeducational programs, and improved access to health care professionals who provide symptom management and end-of-life care.

Family grief therapy during the palliative phase of illness has also improved the psychosocial quality of life of caregivers. Kissane and colleagues[58] used a screening tool to identify dysfunctional family members and relieve distress through a model of family grief therapy sessions. Smeenk and colleagues[59] demonstrated improved quality of life of direct caregivers after implementation of a transmural home care intervention program for terminal cancer patients. Macdonald[60] demonstrated that massage as a respite intervention for caregivers was successful in reducing physical and emotional stress, physical pain, and sleep difficulties. This nonpharmacological and noninvasive intervention is highly valued and accepted by caregivers because of its simplicity and beneficial effects.

Pharmacological Considerations

Pharmacological intervention is the mainstay of treatment for symptom management in palliative care of the elderly patient. Knowledge of the parameters of geriatric pharmacology can prevent serious morbidity and mortality when multiple drugs are used to treat single or multiple symptoms, or when, in the practice of chronic pain management, trials of sequential opioids (opioid rotation, or opioid switch) are used.

Pharmacokinetics

The four components of pharmacokinetics are absorption, distribution, metabolism, and excretion. In the absence of malabsorption problems and obstruction, oral medications are well tolerated in the elderly population. With aging, there is some decrease in gastric secretion, absorptive surface area, and splanchnic blood flow. Most studies show no difference in oral bioavailability—the extent to which a drug reaches its site of action. There is little literature on the absorption of long-acting drugs in the elderly, including controlled or sustained-release opioids, and transdermal opioids commonly used in the treatment of chronic cancer pain in the elderly patient. Controlled-release dosage forms are generally more appropriate with drugs that have short half-lives (less than 4 hours) and include many of the shorter-acting opioids, including morphine and hydromorphone. Generally, it is safer to use opioids that have shorter half-lives in the elderly cancer patient.

Distribution refers to the distribution of drug to the interstitial and cellular fluids after it is absorbed or injected into the bloodstream. There are several significant physiological factors that may influence drug distribution in the elderly palliative care patient. An initial phase of distribution reflects cardiac output and regional blood flow. The heart, kidneys, liver, and brain receive most of the drug after absorption. Delivery to fat, muscle, most viscera, and skin is slower; it may take several hours before steady-state concentrations are reached. Although cardiac output does not change with age, chronic conditions, including congestive heart failure, may contribute to a decrease in cardiac output and regional blood flow.

This second phase of drug distribution to the tissues is highly dependent upon body mass. Body weight generally decreases with age, but more importantly, body composition changes with age. Total body water and lean body mass decrease, while body fat increases in proportion to total body weight. The volume-of-distribution changes are mostly for highly lipophilic and hydrophilic drugs, and the elderly are most susceptible to drug toxicity from drugs that should be dosed on ideal body weight or lean body weight. Theoretically, highly lipid-bound drugs, for example, long-acting benzodiazepines and transdermal fentanyl, both commonly prescribed to elderly patients, may have an increased volume of distribution and a prolonged effect if drug clearance is constant.[61] Water-soluble drugs (e.g., digoxin) may have a decreased volume of distribution and increased serum levels and toxicity if initial doses are not conservative. To avoid possible side effects in a frail elderly patient, it may be safe to start with one half the dose usually prescribed for a younger patient.

Another host factor that influences drug distribution is plasma protein concentrations.[62,63] Most drugs, including analgesics, are extensively bound to plasma proteins. The proportion of albumin among total plasma proteins decreases with frailty, catabolic states, and immobility, commonly seen in many elderly patients with chronic conditions. A decrease in serum albumin can increase the percentage of free (unbound) drug available for pharmacological effect and elimination. In this setting, standard doses of medications lead to higher levels of free (unbound) drug and possible toxicity.

The liver is the major site of drug metabolism. Hepatic metabolism of drugs is dependent on drug-metabolizing enzymes in the liver. The hepatic microenzymes are responsible for this biotransformation. With advanced age, there is a decrease in liver weight by 20% to 50% and liver volume decreases by approximately 25%.[64] In addition, a nondrug marker for hepatic functional mass, galactose clearance, is decreased by 25% in advanced age. Associated with these changes in liver size and weight is a decrease in hepatic blood flow, normalized by liver volume. This corresponds to a decrease in liver perfusion of 10% to 15%. Drugs absorbed from the intestine may be subject to metabolism and the first-pass effect in the liver, accounting for decreased amounts of drug in the circulation after oral administration. The end result is decreased systemic bioavailability and plasma concentrations.[64]

The process of biotransformation in the liver is largely dependent upon the P-450 cytochrome. During biotransformation, the parent drug is converted to a more polar metabolite by oxidation, reduction, or hydrolysis. The resulting metabolite may be more active than the parent drug. The cytochrome P-450 has been shown to decline in efficiency with age. These altered mechanisms of drug metabolism should be considered when treating the elderly palliative care patient with opioids, long-acting benzodiazepines, and neuroleptics.

The effect of age on renal function is quite variable. Some studies show a linear decrease in renal function, amounting to decreased glomerular function; other studies indicate no change in creatinine clearance with advancing age.[64] Renal mass decreases 25% to 30% in advanced age, and renal blood flow decreases 1% per year after age 50.[64] There are also decreases in tubular function and reduced ability to concentrate and dilute the urine. In general, the clearance of drugs that are secreted or filtered by the kidney is decreased in a predictable manner.

For example, delayed renal excretion of meperidine's metabolite, normeperidine, may result in delirium, central nervous system (CNS) stimulation, myoclonus, and seizures. Meperidine is not recommended for chronic administration in any patient but is of special concern for elderly patients with borderline renal function. Other drugs that rely on renal excretion include nonsteroidal antiinflammatory agents, digoxin, aminoglycoside antibiotics, and contrast media.

Table 35–3
Risk Factors for Medication Problems in the Elderly Palliative Care Patient

1. Multiple health care prescribers (e.g., multiple physicians, nurse practitioners)
2. Multiple medications
3. Automatic refills
4. Age-related physiological pharmacokinetic changes
5. Age-related pharmacodynamic changes
6. Sensory losses: visual, hearing
7. Cognitive defects: delirium, dementia
8. Depression
9. Anxiety
10. Knowledge deficits related to indication, action, dosing schedule, and side effects of prescribed medication
11. Complex dosing schedule or route of administration
12. Comorbid medical conditions: frailty, cerebrovascular disease, cardiac disease, musculoskeletal disorders, advanced cancer
13. Self-medication with over-the-counter medications, herbal remedies
14. Lack of social support or lives alone
15. Alcoholism
16. Financial concerns
17. Illiteracy
18. Misconceptions about specific medications (e.g. addiction)
19. Language barrier

Source: Adapted from Walker et al. (1996), reference 155.

Table 35–4
Medication Assessment in the Elderly Palliative Care Patient

1. Identify prior problems with medications.
2. Identify other health care providers who prescribe medications.
3. Obtain a detailed history of present medication use at all patient contacts. Include over-the-counter and herbal remedies and dosage, frequency, expected effect, and side effects. When assessing efficacy of pain management, ask about PRN "rescue" doses.
4. Identify "high-risk" medications and assess for side effects or drug–drug interactions.
5. Evaluate the need for drug therapy by performing a comprehensive physical examination and symptom assessment, and obtain appropriate laboratory data.
6. Assess functional, cognitive, sensory, affective, and nutritional status.
7. Review patient's and family member's level of understanding about indications, dosing, and side effects.
8. Identify any concerns about medications (cost, fears, misconceptions).
9. Identify presence of caregiver or support person and include in all assessments.
10. Implement strategies to increase support if lacking (e.g., skilled or nonskilled home care nursing support, community groups, other family members, community-based day programs).

Source: Adapted from Walker et al. (1996), reference 155.

Medication Use in the Elderly: Problems with Polypharmacy

Older individuals use three times more medications than younger people do. They account for approximately 25% of physician visits and approximately 35% of drug expenditures. Elderly patients are more likely to be prescribed inappropriate medications than younger patients are.[65] Advancing age alone does not explain the risk of adverse drug reactions, and polypharmacy is a consistent predictor. As noted earlier, in the palliative care setting, elderly patients often have more than one comorbid medical condition, necessitating treatment with many medications, which places them at greater risk of adverse drug reactions. In addition, new medications not only place the elderly at risk of adverse drug reactions, they also increase the risk of significant drug interactions. For example, the addition of an antacid to an elderly patient already on corticosteroids for bone pain may significantly decrease the oral corticosteroid effect due to decreased absorption.

Understanding pharmacodynamics in relationship to age-related physiological changes can assist the clinician in evaluating the effectiveness and side-effect profile in the elderly palliative care patient (Table 35–3). When multiple drugs are used to treat symptoms, the side-effect profile may increase, potentially limiting the use of one or more drugs. For example, when using an opioid and a benzodiazepine in treating chronic pain and anxiety in the elderly patient, excessive sedation may occur, limiting the amount of opioid that can be administered. Table 35–4 outlines the components of a comprehensive medication assessment in the elderly palliative care patient.

Symptom Management During the Last Weeks of Life: Special Concerns

Numerous studies have evaluated symptoms during the last weeks of life and indicate that patients experience a high degree of symptom distress and suffering. In one study by Seale and Cartwright,[66] there were age-related difference in the incidence of mental confusion, loss of bladder and bowel control, as well as seeing/hearing difficulties. There was no age-related difference in patients reporting pain (72%), trouble breathing (49%), loss of appetite (47%), drowsiness (44%), and other symptoms, including sleeplessness, constipation, depression, vomiting, and dry mouth.

Studies have documented the most prevalent and difficult-to-manage symptoms in dying patients, including pain, dyspnea, and confusional states.[67–69] In one evaluation of the symptom burden of seriously ill hospitalized patients in five tertiary care facilities, pain, dyspnea, anxiety, and depression caused the greatest symptom burden.[70] In this study, patients for whom hospital interviews were not available had more dependencies in daily living and more comorbidities, were older, sicker, poorer, and more often had respiratory failure and multiorgan system failure.

The complex symptomatology experienced by elderly patients, especially those with cancer and multiple comorbidities, demands that an aggressive approach to symptom assessment and intervention be used. Devising a palliative plan of care for the elderly patient who is highly symptomatic or who is actively dying requires ongoing communication with the patient and family; assessment of patient and family understanding of goals of care and religious, cultural and spiritual beliefs; access to community agencies; psychological assessment; and patient and family preferences regarding advance directives. Dimensions of a palliative care plan for the elderly are outlined in Table 35–5. The management of three prevalent and distressing symptoms experienced by the elderly at the end of life—dyspnea, pain, and delirium—is discussed below. Each of these symptoms is discussed in greater detail in other chapters.

Dyspnea

Dyspnea may be one of the most frightening and difficult symptoms an elderly patient can experience. A subjective feeling of breathlessness or the sensation of labored or difficult

Table 35–5
Dimensions of a Palliative Plan of Care for the Elderly Patient

1. Assess extent of disease documented by imaging studies and laboratory data.
2. Assess symptoms, including prevalence, severity, and impact on function.
3. Identify coping strategies and psychological symptoms, including presence of anxiety, depression, and suicidal tendencies.
4. Evaluate religious and spiritual beliefs.
5. Assess overall quality of life and well-being. Does the patient feel secure that all that can be done for them is being done? Is the patient satisfied with the present level of symptom control?
6. Determine family burden. Is attention being paid to the caregiver so that burnout does not occur? If the spouse or caregiver is elderly, is he or she able to meet the physical demands of caring for the patient?
7. Determine level of care needed in the home if the patient is dying.
8. Assess financial burden on patient and caregiver. Is an inordinate amount of money being spent on the patient and will there be adequate provisions for the elderly caregiver when the patient dies?
9. Identify presence of advance care planning requests. Have the patient's wishes and preferences for resuscitation, artificial feeding, and hydration been discussed? Has the patient identified a surrogate decision-maker who knows their wishes? Is there documentation regarding advance directives?

Source: Adapted from "Improving care at the end of life" (1997), reference 156.

breathing, dyspnea contributes to severe disability and impaired quality of life. Dyspnea and fear of dyspnea produce profound suffering for dying patients and their families. This section will outline the special needs for elderly patients, with a focus on physiological factors that increase the risk of dyspnea.

Physiological Correlates in the Elderly That Increase Risk of Dyspnea

The effects of aging produce a clinical picture in which respiratory problems can develop. With aging, the elastic recoil of the lungs during expiration is decreased due to less collagen and elastin. Alveoli are less elastic and develop fibrous tissue. The stooped posture and loss of skeletal muscle strength often found in the elderly contribute to reduction in the vital capacity and an increase in the residual volume of the lung. Table 35–6 outlines the pulmonary risk factors for the development of dyspnea in the elderly palliative care patient.

Respiratory muscle weakness may play a major role in some types of dyspnea. Palange and colleagues[71] found that malnutrition significantly affected exercise tolerance in patients with COPD by producing diaphragmatic fatigue. In patients with cachexia, the maximal inspiratory pressure, an indicator of diaphragmatic strength, is severely impaired. Cachexia and asthenia occur in 80% to 90% of patients with advanced cancer, and are also prevalent in elderly patients with multiple comorbid psychiatric and medical conditions. These mechanisms may affect the development of dyspnea and fatigue in the elderly who have advanced nonmalignant and malignant disease. Ripamonti and Bruera[72] have suggested that in some patients, dyspnea may be a clinical presentation of overwhelming cachexia and asthenia.

The multiple etiologies of dyspnea in the dying elderly patient include both malignant (e.g., tumor infiltration, superior vena cava syndrome, pleural effusion), treatment-related (Adriamycin-induced cardiomyopathy, radiation-induced pneumonitis, pulmonary fibrosis), and nonmalignant causes (e.g., metabolic, structural).

Two causes of dyspnea, deep vein thrombosis (DVT) and pulmonary embolism (PE), are prevalent in the elderly and are often unrecognized and undiagnosed. They may present as pleuritic chest pain with or without dyspnea and hemoptysis. The risk factors in the elderly include increased venous stasis in the legs, impaired fibrinolysis, coagulopathies, recent surgery, immobility, and congestive heart failure. Treatment is dependent on accurate diagnosis, and an estimate of risks versus benefits should be considered in deciding on a course of action. Ventilation-perfusion scans are the most reliable indicator of whether a PE has occurred, and the identification of a DVT as the source of the PE can be accomplished through noninvasive Doppler studies of the legs. Whether it is prudent or compassionate to perform these studies in the elderly patient who is dying should be considered. In the elderly patient who is not actively dying, diagnostic tests can be safely performed. Treatment with anticoagulants in addition to supportive symptom management will reduce the symptom burden and suffering.

Treatment of Dyspnea

When possible, relief of dyspnea is aimed at treatment of the underlying disease process, whether malignant or nonmalignant in origin. Symptomatic interventions are used when the process is not reversible. Both pharmacological and nonpharmacological interventions should be employed. One patient may present with multiple etiologies; therefore, multiple interventions are indicated.

Therapeutic interventions are based on the etiology and include pharmacological (e.g., bronchodilators, steroids, diuretics, vasodilators, opioids, sedatives, antibiotics), procedural (e.g., thoracentesis, chest tube placement), nonpharmacological (e.g., relaxation, breathing exercises, music), radiation therapy, and oxygen. At the end of life, the pharmacological use of benzodiazepines, opioids, and corticosteroids

Table 35–6
Risk Factors for Dyspnea in the Elderly Palliative Care Patient

Risk Factor	Comment
Structural Factors	
Increased chest wall stiffness	Increase in the work of breathing
Decrease in skeletal muscle, barrel chest, increase in anteroposterior diameter	Decrease in maximum volume expiration
Decrease in elasticity of alveoli	Decrease in vital capacity
Other Factors	
Anemia	
Cachexia	
Dehydration	Drier mucous membranes, increase in mucous plugs
Ascites	
Atypical presentation of fever	Reduced febrile response, decreased WBC response
Heart failure	
Immobility	Increased risk of aspiration, DVT, PE
Obesity	
Recent abdominal, pelvic, or chest surgery	Increased risk of DVT, PE
Lung disease (COPD, lung cancer)	

Sources: Adapted from Eliopoulos (1996), reference 157, and Palange et al. (1995), reference 71.
COPD, chronic obstructive pulmonary disease; DVT, deep venous thrombosis; PE, pulmonary embolism; WBC, white blood cell.

remain the primary treatment. Many palliative care professionals advocate the use of morphine to control dyspnea at the end of life.[72–76] Often there is reluctance among staff to use opioids and sedatives in the elderly due to unfamiliarity with these medications, lack of experience in treating dyspnea in dying patients, low priority given to this symptom, or fear that these drugs may hasten death in the elderly. Table 35–7 outlines management guidelines based on presenting symptoms. Figure 35–1 reviews the overall assessment and management of dyspnea in the geriatric patient at the end of life.

CASE STUDY

An 80-Year-Old Woman with Metastatic Lung Cancer

An 80-year-old woman with metastatic lung cancer to bone, mediastinum, and lung has persistent dyspnea related to lymphangitic spread of disease. She has received radiation therapy to the mediastinum, and she completed a course of chemotherapy 2 months ago. She is still at home receiving morphine sulfate 30 mg orally every 4 hours, which has been very effective for bone pain. She tried long-acting morphine but did not like the way it made her feel. She is also receiving prednisone 30 mg orally 2 times daily for bronchospasm, and an albuterol inhaler, which she occasionally uses. Physical examination reveals breath sounds decreased bilaterally, occasional rhonchi, but no rales or crackles present. She has no distended neck veins, gallop, or peripheral edema. Her respiratory rate is 24 per minute at rest, and she complains of feeling breathless and anxious. She is also very fatigued and cannot sleep at night. She refuses to go to the hospital and says she wants to die in her own bed at home. She also is refusing further aggressive intervention and has signed a home DNR order.

Suggestions for Assessment and Intervention

What further symptom management can be offered to this patient?

1. Determine the etiology of the dyspnea in this patient. In the terminally ill patient, dyspnea is often due to multiple causes. A thorough history and physical examination should be performed and will assist in determining specific interventions. In this patient, the probable cause of the dyspnea is lymphangitic spread of the malignancy.
2. Excessive fatigue is present in this patient, and a complete blood count will determine if anemia is contributing to fatigue and dyspnea. Consider a trial

Table 35–7
BREATHES Program for Management of Dyspnea in the Elderly Palliative Care Patient

B-bronchospasm. Consider nebulized albuterol and/or steroids.

R-rales/crackles. If present, reduce fluid intake. If patient is receiving IV hydration, reduce fluid intake or discontinue. Consider gentle diuresis with Lasix 20–40 mg PO daily, ± spironolactone (Aldactone) 100 mg PO daily.

E-effusion. Determine on physical examination or chest x-ray. Consider thoracentesis or chest tube, if appropriate.

A-airway obstruction. If patient is at risk or has had aspiration from food, puree solid food, avoid thin liquids, and keep the patient upright during and after meals for at least 1 hour.

T-tachypnea and breathlessness. Opioids reduce respiratory rate and feelings of breathlessness as well as anxiety. Assess daily. If patient is opioid naïve, begin with morphine sulfate 5–10 mg PO q4h and titrate opioids 25%–50% daily/every other day as needed. Consider an anxiolytic such as lorazepam (be aware of potential for paradoxical response) 0.5–2 mg PO b.i.d.–t.i.d. Use of a fan may reduce feelings of breathlessness.

H-hemoglobin low. Consider a blood transfusion if anemia is contributing to dyspnea.

E-educate and support the patient and family during this highly stressful period.

S-secretions. If secretions are copious, consider a trial of a scopalamine patch q72h, atropine 0.3–0.5 mg SC q4h PRN, glycopyrrolate (Robinul) 0.1–0.4 mg IM/SQ q4–12h PRN

Sources: Adapted from Storey and Knight (1996), reference 158, Ripamonti (1999), reference 159; Tobin (1990), reference 160; Kuebler (1996), reference 161.

of a low-dose stimulant such as Ritalin 2.5–5 mg orally daily in the morning. This may decrease fatigue and give her more energy during the day.

3. Infection can be ruled out with a complete blood count. If pneumonia is suspected, try to arrange for a chest x-ray if the patient agrees or empirically initiate a trial of oral antibiotics. Although this patient has no signs of congestive heart failure on physical examination, it should be ruled out.
4. If available, use pulse oximetry to determine benefits of oxygen therapy or try nasal O_2 at 3 L/minute.
5. The patient is presently receiving morphine sulfate for pain. Increase her opioids by 25% to 50% to a dose of 40 to 45 mg orally every 4 hours to assist with tachypnea and anxiety.
6. Consider a trial with an anxiolytic such as ativan 0.5 mg orally every 8–12 hours.
7. Consider increasing the prednisone to treat the bronchospasm.
8. Encourage use of an albuterol inhaler 3 to 4 times a day for bronchospasm.
9. If oral morphine cannot be titrated to effect, consider a trial of nebulized morphine 2.5 to 5.0 mg every 4 hours, as needed, if available.
10. Consider the benefit versus burden of additional interventions that are employed. The patient has stated that no further interventions are to be used. Review the goals of care with the patient and family members.
11. Assess functional status and reduce the need for physical exertion. Provide for assistance with daily activities, positioning techniques, and frequent rest periods.
12. Address anxiety, provide support and reassurance. Determine level of support from family and friends, and spiritual and religious beliefs. Reassure patient that symptoms can be controlled.
13. Incorporate nonpharmacological interventions (e.g., progressive relaxation, guided imagery, and music therapy).

Pain

The physiological changes accompanying advanced age have been discussed in this chapter; however it is important to emphasize that the elderly are more sensitive to both the therapeutic and toxic effects of analgesics. The principles of drug selection, route of administration, and management of side effects are the same in the elderly population as for younger adults.

Acetaminophen

Acetaminophen is one of the safest analgesics for long-term use in the older population and should be used for mild to moderate pain. It is particularly useful in the management of musculoskeletal pain and is often used in combination with opioids. In older patients with normal renal and liver function, it can be

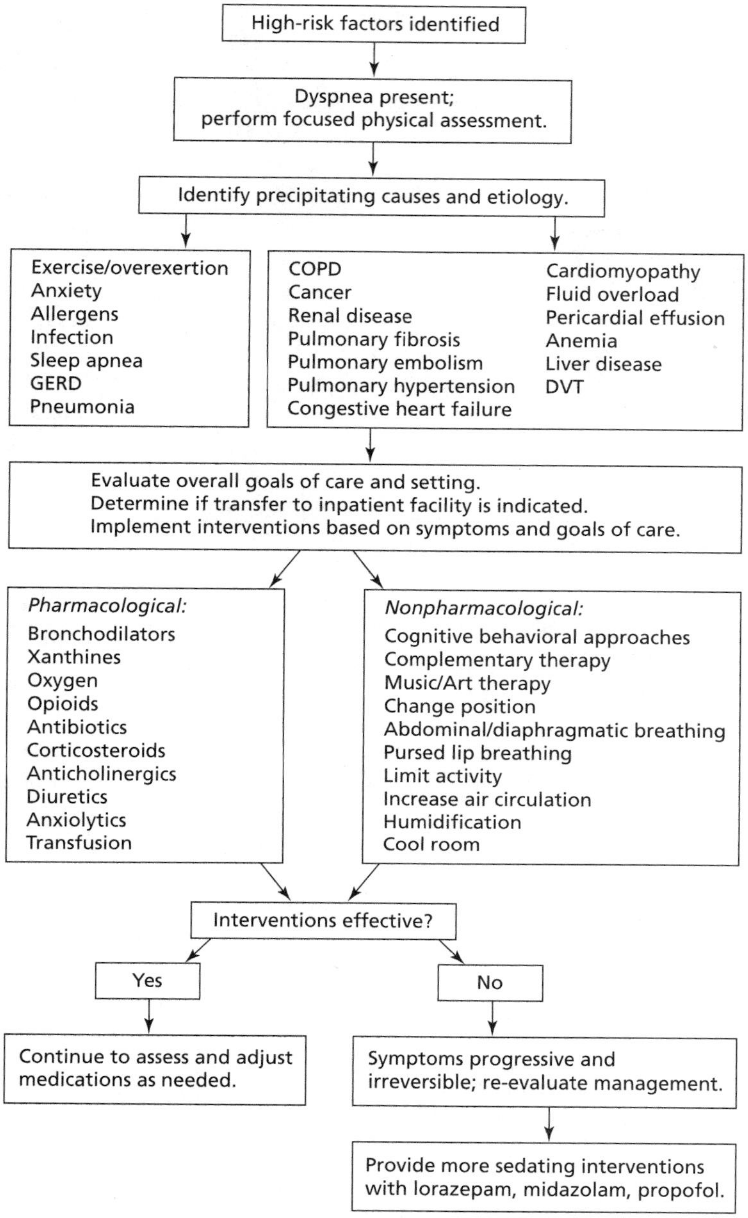

Figure 35–1. Dyspnea management in the geriatric patient at the end of life.

used safely and is highly effective for the treatment of osteoarthritis. In the setting of renal insufficiency, hepatic failure, or with patients who are drinking heavily or have a history of alcohol abuse, avoidance of acetaminophen is recommended.

Nonsteroidal Antiinflammatory Drugs

Nonsteroidal antiinflammatory drugs (NSAIDs) are useful as initial therapy for mild to moderate pain and can be used as an additive with opioids and nonopioids. In particular, NSAIDs are useful in the treatment of nociceptive pain related to bone or joint disease. When used concurrently with opioids, lower doses of opioids may be an additional benefit. NSAIDs are useful as initial therapy for mild to moderate pain and can be used as an additive with opioids and nonopioids. NSAIDs affect analgesia by reducing the biosynthesis of prostaglandins, thereby inhibiting the cascade of inflammatory events. They also have effects on pain receptors, nerve conduction, and may have central effects.[77] The long-term use of traditional NSAIDs, aspirin and ibuprofen, are associated with gastrointestinal ulceration, renal dysfunction, and impaired platelet aggregration.[78,79] The cyclooxygenase-2 (COX-2) enzymatic pathway is induced by tissue injury or by other inflammation-inducing conditions.[80] There appears to be less risk of gastrointestinal bleeding with short-term use of the COX-2 selective NSAIDs.[81] In particular,[82–85] NSAIDs are useful in the treatment of nociceptive pain related to bone or joint disease. When used concurrently with opioids, lower doses of opioids may be an additional benefit.

Elderly patients with a history of ulcer disease are most vulnerable to the side effects of these drugs, which can cause renal insufficiency and nephrotoxicity. Cognitive dysfunction has been reported with the use of salicylates, indomethacin, naproxen, and ibuprofen. Also, NSAIDs are problematic in elderly patients with congestive heart failure, peripheral edema, or ascites. In the palliative setting, consideration of the risks versus the benefits to the elderly patient should be done. If, for example, the use of NSAIDs provides effective analgesia, and the life expectancy of the patient is limited (days to weeks), it is probably prudent to initiate this therapy.

Opioids

In older patients with moderate to severe pain who have limited prior treatment with opioids, it is best to begin with a short-half-life agonist (morphine, hydromorphone, oxycodone). Shorter-half-life opioids are generally easier to titrate than longer-half-life opioids such as levorphanol or methadone, and in the elderly may have fewer side effects. Recent research has demonstrated the importance of both liver biotransformation of metabolites and renal clearance of these metabolites. Most opioids are converted to substances that may have a higher potency than the parent compound or produce more adverse effects with repeated dosing and accumulation.[86] Table 35–8 outlines the most commonly used opioids and their metabolites.

When prescribing opioids in the older population, it may be helpful to obtain baseline renal function studies. A normal serum creatinine does not indicate normal renal function; it is prudent to obtain a 24-hour creatinine clearance to accurately determine renal function.

Morphine is the most commonly prescribed opioid because of its cost and ease of administration. Morphine can be administered as an immediate-release tablet or a liquid formulation, in a controlled-release tablet administered every 8 to 12 hours (MS Contin), or every 24 hours (Avinza, Kadian). Plasma clearance of morphine decreases with age.[87]

When administering morphine for long-term use, the metabolites of morphine—morphine-3 and -6 glucuronide—may accumulate with repeated dosing, especially in the setting of impaired renal or hepatic function.[86,88,89] If, after several days of treatment with morphine, the elderly patient develops side effects that include sedation, confusion, or respiratory depression, it may mean that there is an accumulation of these metabolites, and the opioid should be changed.

Hydromorphone (Dilaudid) is available in oral tablets, liquids, and parenteral formulations and will soon be available in a long-acting preparation. The main metabolite of hydromorphone (H3G) may lead to the same toxicity as seen with morphine—myoclonus, hyperalgesia, and seizures, especially in the setting of renal failure.[90]

Oxycodone is a synthetic opioid available in a long-acting formulation (OxyContin), as well as immediate-release tablets and a liquid preparation. In the oral formulation, it is one third to one half more potent than oral morphine. The cost of OxyContin may be prohibitive to some patients on limited incomes.

Table 35–8
Common Opioids and Their Metabolites

Opioid	Metabolite	Comment
Codeine	Codeine-6 glucuronide	May cause more nausea, vomiting, and constipation than other opioids
Oxycodone	Noroxycodone, oxymorphone	
Dextropropoxyphene	Norpropoxyphene	Routine use is not advised because metabolites can accumulate with repetitive dosing.
Methadone	Metabolite inactive	Pharmacokinetics are variable. Renal excretion is pH dependent; fecal excretion accounts for the greatest part of clearance.
Hydromorphone	H3G, H_6G	Eliminated by the kidney
Fentanyl	Inactive and nontoxic metabolites	Highly lipophilic, which enables it to be absorbed through the skin Less than 10% excreted in the urine
Morphine	M3G, M6G	M6G accumulates in the blood and crosses the blood–brain barrier.
Meperidine	Normeperidine	Half as potent an analgesic as meperidine and 2–3 times more potent as a convulsant; toxicity is not reversed by naloxone; avoid chronic use because normerperidine accumulates with repeated dosing

Fentanyl is a highly lipophilic soluble opioid, which can be administered spinally, transdermally, transmucosally, and intravenously. Transdermal fentanyl (Duragesic) is especially useful when patients cannot swallow, have difficulty adhering to an oral regimen, or have side effects to other opioids. There is some suggestion that transdermal fentanyl may produce less constipation when compared with long-acting morphine. Fever, cachexia, obesity, and ascites may have a significant effect on absorption, predictability of blood levels, and clinical effects.[91,92] The fentanyl patch can be used safely in the older patient, but patients should be monitored carefully. It might be helpful when initiating therapy with the transdermal patch to begin with a short-acting opioid, oxycodone 5 mg every 4 hours, to monitor the patient over 5 to 7 days. If this dose is tolerated, conversion to a fentanyl 25-mcg patch can be safely done. If, after initiation with the fentanyl patch, side effects develop, it is important to remember that they may persist for long periods (hours or even days) after the patch is removed. The frail elderly, however, who have experienced multiple side effects from opioids, may not do well with this route of administration. If this is the case, oral transmucosal fentanyl citrate (OTFC or Actiq) may be tried; it is composed of fentanyl on an applicator that patients massage or rub against the oral mucosa. Absorption occurs rapidly, and many patients begin to have relief after 5 to 10 minutes. This formulation is especially useful in settings where rapid onset of analgesia is needed, such as with severe breakthrough pain, or during a procedure or dressing change. This formulation is only to be used in opioid-tolerant patients who are already receiving an around-the-clock opioid to manage baseline pain. Adults should start with 200 mcg, and the dose should be titrated as needed.[93]

Methadone can be safely used in the older adult, provided they are carefully monitored. The half-life of methadone can be 24 to 72 hours and allows for prolonged dosing intervals. The long half-life increases the potential for drug accumulation and side effects before the development of steady state blood levels, thus placing the patient at risk for sedation and possible respiratory depression. Because of this possibility, close monitoring of these patients should be done during the first 7 to 10 days of treatment. When using high doses or when initiating the IV route, obtaining a baseline EKG is recommended because of the possibility of QT wave abnormalities.[94] Methadone may bind as an antagonist to the NMDA receptor, which may be useful in the management of neuropathic pain.[95] From a cost perspective, it is one of the less costly opioids, making it appealing to some patients on limited incomes.

As in younger individuals, the use of meperidine for the management of chronic cancer pain is not recommended. The active metabolite of meperidine is normeperidine, which is a proconvulsant. The half-life of normeperidine is 12 to 16 hours. With repeated dosing, accumulation of normeperidine can result in CNS excitability, with possible tremors, myoclonus, and seizures. Table 35–9 outlines guidelines for opioid use in the elderly patient.

Parenteral routes of administration should be considered in elderly patients who require rapid onset of analgesia, or require high doses of opioids that cannot be administered orally. They may be administered in a variety of ways, including the IV and subcutaneous route, using a patient-controlled analgesia (PCA) device. A careful evaluation of the skin in the elderly patient should be done before initiation of subcutaneous administration. If the patient has excessive edema, a very low platelet count, or skin changes related to chronic steroid use, absorption may be impaired or subcutaneous tissue may not sustain repeated dosing, even with a permanent indwelling butterfly catheter. Infusion devices with the capability of patient-administered rescue dosing can be safely used in the elderly cancer patient. It is important to remember that severe cognitive impairment should not deter the use of IV administration, especially in the elderly patient at the end of life. Choice of analgesics and routes of administration must be based on individual assessment of each patient. Table 35–10 outlines indications for a subcutaneous or IV PCA pump.

Table 35–9
Opioid Use in the Elderly Patient at the End of Life

Opioid	Comments
Morphine	Observe for side effects with repeated dosing; continuous or sustained release may not be tolerated even after a trial with immediate release
Hydromorphone (Dilaudid)	Short half-life; may be safer than morphine
Propoxyphene (Darvon, Darvocet)	Avoid use—metabolite causes CNS and cardiac toxicity
Codeine	May cause excessive constipation, nausea and vomiting
Methadone	Use cautiously, long half-life may produce excessive side effects; requires careful monitoring, especially during first 72 hours after initiation. If it is indicated, it may be safer to use a short-acting opioid as a rescue dose.
Pentazocine (Talwin)	Opioid agonist/antagonist should not be used; may cause CNS side effects (delirium, agitation)
Transdermal fentanyl patch	Long half-life (12–24 h) is used cautiously in the frail elderly or in elderly with multiple comorbid conditions; cannot titrate easily. If side effects develop, will last at least 12–24 hours after patch is removed
Meperidine	Avoid use in elderly due to CNS toxicity
Oxycodone	Useful for moderate to severe pain control

Source: Adapted from McCaffery and Pasero (1999), reference 162.

Table 35–10
Indications for a Subcutaneous or Intravenous PCA Pump

- Oral route not tolerated—patient cannot swallow (postop, nausea/vomiting)
- Oral absorption impaired or variable
- Bowel obstruction—partial or complete
- Escalating pain that needs to be managed quickly
- Severe breakthrough or incident-related pain
- Dose-limiting side effects with other routes of administration exist
- When managing pain and other symptoms at the end of life
- Suspected misuse/abuse of other opioids via other routes of administration

Dose Titration. After initiation with an opioid, a stepwise escalation of the opioid dose should be done until adequate analgesia or intolerable side effects develop. The increased sensitivity of the elderly to opioid side effects suggests that careful titration and escalation should be performed.[96] It is generally safe to begin with a dose 25% to 50% less than the dose for a younger adult, especially if the elderly patient is frail or has a history of side effects from prior opioid use. Generally, it is safe to titrate opioids 25% to 50% every 24 to 48 hours, although a less aggressive approach may be necessary in elderly patients.

CASE STUDY
An 80-Year-Old Man with Bladder Cancer

An 80-year-old man with bladder cancer and extensive intraabdominal and pelvic disease is receiving hydromorphone 6 mg orally every 4 hours and is reporting inadequate pain relief, with a pain intensity of 7/10. He also is having intermittent nausea and vomiting. He has been on this dose for about 6 weeks and is reporting having some confusion for the past week, which his wife has corroborated. He is also having periods of severe incidental pain related to movement. He has no "as needed" rescue doses ordered. For the past 2 weeks, he has been in bed most of the time. He also reports constipation, with no bowel movement for 5 days.

Case Analysis. What evaluation of this patient should be done and what changes in his opioid regimen should be made?

1. The etiology of the confusion should be determined. A careful review of all medications should be done, and all centrally acting medications discontinued. In this patient, his only additional medication is digoxin.
2. A digoxin level and appropriate laboratory data should be obtained to determine if he is digoxin toxic and if there is any metabolic etiology for his confusion. His digoxin level is normal, and his electrolytes and renal and liver function studies are normal.
3. A change in opioid is indicated, because this may be contributing to his confusion.
4. An evaluation for the etiology of the nausea and vomiting should be done. A history of onset, duration, temporal characteristics, and exacerbating/relieving factors should be obtained. A thorough physical examination is performed, with special attention to the abdominal and rectal examination. The physical examination reveals that bowel sounds are present, and the rectal exam reveals retained feces in the rectal vault.
5. An abdominal x-ray is done and shows extensive retained feces but no bowel obstruction. An abdominal CAT scan done 1 month previously revealed extensive intrapelvic and intraabdominal disease.
6. It has been determined that the etiology of the nausea and vomiting is related to severe constipation and may be worsened by intermittent extrinsic compression of the bowel by tumor infiltration.
7. The severe constipation may also be contributing to the development of confusion.
8. The decision is made to switch the patient to another opioid. In selecting another opioid, factors to consider include half-life, duration of action, and route of administration. The decision is made to start the patient on a continuous infusion of morphine until the nausea and vomiting resolve and then convert the patient to oral morphine. The equianalgesic dose table should be used as a guide. Because of the existence of incomplete cross-tolerance between drugs, advanced age, and cognitive changes, the alternative opioid should be reduced by 50% to 75%.
9. Disimpaction was attempted but could not be tolerated. A bowel regimen of an oil-retention enema followed by a Fleets enema was tolerated, and the patient had a large bowel movement. The patient was also started on an oral regimen of Senokot 2 tabs orally twice a day and Colace 300 mg orally daily.

Management of Side Effects Related to Opioids. The elderly with multiple medical conditions, who are frail and bedbound, are at greatest risk for potential side effects of opioids due to age-related alterations in pharmacokinetics, specifically distribution and elimination. Avoiding side effects by "starting low and going slow" is common advice given to many clinicians when treating elderly patients, but this advice may run the risk of undertreatment of pain. Careful monitoring and frequent assessment can prevent a minor side effect from becoming life-threatening in the elderly.

For mild nausea, vomiting, sedation, or confusion, it might be helpful to decrease the 24-hour total dose by 25% if the patient has adequate analgesia and is taking only a minimal number of "as needed" rescue doses in a 24-hour period. This strategy avoids a complete change in opioid, although anecdotally, this approach may be useful for a limited time only; if the pain escalates, this will necessitate a titration of the opioid, and the side effects will return.

Nausea and vomiting are common with some opioids and are due to activation of the chemoreceptor trigger zone in the medulla, vestibular sensitivity, and delaying gastric emptying.[97] If nausea and vomiting occur at the initiation of therapy, it is usually transient and self-limiting. Patients should be prescribed antiemetics on an as-needed basis. Nausea and vomiting should be aggressively treated in the older adult because of the dangers of dehydration and the need for hospitalization.

Treating the side effect can be effective but the risk of polypharmacy remains. If, for example, the elderly patient is experiencing sedation from the opioid, it may be wiser to decrease the 24-hour total dose rather than add a psychostimulant, which can produce irritability, tremors, anxiety, and insomnia. If decreasing the dose cannot be done, a small dose of a psychostimulant such as Ritalin 2.5 mg orally twice a day, or Provigil 100 mg orally twice a day can be effective in controlling daytime sedation.[98] Changing the opioid can be another strategy to minimize or treat side effects. This intervention can be effective in the management of opioid-induced nausea and vomiting, especially if the patient has had limited exposure to opioids. Again, this strategy eliminates the use of an additional medication with its own potential side effects.

The addition of an adjuvant such as an NSAID has been shown to be effective in reducing the opioid requirement, thus allowing a reduction in the 24-hour opioid dose. Use of adjuvants will be discussed in the next section.

The elderly are particularly susceptible to opioid-induced constipation, and laxative and stool softener should be prescribed whenever an opioid is prescribed.[99] Tolerance to the constipating effects of opioids does not occur, and patients need to be instructed regarding the ongoing need for laxatives and stool softeners. Constipation can be life-threatening in the debilitated elderly patient, especially if it is unrecognized and untreated. The initial presentation of opioid-induced constipation may be confusing. Abdominal signs and symptoms including pain, distension, and nausea may be absent, and the patient may present with confusion, depressed mood, and loss of appetite. Assessment of the elderly patient should include all medications including over-the-counter drugs—iron preparations, antacids, and drugs with anticholinergic properties. A bowel regimen should be routinely prescribed including senna stool softeners. Fluids should be encouraged, but maintaining adequate hydration may be difficult for some older patients. In addition, the intake of fluids may further worsen other symptoms, including peripheral edema, dyspnea, ascites, and other sites of third spacing.

Adjuvant Analgesics and Treatment

Several nonopioid medications have been found to be analgesic. These drugs alter, attenuate, or modulate pain perception. They may be used alone or in combination with opioids or nonopioid analgesics to treat many different pain syndromes, including neuropathic pain. Included in this category are antidepressants, anticonvulsants, *N*-methyl-D-aspartate (NMDA) antagonists, corticosteroids, and local anesthetics. All of these medications have side-effect profiles that can be especially harmful to the older patient, and careful monitoring is required.

Tricyclic antidepressants (TCAs) have been the most widely studied class of adjuvant medications for neuropathic pain. The action of these drugs is probably due to interruption of norepinephrine and serotonin-mediated mechanisms in the brain.[101] Side effects, namely the anticholinergic side effects, often limit the use of these medications. Dry mouth, urinary retention, constipation, blurred vision, tachycardia and delirium are some of the more common side effects. Nortriptyline, a secondary amine, may be preferred in the older adult because it produces less orthostatic hypotension than amitriptyline, and desipramine may have lesser anticholinergic side effects than amitriptyline. TCAs are contraindicated in patients with coronary artery disease, narrow-angle glaucoma, and significant prostatic hyperplasia. When initiating therapy, start the dose low, monitor patients, and titrate the dose in 10-mg increments every 7 to 10 days because tolerance to side effects develops.

Anticonvulsants are used to control sharp, shooting, burning, electric, and stabbing pain, typical sensations found in patients with neuropathic pain. Their analgesic effect is believed to be related to the slowing of peripheral nerve conduction in primary afferent fibers.[102] Several different anticonvulsants are useful for neuropathic pain, including carbamazepine, gabapentin, phenytoin, and valproic acid. Carbamazepine should be used cautiously because of the side-effect profile—blood dyscrasias can occur.[103] Gabapentin is thought to have several different mechanisms of action, including having NMDA antagonist activity. The most effective analgesic doses range from 900 mg to 3600 mg/day, in divided doses every 8 hours.[104–105] Evidence supports the efficacy of gabapentin in several painful disorders, including diabetic neuropathy,[104] postherpetic neuralgia,[105] thalamic pain, spinal cord injury,[106] and restless legs syndrome.[107] The starting dose in elderly patients can begin as low as 100 mg a day, titrated by 100 mg a day every 3 days, until the onset of analgesia. The most commonly reported side effects of gabapentin are somnolence, dizziness, ataxia, tremor, and fatigue. Other anticonvulsants that have been used in the management of neuropathic pain include lamotrigine (Lamictal), topiramate (Topamax), zonisamide (Zonegran), and levetiracetam (Keppra), although no randomized controlled studies are available.

NMDA antagonists are believed to block the binding of excitatory amino acids, such as glutamate, in the spinal cord. Medications that inhibit this receptor interfere with the transmission of pain across the synaptic area. Methadone, ketamine, and dextromethorphan are all NMDA antagonists thought to have analgesic effects in the management of neuropathic pain.[108,109] Ketamine should be used with caution because of its psychomimetic effects, and routine use is not recommended. At the end of life, it has been used in the management of refractory neuropathic pain.[110]

Corticosteroids have specific and nonspecific effects in managing pain, including treatment of painful nerve or spinal cord compression, reducing tissue edema and inflammation, and by lysis of some tumors. The mechanism of effect is by inhibition of prostaglandin synthesis and decreasing edema surrounding neural tissues.[111] Corticosteroids are the standard treatment for malignant spinal cord compression (dexamethasone 16 to 96 mg/day). They may be useful in the management of painful malignant lesions involving the brachial or lumbosacral plexus, hepatic enlargement, distension, and pain.[112,113] Corticosteroids are also helpful in the management of bone pain as well as in the treatment of bowel obstruction.[114,115] Corticosteroids may also be useful in the management of nausea and vomiting. In the older adult, corticosteroids should not be used concurrently with NSAIDs due to the potential increased risk of bleeding.

Local anesthetics have been shown to relieve pain when administered orally, topically, intravenously, and intraspinally. Mexiletine has been useful when anticonvulsants have failed.[116] Topical local anesthetic gels and topical Lidoderm patches have been useful in the management of postherpetic neuropathy[117] and other neuropathic pain syndromes, including peripheral neuropathy, postthoracotomy pain, stump neuroma, complex regional pain syndrome, radiculopathy, and postmastectomy pain.[118] Lidoderm patches 5% should be applied 12 hours on/12 hours off, within a 24-hour period. They have an excellent safety profile; systemically active serum levels of lidocaine do not occur, and patients can cut the patches to fit small areas. In many older patients, the patches may provide an opioid-sparing effect—the patient may use less opioid analgesia within a 24-hour period. IV lidocaine boluses at doses of 1 to 5 mg/kg, maximum 500 mg, administered over 1 hour, followed by a continuous infusion of 1 to 2 mg/kg/hr has been reported to reduce intractable neuropathic pain in the palliative care and hospice setting.[119]

Bisphosphonates inhibit osteoclast–mediated bone resorption and alleviate pain from metastatic bone disease and multiple myeloma.[120,121] Analgesic effects can occur in 2 to 4 weeks, and, for this reason, might not be suitable for patients at the end of life. Pamidronate disodium and zoledronic acid are used in patients with metastatic lesions from breast and prostate cancer. Pamidronate sodium has been shown to reduce pathological fractures in patients with breast cancer.[122] Patients should be monitored with serum calcium levels because hypocalcemia can occur.

Calcitonin may be given subcutaneously or intranasally to relieve pain associated with osteoporotic fractures.[123] Usual doses are 100 to 200 IU/day and are usually well tolerated. At the end of life, this is probably not a practical or helpful intervention.

Radiation therapy is extremely helpful in relieving painful bone lesions. In many instances, single-fraction external beam therapy can be used. Onset of relief can be fairly rapid, often within days of treatment and may be a helpful intervention when patients are having side effects to opioid therapy. Unless a single fraction is considered, at the end of life it is not a practical intervention.

Radionuclide therapy is often helpful when there is widespread bony metastatic disease that cannot be easily targeted with localized radiotherapy.[124] Strontium (Metastron) is a radiopharmaceutical calcium analogue taken up by the skeleton into active sites of bone remodeling and metastasis. A large clinical trial demonstrated that strontium was an effective adjuvant to local radiotherapy, and that it reduced disease progression, decreased new sites of pain, and decreased systemic use.[124] The latency of response can be as long as 2 to 3 weeks, and patients should continue their opioid therapy. Because of this delayed onset of analgesia, patients who are actively dying are not candidates. Side effects associated with strontium use include thrombocytopenia and leucopenia. Samarium lexidronam (Quadramet) is a radiopharmaceutical that has an affinity for bone, and concentrates in areas of bone turnover with hydroxyapatite, which is useful for metastatic bone pain. Patients should also be instructed that a transitory pain flare can occur, and analgesics may need to be titrated.

Invasive Approaches

Anesthetic and neurosurgical approaches are indicated when conservative measures using opioids and adjuvant analgesics have failed to provide adequate analgesia, or when the patient is experiencing intolerable side effects. The use of these approaches is not contraindicated in the older adult. The clearest indication for these approaches is intolerable CNS toxicity. These procedures include regional analgesia (spinal, intraventricular, and intrapleural opioids), sympathetic blockade and neurolytic procedures (celiac plexus block, lumbar sympathetic block, cervicothoracic [stellate] ganglion block), or pathway ablation procedure (chemical or surgical rhizotomy, or cordotomy). At the end of life, these approaches may be useful in some older patients who have intractable pain that cannot be managed with systemic treatment.

Nonpharmacological Approaches: Complementary Therapies

Physical and psychological interventions can be used as an adjunct with drugs and surgical approaches to manage pain in the older adult. These approaches carry few side effects and, when possible, should be tried along with other approaches. In selecting an approach in the dying patient, factors that should be considered include physical and psychological burden to the patient, efficacy, and practicality. If the patient has weeks to live, these strategies may allow for a reduction in systemic opioids and diminish adverse effects.

Cognitive-behavioral interventions include relaxation, guided imagery, distraction, and music therapy. The major advantages of these techniques are that they are easy to learn, safe, and readily accepted by patients. Cognitive and behavioral interventions are helpful to reduce emotional distress, improve coping, and offer the patient and family a sense of control. Other physical interventions such as reflexology and massage therapy have been shown to relieve pain and produce relaxation.[125,126]

The Cognitively Impaired Elderly: Problems in Assessment and Fear of Treating Pain and Other Symptoms

Cognitively impaired nursing home residents present a special barrier to pain assessment and management.[127–131] Residents of nursing homes exhibit very high rates of cognitive impairment.[132] Most studies of nursing home residents reveal that cognitively impaired nursing home residents are prescribed and administered significantly less analgesic medication, both in number and in dosage of pain drugs, than their more cognitively intact peers.[132,133]

Assessment of pain in cognitively impaired elderly at the end of life remains a special challenge. Mild to moderate cognitive impairments seem to be associated with a decrease in propensity to report pain.[132] In severely cognitively impaired individuals, assessment is often difficult because these individuals frequently cannot verbalize their reports of pain. Ferrell and colleagues[134] found in their evaluation of 217 elderly patients with significant cognitive impairment that 83% could complete at least one pain scale, with the McGill Present Pain Intensity Scale having the highest completion rate, and 32% were able to complete all of the scales presented.

The best way to assess pain is to ask the individual. In the cognitively impaired elderly, it is difficult to assess pain. The ability of caregivers, either family or staff, to assess pain in this population is crucial. In one study of caregiver perceptions of nonverbal patients with cerebral palsy, more than 80% of the caregivers used aspects of crying and moaning to alert them to a pain event.[135] In another study evaluating a measurement tool for discomfort in noncommunicative patients with advanced Alzheimer's disease, indicators of pain included noisy breathing, negative vocalizations, facial expression (content, sad, or frightened), frown, and body language (relaxed, tense, or fidgeting).[127]

There is some evidence that cognitively impaired elderly individuals' facial expressions of pain depend on the cause of the underlying cognitive disorder, including hemispheric dysfunction and type of dementia; however, facial expressions and body language can be very useful indicators of pain.

Delirium at the End of Life

Prevalence. Delirium is a frequently occurring consequence of advanced cancer and is characterized by disturbances in arousal, perception, cognition, and psychomotor behavior.[136,137] In all settings, delirium is a common symptom in the elderly medically ill and cancer patient. The presence of delirium contributes significantly to increased morbidity and mortality. Estimates of the prevalence of delirium range from 25% to 40% in cancer patients at some point during their disease, and in the terminal phases of disease, the incidence increases to 85%.[89,136–138] In elderly hospitalized patients, delirium prevalence ranges from 10% to 40%, and up to 80% at the end of life. One of the major problems in the treatment of delirium in the elderly patient is lack of assessment by hospital staff, especially if the patient is quiet and noncommunicative.

Predisposing and Etiological Factors. The etiology of delirium in the medically compromised and dying elderly patient is often multifactorial and may be nonspecific. In an elderly patient, delirium is often a presenting feature of an acute physical illness or exacerbation of a chronic one, or of intoxication with even therapeutic doses of commonly used drugs.[139] A number of factors appear to make the elderly more susceptible to the development of delirium (Table 35–11).

Delirium can be due to the direct effects of the disease on the CNS, metabolic reasons including organ failure, electrolyte imbalance, infection, hematological disorders, nutritional deficiencies, paraneoplastic disorders, hypoxemia, chemotherapeutic agents, immunotherapy, vascular disorders, hypothermia, hyperthermia, uncontrolled pain, sensory deprivation, sleep deprivation, medications, alcohol or drug withdrawal, diarrhea, constipation, or urinary retention. A variety of drugs can produce delirium in the medically ill or elderly patient (Table 35–12). In the palliative care setting, multiple medications are generally required to control symptoms at the end of life. In patients with advanced cancer, prospective data suggest a prevalence of delirium in 28% to 42% on admission to a palliative care unit.[140] Given the projected increase in the numbers of elderly patients, health care providers will encounter the need for management of delirium in the elderly more frequently.

Other risk factors for the development of delirium include advanced age, cancer, preexisitng cognitive impairment, hip fractures, and severe illness.[141–143] In cancer patients, risk factors that have been identified include advanced age, cognitive impairment, low albumin level, bone metastases, and the presence of hematological malignancy. In one study that determined risk factors for delirium in oncology patients, specific etiological factors in the elderly were identified and include reduced cholinergic reserves of the brain, high prevalence of cognitive impairment and comorbid disease, visual and hearing loss, and impaired metabolism of drugs.[144,145]

The diagnosis of delirium in an elderly patient carries with it serious risks. Delirium produces distress for patients, families, and health care providers. Depending on the severity of symptoms (fluctuating cognitive changes, hallucinations, agitation, or emotional lability), patients often require one-to-one observation, chemical, and, rarely, physical restraints. Falls and pressure ulcers are associated with the hyperactive and hypoactive subtypes.[146]

Table 35–11
Factors Predisposing the Elderly to Delirium

Factor	Comments
Age-related changes in the brain	Atrophy of gray and white matter
	Senile plaques in hippocampus, amygdala, middle cerebral cortical layers
	Cell loss in frontal lobes, amygdala, putamen, thalamus, locus ceruleus
	Alzheimer's disease, cerebrovascular disease
Brain damage	
Reduced regulation and resistance to stress	Visual, hearing loss
Sensory changes	Prolonged immobility, Foley catheters
Infection	
Intravenous lines	Pulmonary and urinary tract infections
	Reduced ability to metabolize and eliminate drugs
Impaired pharmacokinetics	Vitamin deficiency as a result of prolonged illness
Malnutrition	Folate deficiency may directly cause delirium
Multiple comorbid diseases	Cancer and cardiovascular, pulmonary, renal, and hepatic disease
	Endocrine disorders, including hyperthyroidism and hypothyroidism
	Fluid and electrolyte abnormalities
Reduced thirst	Hypovolemia
Reduction of protein-binding of drugs	Enhanced effect of opioids, diuretics
Polypharmacy	Use of sedatives, hypnotics, major tranquilizers

Sources: Adapted from Lipowski (1989), reference 139, and Inouye et al. (1996), reference 141.

Given the projected increase in the numbers of elderly patients, health care providers will encounter management of delirium in the elderly more frequently. To reduce the risk of polypharmacologically induced delirium, it is prudent to add one medication at a time, evaluating its response, before adding another medication.

Delirium in the elderly patient is often undertreated for several reasons, including lack of assessment tools, inadequate knowledge of early signs of confusion, and inadequate time spent with the patient to determine cognitive function—all factors that lead to underdiagnosis. In addition, behavioral manifestations of delirium may include a variety of symptoms that may be interpreted as depression, or dementia.

A multifactorial model of delirium in the elderly, with baseline predisposing factors and the addition of various insults, has been established by Inouye.[141] The factors that have been identified to be contributory to baseline vulnerability in the elderly include visual impairment, cognitive impairment, severe illness, and an elevated blood urea nitrogen/creatinine ratio of 18 or greater. Other factors that have been identified in the elderly include advanced age, depression, electrolyte imbalance, poor functional status, immobility, Foley catheter, malnutrition, dehydration, alcohol, and medications, including neuroleptics, opioids, and anticholinergic drugs. Lastly, delirium in an elderly patient is often a precursor to death and should be viewed as a grave prognostic sign.[147]

Alcohol withdrawal may be the cause of delirium in the elderly. In one study, organic mental syndromes were diagnosed in more than 40% of elderly alcoholics admitted for alcohol abuse, and delirium was found in about 10% of these.[148] Illness, malnutrition, concurrent use of a hepatotoxic drug, or one that is metabolized by the liver may result in increased sensitivity of the elderly to alcohol. Alcohol, combined with other medications, especially centrally acting medications, can produce delirium in the elderly.

The diagnosis of delirium in an elderly patient carries with it serious risks. An agitated delirious patient may climb out of bed; pull out Foley catheters, IV lines, and sutures; and injure staff in an attempt to protect himself from perceived threat. Mental status questionnaires are relatively easy to administer, and an examination should be performed on all patients with mental status changes. The Mini-Mental State Exam, a 10-item test, is easy to administer to an elderly patient.[149]

Table 35–12
Drugs Commonly Causing Delirium in the Elderly

Classification	Example
Antidepressants	Amitriptyline, doxepin
Antihistamines	Chlorpheniramine, diphenhydramine, hydroxyzine, promethazine
Diabetic agents	Chlorpropamide
Cardiac	Digoxin, dipyridamole
Antihypertensives	Propranolol, clonidine
Sedatives	Barbiturates, chlordiazepoxide, diazepam, flurazepam, meprobamate
Opioids	Meperidine, pentazocine, propoxyphene
Nonsteroidal antiinflammatory agents	Indomethacin, phenylbutazone
Anticholinergics	Atropine, scopolamine
Antiemetics	Trimethobenzamide, phenothiazine
Antispasmodics	Dilomine, hyoscyamine, propantheline, belladonna alkaloids
Antineoplastics	Methotrexate, mitomycin, procarbazine, Ara-C, carmustine, fluorouracil, interferon, Interleukin-2, L-asparaginase, prednisone
Corticosteroids	Prednisone, dexamethasone
H_2-receptor antagonists	Cimetidine
Lithium	
Acetaminophen	
Salicylates	Aspirin
Anticonvulsant agents	Carbamazepine, diphenylhydantoin, phenobarbital, sodium valproate
Antiparkinsonian agents	Amantadine, levodopa
Alcohol	

Source: Adapted from Lipowski (1989), reference 139.

Delirium and Dementia

Delirium may often be superimposed upon dementia in the elderly patient. In clinical practice, it is important to distinguish whether the delirious patient has an underlying dementia. When an elderly demented patient becomes delirious, it should be assumed that an organic precipitating factor—metabolic, drug-induced, acute illness—is the cause, and the patient should be evaluated for the etiology and treated. The distinction is not always apparent. Both delirium and dementia feature global impairment in cognition. Obtaining a careful history from family members or caregivers to learn about the onset of symptoms is probably the most important factor in making the distinction. In general, acute onset of cognitive and attentional deficits and abnormalities, whose severity fluctuates during the day and tends to increase at night, is typical of a delirium. Delirium, in general, is a transient disorder that seldom lasts for more than a month, while dementia is a clinical state that lasts for months or years.[139] Dementia implies impairment in short- or long-term memory associated with impaired thinking and judgment, with other disturbances of higher cortical function, or with personality change.[150] The presence and severity of cognitive deficits and attentional disturbances should be further established by a comprehensive mental status examination.

Treatment of Delirium

Treatment of delirium includes an identification of the underlying cause, correction of the precipitating factors, and symptom management of the delirium. In the very ill or dying patient, however, the etiology may be multifactorial, and the cause is often irreversible.

If delirium is occurring in the dying elderly patient and the goal of care has been identified as the promotion of comfort and relief of suffering, diagnostic evaluations (imaging and laboratory studies) would not prove beneficial.

Interventions that may be helpful include restoration of fluid and electrolyte balance, environmental changes, and supportive techniques such as elimination of unnecessary stimuli, provision of a safe environment, and measures that reduce anxiety. In many cases, the etiology of delirium may be pharmacological, especially in the elderly patient. All nonessential and CNS-depressant drugs should be stopped. Figure 35–2

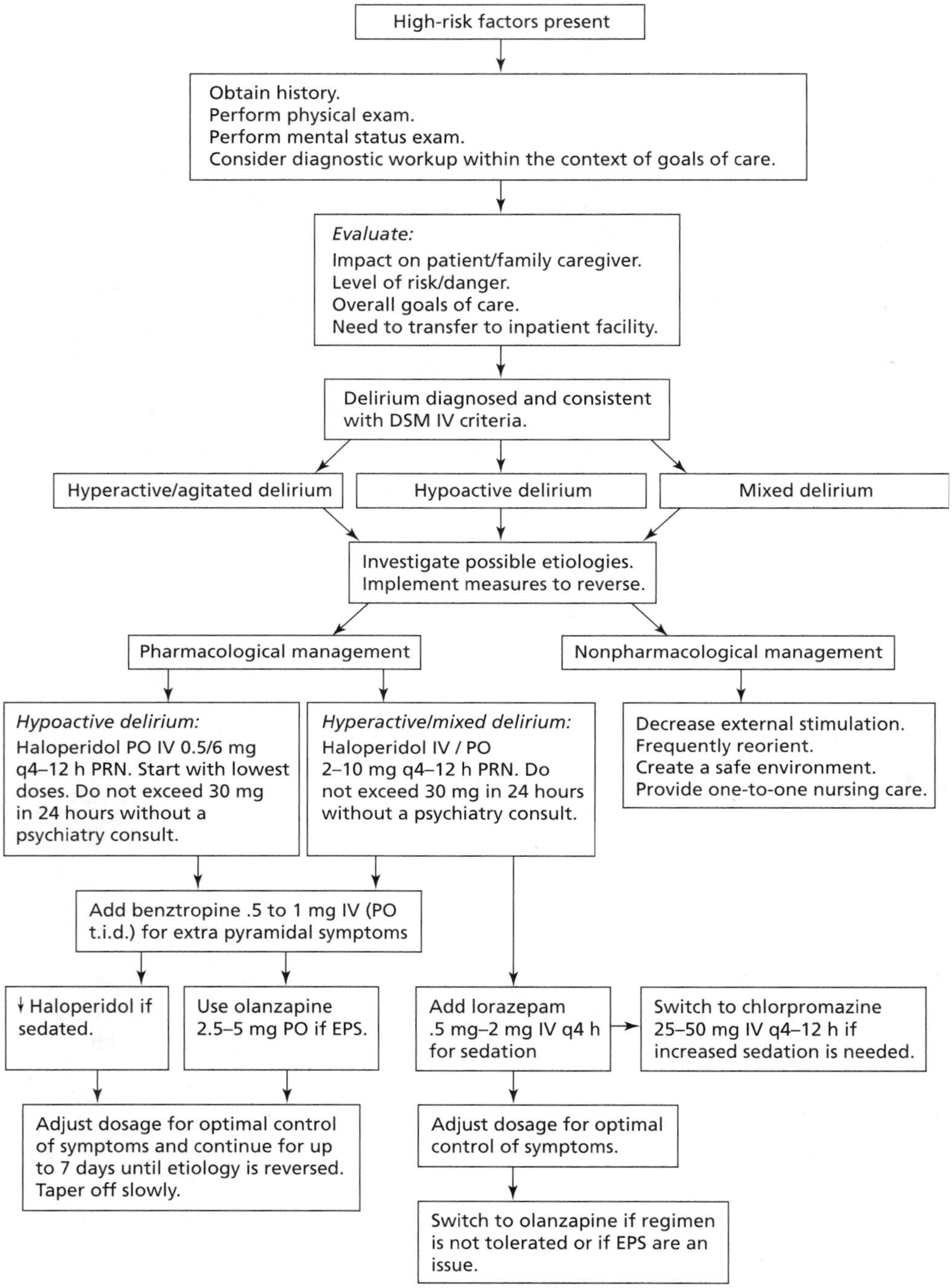

Figure 35–2. Delirium management in the geriatric patient at the end of life. *Source:* Adapted from Memorial Sloan-Kettering Cancer Center algorithm for pharmacologic management of delirium (August 14, 2001).

reviews the overall assessment and management of delirium in the geriatric patient at the end of life.

Pharmacological treatment includes the use of sedatives and neuroleptics. Breitbart and Jacobsen[151] have demonstrated that the use of lorazepam alone in controlling symptoms of delirium was ineffective and contributed to worsening cognition. These authors advocate the use of a neuroleptic such as haloperidol, along with a benzodiazepine, in the control of an agitated delirium. Other neuroleptics, risperidone and olanzapine, have also been used to treat delirium in the elderly, and may have fewer side effects. The oral route is preferred, although in cases of severe agitation and delirium, the parenteral route should be used. In one study by Breitbart, 79 cancer patients were treated for delirium with olanzapine and age over 70 years was found to be the most powerful predictor of poorer response to olanzapine treatment. Other factors included history of dementia, CNS spread of disease, and hypoxia as delirium etiologies.[152] See Chapter 20 for more information on delirium and dementia.

Summary

Elderly patients who are dying should be able to receive skillful and expert palliative care. This means that caregivers must become knowledgeable about the aging process—the physiological changes that normally occur with aging and the impact of progressive disease on an already frail system. Management of symptoms at the end of life in the elderly patient is different from the younger age group because of their altered response to medications, their fear of taking medication, and the need to involve and educate informal and formal caregivers, who are often elderly themselves.

Pain, respiratory distress, and delirium are the three most common symptoms in the elderly patient who is dying. Relief of these symptoms is a basic priority for care of the dying elderly patient. Continued assessment of the patient will allow for drug changes, dose adjustments, and relief of distressing symptoms. Providing relief from these symptoms will help facilitate a peaceful death, one that is remembered as such by family and friends.

REFERENCES

1. Rabin D, Stockton P. Long-Term Care of the Elderly: A Factbook. New York, Oxford University Press, 1987.
2. National Center for Health Statistics Advance report of final mortality statistics, 1987. Monthly Vital Statistics Reports 1989; 38(Suppl 5).
3. Federal Interagency Forum on Aging-Related Statistics. Older Americans 2000: key indicators of well-being. Washington, D.C.: 2002, http://www.agingstats.gov (accessed January 29, 2005).
4. Foley D, Brock D. Demography and epidemiology of dying in the U.S. with emphasis on deaths of older persons. Hosp J 1998; 13:49–60.
5. National Center for Health Statistics. Monthly Vital Statistics Report 1995;43.
6. Grulich A, Swerdlow A, Dos Santos Silva I, Beral V. Is the apparent rise in cancer mortality in the elderly real? Analysis of changes in certification and coding of cause of death in England and Wales, 1970–1990. Int J Cancer 1995;63:164–168.
7. National Center for Health Statistics Moss A, Parson V. Current estimates from the National Health Interview Survey, United States 1985. In: Vital Health Statistics, ser. 10, no. 160. DHHS Pub. No. (PHS) 860-1588. Washington, DC: Public Health Service, 1986:13, 82–83, 106, 118.
8. Foley DJ, Miles TP, Brock DB, Phillips C. Recounts of elderly deaths: endorsements for the Patient Self-Determination Act. Gerontologist 1995;35:119–121.
9. Seeman I. National Mortality Followback Survey: 1986 summary. United States. Vital Health Statistics, ser. 20, no. 19. DHHS Pub. No. (PHS) 92-1656. Hyattsville, MD: National Center for Health Statistics.
10. Foley D, Brock D. Demography and epidemiology of dying in the U.S. with emphasis on deaths of older persons. Hosp J 1998;13:49–60.
11. Wallace R, Woolson R, eds. The Epidemiological Study of the Elderly. New York: Oxford University Press, 1992.
12. Fried T, Pollack D, Drickamer M, Tinetti M. Who dies at home? Determinants of site of death for community-based long-term care patients. J Am Geriatr Soc 1999;47:25–29.
13. Groth-Janucker A, McCusker J. Where do elderly patients prefer to die? Place of death and patient characteristics of 100 elderly patients under the care of a home healthcare team. J Am Geriatr Soc 1983;31:457–461.
14. McWhinney IR, Bass M, Orr V. Factors associated with location of death (home or hospital) of patients referred to a palliative care team. CMAJ 1995;152:361–367.
15. Townsend J, Frank A, Fermont D, Dyer S, Karran O, Walgrove A, Piper M. Terminal cancer and patients' preference for place of death: a prospective study. BMJ 1990;301:415–417.
15a. National Institute of Aging. The Health and Retirement Study (NIA U01AG0974), 2005, http://hrsonline.isr.umich.edu (accessed January 19, 2005).
16. Kemper P, Murtaugh CM. Lifetime use of nursing home care. N Engl J Med 1991;324:595–600.
17. Stein WM, Ferrell BA. Pain in the nursing home. Clin Geriatr Med 1996;12:601–613.
18. Ferrell BA, Ferrell BR, Osterweil D. Pain in the nursing home. J Am Geriatr Soc 1990;38:409–414.
19. Singer P, Martin DK, Kelner M. Quality end-of-life care. Patient's perspective. JAMA 1999;281:163–198.
20. Bernabei R, Gambassi G, Lapane K, et al. Management of pain in elderly residents with cancer. JAMA 1998;279:1877–1882.
21. Castle N. Innovations in dying in the nursing home: the impact of market characteristics. Omega 1998;36:227–240.
22. Ferrell B. Pain evaluation and management in nursing homes. Ann Intern Med 1995;123:681–687.
23. Hanson LC, Henderson M. Care of the dying in long-term care settings. Clin Geriatr Med 2000;16:225–237.
24. Institute of Medicine. Approaching Death: Improving Care at the End of Life. Washington, DC: National Academy Press, 1997.
25. Teno J. Looking beyond the "form" to complex interventions needed to improve end-of-life care. J Am Geriatr Soc 1998;46: 1170–1171.

26. Miller SC, Mor V, Wu N, Gozalo P, Lapane K. Does receipt of hospice care in nursing homes improve the management of pain at the end of life? J Am Geriatr Soc 2002;50:507–515.
27. Travis SS, Bernard M, Dixon S, McAuley WJ, Loving G, McClanahan L. Obstacles to palliation and end-of-life care in a long-term care facility. Gerontologist 2002;42:342–349.
28. Teno JM, Branco KJ, Mor V, et al. Changes in advance care planning in nursing homes before and after the Patient Self Determination Act: report of a five state survey. J Amer Geriactr Soc 1997;45:939–944.
29. Castle N, Mor V. Advance care planning in nursing homes. Pre- and postpatient self-determination act. Health Serv Res 1998;33:101–124.
30. Wagner L. Providing comfort to dying residents. Provider 1999;25:52–54, 57–58, 61–65.
31. Smith GE, Kokmen E, O'Brien PC. Risk factors for nursing home placement in a population-based dementia cohort. J Am Geriatr Soc 2000;48:519–525.
32. Morris JN, Hawes C, Fries BE, et al. Designing the national resident assessment instrument for nursing homes. Gerontologist 1999;30:293–307.
33. Hawes C, Morris JN, Phillips CD, Mor V, Fries BE, Nonemaker S. Reliability estimates for the minimum data set for nursing home resident assessment and care screening (MDS). Gerontologist 1995;35:172–178.
34. Mitchell SL, Kiely DK, Lipsitz LA. The risk factors and impact on survival of feeding tube placement in nursing home residents with severe cognitive impairment. Arch Intern Med 1997;157:327–332.
35. Gornick M, McMillan A, Lubitz J. A longitudinal perspective on patterns of Medicare payments. Health Aff (Millwood) 1993;12: 140–150.
36. Perls TT, Wood ER. Acute costs and the oldest old. Arch Intern Med 1996;156:759.
37. Riley G, Potosky A, Lubitz J, Kessler L. Medicare payments from diagnosis to death for elderly cancer patients. Med Care 1995;33:828–841.
38. Riley G, Lubitz J, Prihoda R, Rabey E. The use and costs of Medicare services by cause of death. Inquiry 1987;24:233–244.
39. Knaus W, Wagner DP, Draper EA, Zimmerman JE, Bergner M, Bastos PG, Sirio CA, Murphy DJ, Lotring T, Damiano A. The APACHE prognostic system: risk prediction of hospital mortality for critically ill hospitalized adults. Chest 1991;100: 1619–1636.
40. Christakis NA, Escarce JJ. Survival of Medicare patients after enrollment in hospice programs. N Engl J Med 1996;18;335: 172–178.
41. Rosenthal MA, Gebski VJ, Keffors RF, Stuart Harris RC. Prediction of life-expectancy in hospice patients: identification of novel prognostic factors. Palliat Med 1993;3:199–204.
42. Bruera E, Miller M, Kuehn N, MacEachern T, Hanson J. Estimate of survival of patients admitted to a palliative care unit: a prospective study. J Pain Symptom Manage 1992;7:82–86.
43. Emanuel L, Madelyn I, Webster JR. Ethical aspects of geriatric palliative care. In: Geriatric Palliative Care, Morrison RS, Meier DE. New York: Oxford University Press, 2003.
44. Phipps E, True G, Harris D, Chong U, Tester W, Chavin I, Braitman LE. Approaching the end-of-life: attitudes, preferences and behaviors of African-American and White patients and their family caregivers. J Clin Onc 2003;21:549–554.
45. McAuley WJ, Travis SS. Advance care planning among residents in long-term care. Am J Hos Palliat Care 2003;20:529–530.
46. Danis M, Garrett J, Harris R, Patrick DL. Stability of choices about life-sustaining treatments. Ann Int Med 1994;120:567–573.
47. Emanuel LL, Emanuel EJ, Stoeckle JD, et al. Advanced directives. Stability of patient's treatment choices. Arch Int Med 1994; 154: 209–217.
48. Rosenfeld KE, Wenger NS, Phillips RS, et al. Factors associated with change in rescuscitation preference of seriously ill patients. The SUPPORT Investigators. Study to Understand Prognoses and Preferences for Outcomes and Risks of Treatment. 156:1558–1564.
49. McParland E, Likourezos E, Chichin E, Castor T, Paris BEC. Stability of preferences regarding life-sustaining treatment: a two-year perspective study of nursing home residents. Mount Sinai J Med 2003;70:85–92.
50. Otten A. About 15% of U.S. adults care for ill relatives. Wall Street Journal, April 22, 1991, B1.
51. Stone R, Cafferata GI, Sangl J. Caregivers of the frail elderly: a national profile. Gerontologist 1987;27:616–626.
52. National Center for Health Statistics. National home and hospice care data. Hyattsville, MD: U.S. Department of Health and Human Services, 2000.
53. Schott-Baer D, Fisher L, Gregory C. Dependent care, caregiver burden, hardiness, and self-care agency of caregivers. Cancer Nurs 1995;18:299–305.
54. Weitzner MA, McMillan S, Jacobson P. Family caregiver quality of life: differences between curative and palliative cancer treatment settings. J Pain Sympt Manage 1999;17:418–428.
55. Burton LC, Zdaniuk B, Schulz R, Jackson S, Hirsch C. Transitions in spousal caregiving. Gerontologist 2003;43:230–241.
56. Schulz R, Mendelsoohn AB, Haley WE, Mahoney D, Allen RS, Zhang S, Thompson L, Bell SH. Resources for Enhancing Alzheimer's Caregiver Health Investigators. N Engl J Med 2003; 349:1936–42.
57. Ferrell BR, Grant M, Borneman T, Juarez G, Ter Veer A. Family caregiving in cancer pain management. J Palliat Med 1995;2: 185–195.
58. Kissane DW, Block S, McKenzie M, McDowell AC, Nitzan R. Family grief therapy: a preliminary account of a new model to promote healthy family functioning during palliative care and bereavement. Psychooncology 1998;7:14–25.
59. Smeenk FW, de Witte LP, Van Haastregt JC, Schipper RM, Biezeman HP, Crebolder HF. Transmural care of terminal cancer patients. Nurs Res 1998;47:129–136.
60. Macdonald G. Massage as a respite intervention for primary caregivers. Am J Hosp Palliat Care 1998;15:43–47.
61. Greenblatt DJ, Harmatz JS, Shader RI. Clinical pharmacokinetics of anxiolytics and hypnotics in the elderly: therapeutic considerations. Clin Pharmacokinet 1991;21:165–177, 262–273.
62. Vestal RF, Montamat SC, Nielson CP. Drugs in special patient groups: the elderly. In: Melmon KL, Morrelli HF, Hoffman BB, Nierenberg DW, eds. Clinical Pharmacology: Basic Principles in Therapeutics, 3rd ed., New York: McGraw-Hill, 1992:851–874.
63. Avorn J, Gurwitz HH. Principles of pharmacology. In: Cassel CK, Cohen HJ, Larson EB, Meier DE, Resnick NM, Rubenstein LZ, Sorenson LB, eds., Geriatric Medicine, 3rd ed., New York: Springer, 1997:55–70.
64. Vestal RE. Aging and pharmacology. Cancer 1997;89:1302–1310.
65. Aparasu RR, Sitzman SJ. Inappropriate prescribing for elderly outpatient. Am J Health Syst Pharm 1999;56:433–439.
66. Seale C, Cartwright A. The Year Before Death. Brookfield, VT: Ashgate Publishing Company, 1994.

67. Fainsinger R, Miller MJ, Bruera E. Symptom control during the last week of life on a palliative care unit. J Palliat Care 1991;7:5–11.
68. Ventafridda V, Ripamonti C, DeConno F, Tamburini M, Cassileth BR. Symptom prevalence and control during cancer patients' last days of life. J Palliat Care 1990;6:7–11.
69. Coyle N, Adelhardt J, Foley K, Portenoy R. Character of terminal illness in the advanced cancer patient: pain and other symptoms during the last four weeks of life. J Pain Symptom Manage 1990;2(5):83–93.
70. Desbiens NA, Mueller-Rizner N, Connors AF, et al. The symptom burden of seriously ill hospitalized patients. J Pain Symptom Manage 1999;17:248–255.
71. Palange P, Forte S, Felli A, et al. Nutritional state and exercise tolerance in patients with COPD. Chest 1995;107:1206–1212.
72. Ripamonti C, Bruera E. Dyspnea: pathophysiology and assessment. J Pain Symptom Manage 1997;13:220–232.
73. Cowcher K, Hanks GW. Long-term management of respiratory symptoms in advanced cancer. J Pain Symptom Manage 1990; 5:320–330.
74. Farncombe M, Chater S. Case studies outlining use of nebulized morphine for patients with end-stage chronic lung and cardiac disease. J Pain Symptom Manage 1993;8:221–225.
75. Fishbein D, Kearon C, Killian KJ. An approach to dyspnea in cancer patients. J Pain Symptom Manage 1989;4:76–81.
76. Allard P, Lamontagne C, Bernard P, Tremblay C. How effective are supplementary doses of opioids for dyspnea in terminally ill cancer patients? A randomized continuous sequential clinical trial. J Pain Symptom Manage 1999;17:256–265.
77. Vane JR, Botting RM. Anti-inflammatory drugs and their mechanism. Inflamm Res 1998;47(Suppl 2):S78–87.
78. Mercandate S. The use of anti-inflammatory drugs in cancer pain. Cancer Treat Rev 2001:27:51–61.
79. Perez Gutthann S, Garcia Rodriguez LA, Raiford DS, Duque Oliart A, Ris Romeu J. Nonsteroidal anti-inflammatory drugs and the risk of hospitalization for acute renal failure (comment). Arch Intern Med 1996;156:2433–2439.
80. Cryer B, Feldman M. Cyclooxygenase-1 and cyclooxygenase-2 selectivity of widely used nonsteroidal anti-inflammatory drugs. Am J Med 1998;104:413–421.
81. Simon LS, Weaver Al, Graham DY, Kivitz J, Lipsky PE, Hubbard RC, et al. Anti-inflammatory and upper gastrointestinal effects of celecoxib in rheumatoid arthritis: a randomized controlled trial. JAMA 1999;282:1921–1928
82. Juni P, Rutjes AW, Dieppe PA. Are selective COX-2 inhibitors superior to traditional nonsteroidal anti-inflammatory drugs? BMJ 2002;324(7353):1538, erratum.
83. Juni P, Dieppe P, Egger M. Risk of myocardial infarction associated with selective COX-2 inhibitors: questions remain. (comment). Arch Intern Med 2002:162:2639–2640, author reply 2640.
84. Wright JM. The double-edged sword of COX-2 selective NSAIDs. (comment) Can Med Assoc J 2002;167:1131–1137.
85. Peterson WL, Cryer B. COX-1-sparing NSAIDs—is the enthusiasm justified? (comment). JAMA 1999;282:1961–1963.
86. Mercadante S, Arcuri E. Opioids and renal function. J Pain 2004;5:2–19.
87. Kaiko RF, Wallenstein SL, Rogers AG, et al. Narcotics in the elderly. Med Clin N Am 1982;66:1079–1089.
88. Anderson G, Jensen NH, Christup L, Hansen SH, Sjogren P. Pain, sedation and morphine metabolism in cancer patients during long-term treatment with sustained-release morphine. Palliat Med 2002;16:107–114.
89. Smith MT. Neuroexcitatory effects of morphine and hydromorphone: evidence implicating the 3-glucuronide metabolites. Clin Exp Pharmacol Physiol 2000;27:524–528.
90. Wright AW, Mather LE, Smith MT. Hydromorphone-3-glucuronide: a more potent neuroexcitant than its structural analogue, morphine-3 glucuronide. Life Sci 2001;69:409–420.
91. Menten J, Desmedt M, Lossignol D, Mullie A. Longitudinal follow-up of TTS-fentanyl use in patients with cancer-related pain: results of a compassionate–use study with special focus on elderly patients. Curr Med Res Opin 2002:18:488–498.
92. Radbruch L, Sabatowski R, Petzke F, Brunsch-Radbruch A, Grond S, Lehman KA. Transdermal fentanyl for the management of cancer pain: a survey of 1005 patients. Palliat Med 2001;15:309–321.
93. Coluzzi PH, Schwartzberg L, Conroy JD, Charapata S, Gay M, Busch MA, et al. Breakthrough cancer pain: a randomized trial comparing oral transmucosal fentanyl citrate (OTFC) and morphine sulfate immediate release (MSIR). Pain 2001;91:123–130.
94. Korrnick CA, Kilborn MJ, Santiago-Palma J, Schulman G, Thaler HT, Keefe DL, et al. QTC interval prolongation associated with intravenous methadone. Pain 2003;105:499–506.
95. Morley JS, Bridson J, Nash TP, Miles JB, White S, Makin MK. Low-dose methadone has an analgesic effect in neuropathic pain: a double-blind randomized controlled crossover trial. Palliat Med 2003;9:73–83.
96. Popp B, Portenoy RK. Management of chronic pain in the elderly: pharmacology of opioids and other analgesic drugs. In: Ferrell BR, Ferrell BA, eds. Pain in the Elderly. Seattle: IASP Press, 1996:21–34.
97. Hanks G, Cherny N, Fallon M, eds. Opioid analgesic therapy. In: Oxford Textbook of Palliative Medicine, 3rd ed., Oxford: Oxford University Press, 2004:316–342.
98. Bruera E, Driver L, Barnes EA, Wiley J, Shen L, Palmer JL, et al. Patient-controlled methylphenidate for the management of fatigue in patients with advanced cancer: a preliminary report. J Clin Oncol 2003;21:4439–4443.
99. Derby S, Portenoy R. Assessment and management of opioid-induced constipation. In: Portenoy RK, Bruera E, eds. Topics in Palliative Care, Vol. 1. New York: Oxford University Press, 1997: 95–112.
100. American Geriatric Society. The management of persistent pain in older person. 2002. AGS panel on persistent pain in older person. J Am Geriatr Soc 2002;50:S205-S224.
101. Max MB. Antidepressants and analgesics. In: Fields HL, Liebeskind JC, eds. Progress in Pain Research and Management, Vol 1. Seattle: IASP Press, 1994:229–246.
102. Leo RJ, Singh A. Pain management in the elder: Use of psychopharmacologic agents. Ann Long-Term Care 2002;10:37–45.
103. Lipman AG. Analgesic drugs for neuropathic and sympathetically maintained pain. Clin Geriatr Med 1996;12:501–515.
104. Lipman AG. Analgesic drugs for neuropathic and sympathetically maintained pain. Clin Geriatr Med 1996;12:501–515.
105. Rowbotham M, Harden N, Stacey B, Bernstein P, Magnus-Miller L. Gabapentin for the treatment of postherpetic neuralgia: a randomized controlled trial. JAMA 1998;280:1837–1842.
106. Ahn SH, Park HW, Lee BS, Moon HW, Jang SH, Sakong J, et al. Gabapentin effect on neuropathic pain compared among patients with spinal cord injury and different durations of symptoms. Spine 2003;28:341–346; discussion 346–347.

107. Garcia-Borreguero D, Larrosa O, de la Llave Y, Verger K, Masramon X, Hernandez G. Treatment of restless legs syndrome with gabapentin: a double-blind, cross-over study. (comment). Neurology 2002;59:1573–1579.
108. Portenoy RK, Prager G. Pain management: pharmacological approaches. In: von Gunten CF, ed., Palliative Care and Rehabilitation of Cancer Patients. Boston: Kluwer Academic Publishers, 1999:1–29.
109. Nelson KA, Park K, Robinovitz E, Tsigos C, Mas MB. High-dose oral dextromethorphan versus placebo in painful diabetic neuropathy and postherpetic neuralgia. Neurology 1997;48: 1212–1218.
110. Coyle N, Layman-Goldstein M. Pain assessment and management in palliative care. In: Matzo M, Sherman D, eds., Palliative Care Nursing: Quality Care to the End of Life. New York: Springer, 2001:422.
111. Watanabe S, Bruera E. Corticosteroids as adjuvant analgesics. J Pain Symptom Manage 1994;9: 442–445.
112. Mercadante S, Fulfaro F, Casuccio A. The use of corticosteroids in home palliative care. Support Cancer Care 2001;9:386–389.
113. Woolridge JE, Anderson CM, Perry MC. Corticosteroids in advanced cancer. Oncology (Huntington) 2001;15:225–234; discussion 234–236.
114. Ettinger AB, Portenoy RK. The use of corticosteroids in the treatment of symptoms associated with cancer. J Pain Symptom Manage 1988;3:99–103.
115. Feuer DJ, Broadley KE. Corticosteroids for the resolution of malignant bowel obstruction in advanced gynaecological and gastrointestinal cancer. Cochrane Database Syst Rev. 2000: CD001219.
116. Sloan P, Basta M, Storey P, von Guten C. Mexiletine as an adjuvant analgesic for the management of neuropathic pain. Anesth Analg 1999;89:760–761.
117. Galer BS, Jensen MP, Ma T, Davis PS, Rowbotham MC. The lidocaine patch 5% effectively treats all neuropathic pain qualities: results of a randomized, double-blind, vehicle-controlled, 3-week efficacy study with use of the neuropathic pain scale. Clin J Pain 2002;Sept–Oct:297–300.
118. Devers A, Galer BS. Topical lidocaine patch relieves a variety of neuropathic pain conditions; an open label study. Clin J Pain 2000;Sep 16:205–208.
119. Ferrini R, Paice JA. Infusional lidocaine for severe and/or neuropathic pain. J Support Oncol 2004;2:90–94.
120. Walker K, Medhurst SJ, Kidd BL, Glatt M, Bowes M, Patel S, et al. Disease modifying and anti-nociceptive effects of the bisphosphonate, zoledronic acid in a model of bone cancer pain. Pain 2002;100:219–229.
121. Rizzoli R. Bisphosphonates and reduction of skeletal events in patients with bone metastatic breast cancer. Ann Oncol 2004; 15:700–701.
122. Hortobagyi GN, Theriault RL, Porter L, Blayney D, Lipton A, Sinoff C, Wheeler H, Simeone JF, Knight RD. Efficacy of pamidronate in reducing skeletal complications in patients with breast cancer and lytic bone metastases. Protocol 19 Aredia Breast Cancer Study Group. N Engl J Med 1996;335:1785–1791.
123. Gennari C, Agnusdei D, Camporeale A. Use of calcitonin in the treatment of bone pain associated with osteoporosis. Calcif Tissue Int 1991;49(Suppl 2):s9-s13.
124. Giammarile F, Mognetti T, Resche I. Bone pain palliation with strontium-89 in cancer patients with bone metastases. Q J Nucl Med 2001;45:78–83.
125. Rhiner M, Ferrell BR, Ferrell BA, Grant MM. A structured nondrug intervention program for cancer pain. Cancer Pract 1993; 1:137–143.
126. Weinrich SP, Weinrich MC. The effect of massage on pain in cancer patients. Appl Nurs Res 1990;3a:140–145.
127. Farrell MJ, Katz B, Helme RD. The impact of dementia on the pain experience. Pain 1996;67:7–15.
128. Hurley AC, Volicer BJ, Hanrahan PA, et al. Assessment of discomfort in advanced Alzheimer patients. Res Nurs Health 1992; 15:369–377.
129. Porter FL, Malhotra KM, Wolf CM, et al. Dementia and response to pain in the elderly. Pain 1996;68:413–421.
130. Sengstaken EA, King SA. The problem of pain and its detection among geriatric nursing home residents. J Am Geriatr Soc 1993; 41:541–544.
131. Stein WM, Ferrell BA. Pain in the nursing home. Clin Geriatr Med 1996;12:601–613.
132. Kaasalainen S, Middleton J, Knezacek S, et al. Pain and cognitive status in the institutionalized elderly: perceptions and interventions. J Gerontol Nurs 1998;24:24–31.
133. Parmelee A. Pain in cognitively impaired older persons. Clin Geriatr Med 1996;12:473–487.
134. Ferrell BA, Ferrell BR, Rivera L. Pain in cognitively impaired nursing home patients. J Pain Symptom Manage 1995;10:591–598.
135. Ferrell BR, Grant M, Chan J, Ahn C, Ferrell BA. The impact of cancer pain education to family caregivers of elderly patients. Oncol Nurs Forum 1995;22:1211–1218.
136. Breitbart W, Bruera E, Harvey C, Lynch M. Neuropsychiatric syndromes and psychological symptoms in patients with advanced cancer. J Pain Symptom Manage 1995;10:131–141.
137. Massie MJ, Holland J, Glass E. Delirium in terminally ill cancer patients. Am J Psychiatry 1983;140;1048–1050.
138. Foreman MD. Acute confusion in the elderly. Ann Rev Nurs Res 1993;11:3–30.
139. Lipowski Z. Delirium in the elderly patient. N Engl J Med 1989;2:578–582.
140. Bruerea E, Miller L, McCallion J, Macmillan K, Krefting L, Hanson J. Cognitive failure in patients with terminal cancer: A prospective study. J Pain Symptom Manage 1992;7:192–195.
141. Inouye S, Charpentier PA, et al. Precipitating factors for delirium in hospitalized elderly persons: predictive model and interrelationship with baseline vulnerability. JAMA 1996;275:852–857.
142. Francis J, Martin D, Kapoor WN. A prospective study of delirium in hospitalized elderly. JAMA 1990;267:827–831.
143. Rockwood K. Acute confusion in elderly medical patients. J Am Geriatric Soc 1989;37:150–154.
144. Schor JD, Levkogg SE, Lipsitz LA, et al. Risk factors for delirium in hospitalized elderly. JAMA 1992;267:827–831.
145. Ljubisavljevic V, Kelly B. Risk factors for development of delirium among oncology patients. Gen Hosp Psychiatry 2003;25:345–352.
146. O'Keefe ST, Lavan JN. Clinical significance of delirium subtypes in older people. Age Ageing 1999;28:115–119.
147. Lawlor PG, Fainsinger RL, Bruera ED. Delirium at the end of life: critical issues in clinical practice and research. JAMA 2000; 284:2427–2429.
148. Finlayson RE, Hurt RD, Davis LJ Jr, Morse RM et al. Alcoholism in elderly persons: a study of the psychiatric and psychosocial features of 216 inpatients. Mayo Clin Proc 1988;63:761–768.
149. Folstein MF, Folstein SE, McHugh PE. "Mini-Mental Status": a practical method for yielding the cognitive state of patients for clinicians. J Psych Res 1975;12:189–198.

150. Costa PT, William TF, Somerfield M, et al. Recognition and Initial Assessment of Alzheimer's Disease and Related Dementias. Clinical Practice Guideline No. 19. Pub. No. 97–0702. 1996. Rockville, MD: U.S. Department of Health and Human Services, Public Health Service, Agency for Health Care Policy and Research.
151. Breitbart W, Jacobsen PB. Psychiatric symptom management in terminal care. Clin Geriatr Med 1996;12:329–347.
152. Breitbart W, Tremblay A, Gibson C. An open trial of olanzapin for the treatment of delirium in hospitalized cancer patients. Psychosomatics 2002;43:175–182.
153. Seeman T, Guralnik J, Kaplan G, Knudsen L, Cohen R. The health consequence of multiple morbidity in the elderly. The Alameda County Study. J Aging Health 1989;1:5066.
154. Stein W. Barriers to effective pain management in the nursing home. In: Ferrell B, ed. Pain in the Nursing Home. Clinics in Geriatric Medicine Pain Management. Philadelphia: W.B. Saunders, 1996:604.
155. Walker MK, Marquis DF, NICHE Faculty. Ensuring medication safety for older adults. In: Abraham I, Bottrell M, Fulmer T, Mezey MD, eds. Geriatric Nursing Protocols for Best Practice. New York: Springer Publishing Co., Inc., 1996:131–144.
156. Field M, Cassel C, Committee on Care at the End of Life, Institute of Medicine. Approaching Death: Improving Care at the End of Life. Washington, DC: National Academy Press, 1977:50–86.
157. Eliopoulos C. Respiratory problems. In: Gerontological Nursing, 4th ed. Philadelphia: J.B. Lippincott, 1996:277–290.
158. Storey P, Knight CF, Unipac Four. Management of selected non-pain symptoms in the terminally ill. A self-study program. Gainesville, FL: American Academy of Hospice and Palliative Medicine, 1996:25–32.
159. Ripamonti C. Management of dyspnea in advanced cancer patients. Support Care Cancer 1999;7:233–243.
160. Tobin M. Dyspnea: pathophysiologic basis, clinical presentation, and management. Arch Intern Med 1990;150:1604–1613.
161. Kuebler KK. Hospice and Palliative Care Clinical Practice Protocol: Dyspnea. Hosp Nurs Assoc 1996:1–28.
162. McCaffery M, Pasero C. Pain: Clinical Manual. St. Louis: Mosby, 1999:179–180.

36

Anne Hughes

Poor, Homeless, and Underserved Populations

Last year at this time I was locked up in a psych ward because I'd tried to kill myself and today I'm fighting for my life. Isn't that ironic?—Matt, a 58-year-old man recently diagnosed with stage IV squamous cell cancer of the hypopharynx, who just completed chemotherapy and radiation therapy after surgery, and refused hospice referral

- ***Key Points***
- *Poor people are at risk for a bad death.*
- *People whose lives have been filled with physical and emotional deprivation may be suspicious of attempts to engage them in "shared" decision-making to limit therapy, regardless of its likely benefits or burdens.*
- *Some poor people have comorbidities (e.g., mental illness, substance abuse, and other chronic diseases) and other social characteristics that have marginalized them in society.*
- *Poor people's interactions with the health care system are frequently marked by rejection, shame, and lack of continuity of care.*

Poverty is inextricably linked to increased morbidity, premature mortality, and limited access to both preventive health care and ongoing medical care. Beyond the medical outcomes of poverty, the individual and community costs are substantial and often invisible. People who are poor constitute a vulnerable population, a term used in community health to describe social groups at greater risk for adverse health outcomes. The root causes of this vulnerability typically are low socioeconomic status and a lack of access to resources.[1] The Institute of Medicine's report, which evaluated racial and ethnic disparities in health care, failed to address the role of poverty in disparities.[2] However, the role of poverty in contributing to inequalities, independent of race and ethnicity, is difficult to decipher because class and race are often closely intertwined.[3,4] Some believe poverty may be most responsible for disparities in health care.[4]

While much has been written about end-of-life care in the United States,[5–8] with some recent exceptions, little has been said about those in our society who live at its margins, such as the urban poor.[9–12a] To be poor and to have a progressive, life-threatening illness presents more challenges than either one of these conditions alone. As Taipale elegantly notes, "Poverty means the opportunities and choices most basic to human development are denied [p. 54]."[13] Consider the following questions: What type of death would a person hope for who doesn't have a home or lives in a room without a phone or a toilet or a kitchen? What are the meanings of life-threatening illness and death when premature death is an all-too-common part of life? What matters at the end of life if most of your life has been spent trying to survive day to day? All of these questions, in part, introduce us to the worlds of the poor who are confronting a life-threatening illness. Physical, psychological, and spiritual deprivation isn't all that poor people contend with—deprivation also harms the moral self and the ability both to act and to live autonomously.[14]

The purpose of this chapter is to examine the characteristics of the poor as an underserved population that place them at particular risk when palliative care is needed. In particular, this chapter looks at a subset of the poor who are homeless or marginally housed, and how this affects both access to and quality of care at the end of life. The experience of being poor is not a single experience, as poor persons are as diverse a population as the nonpoor. The discussion in this chapter focuses on inner-city or urban poor, who are often marginally housed or homeless. Case studies are used to illustrate the concepts discussed and to demonstrate the need for the more research to guide practice. The cases described are composite and reflective of the author's practice in a metropolitan-area public health system that is greatly impacted by HIV/AIDS and by homelessness. As a result, these cases are not generalizable to all the poor or even to all the homeless. Being poor is only one of several characteristics that affect health status and limit access to resources. Persons with many vulnerabilities (e.g., being poor AND a member of a minority community, elderly, or having other medical problems) are at the greatest risk for adverse outcomes at the end of life.[15]

Epidemiology of Poverty in the United States

More than 34 million Americans are poor. The poverty line established by the federal government is based on annual income. In 2002, a single adult was considered poor if his or her income was less than $9,359, and a family of four (with 3 children under 18 years) was considered poor if their annual income was less than $18,307.[16] Thirty-four million Americans represent just over 12% of the entire population of the United States. Table 36–1 lists states whose poverty level exceeds the national average. Many poverty experts, however, believe the federal definition of poverty underestimates the true prevalence of poverty in the United States. For example, the poverty line (annual income) does not capture cost-of-living differences across the country or out-of-pocket medical costs.

The faces of the poor in the United States disproportionately include persons of color, children, and female-headed families.[16] African Americans have the highest rates of poverty in the United States (24.1%), followed by Hispanics (21.8%), Asian/Pacific Islanders (10.3%), and whites (8.0%) according to the U.S. Census Bureau Report for 2002.[16] Children have greater rates of poverty than young and middle-aged adults and the elderly. Almost 50% of the families living in poverty in the United States are headed by a woman.[16]

While poverty is not confined to urban areas, as evident in Table 36–1, 78% of the poor live in or near the more populous metropolitan areas, and 40% of all the poor live in inner (or central) cities.[16] Most of the poor have access to some type of housing or shelter, even if the basic accommodations (telephone, cooking and refrigeration, heat, water, private toilet, and bathing facilities) are inadequate. However, for a small subset, housing is marginal or unavailable. This subset is the focus of the following discussion.

Table 36–1
States Whose Poverty Rates Exceed National Average

State	People in Poverty (%)
Alabama	14.6
Arizona	13.3
Arkansas	18
California	12.8
District of Columbia	16.8
Kentucky	13.1
Louisiana	17
Mississippi	17.6
Montana	13.7
New Mexico	17.8
New York	14
North Carolina	13.1
Oklahoma	14.7
South Carolina	13.5
Tennessee	14.2
Texas	15.3
West Virginia	16

Source: Proctor & Dalaker (2003), reference 16.

Definition and Prevalence of Homelessness

Homelessness is defined in the Stewart McKinney Homeless Act as a condition under which persons "lack fixed, regular and adequate night-time residence" or reside in temporary housing such as shelters and welfare hotels.[17] Calculating the number of Americans homeless or marginally housed is extremely difficult. Most cross-sectional studies fail to capture persons transiently homeless, the hidden homeless staying with family members, those living in cars or encampments, and others living in single-room occupancy hotels (SROs), sometimes known as welfare hotels. Additionally many of the poor and, in particular, the homeless, avoid contact with social and health services.

According to the National Coalition for the Homeless, every night between 400,000 to 800,000 Americans are homeless; 3.5 million Americans experience homelessness in a given year.[18] Persons who are homeless are not members of a homogenous group. Some are street people and chronically homeless, while others are homeless because of a financial crisis that put them out of stable housing. Street people may be more reluctant to accept services and may have much higher rates of concurrent substance abuse and mental illness, that is, the so-called dual diagnosed.[19] Homeless persons frequently are also persons of color, veterans, victims of domestic violence, the mentally ill, and substance abusers.[20] While the rates of mental illness and substance abuse are higher in the homeless than persons who are stably housed, assuming that all the poor, or, for that matter, all homeless suffer from these problems leads only to stereotypes. Domestic violence, mental illness, and substance abuse are not confined to the poor; hence, poverty does not cause these problems, although it may exacerbate them.

Health Problems Associated with Homelessness and Poverty

A number of health problems are associated with homelessness. Many of these problems are related to environmental factors such as exposure to weather conditions, poorly ventilated spaces, unsafe hotels and street conditions, and high-crime neighborhoods, where the poor tend to live.[21] These health problems (Table 36–2) include malnutrition, lack of access to shelter and bathing facilities, problems related to drug and alcohol use, chronic mental illness, and violence-related injuries. One fifth of the homeless have a major psychiatric illness.[20] About one in three homeless persons abuse drugs and alcohol.[20] Drugs and alcohol are sometimes used to self-medicate distressing psychiatric symptoms (e.g., anxiety, depression).

A recent meta-analysis of the influence of income inequality and population health concluded that although the direct effects of poverty on population health were not evident, the individual effects of poverty on health status are irrefutable.[22] Consider the case of coronary artery disease (CAD): the link between onset of CAD and low socioeconomic status (SES) has been established and is believed to be related to lifestyle factors, such as dietary habits, smoking, and physical activity.[23] Recent research suggests that poor cardiac outcomes among the poor may also be related to limited access to standard medical care.[23,24] Persons who are poor, on average, have shorter life expectancies than those whose incomes are higher.[25] Men in Harlem have life expectancy rates comparable to those living in developing countries, such as Bangladesh.[4]

Poverty, Life-Threatening Illness, and Quality of Life

Poor people endure a heavier burden of cancer according to a report from the American Cancer Society.[4] The key findings of the impact of poverty on cancer care, irrespective of race and ethnicity, are listed in Table 36–3. In general, poor people encounter substantial barriers to obtaining quality cancer care, experience more pain and suffering, and are more fatalistic about cancer.

Understanding the role race and ethnicity play in the end-of-life experience of the urban poor is complex. Nevertheless, three studies examined the impact of economic resources on quality of life for persons with life-threatening illnesses.[26-28] Being poor (defined as having an annual income of less than $20,000) negatively affected the quality of life reported by mostly white (85%) men newly diagnosed with prostate cancer, though low income was not related to quality of life over time. However, the lack of health insurance did predict worse quality of life for men with prostate cancer over time but not at baseline.[27] In a qualitative study of heterosexual couples in which only one partner was HIV-positive, the investigators were surprised to learn the "benefits" of having AIDS in providing poor persons with access to subsidized housing, food, and other social services.[26] Indeed, these researchers noted that, given policy changes in welfare programs, having an AIDS diagnosis was a commodity that brought with it benefits

Table 36–2
Health Problems Associated with Homelessness

Causes	Manifestations
Malnutrition	Dental problems, tuberculosis, wasting
Lack of shelter and access to bathing facilities	Skin infections, lice, cellulitis, podiatric problems, hypothermia, tuberculosis
Drug and alcohol use	Overdose, seizures, delirium, sexually transmitted infections (such as HIV, hepatitis B, hepatitis C), trauma, falls, cirrhosis, heroin nephropathy, esophageal varices
Chronic mental illness	Paranoid ideation, antisocial behaviors, psychosis, suicide
Violence-related injuries	Assaults, homicides, rape

Table 36–3
Poverty and Cancer: Findings from an American Cancer Society Report

- Poor people lacking access to quality health care are more likely to die of cancer than nonpoor.
- Poor people experience greater cancer-related pain and suffering.
- Poor people facing significant barriers to getting health insurance often do not seek necessary care if they are unable to pay for it.
- Poor people and their families make extraordinary sacrifices to obtain and pay for care.
- Cancer education and outreach efforts are insensitive and irrelevant to the lives of many poor people.
- Fatalism about cancer is common among the poor and often prevents them from accessing care.

Source: Adapted from Freeman (2004), reference 4.

that the poor were otherwise ineligible to receive. In other words, for poor people, having AIDS improved their quality of life. In a cross-sectional study of 212 adults with heart failure who were predominantly female (68%) and black (53%), quality of life was not related to physiological measures of heart function, but was correlated with greater income, social support, and positive health beliefs.[28] Economic resources were associated with improved quality of life.

In his recently published book, *Dancing with Broken Bones: Portraits of Death and Dying Among Inner City Poor*, Moller poignantly recounts the stories of poor patients followed by an oncology clinic in a midwest city. His insights about the suffering of the urban poor are exquisite: ". . . the dying poor are the quintessential violators of the American dream; they live in the shame of poverty and with the unpleasantness of dying [p. 10]."[10] Since much of a person's "worth" in American society is connected with social status indicators such as occupation and income, the poor represent those who haven't made it. Being poor becomes a matter of personal failure rather than a social problem.[29] From Moller's longitudinal qualitative study of poor inner-city patients, their families, and their health care providers, the researcher drew a number of conclusions that are listed in Table 36–4. His work can perhaps be summed up by saying that the indignities of being poor in America are only intensified when that person is also dying. Unlike persons who are not poor, dying is not always feared in the same way, as it may represent freedom from the misery of living.

Table 36–4
Insights About the Dying Poor

- Poverty inflicts substantial harm throughout life.
- Poverty exacerbates indignity and suffering throughout dying.
- Patients/families are often mistrustful and angry about the care received.
- Patients, at the same time, are often grateful for the care received.
- Spirituality plays an important role in providing strength and resilience when dying.
- Social isolation increases suffering.
- Hidden and sometimes unexpected sources of support can emerge from family and community.
- The emergency room is the front door to health care.
- The organization of medical care is frequently fragmented and lacks continuity.
- Funerals are important rituals, and their cost creates enormous stress for survivors.

Source: Dancing with Broken Bones: Portraits of Death and Dying Among Innercity Poor by David Wendell Moller, © 2000 by Oxford University Press, Inc. Used by permission of Oxford University Press, Inc.

Clinical Presentations of Advanced Disease in the Poor

Persons who are poor frequently present with advanced disease. In addition to the late-stage disease presentation, many have significant comorbidities that affect both the palliation of symptoms and the course and treatment of underlying illnesses. These clinical management issues usually occur within the context of complex psychosocial situations, as the following case illustrates:

CASE STUDY
Lana, a Patient with AIDS

Lana, a 43-year-old white woman, has been living in a shelter since her boyfriend died 18 months ago. She was diagnosed with AIDS 4 years ago after a hospitalization for *Pneumocystis carinii* pneumonia. Lana was shocked and ashamed by this diagnosis because she didn't suspect she was HIV positive. Since that time, she has had repeated hospitalizations, including several for delirium secondary to crack and alcohol use. Currently Lana is taking four antiretroviral medications through a directly observed therapy program (DOT) arranged by her case manager. In addition to AIDS and alcohol and crack abuse, her medical problems include seizure disorder, depression, liver disease, hepatitis B and C infections, and chronic pain from a motor vehicle accident, which fractured her cervical spine and required a metal plate to stabilize the fracture. Lana has lost touch with her family; she is one of 8 children who grew up in the Midwest. Her father was an alcoholic; both of her parents died years ago. Lana had a daughter when she was 15 years old but hasn't seen her daughter in 14 years, when Lana was put in jail for drug use. She doesn't know where her daughter is living. None of her family members know about Lana's lifestyle or about her AIDS diagnosis, and she is adamant that they not be told.

Comorbidities, especially those related to drug use, complicate symptom management and other medical management.[30] As Lana's case study points out, there were several competing factors that may influence her providers' willingness to aggressively manage her pain. Persons known to be chemically dependent are often denied treatment for pain because of providers' concerns of aberrant or drug-hoarding behaviors. Will Lana take the medication as ordered? Is she likely to sell her opioids for cocaine? Are her medications safe in the shelter? Does she have a place to keep them or are others likely to steal them? Some providers even question the use of opioids for any nonmalignant pain syndrome. Who will prescribe opioid medications? If Lana is seen in a teaching clinic, will she need to negotiate the need for analgesia with each new doctor that rotates through? Does she have money or insurance to pay for the medications? Is there a pharmacy near the shelter that carries them? According to a study by Morrison and colleagues,[31] pharmacies in predominantly nonwhite neighborhoods in New York City were less likely to carry opioids for pain management than were pharmacies in neighborhood serving predominantly white communities. Most shelters are located in inner cities, not in middle class or affluent communities, where more whites live. Poor social conditions, criminal activity, and the threat of violence are significant barriers to effective pain management for persons with life-threatening illnesses.[12] Lana is receiving DOT antiretroviral therapy, and, therefore, she is being followed carefully. Perhaps this support system could be enlisted to oversee her pain management and her overall safety and well-being.

Access to treatment is a significant factor that influences symptom management for this population. For example, if an antiemetic prescribed to relieve the chronic nausea experienced by a poor person with pancreatic cancer is not covered on the Medicaid formulary, or the person is not eligible for any drug-assistance program, the range of medications used to manage the nausea will be severely limited. Additionally, use of high-tech methods to control symptoms are probably not an option for the person who lives in a tent encampment. Most poor persons are institutionalized to manage uncontrolled symptoms and terminal care that cannot be managed sufficiently on the street or in the shelter.[10]

The management of symptoms associated with progressive illness is further complicated by end-organ diseases, such as liver or renal disease, that may alter the pharmacokinetics of medications used to palliate symptoms. Clinically significant drug–drug and drug–nutrient interactions are common with antiretrovirals that Lana is taking. Determining whether a patient is experiencing an adverse drug reaction is not easy when the person has comorbidities, has rapidly progressive disease, is malnourished, or may be continuing to use alcohol or other substances.

Comorbidities also affect the health care providers' ability to realistically estimate prognosis and the nature of symptoms or problems that might occur down the road. Charting the dying trajectory for the chronic progressive illness may be conceivable, but superimposing the acute illnesses and injuries that the very poor live with and manage creates jagged peaks and valleys in a downward course. How quickly the life-threatening illness will progress becomes a prognostication puzzle; some persons living on the street truly seem to have had nine lives. In addition to HIV disease, Lana's liver disease may limit her survival. If she resumes using drugs and alcohol, her addiction could also hasten her death.

There is another issue to consider with Lana— adherence to treatment. Despite the prevalence of substance abuse among the poor, lack of attention to self-care activities cannot be assumed in all drug users. Some homeless persons who use drugs manage complex HIV antiretroviral regimens that require scrupulous attention to when to eat, which other medications may or may not be taken at the same time, and the necessary several-times-a-day dosing.[32] Race, class, and housing status cannot be used as surrogate predictors of who abuses drugs and alcohol or who will adhere or not adhere to treatment demands.

Psychosocial Factors Influencing Palliative Care Available to the Poor and Homeless

Health care professionals committed to supporting patients' right to a "good death" may be challenged when working with the poor and the homeless. The good death is described as: (1) free from avoidable distress and suffering, (2) in accord with the patient and family's wishes, and (3) consistent with clinical, cultural, and ethical standards.[5] Bad deaths, in contrast, are accompanied by neglect, violence, or unwanted and senseless medical interventions.[5] Persons who are poor or homeless are at risk for bad deaths. Many persons have had episodic contact with the health care system during acute illnesses or life-threatening trauma and may wind up receiving life-saving therapies such as mechanical ventilation, vasopressors, dialysis, and other therapies. All too often, the client does not have an advance directive or a surrogate decision-maker to articulate his or her wishes. Furthermore, in the absence of a competent patient or family directing otherwise, the technological imperative of hospitals and physicians in training may see saving a life at any cost of greater value.[5] Nevertheless, what constitutes a good or bad death is a question that can only be answered by the individual person and cannot be predicted based on group membership or economic resources.[33]

Basic survival needs (food, shelter, clothing, protection) are of primary concern to the poor, often of greater and more pressing importance than the existential crisis of facing one's own mortality. Seeing others die prematurely, often under violent or disturbing circumstances, may be an all-too-common experience for this population.[34] Table 36–5 lists challenges to providing a good death in this population. The lack of resources, both economic and human, limit the palliative options available to the person who is poor. In the movie *The Wizard of Oz*, Dorothy's refrain, "There's no place like home, there's no place like home," speaks of an almost faraway magical experience that many who are poor and dying cannot even imagine. Housing is so essential to health that, for those of us who do not worry about having a roof over our heads at night, its importance is taken for granted. Many persons who are poor and don't have enough to get by are often trying to figure out how to find a place to stay. And for those with a place, the concerns may be keeping the utilities (lights, heat, water) on and having enough money for other needs.

In addition to basic survival needs of the poor that influence their end-of-life experiences are their relationships with the health care professionals who take care of them. Health care professionals can and often do stigmatize patients for their appearance or lack of hygiene. Sometimes the presence of

Table 36–5
Psychosocial Challenges in Providing Palliative Care to the Poor

- Patient is homeless or has unstable or unsafe housing, with inadequate basic facilities (phone, private bathroom, refrigerator, and cooking facilities).
- Getting to appointments is difficult without reliable transportation.
- Lack of money limits options and often contributes to chaotic lives.
- Patient has fragile or nonexistent support system (e.g., no primary caregiver, caregiver who is unable to provide necessary care, caregiver also sick, no surrogate or proxy decision-maker, estranged from family, history of family violence or abuse).
- Many poor people who have encountered rejection or shame when accessing health care services avoid contact and are slow to trust even well-meaning health care professionals.
- Poor people who obtain health care usually do so without benefit of a long-term relationship with a primary care provider or a case manager familiar with their history can help them navigate a complex care-delivery system.
- Most health care or specialized palliative care services are geographically remote from where poor people live. Some service providers curtail services to the poorest communities because of concerns about staff safety.
- Behavioral problems (e.g., drug hoarding, selling prescriptions, hostility, psychiatric illness, substance abuse) can affect patient relationships with health care providers.
- It is difficult to assess the decision-making capacity and goals of patients who are cognitively impaired, intoxicated, or brain injured.
- Many patients, including the poor, are asked to make treatment decisions without sufficient information about the implications of the decisions, and in the context of a patient–provider relationship that has enormous power inbalances.
- There is little evidence available on which to base therapeutic interventions because this population is not included in clinical trials.

Source: Adapted from Moller (2004), reference 10.

body odor leads to rejection. Historical events and power differential in patient-provider roles can also affect such relationships. For example, the African-American experience with the medical care system includes the Tuskegee experiment and other instances of abuse. Many African Americans feel betrayed by the predominantly white medical care system and believe their trust in the system has been violated.[35]

Many of the poor receive care in public health care systems or indigent care settings that often serve as teaching hospitals, and where continuity of care is an illusion.[10] Additionally, discussions about limiting therapy or do-not-resuscitate (DNR) decisions may be regarded as an attempt by the dominant culture to withhold possibly life-sustaining therapy. Some individuals and communities fear being treated "like a guinea pig" and refuse to participate in clinical trials when offered. The sometimes conflicted relationships that poor people have with health care providers and systems related to care at the end of life is again powerfully captured by Moller:

> . . . Perhaps even more poignant than the anger and disappointment of dissatisfied patients is the absence of resentment on the part of those who have every reason to be upset with the care they receive. It is fair to suggest that, for some, this lack of assertiveness and anger has its roots deep within the experience of poverty. Living every day with chaos, stress, and the indignity of inner-city poverty creates, for many, a level of tolerance that most of us would find intolerable. In this regard, it is not unusual for patients to accept care with which they are unhappy because they have accepted a lifetime of economic and social indignities about which they are unhappy. In a strange sense, many patients often felt their suffering in the face of disease was just, "one more bad thing to endure." Thus despite many variations in form and meaning, disease and dying are often borne with a sense of equanimity that flows from constant adjustments required by a life lived in poverty [p. 1].[10]

CASE STUDY
Matt, a Patient with Squamous Cell Cancer

Matt, a 58-year-old African-American man, grew up in Georgia. He was drafted after high school. When he finished his military service in Vietnam, he settled in a West Coast city far away from his family. He lost touch with his family after years of "serious" alcohol and drug abuse, despite periods of sobriety. Matt's other medical problems include hypertension, posttraumatic stress disorder, and an 80-pack-year history of smoking. Matt had been sober for 5 years until he experienced flashbacks of Vietnam following the invasion of Iraq, at which time he tried to hang himself. He was hospitalized in a psych unit and responded to antidepressants and group therapy. Six months later, after persistent sore throat, difficulty swallowing, and weight loss, he went to a drop-in clinic at the food bank. He was sent to the emergency room at a teaching hospital and was eventually diagnosed with stage IV squamous cell cancer of the hypopharynx. Matt had a radical neck dissection, chemotherapy, and radiation therapy. He agreed to placement in a nursing home while he was receiving chemotherapy and radiation therapy (RT). Matt returned to the oncology clinic for follow-up for an enlarged neck mass, and the white oncology fellow told him that he suspected tumor recurrence and wondered if Matt had thought about hospice. Matt became angry and expressed doubt that this doctor knew what he was doing, because the ENT doctor (also white) had told him the mass may be inflammation caused by the RT. He was clear that he was not ready to die and insisted that he was not afraid. Matt felt like he had gotten his life back and wasn't ready to "cash it in yet—I don't want anything to do with hospice." His supports included a local church that ministers to the urban poor, his AA sponsor, and a case manager who has followed him since his hospitalization.

Matt's story raises a number of complex issues influenced by culture, historical discrimination, and the process of end-of-life decision-making. For some African Americans, according to Crawley, death is seen as a struggle to overcome and, for others, a welcomed friend that precedes going home to heaven.[35] Matt was not ready to go home; while his church and religion were sources of support, he regarded death as a struggle to be overcome. Matt received care in a public hospital from an oncology fellow whose different race, education, and occupation may have contributed to different world views. When to introduce the option of hospice is difficult. For some patients, poor and nonpoor alike, hospice is equated with giving up, with not having hope. Would Matt's response had been different if the fellow had conferred with the ENT physician about his prognosis, and Matt was receiving one message about his progress? What did Matt understand the goals of treatments to be when he agreed to chemo and RT after surgery? Not surprisingly, Matt held onto the contradictory assessment of the ENT physician, who was more hopeful that the mass may be a complication of radiation therapy. Who would not hold onto hope in a situation of advanced disease? Matt is in the curious position of having been ambivalent about living. One year earlier, he had attempted to commit suicide, and now his goal was to live, surely not to die gently. How does a person who has been receiving aggressive treatment to control disease shift to an approach whose goal is a peaceful and dignified death? Many of these questions are not unique to the poor who are dying. Finally, hospice services, while recognized as the standard for end-of-life care, are infrequently used by African Americans.[6]

Where and How Homeless People Die

Limited data are available regarding the socioeconomic factors, places of death, and immediate causes of death of the homeless.[36–38] Most poor people, like those who are not poor, die in institutions. For those who are homeless, dying on the street or in jail is another fact of life.[39]

In 2003, 169 homeless persons died in San Francisco.[38] The profile of the homeless who died were: male (85%), average age of 42 years, and disproportionally more whites and African Americans than live in San Francisco.[36] Drug and alcohol were directly associated with 60% of these deaths. Chronic alcohol abuse and acute alcohol intoxication were also listed as causes of death in the homeless in Georgia.[40] Hypothermia was also noted as a cause of death among the homeless in Chicago and in Georgia.[40,41] Accidental deaths due to fires, falls, and pedestrian–motor vehicle accidents, plus drowning and violent deaths related to homicide and suicide were also reported in the homeless.[40]

Researchers in Boston studied the use of health care by the homeless for the year prior to their deaths.[37] Chart reviews were completed for all patients reported to the state death registry who had participated in a health care program for the homeless. The actual circumstances of the death were not studied; however, the causes of death as listed on death certificates were noted. For the 5-year study period, 558 deaths were reported. Unlike the previous results, which looked at coroner's cases, 81% of the deaths were attributed to natural causes (such as HIV-/AIDS-related conditions, heart disease, cancer, and other unspecified causes), and only 19% were due to external causes such as homicide, suicide, motor vehicle injuries, and drug overdoses.[37] Similar to the homeless who died in San Francisco, most were male (86%), between 25 and 44 years of age (56%), white (59%), and had a history of substance abuse (76% used alcohol). In addition, 28% were mentally ill.[37]

Palliative Care Models for Working with the Poor

Several hospitals serving the urban poor have developed palliative care programs to address their specific needs.[42–44] The longest-running program (since 1986) is a nurse-directed program that serves critically ill patients who are unlikely to survive hospitalization in a trauma level I hospital in the Midwest. This supportive care team has documented decreased use of health care resources and family satisfaction.[42] Another program, an interdisciplinary palliative care service based in a public hospital, follows patients and their families in the community and serves as a bridge when the patient is transferred to a nursing home or hospice for continuing care.[43] The third program was an interdisciplinary palliative care inpatient consult service that served a racially and ethnically diverse community (with many non-English–speaking patients). Despite achieving improved symptom management, increased patient/family participation in decision-making, and documentation of barriers to optimum end-of-life care, this program was eliminated because it was not able to generate sufficient revenue to sustain itself.[44]

Strategies for Working with the Poor and Homeless Who Happen to Be Dying

Working with the very poor can be challenging. Generations of internalized hopelessness, poor self-awareness, differing perceptions of time (everything seeming to take much longer), and difficulties navigating the many bureaucracies necessary to obtain services surely frustrate patients and caregivers alike.[45] Some have suggested modifying expectations to these realities and recognizing small successes as strategies to address these factors.[45]

On the other hand, for many persons who live on the street, survival skills are keenly developed. Knowing when a food bank opens, where to get clothing, when shelter-bed waiting lines begin to form, or how to get benefit checks without an address requires remarkable ingenuity and discipline. Needless to say, as with persons who are not poor, wide variations in abilities, resources, and relationships with health care professionals exist.

Obviously, stable housing is critical to providing palliative care. Researchers noted the benefits of supportive housing to minority elders in East Harlem, including better psychological outcomes and increased use of informal supports.[46] In a qualitative study of nurses who care for persons who are disenfranchised, the researcher used the metaphor of a wall to describe the separation that nurses believed their clients experienced from society.[47] The disenfranchised in this study included the poor, mentally ill, immigrants, persons with substance abuse, and/or those with stigmatizing life-threatening illness. The nurses described three key themes in how they engaged their disenfranchised clients: (1) making a human connection with the client, (2) creating a community connection for their disconnected clients, and (3) making self-care possible.

In summary, developing therapeutic relationships with the poor and homeless requires (1) expecting the person's trust to be earned over time (sometimes a long time) and not be taken for granted; (2) respecting the person's humanity, no matter how they look, what they say, and what feelings in us they evoke; (3) appreciating the person's unique story as influencing his/her response to illness and death; and, finally, (4) recognizing and addressing maladaptive behaviors.[29,39,48] Table 36–6 includes a list of helpful suggestions to reach a difficult-to-engage client.

Table 36–6
Helpful Suggestions When Engaging a Difficult-to-Engage Client

- Address anyone over 40 years of age by the title of Mr. or Ms. Ask permission to be on a first-name basis.
- Do not hestitate to shake hands.
- Be prepared to meet people who are more intelligent, more perceptive, and more wounded than you expect.
- Be tolerant. How would you react if you were in that situation?
- Don't make promises you can't keep.
- Don't take it personally.
- Taking time out helps prevent burnout.
- Get to know the community.
- If you feel you have to save the human race, do it one person at a time.
- Providing material assistance (e.g., clean socks, food, hygiene kits) opens people up.
- Usually the most difficult clients are those most in need. Throw the word *noncompliant* out of your vocabulary.
- Make eye contact. If the person does not like eye contact or becomes agitated, avoid using it.
- Keep in mind that people who live intense lives may not particularly like unasked-for physical contact.
- Don't be afraid to ask "stupid" questions; patients' answers are better than your assumptions.
- Adjust your expectations and accept small victories with satisfaction.

Source: Patchell (1997), reference 48.

In addition to the interpersonal interventions to engage the client in a therapeutic interaction, nurses are often required to become knowledgeable about the availability of and the services provided by community agencies. Knowing which agencies or services are involved with a client and communicating with them assures consistency of approach and continuity of care. Advocacy is often required to access services such as pain management, substance abuse treatment, mental health services, and social services for housing and money management. To truly improve end-of-life care for the poor, nurses need to advocate for public policies that assure access to safe and stable housing, health insurance, and client-centered, community-based primary care.

Conclusion

Providing palliative care to the poor, especially the homeless, is extremely challenging. Comorbid illnesses, illnesses associated with poverty, and clarifying the etiology of presenting symptoms may seem almost impossible at times. Psychosocial risk factors and strained relationships with health care providers sometimes result in the client receiving futile or unwanted medical interventions at an advanced stage of illness. Clarifying with a patient what constitutes a good death for him or her can be humbling when the patient tells you he or she wants simply to have shelter and to feel safe. Meeting the palliative care needs of this vulnerable population will require innovative practice and education models.

The author gratefully acknowledges the financial support of the American Cancer Society Doctoral Scholarship in Nursing, #DSCN-01-202-01-SCN and the National Institute of Nursing Research/NIH 1F31 NR079923.

REFERENCES

1. Flaskerud JH, Winslow BJ. Conceptualizing vulnerable populations health-related research. Nurs Res 1998;47:69–78.
2. Smedley BD, Stith AY, Nelson AR. Unequal Treatment: Confronting Racial and Ethnic Disparities in Health Care. Washington, D.C.: National Academy Press, 2002.
3. Koenig BA, Gates-Williams J. Understanding cultural differences in caring for dying patients. West J Med 1995;163:244–249.
4. Freeman HP. Poverty, culture and social injustice: determinants of cancer disparities. CA: A Cancer Journal for Clinicians 2004; 54:72–77.
5. Field MJ, Cassel CK. Approaching Death: Improving Care at the End of Life. Washington, D.C.: National Academy Press, 1997.
6. Foley KM, Gelband H. Improving Palliative Care for Cancer. Washington, D.C.: National Academy Press, 2001.
7. Krakauer EL, Crenner C, Fox K. Barriers to optimum end-of-life care for minority patients. J Am Geriatr Soc 2002;50: 182–190.
8. SUPPORT. A controlled trial to improve care for seriously ill hospitalized patients: the study to understand prognoses and preferences for outcomes and risks of treatment (SUPPORT). JAMA 1995;274:1591–1598.
9. Gibson R. Palliative care for the poor and disenfranchised: a view from the Robert Wood Johnson Foundation. J R Soc Med 2001;94:486–489.
10. Moller DW. Dancing with Bones: Portraits of Death and Dying Among Inner-City Poor. New York: Oxford University Press, 2004.
11. O'Neill JF, Romaguera R, Parham D, Marconi K. Practicing palliative care in resource-poor settings. J Pain Symptom Manage 2002;24:148–151.
12. Soares LGL. Poor social condition, criminality and urban violence: unmentioned barriers for effective cancer pain control at the end of life. J Pain Symptom Manage 2003;26:693–695.
12a. Hughes A. Poverty and palliative care in the US: issues facing the urban poor. Int J Pall Nurs 2005;11:6–13.
13. Taipale V. Ethics and allocation of health resources: the influence of poverty on health. Acta Oncol 1999;38:51–55.
14. Blacksher E. On being poor and feeling poor: low socioeconomic status and the moral self. Theor Med Bioeth 2002;23:455–470.
15. Aday LA. At Risk in America: The Health and Health Care Needs of Vulnerable Populations, 2nd ed. San Francisco: Jossey-Bass, 2001.
16. Proctor B, Dalaker J. Poverty in the United States: 2002 (Current Population Reports P60-222.): U.S. Census Bureau. Washington, D.C., U.S. Department of Commerce, 2003.
17. National Coalition for the Homeless. (1999, April). The McKinney Act Fact Sheet. Available at: http://www.nationalhomeless.org (accessed December 27, 2004).
18. National Coalition for the Homeless. (2002a, September 2002). How many people experience homelessness fact sheet. Available at: http://www.nationalhomeless.org/ (accessed December 27, 2004).
19. Fellin P. The culture of homelessness. In: Manoleas P, ed., Cross-Cultural Practice of Clinical Case Management in Mental Health New York: Haworth Press, 1996:41–77.
20. National Coalition for the Homeless. (2002b, September 2002). Who is homeless fact sheet. Available at: http://www.nationalhomeless.org (accessed December 27, 2004).
21. Strechlow AJ, Amos-Jones T. The Homeless as a vulnerable population. Nurs Clin N Am 1999;34:261–274.
22. Lynch J, Davey Smith G, Harper S, Hillemeier M, Ross N, Kaplan GA, Wolfson M. Is income inequality a determination of population health? Part I. A systematic review. Millbank Q 2004a;82:5–99.
23. Horne BD, Muhlestein JB, Lappe DL, Renlund DG, Bair TL, Bunch TJ, Anderson JL. Less affluent area of residence and lesser-insured status predict an increased risk of death or myocardial infarction after angiographic diagnosis of coronary disease. Ann Epidemiol 2003;14:143–150.
24. Fang J, Alderman MH. Is geography destiny for patients in New York with myocardial infarction? Am J Med 2003;115:448–453.
25. Lynch J, Davey Smith G, Harper S, Hillemeier M. Is income inequality a determinant of population health? Part 2. U.S. national and regional trends in income inequality and age- and cause-specific mortality. Millbank Q 2004b;82:355–400.
26. Crane J, Quirk K, van der Straten A. "Come back when you're dying," the commodification of AIDS among California's urban poor. Soc Sci Med 2002;55:1115–1127.
27. Penson DF, Stoddard ML, Pasta DJ, Lubeck DP, Flanders SC, Litwin MS. The association between socioeconomic status, health insurance coverage, and quality of life in men with prostate cancer. J Clin Epidemiol 2001;54:350–358.

28. Clark DO, Tu W, Weiner M, Murray MD. Correlates of health-related quality of life among lower income, urban adults with congestive heart failure. Heart Lung, 2003;32:391–401.
29. Kiefer CW. Health Work with the Poor: A Practical Guide. New Brunswick, NJ: Rutgers University Press, 2000.
30. O'Connor PG, Selwyn PA, Schottenfeld RS. Medical care for injection drug users with human immunodeficiency syndrome. N Engl J Med 1994;331:450–459.
31. Morrison RS, Wallenstein S, Natale DK, Senzel RS, Huang LL. "We don't carry that"— failure of pharmacies in predominantly nonwhite neighborhoods to stock opioid analgesics. N Engl J Med 2000;342:240–248.
32. Bangsberg D, Tulsky JP, Hecht FM, Moss AR. Protease inhibitors in the homeless. JAMA 1997;278:63–65.
33. Tong E, McGraw SA, Dobihal E, Baggish R, Cherlin E, Bradley EH. What is a good death? Minority and non-minority perspectives. J Palliat Care 2003;19:168–175.
34. Kozol J. Amazing Grace: The Lives of Children and the Conscience of a Nation. New York: Perennial Publishers, 1995.
35. Crawley L, Payne R, Bolden J, Payne T, Washington P, Williams S. Palliative and end-of-life care in the African American community. JAMA 2000;284:2518–2521.
36. Bermudez R, von der Werth L, Brandon J, Aragon T. San Francisco Homeless Deaths Identified from Medical Examiner Records: December 1997–November 1998. San Francisco: Department of Public Health, 1999.
37. Hwang SW, O'Connell JJ, Lebow JM, Bierer MF, Orav EJ, Brennan TA. Health Care Utilization Among Homeless Adults Prior to Death. J Health Care Poor Underserved 2001;12:50–58.
38. Dineen JK. Increase in homeless death rate on city's streets. San Francisco Examiner, August 28, 2003. Available at: http://www.examiner.com/article/index.cfm/i/082803n_homeless (accessed December 27, 2004).
39. Patchell T. Nowhere to run: portraits of life on the street. Turning Wheel: Journal of Socially Engaged Buddhism 1996;Fall:14–21.
40. CDC. Deaths among the homeless- Atlanta, Georgia. Morbidity and Mortality Report 1987;36:297–299.
41. CDC. Hypothermia-related deaths—Cook County, Illnois. Morbidity and Mortality Report 1991;42:917–919.
42. Campbell ML, Frank RR. Experience with an end-of-life practice at a university hospital. Crit Care Med 1997;25:197–202.
43. Gramelspacher GP. (2001). End-of-life ethics. American Medical Association. Available at: http://www.ama-assn.org/ama/pub/category/5145.html (accessed December 27, 2004).
44. Ryan A, Carter J, Lucas J, Berger J. You need not make the journey alone: overcoming impediments to providing palliative care in a public urban teaching hospital. Am J Hospice Palliat Care 2002;19:171–180.
45. Kemp C. Terminal Illness: A Guide to Nursing Care, 2nd ed. Philadelphia: Lippincott Williams & Wilkins, 1999.
46. Cleak H, Howe JL. Social networks and use of social supports of minority elders in East Harlem. Social Work Health Care 2002; 38:19–38.
47. Zerwekh JV. Caring on the ragged edge: nursing persons who are disenfranchised. Adv Nurs Sci 2000;22:47–61.
48. Patchell T. Suggestions for Effective Outreach. San Francisco: San Francisco Department of Public Health, Homeless Death Prevention Project, 1997.

37

Deborah Witt Sherman

Patients with Acquired Immunodeficiency Syndrome

I thank God that there are medications to treat AIDS, but there are serious side effects and they can make you feel quite sick. Yet, I want to live and I will do everything possible to stay alive. Some people say AIDS is now a chronic disease. There are other medications to treat my symptoms, and there is my belief in God that lifts my spirit. My family helps me care for my kids, but it is hard on everyone. We all need support because we are all suffering one way or another.—A patient

- ***Key Points***
- *With HIV/AIDS, the severity, complexity, and unpredictability of the illness trajectory have blurred the distinction between curative and palliative care.*
- *The focus of AIDS care must be on improving quality of life by providing care for the management of pain and other symptoms, while addressing the emotional, social, and spiritual needs of patients and their families throughout the illness trajectory.*
- *With up-to-date knowledge regarding HIV disease, including changes in epidemiology, diagnostic testing, treatment options, and available resources, nurses can offer effective and compassionate care to patients and families at all stages of HIV disease.*

In 20 years, acquired immunodeficiency syndrome (AIDS) has escalated from a series of outbreaks in scattered communities in the United States and Europe to a global health crisis.[1] Although the emerging biomedical paradigm of highly active antiretroviral therapy (HAART) has significantly reduced the mortality from human immunodeficiency virus (HIV) in the developed world and has transformed AIDS into a manageable chronic illness, the reality worldwide is that people are not "living with AIDS," but, rather, "dying from AIDS" due to a lack of access to medications and appropriate health care.[2] Even in developed countries, AIDS remains the leading cause of serious illness and death for young adults, and at this point in time, there is a false dichotomy created between disease-specific, curative therapies and symptom-specific palliative therapies.[3] AIDS has stimulated the need to evaluate clinical practice when curative and palliative care interface and raises some interesting and interconnected issues about the care of individuals with life-threatening, progressive illnesses.[4] Both the public and health professionals have been troubled by the reality of overtreatment and undertreatment of pain and symptoms in individuals with life-threatening illnesses, particularly at the end of life.[5] Such concern extends to the care of patients with HIV and the resultant illness of AIDS because no cure has yet been found. The focus of care must, therefore, be on improving quality of life by providing palliative care for the management of pain and other physical symptoms while addressing the emotional, social, and spiritual needs of patients and their families throughout the illness trajectory. Even though current therapies have increased the life expectancy of people with HIV/AIDS, the chance of their experiencing symptoms related not only to the disease but to the effects of therapies also increases. Furthermore, palliative measures can be beneficial in ensuring tolerance of and adherence to difficult pharmacological regimens.[6]

Although little attention has been given in the past to palliative care as a component of AIDS care, it is now realized that the palliation of pain, symptoms, and suffering must occur throughout the course of a life-threatening disease, not just in the final stages near the end of life. Because patients are surviving longer in the latter stages of illness, an integrated model must be developed to provide comprehensive care for patients with advanced AIDS and their families.[3] This chapter provides an overview and update of the comprehensive care related to HIV/AIDS and addresses the palliative care needs of individuals and families living with and dying from this illness. With this information, nurses and other health care professionals will gain the knowledge to provide effective and compassionate care, recognizing the need for both curative and aggressive care as well as supportive and palliative therapies to maximize the quality of life of patients and their family caregivers.

Overview and Update: Incidence, Historical Background, Epidemiology, and Pathogenesis

Incidence of HIV/AIDS

HIV/AIDS is a worldwide epidemic affecting more than 40 million people. An estimated 5 million acquired HIV in 2003, with an estimated 3 million people dying from AIDS.[7] The Centers for Disease Control and Prevention (CDC) in 2004 reported that through December 2002, there were more than 877,275 reported cases in the United States since the beginning of the epidemic. 718,002 cases were males, 159,271 cases females, and 9,300 cases estimated in children under age 13.[7] In the United States, the estimated number of deaths of persons with AIDS is 501,669, including 496,354 adults and adolescents, and 5,315 children under age 15.[7] HIV is the leading cause of death of all Americans between the ages of 25 and 44 years, with the highest incidence and prevalence now among African Americans, women, and heterosexuals.[7] Given that there are no approved vaccines against HIV/AIDS or cures for the disease, AIDS remains a life-threatening and progressive illness that marks the final stage of a chronic viral illness, identified by the occurrence of particular opportunistic infections, cancers, and neurological manifestations.[8]

Historical Background of HIV/AIDS

In the early 1980s, cases were reported of previously healthy homosexual men who were diagnosed with *Pneumocystis carinii* pneumonia and an extremely rare tumor known as Kaposi's sarcoma (KS). The number of cases doubled every 6 months, with further occurrence of unusual fungal, viral, and parasitic infections, and it was realized that the immune systems of these individuals were being compromised. Over time, the CDC learned that a complex of diseases producing immunocompetence was experienced outside the homosexual community, among heterosexual partners, intravenous (IV) substance users, persons with hemophilia, individuals receiving infected blood products, and children born to women with the disease. These epidemiological changes alerted health professionals to the existence of an infectious agent transmitted via infected body fluids, particularly through sexual transmission and blood products.[9]

Origins of HIV can be traced through serum studies to 1959, when crossover mechanisms between humans and primates via animal bites or scratches in Africa led to HIV transmission. In 1981, the virus was identified and named lymphadenopathy-associated virus (LAV). By 1984, the term had been changed to human T-lymphocytic virus type III (HTLV-III), and in 1986 renamed the human immunodeficiency virus type 1 (HIV-1). HIV-1 accounts for nearly all the cases reported in the United States, while a second strain, HIV-2, accounts for nearly all the cases reported in West Africa. There have only been 17 cases of HIV-2 reported in the United States, the majority being immigrants from Africa.

Globally, AIDS is characterized as a volatile, unstable, and dynamic epidemic, which has spread to new countries around the world. It has become increasingly complex due to the viruses' ability to mutate and crosses all socioeconomic, cultural, political, and geographic borders.[10] To date, scientific progress has been made in combating the infection: (1) the virus has been identified; (2) a blood-screening program has been implemented; (3) vaccines are being tested; (4) biological and behavioral cofactors have been identified related to infection and disease progression; (5) prophylactic treatments are available to prevent opportunistic infections; (6) newly developed HIV RNA quantitative assays, which measure viral load (VL), have become available to guide the treatment of the disease; and (7) the latest advances in treatment involve the use of combination antiretroviral therapies.[10] However, epidemiological evidence heightens concern regarding changes in the population affected and the morbidity and mortality still associated with the disease.

HIV Epidemiology

Epidemiological studies confirm that HIV-1 is transmitted through semen, cervical and vaginal secretions, breast milk, contaminated drug equipment, transfusions and blood products, tissue transplants, perinatal exposure, and occupational exposure in health care settings.[10] Although HIV diagnosis has remained stable in the United States from 1999 to 2002, the rate of HIV infection has dramatically increased among African Americans (75.6 per 100,000), compared with Hispanics (29.3 per 100,000) and Caucasians (8.0 per 100,000). Diagnosis rates remain higher among males (27.7 per 100,000) than females (10.7 per 100,000). Furthermore, the rate of HIV diagnosis rose 5% per year among men who have sex with men of all races, and remains stable among heterosexuals and IV substance abusers.[11] In the HAART era, there has been a decrease in the incidence of KS and cervical cancer, although the incidence of non-Hodgkin's lymphoma has not decreased. In contrast, in the HAART period, the incidence of lung cancer, Hodgkin's disease, anorectal cancer, melanoma, and head and neck cancers has increased.[11]

Until a vaccine is available, sex education, the use of condoms, and drug-abuse treatment, including the provision of clean needles, have been shown to limit the horizontal spread of HIV/AIDS to other adults. However, personal, social, political, and cultural barriers in almost all countries and governments prevent the widespread implementation of these interventions. In underdeveloped countries, such as those in sub-Saharan Africa, where a large proportion of the adult population is infected with HIV/AIDS, and there is a high burden of suffering and death, it is believed that prevention alone is inadequate. Treatment must be available to preserve the human infrastructure of society, and it is thought that this will increase voluntary testing, break the silence, and offer a powerful life-or-death incentive for people to be tested.[12]

HIV Pathogenesis and Classification

Like all viruses, the HIV virus survives by reproducing itself in a host cell, usurping the genetic machinery of that cell, and eventually destroying the cell.[13] The HIV is a retrovirus whose life cycle consists of (1) attachment of the virus to the cell, which is affected by cofactors that influence the virus's ability to enter the host cell; (2) uncoating of the virus; (3) reverse transcription by an enzyme called reverse transcriptase, which converts two strands of viral RNA to DNA; (4) integration of newly synthesized proviral DNA into the cell nucleus, assisted by the viral enzyme integrase, which becomes the template for new viral components; (5) transcription of proviral DNA into messenger RNA; (6) movement of messenger RNA outside the cell nucleus, where it is translated into viral proteins and enzymes; and (7) assembly and release of mature virus particles out of the host cell.[14]

The host cell therefore produces viral proteins instead of the cell's normal regulatory proteins, resulting in the eventual destruction of the host cell. Given that the virus has an affinity for CD4 molecules, any cells that have the CD4 molecule on their surface, such as T lymphocytes and macrophages, become major viral targets. Recently, research has identified that chemokines and chemokine receptors play important roles in HIV pathogenesis by inhibiting HIV infection. Because CD4 cells are the master coordinators of the immune response, chronic destruction of these cells severely compromises individuals' immune status, leaving them susceptible to opportunistic infections. Macrophages are also directly targeted by the virus and may serve as reservoirs for the virus for months after initial infection, as well as contributing to HIV-related dementias and other neurological syndromes.[14] HIV and AIDS are not synonymous terms but, rather, refer to the natural history or progression of the infection, ranging from asymptomatic infection to life-threatening illness characterized by opportunistic infections and cancers. This continuum of illness is associated with a decrease in CD4 cell count and a rise in HIV-RNA VL.[15] In monitoring disease progression, it should be noted, however, that although low CD4 cell counts are generally correlated with high VLs, some patients with low CD4 counts have low VLs and vice versa. The most reliable current measurement of HIV activity, therefore, is the VL, and the more consistent surrogate marker is the percentage of lymphocytes that are CD4 cells, rather than the absolute CD4 cell count.[16]

In 1993, the CDC reclassified HIV disease according to the CD4 T lymphocyte count and clinical conditions associated with HIV infection. The classification of HIV disease is as follows:[10,13] Primary or acute infection occurs when the virus enters the body and replicates in large numbers in the blood. This leads to an initial decrease in the number of T cells. Viral load climbs during the first 2 weeks of the infection. Within 5 to 30 days of infection, the individual experiences flulike symptoms characteristic of a viremia such as fever, sore throat, skin rash, lymphadenopathy, and myalgia. Other manifestations of primary HIV infection include fatigue, splenomegaly, anorexia, nausea and vomiting, meningitis, retro-orbital pain, neuropathy, and mucocutaneous ulceration.[17] The production of HIV antibodies results in seroconversion, which generally occurs within 6 to 12 weeks of the initial infection. The amount of virus present after the initial viremia and the immune response is called the viral set point.

Clinical latency refers to the chronic, clinically asymptomatic state in which there is a decreased VL and resolution of symptoms of the primary infection. It was previously thought that in this period, the virus lay dormant in the host cells for a period of 5 to 7 years. However, recent advances in the understanding of the pathogenesis of the virus reveal that there is continuous viral replication in the lymph nodes. Because more than 10 billion copies of the virus can be made every day during this period, early medical intervention with combination antiretroviral therapy is recommended.[18]

Early symptomatic stage occurs after years of infection and is apparent by conditions indicative primarily of defects in cell-mediated immunity. Early symptomatic infection occurs when CD4 counts fall below 500 cells/mm^3 and the HIV VL copy count increases above 10,000/mL up to 100,000/mL, which indicates a moderate risk of HIV progression and a median time to death of 6.8 years. There are frequently mucosal clues, ranging from oral candidiasis and hairy leukoplakia to ulcerative lesions. Gynecological infections are the most common reasons women have a medical examination. There are also dermatological manifestations, which include bacterial, fungal, viral, neoplastic, and other conditions such exacerbation of psoriasis, severe pruritus, or the development of recurrent pruritic papules.[17]

Late symptomatic stage begins when the CD4 count drops below 200 cells/mm^3 and the VL increases above 100,000/mL. This CD4 level is recognized by the CDC as the case definition for AIDS. Severe opportunistic infections or cancers characterize this stage and result in multiple severe symptoms. In addition to such illnesses as KS, *Pneumocystis carinii* pneumonia, HIV encephalopathy, and HIV wasting, diseases such as pulmonary tuberculosis, recurrent bacterial infections, and invasive cervical cancer have been added to the list of AIDS-indicative illnesses.[7] Advanced HIV disease stage occurs when the CD4 cell count drops below 50 cells/mm^3 and the immune system is so impaired that death is likely within 1 year. Common conditions are central nervous system (CNS) non-Hodgkin's lymphoma, KS, cytomegalovirus (CMV) retinitis, or *Mycobacterium avium* complex (MAC).[17] Unfortunately, persons with advanced HIV disease diagnosed with AIDS increasingly represent persons whose diagnosis was too late for them to benefit from treatment, persons who either did not seek or had no access to care, or persons for whom treatment failed.[7] In the late stages of the disease, most individuals have health problems such as pneumonia, oral candidiasis, depression, dementia, skin problems, anxiety, incontinence, fatigue, isolation, bed dependency, wasting syndrome, and significant pain.[18] Research regarding AIDS patients experiencing advanced disease confirms the multitude of patient symptoms and factors that contribute to mortality. In a study of 83 hospitalized AIDS patients, factors contributing to higher mortality include the type of opportunistic infections, serum albumin level, total lymphocyte count, weight, CD4 count, and neurological manifestations.[19] Of 363 patients with AIDS referred to community palliative care services, the most severe problems throughout care were patient and family anxiety and symptom control.[20] In the last month of life, a retrospective study of 50 men who died from AIDS indicated that the most distressing symptoms included pain, dyspnea, diarrhea, confusion, dementia, difficulty swallowing and eating, and loss of vision. Dehydration, malnutrition, and peripheral neuropathy were also important problems.[21]

Palliative Care as a Natural Evolution in HIV/AIDS Care

From the earliest stages of HIV disease, symptom control becomes an important goal of medical and nursing care to maintain the patient's quality of life. Palliative care for patients with HIV/AIDS should therefore be viewed not as an approach to care only in the advanced stage of the illness, but as an aspect of care that begins in the early stage of illness and continues as the disease progresses.[22]

With the occurrence of opportunistic infections, specific cancers, and neurological manifestations, AIDS involves multiple symptoms not only from the disease processes but also from the side effects of medications and other therapies. Patients with AIDS present with complex care issues because they experience bouts of severe illness and debilitation alternating with periods of symptom stabilization.[23] In one model of care, AIDS palliation begins when active treatment ends. Although this model limits service overlap and is economical, it creates not only the ethical issue of when to shift from a curative to a palliative focus, but also promotes discontinuity of care and possible discrimination. In contrast, a second model of AIDS care recognizes that AIDS treatment is primarily palliative, directed toward minimizing symptoms and maximizing the quality of life, and necessitates the use of antiretroviral drugs, treatment of infections and neoplasms, and provision of high levels of support to promote the patient's quality of life over many years of the illness.[24] Selwyn and Rivard[25] emphasize that although AIDS is no longer a uniformly fatal disease, it is an important cause of mortality, particularly for young adults and ethnically diverse populations with comorbidities such as hepatitis B and C, end-organ failure, and various malignancies.

Although thousands of individuals have suffered and died from AIDS each year, the palliative care needs of HIV/AIDS patients have been largely neglected by organizations involved in medical care.[26] This has occurred because the division between curative–aggressive care and supportive–palliative care is less well defined and more variable than in other life-threatening illnesses such as cancer.[18] With HIV/AIDS, the severity, complexity, and unpredictability of the illness trajectory have blurred the distinction between curative and palliative care.[27] Other challenges associated with HIV/AIDS are the societal stigmatization of the disease and, therefore, the greater emotional, social, and spiritual needs of those experiencing the illness, as well as their family and professional caregivers who experience their own grief and bereavement processes.

Resources aimed at prevention, health promotion and maintenance, and end-of-life care must be available through health care policies and legislation.[28] Not only the treatment of chronic debilitating conditions, but also the treatment of superimposed acute opportunistic infections and related symptoms is necessary to maintain quality of life. For example, IV therapy and blood transfusions, as well as health prevention measures such as ongoing IV therapies to prevent blindness from CMV retinitis, must be available to patients with AIDS to maintain their quality of life.

Palliative care is therefore a natural evolution in AIDS care. Core issues of comfort and function, fundamental to palliative care, must be addressed throughout the course of the illness, and may be concurrent with restorative or curative therapies for persons with AIDS.[23] The management decisions for patients with advanced AIDS will revolve around the ratio between benefits and burdens of the various diagnostic and treatment modalities, and the patient's expectations and goals, as well as anticipated problems.[29] In the face of advanced HIV disease, health care providers and patients must determine the balance between aggressive and supportive efforts, particularly when increasing debility, wasting, and deteriorating cognitive function are evident.[30] At this point, the complex needs of patients and families with HIV/AIDS require the coordinated care of an interdisciplinary palliative care team, involving physicians, advanced practice nurses, staff nurses, social workers, dietitians, physiotherapists, and clergy.[6,31] Given that in palliative care the unit of care is the patient and family, the palliative care team offers support not only for patients to live as fully as possible until death, but also for the family to help them to cope during the patient's illness and in their own bereavement.[32] Palliative care core precepts of respect for patient goals, preferences, and choices, comprehensive caring, and acknowledgment of caregivers' concerns[33] support the holistic and comprehensive approach to care needed by individuals and families with HIV/AIDS. The components of high-quality HIV/AIDS palliative care, as identified by health care providers, include competent, skilled practitioners; confidential, nondiscriminatory, culturally sensitive care; flexible and responsive care; collaborative and coordinated care; and fair access to care.[34]

Although the hospice and palliative care movement developed as a community response to those who were dying, primarily of cancer, the advent of the AIDS epidemic made it necessary for hospices to begin admitting patients with AIDS. This meant applying the old model of cancer care to patients with a new infectious, progressive, and terminal disease.[35] Unlike the course of cancer, which is relatively predictable once the disease progresses beyond cure, AIDS patients experience a series of life-threatening opportunistic infections. It is not until wasting becomes apparent that the course of AIDS achieves the predictability of cancer.[35] Furthermore, while the underlying goal of AIDS care remains one of palliation, short-term aggressive therapies are still needed to treat opportunistic infections.[36] Also, unlike cancer palliation, AIDS palliation deals with a fatal infectious disease of primarily younger people, which requires ongoing infection control and the management of symptoms.[37]

Barriers to Palliative Care

The neglect of the palliative care needs of patients with HIV disease also relates to certain barriers to care, such as reimbursement issues. Specifically, public and private third-party payers have reimbursed end-of-life care only when physicians have verified a life expectancy of less than 6 months to live.[38] Given the unpredictability of the illness trajectory, many patients with AIDS have been denied access to hospice care. Currently, these policies are under review, and the 6-month limitation is being extended so that patients with AIDS will be eligible for comprehensive care, with control of pain and other symptoms along with psychological and spiritual support offered by hospice/palliative care.

As a second barrier to hospice/palliative care, patients with AIDS have been denied, until recently, access because of the need to continue antiretroviral therapies and other medications to prevent opportunistic infections. Given that the estimated cost of treatment for AIDS patients in hospices could amount to twice the cost of treating patients with cancer, particularly when the costs of medications are included, cost remains an important issue for hospices.[32] Financing of such therapies for patients with AIDS is now being addressed by hospice/palliative care organizations.

The third barrier to palliative care is the patients themselves, many of whom are young, clinging to the hope of a cure for AIDS and unwilling to accept hospice care. However, the current emphasis on beginning palliative care at the time of diagnosis of a life-threatening illness may shift the perception of palliative care as only end-of-life care, and help promote palliative care as an aggressive approach to care throughout the course of the illness to ensure their quality of life. Indeed, media and Internet coverage of government and private initiatives to improve the care of the seriously and terminally ill in the United States is informing patients, families, and nurses of the philosophy and precepts of palliative care, the availability of palliative care for life-defining illnesses, and the rights of patients to receive excellent end-of-life care, as well as the obligations of health professionals to provide such care across health care settings.

Criteria for Palliative Care

Grothe and Brody[35] suggest that four criteria be considered regarding the admission of AIDS patients to hospice: functional ability, statistical prognosis, CD4 count and VL, and history of opportunistic infections. These criteria give a better understanding of the patient's prognosis and needs. The complex needs of patients with advanced AIDS also indicate the need for an interdisciplinary approach to care offered by hospice/palliative care. Bloom and Flannery[39] encourage the continual review of hospice policies in accordance with the changes in the disease and encourage change in the community to provide an effective continuum of care. Indeed, developing different models of care such as enhanced home care, hospice care, day care, or partnerships with community hospitals or agencies and conducting cost-benefit analysis will be important in meeting the health care needs of patients with AIDS and their families in the future.[18]

Important advances are currently being made in the field of palliative medicine and nursing, involving an active set of behaviors that continue throughout the caregiving process to manage the pain and suffering of individuals with HIV/AIDS. Health professionals have the responsibility to be knowledgeable about the various treatment options and resources available for pain and symptom management. They must know about pharmacological agents' actions, side effects, and interactions, as well as alternative routes of medication administration. And they must be able to inform patients of their options for care—documenting their preferences, wishes, and choices; performing a complete history and physical assessment; and collaborating with other members of the interdisciplinary team to develop and implement a comprehensive plan of care.[31]

Health Promotion and Maintenance in Promoting the Quality of Life of Persons with HIV/AIDS

As palliative care becomes an increasingly important component of AIDS care from diagnosis to death,[28] and given the definition of palliative care as the comprehensive management of the physical, psychological, social, spiritual, and existential needs of patients with incurable progressive illness,[33] palliative care must involve ongoing prevention, health promotion, and health maintenance to promote the patient's quality of life throughout the illness trajectory. With HIV/AIDS, health promotion and maintenance involves promoting behaviors that will prevent or decrease the occurrence of opportunistic infections and AIDS-indicator diseases, promoting prophylactic and therapeutic treatment of AIDS-indicator conditions, and preventing behaviors that promote disease expression.[5]

With no current prospect for cure, the health management of patients with HIV/AIDS is directed toward prolonging survival and maintaining quality of life.[40] Nurses generally refer to quality of life as the impact of sickness and health care on an ill person's daily activities and sense of well-being.[41] Furthermore, quality of life varies with disease progression from HIV to AIDS. To understand quality of life means to understand the patient's perceptions of his or her ability to control the physical, emotional, social, cognitive, and spiritual aspects of the illness.[42] Quality of life is therefore associated with health maintenance for individuals with HIV/AIDS, particularly as it relates to functioning in activities of daily living, social functioning, and physical and emotional symptoms.[43] In a study regarding the functional quality of life of 142 men and women with AIDS, Vosvick and colleagues[44] concluded that maladaptive coping strategies were associated with lower levels of energy and social functioning and that severe pain interfered with daily living tasks and was associated with lower levels of functional quality of life (physical functioning, energy/fatigue, social functioning, and role functioning). Therefore, health promotion interventions should be aimed at developing adaptive coping strategies and improving pain management.

Health promotion and maintenance for patients with HIV/AIDS must acknowledge patients' perceived health care needs. Based on a study of 386 HIV-infected persons, it was determined that the health care challenges perceived by patients with HIV/AIDS across hospital, outpatient, home, and long-term care settings included decreased endurance, physical mobility, and sensory perception, as well as financial issues—specifically lack of income and resources to cover living and health care expenses.[45] Furthermore, Kemppainen[46] reported, based on a sample of 162 hospitalized men and women with AIDS, that the strongest predictor of decreased quality of life was depression, which accounted for 23% of the variance, with symptoms accounting for 9.75% and female gender accounting for an additional 8%. In addition, active involvement in the process of nursing care contributed 13.4% to the variance in quality of life. These results indicate the health care challenges and physical, emotional, and interactional needs of patients with AIDS and, that in addition to managing pain and other symptoms, a comprehensive and compassionate approach to care is necessary as the illness progresses. Furthermore, enhancing immunocompetence is critical at all stages of illness, as well as treating the symptoms brought on by the disease or related to prophylactic or treatment therapies. Palliation of physical, emotional, and spiritual symptoms, particularly as experienced in the late symptomatic and advanced stages of HIV disease, is considered the final stage of a health-and-disease-prevention approach and will be discussed later in this chapter.[10]

Through all stages of HIV disease, health can be promoted and maintained through diet, micronutrients, exercise, reduction of stress and negative emotions, symptom surveillance, and the use of prophylactic therapies to prevent opportunistic infections or AIDS-related complications.

Diet

A health-promoting diet is essential for optimal functioning of the immune system. Deficiencies in calorie and protein intake impair cell-mediated immunity, phagocytic function, and antibody response. Therefore, an alteration in nutrition is associated with impaired immune system function, secondary infections, disease progression, psychological distress, and fatigue. In patients with AIDS, common nutritional problems are weight loss, vitamin and mineral deficiencies, loss of muscle mass, and loss or redistribution of fat mass. The redistribution of fat is characterized by increased abdominal girth, loss of fat from the face, and a "buffalo hump" on the back of the neck, which may be due to the administration of protease inhibitors.[47] Patients with HIV/AIDS often have reduced food or caloric intake, malabsorption, and altered metabolism. Reduced food or caloric intake is frequently due to diseases of the mouth and oropharynx, such as oral candidiasis, anular cheilitis, gingivitis, herpes simplex, and hairy leukoplakia.[48] Incidence of diseases of the gastrointestinal (GI) tract that can cause malabsorption, such as CMV, MAC, cryptosporidiosis, and KS increases for individuals with CD4 counts of 50 or less, and may adversely affect their nutritional status.[49] Metabolic alterations may be due to HIV infection or secondary infections, as well as abnormalities in carbohydrate, fat, and protein metabolism.[47] The Task Force on Nutrition in AIDS (1989) recommended that the goals of sound nutritional management should include: (1) provision of adequate nutrients; (2) preservation of lean body mass; and (3) minimization of symptoms associated with malabsorption. Hussein[50] believes that a good diet is one of the simplest ways to delay HIV progression and will bolster immune system function and energy levels and help patients live longer and more productive lives. A diet with a variety of foods from the five basic food groups, including 55% of calories from carbohydrates, 15% to 20% of calories from proteins, and 30% of calories from fats, is important in supporting immune function.[51] It is recommended to have two or three servings daily from the protein and dairy groups, seven to 12 servings from the starch and grain group, two servings of fruits and vegetables rich in vitamin C, as well as three servings of other fruits and vegetables.[10]

Micronutrients

Research has indicated that HIV-infected individuals have lower levels than noninfected individuals of magnesium, total carotenes, total choline, and vitamins A and B_6, yet higher levels of niacin.[52] A linkage has been reported between vitamin A (beta carotene) deficiency and elevated disease progression and mortality.[53] Correcting both vitamin A and B_6 deficiencies has been hypothesized to restore cell-mediated immunity, and vitamin-supplement trials are underway. Current research supports the increase in dietary intake of n-3 polyunsaturated fatty acids, arginine, and RNA to increase body weight and stave off wasting due to malabsorption. Increase in concentrations of amino acids such as arginine has also been found to preserve lean muscle mass.[52]

Exercise

A consistent outcome of the effects of exercise on immune function is the increase in natural killer-cell activity, though variable results are reported on the effects of exercise on neutrophil, macrophage, and T and B cell function and proliferation.[54] In a review of exercise studies, LaPerriere and colleagues[55] reported a trend in CD4 cell count elevation in all but one study, with the greatest effect from aerobic exercise and weight training. The CDC[56] recommend a physical exercise program of 30 to 45 minutes four or more times a week as a health-promoting activity to increase lung capacity, endurance, energy, and flexibility, and to improve circulation.

Massage has also been linked to natural killer-cell activity and overall immune regulation as reported in a research study of 29 HIV-infected men who received daily massages for 1 month.[57] Patient reports of less anxiety and greater relaxation related to exercise and massage are regarded by both patients and practitioners as important laboratory markers.[52]

Stress and Emotions

Stress and negative emotions have also been associated with immunosuppression and vulnerability to disease. In a study of 96 HIV-infected homosexual men without symptoms or antiretroviral medication use, Leserman and colleagues[58] reported that higher cumulative average stressful life events, higher anger scores, lower cumulative average social support, and depressive symptoms were all predictive of a faster progression to both the CDC AIDS classification and a clinical AIDS condition. Stress of living with HIV/AIDS is related to the uncertainty regarding illness progression and prognosis, stigmatization and discrimination, and financial concerns as disabilities increase with advancing disease. Persons with AIDS frequently cite the avoidance of stress as a way of maintaining a sense of well-being.[59] The use of exercise and massage and other relaxation techniques, such as imagery, meditation, and yoga, are reported as valuable stress-management techniques.[60] Cognitive-behavioral interventions have also been shown to improve certain aspects of quality of life of women with AIDS ($n = 330$), specifically in terms of cognitive functioning, health distress, and overall health perceptions. However, no changes were observed in energy/fatigue, pain, or role or social functioning.[61]

Health promotion also involves health beliefs and coping strategies that support well-being despite protracted illness. A study of 53 patients diagnosed with AIDS demonstrated that long-term survivors used numerous strategies to support their health, such as having the will to live, positive attitudes, feeling in charge, a strong sense of self, expressing their needs, and a sense of humor. Other health-promotion strategies frequently used by these patients included remaining active, seeking medical information, talking to others, socializing and pursuing pleasurable activities, good medical care, and counseling.[62] Cohen[63] examined the relationship between the use of humor to cope with stress (coping humor) and perceived social support, depression, anxiety, self-esteem, and stress, based on a sample of 103 HIV/AIDS patients. The results indicated that patients who used more coping humor were less depressed, expressed higher self-esteem, and perceived greater support from friends. However, the use of coping humor did not buffer stress, anxiety, or immune-system functioning. Stress can also be associated with the financial issues experienced by patients with HIV/AIDS. Therefore, health promotion may involve financial planning, identification of financial resources available through the community, and public assistance offered through Medicaid.

It must also be recognized that additional physical and emotional stress is associated with the use of recreational drugs such as alcohol, chemical stimulants, tobacco, and marijuana because these agents have an immunosuppressant effect and may interfere with health-promoting behaviors.[64] The use of such substances may also have a negative effect on interpersonal relationships and are associated with a relapse to unsafe sexual practices.[65] Interventions for health promotion include encouraging patients to participate in self-health groups and harm-reduction programs to deal with substance-abuse problems.

Symptom Surveillance

Throughout the course of their illness, individuals with HIV disease require primary care services to identify early signs of opportunistic infections and to minimize related symptoms and complications. This includes a complete health history, physical examination, and laboratory data including determination of immunological and viral status.

Health History. In the care of patients with HIV/AIDS, the health history should include the following[16]:

- History of present illness, including a review of those factors that led to HIV testing
- Past medical history, particularly those conditions that may be exacerbated by HIV disease or its treatments, such as diabetes mellitus, hypertriglyceridemia, or chronic or active hepatitis B infection
- Childhood illnesses and vaccinations for preventing common infections such as polio, DPT, or measles
- Medication history, including the patient's knowledge of the types of medications, side effects, adverse reactions, drug interactions, and administration recommendations
- Sexual history, regarding sexual behaviors and preferences and history of sexually transmitted diseases, which can exacerbate HIV disease progression
- Lifestyle habits, such as the past and present use of recreational drugs, including alcohol, which may accelerate progression of disease; cigarette smoking, which may suppress appetite or be associated with opportunistic infections such as oral candidiasis, hairy leukoplakia, and bacterial pneumonia
- Dietary habits, including risks related to food-borne illnesses such as hepatitis A
- Travel history, to countries in Asia, Africa, and South America, where the risk of opportunistic infections increase
- Complete systems review, to provide indications of clinical manifestations of new opportunistic infections or cancers, as well as AIDS-related complications both from the disease and its treatments

Physical Examination. A physical exam should begin with a general assessment of vital signs and height and weight, as well as overall appearance and mood. A complete head-to-toe assessment is important and may reveal various findings common to individuals with HIV/AIDS such as[16]:

- Oral cavity assessment may indicate candida, oral hairy leukoplakia, or KS.
- Funduscopic assessment may reveal visual changes associated with CMV retinitis; glaucoma screening annually is also recommended.
- Lymph node assessment may reveal adenopathy detected at any stage of disease, yet is indicative of disease progression.
- Dermatological assessment may indicate various cutaneous manifestations that occur throughout the course of the illness such as HIV exanthema, KS, or infectious complications such as dermatomycosis.
- Neuromuscular assessment may indicate various central, peripheral, or autonomic nervous systems disorders and signs and symptoms of conditions such as meningitis, encephalitis, dementia, or peripheral neuropathies.
- Cardiovascular assessment may reveal cardiomyopathy related to the use of antiretroviral therapy.
- GI assessment may indicate organomegaly, specifically splenomegaly or hepatomegaly, particularly in patients with a history of substance abuse, as well as signs related to parasitic intestinal infections; annual stool of guaiac and rectal examination, as well as sigmoidoscopy every 5 years, are also parts of health maintenance.
- Reproductive system assessment may reveal occult sexually transmitted diseases or malignancies, as well vaginal candidiasis, cervical dysplasia, pelvic inflammatory disease, or rectal lesions in women with HIV/AIDS, as well as urethral discharge and rectal lesions or malignancies in HIV-infected men. Health maintenance in individuals with HIV/AIDS also includes annual mammograms in women, as well as testicular exams in men and prostate-specific antigen (PSA) annually.

Laboratory Data. CD4 counts, both the absolute numbers and the CD4 percentages, should be evaluated to assist the health practitioner in therapeutic decision-making about treatments of opportunistic infections and antiretroviral therapy. Quantitative RNA determination or VL is also an important marker for disease progression and to measure the effectiveness of antiretroviral therapy.[16] The DHHS's Panel on Clinical Practices for the Treatment of HIV recommends that VLs be measured upon diagnosis and every 3 to 4 months subsequently. CD4 cell counts should also be measured at the time of diagnosis in an untreated patient and every 3 to 6 months afterward.[66] Immediately before a patient is started on HAART, the patient's HIV-RNA (VL) should be measured, and again 2 to 8 weeks after treatment is initiated, to determine the effectiveness of the therapy. With adherence to the medication schedule, it is expected that the HIV-RNA will decrease by approximately 1.0 $\log_{10}$ and will continue to decline over the next 16 to 20 weeks until the VL has reached undetectable levels (<50 copies/mL).[66] If a patient does not significantly respond to therapy, the clinician should evaluate adherence, repeat the test, perform a genotyping or phenotyping resistance assay, and rule out malabsorption or drug interactions. It is anticipated that patients with low VLs and high baseline CD4 cell counts will respond positively to therapy.[67]

The decision regarding laboratory testing is based on the stage of HIV disease, the medical processes warranting initial assessment or follow-up, and consideration of the patient-benefit-to-burden ratio. Complete blood counts are often measured with each VL determination or with a change of antiretroviral therapy, particularly with patients on drugs known to cause anemia. Chemistry profiles are done to assess liver function, lipid status, and glycemia every 3 to 6 months or with a change in therapy, and are determined by the patient's antiretroviral therapy, baseline determinations, and co-infections. Abnormalities in these profiles may occur as a result of antiretroviral therapy. Increasing hepatic dysfunction is evident by elevations in the serum transaminases (AST, ALT, ALP, LDH). Blood work should also include hepatitis C serology (antibody), hepatitis B serology and *Toxoplasma* IgG serology.[67]

Urine analysis should be done annually unless the person is on antiretroviral therapy, which may require more frequent follow-up to check for toxicity. Annual Papanicolaou (Pap) smears are also indicated, with recommendations for Pap smears every 3 to 6 months in HIV-infected women who are symptomatic. Syphilis studies should be done annually; however, patients with low positive titers should have follow-up testing at 3, 6, 9, 12, and 24 months. Gonorrhea and chlamydia tests are encouraged every 6 to 12 months if the patient is sexually active. In addition, CMV serology for patients with CD4 cell counts under 100 cells/mm^3 should be measured every 6 months.[16] Individuals with CD4 cell counts below 100 cells/mm^3 and who had negative toxoplasmosis antibodies at baseline should also be tested and started on TMP-SMZ (Bactrim) for prophylaxis.

Annual tuberculin skin testing (TST) is also important for HIV-infected individuals. A TST is considered positive in patients with induration of greater than or equal to 5 mm. With a positive TST, a yearly chest radiograph is warranted.

Prophylaxis

The primary strategy to prevent the development of opportunistic infections is to avoid exposure to microorganisms in the environment. Secondly, the immune system can be supported and maintained through the administration of prophylactic and/or suppressive therapies, which decrease the frequency or severity of opportunistic infections.[68] Primary prophylaxis is the administration of a pharmacological agent to prevent initial infection, while secondary prophylaxis is the administration of a pharmacological agent to prevent future occurrences of infection.[69] However, due to the effectiveness of HAARTs, there has been a significant decrease in the incidence of opportunistic infections. As a result, prophylaxis for life for HIV-related co-infections is no longer necessary in many cases.[67] If HAART restores immune-system function as evident by a rise in CD4 counts, clinicians may stop administering primary prophylaxis under defined conditions.[67] The advantages to ending preventive prophylaxis for opportunistic infections in selected patients is a decrease in drug interactions and toxicities, lower cost of care, and greater adherence to HAART regimens.[67] Table 37–1 describes the common opportunistic infections and recommended prophylactic and alternative regimens that have been updated by the U.S. Public Health Service in 2002. In the late symptomatic and advanced stages of HIV disease, when CD4 counts are low and VL may be high, prophylaxis remains important to protect against opportunistic infections. Therefore, throughout the illness trajectory, and even in hospice settings, patients may be taking prophylactic medications, requiring sophisticated planning and monitoring.[35]

In addition, HIV-infected individuals are at risk for severe diseases that are vaccine preventable, such as hepatitis A and B, tetanus, influenza, pneumococcal and measles, rubella and mumps. Table 37–2 presents vaccine-preventable illness and interventions. Von Gunten and colleagues[70] suggest the continuation of prophylaxis in hospice and palliative care settings for patients with AIDS as long as patients are able to take oral medications. This is because there is a high risk of reactivation and dissemination of diseases that can result in a high number of symptoms. Suppressive therapy for herpes infections is also continued to prevent painful lesions. Von Gunten and colleagues[70] also recommend the following plan regarding prophylaxis and suppressive therapy in hospice/palliative care:

1. If the patient is clinically stable and wants to continue prophylaxis, continue drug therapy.
2. If side effects occur, and the patient continues to be otherwise stable, consider alternative regimens.
3. If patient is intolerant of prophylaxis and/or the regimens are burdensome, discontinue medications.

Although these recommendations were made in 1995, they are still applicable to patients with AIDS who are enrolled in hospice.

Indications for Antiretroviral Therapy Across the Illness Trajectory. Without a cure for HIV disease, all treatments are essentially palliative in nature to slow disease progression and limit the occurrence of opportunistic infections, which adversely affect quality of life. The CD4 cell count and VL are used in conjunction to determine the initiation of antiretroviral therapy.

The goal of initiating HAART is to achieve maximum long-term suppression of HIV RNA and to restore or preserve immune system function and thereby reduce morbidity and mortality and promote quality of life.[67] The potential risks versus benefits of early or delayed initiation of therapy for asymptomatic patients must be considered. The benefits of early therapy include earlier suppression of viral replication, preservation of the immune system functioning, prolongation of disease-free survival, and a decrease in the risk of HIV transmission.[67] However, the risks of early therapy initiation include lower quality of life due to the adverse effects of therapy, problems with adherence to therapy, and subsequent drug resistance, with the potential limitation of future treatment options as a result of premature administration of available drugs. There is further concern regarding the risks of severe toxicities associated with certain antiretroviral medications, such as elevations in serum levels of triglycerides and cholesterol, alterations in fat distribution, or insulin resistance and diabetes mellitus.[66] Given the available data in terms of the relative risk for the progression to AIDS, the evidence supports the initiation of therapy for asymptomatic HIV-infected patients with a CD4 T cell count of <350 cell/mm^3 or a VL of >55,000 copies/mL. If a patient has a CD4 count >350 cell/mm^3, arguments can be made for both conservative and aggressive approaches to therapy. The conservative approach is based on the belief that a significant immune system reconstitution occurs for patients who initiate therapy in the 200–350 cells/mm^3 range. However, the decision to start therapy for the asymptomatic patient in this range involves discussion with the patient of his or her willingness, ability, and readiness to begin therapy, and the risk for disease progression given the VL as well as CD4 count. The aggressive approach to initiating therapy early is supported by studies that indicate suppression of plasma HIV-RNA is easier to maintain when CD4 counts are higher and VLs are lower.[66]

It is further recommended that all patients with advanced AIDS be treated with antiretrovirals regardless of plasma viral levels, as well as all patients with thrush or unexplained fevers. If a patient is acutely ill with an opportunistic infection or other complication of HIV disease, the timing of antiretroviral therapy initiation should be based on drug toxicity, ability to adhere to the treatment regimen, drug interactions, and laboratory abnormalities.[66] However, maximally suppressive regimens should be used, and patients with advanced AIDS should not discontinue therapy during an acute opportunistic infection or malignancy unless there is drug toxicity, intolerance, or drug interactions.[66]

Given that many studies show that baseline levels of HIV RNA may be lower and CD4 cell counts may be higher when AIDS is first diagnosed in women, federal treatment guidelines suggest that clinicians initiate HAART in women even when the CD4 cell counts are higher than 350 cells/mm^3, although a specific threshold has not been established.[66]

Recommended Antiretroviral Therapy. Since the advent of highly active antiretroviral therapy (HAART) in 1995, updated guidelines by the DHHS in July 2003 call for the use of three or more antiretroviral agents. The recommendations are for three alternative HAART regimens that sequence the medications and preserve one class of drug for future use.[67] Currently, triple drug therapy is a first-line option in lowering VL and limiting the destruction of the immune system.[66] Clinical trials indicate that the most effective course of treatment is by combining three or more drugs from the following three categories:

Table 37–1
Opportunistic Infections and Treatments: Prophylaxis to Prevent First Episode of Opportunistic Disease in Adults and Adolescents Infected with Human Immunodeficiency Virus

	Preventive Regimens		
Pathogen	**Indication**	**First Choice**	**Alternatives**
Strongly Recommended as Standard of Care			
*Pneumocystis carinii**	CD4+ count <200/μL *or* oropharyngeal candidiasis	Trimethoprim-sulfamethoxazole (TMP-SMZ), 1 DS PO qd (AI)	Dapsone, 50 mg PO bid *or* 100 mg PO qd (BI); dapsone, 50 mg PO qd *plus* pyrimethamine, 50 mg PO qw *plus* leucovorin, 25 mg PO qw (BI); dapsone, 200 mg PO *plus* pyrimethamine, 75 mg PO *plus* leucovorin, 25 mg PO qw (BI); aerosolized pentamidine, 300 mg qm via Respirgard II nebulizer (BI); atovaquone, 1500 mg PO qd (BI); TMP-SMZ, 1 DS PO tiw (BI)
Mycobacterium tuberculosis Isoniazid-sensitive[†]	TST reaction ≥5 mm *or* prior positive TST result without treatment *or* contact with case of active tuberculosis	Isoniazid, 300 mg PO *plus* pyridoxine, 50 mg PO qd × 9 mo (AII) or isoniazid, 900 mg PO *plus* pyridoxine, 100 mg PO biw × 9 mo (BI); rifampin, 600 mg *plus* pyrazinamide, 20 mg/kg PO qd × 2 mo (AI)	Rifabutin 300 mg PO qd *plus* pyrazinamide, 20 mg/kg PO qd × 2 mo (BIIt); rifampin 600 mg PO qd × 4 mo (BIII)
Isoniazid-resistant	Same; high probability of exposure to isoniazid-resistant tuberculosis	Rifampin, 600 mg *plus* pyrazinamide, 20 mg/kg PO qd × 2 mo (AI)	Rifabutin, 300 mg *plus* pyrazinamide 20 mg/kg PO qd × 2 mo (BIII); rifampin, 600 mg PO qd × 4 mo (BIII); rifabutin, 30 mg PO qd × 4 mo (CIII)
Multidrug (isoniazid and rifampin)-resistant	Same; high probability of exposure to multidrug-resistant tuberculosis	Choice of drugs requires consultation with public health authorities	None
Toxoplasma gondii[§]	IgG antibody to *Toxoplasma* and CD4+ count <100/μL	TMP-SMZ, 1 DS PO qd (AII)	TMP-SMZ, 1 SS PO qd (BIII): dapsone, 50 mg PO qd *plus* pyrimethamine, 50 mg PO qs *plus* leucovorin, 25 mg PO qw (BI); atovaquone, 1500 mg PO qd with or without pyrimethamine, 25 mg PO qd *plus* leucovorin, 10 mg PO qd (CIII)
Mycobacterium avium complex[¶]	CD4+ count <50/μL	Azithromycin, 1200 mg PO qw (AI), or clarithromycin, 500 mg PO bid (AI)	Rifabutin, 300 mg PO qd (BI); azithromycin, 1200 mg PO qw *plus* rifabutin, 300 mg PO qd (CI)
Varicella-zoster virus (VZV)	Significant exposure to chickenpox or shingles for patients who have no history of either condition or, if available, negative antibody to VZV	Varicella-zoster immune globulin (VZIG), 5 vials (1.25 mL each) IM, administered ≤96 h after exposure, ideally within 48 h (AIII)	
Generally Recommended			
*Streptococcus pneumoniae***	All patients	Pneumococcal vaccine, 0.5 mL IM (CD4+ ≥200/μL [BII]; CD4+ <200/μL [CIII])—might reimmunize if initial immunization was given when CD4+ <200/μL and if CD4+ increases to >200/μL on HAART (CIII)	None

Table 37–1
Opportunistic Infections and Treatments: Prophylaxis to Prevent First Episode of Opportunistic Disease in Adults and Adolescents Infected with Human Immunodeficiency Virus *(continued)*

	Preventive Regimens		
Pathogen	**Indication**	**First Choice**	**Alternatives**
Hepatitis B virus (HBV)††	All susceptible (anti-HBc-negative) patients	Hepatitis B vaccine: 3 doses (BII)	None
Influenza virus††	All patients (annually, before influenza season)	Whole or split virus, 0.5 mL IM annually (BIII)	Rimantadine, 100 mg PO bid (CIII), or amantadine, 100 mg PO bid (CIII)
Hepatitis A virus (HAV)††	All susceptible (anti-HAV-negative) patients with chronic hepatitis C	Hepatitis A vaccine: 2 doses (BIII)	None
Not Routinely Indicated			
Bacteria	Neutropenia	Granulocyte colony-stimulating factor (G-CSF), 5–10 μg/kg SC qd × 2–4 wk or granulocyte-macrophage colony-stimulating factor (GM-CSF), 250 μg/m² IV over 2 h qd × 2–4 wk (CII)	None
Cryptococcus neoformans§§	CD4+ count < 50/μL	Fluconazole, 100–200 mg PO qd (CI)	Itraconazole, 200 mg PO qd (CIII)
Histoplasma capsulatum§§	CD4+ count < 100/μL, endemic geographic area	Itraconazole capsule, 200 mg PO qd (CI)	None
Cytomegalovirus (CMV)¶¶	CD4+ count < 50/μL and CMV antibody positivity	Oral ganciclovir, 1 g PO tid (CI)	None

Notes: Information included in these guidelines might not represent Food and Drug Administration (FDA) approval or approved labeling for the particular products or indications in question. Specifically, the terms "safe" and "effective" might not be synonymous with the FDA-defined legal standards for product approval. The Respirgard II nebulizer is manufactured by Marquest, Englewood, Colorado. Letters and Roman numerals in parentheses after regimens indicate the strength of the recommendation and the quality of evidence supporting it.

Abbreviations: Anti-HBc = antibody to hepatitis B core antigen; b.i.w. = twice a week; DS = double-strength tablet; HAART = highly active antiretroviral therapy; IgG = immunoglobalin G; q.d. = daily; q.m. = monthly; q.w. = weekly; SS = single-strength tablet; t.i.w. = three times a week; and TST = tuberculin skin test

* Prophylaxis should also be considered for persons with a CD4+ percentage of <14%, for persons with a history of an AIDS-defining illness, and possibly for those with CD4+ counts >200 but <250/μL. TMP-SMZ also reduces the frequency of toxoplasmosis and some bacterial infections. Patients receiving dapsone should be tested for glucose-6 phosphate dehydrogenase deficiency. A dosage of 50 mg q.d. is probably less effective than that of 100 mg q.d. The efficacy of parental pentamidine (e.g., 4 mg/kg/mo) is uncertain. Fansidar (sulfadoxine-pyrimethamine) is rarely used because of severe hypersensitivity reactions. Patients who are being administered therapy for toxoplasmosis with sulfadiazine-pyrimethamine are protected against *Pneumocystis carinii* pneumonia and do not need additional prophylaxis against PCP.

† Directly observed therapy is recommended for isoniazid, 900 mg b.i.w.; isoniazid regimens should include pyridoxine to prevent peripheral neuropathy. Rifampin should not be administered concurrently with protease inhibitors or nonnucleoside reverse transcriptase inhibitors. Rifabutin should not be given with hard-gel saquinavir or delavirdine; caution is also advised when the drug is coadministered with soft-gel saquinavir. Rifabutin may be administered at a reduced dose (150 mg q.d.) with indinavir, nelfinavir, or amprenavir; at a reduced dose of 150 mg q.o.d. (or 150 mg t.i.w.) with ritonavir; or at an increased dose (450 mg q.d.) with efavirenz; information is lacking regarding coadministration of rifabutin with nevirapine. Exposure to multidrug-resistant tuberculosis might require prophylaxis with two drugs; consult public health authorities. Possible regimens include pyrazinamide plus either ethambutol or a fluoroquinolone.

§ Protection against toxoplasmosis is provided by TMP-SMZ, by dapsone plus pyrimethamine, and possibly by atovaquone. Atovaquone may be used with or without pyrimethamine. Pyrimethamine alone probably provides little, if any, protection.

¶ See footnote † regarding use of rifabutin with protease inhibitors or nonnucleoside reverse transcriptase inhibitors.

** Vaccination should be offered to persons who have a CD4+ count <200/μL, although the efficacy might be diminished. Revaccination 5 years after the first dose, or sooner if the initial immunization was given when the CD4+ count was <200/μL and the CD4+ count has increased to >200/μL on HAART, is considered optional. Some authorities are concerned that immunizations might stimulate the replication of HIV. However, one study showed no adverse effect of pneumococcal vaccination on patient survival (McNaghten et al. (1999), reference 134).

†† These immunizations or chemoprophylactic regimens do not target pathogens traditionally classified as opportunistic but should be considered for use in HIV-infected patients as indicated. Data are inadequate concerning clinical benefit of these vaccines in this population, although it is logical to assume that those patients who develop antibody responses will derive some protection. Some authorities are concerned that immunizations might stimulate HIV replication, although for influenza vaccination, a large observational study of HIV-infected persons in clinical care showed no adverse effect of this vaccine, including multiple doses, on patient survival (J. Ward, CDC, personal communication). Hepatitis B vaccine has been recommended for all children and adolescents and for all adults with risk factors for HBV. Rimantadine and amantadine are appropriate during outbreaks of influenza A. Because of the theoretical concern that increases in HIV plasma RNA after vaccination during pregnancy might increase the risk of perinatal transmission of HIV, providers may wish to defer vaccination until after antiretroviral therapy is initiated. For additional information regarding vaccination against hepatitis A and B, and vaccination and antiviral therapy against influenza, see-CDC. Prevention of hepatitis A through active or passive immunization: recommendations of the Advisory Committee on Immunization Practices (ACIP). MMWR 1996;45(No. RR-15); CDC. Hepatitis B virus: a comprehensive strategy for eliminating transmission in the United States through universal childhood vaccination: recommendations of the Advisory Committee on Immunization Practices (ACIP). MMWR 1991;40(No. RR-13); and CDC. Prevention and control of influenza: recommendations of the Advisory Committee on Immunization Practices (ACIP). MMWR 1999;48(No. RR-4).

§§ In a few unusual occupational or other circumstances, prophylaxis should be considered; consult a specialist.

¶¶ Acyclovir is not protective against CMV. Valacyclovir is not recommended because of an unexplained trend toward increased mortality observed in persons with AIDS who were being administered this drug for prevention of CMV disease.

Source: U.S. Department of Health & Human Services (2001), reference 135.

Table 37–2
Vaccine-Preventable Illness

Condition	Evidence Requiring Intervention	Intervention
Hepatitis A *consider in nonimmune sexually active patients*	Hepatitis A antibody-negative	Hepatitis A vaccine. Doses given at 0 and 6 mo
Hepatitis B	Hepatitis B antibody-negative	Hepatitis B vaccine. Doses given at 0, 1, and 6 mo
Tetanus	No serological test available	Consider booster if not vaccinated within 10 y
Hib	No serological test available	Routine vaccination has not been demonstrated to be beneficial; however, vaccine is inexpensive
Influenza	No serological test available	Vaccine should be offered annually in the fall
Pneumococcal	No serological test available	Vaccine is given at baseline and every 6–8 y
MMR	Measles, rubella, and mumps titer-negative or nonimmune	Vaccination not routinely given but may be required in those never immunized, particularly students, teachers, health care workers, and other care providers

Source: Adapted from Centers for Disease Control and Prevention (1993), reference 131.

- Nucleoside-analog reverse transcriptase inhibitors (NRTIs)
- Nonnucleoside reverse transcriptase inhibitors (NNRTIs)
- Protease inhibitors (PIs)

The NRTIs were the first class of antiretroviral agents approved for the treatment of HIV disease and included the drug known as AZT, also known as zidovudine. NRTIs limit HIV replication early in the HIV life cycle by inhibiting the enzyme reverse transcriptase, necessary for transcription of viral RNA into DNA. For many years, zidovudine was used as monotherapy, but this is no longer the accepted standard of care. NRTIs include zidovudine (AZT, ZVD, Retrovir), didanosine (ddi, Videx), zalcitabine (ddC, Hivid), stavudine (d4T, Zerit), lamivudine (3TC, Epivir), abacavir (Ziagen), tenofovir (Viread), and emtricitabine (Emtriva).[67] The NRTI abacavir, in combination with ZDV and 3TC, appears to suppress VL to a similar degree when compared to a PI plus two NRTIs after 48 weeks of follow-up. However, abacavir is associated with potentially life-threatening hypersensitivity syndrome.[71]

To limit the number of medications taken, thereby promoting medication adherence, a combination antiretroviral drug called Combivir, which combines two NRTIs, lamivudine 150 mg and zidovudine 300 mg, is available as a single tablet. Combivir is often taken with a PI.

The second category of antiretrovirals developed were the NNRTIs. Like the NRTIs, they function by inhibition of the enzyme reverse transcriptase. Because of the potential risk of resistance, these drugs are not recommended for monotherapy, but can be used as triple drug therapy along with an NRTI and a PI. The NNRTIs are nevirapine (Viramune), delavirdine (Rescriptor), and efavirenz (Sustiva). However, not all PIs can be given with NNRTIs; for example, saquinavir should not be given with efavirenz.

The third category of antiretrovirals are the PIs, which are highly potent with limited toxicity. PIs function by inhibiting the action of protease by binding to the cleavage site of replicating HIV and halting the production of new infectious virions. The PIs include saquinavir (Invirase, Fortovase), nelfinavir (Viracept), ritonavir (Norvir), indinavir (Crixivan), amprenavir (Agenerase), atazanavir (Reyataz), and lopinavir/ritonavir (Kaletra).

The fourth category of antiretrovirals are the viral entry inhibitors, which inhibit the fusion of HIV-1 with CD4 T cells by binding to a region of the cell envelope that is involved with the fusion process. Enfuvirtide (Fuzeon) is the first approved viral entry inhibitor.[67] A summary of the current antiretroviral medications is presented in Table 37–3.

To achieve maximal viral suppression, treatment with one potent PI and two NRTIs has proven effective in initial therapy. The NNRTI efavirenz used in combination with two NRTIs

Table 37–3
Antiretroviral Medications

Name	Dosage	Common Side Effects	Special Instructions	Drug Interactions
Nucleoside Reverse Transcriptase Inhibitors (NRTIs)				
Zidovudine (ZVD, AZT, Retrovir)	200 mg tid or 300 mg bid (higher doses may be necessary for neurologic disease)	Neutropenia, anemia, nausea, myalgia, malaise, headache, insomnia	Take with meals to decrease nausea, and myalgias	Increased risk of neutropenia with ganciclovir and trimethoprim-sulfamethoxazole. Methadone increases blood levels. Stavudine may decrease effectiveness. Phenytoin alters metabolism (may increase or decrease levels).
Didanosine (ddI, Videx)	EC capsules: 400 mg PO qd or chewable tablets 200 mg bid	Peripheral neuropathy, abdominal pain, dry mouth, altered taste, diarrhea, pancreatitis, rash	Always take both tablets or all the powder to ensure correct dosage. Take with about 4 oz of water. Should be taken on an empty stomach (1/2 hr before meals or 1–2 hr after a meal). Avoid alcohol. Dapsone, ketoconazole, itraconazole should be taken 2 hr after didanosine. Report any numbness, burning, or tingling. Tetracycline and fluoroquinolone should be administered 2 hr before or after ddI. Indinavir should be administered at least 1 hr before or after ddI on an empty stomach. Ritonavir should be administered at least 2 hr before or after ddI.	Buffer affects dapsone, ketoconazole, protease inhibitors, and quinolones. Ganciclovir increase blood levels. Concomitant administration of pentamidine increases the risk of pancreatitis.
Zalcitabine (ddC, Hivid)	0.75 mg tid	Peripheral neuropathy, pancreatitis, rash, fever, aphthous ulcer, anemia, elevated liver enzymes	Avoid alcohol. Report any numbness, burning or tingling. Should be taken on an empty stomach.	Similar toxicity to didanosine and stavudine.
Stavudine (D4T, Zerit)	>60 kg: 40 mg bid	Peripheral neuropathy, elevated liver enzymes, nausea, diarrhea, myalgia	Avoid alcohol. Report any numbness, burning, or tingling.	Similar toxicity to zalcitabine and didanosine.
Lamivudine (3TC, Epivir)	150 mg bid or 300 mg qd	Mild rash, headache, diarrhea, hair loss, neutropenia	Can be taken with food.	Trimethoprim-sulfamethoxazole increases blood levels.
Abacavir (Ziagen)	300 mg bid	Fatal hypersensitivity reactions. Common side effects: nausea, vomiting,diarrhea, anorexia, insomnia,fever, headache, skin rash.	Take with or without food.	Alcohol decreases the elimination of abacavir, causing an increase in overall exposure.

(continued)

Table 37–3
Antiretroviral Medications *(continued)*

Name	Dosage	Common Side Effects	Special Instructions	Drug Interactions
Tenofovir (Viread)	300 mg qd	Asthenia, nausea, vomiting, diarrhea, flatulence, may be transient renal toxicity	Take with food.	
Emtricitabine (Emtriva)	200 mg qd	Skin discoloration, hyperpigmentation of palms &/or soles of feet	Take with or without food.	
Lamivudine/zidovudine (Combivir, Trizivir)	1 tab bid (150 mg of lamivudine and 300 mg of zidovudine per tablet)	Headache, malaise, fatigue, nausea, diarrhea, cough	Can be taken with food to decrease nausea.	Co-administration of ganciclovir, interferon-alpha or other bone-marrow-suppressive or cytotoxic agents may increase the hematoxicity of ZVD.
Nonnucleoside Reverse Transcriptase Inhibitors (NNRTIs)				
Nevirapine (Viramune)	200 mg, every day for 2 weeks, then 200 mg every 12 hr or 400 mg qd	Rash, pruritus, fever, thrombocytopenia, elevated liver enzymes	Discontinue if severe rash develops. Monitor liver function tests. Should not be used concurrently with hormonal contraception.	Decreases protease inhibitor levels (induces cytochrome P450 enzymes)
Delavirdine (Rescriptor)	400 mg tid or 600 mg bid	Rash, fever, elevated liver enzymes	Take on an empty stomach. Monitor liver function test. Should be taken 1 hr before or after ddI or antacids.	Increases protease inhibitors, clarithromycin, dapsone, rifabutin, ergot alkaloids, dihydropyrides, quinidine, and warfarin levels (inhibits cytochrome P450 enzymes).
Efavirenz (Sustiva)	600 mg PO with protease inhibitor or NRTI	Psychiatric and nervous system symptoms such as dizziness, abnormal dreams, impaired concentration, delusions, insomnia, abnormal behavior, and rash	Taken with or without food. If taken with food, a high-fat meal should be avoided. If taken at bedtime,there is improved tolerability of nervous system side effects.	Drugs that induce CYP3A4 activity such as phenobarbital, rifampin, and rifabutin, would be expected to increase the clearance of efavirenz, therefore resulting in lower plasma concentrations. Warfarin plasma concentrations and effects are potentially increased or decreased with efavirenz. The dose of indinavir should be increased from 800 mg to 1000 mg if co-administered with efavirenz. Saquinavir and clarithromycin plasma concentrations are decreased by efavirenz

Protease Inhibitors (PIs)				
Indinavir (Crixivan)	800 mg tid	Nephrolithiasis, hyperbilirubinemia, fatigue, headache, nausea, abdominal pain	Lactose-intolerant patients should take with Lactaid tablets. Should be taken on an empty stomach or with light, low to nonfat meal. Increase water intake each day (at least 48 oz of fluid in adults). Never take double doses unless instructed.	Inhibits cytochrome P450. Ketoconazole increases blood levels; rifabutin and rifampin decrease blood levels; astemizole, terfenadine, cisapride, and triazolam increases the risk of dysrhythmias.
Nelfinavir (Viracept)	750 mg tid	Mild diarrhea, elevated liver enzymes	Never take double doses unless instructed. Should be taken with a meal or light snack. Should be administered 2 hr before of 1 hr after ddI.	Inhibits cytochrome P450. Rifabutin and rifampin decrease blood levels; astemizole, and cisapride increase risk of dysrhythmias.
Ritonavir (Norvir)	600 mg bid	Nausea, vomiting, diarrhea, taste alterations, paresthesias (hands, feet, and lips), elevated triglycerides	Therapy should be started at a low dose and increased over 5 days to decrease nausea. Never take double doses unless instructed. Monitor liver function test. Evaluate patient's medications profile before administering.	Inhibits cytochrome P450. Numerous drug interactions.
Amprenavir (Agenerase)	1,200 mg bid oral solution 1,400 mg bid	Increased LFTs, oral paresthesias, transient rash.	Avoid high fat meals.	If patients have sulfa allergy, higher incidence of amprenavir skin reactions.
Atazanavir (Reyataz)	400 mg qd	Hyperbilirubinemia; lower hypertriglyceridemia than other protease Inhibitors	Take with food.	
Lopinavir/ritonavir (Kaletra)	3 capsules (LPV 400 mg/RTV 100 mg)	Elevated transaminase levels	Take with food.	
Viral Entry Inhibitors				
Enfuvirtide (Fuzeon)	90 mg sc bid	Cardiac conduction abnormalities		
Saquinavir (Invirase [hard gel capsule] and Fortovase [soft gel capsule]).	600 mg tid	Headache, nausea, diarrhea	Should be taken within 2 hr of a full meal. Never take a double dose unless instructed. Lactose intolerant patients should take with Lactaid tablets.	Inhibits cytochrome P450. Rifabutin and rifampin decrease blood levels; ketoconazole, itraconazole, and ritonavir increase blood levels; terfenadine and astemizole increase risk of dysrhythmias.

Source: Adapted from Murphy & Flaherty (2003), reference 67, and Porche (1999), reference 69.

has also been shown to produce maximal viral suppression.[71] The three alternative HAART regimens include:

- Triple NRTIs combination
- One NNRTI (Nevirapine) plus two NRTIs
- A combination of one PI, one NNRTI, and one NRTI[67]

The advantages of class-sparing regimens, such as a regimen that is PI based and NNRTI sparing, is that clinical and virological efficacy is well documented, CD4-count increases are more robust than with other approaches, two steps of the viral replication process are targeted, and resistance requires multiple mutations. The disadvantages may be related to adherence and long-term side effects such as lipodystrophy, hyperlipidemia, and insulin resistance, as well as increases in cardiovascular disease and bone abnormalities (osteonecrosis, osteoporosis, and osteopenia).[67] Other adverse effects associated with HAART include hepatotoxicity, hepatic stenosis, lactic acidosis, and skin rash.[67] Change from one potent induction regimen to another potent regimen may be necessary if the patient's triglyceride and cholesterol levels become elevated, as lipodystrophy can be induced by protease inhibitors. Although the addition of hydroxyurea to certain antiretroviral regimens may enhance the activity of these agents, the role of hydroxyurea in HIV treatment remains uncertain given the relative lack of information from controlled trials and the number of toxicities.[71]

New Treatment Strategies. In addition to the newly approved viral entry inhibitors, new treatment strategies include mega HAART, structured treatment interruptions (STI), and immune-based therapies.[67] Mega-HAART has been successful in achieving viral suppression in individuals with extensive resistance to antiretroviral medications. In mega-HAART, up to 9 antiretroviral medications are administered. It is believed that no single virion is resistant to all nine drugs and, therefore, these drugs may reduce VL. However, given the drug toxicities and expense, most patients cannot tolerate this regimen for extended periods.[67] Although it was believed that individuals who have a significant antiretroviral drug resistance would benefit from interruptions of all antiretroviral medications to allow for a more drug-sensitive strain of HIV-RNA to emerge, current federal guidelines do not recommend the use of STIs in individuals with advanced illness until further research can be done. This is because STI are associated with a significant increase in VL, a significant decline in CD4 counts, and clinical disease progression.[67] In addition, there is intense investigation of immune-based therapies such as cytokines, particularly interleukin-2, which is used in combination with antiretroviral therapies to boost the immune system and increase CD4 cell counts.[66]

Reasons to Change a Regimen. A change in regimen may be necessary due to insufficient viral suppression evident by an increase in VL, inadequate increase in CD4 cell counts, or evidence of disease progression, as well as adverse clinical effects on the patient, or compromised adherence caused by the inconvenience of difficult regimens. However, the decision to change therapy should take into account whether other drug choices are available because another regimen may also be poorly tolerated or fail to result in better viral suppression, and such a change may limit future treatment options.[67] The criteria for considering changing a patient's antiretroviral regimen include:

- Less than a 0.5 to 0.75 $\log_{10}$ reduction in plasma HIV-RNA by 4 weeks after initiation of therapy or less than a 1.0 $\log_{10}$ reduction in 8 weeks
- Failure to suppress plasma HIV RNA to undetectable levels within 4 to 6 months after initiating therapy
- 3-fold or greater increase from the nadir of plasma HIV-RNA not attributable to intercurrent infection, vaccination, or test methodology
- Persistent decline in CD4 cell numbers measured on two separate occasions
- Clinical deterioration[66]

Clinicians should consult with HIV/AIDS specialists when considering a change in regimen. Furthermore, the change in an antiretroviral regimen can be guided by drug-resistance tests, such as genotyping and phenotyping assays. Drug resistance is a major short-term risk associated with any level of viral replication.[67]

Concern Regarding Drug Interactions. Considerations are also to be given to possible drug interactions such as pharmacokinetic interactions, which occur when administration of one agent changes the plasma concentration of another agent, and pharmacodynamic interactions, which occur when a drug interacts with the biologically active sites and changes the pharmacological effect of the drug without altering the plasma concentration. For example, in palliative care, drug interactions have been reported for patients who are receiving methadone for pain management and who begin therapy with an NNRTI, nevirapine. These individuals have reported symptoms of opioid withdrawal within 4 to 8 days of beginning nevirapine due to its effect on the cytochrome P-450 metabolic enzyme CYP3A4 and its induction of methadone metabolism.[72] See Table 37–3 on antiretroviral medications for dosages, common side effects, special instructions, and drug interactions.

Use and Continuation of Antiretrovirals in the Hospice/Palliative Care Setting and in Patients with Organ Failure. At present, the aims of antiretroviral therapy are to prevent progression to AIDS, prevent the direct effects and symptoms of HIV disease, such as dementia, neuropathy, and diarrhea, and prevent the complications of AIDS. According to Von Gunten and colleagues,[70] the continuation of antiretroviral therapy in hospice or palliative settings is often contingent on the feelings of patients regarding the therapy. Patients can be asked, "How do you feel when you take your antiretroviral medications?" Because medications may still symbolize hope, patients who enter hospice may have a greater acceptance of their mortality and wish to stop antiretrovirals because of the side effects. Other patients may wish to continue antiretroviral therapy because of its symptom relief and the prevention of future symptoms related to opportunistic infections. Von Gunten and colleagues[70] suggest the following plan:

1. If the drug causes burdensome symptoms, discontinue.
2. If the patient no longer wants the drug, discontinue.
3. If the patient is asymptomatic and wants the drug, continue with close clinical assessment.
4. Discontinue the measurement of VLs and CD4 counts and help the patient focus on relief of symptoms.

In the hospice and palliative care settings, it is important for clinicians to discuss with patients and families their goals of care to make important decisions regarding the appropriateness of curative, palliative, or both types of interventions. More specifically, examples of clinical decisions about palliative or disease-specific care include[73]:

- The use of blood transfusions, psychostimulants, or corticosteroids to treat fatigue in patients with late-stage AIDS
- Aggressive antiemetic therapy for PI-induced nausea and vomiting, or discontinuation of such antiretroviral therapies, given severe side effects
- Continued suppressive therapy for CMV retinitis to prevent blindness, or use of amphotericin B for azole-resistant candidiasis for patients who wish to continue eating, or other prophylactic medications in dying patients
- Palliative treatment of disseminated MAC in patients with advanced disease who are unwilling to take anti-infectives or withdrawal of MAC or PCP prophylaxis in patients who are expected to die soon
- Use of HAART for short-term palliation of symptoms related to high VLs, or withdrawal of HAART after evident treatment failure, with assessment of medical risk-benefit and emotional value of therapy
- Decisions to initiate HAART in newly diagnosed late-stage patients

Selwyn and Rivard[73] suggest that decisions regarding these issues need to be based on the specific goals of care, such as quality of life or life prolongation, the use of palliative care interventions to relieve the side effects of other medications, and the use of certain disease-specific therapies to enhance quality of life, as well as the decision to not prolong life when a certain threshold is met, such as progressive dementia.

The use of antiretrovirals must also be seriously considered for patients who have organ dysfunction or failure, given changes in hepatic and renal function and the effects on drug elimination. For example, patients with renal impairment may be at greater risk for zidovudine-induced hematological toxicity due to lowered production of erythropoietin. In addition, because of the markedly decreased clearance of ZVD and increased drug half-life, it is recommended that the daily dosage of ZVD be reduced by approximately 50% in patients with severe renal dysfunction (CrCL, 25 mL/min), for those receiving hemodialysis, and for those with hepatic dysfunction.[74] In addition, due to reduced drug clearance, patients should be monitored for ZVD-related adverse effects.

Although specific dosage recommendations are available for some of the early developed antiretrovirals for patients with organ dysfunction or failure, there are no specific studies that provide guidelines for the dosing of many of the new antiretroviral agents. As many of the antiretroviral agents are metabolized by the liver and excreted by the kidney, knowledge of pharmacokinetic properties of antiretroviral drugs is recommended to monitor drug therapy for efficacy and safety.[74] The suggested dosing recommendations for antiretroviral agents in patients with organ dysfunction are presented in Table 37–4.

Adherence to Therapy. Adherence, which is "the extent to which a person's behavior coincides with medical and health advice,"[75] is essential to health maintenance for patients with HIV/AIDS because nonadherence to antiretroviral therapy may lead not only to resistance to a whole class of drug, especially PIs, but also may affect systemic drug concentration, intracellular drug concentration, drug potency, viral resistance, and viral inhibition.[76]

Medication adherence is defined as the ratio of medication doses taken to those prescribed with a cutoff of 80% to categorize the patient as adherent.[76] However, there is concern that with HAART therapy optimal viral suppression requires 90% to 95% adherence.[67] Simplifying the patient's HAART regimen to decrease the number of medications taken and the number of times the patient has to take medications can improve adherence.[67] Assessment of adherence is most often done by self-report, with studies showing that it is a valid indicator of adherence.[77] Asking patients to bring their medications to a health visit, to describe their pill-taking regimens, to review the number of doses taken in 24 hours, and to ask about problems taking the medications and effects of the medications are important aspects of assessment.[76] Factors not predictive of adherence include age, sex, race, education, occupation, and socioeconomic status,[78] while factors predictive of adherence include[79]:

- Patient characteristics, such as physical and emotional health, material resources, cultural beliefs, self-efficacy, social support, personal skills, and HIV knowledge
- Clinician factors, including interpersonal style, availability, as well as assessment, communication, and clinical skills
- Medication regimen factors, such as frequency, number, and size of pills, taste of pills, storage, side effects, effectiveness, and cost
- Illness factors, including symptoms duration, severity, and stigma

Table 37–4
Dosing Recommendations for Antiretroviral Agents in Patients with Organ Dysfunction

	Renal Dysfunction Creatinine Clearance (mL/min)					
Drug and Body Weight	≥50	26–49	10–25	<10	Hemodialysis	Hepatic Dysfunction
Zidovudine	200 mg q8h	200 mg q8h	100 mg q8h	100 mg q8h	100 mg q8h	100 mg q8h
Didanosine						
≥60 kg	200 mg q12h	200 mg q24h	100 mg q24h	100 mg q24h	100 mg q24h*	Consider empiric dosage reduction in moderate to severe disease†
<60 kg	125 mg q12h	125 mg q24h	50 mg q24h	50 mg q24h	50 mg q24h*	
Zalcitabine	0.75 mg q8h	0.75 mg q12h	0.75 mg q12h	0.75 mg q24h	0.75 mg q24h*	0.75 mg q8h
Stavudine						
≥60 kg	40 mg q12h	40 mg q24h	20 mg q24h	20 mg q24h	20 mg q24h*	40 mg q12h†
<60 kg	30 mg q12h	30 mg q24h	15 mg q24h	15 mg q24h	15 mg q24h*	30 mg q12h†
Lamivudine	150 mg q12h	150 mg q24h	150 mg × 1, then 100 mg q24h	150 mg × 1, then 25–50 mg q24h	150 mg × 1, then 25–50 mg q24h*	150 mg q12h†
Nevirapine	200 mg q12h	200 mg q12h	200 mg q12h	200 mg q12h	NR*	Consider empiric dosage reduction†
Delavirdine	400 mg q8h	400 mg q8h	400 mg q8h	400 mg q8h	NR*	Consider empiric dosage reduction†
Efavirenz	600 mg q24h	600 mg q24h	600 mg q24h	600 mg q24h	NR*	Consider empiric dosage reduction†
Saquinavir§	600 mg q8h	600 mg q8h	600 mg q8h	600 mg q8h	NR*	Consider empiric dosage reduction†
Ritonavir	600 mg q12h	600 mg q12h	600 mg q12h	600 mg q12h	NR*	Consider empiric dosage reduction†
Indinavir	800 mg q8h	800 mg q8h	800 mg q8h	800 mg q8h	NR*	Mild to moderate: 600 mg q8h Severe: consider further dosage reduction†
Nelfinavir	750 mg q8h	750 mg q8h	750 mg q8h	750 mg q8h	NR*	Consider empiric dosage reduction†

*Administer daily dose after completion of hemodialysis.
†No specific recommendations available. Patients should be carefully monitored for adverse effects.
§Data shown for hard gelatin capsule formulation. Dosage for soft gelatin capsule is 1200 mg q8h.
NR = No recommendations.
Source: Hilts and Fish (1998), reference 74.

Table 37–5
Interventions to Improve Antiretroviral Medication Adherence

Type of Intervention	Specific Examples
Interventions addressing the patient	
Key patient education topics	Dynamics of HIV infection Purpose of antiretroviral therapy All names of medications Reasons for dose and administration requirements Potential side effects Techniques for managing side effects
Cues and reminders for patient	Detailed daily schedule Doses planned to coincide with daily habits (favorite TV program, morning news) Medication boxes and timers (available from some pharmaceutical companies) Prepoured medications Unit-of-use packaging
Patient involvement in therapeutic plan	Contributes to choice of antiretroviral combination Self-control of medications for side effects Anticipatory planning for weekends, vacations
Rewards and reinforcements	Positive feedback: falling HIV RNA level, rising CD4+ cell count, fewer clinic appointments
Social support for adherence	Involvement of significant others Support groups Peer counseling and buddy plans Treatment of concomitant conditions such as substance abuse, depression Case management and financial assistance Home visits and telephone follow-up
Interventions addressing the clinician	
Continuing education regarding	Importance of adherence Factors associated with adherence Techniques to increase adherence Teaching skills Communication skills Effective management of side effects
Cues and reminders for the clinician	User-friendly medication review forms Tables and checklists in the clinical chart Patient teaching tools
Social support	Involvement of colleagues Team approach Administrative approval for additional time spent with patient on adherence concerns
Interventions addressing the regimen	Once- or twice-a-day dosing regimens Use of fewer pills per day Use of smaller pills or capsules Improved taste Simpler storage requirements Fewer side effects Increased effectiveness Decreased cost

Source: Williams (1999), reference 76. Copyright 1999 with permission from Elsevier.

Adherence to medication regimens can be improved through educational, behavioral, and social interventions, specific to the patient, clinician, and medication regimen (Table 37–5).[76] An established partnership and an open, trusting, and supportive relationship between patient and clinician remain key factors in promoting not only adherence to medication regimens, but support of all health-promotion and management initiatives to delay disease progression and AIDS-related complications.

AIDS-Related Opportunistic Infections and Malignancies

Opportunistic infections are the greatest cause of morbidity and mortality in individuals with HIV disease. Given the compromised immune system of HIV-infected individuals, there is a wide spectrum of pathogens that can produce primary, life-threatening infections, particularly when the CD4 cell counts fall below 200 cells/mm^3. Given the weakened immune systems of HIV-infected persons, even previously acquired infections can be reactivated. Most of these opportunistic infections are incurable and can at best be palliated to control the acute stage of infection and prevent recurrence through long-term suppressive therapy. In addition, patients with HIV/AIDS often experience concurrent or consecutive opportunistic infections that are severe and cause a great number of symptoms. In Table 37–6, the various categories of opportunistic infections and malignancies are reviewed with regard to epidemiology/pathogenesis, presentation and assessment, diagnosis, and interventions.[10,13]

Pain and Symptom Management in HIV Disease

Patients with HIV/AIDS require symptom management not only for chronic debilitating opportunistic infections and malignancies, but also for the side effects of treatments and other therapies. There are five broad principles fundamental to successful symptom management: (1) taking the symptoms seriously, (2) assessment, (3) diagnosis, (4) treatment, and (5) ongoing evaluation.[80]

- Taking the symptoms seriously implies that symptoms often are not observable and measurable. Therefore, self-report of the patient should be taken seriously by the practitioner and acknowledged as a real experience of the patient. An important rule in symptom management is to anticipate the symptom and attempt to prevent it.[38] Assessment and diagnosis of signs and symptoms of disease and treatment side effects requires a thorough history and physical examination. Questions as to when the symptom began and its location, duration, severity, and quality, as well as factors that exacerbate or alleviate the symptom, are important to ask. Patients can also be asked to rate the severity of a symptom by using a numerical scale from 0 to 10, with 0 being "no symptom" to 10 being "extremely severe." Such scales can also be used to rate how much a symptom interferes with activities of daily life, with 0 meaning "no interference" and 10 meaning "extreme interference."
- Many patients seek medical care for a specific symptom, which requires a focused history, physical exam, and diagnostic testing. Throughout the continuum of HIV disease, CD4 counts and percentages, VLs, and blood counts and chemistries may provide useful information for the management of the disease and its symptoms. Assessment of current medications and complementary therapies, including vitamin therapy, past medical illness that may be exacerbated by HIV disease, and the administration regimen of chemotherapy and radiation therapy should also be ascertained to determine the effects of treatment, side effects, adverse effects, and drug interactions. However, when treatment is no longer effective, as in the case of extremely advanced disease, practitioners must reevaluate the benefits versus burden of diagnostic testing and treatments, particularly the need for daily blood draws or more invasive and uncomfortable procedures. When the decision of the practitioners, patient, and family is that all testing and aggressive treatments are futile, their discontinuation is warranted.
- Treatment of opportunistic infections and malignancies often requires support of the patient's immune system, antiretroviral therapy to decrease the VL and improve CD4 cell counts, and medications and therapies to cure the patient of opportunistic infections or merely palliate the associated symptoms. Indeed, the treatment of symptoms to improve quality of life plays an important role in the management of HIV disease throughout the course of the illness.[22] In the case of many infections, acute treatment is followed by the regular dosing or maintenance therapy to prevent symptom recurrence. To maximize the quality of life, each patient's treatment regimen and plan of care should be individualized, with documentation of the treatment response and ongoing evaluation.
- Ongoing evaluation is key to symptom management and to determining the effectiveness of traditional, experimental, and complementary therapies. Changes in therapies are often necessary because concurrent or sequential illness or conditions occur.[80]

In an article regarding the symptom experience of patients with HIV/AIDS, Holzemer[81] emphasizes a number of key tenets, specifically: (1) the patient is the gold standard for understanding the symptom experience; (2) patients should not be

Table 37–6
Opportunistic Infections and Malignancies Associated with HIV/AIDS

Types of Infections and Malignancies	Epidemiology/Pathogenesis	Presentation and Assessment	Diagnosis	Interventions
Fungal Infections				
Candida albicans	Ubiquitous organism. Occurs with immunosuppression/alteration in mucous membranes or skin. Early manifestation of HIV. Predictor of disease progression. Human-to-human transmission possible. Oropharyngeal candidiasis common.	Oral *Candida* manifests as pseudomembranous white patches, easily removed, leaving erythematous or bleeding mucosa. Vaginal candidiasis manifests with pruritus and curdlike vaginal discharge. Esophageal candidiasis manifests with dysphagia. *Candida* leukoplakia cannot be removed.	Often presumptive by tissue inspection. Wet mount and/or potassium hydroxide (KOH) smear showing budding hyphae. Esophageal diagnosis by endoscopy with biopsy. Diagnosis by culture is unreliable.	Mucotaneous infection treated locally with clotrimazole troches, nystatin suspension, fluconazole, miconazole, or amphotericin B
Coccidioides immitis (Coccidioidomycosis)	Endemic to south western United States. Acquired by inhalation of spores. Occurs with CD4+ count <250 μL.	May be asymptomatic or with progressive signs of fever, malaise, weight loss, cough, fatigue.	Chest radiographs may show diffuse interstitial or nodular infiltrates. Definitive diagnosis by culture or direct visualization of the organism in sputum, urine, or CSF.	System amphotericin B, followed by lifelong suppressive therapy with oral fluconazole
Cryptococcus neoformans (Cryptococcosis)	Ubiquitous organism. Aerosolized and inhaled. Most common life-threatening infection in AIDS. *Cryptococcus* meningitis has a high mortality rate.	Meningitis is most common clinical manifestation, with headache, fever, stiff neck, photophobia, lethargy, and confusion. Symptoms develop over 2–4 wk. Cranial nerve palsies occur. Decreased vision; can lead to blindness. Cryptococcal pneumonia may present with cough, dyspnea. Infection may disseminate to bone marrow, kidney, liver, spleen, lymph nodes, heart, oral cavity, and prostate.	Serum cryptococcal antigen is 99% indicative. Examination of CSF. Infection of extrameningeal sites diagnosed with India ink and culture of tissues and specimens. MRI or CT scan can show cryptococcoma. Chest radiographs show diffuse or focal infiltrates with or without mediastinal adenopathy.	Acute therapy with amphotericin B with or without fluconazole, then lifelong suppression with fluconazole
Histoplasma capsulatum	Endemic to midwest and south central United States. Spores are inhaled. Occurs with CD4+ counts <100 μL.	Cough with fever. Often disseminated disease rather than pneumonitis. Signs and symptoms include fever, weight loss, night sweats, nausea, diarrhea, abdominal pain.	Chest radiographs show diffuse bilateral interstitial infiltrates. One third have normal chest radiograph; 5–10% have cutaneous lesions	Amphotericin B for serious illness or itraconazole or fluconazole for mild disease. Lifelong therapy of itraconazole or fluconazole

(*continued*)

Table 37–6
Opportunistic Infections and Malignancies Associated with HIV/AIDS *(continued)*

Types of Infections and Malignancies	Epidemiology/Pathogenesis	Presentation and Assessment	Diagnosis	Interventions
Mycobacterial Infections				
Mycobacterium tuberculosis (TB)	Increase in infections attributable to the high incidence of HIV infection. HIV infection may lead to reactivation of latent TB infection. Outbreaks of multidrug-resistant TB. Caused by inhalation of infectious particles that are aerosolized. Can have latent infection with no symptoms of active TB. Extrapulmonary TB may occur in 70% of HIV-infected patients; TB decreases CD4+ count and increases viral load.	Fever, weight loss, night sweats, and fatigue are initial complaints. With pulmonary TB, dyspnea, hemoptysis, and chest pain may occur. Extrapulmonary sites such as lymph nodes, bones, bone marrow, joints liver, spleen, skin, and CSF may show TB.	Positive PPD is defined as >5 mm of induration at 48–72 h using Mantoux intradermal method. Check for anergy with use of mumps and *Candida*. Chest radiographs show apical or cavitary infiltrates, and may show intrathoracic adenopathy. Diagnosis confirmed by sputum for acid-fast bacilli (AFB) stain. Blood cultures for AFB should be obtained.	Four-drug regimen with isoniazid, rifampin, pyrazinamide, and either streptomycin or ethambutol. Prophylaxis with isoniazid or rifampin for individuals without current active TB.
Mycobacterium avium intracellulare (MAC)	Composed of *M. avium* and *M. intracellulare*, two related species. Exists in water, soil, and foodstuffs. Person-to-person transmission is not likely. Most common cause of systemic bacterial infection in AIDS. Disseminated disease frequently the cause of mortality in advanced HIV disease.	Respiratory symptoms uncommon. MAC bacteremia is the most common syndrome. Fever, fatigue, weight loss, anorexia, nausea and vomiting, night sweats, diarrhea, abdominal pain, hepatosplenomegaly, and lymphadenopathy are common symptoms.	Positive cultures from normally sterile sites (e.g., blood, bone marrow, lymph nodes). Confirmed by biopsy with AFB stain. Lab studies usually demonstrate anemia and elevated alkaline phosphatase.	Macrolide (clarithromycin or azithromycin) and rifabutin and ethambutol for acute treatment. Prophylaxis with rifabutin or clarithromycin or azithromycin
Viral Infections				
Cytomegalovirus (CMV)	Ubiquitous, human herpesvirus. Most common cause of serious opportunistic disease in AIDS. May have contracted primary infection in childhood or young adulthood. Occurs in >40% of patients with CD4+ count <50/μL.	CMV retinitis most common form; if untreated, can quickly lead to blindness. May be asymptomatic or with painless loss of visual acuity and symptoms of floaters or visual field defects, or conjunctivitis. GI tract is second most common site, with symptoms of dysphagia, abdominal pain, odynophagia, fever, bloody diarrhea, and colitis.	CMV retinitis on ophthalmoscopic exam shows creamy yellow-white exudate with retinal hemorrhage. GI CMV is demonstrated by endocscopy showing ulceration and tissue biopsy.	High doses of ganciclovir or foscarnet, followed by lifelong daily IV infusions, with maintenance doses of one of these two medications

Herpes simplex virus (HSV)	HSV-1 transmitted primarily by contact with mucous membranes and salivary secretions. HSV-2 spread by sexual transmission. Risk with CD4+ count <100/μL.	Cutaneous ulcerative, vesicular painful lesions on any part of the body, particularly face, genitals, or perianal area. May cause esophagitis with dysphagia and odynophagia.	Visual infection with confirmation by viral swab culture. If vesicle is present, it should be unroofed with 18-gauge needle and swabbed over the base of the ulcer.	Acyclovir is used in primary therapy. IV acyclovir for severe HIV infection or HSV encephalitis. Topical acyclovir ointment to relieve subjective symptoms. Maintenance therapy with acyclovir to prevent reactivation.
Varicella-zoster virus (VZV) (herpes zoster—shingles)	Herpesvirus; may be initial presentation of HIV infection. Recurrent or disseminated VZV is seen with advanced HIV disease. Primary VZV is chickenpox.	Radicular pain, a localized burning, followed by localized maculopapular rash along a dermatome progressing to fluid-filled continuous vesicles. Postherpatic neuralgia may persist for months after lesions have healed. Visceral dissemination to lung, liver, or CNS is life threatening.	Clinical appearance. Cutaneous scrapings stained with fluorescein-conjugated monoclonal antibodies to confirm presence of VZV antigens.	Acyclovir, famciclovir, ganciclovir, or foscarnet for acute treatment
Human papilloma virus (HPV)	Most prevalent STD. Occurs with increased frequency in immunocompromised patients	Genital and perianal warts in men and women. Internal warts may also occur.	Cytological dysplasia evident on smears.	Trichloroacetic acid 50% or podophyllin 25% or podofilox or 5-fluorouracil cream for acute treatment. Electrosurgery or surgical excision
Protozoal Infections				
Cryptosporidium parvum	Transmitted through fecally contaminated water or food. May spread person-to-person in HIV-infected individuals. Oocyts can remain active outside the body for 2–6 mo. Major cause of diarrhea when CD4+ count <200/μL.	Profuse watery diarrhea, severe crampy abdominal pain, nausea, flatulence, weight loss, electrolyte imbalance, dehydration. May lead to malabsorption and wasting syndrome.	Confirmed by modified acid-fast or fluorescent antibody stain of stool specimen or small bowel biopsy.	Restore immune system with HAART. No currently approved specific agent. Paromomycin or nitrazoxanide may be beneficial
Toxoplasma gondii	Occurs worldwide in humans and domestic animals, particularly cats. Oocyts transmitted in infected meats, eggs, vegetables, and other food products. Major cause of neurological morbidity and mortality, especially in individuals with CD4+ count <100 μL.	Toxoplasmosis encephalitis most common with headache, fever, altered mental status, focal neurological deficits, and seizures.	Laboratory studies nonspecific. CT scan with contrast or brain MRI shows multiple diffuse mass lesions with edema. Examination of CSF usually is not helpful.	Pyrimethamine and folinic acid as first-line treatment for acute infection. Second-line treatment with clindamycin or atovaquone-oneor clarithromycin or mycin. Lifelong prophylaxis with TMP-SMX for those with CD4+ count <100/μL.

(continued)

Table 37–6
Opportunistic Infections and Malignancies Associated with HIV/AIDS *(continued)*

Types of Infections and Malignancies	Epidemiology/Pathogenesis	Presentation and Assessment	Diagnosis	Interventions
Isospora belli	Distributed throughout the animal kingdom and endemic to parts of Africa, Chile, and Southeast Asia. Transmission through direct contact with infected animals, persons, or contaminated water. Shed in the stool of humans or host animals. Latino and foreign-born persons are at greater risk.	Profuse watery, diarrhea, with stool output averaging 8–10 bowel movements per day, steatorrhea, headache, fever, malaise, abdominal pain, vomiting, dehydration, and weight loss.	Identification of oocytes in the stool. Suggest minimum of four stool specimens taken for patients with AIDS. A rapid autofluorescence technique may help in making a more rapid and reliable diagnosis.	TMP-SMX or pyrimethamine for acute treatment. Maintenance treatment with either agent.
Microsporidia	Includes multiple species that are pathogenic to humans. Worldwide distribution. Occurs with CD4+ count <100 μL. Fecal–oral transmission by ingestion of spores. Can live outside body for for up to 4 months	Profuse watery diarrhea, with crampy abdominal pain, malabsorption, weight loss, and wasting.	Poor staining qualities. Detection requires endoscopy with small bowel biopsy.	HAART has led to the resolution of this infection. Albendazole and octreotide have proved beneficial.
Bacterial Infections				
Streptococcus pneumoniae and *Haemophilus influenzae* (community acquired)	Most common causes of bacterial pneumonia in HIV-infected individuals. Occurs five times more frequently with CD4+ <200 μL. Reaches the lungs through inhalation, aspiration of secretions from mouth or oropharynx, or spread by blood from another site.	Abrupt onset with fever, cough with purulent sputum, and systemic toxic effects.	Chest radiograph shows dense segmental or lobar consolidation. Chest radiograph may show nodular patterns or diffuse interstitial infiltrates.	Clarithromycin or azithromycin used to treat or prevent infection. Low-dose TMP-SMX as secondary prophylaxis for sinopulmonary infections. Vaccination against *H. influenzae* in persons with HIV infection.
Pseudomonas aeruginosa	Important pathogen in late HIV disease. Isolated from soil, water, plants, and animals. Most frequently acquired nosocomial pulmonary or cutaneous infection. High rate of relapse in those who survive initial infection.	Fever, cough, dyspnea, chest pain, sinusitis. May have recurrent cellulitis.	Blood and sputum cultures. Focal chest radiograph similar to other bacterial pneumonias	Optimize immunological status because PCP or MAC prophylaxis is not effective in prevention of *Pseudomonas*. Treatment requires two or more anti-pseudomonal agents.

Salmonella species	Gram-negative bacteria pathogenic in both animals and humans. *Salmonella typhi* causes thypoid fever. Nontyphoid *Salmonella* species cause infection in patients with AIDS. Transmitted person to person by oral–fecal route, and by infection in animals such as chickens. *Salmonella* gastroenteritis results from exposure to infected pets or animal-derived foodstuffs such as poultry or eggs. HIV-infected patients are at risk for *Salmonella* bacteremia with or without GI disease.	Bacteremia without signs of localizing infection and nonspecific signs of septicemia. GI presentation includes diarrhea or abdominal pain.	Bacterial culture of blood. *Salmonella* enteritis is diagnosed by positive stool cultures. Other localized disease is diagnosed by culture of CSF or aspirated fluid.	Ampicillin, fluoroquinolone, ciprofloxacin, cefotaxime, ceftriaxone, or TMP-SMX for acute treatment. TMP-SMX or amoxicillin for maintenance treatment.
Pneumocystis Infections				
Pneumocystis carinii	One of most common opportunistic infections in HIV infection. Most common cause of pulmonary disease. Without prophylaxis, occurs with CD4+ count <200 μL.	Fever, dyspnea, a nonproductive cough; 2% of patients develop spontaneous pneumothorax.	Sputum induction, bronchoalveolar lavage. Arterial blood gases show hypoxia. LDH elevated.	TMP-SMX or dapsone as first-line treatment. Pentamidine or clindamycin as second-line therapy. TMP-SMX for prophylaxis.
Malignancies				
Non-Hodgkin's lymphoma (NHL)	Rate of NHL is 73 times higher in HIV-infected individuals than in the general population. Greater chance of NHL with CD4+ count <50/μL and in older white men. Caused by uncontrolled proliferation of lymphatic tissue, usually arising in the lymph nodes, spleen, liver, and bone marrow. Brain is the most common site of involvement. In patients with HIV disease, 80%–90% of the NHL is extranodal, making lymph node–based tumors uncommon.	Nonspecific symptoms of unexplained fever, weight loss, and night sweats. Elevated serum LDH. Localizing symptoms depend on site of tumor. Neurological deficits if NHL of the brain. NHL of GI tract manifests with abdominal pain, weight loss, or GI bleeding. Small-bowel lymphoma may lead to obstructive jaundice and small-bowel intussusception.	Biopsy of specimens or cytological examination of tissue fluid. CT scan of brain or abdomen.	CNS lymphoma treated with radiation with poor survival (3 mo.). Disease outside CNS treated with chemotherapy. Assess and treat for neutropenia secondary to chemotherapy. Antiretroviral agents may enhance clinical response to chemotherapy.

(*continued*)

Table 37–6
Opportunistic Infections and Malignancies Associated with HIV/AIDS *(continued)*

Types of Infections and Malignancies	Epidemiology/Pathogenesis	Presentation and Assessment	Diagnosis	Interventions
Kaposi's sarcoma (KS)	Classic KS is a rare, unusual neoplasm that usually affects older men of Jewish and Mediterranean ancestory; it is different from KS of HIV infection, which is most frequently seen in HIV-infected men, who have sex with men, and is the most common HIV-associated malignancy. It is associated with specific sexual practices and geographic locations.	Seen in any tissue but most often found in GI tract, mucous membranes, lymph nodes, and skin. Identified as patch, plaque, and/or nodular lesions of any size, color or configuration on the trunk, arms, head, or neck. Lesions in GI tract may be associated with bleeding pain, weight loss, and diarrhea.	GI lesions are visualized by barium studies and are best evaluated endoscopically. Histological examination of tissue biopsy to confirm the diagnosis.	Treatment based on immunological status and symptoms. KS lesions are highly sensitive to radiation therapy. Isolated KS lesions can be treated with cryotherapy or laser surgery. Interferon-alpha with antiretroviral agents may be beneficial, as may single agent or combination chemotherapy.
Cervical invasive cancer	HIV-infected women have a 7-to-10 greater chance of developing precancerous or cancerous cervical lesions and a higher rate of recurrence after cervical intraepithelial neoplasia (CIN) excisions. Progression of CIN (cervical dysplasia) to carcinoma of the cervix is slow in immunocompromised women. Incidence of AIDS-defining cervical cancer appears to be higher in women who are injecting substance users, are black, and live in the southern United States.	Early stages are asymptomatic and usually identified by PAP smear. Vaginal bleeding, usually postcoital, is most common symptom. Metrorrhagia and malodorous, blood-tinged vaginal discharge may be present. Advanced disease may cause pelvic, back or leg pain, hematuria, rectal bleeding, or bladder and bowel involvement.	PAP smear to determine the presence of abnormal cells, visible lesions, or both. Recommended that HIV-infected women have a PAP smear twice in the first year after diagnosis. If both are negative then a yearly PAP smear is recommended. If PAP smear is abnormal than a colposcopy is recommended.	Treatment of CIN and cervical cancer is carbon dioxide laser therapy, conization, cryosurgery, or electrocautery. Treatment of invasive cancer depends on the stage of the disease and may include surgery, radiation, or chemotherapy

Sources: Ropka and Williams(1998) reference 13; Flaskerud and Ungvarski (1999) reference 10; Murphy and Flaherty (2003), reference 67.

labeled "asymptomatic" early in the course of the infection because they often experience symptoms of anxiety, fear, and depression; (3) nurses are not necessarily good judges of patients' symptoms, as they frequently underestimate the frequency and intensity of HIV signs and symptoms; however, following assessment, they can answer specific questions about a symptom, such as location, intensity, duration, etc.; (4) nonadherence to treatment regimens is associated with greater frequency and intensity of symptoms; (5) greater frequency and intensity of symptoms leads to lower quality of life; (6) symptoms may or may not correspond with physiological markers; and (7) patients use few self-care symptom management strategies other than medication.

Pain Management. Pain management must become more integrated in the comprehensive care offered to patients with AIDS because nearly two thirds of patients with HIV/AIDS report increasing pain as the disease progresses.[82] General estimates of the prevalence of pain in HIV-infected individuals range between 25% and 80%, which is associated with psychological and functional morbidity.[83] Shofferman and Brody[84] reported that more than half of the patients cared for in hospice with advanced AIDS experienced pain. In a study by Breitbart and colleagues,[85] only 8% of patients who reported severe pain (score of 8–10 on a pain intensity scale) in an AIDS-patient cohort received a strong opioid, as recommended by the World Health Organization (WHO) pain-management guidelines. Cleeland and colleagues[86] also reported significant undermedication of pain in AIDS patients (85%), far exceeding the published reports of undertreated pain in cancer populations. In a longitudinal study of 95 patients with AIDS, Frich and Borgbjerg[87] reported that the overall incidence of pain was 88%, and 69% suffered constant moderate to severe pain that interfered with daily living. The most common pain locations were the extremities (32%), head (24%), upper GI tract (23%) and lower GI tract (22%). Pain was associated with opportunistic infections, KS or lymphoma, as well as neuropathic pain in the extremities. The number of pain localizations increased significantly as death approached.

The inadequate assessment and treatment of pain often occurs because of societal, practitioner, and patient barriers and limitations. For example, with regard to pain management, society fears addiction to opioids and has not distinguished between the legitimate and illegal use of drugs. Practitioners may have inadequate knowledge and misconceptions about pain management, while patients often fear pain as suggesting advanced disease and are reluctant to report pain, desiring to be perceived as "good" patients.[32]

Pain syndromes in patients with AIDS are diverse in nature and etiology. For patients with AIDS, pain can occur in more than one site, such as pain in the legs (peripheral neuropathy reported in 40% of AIDS patients), which is often associated with antiretroviral therapy such as AZT, as well as pain in the abdomen, oral cavity, esophagus, skin, perirectal area, chest, joints, muscles, and headache.[27] Pain is also related to HIV/AIDS therapies such as antiretroviral therapies, antibacterials, chemotherapy such as vincristine, radiation, surgery, and procedures.[83] Following a complete assessment, including a history and physical examination, an individualized pain management plan should be developed to treat the underlying cause of the pain, often arising from underlying infections associated with HIV disease.[88]

The principles of pain management in the palliative care of patients with AIDS are the same as for patients with cancer, and include regularity of dosing, individualization of dosing, and using combinations of medications.[27] The three-step guidelines for pain management as outlined by WHO should be used for patients with HIV disease.[89] This approach advocates for the selection of analgesics based on the severity of pain. For mild to moderate pain, antiinflammatory drugs such as NSAIDs or acetaminophen are recommended. However, the use of NSAIDs in patients with AIDS requires awareness of toxicity and adverse reactions because they are highly protein-bound, and the free fraction available is increased in AIDS patients who are cachetic or wasted.[83] For moderate to severe pain that is persistent, opioids of increasing potency are recommended, beginning with opioids such as codeine, hydrocodone, or oxycodone (each available with or without aspirin or acetaminophen), and advancing to more potent opioids such as morphine, hydromorphone (Dilaudid), methadone (Dolophine), or fentanyl either intravenously or transdermally. In conjunction with NSAIDs and opioids, adjuvant therapies also recommended are:[83]

- Tricyclic antidepressants, heterocyclic and noncyclic antidepressants, and serotonin reuptake inhibitors for neuropathic pain
- Psychostimulants to improve opioid analgesia and decrease sedation
- Phenothiazine to relieve anxiety or agitation
- Butyrophenones to relieve anxiety and delirium
- Antihistamines to improve opioid analgesia and relieve anxiety, insomnia, and nausea
- Corticosteroids to decrease pain associated with an inflammatory component or with bone pain
- Benzodiazepines for neuropathic pain, anxiety, and insomnia

Caution is noted, however, with use of PIs because they may interact with some analgesics. For example, Ritonavir has been associated with potentially lethal interactions with meperidine, propoxyphene, and piroxicam. PIs must also be used with caution in patients receiving codeine, tricyclic antidepressants, sulindac, and indomethacin to avoid toxicity. Furthermore, for patients with HIV disease who have high fevers, the increase in body temperature may lead to increased absorption of transdermally administered fentanyl.[90]

To insure appropriate dosing when changing the route of administration of opioids or changing from one opioid to another, the use of an equianalgesic conversion chart is suggested. As with all patients, oral medications should be used if possible, with round-the-clock dosing at regular intervals, and the use of rescue doses for breakthrough pain. Often, controlled-released morphine or oxycodone are effective drugs for patients with chronic pain from HIV/AIDS. In the case of neuropathic pain, often experienced with HIV/AIDS, tricyclic antidepressants such as amitriptyline, or anticonvulsants such as Neurontin can be very effective.[27] However, the use of neuroleptics must be weighed against an increased sensitivity of AIDS patients to the extrapyramidal side effects of these drugs.[83] If the cause of pain is increasing tumor size, radiation therapy can also be very effective in pain management by reducing tumor size, as well as the perception of pain. Tables 37–7 and 37–8 present the nonopiate analgesics for pain management in patients with AIDS and opioid analgesics for the management of mild to moderate pain and from moderate to severe pain in patients with AIDS, respectively.

Tolerance, Dependence, and Addiction. Physiological tolerance refers to the shortened or diminished effect of a drug due to exposure to the drug, and, therefore, the need for increasing doses to maintain effect. In the case of opioids, tolerance to analgesic properties of the drug appears to be uncommon in the clinical setting, while tolerance to adverse effects such as respiratory depression, somnolence, and nausea is common and favorable. Most patients can remain on stable doses of opioids for prolonged periods of time. If an increase in opioid dosage is needed, it is usually because of disease progression. Another expected physiological response to opioids is physical dependence, which occurs after 3 to 4 weeks of opioid administration, as evidenced by withdrawal symptoms after abrupt discontinuation. If a drug is to be discontinued, halving the daily dose every 1 to 2 days until the dose is equivalent to 15 mg of morphine will reduce withdrawal symptoms.[32] Tolerance to opioids does not imply addiction, as addiction is a compulsive craving for a drug for effects other than pain relief and is extremely uncommon in patients who are terminally ill. Furthermore, studies have demonstrated that although tolerance and physical dependence commonly occur, addiction (psychological dependence) is rare and almost never occurs in individuals who do not have histories of substance abuse.[83] However, it should be noted that a certain percentage of patients with HIV/AIDS will have a history of substance abuse, either past or current, that needs to be recognized so that their pain can be managed appropriately, as well as other symptoms for which they are self medicating. Health care providers in palliative care are often concerned with the administration of opioids to patients who have a history of substance abuse, who are in methadone maintenance programs, or who currently are abusing drugs. As a result, these patients often receive ineffective pain management. Consistent use of a standard pain scale and regular monitoring of drug consumption by one nurse and one physician can be helpful in ongoing assessment and pain management because it limits potential abuse. Oral administration of medications also lowers abuse potential. Given that substance-abusing patients have greater tolerance to morphine derivatives and benzodiazepines because of previous exposure to these drugs, increased dosage may be necessary for effective pain management, or the interval between doses should be shortened. Furthermore, the dosages of medications should be carefully monitored to avoid overdosing, given the possibility of hepatic failure in substance-abusing patients. Simultaneous use of agonists and antagonists are avoided in all populations because they provoke withdrawal symptoms.

Alleviating Opioid Side Effects. Although opioids are extremely effective in pain management for patients with HIV disease, their common side effects must be anticipated and minimized.

Table 37–7
Nonopioid Analgesics for Pain Management in Patients with AIDS

Analgesic Nonopiate	Starting Dose (mg/d)	Plasma Duration (hours)	Half-life (hours)	Comments
Aspirin	650	4–6	3–12	The standard for comparison among nonopioids. GI toxicity. May not be as well tolerated as some newer analgesics.
Ibuprofen	400–600	4–8	3–4	Can inhibit platelet function.
Acetaminophen	650	4–6	2–4	Overdosage produces hepatic toxicity. Not antiinflammatory. Lack of GI and platelet toxicity.
Choline magnesium trisalicylate	700–1500	12	8–12	Believed to have less GI toxicity than other NSAIDs. No effect on platelet aggregation.
Naproxen	250–500	8–12	13	Lower incidence of side effects than other agents.
Indomethacin	25–75	8–12	4–5	Available in sustained release in the United States.
COX-2 inhibitor: Celecoxib	100–200 mg q.d. or bid	3–5	11	Not used for patients <18 y. Maximum daily dose is 400 mg. Growing concern regarding cardiac toxicities, especially with long term use.

Source: Portenoy (1997), reference 132.

Table 37–8
Opioid Analgesics for Mild to Moderate to Severe Pain in Patients with AIDS

	Recommended Dose (mg)	Peak Effect (hours)	Duration (hours)	Plasma Half-Life (hours)	Comments
For Mild to Moderate Pain					
Codeine (with or without acetaminophen) Tylenol #2 acetaminophen 300 mg + codeine 15 mg Tylenol #3 acetaminophen 300 mg + codeine 30 mg Tylenol #4 Acetaminophen 300 mg + codeine 60 mg	30–60 PO	1–2	3–4	2–3	Metabolized to morphine; often used to suppress cough. When acetaminophen is added, there is a ceiling dose of 4 g/d.
Hydrocodone (with acetaminophen combinations in Lorcet, Lortab, Vicodin, others)	30 PO	1–2	3–6	2–4	When acetaminophen is added, there is a ceiling dose of 4 g/d.
Oxycodone (with or without acetaminophen) Roxicodone (a single-entity oxycodone) Percoset (oxycodone 5 mg + acetaminophen 325 mg) Roxicet (oxycodone 5 mg + acetaminophen 500 mg)	20–30 PO	1–2	3–6	2–3	Toxicity is the same as morphine. Used with acetaminophen for moderate pain. Available as a single agent for severe pain. Equianalgesic to morphine when not combined with acetaminophen
Oxycodone (sustained release)—oxycodone SR	20–40 PO	1	8–12	2–3	—
Oxycodone (controlled release)—OxyContin	20–30 PO	3–4	8–12	2–3	—
For Moderate to Severe Pain					
Morphine (immediate release)	20–60 PO 10 IM, IV, SC	1–2 0.5–1	3–6 3–4	2–3 2–3	Standard of comparison for the opioid analgesics. Constipation, nausea, and sedation are common side effects. Respiratory depression is rare.
Morphine (controlled release)—MS Contin	20–60 PO	3–4	8–12	2–3	—
Morphine (sustained release)—Kadian, Oramorph SR	20–60 PO	4–6	24	2–3	Kadian is only QD dosing.
Hydromorphone (Dilaudid)	7.5 PO	1–2	3–6	2–3	Short half-life
Hydromorphone (sustained release)—Palladone	1.5 IM, IV	0.5–1	3–4	2–3	Toxicities similar to other opioids
Methadone (Dolophine)	20 PO 10 IM	1–2 0.5–1.5	4–>8 4–>8	12>150 12>150	Requires close monitoring for toxicity due to long half-life and careful titration.
Levorphanol (Levo-Dromoran)	4 PO 2 IM	1–2 0.5–1	3–6 3–6	12–15 12–15	Long half-life requiring careful titration in the first week

(continued)

Table 37–8
Opioid Analgesics for Mild to Moderate to Severe Pain in Patients with AIDS *(continued)*

	Recommended Dose (mg)	Peak Effect (hours)	Duration (hours)	Plasma Half-Life (hours)	Comments
Fentanyl	—	—	—	7–12	Can be administered as a continuous IV or SC infusion; 100 mcg/h is roughly equianalgesic to morphine 4 mg/h
Fentanyl transdermal (Duragesic)	—	—	48–72	16–24	100 mcg transdermal system is approximately equianalgesic to morphine 4 mg/h. Not suitable for rapid titration. If patient has pain after 48 h, increase the dose or change the patch every 48 h.
Fentanyl transmucosal (Actiq)	200 mcg (1–2 units) q3h PRN but no more than 4 units/d. The unit is to be sucked and not chewed. Redosing within a single pain episode can occur 15 min after the previous unit has been completed or 30 min after the start of the previous unit.	0.5	—	7	Unit is administered as a "lozenge" on a stick that is to be sucked. Used for breakthrough pain as a rescue dose for cancer patients. Not to be used with opioid-naïve patients due to life-threatening hypoventilation. Recent research findings suggest that the onset of effect is faster than oral morphine and the same as IV morphine.

Source: Portenoy (1997), reference 132.

In medically fragile populations, such side effects may also result from other comorbid conditions rather than from opioid analgesia itself; therefore, a complete assessment is warranted. Medications and treatments to alleviate opioid side effects include:

- Nausea and vomiting, treated with prochlorperazine (Compazine), metoclopramide (Reglan), haloperidol (Haldol), granisetron (Kytril), and ondansetron (Zofran). A change in the opioid may also be necessary.
- Constipation, treated by increasing fiber in the diet, stimulating cathartic drugs such as bisacodyl or senna, or hyperosmotic agents such as sorbitol or lactulose
- Sedation, treated by reducing the opioid in each dose or decreasing the frequency, as well as the ingestion of caffeine, and administration of dextroamphetamine or methylphenidate. Again, a change in the opioid may be warranted.
- Confusion, treated by lowering the opioid dose, changing to a different opioid or Haldol
- Myoclonus, treated with clonazepam (Klonopin), diazepam (Valium), and baclofen (Lioresal), or a change in the opioid
- Respiratory depression, prevented by starting at a low dose in opioid-naïve patients, and being aware of relative potencies when changing opioids, as well as differences by routes of administration. Naloxone (Narcan) may be administered to reverse respiratory depression but should be used with caution in patients who are opioid tolerant because of the risk of inducing a withdrawal state. Dilute one ampule of naloxone (0.4 mg) in 10 mL of normal saline and titrate to the patient's respirations.[83]

Management of Other Symptoms Experienced with HIV Disease. For patients with HIV/AIDS, suffering occurs from the many symptoms experienced at the various stages of the illness. Based on a sample of 1128 HIV-infected patients, Fantoni and colleagues[91] reported that the most commonly experienced symptoms were fatigue (65%), anorexia (34%), cough (32%), and fever (29%). In a study to assess the predominant symptoms

Table 37–9
Selected Symptoms Associated with HIV/AIDS

Symptom	Cause	Presentation	Interventions
Fatigue (asthenia)	HIV infection Opportunistic infections AIDS medications Prolonged immobility Anemia Sleep disorders Hypothyroidism Medications	Weakness Lack of energy	Treat reversible causes. Pace activities with rest periods/naps. Ensure adequate nutrition. Use relaxation exercises and meditation. Take warm rather than hot showers or baths. Use cool room temperatures. Administer dextroamphetamine 10 mg/d PO.
Anorexia (loss of appetite) and cachexia (wasting)	Metabolic alterations caused by cytokines and interleukin-1 Opportunistic infections Nutrient malabsorption from intestines Chronic diarrhea Depression Taste disorders	Diminished food intake Profound weight loss	Treat reversible causes. Consult with dietitian about choice of food. Make food appealing by color and texture. Avoid noxious smells at mealtime. Avoid fatty, fried, and strong-smelling foods. Offer small, frequent meals and nutritious snacks. Encourage patients to eat whatever is appealing. Provide high-energy, high-protein liquid supplements. Use appetite stimulants such as megesterol acetate 800 mg/d PO or dronabinol 2.5 mg PO qd or bid. Testosterone administered by 5 mg transdermal patch to increase weight gain and muscle mass.
Fever (elevated body temperature)	Bacterial toxins Viruses Yeast Antigen–antibody reactions Drugs Tumor products Exogenous pyrogens	Body temperature >99.5°F (oral), 100.5°F (rectal), or 98.5°F (axillary) Chills, rigor Sweating, night sweats Delerium Dizziness Dehydration	Treat reversible causes. Maintain fluid intake. Use loose clothing and sheets, with frequent changing. Avoid plastic bed coverings. Exceptionally high temperature may require ice packs or cooling blankets. Administer around-the-clock antipyretics such as acetaminophen or ASA, 325–650 mg PO q6–8 h.
Dyspnea (shortness of breath) and cough	Bronkospasm Embolism Effusions Pulmonary edema Pneumothorax Kaposi's sarcoma Obstruction Opportunistic infections Anxiety Allergy Mechanical or chemical irritants	Productive or nonproductive cough Crackles Stridor Hemoptysis Inability to clear secretions Wheezing Tachypnea Gagging Intercostal retractions Areas of pulmonary dullness	Treat reversible causes. Elevate bed to Fowler's or high Fowler's position. Provide abdominal splints. Administer humidified oxygen therapy to treat dyspnea. Use fans or open windows to keep air moving for dyspnea. Remove irritants or allergens such as smoke. Teach pursed-lips breathing for patients with obstructive disease.

(*continued*)

Table 37–9
Selected Symptoms Associated with HIV/AIDS *(continued)*

Symptom	Cause	Presentation	Interventions
	Anemia	Anxiety	Use frequent mouth care to decrease discomfort from dry mouth. Treat bronchospasm. Suppress cough with dextromethorphan hydrobromide 15–45 mg PO q4 h PRN, or opioids such as codeine 15–60 mg PO q4 h even if taking other opioids for pain, or hydrocodone 5–10 mg PO q4–6 h PRN, or morphine 5–20 mg PO q4 h PRN (may be increased) to relieve dyspnea, cough, and associated anxiety. For hyperactive gag reflex use nebulized lidocaine 5 mL of 2% solution (100 mg) q3–4 h PRN.
Diarrhea	Idiopathic HIV enteropathy Diet Bowel infections (bacteria, parasites, protozoa) Chronic bowel inflammation Medications Obstruction with overflow incontinence Stress Malabsorption	Flatulence Multiple bowel movements/day Cramps/colic Hemorrhoids	Treat reversible causes. Maintain adequate hydration. Replace electrolytes by giving Gatorade or Pedialyte. Give rice, bananas, or apple juice to reduce diarrhea. Increase protein and calories. Avoid dairy products, alcohol, caffeine, extremely hot or cold foods, spicy or fatty foods. Maintain dignity while toileting. Provide ready access to bathroom or commode. Maintain good perianal care. Administer medications such as Lomotil 2.5–5.0 mg q4–6 h; Kapectolin 60–120 mL q4–6 h (max 20 mg/d); Imodium 2–4 mg q6 h (max 16 mg/d); or aregoric (tincture of opium) 5–10 mL q4–6 h.
Insomnia (inability to fall asleep or stay asleep)	Anxiety Depression Pain Medications Delirium Sleep disorders such as sleep apnea Excess alcohol intake Caffeine	Early morning awakening Nighttime restlessness Fear Nightmares	Treat reversible causes. Establish a bedtime routine. Reduce daytime napping. Avoid caffeinated beverages and alcohol. Take a warm bath 2 h before bedtime. Use relaxation techniques. Provide an environment conducive to sleep (dark, quiet, comfortable temperature). Administer anxiolytics such as benzodiazepines (use for <2 wk because of dependency), antidepressants (helpful over long term), or other sedatives such as Benadryl.

Table 37–9
Selected Symptoms Associated with HIV/AIDS *(continued)*

Symptom	Cause	Presentation	Interventions
Headache	Infections such as encephalitis, herpes zoster, meningitis, toxoplasmosis Sinusitis	Pain in one or more areas of the head or over sinuses	Treat reversible causes. Suggest chiropractic manipulation. Provide message therapy. Use relaxation therapy. Apply TENS. Use stepwise analgesia. Administer corticosteroids to reduce swellings around space-occupying lesions.

Sources: Ropka and Williams (1998), reference 13; Unzarski and Flaskerud (1999), reference 10; Coyne et al. (2002), reference 133.

in 72 patients with AIDS, the most common symptoms were pain (97%), weakness (78%), and weight loss (53%).[78] Based on a sample of 207 patients with AIDS, Holzemer and colleagues[92] also found that 50% of the participants experienced shortness of breath, dry mouth, insomnia, weight loss, and headaches. The records of 50 men who died of AIDS between 1988 and 1992 indicated the distressing symptoms of dyspnea, diarrhea, confusion, dementia, difficulty eating, and swallowing. Therefore, care in the last month of life was often directed at the palliation of symptoms.[21] Indeed, the last stage of HIV infection is often marked by increasing pain, GI discomfort, and depression.[10] Patients may be suffering from inflammatory or infiltrative processes and somatic and visceral pain. Neuropathic pain is commonly a result of the disease process or the side effect of medications[93] Avis, Smith, and Mayer[94] also reported, based on a sample of 92 HIV-positive men, that quality of life was more related to symptoms as measured by the Whalen's HIV Symptom Index than CD4 counts or hemoglobin. With the myriad of symptoms experienced by patients with HIV disease across the illness trajectory, health care practitioners need to understand the causes, presentations, and interventions of common symptoms, as presented in Table 37–9, to enhance the quality of life of patients.

Nonpharmacological Interventions for Pain and Symptom Management. Nonpharmacological interventions for pain and symptom management can also be effective in the care of patients with HIV disease. Bed rest, simple exercise, heat or cold packs to affected sites, massage, transcutaneous electrical stimulation (TENS), and acupuncture can be effective physical therapies with this patient population. Psychological interventions to reduce pain perception and interpretation include hypnosis, relaxation, imagery, biofeedback, distraction, and patient education. In cases of refractory pain, nerve blocks and cordotomy are available neurosurgical procedures for pain management. Increasingly, epidural analgesia is an additional option that provides continuous pain relief.[83]

The 10 most commonly used complementary therapies and activities reported by 1106 participants in the Alternative Medical Care Outcomes in AIDS study were aerobic exercise (64%), prayer (56%), massage (54%), needle acupuncture (48%), meditation (46%), support groups (42%), visualization and imagery (34%), breathing exercises (33%), spiritual activities (33%), and other exercise (33%).[95] Clearly, patients with HIV disease seek complementary therapies to treat symptoms, slow the progression of the disease, and enhance their general well-being. Nurses' knowledge, evaluation, and recommendations regarding complementary therapies are important aspects of holistic care.

Psychosocial Issues for Patients With HIV/AIDS and Their Families

Uncertainty is a chronic and pervasive source of psychological distress for persons living with HIV disease, particularly as it relates to ambiguous symptom patterns, exacerbation and remissions of symptoms, selection of optimal treatment regimens, the complexity of treatments, and the fear of stigma and ostracism. Such uncertainty is linked with negative perceptions of quality of life and poor psychological adjustment.[96] However, many practitioners focus on patient's physical functioning and performance status as the main indicators of quality of life, rather than on the symptoms of psychological distress such as anxiety and depression.[97,81] Farber and colleagues[98] reported, based on a sample of 203 patients with HIV/AIDS, that positive meaning of the illness was associated with a higher level of psychological well-being and lower depressed mood, and contributed more than problem-focused coping and social support to predicting both psychological well-being and depressed mood. During the late stage of AIDS, minority women (n = 220) expressed high levels of psychological disturbance on the Psychiatric Symptom Index (PSI), which were significantly related to their mothers' reports of having non-HIV related medical conditions, spending time in bed during the past 2 weeks, having more activity restrictions, and having difficulty caring for her child due to ill health.[99] In a study of the problems and needs of HIV/AIDS patients during the last weeks of life, Butters and colleagues[100] determined, based on the Support Team Assessment Schedule

(STAS), that symptom control, patient and family anxiety, spiritual needs, and communication between patient and family were their greatest needs. Furthermore, Friedland and colleagues[101] identified the determinants of quality of life in a sample of 120 individuals with HIV/AIDS. Income, emotional support, and problem-oriented and perception-oriented coping were positively related to quality of life, while tangible support and emotion-focused coping were negatively related.

Ragsdale and Morrow[41] emphasized the importance of focusing on the psychosocial aspects of life in patients with HIV/AIDS because patients reported a repetitive cycle of emotional changes with slight physical changes. Disfigurement, the symptoms associated with the disease and its treatment, and the contagious nature of the disease add to the psychological distress associated with HIV/AIDS.

Nurses must also be cognizant of such issues as the experience of multiple losses, complicated grieving, substance abuse, stigmatization, and homophobia, which contribute to patients' sense of alienation, isolation, hopelessness, loneliness, and depression. Such emotional distress often extends to the patient's family caregivers as they attempt to provide support and lessen the patient's suffering, yet are often suffering from HIV disease themselves. Reciprocal suffering is experienced by family caregivers as well as patients, and there is the need to improve their quality of life through palliative care.[102]

Psychosocial Assessment of Patients with HIV Disease

Psychosocial assessment of patients with HIV disease is important throughout the illness trajectory, particularly as the disease progresses and there is increased vulnerability to psychological distress. Psychosocial assessment includes the following:

- Past social, behavioral and psychiatric history, which includes the history of interpersonal relationships, education, job stability, career plans, substance use, preexisting mental illness, and individual identity
- Crisis points related to the course of the disease as anxiety, fear, and depression intensify, creating a risk of suicide
- Life-cycle phase of individuals and families, which influences goals, financial resources, skills, social roles, and the ability to confront personal mortality
- Influence of culture and ethnicity, including knowledge and beliefs associated with health, illness, dying, and death, as well as attitudes and values toward sexual behaviors, substance use, health promotion and maintenance, and health care decision-making
- Past and present patterns of coping, including problem-focused and/or emotion-focused coping
- Social support, including sources of support, types of supports perceived as needed by the patient/family, and perceived benefits and burdens of support
- Financial resources, including health care benefits, disability allowances, and the eligibility for Medicaid/Medicare

Depression and Anxiety in Patients with HIV Disease

Because AIDS is a life-threatening, chronic, debilitating illness, patients are at risk for such psychological disorders as depression and anxiety. Among persons living with HIV/AIDS, the prevalence of depression has been estimated at 10% to 25%,[103] and is characterized by depressed mood, low energy, sleep disturbance, anhedonia, inability to concentrate, loss of libido, weight changes, and possible menstrual irregularities.[104] It is also important to assess whether depressed patients are using alcohol, drugs, and opioids.

Patients with HIV disease who are diagnosed with depression should be treated with antidepressants that target their particular symptoms. For example, tricyclic antidepressants are indicated for anxious depression, insomnia, low daytime energy, and neuropathic pain; selective serotonin reuptake inhibitors (SSRIs) are indicated for lethargy, hopelessness, and hypersomnia; and stimulants are indicated for fatigue, hypersomnia, poor appetite, and improvement of cognitive function.[105] It is noted that monoamine oxidase inhibitors (MAOIs) may interact with multiple medications used to treat HIV disease and, therefore, should be avoided.

Given that depression is a common symptom in patients with HIV/AIDS, research studies have also focused on other factors that relate to depression in this patient population. Schrimshaw[106] examined whether the source of unsupportive social interactions had differential main and interactive relations with depressive symptoms among ethnically diverse women with HIV/AIDS (n = 146). After controlling for demographic variables, it was found that unsupportive social interactions with family had a major effect in predicting more depressive symptoms, and that there was a significant interaction between unsupportive interactions from a lover/spouse and friends, which predicted high levels of depressive symptoms. Arrindell[107] examined differential coping strategies, anxiety, depression and symptomatology among African American women with HIV/AIDS ($n = 30$). The results indicated that the majority of women used emotion-focused coping; however, there were no main effects for coping strategies on psychological distress and no significant difference between symptomatology and coping strategies. An inverse relationship was reported between psychological distress and social support, with less distress reported when women had financial assistance from their family and friends. There was a relationship reported between symptomatology and anxiety, with those who were asymptomatic reporting no anxiety.

Anxiety is often associated with the stresses of HIV, or may result from the medications used to treat HIV disease, such as anticonvulsants, sulfonamides, NSAIDs, and corticosteroids.[107] Generalized anxiety disorder is manifested as worry, trouble falling asleep, impaired concentration, psychomotor agitation, hypersensitivity, hyperarousal, and fatigue.[108]

The treatment for patients with anxiety is based on the nature and severity of the symptoms and the coexistence of other mood disorders or substance abuse. Short-acting anxiolytics, such as lorazepam (Ativan), and alprazolam (Xanax) are beneficial for intermittent symptoms, while buspirone (BuSpar), and clonazepam (Klonopin) are beneficial for chronic anxiety.[105]

For many patients experiencing psychological distress associated with HIV disease, participation in therapeutic interventions such as skills building, support groups, individual counseling, and group interventions using meditation techniques can provide a sense of psychological growth and a meaningful way of living with the disease.[108–110] Such interventions are particularly helpful for patients with HIV/AIDS who may not have disclosed their sexual orientation or substance-abusing history to their families. Often, significant stress is associated with sharing such information, particularly when such disclosures occur during the stage of advanced disease. However, the need for therapeutic communication and support from all health professionals caring for the patient and their family exists throughout the illness continuum. Furthermore, fear of disclosure of the AIDS diagnosis and stigmatization in the community often raises concern in the family about the diagnosis stated on death certificates. Practitioners may therefore write a nonspecific diagnosis on the main death certificate and sign section B on the reverse side to signify to the registrar general that further information will be provided at a later date.

Often many members of a single family are infected and die because of the transmission of the disease to sexual partners and through childbirth. In the homosexual community and substance-abusing community, multiple deaths have also resulted in complicated mourning. The anxiety, depression, sadness, and loneliness associated with these multiple deaths and unending experiences of loss must be recognized and support offered. Community resources and referrals to HIV/AIDS support groups and bereavement groups are important in emotional adjustment to these profound losses.

Spiritual Issues in AIDS

The spiritual care of the patient and the ability of the community to support patients with HIV/AIDS may be unique opportunities for both personal and societal growth and transcendence. Mellors and colleagues[111] examined the relationship of self-transcendence and quality of life in a sample of 46 individuals with HIV/AIDS. The results demonstrated that overall self-transcendence for this sample was relatively high. Quality of life was higher than reported in previous research, yet those with disease progression, evident by the diagnosis of AIDS, had lower quality of life than those who were asymptomatic or symptomatic with CD4 counts greater than 200 cells/mm^3. There was no significant difference in self-transcendence between groups, but those with AIDS were more inclined to accept death and refrained from dwelling on the past or unmet dreams. There was a moderate positive correlation between self-transcendence and quality of life.

As health professionals, assessment of patient's spiritual needs is an important aspect of holistic care. Learning about patients' spiritual values, needs, and religious perspectives is important in understanding their perspectives regarding their illness and their perception and meaning of life and its purpose, suffering, and eventual death. According to Elkins and colleagues,[112] spirituality is a way of being or experiencing that comes about through an awareness of a transcendent dimension and identifiable life values with regard to self, others, nature, and God. An understanding of the patient's relationship with self, others, nature, and God can inform interventions that promote spiritual well-being and the possibility of a "good death" from the patient's perspective.

Patients living with and dying from HIV disease have the spiritual needs of meaning, value, hope, purpose, love, acceptance, reconciliation, ritual, and affirmation of a relationship with a higher being.[105] Assisting patients to find meaning and value in their lives, despite adversity, often involves a recognition of past successes and their internal strengths. Respectful behavior toward patients demonstrates love and acceptance of the patient as a person. Encouraging open communication between the patient and family is important to work toward reconciliation and the completion of unfinished business.

CASE STUDY

Will Stillers, a Patient with MAC

Will Stillers, a 28-year-old homosexual male, was admitted to the inpatient palliative care unit for fever, fatigue, anorexia, nausea and vomiting, and weight loss. He had 20 episodes of liquid diarrhea each day. As a differential diagnosis, he was tested for HIV disease. Findings indicated a CD4 count of 45 cells/mm^3 and a VL of 142,000 mL, indicative of the advanced stage of HIV disease. His laboratory work indicated anemia and an elevated alkaline phosphatase. *Mycobacterium avium intracellulare* (MAC) was confirmed by biopsy with AFB stain. Physical examination revealed hepatosplenomegaly and inguinal lymphadenopathy.

Will was begun on azithromycin and rifabutin to treat MAC, as well as on a highly active antiretroviral (HAART) regimen of one potent PI and two NRTIs, specifically ritonavir (PI), and zidovudine and didanosine (ddI)(both NRTIs) to treat his advanced stage of AIDS. Will had been estranged from his mother and sister, who lived on the West Coast. However, he had a very close friend, Carl, who viewed himself as Will's guardian given that he had known Will for many years, and his mother was friends with Will's mother when she lived in New York. Will lived with Carl and was considered a family member. After Will's infection improved, he returned to Carl's 4th-story walk-up. Will still had difficulty "holding down" food but ate small frequent meals, which he prepared for Carl and himself. Will's only interest was in cooking because he was trained as a chef. He was very weak but enjoyed cooking as his creative outlet, and viewed it as an opportunity to contribute to the household.

The diarrhea improved with medications, but Will was still too insecure to leave the house because he was more comfortable having immediate access to a toilet. He still felt very weak and was also concerned about his ability to climb stairs. Within the month, Will became more depressed and isolated. Although a home health aide visited for a few hours each day, there was minimal verbal interaction between them. Will began to stay in bed for long periods of time during the day. He wondered if he was ever going to recover but hoped some day to get his own apartment and be well enough to work. Will as treated with an antidepressant and within weeks his mood improved. His appetite increased and his physician was encouraged by his response to the HAART therapy. His physician discussed advance directives and Will asked Carl to be his health care proxy, as Carl knew Will's wishes and preferences.

Over the next 2 months, Will's quality of life improved because he was free of opportunistic infections and, although unemployed, he kept busy with household activities. Carl and Will had a wide circle of friends, but unfortunately many were also living with HIV/AIDS. Over the next 3 months, three of their friends died. Will understood the fragility of his condition and was adherent to his medication regimen. However, night sweats, fever, and diarrhea returned, and he was readmitted to the hospital within 6 months of his initial hospitalization with an exacerbation of MAC and severe dehydration. The palliative care team was asked for a consultation by the AIDS specialist. The advanced practice nurse developed a very supportive relationship with Will and Carl. She listened attentively to his fears and concerns and provided a caring presence that helped him to relax. They discussed his relationship with his mother and sister, and he asked the nurse to call his sister and tell her about his hospitalization. Will was coming to terms with his diagnosis and was ready to move beyond old hurts in his relationship with his family. Although he did not have a strong religious faith, Will asked for the chaplain to visit because he was trying to come to terms with his own suffering and the death of his friends.

Over the next few weeks, Will's infection began to resolve, and the advanced practice nurse promised him that when he felt better, she would bring him a meal from his favorite "soul food" restaurant where he once worked. Will's sister and mother asked to come to see him. On the day they arrived, Will's condition took an unexpected turn for the worse. With Carl and his family at his side, Will's fever began to rise and he became delirious. Several tests were conducted to identify other potential sources of the infection, and other possible reasons for the delirium. His symptoms were treated with Haldol and antipyretics. However, within the next day, Will slipped into a coma and died. In a letter found at his bedside, Will thanked his physicians and the members of the palliative team for their care. He said that without their support, he never would have reconciled with his mother and sister. He knew that his illness was advanced and did not expect to regain his health. He thanked Carl for his unconditional friendship and care. He said "I feel that you are my older brother whom I could always count on–no matter what." Members of the palliative care team were surprised at his sudden death but also understood the uncertainty of living with advanced AIDS. In a celebration of his life, the palliative care team brought Will's favorite foods from the restaurant where he worked, and asked Will's family to join them to celebrate his loving spirit and his life. In remembrance, tears were shed because of the tragic death of this promising young man who had touched their hearts, yet the importance of unconditional love, caring presence, and the joys of everyday life, such as sharing a meal, were reinforced by the message he left.

As with many life-threatening illnesses, patients with AIDS may express anger with God. Some may view their illness as a punishment or are angry that God is not answering their prayers. Expression of feelings can be a source of spiritual healing. Clergy can also serve as valuable members of the palliative care team in offering spiritual support and alleviating spiritual distress. The use of meditation, music, imagery, poetry, and drawing may offer outlets for spiritual expression and promote a sense of harmony and peace.

In a grounded-theory study of hope in patients with HIV/AIDS, Kylma and colleagues[113] found that patients had an alternating balance between hope, despair, and hopelessness based on the possibilities of daily life. They experienced losses such as loss of joy, carefree time, safety, self-respect, potential parenthood, privacy, and trust in self, others, systems, and God. However, there was hope as they received strength by seeing their life from a new perspective, and an acceptance of the uncertainty of life and the value of life. Hope was described as a basic resource in life and meant the belief that life is worth living at the present and in the future, with good things still to come. Despair meant losing grip, unable to take hold of anything, while hopelessness implied giving up in the face of an assumably nonexistent future, which was the opposite of hope.

For all patients with chronic, life-threatening illness, hope often shifts from hope that a cure will soon be found to hope for a peaceful death with dignity, including the alleviation of pain and suffering, determining one's own choices, being in the company of family and significant others, and knowing that their end-of-life wishes will be honored. Often, the greatest spiritual comfort offered by caregivers or family for patients comes from active listening and meaningful presence by sitting and hold their hands and knowing that they are not abandoned and alone.

Spiritual healing may also come from life review, as patients are offered an opportunity to reminisce about their lives, reflect on their accomplishments, reflect on their misgivings, and forgive themselves and others for their imperfections. Indeed, such spiritual care conveys that even in the shadow of death, there can be discovery, insight, the completion of relationships, the experience of love of self and others, and the transcendence of emotional and spiritual pain. Often, patients with AIDS, by their example, teach nurses, family, and others how to transcend suffering and how to die with grace and dignity.

Advanced Care Planning

Advanced planning is another important issue related to end-of-life care for patients with HIV/AIDS. Most patients with AIDS have not discussed with their physicians the kind of care they want at the end of life, although more gay men have executed an advance directive than injection-drug users or women.[114] Nonwhite patients with AIDS report that they do not like to talk about the care they would want if they were very sick, and are more likely to feel that if they talk about death, it will bring death closer. In contrast, white patients were more likely to believe that their doctor was an HIV/AIDS expert and good at talking about end-of-life care, and recognize they have been very sick in the past, and that such discussions are important.[114] According to Ferris and colleagues,[115] health care providers can assist patients and families by (1) discussing the benefits of health care and social support programs, unemployment insurance, worker's compensation, pension plans, insurance, and union or association benefits; (2) emphasizing the importance of organizing information and documents so that they are easily located and accessible; (3) suggesting that financial matters be in order, such as power of attorney or bank accounts, credit cards, property, legal claims, and income tax preparation; (4) discussing advance directives or power of attorney for care and treatment, as well as decisions related to the chosen setting for dying; and (5) discussing the patient's wishes regarding their death—Whom does the patient want at the bedside? What rituals are important to the dying patient? Does the patient wish an autopsy? What arrangements does the patient want regarding the funeral services and burial? Where should donations in remembrance be sent? It is important to realize that these issues should be discussed at relevant stages in the person's illness, in a manner that is both respectful to the patient's wishes and strengths and that promotes the patient's sense of control over his or her life and death.

Health care providers must also understand the concept of competency, a "state in which the person is capable of taking legal acts, consenting or refusing treatment, writing a will or power of attorney."[115] In assessing the patient's competency, the health provider must question whether the decision maker knows the nature and effect of the decision to be made and understands the consequences of his or her actions, and determine if the decision is consistent with an individual's life history, lifestyle, previous actions, and best interests.[115]

When an individual is competent, and in anticipation of the future loss of competency, he or she may initiate advance directives such as a living will and/or the designation of a health care proxy, who will carry out the patient's health care wishes or make health care decisions in the event that the patient becomes incompetent. The patient may also give an individual the power of attorney regarding financial matters and care or treatment issues. Advance directives include the patient's decisions regarding such life-sustaining treatments as cardiopulmonary resuscitation, use of vasoactive drips to sustain blood pressure and heart rate, dialysis, artificial nutrition and hydration, and the initiation or withdrawal of ventilatory support. The signing of advance directives must be witnessed by two individuals who are not related to the patient or involved in the patient's treatment. Individuals who are mentally competent can revoke at any time their advance directives. If a patient is deemed mentally incompetent, state statutes may allow the court to designate a surrogate decision-maker for the patient.

Palliative Care Through the Dying Trajectory

Death from AIDS is usually due to multiple causes, including chronic infections, malignancies, neurological disease, malnutrition, and multisystem failure.[116] However, even for patients with HIV/AIDS for whom death appears to be imminent, spontaneous recovery with survival of several more weeks or months is possible. The terminal stage is often marked by periods of increasing weight loss and deteriorating physical and cognitive functioning.[30] The general rule related to mortality is that the greater the cumulative number of opportunistic infections, illnesses, complications, and/or deviance of serological or immunological markers in terms of norms, the less the survival time.[27] Survival time is also decreased by psychosocial factors such as a decrease in physical and emotional support as demands increase for the caregivers, feelings of hopelessness by the patient, and older age (>39 years).[117] In the terminal stage of HIV disease, decisions related to prevention, diagnosis, and treatment pose ethical and clinical issues for both patients and their health care providers because they must decide on the value and frequency of laboratory monitoring, use of invasive procedures, use of antiretroviral and prophylactic measures, and patients' participation in clinical trails.[27]

The dying process for patients with advanced AIDS is commonly marked by increasingly severe physical deterioration, leaving the patient bedbound, experiencing wasting, dyspnea at rest, and pressure ulcers. Ultimately, patients become dependent on others for care. Febrile states and changes in mental status often occur as death becomes more imminent. Maintaining the comfort and dignity of the patients becomes a nursing priority. Symptomatic treatments, including pain management, should be continued throughout the dying process, since even obtunded patients may feel pain and other symptoms.

The end of life is an important time for individuals to accept their own shortcomings and limitations and differences with significant others so that death may be accepted without physical, psychosocial, and spiritual anguish.[31] At the end of life, patients with AIDS may have a desire for hastened death. Pessin,[118] based on a sample of 128 terminally ill patients with

AIDS who were receiving palliative care, found that there was a significant association between desire for a hastened death and cognitive impairment, with memory impairment providing an independent and unique contribution to desire for hastened death. Curtis and colleagues[119] also examined the desire of AIDS patients for less life-sustaining treatment as associated with the medical futility rationale. It was reported that 61% ($n = 35$) of patients with advanced AIDS accept the medical futility rationale as it may apply to their medical care at the end of life, including the use of mechanical ventilation. However, because 26% ($n = 15$) thought the medical futility rationale was probably acceptable and 10% ($n = 5$) said it was definitely not acceptable, clinicians invoking the medical futility rationale should consider the diversity of these patient attitudes toward care at the end of life. Through an interdisciplinary approach to care, health professionals can assist patients with the following: reducing their internal conflicts, such as fears about the loss of control, which can be related to a desire for hastened death; making end-of-life decisions regarding medical treatments that are consistent with their values, wishes, and preferences; promoting the patient's sense of identity; supporting the patient in maintaining important interpersonal relationships; and encouraging patients to identify and attempt to reach meaningful though limited goals.

Because palliative care also addresses the needs of family, it is important to consider the vulnerability of family members to patients' health problems at the end of life. In a study of the health status of informal caregivers ($n = 76$) of persons with HIV/AIDS, Flaskerud and Lee[120] found that caregiver distress regarding a patient's symptoms, anxiety, and education was related to depressive symptoms and that depressive symptoms, anger, and functional status of patients with AIDS were related to poorer physical health of informal caregivers. Therefore, members of the palliative care team can provide much-needed assistance not only to patients but their families.

As illness progresses and death approaches, health professionals can encourage patients and loved ones to express their fears and end-of-life wishes. Encouraging patients and families to express such feelings as "I love you," "I forgive you," "Forgive me—I am sorry," "Thank you," and "Good-bye" is important to the completion of relationships.[121] Peaceful death can also occur when families give the patient permission to die and assure them that they will be remembered.[6]

Loss, Grief, and Bereavement for Persons with HIV/AIDS and Their Survivors

Throughout the illness trajectory, patients with HIV disease experience many losses: a sense of loss of identity as they assume the identity of a patient with AIDS; loss of control over health and function; loss of roles as the illness progresses; loss of body image due to skin lesions, changes in weight, and wasting; loss of sexual freedom because of the need to change sexual behaviors to maintain health and prevent transmission to others; loss of financial security through possible discrimination and increasing physical disability; and loss of relationships through possible abandonment, self-induced isolation, and the multiple deaths of others from the disease.[122] In a study of AIDS-related grief and coping with loss among HIV-positive men and women (n = 268), Sikkema and colleagues[123] reported that the severity of grief reaction to AIDS-related losses was associated with escape-avoidance and self-controlling coping strategies, the type of loss, depressive symptoms, and history of injection drug use. For health care professionals, each occurrence of illness may pose new losses and heighten the patient's awareness of his or her mortality. Each illness experience is therefore an opportunity for health professionals to respond to cues of the patients in addressing their concerns and approaching the subject of loss, dying, and death. Given that grief is the emotional response to loss, patients dying from AIDS may also manifest the signs of grief, which include feelings of sadness, anger, self-reproach, anxiety, loneliness, fatigue, shock, yearning, relief, and numbness; physical sensations such as hollowness in the stomach, tightness in the chest, oversensitivity to noise, dry mouth, muscle weakness, and loss of coordination; cognitions of disbelief, confusion; and behavior disturbances in appetite, sleep, social withdrawal, loss of interest in activities, and restless overactivity.[124]

Upon the death of the patient, the patient's family and significant others enter a state of bereavement, or a state of having suffered a loss, which is often a long-term process of adapting to life without the deceased.[124] Family and significant others may experience signs of grief, including a sense of presence of the deceased, paranormal experiences or hallucinations, dreams of the deceased, a desire to have cherished objects of the deceased, and to visit places frequented by the deceased. The work of grief is a dynamic process that is not time-limited and predictable.[125] It may be that those left behind never "get over" the loss but, rather, find a place for it in their life and create through memory a new relationship with their loved one.

Families and partners of patients with AIDS may experience disenfranchised grief, defined as the grief that persons experience when they incur a loss that is not openly acknowledged, publicly mourned, or socially supported.[126] Support is not only important in assisting families in the tasks of grieving, but is also important for nurses who have established valued relationships with their patients. Indeed, disenfranchised grief may also be experienced by nurses who do not allow themselves to acknowledge their patient's death as a personal loss, or who are not acknowledged by others, such as the patient's family or even professional colleagues, for having suffered a loss.

For all individuals who have experienced a loss, Worden[127] has identified the tasks of grieving as (1) accepting the reality of the death; (2) experiencing the pain of grief; (3) adjusting to a changed physical, emotional, and social environment in which the deceased is missing; and (4) finding an appropriate emotional place for the person who died in the emotional life of the bereaved.

To facilitate each of Worden's tasks, Mallinson[125] recommends the following nursing interventions:

- Accept the reality of death by speaking of the loss and facilitating emotional expression.
- Work through the pain of grief by exploring the meaning of the grief experience.
- Adjust to the environment without the deceased by acknowledging anniversaries and the experience of loss during holidays and birthdays; help the bereaved to problem solve and recognize their own abilities to conduct their daily lives.
- Emotionally relocate the deceased and move on with life by encouraging socialization through formal and informal avenues.

The complications of AIDS-related grief often come from the secrecy and social stigma associated with the disease.[128] Reluctance to contact family and friends can restrict the normal support systems available for the bereaved.

In addition to a possible lack of social support, the death of patients with AIDS may result in complicated grief for the bereaved, given that death occurs after lengthy illness, and the relationships may have been ambivalent. Through truthful and culturally sensitive communication, health professionals can offer families support in their grief and promote trust that their needs are understood and validated. Further bereavement and related nursing interventions are discussed in Chapter 27.

Conclusion

The care of patients with HIV/AIDS requires both active treatment and palliative care throughout the disease trajectory to relieve the suffering associated with opportunistic infections and malignancies. With up-to-date knowledge regarding HIV disease, including changes in epidemiology, diagnostic testing, treatment options, and available resources, nurses can offer effective and compassionate care to patients, alleviating physical, emotional, social, and spiritual suffering at all stages of HIV disease. Patients can maintain a sense of control and dignity until death by establishing a partnership with their health care professionals in planning and implementing their health care, as well as through advanced care planning to insure that their end-of-life preferences and wishes are honored. The control of pain and symptoms associated with HIV/AIDS enables the patient and family to expend their energies on spiritual and emotional healing, and the possibility for personal growth and transcendence even as death approaches. Palliative care offers a comprehensive approach to address the physical, emotional, social, and spiritual needs of individuals with incurable progressive illness throughout the illness trajectory until death. Palliative care therefore preserves patients' quality of life by protecting their self-integrity, reducing a perceived helplessness, and lessening the threat of exhaustion of coping resources.[129] Through effective and compassionate nursing care, patients with AIDS can achieve a sense of inner well-being even at death, with the potential to make the transition from life as profound, intimate, and precious an experience as their birth.[121]

REFERENCES

1. Sepkowitz A. AIDS—The first 20 years. N Engl J Med 2001;344:1764–1772.
2. Watt G, Burnouf T. AIDS—Past and future. N Engl J Med 2002;346:710–711.
3. Selwyn P, Forstein M. Overcoming the false dichotomy of curative vs palliative care for late-stage HIV/AIDS: "Let me live the way I want to live, until I can't." JAMA 2003;90:806–814.
4. George RJ. Palliation in AIDS: where do we draw the line? Genitourinary Med 1991;67:85–86.
5. Knaus W, et al. A controlled trial to improve care for seriously ill hospitalized patients. JAMA 1995;274:1591–1598.
6. O'Neill J, Alexander C. Palliative medicine and HIV/AIDS. HIV/AIDS Management in Office Practice 1997;24:607–615.
7. Centers for Disease Control and Prevention. National Center for HIV, STD, and TB prevention: HIV/AIDS surveillance report (2002). Available at: http://www.cdc.gov/hiv/stat-trends.htm. Accessed January 13, 2005.
8. Goldstone I. Trends in hospital utilization in AIDS care 1987–1991: Implications for palliative care. J Palliat Care 1992;8:22–29.
9. Sherman DW, Ouellette S. Moving beyond fear: lessons learned through a longitudinal review of the literature regarding health care providers and the care of people with HIV/AIDS. In: Sherman DW, ed. HIV/AIDS Update Nursing Clinics of North America. Philadelphia: W.B. Saunders, 1999:1–48.
10. Flaskerud JH, Ungvarski P. (1999). HIV/AIDS: A guide to primary care management. Philadelphia: W.B. Saunders, 1999.
11. Saag M. 11th Conference on Retroviruses and Opportunistic Infections (2004). Available at: http://www.uab.edu/cme. Accessed January 13, 2005.
12. Berkman A. Confronting global AIDS: prevention and treatment. Am J Public Health 2001;91:1348–1349.
13. Ropka ME, Williams AB. HIV nursing and symptom management. Sudbury, MA: Jones & Bartlett Publishers, 1998.
14. Andrews L. The pathogenesis of HIV infection. In: Ropka ME, Williams, AB, eds. HIV Nursing and Symptom Management. Sudbury, MA: Jones & Bartlett Publishers, 1998:3–35.
15. Melroe NH, Stawarz KE, Simpson J. HIV RNA quantitation: marker of HIV infection. J Assoc Nurses AIDS Care 1997;8:31–38.
16. Kirton CA, Ferri RS, Eleftherakis V. Primary care and case management of persons with HIV/AIDS. In: Sherman DW, ed. HIV/AIDS Update. Nurs Clin North Am 1999:71–93.
17. Orenstein R. Presenting syndromes of human immunodeficiency virus. Mayo Clin Proc 2002;77:1097–1102.
18. Foley FJ, Flannery J, Graydon D, Flintoft G, Cook D. AIDS palliative care: challenging the palliative paradigm. J Palliat Care 1995;11:19–22.
19. Gerard L, Flandre P, Raguin G, Le Gall JR, Vilde JL, Leport C. Life expectancy in hospitalized patients with AIDS: prognostic factors on admission. J Palliat Care 1996;12:26–30.
20. Butters E, Webb D, Hearn J, Higginson I. Prospective audit of eight HIV/AIDS community palliative care services. International

Conference on AIDS 11(2):223(abstract no. TH.B. 190); 1996. Unique Identifier: AIDSLINE MED/96924269.

21. Malcolm J, Dobson P. Palliative care of AIDS: the last month of life. Annual Conference of the Australias Society of HIV Medicine 1994;6:266.
22. Barnes R, Barrett C, Weintraub S, Holowacz G. Hospital response to psycho-social needs of AIDS inpatients. J Palliat Care 1993; 9:22–28.
23. Bloomer S. Palliative care. J Assoc Nurses AIDS Care 1998;9: 45–47.
24. Malcolm JA. What is the best model for AIDS palliative care? Annual Conference of the Australias Society of HIV Medicine 1993;5:60 (abstract no. Spa1). Unique Identifier: AIDSLINE ASHM5/94349010.
25. Selwyn P, Rivard M. Palliative care for AIDS: challenges and opportunities in the era of highly active anti-retroviral therapy. J Palliat Med 2003;6:475–487.
26. Walsh TD. An overview of palliative care in cancer and AIDS. Oncology 1991;6:7–11.
27. Kemp C, Stepp L. Palliative care for patients with acquired immunodeficiency syndrome. Am J Hospice Palliat Care 1995;9: 14–27.
28. Higginson I. Palliative care: a review of past changes and future trends. J Public Health Med 1993;15:3–8.
29. Sherman DW. Palliative care. In: Kirton C, Talotta D, Zwolski K, eds. Handbook of HIV/AIDS Nursing. Philadelphia: W.B. Saunders, 2001:173–194.
30. Glare PA. Palliative care in acquired immunodeficiency syndrome (AIDS): problems and practicalities. Ann Acad Med 1994; 23:235–243.
31. Post L, Dubler N. Palliative care: a bioethical definition, principles, and clinical guidelines. Bioethics Forum 1997;13:17–24.
32. Bone R. Hospice and palliative care. Disease-a-Month 1995;61: 773–825.
33. Last Acts Palliative Care Task Force. Palliative Care Core Precepts. Princeton, NJ: Last Acts Palliative Care Task Force, 1997.
34. Armes P, Higginson I. What constitutes high-quality HIV/AIDS palliative care? J Palliat Care 1999;15:5–12.
35. Grothe TM, Brody RV. Palliative care for HIV disease. J Palliat Care 1995;11:48–49.
36. Fraser J. Sharing the challenge: the integration of cancer and AIDS. J Palliat Care 1995;11:23–25.
37. Malcolm JA, Sutherland DC. AIDS palliative care demands a new model. Med J Aust 1992;157:572–573.
38. Walsh TD. An overview of palliative care in cancer and AIDS. Oncology 1991;6:7–11.
39. Bloom JA, Flannery J. Problems in an AIDS hospice setting. International Conference on AIDS 1989;414 (abstract no. W.B.P. 378). Unique Identifier: AIDSLINE ICA5/00210489.
40. O'Keefe EA, Wood R. Quality of life in HIV infection. Scan J Gastroenterol 1996;31:30–32.
41. Ragsdale D, Morrow J. Quality of life as a function of HIV classification. Nurs Res 1992;39:355–359.
42. Ragsdale K, Kortarba J, Morrow J. Quality of life of hospitalized persons with AIDS. Image 1992;24:259–265.
43. Nichel J, Salsberry P, Caswell R, Keller M, Long T, O'Connell M. Quality of life in nurse case management of persons with AIDS receiving home care. Res Nurs Health 1996;19:91–99.
44. Vosvick M, Koopman C, Gore-Felton C, Thoresen C, Krumboltz J, Spiegal D. Relationship of functional quality of life to strategies for coping with the stress of living with HIV/AIDS. Psychosomatics 2003;44:51–58.
45. Baigis-Smith J, Gordon D, McGuire DB, Nanda J. Healthcare needs of HIV-infected persons in hospital, outpatient, home, and long-term care settings. J Assoc Nurses AIDS Care 1995; 6:21–33.
46. Kemppainen J. Predictors of quality of life in AIDS patients. J Assoc Nurses AIDS Care 2001;12:61–70.
47. Keithley J, Swanson B, Murphy M, Levin D. (2000). HIV/AIDS and nutrition implications for disease management. Nurs Case Manag 2000;5:52–62.
48. Greenspan JS, Greenspan D. Oral complications of HIV infection. In: Sande MA, Volberding PA, eds. The Medical Management of AIDS. Philadelphia: W.B. Saunders, 1997:224–240.
49. Rene E, Roze C. Diagnosis and treatment of gastrointestinal infections in AIDS. In: Kotler D, ed. Gastrointestinal and Nutritional Manifestations of AIDS. New York: Raven Press, 1991: 65–92.
50. Hussein R. Current issues and forthcoming events. J Advan Nurs 2003;44:235–237.
51. Aron J. Optimization of nutritional support in HIV disease. In: Watson RR, ed. Nutrition and AIDS. Boca Raton, FL: CRC Press, 1994:215–233.
52. Freeman EM, MacIntyre RC. Evaluating alternative treatments for HIV infection. Nurs Clin North Am 1999:147–162.
53. Semba R, Graham P, Caiaffa J. Maternal vitamin A deficiency and mother-to-child transmission of HIV-1. Lancet 1994;343: 1593–1597.
54. Nieman D. Exercise immunology: practical applications. Int J Sports Med 1996;18:91–100.
55. LaPerriere A, Klimas N, Fletcher M, et al. Change in CD4 cell enumeration following aerobic exercise training in HIV-1 disease: possible mechanisms and practical applications. Int J Sports Med 1997;18:56–61.
56. Centers for Disease Control and Prevention. Physical activity and health: a report of the surgeon general. Morb Mortal Wkly Rep 1996;45:591–592.
57. Ironson G, Field T, Scafidi F, et al. Massage therapy is associated with enhancement of the immune system's cytotoxic capacity. Int J Neurosci 1996;84:205–217.
58. Leserman J, Petitto J, Gaynes B, Barroso J, Golden R, Perkins D, Folds J, Evans D. Progression to AIDS, a clinical AIDS condition and mortality: psychosocial and physiological predictors. Psychol Med 2002;32:1059–1073.
59. Sherman DW, Kirton C. Hazardous terrain and over the edge: the survival of HIV-positive heterosexual minority men. J Assoc Nurses AIDS Care 1998;9:23–34.
60. Eller LS. Effects of two cognitive-behavioral interventions on immunity and symptoms in persons with HIV. Ann Behav Med 1995;17:339–344.
61. Lechner S, Antoni M, Lydston D, LaPerriere A, Ishii M, Devieux J, Stanley H, Ironson G, Schneiderman N, Brondolo E, Tobin J, Weiss S. Cognitive-behavioral interventions improve quality of life in women with AIDS. J Psychosom Res 2003;54:252–261.
62. Remien RH, Rabkin JG, Williams JBW. Coping strategies and health beliefs of AIDS longterm survivors. Psychol Health 1992; 6:335–345.
63. Cohen M. The use of coping humor in an HIV/AIDS population. Dissertation Abstracts International 2001;61:4976.
64. Casey K. Malnutrition associated with HIV/AIDS. Part one: definition and scope, epidemiology, and pathophysiology. J Assoc Nurses AIDS Care 1997;8: 24–34.
65. Sherman DW, Kirton CA. Relapse to unsafe sex among HIV-positive heterosexual men. Appl Nurs Res 1999;12:91–100.

66. U.S. Department of Health and Human Services. Guidelines for using antiretroviral agents among HIV-infected adults and adolescents. Morbidity and Mortality Weekly Report 2002;51:1–56.
67. Murphy R, Flaherty J. Contemporary Diagnosis and Management of HIV/AIDS Infections. Newtown, PA: Handbooks in Health Care Co., 2003.
68. Kaplan J, Masur H, Holmes K. USPHS/IDSA guidelines for the pre-opportunistic infections in persons infected with human immunodeficiency virus: introduction. Clin Infect Dis 1995;21: S1–S11.
69. Porche D. State of the art: antiretroviral and prophylactic treatments in HIV/AIDS. Nurs Clin North Am 1999;34(1):95–112.
70. Von Gunten CF, Martinez J, Neely KJ, Von Roenn JH. AIDS and palliative medicine: medical treatment issues. J Palliat Care 1995;11:5–9.
71. Institutional AIDS Society. Antiretroviral therapy in adults: updated recommendations. JAMA 2000;283:381–390.
72. Klaus BD, Grodesky MJ. Update from the 6th Conference on Retroviruses and Opportunistic Infections. Nurse Practitioner 1999;24:117–121.
73. Selwyn P, Rivard M. Palliative care for AIDS: challenges and opportunities in the era of highly active anti-retroviral therapy. J Palliat Med 2003;6:475–487.
74. Hilts AE, Fish DN. Antiretroviral dosing in patients with organ dysfunction. AIDS Reader 1998;8:179–184.
75. Haynes, R. B., Taylor, D. W., and Sackett, D. L. Compliance in Health Care. Baltimore: Johns Hopkins University Press, 1979.
76. Williams, A. B. Adherence to highly active antiretroviral therapy. Nurs Clin North Am 1999; 34:113–127.
77. Chesney, M. Adherence to HIV/AIDS treatment. In Program of Adherence to New HIV Therapies: A Research Conference. Office of AIDS Research, Washington, DC: National Institutes of Health, 1997.
78. Meichenbaum, D. and Turk, C. Facilitating Treatment Adherence: Practitioner's Guidebook. New York: Plenum, 1987.
79. Haynes RB, McKibbon KA, Kanani R. Systematic review of randomized trials of interventions to assist patients to follow prescriptions for medications. Lancet 1996;348:383–389.
80. Newshan G, Sherman DW. Palliative care: pain and symptom management in persons with HIV/AIDS. Nurs Clin North Am 1999;34(1):131–145.
81. Holzemer W. HIV/AIDS: The symptom experience: what cell counts and viral loads won't tell you. Am J Nurs 2002;102:48–52.
82. Singer EJ, Zorialla C, Fay-Chandon B, Chi D, Syndulko K, Tourtellotte WW. Painful symptoms reported in ambulant HIV-infected men in a longitudinal study. Pain 1993;54:15–19.
83. Breitbart W, McDonald M. Pharmacologic pain management in HIV/AIDS. J Int Assoc Physicians in AIDS Care 1996;7:17–26.
84. Shofferman J, Brody R. Pain in far advanced AIDS. In: Foley KM et al., ed. Advances in Pain Research and Therapy, vol. 16. New York: Raven Press, 1990:379–386.
85. Breitbart W, Passik S, Rosenfeld B, McDonald M, Thaler H, Portenoy H. Undertreatment of pain in AIDS. (abstract) American Pain Society, 13th Annual Meeting, November 10–14, 1994.
86. Cleeland CS, Gonin R, Hatfield AK, Edmonson JH, Blum RH, Stewart JA, Pandya KJ. Pain and its treatment in outpatients with metastatic cancer: the eastern co-operative group's cooperative study. N Engl J Med 1994;300:592–596.
87. Frich L, Borgbjerg F. Pain and pain treatment in AIDS: a longitudinal study. J Pain Sympt Manage 2000;19:339–347.
88. American Pain Society. Principles of Analgesic Use in the Treatment of Acute Pain and Cancer Pain, 3rd ed. Skokie, IL: American Pain Society, 1992.
89. Jacox A, Carr D, Payne R, Berde CB, Breitbart W. Clinical Practice Guideline Number 9: Management of Cancer Pain. Washington, DC: U.S. Department of Health and Human Services, Public Health Service, Agency for Health Care Policy and Research (Pub. No. 94–0592), 1994:139–141.
90. Hughes AM. HIV-related pain. Am J Nurs 1999;99:20.
91. Fantoni M, Ricci F, Del Borgo C, Izzi I, Damiano F, Moscati A, Marasca G, Bevilacqua N, Del Forno A. Multicentre study on the prevalence of symptoms and somatic treatment in HIV infection. Central Italy PRESINT Group. J Palliat Care 1997;13:9–13.
92. Holzemer W, Henry S, Reilly C. Assessing and managing pain in AIDS care: the patient perspective. J Assoc Nurses AIDS Care 1998;9:22–30.
93. Reiter G, Kudler N. Palliative care and HIV. Part II: Systemic manifestations and late stage illness. AIDS Clin Care 1996;8: 27–30.
94. Avis N, Smith K, Mayer K. The relationship among CD4, hemoglobin, symptoms, and quality of life domains in a cohort of HIV-positive men. International Conference on AIDS 11:116 (abstract), 1996.
95. Greene KB, Berger J, Reeves C, Moffat A, Standish LJ, Calabrese C. Most frequently used alternative and complementary therapies and activities by participants in the AMCOA study. J Assoc Nurses AIDS Care 1999;10:60–73.
96. Brashers DE, Neidig JL, Reynolds NR, Haas SM. Uncertainty in illness across the HIV/AIDS trajectory. J Assoc Nurses AIDS Care 1998;9:66–77.
97. Grassi L, Sighinolfi L. Psychosocial correlates of quality of life in patients with HIV infection. AIDS Patient Care and STDs 1996; 10:296–299.
98. Farber E, Mirsalimi H, Williams K, McDaniel J. Meaning of illness and psychological adjustment to HIV/AIDS. Psychosomatics 2003;44:485–491.
99. Silver E, Bauman L, Camacho S, Hudis J. Factors associated with psychological distress in urban mothers with late-stage HIV/AIDS. AIDS & Behavior 2003;7:421–431.
100. Butters E, Higginson I, George R. Palliative care needs of patients referred to two HIV/AIDS community teams. International Conference on AIDS, 1993, 9(1), 522 (abstract no. PO-B34–2322). Unique Identifier: AIDSLINE ICA9/93335959.
101. Friedland J, Renwick R, McColl M. Coping and social support as determinants of quality of life in HIV/AIDS. AIDS Care 1996; 8:15–31.
102. Sherman DW. Reciprocal suffering: the need to improve family caregiver's quality of life through palliative care. J Palliat Med 1998;1:357–366.
103. Atkinson JH, Grant I. Natural history of neuropsychiatric manifestations of HIV disease. Psychiatr Clin North Am 1994;17:33.
104. McEnany GW, Hughes AM, Lee KA. Depression and HIV. Nurs Clin North Am 1996;31: 57–80.
105. Flaskerud JH, Miller E. Psychosocial and neuropsychiatric dysfunction. In: Flaskerud JH, Ungvarski P, eds. HIV/AIDS: A Guide to Primary Care Management. Philadelphia: W.B. Saunders, 1999:225–291.
106. Schrimshaw R. Relationship-specific unsupportive social interactions and depressive symptoms among women living with HIV/AIDS: direct and moderating effects. J Behav Med 2003; 26:297–313.

107. Arriendel J. Differential coping strategies, anxiety, depression, and symptomatology among African-American women with HIV/AIDS. Dissertation abstracts International. Section B: The Sciences & Engineering. 2003;64:1481. US: Univ MicroFilms International.
108. Capaldini L. HIV disease: psychosocial issues and psychiatric complications. In: Sande MS, Volberding PA, eds. The Medical Management of AIDS. Philadelphia: W.B. Saunders, 1997:217–238.
109. Chesney MA, Folkman S, Chambers D. Coping Effectiveness training decreases distress in men living with HIV/AIDS. International Conference on AIDS, Vancouver, July 7–12, 1996;11:50.
110. Kinara, M. Transcendental meditation: a coping mechanism for HIV-positive people. International Conference on AIDS, 1996; 11:421.
111. Mellors M, Riley T, Erlen J. HIV, self-transcendence and quality of life. J Assoc Nurses AIDS Care 1997;8:59–69.
112. Elkins D, Hedstrom LJ, Hughes L, Leaf JA, Saunders C. Towards a humanistic-phenomenological spirituality. J Humanistic Psychol 1998;28:5–18.
113. Kylma J, Vehvilainen-Julkunen K, Lahdevirta J. Hope, despair and hopelessness in living with HIV/AIDS: a grounded theory study. J Adv Nurs 2001;33:764–775.
114. Curtis R, Patrick D, Caldwell E, Collier A. Why don't patients and physicians talk about end of life care?: barriers to communication for patients with acquired immunodeficiency syndrome and their primary care clinicians. Arch Intern Med 2000;160: 1690–1696.
115. Ferris F, Flannery J, McNeal H, Morissette M, Cameron R, Bally G. Palliative care: a comprehensive guide for the care of persons with HIV disease. Toronto, Ontario: Mount Sinai Hospital/Casey House Hospice, 1995.
116. Wood C, Whittet S, Bradbeer C. ABC of palliative care. BMJ 1997;315: 1433–1436.
117. Goldstone I, Kuhl D, Johnson A, Le Clerc, McCleod A. Patterns of care in advanced HIV disease in a tertiary treatment centre. AIDS Care 1995;7:47–56.
118. Pessin H. The influence of cognitive impairment on desire for hastened death among terminally ill AIDS patients. Dissertation Abstracts International 2001;62:2963.
119. Curtis R, Patrick D, Caldwell E, Collier A. The attitudes of patients with advanced AIDS toward use of the medical futility rationale in decisions to forgo mechanical ventilation. Arch Intern Med 2000;160:1597–1601.
120. Flaskerud J, Lee P. Vulnerability to health problems in female informal caregivers of persons with HIV/AIDS and age-related dementias. J Adv Nurs 2001;33:60–68.
121. Byock I. Dying Well: The Prospect for Growth at the End of Life. New York: Riverhead Books, 1997.
122. Welsby P, Richardson A, Brettle R. AIDS: aspects in adults. In: Doyle D, Hanks G, MacDonald N, eds. Oxford Textbook of Palliative Medicine, 2nd ed. New York: Oxford University Press, 1998:1121–1148.
123. Sikkema K, Kochman A, DiFranceisco W, Kelly J, Hoffman R. AIDS-related grief and coping with loss among HIV-positive men and women. J Behav Med 2003;26:165–181.
124. Rando T. Grief, Dying, and Death: Clinical Interventions for Caregivers. Champaign, IL: Research Press Co., 1984.
125. Mallinson RK. Grief work of HIV-positive persons and their survivors. In: Sherman DW, ed. HIV/AIDS Update. Nurs Clin North Am. Philadelphia: W.B. Saunders, 1999:163–177.
126. Doka K. Disenfranchised Grief: Recognizing the Hidden Sorrow. Lexington, MA: Lexington Books, 1989:.
127. Worden J. Grief Counseling and Grief Therapy: A Handbook for the Mental Health Practitioner. New York: Springer Publications, 1991.
128. Maxwell N. Responses to loss and bereavement in HIV. Prof Nurse 1996;12:21–24.
129. Bayes R. A way to screen for suffering in palliative care. J Palliat Care 1997;13:22–26.
130. Centers for Disease Control and Prevention Guidelines for the Prevention of Opportunistic Infections in Persons with Human Immunodeficiency Virus, Morbidity and Mortality Weekly Report 1999;48(RR-10):40–43.
131. Centers for Disease Control and Prevention. Recommendations of the Advisory Committee on Immunization Practices (ACIP): use of vaccines and immune globulins in persons with altered immunocompetence. Morbidity and Mortality Weekly Report 1993;42(RR-5):5.
132. Portenoy RK. Contemporary Diagnosis and Management of Pain in Oncologic and AIDS Patients. Newtown, PA: Handbooks in Health Care Co., 1997.
133. Coyne P, Lyne M, Watson AC. Symptom management in people with AIDS. Am J Nurs 2002;102:48–57.
134. McNaghten AD, Hanson DL, Jones, JL, Dworkin MS, Ward JW, Adult/Adolescent Spectrum of Disease Group. Effects of antiretroviral therapy and opportunistic illness primary chemoprophylaxis on survival after AIDS diagnosis. AIDS 1999;13:1687–1695.
135. U.S. Department of Health and Human Services. USPHS/IDSA Guidelines for the Prevention of Opportunistic Infections in Persons Infected with Human Immunodeficiency Virus. 2001. Available at: http://aidsinfo.nih.gov/guidelines/ (accessed March 24, 2005).

38

Kenneth L. Kirsh, Peggy Compton, and Steven D. Passik

Caring for the Drug-Addicted Patient at the End of Life

Thank you for doctoring my brother. No one else would take care of him.—Brother of a dying cancer patient who had a comorbid addiction problem, requiring extensive management and unorthodox doses of opioid analgesics. At the end of life, the patient was able to go hunting and spend quality time with his family.

- ***Key Points***
- *Identifying addiction in patients with advanced disease is not an easy task, and old conceptions of addiction such as tolerance and dependence need to be reexamined.*
- *Patients with advanced disease and comorbid addiction are difficult to manage but can be successfully treated with careful documentation and planning.*
- *Remember that the patient with advanced disease and comorbid addiction has two diseases that need treatment: one of drug addiction and one of chronic pain.*

Substance use disorders are a consistent phenomenon in the United States, with estimated base rates of 6% and 15%.[1–4] This prevalence of drug abuse certainly touches medically ill patients and can negatively influence how pain is treated. Because of these issues and despite the fact that national guidelines exist for the treatment of pain disorders such as cancer, pain continues to be undertreated, even at the end of life.[5–7] In cancer, approximately 40% to 50% of patients with metastatic disease and 90% of patients with terminal cancer or other advanced diseases are reported to experience unrelieved pain.[5–7] Furthermore, inadequate treatment of cancer pain is an even greater possibility if the patient is a member of an ethnic minority, female, elderly, a child, or a substance abuser.[8] Thus, for multicultural patients, we sometimes have conflicting multiple biases in pain treatment that can lead to poor management, mutual suspicion and alienation, and suffering unless these biases are adequately addressed.

Incidence of Substance Use Disorders in Patients with Advanced Disease

Although few studies have been conducted to evaluate the epidemiology of substance abuse in patients with advanced illness, substance use disorders appear to be relatively rare within the tertiary-care population with cancer and other advanced diseases. Findings from a consultations review performed by the Psychiatry Services at Memorial Sloan-Kettering Cancer Center revealed that requests for management of issues related to substance abuse consisted of only 3% of the consultations.[9,10]

While the incidence of substance use disorders is much lower in patients with advanced disease than in society at large, in community-based medical populations, and emergency medical departments, this may not represent the true prevalence in the advanced illness spectrum overall. Institutional biases or a tendency for patients' underreporting in tertiary-care hospitals may be reflective of the relatively low prevalence of substance abuse among advanced patients. Social forces may also inhibit patients' reporting of drug use behavior. Many drug abusers are of lower socioeconomic standing and feel alienated from the health care system, and, therefore, may not seek care in tertiary-care centers. Furthermore, those who are treated in these centers may not acknowledge drug abuse for fear of stigmatization.[9–11] Additionally, minority patients are treated in such settings more often than are Caucasians.

Issues in Defining Abuse and Addiction in the Medically Ill

It is difficult to define substance abuse and addiction in patients with advanced illness, since the definitions of both terms have been adopted from addicted populations without medical illness. Furthermore, the pharmacological phenomena of tolerance and physical dependence are commonly confused with abuse and addiction. The use of these terms is so strongly influenced by sociocultural considerations that it may lead to confusion in the clinical setting. Therefore, the clarification of this terminology is necessary to improve the diagnosis and management of substance abuse when treating patients with advanced disease.[10]

Substance abuse concentrates on the psychosocial, physical, and vocational harm that occurs from drug-taking, which makes identifying drug-taking behaviors more difficult in patients with advanced illness who are receiving potentially abusable drugs for legitimate medical purposes. In contrast, substance dependence emphasizes chronicity, and includes the dimensions of tolerance and physical dependence. Due to the possibility that patients may develop these effects due to therapeutic drug use, it is inapplicable to use this terminology in the medically ill. Not only does the existing nomenclature complicate the effort to distinguish the drug-taking behaviors of patients with advanced disease that are appropriately treated with potentially abusable drugs, it also impedes the communication that is fundamental for proper pain management and medical care.[9,10]

Theoretical Problems in the Diagnosis of Substance Use Disorders

Since substance abuse is increasingly widespread in the population at large, patients with advanced disease who have used illicit drugs are more frequently encountered in medical settings. Illicit drug use, actual or suspected misuse of prescribed medication, or actual substance use disorders create the most serious difficulties in the clinical setting, complicating the treatment of pain management. However, the management of substance abuse is fundamental to adherence to medical therapy and safety during treatment. Also, adverse interactions between illicit drugs and medications prescribed as part of the patient's treatment can be dangerous. Continuous substance abuse may alienate or weaken an already tenuous social support network that is crucial for alleviating the chronic stressors associated with advanced disease and its treatment. Therefore, a history of substance abuse can impede treatment and pain management and increase the risk of hastening morbidity and mortality among advanced patients, which can only be alleviated by a therapeutic approach that addresses drug-taking behavior while expediting the treatment of the malignancy and distressing symptoms, as well as addiction.[11]

When assessing drug-taking behaviors in the patient with advanced disease, issues exist that increase the difficulty in arriving at a diagnosis of abuse or addiction. These issues include the problem of undertreatment of pain, sociocultural influences on the definition of aberrancy in drug-taking, and the importance of cancer-related variables.[9,10]

Pseudoaddiction

Various studies provide compelling evidence that pain is undertreated in populations with advanced disease.[5–7] Clinical experience indicates that the inadequate management of symptoms and related pain may be the motivation for aberrant drug-taking behaviors. Pseudoaddiction is the term used to depict the distress and drug-seeking that can occur in the context of unrelieved pain, such as similar behaviors in addicts.[12] The main factor of this syndrome is that sufficient pain relief eliminates aberrant behaviors.

The potential for pseudoaddiction creates a challenge for the assessment of a known substance abuser with an advanced illness. Clinical evidence indicates that aberrant behaviors impelled by unrelieved pain can become so dramatic in this population that some patients appear to return to illicit drug use as a means of self-medication. Others use more covert patterns of behavior, which may also cause concerns regarding the possibility of true addiction. While it may not be obvious that drug-related behaviors are aberrant, the meaning of these behaviors may be difficult to discern in the context of unrelieved symptoms.[9,10]

Distinguishing Aberrant Drug-Taking Behaviors

Whereas abuse is defined as the use of an illicit drug or a prescription drug without medical indication, addiction refers to the continued use of either type of drug in a compulsive manner regardless of harm to the user or others. However, when a drug is prescribed for a medically diagnosed purpose, less assuredness exists as to the behaviors that could be deemed aberrant, thereby increasing the potential for a diagnosis of drug abuse or addiction. Although it is difficult to disagree with the aberrancy of certain behaviors, such as intravenous injection of oral formulations, various other behaviors are less blatant, such as a patient experiencing unrelieved pain who is taking an extra dose of prescribed opioids.[9,10]

The ability to categorize these questionable behaviors as apart from social or cultural norms is also based on the assumption that certain parameters of normative behavior exist. Although it is useful to consider the degree of aberrancy of a given behavior, it is important to recognize that these behaviors exists along a continuum, with certain behaviors being less aberrant (such as aggressively requesting medication) and other behaviors are more aberrant (such as injection of oral formulations). Empirical data defining these parameters does not exist regarding prescription drug use (Table 38–1). If a large portion of patients were found to engage in a certain behavior, it may be normative, and judgments regarding aberrancy should be influenced accordingly.[9,10]

The importance of social and cultural norms also raises the possibility of bias in the determination of aberrancy. A clinician's willingness to classify a questionable drug-related behavior as aberrant when performed by a member of a certain social or ethnic group may be influenced by bias against that group. Based on clinical observation, this type of prejudice has been found to be common in the assessment of drug-related behaviors of patients with substance abuse histories. Regardless if the drug-abuse history was in the past or present, questionable behaviors by these patients may immediately be labeled as abuse or addiction. The possibility of bias in the assessment of drug-related behaviors also exists for patients who are members of racial or ethnic minority groups different from that of the clinician.[9,10] The following case study illustrates the point that aberrant behaviors do not have a universal interpretation (including the illegal and obviously worrisome ones) and must be understood in the context of the patient's care.

Table 38–1
Sample Behaviors More or Less Likely To Indicate Aberrancy

Less Indicative of Aberrancy	More Indicative of Aberrancy
Drug hoarding during periods of reduced symptoms	Prescription forgery
Acquisition of similar drugs from other medical sources	Concurrent abuse of related illicit drugs
Aggressive complaining about the need for higher doses	Recurrent prescription losses
Unapproved use of the drug to treat another symptom	Selling prescription drugs
Unsanctioned dose escalation one or two times	Multiple unsanctioned dose escalations
Reporting psychic effects not intended by the clinician	Stealing or borrowing another patient's drugs
Requesting specific drugs	Obtaining prescription drugs drugs from nonmedical sources

CASE STUDY
A 40-Year-Old Woman with Thymoma and Borderline Personality Disorder

A 40-year-old woman with thymoma and borderline personality disorder, chronic pain, and anxiety was angry and feared abandonment by her psycho-oncologist while he was on vacation. Her covering physician gave her a prescription of 80 alprazolam tablets on the Friday before the Monday of the psycho-oncologist's expected return. The patient impulsively altered the prescription so that, instead of reading "80 tablets," it read "180 tablets." The alteration was detected by a pharmacist, who reported it back to her medical team. In the context of the patient's previously uneventful use of the medicine, her psychiatric diagnosis, and the therapist's vacation, it was agreed that the patient's behavior represented an expression of the psychodynamics of abandonment and a self-defeating expression of rage at the therapist. It was dealt with in detail in her psychotherapy.

Disease-Related Variables

Changes caused by progressive diseases, such as cancer, also challenge the principal concepts used to define addiction. Alterations in physical and psychosocial functioning caused by advanced illness and its treatment may be difficult to distinguish from the morbidity associated with drug abuse. In particular, alterations in functioning may complicate the ability to evaluate a concept that is vital to the diagnosis of addiction: "use despite harm." For example, discerning the questionable behaviors can be difficult in a patient who develops social withdrawal or cognitive changes after brain irradiation for metastases. Even if diminished cognition is clearly related to pain medication used in treatment, this effect might only reflect a narrow therapeutic window rather than the patient's use of analgesic to acquire these psychic effects.[9,10]

To accurately assess drug-related behaviors in patients with advanced disease, explicit information is usually required regarding the role of the drug in the patient's life. Therefore, the presence of mild mental clouding or the time spent out of bed may have less meaning than other outcomes, such as noncompliance with primary therapy related to drug use, or behaviors that threaten relationships with physicians, other health care professionals, and family members.[9,10]

Appropriate Definitions of Abuse and Addiction for Advanced Illness

A more appropriate definition of addiction would exemplify that it is a chronic disorder characterized by "the compulsive use of a substance resulting in physical, psychological, or social harm to the user and continued use despite the harm."[13] Although this definition is not without fault, it emphasizes that addiction is essentially a psychological and behavioral syndrome.[9,10]

A differential diagnosis should also be considered if questionable behaviors occur during pain treatment. A true addiction (substance dependence) is only one of many possible interpretations. A diagnosis of pseudoaddiction should also be taken into account if the patient is reporting distress associated with unrelieved symptoms. Impulsive drug use may also be indicative of another psychiatric disorder, diagnosis of which may have therapeutic implications. On occasion, aberrant drug-related behaviors appear to be causally remotely related to a mild encephalopathy, with perplexity concerning the appropriate therapeutic regimen. On rare occasions, questionable behaviors imply criminal intent. These diagnoses are not mutually exclusive.[9,10]

Varied and repeated observations over a period of time may be necessary to categorize questionable behaviors properly. Perceptive psychiatric assessment is crucial and may require evaluation by consultants who can elucidate the complex interactions among personality factors and psychiatric illness. Some patients may be self-medicating symptoms of anxiety, depression, insomnia, or problems of adjustment (such as boredom due to decreased ability to engage in usual activities and hobbies). Yet others may have character pathology that may be the more prominent determinant of drug-taking behavior. Patients with borderline personality disorders, for example, may impulsively use prescription medications that regulate inner tension or improve chronic emptiness or boredom and express anger at physicians, friends, or family. Psychiatric assessment is vitally important for both the population without a prior history of substance abuse and the population of known substance abusers who have a high incidence of psychiatric comorbidity.[14]

Cultural Issues in the Treatment of Substance Use Disorders

As noted earlier, cancer pain continues to be grossly undertreated despite the availability of guidelines for its clinical management, with patients who are members of an ethnic minority or substance abusers having a greater risk of inadequate treatment of cancer pain.[5–7] In fact, various studies have documented that minority patients receive insufficient pain treatment when compared to nonminority patients when being treated for pain caused by a variety of sources.[15–17] Since minority patients with advanced illness are undertreated for pain, they may be at greater risk of being misdiagnosed if exhibiting behaviors of pseudoaddiction.

Recently, more attention has been given to the significant influence that age, gender, and ethnicity have on the issues and treatment of substance abuse. Certain issues must be considered when implementing substance abuse treatment with the minority patient who is suspected of having a substance use disorder.[18]

First and foremost, it must be recognized that immense diversity exists within the different sociocultural groups themselves. Any given minority patient may possess beliefs, values, or drug-taking behaviors that greatly differ from the majority of the sociocultural group of which the patient is a member. In addition to ethnic orientation, attention must also focus on other sociocultural factors such as age, gender, sexual orientation, income, education, geographic location, and level of acculturation.[18] Ascribing certain cultural characteristics to all patients of a particular minority group may lead to stereotyping, alienating patients, and compromising treatment effectiveness.[19] While the perfect scenario would be to accurately understand all of the possible cultural issues that influence the patient within the context of his or her life circumstances, this is difficult and may be impractical.[1,18] Therefore, it is particularly important to respond to cultural needs in the treatment of substance abuse, because sociocultural factors greatly effect the manifestation of the disease. Consequently, clinicians must often acclimate their therapeutic approaches to accommodate the patient's sociocultural orientation.[18]

Risks in Patients with Current or Remote Histories of Drug Abuse

There is a lack of information regarding the risk of abuse or addiction during or subsequent to the therapeutic administration of potentially abusable drugs to medically ill patients with a current or remote history of abuse or addiction.[9] The possibility of successful long-term opioid therapy in patients with cancer or chronic nonmalignant pain has been indicated by anecdotal reports, particularly if the abuse or addiction is remote.[20–22]

Since it is commonly accepted that the likelihood of aberrant drug-related behavior occurring during treatment for medical illness will be greater for those with a remote or current history of substance abuse, it is reasonable to consider the possibility of abuse behaviors occurring when using different therapies. For example, while no clinical evidence exists to

Table 38–2
Basic Principles for Prescribing Controlled Substances to Patients with Advanced Illness and Issues of Addiction

Choose an opioid based on around-the-clock dosing.
Choose long-acting agents when possible.
As much as possible, limit or eliminate the use of short-acting or "breakthrough" doses.
Use nonopioid adjuvants when possible, and monitor for compliance with those medications.
Use nondrug adjuvants whenever possible (e.g., relaxation techniques, distraction, biofeedback, TNS, communication about thoughts and feelings of pain).
If necessary, limit the amount of medication given at any one time (i.e., write prescriptions for a few days' worth or a week's worth of medication at a time)
Use pill counts and urine toxicology screens as necessary.
If compliance is suspect or poor, refer to an addictions specialist.

support that the use of short-acting drugs or the parenteral route is more likely to cause questionable drug-related behaviors than other therapeutic strategies, it may be prudent to avoid such therapies in patients with histories of drug abuse.[9] A basic set of principles pertaining to prescribing controlled substances to this patient population is presented in Table 38–2.

Summary of Issues

Clinicians should understand that essentially any drug that acts upon the central nervous system or any route of administration has the potential to be abused. Therefore, a more comprehensive approach that recognizes the biological, chemical, social, and psychiatric aspects is necessary to effectively manage patients with substance abuse histories. Using this strategy extends beyond merely avoiding certain drugs or routes of administration—it also affords practical means to manage risk during cancer treatment.[9]

Clinical Management of Advanced-Disease Patients with Substance Use Histories

The most challenging issues in caring for patients with advanced disease typically arise from patients who are actively abusing alcohol or other drugs. This is because patients who are actively abusing drugs experience more difficulty in managing pain.[23] Patients may become caught in a cycle where pain functions as a barrier to seeking treatment for addiction with another addiction, possibly complicating treatment for chronic pain.[24] Also, since pain is undertreated, the risk of bingeing with prescription medications and or other substances increases for drug-abusing patients.[23]

General Guidelines

The following guidelines can be beneficial, whether the patient is actively abusing drugs or has a history of substance abuse. The principles outlined assist clinicians in establishing structure, control, and monitoring of addiction-related behaviors, which may be helpful and necessary at times in all pain treatment.[25]

Recommendations for the long-term administration of potentially abusable drugs, such as opioids, to patients with a history of substance abuse are based exclusively on clinical experience. Research is needed to ascertain the most effective strategies and to empirically identify patient subgroups who may be most responsive to different approaches. The following guidelines broadly reflect the types of interventions that might be considered in this clinical context.[10,25]

Multidisciplinary Approach

Pain and symptom management is often complicated by various medical, psychosocial, and administrative issues in the population of advanced patients with a substance use disorder. The most effective team may include a physician with expertise in pain/palliative care, nurses, social workers, and, when possible, a mental health care provider with expertise in the area of addiction medicine.[10,25]

Assessment of Substance Use History

In an effort to not offend, threaten, or anger patients, clinicians many times avoid asking patients about drug abuse. There is also often the expectation that patients will not answer truthfully. However, obtaining a detailed history of duration, frequency, and desired effect of drug use is vital. Adopting a nonjudgmental position and communicating in an empathetic and truthful manner is the best strategy when taking patients' substance abuse histories.[11,25]

In anticipating defensiveness on the part of the patient, it can be helpful for clinicians to mention that patients often misrepresent their drug use for logical reasons, such as stigmatization, mistrust of the interviewer, or concerns regarding fears of undertreatment. It is also wise for clinicians to explain that in an effort to keep the patient as comfortable as possible, by preventing withdrawal states and prescribing sufficient medication for pain and symptom control, an accurate account of drug use is necessary.[11,25]

The use of a careful, graduated-style interview can be beneficial in slowly introducing the assessment of drug abuse. This approach begins with broad and general inquiries regarding the role of drugs in the patient's life, such as caffeine and nicotine, and gradually proceeds to more specific questions regarding illicit drugs. This interview style can also assist in discerning any coexisting psychiatric disorders, which can significantly contribute to aberrant drug-taking behavior. Once identified, treatment of comorbid psychiatric disorders can greatly enhance management strategies and decrease the risk of relapse.[11,25]

Setting Realistic Goals for Therapy

The rate of recurrence for drug abuse and addiction is high. The stress associated with advanced illness and the easy availability of centrally acting drugs increases this risk. Therefore, total prevention of relapse may be impossible in this type of setting. Gaining an understanding that compliance and abstinence are not realistic goals may decrease conflicts with staff members in terms of management goals. Instead, the goals might be perceived as the creation of a structure for therapy that includes ample social/emotional support and limit-setting to control the harm done by relapse.[11,25]

There may be some subgroups of patients who are unable to comply with the requirements of therapy due to severe substance use disorders and comorbid psychiatric diagnoses. In these instances, clinicians must modify limits on various occasions and endeavor to develop a greater variety and intensity of supports. This may necessitate frequent team meetings and consultations with other clinicians. However, pertinent expectations must be clarified and therapy that is not successful should be modified.[11,25]

Evaluation and Treatment of Comorbid Psychiatric Disorders

Extremely high comorbidity of personality disorders, depression, and anxiety disorders exist in alcoholics and other patients with substance abuse histories.[14] The treatment of depression and anxiety can increase patient comfort and decrease the risk of relapse or aberrant drug-taking.[11,25]

Preventing or Minimizing Withdrawal Symptoms

Since many patients with drug abuse histories use multiple drugs, it is necessary to conduct a complete drug-use history to prepare for the possibility of withdrawal. Delayed abstinence syndromes, such as may occur after abuse of some benzodiazepine drugs, may be particularly diagnostically challenging.[11,25]

Considering the Therapeutic Impact of Tolerance

Patients who are active substance abusers may be tolerant to drugs administered for therapy, which will make pain management more difficult. The magnitude of this tolerance is never known. Therefore, it is best to begin with a conservative dose of therapeutic drug and then rapidly titrate the dose, with frequent reassessments until the patient is comfortable.[9,22]

Applying Pharmacological Principles to Treating Pain

Widely accepted guidelines for cancer pain management must be used to optimize long-term opioid therapy.[26,27] These guidelines stress the importance of patient self-report as the base for dosing, individualization of therapy to identify a favorable equilibrium between efficacy and side effects, and the value of monitoring over time.[25] They also are strongly indicative of the concurrent treatment of side effects as the basis for enhancing the balance between both analgesia and adverse effects.[28]

Individualization of the dose without regard to the size, which is the most important guideline for long-term opioid therapy, can be difficult in populations with substance abuse histories.[25] Although it may be appropriate to use care in prescribing potentially abusable drugs to these populations, deciding to forego the guideline of dose individualization without regard to absolute dose may increase the risk of undertreatment.[29] Aberrant drug-related behaviors may develop in response to unrelieved pain. Although these behaviors might be best understood as pseudoaddiction, the incidence of such behaviors serves to verify clinicians' fears and encourages greater prudence in prescribing.[25]

Another common misconception is the use of methadone. Clinicians who manage patients with substance abuse histories must comprehend the pharmacology of methadone due to its dual role as a treatment for opioid addiction and as an analgesic.[30,31] Methadone impedes withdrawal for significantly longer periods than it relieves pain. That is, abstinence can be prevented and opioid cravings lessened with a single dose, while most patients appear to require a minimum of three doses daily to obtain sustained analgesia. Although patients who are receiving methadone maintenance for treatment for opioid addiction can be administered methadone as an analgesic beyond the guidelines of the addiction treatment program, this usually necessitates a substantial modification in therapy, including dose escalation and multiple daily doses.[11,25]

From a pharmacological stance, the management of such a change does not pose difficult issues. It can, however, create substantial stress for the patient and clinicians involved in the treatment of the addiction disorder. Because the drug has been classified as addiction therapy, as opposed to pain therapy, some patients express disbelief in the analgesic efficacy of methadone. Others wish to continue the morning dose for addiction even if treatment throughout the remainder of the day uses the same drug at an equivalent or higher dose. Some clinicians who work at methadone clinics are willing to continue to be involved and prescribe opioids outside the program, and others wish to relinquish care.[25]

Selecting Appropriate Drugs and Route of Administration for the Symptom and Setting

The use of long-acting analgesics in sufficient amounts may help to minimize the number of rescue doses needed, lessen cravings, and decrease the risk of abuse of prescribed medications, given the possible difficulty of using short-acting formulations in patients with substance abuse histories. Rather than being overly concerned regarding the choice of drug or route of administration, the prescription of opioids and other potentially abusable drugs should be carried out with limits and guidelines.[11,25]

Recognizing Specific Drug Abuse Behaviors

In an effort to monitor the development of aberrant drug-taking behaviors, all patients who are prescribed potentially abusable drugs must be evaluated over time. This is particularly true for those patients with a remote or current history of drug abuse, including alcohol abuse. Should a high level of concern exist regarding such behaviors, frequent visits and regular assessments of significant others who can contribute information regarding the patient's drug use may be required. To promote early recognition of aberrant drug-related behaviors, it may also be necessary to have patients who have been actively abusing drugs in the recent past submit urine specimens for regular screening of illicit or licit but unprescribed drugs. When informing the patient of this approach, explain that it is a method of monitoring that can reassure the clinician and provide a foundation for aggressive symptom-oriented treatment, thus enhancing the therapeutic alliance with the patient.[11,25]

Using Nondrug Approaches as Appropriate

Many nondrug approaches can be used to assist patients in coping with chronic pain in advanced illness. Such educational interventions may include relaxation techniques, ways of thinking of and describing the experience of pain, and methods of communicating physical and emotional distress to staff members (see Table 38–2). While nondrug interventions may be helpful adjuvants to management, they should not be perceived as substitutes for drugs targeted at treating pain, or other physical or psychological symptoms.[11,25]

Inpatient Management Plan

In designing the inpatient management of an actively abusing patient with advanced illness, it is helpful to use structured treatment guidelines. While the applicability of these guidelines may vary from setting to setting, they provide a set of strategies that can ensure the safety of the patient and staff, control the patient's manipulative behaviors, allow for supervision of illicit drug use, enhance appropriate use of medications for pain and symptom control, and communicate an understanding of pain and substance abuse management.[11,25]

Under certain circumstances, such as actively abusing patients who are scheduled for surgery, patients should be admitted several days in advance when possible to allow for the stabilization of the drug regimen. This time can also be used to avoid withdrawal and to provide an opportunity to assess whether modifications to the established plan are necessary.[11,25]

Once established, the structured treatment plan for the management of active abuse must proceed conscientiously. In an effort to assess and manage symptoms, frequent visits are usually necessary. It is also important to avoid drug withdrawal and, to the extent possible, prescribed drugs for symptom control should be administered on a regular scheduled basis (see Table 38–2). This helps to eliminate repetitive encounters with staff that center on the desire to obtain drugs.[11,25]

Treatment management plans must be designed to represent the clinician's assessment of the severity of drug abuse. Open and honest communication between clinician and patient to stress that the guidelines were established in the best interest of the patient is often helpful. However, in cases where patients are unable to follow these guidelines, despite repeated interventions from the staff, discharge should be considered. Clinicians should discuss this decision for patient discharge with the staff and administration, while considering the ethical and legal ramifications of this action.[11,25]

Outpatient Management Plan

Alternative guidelines may be used in the management of the actively abusing patient with advanced illness who is being treated on an outpatient basis. In some instances, the treatment plan can be coordinated with referral to a drug rehabilitation program. However, patients who are facing end-of-life issues may have difficulty participating in such programs. Using the following approaches may be helpful for managing the complex and more difficult-to-control aspects of care.

Using Written Agreements

Using written agreements that clearly state the roles of the team members and the rules and expectations for the patient is helpful when structuring outpatient treatment. Basing the level of restrictions on the patient's behaviors, graded agreements should be enforced that clearly state the consequences of aberrant drug use.[11,25] A sample contract for the initiation of opioid therapy is provided in Figure 38–1. This template can be modified and structured to fit individual practices and clinics, but it is a good general indication of the responsibilities of the patient as well as the provider.

Guidelines for Prescribing

Patients who are actively abusing must be seen weekly to build a good rapport with staff and afford evaluation of symptom control and addiction-related concerns. Frequent visits allow the opportunity to prescribe small quantities of drugs, which may decrease the temptation to divert and provide a motive for not missing appointments[11,25] (see Table 38–2).

Procedures for prescription loss or replacement should be explicitly explained to the patient, with the stipulation that no renewals will be given if appointments are missed. The patient should also be informed that any dose changes requires prior communication with the clinician. Additionally, clinicians who are covering for the primary care provider must be advised of the guidelines that have been established for each patient with a substance abuse history to avoid conflict and disruption of the treatment plan.[11,25]

Using 12-Step Programs

The clinician should consider referring the patient to a 12-step program with the stipulation that attendance be documented for ongoing prescription purposes. The clinician may wish to contact the patient's sponsor in an effort to disclose the patient's illness and that medication is required in the treatment of the illness. This contact will also help to decrease the risk of stigmatizing the patient as being noncompliant with the ideals of the 12-step program.[11,25]

Urine Toxicology Screens

Periodic urine toxicology screens should be performed for most patients to encourage compliance and detect the concurrent use of illicit substances. This practice, as well as how positive screens will be managed, should be clearly explained to the patient at the beginning of outpatient therapy. A response to a positive screen generally involves increasing the guidelines for continued treatment, such as more frequent visits and smaller quantities of prescribed drugs.[11,25]

Opioid Medication Consent Form

PATIENT NAME: ______________________________ SSN: ____________________

The purpose of this Agreement is to clarify expectations and prevent misunderstandings about certain medicines I will be taking for pain management. This is to help both my doctor and I comply with the law regarding controlled prescription drugs. I understand that this Agreement is essential to the trust and confidence necessary in a doctor/patient relationship and that my doctor will treat me based on this Agreement.

I understand that if I break this Agreement, my doctor may decide to stop prescribing these pain-control medicines. In this case, my doctor may taper off the medicine (i.e., slowly decrease) over a period of several days, as necessary to avoid withdrawal symptoms. Also, a drug-dependence treatment program may be recommended.

GOALS OF OPIOID TRIAL/TREATMENT

The purpose of this medication is to increase your ability to function at work and at home. Success will be measured by your activity level, not your report of pain.

RISKS OF OPIOID TRIAL/TREATMENT

This medication has the potential to cause an addiction. Physical tolerance and dependence occurs with regular use of a narcotic, but this is different from addiction. For a person's health, safety and protection, this medication may be stopped if there is a concern about addiction.

ADDICTION BEHAVIOR
- ❑ a lot of time & energy focused on obtaining medication
- ❑ continuing to take medications despite being told to stop
- ❑ decline in family and/or work functioning
- ❑ loss of interest in other life activities (e.g., hobbies, social activities)
- ❑ consistent misuse of medications (see below)

MISUSE OR ABUSE OF MEDICATION
- ❑ taking more medication than prescribed
- ❑ use of pain medications that have not been prescribed by this program
- ❑ use of alcohol to manage pain
- ❑ high number of emergency room visits seeking medication
- ❑ failing to use other recommended pain management techniques (e.g., physical therapy, relaxation techniques, TNS unit)
- ❑ getting medication from more than one doctor
- ❑ using someone else's opioid medication
- ❑ reports of lost or stolen medication
- ❑ asking only for medications with a high street value

GUIDELINES FOR OPIOID PRESCRIPTIONS

Our Responsibility
- Medication will only be prescribed by a SINGLE PROVIDER.
- Medication will be prescribed on a "by-the-clock" schedule.
- Lost or stolen prescriptions or medications will not be replaced.
- OPIOID MEDICATIONS WILL NOT TYPICALLY BE FILLED OVER THE PHONE.
- If an opioid taper is unsuccessful, medical care will be provided. Referral to facilities specializing in medication detoxification may be necessary.

Figure 38–1. Pain management guidelines: opioid medication consent form.

Family Sessions and Meetings

The clinician, in an effort to increase support and function, should involve family members and friends in the treatment plan. These meetings will allow the clinician and other team members to become familiar with the family and additionally assist the team to identify family members who are using illicit drugs. Offering referral of these identified family members to drug treatment can be portrayed as a method of gathering support for the patient. The patient should also be prepared to cope with family members or friends who may attempt to buy or sell the patient's medications. These meetings will also assist the team in identifying dependable individuals who can serve as a source of strength and support for the patient during treatment.[11,25] A final case study illustrates how a highly complicated patient case, with advanced cancer requiring an unorthodox amount of medication, was managed in cooperation with hospice nurses to treat his pain and control aberrant behavior.

CASE STUDY

A 39-Year-Old Man with Pancreatic Cancer

The patient, a 39-year-old man with pancreatic cancer, was referred to the palliative care program shortly after he had opted to forego chemotherapy and radiation therapy, and it was decided he was not a candidate for surgical resection. The patient had presented with advanced disease and a 40-pound weight loss. He had been suffering with abdominal pain for months but was self-treating with sustained-release oxycodone, which he had been abusing and dealing for the last several years. The patient had a very limited life expectancy when first evaluated, and he was not open to considering other opioids or celiac plexus nerve blocks. He stated that he just wanted to be comfortable enough to play with his 3-year-old daughter until he died. The patient always required high doses of medication for comfort (800-mg sustained-release oxycodone b.i.d.) and did

Opioid Medication Consent Form (Continued)

Your Responsibility

- A person is responsible for his or her medications, and needs to make sure that prescriptions are filled correctly. Therefore, they need to make certain that the pharmacy gives them the correct number prescribed.
- No increases in medication doses will be made without the approval of the prescribing physician.
- If a person takes more medication than is prescribed, he or she will run out of medication before being given more.
- Narcotic medication use questions should be made during normal business hours, Monday through Friday, 8:00 A.M. to 4 P.M.
- Patients are expected to be on time for all appointments including those not related to refills medications. You will be asked to come in before a medication is to be refilled at times.

Informed Consent

- I will communicate fully with my doctor about the character and intensity of my pain, the effect of the pain on my daily life, side effects, and how well the medicine is helping to relieve the pain.
- I may be asked to bring unused medications to clinic with me for a "pill count" to ensure that I am using the medication as prescribed.
- I consent to submit to a blood or urine test if requested by my doctor to determine my compliance with my program of pain control medicine.
- I will not use any illegal controlled substances, including marijuana, cocaine, etc., as these will interact poorly with my pain medications.
- I will not share, sell, or trade my medication with anyone as these are dangerous to use when not under a doctor's care.
- I will not attempt to obtain any pain medicines, including opioid pain medicines, stimulants, or anti-anxiety medicines from any other doctor.
- I authorize the doctor and my pharmacy to cooperate fully with any city, state or federal law enforcement agency, including this state's Board of Pharmacy, in the investigation of any possible misuse, sale, or other diversion of my pain medicine. I authorize my doctor to provide a copy of this Agreement to my pharmacy. I agree to waive any applicable or right of privacy or confidentiality with respect to these authorizations.

If these guidelines are not met, you may be discharged from the program.

I, the undersigned, agree that the above guidelines have been explained to me, and that my questions and concerns regarding this treatment have been adequately answered. I agree to comply with the above guidelines. I have a copy of this document.

Signed: ______________________ Date: ____________

Physician/Clinician: ______________________ Date: ____________

Witness: ______________________ Date: ____________

Figure 38–1. *(continued)*

eventually agree to also take adjuvant analgesics and corticosteroids. He had remarkably good pain and symptom management until his death, and even went deer hunting 2 weeks before he died. The provision of supportive care would have been impossible without the structure provided by hospice nurses, who delivered 1 day's worth of medicine at a time, turned up randomly for pill counts at the patient's home, collected urine for toxicology screens, and otherwise coordinated tremendous levels of family support from those family members who had been assessed and deemed not involved with illicit drug use and sales.

Conclusion

Treating patients who are experiencing chronic pain from advanced illness and a substance use disorder is both complicated and challenging, since each can significantly complicate the other. The management of an advanced patient who is actively abusing drugs and is a member of an ethnic minority is more perplexing due to cultural differences that may exist. Using a treatment plan that involves a team approach that recognizes and responds to these complex needs is the optimum strategy to facilitate treatment. While pain management may continue to be challenging even when all treatment plan procedures are implemented, the health care team's goal should be providing the highest level of pain management for all patients with substance use disorders.

REFERENCES

1. Muirhead G. Cultural issues in substance abuse treatment. Patient Care 2000;5:151–159.
2. Groerer J, Brodsky M. The incidence of illicit drug use in the United States 1962–1989. Br J Addiction 1992;87:1345–1351.
3. Colliver JD, Kopstein AN. Trends in cocaine abuse reflected in emergency room episodes reported to DAWN. Public Health Rep 1991;106:59–68.
4. Regier DA, Myers JK, Kramer M, Robins LN, Blazer DG, Hough RL, Eaton WW, Locke BZ. The NIMH epidemiology catchment area program. Arch Gen Psychiatry 1984;41: 934–941.

5. Ramer L, Richardson JL, Cohen MZ, Bedney C, Danley KL, Judge EA. Multimeasure pain assessment in an ethnically diverse group of patients with cancer. J Transcultural Nurs 1999;10: 94–101.
6. Glajchen M, Fitzmartin RD, Blum D, Swanton R. Psychosocial barriers to cancer pain relief. Cancer Practice 1995;3:76–82.
7. Ward SE, Goldberg N, Miller-McCauley V, Mueller C, Nolan A, Pawlik-Plank D, Robbins A, Stormoen D, Weissman DE. Patient-related barriers to management of cancer pain. Pain 1993;52: 319–324.
8. Joranson DE, Gilson AM. Policy issues and imperatives in the use of opioids to treat pain in substance abusers. J Law Med Ethics 1994;22:215–223.
9. Passik SD, Portenoy RK. Substance abuse issues in palliative care. In: Berger A, Portenoy R, Weissman D, eds. Principles and Practice of Supportive Oncology. Philadelphia: Lippincott Williams & Wilkins, 1998:513–524.
10. Passik SD, Portenoy RK, Ricketts PL. Substance abuse issues in cancer patients, part 1: prevalence and diagnosis. Oncology 1998; 12:517–521.
11. Passik SD, Portenoy RK. Substance abuse disorders. In: Holland JC, ed. Psycho-oncology. New York: Oxford University Press, 1998: 576–586.
12. Weissman DE, Haddox JD. Opioid pseudoaddiction—an iatrogenic syndrome. Pain 1989;36:363–366.
13. Rinaldi RC, Steindler EM, Wilford BB. Clarification and standardization of substance abuse terminology. JAMA 1988;259: 555–557.
14. Khantzian EJ, Treece C. DSM-III psychiatric diagnosis of narcotic addicts. Arch Gen Psychiatry 1985;42:1067–1071.
15. Anderson KO, Mendoza TR, Valero V, Richman SP, Russell C, Hurley J, DeLeon C, Washington P, Palos G, Payne R, Cleeland CS. Minority cancer patients and their providers. Cancer 2000; 88: 1929–1938.
16. Todd KH, Deaton C, D'Adamo AP, Goe L. Ethnicity and analgesic practice. Ann Emerg Med 2000;35:11–16.
17. Todd KH, Samaroo N, Hoffman JR. Ethnicity as a risk factor for inadequate emergency department analgesia. JAMA 1993;269: 1537–1539.
18. Seale JP, Muramoto ML. Substance abuse among minority populations. Substance Abuse 1993;20:167–180.
19. Finn P. Addressing the needs of cultural minorities in drug treatment. J Substance Abuse Treatment 1994;11(4):325–337.
20. Dunbar SA, Katz NP. Chronic opioid therapy for nonmalignant pain in patients with a history of substance abuse: report of 20 cases. J Pain Symptom Manage 1996;11:163–171.
21. Gonzales GR, Coyle N. Treatment of cancer pain in a former opioid abuser: fears of the patient and staff and their influences on care. J Pain Symptom Manage, 1992;7:246–249.
22. Macaluso C, Weinberg D, Foley KM. Opioid abuse and misuse in a cancer pain population [abstract]. J Pain Symptom Manage 1988;3:S24–S31.
23. Kemp C. Managing chronic pain in patients with advanced disease and substance related disorders. Home Healthcare Nurse 1996;14:255–261.
24. Savage SR. Addiction in the treatment of pain: significance, recognition, and management. J Pain Symptom Manage 1993;8:265–277.
25. Passik SD, Portenoy RK, Ricketts PL. Substance abuse issues in cancer patients, part 2: evaluation and treatment. Oncology 1998; 12:729–734.
26. Agency for Health Care Policy and Research and Management of Cancer Pain. Clinical Practice Guideline No. 9. Washington, DC: U.S. Department of Health and Human Services, 1994.
27. American Pain Society. Principles of Analgesic Use in the Treatment of Acute Pain and Cancer Pain, 5th ed. Glenview, IL: Author, 2003.
28. Portenoy RK. Management of common opioid side effects during long-term therapy for cancer pain. Ann Acad Med Singapore 1994;23:160–170.
29. Breitbart W, Rosenfeld BD, Passik SD, McDonald MV, Thaler H, Portenoy RK. The undertreatment of pain in ambulatory AIDS patients. Pain 1996;65:243–249.
30. Fainsinger R, Schoeller T, Bruera E. Methadone in the management of cancer pain: a review. Pain 1993;52:137–147.
31. Lowinson JH, Marion IJ, Joseph H. Methadone maintenance. In: Lowinson JH, Ruiz P, Millman RB, eds. Substance Abuse: A Comprehensive Textbook. Baltimore: Williams & Wilkins, 1992: 550–571.

VI
End-of-Life Care Across Settings

39

Marilyn Bookbinder

Improving the Quality of Care Across All Settings

Never doubt that a small group of thoughtful, committed citizens can change the world. Indeed, that's the only thing that ever has.—Margaret Mead

- ***Key Points***
- *Quality palliative care is a result of intelligent systematic efforts to raise standards of care.*
- *Tools are available to assist in the monitoring and measurement of structure, process, and competency in the delivery of palliative care.*
- *Outcome measures are needed to evaluate the impact of innovative change on patient and family quality of life, health care systems, and professional practice.*

One system for addressing health and end-of-life care is the inclusion of quality methodologies designed to improve education, streamline health care bureaucracies, help measure costs, and even address how people feel about their jobs. Whether or not your organization is accredited by the Joint Commission on Accreditation of Health Care Organizations (JCAHO), mandated to use a quality improvement (QI) methodology, a planned-change approach is needed to achieve positive outcomes and to cultivate an infrastructure that maintains optimal standards of care for those at the end of life.

This chapter provides perspectives on QI-based initiatives in U.S. health care organizations across settings and populations, and discusses their impact on patient, professional, and system outcomes in palliative care. Principles of QI and structural, process, and outcome approaches to conducting QI studies are introduced. A case study is presented of a pathway for the end of life that is now being tested and used to establish the linkages between QI principles and practice to improve end-of-life care. The chapter closes by showcasing nurses within interdisciplinary teams who are providing leadership in the field of palliative care.

The Terminology Turmoil

Quality improvement is increasingly commonplace in the lexicon of industry and government health care systems in the United States. Typically, QI is used to describe a process for improving things. Although the terms vary, distinct vocabulary, tools, and techniques used to conduct QI studies are the same. Other labels include continuous quality improvement (CQI), total quality management (TQM), total quality systems (TQS), quality systems improvement (QSI), total quality (TQ), and performance improvement (PI).[1]

Because consensus regarding these terms is unlikely, it is recommended that each organization define a methodology and terms that apply across the board and be consistent in their use. This will encourage users of QI to read beyond labels and to examine the meaning behind concepts and the value of teamwork in achieving goals. For the purposes of this chapter, QI is defined generically as the label for the philosophy driving a systematic approach to improving clinical practice, systems, issues, education, and research.

Quality Improvement in Health Care

What Is Quality Improvement?

As a philosophy, QI is broadly defined as "a commitment and approach used to continuously improve every process in every part of an organization, with the intent to exceed customer expectations and outcomes." As a management approach, QI is a way of doing business: a way to stimulate employees to become part of the solution by improving the ways care is delivered, identifying the root causes of problems in systems, designing innovative products and services, and evaluating and continuously improving.[2]

The concepts of QI go back to the 1920s, with pioneers in the field such as Deming, Shewhart, Juran, and Ishikawa. W. Edwards Deming, an American engineer and statistician most widely known for his efforts to assist Japan in its quest for quality after World War II, was all but unknown in his own country until the 1980s. In fact, the Deming prize, Japan's highest award for industrial productivity and quality, was first awarded to an American company, Florida Electric and Light Company, in 1989. To date, no health care organizations have received the Deming prize. Joseph Juran, also involved in the Japanese quality transition in the 1940s and 1950s, added the concepts of planning and control to the quality process and addressed the "costs" of poor quality, which includes wasted effort, extra expense, and defects. Readers wanting more detail about the rationale and statistical methods behind QI philosophy and methods are referred to the writings of Deming and others.[3,4]

Although Deming's quality method has been used extensively in industry with much success, it has only been adapted to education and health care since the early 1990s. The U.S. Health Care Reform Act of 1992[5] fueled the need for QI methods and better control over inconsistencies in services. Effects of the reform include: (1) increased managed-care contracts in health systems and reductions in reimbursement; (2) reorganization and downsizing of hospitals and staff; (3) cross-training and the development of multipurpose personnel; (4) shorter hospital stays for patients; and (5) a shift in the provision of services from hospital care to ambulatory and home care.

Table 39–1 describes six key principles of QI, based on the doctrines of W. Edwards Deming. These principles are being applied to a QI project to improve end-of-life care at Continuum's Beth Israel Medical Center (BIMC) in New York City.[6] At BIMC, chart reviews of inpatient deaths and other sources of data provided evidence that end-of-life care could be improved. The purpose of the 1-year pilot study, funded by a New York State Quality Measurement grant, is to create a benchmark for the care of the imminently dying inpatient.

The QI process begins and ends with customers, determining their needs, and creating products that meet or exceed their expectations. To achieve the necessary improvement, multidisciplinary teams are needed to break down barriers between disciplines and departments, promote collaboration and mutual respect among health care workers, and encourage participation from front-line staff. In the BIMC pilot study, to determine the causes of variation in end-of-life (EOL) care, a 28-member team was formed to involve staff integral to the EOL process on five pilot units: oncology, geriatrics, hospice, medical intensive care, and step-down unit. Early in the study, QI techniques of brainstorming and flowcharting were used to identify health system barriers and to identify possible strategies for dealing with them.

QI teams use a systematic, scientific approach and statistical methods to study problems and make decisions. This paradigm encourages an environment of life-long learning and promotes a team approach to identifying and developing the "best practices." The BIMC project identified a critical need for multidisciplinary education and teambuilding. For example, monthly QI meetings included a segment of the American Medical Association's (AMA's) Education for Physicians on End-of-Life Care (EPEC)[7] training program. Discussions, led by Russell K. Portenoy, M.D., a co-investigator for the AMA project and chairperson of the QI team, provided team members fundamental information about the components of good EOL care, as well as opportunities to voice their own ideas and concerns.

The QI team worked in four subcommittees over a 5-month period to reach the implementation schedule of the project. One subcommittee developed the Palliative Care for Advanced Disease pathway (PCAD), which has three parts: a multidisciplinary care path, a flow sheet for daily documentation of care, and a physician's order sheet, that includes suggested medications for treating 15 of the most prevalent symptoms at EOL. The other three subcommittees addressed (1) education of nurses, physicians, other staff, patients, and families; (2) a timeline and detailed plan for implementation, education, and evaluation of PCAD; and (3) tools and methods for evaluating patient, family, staff, and system outcomes of the project.

Effectiveness of Quality Improvement

While many organizations have embraced the notion of using QI to improve cost and quality outcomes, the experience in the United States is relatively new. In fact, a national survey of U.S. hospitals in 1993 found that 69% had adopted or were beginning to implement some form of QI program. Seventy-five percent of hospitals adopting QI had done so within the previous 2 years,[8] studying administrative issues, such as patient scheduling, record-keeping, and billing, rather than clinical practice.

One study provides evidence that quality and outcomes of care can be improved and certain efficiencies achieved through

Table 39–1
Principles of Quality and Application for Improving End-of-Life Care

Principle	Discussion	Application
1. Customer-driven	The focus is on customers, both internal and external, and understanding them. Teams strive to achieve products/services to better meet needs and exceed expectations of customers.	Chart reviews of patient deaths reveal areas to improve: Documentation regarding advance directive discussions, symptom management effectiveness, spiritual and psychosocial care, treatment decisions in last 48 h of life. Focus groups with caregivers reveal need for better communication with health professionals about patient's progress.
2. System optimization and alignment	Organizations/teams are systems of interdependent parts, with the same mission and goals for customers. Optimizing performance of the entire system means aligning the processes, technology, people, values, and policies to support team efforts to continually improve.	Hospital-wide multidisciplinary CQI team is formed to reduce variation in EOL care with three standardized tools that provide guidelines for care (carepath), documentation, and physician orders. Ongoing resources from Pain and Palliative Care available to pilot unit staff (one advanced practice nurse)
3. Continual improvement and innovation	Focus shifts to processes of care and using a systematic and scientific approach. Methods seek to reduce and control unnecessary process variation and improve outcomes.	Flowcharting and brainstorming techniques help identify current activities and unit norms for EOL care regarding establishing goals of care, advance directives, respecting patient and family preferences, and barriers to implementing goals of project.
4. Continual learning	Resources are available to develop a culture in which people seek to learn from each other and access new sources of evidence. Feedback mechanisms support the use of evidence to drive improvements.	Extensive literature searches and team expertise guide development of clinical tools and educational materials. Team members receive education regarding issues in EOL care, viewing of Education in Palliative and End-of-Life Care (EPEC). Adult learning principles guide sequencing and content of educational sessions for unit staff (e.g., physiology of dying).
5. Management through knowledge	Decision-making is based on knowledge, confirmed with facts about what is "best practice," and guided by statistical thinking.	Team uses FOCUS-PDSA methodology to structure study processes. Content experts in EOL, measurement, outcomes, and QI guide sampling, selected outcome measures, and graphic display of data.
6. Collaboration and mutual respect	Organizations/teams engage everyone in the process of improvement and in the discovery of new knowledge and innovations. Mutual respect for the dignity, knowledge, and potential, contributions of others is valued by members.	Team forms subcommittees to develop materials in four areas based on expertise and interest: Carepath development, flow sheet, physicians' orders Implementation (timeline for phases of planning, launching, rollout, evaluation, dissemination, and decisions to adopt practice changes) Education (staff, patient, and family) Outcomes (patient, family, staff knowledge, process audit of new tools)

the application of QI. A review of the literature from 1991 through 1997 revealed 42 single-site and 13 multisite QI studies for examination.[8] Of the 42 single-site studies, nearly 60% focused on two major areas: streamlining surgical or medical procedures and reducing length of stay. Thirteen studies addressed overuse of services (i.e., provision of health services when the risks outweigh the benefits); three looked at underuse (i.e., failure to provide health services when benefits exceed risks); and 23 evaluated misuse (i.e., appropriate health services selected but poorly provided). Only two studies used randomized design, while most used weaker designs, such as pre–post observation.

Of the 13 multisite studies, seven addressed misuse of services (i.e., focusing on improving care without questioning the amount of care provided); four focused on appropriateness of care in terms of underuse (e.g., pediatric immunizations rates, use of guidelines); and two examined overuse of services (e.g., length of stay). Only one multisite study used a randomized design. Although some study outcomes included standards for better pain management, none addressed the application of QI in palliative care or, specifically, end-of-life care.

Given the emphasis in health care on using QI to improve quality and cost in health care, nurses can expect to see increases in accountability in the following areas: performance monitoring, participation in multidisciplinary team meetings, education in quality improvement, implementation of process improvement approaches, use of flowcharts and other tools and techniques for data gathering, restructuring of work flow patterns and removal of barriers to patient care, development and use of quality indicators, and focus on patient and caregiver outcomes.

Quality Improvement in Palliative Care

The World Health Organization defines palliative care as the "the active total care of patients whose disease is not responsive to curative treatment . . . when control of pain, of other symptoms and of psychological, social and spiritual problems is paramount."[9] Palliative care is often referred to as supportive care or comfort care that seeks to prevent, relieve, alleviate, lessen, or soothe the symptoms of disease without effecting a cure.

A valuable resource for those working in end-of-life care is the landmark report published by a committee of the Institute of Medicine (IOM), *Approaching Death: Improving Care at End of Life.*[10] The committee of 12 experts in medical and nursing care for chronically ill and severely ill patients summarized four areas of improvement: the state-of-the-knowledge in end-of-life care, evaluation methods for measuring outcomes, factors impeding high-quality care, and steps toward agreement on what constitutes "appropriate care" at end of life. The four major findings suggest starting points for QI work:

- Patient care: Too many people suffer endlessly at the end of life, both from errors of omission—when caregivers fail to provide palliative and supportive care known to be effective—and from errors of commission—when caregivers do what is known to be ineffective and even harmful.
- Organizations: Legal, organizational, and economical obstacles conspire to obstruct reliably excellent care at the end of life.
- Education: The education and training of physicians and other health care professionals fail to provide them with knowledge, skills, and attitudes required to care well for the dying patient.
- Research: Current knowledge and understanding are inadequate to guide and support consistent practice of evidence-based medicine at the end of life.

Structures for QI and End-of-Life Care

QI Methodologies Provide Structures

Various methodologies can be used as structural elements in a framework designed to support an EOL care program. Such structures also help to explain the interrelationship of parts. One type of structure, a systematic methodology, organizes and guides the activities of people performing QI; a second type assures the validity and appropriateness of a study to improve end-of-life care.

A systematic methodology is needed to conduct a QI study and various models exist, some of them widely recognized in health care. Others have been designed specifically for particular institutions' QI departments. Although QI models may vary, all of them support QI as an unceasing, organization-wide effort that focuses on improving processes of work. They are not intended for policing or blaming people for errors after the fact. Systematic methodologies provide the infrastructure needed to carry out a study that may span a period of years to reach targeted goals.

Ruskin writes, "Quality is never an accident. Quality is always the result of intelligent effort, intent, and vigilance to make a superior thing."[11] One frequently used methodology designed to support "intelligent effort" is the FOCUS-PDSA cycle, which illustrates the BIMC team's application of each step in the cycle (see Appendix 39–1). The details and application of the FOCUS-PDSA cycle and tools and techniques for conducting QI studies have been described elsewhere.[12,13] This is also sometimes referred to as the FOCUS-PDCA cycle, but will be called by its more commonly used name, the FOCUS-PDSA cycle in this chapter.

The FOCUS-PDSA methodology is briefly described below using the BIMC example. Its first five steps are aimed at team building, clarifying the nature and scope of the improvement needed, and gathering information about the culture and setting in which the study will be done.

FOCUS

- Find a process to improve. The focus for the BIMC study was care of imminently dying inpatients on the five hospital units known to have the highest volume of patient deaths. Chart reviews of patient deaths identified the need for the study.
- Organize to improve a process. A 28-member QI team spanned departments and disciplines to address end-of-life issues, such as ethics, social work, chaplains, pharmacists, nurses, and physicians.

- Clarify what is known. Flowcharts were used to map the ideal process of care and increase dialogue among the team about "why" the care varies. The team's four subcommittees on care path development; implementation, education, and evaluation searched internal and external sources for evidence and rationale in end-of-life care.
- Understand variation. Brainstorming techniques helped the team elicit reasons for variations in the care process and identify potential barriers. An Ishikawa diagram (to display cause and effect) was used to show the barriers: materials, methods, people, and equipment categories were used. Subcommittees considered the barriers when planning and developing elements of the program.
- Select a process improvement. Four subcommittees of the QI team developed evidence-based interventions, including the three-part PCAD care path, educational materials, and appropriate tools to measure professional, patient and family, and system outcomes. This step starts the PDSA cycle.

The PDCA Cycle: Plan/Do/Check/Act (also referred to as the Plan-Do-Study-Act [PDSA]). The Shewhart Cycle[3] constitutes the evaluation aspect of the study, and it is repeated until the team reaches its goals. The implementation of these steps during the BIMC pilot follows:

- Plan. In this step, a timeline of activities for the 1-year pilot prepared administration, team members, and others with direction, goals, and resources. The sample timeline in Appendix 39–1 illustrates the various phases involved in launching a project: the planning phase, roll-out or introduction phase, implementation, evaluation, and dissemination and reporting. The study design is created. This includes determination of sample size and selection, what data will be collected and by whom, what tools will be used and when they will be applied, what training will be conducted and by whom, and who will perform data analysis. Table 39–2 outlines principles for assuring the quality of data.

Table 39–2
Principles for Assuring the Quality of Data

Principle	Key Point
Validity/reliability	There is accuracy and consistency in data collection.
Completeness	Measurement system includes a policy for missing data and timeliness of collection.
Sampling method	Sample size is determined by power analysis to ensure representativeness of population.
Outlier cases	Measurement systems make efforts to validate or correct outliers.
Data specification	There are standardized definitions and terminology for transmission/use of data across departments.
Internal standards	Prespecified data-quality standards are tailored for individual performance measures.
External standards	There is a commitment to implementing data sets, codes, methodologies developed by accrediting bodies (e.g., government, professional organizations) for data use across health care systems.
Auditability	Data are traceable to the individual case level.
Monitoring process	Ongoing data-measurement process in place is based on prespecified standards.
Documentation	Data standards and findings are recorded and available for review.
Feedback	Performance systems regularly provide summary reports on data quality to organization leadership.
Education	Performance systems provide support through education, on-site visits, and guidelines to ensure quality data.
Accountability	Measurement systems are responsible for data quality and dissemination to participating members.

- Do. The interventions are implemented and data collection begins. In the BIMC study, several pre-measures were obtained, including baseline knowledge, using the Palliative Care Quiz for Nurses,[14] chart reviews, and focus groups with staff to obtain baseline data.
- Check. The results of data collection are analyzed by the team and the next steps formulated. The BIMC group used the findings from the knowledge pretest to identify areas for continuing education. Through consensus, members agreed that knowledge items answered incorrectly by 15% of staff would be targeted for continued education.
- Act. Action plans are developed. The BIMC team gave feedback to the QI team, pilot units, and the hospital QI department in a quarterly report. Staff requested education in "the physiology of dying."

Standards of Care Provide Structure

Quality care begins in clinical settings with well-defined standards of care that are accepted as authoritative by professionals. Such standards represent acknowledged conditions against which comparisons are made and levels of excellence are judged. They serve to establish consistency, expectations, and patterns for practice. They articulate what health care professionals do and whom they serve, and they define what clinical services and resources are needed. Standards also provide a framework against which quality of care can be measured and constantly improved.

In QI, the term benchmark is used to refer to "the search for the best practices that consistently produce best-in-the-world results"[4]—the gold standard. Standards of care,[15,16] guidelines,[17,18] position papers,[19–22] principles of professional practice,[23–26] and research models for end-of-life care[27,28] are increasingly becoming available to improve appropriateness, effectiveness, and cost-effectiveness of care.

If explicit, guidelines can describe appropriate management of specific symptoms and at the same time provide a basis for assessment, treatment, and possible outcomes. However, if the evidence is weak, as is the case for much of end-of-life care, guidelines or standards need to be supported with recommendations made through consensus.[10]

Processes for QI and End-of-Life Care

Answering the question "What are the processes for giving care to a dying patient?" can generate many ideas for a QI study. Process refers to the series of activities or functions that bring about a result. Nurses' contributions are critical in the processes of assessment, diagnosis, treatment, and evaluation of patients. Pain, dyspnea, agitation, nausea, diarrhea, and constipation are some important symptoms leading to nursing interventions that can reduce the suffering of dying patients.

To meet the health care reform challenges of high quality at lower cost, there has been an explosion of tools designed to reduce variability in the processes of care. Critical pathways and algorithms are two types of tools that provide useful strategies for nurses to monitor and manage the processes of patient care. These tools define desired patient outcomes for specific medical conditions and delineate the optimal sequence and timing of interventions to be performed by health care professionals.

Clinical Pathways

In the QI context, the term *pathways* refers to clinical approaches or critical paths that form a structured, multidisciplinary action plan that defines the key events, activities, and expected outcomes of care for each discipline during each day of care. Pathways delineate the optimal sequence and timing of interventions.[29] The goal of using a pathway is to "reduce variation" in services and practices, thus reducing costs.[30–33] Table 39–3 shows a six-step process for developing pathways. Table 39–4 lists commonly used elements of care and interventions.[29] By acting on these aspects of QI to improve EOL care, the BIMC QI team pilot-tested the pathway in oncology, geriatrics, and the hospice setting.

Pilot-Test of a Pathway to Improve End-of-Life Care. The entire QI team at BIMC designed an evidenced-based PCAD pathway consisting of three parts: (1) a Care Path—the interdisciplinary plan of care; (2) a Daily Patient Care Flow Sheet for documentation of assessments and interventions (includ-

Table 39–3
The Six-Step Process for Developing a Care Path

1. Identify high-volume, high-priority case types, review medical records, review and evaluate current literature to characterize the specific problems, average length of stay, critical events, and practical outcomes.
2. Write the critical path, defining the sequence and timing of functions to be performed by physicians, nurses, and other staff.
3. Have nurses, physicians, and other disciplines involved in the process review the plan of care.
4. Revise the pathway until consensus on care components is reached.
5. Pilot-test the pathway and revise as needed.
6. Incorporate pathway patient management into quality-improvement programs, which include monitoring and evaluating patient care outcomes.

Source: Janken et al. (1999) reference 29.

Table 39–4
Routine Elements of Care Paths

- Physical elements
- Medications
- Nutrition and dietary
- Vital signs, intake and output, weight
- Comfort assessment
- Safety and activity
- Diagnostic lab work
- Intravenous use
- Transfusions
- Diagnostic tests
- Psychosocial and spiritual needs
- Referrals and consultations
- Patient and family counseling and education

Table 39–5
Goals of the Palliative Care for Advanced Disease (PCAD) Pathway

- Respect patient autonomy, values, and decisions.
- Continually clarify goals of care.
- Minimize symptom distress at end of life.
- Optimize appropriate supportive interventions and consultations.
- Reduce unnecessary interventions.
- Support families by coordinating services.
- Eliminate unnecessary regulations.
- Provide bereavement services for families and staff. *or*
- Facilitate the transition to alternate care settings, such as hospice, when appropriate.

ing automatic referrals to social work and chaplaincy); and (3) a standardized Physician Order Sheet, with suggestions for medical management of 15 symptoms prevalent at the end of life (see Appendix 39–1 and http://www.stoppain.org). This three-part pathway was designed to guide interdisciplinary management of the imminently dying inpatient once the patient's primary physician has ordered PCAD (Table 39–5).

Implementation of PCAD in daily care on three units has confirmed the enormous complexity of predicting the timing of a patient's death.[34] Although "imminently dying" was defined for the study as "hours to 2 weeks until death," nurses and physicians reported discomfort about making this decision. Each patient was assessed for eligibility during daily morning report or at weekly discharge planning rounds by answering the question, "Whose death would not surprise you this admission?" Designated nurse leaders on each unit served as the liaison between staff and primary physicians to request a patient's enrollment into PCAD. During the 3-month start-up period, multidisciplinary teams reported that their greatest challenge was identifying patients who were imminently dying. As patients were identified by nurses as candidates, barriers to implementing PCAD began to surface: patients and families wanted "everything done" to continue curative treatment; a physician evaluated a patient as "fragile" and unable to hear "bad news"; a patient's physical status changed dramatically in 24 hours, from dying to "rallying" and preparing for discharge; and a house staff physician felt that he was already prescribing PCAD and could not see the benefit of enrollment.

There were several positive outcomes of the PCAD pilot. Results included: (1) a heightened awareness by staff of the disease trajectory (such as initial diagnosis, curative treatment, life-prolonging treatment, palliative care, symptomatic palliative care, and care of the imminently dying) and patient wishes for this admission; (2) increased discussions about the goals of care and the rationale for treatment orders; and (3) development of a systematic process for recognizing patient's needing referral to hospice and to pain medicine and palliative care for symptom management and family support following discharge.

Debriefing sessions held with staff after a patient died became an important aspect of the PCAD process. Staff were encouraged to discuss their satisfaction or dissatisfaction with the experience of the PCAD pathway. Such questions as "Were the patient's wishes honored?" "Were unnecessary tests/procedures performed?" "Did the patient have a peaceful death?" "Were symptoms controlled?" "What is the family's likelihood for complicated grieving and the need for follow-up?" generated much dialogue and opportunities for teaching and grief resolution. Overall, staff expressed appreciation for the opportunity to talk about experiences of patient care and the personal involvement in caring for a patient and family whom they may have known over several admissions. Another positive outcome for unit nurses was using the PCAD Daily Flow Sheet. Staffs report that it provides them with an easy and comprehensive system for documenting the assessment and intervention of key elements in EOL care: comfort; physical, psychosocial, and spiritual care; and patient and family support.

QI team members identified several areas needing improvement during the pilot period: (1) clearer definition and measure of the concept of "comfort"; (2) identifying the best forum for educating voluntary physician staff, who have less unit/hospital involvement than staff physicians; (3) documentation of spiritual care and issues; (4) systematic identification of families at risk for complicated grieving; and (5) resources about local bereavement services and education for families.

Results of the pilot study suggest that PCAD is a means for: (1) increasing multidisciplinary team discussions of patients' goals of care during hospitalization; (2) reducing the variation in the documentation of care of imminently dying patients, placing emphasis on comfort, patient and family wishes, and closure for caregivers; (3) increasing staff awareness of patients who are imminently dying or in need of palliative care services, long-term care, and hospice; and (4) identifying areas in EOL care for continual improvement in organizational systems, education, practice, and evaluation.[35]

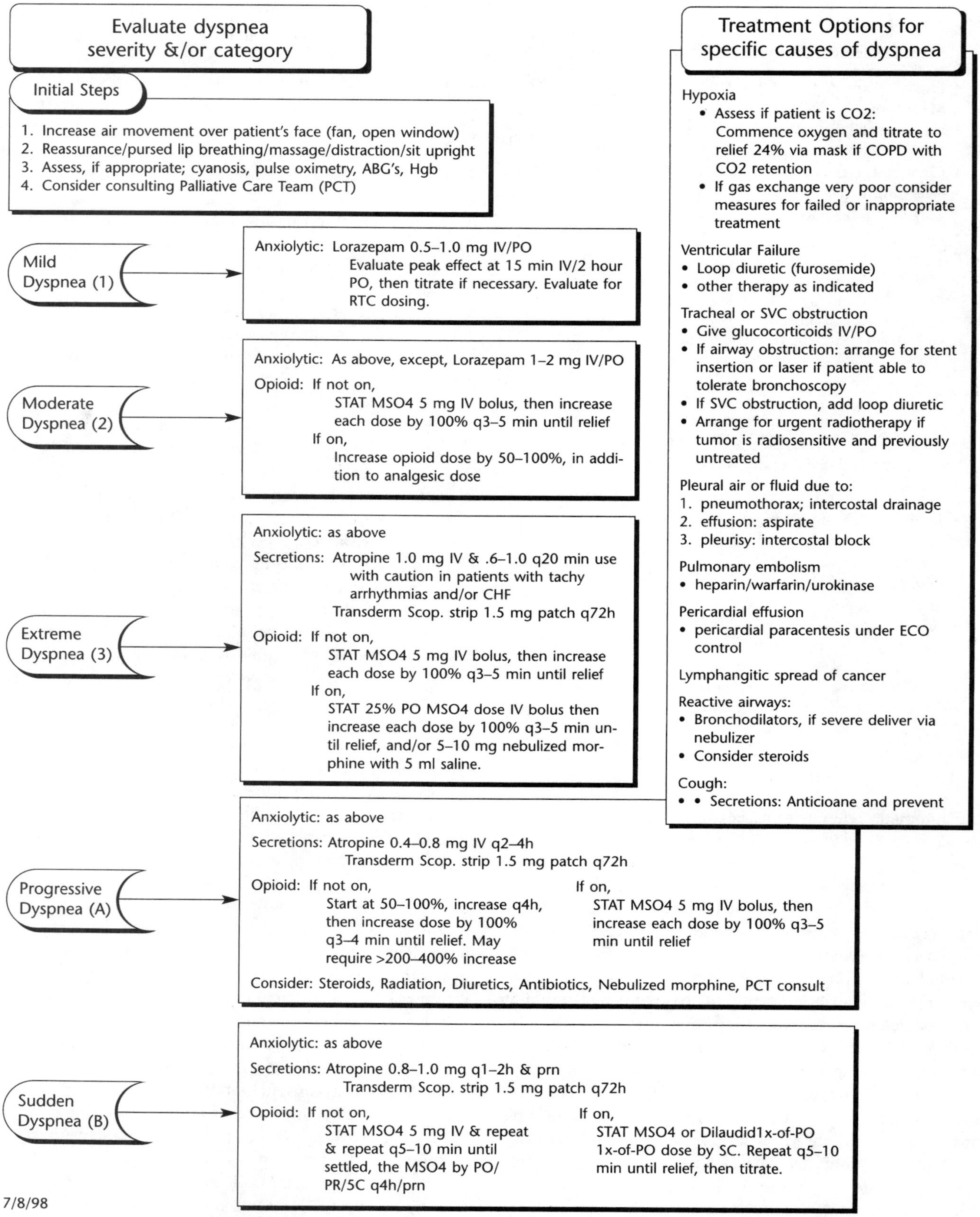

Evaluate dyspnea severity &/or category
Initial Steps
1. Increase air movement over patient's face (fan, open window)
2. Reassurance/pursed lip breathing/massage/distraction/sit upright
3. Assess, if appropriate; cyanosis, pulse oximetry, ABG's, Hgb
4. Consider consulting Palliative Care Team (PCT)
Mild Dyspnea (1)
Anxiolytic: Lorazepam 0.5–1.0 mg IV/PO Evaluate peak effect at 15 min IV/2 hour PO, then titrate if necessary. Evaluate for RTC dosing.
Moderate Dyspnea (2)
Anxiolytic: As above, except, Lorazepam 1–2 mg IV/PO
Opioid: If not on, STAT MSO4 5 mg IV bolus, then increase each dose by 100% q3–5 min until relief
If on, Increase opioid dose by 50–100%, in addition to analgesic dose
Extreme Dyspnea (3)
Anxiolytic: as above
Secretions: Atropine 1.0 mg IV & .6–1.0 q20 min use with caution in patients with tachy arrhythmias and/or CHF
Transderm Scop. strip 1.5 mg patch q72h
Opioid: If not on, STAT MSO4 5 mg IV bolus, then increase each dose by 100% q3–5 min until relief
If on, STAT 25% PO MSO4 dose IV bolus then increase each dose by 100% q3–5 min until relief, and/or 5–10 mg nebulized morphine with 5 ml saline.
Progressive Dyspnea (A)
Anxiolytic: as above
Secretions: Atropine 0.4–0.8 mg IV q2–4h
Transderm Scop. strip 1.5 mg patch q72h
Opioid: If not on, Start at 50–100%, increase q4h, then increase dose by 100% q3–4 min until relief. May require >200–400% increase
If on, STAT MSO4 5 mg IV bolus, then increase each dose by 100% q3–5 min until relief
Consider: Steroids, Radiation, Diuretics, Antibiotics, Nebulized morphine, PCT consult
Sudden Dyspnea (B)
Anxiolytic: as above
Secretions: Atropine 0.8–1.0 mg q1–2h & prn
Transderm Scop. strip 1.5 mg patch q72h
Opioid: If not on, STAT MSO4 5 mg IV & repeat & repeat q5–10 min until settled, the MSO4 by PO/PR/SC q4h/prn
If on, STAT MSO4 or Dilaudid1x-of-PO 1x-of-PO dose by SC. Repeat q5–10 min until relief, then titrate.
Treatment Options for specific causes of dyspnea
Hypoxia
• Assess if patient is CO2: Commence oxygen and titrate to relief 24% via mask if COPD with CO2 retention
• If gas exchange very poor consider measures for failed or inappropriate treatment
Ventricular Failure
• Loop diuretic (furosemide)
• other therapy as indicated
Tracheal or SVC obstruction
• Give glucocorticoids IV/PO
• If airway obstruction: arrange for stent insertion or laser if patient able to tolerate bronchoscopy
• If SVC obstruction, add loop diuretic
• Arrange for urgent radiotherapy if tumor is radiosensitive and previously untreated
Pleural air or fluid due to:
1. pneumothorax; intercostal drainage
2. effusion: aspirate
3. pleurisy: intercostal block
Pulmonary embolism
• heparin/warfarin/urokinase
Pericardial effusion
• pericardial paracentesis under ECO control
Lymphangitic spread of cancer
Reactive airways:
• Bronchodilators, if severe deliver via nebulizer
• Consider steroids
Cough:
• • Secretions: Anticioane and prevent
7/8/98

Figure 39–1. Algorithm designed to improve the management of dyspnea. (Developed at Dartmouth-Hitchcock Medical Center, Lebanon, NH, 1998, used with permission.)

MARY HITCHCOCK MEMORIAL HOSPITAL
Lebanon, NH
Last Breaths (Resource #)
DOCTOR'S ORDERs
DATE/TIME: ____________

Draft

1. **Evaluate severity of dyspnea:** (see reverse side for scale description)

   0 1 2 3 4 5 6 7 8 9 10
   no dyspnea — mild dyspnea — moderate dyspnea — extreme dyspnea

2. **Useful nonpharmacological methods to reduce dyspnea**
   - ❑ Positioning (sit, lean forward, elevate head)
   - ❑ Direct fan toward patient
   - ❑ Breathing strategies (Pursed lip breathing)
   - ❑ Guided imagery, desensitization
   - ❑ Reassurance
   - ❑ Nasal cannula (c O2 ______
   - ❑ Mask (c O2 ______

3. **Medication Categories** — **Dose** — **Route** — **Frequency**

EXPECTORANTS
- ❑ Glycerol Bualacolate ______ ______ ______

MUCOLYTIC AGENTS
- ❑ Acetylcysteine (Mucomyst) ______ ______ ______

OPIOIDS (BE SURE TO FOLLOW-UP WITH BOWEL ORDERS WHEN PRESCRIBING OPIOIDS)
- ❑ Morphine Sulfate ______ ______ ______

SEDATIVES/ANXIOLYTICS
- ❑ Diazepam (Valium) ______ ______ ______
- ❑ Lorazepam (Ativan) ______ ______ ______
- ❑ Midazolam (Versed) ______ ______ ______
- ❑ Promethazine (Phenergan) ______ ______ ______
- ❑ Chlorpromazine (Thorazine) ______ ______ ______

STEROIDS
- ❑ Prednisone ______ ______ ______
- ❑ Dexamethasone (Decadron) ______ ______ ______
- ❑ ______ ______ ______ ______

ANTIMUSCARINICS
- ❑ Atropine ______ ______ ______
- ❑ Scopalamine patch ______ ______ ______
- ❑ Levsin ______ ______ ______

DIURETICS
- ❑ Furosemide (Lasix) ______ ______ ______
- ❑ Bumelanide (Bumex) ______ ______ ______

COUGH SUPPRESSANTS
- ❑ Benzonate (Tessalon) ______ ______ ______
- ❑ Codeine ______ ______ ______

NEUROLEPTICS
- ❑ Haloperidol (Haldol) ______ ______ ______

INHALED MEDS (nebulizer for patients with COPD and hypercapnia should be air and not oxygen)
- ❑ Morphine ______ ______ ______
- ❑ Lidocaine ______ ______ ______
- ❑ Saline ______ ______ ______

BRONCHODILATORS
- ❑ Albuterol ______ ______ ______

______ / ______ / ______
Physician Signature — RN Signature — Secretary Signature

Print Physician Name: ______ Beeper Number: ______

DYSPNEA SCALE

MILD DYSPNEA *(1–3)*
Usually can sit and lie quietly
May be intermittent or persistent
Worsens with exertion
No or mild anxiety during SOB
Breathing not observed as laboured
No cyanosis

MODERATE DYSPNEA (4–7)
Usually persistent
May be new or chronic
SOB worsens if walk or exert; settles partially with rest
Pause while talking q30 sec
Breathing mildly laboured
Cyanosis usual

EXTREME DYSPNEA (8–10)
Agonizing air hunger
Talk only 2–3 words between gasps for air
Very frightened
Exhausted—tries to sit and lean forward, falls back
Total concentration on breathing
Cyanosis usual
+/− resp. congestion
+/− confusion
Maybe cold, clammy

PROGRESSIVE DYSPNEA (A)
Often acute on chronic
Worsening over few days/wks
Anxiety present
Often awaken suddenly with SOB.
+/− cyanosis
+/− onset confusion
Laboured breathing awake & asleep
Pause while talking q15 sec
Cough often present

SUDDEN DYSPNEA (B)
Sudden onset (min. to few hrs.)
High anxiety & fear
Agitation with very laboured respirations
Pause while talking

+/− resp. congestion
~+/− acute chest pain
+/− diaphoresis
+/− confusion

Use incremental titration until, when asked, "Is your breathing easy now?" the patient replies, "Yes."

MEDICATION CATEGORIES	DOSE	ROUTE	FREQUENCY
Acetylcysteine (Mucomyst)	10% 2–20 ml	nebulizer	QID
Albuterol (Proventil, ventolin)	1–2 puffs	MDI	QID
Atropine	0.4–1.0 mg	PO/SC	Q4-12H
Benzonate (Tessalon)	100 mg	PO	Q4-6H
Butemide (Bumex)	0.5–2.0 mg	IV	prn
Chlorpromazine (Thorazine)	25–100 mg	PO	Q4-6H/prn
Codeine	30 mg	PO	Q3-4H
Dexamethasone (Decadron)	1–4mg	PO	QID
Diazepam (Valium)	2–10 mg	FO	prn
Furosemide (Lasix)	20–80 mg	IV	prn
Glycerol guaiacolate	5 ml	PO	Q4H
Haloperidol (Haldol)	.5–30 mg	IV	!6H
Levsin			
Lidocaine 2%	2.5–5 ml	nebulizer	Q6H prn
Lorazepam (Ativan)	1–2 mg	PO	Q8H/prn
Metaproterenol (Alupent)	20 mg	PO	Q6-8H
Midazolam (Versed)	1–10 mg	IV	Q10min
Morphine	5–10 mg	nebulizer	Q4H or 4 hourly prn
Morphine Sulfate	5–10 mg (initial bolus)	1V	Q15 min
	2.5–5 mg/hr (infusion), or		
	5–10 mg, or	PO	Q4H
	2–5 mg	SC	Q4H
Prednisone	10–15 mg	PO	~ TID
Promethazine (Phenergan)	25–50 mg	PO	Q4–6H/prn
Saline	5 ml	nebulizer	Q4H or 4 hourly prn
Scopalamine	1.5 mg	patch	Q72H
Theophylline	100 200 mg	PO	Q6H

Figure 39–1. *(continued)*

Algorithms and Standardized Orders

Algorithms have also become popular tools designed to deliver consistent, timely care, especially symptom management at end of life. Figure 39–1 shows one example of an algorithm developed at Dartmouth-Hitchcock Medical Center, Lebanon, New Hampshire,[36] to improve the management of dyspnea. The tool offers clinicians a methodology for assessing the symptom and its etiology, directing treatment options, and establishing guidelines for pharmacological and nonpharmacological interventions.

The Providence Hospice in Yakima, Washington, is a model program of QI thinking applied in daily practice and service. A pocket-size handbook of standing orders and algorithms, *Symptom Management Algorithms for Palliative Care*,[37] is available for clinicians. The symptom-management algorithms allow for a team approach involving the referring physician, medical director, nurse, pharmacist, patient, and family caregivers. QI results have been positive thus far. In one study, use of an algorithm reduced the turnaround time of medication delivery to home hospice patients from 24–48 hours to less than 2 hours. Other topics in the handbook include algorithms for pain, and other distressing symptoms, such as mucositis, anxiety, and terminal agitation.

Outcomes for QI and End-of-Life Care

Federal and state governments, private purchasers, physicians, nurses, insurers, labor unions, health plans, hospitals, and accreditation organizations, among others, have begun to address some of the significant quality problems in the U.S. health care systems (http://www.ahcpr.gov/qual)[38] by improving the ability to measure and report the quality of care being delivered. Such reporting prompts a closer look at provider and health care practices, both as feedback for clinicians, and as publicly available scorecards for consumer evaluation. Two approaches are described for measuring outcomes in palliative care improvement efforts: using a single indicator of a quality of service or using multiple measures.

QI Indicators: Measures of Organizational Performance

A clinical indicator is defined as a quantitative measure that can be used as a guide to monitor and evaluate the quality of important patient care and support-service activities.[39] Indicators that directly affect quality services include such factors as timeliness, efficiency, appropriateness, accessibility, continuity, privacy and confidentiality, participation of patients and families, and safety and supportiveness of the care environment. Although they are not direct measures of quality, indicators serve as "screens" or "flags" that direct attention to specific performance issues that should be targets for ongoing investigation within an organization.

For institutions that have had a JCAHO survey within the last decade, it is clear that there has been a shift in focus of performance from competence and skills ("Is the organization able to provide quality services?") to productivity and outcomes ("To what extent does the organization provide quality services?"). For example, rather than focusing on whether the institution has a pain management program, surveyors might evaluate whether pain standards have been implemented and if they have had an effect on patients' satisfaction with pain management or patient understanding of side effects associated with specific analgesics.

Indicators reflect a performance measure composed of competence and productivity. Competence means that individuals or the organization have the ability (e.g., education, behavioral skills) to provide quality services; productivity means those abilities are translated into actions that achieve quality outcomes. Indicators also reveal deviations from the norm and may warn of impending problems. The amount and types of resources and expertise available on QI teams will influence the indicators selected to assess quality care. Indicators of care at the end of life, for example, may require a single-item measure, multiple items with a summary score, or multiple tools. Indicators are expressed as an event or ratio (percentage) and can be categorized into structure, process, or outcome indicators that are clinical, professional, or administrative in scope. Three examples are provided below.

1. Structural indicators are derived from written standards of care and need to be in concert with the mission, philosophy, goals, and policies of a department or unit. Structure standards measure whether the rules are being followed. For example, a policy may read that all patients admitted to the hospital require discussion and documentation about advanced directives within 48 hours of admission. A structural indicator might read:

   $$\frac{\text{Number of records with discussion/ Documentation of advanced directives}}{\text{Number of patients who were admitted to the oncology unit}}$$

   A structural indicator used frequently in a rapidly changing health care job market relates to competence. This indicator might require that all staff working on a geriatrics unit pass a written exam and demonstrate behavioral competencies related to end-of life care, including pain management (see Appendix 39–1 for sample knowledge quiz in palliative care). For this indicator, a threshold is determined, such as 90% on the written exam and three return demonstrations in the use of the pathway, for what constitutes successful completion in education in EOL care.
2. Process indicators measure a specific aspect of nursing practice that is critical to patient outcomes. Examples of process indicators might include

screening, assessments, and management of complications. These indicators describe "How care is to be delivered and recorded." Sometimes it may be difficult to separate process indicators from outcome indicators. For example, if an improvement study is directed toward reducing discomfort related to noisy respirations (death rattle) in dying patients, the indicator might involve the process of assessment of respirations, obtaining an order, and giving appropriate medication. The indicator might read that within 2 months' time:

$$\frac{\text{Time medications given to time of relief from noisy respirations (in min)}}{\text{The total time patient experienced noisy respirations (in min)}}$$

3. Outcome indicators[39] measure what does or does not happen to the patient after something is or is not done. More recently, QI teams have strengthened outcome indicators by using research instruments when available. Tools with validity and reliability, for which benchmarking data exist, have a greater potential to predict outcomes and improve practices. For example, an outcome of implementing a multidisciplinary pathway to improve care of dying patients might be to achieve family satisfaction with care at 90% very satisfied, using a 0-to-5 scale (0 = very dissatisfied to 5 = very satisfied). Using one of the items related to satisfaction with care in a standardized tool, an outcome indicator might read that within 6 months' time:

$$\frac{\text{Number of families scoring very satisfied with care}}{\text{Number of families completing satisfaction survey}}$$

Rapid Cycle Testing

The PDSA process is used in several national Improvement for Healthcare Initiative (IHI) collaboratives to improve EOL care. In this model, teams are formed including senior leadership, acknowledging buy-in and support for the effort from the start. Members are coached by IHI faculty. During a year's time, with three 1-day educational sessions, online discussions groups, onsite visits by faculty, and telephone conference calls of frequently discussed topics, such as advance directives, pain and symptom management, and bereavement care. Figure 39–2 shows the general approach to sequential PDSA cycles. Teams are encouraged to take make small changes rapidly, and once met, repeat the PDSA cycle with the next phase of the process or move to another process. This method has helped many achieve positive results within weeks to months. Examples of studies can be found in *Improving Care for the End-of-Life: A Sourcebook for Healthcare Managers and Clinicians.*[13] Encouraging teams to reach their targeted goals quickly reinforces team building and motivates the teams to examine other processes.

Models and Domains to Assess End-of-Life Care

Organizations have shifted their focus from examining the documentation of processes of care to measuring outcomes of care and learning which treatment works best, under what conditions, by which individuals, and at what cost. Although no tested methods currently exist to adequately measure the quality of care at the end of life,[34] efforts are underway to address this need. Results of a controlled trial, the SUPPORT study, support the deficiencies in care, citing the frequency of aggressive medical treatment at end of life (deaths occurring in the ICU) and the lack of adequate symptom management (conscious patients with moderate to severe pain).[40]

Figure 39–3 presents a model used by the BIMC Department of Pain Medicine and Palliative Care for outcomes

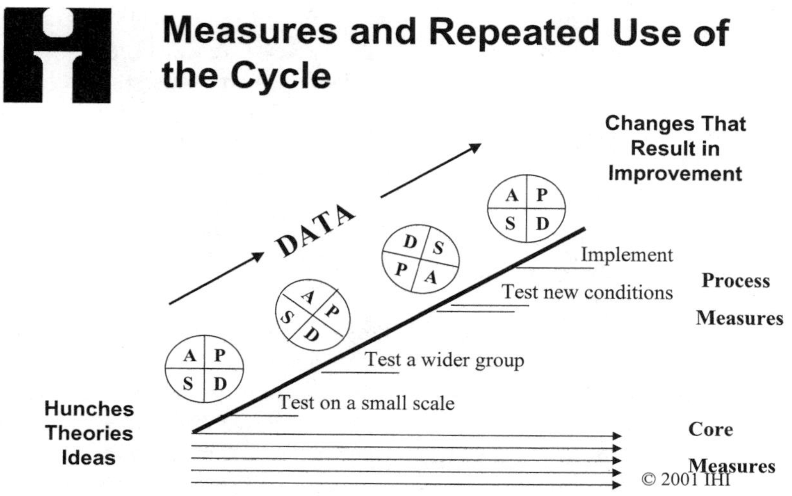

Figure 39–2. General approach to sequential PDSA cycles.

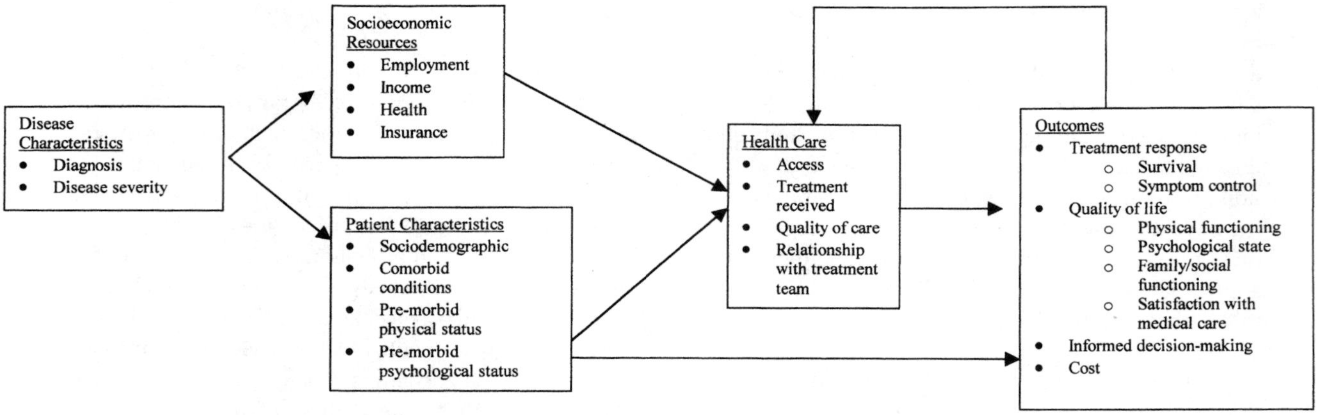

Figure 39–3. Model of outcomes research in the medically ill. (From Kornblith [1999], reference 28, with permission.)

research in the medically ill. The model illustrates the feedback loop between outcomes and health care. Outcomes research requires ongoing data collection and analysis that feeds into the modification of guidelines for clinical practice, resulting in improved patient, caregiver, professional, and systems outcomes, including costs.[27] Appendix 39–1 presents BIMC's Palliative Care Initial Consultation Tool located at http://www.stoppain.org. The tool is used to screen patients for key components of palliative care and resources needed from an interdisciplinary team. The symptom assessment portion of the form is a validated instrument, the Memorial Symptom Assessment Scale-Condensed. This data can be used to evaluate changes in symptoms within individuals and among groups of patients.

The American Geriatrics Society proposes 10 domains to measure performance and assess quality at end of life (Table 39–6).[26] Organizations using the Clinical Value Compass[4] approach to achieve quality and evaluate outcomes use four broad domains that can be applied to EOL care: (1) clinical outcomes, such as pain, dyspnea; (2) functional health status, such as communication with family; (3) satisfaction, such as perceived symptom relief; and (4) costs, such as caregiver out-of-pocket expenses, inpatient charges.

Table 39–6
Areas for Improving Quality Care at the End of Life

1. Physical and emotional symptoms
2. Support of function and autonomy
3. Advance planning
4. Aggressive care near death, including preferences about site of death, CPR, and hospitalization
5. Patient and family satisfaction
6. Global quality of life
7. Family burden
8. Survival time
9. Provider continuity and skill
10. Bereavement

Source: American Geriatrics Society (1996), reference 27.

Outcome Measures to Assess the End of Life

Joan Teno, M.D., of the Center for Gerontology and Health Care Research at Brown University, together with faculty and staff at the Center to Improve Care of the Dying, has assembled a comprehensive annotated bibliography of instruments to measure the quality of care at the end of life. The Toolkit of Instruments to Measure End-of-Life Care (TIME) includes a Patient Evaluation, After-Death Chart Review, and After-Death Caregiver Interview.[41] A recent addition to the toolkit is the mortality follow-back survey of family members or other knowledgeable informants representing 1578 decedents' perceptions of the last place of care.[42] Teno's current research project, *Data Analysis and Reports for Toolkit Instruments* (DART), refines the toolkit and measures for users. Additional outcome measures suggested for improving EOL care are shown in Table 39–7. A review of the current literature related to each tool in the kit can be found at http://www.chcr.brown. edu/Teno.htm. Donabedian[43] stated that "achieving and producing health and satisfaction, as defined for its individual members, is the ultimate validator of the quality of care." There has been limited research to date in examining satisfaction among terminally ill patients and families. Yet, for most dying patients, satisfaction may be the most important outcome variable for themselves and their families.

Professor Irene J. Higginson, Ph.D., a leading researcher for more than 15 years has been using the audit cycle, a feedback process similar to QI methods, to improve outcomes in palliative care. Currently at King's College School of Medicine and Dentistry and St. Christopher's Hospice in London, England, she notes the difficulties in obtaining outcome information, such

Table 39–7
Executive Summary of the Toolkit of Instruments to Measure End-of-Life Care (TIME)

Chart review instrument, surrogate questionnaires, patient questionnaires
Measuring quality of life
Examining advance care planning
Instruments to assess pain and other symptoms
Instruments to assess depression and other emotional symptoms
Instruments to assess functional status
Instruments to assess survival time and aggressiveness of care
Instruments to assess continuity of care
Instruments to assess spirituality
Bibliography of instruments to assess grief
Bibliography of instruments to assess caregiver and family experience
Instruments to assess patient and family member satisfaction with the quality of care

Source: Teno (1998), reference 41.

as quality of life, from the weakest group of patients.[44] She supports the need to test the use of proxies to obtain this important information. One tool currently available for clinicians that is used to measure the quality of life for patients with terminal illness is the Missoula-VITAS quality of life index.[45]

Measures of family satisfaction in palliative care such as the FAMCARE scale[46] are also available. FAMCARE is based on qualitative research that asks family members to list indicators of quality of palliative care from the patient's perspective and their own. A similar instrument, the National Hospice Organization Family Satisfaction Survey,[47] is an 11-item survey that asks about satisfaction with aspects of hospice care.

Summary

Nurses are poised to have pivotal roles in improving the quality of care of the dying in the decade ahead. As nurses, we need to continue to learn what works and what does not work for patients and families in our practice settings, and to stay active in developing and testing QI models, tools, and interventions toward better EOL care. Nurses are providing leadership in areas of clinical practice,[48–52] education,[53–57] and research.[58,59] Nurses are testing interventions for improved symptom management,[60–63] developing models for assuring "best practices" using research,[64,65] and integrating QI methods into palliative care curricula in nurses' education.[56] Nurses will need to strengthen their involvement in national and international efforts that educate professionals and consumers and influence health care policy in EOL care issues.

To survive, health care systems must be able to change and improve. If the quality of EOL care is to improve, nurses will need to have expert knowledge about making change: how to encourage it, and how to manage and to evaluate it within and across organizations and settings. This knowledge needs to be coupled with the methods and know-how to produce change. QI methods and tools are a powerful means for designing and testing strategies to improve EOL care.

REFERENCES

1. George S, Weimerskirch A. Total Quality Management: Strategies and Techniques Proven at Today's Most Successful Companies, 2nd ed. New York: John Wiley & Sons, 1998.
2. Deming WE. Out of the Crisis. Massachusetts Institute of Technology Center for Advanced Engineering Study. Cambridge: MIT Press, 1986.
3. Nelsen EC, Batalden PB, Ryer JC, eds. Joint Commission Clinical Improvement Action Guide. Oakbrook Terrace, IL: Joint Commission on Accreditation of Healthcare Organizations, 1998.
4. Joint Commission on Accreditation of Health Care Organizations. Performance measurement in health care. Available at: http://jcaho.org/pms/index.htm (accessed June 1, 2005).
5. Coile RC, Jr. Health care: top 10 trends for the "era of health reform." Hosp Strategy Rep 1993;5:3–8.
6. Bookbinder MB, Blank AE, Arney E, Wollner D, Lesage P, McHugh M, Indelicato RA, Harding S, Barenboim A, Mirozyev T, Portenoy RK: Improving end-of-life-care: development and pilot-test of a clinical pathway. J Pain Symptom Manage, in press.
7. American Medical Association. Education for Physician's on End-of-Life Care (EPEC). Available at: www.epec.net (accessed May 3, 2005).
8. Shortell S, Bennett C, Byck GR. Assessing the impact of continuous quality improvement on clinical practice: what it will take to accelerate progress? The Milbank Q 1998;76:593–624.
9. World Health Organization. Cancer Pain Relief and Palliative Care. Geneva: WHO, 1989.
10. Institute of Medicine. In: Field MJ, Cassel C, eds. Approaching Death: Improving Care at the End of Life. Committee on Care at the End of Life, Division of Health Care Services, Institute of Medicine. Washington DC: National Academy Press, 1997.
11. American Hospital Corporation. FOCUS—PDCA Methodology. Sponsored by Medical Risk Management Associates Consulting and Software Development Specialists. Available at: http://www.sentinel-event.com/focus-pdca index.htm (accessed January 21, 2005).
12. Bookbinder M, Kiss M, Coyle N, Brown M, Gianella A,Thaler H. Improving pain management practices. In: McGuire D, Yarbro C, Ferrell B, eds., Cancer Pain Management, 2nd ed., Boston: Jones and Bartlett, 1995:321-361.
13. Institute for Healthcare Improvement. Boston, MA. Available at: http://www.ihi.org/ihi (accessed January 21, 2005).
14. Ross M, et al. The palliative care quiz for nurses. J Adv Nurs 1996;23:128–137.
15. National Hospice Organization, National Council for Hospice and Specialists in Palliative Care Services. Making palliative care better: quality improvement, multi professional audit and standards. Arlington, VA: Author, 1997.

16. American Association of Colleges of Nursing (AACN). Peaceful death: recommended competencies and curricular guidelines for end-of-life nursing care. Washington DC: Author, 2002.
17. National Hospice Organization, Working Party on Clinical Guidelines in End-of-Life Care. Changing gears: guidelines for managing care in the last days of life in adults. Arlington, VA: Author, 1997.
18. American Medical Association: Council on Scientific Affairs. Good care of the dying patient. JAMA 1996;275:474–478.
19. Ellershaw J. Care of the dying: clinical pathways—an innovation to disseminate clinical excellence. Innovations in End-of-Life Care 2001;3(4). Available at: http://www2.edc.org/lastacts/ (accessed January 21, 2005).
20. American Academy of Pain Medicine (AAPM). Position Statement: Quality care at the end-of-life. Greenview, IL: Author, 1998.
21. American Society of Pain Management Nurses (ASPMN). Position Statement: End-of-Life Care. Available at: http://www.aspmn.org/html/pseolcare.htm (accessed March 14, 2005).
22. American Nurses Association (ANA). Position Paper: Promotion of Comfort and Relief of Pain in Dying Patients. Available at: http://www.nursingworld.org/readroom/position/index.htm (accessed January 21, 2005).
23. Oncology Nursing Society (ONS). Oncology Nursing Society and Association of Oncology Social Work Joint Position on End-of-Life Care. Revised 10/2003. Available at: http://www.ons.org/publications/positions/EndOfLifeCare.shtml (accessed January 21, 2005).
24. Cassel CK, Foley K. Principles for care of patients at the end-of-life: an emerging consensus among the specialties of medicine. Milbank Memorial Fund: NY, 1999. Available at: http://www.milbank.org/endoflife/ (accessed April 1, 2005).
25. American Association of Colleges of Nursing (AACN) and City of Hope, CA. The End-of-Life Nursing Education Consortium (ELNEC) project. Available at: http://www.aacn.nche.edu/elnec/about.htm (accessed January 21, 2005).
26. Canadian Palliative Care Association. Palliative Care: Towards a Consensus in Standardized Principles of Practice, 1995. Available at: http://www.library.vcu.edu/tml/bibs/nursing.html (accessed January 21, 2005).
27. American Geriatrics Society (AGS). American Geriatrics Society (AGS) Position Statement: The Care of Dying Patients. AGS Ethics Committee, 1996. Available at: http://www.americangeriatrics.org/products/positionpapers/careofd.shtml (accessed January 21, 2005).
28. Kornblith A. Outcomes research in palliative care. Newsletter: Department of Pain Medicine and Palliative Care, Beth Israel Medical Center, New York, NY, 1999;2:1–2.
29. Janken JK, Grubbs JH, Haldeman K. Toward a research-based critical pathway: a case study. Online Journal of Knowledge Synthesis for Nursing. Clinical Column, Document Number 1C, 1999. Available at: http://www.blackwell-synergy.com/links/doi/10.1111%2Fj.1524-475x.1999.00010.x (accessed March 14, 2005).
30. Stair, J. Oncology Critical Pathways. Rockville, MD: Association of Community Cancer Centers, 1998.
31. Blancett SS, Flarey DL. Health Care Outcomes: Collaborative, Path-Based Approaches. Sudbury, MA: Jones and Bartlett, 1998.
32. National Hospice Organization. A pathway for patients and families facing terminal illness. Arlington, VA: Author, 1997.
33. Gordon DB. Critical pathways: a road to institutionalizing pain management. J Pain Symptom Manage 1996;11:252–259.
34. Continuum Health Partners, Inc., Beth Israel Medical Center, Department of Pain Medicine and Palliative Care. Palliative Care for Advanced Disease (PCAD) Care Path. (CQI Team on End-of-Life Care), NY. Available at: http://www.stoppain.org (accessed January 21, 2005).
35. Pirovano M, Maltoni M, Nanni O, Marinari M, Indelli M, Zaninetta G, Petrella V, Barni S, Zecca E, Scarpi E, Labianca R, Amadori D, Luporini G. A new palliative prognostic score: a first step for the staging of terminally ill cancer patients. J Pain Symptom Manage 1999:17:231–247.
36. Dartmouth-Hitchcock Medical Center: Hematology/Oncology Group. A dyspnea algorithm. Lebanon, NH: Author, 1998.
37. Wrede-Seaman L. Symptom Management Algorithms: A Handbook for Palliative Care. Yakima, WA: Intellicard. Available at: http://www.Intelli-card.com (accessed January 21, 2005).
38. Agency for Healthcare Research and Quality (AHRQ). Available at: http://www.ahcpr.gov/qual/-(accessed January 21, 2005).
39. Kirk R. Managing Outcomes, Process, and Cost in a Managed Care Environment. Gaithersburg, MD: Aspen Publishers, 1997.
40. SUPPORT Principal Investigators. A controlled trial to improve care for seriously ill hospitalized patients: The Study to Understand Prognoses and Preferences for Outcomes and Risks of Treatments (SUPPORT). JAMA 1995;274:1591–1598.
41. Teno J. Center to Improve Care of the Dying. Toolkit of instruments to measure end-of-life. 1998. Available at: http://www.gwu.edu/ (accessed January 21, 2005).
42. Teno JM, Clarridge BR, Casey V, Welch LC, Wetle T, Shield R, Mor V. Family perspectives on end-of-life care at the last place of care. JAMA 2004;291:88–93.
43. Donabedian A. Evaluating the quality of medical care. Milbank Q 1996;44:166–203.
44. Higginson IJ, Hearn J, Webb D. Audit in palliative care: does practice change? Eur J Cancer Care 1996;4:233–236.
45. Byock IR. Merriman MP. Measuring quality of life for patients with terminal illness: the Missoula-VITA quality of life index. Palliative Med 1998;12:231–244.
46. Kristjanson LJ. Validity and reliability testing of the FAMCARE scale: measuring family satisfaction with advanced cancer care. Social Science Medicine 1993;36:693–701.
47. National Hospice Organization. Family Satisfaction Survey. Arlington, VA: Author, 1996.
48. Schwarz JK. Assisted dying and nursing practice. Image J Nurs Sch 1999;31:367–373.
49. Lewis AE. Reducing burnout: development of an oncology staff bereavement program. Oncology Nurs Forum 1999;26:1065–1069.
50. The National Consensus Project for Quality Palliative Care (NCP). Available at: http://www.nationalconsensusproject.org/ (accessed January 21, 2005).
51. Volker DL. Assisted dying and end-of-life symptom management. Cancer Nurs 2003:26:392–399.
52. McCaffery M, Pasero C. Pain: Clinical Manual, 2nd ed. St. Louis: Mosby, 1999.
53. Hainsworth DS. The effect of death education on attitudes of hospital nurses toward care of the dying. Oncology Nurs Forum 1996;23:963–967.
54. Ferrell BR, Virani R, Grant M. HOPE: home care outreach for palliative care education. Cancer Pract 1998;6:79–85.
55. Ferrell B, Virani R, Grant M, Coyne P, Uman G. Beyond the Supreme Court decision: nursing perspectives on end-of-life care. Oncol Nurs Forum, 2000;27:445–455.
56. Ferrell B, Virani R, Grant M. Analysis of end-of-life content in nursing textbooks. Oncol Nurs Forum 1999;26:869–876.

57. Matzo M, Sherman D, eds. Palliative Care Nursing: Quality Care to the End of Life. New York: Springer Publishing Co., 2001.
58. Murphy P, Kreling B, Kathryn E, Stevens M, Lynne J, Dulac J. Description of the SUPPORT intervention. J Am Geriatr Soc 2000;48:S54-S161.
59. Schwarz JK. Assisted dying and nursing practice. Image: J Nurs Scholarship 1999;31:367–373.
60. Kirchhoff KT, Beckstrand RL. Critical care nurses' perceptions of obstacles and helpful behaviors in providing end-of-life care to dying patients. Am J Crit Care 2000;9:96–105.
61. Wickham RS. Managing dyspnea in cancer patients. Developments in Supportive Cancer Care 1998;2:33–40.
62. Lynn J, Lynch Schuster J, Kabcenell A. Managing dyspnea and ventilator withdrawal. In: Lynn J, Lynch Schuster J, Kabcenell A, eds. Improving Care for the End of Life. New York: Oxford University Press, 2000:59–72.
63. Elshamy M, Whedon, MB. Symptoms and care during the last 48 hours of life. Quality of Life: A Nursing Challenge 1997;5:21–29.
64. Hospice Nurses' Association (HNA). Hospice and palliative care clinical practice protocol: dyspnea. Pittsburgh, PA: Author, 1996.
65. Miaskowski C, Donovan M. Implementation of the American Pain Society quality assurance standards for relief of acute pain and cancer pain in oncology nursing practice. Oncol Nurs Forum 1992;19:411–415.

APPENDIX 39–1
Sample CQI Study Proposal to Improve End-of Life Care Using FOCUS-PDCA

***F**ind a process to improve.*

Set the boundaries by defining the beginning and end points of the process.

Opportunity statement

An opportunity exists to improve EOL care for the imminently dying inpatient,
(Name the process.)
beginning with a physicians' order for the Palliative Care for Advanced Disease care path
ending with death or discharge to homecare, hospice, or residential facility.
(Set boundaries.)
This effort should improve patient comfort and family satisfaction with EOL care
(Name outcome measure)
for hospitalized oncology, geriatric, hospice, and intensive care unit patients.
(Name the customers.)

The process is important to work on now because good EOL care is an institutional priority, no benchmarks are currently available in the US, and no standard approach is used at BIMC* to assess and treat patients who are imminently dying.
(State significance.)

***O**rganize to improve the process.*

Form a multidisciplinary CQI team; establish roles, rules, and meeting times.

Multidisciplinary Team (22 members)

Department of Pain Medicine and Palliative Care
MDs, nurses, social workers, psychologist, chaplain
Hospital departments
Ethics
Pediatrics
Nutrition
Quality improvement
Pharmacy
Outcomes measurement (research grants and contracts)
Pilot units (Oncology, Geriatrics, Intensive Care, Hospice)
Nurse managers, case managers, clinical nurse specialists

---

* BIMC: Beth Israel Medical Center

Clarify what is known.

FLOWCHART OF PALLIATIVE CARE FOR ADVANCED DISEASE (PCAD) CARE PATH

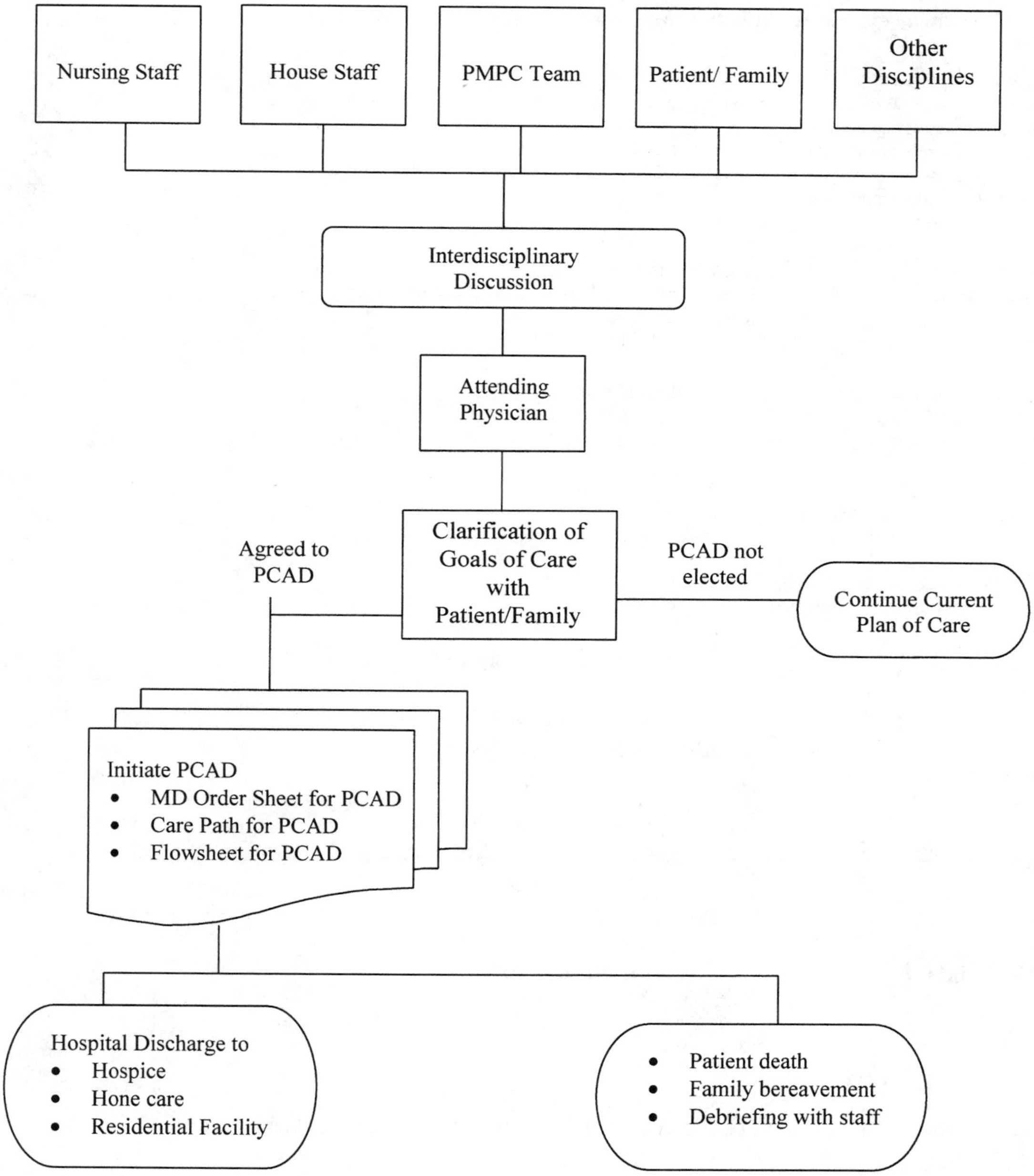

Understand the variation

Brainstorm with those at the grass roots level about why the process varies. Categorize sources of variation by people, materials, methods, and equipment. Display data using a cause-and-effect diagram.

Brainstorming Session with CQI Team on End-of-life (EOL) Care Question:
What barriers could be encountered in implementing an EOL Pathway at BIMC?

EOL awareness/ discomfort/readiness:
- What is "end-of-life care?" When is treatment palliative vs. life ending? How do we choose?
- Patient, family, readiness/awareness of dying
- Physician, family, patient willingness to acknowledge that death is imminent
- Issues of truth telling: family may not know status of patient prior to the pathway
- Physician discomfort with stopping treatment
- Medical uncertainty about when to stop treatment

Team communication:
- Physician and nurse discomfort in discussing change in treatment strategy
- Is it the physician's decision alone? The heath care team as a whole needs to be acknowledged in decision.
- Definition of terms. Need to define who the team is. May need a new model.
- Nurses' comfort—may be put in the middle of team/family attending and decisions.

Unit resistance:
- Resistance of unit teams. May see this project as "another thing to do."
- Large-scale resistance. Some may not see that there is something to "fix."
- Organizational pressure to discharge quickly.

Knowledge deficit:
- Assumptions about pastoral care (patient, family, staff) and what the experience will be.
- Knowledge deficit about medical and nursing interventions
- How to implement the care path and encourage people to speak up front rather than later
- Large cultural diversity at BIMC
- Education needed about biomedical analysis and ethical problems
- Physician/patient and physician/family communication skills

Cause and Effect (Ishikawa) Diagram (Barriers to implementing PCAD)—Themes above

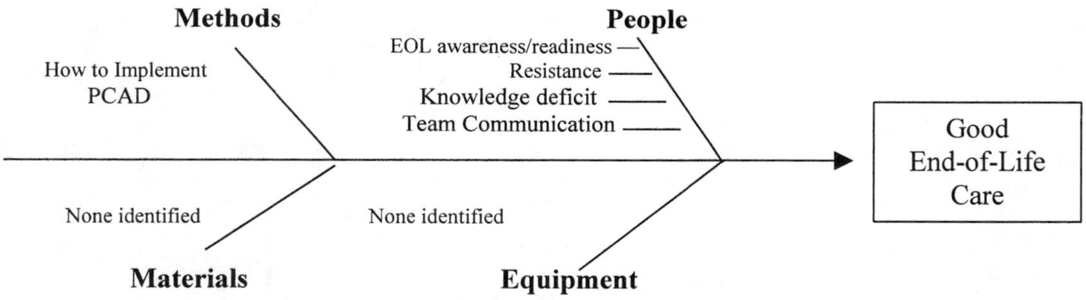

Select the process improvement.

Describe the new intervention in detail. Palliative Care for Advanced Disease (PCAD) Care Path: Care Path, Flow Sheet, and Physicians' Order Sheet **(see following pages)**

BETH ISRAEL HEALTH CARE SYSTEM ☐ **PETRIE DIVISION** ☐ **NORTH DIVISION** ☐ **KINGS HWY DIVISION**

Care Path: ***PALLIATIVE CARE for ADVANCED DISEASE***	**PRE-ADMISSION CONSIDERATION/ ADMISSION CRITERIA** ☐ **Disease at Advanced Stage – limited life expectancy** ☐ **HCP: Agent**____________ ☐ **DNR** ☐ **Primary Caregiver**__________ ☐ **Next of Kin**____________	**DISCHARGE OUTCOMES** ☐ **Discharge to Community:** **_ Hospice _ Home Care** **_ Alternative Care Facility _Home** **or** ☐ **Patient expired/Bereavement resources provided to family**	STAMP ADDRESSOGRAPH NAME OF SERVICE/ATTENDING/ HOUSE MD

PLAN:	**START DATE:**	**ONGOING DAYS:**
TREATMENTS/ INTERVENTIONS/ ASSESSMENTS	1) CLARIFY GOALS OF PALLIATIVE CARE FOR ADVANCED DISEASE (PCAD) WITH PATIENT AND/OR FAMILY 2) FACILITATE DISCUSSION & DOCUMENTATION OF ADVANCE DIRECTIVES: Identify designated individuals & roles in decision-making: 1) Health Care Agent 3) Primary Caregiver 2) Durable Power of Attorney 4) Next-of-kin Identify patient/family preferences regarding: • Health Care Proxy • Resuscitation Status/DNR • Living Will 3) INITIATE PHYSICIAN ORDER SHEET/REVIEW DAILY 4) COMFORT ASSESSMENT to include • Pain and symptom management needs • Psychosocial coping, anticipatory grieving, and social/cultural needs • Spiritual issues and distress 5) VS – None unless useful in promoting pt/family comfort 6) ASSESS FOR AND PROVIDE ENVIRONMENT CONDUCIVE TO MEET PATIENT & FAMILY NEEDS	REPEAT CARE PATH DAILY DOCUMENT IN: DAILY PATIENT CARE FLOW SHEET PROGRESS NOTES
PAIN MANAGEMENT	1) ASSESS PAIN Q 4 HR and evaluate within 1 hr post intervention. Complete pain assessment scale. Anticipate pain needs.	
TESTS/PROCEDURES	1) USUALLY UNNECESSARY for patient/family comfort (All lab work and diagnostic work is discouraged)	
MEDICATIONS	1) Medication regimen focus is the RELIEF OF DISTRESSING SYMPTOMS.	
FLUIDS/NUTRITION	1) DIET: Selective diet with no restrictions • Nutrition to be guided by patient's choice of time, place, quantities and type of food desired. Family may provide food. • Educate family in nutritional needs of dying patient 2) IVs for symptom management only 3) TRANSFUSIONS for symptom relief only 4) INTAKE AND OUTPUT – consider goals of care relative to patient comfort 5) WEIGHTS – consider risks/benefits relative to patient comfort	

ACTIVITY	1) ACTIVITY DETERMINED BY PATIENT'S PREFERENCES AND ABILITY. Patient determines participation in ADLs, i.e., turning and positioning, bathing, transfers	REPEAT CARE PATH DAILY DOCUMENT IN: DAILY PATIENT CARE FLOW SHEET PROGRESS NOTES
CONSULTS	1) INITIATE referrals to institutional specialists to optimize comfort and enhance quality of life (QOL) only.	
PSYCHOSOCIAL NEEDS	1) PSYCHOSOCIAL COMFORT ASSESSMENT of: • Patient • Primary caregiver • Grieving process of patient & family 2) PSYCHOSOCIAL SUPPORT: Referral to Social Work • Offer emotional support • Support verbalization and anticipatory grieving • Encourage family caring activities as appropriate/individualized to family situation and culture • Facilitate verbal and tactile communication • Assist family with nutrition, transportation, child care, financial, funeral issues • Assess bereavement needs	
SPIRITUAL NEEDS	1) SPIRITUAL COMFORT ASSESSMENT • Spiritual supports • Spiritual needs and/or distress 2) SPIRITUAL SUPPORT: Referral to Chaplain • Provide opportunity for expression of beliefs, fears, and hopes • Provide access to religious resources • Facilitate religious practices	
PATIENT/FAMILY EDUCATION	1) ASSESS NEEDS AND PROVIDE EDUCATION REGARDING: • Goals of Palliative Care for Advanced Disease • Physical and psychosocial needs during the dying process • Coping techniques/Relaxation techniques • Bereavement process and resources	
DISCHARGE PLANNING	1) FOR DISCHARGE TO COMMUNITY: Referral to Pain Medicine & Palliative Care/ Hospice/Home Care/Social Work as needed. 2) AT TIME OF DEATH: • Post Mortem care observing cultural and religious practices and preferences • Provide for care of patient's possessions as per family wishes • Bereavement support for family and staff	

This document is to be used as a guideline only. Each case should be evaluated and treated individually based upon clinical findings.

Beth Israel Health Care System

Carepath: Palliative Care for Advanced Disease

DAILY PATIENT CARE FLOW SHEET

ADDRESSOGRAPH

DATE:

☐ DNR ☐ NO DNR ☐ HCP ☐ NO HCP **HCP AGENT:** **CAREGIVER:**

COMFORT ASSESSMENT: Comfort Level Patient states or appears to be
1. Always comfortable 2. Usually comfortable 3. Sometimes comfortable 4. Seldom comfortable 5. Never comfortable

TIME (per MD order)												
PATIENT Comfort Level (Indicate number)												

VITAL SIGNS ONLY AS ORDERED	T												
	P												
	R												
	BP												

PAIN	TIME																
	LOCATION																
	PAIN RATING																
	RELIEF/SEDATION		/		/		/		/		/		/		/		/

PAIN/RELIEF SCALE KEY

NONE ← → WORST

0 1 2 3 4 5 6 7 8 9 10

COMPLETE RELIEF — NO RELIEF

SEDATION SCALE

0 Alert
1 Awake but drowsy
2 Drowsy/Easily awakened
3 Sleeping/Easily awakened
4 Sleeping/Difficult to awaken
5 Unarousable

*** See Progress Note A = Assessment I = Intervention Check mark = present or done * Needs MD Order**

		Time			
EYES	A	Moist/Clear			
		Inflamed			
		Dry/Crusted			
	I	Routine Care			
		__Artificial Tears			
		__Oint/Lubricant			
LIPS	A	Smooth/moist			
		Dry/Cracked			
		Ulcerated			
	I	Routine Care			
		Topical Lubricant			
MOUTH	A	Moist			
		Dry			
		Coated			
		Stomatitis			
	I	Routine Care			
		*Artificial Saliva			
		__Magic Wash			
		Meds as ordered			

		Time			
BREATHING	A	**Rate**: Normal			
		Rapid			
		Slow			
		Rhythm: Reg			
		Irregular			
		Depth: Normal			
		Shallow			
		Labored			
		Secretions: None			
		Mild			
		Copious			
		Breath sounds:			
		Clear			
		Diminished			
		Absent			
		Crackles			
		Wheeze			
		Dyspnea			
	I	None			
		Reposition			
		__O2 via___@___lpm			
		Suctioning q____			
		Trach Care			
		Elevate HOB			
		Fan			
		Meds as ordered			

		Time			
NUTRITION	A	Full meal			
		> 50%			
		< 50%			
		Refused			
		Nausea/vomiting			
		NPO			
		Dysphagia			
	I	Diet as tolerated			
		NG/G tube			
		Enteral feeding			
		Feeding set changed			
		Residual vol-cc's			
		Placement check			
		Meds as ordered			
IV LINES	A	IV site________			
		No S&S infil/phleb			
		Dry & intact			
	I	IV Dsg change			
		IV Tubing change			
		See progress note			
		Cap Change			
		Huber needle change			

		Time			
MOBILITY	A	Bedbound			
		OOB Chair			
		Amb w Assist			
		OOB ad lib			
		BR Privileges			
	I	T&P per pt comfort			
		ROM q___			
		Assistive Device			
		__Ted Stocking(s)			
		Side Rails Up			
ELIMINATION	A	Voiding qs			
		Anuria			
		Incontinent Urine			
		Bowel Movement			
		Incontinent Feces			
		Diarrhea			
		Constipation			
	I	__Foley Catheter			
		Texas Catheter			
		Inc't Pads			
		__Enema			
		Meds as ordered			
SKIN °	A	Normal/Intact			
		Feverish			
		Diaphoretic			
		Pressure Ulcer Stg___			
		Ostomy site D/I			
		Edema___			
		Pruritis			
		Cool/Mottled			
WOUND CARE	I	Site			
		Dressing________			
		Dry & Intact			
		Drain_________			
		Drainage			
		Odor			
		Ostomy site care			
		Tube site care			

		Time			
SLEEP	A	Normal			
		Interrupted Cycle			
		Insomnia			
	I	Modify Environment			
		Relaxation			
		Meds as order			
PSYCHOSOCIAL	A	Awake/alert			
		Responds to voice			
		Resp to tactile stim			
		Unresponsive			
		Oriented			
		Confused			
		Hallucinating			
		Calm			
		Anxiety			
		Agitated			
		Depression			
		Spiritual distress			
	I	Emotional support			
		Verbal/tactile stimulation			
		Social Worker visit			
		Chaplain visit			

		Time			
FAMILY	A	Engaged w pt			
		Coping w loss			
		Distressed			
	I	Goals of care reviewed			
		Encourage verbal & non-verbal communication w pt			
		Family Meeting			
°		Bereavement support			
MISCELLANEOUS		AM Care			
		PM Care			
		PresUlcer Prev Plan			
		Fall Prev Plan			
		Precautions:			
		Isolation:			
		Siderails Up			
		ID Bracelet			
		Allergy Bracelet			
		DNR Bracelet			
		Post Mortem care			

Comments/Progress Notes

PATIENT/FAMILY EDUCATION: **See IPFER**

PCAD Care Path: **Initiated** **Reviewed/Continue With Plan Of Care** **☐ Revised (See Progress Note)**

OTHER NURSING DOCUMENTATION:

☐ I & O SHEET **☐ RESTRAINT FLOW SHEET** **☐ NEURO-ASSESSMENT** **☐ OTHER________________**

SIGNATURE/TITLE	DATE	SHIFT	INITIALS	SIGNATURE/TITLE	DATE	SHIFT	INITIALS
1.				6.			
2.				7.			
3.				8.			
4.				9.			
5.				10.			

Beth Israel Health Care System

DOCTOR'S ORDER SHEET
PALLIATIVE CARE FOR ADVANCED DISEASE

ADMISSION HT_________ ADMISSION WEIGHT________

ADDRESSOGRAPH AREA

ORDERS OTHER THAN MEDICATION/INFUSION	MEDICATION/INFUSION (Specify route & directions)
1 Primary Diagnosis:	1. Assess patient for the following symptoms: Anxiety & Insomnia; Confusion/Agitation; Constipation; Depressed Mood; Diarrhea; Dyspnea; Fever; Hiccups; Nausea/Vomiting; Pain; Pruritis; Stomatitis; Terminal Secretions (Noisy Respirations). *See reverse side for suggestions for pain management and symptom control*
2 Activate PCAD Care Path	
3 Anticipated time on PCAD Care Path: ___ hours ___days ___weeks ___unknown	
4 Allergies:	
5 Diet: ☐ No restrictions (food may be provided by caregiver) ☐ NPO ☐ Other:	
6 Activity: ☐ OOB as tolerated ☐ OOB with assistance	2. DISCONTINUE ALL PREVIOUS MED ORDERS
7 Vital Signs: ☐ Discontinue ☐ Daily ☐ q shift ☐ q ___hours	3. ORDERS:
8 Comfort Assessment: ☐q __ hr ☐q 2 hr ☐q 4 hr ☐q shift	
9 Weight: ☐ None ☐ q ____ day(s)	
10 I & O: ☐ None q ________	
11 Visiting: ☐ Open visiting, nurse-restrictions apply ☐ Per routine policy ☐ Other:	
12 DNR: ☐ Yes ☐ No	
13 PCAD Care Path will include (specify if otherwise): Psychosocial Care – Social Work Referral; Spiritual Care – Chaplaincy Referral	
14 Consults: ☐ Pain Medicine & Palliative Care Consult ☐ Ethics Consult ☐ Hospice Consult ☐ Other:	
15 Labs: ☐ Discontinue all previous standing orders ☐ Continue previous lab orders ☐ Other labs:	
16 Oxygen Therapy: ______L/min via___________	
17 Other orders:	

CLERK	DATE	TIME	NURSE'S SIGNATURE	PRESCRIBER'S SIGNATURE	ID#	DATE	TIME

The following are medications for consideration in treating pain and symptoms of patients on PCAD:

PAIN MANAGEMENT
For Opioid-Naïve Patient:
Morphine Sulfate 15 mg po or 5 mg SQ/IV.
Repeat q 1 hr until pain relief is adequate. Begin Morphine Sulfate 30 mg po or 10 mg SQ/IV q 4 hr ATC or begin IV Morphine Sulfate basal infusion at 2 mg per hour and 2 mg SQ/IV q 1 hr prn.

For Opioid-Treated Patient:
If pain uncontrolled, increase fixed schedule dose by 50%.

Many non-opioid analgesics are available and should be considered after opioid therapy has been optimized. If pain remains uncontrolled, consider consult to Department of Pain Medicine and Palliative Care (Beeper #6702).

ANXIETY & INSOMNIA
Lorazepam 0.5mg po/SQ/IV BID-TID q HS for anxiety.
Temazepam 15 – 30 mg po q HS for anxiety/ insomnia.
Clonazepam 0.5 – 2 mg po BID-TID for anxiety/myoclonus.

CONFUSION/AGITATION
Haloperidol 0.5 mg po/SQ/IV. Repeat q 30 minutes until symptom intensity declines.
Haloperidol 0.5 – 5 mg po/SQ/IV q 4 hr prn.

CONSTIPATION
Lactulose 30 ml po q 2 hr prn until constipation relieved.
When symptom improves, begin Lactulose 30 ml po q 12 hr.
Warm Fleets Enema TIW prn

To prevent constipation:
Senokot 1 – 2 tabs po BID and
Colace 1 – 2 tabs po BID.

SYMPTOMS OF DEPRESSION
If anticipated survival is in weeks:
Begin SSRI, e.g., Paroxetine 20 mg po daily, and titrate to effect.

If anticipated survival is in days:
Methylphenidate 2.5 mg po q morning and at noon and escalate daily to 5 – 10 mg po q morning and at noon or Pemoline 18.75 mg po q morning and at noon and escalate daily to 37.5 mg po q morning and at noon.
Higher doses may be needed.

Consider Liaison Psychiatry consultation

DIARRHEA
Loperamide 4 mg po q 4 hr prn

DYSPNEA
For Opioid-Naïve Patient:
Morphine Sulfate 5 – 15 mg po or 2 – 5 mg SQ/IV. Repeat q 1 hr, if needed. When symptom is improved, begin Morphine Sulfate 30 mg po or 10 mg SQ/IV q 4 hr ATC; or begin Morphine Sulfate basal infusion at 2 mg per hour and 2 mg SQ/IV q 1 hr prn.

For Opioid-Treated Patient:
If dyspnea uncontrolled, increase fixed schedule dose by 50%.
If breathlessness continues, add Lorazepam 0.5mg po or SQ/IV prn. Repeat q 60 minutes if needed until symptom intensity declines, then begin 1 mg po/SQ/IV q 3 hr.

Additional therapies may include:
Dexamethasone 16 mg po/IV, followed by 4 mg po/IV q 6 hr
Albuterol 2.5 mg via nebulization q 4 hr prn if wheezing present

FEVER
Acetaminophen 650 mg po/PR q 4 hr prn, and/or
Dexamethasone 1.0 mg po/SQ/IV q 12 hr prn

HICCUPS
Chlorpromazine 10 – 25 mg po/IM TID prn
Haloperidol 0.5 – 2 mg po/SQ/IV TID – QID

INTRACTABLE SYMPTOMS, MANAGEMENT OF
Consider referral to Department of Pain Medicine & Palliative Care (Beeper # 6702).

IV HYDRATION
Consider decreasing IV rate to 0.5 – 1 liter/24 hr

NAUSEA/VOMITING
Metoclopromide 10 mg po/IV q 4 hr prn, or
Prochlorperazine 10 mg po/IV q 4 hr or 25 mg PR q 8 hr prn with or without Dexamethasone 4 mg po/IVPB q 6 hr

PRURITIS
Diphenhydramine 25 – 50 mg po/IV q 12 hr
Hydrocortisone 1 % cream to affected areas q 6 hr
Dexamethasone 1.0 mg po daily alone or in combination with above

STOMATITIS
Viscous lidocaine 2 % to painful areas prn
Clotrimazole 10 mg troche 5 times daily
Nystatin S & S q 6 hr prn
Magic Mouthwash prn

TERMINAL SECRETIONS (NOISY RESPIRATIONS)
Scopolamine patches 1.5 – 3 mg 72 hr, or
Scopolamine 0.4 mg SQ q 4 – 6 hr

PLAN—DO—CHECK—ACT (the Shewhart cycle)

P lan

Create a timeline of resources, activities, training, and target dates. Develop a data collection plan, the tools for measuring outcomes, and thresholds for determining when targets have been met.

Timeline for One-Year Pilot CQI EOL Project

Phase 0 – Planning

Jan – June	Formalize CQI Team for the development of a clinical pathway. Clarify knowledge of processes: review literature and existing data sources, conduct brainstorming, flowcharting with pilot units. Evaluate and synthesize literature, tools, other data gathered. Identify content for Care Path. Develop and pilot audit tool for chart reviews. Create database, codebook, and scoring guidelines for data entry. Identify patient outcome assessment tools. Identify family outcome assessment tools. Identify staff assessment tools. Refine study tools/procedures. Develop staff education. Develop caregiver educational materials.
June 21	Medical Records review
Aug 2	Tools Committee review
July 3	Committee on Scientific OSA Application and Approval

Phase I – Launching the Project

August 2	Meet with hospital leadership—Introduction to Palliative Care for Advanced Disease Care Path • PCAD Care Path, MD Orders, and Flow sheet • Timeline for Education/Evaluation
August 11	Introduction of PCAD Care Path to medical staff

Phase II – Unit Implementation and Education of PCAD Care Path

	Cohort 1	Cohort 2		Cohort 3
• Meet with unit leaders of pilot units	June 21	September 15	July 21	October 11
• Pre-test	August 23–25	September 27	September 14	TBS
• Unit leadership team meeting	TBS	October 5	October 12	TBS
• Introduction of PCAD Care Path to unit staff	August 31–September 1	September 27–September 30	October 22	TBS
• In-service of unit staff	September 1 September 2 September 3	October 4–October 6	October 25–October 26	TBS TBS TBS
• Rollout of Care Path	September 6	October 11	November 1	TBS
• Brainstorming—educational needs	October 11	November 8	December 13	December 6
• Educational series	September–February	October– March	November–April	November–April
• Focus groups	October & January	November & February	December & March	December & March
• Feedback / closure / continuation	March	April	May	May
• Post-test	March	April	May	May

Phase III – Evaluation

Chart Reviews using Chart Audit Tool (CAT) (Total =330)

June–Aug	• 20 retrospective audits for 5 pilot units	(Total = 100)
Sep 1999–Mar 2002	• 20 retrospective audits for 2 control units	(Total = 40)
	• 10 during implementation audits for 5 pilot units	(Total = 50)
	• 20 post implementation audits for 5 pilot units	(Total = 100)
	• 20 post implementation audits for 2 control units	(Total = 40)
	Each patient on PCAD Care Path as admitted.	
Sep 1999–Mar 2002	Tool: Teno's After Death (interview or mailed survey)	
Dates TBD	Staff survey post-tests (4 mo post-initiation of PCAD) Tool: Palliative Care Quiz	
Sep 1999–Mar 2002	Process Audits (PAT) Ongoing throughout time patient on PCAD Care Path	
Sep 1999–Mar 2002	Brainstorming sessions and focus groups with staff to identify education 1–2 mo after each unit begins PCAD	

Phase IV – Reporting

April 15, 2002 Report to grant agency, hospital, and unit staff

D*o*

Collect data and monitor the intervention until fully implemented.

Palliative Care Quiz for Nurses (PCQN)

Name: ______________________________

Background Information:

Department/ Service

1. Nursing
2. Social work
3. Medicine
4. Pharmacy
5. Surgery
6. Chaplaincy
7. Critical care
8. Other (describe)

Unit: ______________________________

Age: ______________________________

Sex:
1. Male
2. Female

Years of experience in discipline:
1. 0–5
2. 6–10
3. >10

Educational preparation:
1. HS diploma
2. Associate degree
3. Baccalaureate degree
4. Masters' degree
5. Postgraduate degree

Previous education/ training in palliative care:
1. No
2. Yes (describe) ______________________________

____

____

____

____

____

The 20-item survey that follows is used with permission. Ross, M. M., McDonald,B., & McGuinness, J. (1996). The palliative care quiz for nurses (PCQN): the development of an instrument to measure nurses' knowledge of palliative care. Journal of Advanced Nursing, 23:125-137.

Please circle your response to the items below using the following key:

T = True **F = False** **DK = Don't Know**

1. Palliative care is appropriate only in situations where there is evidence of a downhill trajectory or deterioration.	T	F	DK
2. Morphine is the standard used to compare the analgesic effect of other opioids.	T	F	DK
3. The extent of the disease determines the method of pain treatment.	T	F	DK
4. Adjuvant therapies are important in managing pain.	T	F	DK
5. It is crucial for family members to remain at the bedside until death occurs.	T	F	DK
6. During the last days of life, the drowsiness associated with electrolyte imbalance may decrease the need for sedation.	T	F	DK
7. Drug addiction is a major problem when morphine is used on a long-term basis for the management of pain.	T	F	DK
8. Individuals who are taking opioids should follow a bowel regime.	T	F	DK
9. The provision of palliative care requires emotional detachment.	T	F	DK
10. During the terminal stages of an illness, drugs that can cause respiratory depression are appropriate for the treatment of severe dyspnea.	T	F	DK
11. Men generally reconcile their grief more quickly than woman.	T	F	DK
12. The philosophy of palliative care is compatible with that of aggressive treatment.	T	F	DK
13. The use of placebos is appropriate in the treatment of some types of cancer pain.	T	F	DK
14. In high doses, codeine causes more nausea and vomiting than morphine.	T	F	DK
15. Suffering and physical pain are synonymous.	T	F	DK
16. Demerol is not an effective analgesic in the control of chronic pain.	T	F	DK
17. The accumulation of losses renders burnout inevitable for those who seek work in palliative care.	T	F	DK
18. Manifestations of chronic pain are different from those of acute pain.	T	F	DK
19. The loss of a distant or problematic relationship is easier to resolve than the loss of one that is close or intimate.	T	F	DK
20. The pain threshold is lowered by anxiety or fatigue.	T	F	DK

Check

Analyze findings, graph results, and evaluate reasons for variations. If targets are reached, set a date to stop or decrease the frequency of monitoring. Summarize what was learned.

Sample: Results of Palliative Care Knowledge Quiz, Preimplementation of PCAD

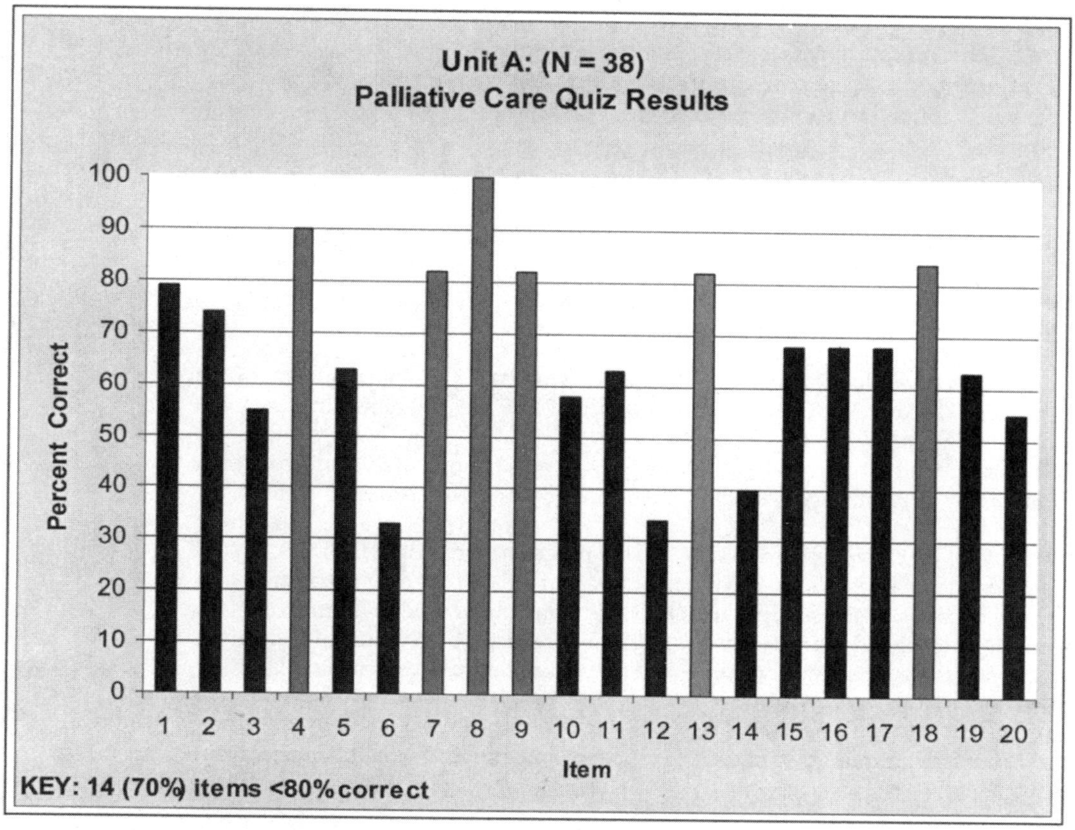

Act

Act on what is learned and determine the next steps. If successful, act to hold the gain achieved and work at making the intervention a part of standard operating procedure.. If not successful, analyze the sources of failure, design new solutions, and repeat the PDCA cycle.

Sample: Quarterly Reporting Form

BETH ISRAEL MEDICAL CENTER
PAIN MEDICINE AND PALLIATIVE CARE
QUALITY IMPROVEMENT STUDY REPORT

Title of Study: Improving End-of-Life Care

Date(s) of study:
1st Quarter ✓ 2nd Quarter__ 3rd Quarter__ 4th Quarter __

Interdisciplinary Team: See listing of CQI Team members.

Sample: The Palliative Care Knowledge Quiz was given to all nursing staff preimplementation of the Palliative Care for Advanced Disease (PCAD) Care Path on three of five planned units thus far.

Findings: In this quarter, we report on the results of knowledge surveys. A total of 90 staff from three units has completed the survey thus far. Analyses have been completed on Unit A described below.

Analysis/interpretation: Unit A, above, is used to describe the process of providing feedback to staff. The threshold for competency was set for 80%. Fourteen of twenty items (70%) are targeted for improvement. No formal education has been given thus far. This data will be used to (a) measure change pre and post an educational series and use of the PCAD in practice, (b) determine levels of competency and targeted areas for continued education, and (c) to stimulate discussion and dialogue with the multidisciplinary team.

Conclusion: Continued education is needed to integrate palliative care principles into the mainstream of daily clinical practice.

Action Plan / Step 1: In-services are scheduled in Quarter 2, 2000. All survey answers will be shared. The Pain Medicine and Palliative Care team will lead a discussion, supported by research results, about the 14 items for which staff answered <80% correctly. Three content areas were identified: end-of-life issues, pain treatment and side effects, and philosophy of palliative care.
Step 2: Based on the dialogue and discussion, subsequent in-services using case-based teaching, will be scheduled. A post-test survey is planned following 6 months of implementation PCAD on each unit.

Follow-up plan: We will report progress at monthly CQI Team meetings. Next report will include chart audit results.

Beth Israel Medical Center-Department of Pain Medicine and Palliative Care

PALLIATIVE CARE CONSULTATION FORM

Patient's Name: ______________________ Date Completed: ____/____/____

Admission Date: ____/____/____ Chart # __________ Date of Follow-up: ____/____/____

Days from Admission: __________ Insurance: __________ Completed by: ______________

I. BACKGROUND

1. Gender: [1] Male [2] Female
2. Age: ________ Date of Birth: ____/____/____
3. Race/Ethnicity: [1] White-Non-Hispanic [2] Black-Non-Hispanic [3] Hispanic-White [4] Hispanic-Black [5] Asian [6] Other
4. Marital Status: [1] Single (*never married*) [2] Married (*living with partner*) [3] Separated [4] Divorced [5] Widowed
5. Household [*circle all that apply*]: [1] Lives Alone [2] Spouse/Partner [3] Children [4] Parents [5] Other Relative
6. Religion: [1] Catholic [2] Protestant [3] Jewish [4] Muslim [5] Hindu [6] Other ____________ [7] None
7. Language: [1] English as primary language [2] Other: ____________, but can speak & understand English [3] Non-English speaking
8. Primary Medical Diagnosis: [1] ______________________
   [2] ______________________
   [3] ______________________
9. Where seen: [1] Inpatient-hospital [2] Inpatient-nursing home [3] Outpatient-office/clinic [4] Home
10. Reason for consult: [1] Pain [2] Other symptoms [3] Management of imminent death [4] Other ____________

SECTIONS II – VII TO BE COMPLETED BY A MEDICAL HEALTH PROFESSIONAL MD/PA/RN

II. COGNITIVE STATUS

11. COGNITIVE IMPAIRMENT
   [1] Normal
   [2] Mild Impairment; some memory loss or cognitive disability, but does not interfere with functioning; some confusion or disorientation, but brief and resolves quickly
   [3] Moderate impairment; memory loss, confusion or disorientation interfering with functioning, but *no* interference with activities with daily living (ADL)
   [4] Severe impairment; confusion, delirium, memory loss interfering with ADL; frank mental retardation.
   [5] Comatose; vegetative state; not conscious

12. DECISIONAL CAPACITY
   [1] Normal – Has decisional capacity
   [2] Cognitively impaired, but has decisional capacity
   [3] Global incompetence, lacks decisional capacity

III. PATIENT SELF-DETERMINATION/ADVANCE DIRECTIVES

13. Circle all treatment preferences/advance directives, with supporting documents
   [1] Living will
   [2] Do not resuscitate (DNR)
   [3] Health care proxy, durable power of attorney
   [4] Court appointed guardian
   [5] Patient chooses not to discuss
   [6] Don't know

   A. If no Health Care Proxy; Who would you like to speak for you if you were not able to speak for yourself?
   Name: ______________________ Phone #: ______________

Beth Israel Medical Center-Department of Pain Medicine and Palliative Care

IV. COMMUNICATION

14. METHOD OF COMMUNICATION
[1] Speaking [2] Language Barrier [3] Sign Language (*for hearing impaired*) [4] Writing Only [5] None

15. DEGREE OF INDEPENDENCE IN COMMUNICATING
[1] Functional; independent with all aspects of communication (speaking, hearing, sight), with or without glasses, hearing aids, or communication devices
[2] Moderate assist; communicates ź 50% of the time
[3] Dependent; unable to communicate with others

V. PHYSICAL/ACTIVITY STATUS

16. PRESSURE ULCERS
[1] None
[2] Mild [Stage I/II]: Injury to skin, Partial loss of skin layers
[3] Severe [Stage III/IV]: Deep craters in skin that extends down to but not through underlying fascia; breaks in skin exposing muscle or bone; extensive destruction, tissue necrosis, or damage to muscle, bone or supporting structures (e.g., tendons)

17. BOWEL AND BLADDER FUNCTION
[1] Independent in bowel and bladder function, with full self-care, including ostomy/catheter, if present
[2] *Not* incontinent, but some assistance needed in managing bathroom or bedpan or ostomy/catheter, if present
[3] Rarely incontinent; requiring substantial assistance in managing bathroom or bedpan or ostomy/catheter, if present
[4] Occasionally incontinent; requires full assistance in managing bathroom or bedpan or ostomy/catheter, if present
[5] Fully incontinent or unable to assist in management of ostomy/catheter, if present
[6] Don't know

18. PERFORMACE STATUS
[0] Normal activity
[1] Capable of all self-care, is ambulatory, but restricted in physicallythan 50% of waking hours strenuous activity, able to carry out work of a light or sedentary
[2] Ambulatory, capable of all self-care activities, but unable to carry out any work activities; up and about more than 50% of waking hours
[3] Capable of only limited self-care; confined to bed greater
[4] Completely disabled; cannot carry on any self-care; nature (e.g., light housework, office work) totally confined to bed/chair

19. NUTRITIONAL INTAKE
[1] Normal
[2] Modified Independent; intake limited, need for modification unknown
[3] Requires diet modification to swallow solid foods and liquids (puree, thickened fluids)
[4] Combined oral and tube feeding
[5] Tube feeding only
[6] No oral intake (NPO) and no tube feeding

20. PRACTICAL SUPPORT WITH ESSENTIAL TASKS (e.g., cooking, cleaning, shopping)
[1] Needs assistance in essential tasks which is not available
[2] Needs assistance in essential tasks which is often unreliable or incomplete
[3] Needs assistance in essential tasks which is sometimes inadequate or available only for less critical tasks such as banking
[4] Needs assistance in essential tasks is usually available; assistance in less critical tasks is incomplete and unreliable; other responsibilities limit helper availability
[5] Assistance is available and adequate for any need

VI. SOCIAL SUPPORT

21. The emotional support I have had from my family and friends has been:
[1] As much as I wanted [2] Very adequate [3] Adequate [4] Inadequate [5] Very Inadequate

Beth Israel Medical Center-Department of Pain Medicine and Palliative Care

VII. SPIRITUALITY (*Skip if Patient is Globally Incompetent*)

22. How important is your religion or spiritual beliefs in your everyday life?
[1] Not at all important [2] A little [3] Somewhat [4] Important [5] Very important

23. During your current illness, how much comfort and strength are you finding from your religion or spiritual beliefs?
[1] None [2] A little [3] Some [4] A lot [5] Great strength/comfort [6] Not religious

NOTES:

SECTIONS VIII - IX TO BE COMPLETED BY PATIENT/FAMILY MEMBER OR HEALTH PROFESSIONAL

VIII. SYMPTOMS (C*MSAS-Condensed* Memorial Symptom Assessment Scale)
If the patient has any of the following symptoms, how severe and distressing are they now?
Specify who is responding: [1] Patient [2] Family member, friend, other [3] Health Care Professional

How much did this symptom bother or distress you in the past 7 days?

Symptom	Present	Not at all	A little Bit	Some what	Quite a bit	Very much
Lack of energy	Y N	0	1	2	3	4
Lack of appetite	Y N	0	1	2	3	4
Pain	Y N	0	1	2	3	4
Dry mouth	Y N	0	1	2	3	4
Weight Loss	Y N	0	1	2	3	4
Feeling drowsy	Y N	0	1	2	3	4
Shortness of breath	Y N	0	1	2	3	4
Constipation	Y N	0	1	2	3	4
Difficulty sleeping	Y N	0	1	2	3	4
Difficulty concentrating	Y N	0	1	2	3	4
Nausea	Y N	0	1	2	3	4

How frequently did these symptoms occur during the last week?

Symptom	Present	Rarely	Occasionally	Frequently	Almost constantly
Worrying	Y N	1	2	3	4
Feeling sad	Y N	1	2	3	4
Feeling nervous	Y N	1	2	3	4

References:

Kaasa, T, Loomis, J, Gillis, K Bruera, E, & Hanson, J. (1997) The Edmonton Functional Assessment Tool: preliminary Development and Evaluation for Use in Palliative Care. JPSM 13(1):10-19.
Coyle, N, Goldstein, M, Passik, S, Fishman, B & Portenoy, R. (1996). Development and validation of a patient needs assessment tool (PNAT) for oncology clinicians. Cancer Nursing. 19(2):81-92.
Oken, M.M, Creech, RH, Tormey, DC, Horton, J, Davis, TE, McFadden, & ET, Carbone, PP. (1982). Toxicity and Response Criteria Of the Eastern cooperative Oncology Group (ECOG). Am J Clin Oncol 5:649-655.
Chang, VT, Hwang, SS, Kasimis, B & Thaler, H. (2004). Shorter symptom assessment instruments: the Condensed Memorial Symptom Assessment Scale (CMSAS). Cancer Invest 22(4):526-36.
National Pressure Ulcer Advisory Panel Report. 1996. Pressure ulcer staging. Wound Ostomy and Continence Society. 4(3).

40

Sarah A. Wilson

Long-Term Care

You know I'm a fighter, and if I wanted to fight I would . . . but I don't want to fight any more. I just want them to leave me alone, no more tests. Don't let them do anything else, please promise me.
—Mother, talking to her daughter

- ***Key Points***
- *The long-term care setting is the home for much of the elderly population and a common setting of end-of-life care.*
- *Unlicensed personnel provide a substantial proportion of long-term care and should be included in palliative care education efforts.*
- *Elderly residents in long-term care settings often have multiple chronic illnesses and complex medication regimens.*

Quality end-of-life care in nursing homes is becoming more important as the number of older adults increases, and managed care continues to minimize hospital stays. Nursing home residents are sicker today and have different care needs. Although nursing homes were not established as sites for terminal care, they are becoming the place where many people do die. Statistics on the place of death tell us little about the environment where someone lived and died. This chapter addresses nursing homes, the environment of nursing homes, the staff, the care of dying residents, and model programs to support dying residents.

The terms *institutional care* and *long-term care* have been used interchangeably in reference to nursing home care, although neither is synonymous with *nursing home care.* Long-term care refers to a continuum of services addressing the health, personal care, and social service needs for persons who need help with activities of daily living due to some functional impairment.[1] Services may be provided in the home, the community, or a nursing home.

Before the late 1970s, nursing homes were the primary source of care that could not be provided by families for persons needing long-term care. Nursing homes have been described as the offspring of the almshouse and boarding house and the stepchild of the hospital.[2] In the mid-19th century, older people who were poor, sick, or disabled and without family support had few options other than the almshouse.[3] Private homes for the aged emerged as an alternative to public almshouses after the passage of the Social Security Act in the 1930s. Women who were caring for their ill family members at home took in other patients to help pay the bills. From these small homes, proprietary nursing homes evolved. When nurses were added to the staff, the homes were referred to as nursing homes, a term that continues to be used today.[4]

Growth of Nursing Homes

The growth of nursing homes from the 1930s to the 1960s was related to six key factors[2]: (1) Old Age Assistance allowed a portion of the elderly to directly purchase services; (2) payments were made directly to facilities for the care of older adults, easing the state's financial obligations and creating a source of payment for care; (3) construction loans and loan guarantees were available through the federal Hill–Burton Act, the Small Business Administration, and the Federal Housing Authority; (4) the Kerr–Mills Program extended financial participation to medically indigent older adults; (5) the American Association of Nursing Homes became a strong lobby for those with interests in the new industry; and (6) the federal government began in a limited way to develop some standards for nursing homes. The growth of nursing homes occurred largely by chance; however, with the passage of Medicare and Medicaid in 1965, nursing homes became an industry.

Nursing homes continue to be a growing industry because people are living longer, with more complex health problems. The latest data (2004) from the National Center for Health Statistics (NCHS) list 18,000 nursing homes, with 1.9 million beds and 1.6 million residents.[5] The majority of nursing homes (66%) are proprietary or profit making.[5] Nursing homes are licensed or certified to designate the level of care provided and method of reimbursement. Approximately 82% of nursing homes are certified by Medicare and Medicaid. Skilled nursing facilities (SNFs) are those certified for Medicare funding. Medicare provides for up to 100 days of skilled care in a nursing home after a 3-day hospitalization. However, reimbursement for nursing home care by Medicare is restricted by narrowly defining what "skilled" is and by limiting the duration of the "skilled" benefit. The cost of nursing home care, averaging $61,320 year, is beyond the means of most Americans.[6] Rates for Medicaid reimbursement vary considerably from state to state. Most elderly who need nursing home care for more than a few weeks spend or liquidate all their resources to qualify for Medicaid.

Population Demographics and Nursing Homes

The population of the United States continues to increase. One of the most significant developments is the growth of the older population. The large number of people who were born between 1946 and 1964, commonly referred to as "baby boomers," contributes to the "graying of America." Statistics from the 2000 census reflect the influence of baby boomers. Thirty million people are over 65 years of age and account for 12.4% of the population.[7] Sixteen percent of the people aged 65 and over are members of minority groups.[7] The fastest growing age group in the United States are people aged 85 and over. The number of centenarians increased 35% between 1990 and 2000. It is projected that by the year 2011, the largest increase will be in the group of people aged 65 to 74 years.[1] The increase in the older adult population will have a major impact on health care in terms of services needed, delivery of health care, and education of health care providers. Older persons have more health problems, use more health services, and are hospitalized more often for longer stays than younger persons.

Five percent is most often cited as the proportion of older adults living in nursing homes. However, this is misleading because the use of nursing homes increases with age. For older adults residing in nursing homes, 34.6% are aged 75 to 84, and 33.8% are aged 85 to 94.[5] The characteristics and needs of nursing home residents have changed with the implementation of the prospective payment system for Medicare. Nursing homes are experiencing changes in the reasons for admissions and discharges. For example, the intensity of care has increased as more people enter nursing homes as a result of early hospital discharge. Some people are entering nursing homes for a relatively short stay and rehabilitation, others are being discharged home, and still others are being transferred to hospitals in the final stages of life and ultimately die there.

Persons who live to age 65 have more than a 40% chance of living in a nursing home before they die, and this is likely to increase to 46% by 2020.[8] Death occurs more frequently among older adults in institutions than at home among family and friends. A widespread belief is that the majority of older people die in hospitals. In fact, the older people are, the more likely they are to die in nursing homes.[8] It is estimated that 40% to 50% of all deaths will occur in long-term care settings by the year 2040.[9] Although nursing homes were not established as places for terminal care, they are increasingly becoming such facilities.

Regulation of Nursing Homes

Nursing homes are highly regulated. The number of rules and regulations have led some to compare the regulations to those of nuclear power plants. The nursing home population is viewed as a population of vulnerable adults who need protection, which, in combination with the history of patient abuse by some providers, has led to a strong tradition of regulation by federal and state governments. Most of the effort in quality assessment has been directed toward detecting problems; less has been devoted to assessing and acknowledging good care.[10]

Almost 2 decades ago, concern with the quality of care in nursing homes led Congress to commission the Institute of Medicine (IOM) to study nursing homes. The recommendations of the IOM Committee on Nursing Home Regulation, as well as many consumer advocacy groups, led Congress to enact major reforms in nursing home regulations as part of the Omnibus Budget Reconciliation Act of 1987 (OBRA 87).[11] The intent of OBRA was to improve the quality of care by establishing a single set of certification conditions for all nursing homes.[12] In addition, these regulations addressed residents' care, rights, and quality of life. A key aspect of OBRA 87 was that residents have the right to be free of physical and chemical restraints. The emphasis of regulations shifted toward addressing outcomes of care. The Minimum Data Set (MDS), a standardized interdisciplinary assessment tool, was mandated for residents within the first 14 days after admission, and whenever there was a significant change in a resident's condition.

Some improvements have been noted in nursing homes since OBRA 87 was implemented.[12] The focus on residents' rights and the empowerment of residents in care decisions have been identified as one of the most significant accomplishments of OBRA.[12] Perhaps most significant, there has been an overall reduction in the use of both physical and chemical restraints. It is significant that OBRA included no provisions for improving reimbursement to increase staffing. The emphasis of OBRA was rehabilitation, restoration, and improvement in function, not the provision of quality end-of-life care.[13]

Accreditation

Nursing homes may apply for voluntary accreditation by the Joint Commission on Accreditation of Healthcare Organizations (JCAHO), an organization created for the accreditation of hospitals that has expanded to include home health agencies and nursing homes, among other health care institutions. The facility pays a fee for the inspection to determine if JCAHO standards are being followed. Some nursing homes that seek JCAHO accreditation believe that it adds to a facility's credibility and makes it more marketable to the consumer.

In summary, growth in nursing homes has been proportionate with the increasing elderly population, and the need for long-term care services will continue to increase as the population ages. Palliative care is an important component of nursing home care. Along with understanding the structure of nursing homes, it is important to consider the sociocultural environment of these institutions.

Sociocultural Environment of Nursing Homes

The sociocultural environment of long-term care differs from that of hospitals. Whereas hospitals must always have physicians present, nursing homes are required only to have physician services available as needed. A medical director, full-time or part-time, is responsible for coordinating and directing resident services.

Physician Involvement

Physician visits to residents in nursing homes are often limited to once every 30 days. Federal regulations require physicians to make at least one visit every 60 days to nursing home residents, in contrast to the acute care environment, where physicians usually see patients every day. The nurse in the nursing home is responsible for communicating any changes in a resident's condition to the physician. If the physician does not respond in a timely manner, the medical director intervenes.

Length of Stay

The length of stay is either short term or long term. In most nursing homes, the length of stay varies, although there is greater movement of residents into and out of nursing homes as a result of early hospital discharges. The short-term resident is usually someone under 75 years of age who stays in the nursing home for 4 to 6 weeks for rehabilitation after an acute illness, such as a stroke or hip replacement. The long-term resident is usually older than 75 and has numerous chronic diseases and functional and cognitive impairments. The average length of stay in a skilled nursing facility is 870 days from admission to discharge.[14] Almost half (47.7%) of all nursing home residents have some form of dementia.[15] The 1999 National Nursing Home Study indicated that the typical resident is a female, 85 years old and older, who needs assistance with one or more activities of daily living and instrumental activities of daily living.[5] The long-term resident is much more likely to die in the nursing home or hospital. Older people who die in a nursing home have dying trajectory of fragility, with 60% having a diagnosis of a stroke or a hip fracture.[16] Between 50% and 60% of all deaths in SNFs are residents with a diagnosis of dementia.[16]

Nursing Home Staff

Nursing homes and hospitals differ in the type of staff employed and in staffing patterns. The acute care hospital has a higher ratio of professional staff to patients than the nursing home. Nursing assistants, the primary caregivers in nursing homes, spend the most time with residents and constitute more than 32% of a nursing home's full-time equivalent (FTE) employees. In comparison, registered nurses (RNs) constitute only 7.6% of the FTE employees.[5] Licensed practical nurses (LPNs) constitute 10.6% of the nursing home's FTE employees.[5] Approximately 50% of SNFs do not have an RN on duty 24 hours a day. Proprietary nursing homes have fewer RNs (6.8%) per 100 beds than nonprofit or government nursing homes (9.1%).[5]

The educational level and preparation of staff in the two types of institutions also differ. The LPN program may be completed in 12 to 24 months and has a limited amount of educational content devoted to geriatrics, palliative care, and death and dying. Most nursing assistants have not completed high school, work for low pay, and receive few benefits. The work assigned to nursing assistants is often difficult and stressful, with little recognition of their contribution to resident care. The IOM committee strongly supports the need to increase the number of professional nurses in nursing homes, noting that there is a clear connection between the RN-to-resident ratio and the quality of nursing care provided.[17]

Public Expectations

The public and the family of nursing home residents may have unrealistic expectations of nursing homes. It is a difficult decision for families to decide on nursing placement. Families expect the same type of care to be provided in the nursing home that was provided in the hospital. For example, families may believe a physician will visit every day instead of once a month. The media reinforces negative images of nursing homes. Cases of abuse and poor management receive more attention in the media than positive images of nursing homes.

The sociocultural environment of nursing homes differs from other health care institutions: the average length of stay is longer, physician visits are less frequent, the primary care providers are nursing assistants, and RNs constitute a small portion of the home's FTE employees.

Studies of Death and Dying in Nursing Homes

Early studies of death and dying focused on hospitals as the place of death. The attitudes of hospital staff toward dying patients, the stresses encountered by nurses in caring for dying patients and families, and communication with dying patients and families were described in these studies.[18–21] More recent studies of death and dying have focused on other settings, including nursing homes. The setting of care has a direct influence on the older adult's quality of life at the end of life.[22] Studies of death and dying in nursing homes have examined family perceptions of care, symptom management, educational needs of staff, and barriers to quality end-of-life care.

Family Perceptions of Nursing Home Care

Teno[23] conducted the first large national study to examine family perspectives on the quality of end-of-life care in institutional settings and home. Family members were surveyed to determine if the adequacy or quality of end-of-life care differed in hospitals, nursing homes, and home. A mortality follow-up survey was used, and 1,578 decedents were represented. Nearly one fourth of all respondents reported the patient did not receive adequate treatmeant for pain and dyspnea. Family members of persons whose last place of care was a nursing home or a home with home health nursing services had higher rates of reported unmet needs for pain compared with persons who had home hospice services. One quarter of the families reported problems with physician communication. Nursing home residents were less likely to have been treated with respect at the end of life. The family members of decedents who received home hospice care were more likely to report a favorable dying expereince.[23]

Wilson and Daley,[24] as a part of larger study of death and dying in nursing homes, interviewed family members whose relatives died in nursing homes. Family members described caring behaviors of staff that were helpful to them. The primary concerns expressed by these family members were lack of spiritual care in some facilities and not being present when their relative died because they were not notified in time by the nursing home staff.

Cartwright[13] reviewed nursing research in nursing homes and assisted-living facilities as places of care for the dying. She noted that a large discrepancy exists between family and staff perceptions of the quality of end-of-life care in nursing homes. Wilson and Daley reported that positive long-term relationships exist between staff, residents, and families in nursing homes.[25] There is clearly a need to examine how these relationships can improve communication and impact the quality of end-of-life care.

Symptom Management

One of the major themes reported in the IOM's study of care at the end of life was that too many people suffer from pain that could be prevented or relieved with the use of existing knowledge and therapies.[26] Several studies have documented the poor control of pain in nursing home residents.[23,27,28] Instruments to assess pain in residents with cognitive impairment are inadequate. Issues related to pain management in nursing homes are reviewed below, and a comprehensive discussion of pain assessment and management are found in Chapters 5 and 6.

Palliative care educational programs have been effective in improving pain mangement in nursing homes.[27,28] Froggatt[27] evaluated an educational program for nursing home staff that included RNs and nursing assistants. Pain management improved; however, the program did not appear to have an impact on institutional practices and policies regarding end of life. Weissman and colleagues[28] designed an educational program to enhance institutional commitment to pain mangement. Multiple facilities (87) participated in the project and sent two or three staff members to full-day education classes on pain management. Participants developed an action plan to change facility practice and policies regarding pain management. Fourteen target indicators, based on standards developed by the American Pain Society and Agency for Health Care Policy and Research, were used to evaluate changes in practice and policy. The indicators included: use of standardized assessment and flow sheets; education of staff, residents and families; establishment of an interdisciplinary pain team; and institutionalization of pain assessment and management polices and quality-improvement standards and processes. Facilities averaged 8.8 indicators in place at the completion of the project. This was a significant improvement from the baseline score of 3.4 indicators. Weissman acknowledged that some indicators were more difficult to change. For example, only 19 facilities had established a pain-education program for staff at the completion of the program.

Educational Needs of Staff

The educational needs of staff have been identified in several studies.[25,27–32] Kayser-Jones and Hanson reported that staff often lack knowledge of how to assess and manage symptoms in nursing homes.[30,31] Wilson and Daley conducted focus group interviews with 155 participants in 11 nursing homes to identify the learning needs of staff.[25] Staff identified the need for education about pain management and comfort measures, grief management, communication skills, and spiritual care. Ersek, Kraybill, and Hansberry[32] reported findings similar to Daley and Wilson in their preliminary studies of educational needs of staff providing end-of-life care in nursing homes.

Daley and Wilson[29] developed a continuing education program to address the learning needs of nursing home staff. One of the content areas dealt with how to communicate with physicians. Nurses were provided with a guide for telephoning physicians about pain that covered how to prepare for the telephone call and what assessment data to report. Steps in preparing to make the call included stating the purpose of the call, enumerating goals for the resident, and defining what they would like to have happen. Assessment data included such information as location, intensity, and quality of pain, what made it better or worse, and what medications had been tried. Nurses were encouraged to develop a standard form to record information. Six to 8 weeks after the continuing education program, participants were asked to describe how they used information from the course. Nurses indicated that they were more comfortable talking to physicians on the phone and used a more assertive approach. Nursing assistants increased their knowledge of what information to report to nurses. Since nursing assistants spend the most time in direct care activities, it is important that they are included in efforts to promote comfort.

Barriers to Quality End-of-Life Care

The nursing home environment has some barriers to quality end-of-life care. Pain management is an area of concern. Physicians are dependent on nurses to assess and to report pain and may be unaware of measures that can be used to control pain in nursing homes. For example, some physicians are unaware that morphine can be given intravenously in many nursing homes. In addition, LPNs receive little education in pain management. Nursing homes are extremely concerned about state and federal regulations and have few protocols for pain management. Pain management is further complicated by the large number of cognitively impaired residents who are unable to communicate if they are in pain.

There is a lack of evidence-based research in the delivery of model programs for quality end-of-life care in nursing homes. Weissman and colleagues' work on building an institutional commitment to pain management in nursing homes is one of the few evidence-based practice studies.[28] Many nursing homes are apprehensive about participating in research studies because of the costs involved, both monetary as well as staff time required. Studies are needed to address issues of protection of study subjects, since many elderly persons in nursing homes are unable to give informed consent. It is important that the researchers clearly explain the purpose(s) of the research and its objectives, the potential benefits to the nursing home, the time and costs involved, and the amount of staff involvement necessary. Researchers should meet with nursing home administration and staff during the course of the study to discuss the study progress and identify any problems. They should also meet with family members to explain the research project. Once the study is completed, the researchers should provide feedback to the nursing home.

In summary, studies of death and dying in nursing homes have described family perceptions of care, the educational needs of staff in providing end-of-life care, and problems with pain management. Further study needs to be done to learn more about the experience of dying in long-term care facilities. Institutional policies and practices need to change to achieve better outcomes in the management of pain.

The next section explores issues related to the care of dying residents in nursing homes, including advance directives, ethical issues, spiritual support, provision of hospice services, support for dying residents and their families, and recognition of the impact of loss on staff.

Caring for Dying Residents

A number of issues relate to providing quality end-of-life care in the nursing home environment. Nursing home staff, especially RNs, can make significant contributions to enhance terminal residents' quality of life.

Advance Directives: Where Are the Letters of Preference?

Nursing home residents have the right to participate in decisions about their care, including end-of-life care. The passage of the federal Patient Self-Determination Act (PSDA) in 1990 required all health care agencies that receive federal funding to recognize advance directives. The purpose of the PSDA was to encourage greater awareness and use of advance directives. OBRA 87 regulations emphasized that residents have the right to self-determination, including the right to participate in care planning and the right to refuse treatments. Residents are usually informed of their rights, including the right to advance directives at the time of admission to the nursing home, a stressful time for both resident and family members. Families report making these decisions in the context of guilt and overwhelming burden related to nursing home admission. There is a large number of nursing homes residents with dementia who have no advance directive or family member to make decisions on their behalf.[33]

When protocols are used to learn what residents want in terms of end-of-life care, there is a decrease in transfer and hospital death at the end of life.[22] Little has been written about the unique situation of chronically seriously ill older adults and their families.[9]

Ethical Issues

Autonomy is based on the assumption that an individual is the best judge of what is in his or her best interest. Nursing homes have been criticized as dehumanizing and promoting dependence. Autonomy gives meaning to one's life and, in relation to nursing homes, it means being able to direct and influence others in decisions regarding daily living situations.[34] The routines, regulations, and restricted opportunities in nursing homes have been described as enemies of autonomy, and the regimentation contributes to a "loss of control." Most nursing homes were designed based on a hospital or medical model of care, which focuses on routines and tasks. The medical model tends to foster a paternalistic approach of "we know what is best." The physical environment of the nursing home also limits autonomy. Space is limited, with most residents sharing a room and toilet facilities that restrict privacy and space for personal possessions. Residents may also wander in and out of others' rooms. The environment could be more individualized by using personal furnishings and creating a homelike common area, such as a dining room.

One of the most difficult and sometimes controversial ethical issues involves decisions regarding food and hydration. Food in all societies is part of the ongoing cycle of daily interaction and activity around which much of family life is organized and which is symbolic of life and caring. Families may continue to try to feed their relatives when they are no longer able to eat. Nursing home staff can assist families by explaining that it is normal to lose appetite at the end of life and that the body only takes in what it needs. Trying to force someone to eat may cause more harm than good. Families should understand that there is a risk of aspiration as a person gets weaker. Nursing staff may encourage families to offer small amounts of liquids, ice chips, or Popsicles.

The following case study illustrates some of the ethical issues at the end of life in nursing homes.

CASE STUDY
Mary's Decision

Mary, an 82-year-old woman, was admitted to Evergreen Nursing Home after a hospitalization for pneumonia. Prior to the hospital admission, Mary lived by herself in an apartment. She has two adult children, one daughter who is single and lives close to Mary, and a son who lives 200 miles away. The daughter either visits or calls Mary every day, and the son calls about once a month and visits infrequently. Mary has had multiple hospital admissions this past year for a variety of health problems, including congestive heart failure, urinary tract infections (UTIs), and dehydration. While in the hospital, Mary received IV antbiotics for UTI and pneumonia. She became very confused in the hopital and, although the confusion decreased after a few days, Mary was much more fragile. She was not able to manage at home by herself, so the decision was made to admit her to Evergreen. Mary has adjusted well to the nursing home admission and continues to have frequent contact with her daughter. She has recently developed a respiratory tract infection and the staff is considering hospital admission. Mary does not want to go to the hospital, and she does not want anything else done. Mary informed her daughter of her decision not to be hospitalized and commented, "I don't want anything done for the sake of prolonging my life . . . God will call me when it's time." The daugher was in agreement with Mary's decision and called her brother to inform him of the decision. The brother was very upset with this phone call and asked how she could agree to this—"everything should be done for Mother." The brother called Evergreen and informed the staff that he was not in agreement with this decision and would visit his mother this weekend.

What are the issues in this case? Who should be involved in making decisions? Why might this be difficult for the son? What are Mary's wishes? What are the the benefits or consequences of this decision? Would the American Nurses Association (ANA) Code of Ethics be useful in making a decision? What are the roles of the nurse and physician in this case? Should anyone else be involved? What needs to be done? What can be learned from this case?

To answer the above questions, consider the following: Is the primary issue whether Mary should go to the hospital for treatment of the respiratory tract infection? What does Mary mean by "I don't want anything done to prolong my life"? Ask her to explain this. Could Mary remain at the nursing home and be given oral antbiotics to treat the respiratory infection? Can a patient who is alert and oriented decide what treatment he or she wants? Would a family conference be helpful to discuss what it means to prolong life and what advance directives are? Could the son have some guilt feelings because he does not see his mother very often? Perhaps the son thinks that not having anything done means no treatment or care. This needs to be explained to him. It would be helpful to clarify what Mary wants to be done. Consider what the outcomes would be if Mary had treatment or did not have treatment. The ANA code of ethics addresses respect for the dignity and worth of all persons, the person's right to self-determination, and the primacy of the patient's interest. How do these principles apply to this case? Consider if Mary wants to discuss this decision with anyone else. Perhaps clergy? Does this case illustrate the importance of advance directives and the need for communication among all involved?

Providing Support to Dying Residents and Their Families

Nursing home staff may provide support to dying residents and their families in coping with the eventual loss of the family member. It is important that nurses communicate openly with families, explain changes in the patient's/resident's condition, and answer questions honestly. Listening is an important communicative skill. Active listening is usually more helpful than judging or giving advice. Effective active listening skills include being able to convey that you want to listen, that you want to be helpful, and that you accept the other's feelings. When communication is a concern for staff, it may be helpful to role-play some representative situations. For example, role-playing can teach what to say on the telephone when informing a family member that their relative is dying and how to help families decide about options.

Families have identified a number of caring behaviors of nursing staff that helped them cope with the eventual loss of their relative.[35] It was important to families for staff to take the time to come to residents' rooms and ask how they were doing. Families also identified that listening to the family's concerns and getting answers to their questions were helpful. Staff also demonstrated concern for families in other ways, such as asking if they would like a cup of coffee or getting a comfortable chair for a family member. Families appreciated the fact that the staff respected their privacy and seemed to know when they wanted to be left alone.

It is important for families to understand the dying process. Staff may explain signs and symptoms of approaching death to families and keep them informed of what is changing and why. If the family is not present, they should be kept informed by telephone. Family decisions, such as being present at the time of death or not being present, should be respected. Every effort should be made to notify families early enough that they may be present at the time of death, if that is their wish. Families may be encouraged to reminisce together. They may participate in providing care by holding a hand or giving a back rub. Staff should remind families that even though the family member cannot respond, the sound of familiar voices may be a source of comfort.

There are some barriers to providing support for dying residents and families in the nursing home environment. The lack of privacy in most nursing homes is a problem, and it is often difficult to find a private area to talk to families and residents. One social worker commented that "dying is almost a public spectacle in the nursing home." Another barrier is the lack of staff time to spend with dying residents and families, as the staffing patterns of most nursing homes do not take into account labor-intensive care at the end of life.

Providing Spiritual Support

An important component of palliative care is spiritual support. Spirituality is often associated with religion, but the two are not identical. Religion is a means of expressing spirituality and refers to feelings, beliefs, and behaviors associated with a faith community. Spiritual needs include the need to see one's self as a person of worth and value, to love and be loved, and to have meaning and purpose in life.[36] Spiritual support is an integral part of supportive care. The search for meaning or spiritual comfort at the end of life is often guided by religious or philosophical beliefs. Spiritual well-being in relation to the end of life has been described as "meaningful existence, ability to find meaning in daily experience, ability to transcend physical discomfort, and readiness for death."[37] Families and residents may fear the future and have questions about life in general. Residents are usually asked about their religious affiliation and the name of their clergy at the time of admission to most nursing homes, but, unfortunately, this may be the only time spirituality is mentioned. Spiritual needs vary and can change at the end of life.

Private, religiously affiliated nursing homes usually have pastoral care available, and most have a room that is designated as a chapel. Many nursing homes have funeral and memorial services for residents. Nonprivate nursing homes usually attempt to make arrangements for pastoral care through volunteer clergy in the community. Some have been successful with these arrangements, but some nursing home staff have stated that it is difficult to find clergy when needed.

Meeting the spiritual needs of dying residents and their families has been identified as an educational need of nursing home staff.[29] Staff often are aware of spiritual needs but are unsure of what to do or say and what would be considered acceptable to their facilities in meeting spiritual needs. Staff may use a number of interventions to provide spiritual care, including praying with the resident and family, reading the Bible or other religious works, singing hymns, and providing therapeutic presence, all of which may help decrease the loneliness and separation persons are experiencing. When a resident is expressing a spiritual need, the following matrix (Table 40–1) may be useful in responding or making suggestions.

Table 40–1
Spiritual Needs: Examples of Needs and Suggested Responses

Need	Danger Sign	Response	Suggestions
To be person of worth	Person says, "I can't even get dressed." "I've made a mess of my life."	"God loves you." "I like you just the way you are."	Address residents with their names to confirm their value and worth.
	Person arranges to get ignored, such as someone who avoids interactions with others or withdraws from interactions.		Spend time with them. Find tasks the resident can do.
Love and to be loved	People who are lonely	Express your feelings to resident.	Help resident recall memories of being loved.
Meaning and purpose	Not being able to do what they used to "Why am I still here?"	Convey that resident did and does make a difference. "You have let me journey with you." "Part of the gift I get is that you let me take care of you and experience you as a person."	Assist resident with other meaningful activities: journaling, helping other residents, praying for others.

With proper staff education and training, most barriers to providing spiritual support in nursing homes can be eliminated. Continuing education programs need to be developed to address staff needs for education on spirituality. Staff need to know the facility's policies regarding spiritual care. Many nursing homes do not have a space designated as a meditation room or chapel. It is important for families and residents to have a private, quiet area where they can meditate. If pastoral care is not available in the nursing home, it may be arranged by contacting local clergy or lay leaders in the community.

Providing Support for Staff

Nursing staff form an attachment to residents that may be defined as a strong emotional bond and connectedness that develops between residents and staff over time.[35] Attachment is fostered by staff efforts to treat residents as "family." The nursing home is "home" for many residents, as some live there for years, so that staff often experience feelings of loss and sadness when a resident dies.

Staff members need to be able to talk about their feelings of loss when a resident dies. It is necessary for nursing homes to develop programs to assist staff in coping with the loss of a resident. Allowing staff time to talk about a resident at staff meetings, sharing memories of a resident, and planning a memorial for residents who have died may be helpful. Other staff members should acknowledge that the loss must be difficult when they know a particular staff member was close to a certain resident.

The loss of a resident may also be stressful for other nursing home residents. Residents develop friendships with other residents over time; they may have shared a room with the resident or sat next to the resident for meals. The death may remind residents of their own mortality. Residents may want to attend the funeral of the deceased resident, or the nursing home may have a memorial service or time of remembrance. Staff should acknowledge the loss and what it means to other residents.

In summary, the nursing home environment influences the care of residents at the end of life. Nursing home staff need to be comfortable talking with residents and families about death and dying. Knowledge of pain management is as important in nursing homes as it is in other settings. Families should be included in the care of dying residents, and their need for privacy should be respected. Several model programs have been developed to address the unique needs of nursing homes, as described in the next section.

Model Programs to Provide Support to Dying Residents

A number of nursing homes throughout the United States have developed model programs to provide support to dying residents and their families. Some of these programs deal with the specific problems of a subset—those nursing home residents who are near death. Exemplar programs are described below.

Kansas City Regional Long-Term Care Ethics Consortium

Ethical issues are encountered by most health care institutions in the delivery of care, and nursing homes are not an exception. When ethical dilemmas do arise, in-house resources may not be available to resolve the issue, and the nursing home may not have an ethics committeee. The Kansas City Regional Long-term Care Ethics Consortium, supported by the Midwest Bioethics Center, developed policy guidelines and ethical consultation and education for long-term care facilities. The mission of the Consortium is to provide a supportive network for people who serve long-term care residents either directly or indirectly. The Consortium has monthly meetings, quarterly case reviews, and educational programs. It provides an opportunity for long-term care professionals to come together and discuss problems and learn from each other. They have been active in advancing palliative care in long-term care. Information about the program may be obtained from http://www.midbio.org.

Abides Ministry

Abides Ministry addresses a variety of the needs of dying residents. It is a model program developed by Luther Manor, a long-term care facility in Milwaukee, Wisconsin. The program was initiated when a group of nurses began talking about how important it was to sit with residents who were dying. Members consist of staff who volunteer after-hours, residents at Luther Manor, and others from the community who want to be present for those who would otherwise die alone.

The Abiders try to anticipate the needs and wishes of dying residents. Abiders sit with a resident and read Bible passages, sings hymns, or most often just hold a resident's hand. Abiders stay with the dying resident 24 hours a day. They also provide relief for family members. Other nursing homes have developed similar programs using volunteers to sit with dying residents.

Palliative Care and Hospice Care in Nursing Homes

Several nursing homes have contracts with hospices for services. Because the nursing home is considered the resident's home, he or she may be eligible for Medicare hospice benefits under home care. The hospice staff is responsible for the plan of care, and any changes in the treatment plan must be discussed with and approved by the hospice case manager. The hospice nurse visits the nursing home, arranges the assessment of the resident, and schedules nursing assistance to provide personal care. The resident is provided with services that would otherwise not be available.

Coordinating hospice care in a nursing home requires good communication between the nursing home staff and hospice staff. Nursing home staff may view the hospice staff as outsiders.

Nursing home staff frequently believe that they know the resident best because they interact and care for the resident every day, whereas hospice staff members may see the resident only two or three times a week. Although hospice care is a benefit to residents, some question why special services are available to one group of residents and not to all residents. Hospice care in nursing homes results in better symptom mangement and improved quality of life at the end of life.[9,13] However, hospice is underutilized in nursing homes.[9] Information on palliative care and hospice care in nursing homes may be found at the National Hospice and Palliative Care Organization website: http://www.nhpco.org.

Hospice Households for Persons with End-Stage Dementia

The Hospice Households Project for persons with end-stage dementia is an example of an innovative approach that applies hospice concepts in nursing homes.[35,39] Although the diagnosis of cancer is one of the common diagnoses of hospice patients, cancer is a less common diagnosis among elderly hospice patients in long-term care. The care of persons with end-stage dementia differs from the care of persons with end-stage cancer in that the course of cancer is more predictable. Persons with cancer often have problems with pain, nausea, vomiting, and breathing. These problems are less common in persons with end-stage dementia. The person with end-stage dementia is unable to communicate needs and has severe impairments in cognitive and social abilities. Careful assessment is essential to determine possible causes of discomfort in persons with end-stage dementia.

Five hospice households were developed in three nursing homes in Milwaukee, Wisconsin for residents with end-stage dementia. The project was guided by the following research question: What is the effect of hospice-oriented care on comfort, physical complications, and behaviors associated with dementia for nursing home residents with a dementing illness?

Residents were eligible to participate in the study if they had a diagnosis of irreversible dementia, had a score on the Short Portable Mental Status Questionnaire that indicated severe cognitive impairment, were unable to participate in group programming for persons with dementia, had a functional behavior profile score of less than 40, and had advance directives that requested no cardiopulmonary resuscitation (CPR) be initiated. The researchers met with family members to explain the study and asked for permission for the relative to participate. Residents who met the criteria for participating in the study were assigned to a treatment group or control group. The treatment group received the intervention and were part of the hospice households.

The hospice households were clustered on six-to-eight-bed areas on units that had 22 to 44 beds. The intention was not to isolate residents on a distant unit. The households were made as homelike as possible by using colorful afghans, pillows, home furniture, and plants. Pictures and biographical sketches of each resident whose guardian consented were displayed in the room. Each facility provided a lounge for the project. Residents ate their meals in the lounge, which became a center for activities.

Case managers for the project were selected by the director of nursing in each facility. The case manager led the interdisciplinary team at the facility and assisted with developing and implementing individualized care plans. Case managers received formal classes in hospice care, care planning, assessment techniques, and case management from the researchers. In addition, an all-day conference was held for all staff involved in the project. Classes focused on hospice concepts, dementia, treatment of behaviors associated with dementia, and activity programming, as well as family and spiritual care. The conference generated interest and enthusiasm for the project.

Five main programs goals were identified that are consistent with hospice goals: comfort, quality of life, dignity, support for family, and support for the staff. The goal for comfort was that staff be able to tell when a resident was experiencing discomfort and when a resident was not. Staff used physical and behavioral assessment skills to recognize discomfort. When a resident displayed a change in behavior, he or she was evaluated for signs of constipation and for signs and symptoms of common infections, such as urinary tract infection using a leukocyte esterase dipstick. Urinary tract infections were common. If the cause for discomfort was not clearly identified, a behavioral intervention, such as distraction, quiet time in the resident's room, or music therapy, was initiated. All residents had orders for Tylenol as needed. If the resident displayed behavior such as agitation or perseverance and behavioral interventions were not effective, nurses were instructed to administer Tylenol rather than a chemical restraint. To promote the goal of quality of life, each resident had a schedule of activities that balanced sensory-calming and sensory-stimulating activities. Staff had identified that residents often received too much stimulation from the environment.

The goal of human dignity was enhanced by treating all residents in a kind and caring manner and respecting resident choices when possible. A written care plan was developed for each resident to aid communication. Interventions were developed to include the goal of the family being an integral part of care planning. Families were surveyed at regular intervals to determine their satisfaction with care. A bulletin board was hung for families to share information, and a periodic family night was held that focused on friendship and support. The final program goal was that staff have an understanding of behaviors associated with dementia and receive support from one another. Staff participated in educational programs, and every effort was made to assure that the project had sufficient staff to achieve its goals.

This project demonstrated that hospice concepts may be incorporated into the care of persons with end-stage dementia with little additional cost to the facility. The facilities that participated in the project did not require any additional staff. A statistically significant difference in levels of discomfort was established between the treatment and control group, and behaviors associated with dementia were lessened in the treatment group, although this difference was not large enough to be statistically significant. Staff reported increased job satisfaction as a result of participating in the project.[35,37]

Recommendations for Change

The quality of end-of-life care in nursing homes can be improved. The following are some recommendations for change: (1) Reimbursement for nursing home care needs to be increased; (2) nursing home staff should include more professional staff, and the ratio of staff to residents should be increased; (3) environmental modifications should be made to improve quality of life and human dignity; and (4) hospice and palliative care concepts should be incorporated in nursing homes.

Reimbursement

Reimbursement and regulations in nursing homes are often impediments to quality end-of-life care. Policy makers and the public need to be educated about the cost of nursing home care. Reimbursement should change from an emphasis on procedures to a focus on continuing comfort measures and palliation. Nursing homes receive most of their revenue from private-pay residents and Medicaid. Medicaid rates need to be increased to reflect the labor-intensive nature of long-term care. The IOM[26] recommends that additional research projects on the use of financial and other resources to improve quality of care and outcomes in nursing homes be funded. An issue closely related to reimbursement is the number and type of staff in nursing homes.

Nursing Home Staff

The relationship between the ratio of RNs to residents and quality of care has been clearly established in nursing homes.[17,22,26] Considering the projected growth in the elderly population, the need for RNs in nursing homes is expected to increase. In addition, nursing home residents will be sicker as a result of shorter hospital stays. A major barrier to increased staffing in nursing homes are the fiscal limits of government support. RN salaries are lower in nursing homes than in hospitals, and vacancy rates are higher.[26] Nursing homes are starting to use advance practice nurses to deal with the complex needs of older adults. Advance practice nurses, geriatric nurse practitioners, and clinical specialists in geriatrics can improve outcomes and contribute to the quality of care.

Nursing assistants provide the most direct care for residents and have the least amount of training. Their work is often difficult, with few rewards—salaries are low and there are few benefits. The care provided by nursing assistants is important to residents' quality of life, yet they are often paid little more than minimum wage. Interaction with professional staff is limited due to the demands of the nursing assistants' work. Nursing assistants should be provided with training for their jobs, and salaries should be increased. Efforts need to be made to include nursing assistants as part of the team.

Environmental Modifications

The environment of nursing homes needs to be changed to promote resident autonomy and quality of life. Residents should be consulted about the type of living arrangement they prefer. For example, some residents may prefer a single room with space for personal belongings, while others may appreciate sharing the room with someone for companionship. Nursing homes should be designed to accommodate residents' preferences. Common areas, such as the dining room and lounge, need to be more homelike, with separate conversational areas. Space should be designated for a meditation room to allow residents and families a quiet place. The elderly in nursing homes are often deprived of natural light. Some simple environmental modifications may improve the older adults' visual abilities—for example, using colors to enhance contrast, using curtains to control glare, and placing chairs in positions to enhance illumination. Biological changes occur within the brain in response to different levels of bright-light exposure, and these biochemical changes may affect hormones and neurotransmitters responsible for regulating mood, energy, sleep, and appetite.[38] Rosenthal's[39] work on seasonal affective disorder describes the effect of seasons and light and dark on a person's mood and energy level. In the fall and winter months, when it's dark and cool, people may be more prone to depression and lethargy. Most people feel better on days when the sun is shining. The nursing home enivironment may be modified to make better use of light by using broad-spectrum fluorescent lights and daylight-simulating lights.

Incorporation of Hospice and Palliative Care Concepts

Palliative care concepts should be an integral part of nursing home care. The emphasis of care should be directed toward the quality of life at the end of life. Both the resident and family should participate in care planning. The nursing home environment should be a therapeutic milieu that addresses the physical, psychological, social, and spiritual needs of all residents. Research by nurses is needed to improve end-of-life care in nursing homes. Nurses can make a difference in the quality of end-of-life care in nursing homes. It is hoped that the reader will incorporate some of the suggestions discussed in this chapter to make a difference in the delivery of end-of-life care for nursing home residents.

REFERENCES

1. Miller CA. Nursing for Wellness in Older Adults: Theory & Practice. Philadelphia: Lippincott Williams & Wilkins, 2004.
2. Kane RL. The evolution of the American nursing home. In: Binstock RH, Cluff LE, Von Mering O, eds. The Future of Long-Term

Care: Social and Policy Issues. Baltimore: Johns Hopkins University Press, 1996:145–168.
3. Holstein M, Cole TR. The evolution of long-term care in America. In: Binstock RH, Cluff LE, Von Mering O, eds. The Future of Long-Term Care: Social and Policy Issues. Baltimore: Johns Hopkins University Press, 1996:19–48.
4. Ignatavicius DD. Introduction to Long-Term Care Nursing: Principles and Practice. Philadelphia: F. A. Davis, 1998.
5. National Center for Health Statistics. Health United States, 2003. DHHS Publication No. 2003-1232. Hyattsville, MD: U.S. Department of Health and Human Services, 2003.
6. Adler, J. Cost of Nursing Home Rooms Jumps. Chicago Tribune. August 31, 2003.
7. U.S. Bureau of the Census: Statistical Abstracts of the United States: 2002. Washington, DC: U.S. Government Printing Office.
8. Spillman BC, Lubitz J. New estimates of lifetime nursing home use: have patterns of use changed? Med Care 2002;40:965–975.
9. Matzo ML, Sherman DW. Gerontological Palliative Care Nursing. St. Louis: C.V. Mobsy Press, 2004.
10. Kane RA. Long-term care and a good quality of life: bringing them closer together. Gerontologist 2001;42:314–320.
11. Institute of Medicine (IOM). Improving the Quality of Care in Nursing Homes. Washington, DC: National Academy Press, 1986.
12. Marek KD, Rantz MJ, Fagin CM, Krecki JW. OBRA '87: has it resulted in better quality care? J Gerontological Nurs 1996;122: 28–36.
13. Cartwright JC. Nursing homes and assisted living facilites as places for dying. Ann Rev Nurs Res 2002;20:231–266.
14. Gabriel CS. Characteristics of elderly nursing home current residents: data from the 1997 National Nursing Home survey. Advance Data 1997;312: 1–16.
15. Magaziner J, German P, Zimmerman SI, Hebel HR, Burton L, Gruber-Baldini AL, et al. The prevalence of dementia in a statewide sample of new nursing home admissions aged 65 and older: diagnosis by expert panel. Epidemiology of dementia in nursing homes research group. Gerontologist 2000;40:663–672.
16. Lunney JR, Lynn J, Hogan C. Profile of older Medicare decedents. J Am Geriatr Soc 2002;50:1108–1112.
17. Mass M, Buckwalter K, Specht J. Nursing staff and quality of care in nursing homes. In: Institute of Medicine. Nursing Staff in Hospitals and Nursing Homes: Is it Adequate? Washington, DC: Academy Press, 1986:361–425.
18. Germain C. Cancer Unit: An Ethnography. Wakefield, MA: Nursing Resources, 1979.
19. Glaser BG, Strauss AL. A Time for Dying. Chicago: Aldine Publishing Company, 1968.
20. Mumma CM, Benoliel JQ. Care, cure, and hospital dying trajectories. Omega 1984;85:275–288.
21. Sundnow D. Passing On: The Social Organization of Dying. Englewood Cliffs, NJ: Prentice-Hall, 1967.
22. Mezey M, Dubler NN, Mitty E, Brody AA. What impact do setting and transitions have on the quality of life at the end of life and the quality of the dying process? Gerontologist 2002;42:54–67.
23. Teno JM, Clarridge BR, Casey V, Welch LC, et al. Family perspective on end of life care in the last place of care. JAMA 2002;291: 88–93.
24. Wilson SA, Daley BJ. Family perspectives of dying in long-term care. J Gerontological Nurs 1999;25:19–25.
25. Wilson SA, Daley BJ. Attachment/detachment: forces influencing care of the dying in long-term care. J Palliative Med 1998;1: 21–34.
26. Institute of Medicine. Approaching Death: Improving Care at the End-of-Life. Washington, DC: National Academy, 1997.
27. Froggatt KA. Evaluating a palliative care education project in nursing homes. Int J Palliative Nurs 2000;6:140–146.
28. Weissman DE, Griffie J, Muchka S, Matson S. Building an institutional commitment to pain management in long-term care facilites. J Pain Symptom Manage 2000;20:35–43.
29. Daley BJ, Wilson SA. Needs assessment in long-term care facilities: linking research and continuing education. J Contin Educ Health Prof 1999;19:111–121.
30. Kayser-Jones J. A case study of the death of an older women in a nursing home: are nursing care practices in compliance with ethical guidelines? J Gerontological Nurs 2000;26(9):48–54.
31. Hanson LC, Henderson M. Care of the dying in long-term care settings. Clin Geriatr Med 2000;16:225–237.
32. Ersek M, Kraybill BM, Hansberry J. Investigating the educational needs of licensed nursing staff and certified nursing assistants in nursing homes regarding end-of-life care. Am J Hospice Palliative Care 1999;16:573–582.
33. Tilly J, Weiner J. Medicaid and end of life care. State initatives in end of life care. Kansas City: Midwest BioEthics Center, 2001.
34. Semradek J, Gammoth L. Prologue to the future. In: Gammoth LM, Semradek J, Tomquist EM, eds. Enchancing Autonomy in Long-term Care: Concepts and Strategies. New York: Springer, 1997.
35. Wilson SA, Kovach CR, Stearns S. Hospice concepts in the care for persons with end-stage dementia. Geriatr Nurs 1996;17:6–10.
36. Weinrich C. Spiritual needs of the dying. In: Wilson SA, Daley BJ, eds. Fostering Humane Care of Dying Persons in Long-Term Care: A Guidebook for Staff Development Instructors. Milwaukee: Marquette University Press, 1997:28.
37. Kovach CR, Wilson SA, Noonan PE. The effects of hospice interventions on behaviors, discomfort, and physical complication of end-stage dementia nursing home residents. Am J Alzheimers Dis Other Demen 1996;11(4):7–15.
38. Rosenthal NE, Wehr TA. Towards understanding the mechanism of action of light in seasonal affective disorder. Pharmacopsychiatry 1992;25:1–62.
39. Rosenthal NE. Diagnosis and treatment of seasonal affective disorder. JAMA 1993;270:217–221.

41

Paula Milone-Nuzzo and Ruth McCorkle

Home Care

I always thought I would want to continue fighting if I had a diagnosis of a terminal illness. Last year, I was diagnosed with terminal lung cancer. The most important thing on my mind was being able to manage the pain. I was less concerned about the disease than the pain. The nurses helped me to manage my pain effectively while being alert enough to interact with and enjoy my family. I am so grateful to have their support.—A terminal cancer patient

- ***Key Points***
- *Home care for terminal patients can be used to improve their quality of life. Often, home care interventions can be provided on a short-term basis when clients experience a crisis that needs focused interventions.*
- *Nurses are the leaders and essential members of the home care team. Advanced practice nurses can have an impact on the cost and quality of care provided to terminally ill patients.*
- *Patients with complex problems need family caregivers who are taught to provide care in the home. Caregiving can be extremely stressful for family members and may adversely effect the health of the caregiver. Home care providers should assist family caregivers to maintain their health.*
- *Palliative home care should be provided by a team of providers, including physicians, mental health workers, therapists, nurses, and paraprofessionals.*

Originally, palliative care in home care nursing was associated with patients who were clearly near the end of life. The contemporary philosophy of palliative care had its beginnings in England in 1967, when Dame Cicely Saunders founded St. Christopher's Hospice. Home and respite care continue to be a major component of that program. Palliative care, by definition, focuses on the multidimensional aspects of patients and families, including physical, psychological, social, spiritual, and interpersonal components of care. These components of care need to be instituted throughout all phases of the illness trajectory and not only at the point when patients qualify for hospice services. Palliative care also needs to be given across a variety of settings and not be limited to inpatient units.

The primary purpose of palliative care is to enhance the quality and meaning of life and death for both patients and loved ones. To date, health professionals have not used the potential of palliative care to maximize the quality of life of patients in their homes. In this chapter, we discuss home care as an environment that provides unique opportunities to promote palliative care for patients and families throughout their illnesses. The chapter gives background information on what home care is, its historical roots, the types of providers available to give services, the regulatory policies controlling its use, examples of models of palliative home care programs, and recommendations to professionals for facilitating the use of home care in palliative care, concluding with a case study illustrating key elements of palliative care provision in the home.

Historical Perspective on Home Care Nursing

The period spanning the middle of the 20th century, during which patients were routinely cared for in acute care hospitals, may turn out to have been but a brief period in medical history. Before that time, patients were cared for primarily at home by their families. Today social and economic forces are interacting to avoid hospitalization if possible and to return patients home quickly if hospitalized. Although at face value these changes seem positive, they have highlighted gaps and deficiencies in the current health care delivery system.

Scientific advances have allowed us to keep patients with diseases such as cancer alive increasingly longer despite complex and chronic health problems. The burden of their care usually falls on families, who often are not adequately prepared to handle the physically and emotionally demanding needs for care that are inherent in chronic and progressive illnesses. In addition, family members often become primary care providers within the context of other demands, such as employment outside the home and competing family roles. The necessity among most of the nation's family members to assume employment outside the home and to alter those arrangements when faced with a sick relative has created an immeasurable strain on physical, emotional, and financial resources. The increasing responsibilities of the family in providing care in the face of limited external support and the consequences of that caregiving for patient and family raise important challenges for clinicians.[1]

The origins of home care are found in the practice of visiting nursing, which had its beginnings in the United States in the late 1800s. The modern concept of providing nursing care in the home was established by William Rathbone of Liverpool, England, in 1859. Rathbone, a wealthy businessman and philanthropist, set up a system of visiting nursing after a personal experience, when nurses cared for his wife at home before her death. In 1859, with the help of Florence Nightingale, he started a school to train visiting nurses at the Liverpool Infirmary, the graduates of which focused on helping the "sick poor" in their homes.[2]

As in England, caring for the ill in their homes in the United States focused, from its inception, on the poor. Compared to the upper and middle class who received frequent visits from the family physician, either in their homes or in the hospital pay wards, treatment of the sick poor seemed careless at best. Visiting nurse associations (VNAs) in the United States were established by groups of people who wanted to assist the poor to improve their health. During 1885 and 1886, visiting nurse services developed in Buffalo, New York, Boston, and Philadelphia that focused on caring for the middle-class sick as well as the sick poor.[2]

During World War II, as physicians made fewer home visits and focused instead on patients who came to their offices and were admitted to hospitals, the home care movement grew, with nurses providing most of the health and illness care in the home. Up until the mid-1960s, not-for-profit VNAs were developed in major cities, small towns, and counties throughout the United States. Under their auspices, nurses focused on providing health services to women and infants and illness care to the poor in their homes, while most acute care was provided to patients in hospitals.

The face of home care in the United States changed dramatically with the passage of an amendment to the Social Security Act that enacted Medicare in 1965. Home care changed from almost exclusively care for well mothers and children and the sick poor to a program that focused on care of the sick elderly in their homes. In 1967, there were 1753 home care agencies, a large percentage of which were not-for-profit VNAs. In 2003, more than 35 years later, there were 7265 home care agencies, with the largest percentage of agencies represented by the proprietary sector.[3] Not only did the types of agencies change, the acuity of patients increased and the development of technology allowed for the delivery of highly complex care in the home setting. The structural changes in the health care delivery system associated with the passage of the Medicare legislation in 1965 provided the foundation for the contemporary practice of home care nursing in the United States.

The 1990s brought a new challenge, managed care, to health care in general and home care specifically in the United States. The most significant impact of managed care on home care was a decline in the number of visits allowed per patient per episode of illness. The result was a decline in the amount of home care patients received, causing a stabilization of the rapid growth in the home care delivery system. The American Balanced Budget Act of 1997 (PL 105–33) mandated the implementation of a prospective payment system for home care for Medicare beneficiaries. In this system, home care agencies receive a designated dollar amount per episode of illness to provide care for a Medicare patient based on the patient's admitting diagnosis and other factors related to physical and functional status. Just as the Diagnostic Related Group (DRG) system caused a significant decline in the number of hospital beds in the 1980s, the prospective payment system for home care has resulted in significant shrinkage of the home health care industry due to patients receiving fewer visits per episode of illness.

Definition of Home Care Nursing

Home care, home health care, and home care nursing can be confusing terms to both providers and consumers, because they are often used interchangeably. Numerous definitions of home care have been provided by the many professional and trade associations that address home care issues (National Association for Home Care, Consumer's Union, American Hospital Association, American Medical Association, Health Care Financing Administration, etc.). Common to all the definitions is the recognition that home care is care of the sick in the home by professionals and paraprofessionals, with the goal to improve health, enhance comfort, and improve the quality of life of clients. Home care nursing is defined here as:

> . . . the provision of nursing care to acute and chronically ill patients of all ages in their home while integrating community health nursing principles that focus on the environmental, psychosocial, economic, cultural, and personal health factors affecting an individual's and family's health status.[4]

Home Care Use in the United States

Home care is a diverse industry that provides a broad scope of care to patients of all ages. In 2000, it was estimated that slightly less than 8 million people received home care services for acute illness, long-term health conditions, permanent disability, and terminal illness.[5] Although home care is provided to a large number of people, it still represents a very small percentage of national health care expenditures. Home care represented only 3% of the total national health expenditure in 2000, while hospital care consumed 40% and physician services 22%,[5] demonstrating the cost-efficient nature of home care practice.

The majority of patients (67.5%) who received home care were discharged primarily to urban home care agencies.[6] As the reimbursement for home care visits decreases and the cost of home visiting in rural areas increases because of increased travel time, many rural home care agencies have been forced to close, limiting access to home care for the population in the region. The federal government has been inconsistent in its payment of the "rural add-on" to home care agencies who provide care in rural settings.

The demographic picture of home health care recipients shows a predominately female (64.8%) and white (75.8%) population. The majority (70.5%) of home care patients are 65 years of age and over, although home care is provided to patients of all ages, from birth to death. The most common primary diagnosis for home care patients is diseases of the circulatory system, most often heart disease. Other common primary diagnoses of patients receiving home care are diseases of the musculoskeletal system and connective tissue, diabetes mellitus, diseases of the respiratory system, injury, and poisoning. A primary diagnosis of malignant neoplasm represents only 5% of home health care patients, while it accounts for 52% of all patients in hospice.[6] Clearly, nonhospice home care has not been used adequately as an integral part of care for cancer patients and families as they endure the physical and emotional demands of complex cancer treatments and move across the acute, chronic, and terminal phases of their disease. This is an ideal context in which the need for palliative care should drive an increased use of home care services.

Types of Home Care Providers

Home care providers are traditionally characterized as either formal or informal caregivers. Informal caregivers are those family members and friends who provide care in the home and are unpaid. It is estimated that almost three-quarters of the elderly with multiple comorbidities and severe disabilities who receive home care rely on family members or other sources of unpaid assistance. More than 75% of those providing informal home care are female, and nearly 33% are more than 65 years of age. Eighty percent of informal caregivers provide assistance 4 hours per day, 7 days per week.[7] The type of care provided by informal caregivers ranges from routine custodial care, such as bathing, to sophisticated skilled care, including tracheostomy care and intravenous medication administration. Informal caregivers assume a considerable physiological, psychological, and economic burden in the care of their significant other in the home. When layered on top of existing responsibilities, caregiver tasks compete for time, energy, and attention. As a result, caregivers frequently describe themselves as emotionally and physically drained.[8] In a qualitative study of 15 family caregivers, Strang and Koop[9] found that several factors facilitated or interfered with caregiver coping. One factor that interfered with caregiver coping is the competence of the formal caregiver. When formal caregivers were less than competent, they added to rather than reduced the caregiving burden. The economic cost of providing informal care in the home also places a significant burden on caregivers. With the shift toward community-based care, a number of costs have shifted to the patient and caregiver. Out-of-pocket financial expenditures include medications, transportation, home medical equipment, supplies, and respite services.[10] These costs are nonreimbursable and often invisible but are very real to families who are trying to provide care on a fixed income.

Formal caregivers are those professionals and paraprofessionals who are compensated for the in-home care they provide. In 1998, an estimated 662,000 persons were employed in home health agencies. In home care, nurses represent 36% of the formal caregivers providing care to patients in Medicare-certified home care agencies. Home health aides also represent a large proportion of the formal caregivers in home care and are expected to increase in number in the upcoming years.[11] The professionals and paraprofessionals who represent the range of home care providers in home health agencies are described in Table 41–1.

Reimbursement Mechanisms

Home health services are reimbursed by both commercial and government third-party payers as well as by private individuals. Government third-party payers include Medicare, Medicaid, CHAMPUS, and the Veterans Administration system. These government programs have specific requirements that must be met for the coverage of services. Commercial third-party payers include insurance companies, health maintenance organizations (HMOs), preferred provider organizations (PPOs), and case management programs. Commercial insurers often allow for more flexibility in their requirements than Medicare. For example, the home care nurse may negotiate with an insurance company to obtain needed services for the patient on the basis of the cost-effectiveness of the home care plan, even though that service may not be routinely covered.

Table 41–1
Types of Providers in Home Care

Type of Provider	Role and Responsibilities
Nurses	
Registered nurses (RNs)	Deliver skilled care to patients in the home. Considered to be the coordinator of care.
Licensed practical nurses (LPNs)	Deliver routine care to patients under the direction of a registered nurse.
Advanced practice nurses (APNs)	Coordinate total patient care to complex patients, supervise other nurses in difficult cases related to their speciality, develop special programs, and negotiate for reimbursement of services. Teach patients and caregivers special skills and knowledge
Therapists	
Physical therapists	Deliver skilled care that includes assessment for assistive devices in the home. Perform therapy procedures with the patient, and teach the patient and family to assist in treatment. Assist patient to improve mobility.
Occupational therapists	Focus on improving physical, mental, and social functioning. Rehabilitation of the upper body and improvement of fine motor ability
Speech therapists	Rehabilitation of patients with speech and swallowing problems
Respiratory therapists	Provide support to patients using respiratoryhome medical equipment such as ventilators. Perform professional respiratory therapy treatments.
Other Clinical Staff	
Social workers	Help patients and families identify needs and refer to community agencies. Assist with applications for community-based services and provide financial assitance information.
Dietitians	Provide diet counseling to patients with special nutritional needs. Direct service of a dietitian is not a reimbursable service in home care.
Paraprofessionals	
Home health aides	Perform personal care, basic nursing tasks (as opposed to skilled), and incidental homemaking.
Homemakers	Perform housekeeping and chores to ensure a safe and healthy home care environment.

Medicare

Medicare is a federal insurance program for the elderly (65 and over), the permanently disabled, and persons with end-stage renal disease in the United States, and is the single largest payer for home health services. To be eligible for this program, an individual or spouse must have paid into Social Security. Medicare is a federal program and, as such, the benefits are the same from state to state. The Centers of Medicare and Medicaid Services (CMS) (formerly called Health Care Financing Administration [HCFA]), a department in the federal government, regulates payments for services under Medicare. The rules developed by CMS that guide the Medicare program are detailed in the Health Insurance Manual-11 (HIM–11). CMS contracts with insurance companies called fiscal intermediaries (FIs) to process Medicare claims that are submitted from home care agencies.

Since agencies are now reimbursed using a prospective payment methodology, home care has gained increased flexibility for the services provided under Medicare. In the former fee-for-service model, designated and specific home care providers were paid for each visit made. Today, home care agencies are responsible for assuring that the patients achieve their health outcomes in the most efficient manner. If a home care agency believes the most effective plan of care would be to integrate alternative and complementary therapies, or mental heath therapy into a patient's plan of care, it will not reduce or increase the amount of payment received from the government.

There are five criteria, summarized in Table 41–2, that a patient must meet for home care services to be reimbursed by Medicare.

Medicare is the main payer of hospice services in the United States under the Medicare Hospice Benefit, which Congress first enacted as part of Medicare Part A in 1982 under the Tax Equity and Fiscal Responsibility Act (TEFRA; P.L. 97–248). The law was in effect from 1983 to 1986, when Congress made hospice a permanent part of the Medicare program.[12] The impetus behind Medicare's hospice benefit came from the recognition that the regulations and restrictions for traditional Medicare were not well suited to meet the needs of terminally ill patients.

Medicare hospice was designed primarily as a home care benefit that included an array of services to assist care providers in the clinical management of the terminally ill in the home.[4] However, the regulations for hospice care also require home care providers to have in-patient hospice beds available for terminally ill patients who are unable to remain in their homes. Recognizing that hospice is a philosophy of care rather than a place for care, it seems appropriate that hospice care is given in a variety of settings.

In order for a patient to elect the Hospice Medicare benefit, the patient must waive the traditional Medicare benefit. By electing the Hospice Medicare benefit, the patient is acknowledging the terminal nature of the illness and opting no longer to have curative treatment.

Medicaid

Medicaid is an assistance program for the poor, some disabled persons, and children. Unlike Medicare, Medicaid is jointly sponsored by the federal government and the individual states. Therefore, Medicaid coverage varies from state to state. These differences can often be dramatic and in some cases dependent on the state's financial solvency. Eligibility for Medicaid is based on income and assets and is not contingent on any previous payments to the federal or state governments.

Unlike the requirements of the Medicare program, Medicaid covers both skilled and unskilled care in the home and usually does not require that the recipient be homebound. To qualify for the home care benefits under Medicaid, patients must meet income eligibility requirements, have a plan of care signed by a physician, and the plan of care must be reviewed by a physician every 60 days.

Commercial Insurance

Many commercial insurance companies are involved in health insurance for individuals or groups. These local or national

Table 41–2
Criteria for Home Care Reimbursement Under Medicare

Criterion	Description
Homebound	A patient is considered homebound if absences from the home are rare and of short duration and attributable to the need to receive medical treatments.
Completed plan of care	A plan of care for home care services must be completed on Health Care Financing Administrating (HCFA) forms 485, 486, and 487. The plan of care must be signed by a physician.
Skilled service	Medicare defines a skilled service as one provided by a registered nurse, physical therapist, or speech therapist. Skilled nursing services include skilled observation and assessment, teaching, direct care and management, and evaluation of the plan of care.
Intermittent and part-time	Part-time means that skilled care and home health aide services combined may not exceed 8 hours per day or 28 hours per week. Intermittent means that skilled care is provided or needed on fewer than 7 days per week or less than 8 hours of each day for periods of 21 days or less, with extensions for exceptional circumstances.
Reasonable and necessary	The services provided must be reasonable for the patient given the diagnosis and necessary to assist the patient to achieve the expected outcomes.

companies often write policies that include a home care benefit. Commercial insurers often cover the same services covered by Medicare in addition to preventive, private duty, and supportive services, such as a home health aide or homemaker. Commercial insurance companies cover patients of all ages, including Medicare patients with supplemental insurance policies that cover health care expenditures not reimbursed by Medicare.

Supplemental insurance policies are a source of confusion and anxiety among home care patients, often when families are under increased stress due to the complexity of the health situation for one of its members. Nurses should encourage families to carefully review the specifics of the supplemental insurance policy, including copays, annual review of benefits, anticipated out-of-pocket costs, and pharmacy costs. Families should recognize that when changing a supplemental insurance carrier, you may also have to change the home care provider, since some supplemental policies state which home care provider will be reimbursed for services.

Commercial insurance often includes a maximum lifetime benefit as part of the policy. The high cost of high-technology care forces a growing number of patients to reach this maximum rather quickly and face the loss of coverage. This has resulted in the development of case-management programs administered by insurance companies. The case manager projects the long-term needs and costs of care for the patient and develops a plan with the patient to meet those needs in a cost-efficient manner. Consideration is given to the life expectancy of the patient in relationship to the maximum lifetime benefit.

Unlike the Medicare program, in which negotiation for services is not an option, it may be important for home care nurses to identify the needed services for a patient with a commercial insurance plan and intervene to obtain funding for those services. When working with an insurance case manager, the home care nurse must be specific about the services the patient will need, the overall cost of those services, and the expected outcome related to the services requested. The more precisely the home care nurse can portray the impact of the care plan on the patient outcomes with objective data, the more inclined the case manager will be to authorize services. Insurance companies are very concerned with the satisfaction of their enrollees. Patients and families should be empowered to make their voices heard about the services they need to remain safe in the home. If out-of-network services or special pricing is negotiated with the insurance case manager, written documentation of the agreement should be included in the patient's record. Ideally, the patient should be given a copy of this agreement in the event that any disputes over payment occur.

The Home Health–Hospice Connection

In order for a patient to receive the full array of hospice services under Medicare, the care must be provided by a certified hospice provider. To be reimbursed, home care agencies that are not certified hospice providers must refer their terminally ill patients to an agency that carries the certification. This regulation affects clinical care in several ways. Home care nurses have a long history of developing strong and intimate bonds with patients and families. As patients progress toward the terminal phase of their illnesses, it is emotionally difficult for home care nurses to refer their patients to hospice providers. At times, it is equally as difficult for a family to accept the referral, knowing that they will have to give up "their nurse." The home care nurse and the family may believe that the relationship that has developed among the patient, the family, and the home care nurse is more important than any additional benefits the hospice might bring.

The greater flexibility in traditional Medicare regulations that came with the resolution of the Duggan vs. Bohan case[13] in 1988 has allowed nonhospice home care agencies to provide extended nursing and home health aide services for patients in the terminal phase of illness. In this legal case, a group of home care agencies challenged the HCFA (now CMS) regarding their strict interpretation of the Medicare regulation on patient qualifications for part-time intermittent care. The suit was won by the home care agencies, requiring HCFA to be more generous in interpreting Medicare regulations. Although families may feel that they are getting sufficient home care, they are not able to take advantage of the prescription drug components of the hospice benefit, which may result in significant financial burden. They also usually do not receive the supportive services, such as pastoral care and bereavement follow-up, that are integral to the hospice program. Because the emotional impact of the patient's death is unknown at the time the patient makes the decision to forego a hospice referral, it is impossible to predict the significance of a service such as bereavement follow-up. Because both the nonhospice home health agency and the hospice provider offer important services, especially nursing care to patients at the end of life, strengthening mechanisms that facilitate transitions between these two types of services is essential. See Chapter 2 for a comprehensive discussion of the hospice admission criteria, including the certification by the physician of a terminal diagnosis and the 6th-month rule.

Cancer as a Prototype for Home Care Use in Palliative Care

Over the years, cancer has shifted from a terminal illness to a chronic disease. Even patients with advanced disease and guarded prognoses initially may be treated as if their disease is curable rather than progressive and terminal. Because the philosophical underpinnings and goals of curative and palliative treatments are quite different, approaching an individual who has advanced disease with a curative stance may have long-term negative effects on physical, social, and emotional functions that ultimately affect the patient's quality of life. Characteristics of advanced cancer that require coordinated palliative care include multiple physical needs, intense emotional distress manifested by anxiety and depression, and complex patient and caregiver needs. The goals of palliative care

are best achieved if care is initiated early on, and one of the most efficient ways of monitoring patients' needs is to coordinate the overall plan of management with home care nursing to decrease fragmentation and promote continuity.

Needs of Cancer Patients

Because of the growing trend to discharge hospitalized patients early, the increasing use of ambulatory care services, and the increasing use of complex therapies, the need for ongoing monitoring and instruction of patients and families has never been greater. Family members, often without the assistance of any formal home care services, are assuming primary responsibility for the care of patients at home.[14–17] This demand on families is not new, although the caregiver role has changed dramatically from promoting convalescence to providing high-technology care and psychological support in the home. Members of a patient's family are of vital importance in meeting the patient's physical and psychosocial needs and accomplishing treatment goals.[18,19] The burden of caring for patients with a diagnosis of cancer, however, may adversely affect families who lack adequate resources or who are insufficiently prepared for this new, complex role. There is mounting evidence that changes in family roles and the burden placed on family caregivers may have negative effects on the quality of life of both cancer patients and their caregivers,[17] particularly during advanced stages of cancer.

Research to identify patient-defined home care needs began in the 1980s and has increased steadily since the 1990s. Evidence suggests that both patients and their families benefit from home care services directed at physical and psychological concerns. An early study[20] identified pain, sleep, and elimination management as major patient needs. Wellisch and his colleagues[21] investigated the types and frequency of problems experienced by two separate groups of seriously ill cancer patients and their families in their homes in the Los Angeles area and explored the types of interventions that helped to reduce the problems. The five most frequent problem categories identified included somatic side effects, including pain; patient mood disturbance; equipment/technology problems; family relationship impairment; and patient cognitive impairment. Interventions reported to be effective included reinforcement to the patient and family, no intervention, and counseling and emotional support. They noted that patients with cognitive deficits had special needs, and their family members were at high risk for ongoing problems.

In Pennsylvania, Houts and colleagues[22] found that the unmet needs of patients with cancer included assistance with emotional problems, transportation, finances, and interactions with medical staff. Wingate and Lackey[23] identified the needs of patients and primary caregivers in the home and compared the priorities between the two. Both identified their psychological distress as their highest priority. For patients, physical and informational needs were next. For caregivers, household management needs, which included direct patient care, were second, followed by informational needs. McCorkle and colleagues[24] followed 233 cancer patients for 6 months after they were hospitalized. Half of the patients were newly diagnosed (n = 115); the other half had had their cancers for more than a year. Patients were discharged with a range of complex problems, including unrelieved symptoms (pain, fatigue, dyspnea, poor appetite), wound care, feeding devices, elimination devices, intravenous medication administration, and other highly technical procedures, such as tracheostomies. The majority of these patients were followed as out-patients and not referred to formal home care services for monitoring, despite their ongoing needs, primarily because they were under 65 years of age. Evers and colleagues[25] assessed whether the needs of younger patients differed from the palliative care needs and experiences of older adults. They found significant differences across age groups on clinical characteristics, advance care planning, and service use. Patients over age 80 had a reduced prevalence of cancer, a higher prevalence of dementia and incapacity, more frequent decisions to withhold life-sustaining treatments, and fewer interventions for symptom management.

Needs of Caregivers

A number of studies have identified the needs of patients and family members who provide care to patients with cancer. A study by Grobe and colleagues[26] described what information was provided to 87 patients in the advanced stages of cancer and their caregivers. This study revealed that families perceived that little, if any, education was provided to them. Hinds[27] conducted a study examining the perceived needs of 83 family caregivers who reported they felt inadequately prepared to provide care for their sick relatives in the home and identified numerous information and skill deficits. Morris and Thomas[28] identified that caregivers are often "tacked on" to patients and seen as co-clients, but unfortunately are not fully recognized and, consequently, do not receive appropriate information or are not taught the skills to provide care to loved ones. Siegel and colleagues[29,30] divided caregiving tasks into categories of personal care, instrumental tasks, and transportation. Each of these areas was associated with greater caregiver demands as patients' physiological factors worsened or if their caregivers associated their care with a high level of burden.

Oberst and colleagues[31] assessed the demands on cancer caregivers, including their perceptions of providing care in the home environment. Caregivers reported that the majority of their time was spent providing transportation, giving emotional support, and maintaining the household. More than one third of the caregivers reported a lack of assistance from health professionals in providing care. In addition, demands on the caregivers escalated as the treatment regimen progressed. Another study lends support to the sense of isolation and the stressful nature of caregiving in that 85% of a sample of cancer caregivers failed to use available resources to assist them in caregiving activities. In addition, 77% of the caregivers reported increased stress, and 28% required medication to help them cope with the burden associated with caregiving.[32]

These accounts present persuasive documentation that caring for a person with cancer is a stressful experience and can have major emotional and physical consequences for caregivers.

In their review of caregiver research, Sales and colleagues[33] concluded that a significant number of cancer caregivers exhibit psychological distress and physical symptoms. Predictors of caregiver distress included a number of patient-related variables, including more advanced stages of cancer, disability, and complex care needs. Given and colleagues[34,35] reported that patients' distress associated with their symptoms, poor mobility, and increased dependency with instrumental activities were linked to significant burdens for family caregivers. They designed a study to test the impact of a 16-week nursing intervention on depressive symptoms of caregivers of patients newly diagnosed with cancer. One hundred twenty-five patient caregiver dyads were recruited and 89 completed the study. The nursing intervention delivered to the experimental group consisted of symptom management and monitoring, education, emotional support, coordination of services, and caregiver preparation to care. Nurses made five home visits and four telephone calls over time. The intervention was effective in slowing the rate of depressive symptoms rather than decreasing the levels of depression in these caregivers. They concluded that the caregivers with higher levels of depression were the ones who withdrew from the study, limiting their effects of the intervention.[36]

Similarly, Carter[37] described sleep and depressive symptoms in 47 caregivers of patients with advanced cancer and found severe fluctuations in sleep patterns. Caregivers reported they suffered progressive sleep deprivation that affected their emotions and ability to continue as caregivers. In another study, caregivers reported that they perceived discomfort in their loved ones who were unresponsive as death was imminent and consequently were at increased risk for psychological problems after the patients' deaths.[38]

In general, the literature on the needs of cancer patients and caregivers of cancer patients highlights: (1) that patients are increasingly being treated in ambulatory clinics and have ongoing, unmet complex care needs with little or no use of home or palliative care referrals; (2) that caregivers are assuming more and more responsibility for monitoring patients' status and providing direct care in the home with no opportunities for respite; (3) that caregivers have a high proportion of unmet needs themselves; (4) that the caregiving experience encompasses both positive and negative elements; and, (5) that the conceptualization of caregiver burden is linked to negative reactions to caregiving.

Models of Palliative Home Care Programs

A number of studies have tested interventions to develop models for palliative home care.[39] Both patients and their caregivers have served as subjects of these studies. Some examples are highlighted.

Patient Programs

Hinton[40] questioned whether home care can maintain an acceptable quality of life for patients with terminal cancer and their relatives. He defined quality-of-life outcomes to include mood, attitude to condition, perceived help, and preferred place of care. The study included 77 randomly selected patients followed by the hospice palliative home care service at St. Christopher's Hospice in England. Overall, the results were extremely positive. Patients' physical symptoms were tolerable, caregivers' depression and anxiety were limited, and the majority of care provided in the home (90%) was complemented by hospitalizations for 1 to 3 days (30%) or longer (41%). Treatment was usually praised by relatives, and at follow-up, relatives approved where patients had received care and had died. In countries other than the United States, home care is an integral part of well-planned palliative care, and a number of palliative home care programs have demonstrated positive patient and caregiver outcomes.

The most recognized model of palliative home care was developed at St. Christopher's Hospice, yet programs in other countries have been equally committed, including programs in the United Kingdom,[41] Canada,[42] Sweden,[43–45] and Italy.[46,47] These programs included hospice-like services, but, more importantly, they were targeted at symptom management and not limited to imminent dying and death. They also encompassed the care of the patient and the family and facilitated transitions from hospitals to homes. In the authors' opinion, the main reasons these programs have been successful have been not only the commitment and passion of nurses, but also the involvement of physicians who recognize their interdisciplinary role in the palliative care component of patients' diseases, and the government reimbursement systems.

In the United States, some attempts have been made by other than traditional home health agencies to integrate palliative care into home nursing care. Martinson's[48,49] seminal study of facilitating the management and death of children in rural Minnesota after discharge from an urban medical center demonstrated that families wanted and assumed the responsibility to provide necessary care with supervision of the specialty nurses from the medical center. Much of the teaching and instruction was provided to families over the telephone.

Yates and his colleagues[50] designed a study to compare two groups of patients with advanced cancer who were treated in rural Vermont. The patients were paired based on population density, distance from the medical center, socioeconomic status, local medical facilities, referral patterns, and local social service resources. The groups were divided into intensive and nonintensive groups. The intensive group received regular home visits by nurse practitioners, and the nonintensive group was not visited by nurses. Both groups received the same multidisciplinary care from the Vermont Regional Cancer Center and monitoring of cancer status through the ambulatory cancer clinic. A total of 199 patients (98 in the intensive group and 101 in the nonintensive group) were followed, and at the end of the 4-year study 139 patients had died. The results were very positive in demonstrating that patients in the intensive group fared better overall than those in the nonintensive group. They demonstrated less need for medical care at the cancer center and greater independence over the course of the study than those in the nonintensive group. Most striking, the home nursing interventions improved individual patient pain management. The authors found that physicians often prescribed pain medications without follow-up monitoring of patient status, whereas the home nurses were vigilant in monitoring patients' comfort. The nurses also improved patient and family negotiations for available community resources. Although the study failed to show a survival difference between the two groups, the researchers did demonstrate cost-effective outcomes. The study demonstrated a decrease in the overall cost of care by facilitating a greater number of home deaths in the intensive group. They concluded that cost savings occurred without sacrifice of patient well-being and with concomitant advantages in patient pain management.

In a statewide study of home care use patterns among cancer patients in Illinois, physicians were found, in general, to be the primary source of patient referral to home health services. More than two thirds of the sample were referred to home services for the purpose of monitoring health status, more often for postsurgical than postmedical treatment effects.[51] Oncology clinical nurse specialists served as consultants to staff nurses in home health agencies in rural Illinois. Both staff and patients reported satisfaction with this model of care delivery. The clinical specialists spent a majority of their time teaching the nurses specific skills and were readily available by telephone to both staff and patients.

McCorkle and her colleagues have completed several studies to test the role of the advanced practice nurse (APN) on patient outcomes in home nursing care.[52,53] The first randomized controlled trial was completed in 1986 to assess the effects of home nursing care on either an oncology home care group (OHC) that received care from oncology home care nurses, a standard home care group (SHC) that received care from home care nurses without oncology training, or an office care group (OC) that received whatever care they needed except home care. One hundred sixty-six patients with lung cancer were entered into the study 2 months after diagnosis and followed for an additional 6 months. Participants experienced significant differences in symptom distress and functional abilities. The two home nursing care groups remained less distressed and more independent 6 weeks longer than the office care group. The home nursing care assisted patients in minimizing distress from symptoms and maintaining their independence longer, in comparison to patients who received no home nursing care. As part of the study, the effects of the three groups (OHC, SHC, and OC) were tested on the spouses' psychological distress during the bereavement period.[54] Of the 100 spouses who participated in the study, 46 patients died. Spouses of the deceased patients were followed for 25 months after the death. Spouses of patients in the OHC group were taught to provide direct care to their loved ones and to sit to be present through the living–dying transition.[55] The OHC nurses served as central coordinators for care and were available 24 hours a day to answer questions, problem solve, and respond to crisis. Spouses' psychological distress was significantly lower 6 months after the patients' deaths and sustained over time in the group cared for by the oncology home care nurses.[54] Findings suggested that the bereaveds' psychological distress was positively influenced and their recovery was hastened by the nursing interventions provided during the terminal phase of illness.[54]

In a second study, McCorkle and her colleagues followed 233 patients who were discharged from seven hospitals with complex care problems requiring home care services. The patients were diagnosed with eight different solid tumors and followed for 6 months. Although all these patients could have benefited from home care, only about half were referred to home care. Patients receiving home care demonstrated improvement in their symptoms, function, and mental health status compared with patients who did not receive home care. Results aided in identifying interventions to help with specific problems related to cancer and treatment effects and were standardized to be tested in a third study.[24]

In the third study, McCorkle and colleagues[56] tested the effect of a standardized nursing intervention protocol (SNIP) on postsurgical cancer patients' outcomes. This study compared the length of survival of postsurgical cancer patients who received specialized home care intervention by APNs after their surgery to the length of survival of those who received the usual follow-up care in ambulatory settings. One hundred ninety patients (50.7%) were in the intervention group and 185 (49.3%) in the usual care group. Patients in the control group received standard postoperative care in the hospital and routine follow-up in outpatient surgical clinics upon discharge. The home care intervention was designed to enhance recovery from surgery and to improve quality-of-life outcomes. The intervention was developed as a protocol that consisted of standard assessment and management guidelines, doses of content, and schedules of contacts. APNs followed specific guidelines to assess and monitor the physical, emotional, and functional status of patients; provided direct care when needed; assisted in obtaining services or other resources from the community; and provided teaching, counseling, and support during the recovery period. Nurses also functioned as liaisons to health care settings and providers, as well as to patients and families in the provision of technical and psychological support.

At the completion of the study, 93 (24.8%) patients had died. Of these, 41 (44%) were from the intervention group and 52 (56%) from the usual care group. For all patients who died, causes of death were documented. Cancer was listed either as the primary or secondary cause on all death certificates. Other causes listed were pulmonary embolus, heart failure, sepsis, and cardiac arrest. Patients receiving the home care intervention had a longer length of survival than the control group. During the first 3 months after discharge, a total of eight patients in the control group died, and one patient from the intervention group died. The intervention, occurring over a period of 4 weeks immediately after surgery and hospitalization, corresponded to a period when the difference in mortality rate between the intervention and control groups was the largest. The combination of physical care and psychosocial support during the acute postoperative period addressed two critical issues. The first was to assist patients and families during the period of transition from hospital to home and to offer education, guidance, and reassurance during high psychological distress and uncertainty. The second was to monitor patients' physical status and offset potential lethal complications that were most prevalent in the acute postoperative period. This study supports the importance of such nursing interventions during the critical diagnostic and surgical treatment phases and is clearly defined within the realm of palliative care, since many of these patients were diagnosed as late-stage.[56]

As part of the third study, Jepson and colleagues[57] examined changes in the psychosocial status of caregivers of postsurgical cancer patients after the patients' discharge. Within a week after being discharged from the hospital, patients were randomly assigned to either the treatment or control condition. Patients in the treatment group received a standardized home care intervention over 4 weeks. The intervention was provided by APNs and consisted of three home visits and six telephone calls. The nursing interventions included problem assessment; monitoring of the patient's condition; symptom management; and teaching caregivers how to problem solve, administer medications, and provide self-care behaviors. Psychosocial status was measured using the Caregiver Reaction Assessment.[35] Overall, caregivers' psychosocial status improved from discharge to 3 months and stabilized thereafter; however, among caregivers with physical problems, the psychosocial status of both patients and caregivers in the treatment group declined over time compared to those in the control group. The researchers concluded that caregivers of cancer patients who have their own physical problems are at risk for psychological morbidity as they assume the caregiving role. They recommended that the health of the caregiver be considered as an essential criteria for the caregiver to assume primary responsibility for the patient's care at home. In the event the caregiver has a compromised health status, then formal home care services are needed.[57] Bradley[58] also recommended that assessments must include caregiver health needs and that for home health care to be effective, nurses must conduct caregiver assessments to identify needs that could impair their caregiving abilities.

Naylor and colleagues[59] studied the effects of comprehensive discharge planning and home visitation by APNs with a population of elderly patients hospitalized for specific medical and surgical problems, including heart disease, orthopedic procedures, and bowel surgery. Some of these patients had cancer diagnoses. The intervention group received standardized comprehensive discharge planning specific for elderly persons at high risk of poor postdischarge outcomes, APN home visits, and telephone calls. The intervention benefitted from the clinical experience of APNs and their abilities in communicating, coordinating, and collaborating with physicians. Outcomes included hospitalization rates, days in the hospital, time to first readmission, functional status, level of depression, patient satisfaction with care, and overall cost of postindex hospitalization health services. Patients in the intervention group were less likely to be readmitted to the hospital, experienced fewer days in the hospital, and had a longer time to the first hospital readmission for any reason. Patients in both groups had improved functional status and depression scores and were satisfied with their care. Overall costs for postindex hospitalization health services for the intervention group were half that of the control group. The results of this study indicated that a comprehensive intervention including home care by an APN has a significant positive effect on patient outcomes and the cost of care for high-risk elderly patients.

Caregiver Programs

There have been a number of programs developed to teach caregivers direct care responsibilities for patients in the home that have had positive outcomes on patients and caregivers.

Ferrell and colleagues[60] examined the impact of cancer pain education on family caregivers of elderly cancer patients. Fifty family caregivers of elderly patients who were at home and experiencing cancer-related pain were recruited for participation in this quasi-experimental study. Outcomes included quality of life, knowledge about pain, and caregiver burden. Caregivers reported significant burden associated with pain management, particularly psychological distress. The pain-education program proved efficacious in improving caregiver knowledge and quality of life. Interventions that teach caregivers to become proficient in the physical aspects of patient care indirectly improve the caregiver's well-being.

A second study that included testing a psychoeducational curriculum intervention was developed by Barg and colleagues.[61] The structured education intervention consisted of 6 to 8 hours of intense educational, skills training, and communication-enhancing strategies, to assist caregivers in being more prepared to care for patients at home. Caregivers reported they were more informed about cancer, its treatment, and symptom control. Part of the content, which focused on expected psychological reactions to cancer and to caregiving, helped normalize distressing emotions that were being experienced by patients and caregivers. These experiences provided a great source of relief for the caregivers. Despite a clear program description and the delineation of measurable outcomes, the researchers reported that a lack of willingness by many cancer caregivers to attend group meetings posed a major obstacle to obtaining a large number of participants. Group-style interventions clearly lend themselves to the study of a self-selected sample. The researchers concluded that caregivers who attended groups most likely were those least in need of intervention, since they demonstrated an ability to use social support and had respite care available, making group attendance possible. Alternatively, individualized strategies are needed to assist caregivers who are unable to participate in groups and feel they cannot leave their loved ones.

In another study, Schumacher and colleagues[62] described the difficulties that patients and family caregivers encountered while participating in a randomized clinical trial related to a nursing pain-control intervention. The intervention group reported they had difficulties in obtaining the prescribed medications, accessing information, tailoring prescribed regimens to meet individual needs, managing side effects, cognitively processing information, managing new or unusual pain, and managing multiple symptoms simultaneously. The researchers concluded that the provision of information about pain management is not adequate to improve pain control in the home, but requires ongoing assistance with problems as they are encountered.

Koop and Strang[63] explored the experience of bereavement following home-based family caregiving of persons with advanced cancer. The caregivers reported both positive and negative outcomes that they attributed to having provided care to their loved one. The positive feelings included feelings of accomplishment and improved family relationships, while the negative feelings included feelings of failure and haunting images of the deceased. Overall positive outcomes outweighed the negative ones and the bereaved family members reported satisfaction with providing care for their loved ones.

Recommendations for Facilitating the Use of Home Care Nursing in Palliative Care

Home care nursing is a logical component of effective palliative care but, for a number of reasons, it has been underused. Patients who need palliative care have complex and often challenging physical and psychological problems. Palliative care for specific types of diseases requires knowledgeable and competent clinicians. It is common for many of the professional staff nurses in home care agencies to lack the knowledge and expertise to manage patients' symptoms and to teach caregivers the skills they need to manage the day-to-day problems they encounter in caregiving. Yet, because of the barriers described to receiving hospice care, home care nurses have to provide much of the palliative care in the community. In addition, for palliative care to be successful in the home, physicians must work collaboratively with nurses and be available to solve problems as they arise. It is often easier for physicians to admit patients to the hospital than to work with home care nurses to keep patients at home.

The state of the science in home care was reviewed for this chapter. Results from these studies have not been systematically incorporated into clinical practice where services are reimbursed. However, we identified critical factors in these studies that, if adopted, could become the basis of successful home care palliative nursing. These include the following:

1. *Staff nurses who are responsible for direct patient care in the home must have contact and access to APNs with specialized knowledge and skills related to the disease-specific needs of patients.* The term "advanced practice nurse" is defined as a professional nurse who has graduated from a master's program in a specialty field such as an oncology advanced practice program, including clinical nurse specialists and nurse practitioners. To assist the staff nurse in dealing with the complexity of palliative care, either a palliative care physician or an APN should serve as a supervisor/consultant to the team and be directly involved in clinical decisions. There may be fewer opportunities for APNs than needed working directly in home care agencies because of the perception that they are too costly to employ. As agencies move to prospective payment and greater efficiency, the role of the APN will factor more prominently in home care agencies. APNs may also work independently and provide care to a group of patients, such as case managers from an ambulatory clinic. As a result of the Balanced Budget Act of 1997 (PL 105–55), APNs, specifically clinical nurse specialists and nurse practitioners, practicing in any setting can be directly reimbursed at 85% of the physician fee schedule for services provided to Medicare beneficiaries. In home care, this change has the potential to facilitate access to care for patients who do not have access to a home care agency or other primary care provider, specifically those in rural and underserved areas.
2. *Because of the barriers to entering hospice care, home care nurses should become knowledgeable and highly skilled in providing palliative care to patients.* This will require not only the development of skills in a new area of clinical expertise but also a paradigm shift in the way home care nurses view the episode of care for home care patients. Home care has traditionally been viewed as a component of the long-term care delivery system. Although the number of home visits per episode of illness has decreased significantly, home visits tend to be spread out over a greater period of time, usually a 60-day certification period. For patients requiring palliation, home care may need to be very intensive over a relatively short period of time (2 to 4 weeks). In this model, the home care nurse can assist the patient and family in methods of managing symptoms and coping with the caregiving role. In the long term, as the patient's disease progresses, the patient and caregivers will need "booster" visits, but the majority of visits and care may be given in short periods of time, when the patient and caregivers are most in need. Telephone visits to provide care have been shown to be an effective strategy for chronic illnesses in which the needs are for support and education. Home care can also be used for short durations in crisis situations. By providing intensive home care for short durations, patients can be helped to address current issues in the most effective way. These short but intensive interventions can improve quality of life

and may also impact survival outcomes for some patients.

3. *Patients are usually hospitalized when symptoms get out of control. When patients are hospitalized, comprehensive discharge planning and follow-up by skilled palliative care nurses is needed to ensure that the plan is implemented, evaluated, and modified as needed.* These nurses may be based in a variety of settings, such as home care agencies, clinics, and private offices. The complexity of symptom management following hospitalization may require the advanced skills of an APN to provide consultation to the palliative care team or to implement a plan of care with a patient and family.
4. *Patients who have complex problems and receive home care nursing need family caregivers who have been taught skills to provide care.* In the event these caregivers are ill themselves, additional or complementary services need to be provided to help with the patients' care. Nurses providing home care for ill patients should conduct ongoing assessments of family caregivers, including their health and demands made upon them. Standardized educational programs to teach family caregivers skills to provide care are needed and should be a part of routine home nursing care.
5. *The use of innovative models must be considered as a strategy for providing care to patients and families.* Telephone visits have been shown to be an effective strategy to help families cope with the caregiver role. Under prospective payment for home care, home care providers are no longer constrained by the per-visit method of reimbursement, and telephone visits can be integrated into the plan of care. The use of alternative and complementary therapy, nutritional counseling or mental health therapies has been made financially reasonable due to the move to prospective payment. Telehealth programs have also been used effectively with patient populations at home. Other technology interventions could include the use of the Internet or E-mail. As the technology becomes less expensive, increased opportunity to implement these strategies will occur.
6. *While nurses are the hub of the palliative care team, professionals from multiple disciplines should provide palliative home care, and physicians must be an integral part of program management.* The multidisciplinary care provided by therapists, nurses, paraprofessionals, and physicians is essential to the development of positive outcomes. Physicians, as members of the multidisciplinary team, must work in collaboration with other professionals to provide comprehensive care to patients and families. Collaboratively, the team determines the amount of care needed, the most appropriate setting for care, and the type of interventions required to improve the quality of life.

A growing number of cancer patients are being discharged from the hospital following surgery or other cancer treatments to be cared for at home by spouses who have chronic illnesses themselves, as described by the following case study.

CASE STUDY

Mr. And Mrs. Rizzi, Patients with Chronic Illnesses

Mr. Rizzi, a 68-year-old Italian retiree, and his wife, Mrs. Rizzi, aged 64, each have a chronic illness. Mr. Rizzi was diagnosed with Stage IIIA non–small-cell lung cancer following 5 months of chest and shoulder pain, fatigue, dyspnea, weight loss, and persistent cough. Despite his medical history, he was physically active until these symptoms, along with his cancer treatment, constrained him. For 50 years before diagnosis, Mr. Rizzi smoked two packs of cigarettes a day. He also had a history of hypertension, osteoarthritis, and a healing duodenal ulcer.

Mrs. Rizzi was a part-time beautician who identified herself as her husband's primary caregiver despite her own comorbidities of hypertension, osteoarthritis, and diabetes. These conditions required regular medical management and caused some physical discomfort and loss of mobility. Mr. Rizzi's treatment included a right upper lobectomy that required chest drainage tubes and subsequent radiation therapy and chemotherapy. He was discharged from the hospital 10 days after surgery. As with many postsurgical patients, Mr. Rizzi went home to be cared for by his wife.

At discharge, Mr. Rizzi's medical care included wound care at the drain site for postsurgical chest tubes and management of symptoms from the disease and from treatment. He was concerned about his ability to recover and anticipated postoperative pain and loss of his independent, active lifestyle. Despite her own chronic illnesses, Mrs. Rizzi reported her overall health as good and considered herself fit to provide home care. She was determined to help her husband with the physical and emotional needs associated with cancer and its treatment. Mrs. Rizzi was unsure of her ability to manage her husband's physical care and doubted her ability to distinguish normal postoperative recovery from more serious complications. She was apprehensive about her new role as manager of the family finances and worried about their ability to pay their bills now that physical limitations prevented part-time employment.

Mr. Rizzi was referred for home care at discharge to the local VNA. This VNA was unique in having an oncology APN on staff to consult with the staff nurses on their cases. Mr. Rizzi's initial assessment visit was conducted within 24 hours following discharge from the hospital. The staff nurse learned that Mr. Rizzi needed wound care and symptom management related to pain control and bowel regimen. She also conducted a family assessment and learned that Mrs. Rizzi had concerns about her role as caregiver. Recognizing the acuity of the problems identified, and after consultation with an APN, the home care nurse scheduled the Rizzis for daily home visits for a week to address the clinical problems of Mr. Rizzi and provide education to Mrs. Rizzi in the caregiver role. Because maintaining the comfort of her husband was Mrs. Rizzi's primary concern, the home care nurse taught her about pain management with medications and alternative comfort measures, such as massage, heat and cold applications, and guided imagery. In addition, the nurse referred the Rizzis to the VNA social worker to assist in dealing with the financial issues associated with Mr. Rizzi's illness. Following the week of intensive home care visits by the nurse, she instituted telephone visits every other day for 2 weeks, followed by weekly telephone calls. Mrs. Rizzi used the telephone calls to discuss changes in her husband's clinical situation and receive advice on how to manage minor clinical problems. They were also a welcome source of support for Mrs. Rizzi as the complexity of the caregiving role increased. As the care of Mr. Rizzi became more complex, the home care nurse spent a great deal of time reassuring Mrs. Rizzi that she was doing a good job.

One of the critical factors in Mrs. Rizzi's ability to perform the role of caregiver was the stability of her own health. Given her comorbidities, Mrs. Rizzi might have fallen ill herself under the additional burden of the caregiver role. Instead, the home care nurse coached Mrs. Rizzi to pay special attention to her own health during these stressful times. On each visit and telephone call, the home care nurse inquired about Mrs. Rizzi's health, making sure she kept her primary care provider appointments and adhered to her medical regimen. Opportunities for respite were arranged so that Mrs. Rizzi could go to get her hair fixed and retain some normalcy in her activities.

As Mr. Rizzi became more ill, Mrs. Rizzi consulted the home care nurse about a hospice referral. The home care nurse consulted with the physician, who agreed that Mr. Rizzi had a prognosis of less than 6 months and was a good candidate for hospice care. Because the VNA did not have a certified hospice program, the home care nurse referred the Rizzis to the local hospice provider in their community. Although it was difficult to discharge the Rizzis from the home care agency, at the hospice, Mr. and Mrs. Rizzi took advantage of the pastoral care services, art therapy program, and the additional resources available under Medicare, such as prescription drug coverage for medications related to the terminal illness. The hospice nurse provided the majority of direct care, with consultation with their APN on the team when Mr. Rizzi's pain increased. Mr. Rizzi died at home following a 2-month service from hospice. The nurse was present with Mr. Rizzi's family at his bedside when he died. The hospice nurse also visited Mrs. Rizzi twice after Mr. Rizzi's death, facilitating Mrs. Rizzi's grief by providing opportunities to review the care her husband received and her responses to his loss.

Conclusion

For palliative care to be a viable component of the service provided by home care agencies, changes are needed in both the structure of home care and the mechanisms for reimbursement. The regulations for the provision of home care under Medicare must be substantively modified to allow increased access to palliative care. Under the current regulations, the physician is the only provider who has the ability to order and to supervise a home plan of care through home care agencies. The literature is consistent in its description of the positive role APNs play in supporting both the patient and family caregivers in the home, yet APNs are not given the authority to direct patient care through home care agencies for patients needing palliation. Exceptions do exist through hospital-based programs. For example, Memorial Sloan Kettering Cancer Center (New York) has a successful hospital-based supportive care program that provides palliative care in the home for patients. This program is directed by an APN, and services are billed through the outpatient service. Regulations that support the critical role APNs play in the clinical management of patients at home who require palliative care and that legitimize the APN's ability to order and to supervise the plan of care are essential. The few successful models in hospital-based and ambulatory clinics should be implemented in home care agencies.

Additionally, the historical structure of Medicare reimbursement was a disincentive for the use of APNs in home care agencies. Because of the regulatory changes in reimbursement to prospective payment, APNs will play an increasingly important role in the delivery of effective home care. As the demographics of the home care population change and the complexity of clinical problems increase, agencies can ill afford to be without expert clinical providers.

The earlier case study had a successful outcome even though the current home care delivery system is fragmented. The need for palliative care to be integrated into both home care as well as hospice care is essential for the provision of a continuum of care to patients at the end of life. For these changes to be integrated into the care delivery system, regulations need to be changed to allow home care nurses to provide end-of-life care in situations in which hospice care is unavailable, or at the request of the patient or family.

In summary, home care is an important component of palliative care. Clinical and regulatory barriers have forced palliative care in the home to be provided by certified hospices at the end of life. Structural changes in home care are needed to fully integrate palliative care into the home care delivery system. Additionally, the role of APNs must be fully developed and reimbursement mechanisms established to integrate palliative care into home care for both patients and home caregivers.

REFERENCES

1. Sarna L, McCorkle R. Burden of care and lung cancer. Cancer Practice 1996;4:245–251.
2. Clement-Stone S, Eigsti D, McGuire S. Comprehensive Health Nursing, 4th ed. St. Louis: Mosby, 1995.
3. National Association for Home Care. Basic Statistics About Home Care, NAHC/GPO. Available at: http://www.nahc.org/nahc/research/04hc_stats.pdf (accessed March 24, 2005).
4. Humphrey C, Milone-Nuzzo P. Manual of Home Nursing Orientation, 2nd ed. Gaithersburg, MD: Aspen, 2000.
5. National Center for Health Statistics. Home Health Care Patients: Data from the 2000 National Home and Hospice Care Survey, Centers for Disease Control. Available at: http://www.cdc.gov/nchs/pressroom/04facts/patients.htm (accessed January 26, 2005).
6. Haupt BJ. An overview of home health and hospice care patients: 1996 National Home and Hospice Care Survey. Washington, DC: Department of Health and Human Services, National Center for Health Statistics, 1998.
7. National Association for Home Care. Basic Statistics About Home Care, GPO. Available at: http://www.nahc.org/Consumer/hcstats.html (accessed January 26, 2005).
8. Chan CW, Chang AM. Managing caregiver tasks among family caregivers of cancer patients in Hong Kong. J Adv Nurs 1999; 29:484–489.
9. Strang V, Koop PM. Factors which influence coping: home-based family caregiving of persons with advanced cancer. J Palliative Care 2003;19:107.
10. McEnroe LE. Role of the oncology nurse in home care: family-centered practice. Semin Oncol Nurs 1996;12:188–192.
11. U. S. Department of Labor, Bureau of Labor Statistics. National Industry-Occupation Employment Matrix: 2000, 2010. Washington, DC: GPO, 2003. Available at: http://ssdc.ucsd.edu/ssdc/bls00002.html (accessed March 24, 2005).
12. U. S. House of Representatives. Committee on Ways and Means, 1998 Green Book. Washington, DC: 105th Congress, 2nd session, 1998.
13. Dombi W. Home care and the law. Caring 1991;10:1.
14. Cawley MM, Gerdts EK. Establishing a cancer caregivers program. An interdisciplinary approach. Cancer Nurs 1988;11:267–273.
15. Conkling VK. Continuity of care issues for cancer patients and families. Cancer 1989;64:290–294.
16. McCorkle R, Given B. Meeting the challenge of caring for chronically ill adults. In: Chin P, ed., Health Policy: Who Cares? Kansas City, MO: American Academy of Nursing, 1991:2–7.
17. McCorkle R, Yost L, Jepson C, Malone D, Baird S, Lusk E. A cancer experience: relationship of patient psychosocial responses to caregiver burden over time. PsychoOncology 1993;2:21–32.
18. Ganz PA. Current issues in cancer rehabilitation. Cancer 1990; 65:742–751.
19. Mor V, Guadagnoli E, Wool M. An examination of the concrete service needs of advanced cancer patients. J Psychosocial Oncol 1987;5:1–17.
20. Googe MC, Varricchio CG. A pilot investigation of home health care needs of cancer patients and their families. Oncol Nurs Forum 1981;8:24–28.
21. Wellisch D, Fawzy F, Landsverk J, Pasnau R, Wocott D. Evaluation of psychosocial problems of the home-bound patient: the relationship of disease and sociodemographic variables of patients to family problems. J Psychosocial Oncol 1983;1:1–15.
22. Houts PS, Nezu AM, Nezu CM, Bucher JA. The prepared family caregiver: a problem-solving approach to family caregiver education. Patient Education & Counseling 1996;27:63–73.
23. Wingate AL, Lackey NR. A description of the needs of noninstitutionalized cancer patients and their primary care givers. Cancer Nurs 1989;12:216–225.
24. McCorkle R, Jepson C, Malone D, Lusk E, Braitman L, Buhler-Wilkerson K, Daly J. The impact of posthospital home care on patients with cancer. Res Nurs Health 1994;17:243–251.
25. Evers MM, Meier DE, Morrison RS. Assessing differences in care needs and service utilization in geriatric palliative care patients. J Pain Symptom Manage 2002;23:424–432.
26. Grobe ME, Ilstrup DM, Ahmann DL. Skills needed by family members to maintain the care of an advanced cancer patient. Cancer Nurs 1981;4:371–375.
27. Hinds C. The need of families who care for patients with cancer at home: are we meeting them? J Adv Pract Nurs 1985;10:575–581.
28. Morris SM, Thomas C. The need to know: informal carers and information. Eur J Cancer Care 2002;11:183–187.
29. Siegel K, Raveis VH, Houts P, Mor V. Caregiver burden and unmet patient needs. Cancer 1991;68:1131–1140.
30. Siegel K, Raveis VH, Mor V, Houts P. The relationship of spousal caregiver burden to patient disease and treatment-related conditions. Ann Oncol 1991;2:511–516.
31. Oberst MT, Thomas SE, Gass KA, Ward SE. Caregiving demands and appraisal of stress among family caregivers. Cancer Nurs 1989;12:209–215.
32. Perry G, Roades de Menses M. Cancer patients at home: needs and coping styles of primary caregivers. Home Healthcare Nurse 1989;7:27–30.
33. Sales E, Schultz R, Biegel D. Predictors of strain in families of cancer patients: a review of the literature. J Psychosocial Oncol 1990;10:1–26.
34. Given BA, Given CW, Helms E, Stommel M, DeVoss DN. Determinants of family care giver reaction. New and recurrent cancer. Cancer Pract 1997;5:17–24.
35. Given CW, Given B, Stommel M, Collins C, King S, Franklin S. The caregiver reaction assessment (CRA) for caregivers to persons with chronic physical and mental impairments. Res Nurs Health 1992;15:271–283.
36. Kozachik SL, Given CW, Given BA, Pierce SJ, Azzouz F, Rawl SM, Champion VL. Improving depressive symptoms among caregivers of patients with cancer: results of a randomized clinical trial. Oncol Nurs Forum 2001;28:1149–1157.
37. Carter PA. Caregivers' descriptions of sleep changes and depressive symptoms. Oncol Nurs Forum 2002;29:1277–1283.
38. Bruera E, Sweeney C, Willey J, Palmer JL, Strasser F, Strauch E. Perception of discomfort by relatives and nurses in unresponsive terminally ill patients with cancer: a prospective study. J Pain Symptom Manage 2003;26:818–826.
39. Smeenk FW, van Haastregt JC, de Witte LP, Crebolder HF. Effectiveness of home care programmes for patients with incurable cancer on their quality of life and time spent in hospital: systematic review. BMJ 1998;316:1939–1944.
40. Hinton J. Can home care maintain an acceptable quality of life for patients with terminal cancer and their relatives? Palliative Med 1992;8:183–196.

41. Corner J, Halliday D, Haviland J, Douglas HR, Bath P, Clark D, Normand C, Beech N, Hughes P, Marples R, Seymour J, Skilbeck J, Webb T. Exploring nursing outcomes for patients with advanced cancer following intervention by Macmillan specialist palliative care nurses. J Adv Nurs 2003;41:561–574.
42. McWhinny I, Bass M, Orr V. Factors associated with the location of death (home or hospital) of patients referred to a palliative care team. Can Med Assoc J 1995;152:361–367.
43. Axelsson B, Sjoden PO. Quality of life of cancer patients and their spouses in palliative home care. Palliative Med 1998;12:29–39.
44. Beck-Friis B, Strang P. The family in hospital-based home care with special reference to terminally ill cancer patients. J Palliative Care 1993;9:5–13.
45. Bostrom B, Hinic H, Lundberg D, Fridlund B. Pain and health-related quality of life among cancer patients in final stage of life: a comparison between two palliative care teams. J Nurs Manage 2003;11:189–196.
46. Peruselli C, Marinari M, Brivio B, Castagnini G, Cavana M, Centrone G, Magni C, Merlini M, Scaccabarozzi GL, Paci E. Evaluating a home palliative care service: development of indicators for a continuous quality improvement program. J Palliative Care 1997;13:34–42.
47. Costantini M, Camoirano E, Madeddu L, Bruzzi P, Verganelli E, Henriquet F. Palliative home care and place of death among cancer patients: a population-based study. Palliative Med 1993;7:323–331.
48. Martinson I. Why don't we let them die at home? RN 1976;39:58–65.
49. Martinson I. Home care for children dying of cancer. Pediatrics 1978;62:1016–1111.
50. Yates J, McKegney P, Kun L. A comparative study of home nursing care of patients with advanced cancer. Proceedings of the American Cancer Society Third National Conference on Human Values and Cancer: Recommendations for Facilitating the Use of Home Care in Palliative Care. Washington, DC: American Cancer Society, 1981.
51. Oleske D, Hauck WW, Heide E. Characteristics of cancer patient referrals to home care: a regional perspective. Am J Pub Health 1983;73:678–682.
52. McCorkle R, Benoliel JQ, Donaldson G, Georgiadou F, Moinpour C, Goodell B. A randomized clinical trial of home nursing care for lung cancer patients. Cancer 1989;64:1375–1382.
53. McCorkle R, Benoliel J, Georgiadou F. The effects of home care on patients' symptoms, hospitalizations and complications. In: Key Aspects of Comfort: Management of Pain, Fatigue and Nausea. New York: Springer, 1989.
54. McCorkle R, Robinson L, Nuamah I, Lev E, Benoliel JQ. The effects of home nursing care for patients during terminal illness on the bereaved's psychological distress. Nurs Res 1998;47:2–10.
55. Tomberg M, McGrath B, Benoliel J. Oncology transition service: partnerships of nurses and families. Cancer Nurs 1984;7:131–137.
56. McCorkle R, Strumpf NE, Nuamah IF, Adler DC, Cooley ME, Jepson C, Lusk EJ, Torosian M. A specialized home care intervention improves survival among older post-surgical cancer patients. J Am Geriatric Soc 2000;48:1707–1713.
57. Jepson C, McCorkle R, Adler D, Nuamah I, Lusk E. Effects of home care on caregivers' psychosocial status. Image: J Nurs Scholarsh 1999;31:115–120.
58. Bradley PJ. Family caregiver assessment. Essential for effective home health care. J Gerontological Nurs 2003;29:29–36.
59. Naylor MD, Brooten D, Campbell R, Jacobsen BS, Mezey MD, Pauly MV, Schwartz JS. Comprehensive discharge planning and home follow-up of hospitalized elders: a randomized clinical trial. JAMA 1999;281:613–620.
60. Ferrell BR, Grant M, Chan J, Ahn C, Ferrell BA. The impact of cancer pain education on family caregivers of elderly patients. Oncol Nurs Forum 1995;22:1211–1218.
61. Barg FK, Cooley M, Pasacreta J, Senay B, McCorkle R. Development of a self-administered psychosocial cancer screening tool. Cancer Pract 1994;2:288–296.
62. Schumacher KL, Koresawa S, West C, Hawkins C, Johnson C, Wais E, Dodd M, Paul SM, Tripathy D, Koo P, Miaskowski C. Putting cancer pain management regimens into practice at home. J Pain Symptom Manage 2002;23:369–382.
63. Koop PM, Strang VR. The bereavement experience following home-based family caregiving for persons with advanced cancer. Clin Nurs Res 2003;12:127–144.

42

Marie Bakitas and Kathleen Daretany

Hospital-Based Palliative Care

We were so grateful that we could bring our dad into the hospital for his last days. We had cared for him at home with the help of hospice for several months. He survived much longer than the doctors and nurses predicted and we just got so tired. At the very end, the Palliative Care team and Hospice helped us to get him admitted to our nearby hospital where they cared for him just like we did at home. He was very comfortable for his last two days of life and they let us stay around the clock. It was a gift to be with him those last days without having to worry about whether we could manage his symptoms and doing all of the physical care.—Family member of man dying of pancreatic cancer

- ***Key Points***
- *The hospital is the appropriate site of care for some dying patients. It is important for all hospitals to develop a minimum standard of palliative care services that are consistent with the agency's care delivery model (e.g. primary, secondary, tertiary care).*
- *Established internal (e.g., Quality Improvement Committee, Ethics Committee) and external (e.g., Joint Commission on Accreditation of Healthcare Organizations, Center to Advance Palliative Care) hospital-based quality improvement resources and committees can assist with the development or improvement of a hospital's palliative care program.*
- *Early introduction of palliative care principles in the disease trajectory and early identification of appropriate palliative care patients allows for planning to meet patient preference for end-of-life care.*
- *It is important to develop infrastructures of care outside the hospital so that alternatives exist to hospital admission at end of life.*

One hundred years ago, the cause, age, and place of death were very different from what they are now, at the turn of the new millennium. Table 42–1 compares some characteristics of dying in 1900 and in 2000. Chronic illness and longer life are the legacy of this century. The hospital is a common location for a good portion of end-of-life (EOL) care in contemporary times, despite Americans' stated preference for death at home.[1,2] An analysis of the experience of dying among Medicare recipients (based on claims data for 1995–1996) demonstrated that the incidence of dying in hospitals varies, but in some regions of the United States it approaches 50% (Figure 42–1).[3] An additional 25% to 35% of the nation's elderly die in nursing homes.[2,4] Although a percentage of patients experience their final admission in the critical care unit, by and large hospital deaths occur in non–critical care units[3] and are likely to be anticipated for hours or days before death actually occurs.[5]

Several investigators have described the quality of dying in the acute care hospital.[6–8] These studies have found that patients experience pain, dyspnea, anxiety, and other distressing symptoms up until the time of death. Table 42–2 summarizes

Table 42–1
Comparison of Death and Dying in 1900 and in 2000

	1900	2000
Life expectancy	47 y	75 y
Usual place of death	Home	Hospital
Most medical expenses	Paid by family	Paid by Medicare
Disability before death	Usually not much	2 y, on average

Source: Lynn and Adamson (2003), reference 1.

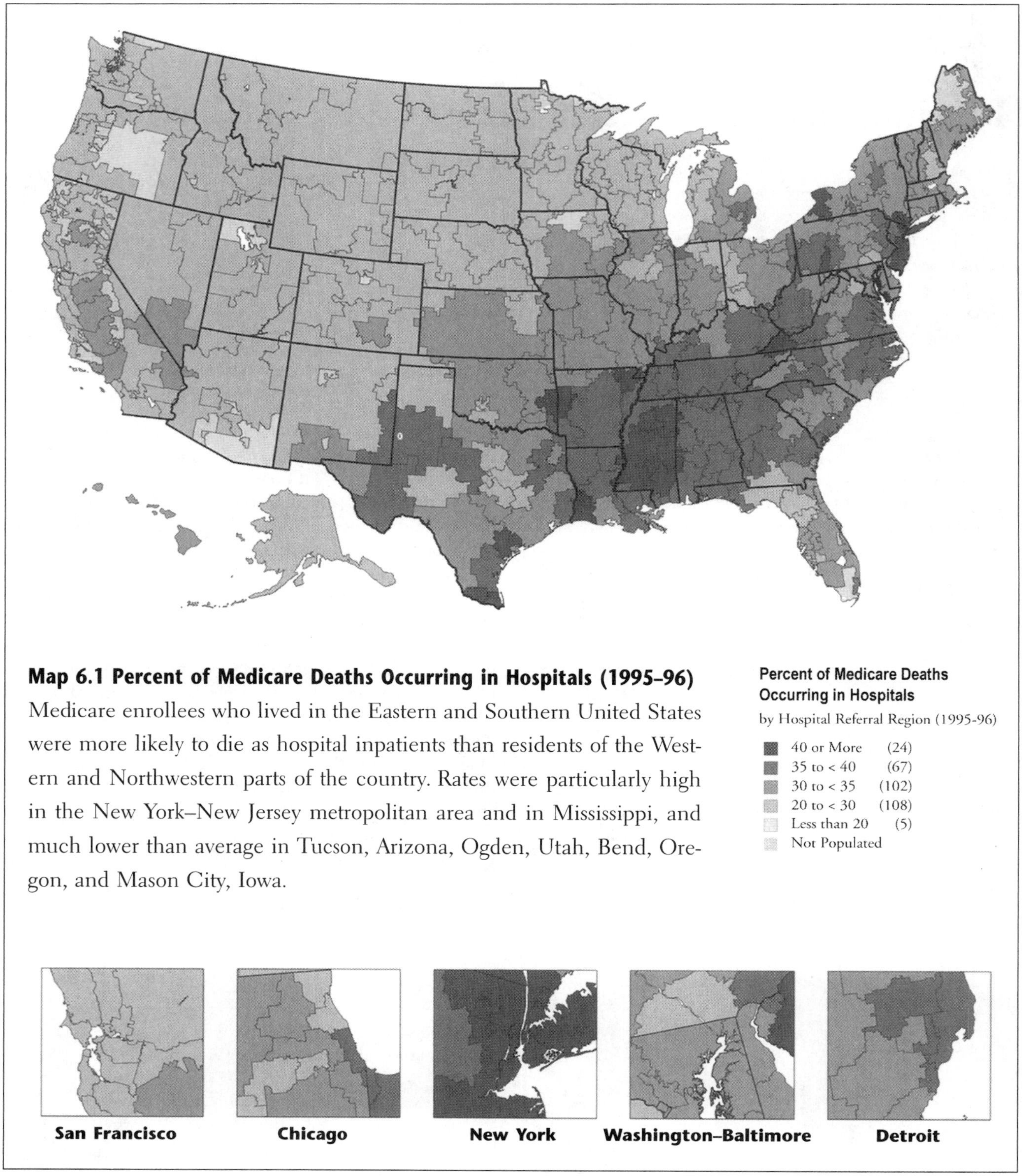

Map 6.1 Percent of Medicare Deaths Occurring in Hospitals (1995–96)
Medicare enrollees who lived in the Eastern and Southern United States were more likely to die as hospital inpatients than residents of the Western and Northwestern parts of the country. Rates were particularly high in the New York–New Jersey metropolitan area and in Mississippi, and much lower than average in Tucson, Arizona, Ogden, Utah, Bend, Oregon, and Mason City, Iowa.
Percent of Medicare Deaths Occurring in Hospitals
by Hospital Referral Region (1995-96)
40 or More (24)
35 to < 40 (67)
30 to < 35 (102)
20 to < 30 (108)
Less than 20 (5)
Not Populated
San Francisco
Chicago
New York
Washington–Baltimore
Detroit

Figure 42–1. Dartmouth Atlas Map of Incidence of Death in Hospital. *Source:* Wennberg J, Cooper M, eds. The Quality of Care in the United States: A Report on the Medicare Program/Dartmouth Atlas of Health. Chicago: AHA Press, 1999. Reprinted by permission.

Table 42–2
Selected Results from the Study to Understand Prognoses and Preferences for Outcomes and Risks of Treatments (SUPPORT)

Study aims

To document and influence patterns of communication (patient/family/health care team), frequency of aggressive treatment, and characteristics of hospital death

Methods

Two-phase study in five academic medical centers

Phase I: 2-year prospective observational study ($N = 4301$)

Phase II: 2-year controlled clinical trial with intervention group ($N = 2652$) and control group ($N = 2152$)

Intervention

A specially trained nurse had multiple contacts with patient/family/health care team to facilitate communications and to provide physicians with accurate information about patients' prognoses and preferences for care.

Main results

There were no differences between the control group and the intervention group on the measures of the study, which included:

- Communication between physician and patients (discussions of CPR preferences)
- Number of days spent in an ICU receiving mechanical ventilation and in coma
- Level of pain reported by patient
- Use of hospital resources

Further, based on interviews with 3357 survivors:

- 40% of patients died in severe pain
- 55% were conscious
- 63% had difficulty tolerating symptoms

Source: Data from Lynn et al. (1997), reference 8.

selected findings of the well-known Study to Understand Prognoses and Preferences for Outcomes and Risks of Treatments (SUPPORT). This multi-hospital, two-phase investigation attempted to alter the quality of the hospitalized adult EOL experience by "reducing the frequency of a mechanically supported, painful, and prolonged process of dying" by increasing communication and improving the provision of information necessary for decision-making among patient, family, and their health care providers.[5]

The discouraging outcomes from SUPPORT and other studies cannot be explained by providers' lack of awareness or inability to relieve symptoms. Many studies in the area of pain management demonstrate that effective methods exist to relieve cancer pain in 90% of patients.[2] It is also not the case that acute care hospitals employ unskilled, insensitive personnel who allow suffering to occur. Rather, the issue appears largely one of system design. Inpatients are cared for in a system that is designed to provide acute, episodic interventions for patients with reversible disorders. This philosophy is exemplified by hospital policies that require all persons having patient contact to be certified in the provision of cardiopulmonary resuscitation (CPR), so as to be able to rescue any patient who experiences cessation of respiration or heartbeat. The application of this death-reversing intervention is applied to all hospitalized inpatients unless specifically ordered to the contrary. Clearly, in such institutions, patients who are dying are viewed as exceptions that require special additional thought, paperwork, and attention to receive a different sort of care.

Implementation of other tenets of palliative and hospice-type care may not be consistent with standard hospital policy. For instance, having family, friends, pets, and familiar items in the immediate patient environment often requires special exceptions or violations of standard hospital protocols. In many institutions, beloved pets, home audio equipment used for listening to special music, or multiple significant others sitting around-the-clock vigils are considered contrary to standard hospital infection control, electrical use rules, and security policies. As stated by Berwick on the nature of system improvement: "Every system is perfectly designed to get the results it gets."[9] In the case of EOL care, it is hard to imagine how hospital-based EOL care could occur any differently than it does. A change in the quantity and quality of deaths in hospital will come about only as a result of fundamental system reform and redesign.[10,11]

This situation ought not to be viewed as discouraging, but rather as a call to action, particularly for nurses. Because people are admitted to hospitals primarily to receive nursing care, much of the care and the system that patients experience can be influenced by nurses at all organizational levels. (Most other types of care, such as physician consultation, diagnostic tests, and pharmaceutical treatments, are available in outpatient or home settings). The information contained in this chapter is usable by all hospital-based nurses, including senior nursing leaders, clinical nurse specialists, nurse practitioners, nurse managers, educators, quality improvement nurses, and especially nurses on the front line at the bedside. Nurses can define, direct, and lead multidisciplinary and interdisciplinary teams and modify efforts at multiple levels of the hospital care system to improve this complex care process.[12,13]

This chapter outlines how nurses and others can take a leadership role in improving the quality of EOL care in acute care hospitals. Some improvements may result from the use of specific "quality improvement" methods, whereas other improvements may not employ this specific process. Although a step-by-step primer on the process of "quality improvement" is beyond the scope of this chapter, a detailed discussion is found in Chapter 39; other excellent sources are also available.[14] In addition, this chapter focuses on methods to reduce hospital admissions at the EOL. Individual and multihospital innovations to improve hospital-based EOL care are described, including examples from hospitals that have used the approach of developing critical pathways and protocols and new services to improve care, such as palliative care consulting teams and inpatient palliative care units (PCUs). In closing, economic issues that influence the quality and quantity of hospital-based palliative care and future directions complete the discussion.

Hospital-Based Palliative Care as a Process

CASE STUDY

Mr. D, a 64-Year-Old Man with Severe Abdominal Pain

The interdisciplinary palliative care consultation team (PCT) was asked by the general internal medicine service to see Mr. D, a 62-year-old man who presented to the emergency room with uncontrollable severe abdominal pain. The patient reported several weeks of anorexia and a 15-pound unintentional weight loss. After a laparotomy and liver biopsy, he was found to have a large pancreatic mass, which was positive for adenocarcinoma and multiple peritoneal metastases. Within 24 hours after diagnosis, the medical team placed concurrent palliative care and oncology consultations. The former requested the need for assistance with uncontrollable pain, symptom management, prognosis/diagnosis explanation, and safe and appropriate discharge; the later requested identification of anticancer treatment options.

The palliative care team's initial assessment revealed that the patient was a retired train operator who lived with his wife. He had two sons who lived within 15 minutes of his home. He had no religious affiliation but identified himself as spiritual and accepted visits from the PCT pastoral care provider. Mr. D's goals were to be free of pain, to be ambulatory, and to go home as soon as possible, so he could finish working on a project he had started for his youngest son's wedding, three months hence. Comprehensive pain assessment revealed constant, gnawing, vague pain with an intensity score of 6 (on a pain scale of 0 to 10). His personal goal for pain relief was a score of 2. Mr. D's pain medication regimen was adjusted by the PCT nurse practitioner to provide pain relief at his tolerable level.

In addition, the PCT organized a patient/family meeting the next day. The meeting was held in the patient's room so that he could participate in the discussions. In attendance from the family were the patient, his wife, and both of his sons. The PCT physician, social worker, nurse practitioner, and a nurse practitioner student were also present. Discussion included the patient's understanding of his diagnosis, prognosis, and the influence and meaning of the disease on his goals of care. Advance directives, health care proxy, and a plan for long-term care at home after discharge were also discussed.

The next day, the patient chose his oldest son as his health care proxy, and his pain was in control under the new regimen. A smooth transition was made to a home hospice agency by the PCT social worker. In addition, the patient decided to follow-up with the outpatient oncology clinic to consider anticancer treatment for symptom relief.

Lessons Learned

- Interdisciplinary PCT is effective in addressing patient/family needs.
- Mandated, ongoing pain assessment practices within the hospital setting supported the ability to rapidly determine a pain relief plan.
- Advance directives are best determined before an emergency or crisis situation occurs.
- Effective palliative care involves the patient and the family.
- Palliative care and disease-modifying treatments can be rendered concurrently.
- The palliative care team's expertise in pain and symptom management can be helpful to the patient and family and to the primary medical team.

CASE STUDY

Mr. F, a 75-Year-Old Man with Bilateral Hip Fractures

Mr. F, a 75-year-old man, was admitted to the medical/surgical unit after a fall at home with bilateral hip fractures. He had undergone open reduction with internal fixation of his hips bilaterally. His past medical history was significant for metastatic lung cancer with bony involvement and chronic obstructive pulmonary disease. Postoperatively, he developed intermittent confusion, cough, and dyspnea. A chest radiograph revealed a right upper lobe infiltrate, and intravenous antibiotics, supportive oxygen therapy, nebulizer treatments, and close observation were instituted.

Mr. F's respiratory status worsened, and he required increasing oxygen via nasal cannula and then via face mask. As his condition declined, he was asked by the intern if he would "like everything done for him." He continuously nodded his head "Yes" to the question. Shortly after this "discussion," Mr. F suffered a respiratory arrest, for which he received CPR, intubation, and mechanical ventilation. He was transferred to the intensive care unit (ICU) in critical condition. No family members could be identified to assist the medical team with decision-making.

While he was in the ICU, a Swan-Ganz catheter and central line were inserted, multiple daily blood draws were taken, and Mr. F was heavily sedated to prevent him from dislodging his tubes. His medical condition progressively deteriorated, and the medical and nursing staff became increasingly frustrated, feeling helpless and not knowing Mr. F's goals of care. After multiple attempts, a neighbor was finally contacted who said he didn't really know the patient well enough to understand what he may have wanted done at this point. After a 2-week ICU stay, Mr. F developed sepsis. Eventually, he died in the ICU.

Lessons Learned

- Discussion of advance directives should take place with patients when they have capacity and are not in crisis.
- Early introduction of palliative care specialists may help to clarify and document patients' goals of care and pain/symptom management preferences.
- Medical and nursing staff education about advance directives, palliative care, and EOL issues can establish baseline competence levels.
- Lack of advance planning can result in health care provider frustration, fatigue, and moral distress.
- Unnecessary patient and staff suffering can be minimized if palliative care education and policies are in place to support patient identification of goals of care.

Both of these cases illustrate ways in which EOL care occurs in hospitals. Each case is followed by "Lessons Learned," which summarize areas of palliative care exemplars and areas ripe for improvement. Table 42–3 outlines a high-level process of care that illustrates "typical" hospital-based EOL care similar to that described in the case of Mr. F. Areas for improvement (some of which were illustrated by the case of Mr. D) are suggested adjacent to the process steps. These issues and cases serve as a basis for the remaining discussion of ways in which hospitals can create care systems that result in improved EOL outcomes for patients requiring hospital-based care.

Avoiding Hospitalized Death

Perhaps one of the most important ways to improve hospital-based palliative care is to develop other infrastructures of care outside the hospital, so that alternatives to inpatient admission at EOL exist. Alternatives such as home hospice care or skilled hospice care within assisted-living centers, free-standing hospices, or specially designated areas in nursing homes or rehabilitation facilities[15] can provide expert palliative and hospice care at the EOL. However, many areas of the United States lack these sorts of options. For instance, in some rural areas, health care services such as visiting nurses or home care are sparse or unprepared to care for people who require intensive EOL care.[16] Some visiting nurse and home care agencies may see so few symptomatic persons at the EOL that it is difficult to maintain adequate palliative care and hospice expertise in these agencies.

To improve the care that nonhospital systems provide, it is imperative that these organizations provide sufficient and appropriate education and training for their staff about the care possibilities at EOL. Organizations should encourage staff

Table 42–3
Process of Care for Seriously Ill Hospitalized Patient at End of Life

Current Process of Care	Possible Areas of Improvement
Symptomatic, seriously ill patient admitted to emergency department (ED)	• Prospective symptom management to avoid hospitalization • Advance care planning communicated to care team
Work up by ED staff	• Direct admission of symptomatic/respite patients
Admission to medical unit	• Availability of palliative care unit/consult team
Diagnostic workup continues with medical house staff	• Minimize/standardize diagnostics to focus on ones that contribute to comfort
Physician notified	• Physician aware and guiding admission process
Initial plan of care determined	• Plan of care states palliative care goals, advance care planning, patient preferences
Treatment is implemented and symptoms managed	• Palliative care pathway and/or standardized symptom assessment
Team acknowledges that patient is dying	• Patient's prognosis and preferences guide palliative care plan from time of admission
"Do-not-resuscitate" (DNR) status determined	• DNR status determined on admission; admission plan of care includes patient's care preferences in addition to DNR status
Comfort measures implemented	• Appropriate comfort care measures implemented at admission
Patient dies in hospital	• Patient dies in preferred site of death • Bereavement care offered to family after the death

members to participate in conferences on EOL and palliative care and also should support them through the continuing education process (e.g., becoming certified in a specialty). Both the nursing and medical professions have embraced the concept of further EOL education and certification. The End-of-Life Nursing Education Consortium (ELNEC) and Education for Physicians on End-of-Life Care (EPEC) are examples of this approach for nursing and medicine, respectively.

The lack of hospice and palliative care expertise outside the hospital can be compounded by another very real problem, reimbursement for out-of-hospital EOL care. This problem must be viewed in the context of the Medicare hospice benefit, which in 2004 provided a standard per diem rate of $118.08 for routine home care; $689.18/d or $28.72/h for continuous care during a crisis to maintain a patient at home; $122.15/d for up to 5 days of respite care; and $525.28/d for hospital, skilled, or free-standing inpatient hospice care for symptom management.[17] These amounts are intended to cover all care needs, including nursing, home health aides, other discipline visits, pharmaceuticals, and medical equipment. For many patients eligible for Medicare hospice care, effective palliative interventions for symptom management (e.g., radiation therapy, chemotherapy, higher-priced supportive care medications for nausea and pain) are costly, given the reimbursement rate. Hence, patients who could otherwise benefit from hospice care are delayed in accessing the benefit until all of the aforementioned palliative treatments have been applied.

It is therefore not only an issue of patient identification, but also one of finance, that is responsible for late hospice referrals. Quality improvement efforts directed at improving EOL care by encouraging earlier referrals to the Medicare hospice benefit that ignore the financial issues are likely to fail. Agencies that place patients on the Medicare benefit despite ongoing expensive treatments are likely to find themselves in a state of financial instability.

Another barrier that must be overcome to realize lower in-hospital death rates is that of home care provision in the current culture of single-parent and two-parent working families. Currently, 75% of women work outside the home, yet they are often the ones called upon to provide care for ailing family members.[18] When patients are enrolled in the Medicare hospice benefit, it is assumed that a family member or other person will be with the patient every day[19] and that hospice staff will visit intermittently. For symptomatic or very ill patients, a family member may need to take a leave of absence or risk jeopardizing employment to provide adequate coverage for home care. Providing EOL care to a family member for an extended period can result in out-of-pocket medical expenses and lost income from both the patient and the caregiver, creating significant financial burdens.[20] In these cases, a "reimbursable" hospital stay may be the only choice for family respite. The Last Acts Workplace Task Force has prepared a report of an employer survey and a set of model activities designed to help caregivers and their families with ill or dependent relatives in need of workplace supports.[21]

Another mechanism to prevent hospital admissions is to develop a system that allows for early identification of patients who are eligible for palliative care and/or hospice care and to identify alternatives to hospitalization in the long-term EOL care plan. Early identification can take place at the beginning of the disease trajectory or at the point of a hospital admission. A good example of putting this concept into practice was illustrated in the first case study in this chapter, that of Mr. D. As soon as the patient was admitted to the hospital and a life-limiting illness was diagnosed, concurrent palliative care and oncology consultation requests were placed.

Early recognition of patients who are eligible for palliative care and prompt referral to experts in the field is a vital step in the process of integrating effective palliative care into hospital care. Putting prospective screening mechanisms in place can reduce the number and type of hospital admissions for palliative care. For instance, consider the situation of discharging a patient with adequate relief of pain but no long-term plan for dealing with worsening disease and increased pain. In this case, neglecting the bigger problem of long-term pain management only postpones the problem until a later date, when pain is likely to increase and the only available solution will be readmission. In addition to creating a long-term plan for already-hospitalized patients, prehospitalization programs that identify elders at home or in nursing homes who do not wish to have their conditions treated in a hospital can preclude undesired admissions.

The Patient Self-Determination Act (PSDA) of 1991 requires that hospitals and other organizations receiving Medicare or Medicaid funding provide written information to patients about their rights to make decisions accepting or refusing medical care.[22] Further, it stipulates that advance directives, including living wills and appointment of a health care proxy, may be used to provide substituted judgment in the event of patients' inability to speak for themselves regarding health care decisions. On the surface, this legislation appeared to be an infrastructure to improve EOL care in hospitals. Theoretically, patients would outline their preferences for certain types of treatments in a document or through a proxy to guide health care providers. For several reasons, however, this legislation has had little impact in defining the type of care received by hospitalized patients.[23] Unfortunately, not all patients actually choose to complete advance directives; the documents apply only if the patients are incapacitated; they may not be specific enough to address the situation in which patients find themselves; and, when they do exist, the health care provider may not be aware of them,[5] or the health care proxy may not interpret them as the patient intended.[24]

Under the Patient Self-Determination Act, institutions are required to ask patients whether they have advance directives and then provide the appropriate information about them. The Act does not stipulate who in the health care agency is to give this information to patients and their families. Often, inexperienced personnel distribute the information without providing appropriate explanation of the documents, leading to lack of completion by patients.

In the second case study, that of Mr. F, there was no evidence of advance care planning before the patient's hospital admission. In this example, the topic of advance directives was introduced too late and inappropriately during the patient's hospitalization. The patient was experiencing respiratory distress and was asked if he "would like everything done" for him. If the topic had been discussed earlier in his admission and he had been provided with comprehensive information regarding his prognosis and probable course of illness, the outcome may have been different. Improving and avoiding hospitalized death requires earlier discussions between patients and their providers regarding the diagnosis and prognosis and intensive health care provider education on the skill of communicating bad news and discussion of CPR.

Recent research and improvement efforts have attempted to study this phenomenon and improve the availability of such information and the consistency between patients' stated preferences and the actual care administered.[14,25] Incorporating such endeavors into quality improvement activities has the potential to influence hospital-based EOL care.[26] An encouraging finding in one chart review of deaths of hospitalized patients indicated an increased implementation of comfort care in patients at the EOL in the minority of patients who had specified a proxy decision-maker, compared with those who had not specified anyone.[27]

Innovative approaches to avoiding unnecessary hospitalization or other undesired care at the EOL are being tested through the Robert Wood Johnson (RWJ) Initiative Promoting Excellence in End of Life Care. (A full description of this program and the specific projects of the grantees is available on the Last Acts website, http://www.edc.org/lastacts/, accessed February 1, 2005.) In demonstration projects, strategies designed to move the knowledge and decision-making about palliative care options earlier in the course of illness than is currently the norm were tested. Four comprehensive cancer centers attempted to integrate palliative care options and approaches at the time of diagnosis of life-threatening, poor-prognosis cancers such as of the lung.[28]

One example, Project ENABLE (Educate, Nurture, Advise Before Life Ends), identified and enrolled all patients with incurable lung cancer, advanced gastrointestinal malignancies, and metastatic or recurrent breast cancers at the time of diagnosis into a program that emphasized palliative care options. The program provided nurse coordination, prospective standardized symptom assessment, and an educational curriculum that focused on topics of empowerment for patient and family decision-making and communication.[29,30] Unlike the nurse coordinator of the SUPPORT study, these advanced practice nurses (and nurse practitioners) were members of the oncology care team and provided non-threatening, expert intervention that had prospectively garnered the support and sanction of the care team. This collaborative approach emphasized shared ownership of the process and, to date, seems to have been successful in influencing and shaping the care trajectory for this population.[31]

Because of the success of the ENABLE project, Dartmouth-Hitchcock Medical Center (DHMC), funded by the National Cancer Institute (NCI), developed a randomized clinical trial, ENABLE II, to test the effectiveness of an intervention to improve quality of life for people with newly diagnosed metastatic or recurrent breast, lung, and gastrointestinal cancers. The intervention was designed to enhance the care that patients already receive at DHMC through nurse educator sessions and Shared Medical Appointments (SMAs) with a palliative care physician and nurse practitioner. The nurse educators in this study are available for resource allocation, education, and care coordination. Patient caregivers are encouraged to participate in the discussions with the patient and the nurse educator. It is hypothesized that, with the addition of the nurse educator and the availability of the SMAs, patients will have an enhanced quality of life and care consistent with their values and preferences.

The first case study, that of Mr. D, demonstrated the importance of early identification of patients so that advance directives and patient/family-centered care could be planned. The introduction of palliative care at the time of diagnosis allowed for appropriate and effective utilization of the palliative care services. If a patient is identified early in the course of illness, the palliative care team can act as a resource, or consultant, to the medical team. At this time, the palliative care specialists can provide information about good symptom and pain management and help with psychosocial issues that may arise. As the patient nears death, and the goal of care becomes focused more on comfort, the palliative care team becomes more prominent in caring for the individual and the family.

Many states laws have provisions for patients at home who are dying and do not want to be resuscitated to use home labeling systems such as a "DNR bracelet," sticker, or forms. Specific details can be obtained in a 138-page report that details the results of a national survey conducted in 1999 of state laws and protocols providing for "do-not-resuscitate" (DNR) orders effective in nonhospital settings.[32] In New Hampshire, before the DNR bracelet for home use was adopted, emergency medical technicians were required to begin resuscitation and transport the patient to a hospital, even if it was clear that this was not the patient's wish. Often, despite teaching, the family faced with a dying loved one panicked as breathing became labored, heart rate slowed or stopped, or bleeding ensued. Even if documents such as living wills and durable powers of attorney for health care were produced, this did not release the emergency medical technicians of the responsibilities of response. In conjunction with New Hampshire Emergency Medical Services, a procedure was developed for outpatients and prehospital care personnel to indicate patient preferences for no emergency care if cardiopulmonary arrest occurs outside the hospital.[33] The DNR bracelet, which looks similar to a typical green hospital bracelet except that it is blue, can be obtained from a local hospital on completion of specific paperwork. In the event of cardiopulmonary arrest at home or in an emergency department, this bracelet releases the responders from providing emergency care other than comfort care, symptom relief, and family support.

Finally, despite the development of nonhospital sites of EOL care, one analysis concluded that the main impetus behind hospital death is the number of hospital beds available in a referral area.[34] This study suggested that, regardless of the availability of out-of-hospital alternatives, hospital deaths will continue at a higher rate in areas that have abundant hospital beds available than in those areas with fewer beds. Since that report was published, another study from Oregon, which has had the lowest in-hospital death rate in the United States (31%), identified factors that facilitate arrangements for death to occur outside the hospital.[35] Many of the factors already mentioned were found to be significant in the Oregon study, as evidenced by the following quotation: "For Oregon, it seems that economic forces and trends, coupled with an array of end-of-life resources, foster an environment in which patients and families more often obtain care during the lasts days of life in the setting they prefer."[35]

Models of Hospital-Based Palliative Care

Promoting palliative care in the acute care hospital requires a myriad of resources. Depending on the model of palliative care being introduced, the required resources can vary greatly. For example, some changes may require financial support via construction or addition of staff, whereas other changes are less resource intensive. Regardless of the hospital and the availability of resources, all health care practitioners have the ability to introduce palliative care concepts and use already established resources to develop or improve their palliative care program. According to von Gunten,[36] "One way that patients and their families will get better care is to ensure that clinical services focusing on the relief of suffering are available in every hospital" (p. 876). He suggested that hospitals consider their mission and level of palliative care delivery—as for other medical specialties (e.g., primary, secondary, tertiary)—and incorporate a model of palliative care resources in accordance with that level.

Primary palliative care refers to a level of care whereby basic skills and competencies are required of all physicians, nurses, and other health care practitioners. All practitioners should be competent at this level. Providers can gain the knowledge, attitudes, and skills needed to provide palliative care to their patients through basic training and clinical practice. Training such as the EPEC and ELNEC programs can provide comprehensive education that is needed at a minimum level.[36] Both educational programs are discussed in more detail later in this chapter.

Secondary palliative care refers to a model in which all providers have a minimum level of competence and in addition have specialists who provide palliative care through consultation services or specialty unit care (or both). The development and success of the consultation team, in most instances, is guided with the training and expertise of hospice organizations.[36] It is not necessary for the team to evaluate every patient with palliative care needs who is admitted to the hospital, but these specially trained clinicians are available as a resource and guide for their colleagues.

Additionally, major teaching hospitals and academic centers with teams of experts in palliative care are classified as tertiary organizations. A tertiary-level practitioner serves as the consultant to the primary and secondary levels in difficult clinical situations. Practitioners and institutions involved at the tertiary level of palliative care are also involved in educational and research activities.[37] It is the responsibility of all hospitals and health care organizations to be competent, at a minimum, at the primary level of palliative care. However, regardless of level, different components of care may be incorporated into the model; some are less resource intense (e.g., care pathways), and others may require additional allocations of budget and personnel. The various levels of hospital-based palliative care and their components are described in greater detail in the following sections.

Primary Palliative Care

Primary palliative care should be available at all hospitals. This level of care requires a minimum of provider education in basics of pain and symptom management. The JCAHO has identified minimum standards that should be present (see later discussion). Additionally, in April 2004, The National Consensus Project for Palliative Care released Clinical Practice Guidelines for Quality Palliative Care. The guidelines, which can be downloaded free of charge from their website (http://www.nationalconsensusproject.org, accessed February 1, 2005), represent a consensus of five major United States palliative care organizations: the American Academy of Hospice and Palliative Medicine, the Center to Advance Palliative Care (CAPC), the Hospice and Palliative Nurses Association, the Last Acts Partnership, and the National Hospice and Palliative Care Organization. The guidelines identify core precepts and structures of clinical palliative care programs. Domains of palliative care from the guidelines are listed in Table 42–4. The domains can serve as a framework for hospitals to develop and evaluate their approach to a comprehensive palliative care program.

Table 42–4
National Consensus Project: Domains of Quality Palliative Care Identified as the Framework for Clinical Practice Guidelines for Quality Palliative Care*

1. Structure and processes of care
2. Physical aspects of care
3. Psychological and psychiatric aspects of care
4. Social aspects of care
5. Spiritual, religious, and existential aspects of care
6. Cultural aspects of care
7. Care of the imminently dying patient
8. Ethical and legal aspects of care

*References supporting the recommendations are included within the guidelines.

Source: http://www.nationalconsensusproject.org/guidelines.pdf (accessed March 14, 2005).

Medical and Nursing Education: A Key Component of Primary Palliative Care

The majority of students in medical, nursing, and other health care disciplines receive clinical training for practice in hospitals. Until recently, with the shift to ambulatory care, the majority of medical and nursing student education was provided in the hospital setting. However, few hospitals provided role models for teaching palliative care practices. The following is one of several comments made by family members about the insensitive way the act of "pronouncing" the death of their loved one was handled by house staff[38]:

> I was holding his hand when he stopped breathing. I called the nurse who called the doctor. He went over and looked at him lying in the bed, listened for a heartbeat with his stethoscope and said, "He's dead," and walked out of the room. That's it, not "I'm sorry," no "Is there anything we can do?" just "He's dead." It was painful—and made us think that the staff didn't care.

It is not surprising that this death occurred at the beginning of July, when interns began their first rotations directly out of medical school. A study by Ferris and colleagues[39] documented that medical schools devote little time to care of dying patients. A survey of medical interns revealed significant concern and fear about providing these services with no or little supervision. Lacking role models, the traditional "See one, do one, teach one" supervisory principle of medical education was ineffective. One resident explained that the pronouncing experience was not one that was perceived as causing harm when performed by the inexperienced. Another stated, "I felt really inadequate, I had absolutely no idea what to do when the nurse called me to pronounce this patient whom I had never met—my first night on call. I was never taught the steps—how long should I listen to the chest to be sure there was no heartbeat; what, if anything else, I should do; what should I say to the family. Thankfully, the death coordinator was there to help me fill out the paperwork." Conversely, in states where nurses are allowed to pronounce deaths, some course work exists to teach a process that gives attention to the family.

Clearly, such a predictable and easily defined process is amenable to quality improvement if it is identified as an educational priority for an institution or health care provider. A sample pocket card developed from multiple data sources of such a project is shown in Figure 42–2. This is printed internally on brightly colored stock on a standard laser printer so that it can be easily modified and so that quantities are readily available. A similar card was developed by others as part of a multimedia packet for resident education, called the Art of Compassionate Death Notification.[40] Other components of this comprehensive program include a facilitator's guide, manuals for learners, and videos demonstrating communication skills.

The problem is further compounded by the lack of EOL content in student curricula[41] and major textbooks.[42,43] These sources have been analyzed and have been found sorely lacking in the content that would inform students about the basics of EOL symptom management, decision-making, and critical communication skills. Until recently, neither textbooks nor clinical experiences were available to provide critical guidance to health professionals in how to provide effective EOL care. On a positive note however, funding is becoming available to study the issue and develop solutions.[44–46]

The introduction of programs in nursing and physician education has provided an important resource in education regarding EOL principles of care. The ELNEC program is partly sponsored by the American Association of Colleges of Nursing. The program is discussed in further detail in Chapter 60, but in brief, it is a curriculum developed to train nurse educators to provide undergraduate and graduate nursing students and practicing nurses with EOL education. The American Medical Association (AMA) and the RWJ Foundation have developed EPEC, a program that addresses similar issues for physicians. Both curricula are widely available as a means to educate nursing and medical staff.

Lastly, nurses have developed a number of other initiatives to advance professional knowledge and competency in EOL care. The American Nurses Credentialing Center (ANCC) administered the first palliative care advance practice nurse certification examination in May 2003.[47] Since the development of the examination, hundreds of advance practice nurses, both nurse practitioners and clinical nurse specialists, have become nationally board certified as palliative care specialists.

Chapter 60 discusses the topic of nursing education in detail. For the purposes of this chapter, it is important to remember to involve students in the process of palliative care education and change. Improvements in hospitals should address the learning environments of students. Specific ideas for improving the interface between education and quality improvement of hospital-based palliative care include the following:

- Arrange for clinician role models to provide lectures to students and faculty.
- Assist with curriculum review of current EOL care training.
- Change elective coursework and clinical work in hospice and palliative care to required status, and include these subjects in other mandatory clinical assignments.
- Use texts that contain clinically relevant palliative care content.
- Include content on ambulatory-based symptom management and decision-making that defines patient preferences for care.
- Encourage students to describe evidence-based approaches to palliative care and to challenge their mentors about approaches and interventions that increase the burden of care without clear patient benefit.
- Encourage students to learn from staff role models appropriate ways of communicating bad news and of presenting options that respect patient preferences and values.

Dartmouth-Hitchcock Medical Center

Quick reference card for: PRONOUNCEMENT OF DEATH

When you are called to pronounce a patient:

- *• **Recognize the extreme emotional significance of the actual pronouncement of death to family members in room.**
- *• Establish eye contact with family member(s) present.
- *• Introduce self to family.
- Examine patient for absence of breath sounds and heart sounds.
- Note time of death.
- After confirmation of death, verbally acknowledge patients death to family.
- *• Communicate condolences verbally (i.e., "I'm sorry for your loss.") or nonverbally.
- Determine legal next-of-kin from chart face sheet.
- Ask legal next-of-kin about autopsy, organ donation, funeral home name (family can call it in later).
- Nurse/secretary will contact Deceased Patient Coordinator (beeper #9399) to help complete the paper work (3 forms).
- Notify attending MD of death.

***DHMC study (Mills, Whedon, et al 1998) revealed these steps were often omitted from the pronouncement process.**

© DHMC End of Life Project June 23, 1998 (Revised 7-7-98)

Figure 42–2. Pronouncement card used as a reference at the time of death. © 1998 DHMC End of Life Project.

- Identify opportunities for undergraduate or graduate fellowships in palliative care.
- As part of quality improvement teams, offer students opportunities to become data collectors from patients, charts, and staff.

Palliative Care Pathways, Standards, and Aggressive Comfort Treatment

Reducing variation is a major strategy used by quality improvement leaders. Variation refers to the fluctuations in a process that can result in delays or unpredictable outcomes.[48] A patient with a serious illness who is experiencing an acute crisis may follow many different paths. Numerous institutions have studied their current processes of care and have created clinical pathways that can help standardize procedures and reduce the variation of care experienced by terminally ill or symptomatic palliative care patients as they traverse the complex health care system.[49,50] Usual components include attention to patient symptoms as well as family needs at system entry and throughout the course of stay until discharge. Assigning time frames to address needs helps in monitoring progress and tracking outcomes that have been met, as well as those that continue to need attention.

Although published guidelines and standards may offer similar suggestions, the road map format of clinical pathways identifies practical and accountable mechanisms to keep patient care moving in the direction of specific identified outcomes. Some pathway forms allow for documentation of variation from the designated path. Analysis of several instances of variation might alert a care team about a potential system "defect" in need of improvement. Additionally, Figure 42–3 illustrates a sample form for a brief, practical, but informative chart review that can be used to evaluate care of patients who died in a hospital environment.

Many institutions have implemented standard orders or evidence-based algorithms to guide various aspects of care pertinent to EOL situations. Some of these include limitations of certain types of therapies such as CPR and blood pressure medications. In addition, preprinted order sheets that outline management of symptoms and side effects such as nausea, constipation, and pain are making it easier for physicians and trainees to reproduce comprehensive plans that do not vary because of individual opinion. These order forms can be valuable teaching tools in a setting of regularly changing care providers. Figure 42–4 shows a sample order sheet and the companion guidelines printed on the reverse for patients who are hospitalized and have a palliative focus of care. Certainly, important considerations in the development of such "recipes" for care include having broad, multidisciplinary, evidence-based input. The process of producing such documents is also potentially a care consensus and learning environment for many teams.

It is perhaps one of the greatest misconceptions that once a person no longer seeks curative treatment "there is nothing more to do." Palliative care is aggressive care directed at comfort. All practitioners are responsible to ensure that, when cure is no longer possible, the patient and family can have confidence that everything will be done to provide pain management and relief of suffering. It is particularly important for health care providers to be cognizant of this fact when caring for individuals in the hospital at the EOL. Nurses in particular can advocate through development of hospital policy, education, and individual practice for aggressive comfort care. The health care team must ensure that a positive approach—focusing on what can be done for dying patients and their families—is implemented.

Hospital-Based Bereavement Programs

Improving the quality of EOL care in hospitals does not end with the development of mechanisms to ensure peaceful, pain-free patient death. Although accomplishing this goal is surely a comfort to family and friends, the aftermath for survivors is an important final step in the process of EOL care. Which families are most in need of specific services? Identifying families at the greatest risk has been the topic of palliative

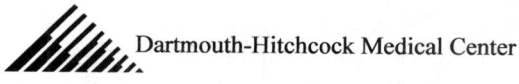

New Hampshire End of Life Care Chart Review

Date: ____________________ Chart Abstractor Name: ________________________________

1. Gender: Female ______ Male ______

2. Religion:
___ Jewish
___ Protestant
___ Roman Catholic
___ Other
___ None/Not Available

3. Primary Insurance
___ Medicare
___ Medicaid
___ Private/Commercial
___ Managed Care/HMO
___ Managed Care/Medicare
___ None/Self Pay
___ Other Insurance
___ Other Hospice Prog
___ Medicare Hosp Bene

4. Marital Status: ___ Never Married ___ Married ___ Widowed ____ Divorced/Separated

5. Next of Kin: ___ Spouse ___ Sibling ____ Son/Daughter ____ Other Unknown

6. _____/_____/_____ Date of Admission
7. _____/_____/_____ Date of Death
8. _____/_____/_____ Date of Birth

9. Unit of Death: ____________________

10. PROBLEMS/SYMPTOMS
Refer to any notes in the chart for the day of death and the day before. Please fill in *Yes* or *No.*

SYMPTOM/PROBLEM	ASSESSED	SYMPTOM PRESENT?	PLAN OF TREATMENT DOCUMENTED?	N/A
Pain/Discomfort				
Confusion/Agitation				
Shortness of breath				
Appetite				
Difficulty swallowing				
Nausea/Emesis				
Fever				
Anxiety Depression				

11. TREATMENTS ADMINISTERED
Refer to any notes in the chart for the day of death and the day before. Please fill in Yes or No.

TREATMENTS	YES	NO
Chemotherapy		
Narcotics (patch/oral/IV)		
Intravenous fluid/non-opioid IV medication		
Enteral tube (NG/peg?G))		
Foley catheter		
Intubation/Ventilator		
Physicial restraints		
Surgery in the OR		
Family emotional needs are noted		
Chaplaincy/Spiritual Consult		

TREATMENTS	YES	NO
Pt. psychosocial support offered		
Palliative Care Cx		
Antibiotics		

12. ICU
Was patient in an ICU at the time of death or within their last 2 calendar days? Yes ____ No ____

If yes, dates in the ICU: ICU Admission Date __________ ICU Discharge Date __________

13. DIRECTIVES
All information should be obtained from notes or orders in the medical chart.

DESCRIPTION	YES	NO	FIRST DATE NOTED IN CHART
Living will			
Values history			
Durable Powers of Attorney for Health Care			
Do not resuscitate (DNR) order			
Do not intubate (DNI) order			
Comfort measures only order			
Physician notes describing DNR discussion.			
Full code per patient preference.			

DHMC version 4/02

Figure 42–3. End-of-Life Hospital Chart Review. *Source*: © 1997 Center to Improve Care of the Dying.

Guidelines for Comfort Measures Orders

D/C ALL PREVIOUS ORDERS- Assess & reorder existing orders effective for comfort.

Activity: Goal is patient comfort. Activity level and hygiene routine should be based on patient's preference.

Hunger: Goal is to respond to patient's hunger, not to maintain a "normal nutritional intake."

Thirst: Goal is to respond to patient's thirst which is best accomplished by oral fluids, sips, ice chips, and mouthcare per patient desires, not IV hydration.

IV Fluids: Goal is to avoid over-hydration which can lead to discomfort from edema, pulmonary, and gastric secretions, and urinary incontinence. A small volume of IV fluid may assist with medication metabolism and delirium.

Dyspnea: Respond to the patient's perception of breathlessness rather than "numerical abnormalities" i.e. oxygen saturation via pulse oximetry. Interventions include medications (e.g. opioids, antianxiety agents, steroids), scopolamine patch and minimizing IV fluids to decrease secretions; oxygen therapy per nasal cannula prn for patient comfort-avoid face mask.
Fans at Bedside – Fans are available for patient comfort and are often more effective for perception of breathlessness than other interventions.

Elimination: Focus on managing distress from bowel or bladder incontinence. Insert Foley Catheter prn – per patient comfort and desire.

Oral Care: Studies show dry mouth is the most common & distressing symptom in conscious patients at end of life.
Ice chips and sips of fluid prn; Humidify oxygen to minimize oral/nasal drying.
Mouth care q 2 hours and prn – sponge oral mucosa and apply lubricant to lips and oral mucosa

Skin Care Air mattress, Pressure Sore Prevention Measures: per DHMC skin care guidelines.
Incontinent care every 2 hours and prn.

Monitoring: Focus monitoring on the patient's symptoms (e.g. pain) & responses to comfort measures.

Psychosocial Consults: Goal is to provide resources and support through the dying process

Medication for Symptom Management (Scheduled & PRN):
Pain Management- scheduled and breakthrough: consider PCA/ IV/SQ/rectal analgesics.
Dyspnea Management: consider opioids, scopolamine patch, atropine for secretions
Anxiety /Agitation Management: consider combination of lorazepam (Ativan) & haloperidol (Haldol).
Myoclonus: consider benzodiazepines &/or opioid rotation for myoclonus.
Depression Management: evaluate for antidepressants or methylphenidate.
Sleep Disturbance Management: consider diphenhydramine (Benadryl).
Pruritus Management: consider diphenhydramine (Benadryl) PO/IV.
Fever Management: consider acetaminophen (Tylenol) PO/ rectal
Nausea/Vomiting Management: consider prochlorperazine (Compazine), metoclopramide; 5-HT3 antagonist PO/IV.
Constipation Management: consider Narcotic Bowel Orders.
Diarrhea Management: consider diphenoxylate/atropine (Lomotil) or loperamide (Imodium).

DARTMOUTH-HITCHCOCK MEDICAL CENTER
One Medical Center Drive
Lebanon, New Hampshire 03756

Physician/ARNP Order Sheet
Comfort Measures

Any order preceded by a check box must have the box checked to enable the order. All other orders will be automatically implemented

☐ **DISCONTINUE ALL PREVIOUS ORDERS**

Activity:	☐OOB as tolerated	☐OOB with assistance	☐ Bedrest
Hunger:	☐Diet as tolerated	☐NPO	☐Other________
Thirst:	☐PO Fluids as tol. **IV Fluids:**	☐ No IVF	☐Yes________
Dyspnea:	☐O_2 prn for patient comfort	☐ No Oxygen	☐ Fan at bedside
Elimination:	☐Insert Foley Catheter prn		
Oral Care:	☐**per guideline (see reverse)**	☐**Other**________	
Skin Care:	☐**per guideline (see reverse)**	☐**Other**________	
Monitoring:			
Vital Signs:	☐ No	☐ Yes - specify ________	
Weight:	☐ No weights	☐ Yes - specify ________	
Labs:	☐ No lab draws	☐ Yes labs - specify________	

Consider Other Consults (if not already involved):☐ Palliative Care ☐Pastoral Care

Medication for Symptom Management
Pain – Scheduled (If PCA use special sheet) :
Pain - Breakthrough:
Dyspnea:
Anxiety/Agitation:
Myoclonus:
Depression:
Sleep Disturbance:
Pruritus:
Fever:
Nausea/Vomiting:
Constipation:
Diarrhea:
Other Orders:

A generic equivalent may be administered when a drug has been prescribed by brand name unless the order states to the contrary.

Physician/ARNP Signature ________ Date/Time ________
Print Physician/ARNP Name ________ Pager or Phone ________
Secretary Transcribing ________

Original to the medical record — Yellow copy to Pharmacy — See Other Side
P&T Committee: 7/15/2004 (P-225) — Medical Records: 08/03/2004 — Form #1826

Figure 42–4. Comfort Measures Physician Orders sheet *(left)* with guidelines for care as reference for house staff education on the back *(right)*. *Source*: © Dartmouth-Hitchcock Medical Center, June 2004; may be reproduced for noncommercial purposes.

care research, particularly in evaluating the quality of palliative care services.[51]

Bereavement services for survivors are an important part of the total care plan after the patient's death (see Chapter 27). Adverse physical and psychological outcomes of unsupported grief are known to occur during the bereavement period. Because of this, bereavement services are a typical component of the services offered to families when patients die as part of a hospice program. Because only 10% of all deaths in the United States have hospice involvement in EOL care, a large portion of families must rely on follow-up offered by other care providers. Few hospitals routinely offer bereavement services to families after patient deaths in hospital.[52]

Evaluation of services during the bereavement period serves two main purposes in quality improvement. First, development of these services by hospitals can address currently unmet needs of survivors, who usually need to discuss their own needs for information and support in order to cope with the loss. Second, this is a time when hospitals can learn more about the effectiveness of their provision of EOL care from the families' perspectives, both what went well and what can be improved. For instance, results of a focus group of bereaved family members indicated that, although the family was quite satisfied with pain management, breathing changes and dyspnea were not anticipated and were very distressing.[53] Another institution determined from a bereavement survey that the institution needed to make improvements in the areas of respecting patient privacy and dignity, family communications, emergency care, advance directives, and bereavement support.[52] See Appendix 42–1 for an example of an questionnaire with which family members can evaluate the EOL care received by their loved one.

After evaluation, hospitals can develop a project to improve and standardize bereavement care and would be well advised to consult with a local hospice program to collaborate on how this might occur. Instituting some very simple, standardized responses to death can vastly improve family satisfaction with care. These actions might include sending a note of sympathy or establishing some other contact from a staff member, mailing a list of local bereavement resources or a pamphlet, and delaying the time before a hospital bill is mailed out to prevent its coinciding with funeral or memorial services.

Secondary and Tertiary Palliative Care

As described previously, some hospitals are able to go beyond minimum palliative care competency and develop additional resources to provide palliative care services. Interdisciplinary consultation teams and units are commonly available to provide more specialized care. A tertiary center also focuses on educating students, developing curricula, performing research that can enhance the evidence base for palliative care, and serving as a role model for other programs. As described later, the AHA has begun to collect data on the number of hospital-based "palliative care programs"; however, these programs can vary, from volunteer personnel focusing on palliative care, to multicomponent programs with many staff and a mission of service, research, and education.

Palliative Care Consultation Teams

A growing literature summarizes the development of palliative care teams within hospitals to offer specialized consultation and expertise to patients, families, and other health care providers. Dunlop and Hockley published a manual in 1990 and a second edition in 1998 describing the experience in England.[54,55] They described the movement as one that tries to take the hospice philosophy of care and bring it into the hospital using a consultancy team. More recently, U.S. and Canadian hospital-based teams have described their experiences.[56–58] Among the components of successful teams are an interdisciplinary approach, strong nursing leadership, physician and nonphysician referral, rapid response to requested consultation, around-the-clock availability, and ability to follow patients through all care settings.[12]

From a quality improvement perspective, these teams can be effective in modeling behaviors that are supportive of appropriate hospital-based palliative care, but they should also recommend infrastructure changes as part of their approach to consultation. For assessment of care and processes to improve, demographic statistics about the location and nature of regular consultations is needed. For instance, if a particular unit or care provider has regular difficulty managing patients with dyspnea, targeted educational approaches and treatment algorithms or standardized orders may help achieve consistent and long-lasting change. Theoretically, a consultancy team could "put itself out of business" with such an approach. However, teams to date have not reported the need to dissolve as an outcome of implementing system changes.

Few studies have examined the impact of a consultation team on the overall care of patients at the EOL. Challenges have included identifying exactly which components or processes of the team are responsible for the outcomes, performing multimethod research (e.g., using both qualitative and quantitative methods) defining outcomes attributable to team intervention, and implementing measures that can validly and reliably capture this information.[59] Establishing an evidence base is paramount to the economic justification and reimbursement mechanisms for many hospitals.

Inpatient Hospice and Palliative Care Units in a General Hospital

Some hospitals, faced with the problem of providing high-quality EOL care in the acute care hospital, have found the development of a specialized unit to be the solution. In the United Kingdom, these units have been developed from preexisting oncology units, as part of another unit, or sometimes in a separate building that is distinct but near the hospital it serves.[55] U.S. hospitals have varying amounts of experience with opening specialized units for the care of patients with

EOL, hospice, or palliative care needs.[55,60–62] This in-hospital approach has some general benefits and burdens.[12] Some of the benefits include the following:

- Patients requiring palliative care have a familiar place to go during the exacerbations and remissions that come with progressive disease.
- Unit staff and policies are under the control and financing of experts trained as a team who are skillful at difficult care and communications.
- Patients may get palliative care earlier if other care teams see the advantages of this approach and trust that patients will receive good care.
- Providers who monitor their patients on these units (if allowed) can learn valuable lessons about palliative care that can be carried forward to future patients. These future patients may not require admission to the PCU for some types of care.

Some of the disadvantages of creating a distinct unit include the following:

- It can prevent others from learning valuable palliative care techniques if the principal staff are seen as "specialized" and are secluded in one area.
- Care providers may come to rely on this expertise instead of learning palliative care techniques themselves.
- If unit transfer includes a transfer of doctors to a palliative care specialist, patients and families may feel abandoned by their primary team in the final hours.
- Hospice providers fear loss of the hospice philosophy when a PCU exists in the context of the general hospital.

Some mature palliative care programs have been able to provide a trinity of services,[12] including a consultancy team, an inpatient palliative care/hospice unit, and a home care program, all under the jurisdiction of a single hospital system. This full-service approach can ease transitions among different levels of care and has the potential to provide the optimum in seamless care for patients at the EOL. Such programs can serve as models and can set standards for other programs to aim for.

A major consideration in the use of such services, regardless of how broadly based, is the barrier to care presented by not recognizing that a patient is dying. Many studies now document health care providers' inaccuracy in predicting prognosis.[2,5,11] As a result, many patients who could benefit from palliative care and hospice services are denied admission. A comprehensive discussion of the reasons for inaccuracy of prognosis is beyond the scope of this chapter, although it remains a major issue that must be addressed within any institution wishing to develop specialty palliative care services. Hospice programs are very familiar with such issues, and palliative care programs would be wise to review lessons learned in providing hospice care earlier in the disease trajectory for patients in need.

Initiatives to Improve Hospital-Based Palliative Care

In 1974, the Royal Victoria Hospital in Montreal, Canada, developed one of the first initiatives in North America to improve hospital-based palliative care. They developed a palliative care service to meet the needs of hospitalized patients who were terminally ill within the general hospital setting.[63] The palliative care service was an integral part of the Royal Victoria Hospital, a 1000 bed teaching hospital affiliated with McGill University, and consisted of five complementary clinical components: (1) the PCU, (2) the home care service, (3) the consultation team, (4) the palliative care clinic, and (5) the bereavement follow-up program. Members of an interdisciplinary team were involved with the care of these patients, and the focus was on holistic care with pain control and symptom management.[63]

These basic palliative care concepts are still not prevalent in many U.S. hospitals. However, positive changes are occurring, as evidenced by data from the AHA, which began to measure hospital-based palliative care in 2000. Table 42–5 summarizes the 2000–2002 AHA survey data on the growth of hospital-based palliative care, hospice, and pain management programs.

Efforts to improve pain management[64] created a foundation for easing the pain of dying patients. However, the improvement strategies implemented in pain management have also been applied to palliative care improvement efforts. The Wisconsin Resource Manual for Improvement[65] and the City of Hope Pain/Palliative Care Resource Center[66] are two examples of pain management efforts that can be expanded to incorporate hospital-based palliative care in general. The City of Hope website (http://www.cityofhope.org/prc/, accessed February 1, 2005) provides articles and tools for pain management, many of which also are useful for palliative care, and an

Table 42–5
Results of American Hospital Association Annual Survey of Hospital-Based Palliative Care Programs, 2000–2002

Type of Program	No. (%) of hospitals with programs 2000	2001	2002
Hospice	1102 (22.7%)	1118 (23.6%)	1134 (23.3%)
Pain management	2052 (42.3%)	2102 (44.5%)	2256 (46.3%)
Palliative care	668 (13.8%)	806 (17.0%)	951 (19.5%)
Total no. of respondents	4856	4728	4876

Source: American Hospital Association. Hospital statistics. Chicago: Health Forum, 2003.

institutional assessment of the quality of pain management.[67] These tools can be easily adapted to help a project team think more broadly about palliative care and symptoms in addition to pain.[68] This section describes other examples of resources for developing or improving hospital-based systems of palliative care.

Center to Advance Palliative Care

One of the major efforts to improve hospital-based palliative care programs in the United States is led by the CAPC. Formed and funded by a 4-year grant from the RWJ Foundation in 2000, the national center was established at Mount Sinai School of Medicine in New York City. The Center, codirected by Christine Cassel, MD, and Diane Meier, MD, has a mission to make information on how to establish high-quality palliative care services available to hospitals and health systems nationwide.[69]

CAPC assists hospitals with the planning, development, and implementation of hospital-based palliative care programs. In addition to assisting hospitals and other health systems in program development, CAPC facilitates collaboration among hospitals, hospices, and nursing homes; promotes educational initiatives in palliative care; and encourages growth and development of new and innovative mechanisms for financing palliative care programs.[69]

CAPC has developed six Palliative Care Leadership Centers (PCLCs) to assist organizations that wish to learn the practical aspects of developing a palliative care program. The six organizations are Fairview Health Services, Minneapolis, MN; Massey Cancer Center of Virginia Commonwealth University Medical Center, Richmond, VA; Medical College of Wisconsin, Milwaukee, WI; Mount Carmel Health System, Columbus, OH; Palliative Care Center of the Bluegrass, Lexington, KY; and University of California, San Francisco, CA. Each represents a different type of health care system and palliative care delivery model. They serve as exemplar organizations offering site visits, hands-on training, and technical assistance to support development of palliative care programs nationwide. Further information regarding the PCLC can be found on the CAPC website[70] (http://www.capc.org, accessed February 1, 2005).

Institute for Healthcare Improvement

In 1997, a quality improvement organization known as the Institute for Healthcare Improvement (IHI) adopted improving EOL care in hospitals and other parts of the health care system as a major mission. As shown in Table 42–6, the structure of the first IHI EOL collaborative and the results of this initiative have been published.[14,26] In brief, the organization provided quality improvement assistance to organizations, and the resulting methods and results constitute a wide variety of outcomes to which almost any hospital or health care agency might aspire.

To assist groups in getting started, a table (Table 42–7) focused on four major issues in EOL care was distributed to encourage organizations to compare their problems and issues ("current practice") with what were proposed as "best" and "optimum" practices. The table included examples of specific, measurable target outcomes that a group might choose to adopt.[26] The four selected areas resulted from brainstorming by the planning group, who were all nationally recognized leaders and clinicians in EOL care. They concluded that the following four areas were most in need of attention and amenable to change:

- Improving the management of pain and other symptoms
- Continuity of care
- Advance directives
- Family support

Each institution sent a team of at least two or more members, representing the key disciplines implementing change in their organizations (e.g., nurses, physicians, chaplains, social workers, administrators) to a series of three meetings between July 1997 and July 1998. Steps to ensure support from senior leaders of each organization were considered vital at the outset. Teams were provided with large-group didactic content and written materials. They also participated in concentrated, small-group meetings to identify what they would do on return to their institutions. Regular progress reports were sent to IHI, monthly conference calls were held, and online discussions were conducted to support the teams and offer advice if particular barriers or issues developed.

These teams were successful in achieving many of their goals, from improving pain relief and dyspnea, reducing hospitalizations, and improving advance care planning, to implementing bereavement services. The experiences of these organizations provide a wealth of practical advice and methods for accomplishing quality improvement in many areas and settings of care and are available on the IHI website (http://www.ihi.org/ihi, accessed February 1, 2005) and in print. Breakthrough improvements achieved by the collaborative are listed in Table 42–8.

In 2003, the IHI, together with the Center for Palliative Care Studies (CPCS), developed a new collaborative focusing on adapting health care systems to meet the challenges of serious chronic illness in the last phase of life. The key goal of the collaborative is to gather information and create a common database that will be used to help improve the dying experience for patients and their families.[71] By participating in this collaborative, organizations have the ability to

- Improve quality of life for people with serious illnesses
- Decrease hospital length of stay
- Enhance use of hospice services
- Meet JCAHO standards
- Build new palliative care programs
- Learn methods to apply quality improvement to real problems

Table 42–6
Structure of the Institute for Healthcare Improvement (IHI) Collaborative: Improving Care at the End of Life*

The Institute for Healthcare Improvement (IHI) is a Boston-based, independent, nonprofit organization working since 1991 to accelerate improvement in health care systems in the United States, Canada, and Europe by fostering collaboration, rather than competition, among health care organizations.

IHI provides bridges connecting people and organizations that are committed to real health care reform and who believe they can accomplish more by working together than they can separately.

Background

Study after study finds that patients, families, doctors, and other professionals want the same qualities of care at the end of life: dignity, comfort, communication, and the company of loved ones. Yet time and again we seem trapped in desperate struggles and wasted energies that help no one. Rational, respectful care at the end of life is possible; now we need to assure it.

Participants

Since July 1997, 48 organizations from throughout the United States and Canada have been working intensively to improve the quality of care at the end of life while also reducing unwanted, nonbeneficial care.

Overall Goals

Reduce incidence of severe pain by 25%.

Increase by 35% the number of patients who have made their wishes known about end-of-life care.

Reduce by 50% the number of patients with transfers in the last 2 weeks of life.

Areas of Focus

Collaborative teams are focusing on the following areas for improving care at the end of life:

- Pain management and palliative care
- Advance care planning for end of life
- Optimizing transfers among care settings
- Family support.

Key Changes

Successful interventions that improve care at the end of life for patients and their families include the following:

- Instituting pain and symptom management protocols.
- Initiating advanced care planning discussions within 24 hours after admission and documenting the plan in a patient's chart. If this is not done, someone other than the patient's physician initiates advanced care planning within 36 hours after admission.
- Increasing 24-hour access to staff, using pagers and other communication devices to decrease hospital emergency room utilization.
- Using a "pull-system"—one-to-one case finding in the hospital to arrange early admission of targeted patients to palliative and hospice care.
- Beginning bereavement assistance and support for the family and friends before the patient dies.

Chair

Joanne Lynn, MD
President, Center for Improving Care of the Dying
George Washington University
Washington, DC

*For more information on IHI collaboratives, see http://www.IHI.org.

Table 42–7
Recommendations for Areas of Focus and Targets for Improvement in Health Care Agencies Involved in IHI Collaborative

Current Practice	Best Practice	Optimum Practice	Proposed Targets (for Your Population)
Pain/Symptoms			
• Most often not assessed/monitored • Routinely treated with predictably inadequate treatment (drugs and dosages) • Usually treated only after established, rather than preventively • Gaps and delays in treatment are agonizing and commonplace • Major symptoms are treatable: pain, dyspnea, depression, anxiety (also nausea, itching, insomnia) • No one held accountable for shortcomings • Patients and families expect severe symptoms	• 100% assessment on a regular, recurrent basis (e.g., "fifth vital sign" or item in nursing home quarterly review) • WHO/APS/AHCPR guidelines for cancer pain • Low rate of use of opioids for breakthrough pain; all opioids on regular dosing • Patients or families in control of dose timing • Coverage doses travel with patient to procedures or during transfers • Serious symptoms considered appropriate for emergency response (stat page, rapid home visit, calling on back-up provider) • Performance routinely reviewed and shortcomings addressed • Patients and families expect comfort	• 100% assessment of pain, depression, dyspnea, and anxiety on appropriate schedule (admission, change in status, and periodically) • Use of all appropriate modalities, often on time-limited trails—including opioids, biofeedback, hypnosis, steroids, neuroablative procedures, stimulants, etc. Severe symptoms always have an appropriately aggressive response • Ready availability of skilled consultants in all settings (including ICU, hospital, nursing home, and home). • Patient and family have expectations of competence, control, comfort and are enabled to be active participants in deciding and providing care • Patient never left suffering due to relocation • Emergency response "on call" for serious symptoms in any setting • Routine care review and routine system feedback for quality improvement, public education, and accreditation	1. Ensure 100% compliance with recurrent assessment protocol. 2. Guarantee initial assessment of serious pain or dyspnea within 5 min in hospital, 15 min in nursing home or at home; initial intervention within 15 min in hospital and 1 h in nursing home or at home. 3. All patients have pain <5 (of 10) in last 2 days of life (by patient or family report). 4. Reduce by 50% the number of patients who report pain >5 (of 10) in any time period or episode of care. 5. All cancer patients with pain >5 (of 10) are on appropriate opioids, and all patients with pain >5 (of 10) are on appropriate analgesics. 6. All patients at risk of severe dyspnea have "standby" plans and needed skills/supplies in place (also advanced care planning goal). 7. Resource people with proven skills in chronic pain management and in management of neuropsychiatric complications of serious illness (depression, psychosis, delirium, anxiety, seizures) are readily available to every patient regardless of setting or insurance. 8. Eliminate times when patient or family reports pain as being overwhelming or out of control. 9. Reduce "prn" for breakthrough pain to less than 20% of opioid use.

(*continued*)

Table 42–7
Recommendations for Areas of Focus and Targets for Improvement in Health Care Agencies Involved in IHI Collaborative *(continued)*

Current Practice	Best Practice	Optimum Practice	Proposed Targets (for Your Population)
			10. All patients/families understand the patient's symptoms and management and can adjust medications within agreed range. 11. All patients with signs of depression have a trial of drug treatment. 12. Individual and regular shortcomings are noted and reviewed in Incident Reports, M&M conferences, QI committee, and credentials review.
Continuity/Transfers			
• Seriously ill persons have no one who stays with them throughout. • Transfers between settings are dictated mostly by utilization and financing issues for the care system, not patient or family preferences. • Transfers among professionals are dictated by professionals' convenience. • Most patients change settings and/or caregivers multiple times in the last few weeks of life. • The fact and the expectation of discontinuity precludes intimacy, empathy, promise-making, and trust. • Many transfers lose settled care plans, treatment schedules, and understandings. • Frequent transfers mean that no one is held accountable for the overall course—or even for there being a standard for a good course. • Transfer to hospice or nursing home is especially discontinuous, and transfer by EMS is routinely maximally life-extending.	• Hospice usually ensures continuity in all settings, once enrolled. • Some nursing homes have developed capacity to care for seriously ill residents on-site, including a hospice-like mode. • Some special "advanced illness" programs coordinate all care out of one office and keep one nurse/social worker/physician in charge of care throughout. • Some programs have coordinated records available at all sites electronically, or have the patient carry the record, or both. • Some nursing home or home care agencies have arranged for special direct hospital or hospice admission to avoid trauma in ambulances and ERs. • Some states and regions have developed accord on orders that reshape EMS services.	• People dying with cancer, advanced old age, or dementia virtually always die where they live. Services are mobilized to these settings. • People dying with strokes and organ system failures die at home (or nursing home) or in a hospital, but in either case under the care of those who know them and with appropriate services. • Utilization-induced transfer almost never happens in the last 2 days of life. • Switching key personnel while a patient is in any one setting is uncommon, viewed as unfortunate, and the subject of careful planning to support patient and family. • Patients dying in ICU, ER, or busy ward settings have more family-attentive settings available for temporary use.	1. >50% of cancer patients are in hospice >4 wk and <20% are in hospice for <2 wk. 2. >60% of those living at home with established fatal disease should die there, with good care. 3. <10% of deaths have change of setting in last 2 days. 4. 90% of families can name the one or two care providers who (together) were constant over the period when their family member was very ill. 5. >80% of those living in nursing homes die there, with good care. 6. >80% of dying persons who have available an integrated care system get all services from that system. 7. >50% of deaths from CHF, COPD, cirrhosis, and stroke have >4 wk in hospice or another special end-of-life program. 8. Serious errors in transfer yield adverse events for all participants: review, payment penalty, QI efforts. 9. DNR orders established in one setting are always transferred to another (and confirmed when appropriate).

(continued)

Table 42–7
Recommendations for Areas of Focus and Targets for Improvement in Health Care Agencies Involved in IHI Collaborative *(continued)*

Current Practice	Best Practice	Optimum Practice	Proposed Targets (for Your Population)
			10. <10% of deaths have change of physician in last 2 days. 11. Written oral care plan moves with or ahead of patient for every change of care setting. 12. 90% of families feel that they know who is "in charge" and how to reach that person at all times.
Advanced Care Planning			
• Very little attention is paid to overall future course—not discussed, articulated, or planned for. • Most people are not even asked to name a surrogate, even when who that would be is quite unclear. • Among persons who have very little chance of surviving CPR and substantial chance of cardiopulmonary arrest, few have discussions about DNR, even when put at special risk by being in hospital. • Most legal advance directives are too nonspecific, unavailable, or inapplicable to direct care, yet patients think they have solved their problems by filling them out. • Almost no care planning deals with the specific drugs, skills, or procedures needed to allow the patient's preferences to be effected. • Some specific documented patient preferences are thoughtlessly abrogated.	• Regularly offering formal written planning opportunities (e.g., Vermont Ethics Network form) • Area-wide advance planning • Emergency kit of drugs and other paraphernalia at home, appropriate to family training and professional availability • Emergency response team to go to home for pain, dyspnea, seizures, family crisis, etc. • Formatted advance planning discussions	• Likely course, including urgent complications and major decision points, is articulated for all chronically ill patients. • "Last phase of life" is noted, negotiated, and shared—among providers, patient and family—for >80% of dying patients. • Plans are written and discussed for likely "urgent complications" and for prolonged incompetence for every "last phase of life." • Plans made in one setting or by one set of providers working with patient and family are honored and confirmed, as appropriate, throughout the care system. • Plans for urgent complications are translated into specific service needs (e.g., drugs, oxygen), and these are put in place in the appropriate settings. • CPR is allowed with strong patient/family preference but is very rare. • Patients and families are not browbeaten into acquiescence with caregivers, nor are they brutalized by having to review painful decisions too often.	1. CPR is attempted at death for <3% of patients who are known to be in the "last phase of life." 2. Decrease unplanned admissions by 50%. 3. A written care plan documents priorities and plans for >80% of patients in "last phase of life." 4. An appropriate surrogate is known (and documented if necessary) for 80% of those in the "last phase of life." 5. 90% of those who die in the system, of chronic disease, are identified as dying 2 months earlier, and 50% are identified 1 year earlier. 6. Patients and families are aware of eventual fatal nature of disease for >75% of those so identified. 7. >80% of patients and families know what to do for worsening pain, dyspnea, or cardiac arrest and know the signs of impending death and what to do. 8. Plans for after death (who should come to share that time, funeral, burial, family support) are made and documented for >50%. 9. ER and 911 use declines by 50% in targeted population.

(continued)

Table 42–7
Recommendations for Areas of Focus and Targets for Improvement in Health Care Agencies Involved in IHI Collaborative *(continued)*

Current Practice	Best Practice	Optimum Practice	Proposed Targets (for Your Population)
			10. 80% of "last phase of life" patients at home have plans documented to shape 911/EMS response.
Support of Family and of Meaningfulness			
• Families are excluded or ignored, granted only the role of veto in care planning. • Families do not know prognosis, uncertainties, desirable timing of behaviors, who to turn to for counsel, or what is reasonably expected of them. • Many opportunities to complete relationship (human or transcendent) are not taken. • Many patients or families do not have opportunity to attend to religious/spiritual issues or meaningful rituals. • Most families have no follow-up in bereavement. • Many dissatisfied or guilt-ridden families are never heard, and some have lives blighted by their experience. • Families and patients have little practice at leave-taking.	• Care in hospice routinely includes family and spiritual concerns. • Hospice and home care agencies sometimes provide brochures and counseling about what to expect and how one might respond. • Hospice and some individual programs routinely follow families in bereavement, providing or referring to services as appropriate. • Some care providers insist on enabling family cohesion and rearrangement, spiritual search for meaning, and culturally meaningful rituals. • Some care settings help patients and families "rehearse" for dying by practicing leave-taking and imagining the time after.	• Center the experience in terms of spirituality and meaning, rather than medical and physiologic issues. • Make human relationships and spiritual issues the central concern, with professional caregiver habits always subservient. • Use episodes of serious illness as "dress rehearsals" for eventual death. • Create rituals that mark stages and ensure reassurance. • Always follow up with family—explain, reassure, counsel. • Learn how to provide care that is death accepting/enhancing, life-prolonging, and physiology-restoring.	1. >90% of families report they would want to be cared for in this way if they were similarly sick. 2. >90% of families report they cannot recall when they were kept "in the dark," an uncaring remark from a caregiver, or a "put down" of their beliefs, practices, or views. 3. All bereaved families get at least one follow-up call from a doctor or nurse who can answer "medical" questions and check for dysfunctional grief. 4. Double the rate at which patients and families agree that "the last few weeks or months were especially meaningful." 5. For chronic organ system failure, develop a care pattern in which 80% of staff and 80% of patients/families feel that staff are pleased and supportive of survival (in an exacerbation) and also supportive of a good dying. 6. >90% of families report that their loved one was given tender care, the family's emotional state was noticed and responded to, and the caregiver said or did something especially meaningful.

APS, American Pain Society; AHCPR, Agency for Health Care Policy and Research; CHF, congestive heart failure; COPD, chronic obstructive pulmonary disease; CPR, cardiopulmonary resuscitation; DNR, do not resuscitate; EMS, emergency medical services; ER, emergency room; ICU, intensive care unit; IHI, Institute for Healthcare Improvement; M&M, morbidity and mortality; QI, quality improvement; WHO, World Health Organization.

Source: Lynn et al. (1997), reference 8. Used with permission of J. Lynn, MD, IHI chair.

Table 42–8
Breakthrough Improvements Achieved in Past CPCS-Led Collaboratives

- 60% reduction in patients with pain greater than 5 on a 10-point scale
- 50% or greater decrease in exacerbations in heart or lung failure
- 90% or greater rates of documented discussion and planning in advance of emergency or incompetence
- Substantial increases in hospice length of stay
- Substantial decline in use of artificial feeding in advanced dementia

CPCS, Center for Palliative Care Studies.
Source: Washington Home Center for Palliative Care Studies. National Medicaring Quality Improvement Collaborative. Available at: http://www.medicaring.org/nc2004/index.html (accessed February 1, 2005).

These two breakthrough series collaboratives have provided resources to hospitals interested in improving EOL care. By participating in the latest collaborative, organizations can expect participation in team learning sessions on improving the quality of care for serious illnesses, telephone and e-mail consultation and feedback from collaborative faculty, and involvement in the improvement process, keeping up with best practices, and mobilizing support for needed changes.[71]

Veterans Health Administration Initiatives

The U.S. Department of Veterans Affairs (VA) health care system has shown leadership in improving EOL care in their hospitals through multiple initiatives that have been designed or implemented since the early 1990s. In 1992, Secretary Jesse Brown mandated that VA medical centers (VAMCs) establish hospice consultation teams to respond to the complex palliative care needs of patients with advanced disease. The VA provided training for team members during 1992 and 1993. One team reported success in pain and cost reduction while also undertaking significant institution-wide improvements through education of nurses and house staff and making pain management resources available.[72]

In 1997, the Veterans Health Administration began an intensive, system-wide, continuous quality improvement (CQI) initiative to improve pain management. This endeavor resulted from a 1997 survey that found both acute and chronic pain management services to be inconsistent, inaccessible, and nonuniform throughout the system. Two major thrusts formed the basis of the initiative: issuing a system-wide mandate and forming a permanent National Pain Advisory Committee to provide direction and encouragement to the development of the program. Thus, this initiative incorporated two essential elements found in all successful system-wide improvement strategies: an influential champion at the highest level of the organization and a mandate for organizational commitment to this activity. The charge document offered a variety of suggestions for system improvement: making pain more visible by enhancing current measurement and reporting methods (using the "Fifth Vital Sign" approach in all patient contacts in the system); increasing access to pain therapy and increasing professional education about pain; adopting the Agency for Health Care Policy and Research and American Pain Society guidelines for pain management; pursuing research on pain therapies for veterans; distributing and sharing pain management protocols via a central clearinghouse; and exploring methods to maintain cost-effective pain therapy.

Also in 1997, the VA incorporated a palliative care measure in the performance criteria of its regional directors. In this program, performance of the directors is evaluated based on the number of charts that contain information about veterans' preferences regarding various palliative care indicators.[73]

In 1998, the RWJ Foundation Last Acts program created a Clinical Palliative Care Faculty leadership program and awarded a 2-year grant to promote development of 30 faculty fellows from VA-affiliated internal medicine training programs. Their goal was to develop curricula to train residents in the care of dying patients, to integrate relevant content into the curricula of residency training programs, and to add internal medicine faculty leaders and innovators to the field of palliative medicine.

In 2001, the VA Hospice and Palliative Care initiative began. This was a two-phase initiative to improve EOL care for veterans. Phase 1 of the project was funded in part by the National Hospice and Palliative Care Organization (NHPCO) and the Center for Advanced Illness Coordinated Care. This phase of the initiative was designed to accelerate access to hospice and palliative care for veterans. A major product of the program was the Hospice-Veteran Partnership Toolkit. It also created 2.5 full-time equivalent employee positions in Geriatrics and Extended Care, to be used for hospice and palliative care presence in the VA system.

In 2004, phase 2 of the project was launched. It was funded in part by Rallying Points and the NHPCO. It builds on the success of phase 1 and aspires to develop a Hospice-Veterans Administration Partnership in every state and to build an enduring infrastructure for the Accelerated Administrative and Clinical Training Program. In a statement made in 2002 regarding the VA national initiatives, the VA made a clear commitment to improving hospice and palliative care for their patients. The Geriatrics and Long Term Care strategic plan is as follows[74]: "All VAMCs will be required to have designated inpatient beds for hospice and palliative care, or access to these services in the community, and an active hospice and palliative care team for consult, care and placement." Together these initiatives address the need for improvement on multiple fronts and create a momentum in the VA system that can set an example for other large hospital-based systems of care.

United Hospital Fund's Hospital Palliative Care Initiative

The multiyear, multihospital research and demonstration initiative of the United Hospital Fund (UHF) sought to improve the quality of hospital care for persons at the EOL. In the first phase of the initiative, 12 hospitals received grants to analyze the institutional, professional, fiscal, and regulatory forces shaping EOL care. In the second phase, 2-year program grants were awarded to the following five New York City hospitals to seek specific goals:

1. Beth Israel Medical Center—To develop an array of new palliative care service delivery and education activities, including the creation of a new position, medical director for palliative care.
2. The Brooklyn Hospital Center—To create a new position of palliative care expert, with responsibility and authority to facilitate the coordinated delivery of palliative care services to a select group of patients and their families.
3. Montefiore Medical Center—To evaluate and improve physician practice patterns concerning EOL care by using evaluative feedback for a 1-year period, focused on five areas of EOL care.
4. The Mount Sinai Medical Center—To create a comprehensive new supportive care service to provide coordinated palliative care services across a range of settings.
5. Saint Vincent's Hospital and Medical Center—To create a new palliative care consulting team to build on the existing outpatient supportive care service and expand them to include physician and psychiatric expertise for a select group of patients and their families in both the inpatient and outpatient settings.

Although not all of these organizations are specifically using quality improvement methods, the outcomes and products to improve palliative care that evolved from these projects can inform other hospitals wishing to replicate their successes.[75]

Since the implementation of the five programs, the UHF has produced a special report, *Building Hospital Palliative Care Programs: Lessons from the Field.* This report can be obtained from the UHF website (http://www.uhfnyc.org/, accessed February 1, 2005) or by calling the organization directly. A major outcome of the initiative was recognition by all involved of the complexity and obstacles to integrating palliative care into hospital systems. Table 42–9 lists the lessons learned from the five-hospital palliative care initiatives and the suggestions for hospitals that are creating palliative care programs in the future.

Table 42–9
The United Hospital Fund—Building Hospital Palliative Care Programs: Lessons from the Field

Lessons learned from five-hospital palliative care initiatives:

- There is no one successful model of palliative care services.
- Initiating palliative care services is extraordinarily demanding of staff time and other resources.
- A key decision is how much authority the palliative care team will have to implement its recommendations after the initial referral.
- Initial resistance among senior primary care physicians should not be underestimated.
- Palliative care teams may make most of their contributions by establishing goals of care, addressing family needs, and resolving conflicts.
- Key departments and their directors must be included early in the planning process.
- It is important to trace the impact on overall hospital and functioning.
- Discharge planning is key to a successful palliative care effort.
- Palliative care services in hospitals are costly and resource demanding.

Next Steps:

- Reach patients earlier in course of illness through the Community Oriented Palliative Care Initiative
- Introduction of palliative care in combination with life-prolonging care
- Provide wider range of services to patients and families
- Decrease the inappropriate use of palliative care service

Source: Hopper SS. Building Hospital Programs: Lessons from the Field. A Special Report. New York, United Hospital Fund of New York, 2001.

The Joint Commission on Accreditation of Healthcare Organizations

The JCAHO is one of the paramount accreditation organizations for hospitals and other health care organizations. The purpose of JCAHO is to continuously improve the safety and quality of care provided to the public. JCAHO is an independent, not-for-profit organization, and perhaps its most important benefit is that JCAHO-accredited organizations make a commitment to continuous improvement in patient care. During an accreditation survey, the JCAHO evaluates a group's performance by using a set of standards that cross eight functional areas[76]: (1) rights, responsibilities, and ethics; (2) continuum of care; (3) education and communication; (4) health promotion and disease prevention; (5) leadership; (6) management of human resources; (7) management of information; (8) improving network performance.

In 2004, a specific palliative care focus was introduced within two standards: (1) rights, responsibilities, and ethics and (2) the provision of care, treatment, and services. The goal of the ethics, rights, and responsibilities standard is to improve outcomes by recognizing and respecting the rights of each patient and working in an ethical manner. Care, treatment, and services are to be provided in a way that respects the person and fosters dignity. The performance standard states that a patient's family should be involved in the care, treatment, and services if the patient desires. Care, treatment, and services are provided through ongoing assessments of care; meeting the patient's needs; and either successfully discharging the patient or providing referral or transfer of the patient for continuing care.[77,78] More detailed information is available by contacting JCAHO or visiting their website at http://www.jcaho.org (accessed February 1, 2005).

The revisions of these standards in 2003 and 2004 incorporated a stronger emphasis on palliative care practices within hospitals. Hence, organizations are being held accountable for the manner in which they provide appropriate palliative care. It is in the public's best interest that JCAHO requires organizations to adhere to these provisions for a successful accreditation. The implementation of specific EOL standards has reinforced the directive that pain and EOL issues must be addressed and health care institutions should strive to maximize performance activities that affect the quality of patient care in this population.

Economic Issues of Hospital-Based Palliative Care

The use of the diagnosis-related group (DRG) system has played a major role in the current provision of hospital-based care. The prospective payment system of Medicare was one of the first economic stimuli that began to shift EOL care out of hospitals. Simultaneously, the Medicare hospice benefit was instituted, which reconfigured financing for hospice care (described earlier) and reimbursed some home care, acute care, and specialized units in nursing homes.[15]

The Health Care Financing Administration (HCFA) uses DRG codes to define Medicare reimbursement, although at present limited mechanisms exist to obtain reimbursement for various types of palliative care in hospitals under Medicare. In response to this limitation, in October 1996 a trial of using the v code 66.7 was initiated as a mechanism to collect data about palliative care being provided in hospitals.[79] At present, this code does not elicit reimbursement but allows for data to be collected about the current nature of palliative care.

Clinicians and administrators may see development of palliative care services as a way to save money as less invasive procedures and tests are recommended, compared with more expensive "curative" care. An evaluation of a high-volume specialty unit and team was able to demonstrate cost savings via cost avoidance in one center. Smith and colleagues[80] evaluated 237 patients housed on the PCU compared with 38 contemporary control patients treated elsewhere in the hospital and determined that PCU patient charges were 59% lower, direct costs 56% lower, and total costs 7% lower. In this case, providing less unwanted care resulted in fewer ICU stays and fewer costly, invasive procedures. However palliative care experts suggest that programs often "rationalize" the use of hospital resources in a way that respects patients' preferences for care. In program development, financial risk–benefit analysis is critical; through CAPC and other resources, tools to assist hospitals wishing to perform such analyses are available.[37]

Although there is a bias against hospital death, because hospital care is associated with high-technology interventions, there are times when dying in the hospital allows for a more comfortable death than at home. In any case, valid reimbursed hospital admissions for palliative care may be difficult to obtain within the current DRG codes. In the best case, the palliative care DRG would remedy this. However, some oppose the creation of a new DRG, because the assignment of the code may only describe what is currently being done, which may not be adequate and hence may not reflect what state-of-the-art palliative care could achieve.

Managed care can influence the quality of EOL care in hospitals in both positive and negative ways. Patients in a managed care plan need approvals and are carefully observed so that they do not spend unnecessary days in the hospital. This approach can be quite restrictive when extra planning time to ensure patient comfort is restricted. On the other hand, several features of managed care make it a potentially positive force for improvement.[81] Anthem Blue Cross and Blue Shield of New Hampshire has implemented an innovative Advanced Disease Care Management approach. In response to identified needs of members, the director of medical management and the clinical quality improvement coordinator (both nurses) redesigned the plan's hospice benefit.[82] Excerpts from the provider/member educational brochure describing their program are shown in Table 42–10. Standards of pain and hospice care were sent to all providers, and a monitoring system was implemented to ensure adherence and to provide for review of situations that were outside the scope of the guidelines. This use of quality improvement methodology outside the hospital to simplify care and hold providers and insurers accountable for a predetermined standard of EOL care proved successful. The approach ultimately benefited plan members by increasing access to appropriate levels of palliative care (including hospital-based care, when appropriate).

Another effort to evaluate how health plans and systems provide EOL care consists of a strategy to measure and compare outcomes across organizations. Funded by the RWJ Foundation in 1997, the Foundation for Accountability (FACCT) assembled an expert panel of EOL clinicians, quality improvement specialists, research scientists, and health plan administrators and held focus groups of high-risk patients to develop a strategy to measure the quality of EOL care in health plans. The intent was to allow for comparisons of plan performance and to help health plans set goals for quality improvement activities at the EOL.[83] The report summarizes distinctions between measures for public accountability and quality improvement, consumer opinion about what is important at the EOL, and important measures and reporting categories for capturing plan performance in eight areas of care within three major categories: steps to good care, results of care, and experience and satisfaction with care. In addition, practical advice about the measurement process and additional areas of needed research are described.[83]

Table 42–10
Anthem Blue Cross and Blue Shield (ABCBS) of New Hampshire Guide to Pain and Symptom Management in Advanced Disease

Goal

- To reach out to the member early in the disease process so that needs can be anticipated and addressed before a crisis occurs.
- Assist members in getting the critical care they need when they are most vulnerable
- Offer Advanced Disease Care Management as one of the proactive Care Management initiatives
- Nurse Care Managers have specialized education and experience to apply knowledge of ABCBS benefits and community resources when working with unique care needs of members, their families, and providers coping with end-of-life issues

Program Components

- Early participation—key to developing a meaningful and trusting relationship between the member and care team
- Participation is appropriate when member is diagnosed with a potentially life-limiting illness: advanced disease, progression is inevitable, function is compromised, and prolonged survival is questionable.
- Appropriate conditions and diseases for the Advanced Disease Care Management program include advanced cancer, end-stage cardiac disease, renal failure, lung or liver disease with no option for transplantation, and advanced neurological disease.
- Oversight by specialized palliative care ABCBS care manager
- Screen for compliance with accepted pain and palliative treatment guidelines

Future Directions

The first and biggest step in improving hospital-based palliative care is to reduce the number of unnecessary acute care in-hospital deaths. Because death in hospitals will never be completely eliminated, the second biggest improvement will come as a result of improved communication among the health team, patient, and family. Strategies can be put into place to identify the goals of hospital care and implement a prompt, effective, holistic plan to meet predetermined values and preferences.

A number of features of hospitals actually make it easier to employ successful full-scale improvements, including the amount of readily available data and regulatory efforts such as those of the JCAHO. Innovations such as palliative care consultation teams, services, units, and pathways have already begun to provide successful models for improvement. A recent study comparing the cost and quality of care for terminally ill patients in PCUs versus regular hospital settings found that patients received better care in these specialized units that also proved to be cost-effective. This example provides a strong case for dedicating specific hospital units and teams to the palliative care population.[80]

Sometimes a disadvantage can really be an advantage. For example, the perceived endless paperwork, rigidity, and regulations common to hospitals may be among the biggest advantages to making improvements in hospital-based EOL care. Extensive and readily accessible databases of variables that reflect the quality of EOL care are available and are the positive side of monumental documentation requirements. Because of this accessibility, the study of the quality of EOL care in hospitals and some areas of quality improvement have been brought to light relatively rapidly, plans for change have been implemented, and results have been monitored. In the context of hospital oversight and regulation, medical professionals have much more control over hospital operations than can ever be expected in the community or home. Improvement of pain relief and palliative care in hospitals is likely to experience a boon under current JCAHO standards.

One of the recommendations of the Institute of Medicine is that all future health care providers and all current practitioners must receive EOL care education.[2] Numerous efforts are being put forth by the medical and nursing communities to provide EOL care and palliative care education for practicing and future nurses and physicians, some of which were discussed in detail earlier in this chapter. Also, the ANCC, in conjunction with the National Board for Certification of Hospice and Palliative Nurses (NBCHPN) and support from New York University, has developed the first advanced practice nursing certification in the specialty of palliative care.[47] However, all health care professionals need to possess a minimum level of palliative care knowledge in order to provide the most effective primary palliative care to patients and their families.

The good news is that there is a growing foundation of resources to assist the clinician or team wishing to apply a quality improvement process to hospital-based EOL care. However, such abundance may overwhelm the beginning clinician, quality improvement personnel, or project team. A mantra from an unknown source on the cover of one quality improvement manual[65] lends heart—"We cannot do everything at once, but we must do something at once." A few key sources provided throughout the chapter describe quality improvement projects, groups, and contacts. Palliative care as a developing specialty lacks an adequate evidence base.[84] However, as more research findings become available, the rapid-cycle improvement infrastructure is one way to quickly test and translate findings into clinical practice. Although funding mechanisms exist for research, fewer funding opportunities exist for quality improvement.

Quality improvement in hospitals has the potential to provide a significant foundation on which to build a larger health care system and culture of humane care at the EOL. Dr. Christine Cassel provides a simple guideline for success in the preface to the National Academy of Sciences Institute of Medicine report entitled *Approaching Death: Improving Care at the End of Life*[2]:

> When medicine can no longer promise an extension of life, people should not fear that their dying will be marked by neglect, care inconsistent with their wishes, or preventable pain and other distress. They should be able to expect the health care system to assure reliable, effective, and humane care giving. If we can fulfill that expectation, then public trust will be strengthened. (p. vii)

ACKNOWLEDGMENTS

The authors acknowledge the following colleagues who provided important information for the development of this chapter: Polly Campion, RN; Marilyn Bedell, RN; Dan Tobin, MD (Department of Veterans Affairs Health Care System); Lisa Morgan (Center for the Advancement of Palliative Care); Yvonne Corbell and Ira Byock, MD (RWJ Promoting Excellence in End-of-Life Care and Section of Palliative Medicine, Dartmouth Hitchcock Medical Center).

REFERENCES

1. Lynn J, Adamson D. Living Well at the End of Life: Adapting Health Care to Serious Chronic Illness in Old Age. RAND Health White Paper WP-137 (2003). Santa Monica, CA: RAND Health Communications, 2003.
2. Field MJ, Cassel CK. Approaching Death: Improving Care at the End of Life. Washington, DC: National Academy Press, 1997.
3. Wennberg J, Cooper M. The Quality of Care in the United States: A Report on the Medicare Program/The Dartmouth Atlas of Healthcare. Chicago: AHA Press, 1999.
4. Brock DB, Foley DJ. Demography and epidemiology of dying in the US with emphasis on deaths of older persons. Hospice J 1998;13(1–2):49–60.
5. SUPPORT Principal Investigators. A controlled trial to improve care for seriously ill hospitalized patients. JAMA 1995;274: 1591–1598.
6. Goodlin S, Winzelberg G, Teno J, Whedon M, Lynn J. Death in the hospital. Arch Intern Med 1998;158:1570–1572.
7. Elshamy M, Whedon MB. Symptoms and care during the last 48 hours of life. Quality of life: A nursing challenge. Quality Assessment 1997;5:21–29.
8. Lynn J, Teno JM, Phillips R, Wu AW, Desbiens N, Harrold J, Claessens MT, Wenger N, Kreling B, Connors AF Jr. Perceptions of family members of the dying experience of older and seriously ill patients. SUPPORT Investigators. Ann Intern Med 1997; 126:97–106.
9. Berwick D. A primer on leading the improvement of systems. BMJ 1996;312:619–622.
10. Miller FG, Fins JJ. A proposal to restructure hospital care for dying patients. N Engl J Med 1996;334:1740–1742.
11. Solomon M. The enormity of the task: SUPPORT and changing practice. Hasting Center Report. 1995;25(6):528–532.
12. Krammer LM, Muir JC, Gooding-Kellar N, Williams MB, von Gunten CF. Palliative care and oncology: Opportunities for oncology nursing. Oncol Nurs Updates 1999;6(3):1–12.
13. Weggel JM. Palliative care: New challenges for advanced practice nursing. Hospice J 1997;12:43–56.
14. Lynn J, Schuster JL. Improving Care for the End of Life: A Sourcebook for Health Care Managers and Clinicians. New York: Oxford University Press, 2000.
15. Castle NG, Mor V, Banaszak-Holl J. Special care hospice units in nursing homes. Hospice J 1997;2:59–69.
16. Ferrell BR, Viriani R, Grant M. HOPE: Home care outreach for palliative care education. Cancer Pract 1998;6:79–85.
17. Department of Health and Human Services Centers for Medicare and Medicaid Services. Program Memorandum Intermediaries—Hospice Payment Rates 2004. Bethesda, MD: DHHS, 2004.
18. Emanuel EJ, Fairclough DL, Slutsman J, Alpert H, Baldwin D, Emanuel LL. Assistance from family members, friends, paid care givers, and volunteers in the care of terminally ill patients. N Engl J Med 1999;341:956–963.
19. Medicare Hospice Benefit: Patient Guide. Publication No. CMS 02154. USDHHS, Centers for Medicare & Medicaid Services, 2003, http://medicare.gov/publications/pubs/pdf/02154.pdf (accessed March 14, 2005).
20. Covinsky KE, Goldman L, Cook EF, Oye R, Desbiens N, Reding D, Fulkerson W, Connors AF Jr, Lynn J, Phillips RS. The impact of serious illness on patients' families. SUPPORT Investigators. JAMA 1994;272:1839–1844.
21. Weinberg M. Research findings from studies with companies and caregivers. In: Last Acts. Princeton, NJ: Robert Wood Johnson Foundation, 1999.
22. Association AN. Position statement on nursing and the self-determination act. Washington, DC: American Nurses Association, 1991.
23. Teno JM, Licks S, Lynn J, Wenger N, Connors AF Jr, Phillips RS, O'Connor MA, Murphy DP, Fulkerson WJ, Desbiens N, Knaus WA. Do advanced directives provide instructions that direct care? SUPPORT Investigators. J Am Geriatr Soc 1997;45:508–512.
24. Sulmasy DP, Terry PB, Weisman CS, Miller DJ, Stallings RY, Vettese MA, Haller KB. The accuracy of substituted judgments in patients with terminal diagnosis. Ann Intern Med 1998;128: 621–629.
25. Hammes B, Rooney B. Death and end-of-life planning in one midwestern community. Arch Intern Med 1998;158:383–390.
26. Lynn J, Schall MW, Milne C, Nolan K, Kabcenell A. Quality improvements in end of life care: Insights from two collaboratives. J Qual Improve 2000;26:254–267.
27. Fins JJ, Miller FG, Acres CA, Bacchetta MD, Huzzard LL, Raplin BD. End of life decision-making in the hospital: Current practice and future prospects. J Pain Symptom Manage 1999;17:6–15.
28. Schapiro R, Byock I, Parker S, Twohig JS. Living and Dying Well with Cancer: Successfully Integrating Palliative Care and Cancer Treatment. Missoula, Montana, 2003, http://www.promotingexcellence.org/downloads/dying_well_cancer.pdf (accessed April 5, 2005).
29. Daubenspeck M. At last . . . Dartmouth Med 2000;24:33–39,53.
30. Bakitas M, Stevens M, Ahles T, Kim M, Skalla K, Kane N, Greenberg ER, The Project Enable Co-Investigators. Project ENABLE: A palliative care demonstration project for advanced cancer patients in three settings. J Palliat Med 2004;7:363–372.
31. Skalla K, Kane N, Roy G. Project ENABLE. Personal communications and unpublished data, 2000.
32. American Bar Association. Commission on the legal problems of the elderly: survey of the state EMS-DNR laws and protocols. Chicago, IL: Author, 1999.
33. Bureau of Emergency Medical Services. New Hampshire prehospital do not resuscitate program physician guidelines.

New Hampshire Chapter of American Medical Directors Advisory Board (ed.). Concord, NH: Bureau of Emergency Medical Services, 1999.

34. Pritchard RS, Fisher ES, Teno JM, Sharp SM, Reding DJ, Knaus WA, Wennberg JE, Lynn J. Influence of patient preferences and local health system characteristics on the place of death. SUPPORT Investigators. J Am Geriatr Soc 1998;46:1242–1250.
35. Tolle SW, Rosenfeld AG, Tilden VP, Park Y. Oregon's low in-hospital death rates: What determines where people die and satisfaction with decisions on place of death? Ann Intern Med 1999;130:681–685.
36. von Gunten C. Secondary and tertiary palliative care in US hospitals. JAMA 2002;287:875–881.
37. Meier D, Spragens LH, Sutton S. Center to Advance Palliative Care. How to establish a palliative care program. CAPC Manual. San Diego: Center for Palliative Studies, San Diego Hospice; and New York: Department of Pain Medicine and Palliative Care, Beth Israel Medical Center, 2001. Available at: http://www.capc.org (accessed March 16, 2004).
38. Bakitas M. Insights from a Family Focus Group on Hospital End-of-Life Care. Unpublished data, Dartmouth-Hitchcock Medical Center, 1999.
39. Ferris TGG, Hallward JA, Ronan L, Billings JA. When the patient dies: A survey of medical housestaff about care after death. J Palliat Med 1998;1:231–239.
40. Art of Compassionate Death Notification [card]. Available at: http://www.bereavementprograms.com/catalog/index (accessed March 16, 2005).
41. Stoehr PJ. The inadequacy of death and palliative care education in the Northeastern University Baccalaureate Nursing Program. Boston: Northeastern University School of Nursing, 1999.
42. Ferrell BR, Virani R, Grant M. Analysis of end-of-life content in nursing textbooks. Oncol Nurs Forum 1999;26:869–876.
43. Carron AT, Lynn J, Keaney P. End-of-life care in medical textbooks. Ann Intern Med 1999;130:82–86.
44. Ferrell BR, Grant M, Virani R. Strengthening nursing education to improve end-of-life care. Nurs Outlook 1999;47: 252–256.
45. American Medical Association The education for physicians on end-of-life care (EPEC) Project. Chicago: AMA, 1992.
46. American Associates of Colleges of Nursing and City of Hope Medical Center. End-of-life Nursing Education. Consortium Training Curriculum (Robert Wood Johnson funded project). Duarte, CA: Authors, 2000.
47. American Nurses Credentialing Center. Collaborative Venture for Advance Practice Palliative Nurse Certification. 2004. Available at: http://www.nursingworld.org/ancc/ (accessed February 1, 2005).
48. Berwick DM. Controlling variation in health care: A consultation from Walter Shewhart. Med Care 1991;29:1212–1225.
49. Stair J. Oncology critical pathways. Palliative care: A model example from the Moses Cone Health System. Oncology 1998; 14(2):26–30.
50. Du Pen S, Du Pen AR, Polissar N, Hansberry J, Kraybill BM, Stillman M, Panke J, Everly R, Syrjala K. Implementing guidelines for cancer pain management: Results of a randomized controlled clinical trial. J Clin Oncol 1999;17:361–370.
51. Kelly B, Edwards P, Synott R, Neil C, Baillie R, Battistutta D. Predictors of bereavement outcomes for family carers of cancer patients. Psycho-oncology 1999;8:237–249.
52. Bilings JA, Kolton E. Family satisfaction and bereavement care following death in the hospital. J Palliat Med 1999;2:33–49.
53. Mulrooney T, Whedon M, Bedell A. Focus group of family members after death of a loved one in the hospital. Dartmouth-Hitchcock Medical Center, unpublished data, 1999.
54. Dunlop RJ, Hockley JM. Terminal Care Support Teams. New York: Oxford University Press, 1990.
55. Dunlop RJ, Hockley JM. Hospital-Based Palliative Care Teams: The Hospital-Hospice Interface, Vol 2, 2nd ed. New York: Oxford University Press; 1998.
56. Bascom PB. A hospital-based comfort care team: Consultation for seriously ill and dying patients. Am J Hospice Palliat Care 1997;14(2):57–60.
57. Weissman DE. Consultation in palliative medicine. Arch Intern Med 1997;157:733–737.
58. O'Neill WM, O'Connor P, Latimer EJ. Hospital palliative care services: Three models in three countries. J Pain Symptom Manage 1992;7:406–413.
59. Teno JM. Palliative care teams: Self-reflection: Past, present, and future. J Pain Symptom Manage 2002;23:94–95.
60. Kellar N, Martinez J, Finis N, Bolger A, von Gunten C. Characterization of an acute inpatient hospice palliative care unit in a US teaching hospital. J Nurs Admin 1996;26(3):16–20.
61. Department of Pain Medicine and Palliative Care, Beth Israel Medical Center. Stoppain.org. http://www.stoppain.org. (accessed April 5, 2005).
62. Regional Palliative Care Program in Edmonton, Alberta. Palliative.org. http://www.palliative.org (accessed April 5, 2005).
63. The Royal Victoria Hospital Manual on Palliative/Hospice Care. Montreal, Canada: Royal Victoria Hospital, 1982.
64. Bookbinder M, Kiss M, Coyle N, Brown M, Gianella A, Thaler HT. Improving pain management practices. In: McGuire D, Yarbro CH, Ferrell BR, eds. Cancer Pain Management, Vol 2. Boston: Jones and Bartlett; 1995:321–345.
65. Gordon DB, Dahl JL, Stevenson KK. Building an institutional commitment to pain management. In: Wisconsin Resource Manual for Improvement. Madison, WI: University of Wisconsin Board of Regents; 2000.
66. City of Hope Pain Resource Center. Duarte, CA: City of Hope/ Beckman Research Institute, http://www.cityofhope.org/prc/ (accessed April 5, 2005).
67. McCaffery M, Pasero C. Building institutional commitment to improving pain management. Pain Clinical Manual. St. Louis: Mosby, 1999.
68. Ferrell BR, Whedon MB, Rollins B. Pain, quality assessment, and quality improvement. J Nurs Care Quality 1999;9:69–85.
69. Robert Wood Johnson Foundation. New National Center Promotes Palliative Care in Hospitals and Health Systems. RWJF News Release, April 24, 2000.
70. Center to Advance Palliative Care. Palliative Care Leadership Centers: Overview. http://www.capc.org (accessed April 5, 2005).
71. Lynn J, Schuster JL. Improving Care for the End of Life: A Sourcebook for Health Care Managers and Clinicians. New York: Oxford University Press, 2000.
72. Abrahm JL, Callahan J, Rossetti K, Pierre L. The impact of a hospice consultation team on the care of veterans with advanced cancer. J Pain Symptom Manage 1996;12:23–31.
73. Hume M. Improving care at the end-of-life. Qual Lett Healthc Lead 1998;10(10):2–10.
74. U.S. Department of Veterans Affairs. Creating and expanding hospice and palliative care programs in VA. 2004. Available at: www.va.gov/oaa/flp/ (accessed February 1, 2005).

75. The Challenge of Caring for Patients Near the End of Life: Findings from the Hospital Palliative Care Initiative Paper Series. Edison, NJ: United Hospital Fund, 1998.
76. Joint Commission on Accreditation of Healthcare Organizations. Joint Commission on Accreditation of Healthcare Organizations Standards for Hospitals, 2004. Available at: http:// www.jcaho.org.
77. Joint Commission on Accreditation of Healthcare Organizations. Provision of Care Standards 06/2003 2003.
78. Joint Commission on Accreditation of Healthcare Organizations. Ethics, Rights, and Responsibilities Standard R1.2.80, 2003. Available at: http://www.jcaho.org.
79. Capello CF, Meier DE, Cassell CK. Payment code for hospital-based palliative care: Help or hindrance? J Palliat Med 1998;1: 155–160.
80. Smith TJ, Coyne P, Cassel B, Penberthy L, Hopson A, Hager MA. A high-volume specialist palliative care unit and team may reduce in-hospital end-of-life care costs. J Palliat Med 2003;6: 699–705.
81. Solomon M, Romer A, Sellers D. Meeting the Challenge: Improving End-of-Life Care in Managed Care—Access, Accountability, and Cost. Newton, MA: Robert Wood Johnson Foundation, 1999.
82. Montan J, Duffy M. NH Blue Cross Blue Shield Report: Insurer's Redesign Hospice Benefit to Improve EOL Care. Tucson, Ariz.: Anthem Blue Cross and Blue Shield of New Hampshire, 1999.
83. Yurk R, Lansky D, Bethell C. Care at the End of Life: Assessing the Quality of Care for Patients and Families. Portland, OR: FACCT—The Foundation for Accountability, 1999.
84. Robbins M. Evaluating Palliative Care: Establishing the Evidence Base. Oxford: Oxford University Press, 1998.

APPENDIX 42–1

Dartmouth-Hitchcock Medical Center Care at the End of Life Questionnaire

Please answer the following questions about your loved one's care during their last hospitalization by putting a check mark next to the response which best describes your opinion. If the question is about something that did not apply to your loved one's last hospitalization, please check the "Does not apply" option. Feel free to use the "Comments" section to give details about your experience that would help us understand your response.

Questions #1-5 are about the care your loved one and your family received.

1. The staff providing care did so in a thoughtful and sensitive manner.

____ Strongly agree ____ Agree ____ Disagree ____ Strongly disagree
____ Does not apply

Comments: ____________________

2. We felt that the doctors and nurses did all they could to carry out the wishes of our loved one and family.

____ Strongly agree ____ Agree ____ Disagree ____ Strongly disagree
____ Does not apply

Comments: ____________________

3. We had enough privacy and space to comfortably stay with our loved one during the last hours of life.

____ Strongly agree ____ Agree ____ Disagree ____ Strongly disagree
____ Does not apply

Comments: ____________________

4. Staff helped to meet our family's needs in a caring and sensitive manner at the time of death.

____ Strongly agree ____ Agree ____ Disagree ____ Strongly disagree
____ Does not apply

Comments: ____________________

5. We felt supported after our loved one's death.

____ Strongly agree ____ Agree ____ Disagree ____ Strongly disagree
____ Does not apply

Comments: ____________________

Questions #6-8 are about pain control. If your loved one did not experience pain during their last hospitalization, please skip to question #9.

6. Our loved one's pain was well controlled prior to their death.

____ Strongly agree ____ Agree ____ Disagree ____ Strongly disagree
____ Does not apply

Comments: ____________________

7. The staff responded quickly to our loved one's needs for pain relief.

____ Strongly agree ____ Agree ____ Disagree ____ Strongly disagree
____ Does not apply

Comments: ____________________

8. There was an acceptable balance between pain relief and side effects of the medication such as drowsiness and/or confusion.

____ Strongly agree ____ Agree ____ Disagree ____ Strongly disagree
____ Does not apply

Comments: ____________________

Questions #9- 10 are about breathing difficulties. If your loved one did not have breathing difficulties during their last hospitalization, please skip to question #11.

9. We were satisfied with the care provided for our loved one's breathing difficulty.

____ Strongly agree ____ Agree ____ Disagree ____ Strongly disagree
____ Does not apply

Comments: ____________________

10. We received enough information about changes in breathing to understand what was happening.

____ Strongly agree ____ Agree ____ Disagree ____ Strongly disagree
____ Does not apply

Comments: ____________________

Questions #11-15 are about communication.

11. We felt there was good communication between:

The doctors at Mary Hitchcock Memorial Hospital and us.

____ Strongly agree ____ Agree ____ Disagree ____ Strongly disagree
____ Does not apply

The nurses at Mary Hitchcock Memorial Hospital and us.

____ Strongly agree ____ Agree ____ Disagree ____ Strongly disagree
____ Does not apply

The doctors and nurses at Mary Hitchcock Memorial Hospital.

____ Strongly agree ____ Agree ____ Disagree ____ Strongly disagree
____ Does not apply

The doctors at Mary Hitchcock Memorial Hospital and our loved one's local doctor.

____ Strongly agree ____ Agree ____ Disagree ____ Strongly disagree
____ Does not apply

Comments: ____________________

12. We received consistent information about our loved one's condition *(reason for hospitalization)* and what to expect.

____ Strongly agree ____ Agree ____ Disagree ____ Strongly disagree
____ Does not apply

Comments: ____________________

13. We felt well informed about what was happening during the last hospitalization prior to death.

____ Strongly agree ____ Agree ____ Disagree ____ Strongly disagree
____ Does not apply

Comments: ____________________

14. We received the information we needed to move forward with funeral arrangements.

____ Strongly agree ____ Agree ____ Disagree ____ Strongly disagree
____ Does not apply

Comments: ____________________

15. Overall, how would you rate the care that your loved one and your family received during their last hospitalization? (1 = the worst possible care and 10 = the best possible care). Please circle one.

1 2 3 4 5 6 7 8 9 10

Please feel free to share any additional comments you may have regarding your loved one's care prior to death. Also, please comment if you have suggestions on how we might improve care to future patients in the hospital who are at their end of life.

43

Kathleen Puntillo and Daphne Stannard

The Intensive Care Unit

I think I'm having a more difficult time than [the patient], because I can see what's going on. I don't know if [the patient] is totally aware of what's going on.—Family member of a critically ill patient[1]

- ***Key Points***
- *Although an intensive care unit is rarely the place where patients would choose to die, transition from aggressive to end-of-life care is a frequent occurrence.*
- *Optimal transitional care in ICUs requires clear communication among patients, family members, and care providers from multiple disciplines.*
- *At the end of life, the appropriateness of procedures should be assessed, unnecessary procedures eliminated, and the pain associated with necessary procedures treated appropriately.*
- *Analgesics should be administered to dying patients in the amounts necessary to decrease pain and symptoms without concern about the milligram dose required.*
- *Pain and symptom assessment and management, although challenging in an ICU setting, are primary roles and contributions of the ICU nurse.*
- *Decisions to forgo life-sustaining therapies are made when the burden of aggressive treatment clearly outweighs the benefits. There are two methods of withdrawing ventilator therapy: immediate extubation and terminal weaning. Guidelines exist for each of these methods of withdrawal.*
- *Caring for families at any point along the dying trajectory encompasses three major aspects: access, information and support, and involvement in caregiving activities.*

An intensive care unit (ICU) is, by tradition, the setting in which the most aggressive care is rendered to hospitalized patients. Patients are admitted to an ICU so that health professionals can perform minute-to-minute titration of care. The primary goals of this aggressive care are patient resuscitation, stabilization, and recovery from the acute phase of an illness or injury. However, many patients die in ICUs. It is estimated that 540,000 people die after admission to ICUs in the United States each year.[2] Stated otherwise, almost one in five Americans receives ICU services before death. ICU deaths account for 59% of all hospital deaths and 80% of all terminal inpatient costs. One third of patients with metastatic cancer who die in hospitals do so in ICUs, as do 85% of patients with acute myocardial infarctions. Therefore, it is clear that management of the process of dying is common in ICUs.[3]

In the high-technology environment of an ICU, it may be difficult for health professionals and families of dying patients to acknowledge that there are limits to the effectiveness of medical care. However, it is important to focus on providing the type of care that is appropriate for the individual patient and the patient's family, be it aggressive lifesaving care or palliative end-of-life care. This chapter discusses the provision of palliative care in ICUs. Specifically, challenges and barriers to providing such care in ICUs are described, and recommendations are offered for the provision of symptom assessment and management. Current issues related to withholding and withdrawing life-sustaining therapies are covered. Recommendations are offered for attending to the needs of families as well as health care providers who care for ICU patients at the end of life. Finally, an international agenda for improving end-of-life care in ICUs is presented.

The Limitations of End-of-Life Care in Intensive Care Units

Although many deaths occur in ICUs, an ICU is rarely the place that one would choose to die.[4] Health professionals in ICUs, frequently uncertain about whether a patient will live or die, are caught between the opposing goals of preserving life and preparing the patient and family for death. It is important for professionals to realize that a patient's death is not necessarily an indication of ineffective care. Yet, there are serious limitations to the care provided to seriously ill and dying patients and their families. Communication between physicians and patients may be poor; physicians often may not implement patients' refusals of interventions; patients may be overly optimistic about the outcomes of cardiopulmonary resuscitation (CPR); and many hospitalized patients die in moderate to severe pain and with other troubling symptoms.[5,6]

In a landmark study, more than 5,000 seriously ill hospitalized patients or their family members were asked questions about the patients' pain.[7] Almost one-half of these patients had had pain during the previous 3 days, and almost 15% had had pain that was moderately or extremely severe and occurred at least half of the time. Of those with pain, 15% were dissatisfied with its control. Other distressing symptoms, such as fatigue, dyspnea, and dysphoria, have been reported by seriously ill and elderly hospitalized patients and their family members.[6] Although patients with colon cancer had the most pain, many of the patients reporting pain had diagnoses that were not surgery or cancer related (e.g., chronic obstructive pulmonary disease, congestive heart failure). These findings stress the importance of attending to the assessment and management of pain and other symptoms in all ICU patients.

Planning Palliative Care for ICU Patients

Providing comfort to patients should accompany all ICU care, even during aggressive attempts to prolong life. However, if a patient is not expected to survive, the focus shifts to an emphasis on palliative care. It is often extremely difficult in an ICU to determine the appropriate time for a change of focus in care. A transition period occurs during which the health professionals, the patient's family, and sometimes the patient recognize the appropriateness of withdrawing and/or withholding treatments and begin to make preparations for death. The transition period (i.e., the time from decision to death) may be a matter of minutes or hours, as in the case of a patient who has sustained massive motor vehicle injuries; or it may be a matter of weeks, as in the case of a patient who has undergone bone marrow transplantation and has multiple negative sequelae while in the ICU. Clearly, this time difference must be recognized as a factor that can influence the experience of a patient's family members. When patients rapidly approach death, their family members may not have time to overcome the shock of the trauma and adjust to the possibility of death. On the other hand, when death is prolonged, family frustration and fatigue may be part of their experience. Health professionals who are sensitive to these different experiences can individualize their approaches and interventions for family members.

However, this transition from aggressive care to death preparation has not been well operationalized. Children who die in ICUs often do so after physician determination that death is imminent and after care has been restricted.[8] The restrictions are usually equally divided among withholding resuscitation, limiting medical interventions in addition to withholding resuscitation, and withdrawing medical interventions.[8,9] In a retrospective study of 300 pediatric patient deaths, the most common mode of death was active withdrawal of support.[10] Usually, physicians raise the issue of restricting care (76% of the time), but sometimes it is the family that initiates these discussions (16% of the time).[8] The unique interdependence between a child and family makes it essential and justifiable for the family to participate in treatment-related decisions[11] during the transition period and throughout the dying process.

The transition period is clearly uncomfortable for many health care professionals. In fact, when scenarios concerning end-of-life decision-making in the absence of patient or family input were presented to more than 1,300 ICU staff, respondents were very confident of their choices less than 30% of the time.[12] Physicians were more confident than nurses, who were more confident than house staff. Although some guidelines exist to assist ICU professionals through the processes of maintaining, limiting, or stopping life-sustaining treatments,[13] there are no well-tested standards to assist in the decision-making process. It is important, therefore, for ICU professionals to consider the following steps when caring for patients at risk for not surviving their ICU course:

1. Identify and communicate the goals of care for the patient at least once a day. Ascertain whether the patient has developed an advance directive, whether a family member has durable power of attorney, and whether the patient has communicated a preference about CPR. Almost half of 960 seriously ill patients who wanted CPR withheld did not have a do-not-resuscitate (DNR) order written during their hospitalization, and almost one third died before discharge.[5]
2. Outline the steps that need to be taken to accomplish the goals of care and evaluate their effectiveness. Technology should not drive the goals of care. Instead, technology should be used when necessary to accomplish the goals, and its use should be minimized when the primary goal is achievement of a peaceful death.
3. Use a multidisciplinary team approach to decision-making regarding transition to end-of-life care. All team members, including the patient's family, should reach a consensus, sometimes through negotiation, that the withdrawal of life support and

a peaceful death are the appropriate patient outcomes.[14]

4. Develop and communicate to professionals and family the palliative care plan, and identify the best persons for implementing the various actions in the plan. End-of-life treatment decisions are particularly complex when the dying patient is an infant or child.[13] De Groot-Bollujt and Mourik[15] provided specific suggestions for involving a child's family members in the dying process. These included offering family members opportunities to participate in preparing the child to die and even holding the child during the dying process.
5. Developing a plan of care may include enlisting the assistance of in-hospital palliative care staff and/or hospice services. If feasible and desired by the family, consideration should be given to transfer of the adult or pediatric patient from the ICU to in-hospital support care services, such as those at Detroit Receiving Hospital.[16] Or, if possible and desired, patients may be transferred to the home or to community hospice services. A major focus in any palliative care plan is on providing optimal symptom management.

Symptom Assessment and Management: An Essential Component of Palliative Care

Pain Assessment

Although pain was identified in the Study to Understand Prognoses and Preferences for Outcomes and Risks of Treatments (SUPPORT) study as one of the most prevalent and distressing symptoms of seriously ill patients dying in large teaching hospitals,[11,13] hospitalized patients continue to receive inadequate pain management.[17] Pain research focusing on dying ICU patients remains scarce, but advances that have been made in the assessment of pain in other critically ill patient populations can be applied to dying patients.[18,19] The patient's self-report continues to be the most valuable indicator of pain.[20] Simple numeric or word rating scales, word quality scales, and body outline diagrams may be offered to patients who are able to point to words, numbers, and figures. It is important to determine the quality, timing, and location of pain whenever possible, so that treatment may be guided by accurate information rather than assumptions. The specificity of the pain presentation guides the selection of optimal treatment interventions.

Often, critically ill patients are unable to self-report because of their disease process, technological treatment interventions (e.g., mechanical ventilation), or the effects of medications (e.g., opioids, benzodiazepines [BZDs]). The use of BZD infusions may make patients too sedated to respond to pain, although pain may still be present. On the other hand, the use of the anesthetic agent propofol or of neuromuscular blocking agents (NMBAs) such as vecuronium may limit or entirely mask the patient's ability to express or show any behavioral signs of pain. It is essential that clinicians understand that propofol and NMBAs have no analgesic properties, even though visible signs of pain disappear during their use. If these agents are used, they must be accompanied by infusions of analgesics, sedatives, or both. In these situations, the nurse may enlist the assistance of family members or friends in their evaluation of the patient's discomfort. The nurse can ask them about any chronic pain experienced by the patient or methods used by the patient at home to decrease pain or stress. This information can then be incorporated into the patient's care plan.

If patients are unable to self-report, the nurse can use a structured, systematic method of pain assessment that includes observation of behavioral and physiological signs of pain. A pain assessment reference guide is one example of a bedside instrument that can assist professionals to perform a multidimensional pain assessment.[21] A behavioral pain scale (BPS) has been developed that quantifies pain in sedated, mechanically ventilated patients.[22] However, further work is necessary to confirm the validity of some of the pain parameters on the BPS (e.g., fighting ventilator) and the usefulness of the BPS in making analgesic decisions. Recently, certain behaviors were documented to be associated with procedural pain experienced by acutely or critically ill patients; these included grimacing, rigidity, wincing, shutting of eyes, verbalization, moaning, and clenching of fists.[23] Patients with procedural pain were at least three times more likely to have increased behavioral responses than patients without procedural pain. These findings provide support to the assessment of specific pain behaviors in patients who are unable to self-report. However, behavioral measures are only proxies for the patient's subjective reports, even though they are frequently the only measures available. As another proxy measure, nurses can use their imaginations to identify possible sources of pain by asking the question, "If I were this patient and had intact sensations, what might be making me uncomfortable?" Even if patients are not exhibiting behavioral or physiological signs of pain, it does not mean that they are pain free.

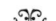

The comfort of 31 adult patients undergoing terminal weaning from mechanical ventilation was assessed by use of behavior observation and physiological measures.[24] Moderate correlations ($r = 5.60$; $P = 0.001$) found between the Bizek Agitation Scale (BAS)[25] and the previously validated COMFORT scale[26] suggested that these observational measures may be able to evaluate responses to pain, distress, or agitation in certain dying ICU patients. Correlations between electroencephalogram (EEG)-derived data, obtained through the use of a cerebral function monitor,[27] and the BAS and COMFORT scales were $r = 5.53$ and $r = 5.58$, respectively ($P = 0.001$). Findings from this study about behavior and physiological measures are preliminary at best. EEG data were derived from only 11 of the 31 patients, because the others had global anoxic encephalopathy. Furthermore, the specific origin or cause of "discomfort"

(e.g., pain, dysphoria) cannot be determined from such global measures. However, the findings show promise for the clinical usefulness of "comfort" assessment measures that can assist clinicians to assess pain and the effectiveness of treatment interventions at the end of life.

Procedural Pain

Before and during the transition from aggressive care to end-of-life care, critically ill patients undergo many diagnostic and treatment procedures. Many of these, such as central, arterial, and peripheral line placements, nasogastric tube placements,[28] chest tube removal,[29,30] and endotracheal suctioning,[31] are quite painful and may be the primary cause of suffering at the end of life.[28] Turning, one of the most ubiquitous procedures performed in acute and critical care settings, was shown to be the most painful of six commonly performed procedures.[31] Other procedures that may be unnecessary, painful, and unpleasant include central line insertions,[22] wound débridement, frequent dressing changes,[31] and the use of sequential compression devices.[22] Paice and colleagues[32] demonstrated through a chart review that 71% to 100% of 57 patients in a medical ICU had numerous procedures during their last 48 hours of life. These procedures included intravenous (IV) medications and fluids, urinary catheters, antibiotics, x-ray studies, enteral feeding tubes, and ventilators. Nurses can act as "gatekeepers" by evaluating the appropriateness of procedures being planned for patients, especially after a decision has been made to end life support, and they can advocate for their omission. Helping patients avoid iatrogenic suffering is a fundamental part of palliative care.[28] The most important procedures for patients to experience at the end of life are those that promote comfort. Yet, when necessary procedures must be performed, the nurse can facilitate pain management before and during procedures.

Pharmacological Management of Pain

Numerous categories of analgesics and types of modalities exist for administration to critically ill patients.[33] As in all situations, the selection of analgesics should depend on the specific pain mechanism, and the route and modality should be matched to their predictability of effectiveness. Although no comprehensive survey of pain management techniques used for dying ICU patients has been reported, the most common analgesic intervention is IV opioids. Use of a continuous infusion of an opioid allows for titration of the drug to a level of analgesic effectiveness and for maintenance of steady plasma levels within a therapeutic range. Foley[18] presented the following recommendations for the use of opioids in dying ICU patients: (1) choose a specific analgesic therapy on the basis of individual patient characteristics; (2) know the equianalgesic dosage of a drug and its route of administration; (3) choose the route of administration that is appropriate to the patients' needs; and (4) develop a dose titration protocol. In addition, health care professionals may consider the administration of intermittent opioid boluses for breakthrough pain (Table 43–1).

Clearly, concerns about patients becoming tolerant of or dependent on opioids are misplaced during terminal care. What is important is that professionals recognize the development of tolerance, which is the need for larger doses of opioid analgesics to achieve the original effect,[34] and increase the dosage as necessary. There is no ceiling effect from opioids; the dose can be increased until the desired effect is reached or intolerable side effects develop. If it is the family's wish to have the opioid infusion decreased in a sedated patient to assess that the patient is able to participate in end-of-life decision-making, this must be done slowly and carefully. Opioid-dependent patients are at high risk of developing withdrawal symptoms,[34] which would seriously increase their discomfort. In this situation, physical dependence can be addressed by gradually lowering the opioid dose while carefully assessing for signs of pain or withdrawal.

Titration of analgesics to achieve the desired effect is one of the most challenging and important contributions that ICU nurses can make to the comfort care of dying patients. The desired effect can often be described as use of the least amount of medication necessary to achieve the greatest comfort along with the optimum level of tranquil awareness.

In ICU settings, concern may arise that administration of analgesics in the amounts necessary to provide comfort could "cause" death. It is essential that ICU health professionals understand the "double-effect" principle. In brief, the double-effect principle states that administration of analgesics to dying patients in the amounts necessary to decrease pain and suffering, although it might have the unintended consequence of hastening death, is a good, ethically sound way to treat a dying patient.[35] This principle, framed in ethics, provides support to such an action when the clinician's moral intent is directed primarily at alleviating suffering rather than intending to kill. In a survey of 906 critical care nurses in the United States, almost all respondents (98%) agreed or strongly agreed with the double-effect principle.[36]

Nonpharmacological Management of Pain

Nonpharmacological interventions for pain management complement, but do not substitute for, the use of pharmacological interventions. Numerous therapies may be used by critical care nurses to augment the administration of medications to promote patient comfort. They include the use of distraction (e.g., music, humor), relaxation techniques (e.g., visual imagery, rhythmic breathing), and massage.[37] Even during occasions when the cognitive status of a somnolent ICU patient is uncertain, the patient can be provided information about activities being done to and around them. Family members can be encouraged to assist with the provision of comfort measures and may welcome this way of participating in care and decreasing their sense of helplessness. Family involvement is discussed in further detail in a later section of this chapter.

Table 43–1
Pharmacologic Symptom Management

Symptom	Drug Type Most Frequently Used	Method of Administration	Usual Dose*
Pain	Opioids (e.g., morphine, fentanyl, hydrocodone, methadone)	Continuous IV infusions with use of intermittent boluses for procedure-related pain or during treatment withdrawal	Continuous infusion: 1–10 mg/h morphine equivalents Bolus: 1–5 mg IV morphine equivalent slow push; titrate to effect
Anxiety/ Agitation	Benzodiazepines (e.g., lorazepam, midazolam)	Same as for opioids	Continuous midazolam infusion: 2–25 mg/h or titrate to effect Bolus midazolam: 5–10 mg IV to augment continuous infusion Continuous lorazepam infusion: 1–5 mg/h or titrate to effect Bolus lorazepam: 1–10 mg IV q6–8h to augment continuous infusion
	Haloperidol	IV boluses	Bolus: 0.5–10 mg IV
	Propofol	Continuous IV infusion	Continuous: 50–300 mg/h
Dyspnea	Oxygen	Multiple methods (e.g., nasal cannula, mask, ventilator)	Concentration as needed
	Opioids (e.g., morphine)	Continuous IV infusion and/or IV bolus; or per nebulizer	See above for IV doses Per nebulizer: 2.5 mg in 3 mL saline (preservative free) or sterile water q4h
	Benzodiazepines	See above	See above
	Bronchodilators (e.g., Alupent)	Per nebulizer	Alupent: 2.5 mL 0.4–0.6% solution
	Diuretics (e.g., Lasix)	IV bolus, slow push	Bolus Lasix: 20–40 mg IV
	Anticholinergics (e.g., atropine)	Per nebulizer	Atropine: 0.025 mg/kg diluted with 3–5 mL saline three or four times daily; doses not to exceed 2.5 mg

*Drug doses are general recommendations. Dosing should be individualized to a particular patient. Under usual circumstances, start with low doses, wait for effect, and titrate to desired effect.

Sources: Govoni et al. (1996), reference 138; Harvey (1996), reference 47; and Kuebler (1996), reference 139.

Anxiety, Agitation, and Sedation

An important part of palliative care in the ICU is assessment and treatment of anxiety and agitation. There are many reasons for a dying patient to be anxious or agitated, or both. Assessment of anxiety and agitation provides the practitioner with information that can guide the use of specific interventions.

Assessment of Anxiety and Agitation

Simple numeric rating scales for anxiety can be used if the patient can self-report to identify how much the patient is psychologically bothered. Critical care clinicians and patients are familiar with the use of the 0-to-10 numeric rating scales for pain. "Anxiety" word anchors can be substituted for pain word anchors so that the numeric rating scales also can be used to quantify the degree of distress.

Common behavioral or physiological signs of anxiety include trembling, restlessness, sweating, tachycardia, tachypnea, difficulty sleeping, and irritability. Several agitation/sedation assessment scales are available (e.g., Jacobi and colleagues[33]). These scales can be printed on the patient flowsheet or on a separate form and used as a bedside assessment tool. Nurses can plan periodic and simultaneous assessments of pain using pain rating scales and agitation scales. The frequency with which the scales are used depends on the patient's condition and the schedule for evaluating treatment interventions.

Pharmacological Management to Promote Sedation in Anxious or Agitated Patients

Along with opioids, other categories of sedating drugs are frequently used in the ICU, especially for patients who are mechanically ventilated. Several guidelines,[33] algorithms,[38] and review articles[39–41] exist regarding the use of analgesics and sedatives. Often, the goal of combined analgesic-sedative therapy is to promote physical and psychological comfort. Practice decisions include choosing the right type and combination of medications; determining whether to use interrupted sedative infusions (which provide opportunities for patient assessment) or continuous infusions[42]; determining appropriate clinical endpoints for pharmacological interventions; and evaluating the effectiveness of sedation protocols on practices and outcomes.[42,43]

The appropriate pharmacological agent to control agitation and anxiety is selected according to the desired effect. For example, uncomplicated anxiety is best treated with BZDs, whereas paranoia, panic, and fear accompanied by delusions and hallucinations may require the addition of antipsychotic agents. BZDs are excellent agents for anxiolysis, but they possess no analgesic or psychological properties. Concomitant use of BZDs, opioids, and certain neuroleptic agents may relieve anxiety-provoking symptoms through a synergistic action.[44,45] When used together, these drugs can be administered in lower doses less frequently, have fewer side effects, and can decrease or delay development of tolerance or dependence through the use of smaller doses of each drug. At lower doses, BZDs reduce anxiety without causing central nervous system sedation or a decrease in cognitive or motor function. With increasing dosages, inhibition of motor and cognitive functions as well as central nervous system depression does occur. Sufficiently high doses can induce hypnosis and coma.[46]

The most frequently used BZDs in critical care are midazolam and lorazepam. When midazolam is used as a continuous infusion, the dose can be 1 to 2 mg/h for mild sedation or as high as 25 mg/h for severe agitation if the patient is mechanically ventilated (see Table 43–1). If the degree of sedation is not adequate, the serum level of midazolam can be raised by one to three small bolus IV injections while simultaneously increasing the infusion rate.[47]

Lorazepam gives effective sedation and anxiety relief over a longer period than does midazolam. Cardiovascular and respiratory effects occur less frequently with this drug than with other BZDs. It may also act synergistically with haloperidol, a neuroleptic agent discussed later in this chapter. Lorazepam can be administered intravenously, intramuscularly, or orally. IV doses may be 1 to 10 mg every 6 to 8 hours. In the critical care setting, it can also be administered as an infusion at 1 to 5 mg/h and titrated to clinical effect.[47]

As with opioids, tolerance to BZD effects can develop in critically ill patients receiving midazolam infusions.[39] In addition, BZD dependence can occur, evidenced by symptoms such as dysphoria, tremor, sweating, anxiety, agitation, muscle cramps, myoclonus, and seizures on abrupt medication withdrawal.[39]

It is important that patients in ICUs be routinely assessed for the presence of delirium.[33] Haloperidol is a frequently used neuroleptic for critically ill patients with delirium. A loading dose of 2 mg can be administered, followed by twice that dose repeated every 15 to 20 minutes while agitation persists. Doses as high as 400 mg have been reported, but adverse effects may occur with these high doses.[33] This drug has few cardiovascular effects unless given rapidly, in which case vasodilation and hypotension may occur. Haloperidol does not depress respirations; rather, it has a calming effect on agitated, disoriented patients, making them more manageable without causing excessive sedation. However, haloperidol has some significant adverse effects, such as reduction of the seizure threshold, precipitation of extrapyramidal reactions, and prolongation of the QT interval leading to torsades de pointes.[39] Once a haloperidol drug dosage has been established, it should not be necessary to increase the dose to obtain the same effect over time, because tolerance should not occur.

Propofol is a highly lipophilic IV sedative/hypnotic agent that has a very rapid onset of action and short duration. It is indicated for use in the ICU to control agitation and the stress response in patients who are mechanically ventilated and those who require deep sedation for procedures.[33] However, propofol has no analgesic properties and must always be used in conjunction with analgesics whenever the patient might experience pain. During initial use of propofol, a drop in systolic blood pressure, mean arterial blood pressure, and heart rate may occur in patients with fluid deficits and in those receiving opioids. The rapid loss of clinical effect of propofol renders it a valuable sedative agent in the critical care environment. Continuous infusion doses may range from 50 to 300 mg/h[47] (see Table 43–1). The short effective half-life of propofol allows rapid clinical evaluation of the patient's level of consciousness and determination of the minimum dose required for effective sedation. This may make it a useful drug during situations in which intermittent interaction with professionals and family members is desired.

Nonpharmacological Interventions for Anxiety and Agitation

Numerous interventions exist that may promote tranquility and sedation in a critical care environment. These include control of environmental noise and the use of clocks, calendars, and personal articles such as pictures from home. Music therapy can be used to decrease anxiety and pain as well as promote sleep. As noted earlier, imagery and relaxation techniques also provide a means of distraction for patients and help to alleviate anxiety.[37]

The act of physically caring for a patient and providing gentle touch is a major source of comfort for patients in critical care. Taking the time to provide simple measures such as back rubs and massages, repositioning the patient, smoothing bed linen wrinkles, removing foreign objects from the bed, providing mouth and eye care, and taping tubes to maintain patency and inhibit pulling effectively promotes comfort and decreases anxiety. Family member participation in caregiving activities, such as bathing, massages, and back rubs, can have a powerful calming effect on patients and promote sleep and psychological integrity.

For alert patients, increasing opportunities for control is a strategy that can reduce the sense of helplessness that often accompanies patients who are critically ill. This sense of control can be promoted by allowing alert patients to make decisions about the timing of interventions. Facilitating contact and communication with clergy, psychologists, or psychiatrists, if appropriate, can help to alleviate the distress experienced by both patients and families.

Other Distressing Symptoms

Scant research has been conducted on symptoms experienced by ICU patients at high risk of dying. A notable exception was the study by Nelson and colleagues.[48] These investigators concentrated on the symptom experiences of ICU patients with current or past cancer diagnoses, because the expectation was that almost half of that group would die during hospitalization. Investigators used a modified Edmonton Symptom Assessment Scale (ESAS) to have patients rate their symptoms. The ESAS was modified by including or substituting symptoms they thought were more relevant to ICU patients and by using a four-point verbal descriptor scale (None, Mild, Moderate, Severe). In a sample of 100 patients who met inclusion criteria, 50% (mean age, 63 years; 64% male) were able to report their symptoms; 60% of these patients were mechanically ventilated. More than 50% of patients reported the following symptoms to be moderate to severe during "daily" assessments (exact number of days not reported): discomfort (75%), unsatisfied thirst (71%), difficulty sleeping (68%), anxiety (63%), pain (56%), and unsatisfied hunger (55%). More than one third of patients reported depression or shortness of breath or both. This study demonstrated that a high proportion of cancer patients at high risk of dying in ICUs experience substantial discomfort. Furthermore, half of the patients in the study were unable to report their symptoms, evidence of the ongoing challenge of symptom assessment in critically ill patients.

ICU nurses play a major role in alleviating distressing symptoms such as thirst, sleeplessness, and general discomfort experienced by patients at the end of life. Because nurses are the health care providers who are constantly at the bedside, they can assess the presence of these symptoms, advocate for effective pharmacological therapy, use additional nursing comfort measures, and provide for continuity of therapy. Symptom management is a special contribution that ICU nurses can make to their patients at the end of life.

End-of-Life Practice Issues: Withholding and Withdrawing Life-Sustaining Therapies

Limiting life-sustaining therapies in an ICU is becoming more common. It is estimated that withholding or withdrawing of life support precedes up to 75% of deaths in ICUs.[49,50] Generally, life-sustaining treatment is withdrawn when death is believed to be inevitable despite aggressive interventions.

The President's Commission for the Study of Ethical Problems in Medicine and Biomedical and Behavioral Research[51] supported the right of a competent patient to refuse life-sustaining and life-prolonging therapy. The Commission also noted that there is no moral difference between withholding and withdrawing therapy. A number of critical care–related professional organizations[52–54] have published position papers in support of the patient's autonomy regarding withholding and withdrawal decisions.

If patients are unable to make treatment decisions, these decisions must be made on the patient's behalf by surrogates or by the health care team.[55] Optimally, patients' living wills or advance directives can provide the direction for decisions related to treatment withholding or withdrawal. Yet, only 10% to 20% of patients complete them.[55] When surrogates are asked to participate in decision-making, it is recommended that the decisions be made based on the following, in order of preference: (1) the patient's previously stated wishes; (2) inferences based on the patient's values or life goals; (3) the patient's best interests, as determined by weighing the benefits and burdens of treatment.[55] Families work with the health care team members caring for their loved ones to arrive at decisions to withdraw life support.[14] They often struggle with concern that they are doing the right thing. Providing clear, consistent information about the patient's prognosis (albeit in the face of prognostic uncertainty) provides support for families in their decision-making.

When a decision to forgo life-saving therapy is made in an acute care setting, there is a common sequence of withdrawal of therapies: blood products, hemodialysis, vasopressors, mechanical ventilation, total parenteral nutrition, antibiotics, IV fluids, and tube feedings.[56] Withdrawal of therapies should be preceded by chart notations of DNR orders and a note documenting the rationale for comfort care and removal of life support.[57] There should be a clear plan of action and provision of information and support to the family. Adequate documentation of patient assessments, withdrawal decisions and plans, therapy withdrawal orders, and patient and family responses during and after withdrawal is essential.[58] There is considerable variability regarding physician documentation of discussions with families regarding withdrawal of life support.[59] This lack of documentation may infer, rightly or wrongly, lack of interactions with families about treatment decisions.

Withdrawal of Ventilator Therapy with Consideration of Analgesic and Sedative Needs

It is important to understand the methods by which mechanical ventilation may be removed. The primary goal during this process should be to ensure that patients and family members are as comfortable as possible, both psychologically and physically. Two primary methods of mechanical ventilation removal exist: immediate extubation and terminal weaning

(Table 43–2). Debates continue as to which of these methods is optimal for the patient, and often the method is determined according to the physician's, patient's, or family members' comfort levels.[60]

Although there is considerable variability regarding the preferred approach to withdrawal,[61] recommendations regarding specific procedures for withdrawal are available.[57,58,60–64] Table 43–3 presents a protocol for withdrawal of mechanical ventilation for the clinician's consideration that includes specific recommendations regarding use of analgesics and sedatives. Consensus guidelines on the provision of analgesia and sedation for dying ICU patients support the titration of analgesics and sedatives based on patient's requests or observable signs indicative of pain or distress.[65] The guidelines emphasize that no maximum dose of opioids or sedatives exists, especially considering that many ICU patients receive high doses of these drugs over their ICU time course. "Anticipatory dosing" (Truog and associates,[61] p. 2339), as opposed to reactive dosing, is recommended by some to avoid patient discomfort and distress.[61,65]

It is important to provide comfort to dying infants, who could experience pain and distress similar as older patients. Opioid analgesia was provided to 84% of 121 infants when life support was withdrawn or withheld in an intensive care nursery.[66] Importantly, there was no difference in time to death according to opioid dose. As with older patients, attention must be paid to involvement of the family in decision-making, providing support to the family, and good documentation of decisions and treatments. However, documentation was found to be lacking for 18 infants who died after ventilator withdrawal.[67] Without proper documentation, evaluation of competent and compassionate care is limited.

Research to guide the practice of ventilator withdrawal is scant. A small group of adult patients ($N = 42$) underwent withdrawal as part of a treatment limitation plan.[68] Clinical data were collected from their medical records, including the specific method of ventilator withdrawal. Twenty-eight patients (85%) died after endotracheal tubes and mechanical support; 10 died with artificial airways in place but mechanical support removed; and 4 died after gradual removal of airway and/or

Table 43–2
Methods of Mechanical Ventilation Withdrawal

Immediate extubation	Terminal weaning
Description	
Abrupt removal of the patient from ventilator assistance by extubation after suctioning (if necessary). Humidified air or oxygen is administered to prevent airway drying.	Physicians or other members of the ICU team (e.g., respiratory therapists, nurses) gradually withdraw ventilator assistance. This is done by decreasing the amount of inspired oxygen, decreasing the ventilator rate and mode, removal of positive end-expiratory pressure (PEEP), or a combination of these maneuvers. Usual time from ventilator to T-piece or extubation: 15–60 min.
Positive aspects	
Patient free of technology; dying process less likely to be prolonged; intentions of the method are clear.	Allows titration of drugs to control symptoms; maintains airway for suctioning if necessary; patient does not develop upper airway obstruction; longer time between ventilator withdrawal and death; moral burden on family may be less because method appears less active.
Negative aspects	
Noisy breathing, dyspnea may be distressful to patient/family.	May prolong dying; patient unable to communicate; machine between patient and family.
Time course to death	
Unpredictable. Usually shorter than with terminal weaning.	Unpredictable

Sources: Faber-Langendoen & Lanken (2000), reference 55; Rubenfeld & Crawford (2001), reference 58; von Gunten & Weissman (2005), references 60, 62, 63; Truog et al. (2001), reference 61.

Table 43–3
A Protocol for the Withdrawal of Mechanical Ventilation

I. Anticipate and prevent distress

A. Review process in advance with patient (if awake), nurse, and family. Identify family goals during withdrawal (e.g., ability to communicate versus sedation). Arrange a time that allows the family to be present, if they wish.
B. Provide for special needs (e.g., clergy, bereavement counselor). Assess respiratory pattern on current level of respiratory support.
C. Use opioids and/or benzodiazepines* to control respiratory distress (i.e., respiratory rate >24 breaths per minute, use of accessory muscles, nasal flaring, >20% increase in heart rate or blood pressure, grimacing, clutching). In patients already receiving these agents, dosing should be guided by the current dose.
D. In the absence of distress, reduce intermittent mandatory ventilation (IMV) rate to less than 10 and reassess sedation.
E. Discontinue therapies not directed toward patient comfort:
   1. Stop neuromuscular blockade after opioids and/or benzodiazepines have been started or increased.†
   2. Discontinue laboratory tests, radiographs, vital signs.
   3. Remove unnecessary tubes and restraints.
   4. Silence alarms and disconnect monitors.

II. Optimize existing function

A. Administer breathing treatment, if indicated.
B. Suction out the mouth and hypopharynx. Endotracheal suctioning before withdrawal may or may not be advisable depending on patient distress and family perception. Consider atropine (1–2.5 mg by inhalation q6h), scopolomine (0.3–0.65 mg IV q4–6h), or glycopyrrolate (1–2 mg by inhalation q2–4h) for excessive secretions.
C. Place the patient at least 30 degrees upright, if possible.

III. Withdraw assisted ventilation‡

A. In general, changes should be made in the following order§:
   1. Eliminate positive end-expiratory pressure (PEEP).
   2. Reduce the fractional oxygen content of inspired air (F_{IO_2}).
   3. Reduce or eliminate mandatory breaths.
   4. Reduce pressure support level.
   5. Place to flow-by or T-piece.
   6. Extubate to humidified air or oxygen.
B. Constant reevaluation for distress is mandatory. Treat distress with additional bolus doses of opioids and/or benzodiazepines equal to hourly drip rate and increase drip by 25–50%.
C. Observe for postwithdrawal distress, a medical emergency. A physician and nurse should be present during and immediately after extubation to assess the patient and to titrate medications. Morphine (5–10 mg IV q10 min) or fentanyl (100–250 μg IV q3–5 min) and/or midazolam (2–5 mg IV q7–10 min) or diazepam (5–10 mg IV q3–5 min) should be administered.

*Drug doses are difficult to specify because of the enormous variability in body weight and composition, previous exposure, and tolerance. In opioid-naïve patients, 2–20 mg morphine or 25–250 μg fentanyl, followed by an opioid infusion of one-half of the loading dose per hour, is a reasonable initial dose.

†Usually the effects of neuromuscular blocking agents (NMBAs) can be reversed within a short period, but it may take days to weeks if patients have been receiving NMBAs chronically for management of ventilatory failure.[61] Neuromuscular blockade masks signs of discomfort. Therefore, clinicians should feel that the patient has regained sufficient motor activity to demonstrate discomfort.

‡There is no one sequence applicable to all patients because their clinical situations are so variable. The pace of changes depends on patient comfort and may proceed as quickly as 5–15 min or, in an awake patient to be extubated, over several hours.

§Patients who require high levels of ventilatory support may die after small adjustments such as reduction or elimination of PEEP or decrease in F_{IO_2} to 21%. In such patients, the physician should be present during and immediately after the change in therapy to assess the patient.

Source: Modified from Prendergast (2000), reference 64, and Prendergast (unpublished guidelines), with author's permission. Also, from Treece et al. (2004), reference 140.

mechanical support. Most of the patients (88%) received morphine during withdrawal. At some time during the withdrawal process, 64% of the patients exhibited at least one sign of distress, most often labored breathing or upper airway noise. The investigators reported that their data suggest that little is gained by gradual withdrawal of respiratory support.

Other investigators evaluated responses of 31 adult patients to rapid terminal weaning from mechanical ventilation.[24] Using both observational and physiological measures, they determined that the predominantly comatose patients in their sample remained comfortable with the use of low doses of morphine and BZDs. A larger, randomized clinical trial of various methods of withdrawal may help to determine whether one method is more efficacious than another. Cumulative morphine doses from 1 to 70 mg/h have been reported to be used for terminal weaning.[24,57,69–71] In a recent study of ventilator withdrawal procedures,[57] bolus doses of opioids or BZDs or both effectively managed two thirds of 21 patients' symptoms, whereas the remaining patients required continuous infusions. These research findings support the need for individualizing pharmacological support during life support withdrawal.

Patients should be withdrawn from NMBAs before withdrawal from life support. The use of NMBAs, such as vecuronium, makes it almost impossible to assess patient comfort; while appearing comfortable, patients may be experiencing pain, respiratory distress, or severe anxiety. The use of NMBAs prevents the struggling and gasping that may be associated with dying, but not the patient's suffering.[72] The horror of such a death can only be imagined. The withdrawal of these agents may take considerable time for patients who have been receiving them chronically, and patients continue to have effects from lingering active metabolites.[61]

Regardless of the method used to withdraw life-sustaining therapies, the critical care nurse plays a major role during the decision and implementation of withdrawal of patients from mechanical ventilation. Increased nursing involvement can help provide optimal care to these patients. Specifically, the nurse can ensure that a rationale for, and all elements of, the plan have been adequately discussed among the team, patient, and family. The nurse can ensure that adequate time is given to families and their support persons, such as clergy, to reach as good a resolution as possible. The family needs reassurance that they and the patient will not be left alone and that the patient will be kept comfortable with the use of medications and other measures. As discussed earlier, opioids, alone or in combination with BZDs, are used during withdrawal to ensure that patients are provided the optimal degree of comfort.

The following case study, reported by a nurse, illustrates important aspects of withholding and withdrawing life-sustaining therapies.*

*The authors thank Julie Waters, RN, for providing the case study. Modifications to Ms. Waters' original case study have been made by the authors.

CASE STUDY

Mr. G, an 84-Year-Old Man with Metastatic Cancer

Mr. G was an 84-year-old Caucasian man who had metastatic cancer. He was admitted to the hospital for aspiration pneumonia. He aspirated shortly after admission, developed respiratory distress, and was intubated and transferred to ICU. The next day, I saw the physician in the hall with the daughter and son, having what appeared to be a very emotional conversation. Shortly after that, the daughter walked into the room and stood by the edge of the bed. The physician came in, and the decision was made to withdraw support. The daughter understood her father's condition: "He wouldn't want this," she said. I quickly arranged for a private area in the ICU room in which to transfer him. After getting the room ready, we moved them back there and I took over care. I tried to find out if there was anything special they wanted to do or needed before we took out the breathing tube. I was pretty sure it wouldn't last long after that.

Morphine had given the patient nightmares in the past, so we started a drip of fentanyl and Versed. This helped to ease the daughter's concerns about what her father was going to experience. After I was sure he had been adequately medicated, I removed the endotracheal tube. It was also very important to the daughter that any lines or tubes that could be removed had been. So the only thing I left was the IV tube to administer the medications. It was hard not to have that rhythm strip showing so that I could tell for sure when things were about to end. But I knew that is what the family wanted. Another nurse stopped in to see how we were doing and asked if they wanted their father shaved. She explained to me it would be nice for the daughter to be able to kiss his smooth face good-bye, especially if that was what she was used to. I was really struck by that idea; it hadn't even crossed my mind. The daughter thought that would be nice, so I got the supplies. It turned out to be a beautiful experience. As I gently warmed his face and shaved him, his daughter told me that she was so glad that he had just been baptized into the Catholic faith and had received communion the previous week. It obviously meant a lot to her. Digging in her purse, she pulled out a Bible and read some scripture to him. She shared other things that she remembered about him, and we laughed together and then just quietly reflected.

His breathing had been a little labored as I began, so I increased his IV dosage. Right after I finished shaving his face the best that I could, the daughter looked at me. "Look at how his breathing relaxed and he calmed down when you did that. Thank you so much." To her, the touch and caring had made the difference.

Finally, his breathing stopped, and I nodded that it was over.

Care for the Family of the Dying ICU Patient

Although the focus of care in many critical care areas is on the critically ill patient, nurses and other clinicians with family care skills realize that comprehensive patient care includes care of the patient's family. A reciprocal and all-important relationship exists between the family and the critically ill family member. A change in one affects the other, and vice versa. Classic and contemporary research that describes the anticipatory and acute grief reactions experienced by family members when their loved one is dying point to this powerful reciprocal relationship.[73–77] Therefore, no discussion of palliative care in the ICU is complete without also discussing care of the dying patient's family. Family is defined here as any significant other who participates in the care and well-being of the patient.

The clinical course of any given critically ill, dying patient can vary tremendously, ranging from a rapid unfolding over several hours to a gradual unfolding over several days, weeks, and even months. How a family copes, of course, is also highly variable. Caring for families at any point along the dying trajectory, however, encompasses three major aspects: access, information and support, and involvement in caregiving activities.

Access

A crucial aspect of family care is ensuring that the family can be with their critically ill loved one. Historically, critical care settings have severely restricted family access and discouraged lengthy family visitation. Commonly cited rationales to limit family access include concerns regarding space limitations, patient stability, infection, rest, and privacy; the negative effect of visitation on the family; and clinicians' performance abilities. Some of these concerns have merit, whereas others, such as adverse patient-related issues and a negative effect on the family, have not been borne out in the research literature.

Many ICUs around the world routinely limit visitors to two at any one time.[78,79] Space limitations in critical care areas can be profound, because most ICUs were designed for efficient use of life-saving machinery and staff and were not intended for end-of-life vigils by large, extended families. Ensuring that all interested family members have access to their loved one's bedside can present challenges to the often already narrow confines of the ICU. However, family members of dying loved ones should be allowed more liberal access (both in visiting time and in number of visitors allowed).[75,80] Patients are confronting what may be the most difficult of life passages and they, therefore, may need support from their family members.

There is a growing body of literature that supports family access to patients during invasive procedures and resuscitation. Facilitating family access during such times has come to be known as facilitating family presence, a practice supported by the Emergency Nurses Association and the American Heart Association.[81,82] Researchers have investigated the impact of family presence on patients and found increased patient comfort and satisfaction.[83,84] Studies examining family satisfaction with family presence have yielded similar results, and one study found no adverse psychological effects on the part of family members after the witnessed resuscitation.[85–87]

Because children as young as 5 years old have been reported to have an accurate concept of death,[88] their visitation needs should also be considered when a family member is dying. Although researchers investigating family presence in pediatric populations have found increased behavioral distress in children when parents were present, both parents and children overwhelmingly prefer family presence.[89,90] With proper preparation and debriefing, children can visit a critically ill family member in the ICU without ill effects.[91]

Finally, caring for the critically ill, dying patient and her or his family can call forth feelings of failure for clinicians bent on cure and force health care providers to reflect on their own mortality.[92] Perhaps this helps to explain why so many health care providers believe that family presence is stressful and disruptive to the health care team caring for the critically ill patient.[86,93–95] Yet, one study found that family presence did not affect self-reported stress symptoms in health care providers participating in the resuscitation events.[96] The emotional burden for health care providers when providing palliative care is discussed later in this chapter.

Information and Support

Information has been identified as a crucial component in family coping and satisfaction in critical care settings.[61,97] Support, in the form of nurses' caring behaviors and interactions, is enormously influential in shaping the critical care experience for both patients and their families.[92,98–100] In the context of caring for a critically ill, dying patient, however, nurses and physicians alike have reported high stress related to "death-telling," or notifying family members of the patient's death or terminal prognosis.[101–104] These same studies point to the fact that few health care providers feel they have the skills and knowledge necessary to counsel families effectively during this emotionally charged time. The ethical principle of honesty and truth-telling collides with the limits of knowing the truth precisely when there is clinical ambiguity and also with the suffering imposed on a family having to face the hard truth. Compassionate truth-telling requires dialogue and relationship, timing, and attunement,[105] all of which are relational aspects that are frequently overlooked in the hectic pace of the ICU. Add patient, family, and health care provider culture to the equation, and one can readily understand why communication between involved parties is a less than perfect science.[106] The educational implications for clinicians are addressed later in this chapter.

Overall satisfaction with end-of-life care has been shown to be significantly associated with completeness of information received by the family member, support and care shown to the patient and family, and satisfaction with the amount or level of health care received.[75,100,107–109] Family conferences have been used extensively as a means to improve communication between health care providers and family members, yet few studies have investigated best practices in relation to the timing, content, and participants necessary for optimal communication during a family conference.[110–112]

Some hospitals have created interdisciplinary teams of helping professionals to work with hopelessly ill patients and their families, in an effort to meet patients' and families' physical, informational, and psychosocial needs.[113–117] Such teams usually include a nurse, physician, chaplain, and social worker. Working in concert with the nurses and physicians at the bedside, these interdisciplinary teams can more fully concentrate on end-of-life issues so that, theoretically, no patient or family needs go unmet during this time.

Finally, because feelings of grief in surviving family members are still commonly unresolved at 1 year after a loved one's death, many critical care units across the lifespan have organized bereavement follow-up programs.[118–122] These programs typically involve contacting the surviving family (by telephone or by mail) monthly for some period of time and at the 1-year anniversary of their loved one's death. In addition to remembering and supporting the family, these programs have also been shown to help health care providers cope with the loss as well.

Involvement in Caregiving Activities

Few interventional studies have examined the effect of family involvement on critically ill patients and their families, yet families should have the opportunity to be helpful.[61] Two studies investigating expert nursing behaviors in caring for the dying patient's family found that expert nurses encouraged family participation in patient care.[118,119] Family involvement in caregiving can range from minor activities (such as assisting with oral care or rubbing the dying patient's feet) to major activities (assisting with postmortem care). This involvement may be helpful for family members in working through their grief by demonstrating their love in caring and comforting ways. Being involved in meaningful caregiving activities can make a family member feel useful rather than useless and helpful rather than helpless.

Although physical death occurs in the dying patient, the social death is felt in the patient's surviving family. Because the perception of death lingers at the family level long after the physical death has occurred, involving family members who are interested in participating in their loved one's care may go far to provide closure, comfort, and connection. Unfortunately, many critical care nurses still feel that families should provide a supportive but nonparticipative role in their loved one's provision of care.[120,121] Nurses' facilitation of family involvement in their dying loved one's care is a practical family intervention which should be more widely employed if humane and comprehensive palliative care is desired.

Care for the Caregiver of the Dying ICU Patient

Numerous studies have described the tension between the cure-oriented critical care setting and palliative care.[92,98,122] The bedside health care provider, typically a nurse, often feels caught between differing perceptions held by physicians and family members concerning patient progress and treatment goals. Facilitating and coordinating dialogue and consensus between these groups as well as caring for the dying patient and family can be physically and emotionally exhausting. If the dying process is prolonged, the nurse can become frustrated and fatigued. Although health care providers often cope with this stress by emotionally disengaging themselves from the charged atmosphere, emotional distancing has been shown to hamper skill acquisition and the development of involvement skills.[123] Involvement skills are defined here as the cluster of interpersonal skills that enable a nurse and the patient and family to establish a relational connection. This section discusses two strategies to help health care providers sustain their caring practices and extend their involvement skills; namely, sharing narratives and death education.

Sharing Narratives

Debriefing, either formally or informally, has been used effectively in many settings to discuss and process critical incidents; analyze health care providers' performance in terms of skill, knowledge, and efficiency; and learn, both personally and institutionally, from mistakes and system breakdown.[92,124–126] Sharing stories or narratives of practice can be used to achieve the same goals, but in addition telling stories from practice enables clinicians to (1) increase their skill in recognizing patient and family concerns; (2) learn to communicate more effectively with patients, families, and other health care providers; (3) reflect on ethical comportment and engaged clinical reasoning; and (4) articulate clinical knowledge development.[123,127]

Creating the interpersonal and institutional space in which to both tell and actively listen to stories from practice also enables health care providers to share skills of involvement and sustaining strategies. These understandings can provide clinicians with guidance—and in some cases, corrective action—to intervene in ways that are true to the patient's condition and to the patient's and family's best interests.[105] Through reflection and dialogue with others, nurses and other health care providers can pool their collective wisdom and extend their care of dying patients and their families.

Death Education

Closely coupled with sharing clinical narratives is the use of seminars and other reflective exercises aimed at preparing nurses and other health care providers for the care of dying patients and their families. Death education often consists of didactic and experiential classes. Participants in these classes are encouraged to reflect on and share their own perceptions and anxieties about death, as well as their attitudes toward care of the dying patient and his or her family. This approach has been used with varying degrees of success with nurses, nursing students, and physicians.[128–130] Because many health care providers feel uneasy and ill-prepared to effectively care for terminally ill patients and their families, this is a promising strategy that deserves more implementation and research.

A "Good Death" in the ICU: A Clinical Example

In this clinical incident,[98] a critical care nurse described a 70-year-old patient who was admitted to the ICU with end-stage liver failure. The patient's son was an ICU nurse himself and was the patient's primary caregiver at home. The nurse described how her relationship with the patient's son developed:

> *Nurse:* [The patient] had diabetes, hepatitis C of unknown etiology, and end-stage liver failure. And the [patient's] son would go to the library and pull up articles on hepatitis C and hepatorenal syndrome. You know, he wanted her started on CVVH (continuous veno-venous hemofiltration) because somebody else was on it and because [the therapy] was a kind of hope. The son was with [the patient] when she was on the ward too, and he pretty much called the shots, or that's the impression I got from the floor nurses. And I guess some nurses in the ICU might have felt that way about him too, but this was his mom, and I guess I can understand his wanting to be involved. That's the only mother he has. Anyway, I guess I don't feel threatened by family members who need to be involved. . . . Over the next 3 weeks, I [involved the son in her care]—he was like my extra pair of hands. I mean, he takes care of her at home and he's a nurse. So, why ignore that part of him—that is him. He takes care of her, she wants him there, she was calmer when he was there, and he wants to help. He helped me turn her, he gave her back rubs, he was just there. And I passed that on from shift to shift. I said, "He wants to help. Let him. Why go look for somebody else when somebody who wants to help is right here?" Being involved gave him a sense of helping and doing something [for his mother]. If everything works out, he'll be caring for her at home. He needs to know what her skin looks like. . . . Another thing about that family, I always take it as a compliment when a family feels they can leave when I'm taking care of their family member.
>
> *Interviewer:* And why is that?
>
> *Nurse:* Because I think that means that they trust me and that it's OK for them to leave. Even after nights and nights of staying with his mother, [the son] was still able to go out and take a break for himself. He knew I would call him on his cellular phone if anything came up. . . . But it was a pretty hopeless situation. She was evaluated for a liver transplant but was not a candidate because of her age and her diabetes. . . . It just got to a point where it looked like [the patient] was suffering so much. She just got more and more bloated, she was like twice the size she normally was. So, we ended up withdrawing support late in the shift. They were short the next shift, so I stayed over with the patient and family for another 4 hours just to kind of finish up with them. I didn't want them to have yet a new face [work with them] for the last hour or two of her life. Nobody who had been following this patient was back on nights, and there were no other co-primaries coming on. And it wasn't that big of a deal, but I guess it was for them. About a week and a half later, the [patient's family] came in and brought me this humongous cake and two dozen roses! So, it was really a good experience, because, even though it was a sad outcome, they felt supported and that was pretty much the only goal I had for them.

This clinical incident illustrates the three major aspects of caring for families of dying patients: access, information and support, and involvement in caregiving activities. The nurse in this situation tailored her family care to match what was both required and desired by the patient's son. Because the son was a nurse himself, he researched his mother's condition extensively and suggested different treatment modalities. Rather than being threatened by the son's interest, the nurse understood and supported him. The nurse ensured that the son had liberal access to his critically ill mother and encouraged hands-on involvement in his mother's care.

The nurse developed a trusting relationship with the son, which enabled him to leave his mother's bedside with confidence, knowing that he would be called with any changes in her status. This trusting relationship also helped, no doubt, when discussions concerning his mother's prognosis arose. Because the son trusted the nurse, one can imagine, for example, that he actively listened to her when the nurse pointed out his mother's bloated condition while they were bathing her together. These daily and often mundane encounters helped to forge the nurse–son relationship, from which both drew great satisfaction.

Once the decision was made to withdraw life support, the nurse stayed past her shift to continue her work with the grieving son. The nurse "stayed over" out of respect for the relationship that had developed, but also to provide the son with a "familiar face" during the uncharted and emotionally charged passage of his mother's life. Because this nurse was bearing witness to the death in particular ways shaped by the nurse–family relationship, a new person would not be able to enter the situation and support the son in the same way. The nurse responded to the ethical responsibility of being in a relationship with the patient's family and, in so doing, facilitated the son's closure with this major family event.

An International Agenda to Improve Care of Dying ICU Patients

Considerable emphasis is now being placed on improving care at the end of life for ICU patients. The first book that comprehensively and specifically addresses ICU end-of-life care has been published.[131] The Society of Critical Care Medicine's 30th Critical Care Congress in 2001 devoted an entire educational track to this topic.[132] A Working Group of experts in critical care and other relevant specialties, whose work was funded in part by the Robert Wood Johnson Foundation, developed a research agenda for end-of-life care in ICUs.[133] A Robert Wood Johnson–sponsored national ICU Peer Workgroup on end-of-life care is conducting several education and research initiatives related to this topic. One of these initiatives is the development of quality indicators for end-of-life care in ICUs.[134] These quality indicators can provide a framework for interventions to improve care of the dying in ICUs. An international consensus conference was held in 2003 to gather the evidence to date on end-of-life care in ICUs and make recommendations for practice and research. Recently published recommendations from this conference provide directions for practice improvements.[135] Currently, the Robert Wood Johnson Foundation is funding demonstration projects in four ICUs in the United States. These demonstration projects are developing palliative care models for ICUs and assessing the impact on the quality of care for patients and their families.[136] It is anticipated that findings from these demonstration projects will guide national and international practice improvements.

Summary

As noted by Todres and colleagues,[13] "There is not one best way to die." However, the authors believe that provision of a pain-free, ethically intact, and dignified death is the right of all ICU patients. Research to date has offered little guidance for managing the issues that surround ICU patient deaths. However, Chapple[137] presented important goals to consider during an ICU patient's dying process: (1) honor the patient's life, (2) ensure that the patient and the family are not abandoned, (3) provide a sense of moral stability, and (4) ensure the patient's safety and comfort. ICU nurses can feel privileged to strive toward the accomplishment of those goals.

REFERENCES

1. Puntillo K. Unpublished data, 2003.
2. Angus DC, Barnato AE, Linde-Zwirble WT, Weissfeld LA, Watson RS, Rickert T, Rubenfeld GD. Use of intensive care at the end of life in the United States: An epidemiologic study. Crit Care Med 2004;32:638–643.
3. Levy M. Dying in America. Crit Care Med 2004;32:879–880.
4. Levetown M. Palliative care in the intensive care unit. New Horizons 1998;6:383–397.
5. The SUPPORT Principal Investigators. A controlled trial to improve care for seriously ill hospitalized patients: The Study to Understand Prognoses and Preferences for Outcomes and Risks of Treatments (SUPPORT). JAMA 1995;274:1591–1598.
6. Lynn J, Teno JM, Phillips RS, Wu AW, Desbiens N, Harrold J, Claessens MT, Wenger N, Kreling B, Connors AF Jr. Perceptions by family members of the dying experience of older and seriously ill patients. Ann Intern Med 1997;126:97–106.
7. Desbiens NA, Wu AW, Broste SK, Wenger NS, Connors AF Jr, Lynn J, Yasui Y, Phillips RS, Fulkerson W. Pain and satisfaction with pain control in seriously ill hospitalized adults: Findings from the SUPPORT research investigations. Crit Care Med 1996;24:1953–1961.
8. Levetown M, Pollack MM, Cuerdon TT, Ruttimann UE, Glover JJ. Limitations and withdrawals of medical intervention in pediatric critical care. JAMA 1994;272:1271–1275.
9. Balfour-Lynn IM, Tasker RC. Futility and death in paediatric medical intensive care. J Med Ethics 1996;22:279–281.
10. Vernon DD, Dean JM, Timmons OD, Banner W, Allen-Webb EM. Modes of death in the pediatric intensive care unit: Withdrawal and limitation of supportive care. Crit Care Med 1993;21:1798–1802.
11. Task Force on Ethics, Society of Critical Care Medicine. Consensus report on the ethics of foregoing life-sustaining treatments in the critically ill. Crit Care Med 1990;18:1435–1439.
12. Walter SD, Cook DJ, Guyatt GH, Spanier A, Jaeschke R, Todd TR, Streiner DL. Confidence in life-support decisions in the intensive care unit: A survey of healthcare workers. Crit Care Med 1998;26:44–49.
13. Todres ID, Armstrong A, Lally P, Cassem EH. Negotiating end-of-life issues. New Horizons 1998;6:374–382.
14. Prendergast TJ, Puntillo KA. Withdrawal of life support: Intensive caring at the end of life. JAMA 2002;288:2732–2740.
15. DeGroot-Bollujt W, Mourik M. Bereavement: Role of the nurse in the care of terminally ill and dying children in the pediatric intensive care unit. Crit Care Med 1993;21:S391.
16. Campbell M, Frank RR. Experience with an end-of-life practice at a university hospital. Crit Care Med 1997;25:197–202.
17. Teno JM, Clarridge BR, Casey V, Welch LC, Wetle T, Shield R, Mor V. Family perspectives on end-of-life care at the last place of care. JAMA 2004;291:88–93.
18. Foley K. Pain and symptom control in dying ICU patients. In: Curtis JR, Rubenfeld GD, eds. The Transition from Cure to Comfort: Managing Death in the Intensive Care Unit. New York: Oxford University Press, 2001.
19. Puntillo KA. The role of critical care nurses in providing and managing end-of-life care. In: Curtis R, Rubenfield G, eds. The Transition from Cure to Comfort: Managing Death in the Intensive Care Unit. New York: Oxford University Press 2001:149–164.
20. Kwekkeboom KL, Herr K. Assessment pain in the critically ill. Crit Care Nurs Clin North Am 2001;13:181–194.
21. Puntillo KA. Pain management. In: Schell HM, Puntillo KA, eds. Critical Care Nursing Secrets. Philadelphia: Hanley and Belfus, 2001.
22. Payen JF, Bru O, Bosson JL, Lagrasta A, Novel E, Deschaux I, Lavagne P, Jacquot C. Assessing pain in critically ill sedated patients by using a behavioral pain scale. Crit Care Med 2001; 29:2258–2263.
23. Puntillo KA., Morris AB, Thompson CL, Stanik-Hutt J, White C, Wild LR. Pain behaviors observed during six common procedures: Results from Thunder Project II. Crit Care Med 2004; 32:421–427.
24. Campbell ML, Bizek KS, Thill M. Patient responses during rapid terminal weaning from mechanical ventilation: A prospective study. Crit Care Med 1999;27:73–77.
25. Bizek KS: Optimizing sedation in critically ill, mechanically ventilated patients. Crit Care Nurs Clin North Am 1995;7:315–325.

26. Ambuel B, Hamlett KW, Marx CM, Blumer JL. Assessing distress in pediatric intensive care environments: The COMFORT scale. J Pediatr Psychol 1992;17:95–109.
27. Aspect Medical Systems. The Aspect A-1000 Bispectral (BIS) Index Manual. Natick, MA: Aspect Medical Systems, 1996.
28. Morrison RS, Ahronheim JC, Morrison GR, Darling E, Baskin SA, Morris J, Choi C, Meier DE. Pain and discomfort associated with common hospital procedures and experiences. J Pain Symptom Manage 1998;15:91–101.
29. Puntillo K. Dimensions of procedural pain and its analgesic management in critically ill surgical patients. Am J Crit Care 1994;3:116–122.
30. Puntillo KA, Ley J. Appropriately timed analgesics control pain due to chest tube removal. Am J Crit Care 2004;13:292–301.
31. Puntillo KA, White C, Morris A, Perdue S, Stanik-Hutt J, Thompson C, Wild L. Patients' perceptions and responses to procedural pain: Results from Thunder Project II. Am J Crit Care 2001;10:238–251.
32. Paice JA, Muir JC, Shott S. Palliative care at the end of life: Comparing quality in diverse settings. Am J Hospice Palliat Care 2004;21:19–27.
33. Jacobi J, Fraser GL, Coursin DB, Riker RR, Fontaine D, Wittbrodt ET, Chalfin DB, Masica MF, Bjerke HS, Coplin WM, Crippen DW, Fuchs BD, Kelleher RM, Marik PE, Nasraway SA Jr, Murray MJ, Peruzzi WT, Lumb PD; Task Force of the American College of Critical Care Medicine (ACCM) of the Society of Critical Care Medicine (SCCM), American Society of Health-system Pharmacists (ASHP), American College of Chest Physicians. Clinical practice guidelines for the sustained use of sedatives and analgesics in the critically ill. Crit Care Med 2002;30:119–141 (erratum in: Crit Care Med 2002;30:726).
34. American Pain Society. Principles of Analgesic Use in the Treatment of Acute Pain and Cancer Pain, 5th ed. Glenview, IL: American Pain Society, 2003.
35. Fohr SA. The double effect of pain medication: Separating myth from reality. J Palliat Med 1998;1:315–328.
36. Puntillo KA, Benner P, Drought T, Drew B, Stotts N, Stannard D, Rushton C, Scanlon C, White C. End-of-life issues in intensive care units: A national random survey of nurses' knowledge and beliefs. Am J Crit Care 2001;10:216–229.
37. Titler MG, Rakel BA. Nonpharmacologic treatment of pain. Crit Care Nurs Clin North Am 2001;13:221–232.
38. Park G, Coursin D, Ely EW, England M, Fraser GL, Mantz J, McKinley S, Ramsay M, Scholz J, Singer M, Sladen R, Vender JS, Wild L. Balancing sedation and analgesia in the critically ill. Crit Care Clin 2001;17:1015–1027.
39. Liu LL, Gropper MA. Postoperative analgesia and sedation in the adult intensive care unit. Drugs 2003;63:755–767.
40. Nickel EJ, Smith T. Analgesia in the intensive care unit. Crit Care Nurs Clin North Am 2001;13:207–219.
41. Savel RH, Wiener-Kronish JP. Analgesia and sedation: What are the best choices for intensive care patients? J Crit Illness 2001; 16:437–444.
42. Kress JP, Pohlman A, O'Connor MF, Hall JB. Daily interruption of sedative infusions in critically ill patients undergoing mechanical ventilation. N Engl J Med 2000;342:1471–1477.
43. Brook AD, Ahrens TS, Shaiff R, Prentice D, Sherman G, Shannon W, Kollef MH. Effect of a nursing-implemented sedation protocol on the duration of mechanical ventilation. Crit Care Med 1999; 27:2609–2615.
44. Guerrero M. Combined pharmacotherapy of anxiety. In: Bone R, ed. Recognition, Assessment, and Treatment of Anxiety in the Critical Care Patient. Proceedings of a consensus conference. Yardley, PA: The Medicine Group, Inc., 1994.
45. Vinik HR, Kissin I. Sedation in the ICU. Intensive Care Med 1991;17:S20–S23.
46. Shelly MP, Sultan MA, Bodenham A, Park GR. Midazolam infusions critically ill patients. Eur J Anaesthesiol 1991;8:21–27.
47. Harvey MA. Managing agitation in critically ill patients. Am J Crit Care 1996;5:7–16.
48. Nelson JE, Meier DE, Oei EJ, Nierman DM, Senzel RS, Manfredi PL, Davis SM, Morrison S. Self-reported symptom experience of critically ill cancer patients receiving intensive care. Crit Care Med 2001;29:277–282.
49. Prendergast TJ, Claessens MT, Luce JM. A national survey of end-of-life care for critically ill patients. Am J Crit Care Med 1998;158:1163–1167.
50. McLean RF, Tarshis J, Mazer CD, Szalai JP. Death in two Canadian intensive care units: Institutional difference and changes over time. Crit Care Med 2000;28:100–103.
51. President's Commission for the Study of Ethical Problems in Medicine and Biomedical and Behavioral Research. Deciding to Forgo Life-Sustaining Treatment: A Report on Ethical, Medical and Legal Issues in Treatment Decisions. Washington, DC: U.S. Government Printing Office, 1983.
52. American Association of Critical Care Nurses. Position Statement: Withholding and/or Withdrawing Life-Sustaining Treatment. Newport Beach, Calif.: AACCN, 1990.
53. Task Force on Ethics, Society of Critical Care Medicine. Consensus report on the ethics of forgoing life-sustaining treatments in the critically ill. Crit Care Med 1990;18:1435–1439.
54. Medical Section, American Lung Association. Withholding and withdrawing life-sustaining therapy. Am Rev Respir Dis 1991; 144:726–731.
55. Faber-Langendoen K, Lanken PN. Dying patients in the intensive care unit: Forgoing treatment, maintaining care. Ann Intern Med 2000;133:886–893.
56. Asch DA, Faber-Langendoen K, Shea JA, Christakis NA. The sequence of withdrawing life-sustaining treatment from patients. Am J Med 1999;107:153–156.
57. O'Mahony S, McHugh M, Zallman L, Selwyn P. Ventilator withdrawal: Procedures and outcomes. Report of a collaboration between a critical care division and a palliative care service. J Pain Symptom Manage 2003;26:954–961.
58. Rubenfeld GD, Crawford SW. Principles and practice of withdrawing life-sustaining treatment in the ICU. In: Curtis JR, Rubenfeld GD, eds. The Transition from Cure to Comfort: Managing Death in the Intensive Care Unit. New York: Oxford University Press, 2001.
59. Hall RI, Rocker GM. End-of-life care in the ICU: Treatments provided when life support was or was not withdrawn. Chest 2000;118:1425–1430.
60. von Gunten C, Weissman DE. Fast Fact and Concept #033: Ventilator Withdrawal Protocol (Part I). End of Life/Palliative Education Resource Center (EPERC), Medical College of Wisconsin. Available at: http://www.eperc.mcw.edu/fastFact/ff_033.htm (accessed February 1, 2005).
61. Truog RD, Cist AFM, Brackett SE, Burns JP, Curley MA, Danis M, DeVita MA, Rosenbaum SH, Rothenberg DM, Sprung CL, Webb, SA, Wlody GS, Hurford WE. Recommendations for end-of-life

care in the intensive care unit: The ethics committee of the society of critical care medicine. Crit Care Med 2001;29:2332–2348.
62. von Gunten C, Weissman DE. Fast Fact and Concept #034: Symptom Control for Ventilator Withdrawal in the Dying Patient (Part II). End of Life/Palliative Education Resource Center (EPERC), Medical College of Wisconsin. Available at: http://www.eperc.mcw.edu/fastFact/ff_034.htm (accessed February 1, 2005).
63. von Gunten C, Weissman DE. Fast Fact and Concept #35: Information for Patients and Families About Ventilator Withdrawal (Part III). End of Life/Palliative Education Resource Center (EPERC), Medical College of Wisconsin. Available at: http://www.eperc.mcw.edu/fastFact/ff_035.htm (accessed February 1, 2005).
64. Prendergast TJ. Withholding or withdrawal of life-sustaining therapy. Hosp Prac 2000;June 15:91–92,95–102.
65. Hawryluck LA, Harvey WRC, Lemieux-Charles L, Singer PA. Consensus guidelines on analgesia and sedation in dying intensive care unit patients. BMC Med Ethics 2002;3(1):3.
66. Partridge JC, Wall SN. Analgesia for dying infants whose life support is withdrawn or withheld. Pediatrics 1997;99:76.
67. Abe N, Catlin A, Mihara D. End of life in the NICU: A study of ventilator withdrawal. MCN Am J Matern Child Nurs 2001;26: 141–146.
68. Daly BJ, Thomas D, Dyer MA. Procedures used in withdrawal of mechanical ventilation. Am J Crit Care 1996;5:331–338.
69. Campbell ML, Carlson RW. Terminal weaning from mechanical ventilation: Ethical and practical considerations for patient management. Am J Crit Care 1992;1:52–56.
70. Daly BJ, Newlon B, Montenegro HD, Langdon T. Withdrawal of mechanical ventilation: Ethical principles and guidelines from terminal weaning. Am J Crit Care 1993;2:217–223.
71. Wilson WC, Smedira NG, Fink C, McDowell JA, Luce JM. Ordering and administration of sedatives and analgesics during the withholding and withdrawal of life support from critically ill patients. JAMA 1992;267:949–953.
72. Rushton, CH, Terry PB. Neuromuscular blockade and ventilator withdrawal: Ethical controversies. Am J Crit Care 1995;4:112–115.
73. Friedman SB, Chodoff P, Mason JW, Hamburg DA. Behavioral observations on parents anticipating the death of their child. Pediatrics 1963;32:616–625.
74. Lindemann E. Symptomatology and management of acute grief. Am J Psychol 1944;101:141–148.
75. Abbott, KH, Sago, JG, Breen, CM, Abernethy, AP, Tulsky, JA. Families looking back: One year after discussion of withdrawal or withholding of life-sustaining support. Crit Care Med. 2001; 29:197–201.
76. Frid I. No going back: Narratives by close relatives of the braindead patient. Intensive Crit Care Nurs 2001;17:263–278.
77. Meert KL, Thurston CS, Thomas R. Parental coping and bereavement outcome after the death of a child in the pediatric intensive care unit. Pediatr Crit Care Med 2001;2:324–328.
78. Miranda DR, Ryan DW, Schaufeli WB, Fidler V. Organisation and Management of Intensive Care: A Prospective Study in 12 European Countries. Heidelberg/New York: Springer Berlin, 1998.
79. Younger SJ, Coulton C, Welton R, Juknialis B, Jackson DL. ICU visiting policies. Crit Care Med 1984;12:606–608.
80. Slota M, Shearn D, Postersnak K, Haas L. Perspectives on family-centered, flexible visitation in the intensive care unit setting. Crit Care Med 2003;31:S362–S366.
81. Emergency Nurses Association. Presenting the Option for Family Presence, 2nd ed. Park Ridge, IL: ENA, 2001.
82. American Heart Association. Guidelines 2000 for cardiopulmonary resuscitation and emergency cardiovascular care [special issue]. Circulation 2000;102:I1–I374.
83. Eichhorn DJ, Meyers TA, Guzzetta CE, Clark AP, Klein JD, Taliaferro E, Calvin AO. Family presence during invasive procedures and resuscitation: Hearing the voice of the patient. Am J Nurs 2001;101:48–55.
84. Shapira M, Tamir A. Presence of family members during upper endoscopy: What do patients and escorts think? J Clin Gastroenterol 1996;22:272–274.
85. Meyers TA, Eichhorn DJ, Guzzetta CE. Do families want to be present during CPR: A retrospective survey. J Emerg Nurs 1998; 24:400–405.
86. Meyers TA, Eichhorn DJ, Guzzetta CE, Clark AP, Klein JD, Taliaferro E, Calvin A. Family presence during invasive procedures and resuscitation: The experience of family members, nurses, and physicians. Am J Nurs 2000;100:32–42.
87. Robinson SM, Mackenzie-Ross S, Campbell Hewson GL, Egleston CV, Prevost AT. Psychological effect of witnessed resuscitation on bereaved relatives. Lancet 1998;352:614–616.
88. Mahon MM. Children's concept of death and sibling death from trauma. J Pediatr Nurs 1993;8:335–344.
89. Foertsch CE, O'Hara MW, Stoddard FJ, Kealey GP. Parent participation during burn debridement in relation to behavioral distress. J Burn Care Rehabil 1996;17:372–377.
90. Gonzalez JC, Routh DK, Saab PG, Armstrong FD, Shifman L, Guerra E, Fawcett N. Effects of parent presence on children's reactions to injections: Behavioral, physiological, and subjective aspects. J Pediatr Psychol 1989;14:449–462.
91. Nicholson AC, Titler M, Montgomery LA, Kleiber C, Craft MJ, Halm M, Buckwalter K, Johnson S. Effects of child visitation in adult critical care units: A pilot study. Heart Lung 1993;22:36–45.
92. Benner P, Hooper-Kyriakidis P, Stannard D. Clinical wisdom and interventions in critical care: A thinking-in-action approach. Philadelphia, Pa.: WB Saunders, 1999.
93. Ellison S. Nurses' attitudes toward family presence during resuscitative efforts and invasive procedures. J Emerg Nurs 2003;29: 515–521.
94. McClenathan BM, Torrington KG, Uyehara CFT. Family member presence during cardiopulmonary resuscitation: A survey of US and international critical care professionals. Chest 2002;122: 2204–2211.
95. Helmer SD, Smith S, Dort JM, Sharpiro WM, Katan BS. Family presence during trauma resuscitation: A survey of AAST and ENA members. J Trauma 2000;48:1015–1024.
96. Boyd R, White S. Does witnessed cardiopulmonary resuscitation alter perceived stress in accident and emergency staff? Eur J Emerg Med 2000;7:51–53.
97. Kristjanson LJ, White K. Clinical support for families in the palliative care phase of hematologic or oncologic illness. Hematol Oncol Clin North Am 2002;16:745–762.
98. Stannard D. Reclaiming the house: An interpretive study of nurse-family interactions and activities in critical care. A dissertation submitted in partial fulfillment of the requirements for the degree of Doctor of Philosophy, University of California, San Francisco. 1997.
99. Buchman TG, Ray SE, Wax ML, Cassell J, Rich D, Niemczycki MA. Families' perceptions of surgical intensive care. J Am Coll Surg. 2003;196:977–983.
100. Curley MA, Meyer EC. Parental experience of highly technical therapy: Survivors and nonsurvivors of extracorporeal

membrane oxygenation support. Pediatr Crit Care Med 2003; 4:214–219.

101. Greenberg LW, Ochsenschlager D, Cohen GJ, Einhorn AH, O'Donnell R. Counseling parents of a child dead on arrival: A survey of emergency departments. Am J Emerg Med 1993;11: 225–229.
102. Field D. Nurses' accounts of nursing the terminally ill on a coronary care unit. Intensive Care Nurs 1989;5:114–122.
103. Swisher LA, Nieman LZ, Nilsen GJ, Spivey WH. Death notification in the emergency department: A survey of residents and attending physicians. Ann Emerg Med 1993;22:1319–1323.
104. Tinsley ES, Baldwin AS, Steeves RH, Himel HN, Edlich RF. Surgeons', nurses' and bereaved families' attitudes toward dying in the burn centre. Burns 1994;20:79–82.
105. Benner P. A dialogue between virtue ethics and care ethics. Theor Med 1997;18:47–61.
106. Nunez GR. Culture, demographics, and critical care issues: An overview. Crit Care Clin 2003;19:619–639.
107. Malacrida R, Bettelini CM, Degrate A, Martinez M, Badia F, Piazza J, Vizzardi N, Wullschleger R, Rapin CH. Reasons for dissatisfaction: A survey of relatives of intensive care patients who died. Crit Care Med 1998;26:1187–1193.
108. Heyland DK, Rocker GM, O'Callaghan CJ, Dodek PM, Cook DJ. Dying in the ICU: Perspectives of family members. Chest 2003; 124:392–397.
109. Warren NA. Critical care family members' satisfaction with bereavement experiences. Crit Care Nurs Q 2002;25:54–60.
110. Curtis JR, Patrick DL, Shannon SE, Treece PD, Engelberg RA, Rubenfeld GD. The family conference as a focus to improve communication about end-of-life care in the intensive care unit: Opportunities for improvement. Crit Care Med 2001;29: N26–N33.
111. Frank RR, Campbell ML. Caring for terminally ill patients: One hospital's team approach. J Crit Illness 1999;14:51–55.
112. Field BE, Devich LE, Carlson RW. Impact of a comprehensive care team on management of hopelessly ill patients with multiple organ failure. Chest 1989;96:353–356.
113. Coolican MB, Pearce T. After care bereavement program. Crit Care Nurs Clin North Am 1995;7:519–527.
114. Hodge DS, Graham PL. A hospital-based neonatal intensive care unit bereavement follow-up program: An evaluation of its effectiveness. J Perinatol 1988;8:247–252.
115. Jackson I. Bereavement follow-up service in intensive care. Intensive Crit Care Nurs 1992;8:163–168.
116. Nesbit MJ, Hill M, Peterson N. A comprehensive pediatric bereavement program: The patterns of your life. Crit Care Nurs Q 1997;20:48–62.
117. Williams R, Harris S, Randall R, Brown S. A bereavement aftercare service for intensive care relatives and staff: The story so far. Nurs Crit Care 2003;8:109–115.
118. Degner LF, Gow CM, Thompson LA. Critical nursing behaviors in care for the dying. Cancer Nurs 1991;14:246–253.
119. McClement SE, Degner LF. Expert nursing behaviors in care of the dying adult in the intensive care unit. Heart Lung 1995;24: 408–419.
120. Hickey M, Lewandowski L. Critical care nurses' role with families: A descriptive study. Heart Lung 1988;17:670–676.
121. Warren N. Bereavement care in the critical care setting. Crit Care Nurs Q 1997;20:42–47.
122. Chambliss DF. Beyond Caring: Hospitals, Nurses, and the Social Organization of Ethics. Chicago: University of Chicago, 1996.
123. Benner P, Tanner CA, Chesla CA. Expertise in Nursing Practice: Caring, Clinical Judgment, and Ethics. New York: Springer; 1996.
124. Isaak C, Paterson BL. Critical care nurses' lived experience of unsuccessful resuscitation. West J Nurs Res 1996;18:688–702.
125. Carelock, J. Critical incidents: Effective communication and documentation. Crit Care Nurs Q 2001;23:59–66.
126. Ihlenfeld JT. Applying personal reflective critical incident reviews in critical care. Dimens Crit Care Nurs 2004;23:1–3.
127. Benner P, Stannard D, Hooper PL. A "thinking-in-action" approach to teaching clinical judgment: A classroom innovation for acute care advanced practice nurses. Adv Prac Nurs Q 1996; 1:70–77.
128. Degner LF, Gow CM. Preparing nurses for care of the dying: A longitudinal study. Cancer Nurs 1988;11:160–169.
129. Hainsworth DS. The effect of death education on attitudes of hospital nurses toward care of the dying. Oncol Nurs Forum 1996;23:963–967.
130. DeVita MA, Arnold RM, Barnard D. Teaching palliative care to critical care medicine trainees. Crit Care Med 2003;31:1257–1262.
131. Curtis JR, Rubenfeld GD. The Transition from Cure to Comfort. New York: Oxford University Press, 2001.
132. Society of Critical Care Medicine 30th International Educational and Scientific Symposium. Crit Care Med 2000;28(12 Suppl):A27–223.
133. Rubenfeld GD, Curtis JR. End-of-life in the intensive care unit: A research agenda. Crit Care Med 2001;29:2001–2006.
134. Clarke EB, Curtis JR, Luce JM, Levy M, Danis M, Nelson J, Solomon MZ; for the Robert Wood Johnson Foundation Critical Care End-of-Life Peer Workgroup Members. Quality indicators for end-of-life care in the intensive care unit. Crit Care Med 2003;31:2255–2262.
135. Carlet J, Thijs LG, Antonelli M, Cassell J, Cox P, Hill N, Hinds C, Pimentel JM, Reinhart K, Thompson BT. Challenges in end-of-life care in the ICU. Intensive Care Med 2004;30:770–784.
136. Promoting Excellence in End-of-Life Care. Grantees: Promoting Palliative Care Excellence in Intensive Care, http://www.promotingexcellence.org/navigate/grantees.html (accessed March 25, 2005).
137. Chapple HS. Changing the game in the intensive care unit: Letting nature take its course. Crit Care Nurse 1999;19:25–34.
138. Govoni LE, Hayes JE. Drugs and Nursing Implications. Norwalk: Appleton & Lange, 1996.
139. Kuebler KK. Dyspnea. Pittsburgh, PA: Hospice and Palliative Nurses Association, 1996.
140. Treece PD, Engleberg RA, Crowley L, Chan JD, Rubenfeld GD, Steinberg KP, Curtis JR. Evaluation of a standardized order form for the withdrawal of life support in the intensive care unit. Crit Care Med 2004;32:1141–1148.

44 The Outpatient Setting

Anna R. Du Pen and Jeanne Robison

I am so glad that you are there for me . . . someone on the other end of the phone who knows what to do when I just can't sort it out.—Annette, 56, colon cancer patient

- ***Key Points***
- *Twenty-four-hour accessibility to health care providers is critical to providing palliative care to outpatients.*
- *Evaluation and management of physical, emotional, and spiritual distress at each office visit are primary components of outpatient palliative care.*
- *Active listening in the office and at telephone triage contributes greatly to individualizing the plan of care.*
- *Providing a sense of control for patients and their families is an integral part of palliative care.*

Dramatic changes over the last two decades have resulted in shorter and shorter hospital stays, longer survival with chronic debilitating disease, and smaller, fractured families—all of which have contributed greatly to increased use of outpatient services. Outpatient care is delivered in private practice offices, free-standing clinics, and hospital-based outpatient settings. Individuals with chronic and terminal illnesses receive care over time in the outpatient clinic or office setting. In these settings, significant long-term relationships develop among providers, patients, and families. As patients move toward the end of life, visits to the clinic provide an excellent opportunity to assess the patient's and family's needs, desires, struggles, and fears.

The months or years spent providing and receiving care in an outpatient setting are fundamental to establishing trust between the care team and the patient. This trusting relationship is vital both early in the disease continuum and at the end of life. Building this relationship is a critical component of the palliative nursing role.[1,2] Unlike in an acute care setting, patients and families have time scheduled with physicians and staff to address their needs. This allows families to avoid the frustration of waiting in a hospital room trying to connect with a physician or nurse to raise issues or ask questions. The patient's and family's questions are answered and processed at one visit, and further clarifying questions and detailed responses can ensue at the next office visit.

In most cases, an outpatient setting is more intimate and less crisis driven than a hospital setting. On the other hand, patients may have excessive time in the waiting room and may be in very different stages of disease than others surrounding them. In the best situation, patients and families meet and support each other and facilities use waiting room space to make educational materials readily available.

There is generally a certain structure to the clinic visit that can lend itself to the integration of palliative care. In addition to taking a history, performing a physical examination, and reviewing medication history, the clinician can effectively integrate a discussion about advance directives into the routine. Treatment plans can be discussed and negotiated with the patient. An assessment of pain and symptoms can be done at the time vital signs are taken or during telephone triage. The pain-related standards for outpatient care of the Joint Commission on Accreditation of Healthcare Organizations (JCAHO) can be used to help incorporate pain and symptom management into the routine documentation of outpatient care.

Challenges in Outpatient Care

A number of challenges associated with the outpatient setting exist. The absence of a strong nursing presence is arguably the most critical barrier to the successful integration of palliative care. For example, ideally, in an outpatient oncology practice, registered nurses would be on staff to administer chemotherapy, to provide patient teaching, and to staff telephone triage systems.[3,4] Assistive personnel are used for non-nursing duties, such as cleaning equipment, stocking, setting up examination rooms, and scheduling.[5] However, with shrinking resources available in all spheres of health care, the use of nonlicensed personnel is expanding, and this trend is not likely to be reversed.

Although it is generally considered preferable for licensed personnel to be responsible for duties such as medication administration and telephone triage, many outpatient settings employ medical assistants or administrative assistants to collect intake data, take vital signs, and answer telephone calls. In many cases, nurses are being asked to do a greater number and variety of treatments, leading to a feeling that there is not enough quality time with individual patients.[6] Some offices have no registered nurse at all in the outpatient setting, causing patients to have to wait for a chance to speak with the doctor before any assistance or suggestions can be offered. This can result in considerable delay in addressing symptom management issues and is clearly less than optimal.

Managed care has played a role in further splintering outpatient care in some medical centers. For example, with a reduction in reimbursement for chemotherapy, patients may be required to receive their treatment at an infusion center, along with patients receiving antibiotic therapy, inhalation therapy, and other treatments, far from the cancer center. Although this is a more cost-efficient way to provide parenteral therapy, it offers less continuity of care over time than does having outpatient cancer center nurses provide all care, from diagnosis through active treatment and on to palliative care.

Although registered nurses in office settings increasingly are being replaced by nonlicensed personnel, the increase in the use of nurse practitioners as physician extenders in outpatient care is a positive development.[7,8] These advanced practice nurses can enable same-day office visits for emergencies or symptoms that require acute management. Many clinics use nurse practitioners to take histories and perform physical examinations for routine admissions to the hospital, while the physician sees patients in the clinic. A new and growing specialty group of acute care nurse practitioners sees very ill or unstable patients in the hospital, again working closely with the physician to balance outpatient and inpatient services. Advanced practice nurses have a higher comfort level with discussing end-of-life issues[9] and maintain a high level of expertise in pain and symptom management (Figure 44–1).

Another area where advanced practice nurses greatly affect care is that of transitions in the goals of care. Clinics have heterogenous populations of patients, whose status may range from the early stages of diagnostic workup all the way through end-of-life care. Taking a lead role in helping to continuously reevaluate the goals of care with patients and families is a key impact area of advanced practice nurses.

One challenge facing advanced practice nurses in some states is the lack of prescriptive authority.[10] In some states, advanced practice nurses, trained and skilled in palliative care management, are allowed to assess pain, address symptoms, and develop treatment plans but may not prescribe controlled medications. This limits patients' access to pain and symptom management and creates a cumbersome process for refilling pain medications and addressing needs for antianxiety agents. These practitioners often become experts at the optimal use of nonsteroidal antiinflammatory drugs (NSAIDs), co-analgesic agents (e.g., tricyclic antidepressants, anticonvulsants), antiemetics, bowel care agents, and a host of other pharmacological therapies.

Several states do allow nurse practitioners full prescriptive authority, which improves access to palliative care.[11] They are able to see patients with pain or symptom problems on the same day and prescribe therapy without the presence of a physician. Patients do not have to wait to receive a written prescription from a physician or travel to an emergency room to be seen by physicians not familiar with their cases.

Finally, another significant challenge in the outpatient setting is managing the increasingly burdensome gatekeeper role. Before a chronically ill patient can be discharged from an acute care setting, arrangements for extended care or home nursing must be made by a hospital discharge planning team. Once this plan of care is established, the outpatient team must coordinate and facilitate the patient's care plan. This can be an overwhelming burden on outpatient nurses, who must constantly field telephone calls and faxes, fill out disability or family leave paperwork, and communicate with caregivers in the community. Balancing the telephone calls that urgently need attention with those of a more bureaucratic nature is a significant problem in many practices. Keeping track of what is happening with outpatients is difficult in the best-staffed clinics and may be overlooked entirely in poorly staffed settings. Return visits to the clinic are vital for evaluating treatment outcomes, assessing ongoing needs of patients, and effectively managing available resources. If clients are unable to travel to the clinic, provider visits to a nursing home, or timely referral to home health care with a focus on continuity of the treatment plan is very important. Incorporating all aspects of the team across inpatient, outpatient, and home care facilitates the best in palliative care outcomes.

Pain and Symptom Management
Waiting Room Checklist

Patient Name: ____________________
Date: ____________

(circle one)
Since you saw your doctor last have you had any "new" pain or symptoms? Yes No

The level of pain is described on a 0 to 10 scale where 0 is no pain and 10 is the worst pain you can imagine. Please circle the number that best indicates the level of pain you have had over the last 24 hours:

0 1 2 3 4 5 6 7 8 9 10

No Pain **Mild** **Discomforting** **Distressing** **Horrible** **Excruciating**

Check the box beside all of the below words that describe your pain

❑ aching ❑ burning ❑ shooting ❑ throbbing

❑ tender ❑ sharp ❑ stabbing ❑ cramping

Please indicate which symptoms you are currently experiencing:

	No	Yes	If yes, is the symptom ✓ Mild	✓ Moderate	✓ Severe	If yes, how long has it been
Nausea						
Hard/infrequent bowel movements						
Drowsiness						
Shortness of Breath						
Dry Mouth						
Feeling Very Tired						
Stomachache after my pills						
Muscle jerking/twitching						
Bad dreams or "seeing things" that are not there						

(circle one)
Are you having any problems with your medications? Yes No

Is there anything that you feel is a priority to discuss at today's clinic appointment? (if yes, please indicate what)

____

____

____

Figure 44–1. Patient waiting room checklist for pain and symptom assessment. The questions relate to pain and any side effects of analgesics—information that can facilitate discussions of symptom management.

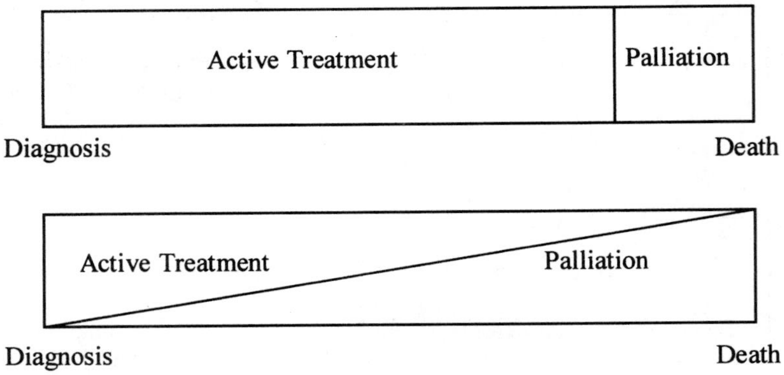

Figure 44–2. Active treatment versus palliative care, depicted in a mutually exclusive "old" model *(top)* and an integrated "new" model *(bottom)*. *Source:* World Health Organization (1995), reference 12.

The two major benefits of the outpatient setting are a more intimate, structured environment and more time to develop long-term relationships. However, the setting also has disadvantages: fewer registered nurses, the increased burden of gatekeeping, and poor access in busy outpatient practices. Providing quality palliative care in the outpatient setting requires creativity and commitment to meeting these challenges.

Integrating Palliative Care into Outpatient Care

A combination of philosophical mission, strategic planning, and bottom-line pragmatism is necessary to integrate palliative care successfully into the current outpatient medical model (Figure 44–2). The philosophical mission must come from the institution and the strategic planning from administration, but the practical, day-to-day implementation occurs in the clinical practice at the hands of nurses and physicians. Integration of palliative care must begin at the initial visit and continue through the ongoing evaluation and management process.

Assessment

Assessment of the patient's and family's goals and preferences begins during the initial meeting. In most outpatient settings, a baseline history, a physical examination, radiographic studies, and laboratory tests should accompany a review of preventive, general, or specialty health care needs during the first few office visits. A routine evaluation of current health needs and preventive health issues can be followed by a review of end-of-life care preferences. If such a discussion is delayed and occurs during a later or exacerbated illness, the patient and family are much more likely to fear that death is imminent or that the doctor is "holding something back." This makes it much more difficult for all involved to reach clarity concerning the patient's goals. A sample clinic conversation is shown in Table 44–1.

If the patient already has a life-threatening diagnosis, it is appropriate early on to establish a routine for assessing pain, fatigue, nausea, and other physical, psychological, and functional parameters. It is critically important to establish a standard approach to assessing the palliative care needs of the patient and family in the outpatient setting. To save time and obtain preliminary information, patients may be given a standard form to fill out before the examination. This can also help narrow down the priority issues for the visit. Increasingly, electronic forms are being used; they may be accessed through a waiting room kiosk or even over the Internet from the patient's home.

Patients and their families should be educated early about the importance of symptom assessment and reporting as well as evaluation of treatment efficacy and side effects. Establishing the patient and family as part of the team improves outcomes. As always, the patient's goals of care become the central focus for facilitating optimized palliative care. A sample dialogue is shown in Table 44–2.

Reassessment of pain and symptoms should occur with new or continuing problems and with a reasonable frequency and method. For example, if a patient with pain level of 7 on a scale of 10 is seen in the office for opioid titration, an explicit follow-up assessment plan should be established before the patient leaves the clinic. Either a clinic nurse should telephone the patient in a day or two, or alternatively, the patient or a family member should call the office nurse if the pain level does not drop below 4 within a day or two. Patient instructions should be specific, such as, "Call the clinic if you go 3 days or longer without having a bowel movement," or "Call the clinic tomorrow if the antinausea medicine is not working." These

Table 44–1
Sample Dialogue for Opening Advanced Directive Discussion

Nurse: Mrs. Jones, have you thought about what you want us to do if your heart stops?

Mrs. Jones: Oh goodness, no. I'm healthy as can be.

Nurse: Do you have a living will?

Mrs. Jones: No. I don't like to think about that sort of thing.

Nurse: It's true that most healthy people don't want to talk about dying, but we need to discuss all aspects of your health care, including end-of-life care, so that we'll be able to do the best job possible of treating you and at the same time respecting your wishes.

Table 44–2
Sample Dialogue for Goal-Oriented Pain Assessment

Nurse: Mr. Edwards, in addition to treating your disease, we also want to be successful at relieving your symptoms. What's your pain level today on the 0 to 10 scale?

Mr. Edwards: Oh, don't worry about my pain—it's only about a 6 today.

Nurse: You mentioned that your pain is 6 out of 10, but I see that you haven't been taking as much pain medicine as the doctor has ordered for you. What level of pain relief would be your goal?

Mr. Edwards: Well, it would be nice to be down around a 4, but the medicine is so darn expensive that I try not to use it unless it gets pretty bad.

Nurse: I see . . . your goal would be to get the pain down to a 4 or so if the cost factor wasn't there . . . is that right? Well, let's ask Dr. Jones if there is a less expensive drug that would work for you. We could also check to see if the drug company has a program to help out with the cost of medication.

Table 44–3
Reminder List

—Any new pain
—Pain that is constantly above a 5 on a 0–10 scale, even with your pain medicine
—Severe episodes of pain, even with your pain medicine
—Stools that are hard and difficult to pass, or if you are moving your bowels only every 2nd or 3rd day or less
—Feeling very drowsy after taking your medicine
—Having bad dreams or "seeing things"
—Nausea, vomiting, or stomachache after taking your medicine
—Muscle twitching or jerking
—Other: 1) *Call the clinic tomorrow if the nausea medicine is not working*
2) *Call the clinic tomorrow if the pain is still >4/10*

instructions may be incorporated into a standard handout for patients and then individualized as needed (Table 44–3).

Because some patients and family members are hesitant to "bother" the clinic with telephone calls, it is often desirable for the reassessment telephone call to be initiated by the clinic. These reassessment, or "check-back," calls can be done by a trained medical assistant or other nonlicensed personnel (Table 44–4). Although the use of nonlicensed personnel is controversial, it is increasingly accepted as part of the priorities for containing spiraling costs. Training in the triage of critical symptom problems is the key to optimal use of nonlicensed staff.

An organized reminder system for callbacks should be instituted. One method is to route a copy of the patient's last

Table 44–4
Sample Dialogue for "Check-Back" Calls: Examples of call-back scripts for follow-up on clinic visits

"Mrs. Edwards, this is Jesse from Dr. Jones' office. I'm calling to check back on Mr. Edwards' constipation since we increased his stool softeners. Has he had a normal bowel movement today?"

"Mr. Smith, this is Jesse from Dr. Jones' office. I'm calling to check back on your nausea. Is that antinausea medicine working for you?"

waiting room checklist (see Figure 44–1) or "Things to Report to the Clinic" sheet to a medical assistant or clerk for follow-up. As with telephone triage, the caller must be given clear criteria for what to do with the information obtained (e.g., document resolved problems, report unresolved problems to the provider). Criteria for further follow-up can be established so that unresolved symptoms identified by the office nurse or medical assistant at telephone triage lead to notification of the physician and further revision of the treatment plan. For example, any new problems should be triaged by a registered nurse or physician. Telephone triage notes can be designed for easy completion, using "check-off boxes" and "circle the symptom" documentation styles (Figure 44–3).

Patients who have a knowledge deficit about their medications or treatment regimen require one or more follow-up calls from a registered nurse or pharmacist. It is extremely helpful to provide the patient with written descriptions of medication changes or significant changes in the plan of care.

Some larger institutions have separate palliative care physicians or nurses who work alongside the primary treatment team and often are called in if a certain symptom (e.g., such as pain consistently >6/10) or a high-risk diagnosis (e.g., amyotrophic lateral sclerosis) is present. These specialty teams work most effectively alongside the primary providers when clear screening guidelines for engaging the service are in place. This is another area in which the advanced practice nurse often plays a role (i.e., early identification and referral for palliative care services).

New or escalating symptoms require timely response by the outpatient team. A reasonable time frame should be set for follow-up of new problems. Ideally, the patient should be seen within 12 hours after the onset of new symptoms—essentially the same day, if possible. This is particularly true for patients with significant symptom management issues, for whom trips to the emergency room or urgent care center would be extremely tiring and would result in the patient's being evaluated without all pertinent data available. Any patient with significant new or escalating symptoms who is seen in an emergency room should be seen again in the outpatient setting within 24 to 48 hours. If the patient receives home care or is involved with a hospice, an initial evaluation can be done at home, with telephone contact with the clinic. If home care or hospice care is not in place, an escalation of symptom management problems often is a very good indication that these resources should be initiated immediately.

Telephone Triage Tool

Patient name ______________________ **Date** __________

Pain/Symptom Assessment

Location: ______________

Intensity (now) - ___/10

Is this a new pain? Yes No

Other Pain Descriptors: (circle) continuous pain, intermittent spikes of pain, pain changes all the time, dull, sharp, radiating, aching, burning, shooting

What pain medicine is ordered? ______________________

What pain medicine is patient actually taking? ______________________

Side effects (constipation, dry mouth, drowsiness, confusion, nausea, vomit)

Treatment Plan

- ❑ Make appointment to come in: ______________________
- ❑ Increase/decrease scheduled/prn opioid dose ______________
- ❑ Change opioid ______________ ❑ Change route
- ❑ Reinforce: take meds on schedule, use prn meds, report unrelieved pain, refills
- ❑ Add tricyclic antidepressant / anticonvulsant: ______________
- ❑ Add NSAID: ______________________
- ❑ Add non-drug intervention: (circle) heat, cold, massage, distraction, relaxation, TENS
- ❑ Treat side effects: (circle) constipation, dry mouth, drowsiness, confusion, nausea
- ❑ Referrals: (circle) social work, psychiatry, physical therapy, anesthesia, radiation

Notes: ______________________

____

Next follow up (phone __________ , visit __________)

Signature ______________________ Date __________

Figure 44–3. Example of a telephone triage tool—a concise assessment and treatment progress note designed for telephone interview for triage of pain and symptoms.

Evaluation and Management

At its core, the outpatient setting is concerned with evaluation and management (E&M). The E&M codes drive reimbursement and consequently dictate documentation requirements. The "evaluate and treat" construct is deeply entrenched in the traditional medical model. However, neither the reimbursement-driven E&M process nor the traditional medical model always supports palliative care. In fact, one of the most persistent problems in palliative care is the "hospice as last resort" assumption of some providers, which causes referrals from the outpatient setting to a home care agency within the last days of life and virtually never before suspension of active treatment. This late utilization of home health resources is further complicated by the "crackdown" on Medicare fraud in home health care and has resulted in drastically reduced home care stays across the country.

Some providers also worry that hospice care will "take over" and that the patient will not have access to appropriate medical oversight. In such cases, the provider essentially "loses" a patient and family with whom he or she has developed a relationship during long-term treatment. In some cases, this concern results in an "us or them" mentality in which everyone loses. Most providers, even if a hospice physician takes over the primary responsibility for managing the patient's care, do stay involved, if only through periodic telephone follow-up.

Many clinicians reject the stark line drawn between active treatment and palliative care and successfully merge these concepts in outpatient care. Conceptually, this model was described by the World Health Organization.[12] The "old" model depicts health care system involvement starting from diagnosis with active treatment and then abruptly, shortly before death, switching to a purely palliative model. The "new" model depicts the health care system using active and palliative care concurrently, with a primarily active treatment focus at diagnosis, integration along the trajectory, and a primarily palliative focus at death (see Fig. 44–2).

Take, as an example, an elderly gentleman with metastatic prostate cancer who has begun hospice care and has developed pain, rated as 9 on a scale of 0 to 10, that begins in his back and

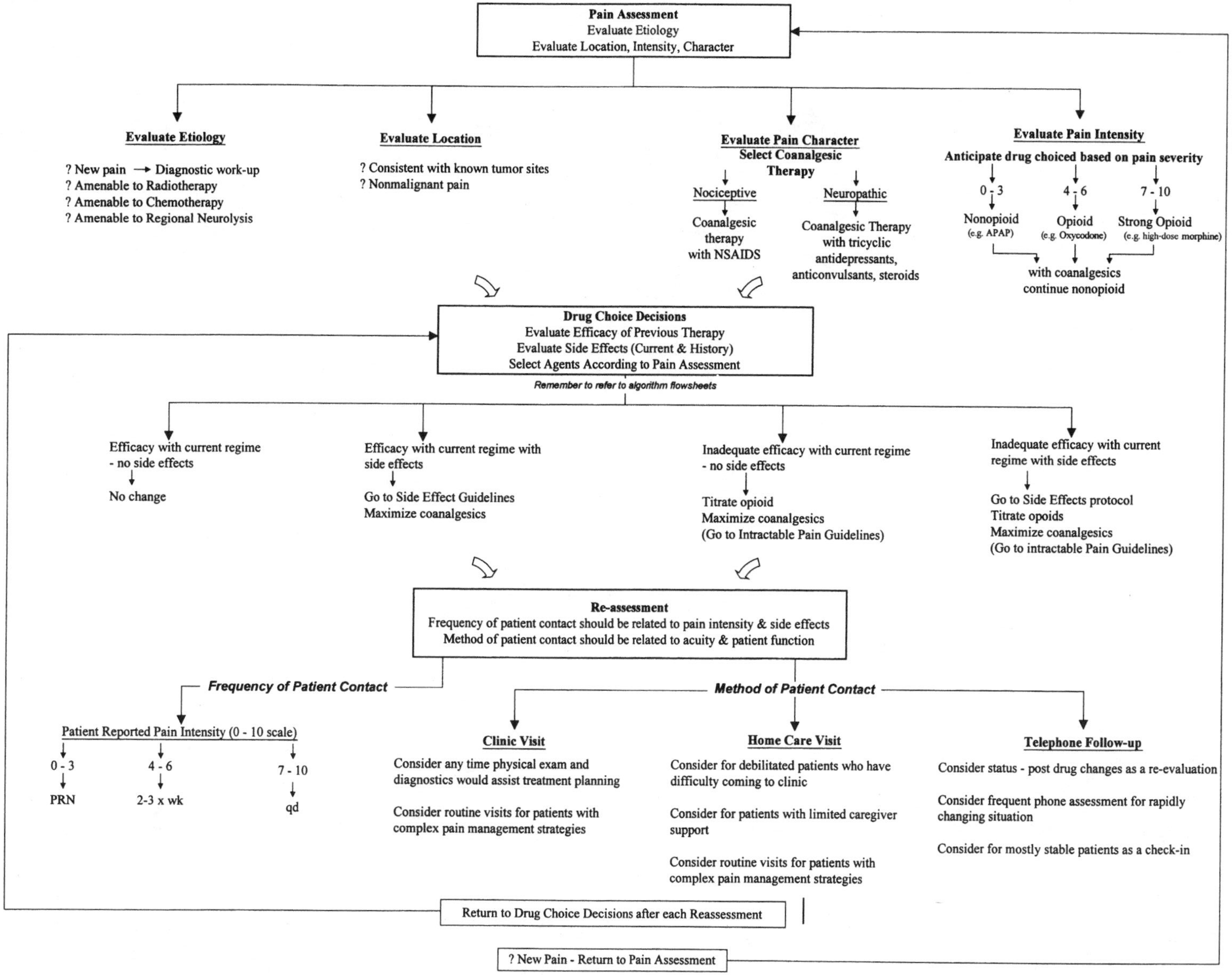

Figure 44–4. The Du Pen Cancer Pain Algorithm—an algorithm designed to aid decision-making in outpatient management of cancer pain. Use of this algorithm in clinical trials produced a significant ($P < 0.02$) reduction from usual pain levels. (*Source:* Adapted from Du Pen S, Du Pen A. Cancer Pain Algorithm Reference Guide. Seattle: Du Pen, Inc., 1998:6–10. © 1998 Swedish Medical Center.)

shoots down his legs. His opioid therapy has been increased aggressively over the past week, and he is now somnolent between periods of extreme pain. His wife also notices he needs more help getting out of bed because his legs "won't hold him up." The patient and his wife explain that their goals are to keep his pain under control and to keep him as functional as possible. This patient may benefit dramatically from steroids and radiation to reduce pain and save the functions of his lower extremities, bowel, and bladder, even though he is receiving hospice care. In such situations, a very clear understanding of the patient's and family's goals of care, well defined and known to both outpatient providers and home care or hospice care providers, facilitates the best possible outcomes.

Treatment algorithms or protocols can promote efficiency in the clinic and enhance outcomes. These tools can be successfully put into place and implemented by both clinic nurses and home care or hospice care nurses. One such algorithm was used in outpatient oncology and resulted in improved pain management.[13] The Cancer Pain Algorithm is a decision tree model for pain treatment that was developed as a practical interpretation of the Agency for Health Care Policy and Research Guidelines for Cancer Pain Management. The algorithm consists of a bulleted set of analgesic "guiding principles" for use with opioids, NSAIDs, tricyclic antidepressants, anticonvulsants and addresses drug side effects. For example, the statement "Titrate to efficacy or side effects" is an underlying principle throughout the algorithm. Drug choice decisions depend on pain assessment data. The flow chart directs the oncology nurse or oncologist to side effect protocols, equianalgesic conversion charts, and a primer for intractable pain.

Figure 44–4 represents the high level algorithm decision-making flow chart. Etiology and location correlate the pain with its known tumor or treatment-related source or indicate the need for further diagnostic work-up. Pain intensity is based on self-report on a scale from 0 to 10, where 0 is no pain and 10 is the worst pain imaginable. Pain character is divided into nociceptive versus neuropathic components; the character of the pain is the primary variable to direct the choice of nonopioid or coanalgesic therapies. The frequency and method of reassessment are outlined for the practitioner based on the results of the last pain assessment contact. An algorithm reference tool contains drug-specific content (e.g., titration parameters, side effect protocols) and a number of highly specific flow charts. The algorithm process is intended as a team effort, relying on the network of physician, clinic nurse, home care nurse, and family caregiver as a cohesive outpatient unit, all applying the principles of the algorithm as they relate to the individual patient.

Another concept now being used in outpatient care is that of the primary nurse "navigator." The navigator takes the concept of case manager a step further, in the sense of acting as a "learned guide" rather than a plan "manager." The navigator is responsible for tracking the course of the patient's care through the myriad of services. A treatment plan becomes a "road atlas," and the nurse navigator steers the patient's care to the key stops along the highway. These stops may be follow-up diagnostic studies, interdisciplinary consultations, hospice referrals, or a variety of other patient-specific services. This model works well for outpatient services that, in general, are disconnected one from another and that might be overlooked under strained resources. The navigator works from critical pathways, or algorithms, and provides feedback to the physician weekly.

Critical Building Blocks for Outpatient Palliative Care

A number of critical elements provide an excellent framework for integrating basic palliative care concepts into almost any outpatient setting. Improving provider accessibility to patients and caregivers, promoting active listening by all staff, providing a sense of control, and continuously assessing psychological and spiritual distress of patients and their families are the building blocks to successful outpatient palliative care.[14–16]

Accessibility

In the outpatient setting, accessibility is critical to the palliative care of patients. Having 24-hour support available to patients and their caregivers helps reduce anxiety and, when necessary, facilitates identification of after-hours problems that need immediate attention, such as escalating pain or shortness of breath.[17] Accessibility is not, of course, only an after-hours issue. A well-organized telephone triage system is necessary to provide access during regular clinic hours.[18] The clerk or other nonlicensed personnel who answer the telephone should receive very clear instructions on how to distinguish problems that need immediate attention. For example, billing questions and insurance issues receive callbacks, whereas pain, shortness of breath, and changes in level of consciousness require a nurse or physician to take the call. These criteria should be agreed upon by all and followed consistently. Calls that require high-level triage should be handled by trained nurses armed with protocols and standing orders that have been approved by the patient's physician. The triage system should include procedures for bringing patients into the clinic for same-day evaluation or for admission to the hospital.[19] Such a system has three main benefits: (1) the patient sees the nurse as a qualified member of the team who is available and ready to assist; (2) the patient and family caregivers become more confident in making adjustments to medications for pain or symptom management, and (3) telephoning allows the nurse to reassess, reassure, and reinforce the teaching that has taken place (see Figure 44–3).

Advanced practice nurses clearly improve accessibility for patients undergoing palliative care management.[8] Many nurse practitioners share on-call responsibilities with physicians, thereby alleviating some of the workload that 24-hour accessibility requires. Flexible scheduling of advanced practice nurses can allow for "same-day work-ins," nursing home visits, or home visits, as circumstances require.

Active Listening

Active listening is a key element to effective communication among patients, the outpatient care team, and the patients' families.[20] This component of palliative care helps to support patients and families who feel physically and emotionally isolated or overwhelmed by a terminal illness. Active listening also leads to more efficient use of time and a stronger relationship with the client,[16] which are important factors in the outpatient setting, both during face-to-face interactions and over the telephone. The astute listener simultaneously watches for nonverbal clues, shows empathy, and assesses the patient's and family's knowledge base. In the outpatient setting, staff become more familiar with the patient and family over months and perhaps years, which makes the process of listening actively and with empathy easier. This ability and opportunity to make assessments over a long period is unique to the outpatient setting.

Oncology nurses are sometimes comfortable opening a dialogue with patients about pain, fatigue, weight loss, and appetite but less comfortable handling conversations about death and dying or loss.[21] If a formerly hopeful patient with a "fighter" attitude responds with "I don't think I can do this anymore," the active listener understands that a transition is occurring. Time must be set aside for this patient, either immediately or with a plan for a follow-up telephone call or family conference. Time spent proactively facilitating these transitions almost always saves crisis-induced time spent later in the patient's course.

Another critical component of active listening involves identifying barriers to effective palliative care. The classic example of a barrier to care is the fear of opioid addiction. A clinic nurse often first identifies the patient's or family member's concern about taking opioids. It is important to discuss this attitudinal barrier early and frequently. Another barrier to pain management at the end of life is the belief that using pain medications hastens death. Because of this belief, family members may resist optimizing opioids and adjuvants at the end of life. In addition to verbal instructions at the time of the clinic visits, written materials on the rationale and role of symptom management in end-of-life care can be extremely helpful.

Another issue that is frequently present and often requires active facilitation by clinic staff is the social context of care. The cost of care is an increasing concern and is an area that patients and families are frequently uncomfortable discussing. This often results in conflicts that are identified only late in the course of care. Distressing issues may arise concerning long-term care and, particularly, the distribution of financial support and caregiving responsibilities among family members. Whenever possible, prompt initiation of family conferences or referrals to social workers are advisable.

Providing a Sense of Control

Helping chronically and terminally ill patients regain a sense of control is a key element in managing the helplessness many patients experience. Within the acute and long-term care settings, "power symbols" exist that shift the locus of control away from the patient.[22] These symbols include the sea of white coats, high-tech equipment, hospital beds that place patients below their professional caregivers, and a general lack of privacy. Interventions that can promote a sense of control in the outpatient setting include allowing patients to remain dressed during most office calls, at least until an examination is required; reducing the clinical, white-coat formality; and providing a safe, nonthreatening, private place for meetings with patients and their families. These accommodations return a sense of control and dignity to the patient with a terminal illness and promote health and well-being.[14] Another critical component of providing a sense of control is having an active patient education component. Giving patients and families the knowledge tools that they need to make decisions is a great empowerment. Practical information regarding how to "negotiate the system," how to get help after hours, and how to communicate with health care professionals in a way that gets them the information they need are all important components of patient education.

Tuning In to Distress

Psychological and spiritual health are often profoundly affected by life-threatening illness. In fact, patients with chronic and terminal illnesses display a high incidence of frank psychiatric morbidity, documented in several studies to range from 40% to 53%.[23,24] Common psychiatric diagnoses among the terminally ill include delirium, amnesia, major depression, and anxiety.[24] However, many patients with significant symptoms of anxiety, depression, and anger do not qualify as having a major psychiatric illness. These symptoms have been described throughout the palliative care literature as distress.[15,24] Identifying distress early in the palliative care continuum allows for early intervention, prevention of comorbid psychological problems, and improved quality of life.

Easy-to-use, inexpensive, brief, noninvasive, and generally well accepted self-reporting questionnaires can be used in the outpatient setting.[25,26] Two good examples are the Hospital Anxiety and Depression Scale (HAD)[28] and the Distress Thermometer.[26,27] The HAD consists of 14 questions to which the client answers yes or no. This tool omits somatic complaints and focuses on questions that can help differentiate anxiety and depression. Despite its title, it has also been successfully used in the outpatient setting.[25]

The Distress Thermometer has been tested in men with prostate cancer.[26,27] It consists of a visual analogue scale made to look like a thermometer, with the bottom of the thermometer reading 1, or no distress; 5 being moderate distress, and 10 (at the top of the thermometer) being extreme distress. Distress is defined in a generic sense of unpleasant stress. This is a simple scale that can be used at the beginning of each office visit or on a regular basis (e.g., quarterly). Responses can be used to open discussions of the symptoms of distress being experienced by a client in the outpatient setting. For example, the clinician may say, "I see that you're feeling a moderate amount of distress. Can we talk about what you're feeling?"

Spiritual distress can be equally devastating to the patient and family. Hearing "What did I do to deserve this?" or "How could God let this happen to my husband?" from a patient or family member is a cue that spiritual support is needed. Some health care systems have chaplains available in the outpatient setting. Many churches and synagogues provide outreach ministries to the gravely ill. Other nontraditional means of spiritual support include meditation and rituals to explore the meaning of events. Whenever possible, the clinic should be given a list of community resources for spiritual support.

The Three C's of Outpatient Palliative Care: Cooperation, Communication, and Closure

At the heart of palliative care in the outpatient setting are the three concepts of cooperation, communication, and closure. The concepts of cooperation and communication are woven throughout this chapter. The outpatient setting is the site of cooperation among patient, family, and outpatient staff. This cooperation expands to the agencies within the community that are caring for the patient. This may include home health care nurses, long-term care staff, local pharmacists, neighbors and friends of the client, and the local church. The physician and advanced practice nurses cooperate to provide easy access to care. The specialist and primary care physician, who both often monitor the patient in the outpatient setting, cooperate. Care in the outpatient setting is not provided in isolation, but by a well coordinated and dedicated community team.

At the heart of this cooperation is good communication. Communication begins with active listening, fostered in the outpatient setting. Efficient and accurate documentation of patient teaching, telephone calls, and interventions is the key to continuity of care. A variety of tools have been developed for use in the outpatient setting to improve this communication.

Not yet addressed, but also important in the outpatient setting, is closure. Bereavement is an issue for nurses, physicians, and staff in the outpatient setting.[29] As patients become sicker and eventually homebound, the outpatient staff is no longer able to see the patients, despite being in close contact with family and home care staff over the telephone. In many cases, this early separation from the patient complicates the ability of the outpatient staff to come to closure with what often has been a long-term relationship with the patient. This abrupt loss of connection can be a significant source of bereavement for staff.

Outpatient nurses may have had years to assess the family or caregivers' previous experiences with death, the support available, and the coping resources of those who have suffered the loss. This familiarity with the family or caregiver helps the nurse in the outpatient setting provide better support to grieving loved ones.

Often, family members or caregivers are drawn back to the outpatient setting to say final good-byes or give gifts of thanks to staff members who may have become as close as family to the patient and caregivers. Staff should be prepared for this visit by being informed of the patient's death. Work should stop for a moment to embrace the returning family members and give them time to tell the story of the death and share feelings of grief and joyful memories of the deceased. Gifts or pictures brought by the family should be accepted graciously. Many offices take time out each month to send cards to families of patients who have died.

Staff of the outpatient clinic, the front desk receptionist, the medical assistant, the nurse, and the physician may experience grief after the loss of a patient. Often, staff require support through the deaths of patients dear to them. It is important to allow for special opportunities to celebrate the lives and mourn the deaths of these patients. Attending funerals, keeping scrapbooks, and having occasional symbolic tributes to patients can help staff through the grieving process. Occasionally, it may be helpful to provide professional counseling or to send staff members on a retreat, where feelings regarding death and loss can be shared. Caregivers, as well as family and friends, need closure when death comes. In the outpatient setting this affords all who have experienced the loss support on the journey toward healing.

Summary

The outpatient setting has both advantages and disadvantages. As more and more patients with end-stage disease choose to remain in their homes, the outpatient clinic has become the main point of contact for care and coordination of resources. The outpatient clinic staff act as gatekeepers, maintaining checks and balances on the home health care system or the long-term care facility. Relationships are developed over many years, creating a sense of trust that fosters the holistic care that is at the heart of palliative medicine.

Strategies for providing palliative care in this setting apply to all diseases. The concepts of active listening, promoting patient control, assessing for distress, and promoting access to care all improve the delivery of palliative care in the outpatient clinic. The use of nurse-staffed telephone triage systems, nurse practitioners, and tools for assessing palliative care needs benefits both the terminally ill patient and the patient with advanced chronic disease. Care algorithms and critical pathways assist staff in implementing research-based interventions to prevent suffering and promote quality of life. Finally, the three C's of outpatient palliative care emphasize the necessity of coordination, communication, and closure.

There is perhaps a fourth quality needed when caring for chronically or terminally ill clients in the outpatient setting—commitment. Through a commitment to alleviate suffering and promote quality of life, caregivers in the outpatient setting assist patients in finding physical, psychological, and spiritual wellness, even at the end of the disease trajectory.

REFERENCES

1. Fitch MI, Mings D. Cancer Nursing in Ontario: Defining nursing roles. Can Oncol Nurs J 2003;13:28–44.
2. Aranda S. Silent voices, hidden practices: Exploring undiscovered aspects of cancer nursing. Int J Palliat Nurs 2001;7:178–185.
3. Cox K, Wilson E. Follow-up for people with cancer: Nurse-led services and telephone interventions. J Adv Nurs 2003;43:51–61.
4. Skalla KA, Bakitas M, Furstenberg CT, Ahles T, Henderson JV. Patients' need for information about cancer therapy. Oncol Nurs Forum 2004;31:313–319.
5. The role of unlicensed assistive personnel in cancer care. Oncology Nursing Society. Oncol Nurs Forum 2001;28:17.
6. O'Leary J, Williamson J. Meeting the challenges in today's outpatient oncology setting: A case study. J Oncol Manage 2003;12:24–26.
7. Bush NJ, Watters T. The emerging role of the oncology nurse practitioner: A collaborative model within the private practice setting. Oncol Nurs Forum 2001;28:1425–1431.
8. Jones A, Ironside V, Jameson G, Leslie M, Sullivan C. A job description for the oncology NP. Nurse Pract 2002;27:61.
9. Sivesind D, Parker PA, Cohen L, Demoor C, Bumbaugh M, Throckmorton T, Volker DL, Baile WF. Communicating with patients in cancer care: What areas do nurses find most challenging? J Cancer Educ 2003;18:202–209.
10. Lynch MP, Cope DG, Murphy-Ende K. Advanced practice issues: Results of the ONS Advanced Practice Nursing survey. Oncol Nurs Forum 2001;28:1521–1530.
11. Hamric AB, Worley D, Lindebak S, Jaubert S. Outcomes associated with advanced nursing practice prescriptive authority. J Am Acad Nurse Pract 1998;10:113–118.
12. World Health Organization. Cancer Pain Relief and Palliative Care, 2nd ed. Geneva: World Health Organization, 1995.
13. Du Pen SL, Du Pen AR, Polissar N, Hansberry J, Miller-Kraybill B, Stillman M, Panke J, Everly R, Syrjala K. Implementing guidelines for cancer pain management: Results of a randomized controlled clinical trial. J Clin Oncol 1999;17:361–370.
14. Fryback PB, Reinert BR. Facilitating health in people with terminal diagnoses by encouraging a sense of control. Med Surg Nurs 1993;2:197–201.
15. Jacobsen PB, Brietbach W. Psychosocial aspects of palliative care. Cancer Control 1996;3:214–222.
16. Straka DA. Are you listening? Have you heard? Adv Pract Nurs Q 1997;3:80–81.
17. Brown C. Health care system changes and nursing. ABNF J 1994;5:41–42.
18. Preston FA. Telephone triage. Clin J Oncol Nurs. 2000;4:294–296.
19. Stacey D, Fawcett L. Telephone triage: An important role for oncology nurses. Can Oncol Nurs J 1997;7:178–179.
20. Srnka QM, Ryan MR. Active listening: A key to effective communication. Am Pharm 1993;NS33(9):43–46.
21. Sivesind D, Parker PA, Cohen L, Demoor C, Bumbaugh M, Throckmorton T, Volker DL, Baile WF. Communicating with patients in cancer care: What areas do nurses find most challenging? J Cancer Educ 2003;18:202–209.
22. Ebersol P, Hess P. Crisis and stress management. In: Ebersol P, Hess P, eds. Toward Healthy Aging, 5th ed. St. Louis: Mosby, 1998, pp 676–701.
23. Derogatis LR, Morrow GR, Fetting J, Penman D, Piassetsky S, Schmale AM, Henrichs M, Carnicke CL Jr. The prevelance of psychiatric disorders among cancer patients. JAMA 1983;249: 751–757.
24. Minagawa H, Uchitomi Y, Vamawaki S, Ishitahi K. Psychiatric morbidity in terminally ill cancer patients: A prospective study. Cancer 1996;78:1131–1137.
25. Moorey S, Greer S, Watson M, Gorman C, Rowden L, Tunmore R, Robertson B, Bliss J. The factor structure and factor stability of the Hospital Anxiety and Depression Scale in patients with cancer. Br J Psychiatry 1991;158:255–259.
26. Roth AJ, Kornblith AB, Batel-Copel L, Peabody E, Scher HI, Holland JC. Rapid screening for psychologic distress in men with prostate carcinoma: A pilot study. Cancer 1998;82:1904–1908.
27. NCCN practice guidelines for the management of psychosocial distress. National Comprehensive Cancer Network. Oncology (Hunting) 1999;13(5A):113–147.
28. Zigmond AS, Snaith RP. The hospital anxiety and depression scale. Acta Psychiatr Scand 1983;67:361–370.
29. Valentino RL. Recognizing and responding to grief: Concepts to guide daily practice. Adv Nurse Pract 2001;9:52–55.

45 Rehabilitation and Palliative Care

Kathleen Michael

I may have cancer, but I have a lot of livin' to do before I go. I have kids to take care of, a house, a job. I have faith that these drugs will help and even if I don't live forever, I still have some livin' to do now and a lot of things to take care of. So I want everything they got to make me strong.
—A patient

- ***Key Points***
- *Rehabilitation principles are applicable to palliative care to enhance quality of life.*
- *Interdisciplinary care is a key concept in rehabilitation.*
- *Rehabilitation in palliative care can prevent disability and complications.*

Even when it is not reasonable to expect cure or reversal of disease processes, or to restore a previous level of functioning and independence, a rehabilitative approach to nursing care adds quality to the experience of life's completion. Grounded in respect for each unique patient, rehabilitation nurses address palliative and end-of life care with concern for preserving hope, human dignity, and autonomy. They involve social, spiritual, and functional support systems. Rehabilitation nursing interventions are designed to help patients and families make the most out of each day in the context of the disease trajectory. The language of rehabilitation nursing is a language shared with those who practice palliative care.

Rehabilitation nurses work with the concepts of independence and interdependence, self-care, coping, access, and quality of life, skillfully weaving them into the assessment, planning, implementation, and evaluation of nursing care.[1,2] Although the focus is on function, fundamental to this practice is the acceptance of varieties of life experiences, including those at life's end.

This chapter applies concepts of rehabilitation to palliative care across settings. Case studies are presented to demonstrate the application of palliative care to patients, even those with life-threatening illnesses. Finally, numerous strategies are discussed for use of rehabilitation techniques to prevent disability and complications in advanced disease.

Rehabilitation Nursing

Rehabilitation nursing in any context concerns itself with adaptation. As life proceeds to its end, adaptation to a new state allows beings to remain whole: to interact with their environments, to experience human relationships, and to achieve personally meaningful goals. Rehabilitation nurses find themselves at work in every phase of growth, development, and dying, as individuals strive to adapt across the continuum of life.

Rehabilitation nurses care for persons with incurable progressive disease states in a variety of settings. Whether care is patient-, provider-, or facility-centered, the merging of rehabilitation and palliative nursing principles is evident.

Acute comprehensive inpatient rehabilitation units are set up in such a way that complex medical-surgical issues may be managed concurrently with the functional processes of comprehensive rehabilitation.[3] For example, patients with metastatic cancer affecting their bones may have significant care needs related to mobility and activities of daily living, well addressed in an inpatient rehabilitation setting.

For many patients with terminal illness, the transition to an acute rehabilitation unit represents a crucial point in their healthcare experience. It is a time when the future comes into focus, and goals are defined based on the likely disease progression. Sometimes a short stay on an inpatient rehabilitation unit makes it possible for patients to return to a home setting, because of the gains in independent function that may be realized. Patients and family members may begin to face limited prognoses, decline in abilities, and changes in roles. Through an interdisciplinary therapeutic process, care needs are clarified, and skills and adaptation strategies are taught to patients and those who will care for them outside of the hospital.

Subacute rehabilitation facilities provide additional therapy activities, such as physical, occupational, or speech therapy, based on patient need, endurance, and tolerance. The pacing and amount of therapy are gauged according to individualized goals. As in comprehensive inpatient rehabilitation units, the aim is to facilitate improved physical function and as much independence as possible, even as the disease process moves the patient toward death. For example, patients with advanced disease who are too frail to participate in a full acute rehabilitation program may benefit from the slower-paced rehabilitation of a subacute setting.

Long-term care settings, such as skilled nursing facilities, are often places where lives are completed. Specialized *geriatric facilities* focus on the care needs of aging persons, often requiring specialized rehabilitation interventions. In both of these settings, rehabilitation nurses may plan and direct care delivery and make sure that patient and family concerns are kept in the forefront. Attention is paid to optimizing function and self-care, as well as addressing physical care issues.

Hospice settings may also provide a venue for a rehabilitative approach to end-of-life care. Careful planning of care to take into account limitations, yet promote function and autonomy, is a key factor in smoothing the transition to an inevitable death. Rehabilitative techniques and strategies make it easier for caregivers to manage increasing deficits, thereby protecting patient comfort and dignity through the dying process.

Pediatric rehabilitation is focused on guiding the development of children to minimize disability and handicap that may result from physical or cognitive impairment. There are situations in pediatric rehabilitation in which palliative care comes into play, and efforts are directed toward enhancing the normal function of both patient and family through the course of disease. For example, the family members of a child with progressive neuromuscular disease may learn how to use adaptive devices to position the child in a wheelchair for comfort and social interaction as well as for physiological function.

In the *insurance industry* and *managed care systems*, rehabilitation nurses have the opportunity to advocate for the needs of persons with disease or disability and to reduce barriers to their access to care and resources. Near the end of a terminal disease course, planning and resource management are essential to ensure optimal care without undue economic and emotional burdens to families. *Case management* is an expanding practice area for rehabilitation nurses, usually with multidisciplinary relationships. Because palliative care needs are unique to individuals and require coordination of the care across disciplines, usual or episodic patterns of delivery and resource use may prove inadequate. The implementation of care pathways in palliative care requires careful and compassionate guidance and evaluation, tailored to meet individual strengths, abilities, needs and preferences.[3,4]

Finally, care of dying patients occurs frequently at *home*. Successful end-of-life care at home is the preference of many patients and families. Such care depends on skill, concern, keen assessment, and creative problem-solving. For the reasons shown in each setting, rehabilitation nursing is well suited to this charge.

Rehabilitation Nursing and Palliative Care

Rehabilitation nursing adds value in the arena of palliative care. As future health care services center on needs, preferences, and informed consent of patients and families in our society, there is less emphasis on cure, illness, paternalism, and prescription. More attention is directed to self-care and client participation, holistic wellness, primary care and prevention, and the quality attributes of care as defined by the consumer.[1]

Patient/family-centered care is clearly appropriate for the unique experience of dying. Enabling a kind of wellness to exist even at the point of death, such as the experience of a "good death," fits with the rehabilitation philosophy. Many rehabilitation nursing actions center on supporting physiological function and preventing complications, goals that are still appropriate at the end of life. Finally, rehabilitation has long been concerned with understanding and measuring quality of life, whether related to physical, psychosocial, or spiritual domains.

The real value of a rehabilitative approach to the nursing care of persons with declining health states lies in the foundations of rehabilitation nursing practice. As defined by the Association of Rehabilitation Nurses in 2004,[4a] rehabilitation nurses

- Attend to the full range of human experiences and responses to health and illness
- Deal with families coping with lifelong issues
- Provide a holistic approach to care
- Facilitate team dynamics and integration
- Educate patients and their families to help them control and manage a wide range of challenges associated with chronic illness or disability
- Form partnerships with patients and other health care providers to attain the best possible outcomes

The hallmark of rehabilitation is interdisciplinary collaboration. The synergy of collaboration enhances the value of rehabilitation nursing interventions and ensures that patient needs are addressed from a variety of perspectives. Typically, the rehabilitation team consists of physicians with specialized training in Physical Medicine and Rehabilitation; rehabilitation nurses; physical, occupational, speech, respiratory, and recreation therapists; exercise physiologists; dietitians; social workers; and others as required to address particular needs (Table 45–1). Effective teamwork requires mutual understanding and synchrony of the roles and responsibilities of each member. When the rehabilitation team works in synergy, it serves patients and families across the continuum of life.

Table 45–1
Role of Interdisciplinary Rehabilitation Team Members

Physiatrists: Direct the rehabilitation team in providing comprehensive, integrated, patient-centered care
Rehabilitation nurses: Address physical care needs, such as mobility, daily living skills, bowel and bladder care, skin care, medications, and pain management, and coordinate the overall rehabilitation process
Physical therapists: Address strength, endurance, mobility, activity level, equipment needs, range of motion, balance and stability, and education about ongoing exercise programs to facilitate independent function
Occupational therapists: Address energy conservation needs, upper-extremity strength and function, self-care and home management skills, need for assistive devices, perceptual evaluation and guidance, and education for adaptation needs
Speech/language pathologists: Address expressive and receptive communication needs as well as eating and swallowing issues
Social workers: Address home care and extended care needs; provide patient and family with counseling and resources.
Rehabilitation psychologists: Address complex emotional and psychological needs of patients and families, guide the team in psychosocial care, and provide comprehensive psychological testing
Vocational counselors: Address concerns and options related to school or work
Recreation therapists: Address adaptation of leisure skills, recreational activities, socialization, stress management, establishment of therapeutic environment, and enhancement of normalization

Conceptual Framework

It is a common view that rehabilitation has a place somewhere between curative and palliative care.[5] Rehabilitation seems not really to fit with curative processes, where care issues resolve with specific treatments and patients' levels of function and independence ultimately return to normal. Nor does rehabilitation seem in keeping with the irrevocable progress toward death, because rehabilitation implies a return to a previous way of living through adaptation. However, rehabilitation has concerns at each point of the continuum from wellness to death. In wellness, the concern is to prevent health problems and reduce factors that might lead to illness and disability. At the end of life, the concern is to promote autonomy and dignity by enhancing function and independence as much as possible.

To conceptualize how rehabilitation nursing fits with care at the end of life, it is helpful to consider a diagrammatic representation (Figure 45–1). In this diagram, curative and palliative care are pictured as two discrete spheres. Rehabilitation overlaps both substantially. In each sphere there is a place for rehabilitation. At the junction between curative and palliative care, rehabilitation may find its greatest impact.

Rehabilitation Principles Applied to Palliative Care

The rehabilitation of patients with palliative care needs should begin as early as possible. As soon as functional deficits are observed or anticipated, appropriate consultation with members of the rehabilitation team should be initiated. Certain diagnoses, such as progressive neuromuscular diseases; malignancies affecting the brain, spinal cord, or skeletal system;

Figure 45–1. A conceptual framework for curative, palliative, and rehabilitative care.

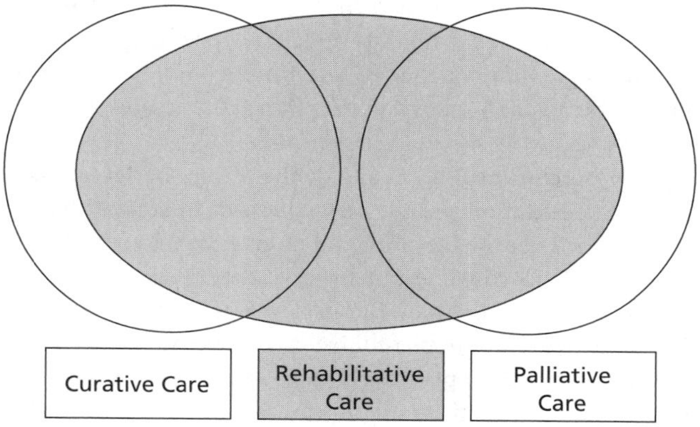

organ failure; and many other conditions that result in functional impairments, should trigger mobilization of the rehabilitation team.

The goals of rehabilitation are to prevent secondary disability, to enhance the functions of both affected and unaffected systems, and to help patients adapt to their physical and social environments by means of physical restoration and adaptive devices.[6]

Rehabilitation nursing strategies focus on

- Caring for whole persons in their social and physical environments
- Preventing secondary disability
- Enhancing function of both affected and unaffected systems
- Facilitating use of adaptive strategies
- Promoting quality of life

To illustrate the rehabilitation strategies as they may be applied in actual palliative nursing care situations, some case studies are offered. The stories serve to illuminate the role of rehabilitation nursing in palliative care and represent issues in common with many rehabilitation patients.

Caring for Whole Persons in Their Social and Physical Environments

Appreciating each person as a unique individual is extremely important to the rehabilitation process. Whereas it may be evident to rehabilitation professionals that certain goals and interventions would suit the patient's needs, even more important is finding congruence with the patient's own perceived and stated goals and values.

CASE STUDY

Edna W, a 60-Year-Old Woman with a Lung Transplant

With a history of rapidly worsening chronic obstructive pulmonary disease, 60-year-old Edna W was faced with few options. As every breath became a struggle, she wondered how she could go on with her life and whether it was worth continuing the fight. She had already lost so much of what was important to her: mobility, independence, and social relationships. Now she found herself homebound, exhausted, and unable to carry on even a telephone conversation with friends and family she so cherished.

After much consultation and deliberation, she agreed that lung transplantation was the only course of treatment that would afford her the function and independence she believed made her life worthwhile. She received the transplanted lungs after a relatively short wait. But her expectations of returning to wellness were not to be fulfilled. Ms. W began an extraordinarily complicated postoperative course and a journey that would lead her to a life's end on which she had not planned.

Initially, Ms. W required prolonged ventilatory support. She struggled with infection and rejection of her new lungs. She experienced shock, sepsis, distress; her records thickened with stories of heroics and near misses, of technology, of miracles, of persistent argument with fate. She had established with her family that she would want everything possible done to preserve her life, and thus the critical balancing act went on for months. Just as her condition seemed to be stabilizing, she had a massive stroke, resulting in dense hemiplegia and loss of speech/language function.

She was admitted to the inpatient rehabilitation medicine service to focus on mobility, self-care, and speech functions in order to help her to return home with her family. She progressed very slowly, with numerous complications related to her pulmonary status, immunosuppression, and cardiovascular deterioration.

A second stroke left her with even more-limited language and cognitive function. She required maximum assistance for all activities of daily living, and she ceased to make progress toward her rehabilitation goals. Her pulmonary function declined. Her family recognized that they would not be able to meet her care needs at home. Further evaluation of her lungs revealed that she had developed a lymphoma, for which, in her case, no treatment could be offered. Her prognosis plummeted, with the likelihood of death in a matter of weeks.

The focus of her rehabilitation care shifted. No longer would it be reasonable to expect her to reach the level of independence she would need to return home. A rigorous exercise program was not going to change the trajectory of her disease and in fact might sap her energies and contribute to more frustration and discomfort.

By talking with family and friends, the rehabilitation team learned that Ms. W was strong-willed, stubborn, difficult, but deeply loved. She was seen as the matriarch of the family. For most of her adult life, she had balanced her responsibilities as a single parent with her work as a postal clerk. She was characterized as determined and cantankerous, impatient, critical, and quick to frustrate. Her family was close and extremely important to her. She had a wide circle of friends. Her four sons took turns visiting her in the hospital and sincerely wanted to get her back home again.

With these facts in mind, the rehabilitation team designed communications and interventions that took into account the personal traits and values that were particular to Ms. W. They knew that she would have difficulty tolerating frustration. They knew that she would need to feel in control as much as possible. They also knew that involvement of her family and friends would be essential. They anticipated the effects of prolonged stress on the family unit and recognized the profound loss the family would sustain as her life concluded.

Rehabilitation nursing actions focused first on communication. Because of her dense aphasia, she was unable to verbalize her thoughts or feelings. Instead, she perseverated on one word, growing increasingly agitated when people were unable to understand her. A speech therapist was involved in setting up nonverbal methods of communication, such as picture boards. As the nursing staff worked with Ms. W, they tuned into behavioral cues and expressions. Family members also helped in the interpretation of her attempts to communicate. Strategies for communication included

- Direct eye contact
- Relaxed, unhurried approach
- Slow, distinct phrases in normal tone of voice
- One thought presented at a time
- Time allowed to process information
- Gestures to convey and clarify meaning

Efforts were directed toward maintaining her comfort and dignity. Whenever possible, she was supported in making her own choices. Occupational and physical therapies concentrated on interventions that would promote her autonomy. Functional activities, such as dressing, grooming, and eating, allowed her opportunities to exercise her independence. Access to her physical environment was accomplished through the use of adaptive devices and wheelchair mobility skills. As her condition deteriorated, it was more difficult to ascertain her desires. Inclusion of family members became more important, both for carrying out her wishes as they knew them and for giving the family the active role in her care that they wanted.

Throughout the course of Ms. W's final illness, spiritual and psychosocial support were priorities. With her ability to communicate so severely impaired, her needs for support might have been misunderstood or overlooked. She was suddenly unable to serve as the source of stability and strength for her family, and roles and expectations were greatly changed. The rehabilitation nurses, the psychologist, the social worker, and the chaplain worked together to counsel and care for both patient and family.

When death came, the family described a mixture of feelings of relief, sorrow, and satisfaction. Through their sadness, they recognized the efforts of the rehabilitation team to preserve Ms. W's uniqueness and integrity as a human being. Thus, they would remember her.

Preventing Secondary Disability

Whatever the disease process, persons in declining states of health are at risk for development of unnecessary complications. Even at the end of life, complications can be prevented, thereby enhancing a person's comfort, function, independence, and dignity. Treatment of one body system must not compromise another. For example, patients who are bed bound are at risk for development of muscular, vascular, integumentary, and neurological compromise, which could result in secondary disability.

CASE STUDY

JB, a Man with Amyotrophic Lateral Sclerosis

JB knew his days were numbered, irrevocably ticking away with the advance of his amyotrophic lateral sclerosis. Bit by bit, his body functions eroded. Weakness began in his lower extremities, then spread to his trunk and upper extremities. He was troubled with spasticity, which soon made ambulation almost impossible. He depended on his wife to help him with all of his daily living activities but continued to get out each day in his electric wheelchair, to work with the city government on disability policies. When he went on the ventilator to support his breathing, he likened his health to driving an old truck down a mountain road: no way to stop, no way to turn around, nothing to do but drive on home.

As JB's disease progressed, he was at risk for the development of secondary disabilities. Concerns included the potential development of edema, contractures, and skin breakdown. JB lacked the normal muscular activity that would promote vascular return, and he developed significant edema in his extremities. Knowing that "edema is glue" when it comes to function, rehabilitation nursing actions included range-of-motion exercises and management of dependent edema with compression and elevation.[1]

Spasticity complicated positioning of JB's limbs. It was important to avoid shortened positions that favored the flexors, because that would allow contractures to occur. Contractures would further limit his mobility and function, so he and his wife were taught a stretching program as well as the use of positioning devices and splints to maintain joints in neutral alignment.

Because of his impaired mobility, JB was at risk for skin breakdown. He enjoyed spending a lot of time in his wheelchair. Although his sensation was basically intact, he was not able to react to the message of skin pressure and change his position. JB learned how to shift his weight in the wheel-chair, by either side-to side shifts or tilt-backs. A small timer helped remind him of pressure releases every 15 minutes when up in his chair. In addition, a special wheelchair cushion protected bony prominences with gel pads.

Enhancing Function of Both Affected and Unaffected Systems

A chief concern in rehabilitative care is enhancing function of both affected and unaffected body systems, thereby helping patients to be as healthy and independent as possible. In palliative care, many care issues involve the interconnections of body systems and the need to enlist one function to serve for another.

CASE STUDY

Mr. O'Neill, a Man with Metastatic Prostate Cancer

Paul O'Neill had been a successful attorney for 30 years. A burly, loud-spoken Irishman, he prided himself in bringing life and laughter everywhere he went. Although diagnosed and treated for prostate cancer, he never slowed the hectic pace of his law practice or his busy social calendar. In fact, he had little time to pay attention to the ominous symptoms that were developing that indicated the advance of his disease.

When he sought medical attention at last, the cancer had metastasized to his spine, resulting in partial paralysis and bowel and bladder impairment. Orthopedic spine surgeons attempted to relieve pressure on his spinal cord with the hope of restoring motor and sensory function. However, when they performed the surgery, they found that the cancer had spread extensively, and they were unable to significantly improve his spinal cord function. Radiation followed, but it had little effect on the spreading cancer.

Mr. O'Neill was stunned. He could not believe the turn his life had taken. Suddenly, nothing seemed to work. He had to depend on others for the first time in his life. He felt like "some kind of freak," unable to move his legs or even manage normal bodily functions. His bulky frame became a heavy burden as he tried to relearn life from a wheelchair. He wrestled with the unfairness of the situation, finally promising himself that he would "go out in style." He wanted to get home as soon as possible, so as not to waste his precious remaining time.

Mr. O'Neill spent 12 days on the inpatient rehabilitation unit, then transitioned to home with continued therapies and nursing care. He died 2 months later, at home with his family present.

In Mr. O'Neill's case, several body systems were at risk for complications, although not all were directly affected by the disease process. Mobility was a critical concern. Bowel and bladder management also presented challenges. His neurological deficits and rapidly progressing disease, combined with his size and the need to learn new skills from a wheelchair level, placed him at risk for development of contractures, skin breakdown, and deep vein thrombosis. Problems with bowel and bladder function put him at risk for constipation, distention, and infection. He experienced severe demoralization. In keeping with his wishes, the rehabilitation nursing staff designed a plan for Mr. O'Neill and his family to follow at home.

Priority rehabilitation nursing issues included

- Managing fatigue related to advancing disease
- Pain control
- Promoting mobility and independence
- Managing neurogenic bowel and bladder
- Alleviating social isolation related to the effects of terminal illness
- Anticipatory grieving and spiritual care

Managing Fatigue Related to Advancing Disease

The rehabilitation team planned Mr. O'Neill's care to protect his periods of rest throughout the day. They knew that his therapy would be more effective and his ability to carry over new learning of functional activities would be better if he were in a rested state. His sleep–wake cycle was restored as quickly as possible. Occupational therapists taught him strategies for energy conservation in his activities of daily living, including the use of adaptive devices, planning, and pacing.

Pain Control

Mr. O'Neill initially described his pain as always with him, dull and relentless, wearing him down. Rehabilitation nurses evaluated his responses in relation to different medications and dosage schedules, as well as nondrug pain control interventions such as positioning and relaxation. The most effective method of pain control for Mr. O'Neill was scheduled doses of long-acting morphine, coupled with short-acting doses for breakthrough or procedural pain. This method of pain management is frequently used in rehabilitation settings, because it does not allow pain to become established, and the patient does not have to experience a certain level of pain and then wait for relief. It also minimizes sedative effects. With his pain under better control, Mr. O'Neill was able to actively participate in his own care and make deliberate decisions about his goals.

Promoting Mobility and Independence

Bed Positioning

Positioning and supporting of the body in such a way that function is preserved and complications are prevented is an important consideration in mobility. As Mr. O'Neill's disease progressed and he experienced increasing weakness and fatigue, he spent more and more time in bed. Teaching of patient and family focused on the techniques of bed mobility and specific precautions to prevent complications.

Supine lying was minimized because of Mr. O'Neill's high risk for sacral skin breakdown. Even with a pressure-reducing mattress, back-lying time needed to be restricted. To reduce shearing forces, the bed was placed in reverse Trendelenburg position to raise the head, rather than cranking up just the head of the bed. Draw sheets were used to move Mr. O'Neill, again to prevent shearing. Shearing is a force generated when the skin does not move as one with the structures beneath it. Stretching and breakage of capillaries and subcutaneous tissues contributes to the potential for deep skin breakdown.

Positioning of the lower extremities is important to prevent complications such as foot drop, skin breakdown, contractures, and deep vein thrombosis. When the patient is supine, care should be taken to support the feet in neutral position. This can be accomplished by using a footboard or box at the end of the bed or by the application of splints. Derotational splints were placed on Mr. O'Neill's lower legs to keep his hips in alignment, to prevent foot-drop contractures, and to reduce the risk of heel breakdown. Range-of-motion exercises were done at least twice daily.

When Mr. O'Neill was side-lying, pillows were employed to cushion bony prominences and maintain neutral joint position. His uppermost leg was brought forward, and the lower leg was straightened to minimize hip flexion contractures. Frequently overlooked as a positioning choice, prone lying offers advantages not only of skin pressure relief and reduction in hip flexion contractures, but also in promoting greater oxygen exchange.[7] Mr. O'Neill's bed position was alternated between back, both sides, and prone at least every 2 hours.

Sitting

There are many physiological benefits of upright posture. Blood pressure, digestive and bowel functions, oxygenation, and perception are geared toward being upright. Weight-bearing helps to avert skeletal muscle atrophy. Sitting, standing, and walking provide for changes in scenery and enhance the ability to socialize. This was an important consideration for Mr. O'Neill, who experienced emotional distress at the social isolation his illness imposed.

It is important to choose seating that supports the patient, avoiding surfaces that place pressure on bony prominences. A seat that is angled back slightly helps keep the patient from sliding forward. Placing the feet on footrests or a small box or stool may add comfort, as may supporting the arms on pillows or on a table in front of the patient. Sitting time should be limited, based on patient comfort, endurance, and skin tolerance. Mr. O'Neill followed a sitting schedule that increased by 15 minutes a day until he was able to tolerate about 2 hours of upright time. That was enough time to carry out many of his personal activities, yet not so much as to overly tire him.

Planning for Mr. O'Neill's return home involved careful assessment of his equipment needs. Physical and occupational therapists conducted a home evaluation to determine how he would manage mobility and self-care activities and what equipment would be appropriate. Family members practiced using equipment and devices under the guidance of the rehabilitation team. The objective was to simplify the care as much as possible, while still supporting Mr. O'Neill's active participation in his daily activities.

Examples of home care equipment often used include commodes, wheelchairs, sliding boards, Hoyer lifts, adaptive devices such as reachers, dressing sticks, long-handled sponges, tub/shower benches, hospital beds, and pressure-relieving mattresses. Examples of home modifications include affixing handrails and grab bars, widening doors, using raised toilet seats, and installing stair lifts and ramps.

Management of Neurogenic Bowel and Bladder

For Mr. O'Neill, the loss of bowel and bladder function was especially distressing. It placed him in a position of dependence and impinged on his privacy. It reinforced his feelings of isolation and being different. The focus of rehabilitation nursing interventions was to mimic the normal physiological rhythms of bowel and bladder elimination. By helping Mr. O'Neill gain control of his body functions, nursing staff hoped to promote his confidence, dignity, and feelings of self-worth.

Bowel regulation and continence were achieved by implementing a classic bowel program routine. Mr. O'Neill was especially prone to constipation due to immobility and the effects of pain medications. The first intervention was to modify his diet to include more fiber and fluids. He also took stool softener medication twice daily. His bowel program occurred after breakfast each morning, to take advantage of the gastrocolic reflex. He was assisted to sit upright on a commode chair. A rectal suppository was inserted, with digital stimulation at 15-minute intervals to accomplish bowel evacuation. The patient and his wife were taught how to manage this program at home. Although reluctant at first, Mr. O'Neill became resigned to the necessity of this bowel program and worked it into his morning routine. His wife, eager to help in any way she could, also learned the techniques. Once a regular pattern of elimination was established, Mr. O'Neill no longer experienced incontinence.

For bladder management, nursing staff implemented a program of void trials and intermittent catheterization. The patient learned to manage his own fluid intake and to catheterize himself at 4-hour intervals, thereby preventing overdistension or incontinence. However, as his disease progressed, he opted for an indwelling urinary catheter because it was easier for him to manage. There is a continuous need to evaluate and individualize rehabilitation goals, and to alter goals as patients experience more advanced disease.

Alleviating Social Isolation Related to the Effects of Terminal Illness

With a history of active social involvement, Mr. O'Neill had great difficulty with the limitations his disease imposed on his energy level and his ability to remain functional. He did not want others to see him as incapacitated in any way. He did not want to be embarrassed by his failing body. The rehabilitation team concentrated on solving the physical problems that could be solved. A recreation therapist assessed his leisure and avocational interests and prescribed therapeutic activities that would build his confidence in social situations. Together, the team helped him learn to navigate around architectural barriers and helped him to practice new skills successfully from a wheelchair level.

Anticipatory Grieving and Spiritual Care

Mr. O'Neill concentrated on making plans and settling financial matters in preparation for his death. He continued to set goals for himself and to maintain hope, but the nature of his goals shifted. Initially, he was concerned with not becoming a burden to his family and focused on his physical functioning. As his mobility and endurance flagged and he had to rely more on others for assistance with basic care needs, he began to change his goals. Some of his stoicism fell away. He revealed his feelings more readily and described the evolution of his emotions. Now the focus became his relationships: an upcoming wedding anniversary, a son's graduation from law school. Rehabilitation nurses, home care nurses, the psychologist, and the social worker supported the patient and his family as they began to grieve the past that would never return and the future that was not to be. Pastoral care was a significant part of the process, as Mr. O'Neill struggled with spiritual questions and sought a peaceful understanding of what was happening to him. The rehabilitation team endeavored to help the patient live all the days of his life, by helping body and soul continue to function.

Facilitating Use of Adaptive Strategies

The ability of patients to continue to participate actively in living their lives has much to do with successful adaptation to changes in function. Even at the end of life, a patient's capacity to adapt remains. Everyday activities may become very difficult to perform with advancing disease. However, rehabilitation nursing actions that promote communication, the use of appropriate tools and equipment, family participation, and modifications to the environment all enhance the process of adaptation.

Communication

Opening the doors to communication is the most important rehabilitation nursing intervention. By removing functional barriers to speech, by teaching and supporting compensatory strategies, and by allowing safe opportunities for patients and families to discuss difficult issues around death and dying, rehabilitation nurses perform a critical function in the adaptation process.

Tools and Equipment

Many adaptive devices are available to patients and families that enhance functional ability and independence. Rehabilitation offers the chance to analyze tasks with new eyes and solve problems with creativity and individuality. Examples of useful tools to assist patients in being as independent as possible include reachers, dressing aids such as sock-starters, elastic shoelaces, and dressing sticks. For some patients, adapted eating utensils increase independence with the activity of eating and thereby support nutritional intake. Modifications to clothing may permit more efficient toileting and hygiene, conserving both energy and dignity.

Family Participation

As illustrated in the previous case studies, the involvement of family and friends has multifaceted benefits. Because of the social nature of humankind, presence and involvement of family and friends has great importance at the end of life. Family members may seek involvement in the caring activities as an expression of feelings of closeness and love. They may try to find understanding, resolution, or closure of past issues. For the person at the end of life, the presence of family, friends, and even pets may be a powerful affirmation of the continuity of life.

Modifications to Environment

Rehabilitation professionals are keenly aware of the effect of the environment of care on function, independence, and well-being. The physical arrangement of furnishings can be instrumental, not only in promoting patient access to the environment, but also in the ease with which others care for the patient. The environment can be made into a powerful tool for orientation, for spatial perception, and for preserving a territorial sense of self.

Light has a strong effect, not only on visual perception, but also on mood and feelings of well-being. Light can be a helpful tool in maintaining day–night rhythms and orienting patients to time and place.[8] Sound is also an important environmental variable. For example, music has been implicated as a therapeutic intervention in both rehabilitation and palliative care.[9]

Promoting Quality at the End of Life

The concept of quality of life is linked to function and independence. Patients often describe their satisfaction with life in terms of what they are able to do. Important determinants of quality of life include (1) the patient's own state, including physical and cognitive functioning, psychological state, and physical condition; (2) quality of palliative care; (3) physical environment; (4) relationships; and (5) outlook.[10] Rehabilitation zeroes in on the essential components of mobility, self-care, cognition, and social interaction, which define what people can do.

CASE STUDY

LN, a 42-Year-Old Woman with a Malignant Brain Tumor

LN, age 42, had just started her own consulting business when she began to experience headaches and visual disturbances. At first, she attributed her symptoms to the long hours and stress related to building her business. But when she experienced weakness of her left side, she knew that something more serious was happening.

She had a glioblastoma multiforme growing deep in her brain. Surgery was performed to debulk the tumor, but in a matter of weeks it was clear that the mass was growing rapidly. A course of radiation was completed to no avail. Her function continued to decline, and it seemed that every body system was affected by the advancing malignancy. Now her left side was densely paralyzed, she had difficulty swallowing and speaking, and her thinking processes became muddled.

Her family was in turmoil. On one hand, they resented the disruption her sudden illness imposed on their previously ordered lives. On the other hand, they wanted to care for her and make sure that her remaining time was the best that it could be. As they watched her decline day by day, ambiguities in their relationships surfaced, and conflicts about what would define quality of life emerged.

Rehabilitation's part in promoting quality of life at the end of life is several-fold. Rehabilitation is a goal-directed process. Realistic, attainable goals based on the patient's own definition of quality of life drive the actions of the team. In the area of physical care, rehabilitation strategies support energy conservation, sequencing and pacing, maintaining normal routines, and accessing the environment. Beyond that, rehabilitation nurses facilitate effective communication and problem-solving with patients and families. They offer acceptance and support through difficult decision-making and help mobilize concrete resources.

When rehabilitation nurses approach care, it is with the goal of enhancing function and independence. In LN's case, the brain tumor created deficits in mobility, cognition, and perception. Also, more subtle issues greatly influenced the quality of her remaining time. It was important to understand how the patient would define the quality of her own life and to direct actions toward protecting those elements.

Promoting Dignity, Self-Image, and Participation

LN's concept of quality of life was evident in how she participated in her care and the decisions that she made about her course of treatment. The rehabilitation team learned that LN's mother had died several years earlier of a similar brain tumor. Caring for her mother had solidified her beliefs about not wishing to burden others. Part of LN's definition of quality of life was that she would not be dependent on others.

LN prided herself on being industrious and self-sufficient. To her, the ability to take care of herself was a sign of success. Rehabilitation nurses and therapists focused on helping to manage symptoms of advancing disease so that she would be able to do as much for herself as possible. This included adaptive techniques for daily living skills, pain management, eating, dressing, grooming, and bowel and bladder management. Even with her physical and cognitive decline, retaining her normal routines helped to allay some feelings of helplessness and to promote a positive self-image.

Control, Hope, and Reality

As her illness progressed, LN felt she was losing control. It became difficult for her to remember things, and expressing herself became more laborious and frustrating. She slept frequently and seemed disconnected from external events. Her family understood her usual desire for control and made many attempts to include her in conversations and to support her in making choices.

At first, her concept of hope was tied to the idea of cure. Radiation therapy represented the chance of cure. When that was completed without appreciable change in her tumor, some of her feelings of hopefulness slipped away. She sank into a depression. Her family was alarmed: LN's psychological well-being was a critical component in her own definition of quality of life. Treating her depression became a priority issue for the rehabilitation team. Through a combination of rehabilitation psychological counseling and antidepressant medications, her dark mood slowly lifted. Hope seemed to return in a different form, less connected to an event of cure and more a part of her interactions with her daughter and sister.

Family Support

Another significant area that related to quality of life for LN had to do with social well-being. She struggled with the idea of becoming a burden to her family and realized that she was losing control over what was happening to her. Her relationships with others in her life were complex, and now they were challenged even further. At the same time, her family members wrestled with memories of the mother's death and feared the responsibilities for care that might be thrust upon them.

The rehabilitation team tried to help the patient and her family work through their thoughts, feelings, and fears, and helped them to find ways to express them. The team arranged several family conferences to discuss not only the care issues but also the changes in roles and family structure. Whenever possible, the team found answers to the family's questions and made great effort to keep communications open. Creating safe opportunities for the family to express their ambivalence and conflict helped move them toward acceptance. The family was able to prepare in concrete ways for the outcome they both welcomed and dreaded.

Understanding Outcomes

In rehabilitation, there is a strong emphasis on the measurement of patient outcomes. Since the 1950s, many functional assessment instruments have been developed and used to help quantify the changes that occur in patients as a result of care

Table 45–2
Measures of Functional Outcomes

Barthel Index[15] (Mahoney 1958)
Dartmouth COOP Functional Health Assessment Charts[16]
Edmonton Functional Assessment Tool[17]
Functional Activities Questionnaire[18,19]
Functional Independence Measure[13,14]
Functional Status Index[20,21]
Index of Independence in Activities of Daily Living (ADL)[22]
Kenny Self-Care Evaluation[23]
Lambeth Disability Screening Questionnaire[24]
Medical Outcomes Study Physical Functioning Measure[25]
Physical Self-Maintenance Scale[26]
PULSES Profile[27]
Rapid Disability Rating Scale[11]
Self-Evaluation of Life Function Scale[28]
Stanford Health Assessment Questionnaire[29]

and recovery. Some instruments to measure functional and physical outcomes are applicable to the assessment of patients within the last month of life.

There are more than a dozen functional outcome measurement tools in common use in rehabilitation settings in the United States and Canada (Table 45–2). Measurement of self-care and mobility are central to rehabilitation, but the functions and behaviors required to lead a meaningful life are much broader. They may include cognitive, emotional, perceptual, social, and vocational function measurements as well.

For measuring function in the last 30 days of life, three scales may be particularly useful. The Rapid Disability Rating Scale (RDRS-2)[11] has a broad scope to include items related to activities of daily living, mental capacity, dietary changes, continence, medications, and confinement to bed. The Health Assessment Questionnaire (HAQ)[12] is a widely used instrument that summarizes the patients' areas of major difficulty. The Functional Independence Measure (FIM) is an ordinal scale that quantifies 18 areas of physical and cognitive function in terms of burden of care.[13,14] These scales are appropriate to palliative care because they focus on specific aspects of function that relate to patients' independence. The scales may be used to determine whether interventions at the end of life serve to foster independence and function for as long as possible.

There is also strong interest in the field of rehabilitation in measuring patients' perceptions of quality of life. When the measured domains are considered, the connection between rehabilitation and end-of life care becomes evident. Most of the measurements of quality of life have to do with physical, cognitive, social, and spiritual function, the chief concerns of the rehabilitation practitioner (Table 45–3).

Table 45–3
Examples of Quality-of-Life Measure

Name of Instrument	Domains Measured
CARES-SF[30]	Rehabilitation and quality of life for patients with cancer
Chronic Respiratory Disease Questionnaire[31]	Measuring outcomes of clinical trials for patients with chronic obstructive pulmonary disease
City of Hope Quality of Life, Cancer Patient Version[32]	Physical well-being, psychological well being, and spiritual well-being
COOP Charts[16]	Screen patients in an outpatient setting
Daily Diary Card-QOL[33]	Changes in quality of life related to symptoms induced by chemotherapy
EORTC QOL-30[34]	Physical function, role function, cognitive function, emotional function, social function, symptoms, and financial impact
FACT-G[35]	Patients undergoing cancer treatment
Ferrans and Powers Quality of Life Index[36]	Satisfaction with and importance of multiple domains
FLIC[37]	Physical/occupational function, psychological state, sociability, and somatic discomfort
HIV Overview of Problems Evaluation Systems (HOPES)[38]	Rehabilitation and quality of life for patients with HIV
Hospice Quality of Life Index—Revised[39]	Physical, psychological, spiritual, social, and financial well-being
McGill Quality of Life Questionnaire[40]	Quality of life at the end of life
Medical Outcomes Study, Short Form Health Survey[25]	Physical functioning, role limitations, bodily pain, social functioning, mental health, vitality, and general health perceptions
National Hospice Study Quality of Life Scale[41]	Quality of life at end of life
Nottingham Health Profile[42]	Physical, social, and emotional health problems and their impact on functioning
Quality of Life Index[43]	General physical condition, important human activities, and general quality of life
Quality of Life for Respiratory Illness Questionnaire[44]	Chronic nonspecific lung disease
Quality of Well-Being Scale[45]	Mobility, physical activity, social activity, and 27 symptoms
Sickness Impact Profile[46]	How an illness affects a person's behavior
Southwest Oncology Group Quality of Life Questionnaire[47]	Function, symptoms, and global quality of life measures
Spitzer QL-Index[48]	Activity level, social support, and mental well-being
VITAS Quality of Life Index[49]	Symptoms, function, interpersonal domains, well-being, and transcendence

Outcome measurements matter because they can reveal a lot about the quality of life experienced by persons near the end of life. For example, by assessing at intervals, it is possible to determine how much function patients retain as they approach death. By identifying and measuring differences in this experience, it is possible to determine the essential interventions and care activities that contribute to the highest levels of functional independence up to the end of life.

Further research is needed to

- Establish norms and indications for the application of rehabilitation in palliative care
- Determine cost-effectiveness of rehabilitation interventions
- Determine optimal time frames for providing rehabilitation services after the onset of disease
- Define variables having the greatest impact on patient outcomes

Conclusion

Rehabilitation nursing approaches have value in palliative care. Regardless of the disease trajectory, nurses can do something more to preserve function and independence and positively affect perceptions of quality of life, even at its end. Rehabilitation nurses facilitate holistic care of persons in their social and physical environments. They direct actions toward preventing secondary disability and enhancing both affected and unaffected body systems. They foster the use of adaptive strategies and techniques to optimize autonomy. The deliberate focus of rehabilitation nurses on function, independence, dignity, and the preservation of hope makes a fitting contribution to care at the end of life.

REFERENCES

1. Hoeman S. Rehabilitation Nursing: Process and Application, 3rd ed. St. Louis: Mosby, 2002.
2. American Nurses' Association. Rehabilitation Nursing—Scope of Practice: Process and Outcome Criteria for Selected Diagnoses. 1988. Kansas City, MO: American Nurses' Association.
3. Doloresco L. CARF: Symbol of rehabilitation excellence. Sci Nurs 2001;18:165,172.
4. Maloof M. The 1989 CARF nursing standards: Guidelines for implementation. Commission of Accreditation of Rehabilitation Facilities. Rehabil Nurs 1989;14:134–136.

4a. Association of Rehabilitation Nurses Position Statements. Available at: http://rehabnurse.org/profresources/pappropr.html (accessed March 7, 2005).

5. Fox E. Predominance of the curative model of medical care: A residual problem. JAMA 1997;278:761–763.
6. Hansen S, Swiontkowski MF. Orthopedic Trauma Protocols. New York: Raven Press, 1993.
7. Ciesla ND. Chest physical therapy for patients in the intensive care unit. Phys Ther 1996;76:609–625.
8. Stewart K, Hayes BC, Eastman CI. Light treatment for NASA shift workers. Chronobiol Int 1995;12:141–151.
9. Halstead MT, Roscoe ST. Restoring the spirit at the end of life: Music as an intervention for oncology nurses. Clin J Oncol Nurs 2002;6:332–336.
10. Cohen SR, Leis A. What determines the quality of life of terminally ill cancer patients from their own perspective? J Palliat Care 2002;18:48–58.
11. Linn M, Linn BS. The Rapid Disability Rating Scale-2. J Am Geriatr Soc 1982;30:378–382.
12. Steen V, Medsger TA. The value of the Health Assessment Questionnaire and special patient-generated scales to demonstrate change in systemic sclerosis patients over time. Arthritis Rheum 1997;40:1984–1991.
13. Stineman M, Shea JA, Jette A, Tassoni CJ, Ottenbacher KJ, Fiedler R, Granger CV. The Functional Independence Measure: Tests of scaling assumptions, structure, and reliability across 20 divers impairment categories. Arch Phys Med Rehabil 1996;77:1101–1108.
14. Granger C, Brownscheidle CM. Outcome measurement in medical rehabilitation. Int J Technol Assess Health Care 1995;11: 262–268.
15. Mahoney FI, Barthel DW. Functional evaluation: The Barthel Index. Md State Med J 1965;14:61–65.
16. Nelson EC, Landgraf JM, Hays RD, Wasson JH, Kirk JW. The functional status of patients: How can it be measured in physicians' offices? Med Care 1990;28:1111–1126.
17. Kaasa T, Loomis J, Gillis K, Bruera E, Hanson J. The Edmonton Functional Assessment Tool: Preliminary development and evaluation for use in palliative care. J Pain Sympt Manage 1997; 13:10–19.
18. Pfeffer R, Kurosaki TT, Harrah CH, Chance JM, Filos S. Measurement of functional activities in older adults in the community. J Gerontol 1982;37:323–329.
19. Pfeffer R, Kurosaki TT, Chance JM, Filos S, Bates D. Use of the mental function index in older adults: Reliability, validity, and measurement of change over time. Am J Epidemiol 1984;120: 922–935.
20. Jette A, Deniston OL. Inter-observer reliability of a functional status assessment instrument. J Chronic Dis 1978;31:573–580.
21. Jette A. Functional capacity evaluation: an empirical approach. Arch Phys Med Rehabil 1980;61:85–89.
22. Katz S, Ford AB, Moskowitz RW, Jackson BA, Jaffe MW. Studies of illness in the aged. The Index of ADL: A standardized measure of biological and psychosocial function. JAMA 1963;185:914–919.
23. Schoening H, Anderegg L, Bergstrom D, Fonda M, Steinke N, Ulrich P. Numerical scoring of self-care status of patients. Arch Phys Med Rehabil 1965;46:689–697.
24. Patrick DL, Darby SC, Green S, Horton G, Locker D, Wiggins RD. Screening for disability in the inner city. J Epidemiol Community Health 1981;35:65–70.
25. Stewart A, Hays RD, Ware JE. The MOS Short Form general health survey: Reliability and validity in a patient population. Med Care 1988;26:724–735.
26. Lawton M, Brody EM. Assessment of older people: Self-maintaining and instrumental activities of daily living. Gerontologist 1969;9:179–186.
27. Moskowitz E. PULSES profile in retrospect. Arch Phys Med Rehabil 1985;66:647–648.
28. Linn M, Linn BS. Self-Evaluation of Life Function (SELF) scale: A short, comprehensive self-report of health for elderly adults. J Gerontol 1984;39:603–612.

29. Fries J, Spitz PW, Young DY. The dimensions of health outcomes: The health assessment questionnaire, disability and pain scales. J Rheumatol 1982;9:789–793.
30. Schag C, Ganz PA, Heinrich RL. Cancer Rehabilitation Evaluation System–Short Form (CARES-sf): A cancer specific rehabilitation and quality of life instrument. Cancer 1991;68:1406–1413.
31. Guyatt G, Berman LB, Townsend M, Pugsley SO, Chambers LW. A measure of quality of life for clinical trials in chronic lung disease. Thorax 1987;42:773–780.
32. Ferrell B, Dow KH, Grant M. Measurement of quality of life in cancer survivors. Qual Life Res 1995;4:523–531.
33. Gower N, Rudd RM, Ruiz De Elvira MC, Spiro SG, James LE, Harper PG, Souhami RL. Assessment of quality of life using a daily diary card in a randomised trial of chemotherapy in small-cell lung cancer. Ann Oncol 1995;6:575–580.
34. Aaronson NK, Ahmedzai S, Bergman B, Bullinger M, Cull A, Duez NJ, Filiberti A, Flechtner H, Fleishman SB, de Haes JC, et al. The European Organization for Research and Treatment of Cancer QLQ-C30: A quality of life instrument for use in international clinical trials in oncology. J Natl Cancer Inst 1993; 85:365–376.
35. Cella D, Tulsky DS, Gray G, Sarafian B, Linn E, Bonomi A, Silberman M, Yellen SB, Winicour P, Brannon J, et al. The Functional Assessment of Cancer Therapy scale: Development and validation of the general measure. J Clin Oncol 1993;11:570–579.
36. Ferrans C, Powers MJ. Quality of life index: Development and psychometric properties. ANS Adv Nurs Sci 1985;8:15–24.
37. Finkelstein D, Cassileth BR, Bonomi PD, Rucksdeschel JC, Ezdinli EZ, Wolter JM. A pilot study of the Functional Living Index–Cancer (FLIC) scale for the assessment of quality of life fore metastatic lung cancer patients. Am J Clin Oncol 1988; 11:630–633.
38. Schag CA, Ganz PA, Kahn B, Petersen L. Assessing the needs and quality of life of patients with HIV infection: Development of the HIV Overview of Problems–Evaluation System (HOPES). Qual Life Res 1992;1:397–413.
39. McMillan SC, Mahon M. Measuring quality of life in hospice patients using a newly developed Hospice Quality of Life Index. Qual Life Res 1994;3:437–447.
40. Cohen S, Mount BM, Strobel MG, Bui F. The McGill Quality of Life Questionnaire: A measure of quality of life appropriate for people with advanced disease. Palliat Med 1995;9:207–219.
41. Greer D, Mor V. An overview of National Hospice Study findings. J Chronic Dis 1986;39:5–7.
42. Hunt SM, McKenna SP, McEwen J, Backett EM, Williams J, Papp E. A quantitative approach to perceived health status: A validation study. J Epidemiol Community Health 1980;34:281–286.
43. Padilla G, Presant C, Grant MM, Metter G, Lipsett J, Heide F. Quality of life index for patients with cancer. Res Nurs Health 1983;6:117–126.
44. Maille A., Koning CJ, Zwinderman AH, Willems LN, Dijkman JH, Kaptein AA. The development of the Quality of Life for Respiratory Illness Questionnaire (QOL-RIQ): A disease-specific quality of life questionnaire for patients with mild to moderate chronic non-specific lung disease. Respir Med 1997;91:297–309.
45. Kaplan RM, Atkins CJ, Timms R. Validity of a quality of well-being scale as an outcome measure in chronic obstructive pulmonary disease. J Chronic Dis 1984;37:85–95.
46. Bergner M, Bobbitt RA, Pollard WE, Martin DP, Gilson BS. The Sickness Impact Profile: Validation of a health status measure. Med Care 1976:14:57–67.
47. Moinpour C, Hayden KA, Thompson IM, Feigle P, Metch B. Quality of life assessment in Southwest Oncology Group Trials. Oncology (Huntingt) 1990;4:79–84,89,104.
48. Spitzer W, Dobson AJ, Hall J, Chesterman E, Levi J, Shepherd R, Battista RN, Catchlove BR. Measuring quality of life of cancer patients: A concise QL index for use by physicians. J Chronic Dis 1981;34:585–597.
49. Byock I, Merriman MP. Measuring quality of life for patients with terminal illness: The Missoula-VITAS quality of life index. Palliat Med 1998;12:231–244.

SUGGESTED READINGS

Association of Rehabilitation Nurses. Rehabilitation Nursing (journal published bimonthly). Glenview, Ill.

Association of Rehabilitation Nurses. Position statements [online], 2004. Available at: http://www.rehabnurse.org/profresources/index.html#positions (accessed February 4, 2005).

Davis MC. The rehabilitation nurse's role in spiritual care. Rehabil Nurs 1994;19:298–301.

Edelman CL, Mandle CL. Health Promotion Throughout the Life-span, 3rd ed. St. Louis: Mosby–Year Book, 1994.

Field MJ, Cassel CK, eds. Approaching Death: Improving Care at the End of Life. Washington, DC: National Academy Press, 1997.

Frank C, Hobbs N, Stewart G. Rehabilitation on palliative care units. J Palliat Care 1998;14:50–53.

Glick OJ. Interventions related to activity and movement. Nurs Clin North Am 1992;27:541–568.

Granger CV, Gresham GE, eds. Functional assessment in rehabilitation medicine. Baltimore, MD: Williams & Wilkins, 1984, pp. 99–121.

Hoeman SP. Pediatric rehabilitation nursing. In: Molnar G, ed. Pediatric Rehabilitation, 2nd ed. Baltimore, MD: Williams & Wilkins, 1992.

Kottke SJ, Stillwell GK, Lehman JS. Krusen's Handbook of Physical Medicine and Rehabilitation, 4th ed. Philadelphia: WB Saunders, 1990.

O'Brien T, Welsh J, Dunn F. ABC of palliative care: Non-malignant conditions. BMJ 1998;316:286–289.

O'Neill B, Fallon M. ABC of palliative care: principles of palliative care and pain control. BMJ 1997;315:801–804.

O'Neill B, Rodway A. ABC of palliative care: Care in the community. BMJ 1998;316:373–377.

Rehabilitation Nursing Foundation. Rehabilitation Nursing—Concepts and Practice: A Core Curriculum, 3rd ed. Glenview, IL: Author, 1993.

Rehabilitation Nursing Foundation. Application of Rehabilitation Concepts to Nursing Practice [independent study program]. Glenview, Ill.: Author, 1995.

Rehabilitation Nursing Foundation. Advanced Practice Nursing in Rehabilitation: A Core Curriculum. Glenview, IL: Author, 1997.

Wood C, Whittet S, Bradbeer C. ABC of palliative care: HIV infection and AIDS. BMJ 1997;315:1433–1436.

RESOURCES

American Academy of Physical Medicine and Rehabilitation (AAPM&R)

One IBM Plaza, Suite 2500, Chicago, IL 60611
http://www.aapmr.org
American Congress of Rehabilitation Medicine (ACRM)
4700 W. Lake Avenue, Glenview, IL 60025
http://www.acrm.org
Association of Rehabilitation Nurses (ARN)
4700 W. Lake Avenue, Glenview, IL 60025–1485
http://www.rehabnurse.org
Commission for the Accreditation of Rehabilitation Facilities (CARF)
4891 E. Grant Road, Tucson, AZ 85712
http://www.carf.org
Rehabilitation Foundation, Inc.
600 S. Washington St. Suite 301A, Naperville, IL 60540
http://www.rfi.org

46

Margaret Campbell and Robert Zalenski

The Emergency Department

We were trained to rescue patients in the ED—I can't just stand by and let someone die.
—Emergency physician and former residency director

- ***Key Points***
- *Each seriously ill person triaged in an emergency department (ED) presents in a crisis that has physical, emotional, social, and spiritual components.*
- *The growing number of patients presenting to the ED at the end of life means an increase in the proportion of patients for whom the default resuscitation approach is less applicable.*
- *Rapid identification of treatment goals with the terminally ill patient or surrogate prevents unwanted resuscitation and application of burdensome life-prolonging therapies.*
- *The most prevalent distressing symptoms that require immediate attention for the patient who is dying in the ED are pain and dyspnea.*
- *Unrestricted access of the family to the dying patient can be successfully implemented in the ED.*
- *An unexpected death in the ED requires a different approach to preparing the body for viewing that consists of minimizing delays and judicious draping.*

Each year, there are 110 million visits to emergency departments (EDs) in the United States, and almost 1% or approximately 1 million of these visits result in death in the ED or hospital.[1] The emergency team in a busy ED typically perform or withholds attempts at resuscitation several times during an 8- to 12-hour shift.

Emergency physicians and nurses traditionally view themselves as foot soldiers in the trenches fighting against the enemy, dying and death. The criterion of success is whether the patient was admitted to the hospital or discharged to the community alive. Death is regarded as failure; it may be blamed on the disease or the patient's response, but must not be blamed on a clinician's lack of willingness to "do everything" to keep the ED patient alive. In this view, every ED case can be dichotomized into success or failure based on whether the patient left the ED with a pulse.

This traditional view of the ED misses the complexity and the reality of life and death. The reality is that each seriously ill person triaged in an ED presents in a crisis that has physical, emotional, social, and spiritual components. Each person who might die soon is at a particular point in his or her life cycle, and for the person and the family, death may be either unexpected or expected. For some of these patients, it would be unthinkable not to have all aggressive efforts to prolong life no matter its quality; for others, the ritualized set of resuscitative procedures before death is considered worse than death itself. In most EDs, there are clinicians who want to know the more complex and vulnerable person beneath the presenting disease label, who are willing to tailor treatment and disposition to the more important needs discovered.

This chapter on palliative care in the ED is designed to assist in recognizing and addressing the needs of irreversibly ill patients and their families. From this perspective, the key questions to be added to the basic ED assessment include the following: Is the patient/family aware of the presence of an incurable illness? What are their preferences for care, and how rapidly can we establish treatment goals? What can be done to relieve distressing symptoms? What can be done to ease the family's distress and meet their needs?

The workload in the ED is such that, for most patients, the "greet, treat, and street" approach must necessarily prevail to prevent gridlock.[2] But for the smaller number of patients who present with severe uncontrolled symptoms and organ failure that is not curable, recommendations made to lessen suffering and respect preferences for care can provide a rewarding sense of satisfaction for provider, patient, and family alike. There are a growing number of elderly persons in this country, and care teams are likely to face an increased incidence of terminally ill patients presenting to the ED who can be guided into the positive outcomes that palliative care can provide.

Recognizing Poor Prognoses

Experienced emergency nurses and physicians are able to recognize the gravely and terminally ill, who arrive with severe distressing symptoms, altered mental status, or imminent death. Examples are an 80-year-old with advanced dementia, decubiti, severe cachexia, and aspiration pneumonia; a 60-year-old with marked cachexia, dyspnea, metastatic non-small-cell lung cancer who has received surgery, radiation, and two courses of chemotherapy; a 50-year-old man with cardiac arrest, in pulseless electromechanical dissociation despite 20 minutes of three rounds of resuscitative therapy; the 60-year-old with severe diabetes and poorly controlled hypertension who has declined dialysis and is now in pulmonary edema with distressing dyspnea.

To help clarify thinking about patients who die, researchers have conceptualized them by placing them on one of five "dying trajectories": (1) terminal illness, such as cancer; (2) sudden death, if younger than 80 years of age and previously healthy; (3) organ failure, such as congestive heart failure (CHF) and chronic obstructive pulmonary disease (COPD); (4) frailty, such as with dementia, bed bound, or with multiple recurrent hospitalizations; and (5) other. Data from Medicare decedents shows that 47% were considered to have died of frailty, 22% were on a cancer-like trajectory, 16% had organ failure, 7% had sudden death, and 8% were in the "other" category.[3]

Within each trajectory, death can be considered expected or unexpected by the provider or patient/family. If death is expected or known by the provider only, this is termed closed awareness; if known by provider and patient, it is called open awareness. Other possibilities are that neither the provider nor the patient is aware that the patient is dying (no awareness), or that the patient is aware but the provider is not, which can be termed "hidden awareness."[4] Assessment here has great implications, because the type of awareness of death (open versus closed versus no) often determines the ability of the provider to render optimal care.

Each trajectory has implications for a palliative approach to the patient. Sometimes such discussions take place in the ED, as they should if the ED clinicians recognize that the reflex curative/restorative ED procedure is in fact the "wrong" thing for the patient and family. More commonly, such decisions are "turfed" to the admitting team by default, although prudence would dictate that ED providers not hand off such discussions on nights or weekends, when the patient might die before others have had a chance to establish or review goals of care.

Patients with terminal illness who present with advanced disease and distressing symptoms should be assessed for their awareness of their prognosis. One approach is to ask the patient, "Tell me what you understand about your cancer." Patients (or surrogates) with open awareness are good candidates to begin a palliative care approach in the ED, rather than resuscitation and admission to the intensive care unit (ICU). Palliative-directed intervention in the ED can help avoid the worst-case scenario: uncomfortable interventions in unrecognized terminal illness that result in a moribund patient who is unprepared for death and unable to make choices to forgo further nonbeneficial interventions.

Patients who die suddenly present a number of challenges to ED clinicians. In general terms, they often leave behind loving family members who are not yet aware of their death. Patients who die unexpectedly of acute renal, respiratory, or heart failure are ideal candidates for the default ED approach and are amenable to all aggressive resuscitative efforts—unless there is an advance directive (AD) to withhold them. When death occurs in the ED after an attempt at resuscitation, the surviving families are ill-equipped to cope with the news and require intensive interventions directed at bereavement care. Studies have revealed that families want to be informed of the death in a compassionate and unhurried manner; to be reassured that the patient's belongings will be properly handled; to be told what to do next (e.g., how to contact a funeral home); and to have the opportunity for follow-up with the hospital to answer unresolved questions.[5–7] Development and implementation of ED-focused bereavement guidelines enhance the quality of care provided to the family after an unexpected loss.[8–10]

Patients with organ failure, notably those with CHF or COPD, are usually resuscitated or pronounced dead in the ED. Because the chance of pulling a patient through one more episode is relatively high, this course of action, conforming to the default ED approach, is often the road of least resistance and the most appropriate course. Inquiring about treatment preferences for resuscitative therapy is important if the patient is still alert or the family is available. Patients who arrive in extremis with clear expressions of their wishes, such as documented and confirmed forgoing of resuscitation, and hospice patients seeking comfort care that outstrips the home's resources should continue to have their preferences honored by the ED team.

Patients dying on the frailty trajectory should have had ample time for their or their surrogate's preferences to be established before the ED visit. As with patients with organ failure, they should have these preferences assessed and their awareness of dying probed. Admission for a palliative care approach rather than ICU admission could be considered.

The fact that growing numbers of patients are presenting to the ED at the end of life means an increase in the proportion of patients for whom the "default" ED approach is less applicable. This calls for a growing sensitivity of ED clinicians for greater skills in palliative care. ED staff must become comfortable with the decisions that patients or their surrogates make regarding forgoing resuscitative interventions and accepting natural death.[11] ED staff are highly trained to rescue and, as with other specialty areas in the hospital, can provide the requisite palliative care interventions to patients and their families who may be dying in the ED.

Establishing Treatment Goals

When the terminally ill patient presents to the ED, rapid identification of treatment goals with the patient or the surrogate of an incapable patient is indicated and may prevent unwanted resuscitation and the application of other potentially burdensome life-sustaining therapies. Likewise, if palliative care treatment goals are established rapidly after an attempt at resuscitation, the patient and family can be afforded a quick transition from resuscitation to comfort by a skilled, compassionate ED intervention to withdraw unwanted life supports. Establishment of palliative care treatment goals in the ED can be inhibited by lack of prognostic information, the lack of any prior relationship with the patient or surrogate, a need for rapid action, and the fear of liability if life is not extended.[12,13] Hopefully, clinicians in EDs will begin to see themselves as ideally positioned to identify and treat palliative care emergencies—such as pain crises—and adopt the goals of prevention of suffering and enabling of a "good death." This development will expand the ED concept of success.

Most physicians (78%) responding to a survey study about cardiopulmonary resuscitation (CPR) indicated that they would honor legal ADs about resuscitation.[12] However, despite more than a decade of experience with the Patient Self-Determination Act,[14] there continues to be a paucity of persons who have completed an AD. In the general U.S. population only 15% of Americans have an AD,[15] but among frail, elderly nursing home residents the prevalence of AD completion increases to 45% to 60%.[15–17]

Even if the AD accompanies the patient to the ED, it may have limited usefulness in guiding emergency management. One study found that, although 44% of nursing home residents seen in the ED had ADs, the ADs frequently addressed only CPR and did not address other life-supporting strategies (e.g., intubation) with the same frequency.[16] Yet, even a limited AD provides the ED clinician with a starting point for a conversation about treatment preferences. The ED clinician can open the discussion with a request for clarification of the preferences expressed in the directive, and the conversation about contemporaneous diagnosis and treatment recommendations and preferences will flow. After ascertaining the patient's or surrogate's understanding about the illness, the clinician might ask, "I see you already have wishes about CPR; will you tell me more about your preferences for treatment?"

In the absence of an AD, or if the AD is ambiguous, the ED staff are obliged to engage in a decision-making process at the earliest opportunity after identifying or inferring the patient's terminal prognosis. This conversation may occur before or after an attempt at resuscitation. A discussion with the patient who has retained decision-making capacity about diagnosis, prognosis, and relevant treatment options is a challenging process in the ED, because the patient may have no prior relationship with the ED staff and may be lacking bonds of trust and rapport. Furthermore, this type of clinician–patient conversation is ideally held in privacy and quiet, and the ED environment is not always a conducive setting. A creative approach to finding a quiet room or screening an area around the patient is needed.

Cognitive impairment is highly prevalent in terminally ill patients, particularly those whose death is imminent, and it may preclude them from having the capacity to make decisions about treatment.[18–20] Reliance on a valid surrogate decision-maker, usually a family member or close friend, becomes necessary. Surrogates appointed by the patient through an AD have pre-eminence in decision-making. In the absence of a patient-appointed proxy, many states have enacted surrogacy statutes, often relying on a next-of-kin hierarchy, to direct clinicians. Clinicians need to know the provisions of their own state when seeking a surrogate decision about treatment. Table 46–1 details the core components of a discussion about end-of-life treatment options.

CASE STUDY

HR, an 88-Year-Old Woman with Dementia

HR is an 88-year-old woman brought to the ED from her nursing home. She is in the terminal stage of dementia by physical examination and report from the nursing home, yet treatment goals have never been established with her only surviving family member, a niece. HR is curled into a fetal position and has stage III and IV sacral, trochanter, and heel decubiti. She is febrile, she has leukocytosis, and her chest radiograph is consistent with aspiration pneumonia. Her respiratory pattern and blood gas analysis predict imminent respiratory failure. The ED staff are in consensus that this patient would benefit from a palliative care approach rather than intubation and admission to the ICU.

The ED social worker calls the patient's niece and asks her to come to the hospital as soon as possible. On her arrival, an ED physician, nurse, and the social worker sit with the niece, discuss the patient's diagnoses and prognosis, and make a recommendation about comfort care. The niece agrees, thanks the team, and reports that no one has ever raised this option with her in the past. She believes that her aunt has "suffered enough" and should "pass naturally and peacefully." The hospital's palliative care service is consulted by the ED for admission, instead of the ICU.

Table 46–1
Core Components of a Discussion about End-of-Life Treatment Goals

Prepare in advance.

- Identify the diagnosis/prognosis.
- Determine what the patient or surrogate already knows.
- Seek assistance from support personnel (e.g., chaplain, social worker, patient advocate).

Establish a therapeutic milieu.

- Identify a private and quiet place in the emergency department where everyone can sit and be seen and heard.
- Minimize interruptions.

Seek patient and surrogate knowledge about diagnosis and prognosis.

- Correct inaccuracies and misconceptions.
- Provide additional information.

Communicate effectively.

- Avoid jargon, slang, and acronyms.
- Demonstrate empathy.
- Be honest and direct.

Make a palliative care treatment recommendation.

- Provide rationale for recommendations.
- Answer questions.

Seek patient or surrogate agreement with recommendation.

Source: Campbell ML. Communicating a poor prognosis and making decisions. In: Foregoing Life-Sustaining Therapy: How to Care for the Patient Who Is Near Death. Aliso Veijo, CA: American Association of Critical-Care Nurses, 1998, pp 19–41.

After the goals of treatment have been determined with the patient or surrogate, the relevant interventions can be identified. A focus on palliation rather than resuscitation indicates that reduction of symptom distress and attention to patient and family grief are the priorities of patient and family care.

Symptom Management: Pain and Dyspnea

The most prevalent symptoms that produce distress in the dying patient and require immediate attention are pain and dyspnea.[21–24] The nursing process (i.e., assessment, planning, intervention, and evaluation) guides effective symptom management in the ED.

The gold standard for pain assessment is the patient's self-report. When the patient is able to self-report, his or her appraisal of pain intensity, location, quality, and possible causes should be sought. A documented trend using a numeric rating or visual analog scale is standard and permits continuous assessment and reevaluation over time and across caregivers. Pain occurs as result of trauma, somatic disorders, and common ED procedures.[25,26]

Critically ill patients and those with cognitive impairments may not be able to provide a self-report in such cases, a combination of measures is used to validate the assessment. Behaviors such as facial grimacing, restlessness, moaning, muscle tension, tachycardia, tachypnea, and diaphoresis may be cues to unrelieved pain.[27–30]

Analgesics are the standard agents for managing pain in the terminally ill patient. Nonsteroidal antiinflammatory drugs have a limited role for treatment of mild to moderate pain and bone pain, and conservative use is recommended in the geriatric patient. Opioids, with the exception of meperidine, are the drugs of choice for moderate to severe pain, and antidepressants or anticonvulsants are used for neuropathic pain.[31,32]

The route is chosen according to patient characteristics and goals of analgesia, including the desired rapidity of response. Intravenous or subcutaneous administration affords the most rapid onset of action. Oral, sublingual, or buccal administration causes the least patient burden when there is an intact oral cavity. Transdermal medication is useful for long-acting, chronic analgesia; it should not be used as the first-line strategy, because of the long delay in onset of action, and or if the therapeutic dose has not been determined, as may be the case with an ED patient. The intramuscular route is discouraged because of poor absorption and patient discomfort.[31,32]

Analgesics are titrated according to the patient's responses; therefore, frequent reassessment to evaluate effectiveness is indicated. Although an individual patient may experience toxicity, there are no dose ceilings when using opioids, and titration to therapeutic effect may require high doses in patients with opioid tolerance or severe pain. Equianalgesia tables and consultation with pain specialists may be used to guide appropriate dosing.[31,32]

Like pain, dyspnea and any associated respiratory distress must be assessed frequently in high-risk patients, because many pulmonary, cardiac, and neuromuscular terminal illnesses produce breathing distress. The gold standard for this subjective experience is the patient's self-report, using either a numeric or a visual analog scale. Behavioral cues are useful if the patient is unable to self-report and include tachypnea, tachycardia, accessory muscle use, a paradoxical breathing pattern, restlessness, nasal flaring, and a fearful facial expression.[33]

Treatment of dyspnea or respiratory distress can be organized into three categories: prevention, treatment of the underlying cause, and palliation of symptom distress. Prevention of dyspnea in the dying ED patient warrants maximizing treatments that have proved beneficial to the patient, including enhancing ventilator synchrony if the patient is going to remain ventilated, avoiding volume overload, and continuing oxygen and nebulized bronchodilators. Measures to correct metabolic acidosis may also be useful to decrease the work of breathing and thereby decrease respiratory distress.

Treating underlying causes of dyspnea may be useful, particularly if the benefit of the treatment is not in disproportion to the burden. If death is not imminent, the patient may benefit from antibiotics, corticosteroids, paracentesis, pleurodesis, or bronchoscopy.

A number of strategies have demonstrated effectiveness for palliation of terminal dyspnea, including optimal positioning, oxygen, and sitting in front of a fan. Upright positioning that affords the patient an optimal lung capacity is useful, especially for patients with COPD.[34,35] Oxygen has been shown to be more effective than air in hypoxemic cancer patients[36,37] and in patients with advanced COPD.[38] However, other investigators reported no difference in cancer patients' respiratory comfort in response to oxygen compared with air,[39] and increased ambient air flow, fans, and cold air have also been found to be therapeutic.[40–43] Oxygen can be more burdensome than beneficial in the patient who is near death, particularly if a face masks is employed, because the mask produces a feeling of suffocation. The individual patient's report or behavior in response to oxygen determines its usefulness. The comatose patient does not require oxygen while dying.

Opioids are the mainstay of pharmacological management of terminal dyspnea, and their effectiveness has been demonstrated in clinical trials. A metaanalysis of 18 double-blind, randomized, placebo-controlled trials of opioids in the treatment of dyspnea from any cause revealed a statistically positive effect on the sensation of breathlessness ($P = 0.0008$). Metaregression indicated a greater effect in studies using oral or parenteral opioids than in studies using nebulized opioids. In subgroup analysis, the COPD studies had essentially the same results as the cancer studies.[44] In the ED, parenteral access is almost universal, obviating the need for other routes of administration except in special or unusual circumstances. Doses for treating dyspnea are patient specific, and, as with opioid use in the management of pain, no ceiling should be placed on dosage. The dose should be rapidly titrated until the patient reports or displays respiratory comfort. Frequent bedside evaluation to assess the efficacy of the medication is essential.

Fear and anxiety may be components of the respiratory distress experienced by the dying ED patient. The addition of a benzodiazepine to the opioid regimen has demonstrated success in patients with cancer[45] and with advanced COPD.[46] As with opioids, these agents should be titrated to effect. Care of the attendant family to reduce their fear, anxiety, and grief warrants as much effort as that directed to the patient's needs.

Family Presence

Studies have consistently demonstrated that families want to be close to their terminally ill loved ones.[47,48] Family access promotes cohesion, affords the opportunity for closure, and may soothe the patient. Unrestricted access of the family to the dying patient is a standard of care in hospitals and nursing homes.[49] The family of the patient who is dying in the ED should be afforded this same benefit. There is growing evidence and support for the successful implementation of families at the side of loved ones during resuscitation and invasive procedures in the ED.[50–53] It follows that if families and patients can be accommodated with open access to one another in the ED during procedures, then unrestricted visiting for the dying patient and grieving family is possible.

Ideally, the patient and family should be separated from the harried milieu of the ED while dying or waiting for a hospital bed, yet still visible and accessible for close monitoring and care. Movement to a quieter area in the ED, such as the observation care unit or an isolation room, may serve this purpose, particularly if there is space for a few chairs and the attendant family. Limiting visitors to only two at a time has no rationale if the patient is dying and there is a large, loving family.

Death Notification and Requests for Organ/Tissue Donation

Delivery of adverse diagnoses and death notification entails all of the communicative skills of the ED staff. A framework for communicating bad news is helpful. There are four temporally ordered segments in the approach to breaking bad news: the preparation, the content, the survivor's response, and the close.[54]

Key elements of the *preparation phase* include a private setting, with determination of what the family already knows about the illness or accident. Important elements of the *content phase* include including a "warning shot." For example, the physician might say, "There has been a factory accident, and I am sorry to say that I have bad news." The news should then be stated clearly: "Your husband died in the accident." Drawn-out deliveries may be more comfortable for the staff, but they are not helpful to the anxious family member.[55]

In order to cast death notification in an easily learned format, similar to the way other procedures are taught, a procedural competency model has been developed.[56] The steps are summarized in Table 46–2.

Deaths that are out of cycle (e.g., death at a young age), out of context (e.g., death was not expected because oncologist overestimated length of life remaining), or sudden are the hardest for families to bear. Ideally, contact information for bereavement counselors or for support groups in the community should be given to the family.

Federal law (Public Law 99-5-9; Section 9318) and Medicare regulations mandate that hospitals give surviving family members the chance to authorize donation of their family member's organs and tissues. Most families are receptive to requests for donation, and many take consolation in helping others despite their own tragic loss. Studies show that it is essential to approach relatives for this purpose only after death notification is completed, allowing a temporal separation between death notification and the request for organs. Also, a higher response rate is obtained if the requesting personnel have received specific training for this purpose.[57,58]

Table 46–2
Elements of an Empathic Death Disclosure

Introduce self/role.

- Sit down.
- Assume comfortable communication distance.
- Tone/rate of speech acceptable.
- Make eye contact.
- Maintain open posture.

Give advance warning of bad news.

- "I'm afraid I have bad news."

Deliver news of death clearly.

- Use direct terms such as "dead" or "died."
- Use no medical jargon.
- Use language that is clear and easily understood.

Tolerate survivor's reaction.

Explain medical attempts to "save" patient.

Offer viewing of deceased.

Offer to be available to survivor.

Conclude appropriately.

- Offer condolences and leave.

Source: Quest et al. (2002), reference 56. Copyright 2002, with permission from The Society for Academic Emergency Medicine.

One of the most difficult tasks caregivers must complete is to witness the acute grief reaction of the family after they have received the news of unexpected death. The newly bereaved is literally broken from the world in which he or she formerly lived. There is often an unreal feeling of disbelief or suspension in time and insulation from place. The bereaved can feel hopeless, frustrated, and oftentimes very angry. It is important for the caregiver to "stay with" the bereaved during this initial grief reaction, which can be brief or last for several minutes. If duties prevent staying put, then the caregiver should most definitely return after the bereaved's initial emotions have subsided. It is only then that the bereaved family member is able to reengage in rational thought, and at that point he or she needs answers to when, where, what, and how questions about the death. Reassurances about the patient's not having suffered, if based in reality, may prove helpful to the bereaved.[59]

A fine tradition from the U.S. military mandates that an officer and aid (a team) stay with the bereaved family until they are released. Although this may be harder to achieve in the ED, the same sense of solemn duty could be embraced by staff members performing death notification. The tone of voice, words, bearing, and demeanor of the individual performing death notification will be seared into the mind and hearts of the bereaved forever. Death notification is an immense responsibility and must be done well. Family witness to resuscitation efforts is an alternative method of death disclosure. The bad outcome and the intensity of life-saving efforts are communicated over a period of 20 minutes rather than 2 minutes.

Care of the Body

It is commonly accepted that long-term outcomes are better for those who are able to see the deceased body of a loved one. Viewing the body helps those who are grieving acknowledge and begin to come to terms with the death.[60] If the death is expected, the body should be bathed and laid out neatly on the stretcher with the eyes closed, and the preparation should be completed before the family arrives. Families who are present at the time of death may want to participate in body preparation. In some cultures, rituals at the time of death require family involvement and should be accommodated within reason in the ED. For example, in some Moslem traditions the body is turned to face east, and persons of the same gender and religion as the deceased perform the postmortem care. Some families may want private time with the body of the deceased, but others may want a supportive person from the hospital staff, such as a nurse, aide, or chaplain, to remain in attendance.[61]

If the death is unexpected, such as from an accident or sudden illness, the family who are arriving at the ED need a different approach to viewing the body. After learning of the death, the family may demonstrate an urgency to see the body, and delays for cleaning and laying out may produce more distress; likewise, not seeing the body because of disfigurement or mutilation causes distress to the bereaved.[60] Seeing the deceased and the evidence of the injury or accident, along with the accoutrements of the attempts at resuscitation, gives a subliminal message to the family that the ED staff did all they could. The ED nurse should allow the family access to the deceased at the earliest possible opportunity and should use judicious draping to cover the most severe disfigurements.

CASE STUDY
HP, a Victim of a Motorcycle Accident

While riding his motorcycle, HP was hit by a truck and dragged. He sustained a closed head injury, a severe scalp laceration, comminuted fractures of both femurs and of the left humerus, rib fractures bilaterally, and a ruptured spleen. He died in the ED during trauma resuscitation.

The frantic family arrived at the hospital shortly after death was pronounced and screamed to see the patient. The resuscitation room looked like a tornado had touched down, with empty supply wrappers, intravenous fluid bags, and soiled dressings on the counters and floor. The deceased was bloody, with his torn clothing partially removed or cut off, and bone was protruding from his left arm and both legs. He had bilateral chest tubes, a Foley catheter, three large-bore Angiocaths, and an endotracheal tube that had to remain in place for the medical examiner.

The nurse recognized the family's need to see the body as quickly as possible. She enlisted a nurse's aide to rapidly reduce the amount of debris on and around the stretcher. She draped the body to cover the worst injuries, including the exposed bones, and washed the deceased's face and hands. A hand towel covered the scalp wound without covering the face. Within five minutes the nurse had prepared the body and room for the family.

The nurse escorted the weeping family to see the body and remained unobtrusively nearby in case anyone fainted. She also answered questions about the injuries and the magnitude of the efforts to resuscitate. Later, after the family was more composed, the nurse explained the procedures for referral to the county medical examiner and the need to identify a funeral home. She also gave the family the business card of a trauma counselor who specialized in bereavement counseling. The nurse found a quiet, private place for the family to wait until they reached an emotional calm that would allow them to drive home safely.

The use of cadavers to practice procedures such as endotracheal intubation in the ED has been commonplace as an integral part of resident training.[62] Current ethical norms do not permit this practice without contemporaneous consent from the surviving family or evidence from a patient's AD that this would be acceptable. Consent is standard elsewhere in health care, and respect for the newly dead and for the survivors warrants this same standard.[63] Recent legal cases have held that families have property rights to the bodies of their loved ones, and the use of cadavers without consent poses a liability risk.[64] Studies show that most patients or families are willing to have procedures performed after death if permission is obtained in advance.[65,66] An empathetic expression of condolences, followed by a sensitive request to permit procedures, may yield the teaching–learning opportunity while demonstrating respect for the deceased and their family.

Summary

Dying care in the ED can be complicated by the milieu and by the usual "resuscitative" expectations of this environment. A default view of ED success is whether the patient left the ED with a pulse. The fact that a growing number of patients are presenting to the ED at the end of life demands palliative care competency by ED staff. In most EDs, there are clinicians who are willing to guide terminally ill patients or their surrogates toward a palliative care approach, in which success is redefined as preventing suffering and enabling a good death.

The paucity of patients with written ADs or advance planning for the terminal illness necessitates rapid establishment of treatment goals with the dying patient or surrogate in the ED. This is accomplished through compassionate communication about diagnosis and prognosis and recommendations for a palliative care treatment focus.

An abundance of evidence about managing pain and dyspnea is available to guide the ED staff in reducing symptom distress. Likewise, optimal caring for the grieving family has been informed by research and includes effective communication about prognosis or death notification and timely access to the patient before or after death.

Personal and professional satisfaction with comprehensive dying care in the ED can be achieved by ED staff. Compassionate recommendations made to decrease suffering and ensure respect for the dying patient afford the survivors a positive experience, even in the face of loss.

REFERENCES

1. Centers for Disease Control and Prevention, National Center for Health Statistics. Health, United States, 2004, With Chartbook on Trends in the Health of Americans. Hyattsville, MD: Author, 2000:293, http://www.cdc.gov/nchs/data/hus/hus04.pdf (accessed March 16, 2005).
2. Karpiel M. Improving emergency department flow: Eliminating ED inefficiencies reduces patient wait times. Healthcare Executive 2004;19(1):40–41.
3. Lunney JR, Lynn J, Hogan C. Profiles of older Medicare decedents. J Am Geriatr Soc 2002;50:1108–1112.
4. Seale CL, Addington-Hall J, McCarthy M. Awareness of dying: Prevalence, causes, and consequences. Soc Sci Med 1997;45:477–485.
5. Fanslow J. Needs of grieving spouses in sudden death situations: A pilot study. J Emerg Nurs 1983;9:213–216.
6. Parrish GA, Holdren KS, Skiendzielewski J, Lumpkin OA. Emergency department experience with sudden death: A survey of survivors. Ann Emerg Med 1987;16:792–796.
7. Walters DT, Tupin JP. Family grief in the emergency department. Emerg Med Clin North Am 1991;9:189–206.
8. Adamowski K, Dickinson G, Weitzman B, Roessler C, Carter-Snell C. Sudden unexpected death in the emergency department: Caring for the survivors. CMAJ 1993;149:1445–1451.
9. Lipton H, Coleman M. Bereavement practice guidelines for health care professionals in the emergency department. Int J Emerg Ment Health 2000;2:19–31.
10. Williams AG, O'Brien DL, Laughton KJ, Jelinek GA. Improving services to bereaved relatives in the emergency department: Making healthcare more humane. Med J Aust 2000;173:480–483.
11. Schears RM. Emergency physicians' role in end-of-life care. Emerg Med Clin North Am 1999;17:539–559.
12. Marco CA, Bessman ES, Schoenfeld CN, Kelen GD. Ethical issues of cardiopulmonary resuscitation: Current practice among emergency physicians. Acad Emerg Med 1997;4:898–904.
13. Marco CA, Larkin GL, Moskop JC, Derse AR. Determination of "futility" in emergency medicine. Ann Emerg Med 2000;35:604–612.
14. Patient Self Determination Act 1990, incorporated into the Omnibus Budget Reconciliation Act 1990, 42 U.S.C. 1395 cc (a).
15. Lynn J, Schuster JL, Kabcenell A. Improving Care for the End of Life. New York: Oxford University Press, 2000.
16. Lahn M, Friedman B, Bijur P, Haughey M, Gallagher EJ. Advance directives in skilled nursing facility residents transferred to emergency departments. Acad Emerg Med 2001;8:1158–1162.
17. McCauley WJ, Travis SS. Advance care planning among residents in long-term care. Am J Hospice Palliat Care 2003;20:353–359.

18. Bruera E, Miller L, McCallion J, Macmillan K, Krefting L, Hanson J. Cognitive failure in patients with terminal cancer: A prospective study. J Pain Symptom Manage 1992;7:192–195.
19. Minagawa H, Uchitomi Y, Yamawaki S, Ishitani K. Psychiatric morbidity in terminally ill cancer patients: A prospective study. Cancer 1997;78:1131–1137.
20. Pereira J, Hanson J, Bruera E. The frequency and clinical course of cognitive impairment in patients with terminal cancer. Cancer 1997;79:835–842.
21. Dudgeon DJ, Kristjanson L, Sloan JA, Lertzman M, Clement K. Dyspnea in cancer patients: Prevalence and associated factors. J Pain Symptom Manage 2001;21:95–102.
22. Hall P, Schroder C, Weaver L. The last 48 hours of life in long-term care: A focused chart audit. J Am Geriatr Soc 2002;50:501–506.
23. Klinkenberg M, Willems DL, van der Wal G, Deeg DJH. Symptom burden in the last week of life. J Pain Symptom Manage 2004;27:5–13.
24. Nelson JE, Meier DE, Oei EJ, Nierman DM, Senzel RS, Manfredi PL, Davis SM, Morrison RS. Self-reported symptom experience of critically ill cancer patients receiving intensive care. Crit Care Med 2001;29:277–282.
25. Morrison RS, Ahronheim JC, Morrison GR, Darling E, Baskin SA, Morris J, Choi C, Meier DE. Pain and discomfort associated with common hospital procedures and experiences. J Pain Symptom Manage 1998;15:91–101.
26. Puntillo KA, White C, Morris AB, Perdue ST, Stanik-Hutt J, Thompson CL, Wild LR. Patients' perceptions and responses to procedural pain: Results from Thunder Project II. Am J Crit Care 2001;10:238–251.
27. Puntillo KA, Morris AB, Thompson CL, Stanik-Hutt J, White CA, Wild LR. Pain behaviors observed during six common procedures: Results from Thunder Project II. Crit Care Med 2004;32: 421–427.
28. Allen RS, Haley WE, Small BJ, McMillan SC. Pain reports by older hospice cancer patients and family caregivers: The role of cognitive functioning. Gerontologist 2002;42:507–514.
29. Krulewitch H, London MR, Skakel VJ, Lundstedt GJ, Thomason H, Brummel-Smith K. Assessment of pain in cognitively impaired older adults: A comparison of pain assessment tools and their use by nonprofessional caregivers. J Am Geriatr Soc 2000;48: 1607–1611.
30. Manz BD, Mosier R, Nusser-Gerlach MA, Bergstrom N, Agrawal S. Pain assessment in the cognitively impaired and unimpaired elderly. Pain Manage Nurs 2000;1:106–115.
31. American Pain Society. Principles of Analgesic Use in the Treatment of Acute Pain and Cancer Pain, 5th ed. Glenview, IL: American Pain Society, 2003.
32. World Health Organization. Cancer Pain Relief and Palliative Care. Geneva: WHO, 1990.
33. Campbell ML. Terminal dyspnea and respiratory distress. Criti Care Clin North Am 2004;20:403–417.
34. Barach AL. Chronic obstructive lung disease: Postural relief of dyspnea. Arch Phys Med Rehab 1974;55:494–504.
35. Sharp JT, Drutz WS, Moisan T, Foster J, Machnach W. Postural relief of dyspnea in severe chronic obstructive lung disease. Ame Rev Respir Dis 1980;122:201–211.
36. Bruera E, de Stoutz N, Velasco-Leiva A, Schoeller T, Hanson J. Effects of oxygen on dyspnoea in hypoxaemic terminal-cancer patients. Lancet 1993;342:13–14.
37. Bruera E, Schoeller T, MacEachern T. Symptomatic benefit of supplemental oxygen in hypoxemic patients with terminal cancer: The use of N of 1 randomized control trial. J Pain Symptom Manage 1992;7:365–368.
38. Swinburn CR, Mould H, Stone TN, Corris PA, Gibson GJ. Symptomatic benefit of supplemental oxygen in hypoxemic patients with chronic lung disease. Am Rev Respir Dis 1991;143: 913–915.
39. Booth S, Kelly MJ, Cox NP, Adams L, Guz A. Does oxygen help dyspnea in patients with cancer? Am J Respir Crit Care Med 1996;153:1515–1518.
40. Burgess KR, Whitelaw WA. Reducing ventilatory response to carbon dioxide by breathing cold air. Am Rev Respir Dis 1984; 129:687–690.
41. Burgess KR, Whitelaw WA. Effects of nasal cold receptors on pattern of breathing. J Appl Physiol 1988;64:371–376.
42. Liss HP, Grant BJB. The effect of nasal flow on breathlessness in patients with chronic obstructive pulmonary disease. Am Rev Respir Dis 1988;137:1285–1288.
43. Schwartzstein RM, Lahive K, Pope A, Weinberger SE, Weiss JW. Cold facial stimulation reduces breathlessness induced in normal subjects. Am Rev Respir Dis 1987;136:58–61.
44. Jennings AL, Davies AN, Higgins JP, Gibbs JS, Broadley KE. A systematic review of the use of opioids in the management of dyspnoea. Thorax 2002;57:922–923.
45. Ventafridda V, Spoldi E, De Conno F. Control of dyspnea in advanced cancer patients. Chest 1990;98:1544–1545.
46. Light RW, Stansbury DW, Webster JS. Effect of 30 mg of morphine alone or with promethazine or prochlorperazine on the exercise capacity of patients with COPD. Chest 1996;109: 975–981.
47. Hampe SO. Needs of the grieving spouse in a hospital setting. Nurs Res 1975;24:113–120.
48. Steinhauser KE, Christakis NA, Clipp EC, MdNeilly M, McIntyre L, Tulsky JA. Factors considered important at the end of life by patients, family, physicians, and other care providers. JAMA 2000;284:2476–2482.
49. Fins JJ, Peres JR, Schumacher JD, Meier C. On the Road from Theory to Practice: A Resource Guide to Promising Practices in Palliative Care Near the End of Life. Washington, DC: Last Acts National Program Office, 2003.
50. Boudreaux ED, Francis JL, Loyacano T. Family presence during invasive procedures and resuscitations in the emergency department: A critical review and suggestions for future research. Ann Emerg Med 2002;40:193–205.
51. Helmer SD, Smith RS, Dort JM, Shapiro WM, Katan BS. Family presence during trauma resuscitation: A survey of AAST and ENA members. J Trauma 2000;48:1015–1021.
52. MacLean SL, Guzzetta CE, White C, Fontaine D, Eichhorn DJ, Meyers TA, Desy P. Family presence during cardiopulmonary resuscitation and invasive procedures: Practices of critical care and emergency nurses. J Emerg Nurs 2003;29:208–221.
53. Williams JM. Family presence during resuscitation: To see or not to see? Nurs Clin North Am 2002;37:211–220.
54. Lamont EB, Christakis NA. Complexities in prognostication in advanced cancer. JAMA 2003;290:98–104.
55. Iverson KV. Grave Words. Tucson, Ariz.: Galen Press Ltd., 1999.
56. Quest TE, Otsuki JA, Banja J, Ratcliff JJ, Heron SL, Kaslow NJ. The use of standardized patients within a protocol competency model to teach death disclosure. Acad Emerg Med 2002;9: 1326–1333.
57. DeJong W, Franz HG, Wolfe SM, Nathan H, Payne D, Reitsma W, Beasley C. Requesting organ donation: An interview

study of donor and nondonor families. Am J Crit Care 1997;7:13–23.

58. Garrison RN, Bentley FR, Rague GH, Polk HC Jr, Sladek LC, Evanisko MJ, Lucas BA. There is an answer to the shortage of donor organs. Surg Gynecol Obstet 1991;173:391–396.
59. Fraser S, Atkins J. Survivors' recollections of helpful and unhelpful emergency nurse activities surrounding sudden death of a loved one. J Emerg Nurs 1990;16:13–16.
60. Haas F. Bereavement care: Seeing the body. Nurs Stand 2003; 17(28):33–37.
61. Campbell ML. Grief: Family needs. In: Campbell ML. Forgoing Life-Sustaining Therapy: How to Care for the Patient Who Is Near Death. Aliso Viejo, CA: American Association of Critical Care Nurses, 1998, pp 123–137.
62. Fourre MW. The performance of procedures on the recently deceased. Acad Emerg Med 2002;9:595–598.
63. Berger JT, Rosner F, Cassell EJ. Ethics of practicing medical procedures on newly dead and nearly dead patients. J Gen Intern Med 2002;17:774–778.
64. Moore GP. Ethics seminars: The practice of medical procedures on newly dead patients—Is consent warranted? Acad Emerg Med 2001;8:389–392.
65. Alden AW, Ward KLM, Moore GP. Should post-mortem procedures be practiced on recently deceased patients? A survey of relatives' attitudes. Acad Emerg Med 1999;6:749–751.
66. Manifold CA, Storrow A, Rodgers K. Patient and family attitudes regarding the practice of procedures on the newly deceased. Acad Emerg Med 1999;6:110–115.

47

Betty R. Ferrell, Gloria Juarez, and Tami Borneman

The Role of Nursing in Caring for Patients Undergoing Surgery for Advanced Disease

At least I'll have a chance of being cancer free. Well, at least somewhat cancer free before the next bombardment, since its obviously, its obviously a virus that I just can't fight off. My immune system has been so compromised that I just can't fight the cancer off. . . . With the surgery, they told me I won't be in remission again. I'll be in transition.—A patient

- ***Key Points***
- *Patients and their family caregivers facing surgery for advanced disease have complex physical and psychosocial problems.*
- *Patients and family members require support as they make decisions regarding the benefits and burdens of treatments for advanced disease.*
- *Palliative surgeries affect physical, psychological, social, and spiritual well-being as well as additional health system outcomes.*

CASE STUDY

Rosa Hernandez, a 38-Year-Old Woman with Cancer of the Gallbladder

Rosa Hernandez is a 38-year-old Hispanic woman who resided in Southern California for the past 8 years, having previously lived her entire life in Mexico. She is married to Juan, and they have four children ranging in age from 6 to 17 years. Three months ago, she began to experience numerous gastrointestinal symptoms including bloating, mild nausea, abdominal pains, and severe indigestion. After trying numerous over-the-counter medications and herbal treatments, she sought medical evaluation and was diagnosed with cholangiocarcinoma. She and her family were drawn to the University Cancer Center, in part because a cousin who had been diagnosed with acute leukemia several years previously had been very successfully treated at this center and cured of his leukemia. They came to the Cancer Center with great confidence that Rosa would also be cured of her disease. The surgeon explained the seriousness of her cancer in the gallbladder and the widespread metastases to the liver. When offered treatment choices, Rosa and Juan as well as their large extended family aggressively voiced their desire for all treatments possible and repeatedly expressed their confidence in the surgical team and staff to save her life.

The surgeon explained that the procedure planned, resection of the tumor and partial liver resection, was not curative but might offer some relief for her symptoms. Juan expressed that they had faith in God and the surgeon. The evening nurse caring for Rosa, Emily James, approached the patient late one evening to discuss the surgical consents for the procedure planned the following day. Rosa told Emily that she had no questions and would sign the consents because she was eager to get rid of the cancer in her body.

This case illustrates the numerous complexities of caring for patients with advanced disease for whom surgical treatment may be an option. The nurse is faced with caring for a patient with advanced cancer and a poor prognosis yet both the patient and family are expecting a "miracle." There are many complex cultural and social factors affecting her decisions for care as well. The nurse is challenged to work with the patient, her family, the physician, and other interdisciplinary colleagues to provide the best information and support for this family, while also anticipating the many immediate postoperative needs as well as the longer-term symptom management and disease issues. This case is but one example of the incredibly complex and challenging needs of patients undergoing surgery for advanced disease.

Decision-Making in Palliative Surgery

Patients facing advanced disease are often in the position of making difficult choices with regard to treatments. Patients often face that critical juncture of determining when they should continue disease-focused treatments such as chemotherapy, radiation, or surgery and when it is time to stop such treatments. Even amid the recognition of advanced disease, patients often seek aggressive treatment with the hope of prolonging their survival, even if only for a matter of months, or of possibly enhancing their quality of life (QOL) through the relief of symptoms.[1–3]

Figure 47–1 is derived from research in the area of palliative surgery conducted at the City of Hope National Medical Center (COH).[4] The model demonstrates that the process of making decisions about palliative surgery often involves influences from the patient, the family, and the health care team. Patients and families must weigh the potential benefit versus the harm of the surgery proposed, while the health care team considers factors such as the difficulty of the procedure, the duration of hospitalization, recovery time, chance of achieving the goal, anticipated durability of the intervention, and anticipated disease progression. It becomes evident in reviewing these factors that much of the decision-making involves great individual variation, so that it is difficult to estimate who might benefit most from more aggressive intervention. For example, the patient with a poor prognosis due to an extremely advanced gastrointestinal tumor, who subsequently lives twice the original duration anticipated, may well have been the patient who

Figure 47–1. Clinical decision-making in palliative surgery. *Source:* Ferrell et al. (2003), reference 4.

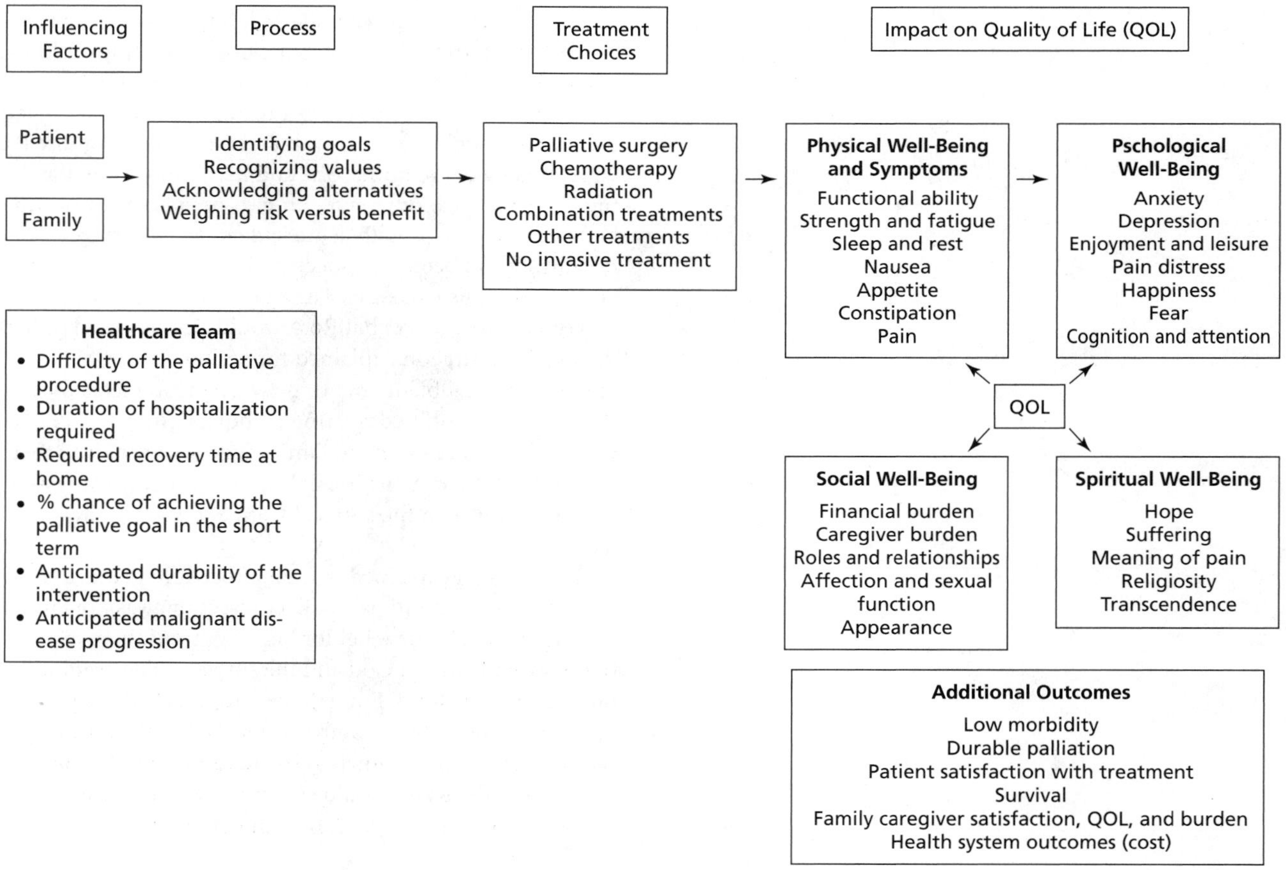

could have benefited from surgery to relieve obstruction for abdominal pressure causing severe nausea, vomiting, or bowel problems.

The process of making decisions involves a focus on goals of care, recognizing the values of the patient, acknowledging alternatives, and always weighing the risks versus benefits.[5,6] As surgeries have become more advanced in technique, it is often possible to do very extensive surgery on an outpatient basis or with very short hospitalization time. This reduced "burden" makes it more likely that patients may opt for surgical procedures. Given the many symptoms or problems resulting from advanced disease, patients consider a variety of treatment choices, including surgery, chemotherapy, radiotherapy, or a combination of treatments.

The outcomes of this process of decision-making are depicted in Figure 47–1 as affecting all dimensions of QOL. Physical well-being and symptoms, as well as function, are almost always affected by treatment choices.[7] Psychological well-being, including anxiety and depression as well as fears, is also influenced by treatment choices.[8] Patients and families have often reflected that, although a particular treatment may have not prolonged survival, it gave them a tremendous sense of assurance that everything possible was being done to treat the illness. In the realm of social well-being, the choices of treatments have very significant impacts on the patient's roles and relationships as well as the burden on caregivers.[9–11]

Although invasive, "high-tech" treatments may often be thought of as adding to the caregiver burden, in advanced disease the failure to aggressively treat problems commonly results in heightened burden. For example, a patient who declines surgery relatively early in the course of an advanced gastrointestinal tumor may then experience much worse nausea, vomiting, diarrhea, and subsequent complications that could result in a more intense caregiver burden than would have been required after earlier surgery.

Finally, spiritual well-being is greatly influenced by decisions regarding palliative surgery, because patients rely upon their faith and religion in making treatment choices.[1,2] One of the strongest themes throughout palliative care research at the COH has been the concept of hope.[2] This concept is covered in greater detail in Chapter 26, but it certainly applies closely to the topic of palliative surgery. Patients may perceive that surgery, even if presented as only palliative in nature, is still potentially curative or life-prolonging, and therefore may opt for surgery with unfounded hope for a cure.[12,13]

The model in Figure 47–1 illustrates how important it is for nurses to provide education, counseling, and support as patients and families wrestle with treatment choices. It also is not uncommon for patients and families to have different perspectives and conflicting opinions. For example, a patient with advanced disease may opt for no further invasive treatments and instead focus on measures of comfort. At the same time, family members may press for the patient to endure continued procedures for even the smallest possibility of prolonged survival.

Research in Palliative Surgery

There has been limited research in the field of palliative care and even far more limited focus on the area of palliative surgery. Recent studies have begun to document both the lack of research in the field and the limitations of existing research.[14–16] Leaders in the field of palliative surgery have documented that few studies evaluating these procedures have included measures of patient QOL, symptom management, or psychosocial concerns.[17–19]

Research in the area of palliative surgery was initiated at the COH in 2000, and since that time a series of studies has been conducted involving collaboration between the Department of Nursing Research and the Department of Surgery. Table 47–1 summarizes phases of this research thus far. The studies have included a review of surgical cases to determine the extent of palliative surgery use at a cancer center, which was followed by a prospective review of cases that led to research evaluating decision-making by patients and family members.[20] In order to broaden understanding of palliative surgery beyond one cancer center, phase III involved a survey of 419 surgeon members of the Society of Surgical Oncology.[21,22] A very important finding of this research was the identification of ethical dilemmas faced by surgeons, such as providing patients with honest information without destroying hope and preserving patient choices.

These early studies have led to clinical investigations exploring symptom management and QOL outcomes, as well as longitudinal measures, in an effort to capture the effects of palliative surgery and its potential impact on symptoms and QOL.[23] These studies have also provided an opportunity to incorporate qualitative methods for exploration of patient and family caregiver experiences.[1,2]

Patient Perspectives

The research at COH has explored patient perspectives of surgery through in-depth individual interviews conducted preoperatively and postoperatively, as well as assessment of symptoms and QOL. Table 47–2 includes some representative comments from patients' perspectives of QOL after surgery. As this study demonstrated, patients may believe that surgery is their only option to avoid progression and eventual death from their disease. The presence of physical symptoms has been found to be a key motivator for seeking surgical intervention. Even those patients who recognize that surgery is not curative may aggressively seek surgical approaches to relieve distressing physical symptoms such as pain, gastrointestinal symptoms, bleeding, odors, and other problems. These studies also demonstrated that tremendous psychological stress and anxiety are induced by the need to make decisions about surgical options. Having surgery in advanced disease seems to be a stark reality given the extent of the disease. Also, it is not uncommon to find evidence during the surgery of far more advanced disease than was originally known.

Table 47–1
Description of Program of Research

Phase I

Surgical Palliation at a Cancer Center (Krouse et al. [2001], reference 25)

Design: Retrospective review of surgical cases ($n = 1915$) during a 1-year period with a 1-year survival follow-up. This descriptive study began exploration of the extent of palliative surgery and identification of patient outcomes.

Key Findings: Palliative surgeries (PS) comprised 240 (12.5%) of 1915 surgical procedures. There were 170 major and 70 minor procedures. Neurosurgical (46.0%), orthopedic (31.3%), and thoracic (21.5%) surgical procedures were frequently PS. The most common primary diagnoses were lung, colorectal, breast, and prostate cancers. Length of hospital stay was 12.4 days (range, 0–99 days). Mortality was 21.9% for surgical procedures classified as major and 10.0% for those classified as minor. The investigators concluded that in significant numbers of PS mortality was high; however, a significant number of patients had short hospital stays and low morbidity. PS should remain an important part of end-of-life care. Patients and their families must be aware of the high risks and understand the clear objectives of these procedures.

Phase II

Advancing the Evaluation of Palliative Surgery for Cancer Patients (Krouse et al. [2002], reference 20)

Design: Prospective review of PS ($n = 50$). Pilot testing of interview guide for use with patients/family caregivers and surgeons to explore decision-making and goals.

Key Findings: Prospective design allowed expansion of outcomes to include quality of life (QOL) and exploration of the involvement of family caregivers.

Phase III

Indications and Use of Palliative Surgery—Results of Society of Surgical Oncology (SSO) Survey (McCahill, [2002a and 2002b], references 21 and 22)

Design: Mailed survey (110 items) of members of the SSO ($n = 419$ responses). This phase was intended to provide a national perspective on the topic of PS and to expand knowledge of surgeons' decision-making.

Key Findings: Surgeons estimated 21% of their cancer surgeries as PS in nature; 43% of respondents believed PS was best defined based on preoperative intent, 27% based on postoperative factors, and 30% on patient prognosis. Only 43% considered estimated patient survival time an important factor in defining PS, and 22% considered 5-year survival rate important. Patient symptom relief and pain relief were identified as the two most important goals in PS, with increased survival the least important. On a scale of 1 (uncommon problem) to 7 (common problem), surgeons reported that the most common ethical dilemmas in PS were providing patients with honest information without destroying hope and preserving patient choice. On a scale of 1 (not a barrier) to 7 (severe barrier), surgeons rated the most severe barriers to optimum use of PS as limitations of managed care and referral to surgery by other specialists. The least severe barriers were surgeon avoidance of dying patients and surgery department reluctance to perform PS.

Phase IV

A Prospective Evaluation of Palliative Outcomes for Surgery of Advanced Malignancies (McCahill, [2003], reference 23)

Design: Prospective evaluation of patients undergoing PS ($n = 59$) with longitudinal measures for 1 year. Outcomes were expanded to provide more detailed evaluation of symptom management and QOL. Qualitative evaluation included in-depth interviews of patients, family caregivers, and surgeons before and after surgery to further describe decisions and outcomes related to surgery.

(continued)

Table 47–1
Description of Program of Research *(continued)*

Key Findings: Preoperatively, surgeons identified 22 operations (37%) as PS, 37 (63%) as curative. Thirty-three patients (56%) were symptomatic preoperatively, and symptom resolution was documented in 79% surviving >30 d. Good to excellent palliation, defined as "more than 70% symptom-free non-hospitalized days relative to postoperative days of life," was achieved in 53% of PS patients. Among patients with postoperative survival <6 mo, 63% had good to excellent palliation. The majority of symptomatic patients undergoing major surgery for advanced malignancies attained good to excellent symptom relief. The researchers concluded that outcome measurements other than survival are feasible and are likely to play an important role in defining surgery as an important component of multimodality palliative care.

Phase V

A Comparison of Resource Consumption in Curative and Palliative Surgery (Cullinane et al. [2003], reference 19)

Design: Prospective evaluations of all surgeries performed over a 3-month period ($n = 302$) with 6-month follow-up. The investigators extended the outcomes of surgery to be evaluated based on Phases I–IV.

Key Findings: Over a 4-month period, the outcome and service needs of 302 consecutive patients with malignancy undergoing surgeon-defined PS or curative surgery were evaluated. Previous treatment history, comorbidities, symptoms, procedures, outcome, and use of supportive services were collected. Patients were monitored for 6 months after the surgical procedures performed for cure (breast or prostate cancer) or for palliation (breast, lung, and bone/soft tissue tumors). There were 3 (1%) curative and 4 (6%) palliative deaths during the surgical admission. Mean hospital stay was 5.1 days (range, 0–58 days) for curative surgery patients and 1.9 day (range, 0–34 days) for PS patients. After discharge, a total of 4690 encounters with the cancer center occurred, including 1676 encounters with surgery, 1595 encounters with medical oncology, 1006 encounters with radiation oncology, 226 visits to medical specialists, and 187 visits with supportive services. Mean number of encounters for curative and PS patients were 15 and 17, respectively, ($P = 0.41$). Curative patients were more likely to have visits with therapeutic intent, including chemotherapy ($P = 0.01$) and radiation ($P = 0.003$). Readmission occurred in 82 (34%) of curative and 28 (48%) PS patients during the 6-month period ($P = 0.04$). PS patients were more likely to be admitted for symptom management ($P < 0.0001$), whereas curative surgery patients were more likely to be admitted for repeat procedures ($P = 0.006$).

Phase VI

Concerns of Family Caregivers of Cancer patients Facing Surgery for Advanced Malignancies (Borneman et al. [2003], reference 1)

Design: Family caregivers were assessed before planned PS and at 2 weeks and 6 weeks after surgery. Quantitative assessment of caregiver QOL occurred at each time point. A subset of nine caregivers also participated in a structured interview before surgery and at 2 weeks after surgery.

Key Findings: The study findings indicate important family caregiver QOL concerns and needs for support at the time surrounding surgery for advanced disease. Psychological issues were most pronounced with common needs of uncertainty, fears regarding the future, and loss. Family caregivers voiced concerns about surgical risks and care after surgery and experienced recognition of the patient's declining status. The investigators concluded that surgery is an important component of palliative care and is an area requiring further research and clinical attention.

Family Caregivers

The palliative surgery research at the COH has also described the concerns of family caregivers of patients undergoing palliative surgeries for advanced malignancies. Family caregivers ($n = 45$) were assessed before planned palliative surgery and at 2 weeks and 6 weeks after surgery.[5] Quantitative assessment of caregiver QOL occurred at each interval. A subset of nine caregivers also participated in structured interviews before surgery and 2 weeks after surgery. Caregiver concerns, QOL, and decision-making were evaluated. Findings of the study indicated that family caregivers have important QOL concerns and needs for support before and after surgery for advanced disease. Psychological issues were most pronounced, and

Table 47–2
Patient Perspectives on Quality of Life and Surgery

Surgery-Only Option

"Because this is one of the slower—slower growing cancers, radiation and chemo wouldn't have helped at all. So there was—there was no option other than—other than the surgery—there was no option."

Gastrointestinal Symptoms

"I used to always, I had the constant urge that I was going to have a bowel movement. Well, I did not have a bowel movement, but, and this urge is so strong I, I'd go in and sit on the toilet. And then, of course, I would pass some mucus and stuff. Um, there for a while before the surgery, oh, it was just terrible. And a lot of it would be quite bloody. And, ah, you know, I had a good day yesterday. I had a good night last night and the night before that I had a good night."

Psychological Well-Being

"But now I feel even the surgery's not complete. I still have my tumor in my kidney. But that is not operable based on what [the doctor] told me. Just, just a few alternatives. You know, it's a surgery, remove the whole kidney? Or do the gene therapy? Or do the freezing or burn technique, you know. So there's still a chance."

Postsurgery Quality of Life

"Yeah. Every time my friend, or whoever, has cancer, I told them don't give up. Find an alternative. If you're rejected by this doctor, don't just give up. Keep on trying whatever possible, whatever you have to go through. So, that's the only way. A lot of my friends are cancer patients. When they come to the end of the tunnel, they don't know how to do and they are so depressed, I say don't worry. We already have the problem. You got to face it. Your worry doesn't help. You know, you got to ask God to give you a day. Use the medical technology available . . . Somebody may save you. You know, a miracle. This could happen to you, too. It happened to me many times."

Source: Ferrell et al. (2003), reference 4.

common concerns included uncertainty, fears regarding the future, and loss.

Family caregivers had concerns about surgical risks and patient care needs after surgery and voiced recognition of the declining status of patients. The needs of family caregivers are multiple and complex, requiring ongoing assessment to provide interventions that help them cope and ultimately improve their QOL. This important topic requires further research and clinical attention.

Table 47–3 includes examples of family caregivers' perspectives provided both preoperatively and postoperatively. Families articulated their concerns about the surgery and its risks and in fact were more concerned than patients about potential negative consequences of surgery.[5] Family members often discussed the benefits of surgery, with a strong sense from both patients and family caregivers that surgery is always a good option because "to take it out" must increase one's chance for survival. For family members, however, the postoperative period was most often one of incredible stress as they faced the reality that the patient's prognosis was not likely to have changed and

Table 47–3
Family Caregivers' Perspectives

Preoperative

Concerns about Surgery and Risks

"I'm scared. I worry about just him getting through it . . . for the first few days, I'll still be worried, and I'll just be glad when he comes home. I'll be glad to do anything, you know, just to have him come home again. I know it's good to know the truth, and I'm glad that [the doctor] was so up front with us. But it's just so hard to deal with. Surgery's very scary. The chemotherapy and radiation was not scary. I knew he would get sick, but I knew that there was no chance of him dying from it. This is a whole different animal."

Benefits of Surgery

"I think it's a good thing. Because, you know, your immune system concentrates on, like, if you have a tumor, they concentrate all over the body. By taking this out, this is a big thing that, you know, it has cancer in it. By taking that out I feel like maybe her body can concentrate on other parts a little bit better than with, you know, with this in her. And then they're going to take the one out of her hip and I, I think it's a good thing. I'm glad that she's having the surgery."

Postoperative

No Change in Prognosis

"It was more of a quality-of-life thing. They'd like to get her eating, like to get her home. Like to get her spending her time in a way that she finds, you know, enjoyable. But, um, they're not planning on curing her or anything like that, I think she is aware of the prognosis. But, you know, like she said, she wants to still be in the treatment category more than, she doesn't want hospice at this point. So, although she knows that, she's not ready to just say that's it and prepare to die. She's wanting to do whatever she can to keep going."

Uncertain Survival

"The last day, of course, he was sleeping. I couldn't stand to even see him because his eyes were all swollen and his face was all swollen. But he never woke up on that second day anyway. That very morning, [the doctor] told me that it would be a long, slow recovery, but he was going to do okay and he had a 50-50 chance that morning. And that was at about 9 o'clock in the morning. And at 7 o'clock that night, [the doctor] told me he wasn't going to make it through the night. Do you know how that can throw a person emotionally? Do you? You have no idea what kind of an emotional roller coaster I was on for those 13 days. One day, everything's looking better. The next day everything was just horrible. I'm surprised I didn't end up having a heart attack myself or a nervous breakdown."

Source: Borneman et al. (2003), reference 1.

that surgery may in fact have revealed more evidence of advanced disease. For many patients, the surgical experience became a "roller coaster," in which they grasped for hope for a cure from surgery, even if intended as palliative, but the hope was balanced by recognition of the patient's decline in status.

Nursing Care of Patients Undergoing Palliative Surgery

The care of patients undergoing palliative surgery is often focused more on the medical aspects, yet nursing care is essential throughout all phases of preoperative, intraoperative, immediate postoperative, and postoperative recovery and discharge. This is a critical time, with numerous transitions between care settings, and nurses can play a vital role in ensuring continuity across settings such as the operating room, intensive care unit (ICU), postoperative surgical unit, and home care. A prime example is the role of nursing in ensuring pain management by assessing a patient's chronic pain problem at the time of admission to plan adequate analgesia as the patient is admitted for surgery. The nurse then works collaboratively with the physician and the pharmacist to plan the analgesic orders for the transition from the oral analgesics used preoperatively to an appropriate regimen after surgery. Additional monitoring is needed, because the patient's pain may escalate after major surgery, and also to ensure the appropriate changes as the patient goes from chronic oral medications at home to parental administration in the postoperative period and in the ICU. Maintaining adequate analgesia after discharge from the ICU, onto the postoperative unit and then to home care, is essential for the patient's timely discharge to home and remains a requirement during recovery. This simple example of just one aspect of care, pain management, illustrates the vital role of nursing during this very acute phase of treatment.

Patients with advanced disease often undergo surgery with the goal of palliation to achieve a longer survival, even when cure is not a realistic goal. The following case illustrates this point:

CASE STUDY

Carl Freedman, a 52-Year-Old Man with Colon Cancer

Carl Freedman is a 52-year-old African American man with stage IV colorectal cancer who has previously undergone surgery for bowel resection followed by chemotherapy. After a prolonged postoperative course and extensive recovery phase, Mr. Freedman was able to resume his work as a maintenance man in a local school. He was admitted to the hospital 2 days ago with signs of bowel obstruction accompanied by symptoms of nausea, vomiting, abdominal pain, and dehydration. On evaluation, Mr. Freedman was found to have a recurrence of the bowel cancer and adhesions with partial obstruction in the bowel. The surgical team meets with Mr. Freedman and his wife to explain the significance of the recurrent cancer and the bowel obstruction and to offer some alternatives for treatment. Because of the location of the obstruction and extent of disease, the surgeon presents nonsurgical approaches, including the use of octreotide and bowel rest, as well as the option of surgery to remove part of the tumor and adhesions. But the surgeon is honest in discussing with Mr. Freedman and his wife the finding that the cancer has metastasized to the liver, that the procedure would not be curative, and, indeed, that his prognosis has now worsened. Mr. Freedman and his wife have a strong faith and believe that "God will guide you, Dr. Barnes, and His hands will help you get the entire tumor." They also say, however, that their most important goal is to see Mr. Freedman live until the graduation of his son from college in 4 months. They explain that this is a particularly significant event, given that their son will be the first in the family to have completed college.

This case illustrates the role of palliative surgery and the benefit of extending patient survival to achieve life goals even if a cure is not possible. Nurses would play a vital role in Mr. Freedman's care, including aggressive management of his existing symptoms and additional psychosocial support required at this critical time in his illness, as he and his family confront the reality of his worsening disease. Continued attention would also be needed after surgery to monitor Mr. Freedman's progress. For example, if his disease progressed more rapidly or if he developed postoperative complications that could lead to shorter survival, it might be necessary to work with the family to realize what choices they could make if indeed he did not live to see the graduation. Supporting Mr. Freedman's faith and the spiritual crisis that might develop if he believed that God had failed him would be essential. This case also illustrates the vital role of nurses in monitoring patients after surgery to assist with transitions to home care/hospice or palliative care programs.

The Goal of Symptom Relief

The following case study illustrates the goal of symptom relief in palliative surgery.

CASE STUDY

Bonnie Crate, an 83-Year-Old Woman with Sarcoma

Bonnie Crate is an 83-year-old Native American woman who was diagnosed with sarcoma approximately 1 year ago. She had experienced severe pain in her shoulder and arm but did not seek medical care; rather, she relied on traditional Native American healers and treatments, believing that her pain was "old age" and arthritis. When she developed severe neuropathy in her hand and was no longer able to cook or care for her grandchildren, she sought medical assistance and was informed of her diagnosis. She opted for supportive care only and initially was not interested in the possibility of surgery or chemotherapy; however, she did want aggressive symptom management with a goal of reducing her pain and maintaining her function "to be a grandmother as long as possible." Bonnie has now moved from her rural tribal community into the home of her daughter in the metropolitan area. Bonnie was seen by the pain and supportive care service at the hospital. However, after numerous attempts at multiple analgesics, treatment of neuropathic pain, unsuccessful attempts at both oral and parenteral analgesics, and a brief trial of epidural analgesia and nerve blocks, the team was unsuccessful in achieving pain relief without excessive side effects.

Bonnie is evaluated by surgery staff, and an option is presented that would involve amputation of her arm for the relief of the pain. On initial presentation of the option her children become extremely agitated saying "Are you crazy?! Why would you take off the arm of an 83-year-old woman?" However, Bonnie tells her children that she will do anything to get some relief from the pain, and with only one arm she could still hold a grandchild. The nurse practitioner in the surgical clinic meets with the patient and family, along with the surgeon, to describe the procedure and the expected postoperative course.

Bonnie undergoes surgery and does extremely well in the postoperative period. She is discharged 1 week later with plans for follow-up evaluation by occupational therapy and return to the pain and symptom clinic for continued monitoring of her symptoms.

This case illustrates the role of surgery in relieving severe symptoms that have been unresponsive to less aggressive means. It also illustrates the importance of evaluating the patient's goals of care and circumstances and that quite often surgical intervention, although considered to be invasive or aggressive, may be the best option even in the face of advanced disease.

Psychosocial Issues Affecting Palliative Surgery

Patients facing advanced disease and critical associated decisions related to treatment options also present with complex psychosocial and spiritual needs. The following case illustrates complex issues in patients who are torn between the desire to survive and weariness and readiness for life's end.

CASE STUDY

Alexandra Nopteski, a 63-Year-Old Woman with Colon Cancer

Alexandra Nopteski is a 63-year-old Russian immigrant residing in Southern California. She and her husband immigrated to the United States approximately 20 years ago and began a janitorial service cleaning office buildings. They are very proud parents of three children, all of whom have completed college. The family has been very prosperous and approximately 5 years ago became U.S. citizens. Three years ago, Alexandra's husband died suddenly from a myocardial infarction. She and the children were devastated, and she has been moderately depressed since that time. Approximately 1 year ago, Alexandra developed cancer of the colon and underwent surgery and radiation therapy, with numerous postoperative complications including a chronic problem with abscess formation and fistulas. She has had a fairly sharp decline in status over the last 6 months.

Alexandra has made her wishes very clear: she does not want life-sustaining treatment and does not want further chemotherapy or radiation therapy. She has felt very sad about the burden that she believes is imposed on her children and wants for them to be able "get on with their lives in America and not be burdened by me." Over the past month, Alexandra has developed heavy rectal drainage which is resulting in constant soiling of her clothing and a very offensive odor. The oncology surgeon has recommended a surgical procedure to remove some of the abscess and fistula areas to eliminate or reduce this problem. Alexandra agrees to the surgery but is somewhat hesitant. She mentions to the nursing assistant that she had hoped that it wouldn't come to this, stating, "I think I'm dying from the inside out." The surgical resident comes to obtain her consent for the surgical procedure. She becomes extremely angry and hostile when the resident informs her that her "do-not-resuscitate" order will have to be rescinded for her to have surgery, because it is the hospital's policy that all patients entering surgery are at full code status. Alexandra tells the resident that she and her deceased husband will haunt him for the rest of his career if he should "rob her the opportunity to die" if God deems it should be so during surgery. The resident leaves very shaken, and the nurse comes to the bedside to talk with her. Alexandra is not to be consoled, saying she still wants the surgery, but she can't imagine that the surgeons would want to resuscitate her if the need should arise during surgery. After she becomes much calmer, she admits to the nurse, "On the other hand, I wish that maybe my heart would stop during surgery so that it would be easier for everyone if I could die quickly rather than prolonging this agony."

The case of Mrs. Nopteski illustrates the complexities of dealing with patients with advanced disease. Cultural, spiritual, and psychosocial issues are important influences. This case also illustrates the importance of nursing leadership in creating policies and procedures that support the goals of palliative care. Many institutions have eliminated their requirement for full code status on patients undergoing surgery and instead now honor the request to avoid resuscitation even if its need should occur during surgery. Mrs. Nopteski's clinical signs of depression are also important to evaluate in considering her overall plan of care. A patient's wish for death should never be dismissed, and such information should be shared with the surgical staff. Instances such as this are also primary examples for incorporating psychiatry or psychology: evaluation of her depression is essential, and attention to her emotions would be needed before the surgery as well as in the follow-up period. Nurses play a critical role in attending to the communication around this issue and in acting as the patient's advocate in all stages of care and across settings.

Summary

Palliative nursing care extends across all treatment modalities, and patients undergoing surgery require intensive support and care. Nurses play a critical role in patient and family communication, establishing goals of care and expert management of symptoms. There is a need for continued research to address this area of palliative care and for continued advancements of clinical nursing expertise to best serve these patients and families.[24–26]

REFERENCES

1. Borneman T, Chu DZJ, Wagman L, Ferrell BR, Juarez G, McCahill LE, Uman G. Concerns of family caregivers of patients with cancer facing palliative surgery for advanced malignancies. Oncol Nurs Forum 2003;30:997–1005.
2. Borneman T, Stahl C, Ferrell BR, Smith D. The concept of hope in family caregivers of patients with cancer at home. J Hospice Palliat Nurs 2002;4:21–23.
3. Angelos P. Palliative philosophy: The ethical underpinning. Surg Oncol Clin North Am 2001;10:31–38.
4. Ferrell BR, Chu DZJ, Wagman L, Juarez G, Borneman T, Cullinane C, McCahill LE. Patient and surgeon decision making regarding surgery regarding advanced cancer. Oncol Nurs Forum 2003;30:E106–E114.
5. Miner TJ, Jaques DP, Shriver C. Decision making on surgical palliation based on patient outcome data. Am J Surg 1999;177: 150–154.
6. Miner TJ, Jaques JP, Shriver CD. A prospective evaluation of patients undergoing surgery for the palliation of an advanced malignancy. Ann Surg Oncol 2002;9:696–703.
7. Burke CC. Surgical treatment. In: Miakowski C, Buchsel P, eds. Oncology Nursing: Assessment and Clinical Care. St. Louis, MO: Mosby, 1999, pp 29–58.
8. Milch RA, Dunn GP. Communication: Part of a surgical armamentiarium. J Am Coll Surg 2001;193:449–451.
9. Andrews SC. Caregiver burden and symptom distress in people with cancer receiving hospice care. Oncol Nurs Forum 2001;28: 1469–1474.
10. Given BA, Gicen CW, Kozachik S. Family support in advanced cancer. CA: A Cancer J Clin 2001;51:213–231.
11. Langenhoff BS, Krabbe PF, Wobbes T, Ruers TJ. Quality of life as an outcome measure in surgical oncology. Br J Surg 2001;88: 643–652.
12. Bottorff JL, Steele R, Davies B, Garrossino C, Porterfiels P, Shaw M. Striving for balance: Palliative care patients' experiences of making everyday choices. J Palliat Care 1998;14:7–17.
13. Bruera E, Sweeney C, Calder K, Palmer L, Benisch-Tolley S. When the treatment goal is not cure: Are cancer patients equipped to make informed decisions? J Clin Oncol 2001;20: 503–513.
14. Velovich V. The quality of quality of life studies in general surgical journals. J Am Col Surg 2001;193:288–296.
15. Dunn GP. The surgeon and palliative care. Surg Oncol Clin North Am 2001;10:7–24.
16. Easson AM, Crosby JA, Librach SL. Discussion of death and dying in surgical textbooks. Am J Surg 2001;182:34–39.
17. American Colleges of Surgeons. Principles of care at end of life. Bull Am Coll Surg 1998;83:46.
18. Cassel C, Foley K. Principles for care of patients at the end of life: An emerging consensus among the specialties of medicine. Report sponsored by The Milbank Memorial Fund. December 1999. Available at: htpp://www.milbank.org/ (accessed February 5, 2005).
19. Cullinane A, Borneman T, Smith DZJ, McCahill L, Ferrell BR, Wagman LD, et al. The surgical treatment of cancer. Cancer 2003;9:2266–2273.
20. Krouse R, Ferrell BR, Nelson RA, Juarez G, Wagman LC, Chu D. Advancing the Evaluation of Palliative Surgery for Cancer Patients. Unpublished manuscript, 2002.
21. McCahill LE, Krouse R, Chu DZJ, Juarez G, Uman GC, Ferrell BR, et al. Indications and use of palliative surgery: Results of Society of Surgical Oncology survey. Ann Surg Oncol 2002a;9:104–112.
22. McCahill LE, Krouse RS, Chu DZJ, Juarez G, Uman GC, Ferrell BR, et al. Decision making in palliative surgery. J Am Coll Surg 2002b;195:411–423.
23. McCahill LE, Smith D, Borneman T, Juarez G, Cullinane C, Chu DZJ, Ferrell BR, Wagman LD. A prospective evalutation of palliative outcomes for surgery of advanced malignancies. Ann Surg Oncol 2003;10:654–663.
24. Foley KM, Gelbrand H. Improving Palliative Care for Cancer. Washington, DC: National Academy Press, 2001.
25. Krouse RS, Nelson RA, Ferrell BR, Grube B, Juarez G, Wagman, LD, Chu DZ. Surgical palliation at a cancer center: Incidence and outcomes. Arch Surg 2001;136:773–778.
26. McCorkle R, Strumpf NE, Nuamah IF, Adler DC, Cooley ME, Jepson C, Lusk EJ, Torosian M. A specialized home care intervention improves survival among older post-surgical patients with cancer. J Am Geriatr Soc 2000;48:1707–1713.

48

Virginia Sun

Palliative Chemotherapy and Clinical Trials in Advanced Cancer: The Nurse's Role

I wanted to give chemo another chance because I am never one to give up easily. This time around, it's not the chemo that scares me; it's what comes along with it—the side effects. I don't want to die from the side effects.—A patient

- ***Key Points***
- *Patients with advanced cancer are often caught between the dichotomy of continuing aggressive treatment and the focus on quality supportive and palliative care.*
- *Faced with difficult decisions, patients and families become especially vulnerable and may experience heightened physical, psychological, social, and spiritual distress.*
- *Palliative chemotherapy uses systemic antineoplastic agents to treat symptoms of incurable malignancies and maintain quality of life.*
- *Nurses can help alleviate suffering by supporting patients and families through changes in treatment intent, the decision-making process, and supportive care needs during palliative chemotherapy.*

Nurses have always been in the forefront of managing treatment-related symptoms. In an ever-changing and complex health care setting, optimal care requires a transdisciplinary approach. This approach is especially valued in an oncology setting, where patients frequently present with complex disease- and treatment-related symptoms. These often debilitating symptoms negatively affect the quality of life (QOL) of patients and their extended families.[1] For patients with advanced cancer, treatment options are often limited. It is usually at this stage of the cancer continuum that discussion of palliative modalities of treatment occurs. These palliative modalities often include, but are not limited to, radiation, surgery, and chemotherapy. It is also during this stage of the continuum that physicians discuss the use of investigational therapeutic agents as an attempt to control the disease. However, it is not uncommon for patients and families to be faced with difficult decisions. Patients with advanced cancer are often caught between the dichotomy of continuing aggressive treatment and the focus on quality supportive and palliative care.[2] The debate of treatment futility often comes into play at this stage of the cancer continuum, because patients and families are faced with a shorter life expectancy and all standard therapeutic regimens have failed to control the spread and proliferation of the tumor itself. Faced with these difficult decisions, patients and families become especially vulnerable and may experience heightened physical, psychological, social, and spiritual distress.[3]

In advanced malignancies, the choice between palliative chemotherapy, clinical trial, or best supportive care may be difficult. This chapter describes the use of chemotherapy and cancer investigational agents as a palliative treatment for patients with advanced cancer. Emphasis is placed particularly on the role of palliative chemotherapy and the dichotomy between clinical trials of cancer investigational therapeutic agents and palliative care. Finally, an in-depth analysis of the role of nurses in supporting patients and families receiving palliative chemotherapy or investigational agents through clinical trials is discussed.

Definitions

Palliative chemotherapy, in its broadest sense, is the use of systemic antineoplastic agents to treat an incurable malignancy.[4] In most medical literature, the efficacy of palliative chemotherapy is reported through data regarding tumor response rate, duration of response, and survival benefit.[5] However, the purpose of these studies usually is not the investigation of these agents for palliation of symptoms, even though most subjects accrued into these clinical trials are deemed incurable.[6] It is only in recent years that symptom palliation has become an important aspect in the design and evaluation of cancer clinical trials. The majority of the symptom palliation research incorporated into therapeutic clinical trials focuses on QOL as a prognostic factor for better patient outcomes.[7] Other, more specific definitions used to describe palliative chemotherapy include the relief of cancer-induced symptoms.[4,8] This refers to the use of antineoplastic agents with the expectation of prolonged survival and improved QOL, which includes the relief and prevention of adverse symptoms that are indicative of advanced malignancies.[4,8]

Curative versus Palliative Chemotherapy

As a primary therapy, chemotherapy may be potentially beneficial in the prolongation of survival in the advanced stages of cancer. However, the majority of malignancies in adults are incurable with chemotherapy. Although the development of adjuvant chemotherapy has resulted in a decrease in recurrence rates, the data show that there is no significant difference in disease-free survival.[4] Therefore, the majority of patients living with cancer will experience recurrence of disease, and it is this population that may also receive palliative chemotherapy.

When the disease has metastasized to other organ systems, the primary goal of using chemotherapy in advanced disease is to control the patient's symptoms and maintain QOL.[8] The rationale for palliating direct or indirect symptoms of cancer is multifaceted, but it is important for practitioners to remember that not all patients are suitable for palliative chemotherapy. Standard chemotherapy should not be offered to all patients with metastatic malignancies. A predicted toxicity of treatment should preclude any consideration for the use of palliative chemotherapy.[4,8] The benefit-to-toxicity ratio of treatment should be seriously considered. Never should subtherapeutic doses of chemotherapy be given to maintain hope in a patient's prognosis.[8] Such a false sense of hope may prove to be even more distressing and may induce tremendous suffering for patients and families.

Several prognostic factors have been used in chemotherapeutic treatments of cancer to determine palliative treatment modality. One of the most important prognostic factors is performance status.[4] A severely debilitated patient with a restricted performance status is more likely to sustain excessive chemotherapy toxicity. The site of metastasis outside the primary tumor can also be prognostic of patient response to symptoms related to treatment.[8] These tumor-specific prognostic factors are crucial because they can assist nurses in defining an incurable disease.

The decision to treat or not to treat is based not only on clinical indicators but also on the patient's perspective. Chemotherapy involves a commitment on the part of the patient and family to travel to the treating institution on a scheduled basis. Repeated hospitalizations, venipunctures, cannulations, investigations, and assessments over and beyond the actual administration of chemotherapy are inevitable routines of cancer treatment. These factors need to be addressed with patients and families in an effort to facilitate the decision-making process.

Quality of Life Concerns in Palliative Chemotherapy

The assessment of QOL has increasingly become a key measure in cancer clinical trials, in conjunction with other measures such as tumor response, disease-free survival, and overall survival.[9] Some of the parameters commonly included in QOL measurement tools are factors that affect the quality of a patient's physical, psychological, social, and spiritual well-being.[4] QOL should be used clinically to weigh the benefit-to-toxicity ratio of palliative chemotherapy. Aside from assessing antitumor effects and the toxicity of chemotherapy, the overall positive or negative impact of the treatment on QOL must also be addressed.[10] An ideal situation in which palliative chemotherapy might be beneficial is one in which the treatment does not alter survival duration but does positively affect QOL.[8]

Very few prospective studies have investigated the QOL benefits of supportive care versus a combination of palliative chemotherapy plus supportive care for the management of advanced, incurable malignancies. The average prolongation of survival with chemotherapy compared with best supportive care has not been fully described in literature. An increasing number of studies have reported the potential palliative benefits of chemotherapy.[11–17] Shanafelt and colleagues[18] performed a systematic analysis of 25 randomized, controlled clinical trials comparing cytotoxic chemotherapy with best supportive care. Sixteen of the clinical trials involved patients with non-small-cell lung cancer. The results indicated that there is a modest relationship between response rate and both median and 1-year survival rate for non-small-cell lung cancer patients treated with cytotoxic chemotherapy.[18]

A meta-analysis of randomized clinical trials of best supportive care versus chemotherapy for unresectable non-small-cell lung cancer was performed to allow for better determination of the actual statistical significance of the treatment effect.[19] There was a survival benefit in the range of 6 to 10 weeks for those patients treated with palliative chemotherapy. However, this benefit was seen only in patients who had an adequate performance status. Patients with Eastern Cooperative Oncology Group (ECOG) performance status of 3 or 4 had no benefit from chemotherapy.[19] In summary, it appears that palliative chemotherapy is effective only for a select group of patients in the lung cancer population. A strong predictor of positive treatment benefit is related to the patient's performance status.[19]

In a study of patients with unresectable metastatic or locally advanced non-small-cell lung cancer, subjects were randomly assigned to receive either best supportive care or two different chemotherapy regimens ($n = 150$).[20] Survival was 8 to 15 weeks longer for the chemotherapy + supportive care arm, but improved survival was observed only in patients who had a high ECOG performance status (0 or 1) and a weight loss of <5 kg. Moreover, about 40% of subjects were judged to have sustained severe, life-threatening, or lethal toxicities.[20] Very few patients showed improvement in performance status or gained weight during chemotherapy treatment.[20]

The QOL of family caregivers was addressed in a study to compare the impact of cancer caregiving in curative and palliative settings.[21] Family caregivers of patients receiving palliative care had significantly lower QOL scores and lower overall physical health scores.[21] There was no additional significant variability in caregiver QOL scores after adjustments for patient performance status and treatment status. These results suggest that patients' poor performance status is a predictor of low QOL in the palliative care setting that also affects caregivers' QOL.[21] The data reinforce the importance of supporting families as well as the impact on their QOL and on the patient's well-being when the treatment intent is palliative.

When and How Long to Treat?

Multiple factors need to direct the decision-making process when considering palliative chemotherapy for patients with advanced cancer. The goal at this juncture in the cancer continuum is to relieve or prevent tumor-induced symptoms, with the potential of prolonging survival.[8] Patients who are symptomatic from malignancy, and those who are expected to be symptomatic soon, are typically considered for treatment initiation within a few days or weeks.[4] This indication for palliative chemotherapy, although proven to be somewhat beneficial for effective palliation in oncologic emergencies, is appropriate for only selected patients.[4] Local treatments with palliative radiation or surgery are also common treatment modalities in advanced malignancies.

A more difficult scenario of whether to delay or begin palliative chemotherapy occurs with patients who are asymptomatic from malignancy. In these circumstances, especially with tumor types that are less responsive to chemotherapy, the general consensus is that the benefit-to-toxicity ratio may be more heavily weighted toward the toxicity side.[4] In such situations, treatment may be withheld and the patient closely monitored until symptomatic progression is evident.

CASE STUDY

Mrs. G, a Patient with Pancreatic Cancer

Mrs. G is a 72-year-old retired special education teacher who was diagnosed with pancreatic cancer 2 months ago. At the time of diagnosis, her disease had metastasized to her liver and lung. She has been fairly asymptomatic except for some dyspnea on exertion, which has caused her to cease her nightly walks around the block with her Chihuahua. She has been wheelchair bound since diagnosis due to her decreasing energy level. Mrs. G's daughter, who lives nearby and visits frequently, and her husband, who last year suffered a severe case of pneumonia, have encouraged her to be aggressively treated. She was started on palliative chemotherapy with weekly gemcitabine. Within 2 weeks, her platelet count dropped, and her energy level significantly decreased to the point where she had trouble with activities of daily living. Her daughter temporarily moved in to assist her in daily tasks. Mrs. G continued on the treatment with dose reductions and schedule changes for another 4 weeks and was then referred to hospice. She passed away at home after 1 week of hospice referral, with her husband, daughter, and dog at her side.

In this case, a focus on watchful waiting or aggressive supportive care was indicated. In general, pancreatic cancer is not a very chemosensitive tumor. Mrs. G's performance status was low; therefore, she could be anticipated to experience more difficulties with treatment side effects. The treatment schedule was also too intense given her performance status. As a result, Mrs. G suffered from a further decrease in functional status and also severe thrombocytopenia. In such cases, the health care team should provide the patient's family with adequate information regarding the pros and cons of palliative chemotherapy at this stage of the cancer trajectory. The team should emphasize that supportive care is aggressive treatment, as well as focusing on symptom management and comfort.

Decision-Making: Accept, Reject, or Continue

After the initial shock of receiving a cancer diagnosis, patients and families must battle anxiety-provoking concerns such as dying from the disease, financial burdens, disease-related pain, and treatment-related toxicities. Chemotherapy is often perceived as an extremely toxic treatment by the general public.[22] These concerns are very much related to patient and family decision-making processes, especially when the intent to treat is to palliate symptoms. Slevin and associates[23] investigated the differences between patients' attitudes to either mild or intensive cancer chemotherapy and the attitudes of health care providers such as physicians and nurses. Cancer patients were more likely to accept intensive treatment with debilitating toxicities in exchange for an extremely small probability of cure, prolongation of life, and symptom relief.[23] Medical oncologists were more likely to accept aggressive treatment than were general practitioners. Oncology nurses, not surprisingly, were more divided on the aggressiveness of treatment. The nurses' perceptions fell between aggressive treatment and wanting more information on the benefit-to-toxicity ratio.[23]

Silvestri and coworkers[24] conducted a study to determine how patients with advanced non-small-cell lung cancer value the tradeoff between the survival benefit of chemotherapy and its toxicities. Data were qualitatively collected through the use of three scripted scenarios. Patients' willingness to accept chemotherapy varied widely ($n = 81$). Many would choose chemotherapy for a likely survival benefit of 3 months only if the treatment positively affected QOL as well.[24] The investigators found that the conflict between patients' preferences and the actual care they received greatly affected their decision-making. It appears that some patients did not receive the treatment they would have chosen had they been fully informed in their previous choice of treatment.[24]

Koedoot and colleagues[25] investigated patient treatment preferences and decision-making processes in regard to palliative chemotherapy or best supportive care. The actual treatment decision was the main outcome of the study. At baseline, the majority of subjects preferred to undergo chemotherapy rather than watchful waiting.[25] The majority of subjects also eventually chose treatment with chemotherapy. Treatment preference and a deferring style of decision-making were predictors of actual treatment choice. Treatment preference is positively explained by striving for length of life and negatively by striving for QOL.[25] The results indicated that it is still questionable whether the purpose of palliative chemotherapy is made clear to patients. This emphasizes the need for health care providers to attach further attention to the process of information-giving and shared decision-making in patients with advanced cancer.[25]

The Role of Nurses in Palliative Chemotherapy

The incorporation of chemotherapy into the palliative care setting has been shown through randomized clinical trials and meta-analyses to have survival benefits for patients with advanced cancer whose disease is incurable. However, these benefits are seen only in patients with higher baseline performance status and in those who are asymptomatic from their metastatic malignancies. Hence, it is evident that palliative chemotherapy, although effective in palliating certain disease-related symptoms, has limited benefits for all advanced cancer patients. Therefore, it is important for nurses, as integral team members in the transdisciplinary approach of oncology palliative care, to support patients and families through the difficult path of answering the quintessential question: to treat or not to treat? Nurses can help alleviate further anguish and suffering for patients with advanced cancer and their families in three crucial areas related to palliative chemotherapy: change in treatment intent, decision-making, and supportive care through treatment choice.

Change in Treatment Intent

When curative intent of treatment becomes impossible, practitioners should begin to address the intent to treat as palliation of disease-related symptoms. This initial communication is traditionally the domain of the treating physician. However, with more and more collaborative practices emerging between nurses, advanced practice nurses (APNs), and physicians, it is becoming apparent that a transdisciplinary approach offers the best support for patients and families during this difficult and vulnerable time.[1] Communication of difficult news should best be conducted in a prearranged consultation session in which the treating physician, nurse, and social worker together deliver the information to the patient, the family, and other individuals who are integral to the decision-making process. Nurses can foster this transdisciplinary approach of delivering difficult news through collaboration and communication with experts across disciplines. Nurses are often the first to recognize the need for dialogue between the health care team and the patient/family regarding treatment intent and prognosis.[26] Hence, nurses can advocate for patients by recommending and organizing these important communication sessions in order to alleviate unnecessary suffering for patients and families.

CASE STUDY
Mr. L, a Patient with Metastatic Esophageal Cancer

Mr. L, a 56-year-old Hispanic man who emigrated from Mexico City to the United States 20 years ago, has metastatic esophageal cancer. He has been treated with first-, second-, and third-line palliative chemotherapy. He wanted to be aggressive with treatment despite his poor prognosis. Functionally, he has been doing well, and his disease- and treatment-related symptoms have been well controlled. He maintains a positive outlook on life and wants to remain functional as long as possible. Mr. L has a G-tube through which he receives all his nutrition and food due to severe dysphagia. A recent computed tomographic scan revealed progressive disease despite third-line palliative chemotherapy. Mr. L speaks some English and is accompanied by his wife, who speaks no English, and his daughter, who speaks fluent English, to talk with the health care team about the next steps in his treatment regimen.

In this case, a consultation session is warranted. The objective of the session is threefold: (1) to present the difficult news of further disease progression and failure of third-line treatment; (2) to reevaluate treatment intent; and (3) to make recommendations for treatment. An interpreter should be at hand during the session to make sure that the patient and the family understand the situation. Before divulging the difficult news, it is important to assess for cultural needs in terms of communicating bad news. The health care team should understand how much information patients want to know and how much they already know. This assessment guides the consultation session. If supportive care experts such as a psychologist or chaplain are not available to be present during the session, it is vital that they be accessible to intervene during this very difficult and sensitive time of the cancer trajectory.

Decision-Making

Once the change in treatment intent has been discussed, the next step is to guide patients and families through an informed decision-making process to either continue on aggressive treatment or focus on symptom relief. Again, this information should be delivered in a setting where all practitioners involved in the care of the patient and family are present. If this scenario is not possible, it is imperative for members of the health care team to communicate and follow-up with each other in regard to details of the information disclosed to the patient and family. In presenting this information, it is important to avoid the use of medical jargon and to use resources such as information leaflets and diagrams to assist the patient and family in informed decision-making.[8] Nurses, having expertise in educating patients and families, can facilitate the availability of these visual resources and present them to patients and families.

Some patients might find it helpful to meet other similar patients or to access supportive care services such as psychology or chaplaincy. Nurses can encourage and facilitate these desires by initiating referrals to these services. A compassionate and ethical approach to review the medical situation with the patient and family is essential to providing them with an informed assessment of possible treatment choices.[4] It is important to include in the treatment choices the use of hospice services and nonchemotherapy palliative care, depending on the patient's individual situation. Another important aspect to consider is the awareness of specific cultural needs and differences. Patient and family desires for open communication and participation in decision-making are greatly influenced by both ethnicity and religion, so it is important to assess these needs and ensure cultural sensitivity before presenting the information.[4]

When discussing the possibility of palliative chemotherapy as a treatment choice, it is essential, before presenting statistical evidence, to learn about other specific factors that may affect the decision-making process. Nurses can facilitate and perform the assessment to obtain this vital information. Questions should focus on the following factors: (1) questions and decisions that need to be addressed in the patient's or family's lives, (2) a special upcoming event or specific unfinished business that must be completed, and (3) fears about dying or spiritual issues that need interventions from other supportive care services.[4] Nurses can play a particularly important role in facilitating information gathering on the third factor: fear of dying and spiritual needs. Fear of dying and spirituality represent a much-ignored area in the general medical literature but have been shown to have significant impact on the QOL of cancer patients, especially when disease is incurable.[27] Nurses can facilitate the patient's and family's search for spiritual understanding of their situation and alleviate existential suffering by first acknowledging patient's fears and distress. Facilitation of open communication regarding existential suffering can help alleviate fears of dying.[27] Nurses must be compassionate listeners and allow patients and families a forum to discuss their deepest fears concerning the seemingly impending and inevitable terminality of their disease.

Supportive Care through Treatment Choice

If palliative chemotherapy is the treatment choice, support for patients and families through treatment becomes the most important objective for nurses. Education regarding the common and expected side effects of the specific chemotherapy regimens can foster a sense of control over symptom management and prevent unnecessary anxiety-provoking episodes related to poorly managed side effects. The use of written materials that list and explain common side effects can be helpful in facilitating the learning process for patients and families. Most importantly, nurses can assist in the continuous assessment of patient and family needs, focusing not only on the physical but also on the psychological, social, and spiritual domains.[26] Communication during this difficult and vulnerable phase of the disease trajectory is key to the success of quality cancer care. Nurses can serve as a bridge of communication by fostering continued dialogue on the goals of treatment between patients/families and the health care team. This bridge of communication, although often difficult to sustain, is essential in a truly transdisciplinary model of care. Open and clear communication among health care team members can guide the assessment of patient and family needs but can also alleviate suffering by maintaining consistency in the amount and types of information provided. Inconsistencies in vital communication factors in palliative chemotherapy, such as treatment intent, often create false hopes and distress for patients and families.[4]

If palliative chemotherapy is not the chosen plan of treatment, patients and families frequently experience a profound sense of abandonment.[4] This sense of abandonment is most often directed toward health care providers. Patients and families, after living through the initial treatment phase of the cancer trajectory wherein follow-up with physicians and nurses is routine, suddenly lose the security of being assessed on a regular basis. Nurses can assist in alleviating this sense of abandonment through reassurance that follow-up care will still be in place. If referral to hospice is warranted, nurses can act as a liaison to attending physicians and hospice services to foster a smooth transition between care settings and maintain continuity of care.

Clinical Trials and Advanced Cancer

Several reports published or commissioned by government advisory boards such as the National Cancer Policy Board and the Institute of Medicine noted that the quality of end-of-life care in the United States is seriously deficient.[6] Many oncology professional organizations assert that hospice is the best-developed model of end-of-life care in the U.S. health care delivery system.[6] Hospice offers quality palliative care using a transdisciplinary approach. With the rising interest in palliative care for terminally ill patients, there has also been a dramatic increase in interest regarding palliative care specifically for advanced cancer patients.

Patients with advanced cancer are often offered the opportunity to enroll in a phase I clinical trial. Although research on new therapeutic agents is crucial to the oncology specialty, it is not uncommon that patients who enroll in phase I trials are forced to forgo the utilization of services such as hospice and palliative care. This dichotomy is primarily a result of U.S. federal policy. Medicare and insurance policies deny hospice coverage to patients with terminal cancer who enroll as participants in phase I studies. Yet, it is precisely this population of cancer patients who would benefit from comprehensive palliative care. It is important to note that phase I studies are designed to determine the toxicity and maximum-tolerated dose of potential treatments, mostly for currently incurable cancers. These studies are not designed, and do not have the intended purpose, to have a therapeutic effect. In fact, studies have shown that therapeutic effects from cancer investigational therapeutic agents occur in only 2% to 4% of subjects enrolled in a phase I clinical trial.[28,29] It is also ironic that the entry criteria for phase I trials is similar to the disease state criteria for admission into hospice—but it is precisely this dichotomy that renders a patient ineligible for the quality palliative care services that hospice provides.[6]

Patients who enter investigational cancer trials participate, in part, because of protocol eligibility such as disease and functional criteria. Many advanced-stage cancer patients who make decisions to participate in cancer clinical trials are also characterized by a highly motivated personality. They feel that active treatment is best for them.[30] Other factors identified with enrollment may include altruism and the influence of the physician.[31] Patient expectations include a response to therapy, a reduction in symptoms, and improved and increased communication with their physicians.[32,33] Therapeutic efforts are often equated with superior QOL and are measured against no other options. By contrast, patients and families believe palliative care is a passive choice, the equivalent of "no care."

When faced with decision-making regarding their plan of care, patients with advanced incurable cancers often do not fully understand the choices that are available to them. Patients who would qualify for hospice services as regulated by Medicare have very little understanding of admission criteria and services rendered.[34] It is unlikely that patients who are potential study participants understand fully that to enroll in a clinical trial means that they must temporarily forgo the opportunity of receiving comprehensive palliative care.[6] Furthermore, there are no informed consent documents that disclose the risk of losing hospice benefits when enrolled in a clinical trial. Within the informed consent documents for cancer investigational therapeutic agents, there are no descriptions in the benefits and risks section that address the risk of temporarily losing hospice eligibility.[35] This loss of eligibility is not permanent; rather, patients and families can enroll and disenroll from hospice benefits whenever they choose. However, with the shortened life expectancy for advanced cancer patients, the decision to forgo palliative care at the initiation of investigational therapeutics is a crucial barrier to accessing aggressive supportive care at a time when patients and families need it the most.

Tensions Between Palliative Care and Clinical Research

Despite significant progress in research and treatments, the diagnosis of cancer creates fear and turmoil in the lives of every cancer patient and the family. Cancer disrupts all components of social integration—family, work, finances, and friendships—as well as the patient's psychological status. Over the extended course of the illness, physical changes and deterioration create multiple and complex demands on the patient and family. These demands, in conjunction with significant financial assaults, generate a negative synergy, which is often ignored in the care of patients with advanced disease.

Patients with advanced, incurable cancers are especially vulnerable and therefore have many unique needs in coping with their disease.[36] Hence, it is helpful to tailor treatment to the specific needs of each individual and family, in order to fulfill personal goals and maintain QOL. This is precisely what a comprehensive palliative care program can provide. At the same time, many patients faced with the terminality of their disease want and seek new innovative therapies. In the absence of further evidence-based and effective standard therapy, clinical trials offer a sense of hope for a potential cure.[36] But for patients who choose to participate in a clinical trial, there are often no guarantees of benefit, and there is the added possibility of harm and discomfort in the form of physical and psychological distress.

The impact of clinical trial participation on physical symptoms related to advanced cancer is complex, and there is a paucity of data regarding the extent of these symptoms.[36] Experimental agents, like standard treatment agents, cause side effects. The difference in the side effect profile of a well-established agent versus an experimental agent lies in the anticipation of symptoms. Well-established agents have well-documented side effect profiles that can be anticipated and predicted and therefore better controlled or even prevented in certain situations. The novelty of experimental agents, however, renders their side effects unpredictable. There is a tremendous amount of uncertainty about what effects an experimental agent might have on a particular patient.

Palliative care stands in contrast to disease-directed therapy at most cancer centers in the United States. The rift between them creates a dissonance for development of clinical research protocols and for recruitment of some groups of patients into cancer clinical trials. Only one third of all cancer patients receive formal palliative care through hospice, and often this occurs only in the final days of life.[37] Although advanced cancer should be a time of refocusing and resolution, the hospice referral process often occurs during crisis situations. As disease advances, a positive relationship exists between increased physiological symptom severity and the patient's level of emotional distress and overall QOL. An inability to complete end-of-life tasks may lead to patient dissatisfaction as well as complicated family/caregiver stress and grief after the death.[38,39] Yet, anecdotal evidence from clinical practice indicates that some patients will participation in investigational therapy precisely because they *do* recognize that QOL is mostly related to functional ability. These patients are unwilling to participate in clinical trials because they perceive that enhanced longevity is unlikely. This cohort of patients, therefore, is lost to clinical research.

Quality of Life Concerns for Clinical Trial Participants

Although the structure and requirement of a clinical trial protocol mandates the inclusion of a plan of action for unexpected physical symptoms, these plans often are focused on pharmacological interventions only. For example, if nausea and vomiting is an anticipated or expected side effect, a protocol of which antiemetic agents to use is written into the clinical trial protocol itself. However, the psychological and social distress from this side effect is not included in the plan. A clinical trial protocol generally does not include plans that specifically state the need for referrals to other allied health professionals such as palliative care specialists and psychologists.[6]

The psychological and cognitive symptoms of patients participating in research studies vary.[36] Some patients may be distressed to be told that they are not eligible for inclusion into clinical trials. Research subjects may also have difficulty when an experimental treatment fails, which often mandates the withdrawal of subjects from the treatment protocol. One potential advantage of enrollment in clinical trials is that several members of the research team care for these patients. There are regularly scheduled visits, and that attention may affect the patient's psychological well being. This added attention might lead to early detection of psychological symptoms that are indicative of depression, sadness, anxiety, or irritability.[36] Subtle changes in psychological effects might be readily detected by research personnel, and nurses are an integral part of this team. However, in order for this added attention to be beneficial to patients and families, it is important for research teams to work collaboratively with allied health professionals and palliative care specialists to address concerns in all areas of patient and family well-being.

Economic demands and caregiving needs may also be affected by clinical trial participation. Financial burdens may be increased for clinical trial participants even if the experimental agents are provided free of charge. The usual intensive monitoring and testing that can sharply increase with participation in clinical trials may not be covered by either the trial budget itself or the patient's insurance. The frequent visits for treatment, physician assessment, and various other procedures that are often mandated in clinical trial protocols may incur further economic burdens in terms of expenses for travel and room and board.[36]

The needs of caregivers and families may also change with clinical trial participation. Families experience tremendous physical, psychological, social, and spiritual concerns that are related to the patient's well-being. Physical symptoms such as fatigue can plague caregivers and families who are faced with the complex care of patients with advanced cancer.[21] The complexity of navigating through the health care and insurance systems can place tremendous burdens on patients and caregivers both. Social exposure may be diminished for caregivers, because much of their days are spent on caring for their loved ones.[21] Finally, the agony of being a witness to a loved one's suffering and the prospect of grief and bereavement in terminal illness may present caregivers with spiritual and existential distress.

Attending to the spiritual and existential needs of patients with advanced cancer is an important factor in the overall experience of patients and families facing the inevitability of terminal illness. It is often at this point in the cancer trajectory that patients experience the needs of altruism.[36] Patients and families who recognize the diminishing hope of survival may find comfort and solace in the possibility of contributing to the advancement of science through participation in clinical trials.[36] Others may choose to focus on using precious time to concentrate on more personal goals, such as unfinished business and QOL.

CASE STUDY

Mr. H, a Patient with Metastatic Colorectal Cancer

Mr. H is a 45-year-old African American real estate agent with metastatic colorectal cancer to the liver. He lives with his partner and primary caregiver, Ms. S, and his 14-year-old adopted son. Ms. S has voiced concerns about Mr. H's comfort, which is worrisome for the whole family. His symptoms primarily involve pain and ascites. Both first-line and second-line chemotherapeutic treatments have failed. Mr. H recently started a clinical trial treatment. Unfortunately, his disease progressed 2 months after initiation of the clinical trial treatment. His ascites has increasingly worsened. Lately, Ms. S has become increasingly tearful while accompanying Mr. H during his clinic visits.

In this case, it is clear that the caregiver is suffering tremendously. After surviving through several bouts of chemotherapy without much effect on the tumor, the impact of repeated discouragement weighs heavily on the patient's and caregiver's hearts. Ms. S has probably witnessed and supported Mr. H through the agonies of treatment and continued progression of disease. One can anticipate that they will experience tremendous difficulties with regard to grief and bereavement, as will their son. It is important, therefore, to recommend or establish support for the family. In this case, referral to supportive care experts might be warranted. The family should be provided with information on other types of support, such as support groups. It might be helpful to connect them with other caregivers, to exchange experiences on caring for a terminally ill loved one, and for the son to connect with other adolescents who have lost a parent.

Simultaneous Care: A Model Linking Palliative Care to Clinical Trials

The Simultaneous Care Model was developed at the University of California Davis as a means to demonstrate that investigational therapy and palliative care can be provided simultaneously.[2] The theoretical framework for this model addresses the flaws in the provision of palliative care for clinical trial patients. In the development of the model, it was hypothesized that the simultaneous delivery of investigational therapy and a structured program of supportive care would result in measurable improvements in predefined outcomes without adverse events for patients, caregivers, or the physician–patient interaction.[2] The model envisions palliative care as timely and team oriented, longitudinal, collaborative, and comprehensive.

A pilot study was conducted to test the feasibility and preliminary efficacy of a problem-solving educational intervention for patients enrolled in clinical trials.[2] All patients entered onto a University of California Davis phase I or phase II cancer investigational therapy protocol were considered eligible for Simultaneous Care protocol entry. Participants in randomized phase III studies were allowed if they compared different chemotherapy regimens for advanced disease.

Consented patients who lived within the service area of the University of California Davis Hospice Program (roughly a 25-mile radius) received Simultaneous Care. Patients who lived outside the service area received Usual Care. The Usual Care or nonintervention group was used as a control cohort in this nonrandomized pilot study.

Simultaneous Care patients were assigned a nurse trained in both cancer chemotherapy and palliative care and a social worker with inpatient, clinic, home health, and hospice patient care experience. The nurse visited the home two to three times a week or as needed, and the social worker visited one to two times a week or as needed. They accompanied the patient and the family to most physician visits. The nurse focused on chemotherapy toxicity, symptom management of advanced cancer, and care coordination. The social worker focused on emotional support issues, family and interpersonal issues, and end-of-life planning.

Sixty-four patients were enrolled into the pilot study.[2] Forty-four patients entered the intervention or Simultaneous care arm, and 20 entered the nonintervention or Usual Care arm. Of 10 physicians eligible to enroll patients, 10 entered patients into the Simultaneous Care protocol. A greater proportion of patients in the Usual Care group had genitourinary tumors (11/20 versus 6/44), whereas non-small-cell lung cancer was more frequent in the Simultaneous Care group (17/44 versus 3/20).[2] No patient disenrolled from Simultaneous Care as a result of discussions of end-of-life issues, palliative care discussions, or conflict between investigational therapy and palliative care goals or providers. The qualitative consensus, derived from physician questionnaires given to each physician for each patient, was that the cancer center personnel not only encouraged Simultaneous Care but also came to expect the nurse and social worker as routine support, potentially redefining Usual Care.[2]

Of the 44 Simultaneous Care patients, 35 died with hospice, 3 died on therapy, 4 died without hospice, and 2 were alive and off therapy without hospice at the time of report. Of the 20 Usual Care patients, 7 died without hospice after therapy was completed, 8 died in a hospice program, and 5 remained alive at the time of report.[2] The median number of days in hospice was the same for both cohorts, but the mean was higher in Simultaneous Care group (54 versus 37 days). Among those who died after completion of therapy, the proportion that entered hospice programs was greater in the Simultaneous Care group 92% versus 53%). Patients in Simultaneous Care received a mean of 3.8 cycles of chemotherapy, and those in Usual Care received a mean of 4.5 cycles.[2]

The results suggest that palliative care can be introduced simultaneously with investigational cancer therapy without adverse events. That is, the introduction of palliative care along with disease-directed therapy neither undermined patient participation in clinical research nor adversely affected the patient/physician relationship.[2] Patients are not asked to choose between two reasonable options, disease-directed therapy and palliative care. Rather, they have an opportunity to receive both, each with a different set of goals, benefits, and burdens. This model of care may also enhance the coordination of care from the home to the clinic or cancer center.[2] The model may assist in the introduction of end-of-life issues early enough for patients and families to benefit fully from specialized supportive care programs including hospice.[2] Currently a multisite, randomized, controlled phase II study of the efficacy of Simultaneous Care is underway, funded by the National Cancer Institute (NCI).

Perspectives Toward Clinical Trials: Patient versus Nurses

The conduct of clinical trials involving human subjects raises ethical concerns for health care professionals. In the process of decision-making in a clinical trial setting for patients with advanced cancer, the impact of nurses presents an additional element.[40] Nurses are involved in clinical trials both as clinical investigators and as caregivers for patients and families undergoing experimental treatments. In the clinical setting, nurses facilitate practitioner–patient communication and also serve as advocates.[40] Nurses often spend a considerable amount of time with patients and their families, and they are acutely aware of attitudes, needs, and concerns regarding participation.

Burnett and coworkers[40] conducted a study to identify nurses' attitudes and beliefs toward cancer clinical trials and their perceptions of the factors influencing patients' participation. A 59-item questionnaire was administered to nurses working in NCI-designated comprehensive cancer centers. Of the 417 nurses who responded, 96% reported that participation is important to improving standards of care, but only 56% believed that patients should be encouraged to participate in these clinical trials.[40] As a group, research nurses were more likely to have favorable views toward clinical trials and also about patient understanding regarding treatment plans and goals. On the other hand, nurses working in intensive care units and bone marrow transplant settings had more concerns regarding patient understanding and patient–physician communication. Ninety-two percent of nurses reported that patients entered a clinical trial with the belief that it would cure their cancer.[40] Sixty-eight percent of nurses reported the belief that patients participate in clinical trials because they hope to receive better medical care. Nurses also indicated their perception that nurses as professionals are more likely to respect patients' wishes and less likely to apply pressure on patients regarding clinical trial participation.[40] These results indicate the concerns that nurses working in oncology settings have toward the informed consent process of clinical trial participation and strongly suggest the need to develop nursing interventions to better support this process.

Aaronson and associates[41] conducted a study to test the efficacy of a telephone-based nursing intervention on improving the effectiveness of the informed consent process in cancer clinical trials. This randomized study compared the effectiveness of this nursing intervention in patients who were randomly assigned to either a standard informed consent procedure based on verbal explanation and written information or the standard informed consent process plus the supplementary telephone intervention (intervention group). Results showed that the intervention group was significantly better informed about the following: (1) the risks and side effects of treatment, (2) the clinical trial context of the treatment, (3) the objectives of the clinical trial, (4) the use of randomization in allocating treatment (if relevant), (5) the availability of alternative treatments, (6) the voluntary nature of the participation, and (7) the right to withdraw from the clinical trial. The intervention did not have any significant effect on patients' anxiety levels or on the rate of clinical trial accrual.[41]

Cox [42] conducted a qualitative study to identify the psychosocial impact of participation in clinical trials, as experienced by the patients themselves. The study sought to interpret patients' ways of coping with their individual situations and also to identify the consequences of trial involvement. Of the 55 patients involved in the study, the offer of a trial treatment was seen as a turning point for patients. Thirty patients (54%) described the offer of participation as being "the light at the end of a tunnel" because they perceived that hope was offered.[42] On the other hand, 58% of subjects described how the trial generated uncertainty, and 54% felt special, privileged, pleased, lucky, and honored to have been offered participation.[42] The majority of patients interpreted the offer of trial participation as being the right plan of action because their physicians offered it. Reasons for patients to accept trial participation included the desire to be in expert hands (54%) and the desire to help others (52%).[42]

As clinical trial initiation began and patients progressed through treatment, an overwhelming sense of being burdened by trial involvement was seen in all cases. These burdens focused on side effects and additional demands such as blood tests and scans.[42] It was evident that these trial burdens were not fully anticipated by patients at the beginning of trial involvement. Nevertheless, most of the patients desired to persevere through treatment instead of withdrawing.

At the conclusion of participation, patients expressed disappointment that the trial drug was not successful. An overwhelming sense of abandonment was a feature in all patients. Subjects were also eager to receive feedback on the trial in which they had participated.[42] Trial withdrawal due to disease progression or toxicity was a common feature for subjects in this study. Trial withdrawal and conclusion was a deeply distressing and stressful time for all patients. In addition to having to confront the realities of having a terminal illness and the lack of response to their last hope for "cure," patients also experienced a dramatic decrease in contact from health care providers, which inevitably led to an overwhelming sense of abandonment.[42] These findings suggest that patients and families need support during and beyond the trial to deal with the major disruption that clinical trial participation might have on the overall dying trajectory. The investigators suggested that one way to overcome these issues is to consider early clinical trials in the context of a continuing palliative care program in which the duty of care extends beyond trial involvement and in which death and dying concerns can be addressed.[42]

The Role of Nurses in Caring for Clinical Trial Patients

Clinical trials of new investigational cancer therapeutics are a necessary component to the process of translating scientific discoveries into standard practice of care.[43] Oncology nurses have many different roles in the conduct of cancer clinical trials. First and foremost, the process of obtaining true informed consent is a critical factor, not only in improving patient accrual into clinical trials but also in the overall well-being of patients and their families. The informed consent process is an opportunity to provide accurate information regarding important factors that affect the patient's and family's decision-making process in advanced cancer. These factors include trial procedures and potential risks and benefits. The initial informed consent process is also a time to correct any misconceptions and allay unfounded fears, and to provide sufficient time for patients and families to thoughtfully consider clinical trial participation.[43] A predecisional support process provided by oncology nurses may influence the soundness of patients' decisions to enroll in clinical trials.[43] Nursing interventions that would assist in well-considered decisions include helping patients gather additional relevant sources of information, describing patients' roles and rights in studies, encouraging patients to define their own reasons for participating in clinical trials, and supporting patients in making decisions that correspond with their personal values and wishes.[44]

Nurses can also assist in educating not only clinical trial patients but also the extended community. Interventions aimed at increasing community awareness can foster better understanding of clinical trials and their importance in the advancement of treatment options and strategies for oncology patients.[43] The formation of clinical trials support groups for patients and families considering enrollment in research is another strategy that may provide necessary education and social support.[43] Strategies such as follow-up phone calls or e-mail messages while patients are considering clinical trials participation can have a positive effect on the decision-making process.[43]

Nurses are in an ideal position to promote awareness of the importance of clinical trials and subsequent improvements in patient care. The three key roles of nurses caring for clinical trial patients and their families are educator, patient advocate, and study coordinator.[45] As patient and family educators, nurses can have a tremendous impact on a patient's experience with clinical trial participation. Nurses are clinical interpreters who provide patients and families with explanations of highly complex and intricate protocols without using medical jargon.[43] Education about the specific protocol process, expectations at each stage, management of side effects, and the importance of communicating changes in health status to practitioners is integral to the oncology research setting.

As patient advocates, nurses play an important role in the critical gateway to clinical trial participation—the informed consent process.[45] Nurses bring to this role a patient-centered, holistic method of support. The nursing perspective is important in that it provides a framework within which patients and families are treated with dignity and respect. Clarification of reasons behind decisions to participate—whether physical, psychological, social, or spiritual—should be encouraged.

APNs such as clinical nurse specialists and nurse practitioners can be an important factor in the conduct of clinical trials. Expertise in symptom management and clinical problem-solving is a key asset for APNs in the research setting. For example, nurse practitioners working in a clinical trials setting have an expanded scope of practice that allows them to perform routine follow-up physical examinations as well as diagnose and manage treatment complications.[26] This level of participation in patient and family care may enhance patient satisfaction, compliance, and retention.

Summary

Of all the topics to which oncology health care providers, palliative care specialists, and ethicists have devoted their attention, few raise as much heated debate as the dichotomy between active treatment and palliative care. The use of palliative chemotherapy and clinical trial participation as a treatment option for advanced cancer patients has been in the heart of this debate for decades. There is a growing movement in the United States to integrate palliative care into clinical trials. However, there is still much work to be done. Frustration lies in the assumption that subjects who are actively treated for symptom palliation, whether through palliative chemotherapy or experimental agents, must forgo a coordinated plan of care that involves quality palliative care.[46] It has become increasingly evident that this dichotomy should not exist; that is, patients and families can simultaneously receive therapy for palliation of symptoms and also have access to quality palliative care. It is also increasingly evident that this quality care can be provided only through a transdisciplinary model of care. Nurses can help alleviate the tension between palliative care and disease-directed therapies through education, advocacy, and coordination of care. It is only by removing this dichotomy that patients with advanced cancer and their families can be provided with the highest quality of information to facilitate their decision-making process.

REFERENCES

1. Joshi TG, Ehrenberger HE. Cancer clinical trials in the new millennium: Novel challenges and opportunities for oncology nursing. Clin J Oncol Nurs 2001;5:147–152.
2. Meyers FJ, Linder J. Simultaneous care: Disease treatment and palliative care throughout illness. J Clin Oncol 2003;7: 1412–1415.
3. Casarett DJ, Karlawish J, Henry MI, Hirschman KB. Must patients with advanced cancer choose between a phase I trial and hospice? Cancer 2002;95:1601–1604.
4. Ellison NM, Chevlen EM. Palliative chemotherapy. In: Berger AM, Portenoy RK, Weissman DE, eds. Principles and Practices of Palliative Care and Supportive Oncology. Philadelphia: Lippincott Williams & Wilkins, 2002, pp 698–709.
5. Peppercorn JM, Weeks JC, Cook EF, Joffe S. Comparison of outcomes in cancer patients treated within and outside clinical trials: Conceptual framework and structured review. Lancet 2004; 363:263–270.
6. Byock I, Miles SH. Hospice benefits and phase I cancer trials. Ann Intern Med 2003;138:335–337.
7. Osoba D. Lessons learned from measuring health-related quality of life in oncology. J Clin Oncol 1994;12:608–616.
8. McIllmurray M. Palliative medicine and the treatment of cancer. In: Doyle D, Hanks G, Cherny N, Calman K, eds. Oxford Textbook of Palliative Medicine. Oxford: Oxford University Press, 2004, pp 229–239.
9. Sloan JA, Cella D, Frost MH, Guyatt G, Osoba D. Clinical Significance Consensus Meeting Group. Quality of life III: Translating the science of quality-of-life assessment into clinical practice—An example-driven approach for practicing clinicians and clinical researchers. Clin Ther 2003;25(Suppl): D1–D5.

10. Osoba D, Slamon DJ, Burchmore M, Murphy M. Effects on quality of life of combined trastuzumab and chemotherapy in women with metastatic breast cancer. J Clin Oncol 2002;20: 3106–3113.
11. Cullen MH, Billingham LJ, Woodroffe CM, Chetiyawardana AD, Gower NH, Joshi R, Ferry DR, Rudd RM, Spiro SG, Cook JE Trask C, Bessell E, Connolly CK, Tobias J, Souhami RL. Mitromycin, ifosfamide, and cisplatin in unresectable non-small-cell lung cancer: Effects on survival and quality of life. J Clin Oncol 1999; 17:3188–3194.
12. Glimelius B, Ekstrom K, Hoffman K, Graf W, Sjoden PO, Haglund U, Svensson C, Enander LK, Linne T, Sellstrom H, Heuman R. Randomized comparison between chemotherapy plus best supportive care with best supportive care in advanced gastric cancer. Ann Oncol 1995;71:587–591.
13. Simmonds PC. Palliative chemotherapy for advanced colorectal cancer: Systematic review and meta-analysis. Colorectal Cancer Collaborative Group. BMJ 2000;321:531–535.
14. Doyle C, Crump M, Pintilie M, Oza AM. Does palliative chemotherapy palliate? Evaluation of expectations, outcomes, and costs in women receiving chemotherapy for advanced ovarian cancer. J Clin Oncol 2001;19:1266–1274.
15. Ellis PA, Smith IE, Hardy JR, Nicolson MC, Talbot DC, Ashley SE, Priest K. Symptom relief from MVP (mitomycin C, vinblastine and cisplatin) chemotherapy in advanced non-small-cell lung cancer. Br J Cancer 1995;71:366–370.
16. Burris HA 3rd, Moore MJ, Andersen J, Gren MR, Rothenberg ML, Modiano MR, Cripps MC, Portenoy RK, Storniolo AM, Tarassoff P, Nelson R, Dorr FA, Stephens CD, Von Hoff DD. Improvements in survival and clinical benefit with gemcitabine as first-line therapy for patients with advanced pancreas cancer: A randomized trial. J Clin Oncol 1997;15: 2403–2413.
17. Cunningham D, Pyrhonen S, James RD, Punt CJ, Hickish TF, Heikkila R, Johannesen TB, Starkhammar H, Topham CA Awad L, Jacques C, Herait P. Randomized trial of irinotecan plus supportive care versus supportive care alone after fluorouracil failure for patients with metastatic colorectal cancer. Lancet 1998; 352:1413–1418.
18. Shanafelt TD, Loprinzi C, Marks R, Novotny P, Sloan J. Are chemotherapy response rates related to treatment-induced survival prolongations in patients with advanced cancer? J Clin Oncol 2004;22:1966–1974.
19. Rapp E, Pater JL, Willan A, Cormier Y, Murray N, Evans WK. Chemotherapy can prolong survival in patients with advanced non small cell lung cancer: Report of a Canadian multicenter randomized trial. J Clin Oncol 1988;6:633–643.
20. Souquet PJ, Chauvin F, Boisel JP, Cellerino R, Cormier Y, Ganz PA, Kaasa S, Pater JL, Quoix E, Rapp E, et al. Polychemotherapy in advanced non-small-cell lung cancer A metaanalysis. Lancet 1993;342:19–30.
21. Weitzner MA, McMillan SC, Jacobsen PB. Family caregiver quality of life: Differences between curative and palliative cancer treatment settings. J Pain Sympt Manage 1999;17:418–428.
22. Comis RL, Miller JD, Aldige CR, Krebs L, Stoval E. Public attitudes toward participation in cancer clinical trials. J Clin Oncol 2003;21:830–835.
23. Slevin ML, Stubbs L, Plant HJ, Wlson P, Gregory WM, Armes PJ, Downer SM. Attitudes towards chemotherapy: Comparing view of patients with those of doctors, nurses, and general public. BMJ 1990;300:1458–1467.
24. Silvestri G, Pritchard R, Welch HG. Preferences for chemotherapy in patients with advanced non-small cell lung cancer: Descriptive study based on scripted interviews. BMJ 1998;317: 771–775.
25. Koedoot CG, de Haan RJ, Stiggelbout AM, Stalmeier PF, de Graeff A, Bakker PJ, de Haes JC. Palliative chemotherapy or best supportive care? A prospective study explaining patients' treatment preference and choice. Br J Cancer 2003; 89:19–26.
26. Aiken JL. Nursing roles in clinical trials. In: Klimaszewski D, Aiken JL, Bacon MA, DiStasio SA, Ehrenberger HE, Ford BA, eds. Manual for Clinical Trial Nursing. Pittsburgh, PA: Oncology Nursing Press, 2001, pp 273–276.
27. Karigan M. Psychosocial considerations. In: Klimaszewski D, Aiken JL, Bacon MA, DiStasio SA, Ehrenberger HE, Ford BA, eds. Manual for Clinical Trial Nursing. Pittsburgh, PA: Oncology Nursing Press, 2001, pp 173–176.
28. Decoster G, Stein G, Holdner E. Responses and toxic deaths in phase I clinical trials. Ann Clin Oncol 1990;1:175–181.
29. Estey E, Hoth D, Simon R, Marsoni S, Leyland-Jones B, Wittes R. Therapeutic response in phase I trials of antineoplastic agents. Cancer Treat Rep 1986;70:1105–1115.
30. Daugherty CK. Impact of therapeutic research on informed consent and the ethics of clinical trials: A medical oncology perspective. J Clin Oncol 1999;17:1601–1617.
31. Daugherty C, Ratain MJ, Grochowski E, Stocking C, Kodish E, Mick R, Siegler M. Perceptions of cancer patients and their physicians involved in phase I trials. J Clin Oncol 1995;13: 1062–1072.
32. Jenkins V, Fallowfield L. Reasons for accepting or declining to participate in randomized clinical trials for cancer therapy. Br J Cancer 2000;82:1783–1788.
33. Yoder LH, O'Rourke TJ, Etnye A, Spears DT, Brown TD. Expectations and experiences of patients with cancer participating in phase I clinical trials. Oncol Nurs Forum 1997;24: 891–896.
34. Oliverio R, Fraulo B. SUPPORT revisited: The nurse clinician's perspective. Study to Understand Prognoses and Preferences for Outcomes and Risks of Treatment. Holistic Nurs Pract 1998; 13:1–7.
35. Horng S, Emanuel EJ, Wilfond B, Rackoff J, Martz K, Grady C. Descriptions of benefits and risks in consent forms for phase I oncology trials. N Engl J Med 2002;347: 2134–2140.
36. Agrawal M, Danis M. End-of-life care for terminally ill participants in clinical research. J Palliat Med 2002;5:729–737.
37. Ferrell BR, Grant MM, Rhiner M, Padilla GV. Home care: Maintaining quality of life for patient and family. Oncology 1992;6 (2 Suppl):136–140.
38. BrintzenhofeSzoc KM, Smith ED, Zabora JR. Screening to predict complicated grief in spouses of cancer patients. Cancer Pract 1999;7:233–239.
39. Schulz R, Beach SR. Caregiving as a risk factor for mortality: The Caregiver Health Effects Study. JAMA 1999;282:2215–2219.
40. Burnett CB, Koczwara B, Pixley L, Blumenson LE, Hwang YT, Meropol NJ. Nurses' attitudes toward clinical trials at a comprehensive cancer center. Oncol Nurs Forum 2002;28: 1187–1192.
41. Aaronson NK, Visser-Pol E, Leenhouts G, Muller MJ, van der Schot A, van Dam F, Keus RB, Koning C, ten Bokkel Huinink W, van Dongen JA, Dubbelman R. Telephone-based nursing intervention improves the effectiveness of the informed

consent process in cancer clinical trials. J Clin Oncol 1996;14: 984–996.
42. Cox K. Enhancing cancer clinical trial management: Recommendations from a qualitative study of trial participants' experiences. Psycho-oncology 2002;9:314–322.
43. Barrett R. A nurse's primer on recruiting participants for clinical trials. Oncol Nurs Forum 2002;29:1091–1098.
44. Sadler GR, Lantz JM, Fullerton JT, Dault Y. Nurses' unique role in randomized clinical trials. J Prof Nurs 1999;15:106–115.
45. Ocker BM, Plank DM. The research nurse role in a clinic-based oncology research setting. Cancer Nurs 2000;23:286–292.
46. Kapo J, Casarett D. Palliative care in phase I trials: an ethical obligation or undue inducement? J Palliat Med 2002;5: 661–665.

VII

Pediatric Palliative Care

49

Melody Brown Hellsten and Javier Kane

Symptom Management in Pediatric Palliative Care

What kind of God would do this to a child?—Mother of a symptomatic pediatric patient with advanced cancer

- ***Key Points***
- *Children are living longer with complex chronic medical conditions.*
- *This life prolongation may be accompanied by multiple acute and chronic health crises and challenges for the child and family.*
- *Symptom management for these children presents a unique challenge to health care providers.*
- *Skilled and compassionate management of symptoms, with a family-centered approach, is an integral part of the care of a chronically ill child.*

Complex chronic conditions of childhood (Table 49–1) are defined as "any medical condition that can be reasonably expected to last at least 12 months, involves either multiple organs or one organ system severely enough to require specialty pediatric care, and some probability of hospitalization at a tertiary care center."[1] Currently, there are limited estimates on the numbers of children living with these disabling and potentially life-limiting complex chronic conditions. Newacheck and Halfon[2] estimated that approximately 4.4 million children in the United States currently live with some level of disabling chronic condition, and that roughly 450,000 of those children have conditions that prevent participation in age-appropriate activities, result in significant limitation in school, and account for increased numbers of hospitalizations and contacts with the health care system. Feudtner and colleagues[3] reviewed death-certificate data from 1979 to 1997 and reported that 21% of the 1.7 million child deaths during that time were the result of a complex chronic condition.

In the past 2 decades, child-mortality trends have shown a decrease in numbers of deaths from complex chronic conditions in middle childhood years, with stable to increased numbers of deaths in late adolescence and early adulthood.[3] This trend most likely reflects the ability of advancing medical science to provide life-prolonging management of children with complex chronic conditions. However, this life prolongation often comes at the cost of multiple acute and chronic health crises and challenges for the child and family, as well as increasing debilitation as the child's condition progresses, thereby increasing the possibility of suffering for the child and family. Medical science therefore must face the challenge of recognizing and attending to suffering as a concurrent obligation to providing scientifically based curative and life-prolonging treatment.[4] Unfortunately, fragmentation of health care, limited acknowledgment of terminal care needs of children, and a paucity of research on the impact of symptoms on quality of life and interventions aimed at managing distressing symptoms all create challenges in alleviating suffering for children with complex chronic conditions.[5]

Table 49–1
Categories of Complex Chronic Conditions of Childhood

Neurological Conditions
Congenital malformations of the brain
Anencephaly
Lissencephaly
Holoprosencephaly
Cerebral palsy/Mental retardation
Neurodegenerative disorders
Muscular dystrophies
Spinal muscular atrophy
Adrenoleukodystrophy
Epilepsy
Cardiovascular Conditions
Malformations of the heart/Great vessels
Cardiomyopathies
Conduction disorders/dysrhythmias
Respiratory Conditions
Cystic fibrosis
Chronic respiratory disease
Respiratory malformations
Renal Conditions
Chronic renal failure
Gastrointestinal Conditions
Congenital anomalies
Chronic liver disease/Cirrhosis
Inflammatory bowel disease
Hematology/Immunodeficiency
Sickle cell disease
Hereditary anemias
Hereditary immunodeficiency
HIV/AIDS
Metabolic Conditions
Amino acid metabolism
Carbohydrate metabolism
Mucopolysaccaridosis
Storage disorders
Genetic Conditions
Trisomy 18
Chromosome 22 deletions
Other congenital disorders
Malignancy
Leukemias/Lymphomas
Brain tumors
Sarcomas
Neuroblastoma

This chapter focuses on issues related to the assessment and management of common nonpain symptoms in children and adolescents with complex medical conditions in the advanced and terminal stages. The unique issues related to children dying in pediatric and neonatal intensive care units are addressed in Chapters 52 and 53, respectively.

Assessing Sources of Suffering in Advanced Childhood Illness

Family-Centered Care

Family-centered care is based on the understanding that the family is the child's primary source of strength and support and that the perspectives and information provided by families, children, and young adults are important in clinical decision-making.[6] In considering symptom management within the context of family-centered care, it is necessary to assess the family system as a whole, as well as its individual members, to identify all sources of suffering that may require intervention. Interdisciplinary collaboration with chaplains, social workers, psychologists, and child-life therapists will contribute to the overall assessment of the ill child, parents, and siblings.

The focus of family-centered care is to develop a process of shared decision-making over the course of the child's and family's illness experience that is based in the interpersonal relationship between the child and family and their health care providers. The physician and health care team must come to know the child and family as individuals and provide diagnostic, prognostic, and treatment information in a manner sensitive to the particular child's and family's experiences, values, beliefs, and available social and spiritual support.[4] Parents and children should be respected as the experts in their illness experience and management, and value must be given to their contribution to the plan of care. The child's and family's illness experience and goals of care, as well as the impact of a particular symptom on suffering and its effect on the child's function and quality of life, will influence the types of interventions considered as symptoms occur.

Illness Experience and Sources of Suffering

Research exploring the experiences of families of children with complex chronic conditions provides a glimpse into their world. Uncertainty prevails as the parents move from the initial suspicion that something is wrong with their child to the confirmation that this is indeed the case.[7–10] Parents struggle to cope with the diagnosis and learn skills necessary to provide technical care and negotiate the health care system for needed services and information.[11–14] Over time, as treatment continues, parents must live with ongoing uncertainty regarding the unpredictability of the illness, the ultimate outcome of their child's treatment, the challenges of parenting a seriously ill child, and the possibility of death.[10,15–19] The child may experience disability, physical pain and other distressing symptoms as a result of the disease and treatments, severe alterations in their social world, and disruption of their developmental process.[20–24] Siblings may experience feelings of anger, guilt, anxiety, depression, and social isolation.[25–29]

While the above picture gives an impression of tremendous struggle and individual distress in the family, there is also research that suggests there are aspects of family functioning that facilitate coping with this new family reality. Parents' adaptation and adjustment to their child's illness is facilitated by several factors, including gaining information regarding the disease, its treatment, and prognosis; good spousal communication, similar coping styles, and means of emotional expression; and sufficient social support.[5,30–32] Factors associated with adaptation of the ill child and siblings include having open communication and emotional support from parents during times of stress, having a wide range of coping skills, seeking information about the disease, and clarifying fears.[33–38]

Assessing and understanding the child's and family's unique experiences during the illness trajectory provides the health care team with insight into what symptoms may contribute to the family's suffering. This assessment involves hearing the child's and family members' "story" as they have lived it during the course of the disease. It is important to elicit care that has been helpful in past experiences with the illness as well as care that was not helpful. Insight into what the family values regarding the role of spirituality or faith in God, the meaning they give to their experience of illness, and what activities or interactions the child and family identify as contributing to quality of life provide a context for identifying and managing symptoms that contribute to suffering for the child and family.

Expectations and Goals of Care

Children with complex chronic conditions are a highly diverse population, with a variety of illness trajectories that are often characterized by prognostic uncertainty, including sudden unexpected death, death from potentially curable disease, death from lethal congenital anomaly, and death from progressive conditions with intermittent health crises. The unpredictability and uncertainty of many of these disease trajectories often result in ongoing medical treatments aimed at cure or aggressive life-prolongation, with little attention to the suffering of the child or family.[5]

In general, goals of care for children with serious, life-threatening, or limiting illness as they progress through their illness trajectory include interventions aimed at cure, life-prolongation with or without aggressive life-sustaining therapies, and care focused solely on interventions aimed at treating discomfort from symptoms as the disease moves into its terminal phase. Ideally, these goals would shift as the child, family, and primary health care team discussed changes in quality of life, symptoms, and prognosis over the disease trajectory. It is very important that interventions aimed at maintaining maximal comfort and quality of life occur throughout the disease trajectory as well as through the terminal stages. Unfortunately, for many families, the presence of a DNR (do not resuscitate) order often leads to health care professionals dismissing treatable illnesses or symptoms as "part of the dying process," thereby contributing to suffering for both the child and family.

The most difficult decision a parent must face is to change the focus of care from cure or aggressive life prolongation to focusing on comfort and terminal care. Wolfe and colleagues[22] reported on disparity between parents and health care providers regarding the realization that a child with progressive cancer had no realistic chance for cure. Parents who came to that realization earlier were more likely to discuss hospice care, to establish a DNR order, and to change the focus of care from cancer-directed therapies to treatments focused on controlling discomfort, and thereby experienced greater quality of home care.

Parents have reported that decisions to forgo further aggressive medical treatments and instead pursue care focused on comfort and quality of life occurred only after realizing that ongoing aggressive treatment would not bring about cure or further life prolongation, and they recognized the physical deterioration and suffering of their child. Once this realization is reached, parents report that the child's wishes and quality of life are major determinants of treatment decision-making.[39–41]

The first step to managing symptoms of children with advanced and terminal illness is a thorough assessment of the child's and family's expectations and goals of care. Interventions aimed at controlling symptoms must be compatible with the family's understanding of where their child is in the disease trajectory and their expectations of care, as well as the child's overall functional status and quality of life. For instance, an adolescent with advanced muscular dystrophy may be attending school and participating in a religious community despite significant physical limitations. This level of function and quality of life may lead the child and family to desire aggressive ventilatory support for life prolongation in the event of an acute respiratory infection, with the hope that the child will be cured of the infection and resume his previous level of functioning. However, if the adolescent were home-bound and seriously debilitated due to progressive respiratory failure, he and his family may choose to pursue home management of respiratory discomfort without the use of ventilatory support to reduce suffering associated with intensive hospital-based interventions. In determining the expectations and goals of care with the child and family, it is important to discuss the balance between relieving and contributing to the child's suffering. The prevailing decision-making framework should not be based on whether an intervention is consistent with a palliative care focus, but, rather, whether the intervention under consideration would provide relief from or contribute to the child's and family's suffering.

Physical Symptoms and Suffering

Children dying as the result of complex chronic conditions experience a number of symptoms throughout their illness trajectory that can contribute to suffering and decreased quality of life (Table 49–2). Wolfe and colleagues[22] reviewed medical

Table 49–2
Symptoms Contributing to Suffering in Advanced and Terminal Disease

General Symptoms
Fatigue
Anorexia
Psychological/Emotional Symptoms
Anxiety/Depression
Neurological Symptoms
Seizures
Somnolence
Respiratory Symptoms
Dyspnea
Gastrointestinal Symptoms
Nausea/Vomiting
Constipation
Diarrhea

records and interviewed 103 parents of children with cancer in a U.S. tertiary-care children's hospital. Generally, most of the children received aggressive life-sustaining treatments at the end of life, contributing to a substantial amount of suffering, primarily from pain and dyspnea. Of the parents surveyed, 89% stated that their child suffered "a lot" or "a great deal" from at least one symptom. However, symptom management was effective in only 27% for pain and 16% for dyspnea.

Similar findings were reported by McCallum, Byrne, and Bruera,[23] who reviewed 30 cancer and noncancer deaths in a Canadian children's hospital. The majority of children died in the intensive care setting despite aggressive measures, and symptoms were inconsistently documented. Little conversation was documented regarding the family's preference for resuscitation or location of death, and only one case documented that the child had been informed of his condition.

Managing these symptoms requires that health care providers remain attentive in their assessment of the child's physical and emotional symptoms. Assessment should include the child's report of symptoms and how distressing he or she finds them, information based on parent observation of their child's condition, and health care provider's knowledge of the pathophysiology of the underlying disease. Diagnostic tests should be considered carefully for the potential discomfort they may cause. Tests should be ordered only if they will help determine an intervention. A test should be questioned for its appropriateness if the results will not change management (e.g., MRI to document growth of known terminal tumor).

As mentioned earlier, symptoms experienced by children with advanced and terminal chronic illnesses are often interrelated. If a child reports a distressing symptom, it is necessary to obtain a thorough assessment regarding the symptom's onset, severity, and effect on function and quality of life. The health care provider must consider the likely cause of the symptom and determine the best course of intervention. For example, pain with urination may be related to an infection and amenable to treatment with antibiotics to cure the infection. Shortness of breath in a child with cystic fibrosis may be related to infection and amenable to treatment with antibiotics, with resolution of the symptom. However, it may also be related to progressive respiratory failure or disease progression. Oxygen therapy, opioids, ventilation and/or energy-conservation techniques may assist in relieving the severity of the symptom, but will not eliminate the underlying cause. This distinction is important to discuss with the child and parent with regard to the goal of treatment and expectation of care in relation to the child's overall condition and quality of life.

Control of present symptoms as well as anticipation of distressing symptoms as disease progresses is imperative in attending to the suffering of children with advanced disease and their families. Following is a discussion of the most common symptoms associated with distress and suffering experienced by children with advanced illness. It is by no means an exhaustive presentation of all symptoms that children with complex chronic conditions may experience. Each symptom is discussed as to its general issues, causes, assessment, and pharmacological and nonpharmacological management. As discussed earlier, there is little evidence-based data on the management of nonpain symptoms in children with advanced disease. Much symptom management in pediatric palliative care is based on empirical approaches and extrapolation from adult hospice and palliative care literature.

An inherent difficulty in pharmacological management in pediatric palliative care is a lack of pharmacological dosing and side-effect information on infants, toddlers, and early school-aged children for many medications. Starting dosages of medications will vary depending on the age, weight, and clinical circumstances of the child. It is incumbent on physicians and nurses to consult with experienced pediatricians and pediatric hospice and palliative care providers for medication choices, appropriate doses, and titration for difficult cases of symptom management. For more information on pediatric pain management, see Chapter 55.

Management of Symptoms During Disease Progression and End of Life

General Systemic Symptoms

Fatigue. The most comprehensive research in fatigue experienced by children with complex chronic illnesses has been in the area of childhood cancer. Fatigue has been described by young children with cancer as a "profound sense of being physically tired, or having difficulty with body movements such as moving legs or opening their eyes"; and as a "changing state of exhaustion that includes physical, mental, and emotional

Table 49–3
Factors Contributing to Fatigue in Children with Advanced Disease

Disease/Treatment
Pain
Unresolved symptoms
Anemia
Malnutrition
Infection
Fever
Sleep disturbance
Debilitation
Psychological Factors
Depression
Anxiety
Spiritual distress

tiredness" by adolescents with cancer.[42–44] Fatigue, lethargy, lack of energy, and drowsiness have been reported in more than 50% of children with cancer, and has been described as moderately to severely distressing.[22,44] There is no clear incidence or prevalence of fatigue or its relation to distress or suffering in children with noncancer advanced illnesses.

Fatigue is a multidimensional symptom that can be related to disease, treatment, or emotional factors (Table 49–3). Assessment requires a multidimensional approach, which includes subjective and objective data to determine the degree of distress and potential causes of the child's fatigue. Subjective assessment involves asking children about their feelings of tiredness or lack of energy, how long they feel tired, when they feel most tired, and how it affected their ability to play or go to school. Objective assessment should include vital signs, presence of other symptoms such as dyspnea or vomiting, evaluation of hydration status, and muscle strength. Laboratory data may include parameters such as oxygen saturation, CBC/differential, and thyroid studies. Management of fatigue will vary depending on the underlying cause and may include both pharmacological and nonpharmacological interventions (Table 49–4). For more information on fatigue, see Chapter 7.

Anorexia/Cachexia. Loss of appetite occurs in nearly all children with terminal illness. Anorexia involves the loss of desire to eat or a loss of appetite, with associated decrease in food intake. Cachexia is a general lack of nutrition that occurs over the course of a chronic progressive disease. Anorexia and cachexia are multidimensional in nature and are influenced by disease, treatment and emotional factors (Table 49–5). These symptoms are particularly distressing to parents of children with illness because they cause concern that the child is "starving to death." Food and meals have a social association with "caring," and is significant in family culture, activities, and ritual. In most instances, children will request favorite foods as a means of comfort and familiarity. It is important to assist parents in understanding their child's changing eating habits and nutritional needs as well as ways to redirect energies toward other caregiving activities. Table 49–6 provides additional suggestions for management of anorexia and cachexia.

Parents and health care providers often struggle with personal and ethical dilemmas regarding fluid and nutrition management for children with terminal illness. The act of withholding medically provided fluids and nutrition (GT feeds, TPN) is legally and ethically permissible for children with irreversible, progressive medical conditions when it is agreed upon by the health care providers and family that such medically provided nutrition will increase the suffering and discomfort of the child and would not alter the progression of the disease or the outcome of death.[45,46] Such decisions are highly individual to the family and influenced by culture, religious tradition, and personal values.

Providing aggressive nutritional support does not usually improve the condition, and, in fact, may add additional symptom burden for the child. Unfortunately, there is no clear data to guide the discussion of the risks/benefits of providing aggressive fluid and nutrition in terminally ill children. When medically provided nutritional interventions are chosen by a family, the challenge is balancing fluid and nutritional supplementation as appetite and metabolic needs decrease with advancing disease. Ideally, as the child's condition progresses, parenteral or enteral supplements can be slowly weaned to promote comfort and decrease symptoms of increased congestion or secretions. For more information on anorexia and cachexia, see Chapter 8.

Psychological/Emotional Symptoms

Anxiety. Children with chronic illness may experience a number of anxiety-provoking events throughout their illness. Episodes of serious illness, hospitalizations, painful procedures, changes in independence and physical abilities, uncontrolled pain and other symptoms, and an uncertain future all can contribute to fear and anxiety.[47] The distinction between childhood fears and anxiety is crucial—childhood fears are specific and developmentally based (e.g., fear of the dark, fear of separation, fear of death), whereas anxiety is a generalized feeling of uneasiness without a known source.[48] Anxiety and depression may be comorbid conditions.

Anxiety in terminal illness is an expected reaction and should be assessed frequently. Toddlers and young children will generally have anxiety reactions that are an extension of the stress and anxiety levels of parents and other family members around them. These reactions may include irritability, clinginess, temper tantrums, and inconsolability. School-aged children and adolescents who can cognitively comprehend their illness and impending death may experience more adult-like symptoms such as chronic apprehension, worry, difficulty concentrating, and sleep disturbance. Chaplains, child-life

Table 49–4
Management of Fatigue in Children With Advanced Disease

Intervention	Dose	Comments
Pharmacological Management		
Blood transfusion	10–15 mL/kg IV over 4 h	Premedicate with diphenhydramine (1 mg/kg/IV/PO, max dose 50 mg), acetaminophen (10–15 mg/kg PO) and hydrocortisone (2 mg/kg IV, max dose 100 mg) prior to transfusion if history of reaction
Psychostimulants		
Methylphenidate	0.3 mg/kg/dose PO bid	Dosage information for ≥6 y. Give doses in AM and early afternoon. May titrate by 0.1 mg/kg/dose to max of 2 mg/kg/d, gauge by child's desired activity level. May decrease appetite.
Dextroamphetamine	6–12 y 5 mg/d. May titrate in 5-mg increments weekly, 12 y 10 mg/d. May titrate in 10-mg increments weekly	Titrate according to child's desired level of activity. Will suppress appetite.
Sleep agents		
Chloral hydrate	20–40 mg/kg/dose PO/PR	Tolerance to hypnotic effect occurs. Maximum of 50 mg/kg/24 h. Not recommended for use >2 weeks or 1 g/dose or 2 g/24 h. Taper dose in situations of prolonged use to avoid withdrawal. Syrup has unpleasant taste, chill or ask pharmacist to mix in flavored syrup.
Diphenhydramine	1 mg/kg IV/PO. Max dose 50 mg/dose	May cause paradoxical excitement, euphoria, or confusion. May use in children as young as 2 y.
Lorazepam	0.03–0.1 mg IV/PO. Max 2 mg/dose	Can cause retrograde amnesia. Taper dose with prolonged use. May use in infants and young children.
Zolpidem	10 mg PO qh	Use for adolescents, young adults. No dosing information in young children.
Nonpharmacological Management		
Nutritional supplementation (e.g., Boost®, Pediasure®, etc.)		
Frequent rest, energy conservation		
Physical/Occupational therapies		
Play therapy		
Exploring fears/anxiety that may interfere with sleep		

Sources: Lacey et al. (2003), reference 29; Hellsten et al. (2000), reference 54.

workers, and social workers are helpful in assessing children's fears, worries, and dreams. Children and adolescents under stress may regress behaviorally and emotionally; therefore, health care professionals should be alert to changes in the child's coping or personality.

Depression. Little is known about the incidence or prevalence of clinical depression in children and adolescents living with chronic illness. Depression can be described as a broad spectrum of responses that range from "expected, transient, nonclinical sadness, to extremes of major clinical depressive disorders and suicidality."[49] Children are unique in their coping abilities, which are influenced by their age and developmental level. Often, during the course of terminal illness, most children remain future focused and continue to plan activities, even in the final days of life.

Risk factors for depression in chronically ill children include frequent disruptions in important relationships, uncontrolled pain, and presence of multiple physical disabilities.[48] Existential factors related to impending death, concern for parents and other family members, and a personal or family history of preexisting psychological problems can also increase the risk for depression in chronically ill children. Suicidal thoughts or wishes are not common in terminally ill children and adolescents, but health care providers should be alert to comments about wishing to die and use social workers or child-life therapists to assist in further assessment and management.

Table 49–5
Factors Contributing to Anorexia/Cachexia in Advanced Disease

Physiological Factors
Uncontrolled pain or other symptoms
Feeding/Swallowing problems
Poor oral hygiene and infections
Mouth sores
Nausea/Vomiting
Constipation
Delayed gastric emptying
Changes in taste
Psychological Factors
Depression
Anger
Stress

Assessment of depressive symptoms must take into account the child's developmental level. Pediatric social workers and child-life therapists are good resources for assessing a child's emotional status. Somatic complaints such as lack of appetite, insomnia, agitation, and loss of energy may be the result of disease and cannot be considered hallmark signs of depression in ill children. More appropriate signs would include a persistent sad face and demeanor, tearfulness, irritability, and withdrawal from previously enjoyed activities and relationships. Siblings may exhibit persistent and significant decrease in school performance, hypersomnolence, changes in appetite or weight, and nonspecific complaints of not feeling well.[48] Parents should be assessed for depressed appearance, fearfulness, withdrawal, a sense of punishment, and mood that cannot be improved with good news, and should be referred for further evaluation as needed.[50]

Pharmacological management of anxiety and depression should be considered if symptoms of anxiety and depression are debilitating. Consultation with appropriate psychiatric specialists for further evaluation and choice of agents is appropriate. Generally, management of anxiety and depression related to terminal illness in children involves nonpharmacological interventions aimed at addressing the underlying issues that are contributing to the symptoms. Both unconditional acceptance of the child's feelings and reassurance are powerful interventions for anxiety and depression. Facilitating open communication between children and their parents may also be helpful. Creative arts therapies, play, relaxation, storytelling, music, and games may assist in helping children begin to talk about their feelings. It is important to recognize that a certain level of anxiety and sadness is normal when facing death. Health care providers must take caution to not be overly "cheerful" or insistent that a child discuss his or her feelings. Calm presence, active listening, and sitting quietly with a child will help to build trust. Adolescents in particular are very private about their thoughts and feelings, and if they choose to share them with a caregiver, confidentiality is an important factor in continuing a

Table 49–6
Management of Anorexia/Cachexia

Intervention	Dose	Comments
Pharmacological Management		
Megestrol	10 mg/kg/dose PO bid	May cause headache, rash, hypertension
Dronabinol	2.5 mg/kg/dose 3–4 times/d	Provides triple effect of antiemetic, appetite stimulant, mood elevation. May be used in young children.
Multivitamins	Infant drops 1 mL PO qd	Anecdotal evidence
Children's chewables	1 tab qd	Suggests B vitamins increase appetite
Nonpharmacological Management		
Prepare small portions of favorite foods.		
Allow child to eat "comfort" foods, don't stress "balanced diet."		
Use thickened liquids or soft foods.		
Offer shakes, smoothies, and other high-calorie foods.		
Provide nutritional drinks as tolerated.		
Assist family in limiting stress over child's eating.		

Sources: Lacey et al. (2003), reference 29; Hellsten et al. (2000), reference 54.

trusting relationship with the adolescent. For more information on depression, see Chapter 19.

Neurological Symptoms

Restlessness/Agitation. Restlessness is a state of hyperarousal in which there is the sensation of not being able to rest or remain in a relaxed position. Agitation in children may present as irritability, combativeness, or refusal of attention or participation. Causes of restlessness and agitation in children with advanced disease can include a variety of physical and psychological causes (Table 49–7).

Assessment should include observing for such behaviors as frequent position changes, twitching, inability to concentrate on activities, inconsolability, disturbed sleep/wake cycles, and moaning. Spiritual distress, disturbing dreams or nightmares, fears, and comorbid anxiety or depression should also be assessed. Treatment for agitation and restlessness should use both age-appropriate pharmacological and nonpharmacological techniques (Table 49–8). Benzodiazepines may be helpful in

Table 49–7
Causes of Agitation/Restlessness in Children

Disease/Treatment-related Causes
Uncontrolled pain or other symptoms
Metabolic disturbances
Infections
Hypoxemia
Constipation
Sleep disturbance
Emotional Causes
Depression/Anxiety
Fear
Change in family routine
Reaction to stress of other family members
Withholding of open information or open discussion with child

Table 49–8
Management of Agitation/Restlessness

Intervention	Dose	Comments
Pharmacological Management		
Lorazepam	0.03–0.1 mg IV/PO q4–6h, may titrate to max 2 mg/dose	Indicated for generalized anxiety
		May increase sedation in combination with opioids
		May use in infants and young children
Midazolam	0.025–0.05 mg/kg/dose IV/SQ	Titrate to effect
	0.3–1 mg/kg (max 20 mg) PR	Indicated for myoclonus related to prolonged opioid use, mild sedation
		Short-acting, quickly reversed if overly sedated
Haloperidol	0.05–0.15 mg/kg/d PO, IV, SQ divided 2–3 times per d	Indicated for agitation not responsive to benzodiazepines
		Monitor for extra-pyramidal symptoms, treat with diphenhydramine as needed
Nonpharmacological Management		
Maximize pain and other symptom assessment and management.		
Decrease environmental stress or stimulation.		
Encourage open communication between child and family.		
Provide relaxation/guided imagery.		
Provide favorite books, videos, or music.		
Encourage cuddling or holding by parents and other significant family members.		

Sources: Lacey et al. (2003), reference 29; Hellsten et al. (2000), reference 54.

reducing mild to moderate agitation and increasing effectiveness of nonpharmacological interventions.

In rare circumstances, children may experience such distressing restlessness or agitation as the result of unrelenting pain or other symptoms that the need for sedation may be considered. Sedation is generally indicated when distress cannot be controlled by any other means either due to limited timeframe or risk of excessive morbidity. Health care professionals must determine what are truly uncontrollable pain or symptoms versus undertreated pain and/or symptoms. Before considering sedation, it is important that all efforts have been made to achieve pain and symptom control. The goal of sedation is to relieve obvious suffering of the child by adding medications to induce sleep, but it is not intended to hasten death.

Presenting the option of sedation to a child and family requires a caring, open relationship between the treating health care professionals and the family. If the child and family are opposed to sedation, they should be reassured that all efforts to relieve distress will continue. If the child and family choose sedation, there are a number of pharmacological agents available to produce the desired level of relief. Consultation with a hospice physician would be appropriate to determine the clinical appropriateness and best agents to use to achieve the desired comfort goals of the child and family.[51]

Seizures. The risk for seizures in advanced and terminal disease is related to the nature of the underlying disease. Children with congenital malformations of the brain such as lissencephaly and congenital hydrocephaly, as well as other neurodegenerative diseases, often have seizures throughout their disease process. Children with malignancies of the central nervous system may experience seizures as an initial presentation of their illness or during disease progression. Children with advanced illnesses may also have seizure activity as a result of metabolic abnormalities, hypoxia, and neurotoxicity from medications. Seizure activity in children can present in a number of ways (Table 49–9). No matter what the cause, uncontrolled seizure is often one of the most distressing symptoms for parents. If a child has any risk for seizure activity at the end of life, emergency medications such as diazepam suppositories should be available in the home. Management involves correcting the underlying cause when possible and adding appropriate prophylactic pharmacological agents such as phenobarbital, clonazepam, or lorazepam (Table 49–10).

Table 49–9
Seizure Patterns in Children

Infants and Neonates
Deviation of eyes
Pedaling or stepping movements of legs
Rowing movements of arms
Eye blinking or fluttering
Sucking or smacking lips
Drooling
Apnea
Tonic/clonic movements
Older Children
Staring spells and deviated gaze
Unilateral or bilateral twitching, tremors
Generalized tonic/clonic movements

Dyspnea. The experience of dyspnea is one of the most common nonpain symptoms reported by children and parents.[22,44,52,53] Dyspnea is the unpleasant sensation of breathlessness and can be particularly frightening for children. Diseases of childhood most associated with dyspnea include cystic fibrosis and other interstitial lung diseases, muscular dystrophy, spinal muscular atrophy, end-stage organ failure, and metastatic cancer. In each of these diseases, there can be a number of underlying causes (Table 49–11) that may be amenable to treatment.

The sensation of dyspnea is a subjective experience, and assessment should include the following: its effect on the child's functional status, factors that worsen or improve dyspnea, assessment of lung sounds, presence of pain with breathing, and oxygenation status. Extent of disease, respiratory rate and oxygenation status may not always correlate with the degree of breathlessness experienced; therefore, patient report is the best indicator of the degree of distress. There is no validated tool to measure dyspnea, however, using a rating similar to a pain scale has proven anecdotally to provide some measure of distress and response to interventions.

Managing dyspnea is dependent on the suspected underlying cause of the symptom. Early in the terminal process, interventions for respiratory discomfort are aimed at improving respiratory effort. Antibiotics, oxygen, chemotherapy, or radiation to decrease tumor burden, and noninvasive ventilation for children with muscular degenerative disease, may be appropriate to treat the underlying cause. As the child becomes increasingly debilitated, the focus is on alleviating anxiety associated with respiratory changes and shortness of breath. There are a number of pharmacological choices for managing respiratory symptoms (Table 49–12). Opioids are the treatment of choice for managing dyspnea, as well as in treating a persistent cough. Anticholinergic medications assist in minimizing secretions. Bronchodilators promote increased air exchange in the lungs, and can be helpful alone or in conjunction with opioids. Anxiolytic drugs can help reduce anxiety related to the feeling of shortness of breath and improve respiratory comfort.[54] As in other discussions of symptom management, it is important to determine with the child and family the level of intervention that is consistent with their perceptions of the child's suffering and quality of life. For more information on dyspnea, see Chapter 13.

Table 49–10
Management of Seizures at End of Life

Intervention	Dose	Comments
Phenobarbitol	*Loading dose:* Children 10–20 mg/kg IV, may titrate by 5 mg/kg increments q15–30 min until seizure controlled or to max of 40 mg/kg/dose *Maintenance dose:* Infants/children 5–8 mg/kg/d in 1–2 divided doses Therapeutic serum levels 1–50 µg/mL	Generalized tonic-clonic seizures Status epilepticus
Carbamazepine	*<6 yrs initial:* 5 mg/kg/d PO, titrate based on serum levels q5–7 d to dose of 10 mg/kg/d, then 20 mg/kg/d if necessary, give in 2–4 divided doses *6–12 yrs initial:* 100 mg/d or 10 mg/kg/d PO in 2 divided doses, increase by 200 mg/d in weekly intervals until therapeutic serum levels reached *>12–Adult initial:* 200 mg PO bid, increase by 200 mg/d in weekly intervals until therapeutic serum levels reached	Partial or complete seizures, generalized tonic-clonic, mixed seizure patterns
Phenytoin	*Loading dose:* Infants/children 15–20 mg/kg IV *Maintenance dose:* 6 mo–3 y: 8–10 mg/kg/d in divided doses; 4 y–6 y: 7.5–9 mg/kg/d in divided doses; 7 y–9 y: 7–8 mg/kg/d in divided doses; 10 y–16 y: 6–7 mg/kg/d in divided doses Therapeutic levels 8–15 µg/mL for neonates, 10–20 µg/mL for children	Generalized tonic-clonic seizures Status epilepticus
Diazapam	2–5 y: 0.5 mg/kg PR 6–11 y: 0.3 mg/kg PR >11 y: 0.2 mg/kg PR May repeat 0.25 mg/kg in 10 min PRN	Status epilepticus

Sources: Lacey et al. (2003), reference 29; Hellsten et al. (2000), reference 54.

Terminal Respirations. In the final days to hours of life, respiratory patterns often change, initially becoming more rapid and shallow, then progressing to deep, slow respirations with periods of apnea, typically know as Cheyne-Stokes breathing. As the body weakens, pooling of secretions in the throat can lead to noisy respirations, sometimes referred to as "death rattle." Often at this point in disease progression, children are somnolent most of the time and do not report distress. However, these symptoms are particularly agonizing for parents and other family members to experience. Assessment should include monitoring changes in heart rate and respiratory rate, observing for distress, stridor, wheezing, and rales/rhonchi. Management should focus on managing family distress by explaining the nature of the dying process, reassuring the family that the child is not suffering, administering appropriate anticholinergic medications to decrease secretions, and decreasing or discontinuing any fluids or enteral feedings that may exacerbate the development of secretions or fluid overload.

Gastrointestinal Symptoms

Nausea/Vomiting. The pathophysiology of nausea and vomiting is often multifactorial, can be acute, anticipatory or delayed, and requires careful assessment to determine underlying causes. Nausea and vomiting can cause extreme exhaustion and dehydration if not well controlled. Underlying causes of nausea and vomiting may include decreased gastric motility, constipation, obstruction, metabolic disturbances, medication side effects or toxicity, and increased intracranial pressure.

A detailed assessment of the onset and duration, as well as the presence of concomitant symptoms (e.g., headache, visual disturbances) must be obtained. Medical management of nausea and vomiting is based on the suspected underlying cause (Table 49–13).

Corticosteroids may be helpful in reducing an intestinal obstruction. Antiemetic medications combined with medications to reduce secretions (e.g., glycopyrrolate) can be helpful

Table 49–11
Causes of Dyspnea

Physiological Causes
Tumor infiltration/compression
Aspiration
Pleural effusion, pulmonary edema, pneumothorax
Pneumonia
Thick secretions/mucous plugs
Bronchospasm
Impaired diaphragmatic excursion due to ascites, large abdominal tumors
Congestive heart failure
Respiratory muscle weakness due to progressive neurodegenerative disease
Metabolical disturbances
Psychological Causes
Anxiety
Panic disorder

in relieving nausea and vomiting related to intestinal obstruction. In cases of severe nausea and vomiting related to obstruction, placement of a nasogastric tube can decompress the stomach and provide comfort. Medications that promote gastric emptying (e.g., metoclopramide) or motility should not be used if obstruction is suspected. Steroids can provide relief from vomiting due to increased intracranial pressure. Nausea and vomiting related to medications or anorexia may be managed by a number of antiemetic medications.[54] Relaxation techniques, deep breathing, distraction, and art therapies may assist in reducing anticipatory nausea. For more information on nausea and vomiting, see Chapter 9.

Constipation. Constipation is a frequent symptom experienced by children with advanced and terminal illness and can occur even in children with limited oral intake. Children and adolescents in particular become embarrassed if asked about bowel habits and will deny problems, leading to a severe problem. It is important to educate the child and family about the potential distress caused by constipation, and determine with the child how to discuss this issue. Constipation occurs due to inactivity, dehydration, electrolyte imbalance, bowel compression or invasion by tumor, nerve involvement, and/or medications. Symptoms include anorexia, nausea, vomiting, colicky abdominal pain, bloating, and fecal impaction. Physical exam may reveal abdominal distension, right lower-quadrant tenderness, and fecal masses. A rectal exam should be done; however, it is important to gain the child's or adolescent's trust before such an invasive assessment. Ask the child which parent he or she would prefer to be present and have that parent sit near the child and provide reassurance and comfort. Assess the rectum for hard impacted feces, an empty dilated rectum, or extrinsic compression of the rectum by a tumor, hemorrhoids, fissures, tears, or fistulas.

Management is aimed at preventing constipation from occurring, but if constipation has occurred, it should be treated immediately to avoid debilitating effects (Table 49–14).

Stool softeners should be given for any child at risk of constipation due to opioid pain management or decreased activity. Softeners are most effective when children are well hydrated, so encourage the child to drink water as tolerated. Stimulant laxatives should be used if a child has not had a bowel movement for more than 3 days past that child's usual pattern. If these measures are not successful, stronger cathartic laxatives (e.g., magnesium citrate) or an enema may be used. If there is stool in the rectum and the child is unable to pass it, digital disimpaction may be necessary. The child should be prepared for the procedure and premedicated with pain and antianxiety medications. For more information on constipation see Chapter 11.

Diarrhea. Although diarrhea is far less common than constipation in children with terminal illnesses, it still may occur and contribute to a diminished quality of life. Diarrhea may be caused by intermittent bowel obstruction, fecal impaction, medications, malabsorption, infections, history of abdominal or pelvic radiation, chemotherapy, inflammatory bowel disease, and foods with sorbitol and fructose (found frequently in juices, gum, and candy).[51] Diseases related to increased risk of diarrhea include HIV/AIDS due to infections, cystic fibrosis related to malabsorption, and malignancies related to disease progression and treatment history.

Assessment should include onset, suddenness, duration and frequency of loose stools, incontinence, and character of the stools (color, odor, consistency, presence of mucus or blood), bowel sounds, presence of palpable masses or feces, abdominal tenderness, and examination of the rectal area. Assessment of dehydration includes observation of mucous membranes for dryness, cracking, poor skin turgor, and generalized fatigue. Diet and medication history should be reviewed for potential causes of diarrhea.

Treatment is aimed at managing the underlying causes and the results of persistent diarrhea (Table 49–15). Dietary intervention should involve continued feeding of the child's regular diet as tolerated, as well as oral rehydration with electrolyte solutions as tolerated.[51] For debilitated children using incontinence garments, attention to skin condition and prevention of breakdown is imperative. For more information on diarrhea, see Chapter 11.

Summary

Symptom management for children with advanced and terminal diseases presents a challenge to health care providers. Suffering from uncontrolled symptoms can be prevented by

Table 49–12
Management of Respiratory Symptoms

Agent	Dose	Comments
Morphine	0.1–0.2 mg/kg/dose IV/SQ	Indicated for dyspnea, cough
	0.2–0.5 mg/kg/dose PO	May need to titrate to comfort
Hydromorphone	15 µg/kg IV q4–6h	
	0.03–0.08 mg/kg/dose PO q4–6h	
Glycopyrrolate	40–100 mg/kg/dose PO 3–4 times/d	Indicated for secretions, congestion
	4–10 µg/kg/dose IV/SQ q3–4h	May give in conjuction with hyoscymine
Hyoscyamine	Infant drops (<2 y) 2.3 kg: 3 gtts q4 h; max: 18 gtt/d 3.4 kg: 4 gtt q4h; 24 gtt/d 5 kg: 5 gtt q4h; max: 30 gtt/d 7 kg: 6 gtt q4h; max: 36 gtt/d 10 kg: 8 gtt q4h; 48 gtt/d 15 kg: 10 gtt q4h; 66 gtt/d	
	2–12 y: 0.0625–0.125 mg PO q4h; max: 0.75 mg/d	
	>12 years: 0.125–0.25 mg PO q4h; max: 1.5 mg/d	
Hydromet (solution combination of hydrocodone and homatropine)	0.6 mg/kg/d divided 3–4 doses/d	
Albuterol	*Oral:* 2–6 years: 0.1–0.2 mg/kg/dose tid; max: 4 mg tid	Indicated for wheezing, pulmonary congestion
	6–12 y: 2 mg/dose 3–4 times/d; max: 24 mg/d	Side effects include increased heart rate, anxiety
	>12 y: 2–4 mg/dose 3–4 times/d; max: 8 mg qid	
	Nebulized: 0.01–0.5 mL/kg of 0.5% solution q4–6h	

Sources: Lacey et al. (2003), reference 29; Hellsten et al. (2000), reference 54.

Table 49–13
Management of Nausea/Vomiting

Agent	Dose	Comments
Ondansetron	0.15 mg/kg/dose IV or 0.2 mg/kg dose PO q4h; max: 8 mg/dose	Indicated for opioid-induced nausea/ vomiting
Metoclopromide	1–2 mg/kg/dose IV q2–4h; max: 50 mg/dose	Indicated for nausea/vomiting related to anorexia, gastroesophageal reflux Can cause dystonia
Promethazine	0.5 mg/kg IV/PO q4–6h; max: 25 mg/dose	Indicated for nausea/vomiting related to obstruction, opioids May increase sedation
Dexamethasone	1–2 mg/kg IV/PO initially, then 1–1.5 mg/kg/d divided q6h; max: 16 mg/d	Indicated for nausea/vomiting related to bowel obstruction, intracranial pressure, medications Side effects include weight gain, edema, and gastrointestinal irritation

Table 49–14
Management of Constipation

Senna
Children <12 y: 1–2 tablets PO qhs
2–4 y: Syrup: ¼–½ tsp PO qhs
4–6 y: Syrup: ½–1 tsp PO qhs
6–10 y: Syrup: 1 tsp PO qhs
Ducosate Sodium
Children <3 y: 10–40 mg/d PO in 1–4 divided doses
3–6 y: 20–60 mg/d PO in 1–4 divided doses
6–12 y: 50–150 mg/d PO in 1–4 divided doses
Older than 12 y: 50–100 mg/d PO in 1–4 divided doses

Table 49–15
Management of Diarrhea

Loperamide
Initial doses: 2–12 y; 2–5 y: 1 mg PO tid; 6–8 y: 2 mg PO bid; 8–12 y: 2 mg PO tid; after initial dose, 0.1-mg/kg doses after each loose stool (not to exceed the initial dose); >12 y: 4 mg PO × 1 dose; then 2 mg PO after each loose stool (maximum dose: 16 mg/d)
Diphenoxylate and atropine
2–5 y: 2 mg PO tid (not to exceed 6 mg/d)
5–8 y: 2 mg PO qid (not to exceed 8 mg/d)
8–12 y: 2 mg PO 5 times/d (not to exceed 10 mg/d)
>12 y: 2.5–5 mg PO 2–4 times/d (not to exceed 20 mg/d)

knowledge of the child's underlying disease process, thorough assessment of the child and family for sources of suffering, advocacy for child and family needs, and the use of an interdisciplinary approach to management that includes appropriate pharmacological and nonpharmacological interventions.

REFERENCES

1. Feudtner C, DiGiuseppe DL, Neff JM. Hospital care for children and young adults in the last year of life: a population based study. BMC Medicine 2003;1:1–9.
2. Newacheck PW, Halfon N. Prevalence and impact of disabling chronic conditions in childhood. Am J Public Health 1998;88: 610–617.
3. Feudtner C, Hays RM, Haynes G, Geyer JR, Neff JM, Koepsell TD. Deaths attributed to pediatric complex conditions: national trends and implications for supportive care services. Pediatrics 2001;107:e99.
4. Kane JR, Brown Hellsten M, Coldsmith A. Human suffering: the need for relationship-based research in pediatric end-of-life care. J Pediatr Oncol Nurs 2004;21:180–185.
5. Field MJ, Behrman RR. When children die: improving palliative and end-of-life care for children and their families. Washington DC: National Academies Press, 2003.
6. Eichner JM, Johnson BH. Family centered care and the pediatrician's role. Pediatrics 2003;112:691–696.
7. Swallow VM, Jacoby A. Mothers' evolving relationship with doctors and nurses during the chronic childhood illness trajectory. J Adv Nurs 2001;36:755–764.
8. Stewart JL, Mishel MH. Uncertainty in childhood illness: a synthesis of the parent and child literature. Scholarly Inquiry for Nursing Practice 2000;14:299–326.
9. Cohen MH. The stages of the prediagnostic period in chronic, life-threatening childhood illness: a process analysis. Res Nurs Health 1995;18:39–48.
10. Cohen MH. The unknown and the unknowable—managing sustained uncertainty. West J Nurs Res 2003;15:77–96.
11. Meleski DD. Families with chronically ill children. Am J Nurs 2002;102(May):47–54.
12. Fisher H. The needs of parents with chronically sick children: a literature review. J Adv Nurs 2001;36:600.
13. Perrin EC, Lewkowicz C, Young MH. Shared vision: concordance among fathers, mothers, and pediatricians about unmet needs of children with chronic health conditions. Pediatrics 2000; 105(Jan):277–285.
14. Satterwhite BB. Impact of chronic illness on child and family: an overview based on five surveys with implications for management. Int J Rehabil Res 1978;1(Jan):7–17.
15. Lewis M, Vitulano LA. Biopsychosocial issues and risk factors in the family when the child has a chronic illness. Child Adolesc Psychiatr Clin N Am 2003;12:389–399.
16. Nereo NE, Fee RJ, Hinton VJ. Parental stress in mothers of boys with Duchenne Muscular Dystrophy. J Pediatr Psychol 2003; 28:473–484.
17. Giammona AJ, Malek DM. The psychological effect of childhood cancer on families. Pediatr Clin N Am 2002;49: 1063–1081.
18. Hodgkinson R, Lester H. Stresses and coping strategies of mothers living with a child with cystic fibrosis: implications for nursing professionals. J Adv Nurs 2002;39:377–383.
19. Steele RG. Trajectory of certain death at an unknown time: children with neurodegenerative life-threatening illness. Can J Nurs Res 2000;32:49–67.
20. Stewart JL. Children living with chronic illness: an examination of their stressors, coping responses, and health outcomes. Ann Rev Nurs Res 2003;21:203–243.
21. Bothwell JE, Dooley JM, Gordon KE, MacAuley A, Camfield PR, MacSween J. Duchenne Muscular Dystrophy—parental perceptions. Clin Pediatr 2002;41:105–109.
22. Wolfe J, Grier HE, Klar N, Levin SB, Ellenbogen JM, Salem-Schatz S, Emanuel EJ, Weeks JC. Symptoms and suffering at the end of life in children with cancer. N Engl J Med 2000; 342: 326–333.
23. McCallum DE, Byrne P, Bruera E. How children die in hospitals. J Pain Symptom Manage 2002;20:417–423.
24. Sourkes BM. Armfuls of Time: The Psychological Experience of the Child with a Life-Threatening Illness. Pittsburgh: University of Pittsburgh Press, 1995.

25. Van Riper M. The sibling experience of living with childhood chronic illness and disability. Ann Rev Nurs Res 2003;21:279–302.
26. Sharpe D, Rossiter L. Siblings of children with a chronic illness: a meta-analysis. J Pediatr Psychol 2002;27:869–710.
27. Foster C, Eiser C, Oades P, Sheldon C, Tripp J, Goldman P, Rice S, Trott J. Treatment demands and differential treatment of patients with cystic fibrosis and their siblings: patient, parent and sibling accounts. Child Care Health Dev 2001;27:349–364.
28. Murray JS. The lived experience of childhood cancer: one sibling's perspective. Issues Comprehen Pediatr Nurs 1998;21:217–227.
29. Lacy CF, Armstrong LL, Goldman MP, Lance LL. Drug Information Handbook, 2003–2004 ed. Canada: Lexi-Comp Inc., 2003.
30. Hendricks-Ferguson VL. Crisis intervention strategies when caring for families of children with cancer. J Pediatr Oncol Nurs 2000;17:3–11.
31. Shapiro J, Perez M, Warden MJ. The importance of family functioning to caregiver adaptation in mothers of child cancer patients: testing a social ecological model. J Pediatr Oncol Nurs 1998;15:47–54.
32. Sheeran T, Marvin RS, Pianta RC. Mothers' resolution of their child's diagnosis and self-reported measures of parenting stress, marital relations, and social support. J Pediatr Psychol 1997;22: 197–212.
33. LeBlanc LA, Goldsmith T, Patel DR. Behavioral aspects of chronic illness in children and adolescents. Pediatr Clin North Am 2003;50:859–878.
34. Ritchie MA. Sources of emotional support for adolescents with cancer. J Pediatr Oncol Nurs 2001;18:105–110.
35. Meijer SA, Sinnema G, Bijstra JO, Mellenbergh GJ, Wolters WH. Coping styles and locus of control as predictors for psychological adjustment of adolescents with a chronic illness. Soc Sci Med 2002;54:1453–1461.
36. Sloper P. Experiences and support needs of siblings of children with cancer. Health Social Care Commun 2000;8(Sept):298–306.
37. Derevensky JL, Tsanos AP, Handman M. Children with cancer: an examination of their coping and adaptive behavior. J Psychosoc Oncol 1998;16:37–61.
38. Murray JS. Social support for siblings of children with cancer. J Pediatr Oncol Nurs 1995;12:62–70.
39. Hinds PS, Oakes L, Furman W, Quargnenti A, Olson MS, Foppiano P, Srivastava DK. End-of-life decision making by adolescents, parents, and healthcare providers in pediatric oncology: research to evidence-based practice guidelines. Cancer Nurs 2001;24:122–134.
40. Vickers JL, Carlisle C. Choices and control: parental experiences in pediatric terminal home care. J Pediatr Oncol Nurs 2000; 17:12–21.
41. Kirschbaum MS. Life support decisions for children: what do parents value? Adv Nurs Sci 1996;19:51–71.
42. Hockenberry-Eaton M, Hinds P, O'Neill J. Developing a conceptual model for fatigue in children. Eur J Oncol Nurs 1999;3:5–11.
43. Hockenberry-Eaton MJ, Hinds PS, Alcoser P. Fatigue in children and adolescents with cancer. J Pediatr Oncol Nurs 1998;15: 172–182.
44. Collins JJ, Devine TD, Dick GS, Johnson EA, Kilham HA, Pinkerton CR, et al. The measurement of symptoms in young children with cancer: the validation of the Memorial Symptom Assessment Scale in children aged 7–12. J Pain Symptom Manage 2002;23:10–16.
45. Carter BS, Leuthner SR. The ethics of withholding/withdrawing nutrition in the newborn. Semin Perinatol 2003;27:480–487.
46. Nelson LJ, Rushton CH, Cranford RE, Nelson RM, Glover JJ, Truog RD. Forgoing medically provided nutrition and hydration in pediatric patients. J Law Med Ethics 1995;23:33–46.
47. Stevens M. Care of the dying child and adolescent: family adjustment and support. In: Doyle D, Hanks G, Cherny N, Calman K, eds. Oxford Textbook of Palliative Medicine. London: Oxford University Press, 2004.
48. Hockenberry M, Wilson D, Winkelstein M, Kline N. Wong's Nursing Care of Infants and Children, 7th ed. St. Louis, MO: Mosby, 2003.
49. Pasacreta J, Minarik P, Nield-Anderson L. Anxiety and depression. In: Ferrell BR, Coyle N, eds. Textbook of Palliative Nursing. New York: Oxford University Press, 2001.
50. Chochinov H, Wilson K, Enns M, Lander S. Depression, hopelessness and suicidal ideation in the terminally ill. Psychosomatics 1998;39:366–370.
51. Hockenberry M, Barrera P, Brown M, Bottomley S, O'Neill J. Pain management in children with cancer. Austin, TX: Texas Cancer Council, 1999.
52. Collins JJ, Byrnes ME, Dunkel IJ, Lapin J, Nadel T, Thaler HT, Polyak T, Rapkin B, Portenoy RK. The measurement of symptoms in children with cancer. J Pain Symptom Manage 2000; 19:363–377.
53. Hunt A, Burne R. Medical and nursing problems of children with neurodegenerative disease. Palliative Med 1995;9:19–26.
54. Hellsten MB, Hockenberry M, Lamb D, Chordas C, Kline K, Bottomley S. End-of-Life Care for Children. Austin, TX: Texas Cancer Council, 2000.

50

Lizabeth H. Sumner

Pediatric Care: The Hospice Perspective

We sit outside at night and we talk about the stupid things people say, like "I know how you feel." Which child of yours is dying of cancer or may die from cancer? If you don't have a child dying from cancer, then you don't know how I feel. You could have lost your husband or your wife or your parents, not your child that you gave birth to. It's not the same game. You can get another husband. Can't get another parent, but you expect your parents to go before you do. You don't expect your children to go before you.—Parent of a child with cancer[1]

Perhaps a simple children's book on the life cycle of nature, Lifetimes, *illustrates it best: "There are lots of living things in our world. Each one has its own special lifetime. All around us, everywhere beginnings and endings are going on around us all the time. So, no matter how long they are, or how short, lifetimes are really all the same. They have beginnings and endings and there is living in between."*[2]

- ***Key Points***
- *Nursing responsibilities in caring for the dying child are extensive.*
- *Specific education and training in symptom management and psychosocial issues are needed.*
- *Unique areas of concern when dealing with a pediatric population are the issues of the parents and those of the siblings.*
- *Improving quality of life for even a brief life can benefit not only the patient but all those affected by the death of a young child including grandparents, other relatives, teachers, school friends, and neighbors, as well as many health care professionals involved in their treatment and care.*
- *Nurses who choose to care for dying infants and children and their families need a significant support system themselves.*

Although much has been written about end-of-life care for adults, far less emphasis has been placed on the needs of dying infants and children. The ongoing painful dilemmas and struggles for families with infants and children who are dying remain hidden from society's view, yet the demands and challenges of caring for a dying child are being addressed within hospitals and homes on a daily basis. Individuals committed to children with life-threatening illnesses and a modest number of hospice programs are making a difference, finding ways to significantly impact the imbalance in addressing the needs of children. The irony for pediatric caregivers is that "end-of-life care" is often necessary at the very beginning of a child's life. Nurses can be instrumental in incorporating this contradiction into a realistic and compassionate framework for the care of children and families dealing with terminal illnesses. The report from the Institute of Medicine, *When Children Die: Improving Palliative and End-of-Life Care of Children and Their Families,* set forward the challenge to improve all aspects of end-of-life care for children and families, including improved quality and access to pediatric hospice.[3] The National Consensus Project Guidelines for Quality Palliative Care published in 2004 also provide direction for pediatric care within the overall perspective of care for all those, adults or children, facing life-threatening illness.[4]

The ultimate goal is not only to promote excellent end-of-life care for these children but also to elevate their status in a health care delivery model. Appropriate hospice care will bring them into the sunlight to be cherished among the living, where they will be removed from the isolating experiences of their dying. Improving quality of life for even a brief life can benefit the patient and all those affected by the death of a young child. Such a powerful wave goes beyond those most obviously affected—the parents and siblings. The rippling effect extends to grandparents, other relatives, teachers, school friends, family friends and neighbors, as well as the many health care professionals

Table 50–1
Children's Hospice International Standards of Hospice Care for Children

Access to Care

Principle

Children with life-threatening, terminal illnesses and their families have special needs. Hospice services for children and their families offer developmentally appropriate palliative and supportive care to any child with a life-threatening condition in an appropriate setting. Children are admitted to hospice services without regard for diagnosis, gender, race, creed, handicap, age or ability to pay.

Standards

A.C.1. Hospice care services are accessible to children and their families in a setting that is desired and/or appropriate for their needs.

A.C.2. The hospice team is available to provide continuity of care to children and their families in the home and/or in an institutional setting.

A.C.3. The hospice program has eligibility admission criteria for the children and families they serve. Care plans are developed which take into consideration the child's prognosis, and the child and family's needs and desires for hospice services. Admission to the hospice care services does not preclude the child and family from treatment choices or hopeful, supportive therapies.

A.C.4. The hospice program provides information to the community and referral sources about the services that are offered, who qualifies, and how services may be obtained and reimbursed.

Child and Family as a Unit of Care

Principle

Hospice programs provide family-centered care to enhance the quality of life for the child and family as defined by each child-and-family unit. It includes the child and family in the decision making process about services and treatment choices to the fullest degree that is possible and desired.

Standards

C.F.U.1. The unit of care is the child and family. Hospice provides family-centered care. The family is defined as the relatives and/or other significant persons who provide physical, psychological, social and/or spiritual support for the child.

C.F.U.2. The hospice program recognizes the unique, personal values and beliefs of all children and families. The hospice respects and maintains, as possible, the wishes and dignity of every child and his or her family.

C.F.U.3. The hospice program encourages that children and their families participate in decisions regarding care, including discontinuation of hospice care at any time, and maintains documentation related to consent, advance directives, treatments, and alternative choices of care.

C.F.U.4. The hospice program provides care that considers each child's growth, development and stage of family life cycle. Children's interests and needs are solicited and considered, but are not limited to those related to their illness and disability.

C.F.U.5. The hospice team seeks to assist each child and family to enjoy life as they are able, and to continue in their customary life-style, functioning and roles as much as possible, especially helping the child to live as normal a life as is possible.

Policies and Procedures

Principle

The hospice program offers services that are accountable to and appropriate for the children and families it serves.

Standards

P.P.1. The hospice program establishes and maintains accurate and adequate policies and procedures to assure that the hospice is accountable to children, their families, and the communities they serve.

P.P.2. The hospice agency is in compliance with all local, state and federal laws and regulations which govern the appropriate delivery of hospice care services.

P.P.3. The hospice program provides a clear and accessible grievance procedure to families outlining how to voice complaints or concerns about services and care without jeopardizing services.

Interdisciplinary Team Services

Principle

Seriously ill children with life-threatening conditions and/or facing terminal stages of an illness and their families have a variety of needs that require a collaborative and cooperative effort from practitioners of many disciplines, working together as an interdisciplinary team of qualified professionals and volunteers.

Standards

I.T.1. The hospice program provides care to the child and family by utilizing a core interdisciplinary team which may include: the child, the family and/or significant others, physicians, nurses, social workers, clergy and volunteers.

I.T.2. Representatives of other appropriate disciplines are involved in the team as needed, i.e., physical therapy, occupational therapy, speech therapy, nutritional consultation, art therapy, music therapy. The team might also include psychologists, child life specialists, teachers, recreation therapists, play therapists, home health aides, nursing assistants, and other specialists or services as needed.

I.T.3. The hospice core team meets on a regular basis and an integrated plan of care is developed, implemented and maintained for every child and family.

Source: Children's Hospice International, http://www.chionline.org. Copyright 1993 Children's Hospice International. Reprinted with permission.

involved in their care and treatment. Each of these may also be deeply influenced by the child's illness and subsequent death. Compared to a terminally ill adult, the comparatively larger number of people affected by a child's illness or impending death is significant. Few, if any, have had any previous experience with the death of a child. Typically, multiple physicians, care providers, suppliers, school professionals, and a variety of family members are involved with these children. Each has unique needs and roles in the child's experience. In addition, knowledge and skills regarding both palliative care and curative care are essential to guide families through this transition in the focus of care.[5]

Hospice care for children has not been well integrated into the existing national guidelines and regulatory standards. When this eventually takes place, the outcome will be a heightened visibility, credibility, and accountability for hospices, allowing home health programs and hospitals to adequately serve dying infants, children, and their families. The National Hospice and Palliative Care Organization (NHPCO) and Children's Hospice International (CHI) trends reveal disheartening underutilization of hospice services for pediatric patients and related health care practitioners. The 1998 CHI survey reported that fewer than 1% of children needing hospice care receive it.[6] Most state hospice organizations do not delineate which programs even serve children. The NHPCO revised its *Hospice Standards of Practice* in an effort to integrate pediatrics into those guidelines. CHI publishes *Standards of Hospice Care*. However, the standards are rarely put into practice at the predominantly adult patient organizations[7] (Table 50–1). The result is an ongoing struggle for professional staff in pediatric care and for families, both of whom are dealing with end-of-life issues, unprepared for the journey they are embarking upon together. Calls for help and consultation come on a weekly basis to the author from health care professionals expressing concern and inadequacy regarding their ability to meet the demands and challenges of these young patients, their families, the schools to which they are connected, and the increasing complexity of their care.

Adult-focused programs and staff are typically unprepared to respond to the infrequent pediatric referrals, and also lack connections to pediatric providers to assist them in providing safe, appropriate hospice care. Treating children as small adults can be risky and is misguided for the patient, the family, and the staff.

The NHPCO developed four end-result patient/family outcomes that it requests hospice programs to use to measure their own effectiveness. These outcomes create goals on which all care and interventions should be based, thus creating opportunities for patients and families to achieve optimum care. The outcome measures are: (1) safe dying, (2) comfortable dying, (3) self-determined life closure, and (4) effective grieving.[8] Although these outcome measures were not specifically intended for the hospice pediatric population, they remain highly relevant and are intended to apply to the patient and caregiving family. Hospice programs are encouraged to use these measures as the foundation for the philosophy and clinical practice behind their service delivery. For example, dying children frequently have specific goals and ideas about what would be important for self-determined life closure (e.g., reaching a milestone of completing a grade level, celebrating a holiday/birthday early, a desire regarding place of death expressed by child and/or parent). The many ways in which the child and parents desire to remain in control over several aspects of their lives can be woven into interventions so that each feels successful.

The Underutilization of Hospice for Infants and Children

A review of local (San Diego County, CA; Table 50–2) and national (United States; Table 50–3) death statistics illustrates the potential diagnoses considered appropriate for pediatric hospice care. Traditionally, cancer diagnoses have dominated the list of relevant diseases for hospice eligibility. Data related to the neonatal and infant (less than 1 year) age group were compelling. Causes of death in this category include prematurity, genetic/chromosomal anomalies, hydrocephaly, anencephaly, severe cardiac anomalies, cerebral palsy, gastroschisis, rare syndromes, and more, many of which were expected to be life-limiting in nature. Until recently, most pediatric patients served by hospices predominantly had cancer diagnoses, congenital anomalies, or acquired immunodeficiency syndrome (AIDS). National data, however, indicate other life-threatening diagnoses, including heart diseases, central nervous system disorders, degenerative disorders, mucopolysacchariduria, degenerative neuromuscular disorders, cystic fibrosis, liver and heart failure, and death-inducing trauma (e.g., drowning, motor vehicle accident, etc.).[9]

These less "traditional" patients include: children discontinued from ventilators following a motor vehicle accident or in the perinatal period who are not expected to survive; drowning accident victims who have not died immediately; chronically ill children with a progressive decline; babies who are "born dying," i.e., transferred from a neonatal intensive care unit (NICU) to home or inpatient hospice care; children with rare and unusual syndromes; and those at any age for whom aggressive care has been withdrawn.

In addition to the above underserved pediatric patients, some circumstances also lead to other categories of underserved children, including those without insurance coverage for hospice care, those with an uncertain prognosis, chronically ill deteriorating children, children cared for by unprepared adult hospice staff, home health patients undertreated for holistic needs, and children of adult hospice patients (Table 50–4). Increased outreach to the health care specialists who work with these groups has resulted in increased referrals and utilization for consultation/collaboration. The development of the perinatal hospice component has created the opportunity for families to access hospice care during a pregnancy that is anticipated to have a fatal outcome for the baby at or soon after birth (Table 50–5).

On a positive note, progress is being made to address palliative care needs for children and families across settings, including

Table 50–2
1996 Top Causes of Death by Age in San Diego County, California

Cause	Number of Deaths	Cause	Number of Deaths
<1 Year		**5–14 Years**	
Certain conditions originating in the perinatal period	113	Unintentional injury	19
Congenital abnormalities	69	Neoplasms malignant	13
Symptoms, signs, and ill-defined conditions	23	Nervous system and sense organs diseases	5
Respiratory system diseases	6	Congenital abnormalities	2
Infectious and parasitic diseases	4	Homicide	4
Heart disease	2	Respiratory system diseases	3
Nervous system and sense organs diseases	10	Suicide	2
Unintentional injury	3	Heart disease	3
Homicide	4	Other circulatory system disease	3
Digestive system diseases	3	Digestive system diseases	1
Total <1 year	*243*	*Total 5–14 Years*	*58*
1–4 Years		**15–24 Years**	
Unintentional injury	9	Unintentional injury	103
Congenital abnormalities	11	Homicide	35
Homicide	7	Suicide	40
Neoplasms malignant	5	Neoplasms malignant	22
Nervous system and sense organs diseases	4	Heart disease	12
Respiratory system diseases	4	Nervous system and sense organs diseases	6
Infectious and parasitic diseases	2	AIDS	1
Heart disease	1	Symptoms, signs, and ill-defined conditions	9
Endocrine, nutritional and metabolic diseases and immunity disorders	3	Infectious and parasitic diseases	1
Symptoms, signs, and ill-defined conditions	3	Congenital abnormalities	6
Total 1–4 Years	*53*	Endocrine, nutritional, and metabolic diseases and immunity disorders	2
		Total 15–24 Years	*253*
		GRAND TOTAL 0–24 Years	*607*

Source: Death Certificate Records, Health and Human Services Agency, County of San Diego 1996 (Health Status of San Diego County Report 1997), San Diego, California.

the emergency department,[10] intensive care unit,[11] and NICUs.[12] Extending hospice principles to these settings not only improves care while children are in those areas, but also may facilitate referrals to hospice from those settings. There is also tremendous opportunity to extend hospice and palliative care much earlier in the child's illness, beginning at the time of diagnosis.[13]

Barriers to Accessing Hospice Care

Barriers to accessing hospice care for pediatric patients differ from those for adult. Society's belief that "children shouldn't die," along with denial of the process, make end-of-life care for this population a distant and mysterious concept. Within the health care profession, a profound silence of discomfort and denial exists regarding babies and children dying. In some cases, health care professionals' own attitudes and denial become the greatest barrier to their patients'/families' ability to access additional options for expert palliative care and support services. In effect, this denies families the possibility of making an informed decision regarding the range of choices available during a child's illness. Excellence in end-of-life care as part of the continuum of clinical expertise should be readily available for families who may transition or alternate their focus of care from a strictly curative mode to one of comfort and quality of life.

The original hospice demonstration project in the 1980s was designed as a Medicare program for older adults with cancer as

Table 50–3
Leading Causes of Death and Numbers of Deaths, According to Age: United States, 2002*

Rank Order	Cause of Death	Number of Deaths
Under 1 Year		
	All causes	*28,034*
1	Congenital malformations, deformations, and chromosomal abnormalities	5,623
2	Disorders related to short gestation and low birth weight, not elsewhere classified	4,637
3	Sudden infant death syndrome	2,295
4	Newborn affected by maternal complications of pregnancy	1,708
5	Newborn affected by complications of placenta, cord, and membranes	1,028
6	Unintentional injuries	946
7	Respiratory distress of newborn	943
8	Bacterial sepsis of newborn	749
9	Diseases of circulatory system	667
10	Intrauterine hypoxia and birth asphyxia	583
1–4 Years		
	All causes	*4,858*
1	Unintentional injuries	1,641
2	Congenital malformations, deformations, and chromosomal abnormalities	530
3	Homicide	423
4	Malignant neoplasms	402
5	Diseases of heart	165
6	Influenza and pneumonia	110
7	Septicemia	79
8	Chronic lower respiratory diseases	65
9	Certain conditions originating in the perinatal period	65
10	In situ neoplasms, benign neoplasms, and neoplasms of uncertain or unknown behavior	60
5–14 Years		
	All causes	*7,150*
1	Unintentional injuries	2,718
2	Malignant neoplasms	1,072
3	Congenital malformations, deformations, and chromosomal abnormalities	417
4	Homicide	356
5	Suicide	264
6	Diseases of heart	255
7	Chronic lower respiratory diseases	136
8	Septicemia	95
9	Cerebrovascular diseases	91
10	Influenza and pneumonia	91

(continued)

Table 50–3
Leading Causes of Death and Numbers of Deaths, According to Age: United States, 2002*
(continued)

Rank Order	Cause of Death	Number of Deaths
15–24 Years		
	All causes	*33,046*
1	Unintentional injuries	15,412
2	Homicide	5,219
3	Suicide	4,010
4	Malignant neoplasms	1,730
5	Diseases of heart	1,022
6	Congenital malformations, deformations, and chromosomal abnormalities	492
7	Chronic lower respiratory diseases	192
8	Human immunodeficiency virus (HIV) disease	178
9	Diabetes mellitus	171
10	Cerebrovascular diseases	171

*Data are based on death certificates.
Source: National Center for Health Statistics. Health, United States, 2004. Table 32, Leading causes of death and numbers of deaths, according to age: United States, 2002, p 158. Available at: http://www.cdc.gov/nchs/data/hus/hus04.pdf (accessed May 11, 2005).

the "typical" disease process. The constantly changing continuum of needs in the pediatric population, from birth through 21-plus years (including diagnoses, variable prognoses, developmental issues and needs, and varying family situations), has made it difficult to "fit into" the adult-oriented guidelines for admission and standards of care. These only increase the barriers to access to appropriate care for the dying child and his or her support system.

Personal Issues and Biases

Nurses may experience emotional turmoil over their young patients' declining conditions and poor prognoses. The professional role of the nurse may quickly give way to the perspective of a parent, mother, or father toward the child. Expressions of transference may emerge and become problematic to the parents, the child, the nurse, or other team members. In programs

Table 50–4
Children's Program of San Diego Hospice

Pediatric Hospice Patients	Children of Adult Hospice Patients	Community Outreach and Education
Serving infants, children and adolescents, young adults (0–21 years of age)	Counseling, resources, and consultation available for children in the adult San Diego Hospice patients families	Creating a bridge between hospice, the school community, and families
"Early Intervention Program": Perinatal Hospice. Support to families during the pregnancy through birth. Their babies have life-threatening conditions.	For children experiencing the life threatening illness of a parent, grandparent, or other relatives. Guidance and education for adults who care for them.	Individualized presentations or training based on a specific situation or a general request to support the students/faculty
Includes extended support system of patient—outreach to classroom, faculty, school	Children's books, therapeutic games and activities	Collaboration with school nurses, teachers, counselors, school psychologists, and other faculty on issues related to children experiencing loss, grief, serious illness—their own or a loved one
Adults 21+ case by case, based on circumstances	Play therapy	Provide resources and access to materials on the needs and concerns of children experiencing serious illness, loss, and grief
	Art therapy	
	Memory-making/keepsake activities	

Table 50–5
Early Intervention Program at San Diego Hospice: Perinatal Hospice

- Create a birthing plan with parents and other health care providers that may include the family's preference on interventions for the baby at birth, and options for the San Diego Hospice team's involvement with the family.
- Assist parents in identifying resources and psychosocial and spiritual counseling to help their family cope during the pregnancy and after the birth of the baby.
- Address the emotional needs and concerns of other children in the family.
- Provide guidance and encouragement in finding hope and comfort amidst the family's anguish and grief.
- Support the needs of the family and baby, if hospitalized, and assist the inpatient staff in coordinating a plan of care, including discharge planning, if appropriate.
- Assist in creating ways to celebrate and welcome the baby to the family in the hospital or at home.
- Assist in creating special keepsakes, rituals, and treasures before and after the baby's birth (for example, a memory box, handprints of baby and family members, photographs, locks of hair, etc.)
- Provide referrals to support groups and resource materials provide by various community organizations and San Diego Hospice.
- Help in planning final arrangements, memorial services, and good-byes at the hospital or at home, as appropriate.
- Provide bereavement support for all family members and other caregivers for a minimum of 18 months after baby dies.

Source: National Hospice and Palliative Care Organization Compendium of Pediatric Palliative Care Programs and Practices (December 2000). Alexandria, VA: Author.

where nurses are not clinically trained or emotionally prepared to manage pediatric patients, many issues can emerge as a result of their anguish. Previous losses of a similar nature, unresolved grief issues, conflicting beliefs regarding "supportive care only" interventions, and insecurities and self-doubt are all common, even within the hospice setting. The "if it were my child" frame of thinking can even be imposed upon parents who are already desperately struggling with their child's condition and the future that lies ahead for them. Personal and ethical dilemmas can emerge regarding withdrawal of aggressive care or nutritional support. Ethics consultations can bring an invaluable contribution to the decision-making process and often raise the option of a hospice consult or referral to hospice care.

Professional Issues

Nurses may lack pediatric physical assessment and symptom-management skills, as well as knowledge of the diverse disease processes and developmental stages and related needs essential to care for neonatal and pediatric patients. Those with a background in aggressive and curative care may find it difficult to support a family in transition to a palliative focus of care. A struggle for control may erupt between the family, the staff, and the child. By continually asking, "Whose need is this meeting?" one can maintain focus on the patient's care.

Most nursing education programs include little or no emphasis on the care of dying children and their families, death and dying issues, grief and loss (professional and family), perinatal death, or hospice care. A recent study was conducted to determine the amount and types of content regarding pain and end-of-life care included in major nursing textbooks. Three of the 50 books reviewed were pediatric texts. Of those, only two had chapters on end-of-life care for this population. The findings revealed that textbooks had limited content regarding end-of-life care in general, with the pediatric subtopic an even smaller percentage.[14] On a positive note, follow-up by the investigators of that textbook analysis also found that the pediatric texts have been responsive to these findings, making significant improvements in recent editions.

This deficit of information in academic texts explains why many nurses lack a foundation for care of pediatric patients at the end of life. In addition, there may be limited access to pediatric experienced staff of all disciplines to train or offer clinical support to the hospice staff. There also is a significant need to enhance the support provided to nurses working in pediatric hospice and in all pediatric settings caring for seriously ill children.[15]

Uncertainty in Determining the Child's Prognosis

State and federal regulations and standards governing hospice care and the clinical guidelines for ongoing appropriateness (Medicare and Medicaid) did not address pediatric patients when they were developed. Determining the required 6-months-or-less prognosis is extremely difficult for pediatric physicians because of the wide variability of prognoses in children, often varying from days to weeks, or months to years. Referral to hospice care by physicians also may represent to them "giving up" on their young patients. The requirement to certify that the child will be dead in 6 months is often perceived as a direct assault on the practice of physicians. Parents may still wish to continue active treatment, which may, in fact, prolong their child's life to some extent, but typically are not ready to "give up everything." Parents should not be forced to give up all treatment to avail themselves of help and guidance to actually make the transition to comfort care.

Payor or insurance providers may impose restrictions that deny access to hospice care for patients continuing curative treatment, and this is particularly problematic for children and parents. Parents and/or the child may want to pursue options that "buy more time," even if the goal is clearly palliative care, in order to be together longer. These families are not just "waiting longer for death" but intentionally trying to maximize the "living time" they have left. The resiliency of children is often astounding in the face of information that says they should have only hours or days to live. This has led to more pediatric hospice patients being discharged from the program. They have converted to a chronically ill child on a very different illness trajectory. These children are referred to as our "graduates" and the event is celebrated with the family. Adult programs are penalized for patients who do not die fast enough, and the pediatric population is even more difficult to predict. Frequent case review and discussions with parents, physicians, the hospice team, and, if possible, the child, ensure that everyone has the same goals and perceptions of the child's condition and appropriateness of care.

Reimbursement Issues

The cost of caring for this population is often a barrier to pursuing a pediatric hospice program. Pediatric hospice care typically requires longer, more frequent home visits; more coordination of care with multiple physicians, other providers, and insurance companies; visits to schools by members of the team on behalf of the sick child or siblings; and hiring or access to pediatric experienced nurses, social workers, and aides. Ongoing therapies for palliation of distressing symptoms continues longer, typically, for children than adults, including blood transfusions, antibiotics, chemotherapy, and enteral and gavage feedings. The cost and responsibility for covering these therapies may be an additional factor to providers in deciding whether to serve children.

Insurance coverage may be inadequate or nonexistent for hospice services. Many states have waiver programs that provide nursing shift care in lieu of hospitalization or for respite care, but these programs also make the child and family ineligible to receive hospice care, creating an unacceptable conflict of needs. Many programs must raise additional funds to offset the expense of the staff-intensive support required for these families. The caseloads for staff managing this population typically are smaller than in adult hospice programs because of the increased time needed for coordination and care, especially if nurses do their own admissions. Traditional measures of productivity are impacted by these factors as well. The norms for practice with the neonatal and pediatric population stands apart from adult hospice care. Play and settling-in time are inherent to interactions with children, which starkly contrast with the direct care approach for adults.

Lack of Knowledge and Awareness of What Hospice Care Is: Successful Strategies

Physicians and nurses dealing with neonatal and pediatric patients may be completely unaware of the option of hospice/palliative care, how to access it, and the appropriate conditions or diseases for eligibility. In reality, pediatric programs are starting from the ground level, trying to educate and build bridges with "hospice-naïve" health care professionals to insure optimal end-of-life care for infants and children. For many clinical areas in pediatrics, death is an infrequent event; staff may not be particularly adept at managing the needs of dying children and their families due to lack of familiarity and experience. In intensive care settings, a change in focus to comfort care seems, for many, completely contradictory to their "culture of high-tech."

Opportunities for families to receive hospice care begin when a relationship can be developed between a unit or department (e.g., NICU, pediatric ICU, hematology/oncology, labor and delivery, etc.) and the hospice team. Learning the needs and unique issues of each setting facilitates a customized approach to the specific populations served and the professional trust and accountability that are essential components for success. Discussing how to make referrals, adopting techniques for introducing the concept of hospice care to families and staff, exchanging expertise and resources, and providing in-service programs and educational opportunities are all methods to create a partnership between two specialties. This type of partnership can greatly influence the quality of life for patients, their families, and staff.

Participating in community based programs (e.g., Fetal Infant Mortality Review, perinatal nurse groups), coalitions regarding children's health care issues, collaborations on grief and loss of children, and presenting cases at grand rounds and professional meetings are all excellent ways to connect with other providers and develop vital linkages for a thriving pediatric hospice program. Some clinical areas allow a hospice team member to attend patient conferences and rounds to provide input to the team as part of case reviews, or even to be an observer in identifying potential patients. Participating in the "informational only," or evaluation visit with the child, parents, and staff can provide an excellent opportunity for modeling, learning the language of hospice care, and learning how to explain hospice services and roles. Trust is transferred between inpatient and hospice staff as a result of seeing, hearing, and experiencing what the other has to offer. The patients and families become more confident if they sense the confidence in those who make the referral. Many years of experience have revealed a higher level of expected accountability and responsiveness from pediatric caregivers regarding their patients when they are referred to hospice than for typical adult hospice care. Once trust and accountability have been established, they can form a strong and lasting foundation that can be passed on to new members as they join the hospice team. The need for ongoing, honest, and open communication between the two groups is critical.

Myths About Hospice Care for Children

Dispelling myths about hospice care can be helpful in creating an appropriate message about end-of-life or palliative care for pediatric patients. Many misconceptions need to be addressed, such as hospice care equals death; hospice care means giving up; hospice care means no more hope; hospice care means letting go or failure. It is important to clarify the scope and intent of hospice and palliative care and to address false perceptions when developing any collaborative relationship. If health care professionals do not have a clear and factual understanding about what hospice care is and is not, they will pass incorrect perceptions on to each other and to families. In no other area of health care is it more important for parents to know what we do and do not do. They must be aware of the following:

- The team does not come in and force discussions on death and dying.
- The hospice team does not insist that families be in complete acceptance of the fact that their child's condition is terminal.
- No one comes into their home and takes over or interferes with their sense of normalcy.
- The team does not decide what happens when.
- Team members do not get in between parents and their child.
- Team members do not challenge or judge the family's belief system.
- Team members do not discipline the child or children, but only set reasonable limits with parental input.

Each of these issues should be discussed during interactions with patients and families. Parents are entitled to be told these things to dispel the unspoken or as yet unarticulated fears they may have concerning hospice care. The hospice team can make this difficult transition somewhat easier for parents by addressing what parents may fear the team might do with, for, or to their child or to them.

Competition Between Home Health and Hospice Programs

Terminal nursing care and pain management programs are incorrectly equated with the interdisciplinary, holistic approach to end-of-life care that hospice programs can provide. The collaborative model of the interdisciplinary hospice team weaves a stronger, broader safety net of support and care around the family, enhancing their ability to meet the extraordinary challenge of a life-threatening illness.

Agencies are challenged with the moral responsibility to make the right decision for the dying child and his or her family, informing them of all relevant options to best meet the needs of the child. It may be in the child's best interest for a home care agency to refer the child to another, more appropriately qualified provider, such as a hospice program, if the program is better equipped to provide end-of-life care for the child. The multidimensional experience of a terminal illness requires attention to all aspects of the child's, parents', and siblings' needs, including spiritual, physical, emotional, and psychosocial needs. An individual nurse may feel overwhelmed by the enormous burden of trying to meet all those needs alone or may experience intense frustration and helplessness in not being able to do so at all within the limitations of traditional home health care. Difficulties can also arise when a referral to hospice care is offered but refused by families based on unfamiliarity and perhaps dependency on the home health care nurse.

Possible solutions to this situation might be a joint case conference to discuss the family's issues and concerns or making a few joint, overlapping visits to transfer trust and to ease the often well-established relationships to the hospice team. These may be nonreimbursed visits, but they may create an openness between the two programs and increase referrals. These visits may require discussions with the parents regarding their fears and concerns and how their needs might be met.

Staffing Issues

Many hospices are not staffed with nurses who are comfortable dealing with babies, young children, and adolescents who are dying, or with the unique issues of the parents and/or extended family. Because the family's outlook is greatly influenced by the personalities and reactions of the staff, a special degree of confidence and caring is required.[16] After-hours staffing poses a particular challenge, and sometimes a hardship, on the agency and its staff. Adult care staff may be unwilling or incapable of caring for pediatric patients. The most serious outcome would be added stress and uncertainty imposed by the very experts from whom families are seeking refuge and comfort. Partnering with pediatric staff to train other staff, as well as thorough reporting to the after-hours staff are helpful actions. Anticipation of needs and problems with a plan for appropriate treatment can minimize and even prevent symptom crises.

Cultural Issues

Various cultures approach the child with a terminal illness differently. This involves decision-making, communication, openness with the patient, the role of the parents in protecting the child from the truth about his or her condition, the role religion or faith plays in health care issues, and determination of who can translate for the family respectfully. Language barriers and lack of translation options can create great obstacles to providing adequate care. For example, parents may direct staff not to address the dying process with the child so as not to discourage the child. They may believe that in saying "it" aloud, it will cause "it" to come to pass. Or simply speaking of death may be too direct within the context of their culture. Hope is often intertwined in cultural issues and in the expression of that culture within the experience of serious illness. For some families, this may necessitate frequent and ongoing reteaching and subsequent validation that a plan for collaborative care has been respected. These issues of decision-making are of particular relevance to adolescents, as they play a more active role in decision-making regarding illness and end-of-life care.[17]

Stretching the Boundaries of Hospice Care: A Model for a Comprehensive Program for Infants and Children

Since 1987, San Diego Hospice has been serving pediatric patients and striving to integrate pediatrics into the mainstream of the hospice culture and industry. What began as an informal relationship with a hospice staff nurse and the nurses and doctors at Children's Hospital San Diego evolved into "the team," a model for other programs across the country. Through many twists and turns, a vision emerged seeking to broaden the continuum of services for children at San Diego Hospice. The focus shifted from serving only a narrow target of sick and dying children to serving all children under the umbrella of care. This meant adding a component of specialized support and clinical intervention for the children of adult hospice patients (Figure 50–1 and Table 50–6).

Children Dealing With Adult Hospice Patients

Children's Program social workers and, as appropriate, a chaplain, work directly with children who have a loved one, such as a parent, grandparent, aunt, or uncle, dying. Their interventions include opportunities for play and art therapy; rituals and keepsake activities for themselves or the family; therapeutic games; and storybooks on coping with feelings and illness, grief and loss, death and dying, the life cycle of nature, funerals, etc. For this new approach, the entire Children's Program considers the focus of care not to be the "patient and family," but the patient (adult or pediatric), family, and school.

The team extends the circle of care to involve the child's or children's school in its web of support for the family. Typically (with parental permission), the social worker will confer or even meet with the teacher, school counselor, or nurse to include them in the plan of care. The primary hospice team, focused on the adult patient, is kept abreast of their involvement and goals. The aim is to facilitate more involvement of the child in the illness experience before the death occurs, maximizing their support systems as well as their ability to cope with the death when it does occur. A great deal can be done to better prepare children for the death and loss of a loved one by early intervention. Besides anticipatory grieving, many practical issues, fears, and concerns emerge for the children and their caregivers. In addition, the team provides adult caregivers with strategies and education regarding children's needs during the loved one's illness and in bereavement.

The Child as a Hospice Patient

Families are never fully prepared for a child to be gone from their lives. The hospice professional can take steps to assist them down the long road of bereavement by helping them create tangible reminders of and treasures from their child's life, no matter how short or long it is. San Diego Hospice has developed a lengthy profile of activities and rituals for families to consider performing while a child is sick. For example, families might create a memory box with the child of special

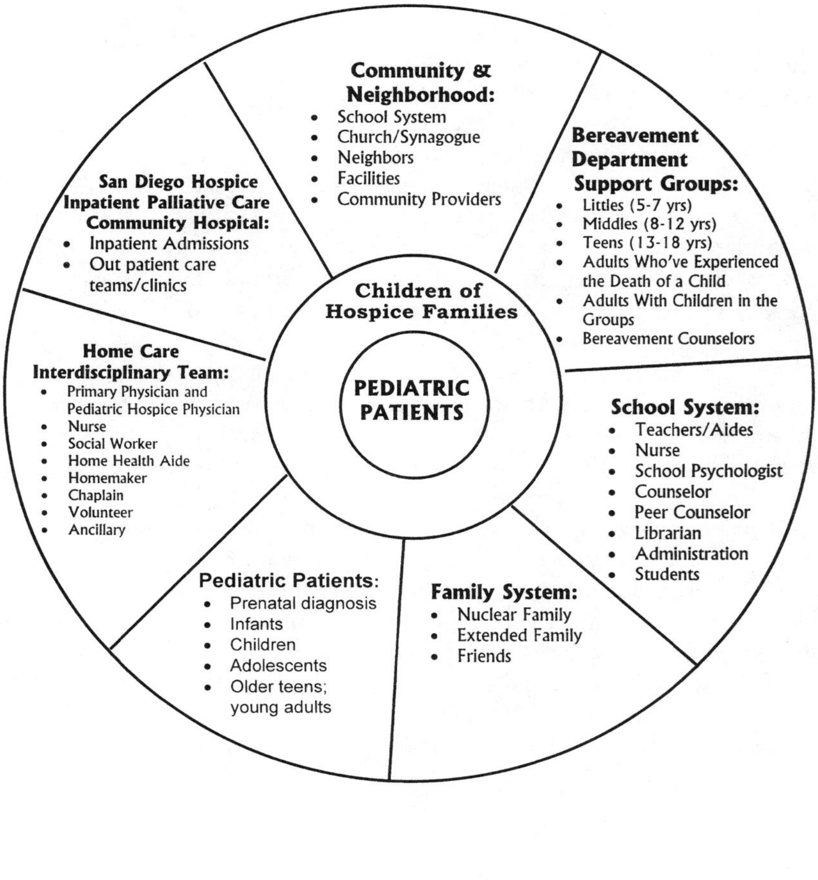

Figure 50–1. A model for a hospice children's program that originated with the San Diego Hospice and has been adopted by many other institutions.

Table 50–6
San Diego Hospice Children's Program: Children in Families of Adult Hospice Patients Served by the Children's Program

1998		1999	
Total by Relationship to Patient		Total by Relationship to Patient	
Children	74	Children	96
Grandchildren	110	Grandchildren	140
Great Grandchildren	0	Great Grandchildren	7
Nephew/Niece	3	Nephew/Niece	4
Other	7	Other	29
TOTAL	194	TOTAL	276

things that remind the child of favorite activities, trips, people, accomplishments—anything that helps to celebrate the child's life. Letters and journals can also be created by parents, the sick child, and siblings and friends. The most popular activity with families is doing handprints. This is done by making handprints of the baby or child, along with parents, siblings, and others, using tempera or poster paint to create a unique family portrait. Ear prints can be taken of a baby with anomalies of the extremities and as another way of preserving something physical of the child. An "All About Me" booklet can be created over time through regular visits of a volunteer or family member, capturing the child's identity before and after the illness and his or her role as part of a family. Schoolmates can send notebooks or letters back and forth to stay connected, and later these can become lovely remembrances of friendships.

The possibilities are endless, and these tangible keepsakes may help siblings and parents stay better connected to memories and significant events as they pass through developmental milestones over the years. These physical tokens may help relatives find their way back to special memories and events concerning their loved one. These treasures may help them to survive their experience a bit more whole, having a "toolbox" to help them integrate this tremendous loss into their being and may help them to create a sense of meaning about the experience over time.

These additional components were added to the Children's Program to meet the needs identified by both the agency and community. The adult hospice patient referrals have been positively influenced by the availability of additional help, specifically for the children in the adult-patient families. The number of these children served by the Children's Program continues to increase dramatically (see Table 50–6).

Local schools began to seek support, training, resources, and family intervention from this team. The next component added to the program became a commitment to assist and support the school community in confronting the illness, death, grief, and loss experiences of their students, families, faculty, and community members.

The first priority was to develop a staffing model for a mixed pediatric patient population. Hospice board and administrative support enhanced resources for handling a growing census and expanded focus. Critical to preserving the stability and integrity of the program was maintaining consistent staff focused on the needs of children, pediatric patient care, and program development. Requiring staff to work on both children and adult care on a constant basis had led to high staff turnover. While creating problems, these changes were essential to increase the visibility and credibility of the program within the community. These changes provided the optimal continuity of care desired by families, staff, and referral sources. It enhanced the ability of the program to meet the enormous demands of educating the hospice-naïve health care professionals throughout the community.

The Children's Program next partnered with the local children's hospital and health care center to become the hospice provider for their entire system. Adding a pediatrician as the children's program medical director has been highly valuable. This role includes building physician relationships in various specialty areas, consulting on potential patients, physician education, identifying potential research, and enhancing clinical practice by hospice nurses.

Overview of Nursing Care Issues for Pediatric Hospice Care

Nursing responsibilities when caring for a dying infant or child are extensive. An awareness of "total suffering" requires that the nurse understand the interconnectedness of the four aspects of the experience of illness and suffering: physical, emotional/psychological, spiritual, and social. Each component greatly affects the others. In the words of Attig, "Suffering is the experience of brokenness. Illness unravels the pattern that belongs uniquely to each child, interrupting the ongoing stories of children's lives."[18] Nurses must assess for imbalances and indications of suffering in each of these areas to appropriately intervene. Without physical comfort, a child has little energy to be "present" to those around him or her and engage in meaningful exchanges. Management of symptoms in children requires the same degree of diligence and aggressive intervention as that used for adult patients.

Symptoms in children are generally similar to those in adults. However, discomfort/seizure management, pain in nonverbal patients, and feeding issues are more common. The age and developmental level of the child directly influence the selection of pain assessment tools, intervention strategies, route of medication, and type of medication. Many excellent resources are available to nurses for gaining competence in pain and symptom management for children. In addition, families require practical help, information, explanations, and support.[19–21] Attention must be paid to the practical issues of preparing for pediatric-appropriate supplies, medications, formulas, feeding tubes, medical equipment, documentation, and teaching tools for parents and children. A gently written, parent-friendly handout on the signs and symptoms of approaching death is an invaluable tool.

Interaction with School

To provide education, support, and resources to classmates, teachers, and other parents, the team goes to the school of the sick child. The bridge developed between the hospice and schools has been a successful addition to the program. This came about in response to an ongoing need identified by the school community to support children during life's challenging experiences.

For example, a child with astrocytoma was still attending school while having intermittent, recurrent seizures despite aggressive pharmacological intervention to control them. The hospice team and supervisor, parents, teachers, school administrator, school nurse, and classroom aide attended a conference at the school to create a plan to respond to her seizures. The need for proper documentation regarding her resuscitation status and hospice involvement had to be kept on hand and accessible in the event of a crisis, since the district was legally required to call 911 despite the parents' wishes. Issues for the other students were addressed and recommendations were made. The emotional reactions of all involved were discussed, and support was offered.

Another example involved a severely disabled child who strongly desired to remain at school as long as possible. A similar conference was held, but with the child in attendance as well. A plan was made among all participants for the hospice staff to visit the patient at school occasionally. Again, a contingency plan was made in the event of an emergency so that the patient's and parents' wishes could be honored. In both situations, the schools were amazed at the collaborative effort and concern demonstrated by the hospice team. To them it seemed extraordinary. When the object of care is a child, a family, and a school, this is the expected standard of excellence.

Support for Siblings

Two unique areas of concern when dealing with a pediatric population are the issues of the parents and those of the siblings. Siblings require explanations along the way and opportunities to be included, not excluded, from these experiences that affect the entire family. Siblings relish the chance to be helpers to nurses and parents as a way to feel important and contribute to the tasks at hand. Helping serves to validate their relationship with the sick child, diminish their feelings of helplessness, and may well affect how they integrate the loss over time.

As mentioned earlier for the children of adult patients, in the same way for siblings, the goal for siblings of terminally ill children is to enhance their feelings of involvement to the greatest degree possible while the sibling is alive to facilitate a healthy grieving process. The attempt to assist in achieving "effective grieving" for the sibling must begin when the sick child is diagnosed, because the family is changed profoundly from that moment on.

Strategies for including siblings in care may be as simple as the nurse including the siblings in his or her visit, asking to see their rooms or favorite toys, or reading a story together. Joint visits with a social worker are highly effective in spreading the attention and interventions among the sick child, siblings, and parents. It is important to repeatedly evaluate the well child's level of understanding about the sibling's condition. Family meetings are also a good setting in which to discuss how everyone is doing, including the patient, how they each perceive the situation, how their needs are (or are not) being met, and how their fears and concerns can be addressed. With parents' permission, an occasional small treat for the sibling is a simple gesture that may help make the well children feel special and included. Hospice volunteers make an excellent addition to the team for the specific role of being available to the sibling for a picnic, playing outside, reading, or a specific project or memory-making activity. Of these, the primary activity of the San Diego Hospice Children's Team is handprinting with the whole family. The sick baby or child is handprinted and the rest of the family's handprints are placed around the child's. The activity lifts the family from focusing on the tasks of the illness to a playful yet reverent level. Subsequently, the print becomes a treasure for the family. The same activity can be done with children of a dying adult as a keepsake for the children. Siblings may wish to have their own set of prints as well. Parents and children are also given "memory boxes" to store treasures in.

Support for Parents

To counterbalance the overwhelming sense of powerlessness and helplessness parents frequently feel, nurses can help to identify ways in which they can feel more in control. For example, with ongoing preparation for anticipated changes in the child's condition, a nurse can have medications in the home or instructions written for whom and when to call for assistance.[22]

Typically, parents of dying children have two overriding concerns: a fear of a sudden or acute increase in pain that they will be unable to manage, especially as death approaches; and fear of a crisis situation or unexpected change in condition, including how and when death may occur. It is critical to address these issues on an ongoing basis.

The need to feel a sense of control is also relevant to the sick child, who may be fearful from experiencing so many physical and emotional changes. Nurses can assist parents with methods to help their child gain control over aspects of his or her experience, retain choices regarding care, and feel comfortable with a daily routine, all of which have great affirmational value. Managing medication regimens and symptoms is a daunting task for parents, having enormous impact on the family.[23] Nurses should consider the overall responsibilities of parents for managing care as well as maintaining family routines when planning medication and treatment regimens with the physician.

Preserving Hope in the Midst of Serious Illness

A common characteristic of pediatric patients and their families is a prevailing sense of hope, evidenced in their language and decision-making. It is important to preserve and nurture hope during all stages of the child's life-threatening illness. No matter how grim the situation, one should always strive to deal with matters in a positive yet realistic manner. The focus of hope inevitably must change over time, for example, from hope for cure, to hope for a longer remission than previously, to hope that the child can continue to be cared for at home, or to hope that the child will die without pain. Hope has a powerful and practical place within these families. With the presence of hope, parents speak of being able to continue their caregiving responsibilities, having the strength to put one foot in front of the other, and being able to carry on in their day-to-day existence. Without hope, the burden of the child's impending death would be utterly paralyzing. Hope offers opportunities for growth for the child and family. Examples of a child's hopes are a wish to return to school once more, to celebrate an important birthday, or to reach a significant milestone or rite of passage. Other expressions of hope include planning for a visit from grandparents, having friends gathered together, or even gaining the understanding that their loved ones will, indeed, survive after they die.

One young boy desperately wanted to be "normal" by continuing to play soccer despite his frail condition. After his blood transfusions, he was able to get out on the field and marvel at his own achievement. He touched many around him. This was a way for him to feel like he was still living with an illness and not just dying from it. Over time, his goals began to change as the benefits from transfusions became negligible, and it became more difficult for him to recover from the activity. He, his father, and the medical team needed assistance from the hospice team to make the transition in his care plan to reduce and finally eliminate the ineffectual blood transfusions. It was an important lesson for many on the changing meaning, purpose, and role the therapies had for the child, his father, and his physicians. The hospice team was able to facilitate that discussion, thus enabling forward movement. Addressing spiritual needs of children and families is an area with great need for improvement.[24]

Hospice Care for Infants

When a dying child is an infant, the need for hope is similar, but time constraints are severe. Parents may need support and encouragement to consider going home with their baby to have the opportunity to "welcome baby home." They may be offered a selection of "keepsake" activities to consider to preserve the presence of their little one's life and record the connectedness they had for such a brief period. For them, it may be a simultaneous greeting and farewell. Strengthening this experience may help diminish long-term psychological implications for parents and siblings. Fortunately, much greater interest is developing in the intervention of palliative care in neonatal intensive care and other settings of infant care.[25–28]

Baby Angel was born with trisomy 18 and not expected to live more than a few days at most. Upon that determination, the NICU social worker referred the family to San Diego Hospice. The team went to the hospital to meet with the young parents, who were weighed down with grief, their dreams and hopes shattered as the new reality for their baby was sinking in. The option of home hospice care seemed overwhelming while still adjusting to the news of their child's impending demise. To ease the potential transition to home care, the parents and their infant were transferred to the Inpatient Hospice Care Center. Angel died within hours of her arrival, with her parents around her. The staff, unaccustomed to the needs of such parents, wondered why she was transferred at all. Was it inappropriate and a waste of effort? According to the parents, it was abundantly clear that it had been worth it and had allowed them to truly feel like parents in a peaceful environment. Compared to the crowded, public, hectic environment of the NICU, they felt peace in the hospice setting. They expressed tremendous gratitude for the efforts made on behalf of Angel's brief life.

In another case, Baby Joseph was born with hypoplastic left ventricle and was, again, not expected to survive more than a few days. His parents were determined to take him home with them for whatever time they could manage and were eager to plan and fulfill this hope. The team worked quickly with the NICU team to arrange for his discharge and to be met at home by a pediatric hospice nurse and social worker. At home, they were admitted to the hospice program and settled in as family gathered to be with Joseph. Together, they created the opportunity to welcome Joseph into the family and into their home. Joseph kept them awake a lot with typical new baby needs. He died quietly in the early morning hours of the following day. Although to many it seemed tragic, his parents were grateful that they had been able to truly be parents for 1 day. In those hours, they were able to etch some precious yet ordinary memories like other parents have and experience the normal stresses as well as provide the comfort all babies need.

The implications for staff in caring for dying infants and children are enormous. Some are more suited for this field than others. Key personal attributes of those identified as successful in this role include a high tolerance for ambiguity and flexibility; an appreciation for individual differences; good external support networks; a realistic awareness of personal limits; a joy for life in general; a sense of humor; an open communication style; a tendency to value self-awareness as an asset; empathy; and a willingness to learn continually. Being able to function in a self-directed mode facilitates using one's own resourcefulness to meet the challenges of an ever-fluctuating schedule.

Perhaps the most basic necessary characteristic is a comfort with death. Only by coming to terms with one's own thoughts and feelings about death is it possible to adapt philosophically to working with children who will die. Swanson-Kauffman[29] developed a model of caring for nurses dealing with perinatal loss. She states that fundamental to caring is understanding the personal meanings of the loss; resonating emotionally with the mother's feelings; offering realistic support, nurture, and protection; facilitating the expression of grief; and helping maintain her faith in her capacity to come through her loss a functioning, whole person.[29] These also apply to the baby's father.

Perinatal Hospice: The Early Intervention Program

In response to a need identified by parents, an innovative addition to the Children's Program was developed as an extension of existing hospice care. This new program grew out of the existing newborns with limited life expectancy described as "babies born dying."

Mothers and parents were coming directly to the hospice for help out of desperation, facing a prenatal diagnosis of a devastating nature for their unborn baby. These parents had decided to continue the pregnancy and treasure their child's life for as long as they could, yet they lacked any ongoing support. Their message was clear: "Finally, someone will just accept our decision and help our family deal with this experience. We don't want to just sit back and wait for our baby's death." Hospice professionals are trained to use an individualized approach to assist patients and families in dealing with life-threatening illnesses and their decisions concerning that experience. This unique group of parents faced the daunting challenge of anticipating and preparing for the birth and death of their baby simultaneously. What they are given, with the help of this unique program, is the opportunity to feel some level of control by making plans based on their individual needs for supporting themselves, their other children, the grandparents, and friends.

The Early Intervention Program provides support to expectant parents through counseling and spiritual guidance for the entirety of the pregnancy, starting prior to and continuing after the delivery. Parents are advised of ways to create a personalized birthing plan that addresses their wishes for themselves and the care of their baby once born. The plan may include specific instructions and preferences for the labor and delivery staff, such as keepsakes and rituals they may wish to create or perform. Some parents await a definitive diagnosis after the baby is born to decide the extent of care to be provided.

The parents' goals and plans are discussed in collaboration with their physician. The physician is kept up to date regarding their psychological state and the development of their birthing plan. Prenatal nursing care is not a part of this program. These women continue their prenatal care under their physician's guidance. The pediatric hospice nurse is involved in educating the parents on the diagnosis, helping them understand what to expect, planning for the possibility of home care, and helping siblings understand the baby's condition.

Perhaps as a reaction to the lack of responsiveness by the health care system and society in general toward perinatal loss, these parents have found ways to support each other. They have truly disenfranchised grief, one not recognized as equal to the grief experienced with other types of death. The Internet is rich with amazing and profoundly intimate resources and ideas, shared experiences, practical help, opportunities to gain support, and even memorials to lost children. These parents have discovered help from within their isolation from others like themselves. Hospice professionals can gain valuable insight from their perspectives and excellent ideas on ways to improve support for these parents.

Initial feedback from the hospice bereavement counselors who work with these parents has highlighted the potential and anticipated impact of the perinatal hospice service. The bereaved parents who received help through the Early Intervention Program demonstrated the following: they were more emotionally and spiritually prepared for their infant's death; they experienced less intense despair/sadness; they had better marital relationship communication and support; and they felt fewer "raw" intense emotions such as anger, rage, and uncertainty regarding the cause of death. The parents without hospice care during pregnancy and after birth seemed to demonstrate a more intense grieving experience, whereas the others expressed a sense of gratitude and peace surrounding the brief life of their child. Parents have told us that they are able to be fully present for their baby when he/she is born due to the planning and guidance beforehand. It also allowed them to maximize the limited time to truly celebrate and to welcome the baby before they had to say goodbye—an essential ingredient to their healing process.

Over time, the keepsakes accumulated during the pregnancy and birth—photographs and other objects—can assist young siblings and parents to integrate the loss of the child into their family experience. Before delivery, a family picture can be taken with the family gathered closely around the mother, all hands placed gently on her abdomen. Because the baby may die in utero or at birth, this earlier image may be helpful in recording and preserving his or her presence in their lives. The team provides paint, poster board, and a memory box, then assists in obtaining handprints of the baby as well as of the entire family at the hospital to create another "family portrait." Because almost all NICUs and labor/delivery areas have developed procedures and activities for the experience of infant death, the hospice team works with the inpatient staff as a bridge of continuity in the parents' experience. Planning the "who, what, when, and where" for the delivery and beyond is important. If this information is not shared with the hospital staff, time may be lost and opportunities missed forever for some critical experiences for the family.

Making both the pregnancy and the death more real helps reduce denial of the loss. Mourning the dead child is facilitated by visual reminders over which families can grieve.[30] The social worker can provide parents with ideas for memorial services or assistance with final arrangements. The chaplain can assist them in personalizing these arrangements, helping to create the theme that reflects their beliefs and desires, and even helping to facilitate their wishes. Even a brief life is mourned for a very long time. Seeds for more effective grieving may be planted for the long journey ahead to recovery and healing.

Acculturating an Agency to a Program to Serve Children

Integrating the Children's Program into the culture and values of San Diego Hospice is a goal in progress. Similarly, efforts continue on a national level to integrate pediatrics into the NHPCO's infrastructure and scope. Internal education and ongoing discussions were the first steps toward creating awareness of the service needs related to this unique population. Just as hospices initially had to confront issues of discomfort, fear, and personal barriers when caring for AIDS patients, the same must be done regarding pediatric patients. Admitting dying infants and children into programs poses an equally challenging situation for both clinical and nonclinical staff. The challenge is to normalize children as part of who is served by hospice care providers. As an industry, hospice and palliative care must commit to serving dying patients across the entire lifespan so that all families may receive this help as they face end-of-life care. Only then will it become integrated into more individual programs.

Ongoing efforts are needed for addressing the ethical issues related to removing life support, discontinuing aggressive care with a dying child, maintaining confidentiality, and incorporating the child's or sibling's school into the plan of care. Prospective hospice employees, both clinical and nonclinical, are informed that infants, children, and young parents are part of the continuum of care. A detailed description of pediatric hospice care during staff interviews and hiring constitutes "informed consent" that the prospective employee acknowledges that these issues will be encountered within the agency. From the education committee to new-hire orientation, and from the ethics committee to business development and marketing, the message is reiterated that children are part of the organizational mission and service population in a variety of ways. If left as the responsibility solely of the Children's Program staff, the potential may be diminished to truly foster an emphasis on children's issues in agency philosophy and practice.

Perhaps with this model as an example, other hospice programs and providers will examine how they might better address the needs of children and enhance their capacity to integrate the very young into their existing services. There is much to be done to support these families and advance the quality of end-of-life care for infants and children. Each step toward increasing awareness regarding these issues is a step forward on behalf of the children who are dying without access to all the resources available to them and their loved ones.

Nurses who choose to care for dying infants and children and their families need a significant support system themselves to maintain the difficult and delicate task of balancing perspectives. However, in doing so, nurses receive a spiritual treasure that only comes from experience with these children, parents, siblings, and others around them—heightened awareness of how very precious life is. Families share their wisdom from their tragedy, urging others to make the most of each moment in their own lives with their own loved ones. The courage and strength observed in families on this pilgrimage is humbling and strengthening at once. The staff of the Children's Program cherish and are grateful for the opportunity to be eyewitnesses to one of life's most intimate and powerful experiences.

Attempts to enhance end-of-life care for infants and children are gaining momentum, as evidenced by recent efforts to create a demonstration project with the Health Care Finance Administration, CHI, and NHPCO. Their effort aims to redesign the model of hospice care to more appropriately meet the needs of young patients and families. It will allow hospices to care for them through a model that begins at diagnosis of a terminal condition and continues through bereavement for the family. Through a collaborative effort with leaders in hospice care, pediatric hospice care, children's health care, and various branches of government, plans are moving forward for appropriations and site applications for the demonstration project. The Children's International Project on Palliative/Hospice Services (ChIPPS) is an international work group that represents the work of experts and leaders in the field of pediatric hospice care. The group is developing a variety of research plans and identifying "best practice" examples and models of care for a compendium of resources to assist hospice programs more quickly to develop services for infants and children.

Hospice care for infants, children, and those around them focuses on living as fully and as normally as possible within the context, limitations, and opportunities that come with life-threatening illnesses.[31,32] It seeks to provide children and their families with the means and opportunities to achieve self-directed life closure in a manner that they themselves define. Pediatric hospice care aims to raise the consciousness of our society that claims to value children as a treasured resource. If this is so, then we must treasure them and honor them in sickness and in health, in living and dying, until death do they part from us.

REFERENCES

1. Ferrell BR, Rhiner M, Shapiro B, Dierkes M. The experience of pediatric cancer pain, Part I: Impact of pain on the family. J Pediatr Nurs 1994; 9:369–378.
2. Mellonie B, Ingpen R. Lifetimes: A Beautiful Way to Explain Death to Children. Toronto: Bantam, 1983.
3. Field MJ, Behrman RE. When Children Die: Improving Palliative and End-of-Life Care for Children and Their Families (Report of the Institute of Medicine Task Force). Washington, DC: National Academy Press, 2003.
4. National Consensus Project Guidelines for Quality Palliative Care. (2004). Available at: http://www.nationalconsensusproject.org (accessed February 7, 2005).
5. Stevens M, Jones P, O'Riordan E. Family responses when a child with cancer is in palliative care. J Palliative Care 1996;12:51–55.
6. CHI 1998 Survey. Hospice Care for Children. Executive Summary Report, Alexandria, VA: Author, June 1999.
7. Hospice Standards of Practice: Draft. Alexandria, VA: Standards and Accreditation Committee, National Hospice Organization, July, 1999.
8. Ryndes T. A Pathway for Patients and Families Facing Terminal Illness. Alexandria, VA: Standards and Accreditation Committee, National Hospice Organization, 1997.
9. Kaye P. Notes on Symptom Control in Hospice and Palliative Care. Essex, CT: Hospice Education Institute, 1994:67–70.
10. American Academy of Pediatrics & American College of Emergency Physicians. Death of a child in the emergency department: joint statement. Pediatrics 2002;105:454–461.
11. Burns JP, Mitchell C, Griffith JL, Truog JD. End-of-life care in the pediatric intensive care unit: attitudes and practices of pediatric critical care physicians and nurses. Crit Care Med 2001; 29:658–664.
12. Catlin A, Carter B. Creation of a neonatal end-of-life palliative care protocol. J Perinatol 2002;22:184–195.
13. Dixon-Woods M, Findlay M, Young B, Cox H, Heney D. Parents' accounts of obtaining a diagnosis of childhood cancer. Lancet 2001;357:670–674.
14. Ferrell B, Virani R, Grant M. Analysis of end of life content in nursing textbooks. Oncol Nurs Forum 1999;26:869–876.
15. Barnes K. Staff stress in the children's hospice: cause, effects, and coping strategies. Int J Palliative Nurs 2001;7:239–254.
16. Stevens M. Psychological adaptation of the dying child. In: Doyle D, Hanks GWC, Cherny N, Calman K, eds. Oxford Textbook of Palliative Medicine, 3rd ed. Oxford: Oxford University Press, 2004;798–806.
17. Edwards J. A model of palliative care for the adolescent with cancer. Int J Palliative Nurs 2001;7:485–488.
18. Attig T. Beyond pain: the existential of children. J Palliative Care 1996;12:20–23.
19. Jordan-Marsh MA, Sutters K, Sumner L. Pediatric pain management. In: Volker B, eds. Comprehensive Pain Management in Terminal Illness. Sacramento, CA: California State Hospital Association, 1996;62–93.
20. Quick Reference Guide. Acute pain management in infants, children and adolescents; operative and medical procedures. Quick Reference Guide for Clinicians. Rockville, Maryland: Agency for Health Care Policy and Research, U.S. Department of Health and Human Services, 1993.
21. McGrath P, Brown S. Pain control. In: Doyle D, Hanks GWC, Cherny N, Calman K, eds. Oxford Textbook of Palliative Medicine, 3rd ed. Oxford: Oxford University Press, 2004:775–789.
22. Laasko H, Paunonen-Illonen M. Mothers' experience of social support following the death of a child. J Clin Nurs 2002;11: 176–185.
23. Ferrell BR, Rhiner M, Shapiro B, et al. The Family experience of cancer and pain management in children. Cancer Pract 1994; 2:441–446.
24. Davies B, Brenner P, Orloff S, Sumner L, Worden W. Addressing spirituality in pediatric hospice and palliative care. J Palliative Care 2002;18:59–67.
25. Glicken AD, Merenstein GB. A neonatal end-of-life palliative care protocol——an evolving new standard of care? Neonatal Network 2002;21:35–36.
26. Kane J, Barber RB, Jordan M, Tichenor KT, Camp K. Supportive/palliative care of children suffering from life-threatening and terminal illness. Am J Hospice Palliative Care 2000;17:165–172.
27. Leuthner SR, Boldt AM, Kirby RS. Where infants die: examination of place of death and hospice/home health care options in the state of Wisconsin. J Palliative Med 2004; 7:269–277.
28. Pierucci RL, Kirby RS, Leuthner SR. End-of-life care for neonates and infants: the experiences and effects of a palliative care consultation service. Pediatrics 2001;108:653–660.
29. Swanson-Kauffman K. Caring in the instance of unexpected early pregnancy loss. Top Clin Nurs 1986;8:37–46.
30. Leon IG. Perinatal loss: a critique of current hospital practices. Clin Pediatr 1992;366–374.
31. Himelstein BP, Hilden JM, Boldt AM, Weissman D. Medical progress: pediatric palliative care. N Engl J Med 2004;350: 1752–1762.
32. Last Acts Palliative Care Task Force. (2002). Precepts of palliative care for children, adolescents and their families, http://www.apon.org/files/public/last_acts_precepts.pdf (accessed June 27, 2005).

51

Marcia Levetown

Pediatric Care: Transitioning Goals of Care in the Emergency Department, Intensive Care Unit, and In Between

We are in need of medicine with a heart . . . The endless physical, emotional, and financial burdens that a family carries when their child dies . . . makes you completely incapable of dealing with incompetence and insensitivity.—Salvador Avila, 2001[1*]

Every word that was said the day Becky died is indelibly etched in my mind. I have replayed the words in my mind a million times. It's a never-ending tape.—Pam Borchart[1a]

- ***Key Points***
- *Pediatric palliative care often occurs in the intensive care unit (ICU) and the emergency department (ED), unlike adult palliative care.*
- *Compassionate, effective, and consistent anticipatory communication with the family and the patient is critical to appropriate planning and to the prevention of suffering.*
- *Attention must be paid to the child's and family's perspectives and goals.*
- *Parents' roles are severely challenged by the illness and potential death of the child, rendering decision-making much more difficult.*
- *Meticulous assessment of and relief of symptoms is critical to engender confidence and to prevent unnecessary suffering; pediatric-specific tools and protocols must be used.*
- *Grief and loss of the child on the part of the parents, family, and health care personnel must be addressed.*

Palliative care is comprehensive, interdisciplinary care focused primarily on promoting quality of life for patients and families living with a life-threatening illness.[2] It can and should occur from the earliest recognition of a life-threatening condition and can be concurrent with efforts to prolong life.[1,3] Palliative care is as applicable in the ED and in the ICU setting as it is in the home.[4–6] This is a critically important issue for children who die, since the vast majority of childhood deaths occur in an ICU setting. In fact, Wanzer and colleagues[7] state:

> As sickness progresses toward death, measures to minimize suffering should be intensified. Dying patients may require palliative care of an intensity that rivals that of curative efforts. Even though aggressive curative techniques are no longer indicated, professionals and families are still called on to use intensive measures—extreme responsibility, extraordinary sensitivity, and heroic compassion.

Approximately 50,000 children die annually in the United States.[8] Infants (<1 year of age) die primarily of congenital defects and prematurity; however, sudden infant death syndrome (SIDS) and trauma (including accidents and homicide) account for 12% of infant deaths. For children (age 1 year–24 years), 72% of deaths are the result of trauma, while the remaining 28% are due primarily to cancer, congenital anomalies, and heart disease. Trauma occurs in previously healthy children who are suddenly injured, and, in most cases, for whom resuscitative measures are initially called for. In addition, some previously healthy children become suddenly ill from an overwhelming illness, such as a viral cardiomyopathy. Thus, the vast majority of children who die are appropriately cared for, at least initially, in the ED and ICU settings. Most children who die of these conditions currently die in the ED or ICU as well. Even children with chronic illnesses and anticipated deaths often die in the ICU, though this may be due less to need or preferability than to the lack of alternatives or effective family counseling and advance planning. In fact, 4.6% of pediatric ICU admissions end in death.[9–11] However, few ICUs or EDs are places that one would choose to die. Most children and adults, when asked, prefer to die at home.[12,13] ICUs and EDs are not "homey."

There are a lot of rules that keep the ED and ICU safe and efficient; these same rules may interfere with simultaneous visits from extended family and friends as a child's life draws to a close. ICUs and EDs are in the business of saving lives; scrupulous attention to communication, symptom control, and grief management have not been a traditional focus of training for health care delivery or personnel.[14] Yet, children and neonates will continue to die in ICUs and EDs.[15] There are ways to meet these patients' and their families' needs for a peaceful, family-centered death, even in these circumstances.[6,16] Specific suggestions for care in the ED have recently been published.[17,18]

While individuals and families differ in the details and nuances of what their conception of a good death is, common themes emerge. Just as with adults, chronically ill children's biggest fears are abandonment by their medical caregivers and families.[19] It is often observed that children will endure treatments they no longer value to protect and not disappoint their parents and doctors. However, children also have needs and priorities in their final days and months that are determined to a large extent by their developmental maturity. For infants, this includes the physical presence of their family. The smell and feel of familiar people provide essential comfort. For toddlers, routines and familiar people and objects assume great importance; for older children, it is social contacts; and for teens, the ideals of having left a legacy and having peer support are critical. The common ICU policy of limiting visitation can interfere with these aspects of achieving a "good death."

Most children and their families want as much honest information regarding prognosis, clearly and empathically communicated, as they can get, beginning as early as possible in the course of illness, followed by regular updates as the prognosis changes.[20–22] This allows rational decisions to be made based on the facts and on the values of the child and his or her family. Patients and families need to understand the anticipated disease trajectory and its associated symptoms and feel confident that they can manage them. They need to understand realistic options for medical care goals and the projected benefits and burdens of each option. Parents need to feel that they have done everything that is "appropriate"; that they have been good, brave, and loving parents; and that the child has "been a fighter."

> It was terribly important for us to do exactly what was right and necessary to help our daughter . . . Our nurse and social worker made us feel that we WERE, in fact, doing everything in our power to take care of our daughter.—Kathleen and James Bula, parents[1]

They need to know what care venues are available to them and how to access them to avoid recurrent, nonbeneficial ICU admissions in the setting of chronic illness. Children with terminal conditions and their families often want spiritual consultation and guidance since it is very hard to understand why so tragic a thing as a child's death has to occur. Above all, children and their families want to feel valued as individuals, with the awesomeness of the impending death duly noted and the opportunity for closure and growth at the end of life to be realized to the greatest extent possible.[19,23–25] If end-of-life care is properly provided, more children with chronic, life-threatening conditions will have the opportunity to die outside the ICU, in a setting they or their family prefer. Avoidable ICU deaths are taxing to the patient and family as well as to the ICU personnel, who often begin to ask, "Are we doing this *to* the child or *for* the child?"

Nevertheless, since a large proportion of children who die do so of acute conditions in the ICU, consideration of palliative care issues must be a part of the care plan.[26,27] This chapter delineates the topics to be considered, explicates concrete suggestions for implementation, and provides case examples in a university hospital system that has instituted some of these strategies in the care of infants and children.

Communication

Clear, honest, open communication is as critical a factor in the care of terminally ill infants and children as any other factor.[28] It may be even more significant because of the sensitivity required to assess the cognitive development of young patients. Some of the factors involved in achieving good communication during the terminal illnesses of children are covered in the following sections.

Preparation and Adherence to Advance Directives

Families and children need and usually want honest information to assist in making good decisions regarding the goals of medical care. Children have a right to be offered information about their treatment options and the associated benefits and burdens.[7,29–32] This information must be presented in a manner consistent with the child's developmental capacity.[33] Ideally, a patient with a chronic, progressive, and ultimately fatal illness would be provided information gradually and recurrently, in an outpatient setting, tailored to the child's particular condition and the family's value system, orchestrated by a long-standing primary care physician.[34–37]

A suggested format for initiating the discussion of advance care planning appears below:

> I would like to take a few minutes to talk about some decisions about treatment for Maia that may come up in the future. As you know, it is possible that Maia's condition will get worse and that she may die. We are doing all we can to prevent that, but if that time comes, you and Maia may want to change the way she receives

care. [*Pause for response.*] For instance, you may want to avoid a lot of procedures and time in the hospital, and you may choose to take her home and receive help to make her comfortable there. Maybe you are ready to talk about these kinds of things today, but it may take some time before you're ready. [*Pause for response.*] That's okay. I just want to let you know that I'm ready to talk about those kinds of things whenever you feel ready.

Other families have told me that it can be very difficult to think and talk about decisions related to dying when they're still hoping for a cure. But the families whose children have died tell me that, when the time came, they were very glad they had considered and talked about those decisions beforehand. We can start talking now about the issues that may come up if your child's condition gets worse, but we don't have to make any of the decisions right now. You can think about it all, talk with your family, friends, spiritual adviser, family doctor, or whomever else you want. Then we can make the decisions bit by bit, as we go along.

As we go along, it's really important that you ask whatever questions you have on your mind, even if you think they might be obvious or very difficult to ask. Just to give you an example, some parents who are thinking about taking their child home for care at the end of life want to know who they are supposed to call at the time of death. It's very difficult for them to ask about that but it's very important information for them to know. So whenever you have questions, about *anything*, please just ask. We will do our best to answer them.[159*]

Most state advance directive laws do not specifically mention children. However, while there is no mandate to address the issues of prognosis or future anticipatable medical interventions and their expected benefits and burdens for chronically ill children, the intent of advance directives applies equally to children with decision-making capacity as it does to adults.

Unfortunately, even when advance directives have been thoughtfully crafted and executed, there are rarely mechanisms in place to honor these decisions. In addition, parents may feel too guilty and too unprepared to follow through with their decisions to limit medical intervention. All too often, when the child begins to have the predicted deterioration, symptoms are inadequately controlled because no palliative care plan is in place and the patient appears in the emergency room *in extremis.*

On arrival at the emergency room, the family is often asked: "Do you want us to do 'everything'?" "Everything" and its possible outcome is not further explained, so there is no reasonable answer but "Yes!" However, to the child and his or her family, "everything" may mean everything to make the child comfortable, whereas to the physician it may mean everything to prolong survival, regardless of the extent of suffering. Assumptions should not be made; clarification of ambiguous terms must be accomplished to ensure that the care rendered is the care desired.[38]

In addition, if the child's symptoms are aggressively controlled in the ER, more rational decision-making can take place. The family could, for example, choose to have the child intubated for respiratory distress or to accept comfort management outside the ICU if extended survival is unduly burdensome for the child as an individual. Moreover, many families harbor significant misconceptions regarding the outcomes of life-sustaining treatments.

A child with long-standing persistent vegetative state, seizures, and gastroesophageal reflux (despite a fundoplication and two antireflux medications) came to the PICU with his fourth full cardiac arrest that year, as a result of yet another aspiration episode. He was admitted through the ED and brought to the PICU on a ventilator, with pressor agents being infused. When his caregiving grandparents were asked about what they hoped we could accomplish with our medical care, they replied, "We want him to be better." When prompted to further clarify their expectations, they replied, "We want him to be like his brothers; to walk, talk, and go to school." Once informed that this was, unfortunately, not possible, they revised the goals of care, dramatically changing the care plan.

In particular, the misperceptions of a high likelihood of survival following CPR and the lack of awareness of the potential to develop significant disability after cardiac arrest have been documented.[39,40] The impact of accurate information on the increased likelihood to forgo CPR has also been proven.[41,42] Children have a particularly poor outcome from true cardiac arrest.[43–47] In the absence of intoxication and congenital heart disease, primary cardiac causes of arrest are exceedingly rare. Children have very healthy hearts. Thus, if cardiac arrest has occurred, it indicates that there is severe multi-organ dysfunction or that there has been a prolonged hypoxemia; neither of these underlying causes of arrest are amenable to medical treatment. Resuscitation in these settings does not commonly lead to intact survival. However, this is not the message that families understand when they are asked, "Do you want us to restart his heart?"

Similarly, seemingly benign comments, such as "He is stable," can be misinterpreted by families of dying children to mean "He is going to be all right." "She has gained weight" may mean the child's condition is worsening if the infant has heart failure, but is universally interpreted as good news by parents of infants. It is critical that members of the health care team communicate effectively with each other and that they give clear and consistent messages to the family.[48] Participation of the bedside nurse in daily rounds and in family meetings makes this process smoother. The information that nurses gather from patients and parents at the bedside is critically important to the entire team in understanding what the

*From McConnell Y, Frager G, Levetown M. Decision-making in pediatric palliative care. In: Carter B, Levetown M. Palliative Care for Infants, Children and Adolescents: A Practical Handbook. Baltimore: Johns Hopkins University Press, 2004: Ch. 4. Used with permission.

patient and family already know, what questions they have, and what further explanations or discussions are needed. In addition, there is a need for excellent communication between nurses at shift change about what the family has been told and what they seem to understand. Parents often call at night to check on their children and get confused by conflicting messages.

It is important to realize that the role of parents as protectors is threatened by the possibility of the death of their child[49]; this occasionally renders them unable to acknowledge or to notice the suffering involved in the ongoing attempts to prolong life. For this reason, whenever possible, the knowing child (who may be as young as 3 years if he or she has been chronically ill)[19] should have a voice in the discussion of the goals of medical intervention.[26,50,51] In addition, the issues of parental guilt ("I can't let my child go—it would mean I failed as a parent.") and family suffering should be frankly discussed. In the author's experience, reassuring parents that letting go is a loving decision has been helpful.

When discussing the choice to forgo life-sustaining medical intervention, the topic of current burdens of therapy as well as the probability of the hoped-for benefits must be clearly explained. Suggested ways of approaching these issues with parents, can be found in Table 51–1.

Nurses, who are often the most trusted member among the caregiving team and who have the longest exposure to parents in the inpatient setting, are in an excellent position to ask many of these questions. Ineffective therapies must not be offered. Common misperceptions about the effectiveness of CPR must be proactively addressed. The proposal to forgo further attempts to prolong life should be presented as a recommendation, not a choice for the family to make alone. The benefits of stopping life-sustaining treatments can be presented as the benefit of dying at home, where possible, or, more commonly, increasing the chances of dying in the hospital at a time when the family is all there together to support the child and each other instead of at some unpredictable time in the middle of the night with no one around. Presenting the option inaccurately as "stopping care" is, not surprisingly, usually rejected. This short-hand phraseology is perceived as painful and unloving. Patients and families fear abandonment above all else.[52,53] A more accurate description is to recommend stopping ineffective interventions, stopping unduly burdensome treatments, changing the goals of care to better meet the needs of the patient in the face of having proven that life-prolonging measures are failing to work. One of the most damaging sentences uttered in the context of irreversible illness is "There is nothing more that we can do." Above all, it is patently untrue. Despite our inability to cure or prolong life at all times, we always have something to offer, even if it is only ourselves.[54] Most important are the promises to care; to aggressively control symptoms; to be available; to assist (as a multidisciplinary team) in the arrangement of visits of family and friends; to facilitate the observation of important rituals; to provide spiritual guidance (when desired); and to transfer to alternate settings (according to the patient's and family's wishes).[55,56] One suggested phrase that captures the essence of intensified caring with new goals is: "We will help your child live to his fullest to the very last moment, regardless of when that is. His comfort and yours are our top priority." The family may also need assistance with funeral arrangements and will benefit from bereavement follow-up provided by direct caregivers.

Table 51–1
Helping Families with Difficult Decisions

- Please tell me in your own words what you understand about your child's condition.
- Please tell me in your own words what you understand about the care being provided to your child at the moment.
- What things have you found particularly difficult to deal with during your child's illness? Who or what has helped you through them? What kinds of additional help do you need, if any?
- How have you been involved in decision-making about your child's care up to this point? How have you felt about that involvement? How would you like to be involved?
- How have other members of your family (for example, your child's siblings or grandparents) been involved in discussions and decision-making up to this point?
- What are your wishes about the care being provided to your child?
- If we were looking at a time when your child may not be able to get through the illness, can you tell me some of your wishes about that time? How would you like things to be?
- Do you have any particular worries about the time when your child may not be able to live through this illness?
- What are your fears or concerns about what your child is experiencing now? In the future?
- What are the most difficult things you are facing at this time? What do you think you might need to help you get through this time?
- What are your fears or concerns about what your child may experience if he or she is unable to live through this illness?
- Is there something that I could do, or avoid doing, to better help you and your family through this time?
- Is there something you can think of that would best help your child through this time?

Source: Adapted from McConnell Y, et al. (2004), reference 159.

Time-Limited Trials

Once the child is in the ICU receiving life-sustaining care, it is helpful to review the patient's progress continuously, monitoring the "big picture" of whether the patient is progressing along the hoped-for trajectory of illness or whether he or she is deteriorating despite the best medical management. Daily updates of this clinical information provided to the patient (when possible and appropriate) and the family can facilitate reasonable decision-making, thereby avoiding burdensome and unhelpful care and diminishing the element of surprise on the day the patient dies. Letting the parents know when the child should reasonably be expected to show a response to treatment and agreement to meet again at that time to discuss how it is going is an effective tool and provides a timeframe for the family to gather their supporters for the news, good or bad.

Breaking Bad News: The Nurse's Role

While breaking bad news is difficult and stressful for everyone, being uninformed is even more stressful for patients and families. One of the most common complaints of patients and

Table 51–2
Breaking Bad News

1. Provide a "warning shot" or an introductory sentence before presenting the distressing information: "I am sorry that I have some bad news to tell you."
2. Provide an opportunity for supportive friends or family to be present when the information is shared: "Would you like to call someone to be with you when we talk?"
3. Tell the news in a private setting, with the physician, nurse, and social worker present. Bring the family (generally parents without the child first, depending on relationships and preferences) to a private conference room rather than speaking to them in the waiting room or the hall. Bring tissues. If appropriate and desired by the family, assist them in telling their children (patient and siblings) afterwards.
4. Sit down near the family, not across a table. Do not stand. Children and families want to be on an even plane with their caregivers. Look the family members in the eye to engender trust unless this is culturally undesirable. Ask them to tell you about their child and about any consistent values of the child and about the things that give him or her pleasure. Ask how much they want to know about his or her medical condition and prognosis. Ask them what they understand is happening. Clarify misconceptions, particularly about the cause of the problem, and attempt to assuage any guilt that may derive from having an inherited or developmental problem ("You did not wish for your child to have this") or from trauma or other causes. Then, let them know this news is difficult for you as well. Nurses can help guide the physician to present the truth in a jargon-free manner that is consistent with the family's educational level, sophistication, and stated desire for knowledge. Ask the family to explain what they understood was said. Clarify misconceptions. Then, solicit additional questions.
5. Be unhurried. If there is only a limited time available for the physician, let the family know: "I'm sorry the doctor only has 15 minutes now, but I will stay with you and answer any questions I can, and the doctor will be back later this afternoon to answer anything I can't and to update you." Don't look at your watch. Have the charge nurse or another nurse care for your patients while you sit with the family. Remind the other team members to give their beepers to someone else during the family meeting, when possible; otherwise, switch the beepers to vibrate mode.
6. Ideally, members of the multidisciplinary team participate as full members during the family conference.[48] The bedside nurse, chaplain, and social worker benefit from hearing the physician–family interaction. They can solicit questions, clarify misconceptions during the meeting and after the physician leaves, and address other facets of the patient's situation that the conversation with the physician evokes. Team members can also give the physician feedback regarding his or her communication with the patient and family, such as words they did not understand, and can help the physician address any unresolved issues at the next meeting. This technique requires interdisciplinary respect and cooperation, which are essential to successful, comprehensive end-of-life care; it prevents divisive misunderstandings between disciplines regarding suspected coercion or other undesirable communication.
7. Bring trainees to the family meeting. This allows the assigned nursing or medical student and resident to learn from directly observing the interdisciplinary critical care team, as well as the patient and family responses. It keeps trainees informed so that unnecessary and often damaging miscommunications do not occur. Trainees often get lost in the minutiae of the patient's laboratory values and vital signs and may unwittingly provide contradictory information to the family. However, do not overwhelm the family with white coats—have trainees take turns attending family meetings.
8. Be specific. The physician should present the options, include a description of life-sustaining treatments, the child's current status, the chance of survival, the probability of full recovery (and the probability of significant disability), and the possible effects of the child's long-term survival on the family.

families is the lack of accurate and clearly communicated information.[20–22,28,57–64] Accompanying comments indicate a willingness and desire to receive bad news as long as it is empathically communicated. The diagnosis and prognosis associated with chronic conditions often provide confirmation of what was already suspected, thus frequently resulting in relief and reduction of anxiety. Reactions to bad news in the setting of an acute event are much more dramatic.[4,5] In either case, accurate information allows the goals of medical intervention to shift and allows family and friends time to plan for gathering in a timely fashion to honor the dying child. Effective and compassionate communication may even allow the child to be discharged from the ICU, when desired, to die at home, or to die in a more private area of the hospital.[1,55,61]

Sometimes, in response to our own pain, medical caregivers communicate the news of a bad prognosis in a brief encounter and may use technical terms to "soften" the blow, or to avoid the conversation altogether or wait until the child is unconscious.[35,62] Research on breaking bad news does not support these techniques.[65,66] Suggestions for breaking bad news in a way that is sensitive to the needs of the child and family, as well as the medical caregivers, are suggested in Table 51–2.

Recommendations for the next step should be presented, based on the team's experience and on the goals and values of the patient, as well as the observations of patient and family members during the meeting and the hospitalization overall. Be sure that the benefits and burdens (including prolongation of suffering) of each potential care plan, the potential reversibility or irreversibility of the conditions being treated, the time frame for reevaluation, the projected future quality of life, and the comfort measures available if the ICU interventions are curtailed or discontinued are explained to the family in a manner they can and do understand (Table 51–3). Give reassurances that, if life-sustaining medical interventions are discontinued, the child will continue to receive attentive care for the relief of symptoms; describe the procedures to be undertaken, including the opportunities to observe important customs and rituals and the visitation allowances.[26]

It is the author's impression that most communication about forgoing life support concentrates on what will be stopped and not what will be added. It is my practice to suggest that, while we cannot help your child live longer, we can help you properly celebrate the wonder of this child, his relationships, his value, and the impact he has had on the world. Suggestions for accomplishing this celebration of life are offered, such as inviting friends and extended family, bringing the child's own clothing and dressing him or her after a bath (the parent may choose to do this or ask to have the nurse do this) as well as removing unneeded medical devices ("To make him your child again, and not a patient"), making a 3D plaster hand mold ("so you will always have your child's hand to hold"), bring in photo albums to remember the good times that were had, bring a camera or video to commemorate the celebration, bring members of the congregation to provide spiritual support and guidance, bring the child's favorite music, toys, videos, or other means of demonstrating the child's specialness. One family brought balloons and a sheet cake; another brought in the teen's make-up and favorite cologne; a third played videos of the teen's victorious football game. Have easy access to a rocking chair or couch for the parent to hold the child (no matter how large the child). Offer unlimited coffee and drinks. Offer to transfer the child to a more comfortable setting, where more supporters can comfortably be present. However, this agreement must usually be predicated by an agreement to terminate the ventilator within hours of transfer.

Avoidance of the topic of a poor prognosis and the performance of "slow codes" are ethically unjustifiable actions.[67,68] They deprive the family and patient of the potential for peaceful and final goodbyes, a commonly lamented missed opportunity. We have so much to share and so much healing to offer if we would just be honest and compassionate with our families. Death is inevitable. Missed goodbyes are not.

Table 51–3
Evaluating Treatment Options

- How realistic is it that the intervention will cure the disease?
- If not able to cure the disease, will the intervention prevent progression of the disease?
- Will the intervention improve the way the child feels?
- Could the intervention make the child feel worse? If so, for how long?
- What will it be like for this child to go through this treatment?
- What is likely to happen without the intervention?
- Will the intervention change the outcome for the child?
- What is the likely impact of this decision on the family?

Source: McConnell Y, et al. (2004), reference 159.

Aggressive Symptom Management

The symptoms most commonly suffered by dying children are poorly documented but include pain, seizures, problems with secretion control, dyspnea, vomiting;[69] perceptions of isolation and abandonment;[19] existential pain ("What did my existence mean to the world?"[70]); relational pain ("I was mean to my brother and I need to say I'm sorry"); and spiritual pain ("What could I have done to deserve this?"). In the ICU setting, where life-supporting technologies are nearly always in use at the time the decision to forgo further life-sustaining measures is made, the most common symptom-distress risks are dyspnea, pain, and seizures (personal observation). Thus, meticulous care at the time of ventilator withdrawal, including the continuous presence of the physician and/or nurse, and protocols for symptom management are key to the effective prevention or immediate management of symptom distress.[71]

It is helpful to most families to affirm their decision and to explain the expected events in advance of their occurrence.

> You are a brave and loving family. You have recognized that we cannot keep Brandon alive and have opted not to prolong his death, but, rather, give him a proper goodbye, surrounded by love, friends, and family. I know this is the hardest thing you have ever done. Brandon is lucky you are willing to do this for him. Do you have any concerns or questions I can address? If not, let me go over the procedure for tomorrow. In order to keep Brandon comfortable, we will discontinue his IV fluids the evening before so that he is not gurgling. We will move him to the larger room in the morning. After your family and friends celebrate Brandon's life, when you and your family are ready, we will suction Brandon's breathing tube and then remove it from his windpipe. We will also stop the blood pressure medication. Brandon may breathe in a funny pattern—sometimes shallow and quick, sometimes like a yawn or hiccup, and sometimes not at all. We will stay with you; if he looks uncomfortable, we will give him medications every 5 minutes until he looks more comfortable according to you and to me. I will not leave your side until he is looking as comfortable as possible.

The SUPPORT (Study to Understand Prognoses and Preferences for Outcomes and Risks of Treatment) trial demonstrated that current adult ICU practice does not address the issue of discontinuation of life support adequately;[72,73] it is unlikely that pediatric and neonatal ICUs do any better. In fact, a recent paper[74] demonstrates that even the most respected institutions frequently fail to effectively manage pain. When attended to by a skilled multidisciplinary team that focuses on these issues as primary concerns, these symptoms are usually successfully addressed. (For more in-depth explanations of the management of these symptoms, see Part II, Symptom Assessment and Management.) A few overarching principles deserve further mention, however.

Pain

Pain is a subjective phenomenon. It is not measured by vital signs, presence or absence of sleep, blood or imaging tests, or the size of an incision. Pain severity is most accurately assessed when measured by patient self-report.[75–77] Several tools exist to facilitate a child's pain self-report, including a visual analogue scale (a 10-cm line ranging from "no pain = 0 to the worst pain you can imagine = 10. Mark the amount of pain you are experiencing."); the categorical scale (no pain, a little pain, medium pain, and very, very bad pain); and the numerical scale ("0–5, 5 is the worst pain you can imagine"). Children 4 to 7 years of age respond well to the faces scale (categorical, with face cartoons to illustrate), the best validated being the Bieri scale,[78] which has too many choices for very young children. Other options include the Oucher scale,[79] Eland color tool,[80] and Wong–Baker faces scales,[81] among others.[82] Of course, when children are sedated or unable to communicate because of developmental immaturity, caregivers need to interpret the child's pain. There are a number of scales validated for the pediatric ICU patient, including the Premature Infant Pain Profile (PIPP), children's pain checklist, FLACC (Face, Legs, Activities, Cry, and Consolability) and Comfort scales.[83–86] Primary nursing assignments facilitate this assessment. Parents also are important resources for pain assessment.

The severity of reported pain dictates the category of pain relievers needed to relieve the pain, irrespective of etiology. For example, according to the World Health Organization (WHO) pain management guidelines for children, severe pain, regardless of etiology, demands prompt treatment with a "strong opioid," such as morphine, hydromorphone (Dilaudid), fentanyl, or methadone.[77] In the vast majority of cases, pain can be controlled.[87]

Dying adult patients often have pain. The occurrence of pain is not well documented in the terminally ill pediatric patient, but suspicion of pain must remain high, and presumptive treatment should occur if there are indications it is present. Where possible, each pain needs to be categorized not only by severity, but also by character (burning, gnawing, throbbing, sharp, crampy), location and radiation, duration, continuous or intermittent nature, and precipitating and relieving factors. The quality and timing of the pain suggest the etiology of the pain and dictate the most efficacious treatment. This ideal is very difficult to achieve in young or developmentally disabled children and in sedated or intubated patients. An empirical judgment of the etiology and physiology of the pain often dictates the choice of intervention in the ICU setting.

Constipation, a common problem in the ICU setting, may present with intermittent, poorly localized, crampy abdominal pain. Treatment with opioids would not be as beneficial as a heating pad and a laxative or, when needed, an enema. Burning pain in a patient who received neurotoxic chemotherapy is a sign of neuropathic pain, that is, pain related to nerve injury. This pain is best treated with "adjuvant pain relievers" (medications most often used for other purposes, but which are effective in the relief of certain types of pain), such as tricyclic antidepressants and anticonvulsants along with "traditional" pain-relieving agents, in addition to stopping the offending agent if it is still in use. Unfortunately, in the ICU setting, some adjuvants may not be of benefit because they must be given for at least 1 week to achieve effectiveness, or they are only available as tablets and capsules. Thus, depending on the patient's circumstance, the best pain management may be the use of nonpharmacological techniques, surgical, and anesthetic techniques where indicated,[88] and aggressive use of traditional pain relievers, including opioids and topical agents, such as topical lidocaine patches.

Concerns about addiction, a psychological phenomenon of craving a drug despite harm to oneself (which has been shown to be rare in the medical use of opioids), are inappropriate in the ICU. Around-the-clock analgesics should be provided, particularly in the setting of surgery, multiple trauma, and recurrent procedures. Medications should be titrated to pain control using acetaminophen or nonsteroidal antiinflammatory medications as background pain relief unless contraindicated, in addition to opioids for more severe pain, opioids and local anesthetics for procedure-related pain, and "adjuvant" analgesics for neuropathic pain. "As needed" or PRN medications should be ordered for the alleviation of increased pain as well as the expected side effects of opioids, such as nausea, pruritus, urinary retention, and somnolence (when it is undesirable). Constipation is a predictable side effect of opioid analgesia that does not resolve, but it is less of an issue in a child who is expected to die within 24 hours, as do most ICU patients undergoing the withdrawal or withholding of life-sustaining medical intervention.[15,73] Changing the specific opioid used[89] may also be considered for the management of refractory opioid-induced side effects when the child's expected survival is longer. Alternative routes of pain relief, such as epidurals for children who are excessively somnolent or who become delirious with systemically administered opioids, may be of benefit in some cases.

Respiratory depression in the face of pain is an uncommon occurrence, despite aggressive use of opioids for pain relief.[90,91] Irregular breathing caused by pain can often be smoothed and regulated to promote optimal gas exchange when pain is relieved. Pupillary size can help in the assessment of the opioid titration of preverbal or nonverbal patients (personal observation).

Pain can be treated effectively only if the results of the intervention are reassessed at the appropriate interval, based on the pharmacokinetics of the medication and route used.[75,77] If pain relief is not achieved, an additional intervention should be undertaken immediately, not at the next timed dosage. For instance, if the patient reports severe pain (a score of 10/10) and morphine is administered intravenously (IV), the child should be reassessed in 15 minutes. If the report remains the same ("severe pain, pain scale score 8/10"), an additional dose of morphine should be administered immediately. This process should continue until the child is comfortable. There is no maximum dose of pure opioids. The proper dose is the dose that controls the pain. The goal is not to sedate the child unless the child desires this; the goal is to relieve the pain. On occasion, pain can be relieved only with aggressive analgesia and sedation.[92]

Medication for consistent pain should be administered on a schedule, around the clock, or by constant infusion (not PRN). Additionally, medication for breakthrough pain (pain occurring despite the regular administration of medication) should be prescribed. The reader is referred to the Agency for Health Care Policy and Research (AHCPR) guidelines for pain management,[76] available from the U.S. federal government online, as well as other standard pain references,[93,94] and to Chapters 6 and 55 for further details regarding pain management. Successful pain management cannot occur unless pain is regarded as a priority, pain is regularly assessed and reassessed,[95] and pain scale scores are documented routinely.[96]

Dyspnea

Often children or their families prefer to forgo mechanical ventilation if there is no reasonable expectation of improvement or cure, with the exception of some patients with neuromuscular disorders who are still young and intellectually intact. When the choice is to discontinue or to not initiate mechanical ventilation, scrupulous attention to the management of dyspnea must be explained and promised to the child (if capable of participating) and the family, and the promise must be realized. The idea that there may be a trade-off between relief of dyspnea and sedation, or even a slightly earlier death, must also be broached and preferences elicited. Most families express preferences for enhanced comfort even in the face of a potentially foreshortened survival. However, this is not a foregone conclusion and, as has been previously reported,[97] patients occasionally are much less distressed than anticipated and are able to enjoy a few hours or even days with carefully titrated opioids, as needed.

In the few studies reviewing duration of survival related to the administration of morphine during withdrawal of mechanical ventilation, however, patients of all ages actually survive longer when liberal doses of morphine are used to ease the dyspnea.[91,97,98] The goals of care must be clear in everyone's mind before proceeding, lest the tragedy of perceptions of wrongdoing plague survivors.[99]

Dyspnea is a symptom that is even more distressing than pain to experience or witness. It is difficult to control and requires intensive hands-on management and reassessment. Several nonpharmacological approaches can be helpful, such as sitting the child upright, having a parent or other close family member or friend present, saying soothing words, and touching the child. In addition, having a small fan blow air across the child's face has been helpful in the hospice setting.

There are no published data on the treatment of dyspnea in children; the few small controlled studies done support the use of opioids as the pharmacological agents of choice in the management of dyspnea.[100] Clinical experience has shown efficacy of opioids in alleviating dyspnea as well.[101,102] The dose of opioids that is optimal is the dose that effectively relieves the dyspnea. This dose must be established by titration to clinical effect. Again, there is no maximal dose.

Various recommendations for the pharmacological management of dyspnea exist.[98,101–103] Regardless of the protocol used, it is imperative that the child be continuously observed and repeatedly treated until symptom relief is achieved. The dose should be rapidly and aggressively escalated if ineffective. The author's preference is to use IV preparations in the setting of extubation to gain rapid control. For example, if the child is receiving 5 mg of morphine IV per hour, the bolus dose would be 5 mg if dyspnea occurred at extubation. If the initial dose is totally ineffective, the next dose should be 50% to 100% higher, 7.5 to 10 mg. If, 5 minutes later, the patient is still *in extremis*, the next dose would be 50% to 100% higher. Often, children respond to these first few doses, and the dyspnea is controlled without loss of consciousness. The expected response to opioids is gradual slowing of respirations to a more normal level; respirations do not suddenly cease unexpectedly. Reversal with naloxone or other opioid antagonists should rarely, if ever, be undertaken. The recommended procedure, when done, is to dilute the naloxone 1:10 and administer it very slowly, repeating every few minutes as needed.

Benzodiazepines alleviate the breathlessness associated with anxiety but not the sensation of dyspnea itself. Administration of diuretics to children with pulmonary edema, withholding IV fluids or enteral feedings, or adding anticholinergic agents may decrease excess secretions. Thorough suctioning of endotracheal tubes before extubation of mechanically ventilated children is helpful as well. For more information on dyspnea, the reader is referred to Chapter 13.

Palliative Sedation

Occasionally, a technique known as terminal sedation is necessary to control symptoms, most often pain, dyspnea, and intractable seizures. Within the palliative care community, palliative sedation has become a generally accepted plan of care for adults in the case of otherwise uncontrollable symptoms, though somewhat more reluctantly so for children who cannot always independently consent in advance.[92] Although considered an "acceptable and justifiable form of euthanasia or physician-assisted suicide" (PAS) by some,[104–106] others see palliative sedation as the extension of the tenet that, above all, the health care provider's duty is to relieve suffering. The intention is not to bring about the demise of the child (as in the case of PAS and euthanasia),[107,108] but rather to control the symptom, even at risk of death (principle of double effect).

Regardless of the philosophical underpinnings that lead to the practice, palliative sedation is widely regarded as the only humane solution to an otherwise uncontrollable and severely distressing problem. It is only undertaken after all other attempts at symptom control have failed and with the full agreement of the child and family.[92] Full explanations of the inability to reverse the underlying process must precede this decision. Some practitioners also use barbiturates, particularly helpful in relieving labored or agonal respirations, for the management of terminal dyspnea and pain.[103]

Unfortunately, significant discomfort and uncertainty on the part of many critical care practitioners impede the availability of these therapeutic strategies. Clinicians fear being perceived as the proximate cause of death due to the administration of opioids,[97] despite numerous well-known ethical opinions that the relief of symptoms is the primary obligation to the dying patient. Critical care nurses giving opioids to terminally ill patients withdrawn from mechanical ventilation reported that they believed they were engaging in euthanasia.[109] On the other hand, the administration of neuromuscular blocking agents, impeding the ability to assess dyspnea, can constitute euthanasia and should be avoided whenever possible.[110]

Extubation Technique

Prior to extubation, engaging in family-centered rituals is important (see Case Studies below). This allows unhurried family time while the child is still pink and breathing. As the family is approaching readiness to extubate, they should be informed about what they can expect after extubation, making this difficult time easier. ("He may turn blue; we will treat this with morphine and oxygen if he looks uncomfortable. He may not breathe at all or may breathe comfortably for some time. I do not know how long he will live, but I expect it will be on the order of (minutes, hours, days). I will stay with you until he is comfortable.") Positive thoughts about extubation are important to share as well. ("This will be the first time you see your daughter's beautiful face without tape and a tube interfering"; "I am giving you back your son as a child, not as a patient"; "You may be able to hear his voice for the first time in a while," depending on the age and circumstances of the child.)

The author's practice, both as an intensivist and as a palliative care physician tending primarily to pediatric ICU patients, is to avoid "terminal weaning," or the gradual decrease of mechanical ventilation support. Terminal weaning allows the child to be dyspneic as well as to have the discomfort of the tube on the nasal mucosa and pharynx until he or she becomes unconscious, either from sedatives or carbon dioxide narcosis. Continued intubation also masks the severity of the child's distress and may lead to inadvertent undermedication. Thus, my practice is to extubate without weaning and provide "blow-by" oxygen as desired. It is critical to constantly assess discomfort and take steps to alleviate it, whether this consists of the simple act of having a loved one stroke the child's hand, giving reassurances of love, or rapidly increasing dosages of opioids or other interventions. The policy of decreasing supplemental oxygen in hypoxic children puts them at increased risk of discomfort. On the other hand, nonhypoxic children do not require the inconvenience and discomfort of supplemental oxygen. Another reason to prefer rapid extubation is that the tape and endotracheal tube create physical barriers between the child and family, who otherwise may feel more freedom to ply the child with kisses, indicating continued love and devotion, attending the devastating symptom of perceived abandonment.

Children with significant central nervous system compromise may have noisy respirations due to floppy pharyngeal soft tissues. The family needs to be made aware of this possibility before extubation. Management strategies include repositioning, discontinuation of IV fluid or enteral intake well in advance of extubation, administration of diuretics and/or anticholinergic medications, aggressive suctioning of artificial airways before removal, or placement of a nasal trumpet. The latter, however, creates a physical wedge between the child and family and should be avoided when possible.

Child Preferences and Critical Care Practices of Withholding or Withdrawing Medical Interventions

Physician indoctrination of the imperative to preserve life at all costs must not override patients' values. Most studies indicate that, in practice, the justification for forgoing life-sustaining medical intervention (LSMI) in ICUs, whether the patient is a child[11] or an adult,[111] is physician assessment of poor prognosis for survival rather than quality-of-life considerations.[112–117] Reassessing the goals of treatment only when the child is dying deprives the patient of choices that the child and family may make earlier to enhance the quality of life rather than extend the duration of life.[26,58] Children who cannot be cured and their families often have preferences regarding medical interventions. Their opinions are not knowable by the medical team a priori; they must be actively solicited.[118–122] In addition, the child's perceptions of discomfort relative to various medical interventions may be very different than the medical caregivers' perceptions. In fact, regardless of the presence of a terminal prognosis, patients and their surrogates have the right to forgo LSMI.[123–125]

Thus, the current practice of withholding discussions regarding burdens and benefits of ongoing LSMI is insupportable. Refusing to honor a child's[126] or surrogates' requests to stop LSMI until the child is certain to die is even worse.[127–129] Patient suffering must play a much more prominent role in the decision-making process if "good deaths" are to be attained for a higher proportion of patients.[111,130] On the other hand, physicians' personal biases regarding quality of life and economic motivations for the withdrawal of LSMI should not play any role in the decision to forgo treatment.[118,131]

Finally, it has been shown that physicians' practices in withdrawing medical interventions are more determined by personal idiosyncrasy[118,132] and fears of litigation or accusation of wrongdoing than by the patient's comfort.[133,134] In several studies, vasopressors were withheld first, oxygen next, and mechanical ventilation next. However, oxygen supplementation and extubation may be preferred and more comfortable. In addition, withholding antibiotics and allowing the peaceful death associated with sepsis, without a trip to the ICU, may be the most humane option available for some children. In other cases, forgoing nutrition may ease nausea, and forgoing hydration may decrease the discomfort of renal failure or congestive heart failure.[135,136] Obviously, much depends on the child's symptoms, the clinical situation, and the child's and family's values and preferences. Effecting a philosophical change among medical decision-makers to proactively solicit children's and families' perspectives may be accomplished by educational intervention, although it is likely that cultural changes within institutions and protocol-driven practice may have more promise.[61]

Review of the Patient Care Plan

After it has been determined that the child and family no longer subscribe to the goal of prolongation of life, because either the burdens are too great or the effort is "futile," the care plan must be reviewed in detail. The likely mechanisms of death must be determined and plans should be made to ameliorate associated symptoms of these mechanisms. It is not uncommon for the child to have several potential mechanisms for death; often, one route can be anticipated to be the most comfortable, such as dying from hyperkalemia or sepsis as opposed to hypoxemia. In this case, Kayexalate or dialysis as well as antibiotics should be discontinued, whereas oxygen by nasal cannula or "blow-by" if possible should be continued.

Anticipation of likely symptoms and care plans that address them proactively are essential.[137] For instance, if the child is likely to have seizures but cannot swallow, rectal or parenteral rapid-onset anticonvulsants should be written as a PRN order. Developmentally appropriate explanations about the possible course of events should be given to the child and family unless they refuse this information. It is unwise to predict an exact time of death, but approximations (with significant margin for error, e.g., minutes to hours, hours to days, days to weeks) are helpful for the family to arrange for the child's other loved ones' and friends to visit before or be present at death.

All interventions that either interfere with comfort or that do not enhance it should be discontinued. For instance, laboratory tests are not designed to enhance comfort. Sometimes in clinical practice, laboratory parameters, such as platelet counts, are monitored to prevent symptoms such as bleeding from arising. However, it is just as efficacious and less intrusive to monitor the patient for clinical bleeding and treat if and when it arises, if desired. Medications that do not enhance comfort, often including antibiotics, should be considered for discontinuation. Even feeding and IV fluids may interfere with comfort if the child has pulmonary edema, heart failure, or renal failure; a decrease in or cessation of these therapies may enhance the child's comfort.

Monitors, such as pulse oximeters, cardiorespiratory monitors, and the like should be removed. They create physical barriers to the closeness of loved ones with the child, distract them from attending to the child with their color displays and flashing lights, create distressing alarms that all have agreed not to respond to, and create a reason for the health care team not to enter the room. (However, some families become so attached that removing these devices seems to them to be a form of abandonment and should not be carried out). Visitation restrictions and many of the usual rules should be reconsidered. Maximization of holding the child or even invitations to family members to climb in bed with the child should be facilitated. Letting the family bathe the child and dress him or her in clothing of the child's or family's choice is often helpful. Other special requests should be honored if at all possible.

Transfer to Alternative Care Settings

When children are acknowledged to be dying, it is common for large numbers of loved ones to gather. They need to support the child, parents, siblings, and each other. Sometimes they may desire to perform rituals that may be difficult to accommodate in the ICU setting. Thus, consideration for transfer to an alternate care setting should be made. If the child is anticipated to live for a few days once ICU interventions are discontinued, referral to hospice in the home care setting may be an option. Usually a 1- to 2-day stay in the hospital to ensure "stability" and to provide family caregiver teaching is needed.

Alternatively, if the child will have significant distress in his or her final days, or the child and/or family prefer to stay in the hospital, admission to the floor, or preferably a palliative care unit, may be the best plan.[1,55,131,132] As large a room as is needed to accommodate the child and his or her loved ones should be provided, if possible.

The Butterfly Room

At the University of Texas Medical Branch at Galveston, we have created an alternative care unit for children with life-threatening conditions called the Butterfly Room.[138] It is a homelike setting distinctly different from any other room in the hospital, with carpeting, wallpaper with butterflies, a kitchenette, TV, Nintendo and VCR, pull-out sofa beds and chairs, padded window seats overlooking the Gulf of Mexico, and storage, as well as a place for the child to sleep. It is as large as two semiprivate rooms and is designed to accommodate the entire family.

One use of the room is for ICU patients who are expected to die within minutes to days following extubation, and who are thus generally not candidates for transfer home. After consultation with the family, it is our practice to review the medical orders and discontinue all laboratory tests, all invasive equipment (extra IV sites, nasogastric tubes, urinary catheters, etc.), all monitors (including the recording of vital signs, fluid balance, and weights), and all medications other than those contributing to the comfort of the patient. Orders not to resuscitate (DNR) are written with the family's agreement. The child, who is still being mechanically ventilated, with vasopressors infusing as needed, is then moved from the ICU to the Butterfly Room. Resuscitative medications, such as atropine and epinephrine, are brought in the elevator for unstable patients to ensure that the family will have a chance for final togetherness, but these medications have never been used. Cardiopulmonary resuscitation beyond these medications would not be done, however.

In the Butterfly Room, the child's loved ones are invited to sit in a rocking chair, or, in the case of an older child, they are invited to sit on a couch and hold the child. Even young siblings participate in this activity. Usually, each family member in turn will whisper loving thoughts and memories to the dying child. Numerous photographs are taken in most cases. The family is offered the opportunity to bathe the child, make handprints, footprints, or handmolds and dress the child in clothing of their choice. Other rituals specific to the family or their heritage may be undertaken. Once these events have taken place, with the family's acknowledgment of readiness, the child is extubated. Opioids, benzodiazepines, and blow-by oxygen are immediately available. The multidisciplinary hospice team, including a spiritual leader of the family's choosing, if desired, a social worker, a child life therapist for siblings, and the nurse and physician remain either in the room or close by, often mingling among the distressed relatives and listening to their concerns, as well as attending to the patient's symptoms.

Consideration of Suffering and Future Quality of Life

It has been documented that, against the legal and ethical principles currently in place, physicians often refuse requests to forgo life-sustaining treatment.[124] Since discontinuation of LSMI often leads to the patient's death, this action must be undertaken with caution, ensuring that the child is not making decisions on the basis of depression or the family making decisions based on exhaustion or financial pressures. However, refusal of LSMI may well represent the child's and family's assessment of future quality of life, often based on the experience of lived, progressive disability and chronic illness, or on long-held values.

Surrogates' (or parents') duties are to act on the child's wishes and in his or her best interests.[120–123,139–142] This role is often not clear and requires explanation. Surrogates, in the author's experience, more often request prolongation of a child's death due to guilt and fear, rather than discontinuation of LSMI too prematurely. Thus, overriding requests to terminate LSMI must also be done with significant forethought and analysis. In addition, the motivation for requests to continue LSMI in the face of an extremely small likelihood of survival, or very large chance of a significantly poor quality of life, must be explored fully. Issues of guilt ("What do you think caused his problems? You were away at work when the accident happened?") and loss ("Tell me about what has happened to your family as a result of your child's condition?" "It sounds like you've been through a lot. I wish I could make your child healthy and make it all OK again but unfortunately, there are limits to what medicine can do. The best we can reasonably hope for, medically, is . . . . Does that change your perspective on treatment options? Our recommendation, based on all you've told us and our assessment of your child's condition is . . ."). Eliciting and demonstrating respect for the family's and child's (where applicable) values can be helpful in resolving these dilemmas.

Notification of Death

Unless there are extremely extenuating circumstances, even if the death is expected, most experts strongly encourage that the notification of death be done in person. ("Mrs. Smith, I am afraid I have some bad news. Could you come in to discuss it?") Empathy can be more easily expressed in person by sitting close to the parents and siblings at the time of the discussion, perhaps even giving the bereaved a hug, or shedding a genuine tear. These small tokens of warmth and understanding help the family to know that the medical team cared about the child as a person. Additionally, insistence that the family come in allows them to see the dead child, which facilitates the acceptance of the fact that death has occurred and allows the family to participate in important rituals, such as bathing the dead, sometimes assisting in the removal of equipment, or sitting vigil as some cultures require. These efforts result in improved bereavement outcomes, particularly for siblings, who often imagine the child has not actually died.

Bereavement Follow-Up

Studies have repeatedly shown an increased mortality rate of surviving spouses in the year following death.[143–145] A recent study of bereaved parents in Denmark showed a marked increase in mortality from natural (maternal) and unnatural causes (maternal and paternal),[146] though no similar study of siblings has been undertaken. The divorce rate among parents the first year after a child's death is higher than the national average. (Over the long term, however, the proportion returns to the national average of 50%.) It is not yet known what interventions are most effective for bereaved parents. However, a recent study indicates that a caring attitude of the ICU staff has short-term and long-term impact on parental adaptation to their loss.[147] Moreover, even for parents whose child died a violent death, attendance at a support group and maintenance of religious connection can enable better adaptation in the long term.[148] In addition, some lessons may be derived from studies of bereaved spouses.

A simple strategy of routinely sending a bereavement card 2 weeks following the death of a hospitalized patient was investigated. One year later, the bereaved survivors could consistently and without warning retrieve the card, indicating the importance to them of such a gesture. Remarks of survivors of patients who had died in the ER included, "At least I know my husband died among caring people."[149] Attending the deceased's funeral is an even more powerful demonstration of caring and may provide relief for the medical caregiver as well.[150]

If an autopsy was performed, families need a face-to-face appointment (autopsy conference) with the treating physician to explain the autopsy findings in understandable terms[151,152] Often, this explanation gives the bereaved family a profound sense of peace by affirming the cause of death, affirming the irreversibility of the problems, or determining a cause of death that was unknown antemortem. It is particularly important to rule out heritable conditions that may affect surviving or future siblings. This process has even been found to improve adaptation to loss. The autopsy visit also allows monitoring of the family's grieving process and provides the opportunity for referral to counseling, if needed, for pathological grief reactions. In the absence of a face-to-face session, families consenting to an autopsy often complain that they had no follow-up and express anger and suspicion about the motivations for the autopsy. This postdeath conference is also helpful for families who did not consent to autopsy, to answer questions and monitor for adaptive grieving. Referrals can be made for families needing counseling or other assistance.

A memorial service may also be offered. This may take several forms; two are particularly suggested for the ICU. Some children's families who have either come to the ICU recurrently, or others who have particularly bonded with the staff due to a child's prolonged stay or for other reasons, may be invited back to the unit with the families of a few other children who have died within the last month or 6 weeks for a ceremony of sharing. The family may bring a picture of the child, and the family and staff can exchange memories of the child. Songs may be sung, poems may be read, and prayers may be shared. Gratitude and admiration may be exchanged. In addition, all families bereaved of children could be invited to a group memorial service conducted on an annual or more frequent basis. One study of the bereavement care of families grieving a child's traumatic death included family contact at the hospital after discharge from the ED, attendance at the funeral home, a home visit, a meeting at a restaurant with the parents and 15 parental supporters 2 months following the death, and a parental interview approximately a year after the death. The latter were for the purpose of educating parental supporters about the course of grief and the need for longer-term support.[153] Even a simple phone call would be appreciated but is rarely received.[17]

Grief of Medical Caregivers

Not only do children suffer and families and loved ones grieve, but we as medical caregivers grieve for our patients, their families, and ourselves. We are exposed to pain and grief both vicariously and in empathy and are forced to confront the certainty of our own and our fellow humans' mortality on a daily basis. In caring for dying children, we are threatened by the reality that our own children, too, could die. The ability to share these feelings in a supportive environment, without sanction, and the ability to take leave to attend funerals can assist in increased job satisfaction and retention of highly skilled critical care personnel. It can also help to reinforce the humanity that makes us the medical caregivers we can be.

Palliative Care for All Patients

The focus on prevention of suffering and on the person as a whole should not be reserved solely for the dying child. All children, from clinic patients to ICU patients to dying children, should have access to the best that medicine has to offer. As a wise man stated very long ago, "The medical care provider's duty is to cure sometimes, to relieve often, and to comfort always."[154]

Teaching End-of-Life Care

Once palliative care philosophy and methods are embraced, they should extend beyond the ICU. Ongoing efforts to teach the principles and practice of palliative medicine must occur to ensure that our trainees are as capable as possible of carrying on the tradition of humane and person-centered end-of-life care. Several courses are described in the literature and could easily be adapted for use in other settings.[155–158] In the absence of training, our trainees will inadvertently contribute to the already unimaginable pain of a child's death.

> The medical student population is probably the one that on a daily basis, offend the parents the most . . . I have been vocal with residents, like this person needs 101 in how to work with a parent . . . . But there is no real formal process set up for that feedback.
> —Tina Heyl-Martineau, parent, 2001 (in Field & Behrman [2002], reference 1, p. 328)

Recommendations For Implementation

Improved end-of-life care begins with more highly focused attention on the individual child and his or her preferences and values. Pediatric and neonatal ICU practitioners are the caregivers for the vast majority of children who die; thus, they must have expertise in palliative care. Some recommendations to enhance end-of-life care in the pediatric and neonatal ICU setting are:

- Admission procedures should include a values history; solicitation of any advance directives for older, chronically ill children; and discussion of expressed preferences in light of the child's current situation. This should not be reserved only for imminently dying children. Waiting until that time only increases the chances that the child's preferences will never be known and the family's guilt will be unnecessarily increased in the event they are later called upon to consent to the withdrawal of life-sustaining medical interventions. Good coordination with primary care providers and specialists who have cared for the chronically ill child can be enormously helpful.
- Attention to pain and the relief of other symptoms, both during procedures and more generally, must become a priority for all children. This can be accomplished only with training and appropriate documentation procedures, as well as emphasis by supervisors and attending physicians.
- Improved communication techniques must be employed that allow children or their surrogates to understand their options in a supportive and unbiased way. Guilt, missed opportunities, love, and existential and spiritual issues should be included in these discussions. Again, training must be developed and carried out. The importance of these issues must be emphasized, demonstrated, and reflected in the practices of the opinion leaders within the unit.
- Cooperation, respect, and regular interdisciplinary rounds among the disciplines of nursing, medicine, social work, pastoral care, and, possibly, palliative care (and others as indicated, such as pharmacy, occupational therapy, physical therapy, child life) will enhance the larger understanding of the child and his or her needs and facilitate the team's ability to assist the child with the accomplishment of his or her goals.
- Establishment of a bereavement follow-up program, including the mailing of bereavement cards, autopsy debriefing or postdeath sessions, "sharing sessions," and memorial services will improve the bereavement outcome for surviving loved ones and ICU staff.
- Excused paid absences for funeral attendance and staff support sessions will prevent burnout and turnover and allow the retention of the ideals and values that brought each staff member to the healing professions.

Summary

Infants die primarily of congenital defects, prematurity, and SIDS. Children older than 1 year of age die primarily from trauma, thus predisposing them to die in ICU settings. The principles of palliative care must be applied to all children, even those whose fate is to die in the ICU. Our challenge, as practitioners of emergency and pediatric critical care medicine, is to provide each of these children a "good death." This can be achieved by intensive attention to the child's and family's perspectives and goals, communication within the team and with the child and his or her loved ones, dedication to the meticulous management of symptoms, particularly during procedures—the most common source of discomfort in ill children—and effective bereavement follow-up.

CASE STUDY
FL, a Near-Drowning Victim

FL, a 14-year-old Pakistani boy, suffered a near-drowning episode that compromised his central respiratory drive mechanism and left him neurologically devastated. His family was informed that life-sustaining medical interventions were futile. They agreed to move him to the Butterfly Room to achieve a family-centered death. Orders not to resuscitate were written in a clear and detailed manner. All laboratory analyses were discontinued and all monitors were removed. Medications were reviewed and all were discontinued. Morphine and lorazepam were added for the management of dyspnea, IV fluids were discontinued, and scopolamine was administered for terminal secretions. One IV catheter was left intact, but all other invasive monitors, such as nasogastric tubes, urinary and arterial catheters, etc., were removed. During his transfer from the ICU to the Butterfly Room, FL remained mechanically ventilated.

Although FL had a small family, he belonged to a close-knit community. Thirty people of all ages came to be with him on his final day of life. They encircled the boy's bed, chanting but not touching him. After approximately 30 minutes, they approached the team and announced their readiness for the discontinuation of mechanical ventilation. One caregiver stated that she was unfamiliar with Pakistani traditions and customs, but had not observed anyone touching FL. She suggested that if touching was allowable and desirable for them, they were welcome to do so. The whole spirit of the group changed, with the circle drawing nearer the bed and men openly grieving and weeping, holding the boy and their wives, as well as each other. People stroked FL's face and body. After an hour, they again informed the team that they were now ready to have the mechanical ventilation discontinued.

FL was suctioned and extubated and needed little pharmacological intervention. His loved ones chanted from the moment the endotracheal tube was removed. Each visitor, in turn, put small amounts of holy water in his mouth. Although the water bubbled out of his nose, a caregiver wiped it away, giving "permission" for the next person to engage in the ritual. After 27 minutes of nonstop chanting, FL died. A peaceful hush fell over the room, and all eyes turned to the same window leading to the outside.

CASE STUDY

LF, a Newborn with Hypoplastic Left Heart Syndrome

LF, a newborn, was diagnosed with hypoplastic left heart syndrome. After a full explanation of the surgical options, the family opted for palliative care. The mother preferred never to see the baby again, because she feared bonding with her child. The baby was in the ICU but, because of her parents' decision, was not receiving ICU interventions. The parents were approached about the Butterfly Program, providing surrogate parents, and moving the baby to the Butterfly Room; they agreed. They decided to visit the baby the next day. She was wearing normal baby clothes, being cared for and appearing like any other baby. When they saw that the baby did not need highly skilled care, they felt that they could care for her themselves at home with the help of the Butterfly Program. The next day, the parents took their daughter home. LF lived well there and visited many churches for blessings, went to numerous restaurants, had house guests, received several hospice visits, and was asymptomatic until her final day at 2 weeks of age, when she began to vomit and become intermittently cyanotic. The Butterfly Team (nurse, social worker, and physician) was summoned to the home. Additional explanations of what was happening and assurances of the child's comfort were provided. The baby received one dose of morphine, but the family assessed that she did not need more. She died in her mother's arms 8 hours after the first cyanotic episode.

CASE STUDY

GG, a 7-Day-Old Infant with Anuria

GG, a 7-day-old male infant, was anuric and referred from a hospital located 3½ hours away by ground transport from the tertiary care hospital. Diagnostic studies showed complete absence of a urinary collecting system and hypoplastic lungs. He underwent intubation for acidosis and respiratory insufficiency; meanwhile, the implications of the findings were communicated to his parents.

GG's 7-year-old brother had begged his parents for a new baby, resulting in GG's birth. He had seen "his baby" for a total of 20 minutes; now the baby was far away and dying. It was unlikely that GG could live long enough to be transported home without life support. The extended family and friends were unable to arrange transportation to the hospital in a timely manner. In addition, they preferred GG to die at home, if at all possible.

The ICU social worker arranged for Medicaid to cover the ambulance expenses of transporting the intubated patient to his home. The Butterfly Team arranged for the ambulance to be met at the house by a local hospice team, which had orders to extubate on arrival, and had medications for dyspnea. The baby was taken to the living room, where his brother and family awaited him. His brother was the first person to hold him. A peaceful 3 hours were spent, and the baby died at home with minimal symptoms.

CASE STUDY

EC, a 7-Month-Old Infant with Severe Neurological Compromise

EC, a 7-month-old infant, had a rare chromosomal anomaly resulting in severe neurological compromise. He had unrelenting gastroesophageal reflux, causing recurrent pneumonia and ICU admissions, and, according to his parents, constant sensations of choking. His family agreed to a fundoplication to enhance his daily comfort rather than to extend his life. The family realized that he would not live very long because, during his entire lifetime, he had spent a total of 7 weeks out of the hospital.

Five days postoperatively, the fundoplication dehisced, and EC developed peritonitis. The family interpreted this as a sign to stop interfering with their son's dying process. They accepted antibiotics but refused further surgery. After 2 days, they chose to take him home. Within 2 hours, he was on a commercial jet to his home, an 8-hour drive away. A hospice team met the family on the tarmac and drove behind them with medications. He arrived safely home and spent 3 days with his family, with frequent visits from the hospice team to ensure his and his family's comfort. He is buried on the family property with a ring of evergreens surrounding his grave. His older sister wrote a poem about him. The family adopted a needy Mexican infant 2 years later. They are doing well.

CASE STUDY

DC, a 5-Week-Old Infant with Intraventricular Hemorrhages

DC was born after a 25-week gestation to a 41-year-old mother who had cervical incompetence. The mother underwent a tubal ligation at the time of DC's birth. Her first child was born at 30 weeks' gestation and had done well. Both parents were schoolteachers of young, disabled children.

DC suffered bilateral grade IV intraventricular hemorrhages early in his course. His parents did not understand the implications of this initially, and he continued an unstable course, with the development of severe bronchopulmonary dysplasia and frequent desaturation episodes. He also developed hydrocephalus. The prognosis became clear to the parents when DC was 5 weeks old, and they requested discontinuation of his life support. He was transported to the Butterfly Room and intubated. The family requested a rabbi and support from the Butterfly Team.

No one in his family had ever held DC because the referring neonatal team had felt that he was "too unstable." When his mother held him to her chest and stroked her son for the first time, he became pink and his heart rate decreased from 180 to 140 beats per minute. The infant's 20-month-old brother sat with him and had photographs taken. DC remained stable.

After some time, a conversation with the parents and aunts confirmed that they were making the decision to stop life support out of love for their child and concern for his suffering, that they had been good parents to him, and that their other son would always be a brother. The rabbi affirmed that their religion supported their decision. A description of what might happen postextubation was offered. The family understood and requested that the ventilator be discontinued. The mother held her son without the impediment of medical equipment, crying quietly to herself and rocking him with her husband, son, and sisters at her side until DC's death 26 minutes later.

Over the ensuing months, the family frequently called the Butterfly Program social worker for counseling, and occasionally they met for lunch. They have been lost to long-term follow-up.

CASE STUDY

KD, a Child with Multisystem Organ Dysfunction

KD, a 2½-year-old boy, had one of 20 world-reported cases of a syndrome that caused multisystem organ dysfunction, primarily liver and digestive, as well as bone marrow. For most of his life, KD was hospitalized an average of 2 to 3 days per month for diarrheal or infectious episodes. He was extremely small for his age (one medical student estimated he was 6 months old on his last admission) but was alert, interactive, and able to talk, although assessed to be "delayed." He enjoyed music and playing "air guitar." His family loved him dearly and had made many sacrifices to ensure his well-being. His mother, the main wage earner, quit her job, and her husband became the sole source of family income. The family had to move to a new neighborhood.

During his last 2 months, KD was continuously hospitalized for severe diarrhea. After 1 month, KD began to require ICU interventions for sepsis episodes. After four episodes in the ICU over the course of 3 weeks, his parents approached the ICU team because they felt that KD, who was intubated for fungal sepsis and general debility, was not going to get better; they requested comfort measures only. They felt that their boy was not benefiting from life-sustaining medical interventions. This was difficult for his medical care team to accept.

KD and his family were moved to the Butterfly Room, where they were joined by an extended family and a circle of friends, a total of 45 people. All monitors were discontinued, and all laboratory testing was discontinued. The desired limitations of medical interventions were documented in the chart.

A discussion with the extended family affirmed that the decisions made for KD were loving decisions. Their chaplain visited and affirmed their choices and the support of the church. Then, a discussion of what KD might look like after extubation, the uncertain time course to death, methods of controlling symptoms, and the principle of double effect were explained. Handprints and footprints of KD were made, his mother and father bathed him, and he was dressed in an outfit that the family had brought from home.

KD was held by everyone in a rocking chair; some people, such as his 7-year-old sister, needed to hold KD several times before they were ready. The family took as much time as they needed while the Butterfly Team (nurse, social worker, child life specialist, and physician) circulated among the group, listening with empathy and encouraging communication. The family was reluctantly ready to stop the ventilator after 4 hours of rocking. As usual, the care team stayed with the family.

KD immediately turned cyanotic and was gasping postextubation; 100% blow-by oxygen was administered, as well as 0.1 mg/kg. IV of morphine. After 5 uncomfortable minutes and no effect on his breathing effort, 0.2 mg/kg of morphine was given. Again, 5 minutes passed with no change; the morphine was again doubled. This process continued until KD relaxed and no longer seemed to be dyspneic. He remained cyanotic, which, despite forewarning, was upsetting to his family. He died 2½ hours postextubation.

Bereavement follow-up included attendance at KD's visitation and funeral by members of the care team; donations by a local service group of a truckload of clothing, paper goods, and shelf food, as well as Christmas presents; phone calls and mailings; and invitations to a yearly memorial service, as well as to support groups. Three years later, the family is doing well.

REFERENCES

1. Field MJ, Behrman RE, eds. When Children Die: Improving Palliative and End-of-Life Care for Children and Their Families. Washington, DC: National Academy Press, 2002.

1a. Maruyama N. Cited by: Field MJ and Behrman RE. Your child is dead. Am Coll Emerg Med News, Oct. 18, 1997. (Ref. 1, p. 113).

2. Billings JA. What is palliative care? J Palliative Med 1998;1:73–81.
3. American Academy of Pediatrics Committee on Bioethics and Committee on Hospital Care. Pediatric palliative care. Pediatrics 2000;106;351–357.
4. Levetown M. Breaking bad news in the emergency department: when seconds count. Top Emerg Med 2004;26:35–43
5. Jurkovich GJ, Pierce B, Pananen L, Rivara FP. Giving bad news: the family perspective. J Trauma 2000;48:865–873.
6. Mosenthal A, Murphy PA. Trauma care and palliative care: time to integrate the two. J Am Coll Surg 2003;197:509–516.
7. Wanzer SH, Federman DD, Adelstein SJ, Cassell CK, Cassem EH, Cranford RE, et al. The physician's responsibility toward hopelessly ill patients: a second look. N Engl J Med 1989;320:844–849.
8. Kochanek KD, Smith BL. Deaths: preliminary data for 2002. National vital statistics reports; Vol. 52, no. 13. Hyattsville, MD: National Center for Health Statistics, 2004.
9. Prendergast TJ, Luce JM. A national survey of withdrawal of life support from critically ill patients. Abstr. Am J Respir Crit Care Med 1996;153:A360.
10. Koch KA, Rodeffer HD, Wears RL. Changing patterns of terminal care management in an intensive care unit. Crit Care Med 1994;22:233–243.
11. Levetown M, Pollack MM, Cuerdon TT, Ruttimann UE, Glover JJ. Limitations and withdrawals of medical intervention in pediatric critical care. JAMA 1994;272:1271–1275.
12. Gallup Organization. Knowledge and Attitudes Related to Hospice Care. Arlington, VA: National Hospice Organization, 1996.
13. The George H. Gallup International Institute. Spiritual Beliefs and the Dying Process: Key Findings from a National Survey Conducted for the Nathan Cummings Foundation and the Fetzer Institute. Life at Risk, December 1997.
14. Sullivan AM, Lakoma MD, Block SD. The status of medical education in end-of-life care: a national report. J Gen Intern Med 2003;18:685–695
15. McCallum DE, Byrne P, Bruera E. How children die in hospitals. J Pain Symptom Manage 2000;20:417–423.
16. Carter BS, Levetown M. Palliative Care for Infants, Children and Adolescents: A Practical Handbook. Baltimore: Johns Hopkins University Press, 2004: Chapters 10 (NICU), 11 (PICU).
17. Ahrens W, Hart R, Maruyama N, Pediatric death: managing the aftermath in the emergency department. J Emerg Med 1997;15: 601–603.
18. Cook P, White DK, Ross-Russell RI. Bereavement support following sudden and unexpected death: guidelines for care. Arch Dis Child 2002;87:36–38.
19. Bluebond-Langner M. The Private Worlds of Dying Children. Princeton: Princeton University Press, 1978.
20. Contro N, Larson J, Scofield S, Sourkes B, Cohen H. Family perspectives on the quality of pediatric palliative care. Arch Pediatr Adolesc Med 2002;156:14–19.
21. Meyer EC, Burns JP, Griffith JL, Truog RD. Parental perspectives on end-of-life care in the pediatric intensive care unit. Crit Care Med 2002;30:263–265.
22. Field MJ, Behrman RE. Communication, goal setting and care planning. In: Field MJ, Behrman RE, eds. When Children Die: Improving Palliative and End-of-Life Care for Children and Their Families. Washington, DC: National Academy Press, 2002:104–140.
23. Webb M. The Good Death: The New American Search to Reshape The End of Life. New York: Bantam Books, 1997.
24. Byock I. Dying Well: The Prospect for Growth at the End of Life. New York: Riverhead Books, 1997.
25. Goldman A. Care of the Dying Child. New York: Oxford University Press, 1994.
26. Levetown M. Ethical aspects of pediatric palliative care. J Palliat Care 1996;12:35–39.
27. Phipps EJ, Cooper MR, Greenstein S. The last days of life: a retrospective study of when resuscitation decisions are made. Fam Syst Med 1993;11:83–88.
28. Levetown M and the Committee on Bioethics. Communicating with children and families: from everyday interactions to skill in conveying distressing information. Pediatrics, in press.
29. Committee on Bioethics, Committee on Hospital Care, American Academy of Pediatrics. Palliative Care for Children. Pediatrics 2000;106:351–357.
30. United Nations Children's Fund. First Call for Children: World Declaration and Plan of Action from the World Summit for Children, and Convention on the Rights of the Child. New York: UNICEF, December, 1990.
31. Dreyer DR. Care of the dying adolescent: special considerations: Pediatrics 2004;113:381–388.
32. Rushforth H. Practitioner review: communicating with hospitalised children: review and application of research pertaining to children's understanding of health and illness. J Child Psychol Psychiatr 1999;40:683–691.
33. McCabe MA. Involving children and adolescents in medical decision-making: developmental and clinical considerations. J Pediatri Psychol 1996;21:505–516.
34. Hofmann JC, Wenger NS, Davis RB, Teno J, Connors AF, Desbiens N, et al. Patient preferences for communication with physicians about end-of-life decisions. Ann Intern Med 1997; 127:1–12.
35. Johnston SC, Pfeifer MP, McNutt R. The discussion about advance directives: patient and physician opinions regarding when and how it should be conducted. Arch Intern Med 1995; 155:1025–1030.
36. Gordon M. Decisions and care at the end of life. Lancet 1995;346: 163–166.
37. Spinetta JJ, Masera G, Eden T, Oppenheim D, Martins AG, van Dongen-Melman J, et al. Refusal, non-compliance, and abandonment of treatment in children and adolescents with cancer: a report of the SIOP Working Committee on Psychosocial Issues in Pediatric Oncology. Med Pediatr Oncol 2002;38:114–117.
38. Tolle SW. Care of the dying: clinical and financial lessons from the Oregon experience. Ann Intern Med 1995;128:567–568.
39. FitzGerald JD, Wenger NS, Califf RM, Phillips RS, Desbiens NA, Liu H, et al. Functional status among survivors of in-hospital cardiopulmonary resuscitation. Arch Intern Med 1996;156: 72–76.

40. Diem SJ, Lantos JD, Tulsky JA. Cardiopulmonary resuscitation on television: miracles and misinformation. N Engl J Med 1996; 334:1604–1605.
41. Murphy DJ, Burrows D, Santilli S, Kemp AW, Tenner S, Kreling B, et al. The influence of the probability of survival on patients' preferences regarding cardiopulmonary resuscitation. N Engl J Med 1994;330:545–549.
42. O'Donnell H, Phillips RS, Wenger N, Teno J, Davis RB, Hamel MB. Preferences for cardiopulmonary resuscitation among patients 80 years or older: the views of patients and their physicians. J Am Med Dir Assoc 2003;4:139–144.
43. Slonim AD. Cardiopulmonary resuscitation outcomes in children. Crit Care Med 2000;28:3364–3366.
44. Sichting K, Berens R. Outcomes following resuscitations at Children's Hospital of Wisconsin. Crit Care Med 1997;25:A61.
45. Lantos JD, Miles SH, Silverstein MD, Stocking CB. Survival after cardiopulmonary resuscitation in babies of very low birth weight. N Engl J Med 1998;318:91–95.
46. Torres A, Pickert CB, Firestone J, Walter WM, Fiser DH. Long-term functional outcome of in-patient pediatric cardiopulmonary resuscitation. Pediatr Emerg Care 1997;13:369–373.
47. Schindler MB, Bohn D, Cox PN, McCrindle BW, Jarvis A, Edmonde J, et al. Outcome of out-of-hospital cardiac or respiratory arrest in children. N Engl J Med 1996;335:1473–1479.
48. Curtis JR, Patrick DL, Shannon SE, Treece PD, Engelberg RA, Rubenfeld GD. The family conference to improve communication about end-of-life care in the intensive care unit: opportunities for improvement. Crit Care Med 2001;29(Suppl):N26–N33.
49. Meyer EC, Snelling LK, Myren-Manbeck LK. Pediatric intensive care: the parents' experience. AACN Clin Issues 1998;9:64–74.
50. Wier R. Affirming the decisions adolescents make about life and death. Hastings Cent Rep 1997;27:29–40.
51. Doig C, Burgess E. Withholding life-sustaining treatment: are adolescents competent to make these decisions? CMAJ 2000;162: 1585–1588.
52. Quill TE. Nonabandonment: a central obligation for physicians. Ann Intern Med 1995;122:368–374.
53. Pellegrino ED. Nonabandonment: an old obligation revisited. N Engl J Med 1995;122:377–378.
54. Lynch J. Regaining compassion. JAMA 1998;279:1422.
55. Miller FG, Fins JJ. A proposal to restructure hospital care for dying patients. N Engl J Med 1996;334:1740–1742.
56. Greig-Midlane H. The parents' perspective on withdrawing treatment. BMJ 2001;323:390.
57. Greisinger AJ, Lorimor RJ, Aday LA, Winn RJ, Baile WF. Terminally ill cancer patients: their most important concerns. Cancer Pract 1997;5:147–154.
58. Nitschke R, Humphrey GB, Sexauer CL, Catron B, Wunder S, Jay S. Therapeutic choices made by patients with end-stage cancer. J Pediatr 1982;101:471–476.
59. Vohra S, Camfield P, Camfield C. Assessing communication after the death of a child. Can J Paediatrics 1994;1:208–211.
60. Adams DW, Deveau EJ. Helping dying adolescents: needs and responses. In: Corr CA, McNeil JN, eds. Adolescence and Death. New York: Springer, 1986:76–96.
61. Solomon MZ. The enormity of the task: SUPPORT and changing practice. Hastings Cent Rep Special Supplement 1995;25: S28–S32.
62. The Society of Critical Care Medicine Ethics Committee. Attitudes of critical care medicine professionals concerning forgoing life-sustaining treatments. Crit Care Med 1992;20: 320–326.
63. Levi RB, Marsick R, Drotar D, Kodish ED. Diagnosis, disclosure, and informed consent: learning from parents of children with cancer. Int J Pediatr Hematol Oncol 2000;22:3–12.
64. Levinson W. Doctor-patient communication and medical malpractice: implications for pediatricians. Pediatr Ann 1997;26: 186–193.
65. Division of Mental Health, World Health Organization. Communicating Bad News. Geneva, Switzerland: Behavioural Science Learning Module, 1993.
66. Lo B. Caring for patients with life-threatening or terminal illness. In: Lipkin M, Putnam SM, Lazare A, eds. The Medical Interview: Clinical Care, Education and Research. New York: Springer, 1995:303–315.
67. Gazelle G. The slow code—should anyone rush to its defense? N Engl J Med 1998;338:467–469.
68. Billings JA, Block SD. Opportunity to present our observations and opinions on slow euthanasia (letter). J Palliat Care 1997;13: 55–56.
69. Hunt AM. A survey of signs, symptoms and symptom control in 30 terminally ill children. Dev Med Child Neurol 1990;32:341–346.
70. Attig T. Beyond suffering: the existential suffering of children. J Palliative Care 1996;12:20–23.
71. Truog R, Cist AFM, Brackett SE, et al. Recommendations for end-of-life care in the intensive care unit: the ethics committee of the Society for Critical Care Medicine. Crit Care Med 2001;29: 2332–2348.
72. Lynn J, Teno JM, Phillips RS, et al. Perceptions by family members of the dying experience of older and seriously ill patients. Ann Intern Med 1997;126:97–106.
73. The SUPPORT Principal Investigators. A controlled trial to improve care for seriously ill hospitalized patients: the study to understand prognoses and preferences for outcomes and risks of treatment (SUPPORT). JAMA 1995;274:1591–1598.
74. Wolfe J, Grier HE, Klan N, Levin SB, Ellenbogen JM, Salem-Schatz S, et al. Symptoms and suffering at the end of life in children with cancer. N Engl J Med 2000;342:326–333.
75. American Pain Society Quality of Care Committee. Quality improvement guidelines for the treatment of acute pain and cancer. JAMA 1995;274:1874–1880.
76. Carr DB, Jacox AK, Chapman CR, et al. Acute pain management: operative or medical procedures and trauma, clinical practice guideline. In: AHCPR Publication No. 92–0032. Rockville, MD: US Public Health Service, Agency for Health Care Policy and Research, 1992.
77. World Health Organization and International Association for the Study of Pain. Cancer Pain Relief and Palliative Care in Children. Geneva: 1998.
78. Bieri D, Reeve RA, Champion GD, et al. The faces pain scale for the self-assessment of pain experiences by children: development, initial validation and preliminary investigation for ratio scale properties. Pain 1990;41:139–150.
79. Beyer JE, Villarruel AM, Denyes M. The Oucher: Technical Report and User's Manual. Bethesda, MD: Association for the Care of Children's Health, 1995.
80. Eland JM. Minimizing pain associated with prekindergarten intramuscular injections. Issues Compr Pediatr Nurs 1981;5: 361–372.
81. Wong DL, Baker CM. Pain in children: comparison of assessment scales. Pediatr Nurs 1998;14:9–17.
82. McGrath PA. Pain in Children: Nature, Assessment and Treatment. New York: Guilford Publishing, 1998.

83. Stevens B, Johnston C, Petryshen P, Taddio A. Premature infant pain profile: development and initial validation. Clin J Pain 1996;12:13–22.
84. Breau LM, Finley GA, McGrath PJ, Camfield CS. Validation of the non-communicating Children's Pain Checklist—post-operative version. Anesthesiology 2002;96:528–535.
85. Voepel-Lewis T, Merkel S, Tait AR, Trzcinka A, Malviya S. The reliability and validity of the Face, Legs, Activity, Cry, Consolability observational tool as a measure of pain in children with cognitive impairment. Anesth Analg 2002;95(Nov): 1224–1229.
86. van Dijk M, de Boer JB, Koot HM, Tibboel D, Passchier J, Duivenvoorden HJ. The reliability and validity of the COMFORT scale as a postoperative pain instrument in 0- to 3-year-old infants. Pain 2000; 84(Feb):367–377.
87. Berde C, Sethna NF. Analgesics for the treatment of pain in children. N Engl J Med 2002;347:1094–1103.
88. Collins JJ. Intractable cancer pain in children. Child Adolesc Psych Clin N Am 1997;6:879–888.
89. de Stouz ND, Bruera E, Suarez-Almazor M. Opioid rotation for toxicity reduction in terminal cancer patients. J Pain Symptom Manage 1995;10:378–384.
90. Citron ML, Johnson-Early A, Fossieck BE Jr., Krasnow SM, Franklin R, Spangnolo SV, et al. Safety and efficacy of continuous morphine for severe cancer pain. Am J Med 1984;77:199–204.
91. Partridge JC, Wall SN. Analgesia for dying infants whose life support is withdrawn or withheld. Pediatrics 1997;99:76–79.
92. Kenny NP, Frager G. Refractory symptoms and terminal sedation of children: ethical and practical management. J Palliative Care 1996;12:40–45.
93. Wall PD, Melzack R, eds. The Textbook of Pain, 3rd ed. New York: Churchill Livingstone, 1994.
94. Schechter NL, Berde CB, Yaster M. Pain in infants, children and adolescents. Baltimore: Williams and Wilkins, 1993.
95. Allegaert K, Tibboel D, Naulaers G, Tison D, DeGonge A, Van Dijk M, et al. Systematic evaluation of pain in neonates: effect on the number of intravenous analgesics prescribed. Eur J Clin Pharmacol 2003;59:87–90.
96. Walco GA, Cassidy RC, Schechter NL. Pain, hurt and harm: the ethics of pediatric pain control. N Engl J Med 1994;331: 541–544.
97. Daly BJ, Thomas D, Dyer MA. Procedures used in withdrawal of mechanical ventilation. Am J Crit Care 1996;5:331–338.
98. Wilson WC, Smedira NG, Fink C, McDowell JA, Lua JM. Ordering and administration of sedatives and analgesics during the withholding and withdrawal of life support from critically ill patients. JAMA 1992;267:949–953.
99. Campi CW. When dying is as hard as birth. The New York Times, Jan. 5, 1998.
100. Bruera E, Macmillan K, Pither J, et al. Effects of morphine on the dyspnea of terminal cancer patients. J Pain Symptom Manage 1990;5:341–344.
101. Campbell ML. Managing terminal dyspnea: caring for the patient who refuses intubation or ventilation. Dimensions Crit Care Nurs 1996;15:4–11.
102. Cohen MH, Anderson AJ, Krasnow SH, Spagnolo SV, Citron ML, Payne M, et al. Continuous intravenous infusion of morphine for severe dyspnea. South Med J 1991;84:229–234.
103. Truog RD, Berde CB, Mitchell C, Grier HE. Barbiturates in the care of the terminally ill. N Engl J Med 1992;327:1678–1682.
104. Billings JA, Block SD. Slow euthanasia. J Palliative Care 1996; 2:21–30.
105. Quill TE, Lo B, Brock DW. Palliative care options of last resort: a comparison of voluntarily stopping eating and drinking, terminal sedation, PAS, and voluntary, active euthanasia. JAMA 1997;78:2099–2104.
106. Quill TE, Dresser R, Brock DW. The rule of double effect—a critique of its role in end-of-life decision making. N Engl J Med 1997;37:1768–1771.
107. Mount B. Morphine drips, terminal sedation and slow euthanasia: definitions and facts, not anecdotes. J Palliative Care 1996;2:31–37.
108. Roy DJ. On the ethics of euthanasia. J Palliative Care 1996;12:3–5.
109. Asch DA. The role of critical care nurses in euthanasia and assisted suicide. N Engl J Med 1996;334:1374–1379.
110. Rushton CH, Terry PB. Neuromuscular blockade and ventilator withdrawal: ethical controversies. Am J Crit Care 1995;4:112–115.
111. Keenan SP, Busche KD, Chen LM, McCarthy L, Inman DK, Sibbald WJ. A retrospective review of a large cohort of patients undergoing the process of withholding or withdrawal of life support. Crit Care Med 1997;25:1324–1331.
112. Liben S. Pediatric palliative medicine: obstacles to overcome. J Palliative Care 1996;2:24–28.
113. Smedira NG, Evans BH, Grais LS, Cohen NH, Lo B, Cooke M, et al. Withholding and withdrawal of life support from the critically ill. N Engl J Med 1990;322:309–315.
114. Stinson R, Stinson P. The Long Dying of Baby Andrew. Boston: Little, Brown, 1983.
115. Lantos JD, Tyson TE, Allen A, Frader J, Hack M, Korones S, et al. Withholding and withdrawing life-sustaining treatment in neonatal intensive care: Issues for the 1990's. Arch Dis Child 1994;71: F218–F223.
116. Luce JM. Withholding and withdrawal of life support: ethical, legal and clinical aspects. New Horiz 1997;5:30–37.
117. Solomon MZ, O'Donnell L, Jennings B, Guilfory V, Wolf SM, Nolan K, et al. Decisions near the end of life: professional views on life-sustaining treatment. Am J Public Health 1993; 83:14–23.
118. Hardart GE, Truog RD. Attitudes and preferences of intensivists regarding the role of family interests in medical decision-making for incompetent patients. Crit Care Med 2003;31:1895–1900.
119. Freyer DR. Children with cancer: special considerations in the discontinuation of life-sustaining treatment. Med Pediatr Oncol 1992;20:136–142.
120. Doyal L, Henning P. Stopping treatment for end-stage renal failure: the rights of children and adolescents. Pediatr Nephrol 1994; 8:768–791.
121. Committee on Bioethics, American Academy of Pediatrics. Informed consent, parental permission and assent in pediatric practice. Pediatrics 1995;95:314–317.
122. Committee on Bioethics, American Academy of Pediatrics. Guidelines on forgoing life-sustaining medical treatment. Pediatrics 1994;93:532–536.
123. President's Commission for the Study of Ethical Problems in Medicine and Biomedical and Behavioral Research. Deciding to Forgo Life-Sustaining Treatment: Ethical, Medical and Legal Issues in Treatment Decisions. Washington, DC: US Government Printing Office, 1983.
124. The Hastings Center. Guidelines on the Termination of Life-Sustaining Treatment and the Care of the Dying. Bloomington, IN: Indiana University Press, 1987.
125. Council on Ethical and Judicial Affairs, American Medical Association. Withholding or withdrawing life-prolonging medical treatment. In: Code of Medical Ethics, Current Opinions. Chicago: American Medical Association, 1992.

126. Dreyer DR. Care of the dying adolescent: special considerations. Pediatrics 2004;113:381–388
127. Asch DA, Hansen-Flaschen J, Lanken PN. Decisions to limit or continue life-sustaining treatment by critical care physicians in the United States: conflicts between physicians' practices and patients' wishes. Am J Respir Crit Care Med 1995;151: 288–292.
128. Nelson LJ. Forgoing treatment of critically ill newborns and the legal legacy of Baby Doe. Clin Ethics Rep 1992;6:1–6.
129. Traugott I, Alpers A. In their own hands: adolescents' refusals of medical treatment. Arch Pediatr Adolesc Med 1997;151: 922–927.
130. Battle CU. Beyond the nursery door: our obligation to the survivors of technology. Clin Perinatol 1987;14:417–427.
131. Luce JM. Making decisions about the forgoing of life-sustaining therapy. Am J Respir Crit Care Med 1997;156:1715–1718.
132. Randolph AG, Zollo MB, Wigton RS, Yeh TS. Factors explaining variability among caregivers in the intent to restrict life-support interventions in a pediatric intensive care unit. Crit Care Med 1997;25:435–439.
133. Alpert HR, Emanuel L. Comparing utilization of life-sustaining treatment with patient and public preferences. J Gen Intern Med 1998;13:175–181.
134. Christakis NA, Asch DA. Biases in how physicians choose to withdraw life support. Lancet 1993;342:642–646.
135. Nelson LJ, Rushton CH, Cranford RE, Nelson RM, Glover JJ, Truog RD. Forgoing medically provided nutrition and hydration in pediatric patients. J Law Med Ethics 1995;23:33–46.
136. Levetown M, Carter MA. Child-centred care in terminal illness: an ethical framework. In: Doyle D, Hanks GWC, MacDonald N, eds. Oxford Textbook of Palliative Medicine, 2nd ed. Oxford: Oxford University Press, 1998.
137. Horsburgh CR, Jr. Healing by design. N Engl J Med 1995;333: 735–740.
138. Levetown M. Different and needing to be more available. Hospice Magazine 1995;Winter:15–36.
139. Leikin S. The role of adolescents in decisions concerning their cancer therapy. Cancer 1993;71:3342–3346.
140. King NMP, Cross AW. Children as decision-makers: guidelines for pediatricians. J Pediatr 1989;115:10–16.
141. Leikin S. A proposal concerning decisions to forgo life-sustaining treatment for young people. J Pediatr 1989;115:17–22.
142. Grisso T, Vierling L. Minors' consent to treatment: a developmental perspective. Professional Psychology 1978;9:412–427.
143. Helsing KJ, Szklo M. Mortality after bereavement. Am J Epidemiol 1981;114:41–52.
144. Clayton PJ. Mortality and morbidity in the first year of widowhood. Arch Gen Psychiatry 1974;30:747–750.
145. Parkes CM, Brown RJ. Health after bereavement: a controlled study of young Boston widows and widowers. Psychosom Med 1972;34:449–461.
146. Li J, Precht DH, Mortensen PB, Olsen J. Mortality in parents after death of a child in Denmark: a nationwide follow-up study. Lancet 2003;361:363–367.
147. Meert KL, Thurston CS, Thomas R. Parental coping and bereavement outcome after the death of a child in the pediatric intensive care unit. Pediatr Crit Care Med 2001;2: 324–328.
148. Murphy SA, Johnson LC. Finding meaning in a child's violent death: a five-year prospective analysis of parents' personal narratives and empirical data. Death Stud 2003;27:381–404.
149. Tolle SW, Bascom PB, Hickam DH, et al. Communication between physicians and surviving spouses following patient deaths. J Gen Intern Med 1986;1:309–314.
150. Irvine P. The attending at the funeral. N Engl J Med 1985;312: 1704–1705.
151. McHaffie HE, Laing IA, Lloyd DJ. Follow up care of bereaved parents after treatment withdrawal from newborns. Arch Dis Child Fetal Neonatal Ed 2001; 84:F125–F128.
152. Rankin J, Wright C, Lind T. Cross-sectional survey of parents' experience and views of the postmortem examination. BMJ 2002;324:816–818.
153. Oliver RC, Sturtevant JP, Scheetz JP, Fallat ME. Beneficial effects of a hospital bereavement intervention program after traumatic childhood death. J Trauma 2001;50:440–446.
154. Anonymous. 16th century aphorism, quoted from MacDonald N. The interface between oncology and palliative medicine. In: Oxford Textbook of Palliative Medicine, 2nd ed. Oxford: Oxford University Press, 1998: Section 2.1, 11.
155. Goldschmidt RH, Hess PA. Telling the patient the diagnosis is cancer: a teaching module. Fam Med 1987;19:302–304.
156. Wolraich M, Albanese M, Reiter-Thayer S, Barratt W. Teaching pediatric residents to provide emotion-laden information. J Med Educ 1981;56:438–440.
157. Gordon GH, Tolle SW. Discussing life-sustaining treatment: a teaching program for residents. Arch Intern Med 1991;151: 567–570.
158. Bagatell R, Meyer R, Herron S, Berger A, Villar R. When children die: a seminar series for pediatric residents. Pediatrics 2002;110 (2 Pt 1):348–353.
159. McConnell Y, Frager G, Levetown M. Decision-making in pediatric palliative care. In: Carter B, Levetown M. Palliative Care for Infants, Children and Adolescents: A Practical Handbook. Baltimore: Johns Hopkins University Press, 2004: Ch. 4.

52

Pamela S. Hinds, Linda Oakes, and Wayne L. Furman

End-of-Life Decision-Making in Pediatric Oncology

I watched the monitors for his blood pressure and his pulse. It was taking more medicines to keep those stable. Every day I would look at those numbers and I recognized it was getting harder and harder. His heart was not really pumping on its own. It was really just those medicines. I said, "This is too hard on his body and I don't think we should continue." The doctor said to me, "You are making the right decision." I said to myself, "God gave me my kid to watch over. I am here to see that nothing happens to him that is bad. I am here to watch over his best interests, and I am not going to make him fight through this just because of my selfishness."—Father who had decided to withdraw life support on behalf of his 17-year-old son dying of leukemia

- ***Key Points***
- *Decision-making for parents facing the terminal illness of a child is, in many cases, extraordinarily difficult.*
- *Personal and professional caregivers can influence the extent to which patients and parents participate in end-of-life decision-making.*
- *Children and adolescents may need assistance making decisions based on their cognitive development, and each patient should be assessed as an individual to determine his or her competence.*
- *Preferences for treatment should be balanced between the child or adolescent patient and the caregiver or surrogate.*
- *Nurses have a professional responsibility to facilitate informed patient decisions at the end of life.*

Deciding to end a child's life, and involving a child in the decision to end his or her life, are startling phrases, but we in pediatric oncology participate in those considerations with parents, patients, and other members of the health care team as a part of providing the highest-quality care for the child or adolescent with incurable cancer. Participating in end-of-life decisions is life altering for the child or adolescent and for the family, but it can also be life altering for the health care provider. Clinical anecdotes suggest that the way in which patients, family members, and health care providers complete end-of-life decision-making can color all of their preceding treatment-related interactions, and may influence how well parents emotionally survive the dying and death of their child. The manner in which end-of-life decision-making processes are completed may also contribute to the survival of health care providers as compassionate and fully competent professionals.

Despite the significant immediate and longer-term impact of participating in end-of-life decision-making for a child or adolescent with incurable cancer, guidelines for making or for facilitating such decisions have only recently become available.[1] Preparation for participating in end-of-life decision-making is rarely a formal part of a health care provider's education and is rarely addressed in preceptoring or mentoring relationships. There is clearly a great need for information that can be used to further develop, test, and refine such guidelines. The purposes of this chapter are (1) to offer a review of the current literature (both clinical and research-based) on end-of-life decision-making in pediatrics, with a special emphasis on pediatric oncology, and (2) to offer guidelines for the use of health care professionals in assisting children, adolescents, their parents, and other health care professionals in making such decisions. Table 52–1 defines key terms used in this chapter.

Table 52–1
Key Terms Used in This Chapter

Decision—The final choice between two or more treatment-related options

Phase I study—The initial stage of human testing of a drug, in which the maximum tolerated dose is established; in oncology, the subjects are usually patients who have refractory disease

Do not resuscitate—An order written in the medical record directing that no cardiopulmonary resuscitation is to be performed in the case of an acute event such as cardiac, respiratory, or neurological decompensation

Withdrawal of life-support—Stopping a life-sustaining medical treatment such as mechanical ventilator therapy, pharmacological support of blood pressure, or dialysis, and vasoactive infusions

Life-sustaining medical treatment—Interventions that may not control the patient's disease but may prolong the patient's life; these may include not only ventilator support, dialysis, and vasoactive infusions, but also antibiotics, insulin, chemotherapy, and nutrition and hydration provided by tubes and IV lines

Supportive care—Comfort measures that exclude curative efforts but could include symptom management (such as pain relief and hydration) or symptom prevention (such as limited blood product support)

Background

Advances in pediatric oncology have significantly increased the survival rates of patients during the past decade. The disease once thought to be universally fatal for children and adolescents is now viewed as a life-threatening, chronic illness that is potentially curable for many.[2–4] However, cancer remains the leading disease-related cause of death in children and adolescents, as ultimately 25% to 33% will die of their disease.[5–8] Indeed, approximately 2200 children and adolescents die of cancer in the United States on an annual basis.[7,9] With treatment advances come more treatment options and more treatment-related decisions for patients, their parents, and their health care providers.[10] Although certain decisions, such as whether to have a permanent venous access device implanted and which type to use, are made early in treatment, parents and health care providers report that the most challenging decision-making in pediatric oncology occurs when efforts to cure the cancer have failed.[11] A few parents report that end-of-life decision-making was not complicated for them because they had already decided what they would do if their child's cancer did not respond to treatment. However, the majority of parents and health care providers involved in the decision process describe this time as extraordinarily difficult. They attribute the difficulty to multiple and complex factors that must be considered, including the differing preferences of those involved in the actual decision-making or affected by it, and to intense emotions at a time when the parents' energy is depleted.

Neonatal and Other Pediatric Specialties

End-of-life decision-making in pediatric oncology has been influenced by clinical and research reports from neonatal and other pediatric specialties and organizations. The growing commitment by professional associations to include pediatric patients and parents in end-of-life decisions marks a notable shift in care philosophy. Expectations that patients and their parents should be involved in these decisions have been formalized in policy statements of organizations such as the American Academy of Pediatrics,[12] the American Nurses Association,[13] the American Association of Critical Care Nurses,[14] the United Hospital Fund in its report on end-of-life care in New York,[15] the International Society of Pediatric Oncology (SIOP),[16] and most recently from the Institute of Medicine.[9] In these published statements, the recommended patient and parental involvement is described as participative and mutual with health care providers. Legislative rulings and legal decisions in some states and Canadian provinces support the participation of adolescents or mature minors in medical decision-making and in creating advance directives.[17–21] It is likely that in the next decade, regulatory bodies such as the JCAHO will become involved in directing or evaluating end-of-life care,[22] including patient and parental involvement in end-of-life decision-making. It is also likely that such involvement will be considered an indicator of the quality of end-of-life care and be linked to reimbursement for such care as is now being proposed for adult cancer patients.[23]

The actual extent to which patients and parents participate in end-of-life decision-making varies and can be influenced by the personal and professional preferences of the health care provider.[24,25] For example, the way the health care provider frames or words information about treatment options may influence the way a patient and family perceive the available alternatives.[26,27] Some advocate that the physician should assume the final responsibility for the decision,[28–30] whereas others believe that the parents should be the primary decision-makers.[31–33] Yet another view, which is not espoused by many authors, is that the adolescent patient should be the primary decision-maker, with his or her parents serving as consultants.[34] Even fewer sources advocate that children should be the primary decision-makers, but several advocate that children as young as 6[35,36] or 7[17] should be involved in the decision-making.

The available reports on end-of-life decision-making that involves parents and health care providers are predominantly from neonatal settings. End-of-life decisions in these settings often reflect the presenting condition of the infant. The decisions primarily considered include (1) limiting care, (2) withdrawing life-support, or (3) withholding life-support for infants who are extremely premature or have severe congenital abnormalities.[37–42] Most reports describe the decision-making as having been initiated when the intensivist determined that the infant had no chance for survival or no chance for quality of life. In most cases, parents agreed with the recommendations of the intensivist or the infant's attending physician. These descriptive reports are based on review of medical records. No information was obtained from parents about the factors they considered when making an end-of-life decision on behalf of their infant.

Two notable exceptions exist. In the first, Able-Boon and colleagues[43] interviewed parents and health care providers of seriously ill infants regarding medical decision-making and the provision of health care information. The parents emphasized their need and desire to be honestly informed of their child's health status. They expressed special appreciation of health care professionals who drew pictures to convey technical information rather than relying only on words. Parents also expressed a strong need for information that is coordinated by the health care team so that it is not confusing or contradictory.

The second study that recorded the values of parents in end-of-life decisions is the grounded-theory study in which Rushton[44] interviewed 31 parents of 20 hospitalized neonates with life-threatening congenital disorders about their decisions for or against implementing or continuing life-sustaining measures for their infants. Rushton concluded that the parents made these decisions based on their understanding of what it means to be a "good parent" for a neonate with a life-threatening congenital disorder. According to these parents, the characteristics of good parents for such neonates include putting the needs of the neonate first, not giving up, not taking the "easy" way out despite the self-sacrifice involved, and courage to pursue a "good" outcome for the child.

Reviews of the medical records of patients who have died in pediatric intensive care units (PICUs) show that withdrawal of life-support was chosen in 8% to 54% of cases,[45–48] and that limitation of supportive care (described as not escalating care efforts but providing hydration and pain comfort measures) was chosen in 26% to 46% of cases.[45,47] The wide range of these percentages may reflect cultural, ethnic, or religious differences: the lowest rate of withdrawal of life-support reported was from a PICU in Malaysia and the highest rates were from PICUs in Europe, the United States, and the United Kingdom. Even within a single PICU setting, decision-making can reflect cultural differences. For example, the report from the Malaysian setting noted that Muslim parents declined end-of-life options at significantly higher rates than did non-Muslim parents.[45] Reports may also reflect the research method used. For example, Meyer and colleagues[49] relied upon surveys completed by parents to assess parental perceptions of pain control, decision-making, and social supports during their child's dying in a PICU. Parents reported that in most cases ($n = 56$; 90%), the physician initiated the end-of-life discussion but in approximately half of those cases, parents had been privately considering an end-of-life decision. Factors identified by parents as influencing their decision-making included concerns about their child's quality of life, their child's chance of getting better, their child's pain or discomfort, advice of hospital staff, attitudes of hospital staff, and advice of friends or family members. Several medical record reviews of end-of-life characteristics of children dying of cancer have been recently completed. In general, the majority of these children and adolescents die of progressive disease with a medical order not to resuscitate (DNR). These characteristics indicate the child's likely death had been discussed with parents or family members. However, despite parental involvement in decision-making, the factors that influenced the decision-making and how the end-of-life discussions were initiated or facilitated were not included in the published reports.

Participation of Children and Adolescents

Children and adolescents have not routinely been involved in making end-of-life decisions on their own behalf, largely because of doubt on the part of parents and health care providers that the child or adolescent has sufficient understanding of the clinical situation.[50–53] This doubt is based in part on adults' belief that children and adolescents are unable to appraise their well-being and are unaware of their life goals and values.[31] Buchanan and Brock[50] described children who are 9 years or older as competent to make certain decisions, but they did not study children's competence in end-of-life decision-making. The same authors also indicated that children of that age may be competent to make some decisions but not others, and that competence thus depends on the specific decision. According to Ariff and Groh,[54] a child's competence to make medical decisions is an ongoing developmental process that parallels other cognitive, moral, and emotional processes and is influenced by environment and by physical and mental illness. The capacity to make an end-of-life decision cannot be determined, then, on the basis of the child's or adolescent's competence in a different situation or decision. Instead, competence must be determined for each specific decision at a defined time point and under specific circumstances.[17] Recent cognitive studies on adolescent decision-making indicate that although adolescents are able to make decisions, they may be unaware of all possible options or may be unable to identify all possible consequences of those options.[55] Therefore, adolescents may need assistance in identifying, considering, and selecting end-of-life options.

Experiencing a life-threatening illness such as cancer and seeing others suffer and die from it may help a child to understand death and his or her own end-of-life circumstances.[21,56,57] Although they acknowledged that the competence to participate in decision-making differs with age and cognitive abilities, Burns and Truog[58] recommended that children and adolescents be involved early in the process of medical decision-making, including end-of-life decisions. In fact, Burns and Truog warned that if a child or adolescent is not involved early in the decision-making process, his or her ability to express an opinion may be lost before it can be exercised. Leikin[59] theorized that adolescents who have been treated for cancer have a clearer idea of the burdens and benefits of treatment options that are most acceptable to them. The ethical perspective is that adolescents have a conception of what is good for themselves. The treatment experience itself contributes to the adolescents' abilities to participate in end-of-life decision-making.

Our combined clinical and research experiences have convinced us that, as a general rule, seriously ill patients aged 10 years and older are able to understand that they are participating in decisions about their cancer-related treatment and their lives, and are able to understand the options and the likely outcomes. Of course, some younger patients may also understand these issues and be competent to participate in end-of-life decisions, whereas some older patients may be less competent. Because of these very possible differences in understanding, each child needs to be individually assessed for his or her competence to participate. An assumption that a child is or is not competent to participate made without the assessment is not in the child's best interest.

Others have provided compelling support for the involvement of younger children in end-of-life decision-making. Nitschke and colleagues[35,36] reported that patients as young as 6 years of age participated in end-of-life discussions in their pediatric oncology treatment setting. They described care conferences held with 43 families over a 6-year period in which children and adolescents with end-stage cancer, and their families, participated in discussions of therapeutic options, disease progression, lack of effective therapies, improbability of cure, and imminent death. The patients (who were 6 to 20 years of age) and their parents were offered the choice of Phase II investigational drugs or supportive care. According to this report, it was the patients who most frequently made the final decision. Fourteen chose further chemotherapy, 28 chose supportive care only, and 1 made no decision. Nitschke and colleagues also noted that patients younger than age 9 understood that they were going to die soon of their disease. The authors concluded that children with cancer do have an advanced understanding of death and recommended that children as young as 5 years of age have the capacity to make decisions about whether to continue therapy. This team did not investigate the specific factors considered by the patients, parents, and health care providers and did not describe ways in which providers may have attempted to facilitate patient and parent decision-making.

A health care team member who has established a relationship of trust with the child or adolescent and who has observed the child or adolescent in various challenging clinical situations is likely to be the best judge of competence in end-of-life decision-making. However, before initiating this assessment, the health care team should discuss the purpose and process of the assessment, first as a group and then with the patient's parent or parents, and identify any areas of actual or potential disagreement between the team and the parents. Disagreements should be openly discussed, and participants should be allowed sufficient time to weigh the issues—another reason for initiating the end-of-life discussions in a timely manner. After the team and the parents agree on the intent and timing of the competence assessment, the team member, parent(s), and child or adolescent choose the location for the discussion. Most children younger than 11 years of age prefer to have their parents present for this discussion.

Determining the child or adolescent's competence requires establishing whether he or she understands the seriousness of the medical condition and understands that a decision point is at hand. If asked to explain the seriousness of the situation, the child or adolescent will use words or describe events that have personal, symbolic, or literal meaning. The health care team can then use these same words to communicate with the patient about decision-making. Throughout the assessment, the child or adolescent will need reassurance from the health care team member that the serious situation is not the fault of the child or adolescent.[60] The child or adolescent must also be able to indicate an understanding of the choices, including the potential consequences of each. In addition, the child or adolescent must show an understanding of how each choice made now could change future options. As McCabe and colleagues[20] emphasized, the health care team member conducting the assessment must ensure that the child or adolescent does not feel coerced to make a certain choice. The team member should also ensure that the child or adolescent has access to the information needed to make a competent decision.[61] The team member needs to allow repeated opportunities for the child or adolescent to review the options and discuss concerns and to do so in a manner that is not rushed, and to provide different mechanisms (verbal, written, drawing) to facilitate expression of concerns or preferences.[62] It is especially important that the team member assess to what extent the child or adolescent wants to be included in the decision-making. That preference should be honored regardless of the personal preferences of team members.

Our experience is that children (some as young as 7 years of age) have definite preferences regarding whether to participate in a Phase I clinical trial. Preferences most commonly reflect a desire to be home, to play with a sibling or a friend, or to not feel sickly. Preferences regarding DNR status, although quite firmly expressed by some adolescents, tend to require more patient contemplation time. By the time this type of end-of-life decision-making needs to be considered, the members of the health care team are very familiar with the child and the family and already have established a style of interacting. However, it is generally useful to preface the assessment of patient preference with a statement that conveys the important nature of what is about to be said, such as, "May I ask you to be quite serious with me for a few moments? I want to tell you something important about your [insert here the term used by the child when referring to the illness]. And I want you to tell me something, too." If the child conveys an inability to be serious at that moment, the team member needs to clarify whether that means the child only wants the "serious and important" topics to be discussed with the child's family, or if it means the child wants to try to be serious at a later time. Clinicians are encouraged to allow repeated opportunities for the child or adolescent to review the care options or concerns, to provide a variety of mechanisms to facilitate the child's expressions (such as using words, drawing or writing), and to do so in a manner that is not rushed.

Competence of Surrogates

Concern about patients' competence to participate in end-of-life decisions, although valid, may sometimes be exaggerated. As Levetown and Carter[61] wrote, it is relatively easy to usurp the autonomy of children and adolescents in end-of-life decision-making. This threat lends special importance to the use of guidelines for making end-of-life decisions. Guidelines could serve as formal reminders to health care professionals to consider the preferences of children and adolescents to the extent that is possible or advisable. Of equal or greater concern is the competence of parents and health care providers to make such decisions on behalf of the child or adolescent. Making these decisions competently requires an understanding of their own values, the patient's values and goals, the treatment options, the likely outcome of each option, and the nature of the life-threatening illness. This imposes a short-term and a longer-term burden of unknown proportions on the parents and the health care providers.

There are few empirically based or theoretically based guidelines for involving children, adolescents, or their parents in end-of-life decisions. Instead, it is generally assumed that children younger than age 10 years are not competent to participate in such decision-making and that their parents are both competent and attentive to the best interests of their child.[20,31,58] This assumption is crucial, because it tends to ensure that end-of-life decisions are made for seriously ill children and adolescents by their parents and health care professionals. Legal rulings and common health care practices support the role of parents as surrogates in this circumstance; it is rarely challenged, and health care providers or others replace parental authority only in exceptional circumstances.[58] To feel competent, to be competent, and to be satisfied with their performance as surrogate decision-makers, parents and health care providers need opportunities to exchange information about the child's preferences, the family's preferences, the child's chances of survival, the progression of the disease, and the intensity and intrusiveness of life-extending interventions and the likelihood of their effectiveness (including length of time gained). They also need to reflect on previous efforts to achieve cure and to question previous decisions. Competence of surrogates may also be affected by their realization of the likelihood of their child not surviving cancer. In one retrospective, descriptive study that included parent interviews and review of medical records, it was identified that physicians knew up to a year before the parents that the child would not survive.[63] Participating in end-of-life care planning is unlikely if the reality of the child's death is not yet in the parents' or surrogates' awareness. Competence of surrogate participation is also influenced by the challenges faced by health care providers when trying to accurately predict timing of the dying.[64] However, only in a limited number of cases is the child's dying unexpected. Because of that, some degree of planning for preferred model of end-of-life care (home, home with hospice, hospital, hospital with hospice) is possible.[65,66] Matching the surrogates' preferences for end-of-life care might contribute to decreasing the morbidity of bereaved survivors.

Participation of Patients and Parents

Previous studies indicate that the more informed parents become about their seriously ill child's condition, the more they are able to participate in making decisions and advocating for their child.[67,68] Parents report that information is most helpful when it is provided gradually and repeatedly.[69] Stevens[70] recommends that parents be allowed to make tape recordings or bring friends or family members to the treatment-related discussions to help them later recall the details of the discussion. Other investigators suggest that parents differ in how much detailed information they desire[71] and in how much they want to participate in the actual decision-making[72,73] during periods of crisis in their child's illness. However, parental preferences about participation in end-of-life decision-making have not been well studied.

In an international feasibility study, parents from pediatric oncology settings in Australia, Hong Kong, and the United States were interviewed about their decision-making on behalf of their ill child. There were clear differences among the countries in parental preference for involvement in decision-making. Mothers in Hong Kong were reluctant to participate in end-of-life decisions because of either their gender ("Women cannot make these decisions.") or their lack of expert knowledge ("I am only the mother. The doctor is the expert and he should decide.").[74] It remains unknown whether these parental preferences change between diagnosis and end of life. Regardless of their preference, all parents need reassurance from the health care team that their child's condition is not their fault.[70]

The factors that parents consider at decision points in the treatment of their seriously ill child have only recently been studied. Using a phenomenological approach, Kirschbaum[75] interviewed 20 parents of children who had died in the previous 6 to 12 months. The parents had all made life-support decisions on behalf of their ill child. A variety of diagnoses were represented, including trauma, cancer, septic shock, liver failure, and congestive heart disease. Nine factors were identified as having influenced the parental decisions: (1) wanting life as the principal good for their child, (2) avoiding suffering and pain, (3) considering current and future quality of life, (4) respecting the individuality of the child, (5) defining and redefining the family, (6) having spiritual beliefs and explanations, (7) believing in natural or biological explanations, (8) considering the child's unique personality, and (9) having a favorable view of technology in health care.

In a retrospective study that conducted telephone interviews with 39 parents of 37 pediatric oncology patients who had died in the previous 6 to 24 months, Hinds and colleagues[11] were able to identify the factors most frequently considered by parents in end-of-life decision-making. The end-of-life decisions that were reported most frequently by these parents were choosing between a Phase I drug study and no further treatment (n=14), maintaining or withdrawing life support (n=11), and giving more chemotherapy or ending treatment (n=8). The factor most considered in the parents' decision-making was "information received from health care professionals." This information included facts, explanations, and opinions about their child's disease status, likelihood of survival, and complexities of continued care. Other factors parents frequently reported were "feeling supported by and trusting of the staff," which reflected the parents' sense that the health care team listened and responded to their or their child's concerns and respected the parents' decisions, and "making decisions together with my child." This factor reflected the parents' comfort in having known and respected their child's wishes.

The parents also completed a 15-item questionnaire about the importance of each factor considered in their decision-making.

Table 52–2
Guidelines for the Health Care Team to Use in Assisting Parents with End-of-Life Decision Making

1. At the time of diagnosis and throughout treatment, actively seek opportunities to provide information to the parent about treatment and the patient's response to treatment.
2. At the time of diagnosis and throughout treatment, involve the parent in treatment-related discussions and decision-making. Be available to discuss and rediscuss decisions and related concerns.
3. Encourage parents to talk with parents of other pediatric oncology patients.
4. Verbally and nonverbally reassure the parents that they are "good" parents who are committed to the well-being of their child.
5. Give assurances that everything that can be done to help the patient is being done and being done well.
6. As the child's disease progresses, provide clear verbal (and written, if desired by the parent) explanations of the child's status.
7. Inform parents of treatment options as they become available in the treating institution or elsewhere.
8. Include more than one health care team member in end-of-life discussions with the parents.
9. When discussing end-of-life options with parents,
   a. Strongly emphasize the team's commitment to the patient's comfort and to providing expert care at all times.
   b. Offer professional recommendations.
   c. Describe how their child is likely to respond to each option (the child's physical appearance, ability to communicate, etc.).
   d. Give information about other support resources (ethics committees, social services, other health care professionals, etc.).
10. When discussing end-of-life options with parents, anticipate
    a. Parents' vacillation between certainty and uncertainty about the decision.
    b. Parents' need for clarification and additional information to resolve their uncertainties.
    c. Parent's need for practical information about ways to explain the end-of-life decision to other family members.
    d. Being asked to give personal advice.
11. Allow parents private time to consider the options.
12. Maintain sensitivity to any specific ethnic, cultural, or religious preferences during the terminal stage.
13. Convey respect for the parents' right to change decisions, when clinically feasible.
14. Demonstrate commitment to maintaining the child's comfort and dignity, and to affirming the parents' role.
15. Do not question the parents' decision after it has been made.

The parents rated eight items as "very important" at least 50% of the time. The highest rated factors included "recommendations received from health care professionals," "things my child had said about continuing or not continuing treatment," "information received from health care professionals," "my child's breathing problems," and "sensing that my child was no longer himself [herself]." These findings clearly indicate that information and recommendations received from health care professionals are very important to parents who are making end-of-life decisions on behalf of their child, as is feeling certain of their child's desires about treatment.

The same research team has prospectively studied end-of-life decision-making by conducting interviews of parents, physicians, and, when possible, the children or adolescents with incurable disease who had participated in making an end-of-life decision within the past week. The same factors noted in the retrospective study—related to trust, support, information, and advice—were also identified in the prospective study. In addition, parents cited these factors: wishing for the child's survival, reassuring themselves of the correctness of their decisions, questioning certain statements or behaviors of health care professionals, and making decisions that would allow them to maintain communication with their dying child for as long as possible (Table 52–2).

CASE STUDY

A Decision Agreement Between Parents and the Health Care Team

A 12-month-old infant girl has been treated for an aggressive form of leukemia. It is clear that the disease is not responding to chemotherapy. The patient was transferred to the PICU when she began to experience respiratory distress. Initially, oxygen was administered by simple mask, but her breathing difficulties persisted and became more evident within a few hours. The possibility of endotracheal intubation was first discussed among the health care team members and then with the parents. During the meeting with the parents, the current symptoms of the little girl were discussed, the current disease status and its unresponsiveness to treatment were reviewed, and options of intubating or not intubating were considered. The parents then discussed the options privately with each other and in less than 30 minutes reached the decision that ventilatory support not be a part of their daughter's medical care. The parents said that knowing that their daughter was not going to be cured of the leukemia and understanding that the ventilator would help reduce their daughter's respiratory distress but not the leukemia were both factors that assisted them in making the decision. They credited their discussions with the doctors as key: "From the discussion we had with the doctors, we felt if it came to that point, the only reason for using a ventilator would be just to keep her breathing." An additional factor identified by the parents as influencing their decision-making was support from the health care team. "Chaplain X and Dr. Y were real patient with us and understood the situation that we were in and did not seem to put pressure one way or another, or seem to think that we were making the wrong decision one way or another . . . they told us the decision was actually ours. They let us know that, but they were supportive and also gave us their opinions."

CASE STUDY

Disagreement

An adolescent with incurable cancer had been hospitalized for 3 weeks, the past 8 days in the ICU. His physical deterioration and suffering had created anguish in his father and in the health care team. The attending physician discussed with the father the likelihood of the adolescent having a cardiac arrest, described the actions the team would take for a full resuscitation, as well as the varying levels of resuscitation approved by the treatment setting, which included a DNR option, and asked the father to express his preferences regarding resuscitation. The father initially chose the DNR status for his son and completed all of the official paperwork to implement that decision. During the next 12 hours, the father actively solicited from nursing and medical staff their definitions of DNR. He then contacted the attending physician to rescind his decision, choosing instead to have a full resuscitation order in place. He explained his decision change as, "When I saw that the nurses and doctors did not all define resuscitation in the same way, I decided that I would not leave that in their hands. I am my son's father and I will be his father to the end." This new decision was enacted and over the next 4 days, the young patient showed clear signs of dying. His father stayed with him in the ICU and witnessed the changes in his son's physical appearance. He began commenting on those changes and on his son's obvious suffering. Two hours before his son's death, the father told the nurse that he did not want his son to be resuscitated. This information was immediately conveyed to the health care team and a brief discussion with the physician, father, and nurse was convened to affirm this decision.

CASE STUDY

Reluctant Agreement Between Adolescent, Parents, and Health Care Team

A 15-year-old male adolescent and former star pitcher for his high school baseball team had been aggressively treated for Ewing's sarcoma for 13 months. The primary site was his upper right arm, his pitching arm. A limb-sparing procedure had been successfully completed but his disease had recurred and rapidly progressed. His pain was exceedingly difficult to manage and he openly spoke of his readiness to die. His mother continued to press for treatment options. They were advised of an open Phase I trial and were made aware of the experimental agent in the trial, and the toxicity-finding purpose of the trial, but were also advised by the treating team to consider only symptom management care efforts. The mother strongly urged her son to enroll in the Phase I trial. In a private meeting with one of his nurses, the adolescent confided that his personal preference was to go home to die but that he had not told his mother about that because he knew she was not ready yet for his death. The nurse asked for his permission to advocate on his behalf with his mother, but he thoughtfully declined, stating that enrolling in the trial was his final gift to his mother, a gift that he wanted very much to give her. With personal regret, the nurse accepted his choice without discussion with his mother and the adolescent enrolled in the trial and completed three courses before his disease progressed. Although he continued to experience pain during those three courses, he remained certain of the importance of his decision because of its benefit for his mother.

Twenty patients participated in individual interviews about the end-of-life decision they had made. The factors most frequently considered in their decisions included "being influenced by relationships with others," "information from my doctor or my parents," "wanting to be done with treatment," and "worrying about my family." These factors convey the interconnectedness between children or adolescents with incurable diseases and their families and health care providers. All are affected by the decision-making process and the outcomes of the decision. This interconnectedness among the seriously ill child or adolescent, the family, and the health care providers contributes to more agreements on end-of-life decisions than disagreements. Although rare, disagreements between the patient and parent, or between parents and health care providers, do occur and are especially difficult for all involved. Disagreeing with a health care professional who is deemed essential for their child's well-being and with whom a care alliance is desired is at best troubling for parents, but at worst, disruptive to relationships and problem solving. When circumstances exist that allow a delay in the contested decision-making, a consultation with an ethicist or ethics board can facilitate decision-making. Involving the family, the patient who is deemed competent to participate in end-of-life decision-making, and the health care team in the same meeting with the ethicist or ethics board is particularly helpful, as all perspectives can be considered. When a family and a health care team do not have agreement, special measures must be initiated by the team leaders to support team members in their efforts to continue to deliver excellent care to the patient and family. Measures can include brief meetings with an esteemed institutional leader who openly acknowledges the sizable difficulty that the team is facing, having information-sharing or cathartic sessions with the ethicist, and developing strategies for handling similar future difficulties. Likewise, similar support measures need to be implemented for the family. In addition, regular opportunities to interact with the health care team (such as care conferences) need to be established so that trust between the family and team can be fostered.

CASE STUDY

Involving an Ethicist to Assist a Team in Anticipation of, During, or After an End-of-Life Decision

A 7-year-old boy had a second recurrence of acute lymphoblastic leukemia. His leukemia was first diagnosed when he was 19 months old. The first recurrence occurred less than a year after completing the 3-year treatment protocol, and the second recurrence occurred 8 months after completing the treatment for relapsed leukemia. As his mother pointed out to the treating team, her son had had very few months in his life of feeling healthy. She conveyed reluctance to continue any curative efforts, preferring instead to have her son discharged from the inpatient unit so that she could take him home. The attending physician, an internationally recognized expert in the treatment of leukemia, strongly disagreed with the mother's stated preference and offered her information on the likelihood of cure (admittedly low) and emphasized his desire to continue curative efforts. When the mother firmly declined the option of further treatment, the physician told the mother that he considered the discharge to be "against medical orders" and noted that in the medical record. A nurse on the team later approached the physician and proposed a meeting with the team and an ethicist to discuss the decision. The physician agreed and the full team met a week later with an ethicist. The physician honestly acknowledged his sadness about the child's incurable disease, his liking of the child, and his concern that because the mother disagreed with his recommendation of further treatment, the health care team might think less of him as a physician. The team and the ethicist reacted with surprise at the last admission and conveyed instead their strong respect for him and his efforts to be a good doctor and for the mother's efforts to be a good parent. The physician offered to write a letter to the mother expressing the team's support of her and her child and that the child would always have complete access to all of the care setting's resources. The mother telephoned the physician after receiving the letter to express her relief. Three weeks later, the mother brought her son to the hospital to die.

Factors Considered by Health Care Providers

The factors considered by health care professionals in end-of-life decision-making on behalf of children and adolescents reveal important similarities and differences between nurses and physicians. Current reports indicate that nurses are more likely to reflect on the moral balance of the decision, that is, the goodness or lack thereof of extending a child's life if doing so also extends or increases the child's suffering,[76] whereas physicians first consider whether the child's life can be saved.[11] This difference can create tension within the health care team and merits discussion by the team members. Nurses and physicians also identified a factor they both consider frequently in end-of-life decision-making for pediatric oncology patients: "respecting the patient's and family's preferences." This factor reflected the health care professionals' efforts to inform the patient and family of all options and then to respect the choice they made. In a survey completed by 21 health care professionals in pediatric oncology (16 physicians, 3 nurses, and 2 chaplains) regarding end-of-life decisions for patients with incurable cancer, the factors rated as most important included "discussions with the family of the patient," "thinking the patient would never get any better," "the belief that nothing else could help the patient," and "things the patient had said about continuing or not continuing treatment." Most of the participating health care professionals also indicated that they did not make end-of-life decisions alone but sought the input of other team members.[11]

Strategies for Facilitating Child, Adolescent, and Parent Involvement

End-of-life decision-making is a process that very likely begins at the time of diagnosis, when the patient and the parents are exposed to the seriousness of the illness, the possible risks of treatment, and the uncertainty of short-term and long-term treatment outcomes. When faced with the actual decision-making, a few parents and patients express a preference seemingly without hesitation or anguish. They are likely to have gained an earlier understanding of the situation; often, patients and parents who observe others undergoing end-of-life experiences begin to reflect on their own life values. More often, however, patients and parents require time to think after becoming aware of the impending decision point and treatment options.[29] In both the briefer and longer contemplation periods, the decision-making capability evolves as treatment continues and understanding of the patient's situation increases. As noted in the American Academy of Pediatrics guidelines on forgoing life-sustaining treatment,[77] end-of-life decision-making is not a single event or one well-defined point in time.

It is essential that health care providers realize that the end-of-life decision-making process begins early in treatment and evolves with each interaction between the provider, the patient, and the parent, and with each observation of or encounter with other seriously ill patients and their parents (Figure 52–1). Each interaction provides an opportunity for the health care provider to build the patient's and family's trust in him or her as a source of information and support and as a care expert who can be relied on to do what is best for the patient.[11] Each interaction is also an opportunity for the provider to facilitate parents' efforts to function fully as parents—a role that becomes increasingly uncertain as parents deal with unfamiliar decisions. Feeling competent in their parenthood is especially crucial to parents who face end-of-life decisions on behalf of their child. Believing that they have acted as "good parents" in such a situation is likely to be very important to their emotional recovery from the dying and death of their child.

Decision-making by patients and parents is influenced not only by their interactions with the health care team but also by the impressions they form through observations of and encounters with other patients and families in the care setting. As patients and parents learn about the treatment experiences and the positive or negative outcomes of other patients, they

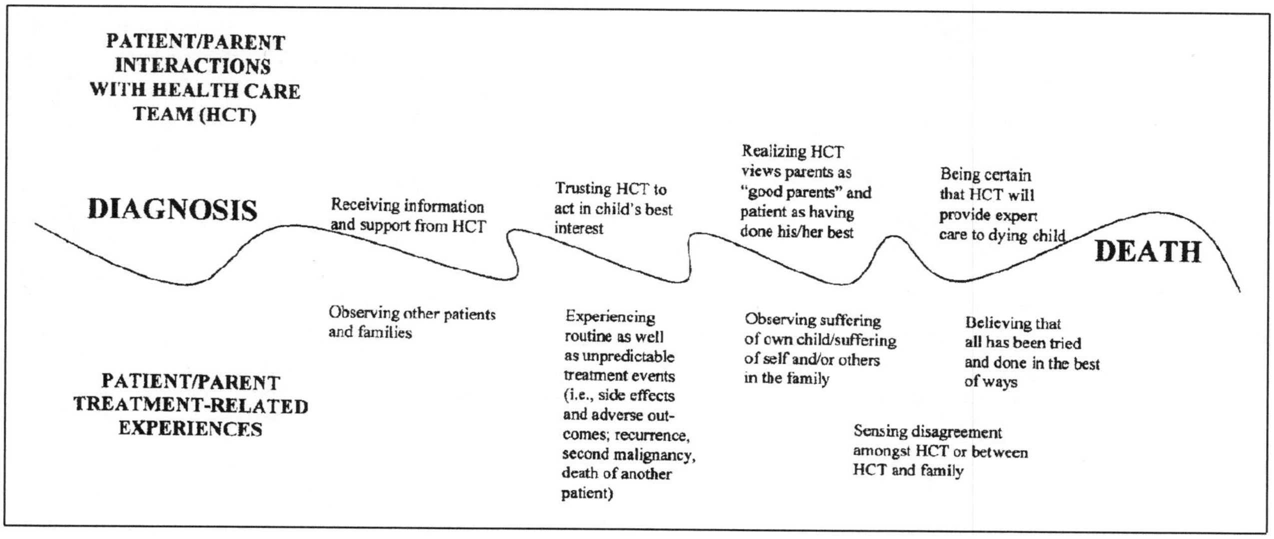

Figure 52–1. The interaction and experiences of pediatric oncology patients, their parents, and the members of their health care team (HCT) from the point of diagnosis forward that influences end-of-life decision-making.

contemplate what it would be like to experience those situations themselves. A second type of personal experience that prompts this kind of reflection is an unexpected negative response to treatment, such as an adverse reaction or even disease progression, after positive responses. When patients and parents feel well informed by health care team members about disease response to treatment and are routinely involved in treatment discussions and other decisions, they are being prepared for end-of-life decision-making, should it become necessary.

A third experience that prepares the patient and parents for end-of-life decision-making is the patient's experience of suffering and the parent's experience of witnessing that suffering and being unable to adequately relieve it. In our research with parents of children and adolescents who are experiencing a first or second recurrence of cancer, parents and guardians are more likely to contemplate ending curative efforts when they see their child in pain, unable to enjoy favorite activities, places, and people, or unable to find comfort.[71,73] Parents may react to the same experiences in different—even opposite—ways. The mother of a child treated for acute lymphocytic leukemia wrote in her guide for parents, friends, and health care providers that an end-of-life decision is an "intensely personal decision."[78] Some parents seek to exhaust all possible treatments, whereas others hope only for sufficient time to prepare themselves and their child for the dying and death. A study by Hollen and Brickle[79] suggested that the socioeconomic status of parents of well adolescents helps to predict the quality of the parents' decision-making about their teenage children. However, no similar data are available that identify relationships between characteristics of parents whose child is seriously ill and their end-of-life decisions on behalf of their child.

The Nurse's Role

The American Nurses Association's Position Statement on Nursing and the Patient Self-Determination Act[13] asserts that nurses have a professional responsibility to facilitate informed decision-making by patients about end-of-life options. The statement does not specify patient age, but other wording, such as that describing the nurse's responsibility for knowing state laws about advance directives, suggests that the statement is oriented toward adult patients. The document also asserts that the nurse is responsible for ensuring that advance directives are current and reflect the patient's choices. The ANA makes equally explicit assertions about the nurse's role in its position statement "Nursing Care and Do-Not-Resuscitate Decisions."[13] That position statement urges nurses to assume principal responsibility for ensuring that competent patients' preferences regarding resuscitation are honored, even if those preferences conflict with those of other health care professionals and family members. Nurses are further urged to facilitate explicit discussions of the resuscitation order with the patient, family members, and health care team, and to document the decisions clearly.

Several general studies about how nurses, physicians, and other health care team members perceive end-of-life decision-making have revealed differences in role responsibilities and interpretations of care priorities.[40,80–84] These differences contribute to tension among team members. It is important that team members be aware of official statements issued by each discipline's professional association about role expectations.

Table 52–3
Guidelines for the Health Care Team to Use in Assisting Each Other with End-of-Life Decision-Making

1. Know the guidelines offered by specific disciplines regarding roles in end-of-life decision-making (i.e., the American Nurses Association's official statements on what the nurse is expected to do to help parents and patients make decisions), because it is possible that the guidelines differ from expectations held by others outside the discipline.
2. Before initiating end-of-life discussions with patients* and parents, all members of the health care team should discuss and agree on
   a. The need for such a discussion.
   b. Which options are appropriate and available.
   c. Whether outside consultants, such as an ethics committee or external oncology expert, are needed to identify which options are in the best interest of the patient.
   d. Which other team members will participate in the discussion with the parents and patient.
   e. The time of the discussion and specific staff members who will participate.
   f. Which staff member will document the discussions in the medical record.
   g. Availability of the appropriate staff time and resources to address any questions parents and patients may have. Communicate to the team members who were not present at the patient-and-parent discussion what specific language was used to provide support to the parents and patient in making this decision.
3. Be available to team members and to the patient and parents to discuss and rediscuss decisions and related concerns.
4. Explore with the team all appropriate options to ensure that all that can be done is being done and being done well.
5. Inform other team members if feedback from or assessment of the patient, parents, or both indicates that any decision needs clarification or reconsideration.

*When considering whether the patient should be present during such discussions, evaluate the developmental stage of the patient and the severity of illness and symptoms at the time of the discussion.

Table 52–4
Guidelines for the Health Care Team to Use in Assisting Pediatric Patients with End-of-Life Decision-Making

1. Seek input of parents as to the timing and extent of information that should be offered to the patient about diagnosis, treatment options, and the likely response to treatment.
2. At the time of diagnosis and throughout treatment, actively seek opportunities to provide information to the child or adolescent that is appropriate to his or her developmental stage.
    a. For a child, assure parental presence during such discussions.
    b. For an adolescent, assure a discussion that includes the parents but offer to discuss with the patient alone as well.
3. Be available to discuss and rediscuss decisions and related concerns in a manner appropriate to the developmental stage of the patient.
4. With parental agreement, encourage the patient to interact with other pediatric oncology patients.
5. Convey verbally and nonverbally the recognition that the patient is trying his or her best and that the health care team is committed to the patient's well-being.
6. Give assurances that everything that can be done to help the patient is being done and being done well.
7. As a patient's disease progresses, provide clear verbal (and written, if desired by the patient) explanations of the patient's status.
8. With parental agreement, inform the patient of treatment options as they become available in the treating institution or elsewhere.
9. Assess patient suffering and the need to change interventions to relieve such suffering.
10. When end-of-life options should be discussed with the patient, consult parents about the appropriate depth and timing of such discussions.
11. After receiving input from the parents and exploring the patient's readiness for information, discuss the end-of-life options, with
    a. A strong emphasis on the team's commitment to the patient's comfort and to providing expert care at all times.
    b. Professional recommendations.
    c. Descriptions about how the the patient is likely to respond to each option (physical appearance, ability to communicate, etc.).
    d. Information about other support resources such as chaplains and ethicists.
12. Include more than one health care team member in end-of-life discussions with the patient.
13. Allow the patient private time to consider the options with his or her parents.
14. Reassess the appropriateness of the chosen end-of-life options on an ongoing basis, remaining aware that patients will
    a. Vacillate between certainty and uncertainty about the decision.
    b. Need clarification and additional information to resolve uncertainties.
15. Convey respect for the patient's right to change decisions, when such changes are clinically feasible.
16. Maintain sensitivity to any specific ethnic, cultural, or religious preferences during the terminal stage.
17. Demonstrate continued commitment to providing symptom management, support of quality of life, and assurance of the parents' well-being.

For example, the *Guidelines on Forgoing Life-Sustaining Medical Treatment* issued by the American Academy of Pediatrics[12] indicates that physicians are expected to provide adequate information to patients, parents, and "other appropriate decision makers" about therapeutic options and their risks, discomforts, adverse effects, projected financial costs, potential benefits, and likelihood of success. In addition, physicians are expected to offer advice about which option to choose and to elicit questions from the patients and parents. Nurses should openly discuss expectations and team functions with other team members (Table 52–3) to prevent misunderstanding or disappointment about their perceived roles.

Guidelines for End-of-Life Decision-making in Pediatrics

End-of-life decision-making for children and adolescents who have been seriously and chronically ill necessitates consistent and careful attention to their most meaningful relationships.[85] The relationships of obvious importance are the relationship of child or adolescent with self and with family. Less obvious but also meaningful relationships are those between the patient and the health care professionals, and between the family and health care professionals (those who provide care for the child or adolescent or for the family). Because of the importance of these relationships in end-of-life decision-making, separate (although overlapping) guidelines are provided addressing how members of the health care team can assist parents, patients (Table 52–4), and each other in making end-of-life decisions. The overlap in the guidelines reflects the parallel, and at times interacting, decision-making processes experienced by children, adolescents, and their parents. Health care professionals will be most effective in implementing these guidelines if they first reflect on their feelings and concerns about the dying and death of children and adolescents and about participating in end-of-life decision-making. Research findings to date consistently indicate that when the child or adolescent participates as fully as possible in end-of-life decision-making, parents and health care providers are more certain and more comfortable about the decision that is made.[10,11,74] Their belief that the decision reflects the child's or adolescent's preferences helps parents and health care providers to make the decision and to recover emotionally from this painful experience.

ACKNOWLEDGMENTS

The authors express sincere appreciation to Linda Watts Parker for her careful formatting of this chapter, to Erin E. Downs, R.N., for her helpful questioning, and to Sharon Naron for her thoughtful editing.

REFERENCES

1. Hinds P, Oakes L, Furman W, et al. End-of-life decision making by adolescents, parents, and healthcare providers in pediatric oncology. Cancer Nurs 2001;24:122–136.
2. United States Department of Education, National Center for Educational Statistics. Youth Indications 1993: Trends in the Well-Being of American Youth. Washington, DC: US Government Printing Office.
3. Karian VE, Jankowski SM, Beal JA. Exploring the lived-experience of childhood cancer survivors. J Pediatr Oncol Nurs 1998;15:153–162.
4. Kazak AE. Psychological research in pediatric oncology (editorial). J Pediatr Psychol 1993;18:313–318.
5. Wolfe J, Grier ME. Care of the dying child. In: Pizzo P, Poplack D, eds., Principles and Practice of Pediatric Oncology, 4th ed. Philadelphia: Lippincott Williams & Wilkins, 2002:1477–1493.
6. Klopfenstein K, Hutchinson C, Clark C, et al. Variables influencing end-of-life care in children and adolescents. Pediatr Hematol Oncol 2001;23:481–486.
7. Ries L, Smith M, Gurney J, Linet M, Tamra T, Young JL, Bunin GR, eds. Cancer incidence and survival among children and adolescents: United States SEER Program 1975–1995. National Cancer Institute, SEER Program, 1999. NIH Pub. No. 99–4649. Bethesda, MD.
8. Wolfe J, Grier H, Klar N, Levin SB, Ellenbogen JM, Salem-Schatz S, et al. Symptoms and suffering at the end of life in children with cancer. N Engl J Med 2000;342:326–333.
9. Institute of Medicine. When Children Die: Improving Palliative and End-of-Life Care for Children and Their Families. Washington DC: National Academy Press, 2003.
10. Hinds P, Oakes L, Quaragnenti A, Furman W, Sandlund J, Bowman L, et al. Challenges and issues in conducting descriptive decision-making studies in pediatric oncology: a tale of two studies. J Pediatr Oncol Nurs 1998;15:10–17.
11. Hinds P, Oakes L, Furman W, Foppiano P, Olson MS, Quargnenti A, Gattuso J, Powell B, Srivastava DK, Jayawardene D, Sandlund JT, Strong C. Decision making by parents and health care professionals for pediatric patients with cancer. Oncol Nurs Forum 1997;24:1523–1528.
12. American Academy of Pediatrics, Committee on Bioethics. Guidelines on foregoing life-sustaining medical treatment. Pediatrics 1994;93:532–536.
13. American Nurses Association, Task Force on the Nurse's Role in End-of-Life Decisions. Compendium of Position Statements on the Nurse's Role in End-of-Life Decisions. Washington, D.C.: American Nurses Association, 1991:1–14.
14. Lindquist R, Banasik J, Barnsteiner J, Beecroft PC, Prevost S, Riegel B, et al. Determining AACN's research priorities for the 90's. Am J Crit Care 1993;2:110–117.
15. Zuckerman C, Mackinnon A. The challenge of caring for patients near the end of life: findings from the Hospital Palliative Care Initiative. New York: United Hospital Fund of New York, 1998: March.
16. Masera G, Spinetta JJ, Jankovic M, Ablin AR, D'Angio GJ, Van Dongen-Melman J, et al. Guidelines for assistance to terminally ill children with cancer: a report of the SIOP working committee on psychosocial issues in pediatric oncology. Med Pediatr Oncol 1999;32:44–48.
17. Awong L. Ethical dilemmas: when an adolescent wants to forgo therapy. Am J Nurs 1988;98:67–68.
18. Kluge EH. Informed consent by children: the new reality. CMAJ 1995;152:1495–1497.
19. Mayo TW. Withholding and withdrawing life-sustaining care: legal issues. In: Levin D, Morriss F, eds. Essentials of Pediatric Intensive Care, Vol. 1. New York: Churchill Livingstone, 1997: 1091–1103.
20. McCabe MA, Rushton CH, Glover J, Murray MG, Leikin S. Implications of the Patient Self-Determination Act: guidelines for involving adolescents in medical decision making. J Adolesc Health 1996;19:319–324.

21. Weir RF, Peters C. Affirming the decisions adolescents make about life and death. Hastings Center Rep 1997;27:29–34.
22. Joint Commission on the Accreditation of Healthcare Organizations. Shared Vision-New Pathways Resources. Available at: http://www.jcaho.org/accredited+organizations/svnp/index.htm.
23. Earle C, Park E, Lai B, et al. Identifying potential indicators or the quality of end-of-life cancer care from administrative data. J Clin Oncol 2003;21:1133–1138.
24. Edwardson SR. The choice between hospital and home care for terminally ill children. Nurs Res 1983;32:29–34.
25. Kollef MH. Private attending physician status and the withdrawal of life-sustaining interventions in a medical intensive care unit population. Crit Care Med 1996;24:968–975.
26. Miller DK, Coe RM, Hyers TM. Achieving consensus on withdrawing or withholding care for critically ill patients. J Gen Intern Med 1992;7:475–480.
27. Overbay JD. Parental participants in treatment decisions for pediatric oncology ICU patients. Dimensions Crit Care Nurs 1996;15:16–24.
28. Campbell A, McHaffie H. Prolonging life and allowing death: infants. J Med Ethics 1995;21:339–344.
29. Nelson L, Nelson R. Ethics and provision of futile, harmful, or burdensome treatment to children. Crit Care Med 1992;20: 427–433.
30. Raffin TA. Withdrawing life support: how is the decision made? JAMA 1995;273:738–739.
31. Rushton C, Glover J Involving parents in decisions to forego life-sustaining treatment for critically ill infants and children. AACN clinical issues. Crit Care Nurs 1990;1:206–214.
32. Rushton C, Lynch M. Dealing with advance directives for critically ill adolescents. Crit Care Nurs 1992;12:31–37.
33. Zaner RM, Bliton MJ. Decisions in the NICU: the moral authority of parents. Child Health Center 1991;20:19–25.
34. Ross LF. Health care decision making by children: is it in their best interest? Hastings Center Rep 1997;27:41–45.
35. Nitschke R, Humphrey G, Sexauer C, Catron B, Wunder S, Jay S. Therapeutic choices made by patients with end-stage cancer. J Pediatr 1982;10:471–476.
36. Nitschke R, Meyer W, Sexauer C, Parkhurst JB, Foster P, Huszh H. Care of terminally ill children with cancer. Med Ped Onc 2000;34: 268–270.
37. Cook LA, Watchko JF. Decision making for the critically ill neonate near the end of life. J Perinatol 1996;16:133–136.
38. De Leeuw R, Beaufort AJ, de Kleine MJ, van Harrewijn K, Kollee LA. Foregoing intensive care treatment in newborn infants with extremely poor prognoses. J Pediatr 1996;129:661–666.
39. Ragatz SC, Ellison PH. Decisions to withdraw life support in the neonatal intensive care unit. Clin Pediatr 1983;22:729–736.
40. Van der Heide A, van der Maas PJ, van der Wal G, de Graaff CL., Kester JG, Kollee LA, et al. Medical end-of-life decisions made for neonates and infants in the Netherlands. Lancet 1997;350: 251–255.
41. Wall SN, Partridge JC. Death in the intensive care nursery: physician practice of withdrawing and withholding life support. Pediatrics 1997;99:64–70.
42. Whitelaw A. Death as an option in neonatal intensive care. Lancet 1986;2:328–331.
43. Able-Boone H, Dokecki PR, Smith MS. Parent and health care provider communication and decision making in the intensive care nursery. Child Health Care 1989;18:133–141.
44. Rushton C. Moral Decision Making by Parents of Infants Who Have Life-Threatening Congenital Disorders. Washington, DC: School of Nursing, Catholic University of America; 1994. PhD dissertation.
45. Goh AY, Lum LC, Chan PW, Bakar F, Chong BO. Withdrawal and limitation of life support in pediatric intensive care. Arch Disabled Child 1999;80:424–428.
46. Lantos JD, Berger AC, Zucker AR. Do-not-resuscitate orders in a children's hospital. Crit Care Med 1991;21:52–55.
47. Vernon DD, Dean JM, Timmons OD, Banner W, Allen-Webb EM. Modes of death in the pediatric intensive care unit: withdrawal and limitation of supportive care. Crit Care Med 1993; 21: 1798–1802.
48. Burns J, Mitchell C, Outwater K, et al. End-of-life care in the pediatric intensive care unit after the forgoing of life-sustaining treatment. Crit Care Med 2000;28:3060–3066.
49. Meyer E, Burns J, Griffith J, et al. Parental perspectives on end-of-life care in the pediatric intensive care unit. Crit Care Med 2002;30:226–231.
50. Buchanan A, Brock D. Deciding for Others: The Ethics of Surrogate Decision-Making. Cambridge: Cambridge University Press, 1989.
51. Foley M. Children with cancer: Ethical dilemmas. Semin Oncol Nurs 1989;5:109–113.
52. Weithorn L, Campbell S. The competency of children and adolescents to make informed treatment decisions. Child Dev 1982; 53:1589.
53. President's Commission for the Study of Ethical Problems in Medicine and Biomedical and Behavioral Research. Deciding to Forego Life-Sustaining Treatment: A Report on the Ethical, Medical and Legal Issues in Treatment Decisions. Washington, DC: U.S. Government Printing Office, 1983:160–170, 197–220.
54. Ariff JL, Groh DH. In the best interests of the child: ethical issues. In: Curley M, Smith J, Moloney-Harmon P, eds. Critical Care Nursing of Infants and Children. Philadelphia: W.B. Saunders, 1996:126–141.
55. Beyth-Marom R, Fischhoff B. Adolescents' decisions about risks: a cognitive perspective. In: Schulenberg J, Maggs J, Hurrelmann K, eds. Health Risks and Developmental Transitions During Adolescence. Cambridge: Cambridge University Press, 1997: 110–135.
56. Hinds P, Martin J. Hopefulness and the self-sustaining process in adolescents with cancer. Nurs Res 1988;37:336–340.
57. Hinds P. Quality of life in children and adolescents experiencing cancer. Semin Oncol Nurs 1990;6:285–291.
58. Burns J, Truog R. Ethical controversies in pediatric critical care. New Horizons 1997;5:72–84.
59. Leikin S. The role of adolescents in decisions concerning their cancer therapy. Cancer 1993;71(Suppl):3342–3346.
60. Goldman A. Life threatening illnesses and symptom control in children. In: Doyle D, Hanks G, MacDonald N, eds. Oxford Textbook of Palliative Medicine, 2nd ed. New York: Oxford University Press, 1998:1033–1043.
61. Levetown M, Carter M. Child-centered care in terminal illness: an ethical framework. In: Doyle D, Hanks G, MacDonald N, eds. Oxford Textbook of Palliative Medicine, 2nd ed. New York: Oxford University Press, 1998:1107–1117.
62. Gowan D. End-of-life issues of children. Pediatr Transplant 2003;7(Suppl 3):40–43.
63. Wolfe J, Klar N, Grier H, Duncan J, Salem-Schatz S, Emanuel FJ, et al. Understanding of prognosis among parents of children who died of cancer: impact on treatment goals and integration of palliative care. JAMA 2000;284:2469–2475.

64. Schmidt L. Pediatric end-of-life care: coming of age? Caring 2003;22:20–22.
65. Rowa-Dewar N. Do interventions make a difference to bereaved parents? A systematic review of controlled studies. Int J Palliative Nurs 2002;8:456–457.
66. Contro N, Larson J, Scofield S, et al. Family perspectives on the quality of pediatric palliative care. Arch Pediatr Adolesc Med 2002;156:14–19.
67. James LS, Johnson B. The needs of pediatric oncology patients during the palliative care phase. J Pediatr Oncol Nurs 1996;14: 85–95.
68. Martinson IM, Cohen MH. Themes from a longitudinal study of family reactions to childhood cancer. J Psychosoc Oncol 1988;6: 81–98.
69. Chesler MA, Barbarin OA. Difficulties of providing help in a crisis: relationships between parents and children with cancer and their friends. J Soc Issues 1984;40:113–134.
70. Stevens MM. Care of the dying child and adolescent: family adjustment and support. In: Doyle D, Hanks G, MacDonald N, eds. Oxford Textbook of Palliative Medicine, 2nd ed. New York: Oxford University Press, 1998:1057–1075.
71. Hinds PS, Birenbaum L, Clarke-Steffen L, Quargnenti A, Kreissman S, Kazak A, et al. Coming to terms: parents response to a first cancer recurrence. Nurs Res 1996;45:148–153.
72. Pyke-Grimm KA, Degner L, Small A, Mueller B. Preferences for participation in treatment decision making and information needs of parents of children with cancer: a pilot study. J Pediatr Oncol Nurs 1999;16:13–24.
73. Hinds P, Birenbaum L, Pedrosa A, Pedrosa F. Guidelines for the recurrence of pediatric cancer. Semin Oncol Nurs 2002; 18:50–59.
74. Hinds PS, Oakes L, Quargnenti A, Furman W, Bowman L, Gilger E, et al. An international feasibility study on parental decision making in pediatric oncology. Oncol Nurs Forum 2000;27: 1233–1243.
75. Kirschbaum MS. Life support decisions for children: what do parents value? Adv Nurs Sci 1996;19:51–71.
76. Davies B, Deveau E, deVeber B, Howell D, Martinson I, Papadatou D, et al. Experiences of mothers in five countries whose child died of cancer. Cancer Nurs 1998;21:301–311.
77. American Academy of Pediatrics, Committee on Bioethics. Informed consent, parental permission, and assent in pediatric practice. Pediatrics 1995;95:314–317.
78. Keene N. Childhood Leukemia: A Guide for Families, Friends and Caregivers. Sebastopol, CA: O'Reilly & Associates, 1997.
79. Hollen PJ, Brickle BB. Quality parental decision making and distress. J Pediatr Nurs 1998; 13:140–150.
80. Phillips RS, Rempusheski VF, Puopolo AL, Naccarato M, Mallatratt L. Decision making in SUPPORT: the role of the nurse. J Clin Epidemiol 1990;43(Suppl):55S–58S.
81. Randolph AG, Zollo MB, Wigton RS, Yeh TS. Factors explaining variability among caregivers in the intent to restrict life-support interventions in a pediatric intensive care unit. Crit Care Med 1997;25:435–439.
82. Randolph AG, Zollo MB, Egger MJ, Guyatt GH, Nelson RM, Stidham GL. Variability in physician opinion on limiting pediatric life support. Pediatrics 1999;103:S43.
83. Solomon MZ, O'Donnell L, Jennings MA, Guilfoy V, Wolf SM, Nolan K, Jackson R, Koch-Weser D, Donnelley S. Decisions near the end-of-life: professional views on life-sustaining treatments. Am J Public Health 1993;83:14–23.
84. Walter SD, Cook DJ, Guyatt GH, Spanier A, Jaeschke R, Todd TR, Streiner DL. Confidence in life-support decisions in the intensive care unit: a survey of healthcare workers. Crit Care Med 1998;26:44–49.
85. Hume M. Improving care at the end of life. Quality Letter for Healthcare Leaders 1998;10:2–10.

53

Carole Kenner and Sylvia McSkimming

Palliative Care in the Neonatal Intensive Care Unit

Why no miracle for my little one, so innocent, so small? Why so much suffering in such a short life? Should I have fought for her or spared her and let her go? The answers to my questions I will never know . . . until we meet again.—Kathleen Petzold, mother

- ***Key Points***
- *Palliative care in the neonatal intensive care unit (NICU) is as much a part of family-centered care as any other aspect of care. Palliative care gives nurses the opportunity to do what nurses do best: nurture and care for the whole infant and family unit at a time of tremendous stress. It is the most intimate time that one can share with a family.*
- *Palliative care incorporates symptom management for the infant, and emotional, psychosocial, and spiritual support for the infant and family members. Family is defined by the parents and may include other children as well as grandparents and other close family members. The support is always provided in a cultural and developmental manner appropriate for each person. Palliative care is provided when a condition is life threatening and may or may not result in death.*
- *Palliative care is the antithesis of what most professionals and families think about within the context of infant care. The primary focus of infant care is and should be life-prolonging care. Yet palliative and end-of-life (EOL) care are a part of neonatal nursing. In 2001 there were 27,568 infant deaths in the United States, with an infant mortality rate of 6.8 per 1000 live births.[1] Neonatal mortality accounts for about 60% of these infant deaths.[2] Thus it is obvious that the death of a newborn can be a part of the nurse's sphere of practice and requires that the nurse develop competencies in providing supportive palliative care, which may lead to a peaceful death.*

American society does not have a word for a parent who has lost a child—another challenge for the nurse. For example, the term "widow" is used for the surviving female spouse, but what do we call the surviving parent? There is no term, but the loss in many cases is more profound than a spousal loss, only because western culture no longer expects children to die before their parents. In fact, the role of parent is often viewed as gone when a baby dies. One nurse, prepared in palliative care, responded to a grieving mother whose baby was not likely to survive to term, "You are a mother now, and you will always be a mother, regardless of whether or not your baby survives. You have a baby and that makes you a mother." While this was comforting to the mother, it points out the lack of good alternative language to describe a parent who has lost a child.

Other cultures may have words or strategies to support parents who have lost an infant, but American culture labels the person a bereaved parent and talks about another child in the parent's future or another child the parent may have.

This chapter presents the core values of palliative care within the context of providing culturally appropriate, individualized, family-centered developmental care (IFCDC) for infants receiving care in the NICU environment. The following case study will act as an exemplar of neonatal/pediatric palliative care.

To illustrate use of palliative care with the neonatal population, the following case study was supplied by team members from the Footprints Program (Continuity of Care Palliative Care Program), SSM Cardinal Glennon Children's Hospital, St. Louis, MO (used with permission).

CASE STUDY

Christian, a Newborn Patient with Holoprosencephaly

March 8, 2001: We arrived at the hospital about 7 AM. Within an hour we were told, "You're going to have a baby today!" During the next 6 hours, everything went spiraling downward.

My doctor discovered I had hemolysis, elevated liver enzyme levels, low platelet count (HELLP) syndrome (my blood wasn't clotting and my liver and kidneys were shutting down). I was prepped for an emergency cesarean section and wheeled into the operating room. My husband, Matt, waited anxiously in the hallway for news of our new baby and my health. I can only imagine the fear he felt as a group of nurses carrying a small bundle rushed out of the operating room. I awoke in the recovery room and asked to see my husband and child. About 30 minutes later, Matt came into the room and bravely told me about our little boy and his problems. Christian was being transferred to SSM Cardinal Glennon Children's Hospital in St. Louis where he could be better evaluated. "Can I see him before he goes?" was all I could ask.

The transport team brought in a tiny 5-pound, 3-ounce, 17-inch baby boy with IVs, an oxygen mask, and monitors. Christian was handed to me and I cradled my son in my arms. Matt said this was the proudest moment of his life. We had our first family photo and handed Christian back to the team after so few minutes. We were supposed to be celebrating the birth of our child but instead were overcome with worry, grief, and fear.

Over the next few days, we talked with many specialists in the NICU at Cardinal Glennon. Christian was diagnosed with holoprosencephaly, a condition in which the brain does not separate into two hemispheres. Christian also had cleft palette, cleft lip, and blindness, and was in constant seizure. We were told he would most likely not live beyond 2 weeks to 2 months, or, if we were lucky, 2 years.

After discussion, we determined we wanted Christian to experience every moment he could while he was alive. First and foremost, we wanted to take him home. Our NICU staff identified a program in the hospital that could help us make that desire a reality. They referred us to the Footprints Program (SSM Cardinal Glennon Hospital, St. Louis, MO); which cares for children with life-threatening and terminal illnesses. The Footprints staff identified a continuity physician who would direct Christian's care and gathered a team of our physicians, nurses, and chaplains to meet with Matt and me and our family members to make plans for Christian's eventual homecoming. Together, we identified our goals and our fears and, with help from the team, developed a plan of care for our son that would give him the best quality of life. While the NICU staff taught us how to care for Christian's basic physical needs, the Footprints staff contacted all of the care providers who would be involved in his care once he was home . . . home health/hospice providers and the emergency medical services (EMS) community in our town. Because we expressed fear at what others might think if Christian died at home so soon after birth, the staff also contacted our local police department to let them know that Christian was seriously ill and not expected to live. A plan was in place! But we had yet to learn that Christian was the strongest person we had ever met!

Christian came home after 13 days in the NICU, and while scary, each day became easier. We focused on Christian and with encouragement from the NICU and Footprints teams made memories that would last forever. We took him outside to experience the wind in his hair, the sun on his face, and cold water on his feet. The next few months brought many changes. We needed to replace the feeding tube with a g-tube. We heard him cry for the first time, and while sad, it also made us smile. We visited the neurologist, and the doctor stated Christian was a "completely different baby than in the NICU." Christian was responding to his surroundings. He became a hospice dropout at the age of 6 months!

The Footprints team stayed very connected with follow-up phone conversations on a regular basis, encouraging us as Christian changed to redefine our goals and our hopes. We knew they were available to answer our questions at any time and always felt supported. We continued to give our son all of life's experiences—trick-or-treating (we ate the candy), snow on his face, and time in church. We were allowed to be Christian's parents and to leave some of the other more technical details to our care team. At a year, we met with the Footprints team and our physicians to reevaluate Christian's care plan, still focusing on the best quality of life we could give him, while keeping him with us as long as possible. We were also more prepared at that time to discuss arrangements for the time of Christian's death. Once again, we had a plan and all caregivers were notified of the revisions and new additions.

In spite of several serious cases of pneumonia, Christian celebrated his 2nd birthday, and he became a big brother. He lived to be 2 years, 8 months, and 2 days. We were able to hold him in our arms as his little body just wore out. His last moments were as we had wished, peaceful and at home with us. We are so glad we had a care plan in place. There were no arguments or questions. Arrangements basically fell into place. Our care plans focused on Christian's quality of life, and helped us to focus on dignity at the time of his death. We were able to celebrate the life of our son each step of the way. The Footprints team continues to support us with phone calls and visits and is always available to help with any questions or issues we might still have.

Christian taught us about strength and hope, and what was truly important in life—love. Our lives are better—we are better—because Christian is a part of our family.
—Jennifer Anderson, Christian's Mom

Case Summary

> We wanted Christian to experience every moment he could while he was alive.

Stated by Christian's mother, this goal is the essence of the best in neonatal palliative care. No one could predict the length of his short life. For this family, his life was much longer than the predicted 2 weeks to 2 months. Thus, his life illustrates that neonatal palliative care must be planned in such a way as to meet the needs of the patient and family for whatever period of life the neonate has, in whatever environment that life is lived. The principles are the same regardless of the length or location of that life. Plan for death, support the parents, provide the best possible symptom relief for the neonate, honor the parents wishes, and at all times honor the life—while at the same time not denying that death is likely to occur prior to a usual lifetime of 70-plus years. With neonatal palliative care, perhaps even more so than adult palliative care, the critical element is for the health care team and family to know the goals for the brief life and not just about advance care planning choices. And as his mother described—create memories of that life lived.

Excellence in palliative care can provide a positive outcome for the family and neonate even though the neonate cannot be cured. Health care professionals can do much to make a difference. Let it never be said that "there is nothing we can do."

Palliative and end-of-life (EOL) care is the antithesis of what most of us expect to provide to newborns. Yet this is a vital part of our neonatal skills. It is a privilege to be a part of birth and death, but it takes a professional who is adept at communicating, anticipating, and nurturing a family under tremendous grief to participate. It also requires acceptance that grief work extends to the health professional, and we must care for ourselves as we care for others.

Table 53–1
Core Principles for Care of Patients (Newborns and Infants)

- Respect the dignity of both child and caregiver.
- Be sensitive to and respectful of the family's wishes.
- Use the most appropriate measures that are consistent with the family's choices.
- Encompass alleviation of pain and other physical symptoms.
- Assess and manage psychological, social, and spiritual/religious problems.
- Ensure continuity of care—the child should be able to continue to be cared for, if so desired, by his/her primary care and specialist providers.
- Provide access to any therapy that may be realistically expected to improve the child's quality of life, including alternative or nontraditional treatments.
- Provide access to palliative care and hospice care.
- Respect the right to refuse treatment that may prolong suffering.
- Respect the physician's professional responsibility to discontinue some treatments when appropriate, with consideration for both child and family's preferences.
- Promote clinical evidence-based research on providing care at the end of life.

Source: Adapted from Cassel & Foley (1999), reference 3.

Core Principles and Philosophy of Care

As this case study points out, a shared interdisciplinary team approach, including the parents as part of the team, can make all the difference in how the end of life is experienced. As with any plan, there must be a shared understanding of how care is to be provided. Just as businesses and other enterprises have moved towards having a mission, vision, and core values or principles, so has palliative care. The mission, for example, of this text is to advance the knowledge of health professionals about palliative and EOL care. The vision of this book is that every individual and family will receive optimal palliative and EOL care. These core principles are the drivers of palliative care. Cassel and Foley[3] present the core principles for care of patients (newborns and infants) that are applicable to the NICU (Table 53–1).

Guiding principles only outline the key features of palliative care. Beyond that the nurse must understand the philosophy of care before employing these guidelines. Americans for Better Care of the Dying formulated seven promises[4] they felt exemplified key aspects of palliative care. These aspects were presented in seven promises designed to constitute a contract between the health professional and the patient and family. These promises were adapted for use by the neonatal nurse. They are as follows:

1. Good Medical Treatment

- Your baby will have the best of medical treatment and nursing care, aiming to prevent illness or disease progression, to promote survival, to encourage growth and development, to prevent known potential complications, and to ensure comfort.
- Your baby will be offered proven diagnoses and treatment strategies that inhibit disease progression, enhance quality of life, and promote living fully even though a condition is life threatening.
- We will use medical and nursing interventions that are in accord with best available standards of care and practice and consistent with your wishes and values.

2. Never Overwhelmed by Symptoms

- Your baby will never have to endure overwhelming pain, severe breathing distress, or other overwhelming symptoms.
- We will anticipate and prevent symptoms when possible. When symptoms occur, we will evaluate and address symptoms promptly.
- We will treat severe symptoms, such as breathing difficulty as emergencies.

- We will use sedation when necessary to relieve symptoms that cannot be relieved in other ways near the end of life.

3. *Continuity, Coordination, and Comprehensiveness*
   - Your baby's care will be continuous, comprehensive, and coordinated.
   - We will be sure knowledgeable, caring, health care professionals care for your baby.
   - We will make sure your baby and your family can count on an appropriate and timely response to needs.
   - We will make sure you can count on access to health care professionals to answer questions.
   - We will try to minimize transitions among services, settings, and personnel; and when transitions are necessary, we will make sure they go smoothly.

4. *Well-prepared, No Surprises*
   - You and your family will be prepared for everything that is likely to happen in the course of your baby's illness.
   - We will let you know what to expect if the illness worsens—and what we expect of you.
   - We will provide you with training and access to the supplies needed to handle your baby's predictable care needs.

5. *Customize Care, Reflecting Your Preferences*
   - Your wishes will be sought and respected and followed whenever possible.
   - We will tell you about the alternatives for care and services for your baby, and support you in making choices that matter to you.
   - If you wish, we will help your child to live out the end of life at home.

6. *Consideration for Patient and Family Resources (Financial, Emotional, and Practical)*
   - We will help you to consider your family's personal and financial resources, and we will respect your choices about their use.
   - We will inform families about services available in the community and the costs of those services.
   - We will discuss and address the concerns of family caregivers. When appropriate, we will make respite, volunteer, and home aide care part of the care plan.
   - We will support families before, during, and after a loved one's death.

7. *Make the Best of Every Day*
   - We will do all we can to see that your baby and your family will have the opportunity to make the best of every day.
   - We will treat your baby as a person, not as a disease. What is important to the baby and family is important to the care team.
   - We will respond to the physical, psychological, social, and spiritual needs of your baby and family members.
   - We will support you before, during, and after your baby's death.

Using the mission, vision, core principles, and philosophy of palliative care as a backdrop, the neonatal and pediatric nursing community felt that the final step in formalizing a structure of care would be to construct precepts for the care. The Association of Pediatric Oncology Nurses (APON), National Association of Neonatal Nurses (NANN), and the Society of Pediatric Nurses (SPN) worked together to adapt the *Precepts of Palliative Care,* developed by the Last Acts Palliative Care Task Force, December, 1997. These precepts were originally written for the adult population and disseminated by the Last Acts Organization. The above organizations felt that newborns, infants, children, and their families represented a unique cohort of care where death was not expected or easily welcomed as a phase of the life cycle. The premise, however, is the same—that palliative care is comprehensive, holistic, and supportive, and it affirms life and regards dying as a profoundly personal process.[5]

So what does this mean for the neonatal nurse confronting a dying newborn or infant? It means that the nurse has to be present—to be fully attentive to the child and family, to separate his/her values regarding birth, life, and death from those of the family, and to clearly ask what it is that they need from their perspective. Of course, it means that the nurse must be ready to break the rules and turn over some control to the family, which is not something that most nurses feel comfortable doing. Nurses must adapt and individualize the care so that there is as much support for the positive development as possible for the infant and family. An IFCDC approach provides the context in which to render palliative and EOL care. This approach reminds the nurse that the families are parents first, and that they want to support their infant's development and preserve their role as parents. It is only after that role is solidified that parents can become the caregiver to a child that may or will die. For culturally competent care to reflect the complexity of care that is much broader than ethnicity, the nurse must be sensitive to cultural, ethnic, and religious values.

Cultural Influences on Care

Cultural values and beliefs, both religious and ethnic, influence the family's view of pain, suffering, and end of life (Table 53–2). The neonatal nurse must incorporate these values and beliefs into the plan of care if it is to be effective. Wong and colleagues[6] and the Texas Children's Cancer Center-Texas

Table 53–2
Religious Influences

Religious Sect	Birth	Death	Organ Donation/Transplantation	Beliefs regarding Medical Care
Baptist	Infant baptism is not practiced. However, many churches present the baby and the parents to the congregation when they attend services for the first time after the birth.	It isn't mandatory that clergy be present at death, but families often desire visits from clergy. Scripture reading and prayer are important.	There is no formal statement regarding this issue. It is considered a matter of personal conscience. It is commonly regarded as positive (an act of love).	Some may regard their illness as punishment resulting from past sins. Those who believe in predestination may not seek aggressive treatment. Fundamentalist and conservative groups see the Bible as the infallible word of God to be taken literally.
Buddhist	Do not practice infant baptism	Buddhist priest is often involved before and after death. Rituals are observed during and after death. If the family doesn't have a priest, they may request that one be contacted.	There is no formal statement regarding organ donation/transplantation. This is seen as a matter of individual conscience.	Believe that illness can be used as a tool to aid in the development of the soul. May see illness as a result of karmic causes. May avoid treatments or procedures on holy days. Cleanliness is important.
Church of Jesus Christ of Latter-day Saints (Mormon)	Infant baptism is not performed. Children are given a name and a priesthood blessing sometime after the birth, from a week or 2 to several months. In the event of a critically ill newborn, this might be done in the hospital at the discretion of the parents. Baptism is performed after the child is 8 years old. Church of Jesus Christ of Latter-day Saints feel that a child is not accountable for sins before 8 years of age.	There are no religious rituals performed related to death.	There is no official statement regarding this issue. Organ donation/transplantation is left up to the individual or parents.	Administration to the sick involves anointing with consecrated oil and performing a blessing by members of the priesthood. While the individual or a member of the family usually requests this if the individual is unconscious and there is no one to represent him or her, it would be appropriate for anyone to contact the church so that the ordinance may be performed. Refusal of medical treatments would be left up to the individual. There are no restrictions relative to "holy" days.
Episcopal	Infant baptism is practiced. In emergency situations, request for infant baptism should be given high priority and could be performed by any baptized person, clergy or lay. Often in situations of stillbirths or aborted fetuses, special prayers of commendation may be offered.	Pastoral care of the sick may include prayers, laying on of hands, anointing, and/or Holy Communion. At the time of death, various litanies and special prayers may be offered.	Both are permitted.	Respect for the dignity of the whole person is important. These needs include physical, emotional, and spiritual.

(continued)

Table 53–2
Religious Influences *(continued)*

Religious Sect	Birth	Death	Organ Donation/Transplantation	Beliefs regarding Medical Care
Society of Friends (Quakers)	Do not practice infant baptism	Each person has a divine nature but an encounter and relationship with Jesus Christ is essential.	No formal statement, but generally both are permitted	No special rites or restrictions. Leaders and elders from the church may visit and offer support and encouragement. Quakers believe in plain speech.
Islam (Muslim/ Moslem)	At birth, the first words said to the infant in his/her right ear are "Allah-o-Akbar" (Allah is great), and the remainder of the Call for Prayer is recited. An *Aqeeqa* (party) to celebrate the birth of the child is arranged by the parents. Circumcision of the male child is practiced.	In Islam, life is meant to be a test for the preparation for everlasting life in the hereafter. Therefore, according to Islam, death is simply a transition. Islam teaches that God has prescribed the time of death for everyone and only He knows when, where, or how a person is going to die. Islam encourages making the best use of all of God's gifts, including the precious gift of life in this world. At the time of death, there are specific rituals (bathing, wrapping the body in cloth, etc.) that must be done. Before moving and handling the body, it is preferable to contact someone from the person's mosque or Islamic Society to perform these rituals.	Permitted. However, there are some stipulations depending on the type of transplant/donation and its effect on the donor and recipient. It is advisable to contact the individual's mosque or the local Islamic Society for further consultation.	Humans are encouraged in the Qu'ran (Koran) to seek treatment. It is taught that only Allah cures. However, Muslims are taught not to refuse treatment in the belief that Allah will take care of them because even though He cures, He also chooses at times to work through the efforts of humans.
International Society for Krishna Consciousness (A Hindu movement in North America based on devotion to Lord Krishna)	Infant baptism is not performed.	The body should not be touched. The family may desire that a local temple be contacted so that representatives may visit and chant over the patient. It is believed that in chanting the names of God, one may gain insight and God consciousness.	There is no formal statement prohibiting this act. It is an individual decision.	Illness or injury is believed to represent sins committed in this or a previous life. They accept modern medical treatment. The body is seen as a temporary vehicle used to transport them through this life. The body belongs to God, and members are charged to care for it in the best way possible.

(continued)

Table 53–2
Religious Influences *(continued)*

Religious Sect	Birth	Death	Organ Donation/Transplantation	Beliefs regarding Medical Care
Jehovah's Witnesses	Infant baptism is not practiced.	There are no official rites that are performed before or after death, however, the faith community is often involved and supportive of the patient and family.	There is no official statement related to this issue. Organ donation isn't encouraged, but it is believed to be an individual decision. According to the legal corporation for the denomination, Watchtower, all donated organs and tissue must be drained of blood before transplantation.	Adherents are absolutely opposed to transfusions of whole blood, packed red blood cells, platelets, and fresh or frozen plasma. This includes banking of ones' own blood. Many accept use of albumin, globulin, factor replacement (hemophilia), vaccines, hemodilution, and cell salvage. There is no opposition to nonblood plasma expanders.
Judaism (Orthodox and Conservative)	Circumcision of male infants is performed on the 8th day if the infant is healthy. The mohel (ritual circumciser familiar with Jewish law and aseptic technique) performs the ritual.	It is important that the health care professional facilitate the family's need to comfort and be with the patient at the time of death.	Permitted and is considered a mitzvah (good deed).	Only emergency surgical procedures should be performed on the Sabbath, which extends from sundown Friday to sundown Saturday. Elective surgery should be scheduled for days other than the Sabbath. Pregnant women and the seriously ill are exempt from fasting. Serious illness may be grounds for violating dietary laws but only if it is medically necessary.
Lutheran	Infant baptism is practiced. If the infant's prognosis is poor, the family may request immediate baptism.	Family may desire visitation from clergy. Prayers for the dying, commendation of the dying, and prayers for the bereaved may be offered	There is no formal statement regarding this issue. It is considered a matter of personal conscience.	Illness isn't seen as an act of God, rather, it is seen as a condition of mankind's fallen state. Prayers for the sick may be desired.
Methodist	Infant baptism is practiced but is usually done within the community of the church after counseling and guidance from clergy. However, in emergency situations, a request for baptism would not be seen as inappropriate	In the case of perinatal death, there are prayers within the United Methodist Book of worship that could be said by anyone. Prayer, scripture, and singing are often seen as appropriate and desirable.	Organ donation/transplantation is supported and encouraged. It is considered a part of good stewardship.	In the Methodist tradition, it is believed that every person has the right to death with dignity and has the right to be involved in all medical decisions. Refusal of aggressive treatment is seen as an appropriate option.
Pentecostal Assembly of God, Church of God, Four Square, and many other faith groups are included	No rituals such as baptism are necessary. Many Pentecostals have a ceremony of "dedication," but it is done in the context of the community of faith/believers (church). Children belong to heaven and only become	The only way to transcend this life; is the door to heaven (or hell). Questions about "salvation of the soul" are very common and important. Resurrection is the hope of those who "were saved." Prayer is	Many Pentecostal denominations have no statement concerning this subject, but it is generally seen as positive and well received. Education concerning wholeness of the person and nonliteral aspects like "heart," "mind," etc., have to	Pentecostals sometimes labeled as "in denial" due to their theology of healing. Their faith in God for literal healing is generally expressed as intentional unbelief in the prognostic statements. Many Pentecostals do not

(continued)

Table 53–2
Religious Influences *(continued)*

Religious Sect	Birth	Death	Organ Donation/Transplantation	Beliefs regarding Medical Care
under this general heading. Pentecostal is not a denomination, but a theological distinctive (pneumatology).	sinners after the age of accountability, which is not clearly defined.	appropriate, so is singing and scripture reading.	be explained. For example, a Pentecostal may have a problem with donating a heart to a "non-believer."	see sickness as the will of God, thus one must "stand firm" in faith and accept the unseen reality, which many times may mean healing. As difficult as this position may seem, it must be noted that, when death occurs, Pentecostals may leap from miracle expectations to joyful hope and theology of heaven and resurrection without facing issues of anger or frustration due to unfulfilled expectations. Prayer, scriptures, singing, and anointing of the sick (not a sacrament) are appropriate/expected pastoral interventions.
Presbyterian	Baptism is a sacrament of the church but is not considered necessary for salvation. However, it is seen as an event to take place, when possible, in the context of a worshipping community.	Family may desire visitation from clergy. Prayers for the dying, commendation of the dying, and prayers for the bereaved may be offered.	There is no formal statement regarding this issue.	Communion is a sacrament of the Church. It is generally celebrated with a patient in the presence of an ordained minister and elder. Presbyterians are free to make their own choices regarding the use of mechanical life-support measures.
Roman Catholic	Infant baptism is practiced. In medical facilities, baptism is usually performed by a priest or deacon, as ordinary members of the sacrament. However, under extraordinary circumstances, baptism may be administered by a layperson, provided that the intention is to do as the church does, using the formula, "I baptise you in the name of the Father, the Son, and the Holy Spirit."	Sacrament of the sick is the sacrament of healing and forgiveness. It is to be administered by a priest as early in the illness as possible. It is not a last rite to be administered at the point of death. The Roman Catholic Church makes provisions for prayers of commendation of the dying, which may be said by any priest, deacon sacramental minister, or layperson.	Catholics may donate or receive organ transplants.	The Sacrament of Holy Communion sustains Catholics in sickness as in health. When the patient's condition deteriorates, the sacrament is given as viaticum ("food for the journey"). Like Holy Communion, viaticum may be administered by a priest, deacon, or a sacramental minister. The church makes provisions for prayers for commendation of the dying that may be said by any of those listed above or by a layperson.

Source: Adapted from Texas Children's Cancer Center—Texas Children's Hospital (2000), reference 7 (pp. 78–79).

Children's Hospital[7] address cultural influence on care by outlining key aspects of health beliefs and practices that must be considered when providing any type of care. (For further information, see References 6 and 7.)

For example, when working with a Native American family, the nurse must consider that they may want to combine healing ceremonies from their tribal rituals with western medicine to alleviate suffering. In this instance, ethnic and religious beliefs are intertwined. But in other instances, religious versus ethnic values must be incorporated into care.

It must be remembered that not every family that identifies themselves as Methodist, for example, strictly adheres to all principles of that faith. The nurse must determine what role religion plays with each family. Additionally, we need to realize that for some cultures there is a biological birth and a social one. Social birth may not occur until it is clear that the infant will survive or until the infant has been given a name. How the family responds to the impending or possible death of the child will differ if the child is not considered a person until after a social birth.[8]

One example of religious belief affecting neonatal palliative care is that of an American Caucasian family strongly tied to the Catholic church. As their infant girl took a turn for the worst, the family was called. They immediately asked that she be baptized. The priest on call was unavailable and the family's priest was 2 hours away. Rather than take the chance that no priest would come before the infant's death, the nurse, a non-Catholic, baptized the baby. When the family arrived, they were reassured that yes, indeed, Angela had been baptized. The infant died peacefully in her parents' arms long before either priest arrived. The family expressed comfort in knowing she was held within the religious arms of the church's beliefs.

Rights of Newborns and Their Families

In today's complex health care delivery system, many families feel they have no rights. The American Hospital Association (AHA) took this to heart and in 1973 developed *A Patient's Bill of Rights.*[9] Keeping this tradition in the adult community, neonatal nurses have long recognized that even the most premature infant has rights, as does the family (Table 53–3). The rights presented here need to be considered whenever neonatal palliative care is being rendered.

Why is it so important to adapt rights to neonates and their families? Because most neonatal health professionals recognize the unique needs of this population—their rights and their care needs. An infant has no history—as one family said, the infant does not know what the future possibilities are; there is no frame of reference. For the family, there are no memories of a past except prenatally, so palliative care is building a lifetime of memories. There are other aspects that are different as well. Table 53–4 summarizes these differences.

Table 53–3
The Rights of the Newborn and Infant

- I have the right to be listened to as a person with rights and am not the property of my parents, medical doctors, nurse practitioners, and society.
- I have the right to cry.
- I have the right to hope.
- I have the right of not being alone.
- I have the right to create fantasies.
- I have the right to interact with my siblings.
- I have the right to have my pain controlled.
- I have the right to have my needs taken care of.
- I have the right to be at home and not in the hospital if my parents choose to have me there.
- I have the right to receive help for my brothers and sisters in dealing with my illness.
- I have the right to comfort care.

Adapted from Palliative Care Center and Hospice of the North Shore (1999), reference 16.

Palliative Care Plan

Catlin and Carter[10] developed a palliative care protocol that has been disseminated widely since 2002 (see Appendix 53–1). Based on their research in neonatal palliative care, it is one of the only evidence-based plans available. It incorporates all of the elements previously discussed in this chapter. This protocol exemplifies the care that was provided in the chapter's opening exemplar—Christian's story. Their respect for the family wishes and alleviation of the pain and suffering were addressed. A team-integrated approach to care was used.

Sometimes we underestimate what toll palliative and EOL care can take on us as caregivers. We often feel torn between spending quality time with a dying child and family and caring for our other patients. We are only human. We need to give ourselves permission to set priorities and to make the most of the time we do have with child and family. Sometimes a word, a gentle touch, a look across the room while providing care for another baby is enough for a parent to know we are there for them. While it is not ideal to be multitasking while caring for a dying child, it is the reality of today's work environment. We also have to realize that sometimes we need to ask for help, to give someone else the opportunity to provide support when we cannot. Try to remember that for some parents this the first time they have lost a family member, let alone a child. They don't know what to expect or if that "ad" in the newspaper with funeral arrangements costs anything. We have to anticipate these questions, but we also have to realize that some days we deal better with these situations

Table 53–4
Differences Between Hospice Care for Newborns/Infants and Adults

Patient Issues

- Patient is not legally competent.
- Patient is in developmental process that affects understanding of life and death, sickness and health, God, etc.
- Patient has not achieved a "full and complete life."
- Patient lacks verbal skills to describe needs, feelings, etc.
- Patient is often in a highly technical medical environment.

Family Issues

- Family needs to protect the child from information about his/her health.
- Family needs to do everything possible to save the child.
- Family may have difficulty dealing with siblings.
- Family feels stress on finances.
- Family fears that care at home is not as good as care at the hospital.
- Grandparents feel helpless in dealing with their children and grandchildren.
- Family needs relief from burden of care.

Caregiver Issues

- Caregivers need to protect children, parents, and siblings.
- Caregivers feel a sense of failure in not saving the child.
- Caregivers feel a sense of "ownership" of children, even at the expense of parents.
- Caregivers have out-of-date ideas about pain in children, especially infants.
- Caregivers lack knowledge about children's disease processes.
- Influence of "unfinished business" on style of care.

Institutional/Agency issues

- There is less reimbursement or none for children's hospice/home care.
- High staff-intensity caring is required for children at home.
- Ongoing staff support is necessary.
- Children's services have immediate appeal to public.
- Special competencies are needed in pediatric care.
- Assess how admission criteria may screen out children.
- Address unusual bereavement needs of family members.

Adapted from Kuebler & Berry (2002), reference 17 (used with permission); and Children's Hospice International, reference 18 (prepared by Paul R. Brenner).

than others. For example, if you have just had a baby yourself, it may be very difficult to care for a newborn who is dying. That is okay. But make sure that someone knows this and, if possible, get reassigned. Communication is the key for others to know what you need—whether it is a new assignment, to have more time with the child and family, or to attend the funeral. You need to make it clear what you need. We practice asking families "Tell me what you need" but often neglect ourselves.

Summary

Neonates who would benefit from excellent palliative care could die minutes, months, or years after birth with a life-threatening anomaly or illness. Because the prognosis is so difficult to predict, the professional is called upon to focus on providing care that is often changing and challenges existing health care system structures. The period of life may be so unpredictable that the focus needs to be on excellent symptom management, while promoting development of the child and family within their community. Families and professionals have the difficult task of helping the child live as fully as possible while preparing for and accepting that the child may not live a long time. This requires a committed interdisciplinary team with community linkages as appropriate.

Regardless of the length of life or the place where that life is lived, excellent palliative care includes optimum symptom relief for the neonate, honoring the parents' wishes, providing ongoing support to parents and family, planning for the death, and honoring the life by creating memories of the life. Even though the neonate cannot be cured, let it never be said that "there is nothing we can do."

APPENDIX 53–1

Neonatal End-of-Life Palliative Care Protocol*

The purpose of this protocol of care is to educate professionals and enhance their preparation and support for a peaceful, pain-free, and family-centered death for dying newborns.

Planning for a Palliative Care Environment

To begin a palliative care program, one must realize that some institutions find it difficult to confront the issue of a dying child. So to begin to create a palliative care environment, there must be staff education and buy-in. This education must address cultural issues that affect caregiving. Ethical issues must be addressed either by the group creating the environment or by consultants who specialize in ethics.

For the family, staff must treat the family as care partners and not visitors. They must recognize that someone needs to be available 24/7 to address issues such as advance directives and symptom and pain management both in the hospital and at home if discharge is possible. There must be a mechanism to prepare the community for the child's entrance home or to hospice. This preparation includes what is appropriate to say to friends, relatives, and visitors.

Prenatal Discussion of Palliative Care

It is essential that fetal development and viability be discussed with all families as a part of prenatal care packages and classes

*This protocol was published in Kenner C, Lott JW. Neonatal Nursing Handbook. St. Louis: Mosby, 2003:506–525. Adapted from Reference 10.

and to all families receiving assisted reproductive therapies. As the course of prenatal care progresses, pregnant women should be made aware that newborns in the very early gestational periods of 22 to 24 weeks and birth weights of less than 500 grams may not be responsive to resuscitation or applied neonatal intensive care.

Physician Considerations

The families need honest, straightforward language. They need to know their options and it is essential that they understand what to expect. Usually the physician delivers this information, but the nurse is generally the one that can help the parents sort through feelings and grasp what they were just told. If this incident is sudden, such as an unexpected premature or complicated birth, then the family's ability to comprehend and retain what is being said is limited. Reinforcement at a later time is advisable.

Family Considerations

Peer support from families that have experienced a similar infant illness or death may help the family cope. If the family finds out that the pregnancy is not viable, then it is up the health care team to help support their needs and to garner resources such as other family members, spiritual counselors, and friends. Helping the family to experience the normal parenting tasks such as naming the baby is very appropriate and helpful. This act helps the family gain some control and to be a parent first and build memories of that experience.

Transport Issues

It is best that mothers not be separated from their newborn infants. Transport is considered both traumatic and expensive, and if the newborn's condition is incompatible with prolonged life, then arrangements to stay in the local hospital may generally be preferred. It is best to avoid transferring dying newborns to Level III NICUs if nothing more can be done there than at the local hospital. The local area is recognized as that location at which parents have their support system, rapport with their established health care providers, a spiritual/religious community, and funeral availability.

The key to whatever decision is made, referral or not, requires good, clear communication with the family and between the two institutions. The family should not feel they are being sent away or given the wrong message by the nature of the transfer, or even return from a tertiary center once a referral is made if there is nothing to be done. The family needs a consistent message if trust is to be developed.

Which Newborns Should Receive Palliative Care?

While many aspects of palliative care should be integrated into the care of all newborns, there are infants born for whom parents and the health care professionals believe that palliative care is the most appropriate form of care. The following list includes categories of newborns that have experienced the transition from life-extending technological support to palliative care. The individual context of applying palliative care will require that each case, in each family, within each health care center, be explored individually. These categories of newborns are provided for educational purposes and may engender discussion at the local institutional level.

- Newborns at the threshold of viability
- Newborns with complex or multiple congenital anomalies incompatible with prolonged life, where neonatal intensive care will not affect long-term outcome
- Newborns not responding to intensive care intervention, who are deteriorating despite all appropriate efforts, or in combination with a life-threatening acute event

Introducing the Palliative Care Model to Parents

Speaking to parents about palliative care is difficult. There is heartache from the staff and heartfelt sympathy for the parents. The following points are offered to help physicians and nurse practitioners facilitate the process:

- Let the family know they will not be abandoned.
- Assist the family in obtaining all of the medical information that they want. Tell them that the entire medical team wishes the situation were different. Let them know you will support them every step of the way and that their infant is a valued and loved member of their family.
- Hold conversations in a quiet, private, and physically comfortable space.
- Give them your beeper number or telephone number to call you after they have digested the information and have more questions. Offer the ability to have a second opinion and/or an ethics consultation.
- Provide parents time to consult the local regional center that works with children with special needs or their area pediatrician, who can provide information on projected abilities and disabilities.
- Offer to introduce them to parents who have been in a similar situation.
- When possible, use lay-person language to clarify medical terms, and allow a great deal of time for parents to process the information.
- The terms "withdrawal of treatment," such as referring to the stopping of life support, or "withdrawal of care," referring to the stopping of feedings or other supportive interventions, should be avoided. The exact treatment or care that is to be terminated should be specifically explained so that the intention is clear.
- Use terms such as "change in care" or "change in treatment."

- Communicate and collaborate with parents at all times. Efforts should be made to clarify mutually derived goals of care for the infant. Give as many choices as possible about how palliative care should be implemented for their infant. Inform the parents of improved access to the infant for holding, cuddling, kangaroo care, and breast-feeding. Use of developmental care approaches such as these promotes the building of a relationship between the infant and parents.
- If the transition in care involves the removal of ventilatory support, explain that the use of ventilators is for the improvement of heart/lung conditions until cure, when cure is a likely outcome.
- Tell the parents that you cannot change the situation but you can support the infant's short life with comfort and dignity. Explain that discontinuing interventions that cause suffering is a brave and loving action to take for their infant.
- Validate the loss of the dreamed-for healthy infant, but point out the good/memorable features he/she has. Help parents look past any deformities and work to alleviate any blame they may express.
- Encourage parents to be a family as much as possible. Refer to the newborn by name. Assist them to plan what they would like to do while the infant is still alive.
- Encourage them to ask support persons to join them on the unit. Facilitate sibling visitation. Support siblings with child-life specialists on staff.
- In daily conversation, avoid terms that express improvement such as "good," "stable," "better" in reference to the dying patient so as not to confuse parents.
- Prepare the family for what may happen as the infant dies.
- Introduce families to the chaplain and social worker early in the process.

Optimal Environment for Neonatal Death

When the decision is made that a newborn infant may be close to death, there are several components to optimizing the care. These include:

- Compassionate, nonjudgmental, consistent staff for each infant, including physicians knowledgeable in palliative care. If consistent staff is not an option in a particular unit, then agreement on the plan of care is essential, with proposed revisions to care discussed with the whole team.
- Nurses and other health care staff educated in providing a meaningful experience for the family while caring for the family's psychosocial needs, including a period of time after the death
- Parents who are educated in what to expect and who are encouraged to participate in, or even orchestrate, the dying process and environment of their infant in a manner they find meaningful
- Flexibility of the facility and staff in responding to parental wishes, such as participation of siblings and other family members, and including wishes of parents and families who do not wish to be present
- Institutional policies that allow staff flexibility to respond to parental wishes
- Providing time to create memories, such as allowing parents to dress, diaper, and bathe their infant, feed him/her (if it is possible), take photos, and hold the infant in their arms. If they wish to take the infant outdoors to a peaceful and natural setting, that should be encouraged.
- Siblings should be made comfortable; they may wish to write letters or draw for the infant. Snacks should be available.
- Allowing the family to stay with the infant as long as they need to, including after death occurs
- The process for treating the dying infant[11–13] is well described in the literature and by the various bereavement programs.
- Parents should be assisted in making plans for a memorial service, burial, etc. Some parents might wish to carry or accompany the infant's body to the morgue, or take it to the funeral home themselves. Issues such as autopsy, cremation, burial, and who may transport the body should be discussed, especially if the parents are far from home and wish to take the body back to their home area for burial. In some states, hospitals may release a body to parents after notifying the county department of vital statistics. The family must sign a form for removal of the body. The quality assurance department should be notified. Further discussion of autopsy and organ/tissue donation issues is included.

Specific skills are needed by the staff to provide palliative care. These include:

- A physician leader of the team who is familiar with family-centered care and the tenets of palliative/hospice care
- A trained nursing staff, clinical social workers, and clergy supportive of this manner of care
- Agreement to cease all invasive care, including taking frequent vital signs, monitoring, medical machinery, and artificial feeding
- Removal of all medications other than those to provide comfort or to prevent or treat a troubling symptom, with continued IV access for pain medication and anxiolytics
- Maintenance of skin care, participation in discussion on the appropriateness of feeding, and prevention of air hunger

- Use of simple blow-by oxygen or suctioning if needed for comfort
- Continuous observation and gentle assessment by nursing staff as individualized by parent wishes
- Physicians' notes describing the need for ongoing physician observation and nursing staff interventions to provide the needed level of care
- Appropriate palliative care orders on the chart

Location for Provision of Palliative Care

Location is not as important as the "mindset" of persons involved in EOL care. The attitude of staff, their desire to care for dying newborns and their families, their training in observation, support, and symptom management, and their knowledge of how to apply a bereavement protocol are more important than the physical location of the patient. Many agree that an active NICU may not be the optimal place for a dying newborn. Whether the infant is moved to a room off of the unit (e.g., a family room), onto a general pediatrics ward, or kept on the postpartum floor, the best available physical space with privacy and comfort should be chosen.

The families need help to make the decision of how and where the infant is to be given care. If families take the infant home, coordination with the EMS personnel may be necessary to prevent undesired intervention. Parents need to be instructed not to call 911 because in some places emergency medical technicians (EMTs) are obligated to provide cardiopulmonary resuscitation (CPR). A letter describing the diagnosis, existence of in-hospital do-not-resuscitate (DNR) order, and hospice care plan for home with the full expectation that the patient will die should be provided to the parents, their primary physician, home-health agency/hospice, and perhaps the county EMS coordinator. Generally, hospice nurses are allowed to confirm a patient's death.

Ventilator Removal, Pain and Symptom Management

At times, cessation of certain technological supports accompanies the provision of palliative care. The following information addresses (1) how to prepare the family, staff, and facility for discontinuation of ventilator support, and (2) the process of removing the ventilator in a manner that minimizes discomfort for the infant and the family. The latter includes who will be present at the time of extubation. A plan must be worked out with the family about what medications and support will be given to alleviate pain and suffering and what they can expect the dying process to be like for their baby. Consideration of developmentally supportive care that is attuned to ambient light and noise as well as comfort measures are important. These should incorporate cultural considerations.

Mementos can be obtained by nurses, such as a lock of hair, hand or footprints in plaster, and photos and/or videotapes of the family together if this is culturally appropriate. If the infant has serious anomalies, photos of hands, ears, lips, feet, can be provided. Ear prints and lip prints are possible. Some parents have indicated that mementos of a newborn who died are not acceptable in their culture.

When Death Does Not Occur After Cessation of Aggressive Support

A private room somewhere in the hospital is recommended where nurses trained in palliative care are available. If the expected time for expiration passes and death does not take place, the infant could be discharged to home for ongoing palliative care services. The parents, NICU staff, and the hospice staff should meet to make plans for home care, including the investigation of what services are offered and what insurance will cover. Continued palliative care/hospice services with home nursing care is essential, including the possibility of ventilator removal at home.

If the infant is to go home, a procedure for dispensing outpatient medications should be in place. All needed drugs and directions for use should be sent along with infant so that parents do not have to go to a pharmacy to fill prescriptions. Identifying and communicating with a community health care provider who will continue with the infant's home care needs is essential.

Some families and health care providers feel dying newborns should be fed, and if unable to suck, should be tube fed. Others feel that artificial feeding is inappropriate. However, withholding of feedings is an ethical dilemma for many health professionals and families and needs careful consideration.[14] Recent research indicates that feeding can be burdensome and that an overload of fluids can impede respirations.[15] In all cases, infants should receive care to keep their mouth and lips moist. Drops of sucrose water have been found to be a comfort agent if the infant can swallow, and they may be absorbed through the buccal membrane.

Parents who feel they cannot take the infant home should be assisted to find hospice care placement.

Discussion of Organ and Tissue Procurement and Autopsy

At some point in the course of care, organ and tissue donation and autopsy will need to be discussed. Prior to discussion with families, the regional organ donation center should be contacted to see if a particular infant qualifies as a potential donor. In some areas, only corneas or heart valves are valuable in an infant under 10 pounds, but in different locations, other organs (e.g., heart) or tissues may be appropriate. It is important to know if a newborn has no potential donor use and to communicate this respectfully. Parents often desire the ability to give this gift and may be doubly hurt if they are hoping for the opportunity to help others and are turned down.

The person who discusses organ/tissue procurement must be specially trained. While the physician usually initiates this, a nurse, chaplain, or representative from donor services may conduct the conversation with tact and compassion. The provider should be aware of cultural, traditional, or religious values that would preclude organ donation for a specific family, as many cultures and religions would consider this desecration of the dead infant.

Suggestions Concerning Autopsy

Requests for autopsies are not required in all states, but may be considered appropriate in many instances of infant death. If the medical examiner or coroner is involved in the case, laws may require autopsy. Some providers feel that asking for an autopsy is important in order to potentially provide parents with some answers regarding their infant's illness and death. The placenta may also be used for testing to provide information. In the discussion, parents may wish to know all or some of the following:

- Autopsy does not cause any pain or suffering to the infant; it is done only after death.
- The body is handled with the ultimate respect.
- Some insurance companies pay for a physician-ordered autopsy.
- Final results are returned in approximately 6 to 8 weeks, at which time the primary physician can meet with the parents, conduct a telephone conference, or communicate by letter to discuss the results.

Family Care: Cultural, Spiritual, and Practical Family Needs

The hospital social worker is an essential component of supportive palliative care. Families may immediately need financial assistance, access to transportation, and a place to stay.

Practical Considerations. Parents of multiples in which some lived and one died will need special attention to validate their bereavement as well as to support their love for their living child(ren).

Time should be permitted for the parents to contact the needed authority in their culture and to plan any necessary ceremony, some of which may require special permission, for example use of incense.

Cultural Sensitivity. These support needs should be anticipated and provided as much as possible.

- When using a translator, simple words and phrases should be used so that the translator can convey the message exactly as it is given. It is most appropriate to use hospital-trained and certified translators to ensure accuracy.
- Whenever possible, written materials should be given in the family's primary language, in an easy-to-read format, culturally and linguistically appropriate for the family.
- Culturally sensitive grief counseling and contact with a support group of other parents who have been through this is helpful.

Family Follow-Up Care

Families who have experienced a neonatal death will likely leave the facility in a shocked state. Families can be best be served by:

- Establishing contact with a social worker, chaplain, or grief counselor prior to discharge
- Receiving an information packet as described and a date for a follow-up discussion with the attending physician (which may be in conjunction with autopsy results)
- Notifying the family's obstetrician of the death no matter how long after delivery it occurred
- A home visit by one of the staff or a public health nurse within a few days
- Phone calls weekly, then monthly, then at 6-month intervals if parents agree. Also providing contact on significant days such Mother's Day, the infant's due date, or anniversary of death
- Invite family to a group memorial service held by the hospital for those who have lost pregnancies or infants in the past year.
- Keep in mind that subsequent pregnancy may be difficult and offer support at that time; include genetic counseling if indicated.
- Keep snapshots and mementos on the unit if parents do not wish to take them at the time, as some parents may reconsider later.

Ongoing Staff Support

The work of providing EOL care for newborns and their families is very intense. Staff needing support must not be limited to the nursing staff, and must include physicians and all health care and ancillary personnel who have interacted with the infant or family. Suggested support includes:

- Facilitated meetings of the multidisciplinary team during the process are needed, especially if some of the team members are reluctant to change to this mode of care.
- Debriefings after every infant's death and after any critical incident will be helpful for the staff.
- Meetings or counseling sessions should be part of regular work hours and not held on voluntary or unpaid time.
- Moral support for the nurses and physicians directly caring for the dying newborn is required from peers as well as the unit director, other neonatologists, chaplain, and nursing house supervisor.
- Nursing staff scheduling should be flexible and allow for overtime to continue with the family or to orient another nurse to take over.
- If they wish, the primary nurse and physician should be called if not present at the actual time of the infant's dying. With permission by the parents,

they should be allowed to attend the funeral if desired and to take time off afterwards if needed.

APPENDIX ACKNOWLEDGMENTS

Catlin and Carter wish to include the following acknowledgments for assistance in the development of this neonatal end-of-life palliative care protocol: We thank our reviewers Alex G. M. Campbell, MD, David Clark MD, Joel Frader, MD, John Lantos, MD and Bill Silverman, MD, and our Delphi methodology consultant, Dr. Carol Lindemann. The project was funded by the American Nurses Foundation Julia Hardy RN Scholar Award, with travel support from the Lambda Gamma Chapter of Sigma Theta Tau. We appreciate support from our institutions, Napa Valley College and Vanderbilt University College of Medicine, and from the IRB at Queen of the Valley Medical Center in Napa, California.

We sincerely thank our 101 participants for their time, wisdom, and commitment. Readers may contact us for participant names as space did not permit listing: acatlin@napanet.net; bcarter@ghsystem.com

REFERENCES

1. Centers for Disease Control and Prevention (CDC). Fast Stats A-Z. Available at: http://www.cdc.gov/nchs/fastats/infmort.htm Accessed February 19, 2005.
2. Rip MR, Dosh, SA. The Neighborhood and Neonatal Intensive Care: A Population-Based Analysis of the Demand for Neonatal Intensive Care in Detroit, Michigan (1984–1988). Available at: http://www.uic.edu/sph/cade/mchepi/meetings/may2001/nicu.ppt (accessed 11/08/03).
3. Cassel CK, Foley KM. Principles of care of patients at the end of life: an emerging consensus among the specialties of medicine. New York: Milbank Memorial Fund, 1999, http://www.milbank.org/reports/endoflife (accessed February 23, 2005).
4. Americans for Better Care of the Dying. Making Promises. Washington, DC: Americans for Better Care of the Dying, 2001, http://www.abcd-caring.org/tools/actionguides.pdf (accessed March 24, 2005).
5. Last Acts Partnership. Precepts of Palliative Care for Children, Adolescents and Their Families, 2003, http://www.apon.org/files/public/last_acts_precepts.pdf (accessed June 11, 2005).
6. Wong D, et al. Nursing Care of Infants and Children, 6th ed. St. Louis: Mosby, 1999.
7. Texas Children's Cancer Center–Texas Children's Hospital. End-of-Life Care for Children. Houston: Texas Cancer Council, 2000.
8. Oosterwal G. Caring for People From Different Cultures: Communicating Across Cultural Boundaries. Portland, OR: Providence Health System, 2003.
9. American Hospital Association (AHA). A Patient's Bill of Rights, http://www.injuredworker.org/Library/Patient_Bill_of_Rights.htm (accessed March 28, 2005).
10. Catlin A, Carter B. Creation of a Neonatal End-of-Life Palliative Care Protocol. J Perinatol 2002;22:184–195.
11. Craig F, Goldman A. Home management of the dying NICU patient. Semin Neonatol 2003;8:177–183.
12. Lundqvist A, Nilstun T, Dykes AK. Neonatal end-of-life care in Sweden. Nurs Crit Care 2003;8:197–202.
13. Milstein JM. Detoxifying death in the neonate: in search of meaningfulness at the end of life. J Perinatol 2003;23:333–336.
14. McHaffie HE, Fowlie PW. Withdrawing and withholding treatment: comments on new guidelines. Arch Dis Child 1998; 79:1–2.
15. Catlin A, Carter B. Creation of a neonatal end-of-life palliative care protocol. J Perinatol 2002;2:184–195.
16. Palliative Care Center and Hospice of the North Shore. Rights of the Newborn and Infant. Evanston, IL: Author, 1999.
17. Kuebler KK, Berry PH. End-of-life care. In: Kuebler KK, Berry PH, Heidrich DE, eds. End-of-Life Care: Clinical Practice Guidelines. Philadelphia: W.B. Saunders, 2002:25.
18. Children's Hospice International, http://www.chionline.org (accessed February 23, 2005).

54

Betty Davies and Juhye Jin

Grief and Bereavement in Pediatric Palliative Care

It's been a challenge for all of us since Sammy died. It's so hard to understand why a child has to die . . . it just doesn't seem right. I still cry a lot, and some days are harder than others. I get a lot of support from my mother and sisters, but my husband doesn't have that kind of support from his family. And he doesn't like to talk much about what happened. I think he works things out on the rugby field. My older daughter (age 8) seems to be doing okay now, but for a while, she wasn't concentrating in school at all, and just didn't seem like herself. The little ones (4-year old twins) . . . well, they ask the hardest questions, like "Will Sammy be here for Christmas?" They are just trying to figure out something that none of us can really figure out.—Mother, age 35, whose 7-year-old died of cancer 18 months ago

- ***Key Points***
- *Bereavement care for all family members is an integral component of pediatric palliative care.*
- *Grieving after a death is a normal process; however, some grief reactions become complicated, and nurses must assess for factors that put family members at risk for such reactions.*
- *Grief assessment begins at the time of diagnosis of a child's life-limiting condition, applies to all family members, and continues into the bereavement period following the child's death.*
- *Nurses have a responsibility to create supportive environments in which family members feel free to express their grief.*
- *Caring for dying children requires nurses to attend to their own personal and professional responses to death, dying, and bereavement as a basis for providing optimal care to families.*

Effective and compassionate care for children with life-threatening conditions and their families is an integral and important part of care from diagnosis through death and bereavement.[1] This guiding principle, one of seven put forth by the Institute of Medicine report on the status of palliative and end-of-life care for children and their families, emphasizes that care continues for the family following the child's death. Though medical science has contributed significantly to the treatment of children with life-limiting illnesses or conditions, children still die from cancer, cardiac disease, respiratory conditions, genetic conditions, and more. Moreover, thousands of neonates die each year and thousands more children of all ages, particularly toddlers and adolescents, die as a result of trauma. Approximately 55,000 children die annually in the United States.[1] Regardless of the cause of death, the death of a child is a tragedy, an incomparable life event that has an impact on all family members, friends of the family, and the community in which the family lives. A child's death also affects the physicians, nurses, social workers, and other health care personnel who provide care for the dying child. The purpose of this chapter is to define common words associated with grief; to describe factors that affect the grief of family members, the effects of grief upon them, and the nurse's role in helping grieving individuals and their families; and to discuss the needs of nurses who work in pediatric palliative care.

Grief as a Process

Death is a part of each individual life, something we all must face though we resist even the thought of our own mortality. The hoped-for pattern is that we experience deaths of others that are easier in earlier life, for us to build the skills to aid us with the more difficult deaths in later life. The death of one's child, though, sits outside of that hoped-for pattern. The grief associated with a child's death begins even before the actual death event, as the child's parents and other family members anticipate the death and experience the child's dying, and their grief continues long past the child's death. Many parents feel they never "recover" from the death of their child. They may resume daily activities, adjust to life without their child's presence, and find new pleasures in life, but most parents feel they remain vulnerable and feel they are not the same people they were before the child's death.[2] The death of a child, or any beloved person, is not something one "gets over"; rather, over time, one learns to integrate the loss into one's life. Indeed, grief is a process that is not always orderly and predictable, and given that grief is the individual experience of each human being, it manifests in many diverse ways.

Grief, Bereavement, and Mourning

The term *grief* is often used to refer to the emotional response to a loss.[3] But grief is much more than emotion—it is an overwhelming and acute sense of loss and despair; it is the personalized feeling and response that an individual makes to real, perceived, or anticipated death; it encompasses feelings, physical sensations, cognitions, and behaviors. Grief encompasses every domain of human life—physical, emotional, psychological, social, and spiritual. Sadness, anger, numbness, sleep and eating disturbances, inability to concentrate, fatigue, existential angst, and tension in interpersonal interactions are among the responses to a loved one's death.

Grief occurs when a loss is deemed as personally significant to the individual. For example, hearing the news about a child's death in a bicycle accident may produce sadness, but not necessarily a grief reaction. However, grief will ensue when it is learned that the child is your nephew. To a certain degree, who or what we consider to be personally significant is culturally defined. For example, in the contemporary United States, the death of one's child is expected to result in profound grief. In fact, a classic research study suggests that grief in response to a child's death is more intense than grief following the death of a spouse or parent.[4]

The term *bereavement* refers to the state of being bereaved or deprived of something. The word derives from an Old English word, "reave," which means to plunder, spoil, or rob.[5] This meaning implies that the loss object is a valued one, together with a suggestion of violence in the way in which the loss occurred. This definition is especially apt for bereaved parents, who often report feeling as if a part of them has been torn away. As the bereaved mother of a 22-month old who died following a brain aneurysm sighed:

> When my son died, it was as if my heart had been stolen from my breast, and my arms that held him ripped from their sockets.

Mourning refers to the outward, social expression of grief, often through ritual and sometimes to the psychological process of adapting to loss.[6] How one expresses a loss may be dictated by cultural norms, customs, and practices, including rituals and traditions. Some cultures may be very emotional and verbal in their expression of loss, others may appear stoic and businesslike. Religious and cultural beliefs may also dictate how long one mourns and how one behaves during the bereavement period. In addition, outward expression of loss may be influenced by the individual's personality and life experiences.[7]

Types of Grief

It is important for nurses' understanding of grief and bereavement and for the implementation of appropriate interventions to be aware of several types, or variations, of grief that have been described in the thanatology literature, including anticipatory grief, disenfranchised grief, and pathological grief reactions or complicated grief. How these concepts apply to pediatric palliative care is particularly important.

Anticipatory Grief

Anticipatory grief often occurs in advance of an expected loss. Rando[8] indicates that anticipatory grief entails grieving not just for future losses, but also for losses that have already occurred and for current losses. It may be associated with the losses of expectations for a "normal" life that are associated with a particular diagnosis, with acute and chronic illness, or with death. For example, parents may fear the potential loss of health in their child when a child is being tested for unusual symptoms. All family members may grieve the expected loss of a part of the child's body, mental function, or self-image; they may grieve the loss of the child's and their own independence, choice, and dreams. Anticipatory grief occurs while the ill child is still alive, and this allows for hope. This is a subtle difference that makes anticipatory grief unique, and helps account for what parents often describe as an "emotional roller coaster," particularly for parents of children with long-term chronic illness. Their experience of witnessing the child's physical deterioration and worsening of symptoms, interspersed with remissions, "good" days, and seeming progress toward health lays fertile ground for emotional ups and downs and hope for the child's recovery. Over time, however, the focus of hope changes, and nurses can play a critical role in facilitating the expression of that hope. Initially, parents of children with cancer, for example, focus their hope on the possibility of cure. Each exacerbation chips away at the hope for the child's full recovery, and family members hope for longer remissions. Eventually, they hope their child will be able to live until he reaches a particular milestone, such as graduation, a special birthday, or the next holiday. As the child's condition worsens, parents may hope that their wish to care for their child at home will be possible, and that their child will not suffer at the end. Hope is life-sustaining; health care providers should support family members in their hope, refraining from crushing hope with overdoses of facts. In response to a mother's proclamation that her child will overcome a serious illness, the nurse can empathize, "I certainly do hope so." The death is anticipated, but it has not occurred, and in the parents' eyes, there is a chance, no matter how small, that it might not occur:

> My son has been to the PICU three times. At his first transfer to the PICU, my sorrow was beyond description. At that time, I thought I would never see him again. But my son has fought against his cancer every time. Whenever he came back to the ward from the PICU . . . I remember recently that day was 3 days before his 13th birthday . . . it was so amazing and I prayed thanks to God for allowing me to hope for his life again.

For more information on hope, the reader is referred to Chapter 26.

Though painful, anticipatory grieving does present an opportunity for families to begin to think about their future without the child. It can help family members begin to face the existential questions that arise when a child is dying. It can help families begin to the process of reorganizing their fractured lives. Anticipatory grieving can also take its toll, especially when the child's illness endures. Rando[9] interviewed parents whose child had died from cancer, and suggests there is an optimal length of anticipatory grief of 6 to 18 months. A shorter time did not give parents enough time to prepare for the loss, and a longer period had a debilitating effect on them.

Unacknowledged grief before the death may inhibit communication and preparation for death which, in turn, may contribute to strong feelings of subsequent guilt and regret.[1] However, anticipatory grief does not mean the grieving that occurs after the child's death is somehow easier or less painful for parents and other family members. Health care providers cannot assume that family members whose child died following a long-term illness grieve "less" than those whose child dies suddenly and unexpectedly. In fact, every child's death is unexpected. Even when parents know their child will die, the actual moment of death is often unexpected, as reflected in parents' words: "*I knew the end was near, but I really thought he would make it until his brother got home from college.*" Or, as the 7-year old sister wept following her brother's death a few days before her birthday: "*But, he was coming to my party.*"

Disenfranchised Grief

Disenfranchised grief acknowledges the social context of grief. It refers to the grief that persons experience when they incur a loss that is not or cannot be openly acknowledged, publicly mourned, or socially supported.[10,11] Those at risk include, for example, classmates, team mates, teachers, coaches, school bus drivers, crossing guards, or past boyfriends/girlfriends of the child or adolescent who died—those whose relationship with the now-deceased child/adolescent is not regarded as significant. Also feeling disenfranchised are those grieving a terminated pregnancy or a neonatal death where the significance of these losses may not even be acknowledged, or if it is, comments such as "You can try again" reflect insensitive misunderstanding of the parents' grief. Families of children with serious cognitive or physical limitations, from progressive neurodegenerative illnesses, for example, may experience disenfranchised grief when others perceive the child's death as a "blessing" rather than a loss for the family. Disenfranchised grief also occurs when bereaved persons are not recognized by society as capable of grief or needing to mourn. Young children, mentally challenged children or adults, and abusing parents whose actions have caused the child's death are often disenfranchised in this way.

Complicated or Troubled Grief

The processes of grief and mourning are normal and healthy aspects of human living. However, all human processes can go awry, especially in particularly difficult situations, and such grief is sometimes referred to as "complicated" grieving. However, as everyone who has experienced the loss of a loved one knows, all grief is complicated. It's just that, sometimes, grief is more complicated than at other times. But common terminology differentiates complicated from uncomplicated grief, with the latter referring to the typical feelings, behaviors, and reactions to loss; complicated grief refers to a response to loss that is more intense and longer in duration than usual.[12] Worden[13] has outlined four basic types of complicated grief: (1) chronic grief is characterized by grief reactions that do not subside and continue over long periods of time; (2) delayed grief is characterized by grief reactions that are suppressed or postponed, and the family member consciously or unconsciously avoids the pain of the loss; (3) exaggerated grief occurs when the family member resorts to self-destructive behaviors such as suicide; and (4) masked grief occurs when the family member is not aware that behaviors that interfere with normal functioning are a result of the loss.

Those who are mourning the loss of a child are at risk for complicated grief. Other risk factors include: preexisting difficulties in the relationship with the deceased (such as between a parent and a delinquent daughter); the circumstances of the death (such as traumatic death through suicide or homicide); chronic illness; the survivor's own history of depressive illness; multiple losses or history of troubled grief reactions to previous deaths; difficulty with the dying process; when the death is socially negated; or a lack of social support system or faith system.

Factors Affecting the Grief Process

Family responses to grief vary widely and depend on a multitude of factors. Some of these factors may be obvious, some less apparent, but all influence how individual family members cope with the pain of a child's death. Influencing factors fall into three broad categories. Individual variables have to do with attributes of the bereaved, including the relationship between the child who died and other family members; environmental factors have to do with the social, familial, and cultural environments; and situational factors pertain to the characteristics of the death. All factors interact with one another to provide the context of grief.

Individual Factors

Individual, or personal, characteristics that affect the grief process may include history and relationship with the child, previous exposure to death, dying, grief and loss, developmental level, and temperament and coping styles.

History and Relationship with the Child. Each parent, sibling, or grandparent has a unique history and relationship with the deceased child. Histories among siblings are closely intertwined because siblings often develop special bonds that are unlike any other. The closer two siblings are to one another before death, the more behavior problems the surviving sibling may have following the death.[14] Similarly, grandparents may be integrally involved in children's lives, whether they live geographically far apart or down the street; in other families, grandparents and children barely know one another. Some histories among the children and other family members will have been predominantly troubled, filled with tension and conflict and others filled with laughter and harmony.

Previous Experience with Death. Past experiences with death and the learned response to loss also affect how each family member will grieve a child's death. Other deaths of a similar nature may have occurred in the family, such as when more than one child suffers from the same life-limiting genetic disorder. How previous losses were handled in the family will influence the current situation.

> In the R. family, for example, when Grandfather R. was 10 years old, his older brother was killed in a car accident. No one explained to the grieving child what had happened, he was not allowed to attend the funeral, and following the death, regretted that he had not been the one to die because he felt his brother was so much smarter than he. As a young boy, he decided unconsciously that he would hide his pain behind a wall of silence; he seldom displayed or talked about emotions. When Mr. R's grandson died from cancer at age 11 years, Mr. R was flooded with memories and sadness. His previously learned coping through silence and withdrawal resulted in his being unprepared for how to help his distraught son and himself with the current loss.

Developmental Level. When we think of "developmental level," we often think only of children and adolescents. But development is a lifelong process; therefore, the developmental level of each grieving individual must be considered. Young parents who are facing the death of their child have not typically experienced many life crises; elderly grandparents may be struggling under the burden of having faced too many. A teenage mother, struggling to be independent from her parents, faces new challenges when she must rely on them for assistance because her baby becomes ill and dies. A midlife father, anxious about his family's financial future following his son's long-term illness, agonizes deeply over the expenses of his son's funeral and feels guilty about his feelings. A grandmother who overcame breast cancer at age 65 laments over why her 20-year old granddaughter was the one to die from cancer.

Personality and Coping Style. Individuals of all ages vary in temperament and personality, and styles of interacting with the world are evident in even the youngest children. Some youngsters are naturally more extroverted; they talk easily with others and eagerly seek out resources and sources of support and comfort. Others are more introverted; they keep their thoughts and feelings to themselves and may prefer the solitude of reading or quiet play. Doka[11] describes styles of grieving among adults that occur along a continuum, with "instrumental" grieving at one end and "intuitive" grieving at the other. Most people fall in the middle, but describing the extremes of the continuum clarifies the differences and may be helpful in understanding how parents and other family members manifest their grief. Intuitive grievers fit the pattern of how we think individuals "should" grieve. They express strong affective reactions, their expression mirrors their inner feelings, and their adaptation involves expression and exploration of feelings. In contrast, the grief experience for instrumental grievers is primarily cognitive or physical, expressed cognitively or behaviorally, and adaptation generally involves thinking and doing. Gender, culture, temperament, and a variety of other factors influence grieving styles. Caution is advised against assuming that mothers are more intuitive in style and fathers more instrumental. Both parents must be assessed individually to determine where on the continuum their style rests. It is important, as well, to remember that these terms represent differences, not deficiencies, in grieving styles. Most parents in pediatric palliative care are young and likely inexperienced with illness, hospitals, technologies, dying, and death. Consequently, they typically have few skills for dealing with significant loss.

Environmental Factors

Environmental factors include the role of the deceased child in the family and various aspects of the family itself.

Role in the Family of the Child Who Died. Ordinal position often defines children's roles in the family. When a child dies, shifts occur among the other children. For example, Jose was the eldest of three sons. When he died, his father told Marco, the middle son, that he was now the "oldest." The three boys had shared very close relationships, and now they felt their father was "forgetting" Jose by no longer regarding him as the eldest son. Children also play particular social, spiritual, and physical roles in the family; the child's absence leaves their role unfilled and resultant adjustments can be difficult for remaining family members. Jose had been the "leader"—Marco did not want to assume his brother's leadership role. As well, how the child defined the other members of the family affects their grieving. Again, Jose particularly liked to joke about his "little" brother who was growing to be taller than Jose. Marco had enjoyed the teasing and did not want to displace his admired older brother. Tension grew between father and sons.

Family Characteristics. Even before their child dies, families have characteristic ways of being in the world, of solving problems, of managing crises, of interacting with one another, and of relating to those outside the family. When a child is seriously ill and dies, families respond in the ways that are typical for how they manage other life events. These ways of coping are more or less functional. Earlier research with families of adult patients[15] and with pediatric patients[14,16] documented eight dimensions of family functioning: communicating openly, dealing with feelings, defining roles, solving problems, using resources, incorporating changes, considering others, and confronting beliefs. These dimensions occur along a continuum of functionality so that family interactions tend to vary along the continuum rather than being positive or negative, or good or bad.[14] In families where thoughts and opinions are expressed freely without fear of recrimination, where a wide range of feelings is expressed and differences tolerated, where roles are flexible, where problem solving instead of blaming is the pattern for dealing with challenges, where families are able to ask for and receive assistance from others, and where beliefs and values are confronted and examined, the children and all family members are better able to manage their grief and support one another. The nurse's role is to assess each family's way of functioning, and to realize that some families are more difficult to assess and work with than others. For example, some families may not wish to share information in the presence of their children, others do not wish to discuss matters with any relatives in the room, while other families include everyone in most discussions. Thus, it is important for the nurse to gather information over time, and to talk with more than one family member to appreciate the varied perspectives. When families are less functional, practitioners may want to offer potential resources one at a time, with considerable attention paid to the possible disruption that would result from each suggestion. In more functional families, a list of possible options can be presented and considered all at once. The vast majority of families value the opportunity to tell their story, and thus listening becomes a central aspect of caring for all grieving families.

Social/cultural Characteristics. No one grieves in isolation from others. Individual responses are shaped by distinct social and cultural circumstances, and, in turn, each grieving person plays many roles in shaping family and community responses. Friends, extended family, and community support also influence how the family unit and individual family members function and come to terms with a child's death. A friend with a sensitive presence and listening ear can be of significant support to a grieving parent or sibling. Or, when grieving parents are challenged by the responsibilities of parenthood, a kind and supportive aunt or uncle can help to maintain a normal routine and a safe and understanding environment for the surviving siblings.

Individuals and families grieve within broader cultural contexts. Some turn to culture and tradition to find support and comfort in the answers, rituals, ceremonies, behavioral prescriptions, and spiritual practices they provide. Others do not strongly identify with the beliefs and mores of their cultures of origin, even when other members of their own family may do so. Too often culture is thought of in prescriptive ways, as if to say that we expect a member of a given community to express and process grief in the manner typical of that group. Surprisingly little attention has been paid to learning about the experiences of families from diverse cultural backgrounds when their child is seriously ill and dies. This seems a remarkable oversight, since it is broadly recognized that cultural values, beliefs, and practices play a central role in shaping how families raise and care for their children not only when they are healthy, but especially when they are seriously ill.[17] It is important to find out what each individual family member believes about the nature of death, the rituals that should surround it, and the expectations about afterlife. As well, we must remember that our modern health care systems, hospitals in particular, have their own cultural mores, which may be in conflict with the cultural beliefs and practices of families in pediatric palliative care.

Watching a child fall sick and die is a crisis of meaning for families, and it is through their cultural understandings and practices that families struggle to explain and make sense of this experience.[18] In fact, though research is sparse on the topic, there are some universal themes across cultures. One is the use of ritual and ceremony, and the other is the struggle for meaning and the questions that come to all bereaved families, whether they are whispered or cried out loud: "Why did my child (my sister, my brother, my grandchild) have to die?" "Where is the child now?" and "Will I ever see her again?"[19] Spiritual or religious rituals may help families find meaning when their child dies, but for some families, some such rituals have the potential to interfere with the expression of grief.

Situational Factors

Situational factors refer to characteristics of the situation or the circumstances surrounding the child's death. These variables include, for example, characteristics of the child's illness, such as its duration, and of the death, such as the cause and place of death, and the extent of involvement in death-related events.

Characteristics of the Child's Illness and Death. Where or when a child died, decision-making about the death, memories of sights and sounds, degree of medical intervention, and the cause of death are all subject matters that families discuss during bereavement while exploring their grief. Ideally, the location (home or hospital) of a child's death is based upon the family's specific needs and requests, but circumstances (insurance issues, nursing shortages, transportation issues) may preclude achieving this goal. Long-term outcomes for bereaved parents and siblings of home-care deaths suggest an early pattern of differential adjustment in favor of home-care deaths.[20,21]

Decisions at the end of life, such as withdrawal of life support, may have been made with parents feeling they had insufficient understanding of the situation. Lasting images or smells may be comforting or concerning to families depending upon their associations. In fact, pain or other distressing symptoms the child might have experienced provide powerful material for families to struggle with during their grief. A full code that ends with the child's death is very different than if a child slips into death from an unconscious state. Years of treatment followed by death is experienced very differently than one in which a child dies quickly.

Involvement in the Illness and Death-related Events. Growing consensus supports informing children about their medical condition and involving them in discussions and decisions about their care, appropriate for their levels of cognitive and emotional maturity.[22–24] The same is true for involving siblings in the care of the ill child and in the events surrounding the death, such as the funeral, memorial service, and burial rituals. In one study, children who were more involved in such activities had fewer behavioral problems following the death.[14] At the same time, practitioners must consider not only the individual child's capacity for involvement, but also the family's values about discussions of death, medical care, and children's roles.

Models and Theories of Grief

From Freud to the current day, several theories and models have been developed that offer conceptual frameworks for how grief manifests in human beings. It is not the purpose of this chapter to provide an in-depth description of these various theories and models, since that content is covered elsewhere within this text. But, since nursing practice is guided by such theories and models, it is important to outline the development of thinking about bereavement as a basis for implementing best practices. Theories and models of grief can be categorized into stages and phase models, medical models, and task models.

Stage and Phase Models of Grief

Models of grief based on stages and phases work on the premise that there is a beginning and an end to the grief process, with some amount of sequential progression through grief. Among stage theorists are Lindemann,[25] Bowlby,[26] Engel,[27] Kubler-Ross,[28] Parkes,[29] and Rando.[30] Common patterns among these theories are the sequential nature they suggest and the emphasis of the physical, emotional, behavioral, social, and intellectual impact of grief.

Medical Models of Grief

Some models of grief liken the process to that of healing secondary to disease, injury, or psychiatric illness. Lindemann,[25] Engel,[27] Parkes,[29] and Rando[30] are among those who discuss issues of symptoms, management, or need for clinical attention with complicated forms of grief. Beverly Raphael[31] urges that although pathological complications in grieving may be more readily equated with illness, the medical analogy is more difficult to sustain with uncomplicated grief. The overall process is articulated as a form of healing that might include issues such as helplessness, resistance to the reality of the death, preoccupation with the deceased, or identification with the deceased.

Stage and medical models have been subject to numerous criticisms in recent years. In particular, they do not capture the diversity of how we experience grief, either from an ethnocultural approach or from the perspective of the individual. Both types of models erroneously suggest that we come to an end in our grieving as we complete uniform or predictable stages or at last recover or reach "acceptance." In truth, the questions of what happens after death or what is the meaning of life are never-ending existential mysteries for all of us. And these models imply that grief is a passive response to loss, when, in fact, grief is hard work.

Task Models of Grief

Lindemann[32] was the first to coin the phrase "grief work," and he identified three tasks: relinquish attachment to the deceased, adjust to life without the deceased, and develop new relationships. Parkes and Weiss[33] and Worden[13] have also developed task models, with a central theme being the need to loosen ties to the deceased. Attig[34,35] describes the work of grieving as an active process of relearning the world, including physical surroundings, social surroundings, aspects of self, and the relationship with the deceased.

Of interest, the only model that specifically addresses grief in children is Bowlby's model, but not only do his three phases suggest a time-limited process, they also downplay the potential long-term impact of childhood bereavement. Attig's model of relearning the world may come the closest to describing how adults, as well as children and adolescents, relearn the world by summing the many smaller tasks that together make up the complex nature of living with grief. A bereaved parent may return to normal life functioning, but is never finished loving or remembering his or her child. Even if the characteristics of that grief modulate over time, there may well be some form of heartache when that child is present in parental thoughts decades after the death. In the words of a bereaved mother, "I buried my child in my heart. I will always be with him anytime and everywhere." Attig asserts that we relearn the world as whole beings, not all at once, but rather piecemeal in distinct and growth-filled encounters. Such a description aptly applies to bereaved children—they cannot take in the whole event at once, and only over time, with their whole beings, do they relearn their worlds.

A central question is how parents and other family members manage the relationship with the child who died. Given that the child is no longer physically present, what do parents, grandparents, aunts, uncles, siblings, or friends do with the bonds, feelings, thoughts, and past experiences with that child? Research studies document that grievers do, indeed, maintain lasting connections with the deceased.[14,34,36] In fact, nurses can do much to facilitate these ongoing connections by offering to assist the family to obtain a memento of their child, such as a lock of hair, a foot or handprint, a photograph taken in the hospital, a piece of artwork, or a poem written by the child.

Impact of Grief and Bereavement on Family Members

Dying Children

Children react to their own dying as they do to most of life's experiences—within their cognitive and emotional capabilities. They live and die as children, but often with much apparent wisdom, sometimes seeming to surpass that of their adult caregivers. One of the earliest studies of seriously ill children indicated that very ill children are, indeed, aware of death and are more anxious than children hospitalized for nonserious illnesses or nonhospitalized children.[37] Bluebond-Langner,[38] based on her ethnographic study of dying children, subsequently described a process of how they become aware of their own impending death (Table 54–1). The children may experience a wide range of feelings, including but not limited to anger, anxiety, sadness, loneliness and isolation, and fear. Behaviors may include avoiding the deceased fellow friends' names or staying away from their belongings; reducing attention to non–disease-related chatter and play; being preoccupied with death and disease imagery, particularly in play; engaging in open talk about the death only with selected persons; feeling anxious about weakened body functions and doubts about going home; evading talk of the future; being concerned with things being done right away; regressing, such as refusing to cooperate with relatively easy, painless procedures; or having estranged relationships with others, demonstrated by anger or silence.

Of course, we need to recognize individual variations within the above patterns, but this work provides some background

Table 54–1
The Process of Children's Perceptions of Their Own Impending Death

Stage I: An ill child's parent is shocked to face the disastrous diagnosis of his or her child. Ill children cannot be answered honestly as to what is happening to them because their parent, and even health care providers, tend to hide the worst information. Children feel that all answers from adults are not fully understandable. Children feel as if they are in the dark—"in a fog." Lastly, ill children conclude that others' responses are not like they were before, when they were sick with a simple disease. They guess themselves that they are "seriously ill," or "very, very sick."
Stage II: When status is uncertain, the children may see their relatives crying even though they are becoming accustomed to the hospitalization with the serious disease. The children also feel that their family members give them special treatment. In addition, they still suffer from some procedural pain. They are less socialized with healthy peers, and they would rather have an opportunity to join a group of ill children in any treatment setting. Through play and talk with fellow patients, they get to learn about their disease and acquire information related to the disease experiences.
Stage III: Based on the characteristics of chronic or life-threatening conditions, children experience remission and recurrence by turns. Every relapse repeatedly baffles them. They may continually take cues from their parents' behavior, often overhearing conversations between health care providers and their parents about their disease process. Their knowledge on the purposes and implications of specific treatment procedures is markedly increased. In particular, health care staffs' refusals to elaborate or vague responses such as "Well, we will see . . ." or "I don't know . . ." erode the provider's credibility. Experiencing several recurrences, many seriously ill children begin to think that their sense of well-being is fading.
Stage IV: They are increasingly aware of being different from their healthy peers. In particular, their world is rapidly transformed by the disease culture due to their disease. The biggest problem to them is the deprivation of the school experience. As sick children, they doubt they will ever get better. To them, the illness is seen as a permanent condition.
Stage V: They know the limitations of medication to cure their disease. Gradually, they can estimate a definite end, death.

Source: Bluebond-Langner M. (1978), reference 38.

for understanding terminally ill children, such as this 14-year-old boy whose death is imminent:

> My mother used to go to church to pray for me early every morning. I also prayed in my bed for my mother to stop her soundless sorrow. We were all sad and we pray separately in different places. Now, I am getting more worried about how sad she will be after my death, and she will feel lonely without me. How can I express my sorrow for her and thank her? She has lost so many things . . . money, time, and smiles, all because of me . . .

Parents

Parent-child relationships are not contractual, but sacred. They are unique and complex. The connectedness between parent and child has its roots in the biological and emotional bonds and attachments that precede birth. It grows as the parent begins to know and care for the child. The child is a parent's link to the future.[39] Parental grief is all-consuming, affecting every aspect of parents' existence.

Parents often struggle with guilt following their child's death due to deep-rooted feelings of responsibility for their child's welfare. Since parents are responsible for protecting and sustaining their children, shielding them from all danger, many parents feel they should have protected their child from illness and death. When children die from an inherited disease such as cystic fibrosis or sickle cell anemia, parents know their child's condition results from their unknowingly passing on the genetic material. When the child dies, parents may still carry the burden of knowing they "gave" their child a terminal illness. Parents whose child died from an accident may also feel guilty for abdicating their protective role. Bereaved parents may cling to irrational guilt since it is often easier to accept blame, with its fantasy of control, than the total loss of control with which they must grapple. Or, they may blame someone else for their child's death. Sometimes this guilt is targeted toward a partner or spouse, another child or family member. Nurses need to be aware of these dynamics and help a family find an appropriate place for their anger and blame.[40]

Parents, as individuals, may have different styles of grieving as described earlier. Nurses can help by acknowledging the "normality" of a variety of grieving styles and encouraging parents to understand each other's ways of grieving. Differences in bereavement response also may lead to a strain on the couple's sexual intimacy. Sexual abstinence is frequently reported by bereaved couples due to a lack of sexual interest; others seek out comfort through sexual intimacy. Again, pointing out that such reactions can be expected may help couples realize the "normalcy" of their reactions. A long-standing myth is that divorce rates among bereaved parents are very high. In fact, it is not higher than the national divorce rate. And, when divorce follows a child's death, it is usually due to problems that existed before the child's illness or death.

Nurses must also be cognizant of the special needs of bereaved parents who cope with additional stressors in their everyday lives. Single parents, or same-sex parents may not have as many options for support as married parents in a heterosexual relationship.

Moreover, nurses must pay attention to the indirect grief of parents who witness or coexperience the death of other terminally ill children in the same clinical setting as their child.[41]

Grandparents

The grief of grandparents is two-fold: they have to bear their own grief, as well as bear the agony of the grief of their own child, the parent of the deceased child. Grandparents can be a source of considerable strength for parents and siblings, or they can be an additional source of stress. Their advice may be sought but then ignored; often their practical help is accepted, but their own grief is barely acknowledged.[2] Grandparents may experience considerable helplessness and frustration; they question the meaning of life as they struggle with the "lack of order" of having the young one precede them in death.

Siblings

Siblings have been called the "forgotten grievers." They have been typically ignored when a brother or sister dies, not for lack of parental concern, but because their parents are so overcome with grief, they have little energy to devote to the needs of their surviving children. The impact of a child's death on surviving siblings is manifested in four general responses, best characterized in the words of the children themselves:[14] "I hurt inside," "I don't understand," "I don't belong," and "I'm not enough." Not all children who have a brother or sister die experience all four responses, but most children through to adolescence demonstrate all responses to varying degrees.

"I Hurt Inside." The first response includes all the emotions typically associated with grief—sadness, anger, frustration, loneliness, fear, guilt, restlessness, and a host of other emotions that characterize bereavement. Unlike adults who are able to talk about their responses, children manifest their responses in various behaviors, such as withdrawing, seeking attention, acting out, arguing, fear of going to bed at night, overeating, or undereating. In response to children who are hurting inside, nurses need to allow, and even encourage, the expression of the hurt the children are feeling. They may endeavor to share their own thoughts and feelings with the children to let them know that they are not alone in this situation. If adults do not allow children to express their feelings, siblings learn there is something wrong with such feelings. When adults are impatient with children, or belittle their expression, siblings learn to stifle their feelings.

"I Don't Understand." Children's difficulty in understanding death is greatly influenced by their level of cognitive development. However, once children know about death, their cognitive worlds are forever altered. If they are not helped to understand what has happened in clear, simple, and age-appropriate ways, children make up their own explanations that usually involve taking responsibility for the death and their parents' distress. Without explanations, they become more frightened and insecure. Nurses must have a solid grasp of children's cognitive development, provide appropriate explanations for events that happen, and be open to questions from children.

"I Don't Belong." A death in the family tears apart the usual day-to-day activities and patterns of living. Parents are overwhelmed with their grief, with making arrangements, and with caring for their other children. Surviving children are overwhelmed with the flurry of activity and the depth of emotion surrounding them. They often feel as if they don't know what to do; they may want to help, but they don't know what to do, or, if they try, their efforts are not acknowledged. They begin to feel as if they are in the way, or as if they are not a part of what is happening. They feel different from their peers as well, and begin to feel as if they don't belong anymore. Nurses can play a critical role in including siblings in illness- and death-related events, such as encouraging or teaching the child to participate in certain treatments (for example, by holding their sibling's hand or blowing bubbles together during painful procedures). After death, the nurse can help the parents by modeling what to say to the children.

"I'm Not Enough." Assuming that they are somehow responsible for their parents' distress, siblings may feel as if they are not enough to make their parents happy ever again. They may feel that their deceased brother or sister was the favorite child, and they should have been the ones to die instead. Some siblings respond by striving to be as good as they can be, trying to prove that they are worthy. They must be made to feel special just for being themselves, and by not comparing them to their deceased brother or sister. Moreover, siblings may not want to burden their parents with their grief, knowing their parents are already overladen. Nurses can assist siblings to feel special by asking them questions about their lives and reassuring them of their value and unique characteristics or abilities.

Adolescents

Teenagers who are dying, or who are the siblings or friends of another child, are often overlooked.[42] They face a particularly complicated situation when they encounter death and bereavement because adolescents are typically engrossed in achieving independence and in proving their invulnerability. Serious illness and grief catches them by surprise, as they seldom have developed the coping skills necessary to deal with their reactions. As well, many adults believe it is difficult to help adolescents cope with death because adolescents are reputed to turn away from adults and to talk only with other adolescents. This is not entirely true, as these young people often seek out and value the input and support of adults they respect, such as a teacher, a nurse, or a friend's parent. Moreover, when adolescents turn to their peers, if they do, they may often find that their peers have no significant resources to offer because they too are inexperienced with death.

Dying adolescents with a terminal disease struggle against physical pain, are sensitive to their parents' reactions, and have a strong desire to have relationships with their friends regardless of their illness status: "I couldn't say anything with my Mom. She pretends to smile to me, but I know how she feels so sad whenever looking at me. I want to come out and share my emotions with my friend at least. But, now there is nobody around me." In such cases, nurses are in a position to help an adolescent's family members to understand adolescent cognitive and psychosocial functioning. Self-help support groups for teens, either in person or via the Internet, often prove valuable to grieving adolescents. Adolescents are often open to writing, art, or music. Adults may come along on such journeys, or share the results, but they should take care to follow the adolescents' lead, respecting confidentiality and permitting them to interpret the significance of their work in their own way.

Assessing Grief

Bereavement care is interdisciplinary in nature, focusing on assessment of the comprehensive pattern and character of the whole family, as well as of individuals within the family. Grief assessment focuses on the ill child, other family members, and their significant others. Grief assessment begins when the child is admitted to the hospital or at the time of diagnosis of acute, chronic, or terminal illness. It is ongoing throughout the course of the child's illness and comes to the forefront during the bereavement period after the death. Nurses, in particular, play a central role in a family's initial bereavement experience. Most children's deaths still occur in the hospital; nurses are most often present at the time of death. If not with the child at the moment of death, the nurse is usually the first one called to the child's bedside. The nurse's words and actions at that time leave indelible imprints upon parents. Even years after their child's death, parents recall vivid memories of the nurse's gentle approach in offering privacy, giving a hug, sharing the sadness, allowing families the amount of time they want with their child before leaving the hospital. Unfortunately, other parents remember the nurse who spoke abruptly to them, or rushed them away because their child's room had to be made ready for the next patient. In even these brief interactions, nurses can do so much to prevent this devastating experience from being any worse than it already is for the family.

In assessing grief, clinicians should keep in mind the range of factors that impact upon the grief of family members, while noting those factors that put individuals and families at risk for disenfranchised or complicated grief. The passage of time is not a useful consideration in assessing grief responses; instead, we must assess the degree of intrusiveness into each individual's life and the extent to which family members can carry out their usual activities.

Helping Bereaved Families

Grief assessment leads to a plan of care with the goal of facilitating and supporting the grieving process. Understanding grief as a normal, human process that is individually expressed enables practitioners to present an accepting, nonjudgmental attitude that helps create a respectful and trusting milieu. The approach to children or other family members experiencing anticipatory grief is the same as for family members whose child has died, but the focus of some interventions may differ. For example, prior to death, families should be offered information about the signs and symptoms of disease progression and the dying process; following death, the focus may be on listening to family members review the course of the child's dying.

Grief Interventions

For Families

Bereaved individuals need an opportunity to express their grief in a supportive environment. Nurses have a responsibility to create such an environment for parents and other family members following a child's death so that they feel it is okay for them to express whatever they are feeling. Such comments as "It must be very difficult for you right now" give permission for expression. The form of expression may vary among family members; some will verbalize, others will cry, some may leave the room. Still others may express anger, and others appreciation.

Nurses may fear "saying the wrong thing" to a family member, or may fear not knowing what to say, or feel they must have the "right thing to say." Attitudes are conveyed through words and more importantly, through actions. Thus, it is usually best to say very little, avoiding clichés and euphemisms that can be so distressing to grieving individuals. It is not appropriate to encourage anyone to "Keep a stiff upper lip" or to "Look on the bright side." It is disrespectful, and even cruel, to say "He is no longer suffering" or "You are young—you will have more children." These messages, whether given directly or indirectly, may compound the pain by making family members think the clinicians do not understand their loss. Instead, sit or stand quietly close to the family, let them know they can stay with their child for as long as they would like, comment on the child's special qualities and acknowledge your own sadness about the child's death. Offering to help in practical and concrete ways is also helpful. However, rather than asking if "there is anything I can help you with," offer to do specific things, such as making phone calls or getting them a glass of water. Most family members have a need to share their story, telling and retelling anecdotes about the child and the events of his living and dying. Listening to their stories is probably the most helpful action. For some families, reviewing what happened with their child with the care providers is critical. Follow-up phone calls or visits with the providers who cared for the child are much appreciated by families.

Many family members who are unaware of the normal manifestations of grief can find some comfort in knowing that their pain is normal. Providing information about the common facts of grief can be helpful; having written materials to send home with families is even better. Understanding that each person's grief experience is unique helps family members understand that there is "no right way to grieve." It also helps them to realize they are not "bad" or "crazy" if they express their grief differently from other family members; it also may prevent family member from telling other family members how they "should" grieve. Clinicians should identify any need for additional assistance and make referrals as needed. For example, a family member may have spiritual concerns that would be best addressed by the pastoral care person; a social worker may assist with funeral arrangements or financial concerns. In addition, the nurse should make referrals to bereavement specialists, psychologists, or physicians as needed.

For Children

Since grief is a human response, children and adults alike feel denial, anger, sadness, guilt, longing in response to a loved one, and experience lack of sleep, lack of appetite, and difficulty concentrating and maintaining usual patterns of interaction with others. However, most children have limited ability to verbalize and describe their feelings; they also have very limited capacity to tolerate the emotional pain generated by open recognition of their loss.[43] Moreover, children's cognitive developmental level interferes with their ability to understand the irreversibility, universality, and inevitability of death, and to understand the reactions of their parents. They also deeply fear being different in any way from their peers, and so are often unable to find comfort, as adults do, in sharing their discomfort with their friends. As play is the work and the language of childhood, children are able to express their feelings through their play, as well as music and art. A summary of grief reactions in children, according to age level, and corresponding suggested interventions, is presented in Table 54–2.

For Parents

Before the child's death, an important emphasis for clinicians is to facilitate connections between the parents and the ill child and their other children, as well by helping them develop memories and keepsakes that they can hold and cherish long after the death. The earlier these can be collected, the better, so they reflect a longer period of time with the child and not simply the final days of life. Facilitating communication between family members and the caregiving staff, as well as among family members themselves, also creates positive memories and optimal coping. Informing parents about the dying process, and helping them with the concept of appropriate death consistent with patient, family, cultural, and spiritual goals is necessary. Assisting with planning funeral or memorial services

Table 54–2
Grief and Bereavement in Children

Characteristics of Age	View of Death and Response	What Helps
Birth to 6 Months		
Basic needs must be met, cries if needs aren't met Needs emotional and physical closeness of a consistent caregiver Derives identity from caregiver Views caregiver as source of comfort and all needs fulfillment Developing trust	Has no concept of death Experiences death like any other separation—no sense of "finality" Nonspecific expressions of distress (crying) Reacts to loss of caregiver Reacts to caregiver's distress	Progressively disengage child from primary caregiver if possible. Introduce a new primary caregiver. Nurture and comfort. Anticipate physical and emotional needs and provide them. Maintain routines.
6 Months to 2 Years		
Begins to individuate Remembers face of caregiver when absent Demonstrates full range of emotions Identifies caregiver as source of good feelings and interactions	May see death as reversible Experiences bona fide grief Grief response only to death of significant person in child's life Screams, panics, withdraws, becomes disinterested in food, toys, activities Reacts in concert with distress experienced by caregiver No control over feelings and responses; anticipate regressive behavior	Needs continual support, comfort Avoid separation from significant others. Close physical and emotional connections by significant others Maintain daily structure and schedule of routine activities. Support caregiver to reduce distress and maintain a stable environment. Acknowledge sadness that loved one will not return—offer comfort.
2 Years to 5 Years		
Egocentric Cause–effect not understood Developing conscience Attributes life to objects Feelings expressed mostly by behaviors Can recall events from past	Sees death like sleep, that is, reversible Believes in magical causes Has sense of loss Curiosity, questioning Anticipate regression, clinging Aggressive behavior common Worries about who will care for them	Remind that loved one will not return. Reassure child that he or she is not to blame. Give realistic information and answer questions. Involve in "farewell" ceremonies. Encourage questions and expression of feelings. Keep home environment stable and structured. Help put words to feelings; reassure and comfort. Reassure children about who will take care of them; provide ways to remember loved one.
5 Years to 9 Years		
Attributes life to things that move; may fear the dark Begins to develop intellect Begins to relate cause and effect; understands consequences Literal, concrete Decreasing fantasy life, increasing control of feelings	Personifies death as ghosts, bogeyman Interest in biological aspects of life and death Begins to see death as irreversible May see death as punishment; may feel responsible Problems concentrating on tasks; may deny or hide feelings, vulnerability	Give clear and realistic information. Include child in funeral ceremonies if they choose. Give permission to express feelings and provide opportunities; reduce guilt by providing factual information. Maintain structured schedule, individual and family activities; needs strong parent. Notify school of what is occurring, gentle confirmation, reassurance.

(*continued*)

Table 54–2
Grief and Bereavement in Children (*continued*)

Characteristics of Age	View of Death and Response	What Helps
Preadolescent through Teens	Views death as permanent	Unambiguous information
Individuation outside home	Sense of own mortality; sense of future	Provide opportunities to express self, feelings; encourage outside relationships with mentors.
Identifies with peer group; needs family attachment	Strong emotional reaction; may regress, revert to fantasy	
Understands life processes; can verbalize feelings	May somaticize, intellectualize, morbid preoccupation	Provide tangible means to remember loved one; encourage self-expression, verbal and nonverbal.
Physical maturation		Dispel fears about physical concerns; educate about maturation; provide outlets for energy and strong feelings (recreation, sports, etc.); needs mentoring and direction.

Source: Fine P. (1998), reference 48. Reprinted with permission.

also can be helpful, particularly for families who have limited support systems.

After the child's death, follow-up by the clinicians who cared for the child is much appreciated by families. Such follow-up also allows ongoing assessment (See Table 54-3 for questions to ask during an initial follow-up telephone call). Parents, overcome with their own grief, may need assistance in dealing with the needs of their other children; encourage parents to enlist the support of aunts, uncles, or good friends in this regard. For parents who are willing and interested in finding additional support, provide a listing of parental support groups and other parent bereavement resources in the community, such as Compassionate Friends, a self-help organization to help parents and siblings after the death of a child (http://www.compassionatefriends.org).

Bereavement Programs

The development of pediatric palliative care programs, including bereavement programs, in health care institutions has increased notably in the past decade despite budget and other resource concerns. Still, the dearth of consistency and excellence in both the training of professionals and the offering of services to families results in many gaps in the experiences of families. Such gaps must be addressed, especially for families of children who had a chronic illness that meant frequent trips to the hospital, sometimes over many years, and resulted in the development of close relationships with staff members. Such families worry that the staff will forget their deceased child; some families want to maintain an ongoing relationship with those who cared for their child. Thus, during the transition after the child's death, families and staff have to navigate the changing relationship.[44] A bereavement program within pediatric palliative care, or as part of an agency-wide program, can be of considerable service to both families and staff. Such

Table 54–3
Questions for an Initial Follow-up Telephone Call to Parents Who Have Experienced the Loss of a Child or Perinatal Loss

"You might recall that you were told that someone from the hospital would call you in (number) weeks . . ."

"Is this a good time to talk?"

"Are there any issues that you have been thinking about that perhaps I could follow-up on for you?"

"Have you been back yet for a postpartum check-up?"

"Some parents have noticed a change in their sleeping or eating habits. Has this been a problem for you?"

"How has (name of other parent) responded to your loss? Sometimes it is hard for both parents to talk about it. How has it been for you?"

"Do you have other family members or friends that you have been able to talk to? What types of things have they been able to do for you?"

"Do you have plans to work outside of your home? The first few days at work can be especially difficult. Have you thought about how it might be for you?"

"Did you receive any information on support groups for parents?"

"Are there any other materials you received in the hospital that you have questions about?"

"Are there any other questions I can answer for you?"

"During the call you stated that . . ."

"I will call you again on (date)."

Source: Friedrichs et al. (2000), reference 49. Permission granted by Baywood Publishing Co., Inc.

a program facilitates referral of families to grief therapists as needed, ensures that all families are made aware of the available services, such as support groups, memorial services, or grief workshops. These services also facilitate bereaved families connecting with the staff who cared for their child, and most importantly, with one another as a source of support. The existence of a bereavement program gives a clear message that an institution and its staff are committed to the care of families.

The Nurse: Death Anxiety, Cumulative Loss, and Grief

Professionals who help children and families with the serious illness and death of a child are witness to numerous heart-wrenching scenes, and are constantly reminded of the frailty and preciousness of life. Working with dying children can trigger nurses' awareness of their own personal losses and fears about their own death, the death of their own children, and mortality in general. Historically, nurses and other health care professionals were taught to desensitize themselves to these experiences and to maintain an "emotional detachment." This approach, which still exists today in many situations, results in the nurses' use of defenses to allay their fears, including focusing only on physical care needs, evading emotionally sensitive conversations with children and families, and talking only superficially about topics that are comfortable for the nurse. These behaviors result in emotional distancing, avoidance, and withdrawal from dying children and their families at a time when children most need intensive interpersonal care and active involvement by the nurse. Death anxiety occurs when clinicians are confronted with fears about death and have few resources or support systems to explore and to express thoughts and emotions about dying and death.[45] Thus, rather than a "desensitization" of oneself, professionals are encouraged to sensitize to this powerful human material. Caring for dying children requires nurses to explore, experience, and express their personal feelings regarding death. Personal death-awareness activities and exercises, discussion of belief systems about death/afterlife with friends and colleagues, self-exploration, and reflection may promote an understanding and acceptance of death as part of life. The process is complicated by cumulative loss, a succession of losses experienced by nurses who work with patients with life-threatening illness and their families, often on a daily basis.[46] When nurses are exposed to death frequently, they seldom have time to grieve one child before another child dies.

Harper[47] has put forth a model of how professional caregivers learn over time to move through the pain of providing this kind of care. Her five-step model (Table 54–4), about caring for dying children, starts with intellectualization of the experience, and is characterized by attainment of knowledge and anxiety about performance. She goes on to describe caregivers moving through emotional survival, depression, and emotional arrival. Finally, and only after working through the personal pain of grief work, caregivers arrive at a place of deep compassion for families, characterized by self-realization and self-actualization on the part of the caregiver. Self-awareness about one's own personal history of loss is necessary to know one's own set of beliefs about death, dying, and the afterlife. Without this awareness, our own beliefs and cultural/spiritual biases can interfere with the experience of the family. For caregivers, strong coping techniques, good self care and ongoing education and support are necessary components to not only do the work, but also to avoid burnout.

Several factors influence nurses' adaptation to the inherent grief in pediatric palliative care. They include the nurses' professional training and other training in dealing with dying, death, and grief; nurses' personal and professional history of loss and possible unresolved issues of dealing with grief; personal and professional life changes; and the presence or absence of support systems.

In one study of nurses' experiences following the death of a child, participants described two types of distress. Moral distress resulted when the nurses knew the child's death was imminent and were required to carry out painful treatments they perceived as unnecessary. Grief distress occurred in response to the child's death. Both types of distress resulted from lack of open communication within the care team and lack of consideration of the nurses' viewpoints.[45] Thus, systems of support are critical to nurses' coping with the stress of working with seriously ill children and their families. In addition to helping bereaved families, as mentioned earlier, institutional bereavement programs also serve the needs of staff. Programs can be structured to offer help in debriefing after a death, validating staff feelings, offering support groups, and encouraging informal support through the one-one-one sharing of experiences with coworkers, peers, or pastoral care workers. The presence of a supervisor, mentor, or instructor during the care of the dying, when a family member visits, or during the time of the child's death can greatly decrease anxiety and provide immense support to the nurse, particularly to novice nurses in pediatric palliative care. Education that enhances knowledge and skills in end-of-life care can promote competence and self-confidence. Education that describes families' experiences can be invaluable because it empowers clinicians to offer care that is more sensitive to the needs of families, more humanistic, and more family centered and thus, more rewarding to staff. Nurses have responsibilities for acknowledging their own personal and professional limitations, seeking assistance, and engaging in self-care activities.

Pediatric palliative care is a challenging field, one that demands finding the balance between providing compassionate quality care and personal satisfaction as a professional nurse. In addition, working with dying children and their families provides meaning to life. Working with these children helps to develop a clear perspective of what is really valuable; it helps us grow as persons and professionals. From the children and their families, we learn that death is part of life, that human beings are remarkably resilient, and that hope is everlasting.

Table 54–4
Coping with Professional Anxiety in Terminal Illness

Stage I 0–3 months: *Intellectualization*	**Stage II** 3–6 months: *Emotional Survival*	**Stage III** 6–9 months: *Depression*	**Stage IV** 9–12 months: *Emotional Arrival*	**Stage V** 12–24 months: *Deep Compassion*
Professional knowledge	Increasing professional knowledge	Deepening of professional knowledge	Acceptance of professional knowledge	Refining of professional knowledge
Intellectualization	Less intellectualization	Decreasing intellectualization	Normal intellectualization	Refining intellectual base
Anxiety	Emotional survival	Depression	Emotional arrival	Deep compassion
Some uncomfortableness	Increasing uncomfortableness	Decreasing uncomfortableness	Increasing comfortableness	Increased comfortableness
Agreeableness	Guilt	Pain	Moderation	Self-realization
Withdrawal	Frustration	Mourning	Mitigation	Self-awareness
Superficial acceptance	Sadness	Grieving	Accommodation	Self-actualization
Providing tangible services	Initial emotional involvement	More emotional involvement	Ego mastery	Professional satisfaction
Utilization of emotional energy on understanding the setting	Increasing emotional involvement	Overidentification with the resident	Coping with loss of relationship	Acceptance of death and loss
Familiarizing self with policies and procedures	Initial understanding of the magnitude of the area of practice	Exploration of own feelings about death	Freedom from concern about own death	Rewarding professional growth and development
Working with families rather than residents	Overidentification with the resident's situation	Facing own death	Developing strong ties with dying residents and families	Development of ability to give of one's self
		Coming to grips with feelings about death	Development of ability to work with, on behalf of and for the dying resident	Human and professional assessment
			Development of professional competence	Constructive and appropriate activities
			Productivity and accomplishments	Development of feelings of dignity and self-respect
			Healthy interaction	Ability to give dignity and self-respect to dying resident
				Comfortableness

Source: Harper, B.C. (1994), reference 47. Reprinted with permission.

REFERENCES

1. Field MJ, Behrman RE, eds. When Children Die: Improving Palliative and End-of-Life Care For Children and Their Families. Washington, DC: Institute of Medicine of the National Academies Press, 2003.
2. Goldman A. Care of the Dying Child. Oxford: Oxford University Press, 1994.
3. DeSpelder LA, Strickland AL. The Last Dance: Encountering Death and Dying, 3rd ed. Mountain View, CA: Mayfield, 1992.
4. Sanders CM. A comparison of adult bereavement in the death of a spouse, child, and parent. Omega 1980;10:303–321.

5. The Compact Edition of the Oxford English Dictionary. Oxford: Oxford University Press, 1971.
6. Silverman PR. Never Too Young to Know: Death in Children's Lives. New York: Oxford University Press, 2000.
7. Corless IB. Bereavement. In: Ferrell BR, Coyle N, eds. Textbook of Palliative Nursing. New York: Oxford University Press, 2001:35.
8. Rando TA. Clinical Dimensions of Anticipatory Mourning. Champaign, IL: Research Press, 2000.
9. Rando TA. Grief, Dying and Death: Clinical Interventions for Caregivers. Champaign, IL: Research Press, 1984.
10. Doka K. Disenfranchised Grief: Recognizing Hidden Sorrow. New York: Lexington Books, 1989.
11. Doka K. Disenfranchised Grief: New Directions, Challenges and Strategies for Practice. Champaign, IL: Research Press, 2002.
12. Prigerson HG, Jacobs SC. Perspectives on care at the close of life. Caring for bereaved patients: "All the doctors just suddenly go." JAMA 2001;286:1369–1376.
13. Worden JW. Grief Counseling and Grief Therapy: A Handbook for the Mental Health Practitioner, 2nd ed. New York: Springer, 1991.
14. Davies B. Shadows in the Sun: The Experience of Sibling Bereavement. Philadelphia: Brunner/Mazel, 1999.
15. Davies B, Reimer J, Brown P, Martens N. Fading Away: The Experience of Transition in Families With Terminal Illness. Amityville, NY: Baywood Publishing, 1995.
16. Davies B, Spinetta J, Martinson I, McClowry S, Kulenkamp E. Manifestations of levels of functioning and grieving families. J Fam Issues 1987;7:297–313.
17. Die Trill M, Kovalcik R. The child with cancer: influence of culture on truth-telling and patient care. Ann NY Acad Sci 1997; 809:197–210.
18. McGrath BB. Illness as a problem of meaning: moving culture from the classroom to the clinic. Adv Nurs Sci 1998;21:17–29.
19. Miller S. Finding Hope When A Child Dies: What Other Cultures Can Teach Us. New York: Simon & Schuster, 1999.
20. Lauer ME, Mulhern RL, Hoffman RG, Schell MJ, Camitta BM. Children's perceptions of their sibling's death at home or hospital: the precursors of differential adjustment. Cancer Nurs 1985; 8:21–27.
21. Mulhern RL, Lauer ME, Hoffman CB. Death of a child at home or in the hospital: subsequent psychological adjustment of the family. Pediatrics 1983;71:743–747.
22. Hilden JM, Emanuel EJ, Fairclough DL, Link MP, Foley KM, Clarridge BC, et al. Attitudes and practices among pediatric oncologists regarding end-of-life care: results of the 1998 American Society of Clinical Oncology Survey. J Clin Oncol 2001; 19:205–212.
23. Hinds PS, Oakes L, Furman W, Quargnenti A, Olson MS, Foppiano P, et al. End-of-life decision making by adolescents, parents, and healthcare providers in pediatric oncology. Cancer Nurs 2001; 24:122–134.
24. Nitschke R, Meyer WH, Huszti HC. When the tumor is not the target, tell the children. J Clin Oncol 2001;19:595–596.
25. Lindemann E. Symptomatology and management of acute grief. Am J Psychiatr 1944;101:141–148.
26. Bowlby J. Attachment and loss. New York: Basic Books, 1969.
27. Engel GL. Grief and grieving. Am J Nurs 1964;64:93–98.
28. Kubler-Ross E. On Death and Dying. New York: Macmillan, 1969.
29. Parkes CM. Bereavement: Studies of Grief in Adult Life, 3rd ed. New York: Routledge, 2001.
30. Rando TA. Parental Loss of a Child. Champaign, IL: Research Press, 1986.
31. Raphael B. The Anatomy of Bereavement. Champaign, IL: Research Press, 1983.
32. Lindemann E. Symptomatology and management of acute grief. Am J Psychiatr 1994;151:155–160.
33. Parkes CM, Weiss R. Recovery From Bereavement. New York: Basic Books, 1983.
34. Attig TW. How We Grieve: Relearning the World. New York: Oxford University Press, 1996.
35. Attig TW. The Heart of Grief: Death and the Search For Everlasting Love. New York: Oxford University Press, 2000.
36. Klass D, Silverman PR, Nickman SL. Continuing Bonds: New Understandings of Grief. Philadelphia: Taylor & Francis, 1996.
37. Waechter EH. Children's awareness of fatal illness. Am J Nurs 1971;71:1168–1172.
38. Bluebond-Langner M. How terminally ill children come to know themselves and their world. In: The Private Worlds of Dying Children. Princeton: Princeton University Press, 1978:166–197.
39. Arnold JH, Gemma PB, eds. A Child Dies: A Portrait of Family Grief, 2nd ed. Philadelphia: The Charles Press, 1994.
40. Worden JW, Monahan JR. Caring for bereaved parents. In: Armstrong-Daley A, Zarbock S, eds. Hospice Care For Children, 2nd ed. New York: Oxford University Press, 2001:137–156.
41. James L, Johnson B. The needs of parents of pediatric oncology patients during the palliative care phase. J Pediatr Oncol Nurs 1997;14:83–95.
42. Christ GH, Siegel K, Christ AE. Adolescent grief: "It never really hit me . . . until it actually happened." JAMA 2002;288:1269–1278.
43. Webb NB. Helping Bereaved Children. New York: The Guilford Press, 2002.
44. McKlindon D, Barnsteiner J. Therapeutic relationships: evolution of the Children's Hospital of Philadelphia Model. Matern Child Nurs 1999;24:237–243.
45. Davies B, Clarke D, Connaughty S, Cook K, MacKenzie B, McCormick J, et al. Caring for dying children: nurses' experiences. Pediatr Nurs 1996;22:500–507.
46. Vachon MLS. The nurse's role: the world of palliative care nursing. In: Ferrell BR, Coyle N, eds. Textbook of Palliative Nursing. New York: Oxford University Press, 2001:647–662.
47. Harper BC. Death: The Coping Mechanisms of the Health Care Professional. Greenville, SC: Southeastern University Press, 1994.
48. Fine P, ed. Processes to Optimize Care During the Last Phase Of Life. Scottsdale, AZ: Vista Care Hospice, Inc., 1998.
49. Friedrichs J, Daly MI, Kavanaugh K. Follow-up of parents who experience a perinatal loss: facilitating grief and assessing for grief complicated by depression. Illness, Crisis & Loss 2000; 8(3):302.

55

Mary Layman Goldstein, Maura Byrnes-Casey, and John J. Collins

Pediatric Pain: Knowing the Child Before You

The worst part of being sick and going to hospital are the needles. I hate needles. . . .—Joey, age 7, receiving treatment for acute lymphoblastic leukemia

- ***Key Points***
- *Pain assessment depends on the child's age and cognitive developmental stage.*
- *Analgesic doses are initiated according to the child's chronological age and body weight (milligrams or micrograms per kilogram).*
- *Pain management plans are based on the child's past experiences, developmental level, present response, and physical, emotional, and cultural factors.*
- *The child and parent are the unit of care. Parental involvement is key to successful interventions. Parents/caregivers must be included in assessment and pain management plans.*

Pain, a source of suffering, is present in many children—those who are facing a potentially life-threatening illness and those who are not. Expert pain management is a necessary part of pediatric palliative care.[1] It is possible for very young children to feel and express pain. A child's ability to communicate pain is influenced by age and cognitive level.[2] Even a preverbal child can communicate pain. To effectively manage an individual child's pain, the nurse first must be aware of the possibility of pain, sensitively observe the child, and use developmentally appropriate, objective assessments. Developmental factors (physical, emotional, and cognitive) play an important role in both pediatric pain assessment and pain management. Through knowledge of these factors and an awareness of how they affect an individual child, it is possible for nurses to effect better management of each child's pain (Table 55–1). Despite a significant increase in interest and in the study of pediatric pain and its control over the last 20 years, there often remains a gap between what is technically possible and what is clinically practiced.[3]

Definitions of Pain and Other Relevant Terms

There are two very useful definitions of pain. The first states that pain is "an unpleasant emotional experience associated with actual or potential tissue damage or described in terms of such damage."[4] The second, which stresses the subjective nature of pain and was stated by Margo McCaffery, RN, in 1968, is that "pain is whatever the experiencing person says it is, experienced whenever they say they are experiencing it."[5]

Nociception is "the perception by the nerves of injurious influences or painful stimuli."[6] This term is frequently used in discussions of pain in the neonate because of the challenges in evaluating the newborn's ability to be conscious to the perception of pain. A neonate is a newborn baby who may be preterm or up to 1 month of age.[7]

Table 55–1
Questions to Answer When Evaluating a Child with Pain

Useful Questions	Clinical Implications of Answers
What is the chronological age of this child?	Age-related physiological development affects pharmacokinetic and pharmacodynamic effects of medications In the neonate, normal neuroanatomical and neurobiological developmental processes occur and allow for transmission of painful stimuli
What is the developmental stage of this child? • Neonate • Infant • Toddler • Preschooler/young child • School-age child • Adolescent	Developmental age helps determine • How a child might express his or her pain • Which assessment tools may be useful • What cognitive-behavioral techniques might be considered
What type of pain does this child have? • Acute pain • Chronic pain • Procedural pain	The particular situation can guide the clinician to a developmentally appropriate assessment tool and a situation-specific pain management plan that includes both pharmacological and nonpharmacological interventions.
Does this child have a chronic illness?	Certain painful conditions have disease-specific, validated pain assessment tools. For example, the Douleur Enfant Gustave Roussy (DEGR) scale is available to assess prolonged pain in 2- to 6-year-olds with cancer*
Is this child neurologically impaired?	Cognitively impaired children may process information and communicate distress differently from normally developed children† Besides knowing the science, and the individual child, it may help to know other children with similar conditions‡ New pain assessment tools for children with intellectual disabilities are being validated to look at generic, procedural, and surgical pain.
Does this child and do the parents of this child speak the same language as the health care providers?	Find ways of obtaining translators Some pain assessment tools are available in translated versions It may be worth having pain assessment tools translated into languages common to certain practice settings.
What is the underlying cause of this pain?	If the underlying cause is treatable, the pain may be reduced or eliminated
What is the weight in kilograms of this child?	Dosage of analgesics is expressed in milligrams or micrograms per kilogram For some medications, the starting dose depends on the child's being larger or smaller than a set weight

(continued)

Table 55–1
Questions to Answer When Evaluating a Child with Pain *(continued)*

Useful Questions	Clinical Implications of Answers
Is the oral route of drug administration used whenever possible?	Besides being a cheaper and less invasive route (with less potential for pain and infection), the oral route in children provides more reliable absorption.
Are there any obvious, outstanding barriers that may be playing a role in this child's pain assessment and management?	Some barriers can be directly and quickly addressed with minimal effect and maximal positive impact.
Have nonpharmacological pain interventions been considered?	Nonpharmacological pain interventions based on the etiology of a child's pain can improve the comprehensiveness and effectiveness of a pain management plan

*Gauvain-Piquard et al. (1999), reference 54.
†Van Dongen et al. (2002), reference 55.
‡Hunt et al. (1995), reference 56.

One term that is frequently encountered in the subject of pediatric pain is procedural pain. Procedural pain is pain that is caused by procedures (e.g., needlesticks, heel punctures, lumbar punctures). All children who interact with the health care system potentially experience procedural pain.

Conscious sedation has been defined by the American Academy of Pediatrics[8] as "a medically controlled state of depressed consciousness that (1) allows protective reflexes to be maintained; (2) retains the patient's ability to maintain a patent airway independently and continuously; and (3) permits appropriate response by the patient to physical stimulation or verbal command" (p. 1110).

Prevalence of Pain in Children

Clinicians working with children in the general pediatric area will encounter pain in children who are undergoing immunizations and procedures and those who have pharyngitis, oral viral infections, otitis media, urinary tract infections, headache, or traumatic injuries. Conditions such as meningitis and necrotizing colitis can cause pain in children. Children who experience chronic diseases such as cancer, human immunodeficiency virus (HIV) infection, sickle cell disease (SCD), juvenile chronic arthritis (JCA), and cystic fibrosis (CF) also will have pain.[6,9] Definitive studies focusing on the prevalence of pain in the pediatric population are lacking. At best, we have studies that look at the incidence of pain in various disease subpopulations. Children with certain conditions are prone to particular pain syndromes. Nurses working with children need knowledge of the pain syndromes they may commonly encounter in the populations they work with and need to feel comfortable assessing and managing those particular pain syndromes.

Etiology of Pain in Children

Neuropathic Pain

Neuropathic pain is less common in children than in adults. Many of the neuropathic pain syndromes seen in adults are not seen as frequently in children. Children may experience neuropathic pain from migraine headaches, scar neuromas after surgery, phantom limb pain after amputations for trauma, tumors, meningococcemia, and complex regional pain syndromes (reported in preteen and teenage girls). Although diabetes is increasing in incidence in the pediatric population, it is rare to see a child who has diabetic neuropathy, a syndrome that takes years to develop. Brachial plexus avulsion, an injury that sometimes occurs to babies during childbirth, is thought by some to be less disabling and painful in babies than when it occurs (for other reasons) in adults. It is not clear whether this is due to inadequate assessment of infants or to the physical developmental functions of babies.[10]

Burns

Burns, thermal injuries caused by hot liquids, flames, and electricity, are among the most common causes of injury to children and are associated with pain. This injury, which destroys the skin, can have significant morbidity and mortality depending on the extent of the burn. Intact skin is necessary for protection against bacterial infection, fluid and electrolyte balance, and thermoregulation. Treatment of severe burns is associated with significant pain. Undertreatment of this pain can make it difficult for the child to cooperate with burn treatment. It is postulated that use in children of an individualized pain management plan with high-quality pain control components, such as intravenous opioids, local block, or even general anesthesia, can avoid the development of a postburn hyperalgesia syndrome caused by continuous or repeated stimulation of nociceptive afferent fibers.[11]

Cancer

As recently as 1998, the World Health Organization (WHO) stated that 70% of children with cancer will experience severe pain during their illness.[12] The types of pain in children with cancer, whether caused by procedures, by the disease or tumor, or by anticancer treatment, have been well described for many years.[12–15] A study by Ljungman and colleagues[16] of children receiving treatment for cancer revealed that procedure- and treatment-related pain were significant problems initially and that procedure-related pain gradually decreased but treatment-related pain remained constant. In addition, children with cancer may have pain for unrelated reasons, such as acute appendicitis.[13]

All children with cancer are at risk for procedural pain. Most procedure-related pain involves needle puncture. This procedure may be necessary for obtaining blood supplies, accessing implanted venous devices, administering intravenous chemotherapeutics, or giving intramuscular or subcutaneous medications. Lumbar punctures (using a spinal needle) or bone marrow aspiration (involving insertion of a large needle into the posterior superior iliac spine) are variations of needle puncture.[13] Some children develop prolonged post–lumbar puncture headaches.[12] Despite significant efforts to avoid needlesticks in the pediatric population, sometimes a needle puncture is necessary and cannot be avoided. Removal of tunneled central venous catheters or implanted ports also causes procedural pain and must be addressed by clinicians caring for the children undergoing this procedure.[13]

For some children, it is the experience of tumor-related pain that leads their parents to seek medical attention and eventual diagnosis. This pain can be nociceptive or neuropathic. Nociceptive pain can be somatic, caused by tumor involvement with bone or soft tissue, or visceral, caused by tumor infiltration, compression, or distention of abdominal or thoracic viscera. Neuropathic pain can be caused by tumor involvement (i.e., compression or infiltration) with the peripheral or central nervous system.

Most children who receive a diagnosis of cancer, no matter what the stage, will receive some sort of anti-cancer treatment. Frequently this treatment causes some sort of pain, either acute or chronic. Surgery leads to acute, postoperative pain. Removal of limbs may lead to the development of phantom limb sensations and pain. This experience is thought to decrease over time in children.[13] Radiation therapy may lead to an acute dermatitis or pain. Children undergoing chemotherapy are at risk acutely for mucositis pain and gastritis from repeated vomiting (if nausea and vomiting are not successfully controlled)[14] and chronically for neuropathic pain from certain chemotherapies. Children who have been treated with high doses of steroids are at risk for development of avascular necrosis, a disabling condition that eventually causes the affected bone to collapse. Some chemotherapies, such as vincristine, asparaginase, and cyclophosphamide, can cause pain or painful conditions such as peripheral neuropathy, constipation, hemorrhagic cystitis, or pancreatitis. Complications of intravenous chemotherapy administration may lead to pain from irritation, infiltration, extravasation, tissue necrosis (if vesicants are used), or the development of thrombophlebitis. Children receiving intrathecal chemotherapy may develop arachnoiditis or meningeal irritation, also painful conditions. The child who is immunocompromised, whether from chemotherapy or from disease, is at risk for infection and infection-related pain. Skin, perioral, and perirectal infections are common. Children seem to be at less risk for acute herpes zoster and its related pain.[13] Bone marrow transplantation may lead acutely to severe mucositis and potentially to chronic graft-versus-host disease, which may manifest as severe abdominal pain if it effects the gastrointestinal system.[13]

Medications used to prevent or modify side effects of primary disease treatment can have painful effects. Use of corticosteroids in disease treatment may lead to bone changes that cause pain.[12] Colony-stimulating factors may lead to medullary bone pain shortly after administration and before the onset of neutrophil recovery.

Nurses caring for patients receiving new treatment protocols need to be alert to the development of pain syndromes associated with particular agents. For example, in recent years, the use of 3F8, an anti-ganglioside monoclonal antibody, in the treatment of advanced neuroblastoma has significantly improved survival but causes an acute episode of neuropathic pain affecting random body parts during infusion.[13] As more is known about the effects of new treatment agents, more effective preventive measures can be taken to improve the quality of life of children undergoing potentially life-sustaining or life-extending therapy.

As children live longer with cancer, they may live longer with pain. Pediatric tertiary care centers, such as Children's Hospital of Boston, have reported a variety of chronic pain problems, including causalgia of a lower extremity, chronic lower extremity pain caused by a mechanical problem with an internal prosthesis, and avascular necrosis of multiple joints in long-term survivors of childhood cancers.[13]

Human Immunodeficiency Virus Infection

Children with HIV infection may experience pain for a variety of reasons, including disease, treatment, and procedures. Some factors are quite similar to those associated with cancer-related pain, and some are unique to HIV disease. For example, children with the acquired immunodeficiency syndrome (AIDS) may have abdominal cramping pain due to AIDS-associated diarrhea.[9]

Sickle Cell Disease (SCD)

One of the most common genetic diseases in the United States, commonly affecting individuals of African, Middle Eastern, Mediterranean, and Indian descent, is highly associated with a variety of painful conditions. SCD is characterized by a predominance of hemoglobin S (HbS), which becomes sickle shaped (as opposed to donut shaped) after deoxygenation. It is this stiff, sickle-shaped red blood cell that becomes trapped in small blood vessels, leading to vaso-occlusion, tissue ischemia, and even infarction.[17]

Some of the many painful states that are commonly associated with SCD include acute painful events, acute hand-foot syndrome, acute inflammation of joints, acute chest syndrome, splenic sequestration, intrahepatic sickling or hepatic sequestration, avascular necrosis of femur or humerus, and priapism. The reader is directed to the American Pain Society's *Guidelines for the Management of Acute and Chronic Pain in Sickle Cell Disease*[18] (pp. 3–7) for a review of the clinical signs and symptoms of these and other common SCD pain states, their underlying causes, and special features or considerations. These episodes can vary in frequency and severity among and within individuals with SCD. Although most would be considered to be frequently recurring acute pain episodes, some, such as those caused by vertebral collapse or avascular necrosis of the femoral or humeral heads, can lead to chronic, debilitating painful conditions. A child with SCD may require hospitalization for pain control. A multicenter study by Platt and associates[19] showed that 39% of patients with SCD had no pain episode that required hospitalization, whereas 1% had to be hospitalized for pain more than six times in a single year. For patients 20 years of age and older, being hospitalized more than three times per year for pain is associated with an increased incidence of death.[18]

Juvenile Chronic Arthritis (JCA)

In 2002, at least 285,000 children in North America were affected by JCA, a condition associated with acute and chronic pain and dysfunction. Disease severity or activity does not predict the intensity of pain that a child with JCA may experience. Children with arthritis may have fewer joints affected and may report less pain, compared with adults. A small percentage may even have painless arthritis. The goal of JCA treatment is to manage the pain and to lessen future problems with joint destruction. A child with JCA may experience procedural pain, acute treatment-related pain (e.g., gastritis), or chronic pain from compression fractures or avascular necrosis.[20] Cassidy reported that chronic pain syndromes in pediatric rheumatology have increased during the last 25 years.[21]

Cystic Fibrosis (CF)

CF, an eventually fatal genetic disease that is diagnosed in 1 of every 3000 live births, has a different trajectory than other lethal childhood diseases. Throughout their lives, children with CF simultaneously receive preventive care to preclude future complications, therapeutic care to reverse the progress of current lung disease, and palliative care to relieve symptoms. Because of advances in medical science, individuals with CF are living longer and longer. Although they are most frequently cared by pediatric specialists, individuals with CF may live to be 20, 30, or even 40 years of age. A study by Robinson and others[22] retrospectively reviewed the care received by 44 patients older than 5 years of age with CF before their deaths from respiratory failure. Thirty-eight patients received opioids for chest pain or dyspnea or both. Although the pain present was not thoroughly described, the fact that it was noted is significant information for those who care for CF populations.

Other Conditions Associated with Pain in Children

Other conditions children experience that may be associated with pain include muscular dystrophy and other degenerative neurological diseases and severe dermatological conditions. Unfortunately, the prevalence, distribution, and description of pain syndromes in many life-threatening illnesses in children have yet to be determined. This shortcoming may be a result of assessment difficulties in infants, preverbal children, and children with communication impairments. Or, it may be a consequence of the often single-minded focus on cure. As clinical interest broadens to also include increased attention to the comfort of these children, it is hoped that the pain and its treatment will be better defined and practiced. [9]

Physiology and Pathophysiology of Pain in Children

Important factors relevant to the physiology and pathophysiology of pain are well covered in Chapter 6. Those working with children need to be aware of the normal neuroanatomical and neurobiological developmental processes that occur in neonates and allow for the development of transmission of painful stimuli (Table 55–2). It is possible to assess the severity of pain and the effects of analgesics in neonates. Neonates who do not cry, move, or show other behavioral response in response to painful stimuli may still be experiencing pain. It has been shown that increased neonatal morbidity may result from prolonged or severe pain. It has been shown that neonates who experience pain may respond differently to pain later on (e.g., pain from inoculation) than do those who have not experienced previous painful events.[7]

Assessment of Pain in Children

The assessment of pain in children is a dialogue between the clinician, the child, and the parents. Through a series of questions, the nurse learns who the child in front of him or her is and how best to address this individual child's pain. To do this, nurses assessing pain in children, from preterm neonates through adolescents, need to be aware of barriers and other

Table 55–2
Pain-Related Developmental Milestones

Age	Development	Assessment and Management Implications
7 wk gestation	Pain receptors present[*]	
20 wk gestation	Full compliment of neurons in cerebral cortex[*] Pain receptors spread to all cutaneous and mucosal surfaces[*]	
26 wk gestation	Can respond to tissue injury as demonstrated by "specific behavioral, autonomic, hormonal, and metabolic signs of stress and distress" (p. 1094) due to sufficient development of peripheral, spinal, and supraspinal afferent pain transmission pathways[†]	
30 wk gestation	Myelination usually complete[*] Slower transmission of pain thought to be offset by decreased distance the impulse must travel[*]	
40 wk gestation	Descending, inhibitory pathways, which alter and modulate pain perception, present[*]	
Neonate (preterm through 1 mo)	Acute pain responses: • Physiological measures, such as increase in vital signs, are similar to those of older children and adults • Behavioral indicators include vocalizations (crying, whimpering, groaning), facial expression changes (grimaces, furrowed brow, quivering chin, tightly closed eyes, squarish open mouth), body movement and posture (thrashing, limb withdrawn, fist clenched, flaccidity), and other behavior changes (sleep/wake cycle, feeding, activity, irritability or listlessness)[*] • Chronic responses can include changes or disruptions in usual feeding, activity, and sleep/wake patterns	• Challenging to differentiate symptoms of pain (a stressful situation) from other life-threatening situations such as hypoxemia[‡] • Validated composite measures include the Neonatal Infant Pain Scale, or NIPS[§]; the CRIES postoperative pain tool[‖] (C = crying; R = requires increased oxygen administration; I = increased vital signs; E = expression; S = sleeplessness) and the Premature Infant Pain Profile, or PIPPS[¶] • One-dimensional pain assessment measure: Neonatal Facial Coding System[#] • Measures do not address neonates with chronic pain, those pharmacologically paralyzed for mechanical ventilation, or those with significant facial deformity[‡]
	Physiological Developmental Issues[†]: • Increased water and volume of distribution for water-soluble medications • Decreased fat and muscle • Immature hepatic enzyme systems, leading to decreased metabolic clearances • Decreased glomerular filtration rates, producing accumulation of renally excreted medications and active metabolites • Many factors in respiratory function lead to increased risk of hypoventilation, atelectasis, or respiratory failure	• Need for increased dosing interval or decreased rates of infusion for many medications[†] • Vulnerable to effects of decreased ventilatory reflexes[†]
Infants (older than 1 mo)	Acute Pain Responses: • Behavioral changes, physiological responses, and facial responses of neonates exhibited[*] • May cry loudly, thrash, arch, or exhibit body rigidity[*] • Local reflex withdrawal of stimulated area in young infants[*] • Deliberate withdrawal of affected area in older infants[*] • Development of stranger anxiety after 7 mo[**]	• Examine infants older than 1 mo in parent's lap[**] • Children's Hospital of Eastern Ontario Pain Scale (CHEOPS)[††]

(continued)

Table 55–2
Pain-Related Developmental Milestones *(continued)*

Age	Development	Assessment and Management Implications
	Physiological Developmental Issues[†]: • Immature hepatic enzyme systems, leading to decreased metabolic clearances • From birth to 7 mo, decreased glomerular filtration rates produce accumulation of renally excreted medications and active metabolites • By 8 to 12 mo, renal blood flow, glomerular filtration, and tubular secretion increase to near adult values • Many factors in respiratory function lead to increased risk of hypoventilation, atelectasis, or respiratory failure	• Need for increased dosing interval or decreased rates of infusion for many medications[†] • Vulnerable to effects of decreased ventilatory reflexes in response to opioids or sedatives[†]
Toddlers	Behavioral changes (such as changes in eating, play/activity, and sleep/wake patterns) and physiological responses as described in neonates[*] May also cry intensely, be verbally aggressive, or withdraw from play or social interaction[*,**] May have words for pain by 18 mo[††] Stranger anxiety persists[**] From age 2 to 6 y, children have a larger liver mass per kilogram of body weight and this is thought to increase metabolic clearance of many medications	Give toddler time to get used to you and build trust[**] Use play and minimized physical contact during physical assessment[**] Language development varies and it is best to use words for pain that are most familiar to a particular child[**] Often it is beneficial to have parents present during assessment and procedures[‡‡] By age 2 y, dosing intervals may be decreased or infusion rates increased because of increased metabolic clearance[†]
Preschooler (young child, age 3–6 y)	Behavioral changes (such as changes in eating, play/activity, and sleep/wake patterns) and physiological responses as described in neonates[*] Developmentally able to give meaningful, concrete information about location and severity of pain[‡,‡‡] Able to anticipate painful events/procedures[*] Behaviors may include clinging, lack of cooperation, attempts to push painful stimuli away before their application[*] "Magical thinking" (mixes facts and fiction)[‡‡] Pain may be viewed as a punishment or as a source of secondary gain[*] From age 2 to 6 y, children have a larger liver mass per kilogram of body weight and this is thought to increase metabolic clearance of many medications	Physical and emotional support by adults present, especially parents, may be comforting Consider building on "magical thinking" abilities when initiating nonpharmacological interventions[‡‡] Offer realistic choices if possible, and provide positive reinforcement[**] By age 2 y, dosing intervals may be decreased or infusion rates increased because of increased metabolic clearance[†]
School-age child	Behavioral changes (such as changes in eating, play/activity, and sleep/wake patterns) and physiological responses as described in neonates[*] May exhibit rigid muscularity (gritted teeth, contracted limbs, stiff body, closed eyes, or wrinkled forehead) May demonstrate more stalling behaviors to delay potentially painful experiences Continued normal cognitive development influences ability to both report and learn information May demonstrate influences of cultural group[*]	Child able to use more objective measures of pain, give more specific and detailed reports Able to use more cognitive coping methods, including educational interventions Cultural beliefs may influence child's pain experience[*]

(continued)

Table 55–2
Pain-Related Developmental Milestones *(continued)*

Age	Development	Assessment and Management Implications
Adolescent	Behavioral changes (such as changes in eating, play/activity, and sleep/wake patterns) and physiological responses as described in neonates* May show more decreased motor activity in presence of pain Continued normal cognitive development Increased influence of peers and cultural group* Increased needs for privacy and independence** Adolescent not legally independent (except in special cases) but needs to have a larger emerging role in his or her care**	May deny pain in presence of peers May be influenced by cultural factors regarding interpretations and expressions of pain*,§§ Parents remain advocate for child but teenagers, if they so desire, need to be involved in decision making**

*Hockenberry et al. (2003), reference 6.
†Berde and Sethna (2003), reference 29.
‡American Academy of Pediatrics (2000), reference 7.
§Lawrence et al. (1993), reference 57.
||Krechel and Bildner (1995), reference 58.
¶Stevens et al. (1996), reference 46.
#Grunau and Craig (1990), reference 59.
**Levetown (2000), reference 60.
††Children's Hospital of Eastern Ontario Pain Scale, reference 61.
‡‡Franck et al. (2000), reference 26.
§§Hockenberry-Eaton et al. (1999), reference 40.

influencing factors that play a role in accurate, developmentally appropriate assessment.

Barriers to pain control in children are similar to those in adults. They primarily relate to (1) lack of assessment; (2) inadequate analgesics; (3) incorrect attitudes or misconceptions by patients, their families, or health care providers about pain and its management; and (4) issues related to systems.[2,23] Table 55–3 reviews these barriers in detail.

To best assess and manage a child's pain, the nurse must ask a series of questions that lead him or her to better know who a particular child is. One of the first questions is, "What is the child's chronological age and what is his or her developmental stage?" Is this child a neonate, infant, toddler, preschooler/young child, school-age child, or adolescent? Nurses who work exclusively with children know that the answers to these questions have a huge impact on how a child is approached. Nurses who do not may find the review of developmental stages and factors relevant to pain useful (see Table 55–2). The following two case studies may also be helpful.

CASE STUDY

Michael, a 7-Month-Old with Severe Mucositis

Michael is a 7-month-old with severe mucositis, and his story illustrates the challenges present in caring for a preverbal child with pain. He is admitted for pain management and total parenteral nutrition (TPN). When the nurse performs the initial assessment, Michael's parents report that they had been giving him acetaminophen when he looked uncomfortable but it didn't appear to help him. Michael is awake, crying in his mother's arms; his mouth is open, and he is drooling thick secretions; he is tachycardic and tachypneic. Michael is prescribed a dose of intravenous morphine. When the nurse assesses him 30 minutes later, he is sleeping and appears to be more comfortable. He is later placed on patient-controlled analgesia (PCA), and after 48 hours he is playful and interactive.

CASE STUDY

Jenna, a 7-Year-Old Undergoing Abdominal Surgery

Older children like Jenna, a 7-year-old who is on day 2 after abdominal surgery, can give more detailed pain-related information during assessment. The nurse is called into Jenna's room because her mother reports that Jenna is experiencing incisional pain. After ascertaining that Jenna is not developmentally delayed, the nurse uses the Numerical Rating Scale to assess her pain. Jenna rates her pain as a 7 out of 10. Her vital signs are within normal limits with the exception of her heart rate, which is 123 bpm. Thirty minutes after receiving the prescribed dose of morphine, Jenna appears

Table 55–3
Pediatric-Specific Barriers to Pain Control

Issue	Barrier/Misconception
Inadequate assessment	*Misconception:* infants and children do not feel pain in the same way as adults do*
	Misconception: Children unable to provide useful, accurate information about the location and severity of their pain†
	Lack of knowledge about how to assess pediatric pain†
	Challenge of pain assessment in preverbal or noncommunicating children
	Choosing the correct population specific tool
Inadequate analgesics ordered or administered	Need for comprehensive assessment with pain etiology and contributing or modifying factors identified
	Need to select most appropriate medications, doses, dosing intervals, and route of administration for situation
	Nurses or parents may not administer the complete dose ordered or as frequently as ordered
	Prescriber's reluctance to send children home with the effective opioids that the child received while hospitalized‡
Incorrect attitudes or misconceptions by patients, families, or health care providers about pain and its management	Pain control in children too difficult or time-consuming*
	Lack of knowledge or incorrect knowledge of pharmacokinetics and pharmacodynamics of analgesics, especially opioids†
	Lack of knowledge of the consequences of unrelieved pain†
	Misconception: Children can tolerate pain better than adults can (this can lead to heightened pain and anxiety about pain control)†
	Misconception: Children are at higher risk for development of chemical dependency from opioid analgesics and the use of opioids should be postponed despite severe pain†
	Fear of opioid-related side effects and lack of knowledge about how to manage them can also prevent appropriate use of opioids in children†
Systems-related issues	Need for systematic re-evaluation and reassessment of pain management plan's effectiveness†
	No systematic, evidenced-based approach to pain management despite rigorous approach to other aspects of a child's care, including disease diagnosis and treatment
	Lack of appropriate use of nondrug therapies to complement or supplement the pharmacological interventions†

(*continued*)

Table 55–3
Pediatric-Specific Barriers to Pain Control *(continued)*

Issue	Barrier/Misconception
	Lack of knowledge by health care professionals of simple and practical physical, cognitive, or behavioral strategies that can give children and their families more control and less anxiety about pain management
	Lack of clear delineation of who is responsible for a particular child's pain control, leading to gaps in management†

*American Academy of Pediatrics (2001), reference 24.
†McGrath and Brown (2004), reference 2.
‡Field and Behrman (2003), reference 9.

comfortable, her heart rate is 100 bpm, and she rates her pain as a 2 out of 10.

Other influencing factors that may make the assessment of pain challenging are language or cultural differences between the child or family and the health care providers; the presence of chronic health conditions, development disabilities, cognitive, sensory, or motor impairments; and severe emotional disturbance.[24] Factors that can complicate the communication between a child and the health care team increase the likelihood of suboptimal pain control.

In learning who an individual child is and what would work best in managing his or her pain, the nurse needs to talk with both the parents and the child. Although parents have varying abilities to recognize pain and its severity in their child, there is probably no one more sensitive to changes in their child's behavior or more motivated in looking out for the health and well-being of a child than his or her parents.[6] Hester and Barcus[25] developed a series of questions for both the child and the parents that reviews the pain experience of a particular child. With the child, the nurse explores what pain or hurt is to this particular child, whether he or she communicates the pain to others, what relieves the pain, what the child finds helpful, what the child wants to avoid from others when he or she is in pain, and anything unique to how the child is when in pain. With the parents, the nurse explores the language a child uses and the behavior the parents observe when their child is in pain. The nurse reviews what painful experiences the child has had, how the child reacts, what tends to relieve a child's pain (including what the child does and what the parents do for the child), and any other special information about the child when he or she is in pain. By using this questionnaire, a nurse is better able to get a complete picture of the child in pain.

Choosing an appropriate tool that will be useful in particular clinical situations can be challenging at best. In choosing a tool, the developmental age of the child should be considered first, and then the type of pain or medical situation or illness that the child will be experiencing. Attempts at measurement of pain include physiological measures, behavioral observations, and self-report measures. Physiological measures may reflect the response to the stress of pain and not the pain itself. Although they are far from ideal, physiological measures are often used in situations in which the child is unable to report pain for himself or herself. Acute pain is often associated with increases of 10% to 20% in noninvasively measured blood pressure, heart rate, or respiratory rate. These changes may not be present in the child with chronic pain.

Observational pain assessment tools, also used when a child cannot self-report pain, are criticized for possibly measuring distress behavior instead of pain behavior.[26] Observational or behavioral scales are most often used in preverbal or cognitively impaired children. The pain behaviors specific to certain conditions may be useful, such as the observation of guarding, bracing, and active rubbing in children with JCA.[20]

Self-report measures, by far the most preferable, can be obtained in some children as young as 3 years of age and generally by 6 years. Most pediatric self-report tools are not multidimensional and measure only pain intensity.[13] To adequately report detailed ratings of pain intensity, a child, usually of school age or older, must understand the concepts of order and numbering. To test this knowledge, a child could be given six different sized pieces of paper and asked to place them in order from smallest to largest.[26] If a 0-to-10 scale is used, with 0 being no pain and 10 being the worst possible pain, older children and adolescents may be asked to rate their pain with an number and then asked, "Do you consider your pain to be none, slight, moderate, severe, or excruciating?" The comparison between the child's numeric pain rating and the categorical pain rating ideally will show some general agreement. Readers attempting to narrow their choices of pain assessment tools are referred to detailed reviews of pediatric pain assessment tools found in several references.[6,26]

In any one practice setting, it may be necessary to use several tools because of the broad range of child development and cognitive disabilities that may be present. In the ongoing stress of pain and illness, a child may regress cognitively and emotionally, which may necessitate the use of a simpler tool. This may also happen when a child is rendered cognitively impaired from medications administered. At present, there is a need for research that can make pain assessment tools more generalizable, with improvement of both specificity and sensitivity.[26]

Assessment for pain begins with screening for the possibility of pain. This can occur in a systematic way every time a child enters a health care system, though the use of documentation tools that ask about the presence of pain. In addition to the collection of this information in an initial nursing database, hospitalized children may be screened more than once a day for the new development of pain or for the presence of unsatisfactory pain control.[27] The so-called QUESTT approach to pediatric pain assessment is a self-explanatory one that summarizes the points stressed in this section and also leads to action and re-evaluation.[28] A slightly adapted version consists of the following:

Question the child and parent.
Use pain rating scales appropriate to developmental stage of the child and to the situation at hand.
Evaluate behavioral and physiological changes.
Secure parents' involvement.
Take the cause of pain into account.
Take action and evaluate results.

In every practice setting, a child with pain needs reassessment on a regular ongoing basis to improve or maintain the management of his or her pain.

Management

No matter what the practice setting, one of the main principles in pediatric pain management is to anticipate and prevent pain whenever possible. If that is not possible, the next principle is to minimize the pain by treating the underlying disease (if possible), using pharmacological and nonpharmacological modalities as appropriate, and choosing the least painful necessary procedures.

Pharmacological Management

Nurses working with children with pain must be aware of age-related physiological trends that are relevant to analgesic action and have an impact on dosage prescribed. The physiological processes that are involved include the body compartments, hepatic enzyme systems for medication metabolism, plasma protein binding, renal filtration and excretion of medications and their metabolites, and metabolic rate, oxygen consumption, and respiratory function.[29] Some of these developmental physiological changes and their clinical implications are presented in Table 55–2. Tables 55–4, 55–5, and 55–6 suggest starting doses for opioids and nonopioids that reflect these developmental aspects of pediatric pharmacology.

Although studies indicate that with proper age-related adjustments and dosing children can safely receive pain medication, it is important to bear in mind that approximately 50% to 75% of medications used in pediatric medicine, including analgesics, have not been adequately studied to provide appropriate labeling information.[30] Clinicians who treat the pain of children have diligently tried to extrapolate data from experience with adults to determine what medications should be used and at what doses in children. This uncontrolled, undocumented, and unsystematic practice of off-label use, although well intended, is a systems problem that does not allow for medications used in children to be studied with sound scientific and ethical principles. It does not allow for the definition of age-dependent differences in pharmacokinetics and pharmacodynamics or for the establishment of which adverse events in children are similar to those in adults and which ones are unique to pediatric patients. This situation frequently occurs because of a result of lack of resources. The pediatric market is but a small segment of the total pharmaceutical market, and there is limited financial incentive to study medications in children.[31]

There are three main groups of medications used to treat pain in children: (1) nonopioids (acetaminophen, nonsteroidal antiinflammatory drugs [NSAIDs], and aspirin), (2) opioids, and (3) adjuvant analgesics. Use of these medications depends on the severity and cause of pain in an individual child. The nonopioids and opioids are most helpful in the treatment of

Table 55–4
Nonopioid Drugs for Relief of Cancer Pain in Children

Drug	Dosage	Remarks
Paracetamol	10–15 mg/kg orally, q4–6h	Has no gastrointestinal or hematological side effects, but lacks antiinflammatory activity
Ibuprofen	5–10 mg/kg orally, q6–8h	Antiinflammatory activity, but may have gastrointestinal and hematological side effects
Naproxen	5 mg/kg orally, q8–12h	Antiinflammatory activity, but may have gastrointestinal and hematological side effects

Source: World Health Organization (1998), reference 12.

Table 55–5
Oral Dosage Guidelines for Commonly Used Nonopioid Analgesics

	Dose			Maximum Daily Dose	
Drug	Child <60 kg	Child ≥60 kg	Interval	Child <60 kg	Child ≥60 kg
Acetaminophen	10–15 mg/kg	650–1000 mg	4 h	100 mg/kg*	4000 mg
Ibuprofen	6–10 mg/kg	400–600 mg†	6 h	40 mg/kg†,‡	2400 mg†
Naproxen	5–6 mg/kg†	250–375 mg†	12 h	24 mg/kg†,‡	1000 mg†
Aspirin	10–15 mg/kg†,§	650–1000 mg†	4 h	80 mg/kg†,‡,§	3600 mg†

*The maximum daily doses of acetaminophen for infants and neonates are a subject of current controversy. Provisional recommendations are that daily dosing should not exceed 75 mg/kg for infants, 60 mg/kg for full-term neonates and preterm neonates of >32 wk postconceptional age. Fever, dehydration, hepatic disease, and lack of oral intake may all increase the risk of hepatotoxicity.

†Higher doses may be used in selected cases for treatment of rheumatological conditions in children.

‡Dosage guidelines for neonates have not been established.

§Aspirin carries a risk of provoking Reye's syndrome in infants and children. If other analgesics are available, aspirin should be restricted to indications for which an antiplatelet or antiinflammatory effect is required, rather than being used as a routine analgesic or antipyretic in neonates, infants, or children. Dosage guidelines for aspirin in neonates have not been established.

Source: Berde and Sethna (2003), reference 29, with permission.

nociceptive pain, and adjuvant analgesics work best for specific neuropathic pain. A general review of these medications and their use is presented in Chapter 6. What follows in this section are factors that are most relevant to the use of these drugs in children.

In 1998, the WHO published guidelines for cancer pain relief and palliative care in children.[12] They stressed four key concepts of analgesic use in children: "by the ladder, by the clock, by the appropriate route, and by the child" (p. 24). "By the ladder" refers to approaching a child's pain based on the presenting severity of pain, with steps clearly delineated for mild, moderate, and severe pain. For mild pain, nonopioids are indicated, with the addition of an adjuvant analgesic if a neuropathic contribution to the pain is suspected. If a child presents with or progresses to moderate pain, the nonopioid is continued (if not contraindicated), an appropriate adjuvant is continued if a neuropathic component is likely, and codeine, a "weak" opioid, is added to the child's analgesic regimen. If this proves ineffective, or if severe pain is present, the codeine is rotated to morphine or another opioid for moderate to severe pain and titrated to effect, with the rest of the regimen continued as appropriate.

"By the clock" reflects the concept that for pain that is almost continuous a child will benefit most from nearly continuous analgesics administered on a regular schedule. This method promotes better pain control and decreases a child's anxiety regarding uncontrolled pain. "By the appropriate route" promotes the administration of analgesics by the simplest, most effective, least painful route. For most children this is the oral route, but for some situations other routes may be more effective. "By the child" indicates the need for individualization of each child's analgesic regimen. Starting doses listed on tables are just that—starting doses. Each child's dose must be titrated up or down based on his or her response. If uncontrolled pain is present, opioids should be titrated upward until analgesic relief is obtained or unmanageable side effects occur.

Although the WHO guidelines were developed for the control of cancer pain, the four concepts can be applied to the use of analgesics in children in other painful circumstances.

Use of Nonopioids in Children

Nonopioids (acetaminophen, NSAIDs, and aspirin) have a ceiling effect and cannot be safely titrated beyond the dose per weight given at drug-specific intervals. Pediatric dosage guidelines for commonly used nonopioid analgesics can be found in Tables 55–4 and 55–5.

Aspirin is not routinely used as an analgesic in infants and children because of the risk of Reye's syndrome associated with its use in this population. The most widely used mild analgesic for children is acetaminophen.[29] The recommended dosing of acetaminophen in children is based on the dose-response for antipyretic effects, because the pediatric analgesic dose response is unavailable.[13] Currently there is no safety data on long-term acetaminophen use in children.[32] NSAIDs have been shown to be safe and effective analgesics for children. Children using NSAIDs have been shown to have greater weight-normalized clearance and volumes of distribution than adults but with similar drug half-lives. Large-scale studies looking at the efficacy and risk-benefit and cost-benefit ratios of selective cyclooxygenase-2 inhibitors in children have yet to be done.[29]

Use of Opioids in Children

It takes until the age of 2 to 6 months for the weight-normalized clearance of many opioids to reach mature levels. Pharmacokinetic studies of morphine show an average serum half-life of

Table 55–6
Opioid Analgesic Dosage Guidelines for Opioid-Naïve Patients*

Opioid (Biological Half-life)	Equianalgesic Doses†		Usual Intravenous or Subcutaneous Starting Dose‡		Parenteral / Oral Dose Ratio	Usual Oral Starting Dose‡	
	Parenteral	Oral	Child <50 kg	Child ≥50 kg		Child <50 kg	Child ≥50 kg
Short-half-life opioids							
Codeine (2.5–3 h)	130 mg	200 mg	N/R	N/R	1:1.5	0.5–1 mg/kg q3–4 h	30 mg q3–4 h
Oxycodone (2–3 h)	N/A	30 mg	N/A	N/A	N/A	0.2 mg/kg q3–4 h	5–10 mg q3–4 h
Pethidine§ N/R (3 h)	75 mg N/R	300 mg N/R	0.75 mg/kg q2–4 h N/R	75–100 mg q2–4h N/R	1:4	1–1.5 mg/kg q3–4 h N/R	50–75 mg q3–4 h N/R
Morphine (2.5–3 h)	10 mg	30 mg	*Bolus dose:* 0.05–0.1 mg/kg IV or SQ q2–4 h *Continuous infusion:* 0.03 mg/kg qh	*Bolus dose:* 5–10 mg IV or SQ q2–4 h *Continuous infusion:* 1 mg/h	1:3	0.15–0.3 mg/kg q4 h	5–10 mg q4 h
Hydromorphone (2–3 h)	1.5 mg	7.5 mg	0.015 mg/kg q2–4 h	1–1.5 mg/kg q2–4 h	1:5	0.06 mg/kg q3–4 h	2 mg q3–4 h
Oxymorphone (1.5 h)	1 mg	N/A	0.02 mg/kg q2–4 h	1 mg q2–4 h	N/A	N/A	N/A
Fentanyl‖ (3 h)	100 mcg single dose	N/A	0.5–2 mcg/kg qh as a continuous infusion	25–75 mcg qh	N/A	N/A	N/A
Long-half-life opioids							
Controlled-release morphine	N/A	N/A	N/A	N/A	N/A	0.6 mg/kg q8h or 0.9 mg/kg q12 h	30–60 mg q12h
Methadone¶ (12–50 h)	10 mg	20 mg	0.1 mg/kg IV or SQ q4–8 h	5–10 mg IV or SQ q4–8 h	1:2	0.2 mg/kg q4–8 h	5–10 mg q4–8 h

N/A, not applicable; N/R, not recommended.
*Important notes:
1. For all drugs for which a distinction is made between children <50 kg and those ≥50 kg, doses should be calculated in milligrams per kilogram for children <50 kg and the "usual adult dose" should be used for those ≥50 kg.
2. When a change is made to short-half-life opioids in an opioid-tolerant patient, the new drug should be given at 50% of the equianalgesic dose (because of incomplete cross-tolerance) and titrated to effect.

†Equianalgesic doses are based on single-dose studies in adults.
‡Usual starting dose is the commonly used standard dose and is not always based on equianalgesic principles (i.e., starting dose of hydromorphone may be 2 mg despite the parenteral ratio of 1:5). For infants <6 mo, starting doses should be ¼ to ⅓ of the suggested dose and titrated to effect.
§Pethidine is not recommended for chronic use because of its long half-life and the possibility of accumulation of a toxic metabolite.
‖Continuous infusion of fentanyl at 100 μg/h is approximately equianalgesic to a morphine infusion of 2.5 mg/h.
¶Methadone may cause irritation when administered SQ. Extreme care is needed when using methadone, both for initiation of therapy and when doses are increased, because of its extremely long biological half-life.
Source: World Health Organization (1998), reference 12, with permission.

9 hours in preterm neonates, decreasing to 6.5 hours in full-term neonates and finally reaching 2 hours in the older infant. If not carefully monitored, neonates may be more likely to develop side effects from morphine due to decreased renal clearance of metabolites. The respiratory reflex response to hypoxemia, hypercapnia, and airway obstruction does not reach full maturity until 2 to 3 months after birth in both full-term and preterm infants. This can lead the nonintubated neonate receiving opioids to be at higher risk for ventilatory depression.[29] Neonates receiving opioids or other agents that can compromise cardiorespiratory function must be continuously monitored in a setting that can quickly provide airway management. Those receiving prolonged opioid therapy may benefit from the use of continuous infusions to avoid the variation

in plasma concentrations that occurs with bolus dosing. In neonates receiving synthetic opioids, the administration of infusions over several minutes or of small, frequent aliquots is recommended to avoid the adverse effects of glottic and chest wall rigidity that are associated with rapid bolus injection of medications such as fentanyl and sufentanil.[7]

When using opioids with infants, children, and adolescents, the goal is to control pain as quickly as possible. Repeated administration of small, ineffective doses that prolong the pain and worsen pain-related anxiety is to be discouraged. For moderate to severe pain, it is appropriate to use opioids such as morphine, fentanyl, and hydromorphone in optimal doses titrated to an individual child's response.[24] Initial pediatric opioid dose guidelines can be found in Table 55–6.

The following case illustrates how opioids can be given and adjusted for the benefit of an individual child.

CASE STUDY

John, a Child with Neuroblastoma

John, age 3 years 6 months, had progressive metastatic neuroblastoma. When his parents were told that his disease had returned and there was an experimental treatment available that would not cure him, they decided against the treatment. Their goal was for John to be comfortable and to keep him at home and hopefully alive until the birth of his new brother. When John started to complain of bone pain, his parents wanted him to receive pain medication. Opioid-naïve, he was started on morphine 0.1 mg/kg intravenously every 3 to 4 hours. As John's disease progressed, so did his pain, and his morphine dose was escalated every 48 to 72 hours. He was eventually started on a morphine PCA pump, with dose escalation every 48 hours. Finally, the day arrived, and John became a big brother. At this point, he slept most the day but had a few good hours of interaction with his family. He was able to hold his brother. His dose of morphine at that time was 200 mg/hour, with rescues of 75 mg every 10 minutes as needed. John died 7 days later, but his parents were thankful that he was relatively comfortable and was able to meet his brother.

Use of Adjuvant Analgesics in Children

Adjuvant analgesics are a heterogeneous group of medications that include psychostimulants, corticosteroids, anticonvulsants, antidepressants, radionuclides, and neuroleptics. Much of the evidence supporting their use in specific targeted pain syndromes comes from the adult literature. However, there has been some initial work looking at the use of adjuvants in children. The use of methylphenidate and dextroamphetamine in adolescents with cancer was reported to be safe, efficacious, and tolerable by Yee and Berde.[33] Intraarticular injection of corticosteroids is one of the mainstays of initial treatment of most children with JCA.[34] Although gabapentin has been studied as an anticonvulsant in children, it has yet to be investigated as an adjuvant analgesic in children despite widespread use as such.[2] It is recommended that a child have baseline hematological and biochemical laboratory studies and an electrocardiogram performed to rule out Wolff-Parkinson-White syndrome and other cardiac conduction defects before initiation of tricyclic antidepressants and at periodic intervals if the child receives long-term therapy or exceeds standard dose/weight guidelines.[32] One case has been reported of the use of 131 iodine-meta-iodobenzylguanidine to treat a boy's bone pain caused by neuroblastoma.[35] Future research in the use of adjuvant analgesics in the pediatric population is needed.

Use of Local Anesthetics and Other Anesthetic Techniques

In the past, local anesthetics were not widely used in children because of concerns regarding cardiac depression and seizures. Today, they can be administered by a variety of routes and have acceptable safety as long as the maximum recommended doses are adhered to. For bupivacaine, with or without epinephrine, the maximum recommended dose is 2 mg/kg for neonates and 2.5 mg/kg for other children. The maximum recommended dose for lidocaine in neonates is 4 mg/kg without epinephrine or 5 mg/kg with epinephrine. For children, the maximum recommended dose of lidocaine with epinephrine is 5 to 7 mg/kg.[29]

Intradermal administration of lidocaine can be used for skin anesthesia if painful punctures will occur. The lidocaine can be buffered with 1 part sodium bicarbonate to 10 parts 1% or 2% lidocaine to avoid the stinging effects of lidocaine administration. Several preparations of local anesthetics can be obtained for topical or transdermal administration to control procedural pain. Of these, eutectic mixture of local anesthetics (EMLA) is available as a cream or anesthetic disc. One hour before puncture, the EMLA cream is placed over the potential site with an occlusive dressing applied to prevent or minimize puncture pain. Lidocaine/adrenaline/tetracaine (LAT) or tetracaine/phenylephrine may be applied to open wounds for suturing, providing skin anesthesia for approximately 15 minutes. LAT, because it contains adrenaline that causes vasoconstriction, must not be placed on distal arteries (located on tip of nose, earlobes, penis, fingers, and toes). "Numby Stuff" is a commercially available product that uses a novel delivery system, iontophoresis, to deliver 2% lidocaine and epinephrine 1:100,000 approximately 10 mm into the skin. It takes approximately 10 minutes of use before dermal anesthesia is achieved. This device may be somewhat frightening to young children, who may not like feeling its mild current.[6]

The use of regional nerve blocks in anesthetized children to provide improved postoperative analgesia has expanded over the last 20 years.[29,36] This technique, which involves the injection of long-acting bupivacaine or ropivacaine into nerves that innervate a designated area, can also be used to provide local anesthesia for surgical procedures such as circumcision or reduction of fractures.[6,24]

Long-acting anesthetics (e.g., bupivacaine, ropivacaine) can be given intraspinally (epidurally or intrathecally) in children. Administration of epidural medications (opioids, local anesthetics, clonidine) can effectively control pain in children, including preterm neonates.[24,29] They are often given for postoperative pain control after specific procedures or in children with chronic pain who have not been helped by effective systemic therapy.[29] The use of epidural analgesia in children requires special education and training on the part of the physicians and nurses. Careful calculation and administration of epidural medications and close postadministration observation are necessary to prevent serious complications. Nurses play a key role in setting the institutional standards for use of intraspinal analgesics in children.[2,7,29]

The following case illustrates the effective use of intraspinal analgesics in an adolescent.

Jacob, a 15-Year-Old with Metastatic Cancer

Jacob, a 15-year-old Orthodox Jewish boy with osteogenic sarcoma metastatic to the spinal nerve roots, was at home receiving hospice care. Because his pain was not well controlled, he was admitted on a Sunday for better pain control. An epidural catheter was placed for severe neuropathic pain, and Jacob became more comfortable. Jacob and his family were eager for him to be discharged home on Friday morning so that they could be together for the Sabbath, which begins at sundown every Friday. His doctors and nurses believed it would be better for him to stay a few more days while they titrated his analgesics. However, because of cultural issues in this family, they agreed to discharge Jacob home to the hospice nurses who were caring for him and his family. Jacob remained at home for the rest of his life, and his parents were grateful for their time with him.

Nonpharmacological Management

Nonpharmacological pain management interventions include psychological, physiatric, neurostimulatory, invasive, and integrative techniques. Components are frequently combined as part of a pediatric pain management plan; they are dependent on the comprehensive pain assessment of an individual child and are based on the presumed etiology of pain. In considering which nonpharmacological interventions might be beneficial, the nurse needs to look at several factors, including the child's and family's past experience with nondrug interventions. What has worked well and what has not? Are there religious or cultural issues or concerns that would make certain interventions not appropriate? Is the proposed intervention consistent with the developmental level of the child? What is the present cognitive status of the child? Has the stress and fatigue from a prolonged illness made it difficult for the child or family members to concentrate, follow directions, or learn new information? Also, the nurse should consider teaching potentially useful techniques before the skills are needed.[37]

Psychological interventions can include patient and family education, cognitive interventions, and behavioral techniques such as writing in a pain diary. Pain diaries may be especially useful in working with children who have recurrent or chronic pain, and their use has some value in pediatric pain research.[38] Children who enjoy writing may benefit from a private place to express themselves. Young children who have not mastered the written word may find drawing about their pain and pain experiences helpful.

The value of cognitive techniques such as distraction and relaxation is well established in children. Across studies, distraction has been shown to reduce children's behavioral distress during procedural pain, although it has a variable effect on pain intensity. Various distractors have been used for children's pain management, including bubble-blowing, party blowers, puppetry, video games, and listening to music. The distractor is more likely to be effective if it is age-appropriate and complementary to the interests and preferences of the individual child.[39] Nurses working with infants and toddlers, to the age of 2 years, may distract them with mobiles, rocking, stroking, or patting. Children from 2 to 4 years of age may find blowing bubbles, breathing, puppet play, or storytelling useful distractions. Four- to six-year-olds like these activities and may also like television shows and talking about favorite places. School-age children can be distracted with these activities and may also be receptive to humor, counting, or thumb squeezing. Progressive muscle relaxation exercise is used most effectively in older children and adolescents but can also be taught to children as young as 5 years of age. Guided imagery, which ideally incorporates all of a child's senses, can help children "escape" to a safe favorite place unique to that child. Sometimes children like to imagine doing a favorite activity, such as swimming or skating.[40]

More research is needed regarding the efficacy and acceptability of the use of some complementary or integrative approaches (e.g., acupuncture) in children with pain before these modalities can be routinely recommended. Such data can potentially establish other credible choices for assisting children with pain as well.[9]

Nurses caring for children with pain have both collaborative and independent functions when implementing nonpharmacological interventions. Psychological interventions that a nurse should feel comfortable initiating include patient family education and cognitive techniques such as distraction, relaxation, positive self-statements, and pain diaries. An individual nurse might initiate the use of music as a relaxation or distraction technique. Independent physiatric interventions can include movement and positioning and swaddling of neonates. Collaborative efforts may involve massage, vibration, or use of superficial heat or cold. (Protecting the child's skin by placing the heat or cold source in commercially available animal wraps or using towels decorated with favorite characters may make the experience more enjoyable for young children.) The nurse needs to know which members of a child's primary team are knowledgeable in the use of nonpharmacological techniques and which special consultants are available to help if needed.[37] Child life specialists can be a resource for employing distraction and other psychological pain management techniques in children.[9] Cognitive techniques such as biofeedback and hypnosis, although potentially useful for children with chronic pain, require the use of trained instructors for initiation.[41]

The resources available to the nurse (including time available to initiate a particular intervention, education in a particular technique, availability of patient/family educational materials, and availability and affordability of particular devices) play a role in what techniques are initiated with an individual child.[40] The Institute of Medicine noted that the teaching of cognitive behavioral techniques, despite their demonstrated effectiveness, is not done in as rigorous or consistent a way as is observed for other clinical modalities.[9] More detailed information regarding the use of nonpharmacological pain relief methods with children can be found in a variety of sources for those wishing to expand their practice.[5,6,41]

Procedural Pain Management

Procedural pain is a widespread experience for most children interacting with the health care system. Nurses who know how to successfully address procedural pain, using both pharmacological and nonpharmacological techniques, can help a very large number of children. Procedural pain is the one area in the pain literature that is much better developed for children than for adults, who may also experience this problem. The goals of successful procedural pain management include minimizing pain, maximizing patient cooperation, and minimizing risk to the patient.[42]

Anticipation is the key word. Having procedures performed by technically competent individuals can reduce both risk of pain and risk of harm. The medical personnel involved must be knowledgeable in both pharmacological and nonpharmacological pain management appropriate to the child and the situation. Both children and parents need appropriate information regarding what will happen and how they can decrease stress.[24]

How pain is avoided or managed the first time a child undergoes a particular procedure influences how the child anticipates and copes with subsequent procedures. It is recommended that pain and anxiety be maximally treated the very first time a child undergoes a procedure.[43] Depending on the procedure and the individual child, this can be as simple as providing information and topical analgesics or vapo-coolant immediately before needle punctures or as complex as administering conscious sedation with the combination of an opioid analgesic and a benzodiazepine. A recent review of the effectiveness of conscious sedation for anxiety, pain, and procedural complications in young children suggests that its use should be considered and advocated if a child is experiencing a heightened stress reaction.[44] It is important to bear in mind that the use of anxiolytics or sedatives alone does not provide analgesia but does render a child unable to communicate distress.[24]

It is useful to discuss coping strategies with the child and parents, if possible, long before the medical procedure. This enables them to mentally rehearse ways in which they can cope with the situation when it occurs.[39] Review of the literature by Christensen and Fatchett[45] revealed that distraction, relaxation, and imagery are effective for children in decreasing anxiety and pain associated with painful procedures. Therapeutic play and orientation to the room and equipment may help to promote patient cooperation. Risk can be minimized by having all equipment, supplies, and staff ready and available for both routine and emergency care.

Other things the nurse can do to facilitate comfort for children during stressful procedures include inviting the caregiver to be present and attending to environmental factors. This includes using a treatment room whenever possible; creating a pleasant environment; minimizing noxious noises, sounds, and sights; and maintaining a calm, positive manner. Attending to these details can not only increase the comfort of the parents and the child but also that of the health care personnel involved.[46] Finally, during and after the procedure, the nurse needs to provide ongoing assessment of pain and anxiety and work to collaborate and modify the treatment plan if suboptimal control of either occurs.

Where Improvement Is Needed

All children are vulnerable to inadequate pain assessment and management. Those most vulnerable include the preverbal child, the cognitively or neurologically impaired child, immigrant children, and children without homes or consistent caregivers. System issues that interact with the barriers discussed earlier also need to be addressed (see Table 55–3).[2] For example, children cared for in pediatric tertiary care centers may find that health care professionals in their home environment lack up-to-date information about pain assessment and comprehensive pain control in children.[9]

Long-term follow-up and outcome expectations and monitoring are important in preventing, anticipating, and alleviating pain in the pediatric population. Implementing a successful pediatric pain management program is more complicated than just selecting a pain assessment tool and requires a commitment of resources.[26] To follow up in a systematic way and promote the timely and adequate use of appropriate medications and behavioral interventions for children, initiatives have been started that work to develop and implement evidence-based pediatric pain assessment and management protocols.[9,47,48] Disease-specific guidelines have been developed for children with SCD[18] and JCA,[20] and a position paper has been published by the Association of Pediatric Oncology Nurses for pain management of the child with cancer at the end of life.[49] It is hoped that pain will receive this kind of attention in other pediatric populations.

To start to improve the process of pain management, it is necessary to collect information about the present process, to develop an awareness of all the various factors that may either promote or deter achievement of the desired outcome. The literature reveals several efforts to collect baseline information about pain management and areas for improvement.[50,51] One area to consider is that of pain medication errors. Sources of errors in pediatric medication administration include dilution errors, milligram-microgram errors, decimal point errors, and confusion between a total daily dose and a fractional dose.[29,52] Through application of the quality improvement process, nurses can play an important role in improving pain control for both the individual children they care for and other children that they may not be directly involved with.

Summary

Despite the significant increase in knowledge about assessment and management of pain in infants and children, too many suffering children do not receive proper treatment. In today's age of "powerful, invasive medicine, we can save more lives, but any wrong choice turns medicine into torture, inflicting avoidable sufferings on patients" (p. 2).[53] To prevent suffering for children and their families, nurses and other health care professionals must apply the most up-to-date techniques of pain assessment and management to all children they care for, especially from the time a child receives a diagnosis of a potentially life-threatening illness through his or her survival or death. By application of an integrated treatment plan that is based on the developmental level of the individual child, involves his or her family, and uses both pharmacological and nonpharmacological interventions, optimal pain control is possible.[2]

REFERENCES

1. Last Acts Palliative Care Task Force. Precepts of palliative care for children/adolescents and their families. 2003. Available at: http://pedsnurses.org/html/LastActsPrecepts03 (accessed March 29, 2005).
2. McGrath PA, Brown SC. Paediatric palliative medicine: 9.1 Pain control. Oxford Textbook of Palliative Medicine, 3rd ed. New York: Oxford University Press, 2004.
3. Walco GA, Cassidy RC, Schechter N. Sounding Board: Pain, hurt, and harm—The ethics of pain control in infants and children. N Engl J Med 1994;331:541–544.
4. Pain terms: A list with definitions and notes on usage. Recommended by the International Association for the Study of Pain Subcommittee on Taxonomy. Pain 1979;6:249–252.
5. McCaffery M, Pasero C. Pain: Clinical Manual, 2nd ed. St. Louis, Mo.: Mosby, 1999.
6. Hockenberry M, Wilson D, Winkelstein M, Kline N. Wong's Nursing Care of Infants and Children, 7th ed. St. Louis, Mo.: Mosby, 2003.
7. American Academy of Pediatrics, Canadian Pediatric Society. Prevention and management of pain and stress in the neonate. Pediatrics 2000;105:454–461.
8. American Academy of Pediatrics. Guidelines for monitoring and management of pediatric patients during and after sedation for diagnosis and therapeutic procedures. Pediatrics 1992;89:1110–1115.
9. Field MJ, Behrman R, eds. When Children Die: Improving Palliative and End-of-Life Care for Children and Their Families. Report of the Institute of Medicine Task Force. Washington, DC: National Academy Press, 2003.
10. Ingelmo PM, Locatelli BG, Carrara B. Neuropathic pain in children. The Suffering Child 2003;2(February):1–15. Available at: http://www.thesufferingchild.net (accessed February 28, 2005).
11. Busoni P, Bussolin L. Pain in acutely burned children. The Suffering Child 2002;1(October):1–7. Available at: http://www.thesufferingchild.net (accessed February 28, 2005).
12. World Health Organization. Cancer Pain Relief and Palliative Care in Children. Geneva, Switzerland: WHO, 1998.
13. Collins JJ, Berde CB. Management of cancer pain in children. In: Pizzo PA, Poplack DG, eds. Principles and Practice of Pediatric Oncology. Philadelphia: Lippincott-Raven Publishers, 1997.
14. Patterson KL. Pain in the pediatric oncology patient. J Pediatr Oncol Nurs 1992;9:119–130.
15. Bossert EA, Van Cleve L, Adlard K, Savedra M. Pain and leukemia: the stories of three children. J Pediatr Oncol Nurs 2002;19:2–11.
16. Ljungman G, Gordh T, Sorensen S, Kreuger A. Pain variations during cancer treatment in children: A descriptive survey. Pediatr Hemacol Oncol 2000;17:211–221.
17. Jakubik JD, Thompson M. Care of the child with sickle cell disease: Acute complications. Pediatr Nurs 2000;26:373–379.
18. American Pain Society. Guidelines for the Management of Acute and Chronic Pain in Sickle Cell Disease. Glenview, IL: APS, 1999.
19. Platt OS, Thorington BD, Brambilla DJ, Milner PF, Rosse WF, Vichinsky E, Kinney TR. Pain in sickle-cell disease: Rates and risk factors. M Engl J Med 1991;325:11–16.
20. American Pain Society. Guideline for the Management of Pain in Osteoarthritis, Rheumatoid Arthritis, and Juvenile Chronic Arthritis, 2nd ed. Glenview, IL: APS, 2002.
21. Cassidy JT. Progress in diagnosis and understanding of chronic pain syndromes in children and adolescents. Adolesc Med 1998;9:101–114,vi.
22. Robinson WM, Ravilly S, Berde C, Wohl ME. End-of-life care in cystic fibrosis. Pediatrics 1997;100:205–209.
23. Nilofer S, Sunil S. Pain in neonates. Lancet 2000;355:932–933.
24. American Academy of Pediatrics. The assessment and management of acute pain in infants, children, and adolescents. Pediatrics 2001;108:793–797.
25. Hester N, Barcus C. Assessment and management of pain in children. Pediatr Nurs Update 1986;1:3.
26. Franck LS, Greenberg CS, Stevens B. Pain assessment in infants and children. Pediatr Clin North Am 2000;47:487–512.
27. Bookbinder M, Coyle N, Kiss M, Layman Goldstein M, Holritz K, Thaler H, et al. Implementing national standards for cancer pain management: Program model and evaluation. J Pain Symptom Manage 1996;12:334–347.
28. Baker C, Wong D. Q.U.E.S.T.: A process of pain assessment in children. Orthop Nurs 1987;6:11–21.

29. Berde CB, Sethna NF. Analgesics for the treatment of pain in children. N Engl J Med 2003;347:1094–1103.
30. Roberts R, Rodriquez W, Murphy D, Crescenzi T. Pediatric drug labeling: Improving the safety and efficacy of pediatric therapies. JAMA 2003;290:905–911.
31. Budetti PP. Ensuring safe and effective medications for children. JAMA 2003;290:950–951.
32. Collins JJ. Palliative care and the child with cancer. Hematol Oncol Clin North Am 2002;16:657–670.
33. Yee JD, Berde CB. Dextroamphetamine or methylphenidate as adjuvants to opioid analgesia for adolescents with cancer. J Pain Symptom Manage 1994;9:442.
34. Cron RQ, Sharma S, Sherry DD. Current treatment by United States and Canadian pediatric rheumatologist. J Rheumatol 1999; 26:2036–2038.
35. Westlin JE, Letocha H, Jakobson S, Strang P, Martinsson U, Nilsson S. Rapid, reproducible pain relief with [131]iodine-meta-iodobenzylguanidine in a boy with disseminated neuroblastoma. Pain 1995;60:111–114.
36. Dalens B. Periperhal blocks in children: Which techniques to begin with? The Suffering Child 2002;1(October):1–24. Available at: http://www.thesufferingchild.net (accessed February 28, 2005).
37. Coyle N, Layman-Goldstein M. Pain assessment and management in palliative care. In: Matzo ML, Sherman DW, eds. Palliative Care Nursing: Quality Care to the End of Life. New York: Springer, 2001:362–486.
38. Palermo TM, Valenzuela D. Use of pain diaries to assess recurrent and chronic pain in children. The Suffering Child 2003; 3(June):1–24. Available at: http://www.thesufferingchild.net (accessed February 28, 2005).
39. Piira T, Hayes B, Goodenough B. Distraction methods in the management of children's pain: An approach based on evidence of intuition? The Suffering Child 2002;1(October):1–10. Available at: http://www.thesufferingchild.net (accessed February 28, 2005).
40. Hockenberry-Eaton M, Barrera P, Brown M, Bottomley SJ, O'Neil JB. Pain Management in Children with Cancer Handbook. Texas: Texas Cancer Council, 1999. Available at: http://www.childcancerpain.org/frameset_nogl.cfm?content=handbook.html (accessed February 28, 2005).
41. Rusy LM, Weisman SJ. Complimentary therapies for acute pediatric pain management. Pediatr Clin North Am 2000;47:589–599.
42. Schecter N, Berde C, Yaster M. Pain in Infants, Children, and Adolescents, 2nd ed. Philadelphia, Penn.: Lippincott, Williams & Wilkins, 2003.
43. American Academy of Pediatrics. Report of the Subcommittee on the Management of Pain Associated with Procedures in Children with Cancer. Pediatrics 1990;86:827.
44. Dresser S, Melnyk BM. The effectiveness of conscious sedation on anxiety, pain, and procedural complications in young children. Pediatr Nurs 2003;29:320–323.
45. Christensen J, Fatchett D. Promoting parental use of distraction and relaxation in pediatric oncology patients during invasive procedures. J Pediatr Oncol Nurs 2002;19:127–132.
46. Stevens BJ, Johnson C, Petryshen P, Taddio A. Premature Infant Pain Profile: Development and initial validation. Clin J Pain 1996; 12:13–22.
47. Jacox A, Carr DB, Payne R, Berde CB, Breibart W, Cain JM, et al. Management of Cancer Pain. Clinical Practice Guideline No. 9. AHCPR publication No. 94-0592. Rockville, Md.: Agency for Health Care Policy and Research, U.S. Department of Health and Human Services, Public Health Service, 1994.
48. Agency for Health Care Policy and Research. Acute Pain Management in Infants, Children, and Adolescents: Operative and Medical Procedures. Quick Reference Guide for Clinicians. Rockville, Md.: U.S. Department of Health and Human Services, 1992.
49. Hooke C, Hellstren MB, Stutzer C, Forte K. Pain management for the child with cancer in end-of-life care: APON position paper. J Pediatr Oncol Nurs 2002;19:43–47.
50. Ellis JA, McCarthy P, Hershon L, Horlin R, Rattray M, Tierney S. Pain practices: A cross-Canada survey of pediatric oncology centers. J Pediatr Oncol Nurs 2003;20:26–35.
51. Ely B. Pediatric nurses' pain management practice: barriers to change. Pediatr Nurs 2001;27:473–480.
52. Levine SR, Cohen MR, Blanchard NR, Frederico F, Magelli M, Lomax C, Greiner G, Poole RL, Lee CKK, Lesko A. Guidelines for preventing medication errors in pediatrics. J Pediatr Pharmacol Ther 2001;6:426–442.
53. Facco E, Giron G. The nature of pain and the approach to the suffering child. The Suffering Child 2003;2(February):1–3. Available at: http://www.thesufferingchild.net (accessed February 28, 2005).
54. Gauvain-Piquard A, Rodary C, Rezvani A, Serbouti S. The development of the DEGR®: a scale to assess pain in young children with cancer. Eur J Pain 1999;2:165–176.
55. Van Dongen KAJ, Abu-Saad HH, Hammers JPF, Zwakhalen SMG. Pain assessment in the intellectually disabled child: the challenges of tool development. The Suffering Child 2002; 1:1–18.
56. Hunt AM, Burne R. Medical and nursing problems of children with neurodegenerative disease. Pall Med 1995;9:19–26.
57. Lawrence J, Alcock D, McGrath P, Kay J, MacMurray SB, Dulberg C. The development of a tool to assess neonatal pain expression. Neonatal Network 1993;12:59–66.
58. Krechel SW, Bildner J. CRIES: a new neonatal postoperative pain measurement tool. Initial testing of validity and reliability. Paediatr Anaesth 1995;5:53–61.
59. Grunau RVE, Craig KD. Facial activity as a measure of neonatal pain expression. In: Tyler EC, Krane EJ (eds). Advances in Pain Research Therapy: Pediatric Pain. Volume 15. New York: Raven Press, 1990.
60. Levetown M (ed). Compendium of Pediatric Palliative Care. Alexandria, VA: National Hospice and Palliative Care Organization, 2000.
61. Children's Hospice of Eastern Ontario Pain Scale. http://www.cebp.nL/media/m333.pdf (Accessed March 29, 2005).

VIII

Special Issues for the Nurse in End-of-Life Care

56

Mary L. S. Vachon

The Experience of the Nurse in End-of-Life Care in the 21st Century

Once you do hospice nursing you are never the same—love it or hate it, it brings mortality straight into your face.—A hospice nurse

- ***Key Points***
- *Hospice palliative care nursing can be both stressful and very rewarding.*
- *Caregivers may see their work as a job, a career, or a vocation, and their perceptions of stressors and ability to cope may vary accordingly.*
- *Hospice palliative care nursing is whole-person care in that the whole person of the patient and caregiver must be considered in the process of truly caring.*
- *To care for others effectively, we must care for ourselves.*

The discipline of hospice palliative care nursing began more than 30 years ago. The author has been involved in the field as a researcher, educator, and practicing clinician since before its early days and has written what might be seen as snapshots of stress and coping in hospice palliative care at various points over the past three decades.[1–7] This chapter focuses on the experience of hospice palliative care nursing at the beginning of the 21st century.

Method

The literature from the first 4 years of the new century was reviewed. Early in 2004, hospice palliative care nurses were interviewed in two settings: an inpatient palliative care unit in a large teaching hospital in Canada ($N=6$) and a free-standing hospice with an inpatient unit, a hospice home care team, a palliative care home care team, and satellite units on the west coast in the United States ($N=16$). The nurses were asked to comment on the stressors and satisfactions of hospice palliative care; how their stress was manifested; what, if any, role spirituality played in their personal lives and clinical practice; and how they coped in their role in hospice palliative care. In addition, nurses on the Canadian Hospice/Palliative Care Nurses Listserv were invited to respond and to describe their experience of palliative care, its stressors, and coping mechanisms they had found to be effective. Between late 2003 and early 2004, 23 nurses and one music therapist responded. Some nurses gave responses from their units or their community practices, as well as personal experiences. Colleagues from abroad wrote, telling some of their stories, and discussions were held with colleagues at the International Workgroup on Death, Dying and Bereavement Meeting in March 2004. To all of these people who shared their experiences and wisdom, the author is deeply grateful. Although not every respondent can be quoted, each interview has contributed to this chapter.

To ground this chapter in the reality of clinical practice and to show the process of the career of practitioners in the field, the chapter opens with excerpts from a letter received in response to the author's request to members of the Hospice/Palliative Care Listserv.

Hello Mary,

. . . It is now 23 years since I first heard you present at a conference (in Calgary). I have been drawn to this work since that life-changing conference, and have been involved directly and indirectly with hospice palliative nursing for over 20 years. But more importantly, I know many nurses and health professionals who have remained active and committed to this work at a front-line level. This is an amazing feat and, to me, flies in the face of prevailing perspectives of death saturation, accumulated losses, and burnout. This phenomenon truly warrants further investigation, discussion, and research.

I was delighted to see a qualitative study by Webster and Kristjanson[8] last year that proposed that hospice palliative care has exhilarating and vitalizing components. I think their research extends our understanding on the nature of palliative practice. Although I have not seen discussion yet in the literature, I suspect that one linkage between the notion of vitalization and hospice palliative nursing is located within nurses' opportunity to bear witness as their dying patients engage in their search for meaning. As Davies and Oberle write,[9] "finding meaning is strength-giving." Indeed it is. I contend it is strength-giving not only for the patient/person who is living with dying, but for the nurse who journeys with that individual and family.

Work-life conditions drove me away from direct care at a hospice, in search of an educator role, and the right to go to bed at night, to preserve my health and sense of well-being. To this day, I mourn the loss of my capacity to directly provide nursing care to dying persons and their family.

As you prepare to update the important chapter on stresses related to hospice palliative nursing, I hope that you can find a way to represent and articulate the other perspective related to the impact of this work: its capacity to inspire and inspirit the palliative care nurse.
—Deanna Hutchings, RN, MN; Victoria, BC

Frameworks for Viewing Hospice Palliative Care

In their powerful book, *Crossing Over: Narratives of Palliative Care*, which describes the experience of palliative care in two settings in the United States and Canada, Barnard and colleagues[10] stated, "Palliative care is whole-person care not only in the sense that the whole person of the patient (body, mind, spirit) is the object of care, but also in that the whole person of the caregiver is involved. Palliative care is, par excellence, care that is given through the medium of a human relationship" (p. 5). These authors documented the experiences of patients, families, and caregivers during some of their finest and not so fine moments. The reader comes to understand the humanity of all involved. Figure 56–1 reminds us that the caregiver as much as the patient will one day also face personal death.

A more recent study of nurses in a European academic palliative care setting[11] ($n = 14$) was undertaken to gain insight into the fact that many nurses were leaving feeling frustrated by the far-reaching medical orientation on the ward and unable to provide the care they wanted to give. These nurses were not neophytes. They were typically oncology nurses, 35 to 55 years of age, who had been working on this unit from 6 months to more than 4 years. They raised questions about the benefits and burdens of the medical treatment with which they collaborated. This study challenges whether the assumptions of Barnard[10] are completely generalizable at this point in time and may shed light on some of the conflicts hospice palliative care nurses are experiencing in the early years of the 21st century.

In order to understand the process that hospice palliative care nurses might experience in adapting to their role, the work of Georges and associates[11] is compared with that of Bernice Catherine Harper.[12] Dr. Harper is a social worker whose initial work involved supervising other social workers at City of Hope Hospital in California. Her model proposes that "learning to be comfortable in working with the dying patient and his family must be preceded by a growth and developmental process or sequence including cycles of productive change, observable behavior, and feeling" (p. 124). The stages of her model are described in depth in Chapter 2 (see Figure 2–1).

Striving to Adopt a Well-Organized and Purposeful Approach versus Striving to Increase the Well-being of the Patient

The study by Georges and associates[11] showed a different pattern of practice from that described by Harper[12] and by Barnard and coworkers.[10] Georges' group observed that the concept of palliative care demands that relationships with dying patients and their family members must be grounded in a real encounter and shared mutual understanding, and not in self-conscious use of

Figure 56–1. The very thing that we fear, we carry within us right now—our corpse. (Milarepa). *Source*: Mary Pocock, http://www.keylight.org (accessed February 28, 2005).

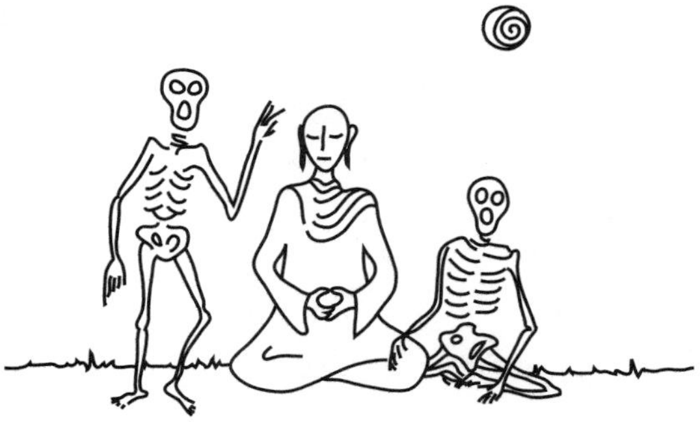

psychosocial skills and techniques. Harper states that health professionals must learn to cope with the anxieties which arise from such interpersonal experiences, coming to grips with their own feelings about mortality—both theirs and the patient's.[13] Palliative care is defined as a moral practice, based on hope and acceptance, that creates freedom and space for individual patients.[14]

That palliative care goes beyond the management of physical symptoms is well known but can be illustrated by the fact that 57% of 814 new referrals to the McMillan Nurses in the United Kingdom were for emotional support.[15]

Georges and colleagues[11] found that on the unit they studied, which was having trouble retaining nurses, two methods of practice described the nurses' actual activity. The first and more prominent method was "striving to adopt a well-organized and purposeful approach as a nurse on an academic ward" ($n=12$); the second was "striving to increase the well-being of the patient" ($n=2$).

Striving to Adopt a Well-Organized and Purposeful Approach in an Academic Setting

Several of the nurses adopted an academic attitude, underpinning their nursing practices with a scientific and professional rationale. They felt that it was important to use a "scientific" classification system of nursing diagnosis, to formulate nursing interventions in relation to the diagnosis, and to work within the limits set by the policy of the ward and the hospital. These nurses were very concerned with appropriate bed utilization and attempted to make discharge arrangements at an early stage in order to avoid unnecessary occupation of beds. The authors noted that, for these nurses, carrying out the nursing process in a professional manner was more important than investing in their relationships with patients.

Developing a Professional Attitude. A professional attitude refers to the rational approach of nurses, which is principally directed to gaining information about patients' symptoms and gaining insight into their problems. These nurses had a more detached attitude and tended to focus on identified tasks and problems. For example, when giving information to patients, nurses may pay much attention to clarity and completeness while failing to consider the emotional impact of the message.

Striving to Remain Objective. These nurses described patients' health problems in a formal language. They avoided speaking about problems that could not be labeled well, because they were not sure members of the multidisciplinary team would understand them. They argued that being objective was more in accordance with current professional developments in the field of nursing. They used diagnostic instruments to establish their observations. This allowed them to feel more comfortable speaking with physicians, to feel they were seen as being more trustworthy, and hence to be involved in the decision-making process. These nurses consciously strived to avoid allowing their feelings to have an impact on the way they responded to situations.

Being Task Oriented. These nurses were mostly committed to improving the situation of patients by solving or reducing their problems. They found it important to see that their interventions actually did improve the situation. If it was not possible to find a solution for patients' problems (e.g., to achieve sufficient symptom control, especially pain) nurses felt powerless and felt that they had not been able to achieve something meaningful for their patients.

Avoiding Emotional Stress. Coping with the emotional aspects of palliative care was a leading theme in the interviews with these nurses. The stress they experienced seemed to be related mainly to their appraisal of, and approach to, palliative care. Some said that the gravity of caring for dying patients would inevitably lead to burnout, so they did not plan to work too long in palliative care. These nurses tended to distance themselves from patients by focusing on tasks and the treatment of symptoms. Some nurses explained that their experience had taught them to remain more professional and detached, while others decided consciously not to invest too much in their relationship with patients because it would be too demanding.

This way of coping is not only found in Europe. Kelly and coworkers[16] wrote of dealing with death on the bone marrow transplantation (BMT) unit. They found that nurses often deny the difficulty of BMT, their emotional attachment to the patient, and the quality of the patient's life. They suggested that denial of emotion, if not appropriately reflected upon as a necessary strategy for dealing with very uncomfortable events, avoids a context in which understanding and ways of coping may be developed.

Embracing a Practitioner-Focused Perspective. It seems difficult for nurses to distance themselves from their own beliefs and to learn to be available to discern the perspective of patients and the meaning of the situation for them. Working in accordance with rules, these nurses emphasized the need to respect important rules of the ward. For example, if patients mentioned that they were considering euthanasia, some nurses explained that they first had to follow the procedures of the organization and then went on to explain them to the patient. "These nurses, by being mainly directed to using a rational and 'scientific' approach to their tasks, could fail to meet the real needs of patients and to pay sufficient attention to the development of a compassionate attitude. This perception, which was very much present on the ward, is mainly characterized by a distant approach towards patients and a well-developed self-awareness to work on one's own development as a professional."[11]

Striving to Increase the Well-being of the Patient

Nurses who practiced under the second model, of striving to increase the well-being of the patient, felt that it was important to use their individual capabilities, such as being sensitive to patients' concerns, and they adapted their approach to individual patients. They found that, when fully aware of the needs of patients, it was not difficult to explain them to other caregivers.

Care appeared to be a central concern for these nurses and a main source of satisfaction. They were aware that, thanks to their caring attitude, they could mean something to patients, even if only for a short time, and they felt this to be rewarding.

Adopting a Humble Attitude. In order to act in accordance with the needs of patients, these nurses tried to put their own considerations aside and to find a way to cope with their own emotions. They strove to adopt an unobtrusive approach and to show their availability to patients without forcing anything, even without expecting patients to answer their "invitation."

Giving Attention to Patients and Their Experiences. The approach of some nurses seemed to be shaped by their sensitivity to the feelings of patients. Being aware of patients' experiences is related to individual efforts to discover and understand what patients experience and why they react as they do. To be conscious of patients' experiences requires being really present. Some nurses, for example, were concerned that giving inadequate or incomplete information to patients could badly affect the direction of their decisions about further treatment. By their sensitivity to the experiences of patients, they became more connected with them and tried to really help them, even if they had to "break the rules."

Being Available. Being available, truly present, appeared to be a major virtue of nurses that allowed them to perceive the troubles and needs of a patient. They spoke about being sensitive to unspoken messages and about trusting their intuition. Being receptive to what is going on helped them see how they could contribute to the well-being of patients.

Valuing a Caring Attitude. The meaning nurses assigned to their work was based mainly on their experience as nurses and on their daily encounters with patient care. They developed a caring attitude based on authentic relationships with patients.

Remaining Attentive and Thoughtful. In order to find solutions to the problems they were confronted with, these nurses used self-reflection, striving to adopt a patient-centered attitude and to improve their caring attitude. They were also attentive to the context of their work, particularly to what should be changed so as to make it easier to express a caring perspective.

Trying to Accept and Cope with Emotional Strain. Nurses recognized that by caring for patients whose life was limited they were exposed to painful moments. However, they tried to accept emotionally difficult situations as a part of their own reality and did not attempt to avoid them. They strove to remain "authentic" and to stay close to patients even if they could not alleviate their problems.

Harper's Model of Cumulative Loss and the Caregiver

Bernice Harper's[12] work has been extensively described in Chapter 2. According to her model, there are six stages of adaptation experienced by the nurse caring for dying patients. These stages include intellectualization, emotional survival, depression, emotional arrival, deep compassion, and the Doer. To view Harper's model, called the "Line of Comfort-ability," the reader is referred to Figure 2–1.

Reflections on a Comparison of the Two Models

A comparison of Harper's work[12] with that of Georges' group[11] shows that, although Harper's model is very useful to describe the career path of some nurses in palliative care, there may be others who do not progress in the manner that Harper describes. From her perspective, these nurses may never have evolved beyond the first stage of comfort-ability. They are still involved in an intellectual approach to their role and are defending against allowing emotions to intrude. However, the nurses in the category striving to increase the well-being of the patient could be seen to be in Harper's stage IV or higher, in which they have "the control to practice the art of one's science" (p. 71).

Part of the reason for the split between the two approaches to nursing may be the bureaucratization of hospice palliative care. As Byock[17] noted, Max Weber, the renowned German sociologist, observed that, although social movements evolve to meet the needs of the time, they continue only through the process of bureaucratization. "Routinization is part and parcel of a social movement's success; with it comes stability, confidence and bureaucracy."[18] Some of the issues being confronted by the nurses in the Georges study[11] can be seen as related to the bureaucratization and standardization of palliative care. Both Doyle[19] and Kearney[20] warned earlier that palliative care specialists needed to avoid becoming merely symptomatologists. The field needed to recognize that

> We are, in the presence of death, working toward health—that balance of body, mind and spirit that is so much more than freedom from disease. For that reason I believe we have no choice but to be alert to and responsive to human spiritual needs.[19] [It is] as though the dragon (that is the patient's distress) also guards a treasure—something essential for that particular individual's healing at that moment in time. It is suggested that if we in palliative medicine fail to accept this view, a view which allows that there may also be a potential in the suffering of the dying process, if we sell out completely to the literalism of the medical model with its view that such suffering is only a problem, we will be in danger of following a pattern which could lead to our becoming 'symptomatologists', within just another specialty.[20]

An alternative explanation for nurses' maintaining distance from patients is that the nurses previously practiced a more patient-centered approach to nursing but stopped doing so because of their emotional reactions, for which they may not have had appropriate help and mentoring.

A nurse with many years of experience felt that she used to get overinvolved with her patients, but now she guards against that happening. She became very involved emotionally with a woman dying of amyotrophic lateral sclerosis:

She asked me to tell her when it was time to let go—when she got real close. One day she was not able to move. She could only blink one eye. She was lying in semi-Fowler's position, keening in her throat. I didn't know if her problems with shortness of breath were because of fear. I got her to the inpatient hospice unit. The next day she was still doing it, so I knew she wasn't there yet. I came out of her room and talked with the doctor and nurse. They planned to increase her morphine. I don't know what was on my face, but the chaplain asked, "Are you OK?" I said, "No." That was the first time it ever hit me like that. The next day she was better. Her breathing was quieter and gentler. Every day I'd go and say good-bye. That was my way of saying that she could let go. After several days she was still there—she had will. I asked the family if they had told her it was OK to go. I guessed that I would have to say it. I bent over and whispered in her ears, "It's OK to go now." She died that night. I had some feeling that maybe I hadn't done it soon enough and I had guilt. I don't want to be God, tell them it's OK to die. I didn't think that was my place, but I did it occasionally.

Now I've changed my job in order to still be able to remain in hospice. I didn't want management, but I had to back off because of several people I became very involved with. I needed to take a breather. I'm breathing here in extended care, with team support. There was an opening on nights. I took it tentatively. It's working for me. I don't have obligations at home, and I enjoy having some time off during weekdays. I'm not trying to escape from the intensity. I still go through intense moments. The intensity is good. . . . Now I've switched to nights. It provides a level of involvement that I can deal with that doesn't drain me so much.

Today some nurses may be straddling the fence between a deep involvement in patient care and feeling challenged by bureaucratic issues; others may be carrying on their practice in the manner that Harper describes, whereas others may be practicing a type of nursing that might be more common to that seen in traditional medical settings. The nurse in the above anecdote had clearly evolved through some of Harper's stages and was able to be a caring hospice palliative care nurse. She had backed off somewhat from her earlier involvement for the sake of her own mental health, and she was somewhat more protective of personal space and involvement. She was fortunate to work in a setting in which she could switch roles to preserve her mental and physical health. It would be interesting to know whether the nurses in the Netherlands palliative care unit had previously "connected" to patients and then distanced, or whether they had been distant all their professional careers.

Dr. Ira Byock speaks of trying to devise a palliative care system that is "cutting edge, medically crisp, but tender and loving."[17] What are some of the issues that keep this from happening?

Meier and colleagues[21] described what might happen in physicians, and these comments hold true for nurses as well (p. 3007):

> Seriously ill persons are emotionally vulnerable during the typically protracted course of an illness. Physicians respond to such patients' needs and emotions with emotions of their own, which may reflect a need to rescue the patient, a sense of failure or frustration when the patient's illness progresses, feelings of powerlessness against illness and its associated losses, grief, fear of becoming ill oneself, or a desire to separate from and avoid patients to escape these feelings. These emotions can affect both the quality of medical care and the physician's own sense of well-being, since unexamined emotions may also lead to physician distress, disengagement, burnout, and poor judgment.

These authors provided a model of reflective practice for physicians to use to increase their awareness and improve their clinical practice.

This next section of this chapter discusses some of the stressors currently experienced in hospice palliative care and the ways in which stress may be expressed.

Stressors in Palliative Care

This letter received from one of the nurses on the Canadian Hospice/Palliative Care Listserv gives a perspective of palliative care in a somewhat rural area of Canada and summarizes much of the stress and satisfaction received by hospice palliative care nurses.

> Well, as I was traveling around over the past two weeks throughout [the area I cover], I asked the nurses what they thought the stresses were in working in palliative care. . . . The community nurses—probably the most unsatisfied of all nurses, due to the awful working conditions [listed the following]:
>
> - No full time positions, therefore no security
> - Limited number of visits [they are allowed to make] . . . even if they think there are more needs
> - Feeling of lack of support by a team; difficult to get together to debrief; isolated practitioners out on the road; no 24-hour care available; difficulty in being able to reach a physician when needed; lack of family doctors, so patients have to go to the hospital
> - Emotional strain and need for more support
> - Need for more pain clinics or access to pain specialists
> - Dying children
> - Families treating them either really nicely or really badly (One nurse told that she was not allowed to heat up her tea in the microwave, sit too close to the patient, etc.)

- Funding issues
- Communication between hospital and community
- Late referrals from city hospitals when patients come back to community means little time to establish relationships and crisis pain management
- Difficulty keeping the family doctor involved during treatment, so that he or she will be up-to-date when the patient is at the end of life

However much as it sounds like their work is terrible, these nurses love their patients. It is just that they have to be so incredibly flexible, astute in their perceptions of the situations and understanding of the difference in families' reactions. This story just recently happened and shows the incredible courage and fortitude of nurses:

A patient had been dying slowly in the hospice suite in the community, but the goal was to go to hospital at the end, because the hospice is not staffed for end-of-life care yet. However, when the time came, the hospital was full and couldn't take her. The hospice nurse found the lady in the emergency department and, when it became inevitable that she couldn't be admitted, told the paramedics to take the lady back to the hospice suite. She got on the phone, notified the physician, called the community agency for any help they could give, rallied her own nurses and volunteers (this meant using up every last cent in her budget), and made the patient comfortable in the lovely environment of the hospice. The community nurse pulled out all the stops and got as much nursing help as she could also. The patient lived for several days, much to the amazement of the staff. One thing that she had requested before she died was to renew her wedding vows, and, sure enough, the staff got that organized very quickly and she died 12 hours later.

What a story of amazing flexibility and drive, all to make the end of life the best they all could for this woman.

Generally speaking, even though these nurses carry many stresses in their palliative care work, there are many dedicated ones who wouldn't work in any other field. Hats off to them, but we as managers and advocates must speak up for them to make their work life better.

A Model for Understanding Occupational Stress

Maslach and associates[22] reviewed the research on burnout over the past three decades. Previous research had focused on the Person-Environment Fit model.[23] More recent research has focused on the degree of match or mismatch between the person and six domains of the job environment. The greater the gap or mismatch between the person and the environment, the greater the likelihood of burnout. The greater the match or fit, the greater the likelihood of engagement with work. Mismatches arise when the process of establishing a psychological contract leaves critical issues unresolved or when the working relationship changes to something that the person finds unacceptable. Mismatches lead to burnout. Six areas of work life come together in a framework that encompasses the major organizational antecedents of burnout.

Workload—Excessive workload exhausts the individual to the extent that recovery becomes impossible. Emotional work is especially draining if the job requires people to display emotions inconsistent with their feelings. Workload relates to the exhaustion component of burnout.

Control—Control is related to inefficacy or reduced personal accomplishment. Mismatches often indicate that individuals have insufficient control over the resources necessary to do their work or insufficient authority to pursue the work in what they believe is the most effective manner.

Reward—Lack of reward may be financial if one does not receive a salary or benefits commensurate with one's achievements, or social, if one's hard work is ignored and not appreciated by others. The lack of intrinsic rewards (e.g., doing something of importance and doing it well) can also be a critical part of this mismatch.

Community—This mismatch arises when people lose a sense of personal connection with others in the workplace. Social support from people with whom one shares praise, comfort, happiness, and humor affirms membership in a group with a shared sense of values.

Fairness—This mismatch arises when there is not perceived fairness in the workplace. Fairness communicates respect and confirms people's self-worth. Mutual respect among people is central to a shared sense of community.

Values—Individuals may feel constrained by their job to do something that is unethical and not in accord with their own values. Alternatively, there may be a mismatch between their personal career goals and the values of the organization. People can also be caught in conflicting values of the organization, as when there is a discrepancy between a lofty mission statement and actual practice, or when the values are in conflict (e.g., high-quality service and cost containment do not always coexist).

Burnout arises from chronic mismatches between people and their work settings in some or all of these areas. Preliminary evidence suggests that the area of values may play a central mediating role for the other areas. Alternatively, individuals may vary in the extent to which each of the six areas is important to them. Some people may place a higher weight on rewards than on values, or some may be prepared to tolerate a mismatch regarding workload if they receive praise and good pay and have good relationships with colleagues.

The recent research on hospice palliative care nursing is now reviewed within this framework.

Workload

Hospice nurses initially prided themselves on having the time to spend with patients that was conducive to the best patient care. Current issues with managed care, the nursing shortage, and fiscal restraint have changed this situation in many settings.[24] A study in the Netherlands found that direct patient-care activities had an impact on stress through a heavy workload of complex care, a shortage of staff, and an experienced lack of competence.[25] Papadatou and colleagues[26] found that nurses working with critically ill and dying children in Hong Kong and Greece felt unable to provide quality care because of the shortage in nursing personnel. This added to their stress. However, in a study of hospice nurses in the United Kingdom, Payne[27] found that, despite that fact that workload was a frequently reported stressor, it was not related to burnout, suggesting that some stress may be necessary for optimal functioning.

Several of the nurses interviewed for this chapter commented on the issue of workload. A selection of comments follows.

A Canadian nurse working in a rural setting stated,

> Stress. . . . . . that's the word of the year, I think. It seems that while the workload is increasing, funds continue to decrease. We are all trying to do more with less . . . and it's beginning to show.

A nurse in a large palliative care program commented,

> I'm stressed out by being overloaded with 14 to 15 patients. There is a high acuity level with each patient. We don't have enough time to deal with each patient. I try not to carry my frustration into the next person. Too much work, not enough time. The workload is unmanageable. I've worked for 10 years in hospice. We have to keep doing more, faster with less. There is a push for productivity, what your case load is, how fast you can work, how little overtime you can bill for.

A palliative care nurse who had worked in many settings commented on the role strain that she had felt in a previous position:

> It would be 3:00 A.M. I'd be driving in west Texas avoiding the cows in the road. There were no streetlights. I would be winging it and praying for good directions. I'd be going to the drug store meeting with the pharmacist in the middle of the night. Hopefully I'd have a good doctor who would cover me. I'd hope and pray that I wouldn't have to go back and pronounce the person soon after I left. I'm a single Mom. I'd bring the kids when I was on call. I'd pile in pillows and the dog and try to make it fun. We'd go to a restaurant or a park. The kids would ask, "Mom, are you on call? Are we going on an 'excavation'?"

Control

Current research suggests that restructuring of high-demand, low-control jobs may enhance productivity and reduce disability costs.[28] Recent practices in hospice led by fiscal constraints have raised increasing concern. Nurses are sometimes expected to perform procedures in the community for which they have not been prepared and for which no supervision is provided. When people are expected to assume responsibility with inadequate training, they have difficulty functioning.

Nurses report being in situations, both in the hospital and in the community, in which they feel responsible for alleviating the pain of a palliative care patient yet do not have a physician willing to order the medication they feel is sufficient to control pain.

> I'm the admitting nurse. I have so many hours to get a patient on the service. I can't predict if the doctor will call back. He may not call back until the next day. It can happen that I am at X Hospital. The patient is going home. I call his doctor and tell him that the patient is short of breath and there isn't an order for Ativan. The doctor may not call back until tomorrow. We could use our hospice doctor, but I don't want to make the referring doctor angry.

In addition, with the earlier discharge of sicker patients, nurses with limited experience may be expected to care for seriously ill palliative care patients in their home, without access to physicians skilled in effective palliative care and symptom management.[29] Dr. Neil MacDonald[30] testified before a Senate Subcommittee on End-of-Life Care in Canada that the opinion of Quebec oncologists and palliative care physicians in one study was that the big problem in managing cancer pain was the reluctance on the part of physicians to use opioids and the misunderstanding of patients about the use of pain medications.

An American nurse said that when she reported that a dying patient was in severe pain and she felt that he needed to have his medication increased, the physician asked who he was treating—the patient or the nurse?

Issues of control can also be related to physical safety. Nurses reported feeling unsafe when they were making visits to deserted country homes in the middle of snowstorms without access to cell phones or other ways of communicating if there is trouble; visiting in unsafe areas of the community, where the nurses do not feel safe during the day, and particularly at night; and visiting in homes where the family dynamics are such that nurses do not feel physically safe. If there are no organizational policies about how to handle these situations, staff can feel quite stressed.[24]

Nurses may also feel out of control if they begin to get emotionally involved with patients and families without sufficient supervision and support. Barnard and coworkers[10] noted the need to give full weight to both the promise and the fear of intimacy in palliative care and referred to palliative care as challenging caregivers to leap into the confrontation with the forces of chaos and disintegration (p. 26):

> We live in the tension between the promise of intimacy and the fear of our own undoing. Surprised by intimacy, we are exhilarated and lifted beyond ourselves, as if we have not only made contact with another person

> but also with another dimension of living. At the same time we are brought face to face with forces of chaos and destructiveness, internal as well as external, and we fear that we ourselves shall be destroyed.

These feelings can lead caregivers to feel out of control and to experience significant role strain.

Nurses also feel out of control because of the timing of patient referrals:

> Patients are referred later and sicker. They are more acute. You don't have the time that you used to have. Ten years ago we had patients for a couple of months on average. Now it is just weeks. The doctors don't refer until later because there is a fear of referring too soon with reimbursement. There are more treatment modalities. Patient's families want them to try more. There is less time for me to do what I need to do, which is (1) palliate symptoms, (2) prepare people for impending death, (3) be a supportive presence so they aren't so afraid, and (4) establish a trusting rapport.

An inpatient male nurse commented:

> Patients come when you can't control it, they poop when you can't control it, want ice when you can't control it. There are other jobs with more control. I came into nursing kicking and screaming to do hospice nursing. I spent a lot of time looking for something fulfilling to do with my life. I thought, "If there is a purpose to life, then I should be able to find it." I came to terms with being a man in nursing. I love my job. I'm here on my day off. There is so much work. Someone poops when I have to do paperwork.

Nurses can also feel out of control if they believe that they do not have the necessary education to handle problems with patients and families. White and colleagues[31] asked respondents to rank-order 12 topics that comprise end-of-life care competency that they wish they had learned in nursing school. Almost two thirds of the respondents ranked one of three competencies highest: how to talk to patients and families about dying (30%), pain control techniques (28%), and comfort care nursing interventions (9%).

Older nurses (born before 1946) were 40% more likely than were nurses born after 1946 to rank how to talk to patients and families about the dying process as number 1. "Baby boomer" nurses (born between 1946 and 1964) were 28% more likely than were the other age groups to rank how to talk to patients and families about the dying process as number 1, followed by "generation X" nurses (born after 1964) at 27%. This difference by age group might be related to the times when these nurses were educated and the prevailing attitudes about nurses' roles in communicating with patients and families about dying. In addition, longer life spans and demands for end-of-life care are greater now than when older nurses received their education. One might have hoped that ongoing education and maturing would have helped the older nurses to be more comfortable dealing with these issues, but that did not seem to be the case.

Reward

Funding issues were a problem for many programs. Participants in the Australian study[8] reported that economic pressures resulted in less staff support, competition between services for funding, inadequate funding to provide services in areas of need, lack of support for psychosocial needs including bereavement care, and experienced staff's leaving palliative care. Nurses in a Canadian study[32] reported difficulty with resource allocation issues, but the majority of their concerns were related to their inability to provide quality care because of financial constraints and staffing cutbacks.

An American nurse noted some of the difficulties with the financial reward of hospice palliative care nursing:

> The money isn't very good in a not-for-profit hospice, but I can cope with the pay. I could make more, though, in a for-profit hospice.

Community

Team communication problems have been a significant part of hospice palliative care and, to a lesser extent, the field of oncology since the early days of these specialties. The research on this subject has been reviewed elsewhere.[5,24] Team issues have been documented in numerous studies and across many cultures.[4,25,26]

Lack of cooperation and discipline occurs when teams have coordination without cooperation. If team members are ordered about without consultation or participation, they will not give their best effort and will fail.[24]

Studying hospice nurses in the United Kingdom, Payne[27] found that dealing with death and dying, inadequate preparation, and workload were slightly more problematic than were conflict with doctors, conflict with other nurses, lack of support, and uncertainty concerning treatment. However, in that study conflict with staff contributed to both the emotional exhaustion and depersonalization subscales of the Maslach Burnout Inventory.[33]

Community can also refer to the community in which caregivers live. Palliative care workers in rural Australia spoke of the difficulty involved in being expected to work beyond normal working hours and of the lack of anonymity in a small rural community.[34]

Fairness

Rivalries between hospice and other settings of care and between different hospice programs have long been an issue.[4,24] Rivalries are encountered as programs try to determine with which agencies, if any, they will have preferred partner arrangements. Other settings have developed palliative care programs in an apparent move to avoid referral to hospice and to gain access to funding that might be made available for dying persons.[24] In addition, there are financial barriers, including reimbursement systems that provide only for the options of cure or certain death.[35,36]

Whedon,[36] an oncology nurse whose practice changed to pain and symptom management, observed (p. 27),

> Patients without a care provider; unwilling to forego beneficial palliative chemotherapy, radiation, or surgery; or with a prognosis that was not absolutely certain to be 6 months or less, were caught in the middle. This part of the path felt treacherous; we had no trail markers, no compass, and darkness was about to fall.

Values

Webster and Kristjanson[8] did a small qualitative study of caregivers in various professions working in palliative care. They spoke of the importance of being allowed to bring personal values to the workplace and of being encouraged in their personal growth.

Oberle and Hughes[32] did a qualitative study of 7 doctors and 14 nurses working in acute care adult medical-surgical areas, including intensive care. The respondents were asked to describe ethical problems that they frequently encountered in their clinical practice. All participants experienced ethical problems related to decision-making at the end of life. The core problem for both doctors and nurses was witnessing suffering, which engendered a moral obligation to reduce that suffering. Uncertainty about the best course of action for the patient and family was a source of moral distress. Competing values, hierarchical processes, scarce resources, and communication emerged as common themes. The key difference between the groups was that doctors are responsible for making decisions and nurses must live with those decisions.

Nurses experienced moral distress in these uncertain situations when they believed that the wrong course of action was being followed and they were contributing to the patient's misery.[32] Nurses tended to judge the doctors' actions as a function of whether they had made the right decision and written the right order. Nurses often had clear ideas about what was acceptable and what was not, reflecting a degree of certainty not evident in the doctors' responses. Distress arose for nurses when they perceived that the patient's suffering was intensified because doctors just could not or would not write the "appropriate" orders. However, paradoxical thinking was evident in many of the nurses' responses. Whereas they expressed concern that the doctor had not made the "right" decision, they also recognized that the decisions were difficult and that outcomes were, indeed, uncertain.

Competing values operated in these situations. Decisions about care and treatment at the end of life are intrinsically value laden, and recognition of this fact raised concerns for all participants. Questions arose about whose values should carry the most moral weight in any given situation and whose values had, or should have had, the most impact on decisions taken. This was particularly problematic if the patient was unable to speak for himself or herself. The value embraced by all participants was the good of the patient. In the absence of a patient voice, patient autonomy was not a realistic goal, but doing "what the patient would want" was a reasonable alternative. Unfortunately, it was seldom clear just what the patient would want, and the parties in discussion about continuing or discontinuing treatment sometimes possessed different beliefs about the patient's wishes.[32]

The authors concluded that observed differences between doctors and nurses were a function of the professional role played by each rather than differences in ethical reasoning or moral motivation. For nurses, ethical problems were related to their "lower" position on the hierarchical structure: not being listened to by doctors; being expected to remain silent even when witnessing wrong choices; being unable to affect decisions despite their professional assessment and detailed understanding of the patient's condition. Again, their problem was with their inability to reduce the patient's suffering, which in turn resulted in their own suffering (experienced as moral distress). Neither group appeared to be aware that hierarchy and a sense of powerlessness were issues for the other.[32]

Georges and coauthors[11] quoted James and Field,[37] who said that when the originating ethics of palliative care are marginalized, the heart and soul of care are endangered. "Expert" values based on medical technologies and psychosocial skills replace the compassionate help. Death is no longer a truth to confront but a process that must be managed as efficiently as possible. Nurses who participated in this study[11] were encouraged in this context to acquire knowledge and skills, whereas development of the moral qualities necessary to care for those who are dying was not addressed. Therefore, they became less sensitive to the moral values in situations. They responded less to problems because their moral values were endangered, mainly because they conflicted with their professional norms and established rules. In situations of pain and suffering, these nurses mainly tried to overcome their powerlessness by a medical approach, overlooking the possibilities of alleviating suffering by an authentic caring attitude based on really meeting with patients.

Studies about the experience of palliative care nurses show that they are looking at patients' problems in a broad way and trying to see them from the patient's point of view, not merely from a medical point of view.[38] Caring has repeatedly been found to be the core value that nurses espouse when caring for the terminally ill.

The findings of George and colleagues[11] illustrate the potential differences between applying palliative care in an academic hospital directed by a predominantly medical approach and applying it in the tradition of the hospice movement, where care is at its most fundamental. Time will tell whether Byock's vision[17] of "cutting edge, medically crisp, but tender and loving care" can be realized.

Issues of Death and Dying

Although the literature has been somewhat divided as to whether care of the dying is a major stressor in hospice palliative care,[4–6] recent research in the burnout area has focused explicitly on emotion-work variables (e.g., the requirement to display or suppress emotions on the job, the requirement to be emotionally empathic) and has found these emotional factors do account for additional variance in burnout scores over and above job stressors.[22]

The most problematic stressor reported by hospice nurses was "death and dying."[27] Greek oncology nurses studied by Georgaki and associates[39] believed that they were not sufficiently trained in communications skills and therefore found it difficult to have an open conversation with a patient about his or her forthcoming death. Although a large percentage of the participant nurses believed that it is essential for a patient to know the truth to accomplish a successful therapeutic relationship, their responses showed that they also believed that too much information may lead the patient to feelings of disappointment, despair, and isolation. The authors concluded that Greek nurses wish to be closer to patients and to communicate and share their thoughts and worries. However, they find it difficult to do so because of inadequate education in communication skills.

The difficulties associated with the care of dying persons may also in part a result of the close connections palliative care nurses often develop with their patients. As has already been noted, palliative care is, par excellence, care that is given through the medium of a human relationship.[10] Barnard and colleagues noted that education for palliative care involves the art of building and sustaining relationships and using the self as a primary instrument for diagnosis and treatment. This involves psychological risk-taking that may be unique in the health field.[10] As was clear from the work of Georges and associates,[11] not all nurses are prepared for this involvement, either personally or through their education, professional training, mentoring, and supervision.

Boston and coworkers[40] noted that dying persons experience disruption of the essence of day-to-day living and challenges to their perception of who they are. Through this process, they gain new wisdom and reshape their sense of meaning in life. A different way of knowing the world evolves, characterized by inner know-how and tacit knowledge that defines the self in relationship to others. Caregivers and others around them "are perceived to be in another place, or don't seem to be there at all" (p. 248). Patients and caregivers may feel that they just don't connect. Boston and coauthors[40] speak of palliative care as taking caregivers into emotional realms that are neither easy nor comfortable. The caregiver may be permanently changed through this encounter.

Staff in an African hospice had a well-established program that had changed over the years as the country had changed. They themselves were being changed and needed to respond in different ways as a result of the encounters they were having. The hospice director spoke of a family she and her staff were dealing with: the father had died of AIDS; the mother was quite sick with AIDS and was being cared for by her 11-year-old son, who was also HIV positive, as was one of his siblings. His 5-year-old sister was HIV negative. The oldest brother went into the city to earn money to help the family and was killed by rebels. The staff seriously wondered what they could do in this situation in which they had to take the least possible goal and try to make things better in whatever way they could (anonymous personal communication).

In a study comparing nurses working with dying children in Hong Kong and in Greece,[26] nurses generally were assigned to work on the unit, rather than choosing this work. They reported helplessness when caring for a dying patient and difficulties in communicating with the children and parents during the terminal phase of the disease. Part of their difficulty related to feeling unable to provide quality care because of the shortage in nursing personnel or feeling unable to alleviate the child's physical and/or emotional suffering or the parents' distress. Occasionally, difficulties were also associated with a desperate need to cognitively make sense of childhood death, which appeared "meaningless" because it reversed the perceived order of nature.

Multiple Losses

One does not have to work very long in palliative care before one begins to feel the accumulation of grief related to the experience of multiple losses. Although Mount wrote of the concept of multiple losses within the context of oncology,[41] the concept became more recognized with the AIDS epidemic. The concept of multiple losses in AIDS caregivers reflected in part the reality that many caregivers were caring for dying patients while partners, friends, and members of their social network were dying at the same time.[24]

Garfield[42] wrote of alternating between numbness and experiencing grief while caring for people dying of AIDS. Papadatou and coworkers[26] reported that the majority of the pediatric nurses working with dying children they studied acknowledged that the impending or actual death of a patient elicits a grieving process, which is characterized by a fluctuation between experiencing and avoiding loss and grief. Greek and Chinese nurses differed in their expression of grief and in how they attributed meaning to childhood death.

Papadatou[43] extended earlier work[4] to note that the losses nurses experience may extend beyond the deaths of their patients. These losses include

- Loss of a close relationship with a particular patient
- Loss due to the professional's identification with the pain of family members
- Loss of one's unmet goals and expectations
- Losses related to one's personal system of beliefs and assumptions about life
- Past unresolved losses or anticipated future losses
- The death of self

Satisfactions in Hospice Palliative Care

Although work in hospice palliative care can be stressful, it also has many rewards. Current research has focused on the experience of job engagement, which is conceptualized as being the opposite of burnout. It involves energy, involvement, and efficacy. Engagement involves the individual's relationship with work. As described by Maslach and colleagues,[22] it involves a sustainable workload, feelings of choice and control, appropriate recognition and reward, a supportive work community, fairness and justice, and meaningful and valued work. Engagement is also characterized by high levels of activation and pleasure. Clearly, for many caregivers, their work in hospice palliative care is very engaging, as was noted in the research reviewed in this section.

Palliative care is a way of living. Vitality—the capacity to live and develop which is associated with energy, life, animation, and importance—is the core meaning of palliative care. This way of living involves unity with self, being touched to the heart, and personal meaning. Caregivers in Webster and Kristjanson's study[8] found that the lessons learned from their work added meaning to their personal and professional lives. Caregivers were animated in describing their work, and they articulated the importance of their experience in terms of personal growth for patients, families, and caregivers. Interactions with patients, families, and colleagues were meaningful, and the workplace was described as being full of fun. Crucial to the experience of palliative care for the participants was patient and family, holistic care, and the interdisciplinary team.[8]

Others have described the satisfactions in palliative care as helping patients to find meaning in suffering[10,44] and experiencing positive relationships and support from colleagues.[45] Despite the difficulties, nurses in units in both China and Greece derived significant rewards from their work with dying children.[26,28] They reported a deep sense of satisfaction from having contributed something significant in the care of each child. They believed they were doing a very difficult but also meaningful job. They often described their role as "unique" or "special" by comparison to the role of nurses who worked in other units. In both units and both cultures, nurses' involvement and intimate encounters with children were recognized and appreciated by the patient's family.[26,28]

The nurses interviewed for this study also validated this concept of engagement in their work. Deanna Hutchings, who was quoted earlier in this chapter wrote in her letter,

> Years ago, I cut a short article by Campion out of the *Globe and Mail.* Her words contain, I believe, seeds of truth that enable us to see hospice palliative practice in new ways. She wrote the following:
>
> "When people work closely with the dying . . . something happens on this intimate journey, with its risks and sadness and fear and joy, with its naked acknowledgment of the mystery of our human existence, that sustains health-care providers far beyond the demands of caring for a particular patient."[46]
>
> Yes, something happens. As nurses, we need to begin to explore and explicate what that sustaining "something" is and how that transformative "something" impacts seasoned nurses in this field.
>
> I liken the importance of identifying the nourishing parts of this work to acknowledging the beautiful moments that commingle with difficult moments in our work, and in our lives. While walking in the Victoria rain yesterday morning, I was treated to a stunning rainbow, and I thought, hospice nursing is like that. We can focus on examining the "rain" of stresses in this work, but we can also look up, and savor the exquisite rainbow of tender moments and courageous acts to which we bear witness in the course of our nursing practice with dying persons. I believe we need to acknowledge the rainbows and inform one another about the rainbows.

Coping in Hospice and Palliative Care

In the author's earlier study of more than 600 caregivers from around the world, the primary personal coping mechanism was a sense of commitment, control, and pleasure in one's work.[4] This characteristic is strongly linked with Antonovsky's sense of coherence,[47] with Kobasa's personality construct of hardiness,[48,49] and with Hirshberg and Barasch's sense of congruence.[50]

Compassionate Caring and Service

More recently, Carolyn Myss[51] has spoken of the difference between a job, a career, and a vocation. She refers to the chakras—sources of energy in the body having to do with various aspects of life.

A job takes care of the lower chakras, the first and second chakras (having to do with safety, security, emotions such as fear and anger, putting a roof over one's head and food into one's body). A career takes care of the third chakra (the ego, one's power source in the universe). A vocation involves the higher chakras, or service to one's soul (the heart chakra, giving and receiving love; the throat chakra, speaking one's truth and getting in touch with one's creativity; the third eye, seeing what we cannot see with our human eyes; and the seventh chakra, connecting with the Divine, or the universe).

Caregivers in hospice palliative care can see their roles as a job, a career, or a vocation. This perspective may further understanding of the different approaches caregivers take. For some, hospice palliative care is a job—simply a way to earn a living. For others, perhaps some of those nurses described by Georges and colleagues,[11] palliative care is a career, feeding their ego. This is not to say that the work they do is not good, but that in some ways the work is more about themselves and their own satisfaction than it is about entering into a deeply caring relationship with patients. These nurses have been taught skills, as opposed to reflecting on values. By mastering nursing diagnosis and being able to speak with physicians in a manner they believe is appropriate to an academic setting, these nurses can derive a great deal of satisfaction. However, some would say that something is missing from their care—which perhaps explains why so many staff were leaving the unit. For many caregivers in hospice and palliative care, their work is a vocation—service to their souls. In truly meeting the needs of others, they are meeting the needs of their own souls.

Dr. Rachel Naomi Remen[52] writes, "Basically service is about taking life personally, letting the lives that touch yours touch you" (p. 197). She contends that service is a relationship between equals. When you serve, the work itself keeps you from burnout. Unless you let the patients touch you, you will never last in this work.[52] Protecting ourselves from loss rather than grieving and healing our losses is one of the major causes of burnout[53]: "We burn out not because we don't care but because we don't grieve. We burn out because we have allowed our hearts to become so filled with loss that we have no room left to care" (p. 52).

Remen speaks of compassion, which, she says, "begins with the acceptance of what is most human in ourselves, what is most capable of suffering. In attending to our own capacity to suffer, we can uncover a simple and profound connection between our own vulnerability and the vulnerability in all others. Experiencing this allows us to find an instinctive kindness toward life which is the foundation of all compassion and genuine service."[52] This concept recognizes the reciprocity that is inherent in the caring relationship. Jean Watson, a nurse theoretician, states, "When both care providers and care receiver are coparticipants in caring, the release can allow the one who is cared for to be the one who cares, through the reflection of the human condition that in turn nourishes the humanness of the care provider. In such connectedness they are both capable of transcending self, time and space."[54]

An image of compassion that has become central to the author's professional work and life is The Man in Sapphire Blue, an illumination that was received by the 12th century mystic, Hildegard of Bingen. Mathew Fox[55] writes of this image and states that the color of the heart chakra is green. Hildegard built her entire theology on *viriditas* or "greening power." She felt that all creatures contained the greening power of the Holy Spirit, which makes all things creative and nourishing. In her picture of the Man in Sapphire Blue, the man's hands are outstretched in front of his chest. This gesture is an ancient metaphor for compassion, because compassion is about taking heart energy and putting it into one's hands—that is, putting it to work in the world. This is the work of healing and assisting. As Fox[55] described the image, "An energy field surrounds the man. Clearly this is a man whose 'body is in the soul' and not whose soul is in the body. Both Hildegard and later, Meister Eckhart, spoke of the body/soul relationship in this imagery of shared energy systems, with the soul energy being the greater entity" (p. 23). In the illumination, there is "an aperture at the man's head, so that this powerful healing energy can leave his own field and mix with others—and vice versa" (p. 23).

Recent 20th century science found "evidence" of this shared energy "seen" by a mystic in the 12th century. Dr. Michael Kearney, a hospice physician, uses concepts in the "new physics"[44] to describe the integration between the traditional medical model and the healing model that can be applied in palliative care and its relevance to the relationship between the caregiver and the patient. "The quantum idea that ours is a participatory universe has implications for carers. Although there are still subjects and objects within the healing model, the boundaries may not be as clear as they were within the medical model. Caring now becomes a dynamic event. While the roles of 'carer' and 'patient' remain, there is also an interweaving of the two. The term 'clinical objectivity' is joined by that of 'clinical subjectivity,' acknowledging a shared dimension to the healing encounter."[44]

Harper[12] says of stage VI in her model "The Doer" (as described in Chapter 2 of this textbook) that to "some extent Doers have learned how to gather from the universe what they need to do their work. Their clients recognize something in them and feed back this information that can then be used to help others" (p. 101). Another example of this is provided by Vachon.[56]

> Several years ago, I was diagnosed with stage 4 non-Hodgkin's lymphoma. My odds of survival were 1:4. This was a spiritually transforming experience which led to many changes in my life, including leaving my position in an academic setting. Through this experience I felt a connection to God, the universe, and the people I had worked with who had gone before me. I started using these new-found insights in my clinical practice through the use of meditation and prayer with clients.

The following story from the author's own experience is used with Andrea's permission.

CASE STUDY
Andrea

At 27, Andrea was diagnosed with soft tissue sarcoma. Within a few months she had a local recurrence, and within another few months she had metastatic disease in her lungs. She was told that she would have chemotherapy, which would probably not work very well because of the nature of her disease. Andrea was told that her disease showed up as a matrix in her lungs and that even if the cancer did disappear it would be hard to see this, because the matrix would continue to be there. At the end of chemotherapy, she would have surgery and would have the remaining cancer removed. She was told that a year later her cancer would recur, and again she would have chemotherapy and surgery. Andrea was understandably very upset by this news. She was referred for help in dealing with this new diagnosis.

We did a series of meditations before and during chemotherapy. After her first chemotherapy treatment, Andrea developed febrile neutropenia and was admitted to a local community hospital. There she became quite ill and during this time saw a vision of the face of God. At around the same time, the author was walking and listening to spiritual tapes including a favorite song with the words, "You shall see the face of God and live." When Andrea returned for her second chemotherapy treatment, her oncologist could not find her previous X-ray films but said that if he didn't know better he would think that her chest X-ray was normal. He would, however, continue with chemotherapy and then she would have surgery at the end of chemo. When chemo finished, there was still no evidence of disease, so there was no surgery. A year and a half later, Andrea is well; she has moved, married, and begun a new career.

Was there a connection between the meditations, the vision, the tape, and the remission? We will never know, but sometimes, as we are able to access some powers beyond our own, such occurrences happen more than they used to before we accessed such powers.

Environmental Coping in Hospice Palliative Care

Despite the fact that the stressors of staff in hospice palliative care have been documented from the beginning of the field,[1–3,57] there is no substantial body of work documenting the impact of programs of intervention. This section reports on some recent research as well as some programs that hold promise.

Teamwork

Chaplain and psychotherapist Peter Speck[58] noted that the ability to "contain" powerful reactions and strong emotions is an essential part of all caring relationships. As quoted by Kearney,[44] "The most significant factor in creating containment for the person in suffering is the web of caring relationships that establish security and trust with that person. However, the containment that is created by interprofessional teamwork does not simply come about because a number of different disciplines happen to be involved in that patient's care and treatment. The container has to be built, a process which involves deliberate and conscious effort" (p. 88). Workers in each discipline involved in the patient's care must have a clear sense of their own professional identity, including their profession's strengths and limitations. There must also be an acknowledgment of and respect for the contributions that other professions have to offer[44]:

> There must also be an awareness of shared areas of care, where close communication and cooperation are essential to avoid duplication of effort, interdisciplinary territorialism, and confusion or 'flooding' of the patient. . . . The process of team self-awareness comes through individual disciplines meeting together and with regular interdisciplinary team meetings. [In addition,] each discipline needs to be fully versed in the Hippocratic approach as it applies to its domain of clinical responsibility and to be effective in its therapeutic task. Such competence helps to create trust with patients, to lessen their sense of fear, and to increase their sense of security. (p. 88)

Kearney[44] suggested that the presence of an outside facilitator, experienced in team management and psychodynamics, can be invaluable in the early stages of team building as well as when dealing with difficult issues arising from the care of a particular patient.

Regular opportunities to meet and talk together can also help teams to develop a respectful understanding of differences in respect to specific situations. For example, Redinbaugh and associates[59] noted that physicians and nurses may prefer different coping strategies and may have different personality structures that lead to differences in response to patient deaths. These authors drew on Holland's theory of occupational interest[60] to propose a model of grief that might help in understanding team differences. Individuals have natural propensities and aversions for minimizing grief reactions. Emotion-focused coping would be used by those with a high "Social" score and low "Realistic" score. They would be likely to talk with others about their grief. Those with a high "Artistic" score with a low "Social" score would attempt to understand their grief through its depiction in literature and the arts. High "Conventional" scores paired with low "Investigative" scores are reflective of those who are less likely to dampen their grief with alcohol or drugs and more likely to use personal faith to resolve their grief.

Both teams and individual caregivers need to find ways to manage their grief in order to survive in this work. The approach each individual uses may be different, but there needs to be a way of grieving the losses that occur.

Models of Team Intervention

The development of supportive, collaborative work relationships is fundamental to enhancement of self-efficacy and self-esteem. It is important that organizations create the opportunity for ongoing support and that nurses have the time to attend support sessions, especially for those working alone in the community. Support may be provided through team meetings, easy access to consultants, a buddy or mentor system for ongoing support, and the opportunity to debrief after critical incidents.[24] Ideally, caregivers would also be provided with supervisors or mentors who could assume a role similar to that which Harper[12] had with the oncology social workers with whom she worked.

Although support groups are recommended almost as a panacea for either team stress or problems with patients, their effectiveness has generally not been well researched. Van Staa and coworkers[25] described an intervention in a new palliative care unit in the Netherlands. A carefully designed training program and staff support activities were meant to enhance personal growth, to give emotional support, and to deal with death and bereavement issues. The interventions did not involve mutual collaboration, practical problems, managerial and communication skills, or the skills needed to deliver complex palliative care. There was a cultural difference between the external consultants, who embraced a relational therapeutic world view, and the hospice staff, who came from a rational, technical, hospital environment. To be successful, the former approach involves complete trust and openness.. Not all staff members were convinced of the value of the nondirective approach. In addition, a therapeutic group is fundamentally different from a group that has to work together after the session. The researchers suggested that future leaders should focus on content as well as process issues. They also suggested that adequate resources, a supportive management structure, an extensive educational training program, and attention to individual needs should accompany support groups. These issues have been identified earlier,[4,5] so it is worth noting that they still exist.[61]

Medland and colleagues[45] described an intervention with 150 members of the multidisciplinary team at Northwestern Memorial Hospital. They noted that, particularly during times of uncertainty and change, social networks played a key role in protecting staff against burnout.[62] Community building in the workplace is touted as a defense against the constantly changing environment, according to Parker and Gadbois,[63] who suggested encouraging "community in the workplace" as a value in creating a meaningful and rewarding work environment. Medland's group[45] suggested that the failure of management to address this "human side of work" and the need for support and a supportive work environment intensify stressors and put employees at risk for developing the burnout syndrome.

Medland and colleagues[45] also described an intervention to interrupt the cycle of turnover on a state-of-the-art oncology unit. The intervention included an array of tactics and strategies, with the development of social support through enhanced collaboration and the cultivation of stress management strategies being high on the list. Other issues addressed included compensation, benefits, flexible scheduling, supportive management, and staffing that is in line with the demands of patient acuteness. Issues surrounding patient intensity exerted the most powerful impact on turnover. The leadership team set out to create a healthier work environment. The goal[45] was to create an environment wherein care providers would be infused with an intense sense of gratification and fulfillment and where a passion for service and excellence would prevail (p. 50).

A series of one-day Circle of Care retreats addressed specific concerns pertinent to improving the psychosocial wellness and skills of care providers. A total of 150 multidisciplinary team members attended this program over five sessions. These workshops were seen to be the first phase of a comprehensive, ongoing psychosocial support program for staff, tailored to address the psychosocial demands of oncology nursing. The day included interactive and informal presentations about staying well, managing losses, developing stress management skills and strategies (e.g. relaxation, journaling), facilitating bereavement, cultivating team effectiveness, group support, story telling, and an art therapy session, called "All Gifts Differing," that offered a reflection of the unique attributes staff members bring to the work setting.

The intervention beyond the Circle of Care workshops used the FISH! management philosophy,[64] which emphasizes the power each person has to improve the work environment.

In addition, the program used the CARES philosophy to provide a framework for incorporating the stress management and self-care skills staff members had learned into their practice. This philosophy involves the following[45]:

C—*creation* of a community of care, as opposed to feeling solely responsible for meeting the needs of clients; *caring* for each team member unconditionally; being *cognizant* that the stress of the day depends more on work group than on patient care assignment

A—*awareness* of the signs and symptoms of stress and burnout in self and others, and a recognition that stress management needs to be as integral a competency as preparing chemotherapy treatments

R—*reinforcement* of the importance of relaxation and rejuvenation as a self-care skill so that the needs of others can be met effectively

E—*emphasis* on regular aerobic exercise and healthy eating

S—*spiritual awareness* and reconnection to whatever is personally meaningful: reconnect to faith and be playful and attentive to the "spirit" at work.

After the Circle of Care retreat session, a Circle of Care Bereavement Council Group composed of alumni was convened to discuss and implement strategies discussed at the retreat and to develop rituals to be associated with bereavement care, for staff as well as bereaved families.

This project has not yet been evaluated, but staff retention has improved. Plans are underway to measure the effectiveness of the program through increased overall patient satisfaction, psychosocial patient satisfaction, and spiritual patient satisfaction scores. Measurement of the level of staff psychosocial wellness, as evidenced by follow-up human services surveys, is planned for the future. Most importantly, staff members will be monitored for changes in behavior that reflect the use of positive coping strategies and constructive self-care behaviors.

Another model for shifting established patterns is being conducted in the European Union, with a goal of improving the interaction between palliative care mobile teams (PCMT) and the hospital staff personnel with whom they interact.[65] In this model, recognizing the full range of convictions held by persons in a hospital setting, the concept of palliative care/terminal care has been bolstered by the concept of "continuous care." Continuous care tends to articulate both curative and palliative procedures rather than setting one form of therapy against the other. Continuous care is a multidisciplinary approach that brings together medical, social, and psychological concepts (as well as spiritual beliefs for some people) in a continuum starting from the time a grave illness is announced and on to the end of life, without any lapse. In that context, the role of the caregiver who is member of a PCMT is often transformed into one of interface and training.

The results analyzed from several studies supported the use of specialist multiprofessional teams in palliative care to improve the quality of life of patients with advanced cancer and their families. However, there were some difficulties in incorporating this concept into general hospital settings. In order to have mutual benefit, this project was undertaken with the following main research objectives[65]:

- Identify the internal and external mode of operation of seven PCMTs in Europe
- Identify the strong values and principles of the hospital PCMTs
- Examine the background and evolution of these teams through their different traditions and in light of the different cultures in Europe
- Identify areas of resistance to the values and principles of palliative care
- Identify the problems of integrating hospital PCMTs
- Update and modify the contents of the philosophy on palliative care in line with the reality of hospital institutions
- Find new organizational and teaching strategies to improve the integration of PCMTs into hospital institutions and to promote continuous care.
- Articulate the tension between the ethical, sociopolitical, and training dimensions of the PCMTs' activities in order to reinforce their impact in the hospitals

This project was envisioned to be the first step in a large European public health campaign to foster research in prevention of suffering. The research project had several unique components, including ethics mediation as a part of the research design. Educational programs involved developing an interactive team learning style based on understanding of the different learning styles of the PCMT and the hospital-based team and learning to communicate in the "other's learning style." The program was developed based on research showing that the PCMTs needed to assume a different learning style with hospital staff. Four months after the educational program was developed, the PCMTs reported improved interaction among themselves and with the hospital staff personnel.[65]

Oberle and Hughes[32] suggested that doctors and nurses need to engage in moral discourse so that each might understand and support the ethical burden carried by the other. Administrators should provide opportunities for discourse to help staff reduce moral distress and generate creative strategies for dealing with this problem.

Educational Interventions

Georgaki and associates[39] suggested that the academic curricula in nursing should be given further attention and reorganization to diminish feelings of insecurity when communicating with palliative care patients and their families. Educational strategies for preparing nursing students to care for patients with cancer should be further explored and addressed. In the future, nurses should be systematically provided with (continuing) training programs in which they learn how to communicate effectively in relation to patients' emotions and feelings and how to integrate emotional care with practical and medical tasks.

Medland and colleagues[45] noted that, "Appreciating oncology nurses as a cherished resource in the healthcare setting mandates a comprehensive approach to their retention, not only by providing for their technical competence and educational needs, but also by including programs that allow them to creatively manage the emotional components of their role and to learn and cultivate life- and practice-enhancing skills. Novice nurses in particular require clinical and psychological mentorship as they work toward becoming oncology nurses and find themselves highly vulnerable to the profession's many intrinsic stressors" (pp. 47–48).

In the United States, White and coworkers[31] studied members of the Oncology Nursing Society in four states. Only 26% said they had an excellent level of preparation to effectively care for a patient and family during the end-of-life period; 54% reported a good level of preparation, 17% indicated a fair level, and 4% reported little preparation. A total of 553 respondents (74%) indicated that they had received continuing education related to end-of-life care in the last 2 years. This training ranged from more than 4 hours (55%) to 1 or 2 hours (17%).

More than half of the 553 respondents who reported receiving some continuing education said that the information they received was useful and current, and the majority indicated that they were able to use the education in their practice. Although most respondents rated their ongoing education as excellent, very good, or good (76%), one fourth of the group rated their education as fair to poor. Combining the latter group with respondents who had no end-of-life continuing education indicates that almost half of the respondents did not participate in end-of-life continuing education or believed it was of dubious quality.

Barnard and colleagues[10] noted that education for palliative care involves the art of building and sustaining relationships and use of the self as a primary instrument for diagnosis and treatment. This involves psychological risk-taking that may be unique in the health field. This is the type of education that must be undertaken for professionals to strive and thrive in palliative care.

Personal Coping Mechanisms

Payne[27] found that two coping strategies were related to reduced burnout: (1) a problem-focused strategy, or planful problem-solving, and (2) an emotion-focused coping strategy, or positive reappraisal, which describes efforts to create positive meaning by focusing on personal growth.

Given that the whole person of the caregiver is involved in palliative care, the caregiver needs to understand how to take care of himself or herself in order to effectively work in the field. With knowledge about oneself and the ways of nurturing oneself, the caregiver can then teach and serve as a role model to patients and families on how to care for themselves.

Webster and Krisjanson[8] found that, in the Australian caregivers they interviewed, palliative care was seen as a way of living. The individual caregivers made a personal connection between the lessons of the workplace and application of these lessons to personal life—making a decision to live one's life congruent with work experience. Of interest is the fact that in a study of people with an unexpectedly good outcome to metastatic cancer, a sense of congruence was found to be important.[50]

Lifestyle Management

Table 56–1 lists a number of lifestyle management techniques that are helpful for continuing to work in stressful situations.

Remember the Serenity Prayer at work: "God grant me the serenity to accept the things I cannot change, the wisdom to change the things I can, and the wisdom to know the difference." Sometimes work-related problems can be solved; at other times, leaving the work environment, taking the wisdom gained, is a good solution.

Space does not allow for the many anecdotes received from participants regarding their ways of coping, so one anecdote is given to illustrate the many creative ways in which caregivers cope:

> This particular nurse was a student of the author's many years ago. We reconnected at a hospice meeting where I was speaking. She reflected that she had hated the course in Psychiatric Nursing that I taught in the early 1970s. However, she had become a psychiatric nurse and then a hospice nurse in a rural community. Now our paths crossed again. "I found a very small space that was being used for storage. It had windows, so I pushed to get it for my office. It has enough room for three chairs, a small desk, and my computer. I filled it with plants that reach to the ceiling. The patients and families love it. When I get fed up with dealing with death, I take a breather and garden. One day, I was making an azalea into a bonsai plant. I was bent over a wastebasket in the coffee room, digging in a pot loosening roots, when I looked up to see my bosses looking at me. I looked up and said, 'OK. I'm fed up with death, so I'm doing life.' "

Many of the lifestyle management techniques listed in Table 56–1 involve some type of energy work—meditation, yoga, qi gong, reiki, nature, and so on. Cumes[66] noted the importance of the caregiver's achieving personal balance so that more effective healing can occur. This process happens in part through intensifying one's own internal energy, to enable one's own Inner Healer. The Inner Healer, who has been wounded through various life experiences from the past as well as through education, clinical encounters, and the workplace, needs to be able to replenish himself or herself in order to bring the caregiver's healing potential into the clinical encounter.

Table 56–1
Lifestyle Management Techniques

Recognize and monitor symptoms.
Practice good nutrition.
Use meditation.
Pay attention to your spiritual life.
Grieve losses, personally and as a team.
Decrease overtime work.
Exercise—aerobic, yoga, qi gong, tai chi.
Spend time in nature—walking, gardening.
Incorporate music—singing, listening to music, playing an instrument.
Try energy work—reiki, healing touch, therapeutic touch.
Maintain a sense of humor.
Balance work and home life to allow sufficient "time off."
Have a good social support system, both personally and professionally.
Discuss work-related stresses with others who share the same problems.
Visit counterparts in other institutions; look for new solutions to problems.
Seek consultation if symptoms are severe.

Spirituality and Religion

Our Inner Healer is enabled if we intensify our internal energy, life force or *Prana* (breath, in yoga), or *Qi* (pronounced "Chi," in Taoist philosophy). In Hebrew, this life force is called *Ruach*, which also means wind, breath of life, soul, or spirit—the mysterious unseen and irresistible presence of the Divine Being or the Spirit of God.[66] This requires some form of inner practice, either physical or mental, such as prayer, meditation, imagery, yoga, tai chi, qi gong, or breath work.

Religion and spirituality have been found to be helpful to caregivers. In a study at Memorial Sloan Kettering Cancer Center,[67] nurses were found to be more religious than other groups. Oncologists were more religious than fellows. Those who were "quite a bit" religious to "extremely" religious had significantly lower scores on diminished empathy or depersonalization and lower emotional exhaustion on the Maslach Burnout scale.[33] In a study of 155 members of the Israeli Oncology Society, spiritual well-being, extrinsic religiosity, and education demonstrated significant direct relationships in a path analysis toward attitudes toward spiritual care. Spiritual well-being of the nurse was the strongest predictor of Israeli oncology nurses' attitudes toward spiritual care.[68]

One of the most important spiritual practices the author uses is the Prayer Wheel, which was developed by Dr. John Rossiter Thornton[69] (Figure 56–2).

Invest in Your Spirit with

THE PRAYER WHEEL™ Program

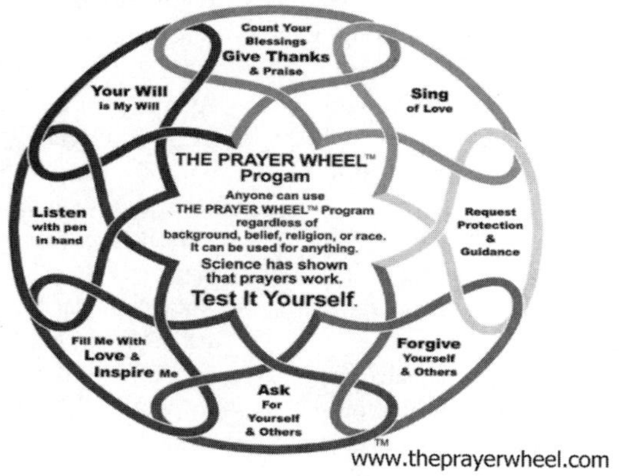

The Prayer Wheel: A Way to Pray

Prayer is a self-help technique that costs nothing, requires no equipment, and can be used in any situation. *Now science has proven that prayer works.* We no longer have to take prayer on faith! The Prayer Wheel can be used by anyone, regardless of background, belief, religion, or race. Starting at the top, going clockwise, use your favorite inspirational stories, songs, poems, or prayers for each segment theme. In the SING segment, sing your favorite love songs to the Maker of Life, instead of to a partner. In the ASK segment, record and date your requests. In the LISTEN segment, simply sit quietly and listen. Should any thoughts, words, or ideas come to your mind at this time, write them down and date them.

The wheel takes 40 minutes using 5 minutes per segment. If you have less time, either shorten the segments or just complete the segments you most need. Do not shorten the LISTEN segment.

You don't have to believe in prayer for it to work, just pray with love in your heart.

Don't take our word for it. **Test it yourself**. Daily use brings amazing results.

Figure 56–2. The Prayer Wheel. (*Source:* Dr. John Rossiter Thornton, © 1999 Rossiter-Thornton Associates, http://www.theprayer wheel.com (accessed June 22, 2005). Used with permission.

Conclusion

Nurses work in palliative care for a variety of reasons. Some may regard the work as simply a job, perhaps to be done for only a few years so as not to become overly involved in the stress associated with caring for dying persons and their families. Others may see hospice palliative care nursing as a career. It may feed their ego to be able to get on top of symptoms, resolve psychosocial issues, communicate well with other disciplines, and perhaps even achieve recognition as an expert in their field. For others, hospice palliative care nursing is about service to their soul. As the Prayer of St. Francis says, "It is in giving that we receive."

To continue to work in this field, however, one cannot focus exclusively on giving, or else one exhausts one resources. To care for others, one must be sure to care for oneself and to nurture the various aspects of one's mind, body, soul, and spirit. Learning to care for oneself so as to care for others—hopefully in a work environment that has a reasonable workload, offers community, is fair, gives one appropriate rewards as well as some control and power, and is congruent with one's values—can be an enriching experience. Organizations will hopefully provide mentoring, education, and supervision to help nurses progress on the path to Harper's Comfort-Ability[12] in hospice palliative care nursing.

Dealing with dying persons and their families can be difficult, but it can be extremely satisfying and rewarding as well. We need to grieve our losses when patients die, but we can also be grateful for having had the privilege of accompanying them on this very special journey, hoping there will be others to accompany us when our time comes, as indeed it will.

REFERENCES

1. Lyall WAL, Rogers J, Vachon MLS. Report to Palliative Care Unit of Royal Victoria Hospital regarding professional stress in the care of the dying. In: Palliative Care Service Report. Montreal: Royal Victoria Hospital, 1976:457–468.
2. Vachon MLS. Motivation and stress experienced by staff working with the terminally ill. Death Educ 1978;2:113–122.
3. Lyall WAL, Vachon MLS, Rogers J. A study of the degree of stress experienced by professionals caring for dying patients. In: Ajemian I, Mount BM, eds. The RVH Manual on Palliative/Hospice Care. Montreal: Royal Victoria Hospital, 1980:498–508.

4. Vachon MLS. Occupational Stress in the Care of the Critically Ill, Dying and Bereaved. Washington, DC: Hemisphere, 1987.
5. Vachon MLS. Staff stress in hospice/palliative care: A review. Palliat Med 1995;9:91–122.
6. Vachon MLS. Recent research into staff stress in palliative care. Eur J Palliat Care 1997;4:99–103.
7. Vachon MLS. Reflections on the history of occupational stress in hospice/Palliative Care. Hospice J 1999;14:229–246.
8. Webster J, Kristjanson LJ. "But isn't it depressing?" The vitality of palliative care. J Palliat Care 2002;18:15–24.
9. Davies B, Oberle K. Dimensions of the supportive role of the nurse in Palliative Care. Oncol Nurs Forum 1990;17:87–94.
10. Barnard D, Towers A, Boston P, Lambrinidou Y. Crossing Over: Narratives of Palliative Care. New York: Oxford, 2000.
11. Georges JJ, Grypdonck M, De Casterle BD. Being a palliative care nurse in an academic hospital: A qualitative study about nurses' perceptions of palliative care nursing. J Clin Nurs 2002;11: 785–793.
12. Harper BC. Death: The Coping Mechanism of the Health Professional, rev. ed. Greenville, SC: Southeastern University Press, 1994.
13. Harper BC. Growth in caring and professional ethics in hospice. Hosp J 1997;12:65–70.
14. Bradshaw A. The spiritual dimension of hospice: The secularisation of an ideal. Soc Sci Med 1996;43:409–419.
15. Skilbeck J, Connor J, Bath P, Beech N, Clark D, Hughes P, Douglas HR, Halliday D, Haviland J, Marples R, Normand C, Seymour J, Webb T. A description of the Macmillan Nurse caseload. Part 1: Clinical nurse specialists in palliative care. Palliat Med 2002;16:285–296.
16. Kelly D, Ross S, Gray B. Death, dying and emotional labour: Problematic dimensions of the bone marrow transplant nursing role. J Adv Nurs 2000;32:952–960.
17. Byock I. Dying in America: Past, Present and Future. Paper presented at The Great Journey—Death, Dying and Bereavement, Tucson AZ, 27 March 2004.
18. Byock I. From innocence to audit: Transatlantic lessons on the routinization of hospice. Am J Hospice Palliat Care 1994; 11:4–7.
19. Doyle D. Have we looked beyond the physical and psychosocial? J Pain Symptom Manage 1992;7:302–311.
20. Kearney M. Paliative medicine: Just another specialty? Palliat Med 1992;6:41.
21. Meier DE, Back AL, Morrison RS. The inner life of physicians and the care of the seriously ill. JAMA 2001;286:3007–3014.
22. Maslach C, Schaufeli WB, Leiter MP. Job burnout. Ann Rev Psychol 2001;52:397–422.
23. French JRP, Rodgers W, Cobb S. Adjustment as person-environment fit. In: Coelho GV, Hamburg DA, Adams E, eds. Coping and Adaptation. New York: Basic Books, 1974:316–333.
24. Vachon MLS. The nurse's role: The world of palliative care nursing. In: Ferrell B, Coyle N, eds. Oxford Textbook of Palliative Nursing. New York: Oxford University Press, 2001:647–662.
25. van Staa AL, Visser A, van der Zouwe N. Caring for caregivers: Experiences and evaluation of interventions for a palliative care team. Patient Educ Couns 2000;41:93–105.
26. Papadatou D, Martinson IM, Chung P, Man MN. Caring for dying children: A comparative study of nurses' experiences in Greece and Hong Kong. Cancer Nurs 2001;24:402–412.
27. Payne N. Occupational stressors and coping as determinants of burnout in female hospice nurses. J Adv Nurs 2001;33:396–405.
28. Yandrick RM. High demand low control. Behavioral Healthcare Tomorrow 1997;6(3):41–44.
29. Coyle N. Focus on the nurse: Ethical dilemmas with highly symptomatic patients dying at home. Hospice J 1997;12:33–41.
30. MacDonald N. Testimony before The Subcommittee to Update "Of Life and Death" of the Standing Senate Committee on Social Affairs, Science and Technology. Ottawa, Ont.: March 28, 2000.
31. White K, Coyne PJ, Patel UB. Are nurses adequately prepared for end-of-life care? J Nurs Schol 2001;33:147–151.
32. Oberle K, Hughes D. Doctors' and nurses' perceptions of ethical problems in end-of-life decisions. J Adv Nurs 2001;33: 707–715.
33. Maslach C, Jackson SE. The Maslach Burnout Inventory (manual), 2nd ed. Palo Alto, Calif.: Consulting Psychologists Press, 1986.
34. McConigley R, Kristjanson LJ, Morgan A. Palliative care nursing in Western Australia. Int J Palliat Care Nurs 2000;6:80–90.
35. Lynn J, O' Mara A. Reliable, high quality, efficient end-of-life care for cancer patients: Economic issues and barriers. In: Foley K, Gelband H, eds. Improving Palliative Care for Cancer: Summary and Recommendations. Washington, DC: National Academy Press, 2001:67–95.
36. Whedon MB. Revisiting the road not taken: Integrating palliative care into oncology nursing. Clin J Oncol Nurs 2002;6:27–33.
37. James N, Field D. The routinization of hospice: Charisma and bureaucracy. Soc Sci Med 1992;34:1363–1375.
38. Cannaerts N, Dierckx de Casterle B, Grypdonck M. Palliatieve zorg: Zorg voor het leven. Een Onderzoek Naar de Specifieke Bijdrage Van de Residentiele Palliatieve Zorgverlening. Gent, Belgium: Academia Press, 2000.
39. Georgaki S, Kalaidopoulou O, Liarmakopoulos I, Mystakidou K. Nurses' attitudes toward truthful communication with patients with cancer: A Greek study. Cancer Nurs 2002;25: 436–441.
40. Boston P, Towers A, Barnard D. Embracing vulnerability: Risk and empathy in palliative care. J Palliat Care 2001;17:248–253.
41. Mount BM. Dealing with our losses. J Clin Oncol 1986;4:1127–1134.
42. Garfield C, Spring C, Ober D. Sometimes My Heart Goes Numb: Love and Caring in a Time of AIDS. San Francisco: Jossey-Bass, 1995.
43. Papadatou D. A proposed model of health professionals' grieving process. Omega 2000;41:59–77.
44. Kearney M. A Place of Healing: Working with Suffering in Living and Dying. Oxford: Oxford University Press, 2000.
45. Medland J, Howard-Ruben J, Whitaker E. Fostering psychosocial wellness in oncology nurses: Addressing burnout and social support in the workplace. Oncol Nurs Forum 2004;31: 47–54.
46. Campion B. Taking the final steps to a "good death." Toronto: Globe & Mail, p. A20, November 19, 1993. Oncol Nurs Forum 2001;28:25–27.
47. Antonovsky A. Health, Stress and Coping. San Francisco: Jossey-Bass, 1979.
48. Kobasa SC. Stressful life events, personality and health: An inquiry into hardiness. J Pers Soc Psychol 1979;37:1–11.
49. Kobasa SC, Maddi SR, Kahn S. Hardiness and health: A prospective study. J Pers Soc Psychol 1982;42:172–177.
50. Hirshberg C, Barasch MI. Remarkable Recovery. New York: Riverhead Books, 1995.
51. Myss C. Advanced Energy Anatomy. Boulder, CO: Sounds True, 2001.
52. Remen RN. My Grandfather's Blessings. New York: Riverhead Books, 2000.

53. Remen RN. Kitchen Table Wisdom. New York: Riverhead Books, 1996.
54. Watson J. Human caring and suffering: A subjective model for health sciences. In: Taylor RL, Watson J, eds. They Shall Not Hurt: Human Suffering and Human Caring. Boulder, Colo.: Colorado Associated University Press, 1989:125–135.
55. Fox M. Sins of the Spirit, Blessings of the Flesh: Lessons in Transforming Evil in Soul and Society. New York: Three Rivers Press, 1999.
56. Vachon MLS. The use of imagery, meditation, and spirituality in the care of people with cancer. In: Murray Edwards D, ed. Voice Massage: Scripts for Guided Imagery. Pittsburgh, PA: Oncology Nursing Society, 2002:21–41.
57. Besterczy S. Staff stress on a newly-developed palliative care service: The psychiatrist's role. Can Psychiatr Assoc J 1977:22: 347–353.
58. Speck P. Unconscious communications [editorial]. Palliat Med 1996;10:273.
59. Redinbaugh EM, Schuerger JM, Weiss L, Brufsky A, Arnold R. Health care professionals' grief: A model based on occupational style and coping. Psycho-Oncology 2001;10: 187–198.
60. Holland JL. Making Vocational Choices: A Theory of Vocational Personalities and Work Environments. Odessa, FL: Psychological Assessment Resources, 1985.
61. Vachon MLS. The stress of professional caregivers. In: Doyle D, Hanks G, Cherny N, Calman K, eds. Oxford Textbook of Palliative Medicine, 3rd ed. Oxford: Oxford University Press, 2004:992–1004.
62. Garrett DK, McDaniel AM. A new look at nurse burnout: The effects of environmental uncertainty and social climate. J Nurs Admin 2001;31:91–96.
63. Parker M, Gadbois S. The fragmentation of community. Part 1: The loss of belonging and commitment at work. J Nurs Admin 2000;30:386–390.
64. Ludin S, Paul H, Christensen J. FISH! New York: Hyperion Press, 2000.
65. How to promote the integration of continuous care into hospital institutions? Palliative care mobile teams as a vehicle for a philosophy of continuous and integrated care. Analysis of medical practice and research into new strategies for integration. Available at: http://www.mobileteam.irisnet.be (accessed May 6, 2005).
66. Cumes D. The Spirit of Healing. St. Paul, MN: Llewellyn Publications, 1999.
67. Kash KM, Holland JC, Breitbart W, Berenson S, Dougherty J, Ouelette-Kobasa S, Lesko L. Stress and burnout in oncology. Oncology 2000;14:1621–1637.
68. Musgrave CF, McFarlane EA. Israeli oncology nurses' religiosity, spiritual well-being, and attitudes toward spiritual care: A path analysis. Oncol Nurs Forum 2004:31:321–327.
69. Rossiter Thornton J. The Prayer Wheel. Available at: http://www.theprayerwheel.com (accessed March 25, 2005).

57 Ethical Considerations

Karen J. Stanley and Laurie Zoloth-Dorfman

The girls and I always knew Mark would be safe if you were taking care of him. The day that he died, we left the hospital with confidence that you would treat his body with as much respect as if he were still alive. You were always straight with us, and our trust in you was more valuable for us than you'll ever understand. . . . We never felt we abandoned him when we left the hospital because you were our eyes and our ears.—A wife writing to her late husband's caregiver

- ***Key Points***
- *The nurse's ethical responsibilities in caring for patients at the end of life are actualized in all dimensions of care.*
- *Acts of truth-telling, respect for autonomy, and nonabandonment reflect the highest standards of nursing care.*
- *Issues of futility and treatment decision-making should be viewed within the context of the patient's goals of care.*
- *The allocation of health care resources has the potential to markedly affect future care.*
- *Nurses must assert their role as full members of the interdisciplinary team in discussions of moral issues.*

Technological advances in the diagnosis and treatment of chronic disease have resulted in longer lifespans and, in many cases, an extended period of dying. This ability to prolong life has been almost seamlessly integrated into the medical profession's philosophical approach to treating disease as an adversary that can and must be conquered. The value of existence for its own sake, a false sense of security about technology's ability to rescue, and the human need to maintain hope and delay the end of life have obscured and postponed the inevitable need to confront critical issues.

Solomon and colleagues[1] demonstrated that physicians frequently recognized that they were overtreating patients at the end of life but did not know how to stop. *Means to a Better End: A Report on Dying in America Today*[2] confirmed that significant numbers of patients continue to end their lives in a hospital setting and that 18% to 34% of patients older than 65 years of age have seven or more days in intensive care units (ICUs) during the last 6 months of life. The ability to prolong life has outpaced medical, philosophical, bioethical, and societal efforts to reach a value-based consensus on the goals of and criteria for care across the illness continuum. Ethical dilemmas on macro and micro levels emerge daily as the debate on extending life versus postponing death continues. These dilemmas are normative over the continuum of care and continue in the palliative care arena, where decisions about life-supporting and life-ending interventions are made on a daily basis.

Palliative care as a viable and worthwhile choice for those at the end of life is often obscured by the focus on technology. From a societal perspective, demographic trends separate the generations, and cultural norms may no longer validate caring for one's aging family members in the home setting. Consequently, many individuals and families have not lived with or cared for a dying person. A generation that has no practical or emotional experience with the act of dying is bound to be uncomfortable with decisions that must be made and insecure about delivering care at home. Patients and families continue to choose interventions that can be delivered only in the acute care setting, as opposed to a death at home under the care of a family member or significant other.[2]

The issues of truth-telling and informed consent, withholding or withdrawing treatment, the definition of ordinary versus extraordinary medical intervention, and the right to assistance in ending one's life because of an unacceptable health condition are becoming further removed from those individuals most effected by the decisions. The argument is persuasive that these issues must be addressed through conversations, debates, and discussion groups in order to clarify individual and societal rights regarding end-of-life care. The inability to agree on a health care decision-making paradigm that allows the expression of diverse values endangers the right of individuals to make personal choices about health care.

The rising costs of medical care have introduced another dilemma central to the whole spectrum of debate. The allocation of health care resources described as finite suggests that there can be limits to medical intervention. The demand that society bear the cost of every possible medical intervention returns the debate to the most basic of issues: Are there circumstances in which existence is no longer intrinsically valuable? Whose values should drive the goals of care? How should these decisions be made, and by whom?[3]

These debates largely began with cases in which patients demanded, first to their doctors and then to the courts, to be rescued from the technological imperative. Karen Ann Quinlan's family contested her life on a ventilator, asking that this "artificial" but life-sustaining intervention be removed.[4] Nancy Cruzan's family requested that a feeding tube delivering enteral nutrition be discontinued.[5] These kinds of cases, in which the patient's wishes were not known or documented or the patient's and family's wishes were not honored without resorting to the courts, were common in the 1970s and 1980s. That ongoing public dialogue and legal activity sensitized the lay public to the concept of autonomy, and health care consumers began to insist on greater control over health care decision-making. The courts redefined what constituted extraordinary treatment and countenanced the wishes of patients and their families if patients were unable to speak for themselves, even to the extent that life-sustaining treatment could be withdrawn.[4,5] Recently, the Terry Schiavo case[5a] reopened the debate about who can make life-ending decisions and under what circumstances.

One's abilities to understand current legal statutes, to comprehend ethical discourse, and to clarify one's personal philosophy can be strengthened by a review of ethical methods and terminology. Nursing is not isolated from bioethical conflicts, and, in fact, nurses have significant responsibility in understanding and articulating an ethical rationale for decision-making and consequent actions.

Traditional Methods of Ethics

Ethics asks these questions: What is the right act, the good human moral gesture, and what makes it so? What is the meaning of a good life, and how is it made? How is justice best achieved among competing moral appeals? Who ought people to be, and how ought they to treat others, and what are the criteria for knowing such things? Ethics seeks to logically justify choices for right behavior, rules, and activities, particularly in situations that challenge established norms of behavior or require new paradigms for judging behavior. It is this understanding of ethics as a methodology that distinguishes it from morality, rules of proper conduct, or descriptions of cultural norms.[6] In its normative capacity, ethics is an applied theory for the practice of medicine (bioethics) and the conduct of research, business, and political actions.

Ethical inquiry, in its interpretation of any act—for example, the judgment that it is "the right thing to do"—traditionally has evaluated (1) the moral agents and their character; (2) the motive for the act itself; or (3) the effects of the action on others, with the assumption that humans are rational beings with the ability to justify their actions. Although this process historically has relied on sociability, accountability, conscience, and rationality, certain assumptions are currently being challenged. For example, Can there be a single standard for rightness of action in a world so profoundly diverse? Can there be, if not agreement on the definitions of a good action, agreement on a common language of ethics?

The various ethical methods[7] have emerged at specific historical periods and are shaped by the culture, class, and gender of the theorists. At best, each is useful as a starting place for defining one's approach to ethical dilemmas.

Virtue theory, the study of character attributes that are necessary for the achievement of a good life, was developed in the Greek philosophic tradition. The virtues described as good include courage, loyalty, and civic friendship. They are developed through training or role modeling a virtuous person's behavior. The theory was expanded to include compassion, merging the Greek ideal with Christian philosophy. Palliative care, with its emphasis on caring, kindness, and respect for another person (virtuous attributes), is well suited to this methodological approach.

Deontological ethics focuses on rules and motives for behavior. It argues that certain qualities that are innate to a human being or a social order require specific obligations or duties. These obligations can be based in God's law—as in rabbinical text, with its emphasis on a life of commands and obligations to those commands—or in essential unconditional imperatives whose moral worth is to be found in the rule itself—for example, Kant's[8] imperative never to lie. This approach incorporates the bioethical requisites to "do no harm" (the principle of nonmaleficence) and to "do that which is good" (the principle of beneficence).

Consequentialism is based in the 19th-century utilitarian philosophic tradition. The virtue of a behavior bears a direct relationship to its outcome. In contrast to deontological theories, which are rooted in commitments, essential obligations, or promises, consequentialist thinkers argue that assessment of a right action should be based on the possible outcomes of that action. In this theory, individual rights are more questionable, and individual freedoms depend on the outcome for the general good, the good for the greatest number,[9] or the avoidance of harm to the most.[10] This approach would argue that a dying individual's right to autonomous choice about assisted death is superseded by concern for society as a whole and the fear of imposing assisted death on those who do not wish for that outcome.

Ethics and Palliative Care

An examination of ethical issues in palliative care requires an articulation of the standard to which all practice is compared. Ethical dilemmas surface as those comparisons draw attention to the inadequacies of practice. For an ethical standard to be meaningful, it must reflect a comprehensive approach that simultaneously allows for each individual's particular needs. The extraordinary spectrum of requisites, from the most basic of physical care concerns to the broad issues of existential distress, reflects the daunting ethical responsibilities that are integral to palliative care.

Cassell[11] succinctly described ethical obligations in health care as accountability for diagnosis and treatment plans made in terms of the patient rather than the disease, balancing quality versus quantity of life, and minimizing suffering for the patient and family. Ferrell's quality-of-life model,[12] which identifies the essential components of physical, psychological, social, and spiritual well-being, is comprehensively reflected in the Five Principles of Palliative Care[13] (Table 57–1). These principles translate larger obligations into specific accountabilities and can serve as a "checklist" for any health care professional caring for persons at the end of life.

The need for improving care at the end of life remains a constant in the midst of any ethically focused discussion. The results of the landmark Study to Understand Prognoses and Preferences for Outcomes and Risks of Treatment (SUPPORT) study,[14] which examined how people died, were discouraging. The majority of people died in the hospital, often alone and uncomfortable, while receiving medical intervention they did not want. The current inadequacy of formal professional training,[15–18] despite excellent supplemental training provided by the Education for Physicians on End of Life Care (EPEC) course for physicians and End of Life Nursing Education Consortium (ELNEC) course for nurses, and the subsequent lack of a cadre of health care professionals with palliative care expertise[2,19–21] impede excellence in care and interfere with the professional's ethical obligation to provide that same excellent care.

These variables have contributed to a decline in the public's belief in the integrity of the medical care system and in confidence that the physician "knows best." The health care team is increasingly being held accountable for the delivery of skilled palliative care. Patients and their families are asking for the information necessary to make informed decisions and the right to be involved in the decision-making process.[22]

Ironically, as this higher standard of accountability for quality care has emerged, end-of-life care is shifting from acute care to outpatient settings. Patients who are no longer candidates for active medical intervention are being discharged with complex care requirements. As a result, patients and their families are assuming responsibility for care that was previously delivered by health care professionals.

Demographic mobility, separation and divorce, changing cultural mores, and a decreasing sense of accountability for the care of elderly parents have altered the definition of family and the availability of support systems. Adequate caregivers for dying persons may not be readily available if their spouses have predeceased them; adult children may be geographically distant and dependent on dual incomes; or the primary caregiver may also have health problems. Even more caregivers will be needed in the future, given increased life expectancy and the aging of the population. Palliative medicine practitioners will continue to be ethically challenged to provide safe care to increasing numbers of patients.

The realities of the current health care delivery system, including a critical nursing shortage, demand even more of nurses. Home health, hospice, and extended care facilities rely heavily on nursing assessment, intervention, and presence to ensure high standards of supportive care. The profoundly existential issues that are the essence of the palliative care experience can be double-edged swords for the nursing profession. Although they present valuable caring opportunities, they may simultaneously generate moral distress—an inability to provide care valued as most appropriate or an inability to "do the right thing."[23] These conflicts may reflect differences in perspective from those of the patient, the family, or other members of the health care team, and they occur, ironically, in the context of providing care that may preserve or lengthen life or, conversely, hasten or end life.

Table 57–1
Five Principles of Palliative Care

1. Respects the goals, likes, and choices of the dying person
2. Looks after the medical, emotional, social, and spiritual needs of the dying person.
3. Supports the needs of family members.
4. Helps gain access to needed health care providers and appropriate care settings.
5. Builds ways to provide excellent care at the end of life.

Source: Five Principles of Palliative Care, Reference 13.

CASE STUDY

Michael, a Man Who Wanted "All the Life He Could Get"

Michael was diagnosed with extensive lung cancer in his mid-forties. He had recently received a significant promotion at work and had two young children. He declared from the beginning that he wanted everything possible done, but the treatment regimen had not slowed disease progression. As he began to deteriorate, he insisted on continued chemotherapy, and his oncologist continued therapy. The nursing staff who were administering the chemotherapy felt very conflicted about this intervention. Although they wanted to honor his wishes, they believed that continued chemotherapy would cause more harm than good. The clinical nurse specialist (CNS) caring for Michael understood his wish to hang on to life and wished it were possible. She had been involved with Michael and his family for several months and felt equally uncomfortable with continued therapy that contributed markedly to the "suffering quotient." Late one night, Michael was open to conversation, and they had a frank discussion about the dilemma at hand. She spoke of quality of life, time at home with his family, and finishing up personal business as valuable goals. He spoke of the future that he wished could be. They collaboratively made a list of possible opportunities for Michael that were not dependent on further therapy. He wavered over the next several days as he continued aggressive supportive therapy, but he was ultimately discharged home that week after talking at length with his physician and his minister. The CNS continued to see him at home and supported him as he made his way through the list of "opportunities." He died, still wishing that more time had been available but thankful he had spent time with his family.

Ethical dilemmas emerge across the spectrum of care as nurses endeavor to provide the best possible physical and psychological care, communicate appropriately and honestly with the patient and family, provide culturally competent care, assist patients and families in making decisions to withhold or withdraw treatment, and respond to requests for interventions that may conflict with their personal value systems. As each patient and significant other confronts the realities of mortality and fragility, and as each nurse intervenes in the crisis, meaning and shape emerge from those choices made at the bedside. How one decides to act in any particular case is really the measure of how far one is willing to explore alternative diagnoses and treatments and of what one considers appropriate at the end of life.

Changing Role of the Nurse

As the health care delivery system has changed, historic role expectations have been adapted to meet the needs of patients and families, professional staff, and the health care delivery system itself. The multidisciplinary approach that is common in the palliative care arena requires that each team member contribute to the overall sum of excellence in patient care. Although traditionally the nurse's role was to carry out the physician's orders, that expectation has been expanded. The varied sites of palliative care, the nurse's primary role in case management, and the changing parameters of the health care delivery system require that nurses be expert practitioners. Assessment, intervention, evaluation, and reevaluation in physical and psychological arenas are accepted nursing roles. It is not unusual for nurses to practice autonomously in providing expert symptom management under established standards of care. Expert nurses adjust medications and dosages, make multidisciplinary referrals, and engage patients at the most existential of levels as part of a normal day's work.

The enlarged arena of nursing responsibility translates into greater ethical obligations as well. The American Nursing Association (ANA) supports the role of nurses in facilitating informed decision-making for patients making choices about end-of-life care.[24] In fact, it is not unusual for nurses to be involved in discussing advance directives, prognoses, do-not-resuscitate (DNR) decisions, and a myriad of other palliative care issues.[25] Distinguishing quality versus quantity of life, providing objective feedback about the patient's current status, articulating outcomes of health care decisions, and offering to be present as health care choices are clarified are activities that demonstrate nurses' commitment to these significant responsibilities.

CASE STUDY

Edgar, a 72-Year-Old Man Undergoing Chemotherapy

Edgar was a 72-year-old man in blast crisis. He was admitted to the hospital on a weekend when his oncologist was out of town. The covering physician was prepared to begin the chemotherapy his colleague had planned; although he had reservations because of the toxicities involved, he did not know the patient and felt uncomfortable changing his colleague's treatment plan. He was also mindful that the hospital had recently been involved in a lawsuit concerning a patient's right to continue therapy despite limited benefits and significant risks. The nurse who was scheduled to administer the chemotherapy conferred with the CNS, expressing her concerns that Edgar did not understand what he was facing. She knew that the high-dose chemotherapy was risky at best and was unlikely to provide much benefit. Although neither the staff nurse nor the CNS knew the patient, they both felt it imperative that someone speak to Edgar and his family about the risks of therapy. The CNS went to Edgar's room, introduced herself, and spoke of the realities of the current circumstances. Her anguish regarding the need to have such a difficult conversation was reflected in her face and the tears in her eyes. Edgar, his wife, and the nurse held hands as the three of them discussed what Edgar wanted. He elected to go home as soon as possible so that he might spend time with his friends, play a few games of checkers, and be with his family.

The opportunity to immerse one's self along with the patient in physical, psychological, social, and spiritual realms is rarely offered as frequently in any other nursing discipline. Establishing a trusting relationship in the midst of a frightening and anxiety-laden time requires effort and a significant investment of one's self but facilitates the transition from that of "kind stranger" to trusted clinician and confidante. This kind of relationship authenticates a partnered experience essential for addressing ethical issues.

As nurses assume increasing responsibility for patients' care and well-being, it is important that they continue to hold themselves and each member of the multidisciplinary health care team accountable for the highest standards of ethical behavior. Open and thorough discussions regarding the rationale for care provide an opportunity for all team members to articulate personal values. This is an opportunity for nurses to role model moral courage.[23] By continuing to articulate concerns about circumstantial realities versus medical intentions and encouraging an ongoing dialogue with the patient and family, the nurse may facilitate the health care team's acknowledgment of its impotence and allow patients greater opportunities for a peaceful and dignified death.

Selected Ethical Issues in Palliative Care

Ethical issues in palliative care involve and affect patients and their significant others, health care providers, the health care delivery system, and society as a whole. Issues central to discussion and debate focus on concerns about individual autonomy versus societal norms or the state's interest; disparity between the patient's goals of care and those of family, friends, and the health care team; adequacy of communication essential for informed decision-making; consistency of care across the illness continuum; and the allocation of health care resources across the wellness–illness continuum. These broader issues are revealed in disputes regarding the appropriate timing of transition from curative to palliative care, withholding and withdrawing treatment, an individual's right to use personal value-based parameters (e.g., quality of life, religious beliefs, cultural norms) as the ultimate arbitrator of the value of existence, and the right to assistance in dying.

Death does not seem to visit us "gently." For many patients and families in the palliative care phase of illness, the simplest of decisions may carry significant consequences. Ethical issues consistently arise as nurses struggle along with patients and their significant others to make realistic yet comforting decisions. Nurses' obligations to individuals at the end of life reflect a wide spectrum of behaviors. Navigating the health care delivery system, with its myriad professionals and sites of care, can be daunting. Patients and families often lose sight of appropriate goals of therapy when multiple clinicians are involved in the plan of care. Once the nurse is assured of informed consent, appropriate interventions include discussions about personal choice, the goals of medical care, and subsequent choices about that care.

Meaningful conversations cannot occur in the midst of unrelieved symptoms. Nurses must advocate for and contribute to effective pain and symptom management. They must become expert practitioners, hold others accountable for that same standard of excellence, and continue to advocate for the patient until symptoms are satisfactorily managed.[26]

Corley[23] identified multiple care scenarios that contribute to nurses' moral distress. She described circumstances in which terminally ill patients were not allowed to die with dignity, critically ill patients were resuscitated without a clear understanding of their circumstances, patients died with inadequate symptom management, and dying patients were kept on life support until death. Although the specifics of patients' and families' wishes regarding care were not identified, what is clear is that nurses experience moral angst about the rightness of their actions.

Nurses must be involved in discussions regarding (1) withholding and withdrawing treatment, (2) providing care demanded by patients but deemed inappropriate by the health care team, (3) patient requests to stop eating or drinking, (4) appropriate criteria for sedation to relieve intractable distress, and (5) patient requests for assisted death. As central providers of palliative care, nurses must serve as a moral voice in these dialogues. In so doing, they are able to honor their commitment to patients and families.

Pain and Symptom Management

Optimal pain and symptom management continues to be a priority and one of the most important ethical issues in palliative care. Patients worry that pain or other symptoms will not be well managed,[26] and they articulate that physical symptoms are far more stressful than the cancer diagnosis itself.[12] Pain, dyspnea, fatigue, nausea, sedation, and confusion are troublesome.[27] These unmanaged symptoms can strip patients of their dignity, impose tremendous professional and ethical burdens on nurses, and destroy the quality of life of both patient and family.[28]

Although all symptoms are deserving of the same meticulous attention, pain continues to be the most prevalent of physical symptoms at the end of life. Overwhelming and unrelieved pain can cause anxiety, irritation, restlessness, sleeplessness, depression, fatigue, emotional withdrawal, and existential distress for both patients and caregivers. Its continued presence can provoke patients to request life-ending measures. Unrelieved pain is both an emergency and an ethical dilemma and demands the full attention of the palliative care team until resolved. This dilemma can be even more pronounced in the home care setting, where nurses work independently with patients.[29] The standard to which all health care team members must be held is adequate pain relief as defined by the patient.

CASE STUDY

Jonathan, a Man with Progressive Lung Cancer

Jonathan had rapidly progressing lung cancer. He was admitted to the hospital for intensive care secondary to obstipation. The pain management nurse saw him on consultation and found him to be a man in extreme pain with orders on the chart for nonsteroidal antiinflammatory drugs and "no narcotics." She determined that Jonathan had been previously discharged on an oral opioid without an accompanying bowel regimen. Three weeks of opioid therapy without any kind of laxative intervention had triggered severe obstipation and ultimately sepsis. Jonathan had been hospitalized for almost 1 month when the pain management consult was written. His physician was reluctant to use opioids for fear of causing the same problem. The nurse discussed the use of opioids in tandem with an aggressive bowel regimen and recommended intravenous opioids immediately, titration to effect, and concurrent titration of an effective bowel regimen.

She spoke to Jonathan, who was frantic for any kind of pain relief, and described what the plan of care would be. As she administered the initial dose of intravenous opioid, tears came into his eyes as he relaxed and allowed the medication to relieve the pain. Over the next few days, the opioid was titrated upward, and a bowel regimen that differed from the norm was instituted. As the nurse prepared Jonathan for discharge, he gave her a napkin on which he had drawn a picture of an angel. "That's how I see you," he said. "Thank you for saving me from hell."

Although aggressive pain management in terminally ill patients rarely causes death, the fear that it will do so continues to be a significant ethical barrier to adequate relief. Many nurses are reluctant to administer the analgesic doses necessary to adequately control pain for fear of causing respiratory depression. The ANA expects nurses to use effective doses of analgesics for the proper management of pain in the dying patient and has stated that increasing titration of medication to achieve adequate symptom control is ethically justified.[26] In 1997, the Supreme Court, although disallowing an individual's right to physician-assisted suicide (PAS), cogently argued that palliative care may and should be aggressive, even if the provision of such care should hasten death.[29a]

An ethical responsibility of advocacy emerges as the nurse anticipates and plans for expected sequelae to both the illness and any side effects of prescribed analgesics. Discussing expected symptoms, and the plan for managing those symptoms should they occur, relieves patients and caregivers, provides an opportunity to articulate other concerns, and reassures patient and their caregivers that future "unknowns" can be expertly handled. Further advocacy responsibilities include suggesting pharmacological and nonpharmacological interventions to other members of the health care team, consulting with the physician for assistance in managing difficult symptoms or side effects, and continuing to attend to those issues until they are satisfactorily resolved.[30]

A genuine collaborative approach to palliative care requires the acknowledgment that no one team member has exclusive domain over specific areas of knowledge. In the absence of a communal collaborative milieu, nurses must continue to advocate for the very best in pain and symptom management; they should role-model appropriate analgesic decision-making and should never apologize for what they know.

The use of placebos is less frequent in today's health care system for the management of cancer pain, but it does still occur. The Oncology Nursing Society (ONS)[31] has issued a position paper on cancer pain management stating that placebo use is appropriate only if a patient has provided informed consent. Placebos should not be used to assess or manage cancer pain. Their use is deceitful, is harmful to both patients and health care professionals who use them in a dishonest way, and can damage or destroy the nurse–patient relationship. Nurses, as moral agents, have an ethical responsibility to avoid the use of placebos and to assist in establishing institutional policies to prevent their use in pain management.

Issues of Truth-Telling

Ethically sound communication is central to the highest standards of palliative care. Issues concerning to every domain of quality of life (i.e., physical, psychological, social, and spiritual) require communication such that goals and expectations can be articulated and those who are cared for can know the comfort that a shared experience provides. Ethical principles are reflected not only in behavior but also in language.[32]

Delivering bad news is an essential part of practice in the palliative care arena, and truth-telling, although viewed as ethically appropriate behavior, can be morally troublesome in a multitude of situations. There is little disagreement in western European cultures that autonomous patients have the right to complete information regarding their illness, potential interventions (including risks and benefits), and prognoses, in order to make informed decisions. However, the ability to function as an "existential advocate"[32] is far more complex than the verbalization of correct information. Issues such as presenting truthful information to both asked and unasked questions without destroying hope, providing information that has been purposefully "filtered" because of the patient's wishes or cultural background, and confronting other members of the health team who obscure information because of their own fears are not uncommon.

Truth-telling should occur in the context of the patient's wishes and emotional status. The nurse should confirm that the patient is ready to hear difficult news while concurrently giving permission to defer the conversation until greater emotional resources are available or family support is present. When difficult questions are asked, one of the authors responds in this manner: "I need to be sure that when you ask what must be very hard questions you want a truthful answer. I am an honest person and would feel I was honoring you by doing so. However, I want to hear from you how you believe these discussions would best be handled."

A reasonable ethical standard requires that patients receive answers to difficult and frightening questions as quickly as possible. Although conveying distressing news has historically been the physician's domain, the multidisciplinary structure of palliative care allows a modification of these role expectations in deference to the patient's best interests. Patients often question nurses regarding test results that could confirm a life-threatening illness or progression of that illness. It has been common practice for the nurse to refer the patient to the physician at such times. But is it appropriate to ask the patient to wait and, of course, worry until the physician arrives? Is it unfair or unkind to postpone for what seems an interminable period answers to questions that carry such grave import? These circumstances offer nurses a unique opportunity. The best possible scenario in such situations would be a rapid resolution of the matter. Table 57–2 summarizes recommendations for a collaborative approach to truth-telling. Appropriate follow-up would include offering to be present when the patient discusses the information with others and leaving the door open to revisit any of the issues raised.

If the physician cannot be reached or a physician unknown to the patient is on call, and the nurse can answer the questions correctly and appropriately, they should be answered. If the nurse has established a close relationship with the patient, it can be argued that it is reasonable to hear difficult news from someone who is known and trusted. Remaining attentive to the primary goal of allowing the patient access to information as quickly and humanely as possible removes the focus from role issues to that of patient interests. However, nurses should not provide information that has not been verified, and they should not feel compelled to answer questions that they are not able to competently address. It is often necessary to provide compassionate understanding of the patient's anxiety regarding undisclosed information, yet defer to the physician to provide the actual information.

Table 57–2
A Collaborative Approach to Truth-Telling: Answering Questions Regarding Diagnostic Results

1. Report the patient's concerns to the physician, emphasizing the urgency of the matter.
2. Determine the physician's availability.
3. If the physician is unavailable for a significant period, offer to discuss the test results with the patient. If the physician is available, plan to be present for follow-up questions and support.
4. Plan with the physician how best to respond regarding the meaning of the diagnostic results and the continued plan of care.
5. Explain to the patient that the physician is not available and is concerned that the information be provided in a timely manner.
6. Ask the patient's permission to discuss the questions asked. If the response is positive, determine which individuals the patient would like to be present and ensure they are there.
7. Use language the patient understands, answering all of the questions.
8. Stay present, both emotionally and physically, until the patient feels the conversation has ended.
9. Provide assurances that the physician will be available for further discussion.
10. Provide a detailed description of the discussion in the medical record and speak personally with the physician about the patient's intellectual and emotional responses to the information.

The patient's wishes regarding access to information about the illness, prognosis, progression of the illness, and plans for care trump everyone else's wishes. However, it is not uncommon for members of the health care team to present an inaccurate, obscure, or overly hopeful description of the current physiological circumstances; to ask colleagues on the team to remain positive about outcomes regardless of current realities; or to ask that the patient not be told of the current realities. Physicians may write a do-not-resuscitate (DNR) order for a patient, without having a previous discussion with the patient and family, because they are uncomfortable with the topic or believe that the patient and or family may refuse such a request. DNR orders, which have been upheld by the courts, disallow heroic measures (at the request of the patient or family) in a multitude of health care circumstances. DNR orders can serve patients well by preventing unwanted and unnecessary interventions, but they may also be improperly and unethically used to unilaterally prevent life-sustaining treatment. In each of the circumstances described, it is the perceived physician–nurse power differential that may provoke a sense of moral distress and impotence in nurses.[23]

The tactic of using technical or purposely obscure language when breaking bad news to a patient is unethical. Patients may be confused, unsure, and reluctant to ask further questions. Family members become uncertain and anxious as well; they should, with the patient's permission, be kept current as to the illness, its status, and expected outcomes.[33] If these behaviors are indicative of the professional's own anxiety and sense of unease, the problem should be openly discussed among members of the multidisciplinary team. Nurses can act as both witness to and translator of the clinical conversation by articulating the inherent lack of understanding that occurs when clinical jargon is used to frame and distance an event.

If other members of the health care team request that the patient not be told, the nurse should ask for the rationale prompting the request. If self-protection or discomfort is evident, it is appropriate to speak to the ethic of truth-telling and offer to assist with the task. These circumstances can be particularly difficult for nurses and require sure knowledge of informed consent, effective advocacy skills, and a genuine sense of the moral weight of truth.

Family or friends may ask that the patient be "protected" from distressing news. A promise to keep silent would interfere with the nurse's truth-telling ethic and potentially compromise the nurse–patient relationship. The request should, however, prompt a frank discussion with concerned family members in a quiet and protected environment. Family concerns and the adverse consequences of well-meaning attempts to protect the patient can be addressed. Potential solutions include "checking in" with the patient about the amount of information wanted in the presence of a family member and offering the services of any member of the health care team to assist the family in difficult discussions with the patient.

CASE STUDY
Margaret, a 72-Year-Old Woman with Advanced Breast Cancer

Margaret was 72 years old when she was diagnosed with widespread breast cancer. Her family asked the health care team to avoid the term "cancer," because, they argued, it would destroy all hope. Despite repeated conversations, the family was adamant that this would be what she wanted. Margaret had not been part of this conversation about what she would want, and the team was uncomfortable about the family's demands. Her family left to get breakfast, and the physician was writing treatment orders, still deliberating how he might best honor Margaret and her family. The nurse was in Margaret's room starting an intravenous line. Margaret grabbed the nurse's hand and said, "I know there's something terribly wrong. I see those fake smiles and hear those words that don't make sense. Surely you can tell me what's wrong with me. I want to know, and I want to know now." Her grip was tight on the nurse's hand. The nurse looked into her eyes and replied, "You have breast cancer that has spread to your bones. Your doctor is planning treatment for you right now. I'll go and get him so that he can give you the details and you can ask as many questions as you want." Oddly enough, she visibly relaxed and said, "I just wanted the truth. It's frightening to be alone in a lie."[34]

An equally complex dilemma arises when the patient's cultural norms are such that it is inappropriate to discuss diagnosis and prognosis. The ONS[34] describes provision of "culturally appropriate and competent" care as a primary right of cancer patients. Clinicians accustomed to the Western model of informed consent feel unsettled when patients abrogate autonomy to family members. However, asking individuals from culturally diverse groups to express their wishes may seem not only bewildering but also unnecessary, distasteful, or even immoral.[35] Cultural values may dictate that the family receive the frightening information and filter it for the patient. Although it is ethically important to honor cultural dictates, it is equally important to query the patient regarding the extent of information desired. Health care team members can wrongly assume that a patient's heritage reflects stereotypical behaviors and beliefs. In fact, individual variation is the norm.

Honoring Patients' Wishes

The SUPPORT study,[14] which examined how and where people died and whether their deaths occurred in line with previously expressed wishes, reflected the gaps in meeting the dictates of the Patient Self-Determination Act (PSDA).[36] The PSDA mandated that health care professionals educate patients about advance directives at the time of hospital admission and document their existence in the medical record. As previously mentioned, advance directives were not common, but a more urgent matter was that physicians routinely did not discuss end-of-life issues, nor did they know patients' preferences for resuscitative measures.

Informed consent in end-of-life care is imperative for reasons beyond the legal requirement. Patients and families considering refusal of further treatment should be told of the consequences of their choice, just as they are informed of the benefits and risks of other interventions. Patients and families encountering the withdrawal of treatment may not have been fully informed of the risks and benefits of therapy at initiation, nor of the possibility that treatment could be discontinued if no longer beneficial to the patient.

When the burdens of continued treatment are known, patients with decision-making capacity may refuse or stop unwanted medical treatment even if such refusal could result in their deaths.[37,38] Those who lack capacity have the same rights, but those rights may be exercised through an authorized surrogate decision-maker.[39,40] This right may be ethically burdensome for nurses if they believe that further intervention would markedly benefit the patient. In these circumstances, nurses are obligated (1) to reaffirm informed consent, (2) to support the patient in the right to make personal choices, and (3) to ensure that the patient is not abandoned, emotionally or otherwise.

The medical, legal, bioethical, and consumer advocacy communities are in agreement that support for and encouragement of individual written directives for health care would serve patients well and prevent needless tragedies. The articulation of health care preferences and identification of a surrogate agent to advocate for those preferences can reduce questions and conflicts about what a patient would want, provide direction to the health care team, and relieve family members of the burden of difficult decision-making.

However, a low completion rate of written (advance) directives, as well as their inability to direct care in actual clinical situations,[41–44] continues to be the norm. Individuals may choose to defer to the health care team for appropriate decision-making, may be reluctant to contemplate the issues at all, may argue that they will complete a written directive when "it is really needed," or may refuse to commit themselves to a specific course of action. If a written directive is actually available in a time of crisis, the language may be too obscure to direct the course of care, or the choices may be challenged by the patient's family or members of the health care team.

It is not surprising, then, that a patient's values and wishes can be compromised in a multitude of ways, both intentional and unintentional. The inability to affirm a patient's care preferences may occur in situations such as the following: (1) providing care that one believes the patient would want based on knowledge of that individual's value structure; (2) changing to a pattern of care that one considers appropriate, but that does not reflect the patient's wishes, after family members have left the clinical setting; (3) allowing family members to speak for a timid patient who has privately expressed health care choices that are at odds with those of the family; and (4) ignoring known preferences or honoring the preferences of assertive family members when the patient can no longer articulate personal wishes. In all of these instances, nurses have an ethical obligation to speak to the truths that exist and to hold all health care providers accountable to those truths. If necessary, the nurse may refer the case to the institution's bioethics committee.

Abandonment

Meaningful relationships require continued presence. The ability to remain available in the midst of considerable anguish, fear, sorrow, or profound grief requires tremendous courage. Nurses must be willing to set aside personal biographies and professional privilege. If nurses allow professional attitudes to distance themselves from the intimacy of the experience, their role is diminished and the relationships lose meaning. Nurses must be able to function in a partnership with patients, recognizing and acknowledging that one of the most meaningful parts of their response to the dying experience is continued presence.[32]

Patients fear abandonment in response to decisions that conflict with those of the health care team. The fear of losing those whom one has known and trusted at a time of crisis can be overwhelming. Moreover, abandonment can be very subtle. If a patient or patient advocate chooses a course of care that is discomforting or unacceptable (i.e., refusing treatment, stopping active treatment, demanding treatment deemed useless by the health care team, or asking for removal of life-prolonging interventions), health care professionals may withdraw in a multitude of ways. Less time may be spent with the patient, or such visits may become less frequent, and direct verbal engagement may become limited. Any of these behaviors may be viewed by the patient and family as emotional withdrawal at the least and abandonment at the worst.

The ethical dilemma is evident: How can one balance one's own moral values and the patient's right to autonomous behavior while remaining available to and supportive of the patient? Nurses are particularly vulnerable. They may feel "caught in the middle" if they are expected to provide care in circumstances that clash with their personal values. While wanting to remain loyal to the patient, they may be conflicted by (1) providing care they deem futile or inappropriate—for example, continuing artificial life support despite a diagnosis of brain death; (2) following orders to provide care that is morally unacceptable—for example, discontinuing hydration or nutrition or removing a patient from a ventilator; or (3) responding to requests from patients that they cannot honor—for example, a request for assisted death.[23]

According to the ANA Code for Nurses,[45] nurses may morally refuse to participate in care, but only on the grounds of patient advocacy or moral objection to a specific type of intervention. Although it is ethically imperative to reassure the patient/family unit that their decisions will be respected and they will not be abandoned if their goals differ from those of the health care team, nurses may remove themselves from the patient's direct care while simultaneously continuing to be available to the patient. These behaviors reflect a continuous partnership and acknowledge the importance of an ongoing personal commitment to caring and problem solving.[46]

CASE STUDY

Caroline, a 60-Year-Old Woman with Leukemia

Caroline and her nurse grew to know each other very well over her weeks of treatment for acute myelogenous leukemia. She was hoping to receive a bone marrow transplant (BMT), which she believed would cure her. She was 60 years of age, was becoming increasingly frail, and had limited functional capacity. The health care team had reservations about the advisability of a BMT but did not discuss those reservations with her. The task at hand was to get her into remission and ready for the transplant. One week after discharge and successful completion of the induction therapy, Caroline returned to the hospital with recurrent disease and in significant pain. She asked her nurse if she would die and how it would be. The nurse told her that another course of chemotherapy would be given, that the odds for cure had decreased markedly with the recurrence, and that the BMT posed grave risks to her life. She also described complications that would occur if the cancer did not respond to treatment and how those symptoms would be managed. The leukemia did not respond to reinduction chemotherapy, and Caroline's pain worsened. In getting out of bed one day, she moved too quickly and suffered a pathological fracture in one of her vertebrae. The pain was severe and not easily managed. It was quiet on the unit early the next evening, and Caroline asked the nurse to sit with her. She seemed so frightened. The nurse sat beside her on the bed and held her hand. Caroline said, "I can't do this anymore. I'm so tired, and I'm afraid of the pain. Please give me a shot and put me to sleep forever." The nurse felt anguish at the request, for she had promised Caroline she would not let her suffer. She felt cowardly and disloyal as she explained why she could not provide the medication. Her moral distress centered on her inability to honor her promise and her mixed feelings about what would be appropriate in those circumstances. She promised Caroline she would stay with her and make sure she was comfortable. She asked whether Caroline wanted her to call someone else to be there with her, but she declined. Caroline died that night, never having spoken another word to the nurse.

This case brings attention to multiple issues that might have led to a better outcome for the patient, family, and health care team. Earlier and frank discussions with the patient and family about the course of the illness, the prognosis, and treatment expectations and realities might have allowed both the patient and family the opportunity to plan for death in a more comprehensive and meaningful way. These discussions might have presented opportunities for understanding the patient's perspective on assisted death and the circumstances that might trigger such a request. Finally, it would have allowed the health care team an opportunity to be clear about the kind of support they could offer.

Futility and Withdrawal of Treatment

Decisions in the clinical arena are increasingly made under a new kind of pressure. With almost every health care delivery institution facing financial constraints, health care providers are experiencing the tensions of "limits" imposed on professional standards of care. A powerful new vocabulary, that of "medical futility," has entered the discourse.

Health care professionals often feel that patient expectations and desire for care are unreasonable, sometimes impossible, and, on occasion, limitless. Nurses may find themselves searching for unilateral solutions to complex problems when historically they have acted in tandem with the patient and family. They may feel that a patient's continued treatment serves no purpose, increases the suffering quotient, and uses increasingly scarce resources. They question what good comes from their actions and ask whether these interventions may be refused. Influenced by outcome-based practice standards, reimbursement formulas, and a growing disenchantment with "hi-tech" interventions, these dilemmas evolve into questions of whether to withhold or withdraw treatment.

But it is often precisely at this moment that patients and families insist on continuation of aggressive treatment and question the health care system's motives, wondering whether the declaration of futility is a cover for cost containment or racial or other prejudice. They feel increasingly alienated from and even abandoned by the health care staff. This dilemma is becoming more common: Is it ever ethical to withdraw care deemed futile by the staff in the face of an intense patient or family desire to continue? A description of the nurse's role in such circumstances can be constructed only after there is a clearer definition of futility and an understanding of the legal and ethical dictates supporting the clinician's right to withdraw treatment.

Many definitions of medical futility have been proposed. Some have defined a futile treatment as one that does not serve a valid goal of medical practice (a standard of medical judgment),[47] with it being the normative professional responsibility of the medical team to decide whether desired treatment courses are realistic. Others have argued for a more precise definition, suggesting that a treatment is futile if it is unsuccessful more than 99% of the time (a standard of efficacy). Still others have indicated that treatment outside accepted community standards could be understood as futile (a standard of communal evaluation).

Rubin[48] suggested that futility exists if the treatment does not achieve the patient's intended goal. As Younger[49] noted early in the debate, futility is a concept that makes no sense standing alone; rather, it is an evaluative judgment based on the worth of possible goals. The value of a treatment would depend on the meaning of the goals and who was empowered to select them, and that same treatment would be futile only if the goals could not be met. With that understanding, the contemporary futility debate could be understood in terms of power: the power to define the acceptable use of medical interventions, to determine whether and under what conditions limits can be appropriately set, and to negotiate the terms of the provider–patient relationship.

The demands of the current health care system ask the health care team to assess a treatment's relative futility even though there is no agreed definition or determined criterion against which it can be measured. Further, they are asked to develop practice standards and institutional policies even though there is no vision of how to set appropriate limits. Worst of all, they are offered the illusory hope that complex ethical dilemmas can be resolved merely by identifying treatments as futile and concluding that they need not be provided or paid for. Reframing the futility discussion in the language of goals is one of the most effective ways of addressing the moral appeals at stake in conflicts between patients and their providers, and, in the authors' opinion, it is the most significant intervention clinicians and ethicists can make when the new language of futility emerges as a way of talking about a case.

In the majority of situations in which death is imminent, consensus is reached and life-sustaining interventions are not provided. Conflicts in which questions of relative value arise do not represent straightforward issues of futility. Examples include life-sustaining interventions for a patient who is in a persistent vegetative state, resuscitation efforts for patients with life-threatening illnesses, use of chemotherapy for patients with extensive metastatic cancer, and use of antibiotics or artificial hydration and nutrition for patients who are in the advanced stages of an illness.

The concept of medical futility is more commonly invoked when values conflict. Those arguing from the provider's perspective believe that the health care team should neither offer nor provide therapy that is unlikely to work or will only diminish quality of life. To do otherwise, they believe, would be to violate professional integrity, offer false hope to patients and families, and inflict harm on patients without the possibility of benefit. Others disagree, wondering why the provider's values should override the values of the patient and family, especially if those values are religiously based. The disagreements that arise are fundamentally moral and not medical in nature.

When a claim of medical futility arises, the investigation should first identify the goals and intentions of treatment and determine whose goals seem to be taking precedence. This offers a more productive method for discussion of concerns and the mutual exploration of goals and their meaning. It also encourages the health care team to consider their ability and commitment to meet goals that differ from their own. If inadequate communication is part of the problem, assessing and responding to misunderstandings by clarifying diagnosis and prognosis, eliminating medical jargon, discussing what "do everything" actually means, and checking for mistaken notions of legal requirements can be extremely helpful. Interpersonal issues such as distrust, grief, guilt, intrafamily issues, secondary gains, differences in values, and religious beliefs may contribute to the conflict and should be explored. The nurse, who is more likely to have developed a close relationship with the patient and family, should be involved at every stage of the futility discussion. Opportune moments may arise when other members of the health care team are not available, and that particular nurse–patient conversation may help to resolve the conflict.

The withdrawal or withholding of life-sustaining treatment is very often at the heart of medical futility conflicts. Withholding or withdrawing life-sustaining medical interventions is considered neither homicide[50] nor suicide.[37] Courts have drawn a distinction between purposefully causing a patient's death and allowing a patient to die after life-sustaining measures are withdrawn. Courts have upheld the validity of DNR and other treatment limitation orders,[51] and there are no limits on the type of treatment that may be withheld or withdrawn. Ventilator withdrawal[4,37] and the withholding or withdrawing of parenteral nutrition and hydration[5] may occur under the same conditions, as any other form of medical treatment.

That moment in nursing that demands an elegant level of practice is the moment when patients and families decide to forgo aggressive care and elect a palliative approach. Patients and their families may need support for such difficult decisions and often require repetitive feedback about medical data, review of past therapies, reconsideration of any potential interventions, and, in some instances, retrospective permission to make that particular choice. Nurses have witnessed the dilemma of physician withdrawal when the medical team painfully confronts its inability to cure. The turn to palliation is not a defeat for the nurse but, rather, an intensification and revaluing of the skills of nursing. The graceful art of deferring to the patient's story and remaining emotionally available in the face of considerable fear and anguish involves interaction on multiple intellectual and emotional levels and enriches the lives of both the patient and the nurse.[32] In this context nothing is futile—no touch, no glance, no offer of assistance, and no silence held in common. The worth of the interaction is always based on nurturing and caring as an end goal. It is a stance that will require fierce protection and defense.

Despite legal support for withholding or withdrawing life-sustaining treatment at the patient or proxy's request, the health care team can find itself at odds with patients and families who become suspicious, fearful, and often unmoving in their opposition when the subject is broached. Ethical differences exist in any pluralistic society, especially one in which resources are increasingly scarce. The desire to struggle aggressively with death is one of the most deeply rooted moral choices an individual can make, and there is little consensus about those choices, as evidenced by the right-to-life and assisted death debates.

Although there are circumstances in which life-sustaining treatment can be stopped over the objections of patients and families—for example, when a patient meets the defined criteria for brain death—consensual standards should be developed after the fullest possible public discussion. Because there is no authoritative legal definition of medical futility or clear resolution in the courts as to its meaning or jurisdiction,[48] the critical voices of physicians, nurses, and patients must be heard. Claims of medical futility cannot be made simply to transfer unwilling patients gratuitously into hospice settings as a cost-saving scheme.

The discussion cannot occur in a piecemeal fashion, at the bedsides of the most vulnerable or in the closed boardrooms of individual institutions. Opening a communal debate rather than closing it with simplistic unilateral solutions is the only defensible decision-making process and the only way out of the futility challenge. Bioethics committees allow for such discourse, and their approach could become the template for (1) discussion of difficult cases, (2) just evaluation of new outcome data, (3) allowing for cultural differences in the selection of goals, and (4) facilitating end-of-life decision-making. This approach would allow for a forum of careful debate before the inevitable crisis emerges, and for an appeals process that would permit a more detailed immersion into the decision-making process. Whenever possible, joint decision-making should occur. If resolution is not forthcoming after careful and deliberate discussion, a step-by-step process of communication and problem-solving has been suggested by the American Medical Association (AMA).[52] See Table 57–3 for a "due process to futility situations" paradigm.

Table 57–3
A Due-Process Approach to Futility Situations: A Paradigm for Preventing and Resolving Conflicts

1. Attempt to negotiate an understanding among patient, surrogate, and the health care team as to what constitutes futile care in advance of the actual conflict.
2. Establish joint decision-making as the goal. Use the assistance of consultants as appropriate.
3. If disagreement persists, suggest use of other consultants, colleagues, and the institution's ethics committee. This provides the maximum possible place for patient autonomy.
4. If institutional review supports the patient's position and the physician is uncomfortable with the decision made, transfer of care may be arranged.
5. If review supports the health care team's position and the patient or surrogate disagrees with the decision, transfer to another institution or provider can be arranged if both parties agree and if possible.
6. If no receiving institution can be found, the problem remains unsolved and further discussion must continue.

Source: American Medical Association (1999). The Education for Physicians on End-of-Life Care (EPEC) Curriculum: © The EPEC Project, 1999, 2003 (reference 52).

CASE STUDY
Matthew, a 42-Year-Old Man with Recurrent Lymphoma

Matthew was 42 years of age when his aggressive form of lymphoma recurred. He was admitted to the ICU insisting that he wanted everything done and adamant that he meant everything. His wife Sue supported him in that decision, but, as the hours passed and he became increasingly ill, she started to question their decision. Sue spoke at length with the nurse about their personal history. This was her second marriage, her first husband having died of cancer. Matthew had promised Sue that he would never leave her, that he would not die before she did. The nurse spoke at length with Sue, reviewing current interventions and Matthew 's prognosis in relation to those interventions. She asked Sue to review their family's goals in light of this difficult prognostic information. Sue agonized about having the conversation with Matthew and expressed concern about feelings of guilt and disloyalty. The nurse continued to encourage her, framing the discussion in terms of goals of care, Matthew 's suffering, and the health care team's commitment to both of them. Sue understood that she would need to give Matthew permission to let go. She could see he was going to die despite the intensive interventions, and she wanted him to have a peaceful death. She did talk with Matthew, and most of the interventions were discontinued after that conversation. The next day, as Sue held him, he died.

Assisted Death

The profound existential issues innate to end-of-life care are no more evident than in discussions regarding assisted death. The adult patient's right to control health care interventions has historically allowed individuals to refuse to seek medical care, refuse recommended care, stop hydration and nutrition and other prescribed recommendations, and forgo or discontinue life support. These historical methods of ending life sooner have become commonplace. They are legally and also morally acceptable to the majority of practitioners and, in fact, have become a standard of practice for patients and the health care team alike.[53,54]

The ability to exercise autonomy in health care decision-making, as reflected in these circumstances, has engendered questions in both the medical and lay communities as to the "rightness" of extending autonomous behavior to other practices that have been described as humane—interventions that would stop or prevent intractable suffering or unacceptably diminished quality of life. Certainly the courts have supported an individual's right to refuse or withdraw from life-sustaining treatment.[4,37,50,51]

It has been argued that withholding or withdrawing treatment and refusing treatment are no different, from a consequential perspective, from PAS, voluntary active euthanasia, or sedation for intractable distress in the dying.[55–59] Others have argued that there is a distinct moral difference.[60,61] Although PAS is a small part of the process of improving care for all dying patients and their families, the current and intense focus on the quality and scope of end-of-life care has added fuel to the debate about it. Scholars, lawyers, ethicists, health care personnel, religious organizations, and consumer organizations have taken varied stances, as reflected in Table 57–4.[61–66]

Professional health care organizations such as the AMA, the ANA, and the Hospice and Palliative Nurses Association (HPNA) have published position statements opposing PAS but strongly supporting excellence in end-of-life care. The position of the ONS on nurses' responsibility to patients requesting assisted suicide[67] recognizes that "individual nurses may encounter agonizing clinical situations and experience both personal and professional tension and ambiguity surrounding a patient's request for assisted suicide."[68] Nurses are urged to explore the rationale for the request, assess and provide for any unmet needs, and resist any behavioral or nonbehavioral indications of abandonment. Schwarz,[69] in a phenomenological study, found that few nurses unequivocally agreed or refused to directly help a patient die. Most grappled in solitary and silent ways to find interventions that would be legally and morally acceptable.

Oregon voters approved PAS in 1994, and the appeal process ultimately sent the question to the United States Supreme Court. In June of 1997, the Supreme Court ruled that an individual does not have a Constitutional right to assistance with dying, nor does a physician have an obligation to provide that assistance.[29a] Subsequent to the Supreme Court decision, in the fall of 1997, the citizens of Oregon again voted and legalized PAS with a 60%/40% majority.[69]

Terminally ill residents of Oregon are able to receive prescriptions from their physicians for lethal medications that may then be self-administered.[69] Criteria to protect citizens from coerced or involuntary action include the following (1) the patient must be an adult able to make and communicate decisions; (2) the terminal illness must be expected to lead to death within 6 months; (3) there must be one written and two oral requests separated by a 2-week period; (4) there must be confirmation of the terminal diagnosis, prognosis, and capability by both the patient's primary physician and a consultant; and (5) there must be referral to counseling if either the primary physician or the consultant believes that the patient's judgment is impaired by depression or some other psychiatric disorder. The primary physician is also responsible for discussing all feasible alternatives with the patient—that is, comfort care, hospice care, and pain-control options.

Many reasons have been postulated as to what might instigate a request for PAS. Inadequacy of pain relief,[70–72] inadequate recognition and management of depression,[73–75] or inadequate management of other symptoms such as dyspnea, intractable nausea, and vomiting or diarrhea[59,76] are believed to be primary causes. In Oregon,[77] the very small number of patient requests were more likely to correlate with strong, vivid personalities characterized by determination and inflexibility; a need to control the timing and manner of death;

Table 57–4
The Debate Concerning Assisted Death

Argument	Pro	Con
Liberty interest vs. state's interest	There is equal protection under the law that allows the right to refuse or withdraw treatment and to commit suicide.	There is constitutional power to override certain rights in order to protect citizens from irrevocable acts.
Autonomy	Every competent person has the right to make momentous decisions based on personal convictions.	Human beings are the stewards but not the absolute masters of the gift of life.
Quality of care	Removal of legal bans would enhance the opportunity for excellent end-of-life care for all patients secondary to statutory requirements that the very best in palliative care be provided.	The aim of medicine should be to facilitate a death that is pain free but also a human experience. A good natural death contributes value to the community.
Nonmaleficence	From the patient's perspective, there is no difference between ending life by providing a lethal prescription and by stopping treatment that prolongs life.	The role of the nurse has been to promote, preserve, and protect human life. Assisted death violates the oath to "do no harm" and destroys trust between the patient and nurse.
Beneficence	More patients could benefit from relief that is now available illegally to many people who have strong relationships with physicians willing to risk assisting them to die.	A misdiagnosis of the illness, inadequate assessment of competence, or pressure from the family or the physician might place patients in jeopardy.
Slippery slope	The states could adopt regulations to ensure informed, competent, and freely made decisions.	Although assisted death might initially be restricted to competent, terminally ill patients, in time many other kinds of patients might be assisted to die in more aggressive ways.

Source: Adapted from references 62–66.

and a desire to avoid dependence on others. In the summative experience with PAS in Oregon, unmanaged symptoms have not been ranked as primary reasons for PAS requests. This may reflect advances in pain management in Oregon, which ranks among the top five states in per capita use of morphine for medical purposes,[78] and the Oregon statute's requirement that the very best in palliative care be provided to this group of patients. Patients with access to a lethal dose of medication report that it provides them the freedom and reassurance to continue living, knowing that they can escape if and when they choose.[79,80]

Inadequate physical or psychological care is most frequently postulated by professional caregivers, and researchers have identified characteristics of those requesting assistance in dying. However, there are sparse data examining the terminally ill individual's reason for asking the question in the first place.[81] An expressed desire for hastened death may not be a literal request but could rather have multiple meanings and uses. Coyle and Sculco[82] discovered additional possible rationales for this "cry for help." They identified such requests as (1) a way of drawing attention to the individual and his or her unique needs so that they might be seen and heard; (2) a gesture of altruism, to relieve the family of further burden; or (3) an attempt to manipulate the family and avoid abandonment. Their research reinforced the need to consider the request in context of the patient's lived experience.

The spectrum of professional and lay responses highlights the intensity of the dilemma. Wolfe and colleagues,[83] in examining the stability of attitudes regarding PAS and euthanasia among oncology patients, physicians, and the general public, found a growing disparity between the public and the medical profession. As laypersons are becoming more comfortable with the concept, physicians are growing less supportive. In 2002, Emanuel[84] reviewed data from surveys of the general public and health care professionals as to attitudes about and experience with PAS and euthanasia. Public support for PAS varied from 34% to 65% and that percentage had not changed over the past several years. Most physicians do not view PAS as ethical, although some have agreed that in some instances suicide may be a rational act. They have consistently indicated that they do not wish to participate in assisted death. There has been a decline in support for PAS on the part of U.S. oncologists that may be due to a more recent focus on end-of-life care and its possibilities. Many studies indicate that a small proportion of U.S. physicians have performed PAS. Requests more frequently come to oncologists, and oncologists generally report having performed PAS more frequently. Of interest is that when physicians encounter such requests, they are very likely to use fewer life-prolonging therapies and to increase interventions aimed at symptom management (e.g., improved analgesic therapy, treatment of depression and anxiety, referral for psychiatric evaluation). Surveys demonstrate that about half of nonphysician health professionals support PAS in some circumstance, but fewer than one third have received requests. Emanuel also reviewed attitudes and practices of U.S. patients. He drew four major conclusions from the data: (1) patients with cancer primarily use PAS; (2) pain does not seem to be a major determinant of interest in or use of PAS; (3) depression, hopelessness, and general psychological distress are consistently associated with interest in PAS; and (4) among terminally ill patients, the extent of caregiving needs was associated with interest in PAS.

In the midst of the ongoing deliberation, nurses daily face ethical dilemmas as to the most appropriate response to patients who ask for such assistance. Matzo and Emanuel,[85] in their survey of oncology nurses, reported that 30% of the respondents (131 nurses) had been asked to assist with a patient's suicide. Historically, nursing surveys have reflected the professional individual's ambiguity about this issue.[85,86] Schwarz[59] and Volker[68] described feelings of conflict, guilt, and moral distress in these circumstances. They saw compelling cases in which patients were devastated physically and emotionally by illness and confronted with the suffering and exhaustion of their families. Personal and professional tension and ambiguity about what is right are bound to occur in such situations. At times, it may be difficult to balance facilitation of a dignified death with preservation of life,[76] and the willingness to consider participation in assisted suicide may be motivated by mercy, compassion, promotion of autonomy, and quality-of-life considerations.[59,68] Dr. Ira Byock, who has publicly spoken out in opposition to PAS, suggests that our responsibilities, if PAS were legalized, would be to stand by the patient and family, whatever their decision, and continue to provide care. Byock also asserts that although patient choices may differ from the provider's preference, there is an obligation to respect those choices and struggle along with them.[87]

Nurses who are asked about PAS or asked to assist with a patient's suicide are ethically bound to (1) respond nonjudgmentally to requests; (2) provide all relevant information about the state's legal restrictions as well as alternative treatments and options; (3) participate with the multidisciplinary team in a thorough evaluation of the patient's rationale for the request; (4) assist in the clarification of goals; and (5) ensure that all symptoms, including depression, are assessed and managed at a level acceptable to the patient and family. Ongoing emotional support and caring for the patient and family can be offered without regard for statutory law.

The Oregon Nurses Association (ONA) has published a white paper[88] on the Oregon Death with Dignity Act[69] that supports the ethical stances of nurses who choose to care for or discontinue involvement in the care of individuals who request PAS. The ONA supports both the patient's right to self-determination and the nurse's right to a professional practice congruent with personal moral values. Oregon nurses who choose to continue caring for a patient requesting assisted suicide may (1) explain the law as it currently exists; (2) discuss and explore options with the patient and make referrals if appropriate; (3) explore reasons for the patient's request, ensuring that depression is thoroughly evaluated and treated if present; (4) maintain patient and family confidentiality; (5) provide care and comfort throughout the dying process; (6) remain present during the patient's self-administration of the medication and subsequent death to console and counsel the family; (7) continue to provide ongoing emotional support; and (8) be involved in policy development within the health care facility or the community. The state expects nurses to respect patient confidentiality and to respect patient choices. Nurses may not inject or administer the medication that will lead to the end of the patient's life, and they may not make unwarranted judgmental comments to other members of the health care team who care for patients who have chosen assisted suicide.

Ethical imperatives for those Oregon nurses who choose not to be involved can offer some guidance for nurses whose legal jurisdiction does not legitimize assisted suicide and who want to respond appropriately and compassionately to the patients they serve. The nurse who feels ethically compromised in caring for a patient who has chosen assisted suicide is obliged (1) to provide for the patient's comfort and safety, (2) to withdraw only if assured that alternative sources of end-of-life care are available to the patient, and (3) to continue to provide ongoing care if unable to transfer that care to another provider. Nurses may not breach confidentiality, subject patients or their peers to judgmental remarks about PAS, or abandon or refuse to provide comfort and safety measures to the patient.

The imperative to explore the rationale for patient's requests needs to be translated into health care policies. Most health care systems do not provide written guidelines for their staff. The Hospice of Boulder County in Boulder, Colorado, has developed guidelines for caring for the patient who expresses interest in hastening death.[89] Modeled after the ONA's white paper, it provides a thoughtful and caring structure for a multidisciplinary response to a distressed patient. Table 57–5 presents a paradigm of this policy.

Table 57–5
Identifying Vulnerability Factors and Responding to Those Patients Who Express Interest in Hastening Death

I. Assessment

A. Patient interview

1. What is happening now that makes you consider this action?
2. If we could relieve that problem, would you still be interested in dying now?
3. Have you thought about a method?
4. What do you know about the consequences of this method for your family?
5. Is this an idea that is yours alone, or has someone suggested that you consider this?
6. Have you discussed this with family members, your doctor, or others who are caring for you?

B. Evaluation

1. Satisfaction with pain and symptom management?
2. Depression? Anxiety?
3. Fears? Anger? Family pressures?
4. Personal and spiritual philosophy?
5. History of depression or mental illness?
6. Weapons on the premises?

II. Intervention

A. Team meeting

1. Physician notification
2. Possible request for ethics committee consultation

B. Response to unmet needs

1. Aggressive efforts made to alleviate any unmet physical, emotional, or spiritual needs
2. Anxiety or depression? Offer pharmacological treatment and/or psychotherapy

C. Response to request

1. Description of current state law, its requisites, and the provider's rights and responsibilities
2. Information and counseling regarding the patient's request
3. Encouragement to discuss with family and others involved in care
4. Removal of weapons from the premises if they present a threat to staff or family
5. Notification of appropriate authorities if violent death (e.g., shooting) occurs

D. Staffing

1. Staff assignments made in terms of comfort/discomfort with patient request
2. Support offered to those who have cared for the patient but choose not to continue after a wish for hastened death has been expressed
3. Review of case by involved staff and volunteers

E. Documentation

1. Assessment
2. Interventions

Source: Adapted from Hospice of Boulder County Ethics Committee (1999), reference 91, and Oregon Nurses Association (1995), reference 90.

CASE STUDY

Josephine, a Patient Seeking to Hasten Death

Josephine was a strong woman. She had emigrated to the United States as a child. When diagnosed with metastatic colorectal cancer, she stoically began treatment. As she and her nurse developed a relationship over time, she mentioned her fears of dependency, of losing her ability to think and communicate clearly, of losing her ability to control her bodily functions. She was absolutely clear that she did not want to die having lost control of her physical or mental abilities. One day she asked her nurse if she would be able to "put her to sleep" when the time seemed appropriate. As the nurse explained why this was not possible, Josephine interrupted her and said, "They treat dogs better than they do human beings." The topic came up frequently over the next few months, and each time the nurse reiterated the difficulties while continuing to remind Josephine that she would be supported with the very best in palliative care in order to ensure a death that was peaceful. Josephine never stopped asking for assistance in dying. She ultimately became very confused in her final days. The nurse was with her when she died, and her last words, jumbled though they were, included the word "dog."

Josephine's experience reflects the conflicts that nurses encounter daily. Many patients express fears as they near the end of life, such as fear of losing control, fear of acting in a way that they regard as undignified, or fear of living beyond the time they consider acceptable. These fears may be at the most existential and intimate of levels and cannot be dismissed with easy answers. And so patients often ask for assistance in dying. The dilemma for the nurse and other members of the multidisciplinary team is how best to resolve the patient's deeply felt fears, how best to identify interventions that have meaning, and how to personally resolve the tensions generated by the inability to respond to another's plea for help. Josephine might have benefited from more detailed discussions of how she could be supported at the end of life and more assistance from the hospice team's social worker in exploring her fears.

Voluntarily stopping eating and drinking (VSED) has been suggested as an acceptable moral alternative to PAS.[90] Although VSED is legally permissible, some patients, families, and members of the health care team may consider this method equivalent to "dehydrating" or "starving" a patient and therefore morally offensive. Ganzini and associates[91] surveyed hospice nurses in Oregon regarding their experiences with patients who chose VSED; 33% of the 307 nurses who returned the questionnaire reported that in the previous 4 years they had cared for a patient who deliberately hastened death by voluntary refusal of food and fluids. Nurses reported that patients chose VSED because they were ready to die, saw continued existence as pointless, and considered their quality of life poor. This choice requires considerable patient resolve, because life may continue for weeks; Ganzini's survey showed that 85% of patients died within 15 days after stopping food and fluids. On a scale from 0 (a very bad death) to 9 (a very good death), the median score for the quality of these deaths, as rated by the nurses, was 8. Should a patient choose this course of action, the nurse should continue meticulous comfort care and may need to implement sedative orders for the management of delirium. The choice to use VSED is based on the patient's values, and it would be egregious if the physician or nurse condemned the patient for this choice. Those health care professionals who believe VSED to be morally impermissible may excuse themselves from care after ensuring a suitable substitute caregiver.

Even with state-of-the-art care, a small number of dying patients will experience suffering that cannot be satisfactorily relieved—such as pain, shortness of breath, intractable nausea or vomiting, and delirium. "Terminal sedation" as a solution to these unmanageable kinds of suffering is a phrase that has appeared in the palliative care literature in the last few years. The U.S. Supreme Court[29a] made terminal sedation legally acceptable in the same opinion that ruled PAS was neither a patient right nor a medical obligation.

However, consensus had not been reached as to a clear definition of terminal sedation.[92] Chater and colleagues[56] suggested the following: "The intention of deliberately inducing and maintaining deep sleep, but not deliberately causing death in specific circumstances[—that is,] for the relief of one or more intractable symptoms when all other possible interventions have failed and the patient is perceived to be close to death and/or for the relief of profound anguish (possibly spiritual) that is not amenable to spiritual, psychological or other intervention and the patient is perceived to be close to death" (p. 257). They also suggested a less pejorative term: "sedation for intractable distress in the dying."

Regardless of the terminology, there continues to be much debate in the bioethical and medical communities about the moral repercussions of sedation for intractable distress.[57–59,76,93] Some have argued that death with sedation for intractable distress is "foreseen" but not "intended," thereby invoking the principle of double effect—that is, the sedation itself is not causing death but is intended to relieve suffering, an accepted aim of medicine.[59,94] Those who take the middle ground allow the possibility that in some cases sedation for intractable distress may be morally acceptable if symptoms cannot be managed otherwise.[56,93,95,96] Finally, others see it as tantamount to euthanasia, because the sedated patient may die from the combination of two intentional acts—the induction of stupor or unconsciousness and the withholding of food and water.[57] The ANA[26] has stated that the risk of hastening death through treatments aimed at alleviating suffering or controlling symptoms is ethically acceptable.

If sedation for intractable distress is evaluated to be necessary in light of current patient circumstances, the health care team must ensure that the patient's decision is informed and voluntary before initiating the intervention. If the patient lacks decision-making capacity and appears to be suffering intolerably, it is essential to discuss with family members or the health care proxy the exhaustion of all other palliative care interventions and to collaboratively determine the current goals of care in relation to the patient's health status.

CASE STUDY

Frank, a Man with Intractable Pain

Frank was an older gentleman with widely metastatic colon cancer. Pain became the formidable adversary of the hospice team. Every possible analgesic intervention was tried, including all atypical analgesics, all anesthetic procedures, including intraspinal analgesia. He continued to experience severe pain and begged to have his life ended. After an emotional but carefully thought out discussion and consultation with the hospital's bioethics committee, the family supported the decision to begin intravenous sedating therapy in order to ensure Frank's comfort. Many of the nurses who had been caring for him believed that this was equivalent to euthanasia and asked to be excused from caring for him. They were forbidden to voice their concerns to Frank and his family but were allowed to offer comforting words and expressions of their feelings for Frank. Those nurses who were morally comfortable with the decision took responsibility for his care.

Ultimately, safeguards must be in place when considering any intervention that might end the patient's life sooner than would be otherwise true. Such safeguards include (1) informed and voluntary consent after detailed discussion, (2) diagnostic and prognostic clarity, (3) an independent second opinion from a consultant with expertise in palliative care, (4) a brief waiting period and reevaluation of the issues with the patient and family, and (5) documentation and review to ensure accountability.

If the goal of care is to manage a symptom, not to hasten death, documentation of the whole process should be meticulous. The goals of care and discussion with the patient and family (i.e., informed consent) should be clearly outlined in the progress notes. Careful documentation is not limited to sedation to relieve intractable distress in the dying. Withholding or withdrawal of treatment and increasing doses of medication for symptom relief that may secondarily shorten life (e.g., opioids for pain relief) must receive the same careful attention.

Allocation of Resources

As health care costs rise, increasing numbers of individuals are without health care insurance, and Medicare reimbursement for older adults changes, questions arise about adequate care for persons at the end of life. Long-term chronic disease has emerged as the primary pathway to dying, representing a prolonged course of increasing disability and illness before death. The financing of end-of-life care largely occurs within Medicare. Of the 2.3 million Americans who died in 1997, roughly 86% were Medicare beneficiaries. End-of-life care represents about 27% of the Medicare budget.[97]

Providers and patients are concerned about care choices and limitations on those choices. Access to care, the site of care, the philosophical approach to care, and the quality of the care provided are troubling issues. Health care researchers have continued to provide valuable information about where people die. Wennberg and coworkers[98] examined the use of health care resources during the last 6 months of life by patients of 77 U.S. hospitals with strong reputations for high-quality care in managing chronic illness. They found that ICU days ranged from 1.6 to 9.5; hospitals days, ranged from 9 to 27; the number of physician visits, ranged from 17 to 76, with 17% to 58% of patients seeing 10 or more physicians; and hospice enrollment varied from 11% to 44% (median, 22% to 32%). Although these data represent a striking variation in the utilization of end-of-life care among those institutions studied, it is a reminder, as was documented in the SUPPORT study,[14] that hospice care is not the normative choice for care in the final days of life.

Bird and colleagues[99] reviewed a random sample of Medicare beneficiaries who died between 1993 and 1998. Medicare expenditures in the last year of life were lowest for decedents in the oldest age group but 70% higher for those in the youngest age group (ages 65 through 69 years). Inpatient expenditures, regardless of age cohort, represented the largest single cost percentage among sites of care.

Cassel and associates[100] examined end-of-life care in ICUs and found that surgeons and intensivists approached care very differently. The former prioritized defeating death as a primary goal, whereas the latter incorporated scarce resources and quality of life as significant variables in the decision-making process. Pekmezaris and coworkers[101] examined the specificity of advance directives in relation to site of death and found that a significantly higher proportion of patients died in nursing homes, as opposed to hospitals, if their advance directives specifically prohibited resuscitation, intubation, artificial feeding and hydration, or hospitalization.

Based on data about where people die, it may be argued that our society's philosophical approach to dying remains grounded in the Western medical model of cure. Selwyn and Forstein[102] described the false dichotomy of curative versus palliative care for patients with late-stage HIV/AIDS. Uncertainties about prognosis and the promise and limitations of rapidly evolving therapies have made decision-making about end-of-life issues more complex. As a result, individuals continue on antiretroviral therapy with its significant side effect burden and in the presence of worsening disease, with the hope that they will improve. Fried and Bradley[103] examined the influences on end-of-life treatment choices in older, seriously ill persons. They found three major influences: treatment burden, treatment outcome, and the likelihood of the outcome. As might be expected, the burden of treatment was bearable if the outcome was desirable, but individuals were less willing to undergo the burden of care for more marginal results. Of interest was a third finding: some participants disclosed that their willingness to tolerate adverse outcomes might increase even as their illness progressed. Although many observers have believed that cancer chemotherapy is overused at the end of life, Emanuel and colleagues[104] were able to confirm this belief. The charts of all Medicare patients who died of cancer in Massachusetts and 5% of Medicare cancer decedents in California in 1966 were examined. Chemotherapy was used frequently in the last 3 months of life, and the cancer's responsiveness to chemotherapy did not seem to influence whether dying patients received chemotherapy during that time.

The high prevalence of death among ICU patients and readmissions to the ICU generate significant cost expenditures.[105] At times of crisis, it is not uncommon for family members to be asked to determine goals of care and to interpret a patient's health care wishes. High levels of stress, complex information, inadequate time, and lack of consistent communication do not adequately prepare families to make such decisions. Ahrens and associates[106] studied the effect of improved communication with family members on length of stay and resource utilization in the ICU. For patients at high risk of death, these researchers compared the length of stay and cost effects of daily family communication by one medical doctor–clinical nurse specialist (MD-CNS) team to the usual communication process. Daily communication in the intervention group focused on daily goals, a discussion of options other than curative care, opportunity to clarify issues, and time to verbalize any thoughts, values, or emotions family members were having. The research team discovered that when families had consistent communication with the MD-CNS team, direct and indirect costs were significantly lower and mortality in the ICU setting was 20% less, compared with the control group. Length of stay in the hospital and in the ICU were significantly lower in the intervention group. This effort demonstrated that appropriate communication that is medically and ethically sound not only represents excellence in care but has a secondary effect of conserving resources.

Many members of the professional and lay communities have expressed grave concerns regarding the impact of managed care on quality care at the end of life. Slutsman and associates[107] compared the experiences of terminally ill patients in managed care and in fee-for-service care. Overall, the two populations were found to have comparable outcomes. Managed care patients were more likely to use an inconvenient hospital but less likely to have unmet care needs for nursing care or homemaking. There were three primary findings of note: (1) access to care was comparable, (2) there were few differences in the quality of the doctor–patient relationship, and (3) experiences as gauged by specific outcome measures were comparable. McCarthy and colleagues[108] reviewed the care of 260,000 Medicare patients in the same two populations. Her team concluded that Medicare beneficiaries enrolled in managed care had consistently higher rates of hospice use and significantly longer hospice stays than those enrolled in fee-for-service systems. Although these differences may reflect patient preferences, there is the possibility that some managed care plans are more successful at facilitating and encouraging hospice use for patients dying with cancer.

Nurses must be vigilant in ensuring access to care for patient who are poor, socially disadvantaged, or marginalized by race, ethnicity, language, or geography. The future of quality health care is uncertain, and nurses are ethically obligated to speak for those who cannot or do not speak for themselves.

The Role of the Nurse in a Bioethical Community

The struggles that surround the level and intensity of treatment are not the only ethical conflicts that emerge in the practice of palliative care. Choices about confidentiality, consent, research dilemmas, and family authority create a series of moral crossroads for the nursing staff. When faced with a conflict of deeply held moral values, the nurse must first consider her or his own role in the clinical setting. Then a thoughtful conversation must begin within the "community" that includes the patient, the family (if the patient so desires), and the entire interdisciplinary health care team. It is at this point that institutions have turned to bioethics committees for the "moral architecture" of the clinical conversation.

As an integral part of the interdisciplinary team, nurses must sit at this table to provide descriptive, specific, and personal perspectives on moral issues; advocate for the patient and family; and immerse themselves in the milieu of accountability. A substantive discussion cannot occur without the clear and courageous voice of the bedside caregiver. Nurses must consider what is at stake in the nurse–patient relationship and the obligations of the role. They must evaluate how their own acts will shape both their characters and future practice. Finally, they must be vigilant for moral breaches in care and refer patients and their circumstances to the bioethics committee if a moral conflict cannot be resolved.

The nurse who is committed to palliative care needs to become comfortable addressing the bioethics committee with his or her concerns and involving the ethicist and committee in troublesome cases. The nurse must have the courage to speak of difficult issues, involve patients and families in the discussions, and develop both the patience and the perspective necessary to genuinely hear all voices.

If there is not yet a committee at the institution (hospital, hospice, or home care agency), nurses should (1) be part of the endeavor to create a committee; (2) identify and recommend other health care providers and consumer and public members for membership; (3) advocate for training in bioethics provided by a qualified ethicist; (4) participate in the training and education; (5) assist in establishing a methodology for consistent, ongoing development and education for committee members, other health care providers, and the institution's lay members; (6) assist in formulating policies regarding treatment issues (e.g., consent for treatment, treatment refusal, withholding and withdrawing of care, withholding nutrition and hydration, requests for assisted death); and (7) assist in formulating policies for education, case consultation, and documentation of the committee's work.[109] Nurses can assist in teaching the health care community about ethical norms and controversies, particularly drawing attention to end-of-life dilemmas.

If conflicts emerge and the patient–family–health care provider triad cannot reach consensus, the bioethics committee first assesses the patient's medical condition and wishes regarding medical intervention. They explore who the patient was before the illness and who the patient currently is, as well as the patient's current circumstances and situation. This "photograph" of the patient allows for a discussion based on the realities of personhood as well as medical facts and allows the nurse an opportunity to provide details that might not be known by other members of the health care team. The nurse

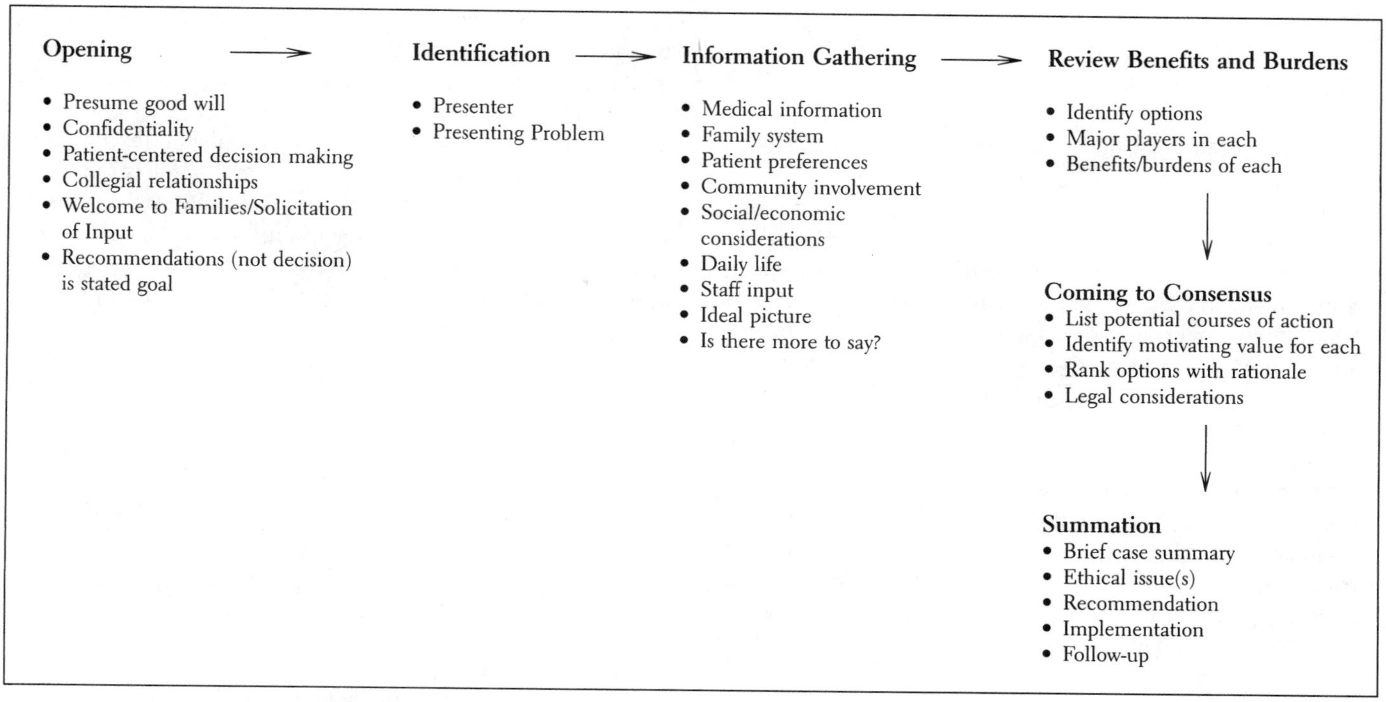

Figure 57–1. An ethics decision-making model. *Source:* Forming a Moral Community: A Resource for Healthcare Ethics Committees. Berkeley, CA: Bioethics Consultation Group, 1992.

must also consider the duties of the nursing profession, including resistance to immoral actions or rules, and assess how the decisions made affect the patient's rights and responsibilities.

Next, the consequences of possible choices are considered. Can harms and wrongs be minimized and happiness maximized? After all the information has been gathered from every possible source, the committee makes a recommendation about the dilemma (Figure 57–1).

As a contributing member of the bioethical community, the nurse will increasingly need to balance autonomy with the issue of justice in the clinical setting, and that will be a challenge. Patients who might reasonably be considered candidates for palliative care may insist on active, aggressive medical intervention. Patients enrolled in hospice programs may demand interventions that would better serve the acute care population. The clinical setting must be a place not only of healing but of fairness, a fact that nurses understand and can articulate.

Inherent Tensions in Meaning, Power, and Moral Agency

Attention to ethical and spiritual issues, as well as issues of justice, allocation, and marketplace *real politic,* shapes the framing of cultural responses to the dying process. In a world focused on productivity, illness and death are viewed as distractions and profoundly personal problems. Limits on nurses' obligations to the dying are formulated within a milieu of legal and fiscal considerations in which health care and illness are viewed as "business." As Congress debates legislation about how to adjudicate treatment constraints, small battles are being waged at the bedside of the dying every day.

As mentioned earlier, nurses find themselves all too often "in the middle" when there are conflicts between providers, patients, and families about the most appropriate kind of care that should be delivered. Inherent in these tensions are actual ethical dilemmas that nurses encounter daily—circumstances in which two competing moral appeals are in conflict. A classic example might be that of struggling to ensure informed consent when a family does not want to understand current realities and believes that information sharing will destroy the patient's hope and cause the patient to "give up" (dilemma of veracity vs. maleficence).

Moreover, individual ethical dilemmas occur when the practitioner's personal values are compromised.[23] As each individual filters circumstantial realities through her or his own "mesh" of values, conflicts arise that may be particular to that person. Clinical issues of withdrawing treatment or providing sedation to relieve intractable distress in the dying can be morally impermissible to some but morally permissible to others. These dilemmas are distinct from legal constraints, fiscal considerations, and cultural implications. Practitioners will continue to struggle as they balance the demands of professional obligation and personal meaning and wonder whether their roles as moral agents will be defended or defeated.

Considerations Regarding the Future Role of Nursing in End-of-Life Care

The responsibilities of the nurse in the future will include not only advocacy for patients but advocacy for the staff and team that support the patient. Discussion of advance directives, to be effective, needs to begin much earlier and should be a comprehensive part of the provider relationship—an admittedly difficult task in a changing health care environment. None of what any ethicist can suggest is revolutionary but rather focuses attention on oft-repeated truths. Advance conversations (not just "directives") about dying and the use of the hospice model merit particular attention.

First, in thinking about advance conversations and end-of-life planning, the professional must incorporate the constellation of friends and colleagues who support the patient. The notion that one is not alone, that one has comradeship and friendship, is embedded in advance conversations. Second, social support for this stage of life must be secured from health care systems that have the ability to provide real options for the dying patient. Nurses must speak strongly and courageously about the need for and value of palliative care to both policy makers and the public. Third, the meaning of the well self versus illness, autonomy versus limits, the importance of control versus the impotence of treatment interventions, the meaning of risk versus the potential for harm, and the place of faith need to be understood by providers before a rigorous discussion with the patient can occur. Nurses, because of their ongoing contact with patients at the end of life, are well positioned to understand the nature of these discussions and to insist on these conversational "gold standards."

The second critical issue in the future will be support for hospice and palliative care. Pioneering efforts by a multitude of practitioners and support from multiple segments of the public and private sectors are allowing robust consideration of a variety of ways to create innovations in care of the dying. The hospice and palliative care movement frames ethical reflections on the dying process. Hospice interrupts death as an unrelenting, fast-moving tragedy and slows the process with friendship, the claims of even the stranger, and a responsive community.

Hospice care resonates with the name itself—way stations for ones who wandered in war, far from family, moving into a wider and unknown world. Modernity necessitates the same passages. It will be the privilege of the nurse to hear the stories that travelers bring and to recognize the importance of each, even the abandoned, as we collectively work to expand the hospice model. Taking on the care of the dying is an extraordinary responsibility, one that calls on the development of a vision of a life of virtue, of serious personal consideration of what obligations the nurse will take on, and of a turn from the objective to the subjective. For such work, nurses will need to resist strong pressures to rescue and fix what cannot be repaired. They will need to learn to turn from the role of hero to the role of witness.

All of this will require a new sort of language, in a population that is fearful of death they find difficult to master. The speech is ordinary and very plain. It is tempting to pretend otherwise and to discuss problems not in terms of befallenness, need, and loss, but in technological detail, the mother tongue of medicine. Not only patients and families but also nurses will need to create internal communities of meaning and conversation. Such moral communities are the place for ethical reflection, conflict debate, closer examination of deep moral discord, and, finally, the development of new ethical visions that enrich the lives of all who participate in the experience.

REFERENCES

1. Solomon MZ, O'Donnell L, Jennings B, Guilfoy V, Wolf SM, Nolan K, Jacson R, Koch-Weser D, Donnelley S. Doctors near the end of life: Professional views on life-sustaining treatments. Am J Public Health 1993;83:14–27.
2. Means to a Better End: A Report on Dying In America Today. Washington, DC: Last Acts, 2002.
3. Stanley KJ. End-of-life care: Where are we headed? What do we want? Who will decide? Innovations in Breast Cancer Care 1998;4(1):3–8.
4. In re Quinlan, 70 NJ 10, 355 A2d 647, cert denied 429 US 922, 97 SCt 319, 50 Led 2d 289 (1976).
5. Cruzan v. Director of Missouri Department of Health, 109 SCt 3240 (1990).
6. Robb CS, Casebolt CJ, eds. Covenant for a New Creation: Ethics, Religion, and a New Public Policy. New York: Orbis Books, 1991.
7. Jonsen AR. The Birth of Bioethics. Oxford, England: Oxford University Press, 1988.
8. Kant I. Fundamental principles of the metaphysics of morals. In Kant's Critique of Practical Reason and Other Works on the Theory of Ethics. London: Longmans, Green, 1898.
9. Mill JS. Utilitarianism. London: Longmans, Green, 1897.
10. Jonsen AR, Toulmin SE. The Abuse of Casuistry: A History of Moral Reasoning. Berkeley: University of California Press, 1990.
11. Cassel EL. The nature of suffering and the goals of medicine. N Engl J Med 1982;306:639–645.
12. Ferrell BR. The quality of lives: 1,525 voices of cancer. Oncol Nurs Forum 1996;23:907–916.
13. Five Principles of Palliative Care. Available at: http://www.ec-online.net/Knowledge/Articles/palliative.html (accessed May 6, 2005).
14. SUPPORT Principal Investigators. A controlled trial to improve care for seriously ill hospitalized patients: The Study to Understand Prognoses and Preferences for Outcomes and Risks of Treatment. JAMA 1995;274:1591–1598.
15. Billings JA, Block S. Palliative care in undergraduate education: Status report and future directions. JAMA 1997;278:733–738.
16. Ferrell B, Virani R, Grant M. Analysis of end-of-life content in nursing textbooks. Oncol Nurs Forum 1999;26:869–876.
17. Herndon CM, Jackson K 2nd, Fike DS, Woods T. End-of-life care education in United States pharmacy schools. Am J Hospice Palliat Care 2003;20:340–344.
18. Schulman-Green D. How do physicians learn to provide palliative care? J Palliat Care 2003;19:246–252.

19. Meraviglia MG, McGuire C, Chesley DA. Nurses' need for education on cancer and end-of-life care. J Contin Educ Nurs 2003;34(3):122–127.
20. Rubenfeld GD, Curtis JR. Improving care for patients dying in the intensive care unit. Clin Chest Med 2003;24:763–773.
21. Rushton P, Eggett D, Sutherland CW. Knowledge and attitudes about cancer pain management: A comparison of oncology and non-oncology nurses. Oncol Nurs Forum 2003;30:849–855.
22. Teno JM, Welch LC, Edgman-Levitan S. Patient-focused, family-centered end-of-life medical care: Views of the guidelines and bereaved family members. J Pain Symptom Manage 2001;23: 738–751.
23. Corley MC. Nurse moral distress: A proposed theory and research agenda. Nurs Ethics 2002;9:636–650.
24. American Nursing Association. Ethics and Human Rights Position Statements: Nursing and the Patient Self Determination Acts. Available at: http://www.nursingworld.org/readroom/position/ethics/etsdet.htm (accessed February 28, 2005).
25. Matzo ML., Sherman DW, Sheehan DC, Ferrell BR, Penn B. Communication skills for end-of-life nursing care: Teaching strategies from the ELNEC curriculum. Nurs Educ Perspect 2003;24:176–183.
26. American Nurses Association. Position Statement: Pain Management and Control of Distressing Symptoms in Dying Patients. Available at: http://www.nursingworld.org/readroom/position/ethics/etpain.htm (accessed February 28, 2005).
27. Cherny N. Challenge of palliative medicine. In: Doyle D, Hanks GWC, Cherny N, Calman K, eds. Oxford Textbook of Palliative Medicine, 3rd ed. New York: Oxford University Press, 2004:7–51.
28. Brant JM. The art of palliative care: Living with hope, dying with dignity. Oncol Nurs Forum 1998;25:995–1004.
29. Schumacher KL, Koresawa S, West C, Hawkins C, Johnson C, Wais E, Dodd M, Paul SM, Tripathy D, Koo P, Miaskowski C. Putting cancer pain management regimens into practice at home. J Pain Symptom Manage 2002;23:369–382.
29a. Vacco v. Quill, 117 SCt 2293 (1997).
30. Hospice and Palliative Nurses Association. Value of the professional nurse in end-of-life care. Available at: http://www.hpna.org/position_NurseValue.asp (accessed February 28, 2005).
31. Oncology Nursing Society. Oncology Nursing Society Position on Cancer Pain Management. Available at: http://www.ons.org/publications/positions/CancerPainManagement.shtml (accessed February 28, 2005).
32. Stanley KJ. The healing power of presence: Respite from the fear of abandonment. Oncol Nurs Forum 2002;29:935–1040.
33. Stanley KJ. Family and caregiver issues. In: Gates RA, Fink RM, eds. Oncology Nursing Secrets, 2nd ed. Philadelphia: Hanley & Belfus, 2001.
34. Oncology Nursing Society. Patient's bill of rights for quality cancer care. Available at: http://www.ons.org/publications/positions/PatientsBillOfRights.shtml (accessed February 28, 2005).
35. Ersek M, Kagawa-Singer M, Barnes D, Blackhall L, Koenig BA. Multicultural considerations in the use of advance directives. Oncol Nurs Forum 1998;25:1683–1690.
36. The Patient Self Determination Act of 1990 (PSDA) (Sections 4206 and 4571 of the Omnibus Budget Reconciliation Act of 1990, PL 101–508). Effective December 1, 1991.
37. Bartling v. Superior Court, 163 CalApp3d 186, 209 Cal Rptr 220 (1984).
38. Bouvia v. Superior Court, 179 CalApp3d 1127, 225 Cal Rptr 297 (1986).
39. Wis Sup Ct Case No 89-1197 4/1/92.
40. In re Jobes, 108 NJ 394 529 A2d 434 (1987).
41. Ditto PH, Smucker WD, Danks JH, Jacobson JA, Houts RM, Fagerlin A, Coppola KM, Gready RM. Stability of adults' preferences for life-sustaining medical treatment. Health Psychol 2003;22:605–615.
42. Hickey DP. The disutility of advance directives: We know the problems, but are there solutions? J Health Law 2003;36:455–473.
43. Mitchell SL, Kiely DK, Hamel MB. Dying with advanced dementia in the nursing home. Arch Intern Med 2004;164:321–326.
44. Pekmezaris R, Breuer L, Zaballero A, Wolf-Klein G, Jadoon E, D'Olimpio JT, Guzik H, Foley CJ, Weiner J, Chan S. Predictors of site of death of end-of-life patients: The importance of specificity in advance directives. J Palliat Med 2004;7:9–17.
45. American Nurses Association. Code for Nurses with Interpretive Statements. Kansas City, MO: American Nurses Association, 1985.
46. Quill TE, Cassell CK. Nonabandonment: A central obligation for physicians. Ann Intern Med 1995;122:368–373.
47. Teno JM, Murphy D, Lynn J, Tosteson A, Desbiens N, Connors AF Jr, Hamel WB, Wu A, Phillips R, Wenger N, et al. Prognosis-based futility guidelines: Does anyone win? J Am Geriatr Soc 1994; 42:1202–1207.
48. Rubin S. When Doctors Say "No." Bloomington, IN: Indiana University Press, 1998.
49. Younger S. Futility: Saying no is not enough. J Am Geriatr Soc 1994;42:887–889.
50. Barber v. Superior Court 147 CalApp3d 1006, 195 Cal Rptr 484. (CalCt.App, 2nd Dist 1983).
51. In re Dinnerstein, 6MassAppCt 466, 380 NE2d 134 (1978).
52. American Medical Association. The Education for Physicians on End of Life Care (EPEC) Curriculum. The EPEC Project, 1999. Available at http://epec.net.
53. Quill TE, Lee BC, Nunn S. Palliative treatments of last resort: Choosing the least harmful alternative. University of Pennsylvania Center for Bioethics Assisted Suicide Consensus Panel. Arch Intern Med 2000;132:488–493.
54. American Nurses Association. Ethics and Human Rights Position Statements: Assisted Suicide. Available at: http://www.nursingworld.org/readroom/position/ethics/etsuic.htm (accessed February 28, 2005).
55. Quill TE, Lo B, Brock DW. Palliative options of last resort: A comparison of voluntarily stopping eating and drinking, terminal sedation, physician-assisted suicide, and voluntary active euthanasia. JAMA 1997;278:2099–2104.
56. Chater S, Viola R, Patterson J, Jarvis V. Sedation for intractable distress in the dying: A survey of experts. Palliat Med 1998; 12:255–269.
57. Orentlicher D. The Supreme Court and physician-assisted suicide: Rejecting assisted suicide but embracing euthanasia. N Engl J Med 1997;337:1236–1239.
58. Rosseau P. Terminal sedation in the care of dying patients. Arch Intern Med 1996;156:1785–1786.
59. Schwarz JK. Understanding and responding to patients' requests for assistance in dying. J Nurs Schol 2003;35:377–384.
60. Pellegrino ED. Compassion needs reason too. JAMA 1993; 270:874–875.
61. Bleich JD. Life as an intrinsic rather than instrumental good: The "spiritual" case against euthanasia. Issues Law Med 1993;9: 139–149.
62. Angell M. The Supreme Court and physician-assisted suicide: The ultimate right. N Engl J Med 1997;336:50–53.

63. Annas GJ. The bell tolls for a constitutional right to physician-assisted suicide. N Engl J Med 1997;327:1098–1103.
64. Brody HR. Assisted death: A compassionate response to a medical failure. N Engl J Med 1992;19:118–124.
65. Rawls J, Thomson JJ, Nozick R, Dworkin R, Scanlon TM, Nagel T. Assisted suicide: The philosopher's brief. The New York Review, March 27, 1997:41–47.
66. Weir RF. The morality of physician-assisted suicide. Law Med Health Care 1992;20:116–126.
67. Oncology Nursing Society. The Nurse's Responsibility to the Patient Requesting Assisted Suicide. Available at: http://www.ons.org/publications/positions/documents/pdfs/AssistedSuicide.pdf (accessed February 28, 2005).
68. Volker DL. Oncology nurses' experiences with requests for assisted dying from terminally ill patients with cancer. Oncol Nurs Forum 2001;28:39–49.
69. Oregon Death with Dignity Act (1997). Oregon Revised Statute 127800-127:897.
70. Meier DE, Emmons CA, Litke A, Wallenstein S, Morrison RS. Characteristics of patients requesting and receiving physician-assisted death. Arch Intern Med 2003;163:1537–1542.
71. Beck AL, Wallace JJ, Starks ME, Pearlman RA. Physician assisted suicide and euthanasia in Washington state: Patient requests and physician responses. JAMA 1996;275:819–825.
72. Cummings NB, Eggers PW. Decision to forgo ESRD treatment. In: Orcopoulos DG, Michelis MF, Mershorn S, eds. Nephrology and Urology in the Aged Patient. Boston: Klower, 1993.
73. Breitbart W, Rosenfeld BD, Passik SD. Interest in physician-assisted suicide among ambulatory HIV-infected patients. Am J Psychiatry 1996;153:238–242.
74. Chochinov HM, Wilson KG, Enns M, Mowchun N, Lander S, Levitt M, Clinch JJ. Desire for death in the terminally ill. Am J Psychiatry 1995;152:1185–1191.
75. Emanuel EJ, Fairclough DL, Daniels ER, Clarridge BR. Euthanasia and physician-assisted suicide: Attitudes and experiences among oncology patients, oncologists, and the general public. Lancet 1996;347:1805–1810.
76. Quill TE, Meler DE, Block SD, Billings JA. The debate over physician-assisted suicide: Empirical data and convergent views. Ann Intern Med 1998;128:552–558.
77. Ganzini, L, Dobscha SK, Heintz RT, Press N. Oregon physicians' perceptions of patients who request assisted suicide and their families. J Palliat Med 2003;6:381–390.
78. Drug Operations Section, Drug Enforcement Agency (2004). ARCOS 2 Quarterly Report. Report 3. Available at: http://www.deadiversion.judoj.gov/arcos/retail_drug_summary/2004/2qtr04rpt3.pdf (accessed April 1, 2005).
79. Quill TE. Death and dignity. N Engl J Med 1991;324:691–694.
80. Rollins B. Last Wish. New York: Warner Books, 1985.
81. Mak Y, Elwyn G. Use of hermeneutic research in understanding the meaning of desire for euthanasia. Palliat Med 2003;17: 395–402.
82. Coyle N, Sculco L. Expressed desire for hastened death in seven patients living with advanced cancer: A phenomenologic inquiry. Oncol Nurs Forum 2004;31:699–709.
83. Wolfe J, Fairclough DL, Clarridge BR, Emanuel EJ. Stability of attitudes regarding physician assisted suicide and euthanasia among oncology patients, physicians, and the general public. J Clin Oncol 1999;17:1274.
84. Emanuel EJ. Euthanasia and physician-assisted suicide: A review of the empirical data from the United States. Arch Intern Med 2002;162:142–152.
85. Matzo ML, Emanuel EJ. Oncology nurses' practices of assisted suicide and patient-requested euthanasia. Oncol Nurs Forum 1997;24:1725–1732.
86. Leiser RJ, Mitchell TF, Hahn JA, Abrams DI. The role of critical care nurses in euthanasia and assisted suicide. N Engl J Med 1996;335:972–973.
87. Hospice News Service. Box 31516. San Francisco, CA 94131. 1995.
88. Oregon Nurses Association. ONA provides guidelines on nurses' dilemma. 1995. Available at: http://www.oregonrn.org/associations/3019/files/AssistedSuicide.pdf (accessed April 1, 2005).
89. Hospice of Boulder County Ethics Committee. Guidelines for Caring for the Patient Who Expresses Interest in Hastening Death. Boulder, CO: Hospice of Boulder County (2825 Marine Street, Boulder, CO 80303), 1999.
90. Holden C. Caring for the patient who has a plan for hastened death. Fanfare 1998;12:5–6.1.
91. Ganzini L, Goy ER, Miller LL, Harvath TA, Jackson A, Delorit MA. Nurses' experience with hospice patients who refuse food and fluids to hasten death. N Engl J Med 2003;349:359–365.
92. Braun TC, Hagen NA, Clark T. Development of a clinical practice guideline for palliative sedation. J Palliat Med 2003;6: 425–427.
93. Sykes N, Thorns A. Sedative use in the last week of life and the implications for end-of-life decision making. Arch Intern Med 2003;163:341–344.
94. Jansen LA, Sulmasy DP. Sedation, alimentation, hydration, and equivocation: Careful conversation about care at the end of life. Ann Intern Med 2002;136:845–849.
95. Lawlor PG, Bruera ED. Delirium in patients with advanced cancer. Hematol Oncol Clin North Am 2002;16:701–714.
96. Lynch M. Palliative sedation. Clin J Oncol Nurs 2003;7:653–657.
97. Medicare Payment Advisory Commission. Improving care at the end of life. In: Report to the Congress: Selected Medicare Issues. Washington, D.C., 1999:Chapter 7.
98. Wennberg JE, Fisher ES, Stukel TA, Skinner JS, Sharp SM, Bronner KK. Use of hospitals, physician visits, and hospice care during last six months of life among cohorts loyal to highly respected hospitals in the United States. BMJ 2004;328:607–611.
99. Bird CE, Shugarman LR, Lynn J. Age and gender differences in health care utilization and spending for Medicare beneficiaries in their last years of life. J Palliat Med 2002;5:705–712.
100. Cassel J, Buchman TG, Streat S, Stewart RM. Surgeons, intensivists, and the covenant of care: Administrative models and values affecting care at the end of life-updated. Crit Care Med 2003;31:1551–1559.
101. Pekmezaris R, Breuer L, Zaballero A, Wolk-Klein G, Jadoon E, D'Olimpio JT, Guzik H, Foley CJ, Chan S. Predictors of site of death of end-of-life patients: The importance of specificity in advance directives. J Palliat Med 2004;7:9–17.
102. Selwyn PA, Forstein M. Overcoming the false dichotomy of curative vs palliative care for late-stage HIV/AIDS. JAMA 2003; 290:806–815.
103. Fried TR, Bradley EH. What matters to seriously ill older persons making end-of-life treatment decisions?: A qualitative study. J Palliat Med 2003;6:237–244.
104. Emanuel EJ, Young-Xu Y, Levinsky NG, Gazelle G, Saynina O, Ash AS. Chemotherapy use among Medicare beneficiaries at the end of life. Ann Intern Med 2003;138:639–643.
105. Hamel MB, Phillips RS, Davis RB, Teno J, Desbiens N, Lynn J, Tsevat J. Are aggressive treatment strategies less cost-effective for older patients? The case of ventilator support and aggressive care for patients with acute respiratory failure. J Am Geriatr Soc 2001;49:382–390.

106. Ahrens T, Yancey V, Kollef M. Improving family communications at the end of life: Implications for length of stay in the intensive care unit and resource use. Am J Crit Care 2003; 12:317–323.
107. Slutsman J, Emanuel LL, Fairclough D, Bottorff D, Emanuel EJ. Managing end-of-life care: Comparing the experiences of terminally ill patients in managed care and fee for service. J Am Geriatr Soc 2002;50:2077–2083.
108. McCarthy EP, Burns RB, Ngo-Metzger Q, Davis RB, Phillips RS. Hospice use among Medicare managed care and fee-for-service patients dying with cancer. JAMA 2003;289:2238–2245.
109. Fletcher J. Clinical Ethics Consultation. Frederick, MD. University Publishing Group, 1997.
110. Forming a Moral Community: A Resource for Healthcare Ethics Committees. Berkeley, CA: Bioethics Consultation Group, 1992.

58

Colleen Scanlon

Public Policy and End-of-Life Care: The Nurse's Role

The public expects nurses to be vigilant in care when they are ill and advocate on their behalf when public policy changes are necessary to promote health. As nurses we are both the professional voice and the voice of the public. We understand the public policy barriers to excellent end-of-life care as we care for others and we understand the barriers as we and our loved ones need care. Because of our unique knowledge, we have a responsibility to inform our communities and policy makers about the possibilities for excellent end-of-life care and identify the barriers to that care. United through our professional organizations we are a powerful voice. We are knowledgeable of both the science of excellent end-of-life care and of the narratives of suffering and healing. Our covenant with the public requires that we speak.—Sylvia McSkimming, PhD, RN, Executive Director, Supportive Care of Dying: A Coalition for Compassionate Care

- ***Key Points***
- *Public policy decisions have the potential to positively impact the quality and availability of palliative care services.*
- *End-of-life care issues have moved to a prominent place on national and state policy agendas.*
- *Public policy initiatives create a unique opportunity for nurses to influence present and future directions in palliative care.*

The convergence of significant trends in clinical, research, social, legal, professional, economic, and political realities has dramatically influenced the evolution of palliative care within the last several decades.[1] It has become clear that end-of-life care is not just the concern of health care professionals, patients, and families. It is also a concern for the public at large and for governmental entities. There has been increasing interest and activity within the public policy arena at the state and federal levels of government that can create needed improvements in end-of-life care.[2] Institutions and individuals also have a responsibility to inform and influence pertinent public policy initiatives. Nurses, as the largest group of health professionals and with a rich history of concern and care for others, have a vital role in advocating for quality of life, particularly at life's end.[3]

The Evolution of Palliative Care

The enormous strides in research, prevention, detection, and treatment of disease have been incredibly promising. Scientific and medical progress has created significant options and desired choices for those facing life-threatening illness, yet these possibilities have also created poignant questions and dilemmas for those at life's end, their families, and health care providers. This reality has drawn the attention and activism of health care professionals, the public, and policy makers.

Although significant changes in health care, including end-of-life care, have occurred, and although these have been mostly positive, it is recognized that there is still a dramatic need for additional improvements. Intersecting trends have propelled palliative care to the forefront of American culture.

Changing Nature of Death and Dying

Significant scientific and technological advances have created the possibility of extending life and delaying death. At times, the desire to preserve life has overshadowed the obligation to provide appropriate, compassionate, and dignified care.[1] With the expansion of technology, there has been growing attention to the acceptability of limiting treatment interventions and focusing on the comprehensive, holistic needs of the person with life-threatening illness. Recent decades have witnessed the affirmation of the decisional authority of the individual, the dominance of self-determination, the acceptability of do-not-resuscitate (DNR) decisions, the use of advance directives, and the acceptance of withdrawal of life-sustaining therapies.

Judicial Decisions

End-of-life care has also been on the nation's judicial agendas. Judicial history is filled with cases, court decisions, and opinions that have influenced directly and indirectly the course of end-of-life care. From the middle of the 1970s, starting with the Karen Ann Quinlan[4] case, through the 1997 United States Supreme Court decision,[5] the judicial system has dealt with complex issues in end-of-life care, including decisional authority, refusal of therapy, and physician-assisted suicide (PAS). Although each of these decisions dealt with discrete legal questions, these and other judicial cases drew notable attention to the broader questions and concerns in end-of-life care.

Research Data

The acquisition of quantitative and qualitative research data has influenced care at life's end and has the potential to shape public policy. Multiple clinical, attitudinal, experiential, and health professional studies have been generated in the last several decades. In addition, public opinion polls and surveys have drawn attention to the challenges in providing quality end-of-life care. Although these projects may generate important information, the ongoing challenge is to ensure that relevant data and knowledge garnered from research is integrated into care improvements that benefit individuals and communities. Research data on quality, cost, access, and utilization are necessary for public policy debate and action on needed reforms in end-of-life care.[6]

The Study to Understand Prognoses and Preferences for Outcomes and Risks of Treatment (SUPPORT) was the largest research project to examine end-of-life care and identify its inherent challenges and deficiencies.[7] SUPPORT was a 10-year project divided into two phases: the first phase focused on assessment of the experience of patients at the end of life, including decision-making and clinical outcomes, and the second phase involved testing of an intervention designed to improve communication and decision-making among patients, families, and physicians. Despite attempts to positively affect clinical outcomes, the conclusions of the study found the interventions to be ineffective in (1) ensuring that patient preferences were known and honored; (2) affecting the incidence and timing of DNR orders; (3) decreasing days in the intensive care unit or on a ventilator before death; (4) improving pain management; and (5) controlling the utilization of hospital resources.[4]

Since the SUPPORT study, numerous other investigational efforts have been initiated. A 2-year comprehensive study conducted by the Institute of Medicine (IOM) concluded that there were serious problems in end-of-life care and delineated steps to address this reality and improve care.[8] One of the committee's tasks was to propose steps that state and federal policy makers and others could take to improve the organization, delivery, financing, and quality of care for persons with terminal illness. An outcome of the study was seven recommendations that could lead to significant improvements and provide a framework for public policy options (Table 58–1).

Also in the late 1990s, the Robert Wood Johnson Foundation, through the Last Acts project, promulgated a set of guiding principles, the "Precepts of Palliative Care," in an effort to explicate the nonnegotiables of palliative care for the professional community and the public.[9] The precepts have been endorsed by numerous national and local organizations and disseminated widely to the public. One precept states that "palliative care relies on the formulation of responsible policies and regulation by institutions and by state and federal governments."[9] The precepts also provide a starting point for needed reform in end-of-life care (Table 58–2).

Table 58–1
Institute of Medicine Recommendations for Improving End-of-Life Care

- Create and facilitate patient and family expectations for reliable, skillful, and supportive care.
- Ask health care professionals to commit themselves to improving care for dying patients and to using existing knowledge effectively to prevent and relieve pain and other symptoms.
- Address deficiencies in the health care system through improved methods for measuring quality, tools for accountability by providers, revised financing systems to encourage better coordination of care, and reformed drug-prescribing laws.
- Develop medical education to ensure that practitioners have the relevant attitudes, knowledge, and skills to provide excellent care for dying patients.
- Make palliative care a defined area of expertise, education, and research.
- Pursue public discussion about the modern experience of dying patients and families and community obligations to those nearing death.

Source: Field and Cassel (1997), reference 8.

Table 58–2
Precepts of Palliative Care

Respecting Patient Goals, Preferences, and Choices

Palliative care . . .

- Is an approach to care that is foremost patient-centered and addresses patient needs within the context of family and community.
- Recognizes that the family constellation is defined by the patient and encourages family involvement in planning and providing care to the extent the patient desires.
- Identifies and honors the preferences of the patient and family through careful attention to their values, goals, and priorities, as well as to their cultural and spiritual perspectives.
- Assists patients in establishing goals of care by facilitating their understanding of their diagnosis and prognosis, clarifying priorities, promoting informed choices, and providing an opportunity for negotiating a care plan with providers.
- Strives to meet patients' preferences about care settings, living situations, and services, recognizing the uniqueness of these preferences and the barriers to accomplishing them.
- Encourages advance care planning, including advance directives, through ongoing dialogue among providers, patient, and family.
- Recognizes the potential for conflicts among patient, family, providers, and payors, and develops processes to work toward resolution.

Comprehensive Caring

Palliative care . . .

- Appreciates that dying, although a normal process, is a critical period in the life of the patient and family, and responds aggressively to the associated human suffering while acknowledging the potential for personal growth.
- Places a high priority on physical comfort and functional capacity, including, but not limited to, expert management of pain and other symptoms, diagnosis and treatment of psychological distress, and assistance in remaining as independent as possible or desired.
- Provides physical, psychological, social, and spiritual support to help the patient and family adapt to the anticipated decline associated with advanced, progressive, incurable disease.
- Alleviates isolation through a commitment to nonabandonment, ongoing communication, and sustaining relationships.
- Assists with issues of life review, life completion, and life closure.
- Extends support beyond the life span of the patient to assist the family in their development.

Utilizing the Strengths of Interdisciplinary Resources

Palliative care . . .

- Requires an interdisciplinary approach drawing on the expertise of, among others, physicians, nurses, psychologists, pharmacists, pastoral caregivers, social workers, ancillary staff, volunteers, and family members to address the multidimensional aspects of care.
- Includes a clearly identified, accessible, and accountable individual or team responsible for coordinating care to ensure that changing needs and goals are met and to facilitate communication and continuity of care.
- Incorporates the full array of interinstitutional and community resources (hospitals, home care, hospice, long-term care, adult day services) and promotes a seamless transition between institutions/settings and services.
- Requires knowledgeable, skilled, and experienced clinicians who are provided the opportunity for ongoing education, professional support, and development.

Acknowledging and Addressing Caregiver Concerns

Palliative care . . .

- Appreciates the substantial physical, emotional, and economic demands placed on families caring for someone at home as they attempt to fulfill caregiving responsibilities and meet their own personal needs.

(continued)

Table 58–2
Precepts of Palliative Care *(continued)*

- Provides concrete supportive services to caregivers, such as respite, around-the-clock availability of expert advice and support by telephone, grief counseling, personal care assistance, and referral to community resources.
- Anticipates that some family caregivers may be at high risk for fatigue, physical illness, and emotional distress, and considers the special needs of these caregivers in planning and delivering services.
- Recognizes and addresses the economic costs of caregiving, including loss of income and nonreimbursable expenses.

Building Systems and Mechanisms of Support

Palliative care . . .

- Requires an environment that supports innovation, research, education, and dissemination of best practices and models of care.
- Needs an infrastructure that promotes the philosophy and practice of palliative care.
- Relies on the formulation of responsible policies and regulations by institutions and by state and federal governments.
- Promotes equitable and timely access to the full array of interdisciplinary services necessary to meet the multidimensional needs of patients and caregivers.
- Demands ongoing evaluation, including the development of research-based standards, guidelines, and outcome measures.
- Ensures that mechanisms are in place at all levels (e.g., systems, direct care services) to guarantee accountability in provision of care.
- Requires appropriate financing, including the development of new methods of reimbursement within the context of a changing health care financing system.

Source: Precepts of Palliative Care (1998), reference 9.

Several years later, Last Acts issued a report, *Transforming Death in America: A State of the Nation Report,* which outlined the current reality of dying in this country, the challenges, and the needed changes.[10] Last Acts' most recent study rated each of the 50 states and the District of Columbia on eight evaluative criteria on end-of-life care and was the first comprehensive measurement "report card"—a catalyst for dialogue and action.[11] Education of policy makers and regulators by individuals and communities is crucial to lay out a roadmap for improvement and action in various areas, including the enactment of needed legislation[10,12] (Table 58–3).

Legislation

Legislative initiatives have significantly influenced end-of-life care. From an historical perspective, one of the most significant pieces of legislation is the Patient Self-Determination Act (PSDA), which provides protection for the decisional authority of individuals.[13] The PSDA was the first federal act to require that all Medicare and Medicaid provider organizations recognize the legal rights of the recipients of care to make decisions about their health care. This monumental legislation provided the impetus for legislative activity at the state level and the widespread acceptance of advance directives.

Simultaneous with legislative proposals related to protecting decision-making authority has been the initiation of legislation regarding DNR orders, financing mechanisms, pain management, surrogate decision-making, and PAS. These are explored further in later sections.

Regulation

Once the legislative process is completed with the passage of a law, there is still the need to provide specificity through regulations and rules. Federal and state administrative agencies (e.g., Health and Human Services, Justice) assume responsibility for adding the needed details of the law so that it can be understood and implemented.[14] Public policy advocacy needs to include knowledge of relevant governmental agencies and access to them.

Generally, agencies release proposed regulations for public comment before the issuance of the final rule. The rule-making process is a critical point of influence in the entire legislative process. Ensuring that regulations include relevant definitions, authority, eligibility, benefits, standards, and quality measures is essential to the delivery and financing of sustainable, efficient, and improved end-of-life care.[15,16] The significance of regulatory bodies and regulations should not be overlooked.

Regulatory influence extends beyond codified regulations and rules to other guidance. The Drug Enforcement Agency (DEA) joined with 21 health care organizations to endorse a statement supporting the medical use of opioids.[17] Although

Table 58–3
Approaching Just Access: Recommendations

1. Health care leaders, policymakers, and key stakeholder groups must come to consensus on the definition of palliative care and develop a framework for greater accountability in palliative care delivery in concert with financing mechanisms.
2. Public policy should expand the scope of hospice services.
3. Policymakers should act immediately to bring about policy reform of the absolute application of an individual's prognosis as a primary criterion for reimbursement of services.
4. Access and delivery of hospice care should be expanded to dying persons residing in long-term care facilities.
5. Leaders in the hospice community and in mainstream medicine must promote hospice–hospital partnerships to meet current and projected needs of the rapidly expanding volume of chronically and terminally ill patients.
6. Telemedicine should be developed to expand access to palliative care.
7. The business community should be engaged.
8. Educational programs should be developed to "reintroduce" hospice and palliative care to the public in light of their new capabilities, flexibility and accessibility.

Source: Jennings et al. (2003), reference 12.

it represented no change in DEA policy, it was an example of a partnership (between regulators and providers) that was aimed at improving end-of-life care by removing barriers to pain management. The Centers for Medicare and Medicaid Services (CMS) released a program memorandum entitled "Hospice Care Enhances Dignity and Peace as Life Nears Its End" to educate providers about the importance of hospice care and CMS' coverage of hospice for patients at the end of life.[18] The guidance was intended to increase awareness of hospice care, to clarify the benefit, and to encourage providers to recommend hospice to those they believe would benefit, without concern about CMS penalties.[18] The Health Resources and Services Administration (HRSA) released *A Clinical Guide to Supportive and Palliative Care for HIV/AIDS* to improve the overall quality of care and life for those living with HIV/AIDS.[19] Each of these documents provided further clarification and guidance for various constituencies.

Framework for the Development of Public Policy

An initial step in the process of developing relevant public policy proposals is to determine and clarify the particular issue or problem that needs to be addressed and to ascertain the perspectives of various stakeholders on the issue. Patients, providers, payers, and governmental entities may have very different goals and ends that they are seeking. The agendas and concerns of the multiple interested parties need to be considered, negotiated, and balanced. Ultimately, a priority issue focus needs to be crafted, messaged, and delivered to any and all audiences with the ability to advance the desired agenda.

Spectrum of Issues Addressed in Palliative Care Public Policy Proposals at the State Level

In almost every state, public interest in improving end-of-life care and the momentum for legislative initiatives at the state level have been growing.[20,21] There are town meetings, state commissions, community projects, grant allocations, seminars, active coalitions, and proposed legislation. Over recent years, statewide coalitions have had a significant role in end-of-life care policy reforms.[2,22] State governors, attorneys general, and the medical community have all begun to initiate activities related to end-of-life care. Recently, the National Association of Attorneys General (NAAG) released a report on the role of attorneys general in improving end-of-life care.[23] The report identified specific areas on which attorneys general can focus, including pain management, advance care planning, education, and leading practices across the country.[23] Although all of these interested parties may share a common goal, the focus can significantly vary from research, public dialogue, and grant projects to legislation.

Some of the impetus for public and professional interest in state policy initiatives may be the presence of controversial issues such as PAS or just a growing awareness of the present deficiencies in end-of-life care. Many, if not most, Americans have directly experienced or heard of the plight of someone facing death.

The overwhelming majority of states have some legislative initiatives proposed within the domain of palliative care. The following are examples of issues that are being addressed at the state level with specific public policy initiatives.

Advance Care Planning

Although all states have some type of advance directive legislation (e.g., living will, durable power of attorney for health care), there continues to be ongoing attention to the area of individual and surrogate decision-making through proposed acts or amendments to existing legislation.[21] Legislative proposals include simplification of form and process, combining approaches into one document, removing preconditions, alternative means of availability (e.g., motor vehicle departments), and creating new approaches such as open-ended, situation-specific response forms. In addition, separate advance directives have been developed for mental health treatment and for long-term care.

A growing trend within the states has been the establishment of some form of surrogate consent provision in legislative codes. Thirty-seven states and the District of Columbia have included some type of surrogate provision in their statutes.[21] Given the paucity of individuals who complete advance directives, this protection of appropriate decisional authority of others becomes increasingly important.[24] Although families have historically been considered the most natural decision makers and their involvement in clinical decisions is generally normative in practice, in many states it is not always legally sanctioned. States have begun to rectify the problems created by this reality with specific legislation.

Pain and Symptom Management

Statutory approaches are another avenue to address concerns about appropriate pain management, and the last decade has seen many positive developments in state pain policies.[25] A state statute can affirm justifiable and legitimate pain management practices, address appropriate disciplinary or prosecutorial actions, and provide guidance to professionals and to the courts.[26]

Several states have proposed intractable pain statutes or amendments to deal with the issue of pain management. The general goal of these state statutes and regulations is to mitigate barriers and improve pain and symptom management by creating a legal affirmation of the physician's appropriate role in prescribing controlled substances to relieve pain without the threat of legal liability.[27,28] Although the specific details of these statutes vary from state to state, they typically provide some level of protection for clinicians from disciplinary action for prescribing controlled substances for intractable pain. These statutes clearly have benefits in recognizing the legitimacy of appropriate pain management with opioids, yet there are some risks related to interpretation and application in varied situations.

States are also addressing legal, regulatory, and other policy barriers that may interfere with the effective management of pain, such as restrictive prescription monitoring laws (e.g., the requirement to use triplicate forms), dosage limitations, and patient reporting.[29] In addition, state proposals have offered resolutions dealing with medical school education, the use of palliative care experts, and medical marijuana referendums.[30,31] If state pain policies are to continue to improve pain management, they will need to remove legislative and regulatory barriers (often focused on controlling substance abuse) that interfere with appropriate clinical care and medical decision-making.[25,32]

Do-Not-Resuscitate (DNR) Orders

Periodically there are initiatives to expand and/or strengthen standard DNR laws (e.g., the definition of a terminal condition) that are used within inpatient settings, but the more significant activity concerns DNR orders in other settings, such as the home. Since the early 1990s, states have begun to address the needs of the seriously ill and dying in the community. An area of particular attention has been the appropriateness of resuscitative interventions by emergency medical service (EMS) teams in the home. Usually, EMS personnel are required to automatically institute cardiopulmonary resuscitation and other advanced lifesaving techniques in a crisis situation for the homebound. Many states have instituted nonhospital DNR orders to protect the wishes of individuals at home and to avoid interventions that are unwanted.[33]

Reimbursement

Financing and reimbursement options are also included in state legislative initiatives. These include expansion of hospice and home health benefits, changes in eligibility requirements, reimbursement rates, medication coverage, Medicaid waivers, long-term care and nursing home reform, and attention to the care of seriously ill children.[22] The different types of payment sources for palliative care services can include Medicare, Medicaid, private insurance, out-of-pocket, and charity care and can vary according to setting and geographic area, making it difficult to understand the actual financing realities.[32,34]

Physician-Assisted Suicide

There has been increasing attention to legislation on PAS. State legislative initiatives started with initial proposals in California and Washington, and those initiatives paved the way for an extensive "right-to-die" campaign.[35] The Oregon "Death with Dignity" bill, the first state legislative initiative to legalize PAS, passed in 1994 and was reaffirmed by public vote again in 1997.[36] Since the emergence of this issue at the state level, a wide spectrum of proposals and perspectives has been offered.[20,31] States have proposals to criminalize or to legalize PAS, and some have both pending simultaneously. The criminal laws of several states have been expanded to include harsher penalties, including civil actions and the revocation of medical licenses.

Although dialogue and legislative action within the states is present, Oregon remains the only state legally allowing PAS, despite ongoing challenges from the U.S. Justice Department. It may be that state legislators and the populace at large wants to continue to evaluate the experience of Oregon before following suit. Oregon's most recent report shows there has been an increase in the number of patients taking lethal medication, but that it is a relatively small number compared to total deaths in the state.[37] There is indication that the existence of legally permissible PAS has led to efforts to improve end-of-life care generally through other options.[37]

Federal Legislative Proposals

As is occurring at the state level, the federal government has been directing attention to issues of end-of-life care. Often, the attention occurs through the budgeting process when funds are allocated for Medicare and Medicaid services (e.g., hospice benefit) and through appropriations for health agencies (e.g., National Institutes of Health). Additionally, governmental entities have begun to address concerns about pain control, advance care planning, and PAS. Through the 1990s and into the early 2000s, many federal legislative proposals were introduced; some had success in one or both congressional bodies (U.S. Senate and House of Representatives), but all ultimately failed to become law.[20] Examples of current federal legislative proposals follow.

Conquering Pain Act of 2003

This legislation was re-introduced with modifications in the House and Senate after receiving very little attention as the Conquering Pain Act of 1999 and 2001. The current bill is intended to establish Family Networks for Pain Management to improve access to and quality of end-of-life care and serve as national models for replication.[38]

National Pain Care Policy Act of 2003

This legislation amends the Public Health Services Act to establish a National Center for Pain and Palliative Care Research within the National Institutes of Health.[39] It is intended to increase awareness, improve, and advance the quality, appropriateness, and effectiveness of pain management and palliative care through research, grants, public campaigns, and education. In addition, the bill includes provisions to improve access to care in federally financed institutions and health plans.

Children's Compassionate Care Act of 2003—Pediatric Palliative Care Act of 2003

This legislation to improve palliative care for children was introduced in both the House of Representatives and the Senate. The content of the two bills is virtually the same, and the aim is to create pediatric palliative care demonstration projects and provide grants to expand services, training, and research.[40,41]

Living Well with Fatal Chronic Illness Act of 2003

This legislation addresses the issues surrounding fatal chronic illnesses by requiring federal agencies to expand and improve research, demonstration projects, education, clinical treatment, and care services.[42] Further, the bill relates to respite services for caregivers, long-term care financing, and home health care.

Life Span Respite Care Act of 2003

This Senate-passed legislation authorizes millions of dollars in competitive grants to states and other qualifying entities to make respite care available to family caregivers.[43] Although the House of Representatives has a companion bill, most efforts are focused on having the Senate bill considered and passed in the House, which could expedite enactment.

Medicare Prescription Drug Improvement and Modernization Act of 2003

After many years of consideration, the "Medicare Prescription Drug Improvement and Modernization Act of 2003" (the "Act") was signed into law (P.L. 108–173) on December 8, 2003.[44] The legislation has drawn attention primarily because of the new Medicare drug benefit, but there are many other significant provisions contained in the Act, including those that benefit the chronically ill and dying. Although many of the accompanying regulations to the legislation have yet to be developed and disseminated, such improvements are lauded among end-of-life advocates. There are several provisions to improve access to hospice care and to make services more available to patients and families earlier in their illnesses. The Act addresses hospice payments for beneficiaries and consultative education, expanded contracting opportunities, and rural hospice care.

The Act also recognizes nurse practitioners in the role of attending physicians to care for hospice patients. Under existing law, only an attending physician, medical director, or other physician at the hospice can certify a patient as terminally ill and determine the medical care to be delivered. The Act now expands the definition of attending physician in hospice to include nurse practitioners, although they are still not permitted to certify a patient as terminally ill for the purposes of receiving the hospice benefit.

Public Policy and Physician-Assisted Suicide

At both the federal and state level, attention to the legalization of PAS has escalated throughout the last decade. Since the early 1990s, the majority of states in this country have grappled with this issue. The highest court, the Supreme Court of the United States, addressed the issue of an individual's right to PAS. The fact that this issue found its way to the nation's highest court is symbolic of the growing acceptability of PAS as a tenable choice.

The Supreme Court reversed the holdings of two lower courts[45,46] and found that there is no constitutionally protected right to PAS on behalf of terminally ill patients.[5] The ruling of the Supreme Court does not prohibit individual states from legalizing such practices in the future. Probably one of the most significant aspects of the Court's decision was the attention directed at the urgent need to improve the quality of end-of-life care.[47] The Court demonstrated enormous sensitivity to the plight of the dying in the present health care system and emphasized the importance of effective pain relief for the dying.[47]

The nursing community became actively engaged in the debate and activities surrounding the PAS issue. Major professional and specialty nursing organizations struggled with the associated complex moral and professional issues. Nurses have invaluable experience and insight into care at the end of life, which informs the assisted suicide debate and guides the profession's response. The development of position statements[48] (Table 58–4) and educational resources, involvement in professional

Table 58–4
Position Statements on the Nurse's Role in End-of-Life Decisions

Active Euthanasia

Summary: The American Nurses Association (ANA) believes that the nurse should not participate in active euthanasia because such an act is in direct violation of the Code for Nurses with Interpretive Statements (Code for Nurses), the ethical traditions and goals of the profession, and its covenant with society. Nurses have an obligation to provide timely, humane, comprehensive, and compassionate end-of-life care.

Assisted Suicide

Summary: The ANA believes that the nurse should not participate in assisted suicide. Such an act is in violation of the Code for Nurses and the ethical traditions of the profession. Nurses, individually and collectively, have an obligation to provide comprehensive and compassionate end-of-life care, which includes the promotion of comfort and the relief of pain, and at times forgoing life-sustaining treatments.

Nursing Care and Do-Not-Resuscitate (DNR) Decisions (Revised 2003)

Summary: Nurses face ethical dilemmas concerning confusing or conflicting DNR orders, and this statement includes specific recommendations for the resolution of some of these dilemmas. Although cardiopulmonary resuscitation has been used effectively since the 1960s,[*] the widespread use and possible overuse of this technique and the presumption that it should be used on all patients has been the subject of ongoing debate.[†,‡] The DNR decision should be directed by what the informed patient wants or would have wanted. This demands that communication about end-of-life wishes occur between all involved parties (patient, health care providers, and family as defined by the patient) and that appropriate DNR orders be written before a life-threatening crisis occurs.

Forgoing Medically Provided Nutrition and Hydration

Summary: The ANA believes that the decision to withhold medically provided nutrition and hydration should be made by the patient or surrogate with the health care team. The nurse continues to provide expert and compassionate care to patients who are no longer receiving medically provided nutrition and hydration.

Nursing and the Patient Self-Determination Act

Summary: The ANA believes that nurses should play a primary role in implementation of the Patient Self-Determination Act, passed as part of the Omnibus Budget Reconciliation Act of 1990. It is the responsibility of nurses to facilitate informed decision-making for patients making choices, particularly at the end of life. The nurse's role in education, research, patient care, and advocacy is critical to the ongoing implementation of the Patient Self-Determination Act within all health care settings.

Pain Management and Control of Distressing Symptoms in Dying Patients

Summary: In the context of the caring relationship[§] nurses perform a primary role in the assessment and management of pain and other distressing symptoms in dying patients. Therefore, nurses must use effective doses of medications prescribed for symptom control, and nurses have a moral obligation to advocate on behalf of the patient if prescribed medication is insufficiently managing pain and other distressing symptoms. The increasing titration of medication to achieve adequate symptom control is ethically justified.

*Kouwenhoven WB, Jude JR, Knickerbocker GG. Closed-chest cardiac massage. AMA 1960;178:84–97.
†Hayward M. Cardiopulmonary resuscitation: are practitioners being realistic? Arch Intern Med 1996;156(7):793, 797.
‡Lederberg MS. Doctors in limbo: the United States DNR debate. Psychooncol 1997;6(4):321–328.
§American Nurses Association Nursing's Social Policy Statement. Washington, DC: Author, 2003.
Source: American Nurses Association (1996), reference 48.

collaborations and end-of-life coalitions, provision of testimony to congressional leadership, and submission of an amicus curiae brief with other health-professional organizations to the Supreme Court of the United States were some of the important activities supported by and engaged in by the nursing profession.[49,50] For more information on PAS, the reader is referred to Chapter 59.

The Role of Nurses in Palliative Care Public Policy

Advocacy is generally considered a prominent component of professional nursing practice. Advocacy is most frequently understood by nurses in their clinical, patient-centered experiences; however, a broader perspective of advocacy is called for. Professional commitment must also express concern for the wider community, for society, and particularly for those who are most vulnerable. The skills that nurses use in their clinical, research, educational, and administrative roles can be extremely valuable and transferable into legislative and political arenas.[51]

Undoubtedly, public policy initiatives will continue to emerge at the state and federal levels, and nurses can assume an important role. Nurses need to remain in the forefront as advocates for improved end-of-life care, and they need to see public policy advocacy as yet another growing opportunity to demonstrate this commitment.

Nurses have most frequently been the professionals who have attempted to provide appropriate, competent, and compassionate care to individuals and families who confront the brevity of life. As the largest group of health professionals and those most connected to the comprehensive needs of the terminally ill and their families, nurses are obligated to provide leadership that advances improvements in end-of-life care.

Nurses, individually and collectively, must be interested in and become involved in the assessment of proposed end-of-life legislation and regulation. A proactive, responsible stance on the part of nurses can influence the creation and evaluation of needed end-of-life initiatives. Nurses bring an understanding of the present state of end-of-life care that helps in the analysis of appropriate public policy options and can craft future initiatives.

The Code for Nurses with Interpretive Statements (Code for Nurses), the profession's code of ethics, directs nurses "to engage in political action to bring about social change."[52] The Code for Nurses affirms the role of professional associations in acting on behalf of nurses to shape health care policy. Ethical values that undergird professional responsibilities, such as respect for autonomy, justice, professional integrity, beneficence, and advocacy, interface with the goals of improving end-of-life care and provide a context for assessment of policy proposals.

Although nurses may individually engage in public policy initiatives, it is most often through their involvement in entities such as professional associations or coalitions that advocacy efforts are effectively advanced. These entities can catalyze and promote concerted action on priority issues.[53] For example, the Hospice and Palliative Nurses Association formed a partnership with other organizations (American Academy of Hospice and Palliative Medicine and National Hospice and Palliative Care Organization) to form the Hospice and Palliative Care Coalition (HPCC) to advocate for improved end-of-life care in this country[54,55] (Table 58–5). Unifying the voices of interested and invested constituencies can have a powerful impact on legislators and regulators. Depending on the importance of a particular issue, the nursing community may assume different roles and levels of activism. At times, the nursing community may act as the leader, advancing a particular public policy concern; at other times, it may choose to provide endorsement or support of an issue.

Nurses can and should become actively involved in the legislative and regulatory processes by gathering necessary information, providing the perspectives of not only professionals but also the recipients of care, evaluating policy proposals, communicating with policy leaders, and lobbying on specific bills.[56–58] The more knowledgeable individuals are about the legislative process, the more effectively they can participate and influence outcomes. Health care policy that is developed without the input of nurses lacks an important influence because of the unique and essential role that nurses have in the care of patients, families, and communities.[59] Involvement by nurses in public policy and political advocacy through various activities is yet another way to demonstrate professionalism and promote improvements in end-of-life care[60] (Table 58–6). Nurses

Table 58–5
National Hospice and Palliative Care Organization Public Policy Agenda

1. Increase access to hospice under Medicare by reducing barriers caused by eligibility criteria and an overly aggressive regulatory environment.
2. Increase resources at the bedside by reducing regulatory burdens.
3. Increase access and the ability of hospices to incorporate current pain and symptom management interventions by updating reimbursement rates originally based in 1983.
4. Make changes to the Medicare Hospice Benefit to assure more comprehensive end-of-life care.
5. Fund research to improve end-of-life care and access to hospice.
6. Educate Americans about hospice and the Medicare Hospice Benefit.
7. Promote end-of-life and hospice education among health professionals.
8. Promote caregiving.
9. Empower Americans with end-of-life care.

Source: National Hospice and Palliative Care Organization Public Policy Agenda (2002), reference 55.

Table 58–6
Dimensions of Advocacy Activities for Nurses

Agenda Setting

- Identify palliative care issues/legislation of greatest importance to the profession and the public (often these are not evident to policy makers).
- Define and prioritize those issues and decide where time and resources will be concentrated.
- Collect relevant data/information to validate the importance of particular health policy issues to the public, health care providers, and legislative leaders.
- Evaluate policy proposals in light of professional goals and values.
- Develop consensus positions and form recommendations on issues of highest priority.
- Formulate new public policy proposals when needed.

Coalition Building

- Identify other groups (e.g., health professionals, special-interest groups, consumers) with similar agendas with whom collaborative and coordinated efforts can be initiated.
- Seek opportunities for combining, allocating, and sharing advocacy work.
- Build grassroots networks within the profession through associations and coalitions such as the American Nurses Association, the Hospice and Palliative Nurses Association, and the Oncology Nursing Society.
- Recognize that, in coalition building, broad policy positions are more successful and compromise may be necessary to advance a proposal.
- Consider involving stakeholders who may not be typical partners in advocacy efforts, such as community members and employees.
- Educate others to the importance of particular palliative care policy proposals.

Political Activism

- Become involved with associations and groups that influence palliative care policy.
- Develop strategic plans for advancing particular policy initiatives.
- Establish and maintain reliable relationships with key legislators and regulatory leaders.
- Mobilize and involve interested individuals in advocacy campaigns, including communicating (via letters, faxes, e-mails, phone calls) and visiting with key contacts.
- Invite policy makers and community leaders to environments where they can learn more about the experience of patients and families receiving palliative care services and the needs of providers.
- Engage the media in efforts through editorials, articles, and press conferences.
- Testify before public policy makers to put a human face on the issue.
- Monitor results of proposed public policy initiatives and communicate them to involved stakeholders.
- Follow up with policy makers, expressing either satisfaction and gratitude or disappointment with public policy outcomes.

Source: Scanlon (2001), reference 60.

can provide a critical and valuable voice in professional, public, and governmental discourse about end-of-life care.

Conclusions

Public policy initiatives at state and federal levels of government can provide another avenue to advance improvements in end-of-life care. Nurses can inform and influence the process of developing, evaluating, and enacting palliative care public policy that benefits individual, family, and community end-of-life care. Involvement in public policy advocacy provides nurses an opportunity to assume their professional citizenship responsibilities and to positively affect the quality of end-of-life care provided throughout the United States.

REFERENCES

1. Scanlon C. Unraveling ethical issues in palliative care. Semin Oncol Nurs 1998;14:137–144.
2. Schuster LJ Jr, Kabcenell A. Improving Care for the End of Life: A Source Book for Health Care Managers and Clinicians. New York: Oxford University Press, 2000.
3. Hospice and Palliative Nurses Association. Value of the Professional Nurse in End-of-Life Care. Position Statement. Pittsburgh, PA: HPNA, October 2003.

4. In re Quinlan, 70 N. J. 10, 355 A.2d 647, 1976.
5. U.S. Supreme Court. (1997, June). No. 96–110, Washington et al., Petitioners v. Glucksberg et al. and No. 95–1858, Vacco et al. v. Quill et al.
6. Kyba FC. Legal and ethical issues in end-of-life care. Crit Care Nurs Clin North Am 2002;14:141–155.
7. SUPPORT Principal Investigators. A controlled trial to improve care for seriously ill hospitalized patients. JAMA 1995;274: 1591–1598.
8. Field MJ, Cassel CK, eds. Approaching Death: Improving Care at the End of Life. Report of the Institute of Medicine Committee on Care at the End of Life. Washington, DC: National Academy Press, 1997.
9. Precepts of palliative care. Developed by the Task Force on Palliative Care, Last Acts Campaign, Robert Wood Johnson Foundation. J Palliat Care Med 1998;1(2):109–112.
10. Metzger M, Kaplan KD. Transforming Death in America: A State of the Nation Report. Washington, DC: Last Acts, June 2001.
11. Last Acts. Means to a Better End: A Report on Dying in America Today. Washington, DC: November 2002.
12. Jennings B, Ryndes T, D'Onofrio C, Ball MA. Access to Hospice Care: Expanding Boundaries, Overcoming Barriers [Summary]. Hastings Cent Rep, March-April 2003.
13. Omnibus Reconciliation Act of 1990. Publ. No. 101–508, Sect 4206, 4751.
14. Habgood CM, Welter CJ. Importance of the regulatory process and regulation. AORN J 2000;March:682–687.
15. Kapp MB. Legal anxieties and end-of-life care in nursing homes. Issues Law Med 2003;19:111–134.
16. Schuster JL, Myers D, Rogers SK, et al. Can we make the health system work? In: Morrison RS, Meier DE, Capello C, eds. Geriatric Palliative Care. New York: Oxford University Press, 2003: 345–356.
17. A Joint Statement from 21 Health Organizations and the Drug Enforcement Administration. Promoting Pain Relief and Preventing Abuse of Pain Medications: A Critical Balance Act. October 23, 2001. Available at: http://www.medsch.wisc.edu/painpolicy/dea01.htm (accessed February 28, 2005).
18. Centers for Medicare and Medicaid. Hospice Care Enhances Dignity and Peace As Life Nears Its End. March 28, 2003. Available at: http://www.cms.hhs.gov/medlearn/hosp_article.pdf (accessed March 1, 2005).
19. Health Resources and Services Administration. A Clinical Guide to Supportive and Palliative Care for HIV/AIDS. February 2003. Available at: http://hab.hrsa.gov/tools/palliative/ (accessed March 1, 2005).
20. Tanner R. Providers Issue Brief: End of Life Issues. Year End Report, 2003. Health Policy Tracking Service. Washington, DC: December 31, 2003:1–19.
21. State Health Decisions Legislative Update. American Bar Association Commission on Law and Aging 2002. Available at: http://www.abanet.org/aging/update.html.
22. State Initiatives in End-of-Life Care. Focus: Community State Partnerships. Midwest Bioethics Center. Kansas City: Issue 19, June 2003.
23. National Association of Attorneys General. Report on End-of-Life Care. July 2003. Available at: http://www.naag.org/publications/naag/end_of_life/pub-end_of_life.php (accessed March 1, 2005).
24. Nolan MT, Bruder M. Patient attitudes toward advance directives and end-of-life treatment decisions. Nurs Outlook 1997;45: 204–208.
25. University of Wisconsin Pain and Policy Studies Group. Achieving Balance in State Pain Policy: A Progress Report Card, September 2003. Available at: http://www.medsch.wisc.edu/painpolicy/2003_balance/ (accessed March 1, 2005).
26. Johnson S. Disciplinary actions and pain relief: Analysis of the pain relief act. J Law Med Ethics 1996;24:319–327.
27. Joransen DE, Gilson AM. State intractable pain policy: Current status. Am Pain Soc Bull 1997;7:7–9.
28. Ramsey G. Legal aspects of palliative care. In: Matzo ML, Sherman DW, eds. Palliative Care Nursing: Quality Care to the End of Life. New York: Springer, 2001:180–216.
29. Joransen DE, Gilson AM. Regulatory barriers to pain management. Semin Oncol Nurs 1998;14:158–163.
30. Sabatino CP. State legislatures address legal issues. Last Acts 1999;6:4.
31. Choice in Dying, Inc. Legislative update. Right-to-Die Law Digest, March 1999.
32. Dahl JL. Working with regulations to improve the standard of care in pain management: The US experience. J Pain Symptom Manage 2002;24:136–146.
33. Merritt D, Fox-Grage W, Rothouse M. State Initiatives in End-of-Life Care: Policy Guide for State Legislators. Washington, DC: National Conference of State Legislatures, 1998.
34. Stelzer L, ed. Major Health Care Policies: Fifty States Profiles, 1998. Washington, DC: Health Policy Tracking Service, 1999.
35. Hoefler J, Kamole B. Deathright: Culture, Medicine, Politics and the Right to Die. Boulder, Colo.: Westview Press, 1994.
36. Oregon Death with Dignity Act. Ballot Measure 16. General Election, November 8, 1994.
37. Oregon Department of Human Services. Sixth Annual Report on Oregon's Death with Dignity Act. Portland, OR: March 10, 2004:1–24.
38. Conquering Pain Act of 2003, 108th Congress, 1st Sess. H.R. 2507 and S. 1278.
39. National Pain Care Policy Act of 2003, 108th Congress, 1st Sess H.R. 1863.
40. Children's Compassionate Care Act of 2003. 108th Congress, 1st Sess S. 1629.
41. Pediatric Palliative Care Act of 2003. 108th Congress, 1st Sess. H.R. 3127.
42. Living Well With Fatal Chronic Illness Act of 2003, 108th Congress, 1st Sess H.R. 2883.
43. Life Span Respite Care Act of 2003, 108th Congress, 1st Sess, S. 538, H.R. 1083.
44. Medicare Prescription Drug, Improvement and Modernization Act of 2003, P.L. 108–173, December 18, 2003.
45. Quill v. Vacco, F3d, 996 US App (2d Cir), 1996.
46. Compassion in Dying v. Washington, F3d, 1996 (9th Cir), 1996.
47. Scanlon C, Rushton C. Assisted suicide: Clinical realities and ethical challenges. Am J Crit Care 1996;6:397–403.
48. American Nurses Association. Position Statements on the Nurses Role in End-of-Life Decisions. Washington, DC: American Nurses Association, 1996.
49. Scanlon C. Assisted suicide: The contemporary controversy. Nurs Trends Issues 1996;4:1–9.
50. Amicus Curiae Brief of the American Medical Association, the American Nurses Association, and the American Psychiatric Association as Amici Curiae in Support of Petitioners (1996, November). Vacco et al. v. Quill et al., United States Supreme Court, No. 95–1858.

51. deVries CM, Vanderbilt MW. The Grassroots Lobbying Handbook: Empowering Nurses through Legislative and Political Action. Washington, DC: American Nurses Association, 1992.
52. American Nurses Association. Code for Nurses with Interpretive Statements. Washington, DC: American Nurses Association, 2001.
53. Cohen N, Judd T. Ally development and coalition-building. In: Kramer T, Pederson W, eds. Winning at the Grassroots: A Comprehensive Manual for Corporations and Associations. Washington, DC: Public Affairs Council, 2000.
54. Coalition Announcement: HPNA Joins with the American Academy of Hospice and Palliative Medicine and the National Hospice and Palliative Care Organization to Launch Hospice and Palliative Care Coalition. January 2003. Available at: http://www.hpna.org/coalition_announcement.asp.
55. National Hospice and Palliative Care Organization. Public Policy Agenda. Alexandria, Va.: NHPCO, December 2002.
56. Aiken TD, Catalano JT. Legal, Ethical and Political Issues in Nursing. Philadelphia: FA Davis, 1994.
57. Davis A, Aroskar M, Liaschenko J, Drought T. Ethical Dilemmas in Nursing Practice, 4th ed. Stamford, CT: Appleton & Lange, 1997.
58. Schulmeister L. The first state-by-state report card on end-of-life care: How did your state do? Clin J Oncol Nurs 2003; 7:131–132.
59. Aroskar M, Moldow D, Good C. Nurses' voices: Policy, practice and ethics. Nurs Ethics 2004;11:266–276.
60. Scanlon C. Public policy and end-of-life care. In: Ferrell B, Coyle N, eds. Textbook of Palliative Nursing. New York: Oxford University Press, 2001:688.

59 Palliative Care and Requests for Assistance in Dying

Deborah L. Volker

I'm not afraid of dying. It's the process of dying. The pain and disorientation, struggling for breath.
—Woman with stage IV breast cancer

- ***Key Points***
- *Palliative care nurses do encounter patient and family questions, concerns, and requests for assisted dying.*
- *Withholding and withdrawing life-sustaining measures and provision of pain relief are* not *acts of assisted dying.*
- *Individuals with life-limiting disease who may consider assisted dying include those experiencing unrelieved pain, depression, hopelessness, psychological distress, spiritual distress, poor social support, poor quality of life, or a perception of being a burden on others.*
- *Nurses should respond to requests for assisted dying in a manner that reflects professional guidelines and a sense of advocacy for patient rights for quality end-of-life care.*

The concept of palliative care, as described by the World Health Organization, is in direct conflict with the idea of deliberately hastening a person's death via the practice of assisted dying (AD). Indeed, palliative care "intends neither to hasten nor postpone death."[1] Yet patients may be fearful of the extreme discomfort they anticipate, or they may simply want some certainty as to the timing or circumstances of death. Nurses who care for patients with life-limiting disease encounter patient and family questions, concerns, and requests for AD. Receiving such a request can represent a morally troubling dilemma in which there is uncertainty about how best to respond. The purpose of this chapter is to review the ethical and legal status of AD, summarize empirical findings regarding both professional and lay opinions and experiences with AD, and offer guidelines for responding to requests for AD.

What Is Assisted Dying?

The term "assisted dying" is typically used to describe an action in which an individual's death is intentionally hastened by the administration of a drug or other lethal substance. This may take the form of either assisted suicide or active euthanasia. *Assisted suicide* is defined as "making a means of suicide available to a patient (e.g., providing pills, weapon) with knowledge of the patient's intention. The patient who is physically capable of suicide subsequently acts to end his or her own life."[2] *Active euthanasia* occurs when "someone other than the patient commits an action with the intent to end the patient's life."[3] Such an action can be voluntary (e.g., requested by a competent individual) or involuntary (administered without the individual's knowledge or consent).

It is important to distinguish between the concept of AD and other actions designed to allow patients to die as comfortably as possible. Withholding and withdrawing life-sustaining measures are actions designed to not interfere with the natural trajectory of an illness. That is, life-sustaining measures such as artificial ventilation, renal dialysis, cardiopulmonary resuscitation, or artificial nutrition and hydration are withheld or stopped; the patient subsequently dies due to the effects of disease. In this instance, the intent of the action is to allow a natural death, and the cause of death is the underlying illness. In AD, the intent of the action is to hasten death, and the cause of death is the lethal drug or other means administered to end life. Intent and causation are the key concepts that differentiate the two actions. Some practitioners worry that administration of sufficient doses of pain medication and other drugs designed to relieve suffering may hasten death and therefore may constitute AD. However, this is *not* an action of AD. It does not qualify as AD because the intent is to relieve suffering, even though there may be a foreseen possibility that the medications could result in a hastened death. This is an example of the ethical principle of double effect, in which a good effect (relief of pain or other symptoms) is the goal despite the possibility of an unintended, harmful effect (a hastened death). The reader is referred to Chapters 6 and 57 for more information on the principles and ethics of proper pain management.

What Are the Ethical and Legal Issues?

The ethical issues associated with AD have been extensively described.[4–6] In essence, those who support the practice cite the patient's right to determine his or her own fate (autonomy), relieve untenable suffering, and maintain control over the end of life. Also relevant is the issue of equity, in that patients who are not dependent on life support do not have the same access to ending life as patients who can deliberately end life by discontinuing a ventilator, for example. Those who believe AD is unethical worry that the practice will erode trust in health care professionals, deny the sanctity of human life, discourage efforts to make palliative care available to all, and initiate a "slippery slope" in which vulnerable, underserved, or disenfranchised patients will feel pressured to take a quick way out with death. The health care professions' ethical codes and position statements uniformly oppose the practice of AD. Table 59–1 summarizes nursing organizations' relevant codes and statements.

Active euthanasia is illegal throughout the United States, whereas the Netherlands and Belgium have legalized both assisted suicide and active euthanasia under certain circumstances.[7] Australia briefly enacted a law that legalized both active euthanasia and assisted suicide; the statute was passed in 1996 and repealed a year later.

Worldwide, the Netherlands has had more experience with the practice of active euthanasia than any other country. Euthanasia was legally sanctioned via a series of court decisions in the Netherlands beginning in the 1970s; euthanasia and physician-assisted suicide were legalized in 2000 by the Dutch parliament.[8] Controversy exists as to whether increasing tolerance of these practices by physicians and the public has led to an increase in their use and a lesser emphasis on palliative and hospice care. Onwuteaka-Philipsen and colleagues[9] studied end-of-life decision-making practices by physicians in the Netherlands in 1990, 1995, and 2001. They concluded that the incidence of physician-assisted death had not risen since 1995. However, they did not evaluate quality of end-of-life care, nor did they obtain views of patients or family members. In an overview of the Dutch experience with euthanasia, Hendin[8] asserted that regulations limiting euthanasia to a voluntary practice are frequently violated and that patients are put to death without their consent. Indeed, he claimed that "euthanasia intended originally for the exceptional case has become an accepted way of dealing with the physical and mental distress of serious or terminal illness" (p. 223). Ongoing study of AD in the Netherlands is anticipated.

Assisted suicide was legalized in Oregon in 1997 with the passage of the Death with Dignity Act via two citizen referenda separated by 3 years. This Act allows a terminally ill person to obtain a prescription for a lethal dose of medication with the prescribing physician's understanding that the intent of the medication is to end life. Eligible patients must meet several criteria, including being at least 18 years of age, an Oregon resident, capable of making health care decisions, and diagnosed with a terminal illness that will cause death within 6 months.[10] The patient who requests a prescription must make two oral requests (separated by at least 15 days) to his or her physician and provide a written request that is signed in the presence of two witnesses. The prescribing physician and a consulting physician must confirm the diagnosis and prognosis and determine whether the patient is competent to make the decision. If either physician believes the patient's judgment is in question, the patient must be referred for a psychological examination. The prescribing physician must discuss alternatives to assisted suicide (comfort care, hospice care, and pain control) with the patient and must request (but not require) that the patient notify next-of-kin of his or her plans.[10] The Act was challenged in 2001 by the U.S. Attorney General, who asserted that physicians who prescribe lethal doses of drugs are violating federal laws regarding controlled substances. To date, the State of Oregon has prevailed in court rulings.[11]

Who Wants Access to Assisted Dying and Why?

It is not unusual for terminally ill people to desire a hastened death. People who have life-limiting diseases such as cancer, degenerative neurological disorders, acquired immunodeficiency syndrome (AIDS), or end-stage cardiovascular or renal disease have been identified as individuals who may be interested in access to AD. A variety of studies reveal characteristics of those who have expressed a desire for hastened death. Meier and coworkers[12] conducted a national survey of physicians who had received requests for assisted suicide to determine the demographic and illness characteristics of patients who had

Table 59–1
Ethical Codes and Position Statements of Nursing Organizations Relevant to Patient Requests for Assisted Dying

Organization	Document	Guidelines
American Nurses Association	*Code of Ethics for Nurses with Interpretive Statements*	"Nurses may not act with the sole intent of ending a patient's life even though such action may be motivated by compassion, respect for patient autonomy and quality of life considerations." (p. 8) Nurses are charged with alleviating suffering and providing supportive care to the dying.
American Nurses Association	*Position Statement on Active Euthanasia*	"Moral opposition to actively taking a human life prohibits the nurse from participating in active euthanasia [but] does not negate the obligation of the nurse to provide proper and ethically justified end-of-life care which includes the promotion of comfort and the alleviation of suffering, adequate pain control, and at times forgoing life-sustaining treatments" (p. 2).
American Nurses Association	*Position Statement on Assisted Suicide*	"The nurse should not participate in assisted suicide" (p. 1). Responses should include a nonjudgmental approach; a search for understanding the meaning of the request and personal discomfort with the request; provision of counsel, support, and palliative care programs to manage chronic, severe bio-psycho-social and spiritual distress; collaboration with other health care team members; and a commitment to nonabandonment.
Oncology Nursing Society	*The Nurse's Responsibility to the Patient Requesting Assisted Suicide*	"Upholding the ethical mandates of the profession while simultaneously seeking to understand the meaning of the request . . . is important" (p. 442). Responses should include "a thorough and nonjudgmental multidisciplinary assessment of the patient's unmet needs, and prompt and intensive intervention for previously unrecognized or unmet needs" (p. 442).
Oregon Nurses Association	*Position Paper on the Nurses' Role in the Death with Dignity Act*	Articulates the patient's right to self-determination and to have decisions regarding end of life be respected. Includes nurses' responsibility to share information about legal choices and right to refuse to be involved in the care of a patient who has chosen assisted suicide (p. 12).
Oregon Nurses Association	*Guidelines for RNs: Death with Dignity Act*	Responses include providing care and comfort to the patient and family throughout the dying process and maintaining confidentiality of patient choice about end-of-life decisions. Allows nurses to be present during a patient's self-administration of a lethal dose of medication. Prohibits patient abandonment by a nurse who does not morally agree with assisted suicide but allows transfer of responsibility for patient's care to another provider (p. 13).

(*continued*)

Table 59–1
Ethical Codes and Position Statements of Nursing Organizations Relevant to Patient Requests for Assisted Dying
(*continued*)

Organization	Document	Guidelines
International Council of Nurses	*The ICN Code of Ethics for Nurses*	Does not specifically address care of the dying but states that the nurse should "provide sufficient information to permit informed consent and the right to choose or refuse treatment" (p. 377).
International Council of Nurses	*Nurses' Role in Providing Care to Dying Patients and Their Families*	Emphasizes the nurse's role in providing skilled care at the end of life and the patient's right to a dignified death. Does not address assisted suicide/active euthanasia.

Source: Volker (2003), reference 33, with permission.

such requests denied or honored. Of the 1902 physicians who responded, 63% described instances of receiving requests, and 80 requests were honored. Requesting patients were seriously ill, suffered from pain and other physical discomfort, and were near death. Physicians who honored requests were more likely to do so if the patient was in severe pain or discomfort, had a life expectancy of less than 1 month, and was not considered to be depressed.

Unrelieved pain is a major risk factor for suicide among cancer patients. Numerous studies have shown that the overwhelming majority of cancer patients who have died by suicide have had poorly controlled and poorly tolerated pain.[13] The role of depression and hopelessness in requests for a hastened death also is well known. For example, in a study of 92 terminally ill cancer patients, Breitbart and colleagues[14] found that depression and hopelessness were the strongest predictors of a wish for a hastened death. Other factors associated with desire for hastened death include psychological distress, spiritual distress, poor social support, poor quality of life, and the perception of being a burden to others. Of note is a study of the will to live in cancer patients in palliative care, in which Chochinov and colleagues concluded that the will to live seems to vary over time and decreases with anxiety, depression, and shortness of breath.[15]

Ganzini and Block[16] asserted that patients with amyotrophic lateral sclerosis (ALS) are more likely than other terminally ill patients to request AD. In a Washington and Oregon study of attitudes of patients with ALS ($n=100$) and their family caregivers ($n=91$) toward assisted suicide, these researchers found that 56% of the patients would consider assisted suicide. Compared with patients who opposed assisted suicide, those who did not were more likely to be male, better educated, and less religious and to have higher levels of hopelessness and a lesser quality of life. Notably, Ganzini and Block asserted that no relationship exists between depression and hopelessness in ALS patients' desire for assisted suicide, and that hopelessness may be a better predictor of interest in AD. They postulated that hopelessness represents feelings about the future and can occur without depression per se. They also speculated that the invariable progression of the disease process, coupled with poor symptom management and substantial family caregiver burden, may contribute to requests for assisted suicide by people with ALS.[16]

Experience with legal assisted suicide in Oregon reveals another picture. During the first 5 years of the Death with Dignity Act, 129 patients took lethal medications to end their lives, whereas 42,274 other Oregonians died from the same underlying illnesses.[10] The characteristics of Oregonians who died from assisted suicide included older age (mean, 69 years), non-Hispanic White race, and college level of education. Most had a diagnosis of either cancer or ALS and were enrolled in hospice care. The most common end-of-life concerns voiced included loss of autonomy, decreased ability to participate in enjoyable activities, and loss of control over bodily functions.[10]

Despite access to legal AD, or perhaps because of it, Oregon has become a national leader in improving planning for end-of-life care. Indeed, Oregon has the lowest rate of in-hospital deaths and high rates of written advance directives and do-not-resuscitate orders.[17] An Oregon physician has speculated that the Death with Dignity Act may have resulted in prevention of some suicides by allowing patients to openly communicate their desire for death, thereby prompting caregivers to address unmet needs.[18]

Recently, Coyle and Sculco[19] conducted a phenomenological study to investigate the meaning and uses of expressed desire for hastened death in seven patients living with advanced cancer. They concluded that expression of desire for hastened death constituted a communication tool used by the patients. Analysis of patient interviews revealed that meanings and uses of expression about desire for hastened death manifested in a variety of ways. Examples included expressions as a manifestation of the will to live, that the dying process itself was so difficult that an early death was preferred, and that the immediate patient situation was unendurable and required immediate action. The investigators observed that a request for hastened death may not be a literal expression of desire for suicide and may take on many meanings and uses for patients. Nurses should listen carefully to patient requests and associated stories to better understand what the patient is asking for.

How Do Nurses Respond to Requests for Assisted Dying?

Given their pivotal role in providing palliative care, nurses often may encounter patient requests for AD. Survey studies have captured nurses' experiences with receiving requests for AD. For example, Matzo and Emanuel[20] surveyed 441 New England oncology nurses and discovered that 30% had received requests for assisted suicide, 1% had engaged in assisted suicide, and 4.5% had injected a drug to intentionally end a patient's life. In a national survey of more than 2333 nurses,[21] 23% had received patient requests for assistance with obtaining a lethal prescription, and 22% had patients who requested that they be injected with a lethal dose of medication.

Qualitative studies have also been conducted to capture nurses' experiences with AD. Volker[22] analyzed 48 anonymously submitted stories of oncology nurses' experiences. Some of the nurses' stories reflected patient's, family's, or health care provider's desires for control over an uncontrollable end-of-life experience. Many stories reflected nurses' moral conflicts over how to respond to patient or family requests for AD; covert communication among nurses, physicians, and family members regarding agreement to intentionally hasten death; and a sense that the experience of receiving such a request had an enduring influence on future practice. Schwarz[23] interviewed 10 nurses from hospice, AIDS, critical care, and spinal cord injury practice settings to discern their experiences with being asked to help someone die. The nurses spoke both of unintentionally hastening death via clinically appropriate symptom management (illustrative of the principle of double effect) and, on occasion, of knowingly intending death. Many expressed feelings of conflict, guilt, and moral distress. Notably, the context of a patient's request for AD shaped the nurses' responses; neither codes of ethics nor professional position statements were used.

The experience of Oregon nurses with hospice patients who requested assisted suicide has also been examined. Of 82 hospice nurses who reported on 82 patients who had died by assisted suicide (in accordance with the Death with Dignity Act), Ganzini and colleagues[24] ascertained that 98% had discussed the patient's request with coworkers; 77% of the requests were discussed at an interdisciplinary patient care conference. The nurses reported that the most frequent reasons patients gave for wanting assisted suicide were the desire to control the circumstances of death, readiness for death, and the desire to die at home. The least frequent reasons were lack of social support, nausea or fear of worsening nausea, and depression or other psychiatric disorder.

How Should Nurses Respond to Requests for Assisted Dying?

Of the myriad communication skills expected of nurses, responding to requests for AD can be the most difficult.[25] Regardless of his or her personal feelings about the moral acceptability of AD, the professional nurse has a responsibility to respond to a patient's request for AD in a compassionate, sensitive way. The patient advocacy role of nursing is central to that response. Table 59–1 summarized the guidelines that professional organizations offer to assist nurses in formulating responses to requests for AD. In particular, the Oncology Nursing Society[26] has emphasized that "requests for assisted suicide should prompt a frank discussion of the rationale for the request, a thorough and nonjudgmental multidisciplinary assessment of the patient's unmet needs, and prompt and intensive intervention for previously unrecognized or unmet needs" (p. 442). Table 59–2 provides guidelines for exploring a request for assisted suicide. Additionally, Scanlon[27] has identified nursing actions that include exploring the patient's treatment goals and options; assessing the patient for depression, decisional capacity (especially regarding informed consent), cognitive function, and spiritual distress; documenting the patient's request; and remaining present with the patient who chooses an assisted suicide. The Oregon Nurses Association[28] has published detailed guidelines for nurses who choose to be involved in an assisted suicide, as well as guidelines for those who choose *not* to be involved (Table 59–3). In either case, nurses may *not* inject or administer medication intended to end life; subject the patient, family, or other health care team members to judgmental comments or actions; or refuse to provide comfort and safety measures to the patient.

Are There Alternatives to Assisted Dying?

The wish for a peaceful, comfortable death is not unreasonable. Given that AD is not a viable moral or legal option for many individuals, what are the alternatives that could fulfill a desire to control the circumstances of the dying process? The obvious answer is universal access to expert palliative care. Indeed, there is strong moral consensus among health care providers that untreated suffering must never be a justification for AD. However, there are legally and ethically sanctioned options other than AD that may be palatable for some individuals. Refusal of medical treatment is a widely respected means for allowing the dying process to unfold unimpeded by treatments that will not fulfill the patient's personal goals for the end-of-life experience. Refusal may be in the form of withholding or withdrawing a life-sustaining treatment.

The individual who is not dependent on medical interventions to sustain life and wishes to control the timing of his or her death is faced with a more perplexing challenge.

Table 59–2
Approach to Exploring a Request for Physician-Assisted Suicide (PAS)

Area of exploration	Potential motivation in request for PAS	Follow-up questions
Expectations and fears	Fears of uncontrolled symptoms Expectation of lingering death Expectation of unrelieved suffering	How do you expect your own death to go? What concerns you most about dying? What are your greatest fears? What's the worst thing that could happen to you as you die? Have other people close to you died? How did their deaths go?
Options for end-of-life care	Lack of knowledge of legally available options Equating PAS and euthanasia Equating PAS and aggressive symptom control (double effect)	What do you understand about your options for end-of-life care? How specifically would you like me to assist you?
Establishing patient goals	Discerning whether PAS contemplated for future use Identifying sources of meaning for the patient	What are your goals for now or whatever time you have remaining to live? What is the most important thing for you right now? If you were to die now, what would be left undone?
Family or caregivers	Family's beliefs may not be congruent with patient's Patient concern about being a burden on family	What does your family think about this decision? How has your illness affected your family? How will your family react if you proceed with PAS?
Relief of suffering or physical symptoms	Patient's unique perspective on experience of suffering	Are you suffering right now? What is your principal source of suffering? What kind of suffering concerns you most? What is your most troublesome symptom right now?
Sense of meaning and quality of life	Understanding patient values	What is your quality of life right now? What gives your life meaning right now? How bad would your quality of life have to become for your life to have no meaning?
Ruling out depression	Presence of treatable depression Patient capacity to make informed decision	Are you depressed? What things in life still give you pleasure? Have you had a good life? Do you have any regrets?

Source: Bascom and Tolle (2002), reference 34, with permission.

Voluntary refusal of food and fluids has been identified as a possible option. Although such action requires no direct participation by the health care team, nurses can support patients who choose this option by ensuring optimal comfort measures and family support. Depending on the patient's underlying condition, death usually occurs within 1 to 3 weeks.[29] Concern has been voiced regarding discomforts that could accompany this action. To evaluate this possibility, Ganzini and associates[30] surveyed hospice nurses who had cared for terminally ill patients who deliberately hastened death by cessation of eating and drinking. Thirty-three percent of their 307 respondents reported that they had cared for such patients. The most common reasons given by patients for this choice were readiness for death, poor quality of life or fear of poor quality of life, view that continued existence was pointless, and desire to die at home. Most

Table 59–3
Oregon Nurses Association Assisted Suicide Guidelines

Nurses who choose to be involved

If, as a nurse, your own moral and ethical value system allows you to be involved in providing care to a patient who has made the choice to end his or her life, within the provisions of the Death with Dignity Act, the following guidelines will assist you.

You may:

- Provide care and comfort to the patient and family through all stages of the dying process.
- Teach the patient and family about the process of dying and what they may expect.
- Maintain patient and family confidentiality about the end-of-life decisions they are making.
- Explain the law as it currently exists.
- Discuss and explore with the patient options with regard to end-of-life decisions and provide resource information or link the patient and family to access the services or resources they are requesting.
- Explore reasons for the patient's request to end his or her life and make a determination as to whether the patient is depressed and whether the depression is influencing this decision; or whether the patient has made a rational decision based on his or her own fundamental values and beliefs.
- Be present during the patient's self-administration of the medication and during the patient's death to console and counsel the family.
- Be involved in policy development within the health care facility and/or the community.

You may not:

- Inject or administer the medication that will lead to the end of the patient's life; this is an act precluded by law.
- Breach confidentiality of patients exploring or choosing assisted suicide.
- Subject your patients or their families to unwarranted, judgmental comments or actions because of the patient's choice to explore or select the option of assisted suicide.
- Subject your peers or other health care team members to unwarranted, judgmental comments or actions because of their decision to continue to provide care to a patient who has chosen assisted suicide.
- Abandon or refuse to provide comfort and safety measures to the patient.

Nurses who choose not to be involved

If, as a nurse, your own moral and ethical value system does not allow you to be involved in providing care to a patient who has made the choice to end his or her life, within the provisions of the Death with Dignity Act, the following guidelines will assist you.

You may:

- Provide ongoing and ethically justified end-of-life care.
- Conscientiously object to being involved in delivering care. You are obliged to provide for the patient's safety, to avoid abandonment, and to withdraw only when assured that alternative sources of care are available to the patient.
- Transfer the responsibility for the patient's care to another provider.
- Maintain confidentiality of the patient, family and health care providers continuing to provide care to the patient who has chosen assisted suicide.
- Be involved in policy development within the health care setting and/or the community.

You may not:

- Breach confidentiality of patients exploring or choosing assisted suicide.
- Inject or administer the medication that will lead to the end of the patient's life; this is an act precluded by law.
- Subject your patients or their families to unwarranted, judgmental comments or actions because of the patient's choice to explore or select the option of assisted suicide.
- Subject your peers or other health care team members to unwarranted, judgmental comments or actions because of their decision to continue to provide care to a patient who has chosen assisted suicide.
- Abandon or refuse to provide comfort and safety measures to the patient.

Source: Oregon Nurses Association (1998), reference 28, with permission.

of the patients had either cancer or a neurological disease; 85% of the patients died within 15 days after ceasing intake of food and fluids. The nurses were asked to rate the quality of these patients' deaths on a scale from 0 (a very bad death) to 9 (a very good death); the median score for this sample was 8. The authors concluded that, from the perspective of the nurse participants, most of the patients died a good or peaceful death. Of note, no family or patient perspectives were obtained in this study. Future research should focus on evaluating these perspectives.

The practice of palliative sedation represents another alternative to AD. Palliative sedation refers to the use of medications to relieve refractory symptoms in the dying patient by causing unconsciousness, but not death.[31] The goal is to relieve suffering, not to cause death. A detailed discussion of this practice is provided in Chapter 24. Palliative sedation may be ethically troubling for both family and professional caregivers, because some do not differentiate between this practice and active euthanasia. Palliative care experts can provide guidance to assist patients, families, and professionals with appropriate use of sedation and to distinguish palliative sedation from hastened death. In addition, some patients may not find this choice acceptable because they view induction of unconsciousness until the time of death as undignified and as prohibiting communication with loved ones in those final days or hours.

CASE STUDY

A Request for Assisted Dying

In the following scenario, a home hospice nurse described an experience of receiving a request for a hastened death from a 25-year-old man with end-stage AIDS.[32]

"I was asked by this patient, 'Can't you do something to end this pain and suffering now? Something that will end my life?' This patient had lived with pneumonia, Kaposi tumors, constant lung infections, skin eruptions, and joint and limb pain. He had spent all his savings, sold most of his furniture, and mortgaged his house to pay for medical expenses. He had not worked for 3 months, and his partner had left him. My response was straightforward and reassuring: 'Pain control starts today, and before I leave you, you will feel less pain.' I could not give him something to end his life. My presence and work is to eliminate as much pain as possible and to keep him comfortable at home. Quick phone calls to the physician for pain relief medication and quick delivery helped. We discussed at length what was causing him to want to die at that moment. Pain was his biggest reason. He was depressed with his circumstances—no money, more than 25 pills a day (when he had never even taken an aspirin when he was healthy), no visits from his friends (even to help him get to the doctor's office), and no way to continue his job. Also, loss of sleep and poor vision were contributors. Once his pain relief was achieved, he was able to sleep. With the hospice team, a social worker, and volunteers to help with his daily needs, my weekly visits were a mixture of comforting and counseling. He asked three times over a month's time to help him 'let go' and die. Each time I tried to identify the current problem and seek some remedy. I believe that his dignity was injured and that he believed a quick death would be his escape."

This case illustrates the devastating consequences of untreated suffering that can occur at the end of life. The patient's cry for AD was the prompt for assessment and intervention to address his needs. The nurse upheld professional standards by refusing to help him end his life and immediately initiated actions to alleviate his suffering. However, her concluding observations about this situation are not unusual for nurses who encounter requests for an assisted death:

"A death of this nature is very difficult for the patient and the nurse. My inner feelings were conflicted. He was going to die; why not let him die by his choosing? My oath to administer to the sick and do no harm must be upheld. How else do we keep a measure of control on end-of-life issues? I feel I did my job correctly, but did I serve this man's needs? I do not know."

Conclusion

Although many requests for AD can be resolved by the application of expert palliative care, a small subset of individuals may seek AD despite such care. Nurses are responsible for responding to patient requests in a manner that reflects professional guidelines and a sense of advocacy for patient rights for quality end-of-life care. Regardless of personal values or discomfort with a request for AD, nurses must apply open communication techniques that allow exploration of patients' needs and fears about the final phase of life.

REFERENCES

1. Sepulveda C, Marlin A, Yoshida T, Ullrich A. Palliative care: the World Health Organization's global perspective. J Pain Symptom Manage 2002;24:91–96.
2. American Nurses Association. Position Statement on Assisted Suicide. Washington, D.C., 1994.
3. American Nurses Association. Position Statement on Active Euthanasia. Washington, D.C., 1994.
4. Ersek M. The continuing challenge of assisted death. J Hospice Palliat Nurs 2004;6:46–59.
5. Kopelman L, De Ville KA. The contemporary debate over physician-assisted suicide. In: Kopelman L, De Ville KA, eds. Physician-Assisted Suicide: What Are the Issues? Boston: Kluwer Academic Publishers, 2001:1–25.
6. Lorenz K, Lynn J. Moral and practical challenges of physician-assisted suicide. JAMA 2003;289:2282.
7. Battle J. Legal status of physician-assisted suicide. JAMA 2003; 289:2279–2281.
8. Hendin H. The Dutch experience. Issues Law Med 2002;17: 223–246.
9. Onwuteaka-Philipsen BD, van der Heide A, Koper D, Keij-Deerenberg I, Rietjens J, Rurup M, Vrakking A, Georges J, Muller M, vander Wal G, van der Maas P. Euthanasia and other end-of-life decisions in the Netherlands in 1990, 1995, and 2001. Lancet 2003;362:395–399.
10. Hedberg K, Kohn M, Hopkins D. Fifth Annual Report on Oregon's Death with Dignity Act. 2003. Available at: http:www.ohd.hr.state.or.us/chs/pas/ar-index.cfm (accessed March 1, 2005).

11. Vollmer V. Recent developments in physician-assisted suicide. March 2004. Litigation. Available at: http://www.willamette.edu/wucl/pas/2004_reports/032004.html (accessed March 1, 2005).
12. Meier DE, Emmons C, Litke A, Wallenstein S, Morrison S. Characteristics of patients requesting and receiving physician-assisted death. Arch Intern Med 2003;163:1537–1542.
13. Breitbart W, Chochinov HM, Passik S. Psychiatric symptoms in palliative medicine. In: Doyle D, Hanks G, Cherny N, Calman K, eds. Oxford Textbook of Palliative Medicine, 2nd ed. Oxford: Oxford University Press, 2003:746–771.
14. Breitbart W, Rosenfeld B, Pessin H, Kaim M, Funesti-Esch J, Galietta M, Nelson CJ, Brescia R. Depression, hopelessness, and desire for hastened death in terminally ill patients with cancer. JAMA 2000;284:2907–2911.
15. Chochinov HM, Tataryn D, Clinch JJ, Dudgeon D. Will to live in the terminally ill. Lancet 1999;354:816–819.
16. Ganzini L, Block S. Physician-assisted death: A last resort? N Engl J Med 2002;346:1663–1665.
17. Tolle SW, Tilden VP. Changing end-of-life planning: The Oregon experience. J Palliat Med 2002;5:311–317.
18. Reagan P, Hurst R, Cook L, Zylicz Z, Otlowski M, Veldink J, van den Berg L, Wokke J. Physician-assisted death: Death with dignity? Lancet Neurology 2003;2:637–643.
19. Coyle N, Sculco L. Expressed desire for hastened death in seven patients living with advanced cancer: A phenomenological inquiry. Oncology Nursing Forum. 2004;31:699–709.
20. Matzo M, Emanuel E. Oncology nurses' practices of assisted suicide and patient-requested euthanasia. Oncol Nurs Forum 1997; 24:1725–1732.
21. Ferrell B, Virani R, Grant M, Coyne P, Uman G. Beyond the Supreme Court: Nursing perspectives on end-of-life care. Oncol Nurs Forum 2000;27:445–455.
22. Volker DL. Oncology nurses' experiences with receiving requests for assisted dying from terminally ill patients with cancer. Oncol Nurs Forum 2001;28:39–49.
23. Schwarz JK. Understanding and responding to patients' requests for assistance in dying. J Nurs Schol 2003;35:377–384.
24. Ganzini L, Harvath T, Jackson A, Goy E, Miller L, Delorit M. Experiences of Oregon nurses and social workers with hospice patients who requested assistance with suicide. N Engl J Med 2002;347:582–588.
25. Sivesind D, Parker P, Cohen L, DeMoor C, Bumbaugh M, Throckmorton T, Volker D, Baile W. Communication with patients in cancer care: What areas do nurses find most challenging? J Cancer Educ 2003;16:202–209.
26. Oncology Nursing Society. The nurse's responsibility to the patient requesting assisted suicide. Oncol Nurs Forum 2001; 28:442.
27. Scanlon C. Assisted suicide: How nurses should respond. Int Nurs Rev 1998;45:152.
28. Oregon Nurses Association. Assisted suicide: ONA provides guidance on nurses' dilemma. 1998. Available at: http://www.oregonrn.org/associations/3019/files/AssistedSuicide.pdf (accessed March 1, 2005).
29. Quill T, Lee B, Nunn S. Palliative treatments of last resort: Choosing the least harmful alternative. Ann Intern Med 2000; 132:488–493.
30. Ganzini L, Goy E, Miller L, Harvath T, Jackson A, Delorit M. Nurses' experiences with hospice patients who refuse food and fluids to hasten death. N Engl J Med 2003;349:359–365.
31. Lynch M. Palliative sedation. Clin J Oncol Nurs 2003; 7:653–667.
32. Volker DL. Oncology nurses' experiences with requests for assisted dying from terminally ill cancer patients. Doctoral dissertation, The University of Texas at Austin, 1999. Dissertation Abstracts International, 61(01), 199B.
33. Volker DL. Assisted dying and end-of-life symptom management. Cancer Nurs 2003;26:392–399.
34. Bascom PB, Tolle SW. Responding to requests for physician-assisted suicide: "These are uncharted waters for both of us. . . ." JAMA 2002;288:91–98

60

Denice K. Sheehan and Betty R. Ferrell

Nursing Education

It is imperative to integrate current clinical practice expertise into education to keep pace with the progression of medical treatments and patient care.—Carol R. Matthews, MSN, CNS, BC-PCM, 1999 graduate of The Breen School of Nursing Palliative Care Masters Program

- ***Key Points***
- *There is a need for palliative care nursing education.*
- *Knowledge deficits exist among nurses regarding palliative care.*
- *Model academic programs are available for education in palliative care nursing.*

One of the earliest responsibilities of the professional nurse was care of the dying. Florence Nightingale and other nurses provided care to soldiers dying on battlefields as well as to civilians dying as a result of epidemics. A major shift in patterns of disease and treatment began in the 20th century as more effective treatment modalities became available. Today, student nurses are exposed primarily to curative-oriented care and are less likely to encounter comfort-oriented care. Although many health care providers work with people at the end of their lives, nurses spend the most time with the dying and their families. Most nurses will provide palliative care to patients and their families no matter where they practice. Therefore, education in palliative care should begin in the nursing schools and extend through clinical inservices, continuing education courses, and professional conferences.

The Need for Improved Palliative Care Nursing Education

It is imperative that nurses learn through both didactic and clinical experiences. Working with a palliative care or hospice team provides the best experience for learning about the interdisciplinary approach to patient care as the team members model excellence in care for the student. Many studies of end-of-life knowledge, attitudes, and skills of nurses provide evidence of the need to improve the education of nursing students, practicing nurses, and nursing faculty.[1–7] This chapter focuses on the role of nursing education in palliative care. An overview of the need to improve palliative care nursing education includes a brief history of nursing care of the dying, knowledge deficits, and the current focus on these deficits. Issues and challenges in palliative care education are discussed. Several models of nursing education programs are presented.

Many people, especially nurses and physicians, have been instrumental in developing a framework for care of the dying and their families. Dame Cicely Saunders is credited as the founder of the modern hospice movement. She was educated first as a nurse and later as a physician in London. Her interest in pain management led her to care of the dying. With support from the community and the national government, she founded St. Christopher's Hospice in Sydenham on the outskirts of London in 1967.[8] At about the same time, Dr. Elizabeth Kubler-Ross, a psychiatrist, began interviewing dying patients in hospitals. She found it difficult to find these patients because doctors and nurses repeatedly told her that there were no dying patients in their hospitals. She later proposed a model that described the five stages of dying.[9]

Jeanne Quint's landmark study in 1967 revealed little emphasis throughout the nursing curriculum on teaching nursing students to care for dying patients.[10] Teaching and support were particularly lacking in the clinical setting. Nursing instructors were inadequately prepared to teach or support the students in care of the dying and were not comfortable with nursing problems associated with dying patients. She recommended that faculty standardize death education curricula so that they could be offered consistently throughout schools of nursing and continuing education.

Recognizing Deficits in Pain Education in the 1980s and 1990s

Many research studies have documented the lack of knowledge about pain management among student nurses, practicing nurses, and nursing faculty.[11–13] Studies have documented serious misconceptions in the assessment and treatment of pain and knowledge deficits in basic areas such as opioid pharmacology, use of adjuvant medications, and treatment of side effects. A recent national report documented poor pain management among nursing home residents and deficits in state pain policies.[3] These studies have been instrumental in encouraging greater emphasis on pain management in nursing education programs and the significant need to provide pain education to practicing nurses.

The awareness of educational deficits in the specific area of pain education extended in the late 1990s to the broader area of end-of-life content in nursing education. Many studies have documented the inadequate preparation of nurses to care for patients and their families at the end of life.[14–20] Several research studies have described important nursing behaviors in the care of the dying.[21,22] Inadequate professional education is often cited as a major barrier to appropriate end-of-life care. In Webster's 1981 study,[22] more than 30% of the student nurses reported that they were not always told which of their patients were expected to die. Additionally, 60% were not told whether the patients knew they were dying. Care of the dying patient was not routinely incorporated into their curriculum. The type and amount of knowledge and support were dependent on the instructor. Although the students may have learned these skills by working with more experienced nurses, observations revealed that 25% of the students worked alone with the dying, and the remaining 75% had only intermittent supervision.

Rittman and colleagues[23] identified five themes that were common among expert oncology staff nurses. They included knowing the patient and the stage of the disease, preserving hope, easing the struggle, providing for privacy, and responding to the spiritual aspects of living and dying. The nurses were able to maintain a high standard of practice by incorporating these themes into their clinical practice to provide for a peaceful death for their patients. They found that nurses who were able to deal with their own mortality became more comfortable with death.

Several studies have analyzed end-of-life content in nursing textbooks.[24,25] Kirchhoff and colleagues[24] analyzed 14 critical care nursing textbooks using the American Association of Colleges of Nursing (AACN) end-of life competencies for undergraduate nursing education as their framework. Four additional end-of-life content areas were identified during the analysis. None of the textbooks contained all of the content areas. Although there was extensive information on ethical and legal issues, organ donation, and brain death in six or seven of the textbooks, the remaining textbooks contained no information on these topics. Pharmacological information was either mentioned briefly or absent. Approximately half of the textbooks had some information on patient/family communication.

Ferrell and colleagues[25] completed an analysis of nine areas of end-of-life content in nursing textbooks. Their review of 50 nursing textbooks revealed that only 2% of overall content was related to end-of-life care, and much of the information was inaccurate (Table 60–1). Deficiencies were found in all areas. Palliative care was usually discussed in terms of the hospice model of care rather than the broader concept of palliative care. There was little information on quality of life, which was surprising in view of the recent explosion of research in this area. Pain was often included in the textbooks, but usually in the context of acute rather than chronic pain. Pain management during the end of life was virtually absent. Major gaps were found in symptom assessment and management. Information about communicating with patients and families at the end of life was also lacking. There was little information about the roles and needs of family caregivers or about issues of policy, ethics, and law. A paucity of information was found about death awareness, anxiety, imminent death, and preparing families for the death. The stages and process of grief were described, but there was little information about nursing interventions or the nurse's personal grief.

Another component of this project was the collaboration with the National Council of State Boards of Nursing, Inc. (NCSBN).[26] The goal of this project was to improve end-of-life content in the national nursing licensure examination for registered nurses (NCLEX-RN). End-of-life content was increased in the NCLEX beginning with the April 2001 examination by incorporating the 15 competencies set forth by the AACN in the *Peaceful Death* document.[27] This was a significant force in increasing end-of-life content in the nursing curriculum.

Table 60–1
Analysis of End of Life (EOL) Content in Nursing Textbooks

Category of Nursing Text	No. of Texts Reviewed	% of Texts	No. of Pages	No. of EOL-Related Pages	No. of Chapters	No. of Chapters Devoted to EOL Content
AIDS/HIV	1	2	526	20	16	0
Assessment/diagnosis	3	6	1783	15.3	80	0
Communication	2	4	767	38	35	0
Community/home health	4	8	3108	21.3	116	0
Critical care	4	8	4116	80.8	181	2
Emergency	4	8	1006	14.5	69	1
Ethics/legal issues	5	10	2018	143	88	4
Fundamentals	3	6	4353	114.9	140	3
Gerontology	3	6	2515	84.8	72	2
Medical-surgical	5	10	9969	146.3	298	2
Oncology	2	4	3264	107.5	149	7
Patient education	2	4	636	8.0	26	0
Pediatrics	3	6	2599	33.5	70.0	2
Pharmacology	4	8	3476	22.0	236	0
Psychiatric	3	6	2886	35.3	127	1
Nursing review	4	8	2661	17.0	47	0
Total	**50**	**100**	**45,683**	**901.9 (2%)**	**1,750**	**24 (1.4%)**

Source: Ferrell (1999), reference 25. Reprinted with permission.

Each of these studies has consistently echoed the strong message that improved patient care is contingent on adequate preparation of nurses. The deficits cited in these studies provide direction for needed areas of education.

The Issues and Challenges in Palliative Care Education

The World Health Organization (WHO) has recognized the need for the development of national policies and programs for palliative care and has issued several recommendations regarding the education and training of health care professionals. In addition, WHO has suggested that palliative care programs be incorporated into the existing health care system.[28]

Another key document, the Institute of Medicine's 1997 report on improving end-of-life care,[4] made several recommendations specific to improving professional knowledge. Three of these related specifically to education:

> *Recommendation 2:* Physicians, nurses, social workers, and other health care professionals must commit themselves to improving care for dying patients and to using existing knowledge effectively to prevent and relieve pain and other symptoms.
>
> *Recommendation 4:* Educators and other health professionals should initiate changes in undergraduate, graduate, and continuing education to ensure that practitioners have relevant attitudes, knowledge, and skills to care well for dying patients.
>
> *Recommendation 5:* Palliative care should become, if not a medical specialty, at least a defined area of expertise, education, and research. Palliative care experts should provide expert consultation; serve as role models for colleagues and students; supply leadership for undergraduate, graduate, and continuing education; and organize and conduct research.

The Institute of Medicine report cited major deficiencies in professional education for end-of-life care. These included the relative absence of death in the curriculum, a lack of educational materials pertaining to the end stages of most diseases and neglect of palliative strategies, and the lack of clinical experiences with dying patients and those close to them. The report[3] suggested that educators could improve care by doing the following:

1. Conferring a basic level of competence in care of the dying patient for all practitioners
2. Developing an expected level of palliative and humanistic skills considerably beyond this basic level
3. Establishing a cadre of superlative professionals to develop and provide exemplary care for those approaching death, to guide others in the delivery of such care, and to generate new knowledge to improve care of the dying.[4]

A recent national report card on dying in America encouraged the development of hospice or palliative care service rotations in nursing education and requirements for continuing nursing education in end-of-life care.[3] Educational programs for nurses in palliative care vary widely throughout the world. There are established courses and programs in palliative care at universities as well as seminars, workshops, and conferences in the Americas, Australia, the United Kingdom, and elsewhere in northern Europe. In other parts of the world, education in palliative care is woven into other courses. Palliative care concepts are taught within oncology courses in Japan and Thailand. Since 1990, the Nairobi Hospice in Kenya has provided palliative care courses for health care professionals and has extended this program to nursing schools throughout Kenya. They are working to incorporate palliative care into the nursing curriculum. An increase in the availability of charitable sources has resulted in support for the development of palliative care in Russia and the Czech republic.[29]

There are many challenges in improving palliative care education. All educators struggle with how best to integrate more content into an already packed curriculum. Nurse educators have described undergraduate programs designed to incorporate end-of-life content into the curriculum through didactic and practicum courses.[30,31] Other academicians have described the process of developing interdisciplinary courses at the graduate level.[32] There also is tremendous need to increase the knowledge of faculty in palliative care so that they can lead the change in curriculum. Faculty also require current teaching guides such as audiovisual materials, case studies, and other resources to present this challenging content.

Teaching palliative care is not only a matter of didactic content. Preparing nurses to care for the terminally ill necessitates attention to the student's values, beliefs, personal experiences, and culture. It is essential that palliative care education not only incorporate knowledge and skills but also strive to identify methods to best enhance compassion, empathy, and the existential aspect or "art" of palliative nursing.[33–37]

The Nursing Profession's Response to the Need for Change

In recent years, major professional nursing organizations have recognized the importance of nursing response to the mandate for improved end-of-life care. In 1997, the International Council of Nurses mandated that nurses have a unique and primary responsibility for ensuring that individuals at the end of life experience a peaceful death.[38] In the same year, the AACN convened a roundtable of expert nurses and other health care professionals to address this topic. The report from that meeting was titled *Peaceful Death*.[27] This document outlined 15 competencies necessary for nurses to provide high-quality care to patients and families during the transition at the end of life. These competencies should be attained before graduation from undergraduate programs of nursing. The group also made recommendations concerning the curriculum content areas in which these competencies could be addressed (Table 60–2).

At about the same time, the Nurses Section of the National Hospice Organization, under the direction of Cindy Yocum Scott and Nancy English, developed the *Guidelines for Curriculum Development on End of Life and Palliative Care in Nursing Education*.[39] Separate guidelines were prepared for undergraduate and graduate nursing programs. They included the biological, psychosocial, and spiritual responses to dying. Theory, assessment, interventions, and clinical placement were addressed within this conceptual framework (Table 60–3).

Dr. Cynda Hylton Rushton, faculty of the School of Nursing of Johns Hopkins University, and colleagues at the Institute for Johns Hopkins Nursing convened a meeting of 23 nursing specialty groups in 1999 to design an agenda for the nursing profession on palliative and end-of-life care.[40] The group, the Nursing Leadership Consortium on End-of-Life Care, consisted of nursing organizations with administration, research, practice, and policy responsibilities and created a priority map for the nursing profession. The Nursing Leadership Academy for Palliative and End-of-Life Care continued the work of the Consortium.[41,42] In 2000, leaders from 22 nursing organizations met for 5 days to develop action plans to address key issues in end-of-life care in their organizations. This effort was repeated with another cohort in 2002, raising the number of participating organizations to 44. The project was funded by Project on Death in America.

In 2001, Dr. Ira Byock convened a group of palliative care advanced practice nurses (APNs) with expertise in clinical practice, education, and research to discuss the state of advanced practice nursing in palliative care in the United States and to make recommendations for the future development of this emerging nursing specialty. They recommended that nurse educators become more familiar with palliative care, develop continuing education to prepare current APNs in palliative care competencies, integrate the competencies into the education of all APNs, and develop clinical tracks for APN students who intend to specialize in palliative care. The Robert Wood Johnson Foundation funded this project through the Promoting Excellence in End-of-Life Care national program.[43,44]

Another group reviewed certification examinations administered by nursing specialty organizations to encourage end-of-life content. The quantity and quality of end-of-life content in certification examination blueprints, specialty nursing scope and standards of practice documents, and specialty nursing core

Table 60–2
Competencies Necessary for Nurses to Provide High-Quality Care to Patients and Families During the Transition at the End of Life

1. Recognize dynamic changes in population demographics, health care economics, and service delivery that necessitate improved professional preparation for end-of-life care.
2. Promote the provision of comfort care to the dying as an active, desirable, and important skill and an integral component of nursing care.
3. Communicate effectively and compassionately with the patient, family, and health care team members about end-of-life issues.
4. Recognize one's own attitudes, feelings, values, and expectations about death and the individual, cultural, and spiritual diversity existing in these beliefs and customs.
5. Demonstrate respect for the patient's views and wishes during end-of-life care.
6. Collaborate with interdisciplinary team members while implementing the nursing role in end-of-life care.
7. Use scientifically based standardized tools to assess symptoms (e.g., pain, dyspnea [breathlessness], constipation, anxiety, fatigue, nausea/vomiting, and altered cognition) experienced by patients at the end of life.
8. Use data from symptom assessment to plan and intervene in symptom management using state-of-the-art traditional and complementary approaches.
9. Evaluate the impact of traditional, complementary, and technological therapies on patient-centered outcomes.
10. Assess and treat multiple dimensions, including physical, psychological, social, and spiritual needs, to improve quality at the end of life.
11. Assist the patient, family, colleagues, and one's self to cope with suffering, grief, loss, and bereavement in end-of-life care.
12. Apply legal and ethical principles in the analysis of complex issues in end-of-life care, recognizing the influence of personal values, professional codes, and patient preferences.
13. Identify barriers and facilitators to patients' and caregivers' effective use of resources.
14. Demonstrate skill at implementing a plan for improved end-of-life care within a dynamic and complex health care delivery system.
15. Apply knowledge gained from palliative care research to end-of-life education and care.

Source: American Association of Colleges of Nursing. (1997), reference 27.

curriculum textbooks were analyzed and found to be lacking. This project, coordinated by the Oncology Nursing Certification Corporation, was designed to promote changes in nursing practice by introducing changes in continuing education materials focused on preparing candidates for the certification examinations and by promoting increasing content on end-of-life care in the examinations.[45]

Involvement of the certification corporations is a vital force in promoting palliative nursing care. In addition to integrating end-of-life content across multiple specialty organizations, the Hospice and Palliative Nurses Association (HPNA) has provided leadership to this evolving discipline. HPNA is the leading nursing organization supporting the development of palliative nursing. This organization provides numerous educational programs, publishes extensive educational materials, and also has a certification arm, the National Board for Certification of Hospice and Palliative Nurses (NBCHPN), that administers the specialty certification in Hospice and Palliative Nursing for registered nurses (Certified Hospice and Palliative Nurse, CHPN), for APNs (Board Certified–Palliative Care Management, APRN, BC-PCM), and for nursing assistants (Certified Hospice and Palliative Nursing Assistant, CHPNA).

Model Nursing Programs

Undergraduate and Graduate Education

The coauthor of this chapter (Sheehan) has identified many important strategies in teaching palliative care to nursing students. It is important to include both didactic and clinical components in both undergraduate and graduate curriculums. An example of an undergraduate model includes content on loss, grief, and bereavement, as well as pharmacological interventions for symptom management, at the sophomore level. Content on the physiology of dying, psychosocial and spiritual issues, and the hospice model of care is presented at the junior

Table 60–3
The Human Response to Dying (Approaching Death)

Level I (entry-level nursing students):
Theory and clinical practice to be integrated within the two years of a generic nursing education curriculum.

Biological Response	Psychosocial Response	Spiritual Response
Theory		
Physiology of dying (physical decline) Adaptive responses to approaching death Palliative nursing care	Family dynamics in crisis Loss–grief continuum Exploration of attitudes regarding death and dying Legal issues: • Advance directives • Proxy decision maker Ethics—Dying Community health nursing aging caregivers Belief systems and cultural customs (rural/urban, minority, etc.)	Death as a final stage of growth Meaning of death from a philosophical view Meaning of the human spirit Meaning of suffering Fears surrounding dying: Loneliness and abandonment Role of hospice interdisciplinary team
Nursing theory		Carative model of nursing practice Role of hospice-caring and comfort The carative role of the nurse Palliative nursing
Assessment/nursing diagnosis		
Nutritional needs Fluid volume needs and processes Elimination needs Skin and tissue integrity Delirium Pain: acute, chronic, terminal Confusion Cycles sleep–rest Cardiovascular processes Respiratory processes: Agitation Anoxia	Coping strategies in response to loss: • Anticipatory grieving • Powerlessness Age-related responses to loss	Patient/family assessment of needs Assess the process: • Spiritual distress • Fear • Anxiety • Ineffective coping, individual/family
Interventions		
Palliative care (symptom management to provide comfort and alleviate suffering) Emphasis on comfort measures Complementary therapies Pain management guidelines	Communication: • Therapeutic vs. nontherapeutic use of reflection storytelling • Empathetic listening	

(*continued*)

Table 60–3
The Human Response to Dying (Approaching Death) *(continued)*

Level I (entry-level nursing students):
Theory and clinical practice to be integrated within the two years of a generic nursing education curriculum.

Biological Response	Psychosocial Response	Spiritual Response
Complementary therapies as a focus of interventions		
		Touch with intent Therapeutic Touch Massage Music therapy Prayer Imagery
Clinical placement		
Nursing care centers (nursing homes) Assisted-living centers Inpatient hospice centers Senior-level optional community health nursing Hospice in the home	Same as those listed under biological responses Psychosocial competencies identified	Same as those listed under biological responses

Level II (Registered Nurses with 6 months to 1 year of experience in clinical nursing):
Time required to complete Level II: three semesters (or four quarters) in a university setting, including at least 12 weeks in a palliative care hospice setting.

Biological Response	Psychosocial Response	Spiritual Response
Theory		
Palliative care: • History and present day • Application in health care Pathophysiology (end-stage disease processes): • Malignancies • Immune deficiency disease • Dementia • Chronic illness Neurophysiological mechanisms of acute/chronic/terminal pain Principle of pain management Physiology of symptoms: • Anoxia • Dyspnea • Fluid volume changes • Changes in antidiuretic hormone and kidney function • Nutritional changes—nausea, constipation • Restlessness Agitation Delirium	Palliative nursing care role Nursing role in hospice: • In-home vs. residential care • Teaching: families, caregivers, and nursing assistants • Liaison with community health organizations/resources Recognition of personal needs and attitudes regarding death/pain/loss Interdisciplinary team Family dynamics—pathological families: • Abuse and neglect • Closed systems • Addictive/manipulative • Enmeshed Cultural differences: • Rituals • Customs • Values • Funeral preparations • Religious influence Symbolic communication Communication/interaction: • Interviewing techniques • Reflection • Empathetic listening • Silence	Philosophical and historical role of healers The spiritual process and spiritual distress: • Religiosity vs. spirituality Meaning of suffering Consciousness and dying Transpersonal meaning of existence Theories of Jung-Cassel Nursing theory Carative model Addressing the intuitive process within the nurse: • Centering • Journaling

(continued)

Table 60–3
The Human Response to Dying (Approaching Death) *(continued)*

Level II (Registered Nurses with 6 months to 1 year of experience in clinical nursing):
Time required to complete Level II: three semesters (or four quarters) in a university setting, including at least 12 weeks in a palliative care hospice setting.

Biological Response	Psychosocial Response	Spiritual Response
Assessment/nursing diagnosis		
Emphasis on physical assessment, symptoms and behaviors in end-stage processes Pain assessment—types and analogies of measurement Age-related pain behaviors: • Infants • Children • Preadolescents • Adolescents • Middle adulthood • Aging	Human response to loss of individual/family Coping strategies: • Denial/anger/bargaining/depression/acceptance • Grief and grieving • Anticipatory grief Bereavement meaning and importance in hospice: • High-risk families Social isolation	Suffering Spiritual distress Hopelessness Powerlessness Anxiety Fear
Interventions		
Palliative nursing role Advanced practice role Common approaches to symptom management: • Pharmacological • Nonpharmacological Complementary therapies Pain management: • Cancer pain • Acute pain • Chronic pain Terminal pain	Therapeutic communication: • Patient/family • Hospice team Crisis intervention Teaching: • Patient/family • Staff • Community Conflict resolution: • Patient/family • Staff • Hospice team Complicated bereavement	Establishing criteria for the efficacy of complementary therapies Scientific and historical evidence in support of complementary therapies • Therapeutic Touch • Massage • Acupressure • Aroma therapy • Music therapy • Guided imagery • Visualization • Prayer • Relaxation techniques • Breathing • Homeopathy
Clinical experience		
Inpatient hospice Assisted living In-home hospice or residential setting Correctional institutional (hospice center)		
Management role of the nurse		
Strategies for reimbursement Health maintenance organization Medicare/Medicaid Regulatory agencies • Federal • State	Supportive intervention for staff Facilitate communication with team members For profit vs. nonprofit hospice Regulations interval • Policy • Procedural guidelines	

(continued)

Table 60–3
The Human Response to Dying (Approaching Death) *(continued)*

Level II (Registered Nurses with 6 months to 1 year of experience in clinical nursing): Time required to complete Level II: three semesters (or four quarters) in a university setting, including at least 12 weeks in a palliative care hospice setting.		
Biological Response	**Psychosocial Response**	**Spiritual Response**
Standards/Accreditation • Joint Commission on Accreditation of Healthcare Organizations (JCAHO) • National Hospice and Palliative Care Organization (NHPCO) • National Consensus Project (NCP) Guidelines[52] Liaison with specialized agencies Quality assurance standards	Education/training • Inservice/staff • Community • Management/leadership training Support and interface with community	

Source: National Council of Hospice Professionals (1997), reference 39.

level, with a minimum of 12 hours with nursing faculty at an inpatient hospice facility. At the senior level, content on the dying child is covered in the Developing Families rotation.

Students tend to learn best during teachable moments. These include real events with real people. For student nurses, this usually means the clinical setting. During the clinical experience, the students work with an experienced hospice nurse. They attend the morning report and choose one or two patients with the guidance of the hospice nurse. The nursing instructor asks questions of the student and hospice nurse to facilitate learning. The instructor also meets with the students as a group early in the day to clarify the assignments for the day and to check on how the students are feeling in this environment.

The instructor brings the students together as specific learning opportunities arise, such as the death of a patient, unusual dressing changes, or pharmacological interventions. The use of reflection is a powerful tool to assist students and faculty to learn about themselves and about their practice from situations they encounter in the clinical setting and to integrate personal and professional learning experiences. For this reason, the students write a reflection on practice for each hospice clinical day. Students are prepared for the hospice experience through a group meeting with the nursing instructor early in the day. The following is an example of instructions for clinical assignments.

Undergraduate Clinical Preparation

1. You may feel exhausted by the end of the day even if you have done very little physical work. You may be emotionally drained.
2. Take time to discuss your fears and experiences with death with your clinical instructor, the hospice nurse, or your peers.
3. You may leave the unit (or classroom) at any time. Please let your instructor know how you are feeling.
4. You will be given the option to see someone who has just died to discuss physical changes in the body and the feeling in the room. You may decline this opportunity.
5. Take time to reflect on your practice.
6. Be open to learning from a variety of people, including patients, families, interdisciplinary team members, peers, and yourself.

Undergraduate Clinical Assignments

1. Listen to the full report on your unit.
2. Review *Patient/Family Guidelines for Signs and Symptoms of Approaching Death.*
3. Make rounds with the hospice nurse to see all of his or her patients.
4. Choose one or two patients with guidance from the hospice nurse.
5. Review patient/family information with the hospice nurse.
6. Assess one specific physical symptom that is most important to the patient. Use the literature to link the diagnosis with the pathophysiology. List the appropriate nursing interventions and expected outcomes. This information will be presented during the clinical conference.
7. Listen to the patient's story throughout the day.
8. Reflection on practice: What happened today that made a difference in the way you will practice nursing?

Madonna University in Livonia, Michigan, was the first institution in the United States to offer interdisciplinary hospice education programs under the direction of Sister Mary

Cecilia Eagan. The hospice education department, under the direction of Kelly Rhoades, PhD, offers associate's, bachelor's, and master's degrees in hospice education. Students in the Master of Science in Hospice (MSH) program complete 30 semester hours of coursework and select one of five cognate specialties in bereavement, pastoral ministry, business, education, or nursing. Students may enroll in certificate programs at both the graduate and undergraduate levels in hospice education or bereavement.

The Breen School of Nursing at Ursuline College in Pepper Pike, Ohio, was the first graduate program in the United States to prepare APNs in palliative care. The Master of Science in Nursing program officially began in August 1998, under the direction of Denice Sheehan, although the first course was offered during the 1998 spring semester. The program builds on the college's mission to provide an education based on values. Contemplation and reflection on practice are hallmarks of this program. The core curriculum of the master's program concentrates on theory, informatics, research, critical thinking, evidence-based practice, and leadership. The APN courses include pathophysiology, pharmacology, and health assessment. Students in the palliative care program also take two specialized palliative care courses and 500 hours in the palliative care practicum. Table 60–4 lists the required courses. A post-master's certificate is offered to nurses with a Master of Science in Nursing (MSN) degree.

Table 60–4
Ursuline College's Master's Degree Program and Post-Master's Certificate

Master's Degree Program

I. Nursing Core: 18 credits
- Health Care Financing
- Concepts and Theories
- Applied Nursing Research I
- Applied Nursing Research II
- Nursing Informatics
- Health Policies, Roles and Issues

II. Advanced Practice Core: 12 credits
- Advanced Physiology and Pathology
- Advanced Pharmacology
- Advanced Health Assessment
- Health Promotion, Maintenance, and Restoration

III. Area of Concentration: 9 credits
- Palliative Care I
- Palliative Care II
- Palliative Care Practicum

Post-Master's Certificate

Nursing Informatics
Advance Physiology, Pathology
Advanced Pharmacology
Advanced Health Assessment
Introduction to Palliative Care and Hospice (web-based)
Palliative Care I
Palliative Care II
Palliative Care Practicum

Table 60–5 summarizes the topical outlines for the palliative care courses in the Breen graduate program. Introduction to Palliative Care and Hospice is an interdisciplinary web-based course. It is the first course offered in the post-master's certificate program. The content is taught in the core courses in the MSN program. This Introduction course provides an overview of palliative care with respect to history, philosophy, the interdisciplinary team model, and reimbursement mechanisms. Students have opportunities to explore personal beliefs, attitudes, and reactions to progressive illness, dying, and death. They discuss ways in which these attitudes can influence the care of people with life threatening illnesses and their families. Ethical issues are explored in relation to treatment decisions and quality of life. Spirituality is explored within a framework of individual values and beliefs. The essence of the self as the physical being deteriorates at the end of life is analyzed. Religious and cultural beliefs, traditions, and rituals are discussed as they pertain to end-of-life issues. Loss, grief, and bereavement are also explored as they relate to the terminally ill person and the family. Communication and counseling techniques are woven throughout this course. Research, case studies, and personal and professional experiences are used to emphasize key concepts. Classical literature is woven throughout this course in the form of case studies. Students participate in virtual rounds using asynchronous learning online. Virtual rounds provide the opportunity to make daily rounds at the hospice without actually being there. The nursing faculty member teaching the course makes rounds with the interdisciplinary team on day 1 to choose a patient to observe over the next 3 days. She presents the patient to the students via the online course on day 1. She returns to the hospice daily. The patient is presented to the students online with specific discussion questions as the case unfolds. Students are expected to make substantive comments supported by the literature and their clinical experiences. Their questions and comments are shared with the interdisciplinary team, and feedback is provided for the students. This technique has been found to be very beneficial to the students and the team. Most of the students in the post-master's certificate program have extensive hospice or palliative care experience and clinical expertise. They live and work in urban and rural areas across the United States. This combination of expertise, diversity, and openness to new ideas creates complex discussions and innovative approaches to care.

In Palliative Care I, students have an opportunity to analyze personal attitudes toward progressive illness, dying, and death and compare their current analysis to that developed in earlier courses. They also continue the discussion about how these attitudes can influence the care of patients with life-threatening

Table 60–5
The Breen School of Nursing: Topical Outlines for Palliative Care Graduate Courses

Introduction to Palliative Care and Hospice
Overview of Palliative Care and Hospice
Personal and Societal Perspectives on Dying
An American Profile on Death and Dying
The History and Philosophy of Palliative Care and Hospice
The Interdisciplinary Team
The Importance of the Narrative
Physiology of Dying
Spirituality, Religiosity, and Culture
Ethical Issues
Legal Issues
Loss, Grief, and Bereavement
Reimbursement Issues
Palliative Care I
Personal Perspectives on Dying
Setting Professional Boundaries
Nursing Standards and Competencies
Communication and Counseling
Nursing Care of the Patient with Selected Symptoms
Clinical Emergencies
Ethical Issues—End-of-Life Decision Making
Palliative Care II
Advanced Practice Nurse Role Development in Palliative Care
Continuous Quality Improvement and Analysis
Impact of Economic and Political Factors on the Delivery of Palliative Care
Resource Management
Enhanced Communication Skills Used in Collaborative Practice
Influencing Legislation Related to Palliative Care and Hospice
Cultural Issues Related to Loss, Grief, and Bereavement
International Perspectives in Palliative Care

illnesses and their families. Ethical issues are explored in relation to treatment decisions and quality of life. This course integrates pathophysiology, pharmacology, psychosocial issues, and spirituality in the assessment and management of symptoms. Current research in palliative care is analyzed and applied in the clinical setting. The practicum may be taken concurrently or after Palliative Care I.

Students in Palliative Care II explore leadership roles for the palliative care APN in administration, education, consultation, and clinical practice. Quality process and measurement is presented within the framework of continuous quality improvement. The impact of economic and political factors on the delivery of palliative care in a variety of settings is analyzed. Students focus on special populations such as prisons and decide on special topics depending on the interests of the group.

During the Palliative Care Practicum, students have opportunities in the clinical area for direct contact with expert palliative care practitioners. This includes direct patient–family contact during home visits, team conferences, and clinical forums with the clinical group and the instructor. The students work with the dying and their families in the home, hospice, and palliative care inpatient facilities, hospitals, and extended-care facilities. Students meet with an assigned faculty member to tailor the practicum to meet the learning needs of the student. The students work with patients and their families through the dying process and participate in grief support groups. They keep a clinical journal, including learning objectives, personal/professional strengths identified during the practicum, and reflections on their thoughts and feelings during the clinical experience. They also participate in team meetings, research, and educational presentations to staff, patients and their families, and the community.

Another model nursing program is located at New York University (NYU) in New York City. NYU was the first institution in the United States to offer a Palliative Care Nurse Practitioner program. Under the direction of Dr. Deborah Sherman, the palliative care program builds on the core curriculum of the master's program, focusing on theory, research, evidence-based practice, critical thinking, human development, cultural competence, community health care systems, and leadership. In addition to advanced science courses in pathophysiology, pharmacotherapeutics, and advanced health assessment, students take five specialized palliative care courses, a role development course, and 610 hours of palliative care practicums. A post-master's certificate is an option for those individuals who already have a master's in nursing. A summary of the curriculum is included in Table 60–6.

Schools of nursing are incorporating palliative care into existing graduate curricula as a subspecialty or focus. Vanderbilt University School of Nursing in Nashville, Tennessee, offers three options at the graduate level to prepare nurses to care for people with life-threatening illnesses and their families across the palliative care trajectory. The first is an adult nurse practitioner program (ANP) with a palliative care focus under the direction of Professor James C. Pace, DSN, MDiv, RN, ANP-CS. Graduate nursing students complete 39 semester hours of coursework and 700 practicum hours in a variety of outpatient clinics, long-term care facilities, and hospice settings. At the conclusion of the program, students are eligible for ANP certification as well as certification in advanced practice palliative care. The second option includes joint degree initiatives leading to either the MSN/MDiv or MSN/MTS degrees offered in cooperation by the Schools of Nursing and Divinity at Vanderbilt University. Students complete individually designed programs of study in both nursing and theology, and course credit is shared between schools. Students can fulfill the 700-hour practicum requirement in the school of nursing and satisfy part of the field work credit required by the

Table 60–6
New York University Master's Degree Program in Palliative Nursing

I.	Nursing Core: 18 credits
	Nursing Science and Unitary Human Beings
	Population Focused Care
	Research in Nursing
	Nursing Issues and Trends Within the Health Care Delivery System
	Nursing Leadership
	Basic Statistics II
II.	Advanced Practice Core: 12–15 credits
	Palliative Care I: Foundations of Palliative Care
	Palliative Care Practicum I: Advanced Comprehensive Health and Physical Assessment
	Clinical Practice: Advanced Practice Roles
	Advanced Pathophysiology
	Clinical Pharmacotherapeutics
III.	Electives: 3 credits
	Nursing or Free Elective or Independent Study
IV.	Area of Concentration: 12 credits
	Palliative Care II: Enhancement of Quality of Life Through the Management of Pain and Suffering
	Palliative Care Practicum II: Comprehensive, Holistic End-of-Life Care
	Palliative Care III: Enhancement of Quality of Life Through Symptom Management
	Palliative Care Practicum III: Advancing Nursing Practice and Leadership in Palliative Care

divinity school. A third option at the graduate level includes two elective courses, "Research in Religion and Health" and "Health and Salvation Themes," which are cotaught by Dr. Pace and Dr. Leonard M. Hummel, Assistant Professor of Pastoral Counseling and Pastoral Theology at The Vanderbilt Divinity School.

Continuing Education

Although palliative care education in undergraduate and graduate programs provides an important foundation for the nursing profession, continuing education is also needed to reach nurses already in practice. Continuing education is needed to reach nurses in all settings involved in end-of-life care. A wide range of methods, including conferences, self-study courses, computer- and web-based approaches, and simulated clinical experiences, are needed.

In 1999, the AACN and the City of Hope National Medical Center initiated collaboration to develop a national education program on end-of-life care for registered nurses. This national project, the End-of-Life Nursing Education Consortium (ELNEC), followed the efforts by the medical profession to address end-of-life care through the Education for Physicians in End-of-Life-Care (EPEC) program. The ELNEC project was funded by The Robert Wood Johnson Foundation (RWJF). The nine components of the ELNEC curriculum included Nursing Care at the End of Life, Pain Management, Symptom Management, Ethical/Legal Issues, Cultural Considerations, Communication, Grief/Loss/Bereavement, Achieving Quality Care, and Care at the Time of Death. The ELNEC project was developed as a 3-day training program that included many educational modalities such as lectures, role-plays, small-group work, case discussion, and other experiences. The "Train-the-Trainers" model was used: individuals attending the ELNEC course were expected to gain knowledge of the content as well as skills in teaching the content. A very extensive application process was designed to ensure that ELNEC participants had established goals for their dissemination of the curriculum before attending the course and had the support of the Dean or administrators to ensure success in their implementation. The RWJF funding provided eight initial courses targeted for 100 participants per course. These courses included five focused on faculty teaching in undergraduate nursing programs and three targeted for continuing education providers. The five training programs were held in 2001 and 2002 and addressed continuing education providers and nurse educators from hospices, palliative care programs, and community agencies. The components of the ELNEC program are listed in Table 60–7.

The ELNEC project subsequently received funding from the National Cancer Institute to reach educators in graduate nursing programs for an APN version of the curriculum, and in 2003 the project received funding to initiate a curriculum

Table 60–7
End-of-Life Nursing Education (ELNEC) Consortium

Module	Description of Content
1. Nursing Care at the End of Life	Goals of care; cost issues in palliative care; use of aggressive interventions, personal death awareness, board review of end-of-life care, to encompass all age groups and across various disease trajectories or acute illness
2. Pain Management	Assessment; pharmacological, nonpharmacological, and complementary therapies
3. Symptom Management	Assessment; pharmacological, nonpharmacological, and complementary therapies
4. Cultural Considerations in End-of-Life Care	Cultural assessment; beliefs regarding death and dying, afterlife, and bereavement
5. Ethical/Legal Issues	Assisted suicide, euthanasia, advance directives, decision-making, advanced care planning
6. Communication	Breaking bad news; communicating with other disciplines; interdisciplinary collaboration
7. Grief, Loss, Bereavement	Assessment; interventions; nurses' experiences with cumulative loss and grief
8. Preparation and Care for the Time of Death	Nursing care at the time of death, including physical care, support of family members, saying good-bye
9. Achieving Quality of Life at the End of Life	Physical, psychological, social, and spiritual well-being; needs of special populations

specific for oncology nurses. The oncology project is conducted in collaboration with the Oncology Nursing Society (ONS). From 2001 to 2003, the ELNEC investigators developed and tested a pediatric version of ELNEC, with the first national training program held in August 2003. Several publications have described the ELNEC project and its curriculum care.[46–48] The reader is directed to the ELNEC website at http://www.aacn.nche.edu/elnec/ for additional information.

Continuing education opportunities are offered by specialty nursing organizations. All of these organizations hold annual conferences and publish palliative care articles in their journals, many with continuing education credit. In addition, the HPNA offers teleconferences online for nurses and nursing assistants. The ONS hosts an annual Institute of Learning and a biennial Cancer Nursing Research Conference. Virtual Sessions uses streaming video to showcase instructional sessions from the ONS Congress and Institutes of Learning. Sigma Theta Tau International offers online sessions in end-of-life care.

Future Directions

Clearly, there is much work to be done to advance nursing education in palliative care. Improving the care of patients will be accomplished only when nursing education within undergraduate, graduate, and continuing education is improved and supported by research. Progress over the next decade will require collaboration internationally and a close commitment by nursing education, research, and practice. Collectively, these efforts can advance the profession of palliative nursing and dramatically improve care at the end of life.

Evaluation of Palliative Care Education

Evaluation of education is a challenge in any program and for any content, but it is a special challenge in palliative care education. As the core content of this education evolves, so will the methods of evaluation. There is a need for standard knowledge assessment measures, as well as means for evaluating clinical skills, decision-making, and a broad range of physical, psychosocial, and spiritual care skills necessary in palliative care.[49–51] New technologies, such as web-based teaching and evaluation tools, will be important resources for educators.

REFERENCES

1. Meraviglia MG, McGuire C, Chesley DA. Nurses' needs for education on cancer and end-of-life care. J Cont Educ Nurs 2003; 34(3):122–127.
2. Durkin A. Incorporating concepts of end-of-life care into a psychiatric nursing course. Nurs Educ Perspect 2003;24(4):184–185.
3. Last Acts. Means to a Better End: A Report on Dying in America Today 2002. Washington, DC: Last Acts.
4. Field MJ, Cassel CK, eds. Approaching Death: Improving Care at the End of Life. Report of the Institute of Medicine Task Force

on End of Life Care. National Academy of Sciences, Washington, DC, 1997.
5. Proctor M, Grealish L, Coates M, Sears P. Nurses' knowledge of palliative care in the Australian Capital Territory. Int J Palliat Nurs 2000;6:421–428.
6. Bowden V. End-of-life care: A priority issue for pediatric nurses. J Pediatr Nurs 2002;17:456–459.
7. Institute of Medicine. Priority Areas for National Action: Transforming Healthcare Quality. National Academy Press, Washington D.C., 2003.
8. Bennahum DA. The historical development of hospice and palliative care. In: Forman WB, Kitzes JA, Anderson RP, Sheehan DK, eds. Hospice and Palliative Care: Concepts and Practice, 2nd ed. Boston: Jones and Bartlett, 2003:1–11.
9. Kubler-Ross E. On Death and Dying. New York: Macmillan, 1969.
10. Quint JC. The Nurse and the Dying Patient. New York: Macmillan, 1967.
11. Hollen CJ, Hollen CW, Stolte K. Hospice and hospital oncology unit nurses: A comparative survey of knowledge and attitudes about cancer pain. Oncol Nurs Forum 2000;27:1593–1599.
12. Grant MM, Rivera LM. Pain education for nurses, patients, and families. In: McGuire DB, Yarbro CH, Ferrell BR, eds. Cancer Pain Management. Boston: Jones and Bartlett, 1995:289–319.
13. Glajchen M, Bookbinder M. Knowledge and perceived competence of home care nurses in pain management: A national survey. J Pain Symptom Manage 2001;21:307–316.
14. Arber A. Student nurses' knowledge of palliative care: Evaluating an education module. Int J Palliat Nurs 2001;7:597–598, 600–603.
15. Field D, Kitson C. Formal teaching about death and dying in UK nursing schools. Nurse Education Today 1986;6:270–276.
16. Pickett M, Cooley ME, Gordon DB. Palliative care: Past, present, and future perspectives. Semin Oncol Nurs 1998;14(2):86–94.
17. Samaroo B. Assessing palliative care educational needs of physicians and nurses: Results of a survey. Greater Victoria Hospital Society Palliative Care Committee. J Palliat Care 1996; 12:20–22.
18. Sellick SM, Charles K, Dagsvik J, Kelley ML. Palliative care providers' perspectives on service and education needs. J Palliat Care 1996;12:34–38.
19. Webber J. New directions in palliative care education. Support Care Cancer 1994;2:16–20.
20. Degner LF, Gow CM, Thompson LA. Critical nursing behaviors in care of the dying. Cancer Nurs 1991;(14)5:246–253.
21. McClement SE, Degner LF. Expert nursing behaviors in care of the dying adult in the intensive care unit. Heart Lung 1995; 24:408–419.
22. Webster NE. Communicating with dying patients. Nursing Times 1981;June 4:999–1002.
23. Rittman M, Paige P, Rivera J, Sutphin L, Godown I. Phenomenological study of nurses caring for dying patients. Cancer Nurs 1997;(20)2:115–119.
24. Kirshhoff KT, Beckstand RL, Anumandla P. Analysis of end-of-life content in critical care nursing textbooks. J Prof Nurs 2003; 19:372–381.
25. Ferrell BR, Virani R, Grant M. Analysis of end of life content in nursing textbooks. Oncol Nurs Forum 1999;26:869–876.
26. Wendt A. End-of-life competencies and the NCLEX-RN examination. Nurs Outlook 2001;3:138–141.
27. American Association of Colleges of Nursing. A Peaceful Death. Report from the Robert Wood Johnson End-of-Life Care Roundtable. Washington, DC, November 1997.
28. World Health Organization. Cancer Pain Relief and Palliative Care. WHO Technical Report Series 804. Geneva: WHO, 1990.
29. Jodrell N. Nurse education. In: Doyle D, Hanks G, MacDonald N, eds. Oxford Textbook of Palliative Medicine, 2nd ed. Oxford: Oxford University Press, 1998:1202–1208.
30. Birkholz G, Clements PT, Cox R, Gaume A. Students' self-identified learning needs: A case study of baccalaureate students designing their own death and dying course curriculum. J Nurs Educ 2004;43:36–39.
31. Pimple C, Schmidt L, Tidwell S. Achieving excellence in end-of-life care. Nurs Educ 2003;28:40–43.
32. Gelfand DE, Baker L, Cooney G. Developing end-of-life interdisciplinary programs in universitywide settings. Am J Hospice Palliat Care 2003;20;201–204.
33. Scanlon C. Unraveling ethical issues in palliative care. Semin Oncol Nurs 1998;14:137–144.
34. Redman S, White K, Ryan E, Hennrikus D. Professional needs of palliative care nurses in New South Wales. Palliat Med 1995; 9:36–44.
35. Sheldon F, Smith P. The life so short, the craft so hard to learn: A model for post-basic education in palliative care. Palliat Med 1996;10:99–104.
36. Vachon ML. Caring for the caregiver in oncology and palliative care. Semin Oncol Nurs 1998;14:152–157.
37. Yates P, Hart G, Clinton M, McGrath P, Gartry D. Exploring empathy as a variable in the evaluation of professional development programs for palliative care nurses. Cancer Nurs 1998; 21: 402–410.
38. International Council of Nurses. Basic Principles of Nursing Care. Washington, D.C.: American Nurses Publishing, 1997.
39. National Council of Hospice Professionals. Guidelines for Curriculum Development on End-of-Life and Palliative Care in Nursing Education. Arlington, VA: National Hospice Organization, 1997.
40. Rushton C, Scanlon C, Ferrell B. Designing an Agenda for the Nursing Profession on End of Life Care. Report of the Nursing Leadership Consortium on End of Life Care. Aliso Viejo, CA: Association of Critical Care Nurses, 1999:1–14.
41. Rushton CH, Spencer KL, Johanson W. Bringing end-of-life care out of the shadows. Nurs Manage 2004;35:34–40.
42. Rushton C, Sabatier K, Gaines J. Uniting to improve end-of-life care. Nurs Manage 2003;34:30–33.
43. Advanced Practice Nurses' Role in Palliative Care: A position statement from American Nursing Leaders, July 2002. Available at: http://www.dyingwell.com/downloads/apnpos.pdf (accessed March 22, 2005).
44. Advanced Practice Nursing. Pioneering practiced in palliative care. Promoting Excellence in End-of-Life Care, July 2002. Available at: http://www.promotingexcellence.org/downloads/apnreport.pdf (accessed March 22, 2005).
45. Esper P, Lockhart JS, Murphy CM. Strengthening end-of-life care through specialty nursing certification. J Prof Nurs 2002; 18:130–139.
46. Sherman DW, Matzo ML, Rogers S, McLaughlin M, Virani R. Achieving quality care at the end of life: A focus of the End-of-Life Nursing Education Consortium (ELNEC) curriculum. J Prof Nurs 2002;18:255–262.
47. Matzo ML, Sherman DW, Mazanec P, Barber MA, Virani R, McLaughlin MM. Teaching cultural considerations at the end of life: End-of-Life Nursing Education Consortium program recommendations. J Cont Educ Nurs 2002;33:270–278.

48. Matzo ML, Sherman DW, Penn B, Ferrell BR. The End-of-Life Nursing Education Consortium (ELNEC) experience. Nurse Educator 2003;28:266–270.
49. MacLeod RD. Education in palliative medicine: A review. J Cancer Educ 1993;8:309–312.
50. Sowell R, Seals G, Wilson B, Robinson C. Evaluation of an HIV/AIDS continuing education program. J Cont Educ Nurs 1998;29:85–93.
51. The SUPPORT Principal Investigators. A controlled trial to improve care for seriously ill hospitalized patients: The Study to Understand Prognoses and Preferences for Outcomes and Risks of Treatments (SUPPORT). JAMA 1995;274:1591–1598.
52. National Consensus Project. Clinical Practice Guidelines for Quality Palliative Care, 2004. Available at: http://www.nationalconsensusproject.org/Guidelines_Download.asp (accessed May 9, 2005).

61

Betty R. Ferrell and Marcia Grant

Nursing Research

From the cellular to the social level, much remains to be learned about how people die and how reliably excellent and compassionate care can be achieved. Important, unanswered questions exist about the fundamental physiological mechanisms of the symptoms that cause so much suffering among dying patients and about the kinds of interventions that will relieve these symptoms. Basic epidemiological information on how people die is limited, and the influence of attitudes and beliefs on people's experience of dying and on caregiving practices is little charted. In addition, a better understanding of the reasons for the inadequate application of existing knowledge would help in identifying organizational, economic, and other incentives for the provision of accessible, effective, and affordable care at the end of life.—Field and Cassel (1997)[1]

- ***Key Points***
- *The goal of nursing research is to improve patient care.*
- *Nurses have been instrumental in the field of palliative care research.*
- *Palliative nursing research includes many sensitive topics such as pain, quality of life, and fatigue.*
- *Nurse researchers face many obstacles in conducting research, such as obtaining informed consent, and openly discussing the end of life with patients and families, as well as facing a high subject attrition.*
- *The interdisciplinary team, as well as caregivers and patients' families, should be involved in nursing research.*

The words of Field and Cassel, from a 1997 report of the Institute of Medicine (IOM) on improving care at the end of life, capture the breadth of palliative care research. Uniform agreement across disciplines and among authors confirms the paucity of palliative care research and the resultant absence of a scientific foundation for practice, which affects the care of patients at the end of life.[2–7] Better patient care depends on both the quantity and the quality of palliative care research.

A major component of palliative care research is nursing research. The patient experience of dying is an ideal health care concern appropriate for nursing inquiry.[8,9] Because nurses are concerned with patient responses to illness, the physical, psychological, social, and spiritual responses of the terminally ill and their families are prime areas for nursing research.

The ultimate goal of nursing research, and indeed of nursing knowledge, is to improve patient care. Palliative care offers a rich opportunity for research to directly influence patient care in areas such as symptom management, psychological responses to a terminal illness, and the family caregiver experience of terminal illness.[10–14]

Some of the earliest contributions to palliative care research were made by nurses. Pioneering work by Jeanne Quint Benoliel and others raised awareness of deficiencies in care of the dying.[15,16] Early descriptive studies documented the influence of nursing attitudes and beliefs about death on the care provided to patients.

From the earliest studies in the 1960s to the "awakening" of attention to palliative care in the late 1990s, research in palliative care has been limited. Nurse investigators have addressed aspects of end-of-life care such as pain management, bereavement, settings of care, and care of special populations such as patients with the acquired immunodeficiency syndrome (AIDS). However, there has been a lack of cohesive commitment to palliative care nursing research.

In 1997, the National Institute of Nursing Research (NINR) led an initiative regarding end-of-life care research across several institutes of the National Institutes of Health (NIH).

Specific recommendations of an NINR-sponsored conference on end-of-life care are described later in this chapter.[17] NINR has been designated as the lead institute at the NIH in the area of end-of-life care. It is appropriate and commendable that the NINR is providing leadership at the NIH in this research agenda.

As has been true in other areas of health care, the research agenda has lagged behind the demands of clinical practice and education. Hospice programs and palliative care settings face increased demands for improved end-of-life care with little scientific knowledge to guide clinical decisions. Nursing schools have begun to develop undergraduate and graduate courses in palliative care, and some have launched degree or certificate programs in palliative care, again with limited research as a scientific foundation of their programs. Obviously, development of a solid research agenda and support of nursing science in palliative care are overdue.

Goals of Palliative Care Research

The goals of palliative care nursing research are similar to goals of other areas of nursing inquiry. Nursing research serves multiple functions, including quantification of information, discovery, description of phenomena, quality improvement, and problem-solving.[9] Quantification is accomplished through descriptive studies or through epidemiologic approaches. For example, there is a need to quantify the symptoms present in terminal illness, as well as their severity and impact. The field of palliative nursing care is relatively unexplored, and therefore there is great opportunity for discovery. What are the greatest needs of terminally ill patients and their family caregivers? What is the unique role of nursing within the interdisciplinary team?

The subjective nature of terminal illness and the existential experience of dying require research methods that describe phenomena. Death, as a subject that has been avoided in society, is still a relatively unknown aspect of life. On a more specific level, palliative care is also a field that would benefit tremendously from research linked to quality improvement. Numerous reports have identified serious deficits in end-of-life care, and efforts to improve the quality of end-of-life care will undoubtedly benefit from research. Finally, a major goal of palliative care research should be basic problem-solving. What drugs are most beneficial for dyspnea or agitation? What is the best treatment for pressure ulcers in a dying patient? What education best prepares family caregivers for signs and symptoms of approaching death?

Ethical and Methodological Considerations in Palliative Care Research

There are many unique aspects of research in palliative care. The multidimensional nature of care at the end of life and the vulnerability of the population are but two examples of factors that pose special challenges to this area of research.

The challenges of nursing research in palliative care should be prefaced by a discussion of the benefits. Although even the mention of conducting research with dying patients and their burdened families immediately creates concerns, there are in fact many benefits to participants. Participating in research, even at this most vulnerable and sensitive time of life, provides the opportunity for research subjects to contribute to others. Research participation often provides an opportunity to derive meaning from illness and to feel that one's suffering will provide benefit to others.[8,18]

In the authors' research at the City of Hope, involving numerous studies in sensitive areas such as pain, quality of life, and fatigue, positive feedback has consistently been received from research subjects. Patients and family caregivers often have thanked the researchers for studying these topics, which they perceive to be of great importance. Subjects have also frequently related that completing written instruments or participating in interviews provided a mechanism for communicating needs that had not previously been voiced.

However, research in palliative care is very challenging and includes many obstacles. Nurses are often conflicted in balancing the role of clinician with that of researcher. For example, in conducting research related to pain in terminally ill cancer patients, the authors have often had to carefully balance these roles. Identifying a patient with severe pain has often meant that the patient's participation in a study must be ended in order to seek treatment for the pain. Research must always respect the more important ethical consideration of protecting the patient's well-being.[18]

Seeking informed consent in rapidly declining, weak patients is a challenge, as is the need to constantly protect patient and family autonomy. Subjects in palliative care research may feel obligated to participate in research, particularly if they have been the recipients of good care. Although all patients in palliative care are considered vulnerable, certain subgroups, such as the cognitively impaired, the poor, and the elderly, are of special concern.[19–23]

The sensitive nature of palliative care research provides inherent challenges. The areas of concern at the end of life are highly emotional and may invoke heightened distress. Exploring areas such as grief, fears, spiritual concerns, family conflict, and other common dimensions of terminal illness is highly challenging. Participation in research can bring to the forefront previously undisclosed problems. The authors have found, in their research experience, that palliative care research necessitates highly skilled research staff. Collecting data from palliative care subjects is very different from research in healthy or chronically ill subjects. Research nurses in palliative care studies must be clinically competent, highly skilled nurses equipped to balance the rigor of research with extreme sensitivity.

Palliative care research, perhaps more than any other field of inquiry, must carefully weigh subject burden. The time required of research subjects in palliative care, a precious commodity for those with terminal disease, must be carefully protected. Special consideration must be given to selection of research instruments and procedures to minimize subject burden.

A useful resource for nurses researchers in palliative care is a "Tool Kit" project, supported by a grant from the Robert Wood Johnson Foundation to researchers at the University of Rhode Island. This project reviewed and compiled a list of research instruments recommended for use in palliative care. The tool kit is available online at http://www.chcr.brown.edu/web-pubs.htm#top (accessed March 1, 2005).

Subject attrition is another common problem area in palliative care research. Higher attrition has serious implications when determining sample sizes and also has budget implications. This problem area becomes an even greater concern in longitudinal studies, which are a definite need in palliative care.[19–23] New approaches to handling data are needed to improve data analysis.

Palliative care research also necessitates diversity in research methods. The authors' experience has been that a combination of qualitative and quantitative approaches is needed.[24] Qualitative approaches are especially important in descriptive studies. Appendix 61–1 includes examples of two qualitative nursing studies that serve as models for application of these methods for palliative care research. Quantitative approaches are essential when studying symptoms, their frequency and nature, and response to treatment.

The authors also have found that nursing research in palliative care is greatly enhanced by interdisciplinary collaboration. The problems studied are multidimensional and are best defined from the viewpoints of various members of the health care team. Participation from colleagues in psychology, theology, social work, and other disciplines has enhanced our work considerably.

A final special consideration in palliative care research is the importance of including family caregivers. Terminal illness is a shared experience, and including family caregivers as subjects enriches the benefits to be derived from the research.[10,12,13]

Table 61–1 summarizes some of the key challenges of conducting palliative care research. Advancement of the nursing profession in palliative care will require attention to overcome these obstacles.

Table 61–1
Barriers to Nursing Research in Palliative Care

- Overall limitations in funding for nursing research and in the limited number of nurse researchers.
- Research establishment and associated funding that has been focused on rehabilitation or cure.
- Lack of political or consumer advocates to promote a research agenda in end-of-life care.
- Limited focus on palliative care in graduate nursing education to promote end-of-life research within master's or doctoral nursing education.
- Few established relationships between nurse researchers and clinical settings of palliative care.
- Ethical considerations of conducting research with vulnerable populations, including issues related to ability to provide consent.
- Rapidly declining status, which limits subject accrual and opportunity for longitudinal measures.
- Lack of conceptual frameworks appropriate for palliative care research.
- Interference with demands of patient care caused by participation in research.
- Late referrals to hospice or palliative care programs, which severely restricts opportunities for accrual to studies.
- Lack of research instruments and methods appropriate for this population.
- Challenge of conducting research in a sensitive area.
- Need to balance demands of rigorous research, such as the need for randomization, with awareness of patient needs.

Sources: Adapted from Field and Cassel (1997), reference 1, and Doyle et al. (2004), reference 29.

A Research Agenda in Palliative Nursing

The IOM report identified priority areas for end-of-life care research, including pain, cachexia-anorexia-asthenia, dyspnea, cognitive, and emotional symptoms. Also addressed was the need for social, behavioral, and health services research. Nursing as a profession has much to contribute to each of these identified priorities.[8,9]

There is a tremendous need to bring together nurse researchers and nurse clinicians in palliative care. Historically, few nurse researchers have focused on palliative care; likewise, few expert clinicians in palliative care have had opportunities or expertise in research.

Although an exhaustive review of research methods or grant writing is not possible in this chapter, a few comments are worthy of attention. Palliative care clinicians are encouraged to seek collaboration with nurse researchers to initiate clinically relevant and scientifically sound studies. Another key issue of advice is to begin small. Conducting small pilot studies is an essential foundation to launching larger-scale studies. Potential sources for funding are found in Table 61–2.

Table 61–3 includes an example of criteria used in evaluating small-scale research projects. These criteria, adapted from

Table 61–2
Funding Sources for Pilot Studies

Hospital Continuous Quality Improvement programs
Oncology Nursing Foundation
Sigma Theta Tau
American Nursing Foundation
American Society of Pain Management Nurses
Local community foundations
Pharmaceutical companies
Hospice and Palliative Nursing Association

Table 61–3
Research Proposal Evaluation Criteria

Abstract

- Abstract accurately reflects the proposal.
- Abstract includes problem statement and purpose.
- Abstract summarizes key variables, sample, and methods.

Study aims, hypotheses, or study questions

- Clearly stated
- Hypotheses or study questions are consistent with the study aim.
- All proposed study procedures and data to be collected are encompassed.

Significance of the study

- The research contributes to the science of palliative nursing care.
- The research has the potential to lead to further investigation.
- The research offers a unique contribution to the literature.
- The research is clinically relevant to end-of-life care.

Literature review

- Relevant and current literature is reviewed.
- Literature primarily includes research rather than opinion.
- Literature is critiqued, synthesized, and analyzed.

Conceptual/theoretical framework

- Framework identified is appropriate to the study and consistent with study questions and methods.
- Framework is consistent with the philosophy of palliative care.

Procedures

- The procedures are feasible.
- Procedures include methods for training and supervision of personnel.
- Procedures provide sufficient description of precisely what will be required of subjects.

Data analysis

- Specific statistical procedures are identified.
- Analysis is appropriate for the type of data and study design and answers the study questions.
- Computer facilities and consultation are described.
- Investigator has sought consultation if necessary in preparing the proposal.

Human subjects considerations

- Institutional Review Board approval is given or documentation of pending review is given.
- The investigator is clearly aware of the impact of participation in the study on the subject.
- The investigator addresses concerns regarding length, intrusiveness, and energy expenditure required.
- The investigator has acknowledged special considerations of terminal illness.

Investigators and research team

- Consultation is available for the less experienced researcher.
- The role of co-investigators or consultants is established.

Overall

- The proposal strictly adheres to format restrictions and page limitations

Source: Adapted from reference 31 (2004).

Table 61–4
General Tips for Preparing Research Proposals

- Grant writing is not a solo activity—seek consultation and collaboration from others. Seek opportunities to involve clinical palliative care settings, such as hospices, in nursing research.
- Have your proposal reviewed by peers before submitting it for funding. A proposal submitted for funding is generally the product of numerous revisions.
- Follow the directions in detail, including margins, page limits, and the use of references and appendices. Communicate directly with the funding source to clarify any directions you are unsure of.
- State ideas clearly and succinctly. Word economy is essential to a fine-tuned proposal.
- Use high-quality printing and use a good-quality copier. Give attention to spelling and grammar.
- Plan ahead and develop a time frame for completing your grant. Avoid the last-minute rush that will compromise the quality of your proposal. It is better to target a future deadline for submission than to compromise your score due to a lack of time for preparation.
- Use appendices to include study instruments, procedures, or other supporting materials. Adhere to funding agency criteria, but maximize the opportunity for a complete proposal.
- Include support letters from individuals who are important to the success of your study. This includes medical staff, nursing administration, consultants, and co-investigators.
- Do not hesitate to contact experts in your subject area to seek their input. They are often able to review your work and direct you toward related instruments or literature.
- Start small. Successful completion of a pilot project is the best foundation for a larger study. Efficient use of small grant funding is influential when seeking larger-scale funding for major proposals.
- Be realistic. Design research projects that can be realistically accomplished within the scope of your other responsibilities and the limitations of your work setting.
- Keep focused on the patient. Design and implement research that is relevant to patient care and improves quality of life at the end of life for patients and families.

Source: Ferrell et al. (1989), reference 30.

the Oncology Nursing Foundation, depict the essential elements of a research proposal. Many professional organizations provide small grant support to novice investigators. Table 61–4 includes some general tips for preparing a research proposal.

Another useful guide for nurses initiating research proposals is included in Table 61–5. This includes the review considerations used by grant reviewers at the NIH. The five criteria of significance, approach, innovation, investigator, and environment can serve as a useful guide in designing research proposals.[17]

Several initiatives have begun to establish an agenda for palliative care research. Topics frequently identified as priority topics for palliative care research include pain, symptom management, epidemiological studies of terminal illness, family caregiver needs, bereavement, cultural considerations, spiritual needs, and health systems considerations such as costs of care.[4,25–27]

At the City of Hope, we have developed a framework of nine areas of palliative nursing care that is used in our nursing education efforts (see Chapter 59). Table 61–6 includes a summary of these nine topic areas, with examples of potential research that is needed.[28]

Another excellent resource for identifying future areas of palliative care research comes from the conference convened by the NINR described previously.[17] An excerpt of the Executive Summary from this NIH research workshop, which focused on symptom management in terminal illness, is included as Appendix 61–2, together with the specific recommendations from that conference, which identified research needs regarding the symptoms of pain, dyspnea, cognitive disturbances, and cachexia.[17]

Summary

Advances in the care of patients and families facing terminal illness is contingent on advances in palliative nursing research. Control of symptoms, comfort for families, and attention to psychosocial and spiritual needs will improve when nurse clinicians have a stronger scientific foundation for practice. Research will require collaboration with other disciplines and unity of nurse clinicians and researchers.

Table 61–5
Review Considerations for Research Sponsored by the National Institutes of Health

Significance

Does this study address an important problem? If the aims of the application are achieved, how will scientific knowledge be advanced? What will be the effect of these studies on the concepts or methods that drive this field?

Approach

Are the conceptual framework, design, methods, and analyses adequately developed, well integrated, and appropriate to the aims of the project? Does the applicant acknowledge potential problem areas and consider alternative tactics?

Innovation

Does the project employ novel concepts, approaches, or methods? Are the aims original and innovative? Does the project challenge existing paradigms or develop new methodologies or technologies?

Investigator

Is the investigator appropriately trained and well suited to carry out this work? Is the work proposed appropriate to the experience level of the principal investigator and other researchers (if any)?

Environment

Does the scientific environment in which the work will be done contribute to the probability of success? Do the proposed experiments take advantage of unique features of the scientific environment or employ useful collaborative arrangements? Is there evidence of institutional support?

Additional Considerations

In addition, the adequacy of plans to include both genders and minorities and their subgroups as appropriate for the scientific goals of the research are reviewed. Plans for the recruitment and retention of subjects is also evaluated.

Source: Adapted from reference 31 (2004).

APPENDIX 61–1

Two Examples of Qualitative Nursing Studies

Interaction Patterns Between Parents with Advanced Cancer and Their Children

Denice Sheehan, RN, MSN
Doctoral Dissertation, University of Akron and Kent State University

The purpose of this project is to develop a theoretical framework to describe interaction patterns between parents with advanced cancer and their children and to identify strategies that parents use to prepare their children for their lives after the parent's death. Most of the published literature about parents with cancer and their children focuses on psychosocial and emotional distress, functional changes within the family, and economic burdens. Few researchers have considered the end of life as an opportunity for growth and healing. Studies are needed to understand the process by which parents with advanced cancer interact with their children, a complex psychosocial process. Therefore, grounded theory methodology is used to develop a theoretical framework. A minimum of 30 participants are recruited. Parents with a diagnosis of advanced cancer who have children younger than 18 years of age are recruited from cancer centers, hospice programs, and support groups. The spouses and children of these informants are also invited to participate, because they are able to offer important perspectives on the ways in which the parent and child interact that may be unknown to the parent with cancer. The primary investigator conducts semi-structured interviews in a private room at the cancer center, hospice facility, or support group site. Findings from this study facilitate nurses to provide optimum support and communication to parents who are faced with the challenge of parenting children while living with their own impending death. Identification of these processes may also inform the development of nursing interventions aimed at assisting parents and children coping with advanced cancer.

Table 61–6
Potential Areas for Research in End-of-Life (EOL) Care

Critical Areas of End-of-Life Care	Examples of Area Content	Examples of Potential Areas of Inquiry
1. The Concept of Palliative Care	A. Importance of palliative care for nurses B. Definitions of palliative care C. Important goals/characteristics of palliative care: 1. Dignity/Respect 2. Relief of symptoms 3. Peaceful death 4. Ethical issues 5. Patient control/choices D. Importance of interdisciplinary collaboration E. Recognition of nurses' own discomfort/anxiety	• Refinement of definitions/criteria for palliative care • Descriptive studies of interdisciplinary involvement and related outcomes • Evaluation of methods to provide staff support in palliative care
2. Quality of Life (QOL) at the EOL	A. Recognition of multiple dimensions of QOL at the EOL 1. Physical well-being 2. Psychological well-being 3. Social well-being 4. Spiritual well-being	• Development/testing of QOL instruments for use in palliative care • Refinement of research methods to decrease patient burden in QOL assessment • Development/testing of QOL instruments for family caregivers
3. Pain Management at EOL	A. Definition of pain B. Assessment of pain C. Assessment of meaning of pain D. Pharmacological management of pain at EOL E. Use of invasive techniques F. Principles of addiction, tolerance, and dependence G. Nonpharmacological management of pain H. Physical pain vs. suffering I. Side effects of opioids J. Barriers to pain management K. Fear of opioids hastening death L. Equianalgesic dosing M. Recognition of nurses' own burden in pain management at EOL	• Methods of assessing pain in the nonverbal or confused patient • Refine methods for pain assessment to decrease patient burden • Development of pain measures that incorporate all dimensions of pain at EOL (e.g., spiritual pain) • Intervention studies to treat common pain syndromes at EOL • Testing of protocols to treat pain at EOL, including changing routes of analgesia • Development/evaluation of teaching programs for patients/families to decrease fears regarding pain management • Development/evaluation of programs to educate/support nurses in managing pain
4. Other Symptom Management at EOL	A. Assessment and management of common EOL symptoms 1. Dyspnea/cough 2. Nausea/vomiting 3. Dehydration/nutrition 4. Altered mental status/delirium/terminal restlessness 5. Anxiety/depression 6. Weakness/fatigue	• Descriptive studies to better understand symptom prevalence and patterns at EOL • Evaluation of pharmacologic treatments for each symptom • Development of patient/family caregiver education for symptom management, including pharmacological and nonpharmacological treatments

(*continued*)

Table 61–6
Potential Areas for Research in End-of-Life (EOL) Care *(continued)*

Critical Areas of End-of-Life Care	Examples of Area Content	Examples of Potential Areas of Inquiry
	7. Dysphagia 8. Incontinence 9. Skin integrity 10. Constipation/bowel obstruction 11. Agitation/myoclonus	• Evaluation of protocols/algorithms to enhance nurses' effectiveness in symptom assessment and management
5. Communication with Dying Patients and Families	A. Definition/goals of communication B. Importance of listening C. Barriers to communication D. Delivering bad news/truth-telling E. Recognizing family dynamics in communication F. Sensitivity to culture, ethnicity, values, and religion G. Discussion of options/decisions with patients/family H. Communication among interdisciplinary team members/collaboration I. Responding to requests for assisted suicide	• Descriptive studies to better determine common areas of concern regarding communication at EOL • Studies that describe the role of nursing in communication • Evaluation of protocols for delivering/ reinforcing bad news • Studies that explore cultural issues influencing communication • Evaluation of methods that support communication (e.g., written materials, family conferences) • Exploration of decision making by patients and family caregivers • Exploration of causes of requests for assisted suicide and preparation of nurses to respond to requests
6. Role/Needs of Family Caregivers in EOL Care	A. The importance of recognizing family and caregivers needs at EOL B. Assessment of family needs C. Family dynamics D. Recognizing ethical/cultural influences E. Coping strategies and support systems	• Descriptive studies to enhance understanding of the family caregiver perspective of terminal illness • Studies that explore family dynamics and the family as a unit rather than focus only on single caregivers • Exploratory studies to enhance understanding of cultural influences
7. Care at the Time of Death	A. The nurse's personal death awareness B. Death as natural process C. Recognizing signs/symptoms of impending death D. Patient/family's fears associated with death E. Preparing for the death event 1. Health care providers 2. Patient 3. Family caregivers F. Physical care at the time of death G. Spiritual care at the time of death	• Evaluation of educational/support approaches to enhance personal death awareness • Evaluation of teaching approaches to prepare families for impending death • Development and evaluation of protocols for care at the time of death—i.e., physical and spiritual care
8. Issues of Policy, Ethics, and Law	A. Patient preferences/advance directives B. Assisted suicide C. Euthanasia D. Withdrawing food/fluids E. Discontinuing life support	• Evaluation of approaches to enhance use of advance directives • Testing of educational methods to enhance nurses' ability to respond to requests for assisted suicide/euthanasia

(continued)

Table 61–6
Potential Areas for Research in End-of-Life (EOL) Care *(continued)*

Critical Areas of End-of-Life Care	Examples of Area Content	Examples of Potential Areas of Inquiry
	F. Legal issues at the EOL G. Need for changes in health policy H. Confidentiality	• Development and evaluation of protocols that promote patient comfort while discontinuing food/fluids and life support • Identification of legal and regulatory barriers to optimal EOL care
9. Bereavement	A. Stages/process of grief B. Assessment of grief C. Interventions/resources D. Recognition of staff grief	• Descriptive studies of grief by patients, families, and staff with attention to cultural considerations • Refinement of efficient methods of grief assessment • Testing of approaches to facilitate staff grieving

Meanings and Uses of an Expressed Desire for Hastened Death in People Living with Advanced Cancer

Nessa Coyle, PhD, RN, FAAN
Memorial Sloan-Kettering Cancer Center

An exploratory qualitative study, using an interpretive phenomenological approach, explored the impact of advanced cancer on seven individuals living with the disease. These individuals had received the majority of their care at an urban research cancer center and had expressed, at least once, a desire for hastened death.[32] The hypothesis was that by providing an individual the space to talk about his or her lived experience through a series of in-depth, semistructured interviews, the grounds for the expression of desire for hastened death for that individual would be uncovered. A total of 25 interviews were held.

Through an interpretive analysis of the narratives of the seven individuals, four themes and two overarching themes were identified. The four themes were "Listen to Me," in which the participants described their relationships to the health care system; "Who Am I Now and Where Do I Belong," in which the participants dealt with changes in themselves and their place in the world; "Up Against the Wall—There Is No Way to Live with Such Pain," in which the participants described their experiences with excruciating or chronically uncontrolled pain; and "The Existential Slap," the moment of realization by the participants that death was imminent. The two overarching themes were "The Hard Work of Living in the Face of Death" and the "Existential Paradox"—that is, that although the participants had expressed at least once a desire for death, what they were seeking was life.

The overarching themes appeared to capture the paradox of an expressed desire for hastened death and informed the interpretive analysis of the narratives—that an expressed desire for hastened death in these participants was a tool of communication reflecting:

1. A manifestation of the will to live
2. That the dying process itself was so difficult that an early death was preferred
3. That the immediate situation was untenable and required immediate action
4. That a hastened death was an option to extract oneself from an unendurable situation
5. A manifestation of the last control the dying can exert
6. A way of drawing attention to "me as a unique individual"
7. A gesture of altruism
8. Manipulation of the family in order to avoid abandonment
9. A despairing cry depicting the misery of the current situation

The overall interpretation was that an expressed desire for hastened death in these individuals was not a literal request for death but a tool of communication to get needs met.

APPENDIX 61–2
NIH Research Workshop on Symptoms in Terminal Illness—Executive Summary

Patients at the end of life experience many of the same symptoms and syndromes, regardless of their underlying medical condition. Pain is the most obvious example, but others are difficult breathing (dyspnea), transient episodes of confusion and loss of concentration (cognitive disturbances and delirium), and loss of appetite and muscle wasting (cachexia), as well as nausea, fatigue, and depression. Taken together, these and other symptoms add significantly to the suffering of patients and their families, and to the costs and burden of their medical care. Yet in many cases the symptoms could be treated or prevented.

Pain, for example, is a multibillion-dollar public health problem in the United States. More than half of all cancer patients experience pain related to their disease or its treatment. Similarly, half of all cancer patients and 70% of all hospice patients experience shortness of breath in the last weeks of life. Yet dyspnea remains underdiagnosed and undertreated. Forty percent of all patients experience cognitive disturbances during the final days of life, and high numbers of terminally ill patients experience cachexia regardless of their primary disease. Significantly, these symptoms occur not in isolation but in clusters, with most patients experiencing combinations of symptoms that vary greatly in their prevalence and severity, as well as in the suffering they cause.

Basic research has improved understanding of the underlying mechanisms of symptoms that are commonly experienced at the end of life, particularly with respect to pain. Clinical research has in some cases translated this knowledge into new drugs and other interventions that can effectively relieve or prevent these symptoms, even if the underlying disease cannot be cured. At present, however, there remain a number of important gaps in knowledge.

Clinical care would benefit from an integrative, multidisciplinary research initiative that brings basic and clinical researchers together to address the constellation of symptoms at the end of life. The following areas should receive priority:

- Epidemiology—There is a need for better data on the incidence and combinations of symptoms that are experienced at the end of life in specific populations. Epidemiological data will demonstrate the magnitude and costs of the problem and suggest specific topics for basic and clinical research.
- Basic research—Additional research is needed on the mechanisms and interactions of these symptoms, including biochemical, neuronal, endocrine, and immune approaches. The possibility of common factors, mechanisms, and pathways across different symptoms should be examined. There is also a need for research on the mechanism of action of successful therapies, with particular attention to the role of opioid receptors. This research could lead to therapies that are better targeted and more selective in their action, and thus produce fewer side effects.
- Clinical research—Because these symptoms have multiple determinants, and occur in clusters, successful interventions will also be multifactorial, including behavioral as well as pharmacological approaches. Combination therapies and off-label drugs should be explored. Researchers should be alert to differences in outcome based on age, gender, and underlying disease. Interventions to mobilize psychosocial and spiritual resources may be of help in mediating the perception and interpretation of symptoms. The goal of research should be to test a wide range of interventions that could be successfully implemented in the home or hospice, as well as in the hospital.
- Methodology—Researchers need better tests for diagnosing and assessing the level of severity of these symptoms, as well as for monitoring the effectiveness of interventions. Standardized terminology and definitions of symptoms should be established. Particular attention should be paid to validating subjective and nonverbal measures. Better data and tools are also needed for evaluating outcomes, in order to determine costs and strengthen accountability for the quality of care at the end of life. It is important to develop and use measures that reflect the subjective experience of the effects of symptoms on quality of life.

Research is also needed on the ethical issues that may be barriers to research at the end of life, including the needs and protection of vulnerable populations, especially the role of privacy during this important phase of life. Attention must be paid to community and individual preferences about the relative value of symptom management at different points in the dying trajectory, and to the development of comprehensive strategies for early detection and treatment of the full range of symptoms at the end of life—an approach that will reduce costs as well as burdens, while preserving the patient's dignity and quality of life.

Recommendations for Research on Specific Symptoms

The following preamble for the recommendations reflected the consensus of the entire workshop:

> To adequately address symptom control in the terminally ill, an important first step is to invest resources in the development of new methodologies for assessing symptoms and evaluating treatments. These tools will allow us to elucidate the extent of the problem and to set national priorities to improve quality of life for those facing life-limiting illness.

Pain

1. Epidemiology—There is still a great need for epidemiological data on the incidence and types of pain at the end of life. Research in this area will provide direction for researchers regarding what specific topics should be tackled next.
2. Treatment—There is a clear need to discover new drugs for the treatment of pain, including analgesic combinations. Neuropathic pain, because of its incidence and burden, should be a particular priority. There should also be studies of the relationship between disease, pain, and suffering at the end of

life, which would also include psychosocial mediators. Clinical Trials Groups should be developed to study promising interventions.

3. Measurement—Methods should be developed for collecting valid data on pain in the home, in nursing homes, and so on, possibly using telephones or computer technology. Measurement of other outcomes of subjective experience, such as the suffering caused by pain, should also be developed and utilized.

Dyspnea

1. Epidemiology—What are the incidence and impact of dyspnea in different populations? There is some information about dyspnea in patients with cancer or chronic obstructive pulmonary disease (COPD), but almost none about patients with cardiac disease or other terminal conditions.
2. Mechanisms—Relatively little is known about the various determinants of dyspnea, including respiratory muscle strength, exercise capacity, respiratory controller, gas exchange, and psychosocial factors. Neurobiological models, like those developed for pain, will be useful, but the overall approach must be integrative. The determinants are almost certainly multifactorial, necessitating multidisciplinary strategies.
3. Measurement—Research is needed to refine available instruments and develop new ones for measuring both the causes of symptoms and the effects of treatments. There is at present no standardized approach for assessing the degree of dyspnea in a given disease (e.g., chronic vs. acute, COPD vs. cancer). The goal would be to formulate guidelines for optimal assessment, which would point to optimal treatment.
4. Treatment—A number of potential treatments are available, but there is little information on their relative effectiveness. Particular attention should be given to the choice and timing of anxiolytics, phenothiazines, oxygen, opiates, and exercise. Attention should also be given to the timing and management of terminal weaning (removal of ventilation), including the role of families.

The collaborative and integrative nature of this research is well suited to sponsorship and funding by NIH. It would be useful, for example, for the various NIH Institutes to sponsor a series of joint workshops that would characterize the clinical experience and impact of therapies on dyspnea in diseases other than lung cancer.

Cognitive Disturbances

There is a considerable amount of epidemiological data on delirium already, and although it might be useful to gather additional information on specific patient populations, this symptom is known to be under recognized and under treated. Consequently, the research priorities in this symptom area are as follows:

1. Measurement—Research is needed to enhance the recognition of delirium in different treatment settings (homes, hospices, hospitals), including common diagnostic criteria and terminology. Also needed are better instruments to describe and rate the severity and course of episodes of delirium. This research will lead to a better understanding of the phenomenology of delirium—its signs, patterns, and subtypes—which in turn should produce benefits in terms of newer, more sensitive, and more effective treatments.
2. Treatment—Two aspects of treatment research deserve simultaneous attention. First, there should be randomized, placebo-controlled trials to systematically assess the efficacy of currently available therapies as well as emerging approaches, including both pharmacological and nonpharmacological strategies. Second, there should be research on the relation between the mechanism of action of these therapies and the underlying pathophysiology of delirium. In both cases, studies should include both random populations and populations with delirium of homogeneous etiology.
3. Epidemiology—Finally, there is a need for additional research on the interactions between delirium and other symptoms at the end of life.

A concurrent policy issue that must also receive priority attention is the need for guidelines for research in patients who are incapable of giving informed consent because of serious medical illness.

Cachexia

1. Epidemiology—High priority should go to epidemiological studies of anorexia-cachexia, to establish the magnitude of the problem, its impact on the patient and family, and its costs to society. However, it is important that cachexia not be studied in isolation from other symptoms. If the ultimate goal of cachexia research is prevention and early intervention, then it would be useful to conduct studies that examine the epidemiology of several related symptoms (e.g., pain, dyspnea, delirium) at an earlier stage in their development.
2. Mechanisms—Basic and clinical research on cachexia should be done in parallel. Basic research should emphasize the interactions among multiple underlying pathophysiological mechanisms, both central and peripheral, including biochemical, neuronal, metabolic, endocrine, and immunological.

Research is also needed on the varying clinical manifestations of these mechanisms, both neuropsychiatric and gastrointestinal. This calls for a multidisciplinary approach.

3. Treatment—Similarly, because it is unlikely that any single therapeutic intervention will be successful, clinical research should emphasize multiple combination therapies that include nutritional, pharmacological, and nonpharmacological components. Combination therapies should be evaluated for their effects on other symptoms such as pain, dyspnea, and delirium. Particular attention should also be paid to differences in outcome based on age, gender, and underlying disease. In considering drug trials, NIH should concentrate on studies that would not otherwise be funded by drug companies.

Given the wide range of mechanisms and therapeutic strategies in cachexia, it would be useful to convene a preliminary, integrative workshop that would include both basic and clinical researchers

Cross-Cutting Recommendations

Methods issues that need to be addressed in all four symptom areas include the following:

1. Statistical handling of missing data.
2. Proxy reporting for subjective symptoms.
3. Outcome measures that indicate quality care.
4. Ethics issues are also important. What are the barriers to research at the end of life, including the needs and expectations of vulnerable populations? What are community and individual preferences with respect to symptom management of dying persons?
5. Economics questions include the direct and indirect costs and burdens of symptoms.

REFERENCES

1. Field M, Cassel C. Approaching death: Improving care at the end of life. Committee on Care at the End of Life. Washington, DC: Institutes of Medicine, National Academy Press, 1997.
2. Field MJ, Behrman DE. When Children Die: Improving Care at the End of Life. Washington, DC: Institute of Medicine, National Academy Press, 2003.
3. Jennings B, Ryndes T, D'Onofrio C, Baily MA. Access to Hospice Care: Expanding Boundaries, Overcoming Barriers. Hasting Center Report 2003; Supplement 33(2).
4. Corner J. Is there a research paradigm for palliative care? Palliat Med 1996;10:201–208.
5. Hearn J, Higginson IJ. Outcome measures in palliative care for advanced cancer patients: A review. J Public Health Med 1997; 19:193–199.
6. Pickett M, Cooley ME, Gordon DB. Palliative care: Past, present, and future perspectives. Semin Oncol Nurs 1998;14:86–94.
7. Richards MA, Corner J, Clark D. Developing a research culture for palliative care. Palliat Med 1998;12:399–403.
8. Kristjanson LJ, Coyle N. Qualitative research. In: Doyle D, Hanks G, Cherny N, Calman K, eds. Oxford Textbook of Palliative Medicine, 3rd ed. Oxford: Oxford University Press, 2004: 138–144.
9. Ferrell BR, Funk B. Hospice research. In: Sheehan DC, Forman WB, eds. Hospice and Palliative Care. Sudbury, MA: Jones and Bartlett, 1996;167–174.
10. Change E, Daly J. Priority areas for clinical research in palliative care nursing. Int J Nurs Pract 1998;4:247–253.
11. King CR, Hinds PS, eds. Quality of Life from Nursing and Patient Perspectives, 2nd ed. Sudbury, MA: Jones and Bartlett, 2003.
12. Dawson S, Kristjanson LJ. Mapping the journey: Family carers' perceptions of issues related to end-stage care of individuals with muscular dystrophy or motor neurone disease. J Palliat Care 2003;19:36–42.
13. Patterson LB, Dorfman LT. Family support for hospice caregivers. Am J Hospice Palliat Care 2002;139(5 Pt 2):410–415.
14. Brazil K, Bedard M, Willison K, Hode M. Caregiving and its impact on families of the terminally ill. Aging Ment Health 2003; 7:376–382.
15. Benoliel JQ. Death influence in clinical practice: A course for graduate students. In: Benoliel JC, ed. Death Education for the Health Professional. Washington, DC: Hemisphere Publishing, 1982;31–50.
16. Benoliel JQ. Health care providers and dying patients: Critical issues in terminal care. Omega 1987;18:341–363.
17. National Institutes of Health. Symptoms in Terminal Illness: A Research Workshop. September 22–23, 1997. Available at: http://www.nih.gov/ninr/end-of-life.htm (accessed March 1, 2005).
18. Casarett D, Ferrell B, Kirschling J, Levetown M, Merriman MP, Ramey M, Silverman P. NHCPO Tast Force Statement on the Ethics of Hospice Participation in Research. J Palliat Med 2001; 4:441–449.
19. Cohen SR, Mount BM. Quality of life in terminal illness: Defining and measuring subjective well being in the dying. J Palliat Care 1992;8:40–45.
20. American Geriatric Society Panel on Chronic Pain in Older Persons. AGS Clinical Guidelines: Management of Persistent Pain in Older Persons. 2002. Available at: http://www.americangeriatrics.org/education/executive_summ.shtml (accessed March 22, 2005).
21. Calman K, MacDonald N, et al. Ethical issues. In: Doyle D, Hanks G, Cherny N, Calman K, eds. Oxford Textbook of Palliative Medicine. Oxford: Oxford University Press, 2004:55–97.
22. Rinck GC, van den Bos GA, Kleijnan J, de Haes HJ, Schade E, Veenhof CH. Methodological issues in effectiveness research on palliative cancer care: A systematic review. J Clin Oncol 1997; 15:1697–1707.
23. Boult L, Dentler B, Volicer L, Mead S, Evans JM; Ethics Committee of the American Medical Directors Association. Position Statement: Ethics and Research in Long-Term Care. J Am Med Dir Assoc 2003;4:171–174.
24. Clark D. What is qualitative research and what can it contribute to palliative care? Palliat Med 1997;11:159–166.
25. Dudgeon DJ, Raubertas RF, Doerner K, O'Connor T, Robin M, Rosenthal SN. When does palliative care begin? A needs assessment of cancer patients with recurrent disease. J Palliat Care 1995;11:5–9.
26. Smith TJ, Coyne P, Cassel B, Penberthy L, Lopson A, Hager MA. A high-volume specialist palliative care unit and team may

reduce in-hospital end-of-life care costs. J Palliat Med 2003;6: 699–705.
27. Lynn J, Nolan K, Kabcenell A, Wessman D, Milne C, Berwick DM; End-of-Life Care Consensus Panel. Reforming care for persons near the end of life: The promise of quality improvement. Ann Intern Med 2002;137:117–122.
28. Ferrell BR, Virani R, Grant M. Analysis of end of life content in nursing textbooks. Oncol Nurs Forum 1999;26:869–876.
29. Doyle D, Hanks G, Cherny N, Calman K, eds. Oxford Textbook of Palliative Medicine, 3rd ed. Oxford: Oxford University Press, 2004.
30. Ferrell BR, Nail IM, Mooney K, et al. Applying for Oncology Nursing Society and Oncology Nursing Foundation grants. Oncol Nurs Forum 1989;16:728–730.
31. NIH announces updated criteria for evaluating research grant applications. Notice Number: NOT-OD-05-002. October 12, 2004. Available at: http://grants.nih.gov/grants/guide/notice-files/NOT-OD-05-002.html (accessed March 22, 2005).
32. Coyle, N. Expressed desire for hastened death in a select group of patients living with advanced cancer: a phenomenological inquiry. Dissertation Abstracts International 2004;63–11B:5156.

IX

Models of Excellence and Innovative Community Projects

62

Ira Byock and Jeanne Twohig

Delivering Palliative Care in Challenging Settings and to Hard-to-Reach Populations

I told him "I love you. Thank you. You can go. I love you." And then he died. It was perfect. It was everything we had done. It was like music ending.—Family member of a patient served by The Comprehensive Care Team, a project of the University of California San Francisco School of Medicine

- ***Key Points***
- *Although high-quality hospice programs represent the gold standard of palliative care, they are often underutilized by or unavailable to special patient populations, prompting consideration of new models of delivering palliative care.*
- *A broad quality improvement strategy emerged in the late 1990s, including new delivery models that offer palliative care simultaneously with cure-oriented care to patients and families.*
- *There are discernible programmatic elements, clinical components, and educational strategies that lead to strong, successful, sustainable palliative care programs.*
- *Preliminary data from The Robert Wood Johnson Foundation's* Promoting Excellence in End-of-Life Care *demonstration projects suggests that the concurrent provision of life-prolonging care and palliative care is feasible, clinically effective, embraced by patients and families, and associated with system efficiencies.*

High-quality hospice programs represent a gold standard for comprehensive care for people who are dying. In the United States, hospice use has increased among cancer patients and other defined patient groups. However, even the most innovative hospice organizations meet barriers in attempting to serve patient populations in acute care hospitals, particularly academic research and teaching hospitals, and in highly technical environments such as renal dialysis units and intensive care units. Hospice is also challenged to deliver care in geographically isolated rural communities and for socioeconomically isolated populations served by "safety net" facilities, such as impoverished inner-city residents, military veterans, and prison inmates.

A Strategic Direction

Clinicians, health care administrators, payers, and consumers all have vested interests in redesigning health care systems to respond to the suffering experienced by patients with advanced, incurable illness. Recognizing the need in the United States for innovative models for delivering palliative care to these underserved patient populations, during the late 1990s clinicians and researchers embarked on strategic efforts to improve care through the end of life, supported by government and private philanthropies. Cognizant of the complexity of achieving necessary systemic and cultural change, they employed a multifaceted approach that simultaneously targeted a range of leverage points (Table 62–1).

This broad quality improvement strategy has at its heart a commitment to position patients and families at the center of the health care goals. Components of this strategic approach include efforts to elucidate clinical practice standards and domains of quality for palliative care, as well as clinician training curricula and continuing education that encompasses the full breadth of patient and family experience and palliative

Table 62–1
A Strategic Plan For Improving Palliative and End-of-Life Care Standards

Education
Measurement
Continuous quality improvement
Accreditation oversight and accountability
Research and development
Public support and stakeholder expectations
Public policy, legislation, reimbursement, and regulation

Source: Byock I. Dying Well in America: What Would Success Look Like? Paper presented at the Leverage Points: A Report Based on the Second Last Acts National Leadership Conference, October 29–30, 1997.

care practice. The strategy also includes development of measurement tools and methodologies applicable to clinician skills, quality of care, and health service delivery that are capable of not only distinguishing the adequate from inadequate, but also the excellent from the merely mediocre. These measurement tools can be applied to performance and outcomes evaluation and to relevant oversight, certification, and accreditation processes. The strategy further calls for research and development of demonstration projects to build and assess innovative models of care delivery. In order for advances in quality and delivery of care to be successfully applied, changes in public policy, health care regulations, and reimbursement are needed. The strategic approach entails public education to raise awareness, along with citizen advocacy and consumer pressure supported by meaningful data on access, quality, and costs of care.

This chapter focuses on the research and development component that creates and tests new models of care delivery, drawing on the experience of a variety of innovative service delivery models developed with support from The Robert Wood Johnson Foundation's *Promoting Excellence in End-of-Life Care* program. These demonstration projects offer programmatic prototypes for delivering palliative care to hard-to-reach patient populations and in challenging clinical settings. These models are designed to offer seriously ill patients and their family members coordinated and continuous attention to their psychosocial and spiritual needs, as well as their physical needs, provided by a skilled team. These characteristics are key principles of palliative care.[1–3]

Unmet Expectations and an Unnecessary Dichotomy

Recent studies indicate an incongruity between what seriously ill people feel is most important and what the current American health care system provides. In qualitative research involving seriously ill patients and recently bereaved family members, as well as experienced clinicians, Steinhauser and colleagues[4] found that patients and their families value pain and symptom management, clear decision-making, preparation for death and life completion, a sense of contributing to others, and affirmation of the patient as a whole person. Similarly, a qualitative study by Wenrich and associates[5] concluded that patients and families value clinicians who talk in honest, straightforward ways about their patients' conditions and who can sensitively break bad news without shirking discussions about death. They want clinicians who encourage questions and are sensitive to when patients are ready to talk about death. Although these values and expectations are reasonable, they are not consistently achieved.

Thirty years ago, life-prolonging and palliative treatments seemed clearly distinct. Advances in the physiology and pharmacology of treatment, particularly in the fields of oncology, cardiology, pulmonology, and neurology, have progressively blurred distinctions between treatments intended to prolong life and those intended to improve a patient's comfort and quality of life. The familiar diagrams in Figure 62–1 illustrate, first, the current dichotomy between life-prolonging and palliative care that results in a sequential model of care, wherein palliative care is initiated only when curative treatment is abandoned. There is broad agreement that a concurrent approach, with palliative care introduced at diagnosis and extended through the course of treatment, decline, death, and grief, would better respond to the needs of seriously ill patients and their families.

In theory, concurrent care should align health service delivery with contemporary clinical realities and the real needs of chronically ill patients and their families. New models of delivering palliative care are emerging to build and test this vision.

Figure 62–1. Comparison of sequential versus integrated models of end-of-life care.

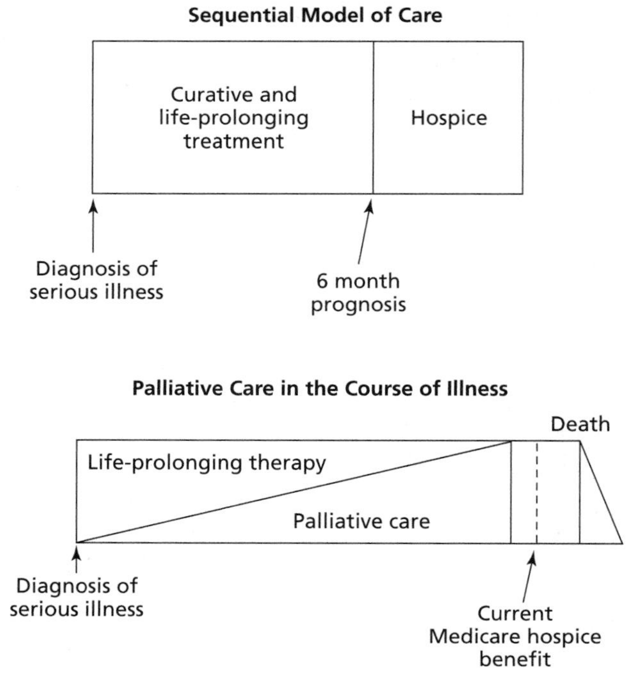

Promoting Excellence in End-of-Life Care: Building Models to Translate Theory into Practice

The Robert Wood Johnson Foundation's *Promoting Excellence in End-of-Life Care* program was created in 1997 to provide grant support and technical assistance to clinician-researchers for development of innovative ways of extending comprehensive, patient- and family-centered palliative care to those living with progressive, incurable conditions, regardless of diagnosis, prognosis, age, socioeconomic status, or venue of care. *Promoting Excellence* sought to identify patient populations and clinical settings in which hospice care was underutilized or unavailable. Setting the best hospice programs and care as gold standards, the *Promoting Excellence* program intended to extend palliative care upstream in the course of illness, concurrent with ongoing life-extending care. Many of the projects collaborated with local hospice programs, and most projects developed a continuum of services that included referral to hospice.

The more than 25 projects were awarded *Promoting Excellence in End-of-Life Care* grants, representing a broad range of patient populations and contexts of care. This diverse array of demonstration projects involved four university cancer centers, tertiary care pediatric hospitals, critical care units in four academic medical centers, a regional set of renal dialysis clinics, and hospice and home health agencies within highly penetrated managed care environments. Several programs served inner-city residents, and others served rural and frontier communities, including projects focused on Native American and Alaska Native populations. Other programs were designed for elderly residents in nursing homes, patients with dementia cared for in a geriatric specialty clinics, and hospice programs based in penitentiaries in four states.

The purpose of building prototypical programmatic models was to determine the feasibility of providing palliative care within these challenging contexts of care and to these patient populations. Demonstration projects represent applied research, the translation of theory into practice, which provides tangible evidence of what is possible—and what is not—from the perspective of provider organizations, clinicians, and the people being served. Prototype projects generate valuable information regarding whether and how well services are valued by the intended population. Successful health service prototypes have potential to stimulate improvements beyond local systems and communities, raising collective expectations and challenging administrators, health planners, and public policy-makers to consider new approaches to existing problems and to aim for higher outcomes than they otherwise might have thought possible.

Elements of Successful Delivery Models

Analysis of prototypical models indicates that there are discernible elements that, when included in the program design, lead to strong, successful, and sustainable programs for delivery of palliative care (Table 62–2). Clinician-researchers have learned that innovative palliative care programs must be anchored in the institution's and local health system's core mission and that *aligning the program with the organizational mission* results in increased receptivity for the initiative by

Table 62–2
Essential Ingredients for Building Successful Palliative Care Programs

A well defined vision that

- Advances the institution's mission
- Encompasses a comprehensive definition of palliative care

A well-planned implementation strategy that is

- Manageable in scope
- Consistent with available human and financial resources

Unwavering support from clinical and administrative leaders willing to

- Champion the program
- Help secure operational resources

Ongoing efforts to bridge the differences between palliative and acute care clinical cultures that

- Entail learning on both sides
- Integrate experienced staff with diverse expertise, including psychosocial and spiritual care

A focus on making "the right way the easy way" by

- Responding to workday needs of time-pressured clinicians and staff
- Redesigning operations to embed and trigger palliative practices in daily routines

Ongoing education, support, and attention to team building for clinicians and system personnel to

- Ease adoption of innovation
- Strengthen clinical interventions

Authority to write orders or working relationship with primary physicians that ensures that palliative care team recommendations are routinely followed

Attention to diverse ethnic and religious cultures of individual patients and families through

- Sensitivity to the uniqueness of individuals and their preferences
- Careful selection of language to convey program elements

A forum for clinicians to discuss problems and ideas for improvement, and safe havens to discuss their feelings associated with providing care for seriously ill patients and their families through death and grief

Targeted data collection focusing on

- Increased access to palliative care
- Improved quality of care
- Resource utilization and cost
- Patient/family/clinician satisfaction

A communications strategy for succinctly presenting relevant data to stakeholders institutional decision-makers. Programs must be *manageable in scope*, allowing nascent initiatives to achieve early successes and earn support from recognized leaders in both clinical and administrative realms. Palliative care teams are more readily integrated into the institution's clinical practice if they are able to *improve the workflow of time-pressured clinicians*, assisting them in addressing patients' and families' psychosocial needs and the personal ramifications of their patients' life-compromising illness. Successful interdisciplinary teams are able to *embed palliative care into routine operations* and have *authority to carry out their recommendations* and interventions for patient care. They earn the confidence of colleagues by skillfully and reliably caring for difficult, complex cases.

In addition to focusing on clinical aspects of integrating palliative care and cure-oriented treatment, sustainable programs *develop business plans* that address economic aspects of operations and service delivery. They also *develop communication plans* that convey cohesive messages, including *salient data* to patients, families, clinicians, health system managers, administrators, and policy-makers about the availability and benefits of palliative care services.

Project Safe Conduct

Project Safe Conduct is a collaborative effort of the Ireland Cancer Center (ICC) and Hospice of the Western Reserve (HWR), both based in Cleveland, Ohio. ICC is a National Cancer Institute designated comprehensive cancer center, and HWR is an independent community-based hospice. Their collaboration exemplifies a model that incorporates these elements into their program design and implementation. The goal of Project Safe Conduct, to create a seamless transition of care for persons with advanced cancer and their families in the ambulatory cancer setting by integrating principles of palliative care, was clearly defined at the onset. The program was initially limited to patients with stage IIIB and IV lung cancer to allow clinician-researchers to test and refine the model with a discrete patient population before considering inclusion of a larger patient group. The project was staunchly supported by administrative and clinical leaders from both institutions, as evidenced by the ICC director's unprecedented decision to close the cancer clinic to enable clinical staff to attend a day-long retreat to discuss and launch Project Safe Conduct.

The Safe Conduct team, comprised of an advanced practice nurse, a social worker, and a spiritual care provider, represents both acute care and hospice care backgrounds. The team was employed by HWR but physically located within ICC, to reinforce the integration of the palliative care team with the cancer care team. The staffing design reflected the belief that care of cancer patients should be managed and supported by their primary oncologist and that oncologists and their patients can benefit from the support and counsel of trained palliative care professionals. Project leadership implemented extensive cross-training to bridge the differing medical cultures of oncology and palliative care and to provide ongoing support to the teams. Interdisciplinary discussions were regularly scheduled to allow a safe haven for conversation among clinicians about issues of death and dying and the quality of the patient's and family's experiences.[6]

Safe Conduct leaders crafted an evaluation plan to collect process and outcome data to assess the impact of the project on the accessibility of palliative care for patients and families; the quality of the care as perceived by patients, families, and clinicians; and resource utilization. Clinician-researchers were able to demonstrate improved pain and symptom management, increased hospice referrals and hospice lengths of stay, diminished hospitalizations, and decreased pharmaceutical costs. These data proved convincing to administrators, who decided to expand Safe Conduct beyond lung cancer patients, extending the service to those with gastrointestinal cancer and other advanced malignancies (see detailed discussion of Project Safe Conduct in Chapter 64).

Clinical Components of Delivery Models

Regardless of the diverse clinical settings in which *Promoting Excellence* projects were created, the clinician-researchers directing these innovative palliative care programs recognized the importance of articulating *whom* the palliative care program was designed to serve, *what* the service package entailed, *where* the services were to be provided, and by *whom.*

Identifying Patients Appropriate for Palliative Care

Promoting Excellence palliative care programs primarily sought to serve seriously ill patients who were of "prehospice" status by current insurance or Medicare criteria but were likely to benefit from the simultaneous provision of disease-modifying treatment and palliative care. At entry into these programs, patients' prognoses were longer than 6 months and/or their mindsets were oriented toward living as long as possible. Clinicians evaluating the benefits of palliative care for a given patient often considered what is termed the "surprise question": "Would you be surprised if this patient died within the next year"?[7] Alternatively, they screened for patients' health service utilization patterns, looking for events such as recurrent hospitalizations and emergency department visits, to identify those who might benefit from typical palliative care services of care management, care coordination, anticipatory guidance, and crisis prevention.

Promoting Excellence projects offer examples of various patient accrual methods, each unique to the goals, parameters, and venues of its particular palliative care program:

- The University of Pennsylvania School of Nursing, in collaboration with Genesis ElderCare, a national nursing home corporation, developed a palliative care assessment tool to identify patients in participating nursing homes who were appropriate for palliative care.

- The Veterans Administration Greater Los Angeles Health Care System used clinical triggers as eligibility criteria to identify patients with lung cancer, congestive heart failure, or chronic obstructive pulmonary disease, who were appropriate for palliative care.[8]
- The CHOICES program of Sutter Visiting Nurse Association and Hospice in northern California developed non-prognosis-based eligibility criteria focusing on diagnosis, clinical state, and utilization patterns. These criteria were designed to identify patients of higher acuteness who had late-stage chronic illnesses but did not necessarily fit the terminal criteria for hospice enrollment.[9]

Palliative Care Services

Comprehensive palliative care programs strive to deliver state-of-the-art clinical care to both patients and their families, with a commitment to respecting the cultural, ethnic, religious, and personal values of those they serve (Table 62–3). The programs emphasize clear communication with patients and families through clinical protocols, education, and quality improvement. Crisis prevention and early crisis management are common components of care planning and practice. Some member of the team who is familiar with the patient and family and knowledgeable about the plan of care is available around the clock. Symptom management for both physical pain and psychosocial distress is conducted in a comprehensive and assertive manner. Symptom management plans are frequently updated to reflect the changing condition of the patient and family. Supportive counseling with patients and families regarding issues of life completion and closure is part of routine anticipatory guidance for these inherently difficult but normal tasks. Families are routinely offered bereavement support after the death of their loved one.[10]

Table 62–3
Typical Services of Palliative Care

Ongoing communication and review of goals of care
Advanced care planning
Formal symptom assessment and treatment
Care coordination
Spiritual care and attention to psychosocial needs
Anticipatory guidance related to adaptation to illness and issues of life completion and life closure
Crisis prevention and early crisis management
Bereavement support
24/7 availability by a familiar and knowledgeable clinician

Palliative Care Personnel

Comprehensive palliative care programs designed to reach patient populations in challenging settings usually have interdisciplinary teams modeled after the structure of hospice clinical teams. These teams frequently include a physician with expertise in palliative care, a specially trained palliative care advanced practice nurse, a social worker, and a pastoral or spiritual care counselor. Core teams are often enhanced by ancillary team members such as psychologists; pharmacists; pain specialists; physical, occupational, and respiratory therapists; and professionals trained in the therapeutic use of art and music. Together with patients and families, these interdisciplinary teams create multifaceted, individualized plans of care that reflect the patient's and family's values and personal preferences.

A near-universal feature of palliative care programs is the presence of one or more "case managers" or "care coordinators." This position is often recognized by team members as a linchpin for ensuring ongoing monitoring of a patient's condition and family living situation, assisting with pragmatic issues of access to needed health services, and coordinating consultations and referrals for both life-prolonging and palliative treatments. The care coordinator oversees the implementation of the plan of care developed by the interdisciplinary team, monitors the patient's and family's status, and typically leads development of a crisis prevention and management plan.

In non–hospital-based programs, interdisciplinary palliative care teams receive medical direction in a variety of ways, often based on the venue of care, the proximity of the primary provider, and the culture of the local institutional and health community. The goal is to provide appropriate care for each patient and family while preserving, to the extent each desires, the relationships between patients and their physicians. To do so, teams must determine the role that each patient's primary care physician expects and ascertain each physician's level of familiarity and comfort with palliative care.

In many practice settings, it is advantageous for the palliative care team to have authority to write orders for diagnostic tests, to adjust medications, and to initiate treatments in accordance with the interdisciplinary plan of care. Some programs reflect a co-management model, wherein the palliative care team assumes primary management in communication and coordination with the patients' primary care providers. In other programs, the primary care physician continues to write orders and prescribe medications, but the recommendations of the palliative care team are routinely incorporated into the patient's overall plan of care. An example of this approach is offered by the Comprehensive Care Team at the University of California San Francisco, where the interdisciplinary team, including a palliative care physician, develops palliative care treatment plans that are then formally recommended to the primary care provider for implementation.[11]

Other palliative care programs provide training in palliative care to the medical specialists who serve as patients' primary

Table 62–4
Overview of Promoting Excellence Models

Project	Institution/Venue	Overview	Patient Identification	Staffing	Services
Helping Hands "Ikayurtem Unatai"	Bristol Bay Area Health Corporation, Dillingham, Alaska Frontier location Home health based	Based in home health service in Dillingham, extending to 32 remote Alaskan villages via training of community health aides in palliative care (PC), using existing health delivery and community for support	Patients of all ages and diagnoses with advanced illness who are likely to die within 2 years	Primary physician in Dillingham oversees plan of care Home health RN/PC coordinator and volunteer coordinator visit the villages Community health aides, family aides and community volunteers in villages All receive PC training	Assessment visit and ongoing visits by RN/PC Coordinator Development of PC plan of care Pain and symptom management, medical and psychosocial Culturally sensitive volunteer support Ongoing community health aide visits
Project Safe Conduct	Collaboration between Ireland Cancer Center (ICC) and Hospice of the Western Reserve (HWR)	Seamless transition from curative care to PC to end-of-life care for patients with advanced lung cancer by integrating a hospice-like team into the care delivered at a cancer center	All patients newly referred to ICC with stage IIIB & IV lung cancer, and those receiving chemotherapy or radiation therapy	Patient's medical oncologist oversees medical management Safe Conduct Team (SCT): advanced practice nurse, social worker, spiritual counselor Additional team members: pain consultant, psychologist	SCT and primary oncologist address physical, psychosocial, spiritual, and economic dimensions of care SCT follows patients/families through therapies SCT assessment provides pain and symptom management in conjunction with hospice medical director and primary oncologist Advanced care planning Psychosocial counseling and life closure discussions Referrals to community services Bereavement support
Palliative Care in Nursing Homes	University of Pennsylvania School of Nursing Genesis ElderCare Six rural and urban Genesis-owned nursing homes in Maryland	Infuse PC practices into the nursing home culture by training and supporting staff in PC concepts and practices and developing a nursing home–based interdisciplinary team	Any resident is considered a potential PC beneficiary Patients are offered PC based on PC assessment and chart review by trained staff	PC nurse consultant trains nursing home staff, provides consultations, assists with plan of care development and problem resolution Nursing home medical director provides oversight All nursing home staff reflect PC ideals	Screening for appropriateness for PC Assessment and management of symptoms, with approval of primary physician and involvement of nurse consultant Advanced care planning with patients and families

providers. This model has been effective with disease-based palliative care programs, such as the Renal Palliative Care Initiative at Baystate Medical Center in Springfield, Massachusetts, where nephrologists and dialysis unit staff, who had established relationships with the patients, became trained in palliative care.

Palliative care teams can extend their ability to meet patient and family needs by integrally involving volunteers in a variety of supportive capacities, as was evidenced by several *Promoting Excellence* grantees:

- Staff at Cooper Green Hospital's Balm of Gilead unit in Birmingham, Alabama, worked with area faith communities to "adopt" a room on the palliative care unit, decorating it and visiting the occupying patients at this public, safety-net hospital.
- Comprehensive Care Team project members, who were faculty at the University of California San Francisco Medical School, created a Community Health elective for pharmacy, social work, and medical students that incorporated visits with terminally ill patients as part of the curriculum.
- Through the Volunteers of America GRACE project, almost 200 prison inmates in four states were trained as "hospice" volunteers to help care for terminally ill fellow prisoners.
- Several Alaska Native communities participating in the Helping Hands project based in Dillingham, Alaska, developed programs in which high school student volunteers lent a helping hand to frail elders and ill members of the community enrolled in the palliative care program.

Table 62–4 provides an overview of the components of models developed by four *Promoting Excellence* grantees.

Educational Components of Palliative Care Models

Education of clinical professionals is a critical component of any strategy to expand access to team-based specialist palliative care programs. The increased awareness achieved through education and training results in increased referrals to palliative care and helps embed attention to comfort and quality of patient and family life within the focus of mainstream practice.

Many *Promoting Excellence* projects incorporated palliative care topics into required educational in-services, grand rounds and other "on-the-job" training for all disciplines. For example, the project director at Cooper Green Hospital incorporated 15-minute lectures on palliative care topics into daily morning rounds with medical residents. At Baystate Medical Center, nephrologists and dialysis staff incorporated palliative care issues into their regular morbidity and mortality conferences, moving discussions beyond the pathophysiology and metabolic chemistry of renal disease to include questions such as, "Did the patient 'die well'?" and "Were preferences known and followed?"

Promising Results

Sound evaluation plans are necessary for innovative palliative care programs to succeed and be sustained within the larger health care system in which they function. Because the *Promoting Excellence* demonstration projects were designed to build programmatic prototypes of health service delivery, evaluations focused on the *feasibility* of the programmatic approach; its *acceptability* among a range of stakeholders, including patients, families, clinicians, and management of the larger health system; and the program's potential for *sustainability*. To the extent possible, the palliative care programs also evaluated whether the expanded *access* to palliative care improved the *quality* of care as perceived by patients, families, and clinicians, as well as the *financial ramifications* of concurrently providing palliative care.

Preliminary data on access, quality, and cost from *Promoting Excellence* projects are exciting and promising. Using various strategies to institute and refine palliative care practices, *Promoting Excellence* programs experienced improved pain and symptom management and increased advance care planning and coordination, with patients and families reporting enhanced quality of life. Data from these prototypical models suggest that concurrent palliative and cure-oriented care is clinically effective and is associated with systems efficiencies and no increase—in fact, in most cases a decrease—in total expenditure of health care resources.

In the United States, complexities in accounting for health care costs abound. The lack of consistency for pricing and charges and the broad array of independent providers of care contribute to the challenges of assessing actual costs of products and services. Accounting limitations often make it difficult to distinguish between cost reductions and cost shifting to other parts of the health service delivery system, or to patients and their families. With these caveats acknowledged, in looking across the experience of *Promoting Excellence* programs, it is possible to offer some observations regarding the impact on patterns of resource use that affect costs.

Patients in *Promoting Excellence* programs often expressed a preference to avoid hospitalization. With good palliative support, their care was typically managed in the home, and crises that might have led to hospitalization were avoided. Expanded access to palliative care teams for consultation and ongoing management was associated with fewer hospital days, fewer unplanned hospitalizations, fewer emergency department visits, and fewer intensive care bed days. The number of hospice referrals and length of service increased; in several programs, days of hospice care doubled or tripled from baseline. More patients spent their last days at home.[6,12,13]

Collaboration, creativity, and flexibility in responding to needs of patients and providers are essential for the alignment of access to services, quality of care, and costs to be realized. Palliative care leaders benefit from exploring partnerships and engaging in dialogue with insurers and insurance regulators to create more flexible management of coverage benefits. *Promoting Excellence* projects found that by loosening restrictions on certain insurance benefits and being responsive to patient and family needs, they were able to effectively deliver care with high customer satisfaction while effectively controlling costs.

CASE STUDY
Pathways of Caring

The experience of the Pathways of Caring project at the Department of Veterans Affairs' (VA) Greater Los Angeles Healthcare System illustrates these results. Although the Pathways project was unique and the number of patients studied was relatively small, the findings exemplify the programmatic experience and trends of other *Promoting Excellence* projects.

Pathways of Caring clinician-researchers were committed to providing side-by-side disease-modifying treatment and palliative care for advanced life-limiting illnesses, to increase comfort and quality of life for veterans diagnosed with lung cancer, advanced congestive heart failure, or chronic obstructive pulmonary disease. The Pathways model began with the identification of patients within the hospital, clinic rolls, and medical records of the VA Greater Los Angeles health system who had poor prognoses and were likely to benefit from comprehensive symptom management. The project's goals extended to ensuring relative comfort for patients, coordinating care through the course of illness, and expanding access to home care and hospice. In the Pathways service model, a nurse case manager educates patients and their families regarding decision-making and symptom self-management and provides continuity of care, while serving as the hub of an interdisciplinary team that also includes a social worker, chaplain, dietitian, and physician.

Preliminary data on 54 participants who died while enrolled in the Pathways of Caring program show dramatic differences, compared with a retrospectively matched control group of patients who did not receive the palliative intervention. Available evidence indicates improvements in the proportion of cases with documented goals of care and completed advance directives. Forty-three percent of patients in the Pathways program were able to die at home, compared with 7% of matched control patients. Forty-five percent of Pathways patients died in a hospital or long-term care facility, compared with 68% of controls.

The Pathways program averaged 3.5 hospital days per patient during the final month of life, compared with 8.2 days for the control group. More striking still, the group of patients who died while served by Pathways spent an average of 0.4 days in intensive care during the last month of life, compared with 4.5 days for those in the group not enrolled. Intervention patients averaged far less time on mechanical ventilators in their final month, just 0.1 days per patient, compared with 3.5 days in the comparison group. As shown in Table 62–5, the program's ability to better manage its patients with life-threatening illnesses in more appropriate and cost-effective settings has important financial ramifications, with overall savings of 45% on the cost of care in the final month of life.

Table 62–5
Pathways of Caring Cost Per Patient in the Final Month of Life

Item	Pathways of Caring	Control Group
Number of patients	54	28
Inpatient costs, mean*	$ 4,416	$ 15,506
Nursing home care unit costs, mean	$ 2,428	$ 1,424
Intensive care unit costs, mean	$ 250	$ 4,871
Outpatient costs, mean	$ 3,069	$ 1,923
Total costs, mean	$ 10,248	$ 18,853

*Does not include long-term care facility costs listed separately.
Source: Department of Veterans Affairs, Greater Los Angeles Healthcare System.

The feasibility of this service delivery model and its acceptance by veterans, their families, and clinicians was clearly evidenced by the appreciation expressed and the steady rise in referrals and caseload. The ability of the Pathways team to document the program's success, including its salutary impact on the system's efficiency and use of health resources, provided a convincing argument for sustaining the program beyond the grant's duration. In fact, the Pathways program has been expanded, with an increased number of case management nurses and palliative care staff physicians, expansion and further integration of the palliative care consultation team, and formalization of an outpatient palliative care clinic.

Discussion

Hospice is acknowledged as a gold standard in the care of patients who are nearing the end of life, yet hospice care is not reliably available to all patients who are dying.[3,14] A dichotomy between life-prolonging care and hospice care exists in the mindset of clinicians as well as patients. In the United States, this dichotomy has been codified under Medicare, the government program that is the predominant payer of health care for people 65 years of age or older. By statute and regulation, Medicare's hospice benefit is available only to recipients who are judged to have a life expectancy of 6 months or less and who are willing to forego disease-modifying care. Yet, the distinction between life-prolonging and palliative interventions is arbitrary and without clinical or ethical basis. Indeed, advances in treatments for late-stage cancer, heart, lung, and neuromuscular diseases continue to blur that distinction. Sometimes treatments primarily intended to prolong life also improve patients' comfort and quality of life. Conversely, sometimes palliative care provided to address symptoms, alleviate suffering, and support patients and families seems to extend patients' lives.

The Institute of Medicine's landmark report, *Approaching Death*,[15] recognized an urgent need to improve care through the end of life. It called for significant improvements in clinical education, health systems design, and service delivery, as well as changes in health care financing, outcomes measurement, quality improvement, and oversight. In order to meet the growing mandate to deliver patient-centered care, health care systems and clinicians must attend to more than the pathophysiology of disease and the physiology and pharmacology of treatment. Patients with advanced, incurable conditions and their loved ones must be able to expect clear communication and shared decision-making about medical treatments and care plans. They should expect effective management of their symptoms, continuity of care, prevention of or early response to crises, and support for families in their caregiving and in their grief. The early clinical and programmatic results of *Promoting Excellence* projects have clearly shown that these reasonable expectations are achievable.

The concurrent delivery of palliative care and life-prolonging care is possible and well accepted across a wide variety of settings for health service delivery and to diagnostically and demographically diverse patient populations. This integration supports a higher quality of care, including smoother transitions of care across settings, and results in improved quality of life for seriously ill patients and families. *Promoting Excellence* projects found that availability of palliative care and enhanced staff training in palliative skills can change the culture of an institution, increasing sensitivity to and ambient skills in management of symptoms and response to the social needs of all patients.

Perhaps the ultimate mark of success of model building in health service delivery is the sustaining or expansion of the projects beyond the duration of grant funding. The large majority of *Promoting Excellence* projects are continuing. Some have evolved into new programs, and others are being expanded. Collectively, these prototype models of health service delivery proved their feasibility and efficiency within their local health care systems and are highly valued by patients, families and providers alike. They demonstrated that it is possible to align health services to meet the needs of seriously ill patients and their families and, notably, to improve outcomes of care, while remaining fiscally responsible for the financial well-being of health care institutions.

Conclusion

The vision of a seamless continuum of care that treats a patient's disease while also addressing physical, psychosocial, and spiritual comfort and quality of life for each seriously ill person and family is no longer an abstract notion or distant dream. The experience of *Promoting Excellence in End-of-Life Care* projects provides real-world experience that concurrent palliative and life-prolonging care is feasible and well accepted within a wide variety of settings and patient populations that span various ages, demographics, and diagnoses. The *Promoting Excellence in End-of-Life Care* web site, http://www.promotingexcellence.org, describes the projects and contains practical clinical, evaluative, educational, and programmatic tools and publications for delivering palliative care in challenging settings and to hard-to-reach populations. (Table 62–6 lists *Promoting Excellence* publications.) The success of these projects demonstrates what can be achieved and challenges clinicians, managers, and payers of health care to set and keep sights high.

The collective programmatic experience of the *Promoting Excellence* service delivery prototypes provides the foundation for future change. The next steps are well-designed population-based demonstration projects to advance delivery and study the outcomes of concurrent palliative and life-prolonging

Table 62–6
Promoting Excellence in End-of-Life Care* Publications

Promoting Excellence in End-of-Life Care: An Interim Report, May 2001
New End-of-Life Benefits Models in Blue Cross and Blue Shield Plans, January 2002
Advanced Practice Nursing: Pioneering Practices in Palliative Care, July 2002
A Position Statement from American Nursing Leaders, July 2002
Completing the Continuum of Nephrology Care: Recommendations to the Field, November 2002
Financial Implications of Promoting Excellence in End-of-Life Care, December 2002
Living and Dying Well with Cancer, April 2003
Accounting for the Costs of Caring Through the End of Life, January 2004
Completing the Continuum of ALS Care: A Consensus Document, February 2004
Lifting the Veil of Huntington's Disease, February 2004
Integrating Palliative Care into the Continuum of HIV Care: An Agenda for Change, April 2004
Journal of Palliative Medicine Series on *Promoting Excellence in End-of-Life Care* Projects, Ongoing since April 2003
New Models—New Markets: Successful Approaches to Delivering Palliative Care, a compact disk developed in partnership with the National Hospice and Palliative Care Organization, September 2003

*Links to these and other *Promoting Excellence in End-of-Life Care* resources are available at http://www.promotingexcellence.org.

care on quality and costs. In this manner, health care systems can evolve to provide excellence in clinical care in an approach that is clinically effective, socially responsible, and culturally affirming.

REFERENCES

1. NHO Committee. A Pathway for Patients and Families Facing Terminal Disease. Arlington, VA: National Hospice Organization, 1997.
2. Last Acts Task Force. Precepts of palliative care. J Palliat Med 1998;2:109–112.
3. Cassel CK, Foley KM. Principles for Care of Patients at the End of Life: An Emerging Consensus among the Specialties of Medicine. New York: Milbank Memorial Fund, 1999.
4. Steinhauser K, Clipp E, McNeilly M, Christakis N, McIntyre L, Tulsky J. In search of a good death: Observations of patients, families, and providers. Ann Intern Med 2000;132:825–832.
5. Wenrich M, Curtis J, Shannon S, Carline J, Ambrozy D, Ramsey P. Communicating with dying patients within the spectrum of medical care from terminal diagnosis to death. Arch Intern Med 2001;161:868–874.
6. Pitorak E, Armour M, Sivec H. Project Safe Conduct integrates palliative goals into comprehensive cancer care. J Palliat Med 2003;6:645–655.
7. Lynn J, Schuster JL, Kabcenell A. Case study: Franciscan Health Care Systems. In: Lynn J, Schuster JL, Kabcenell A. Improving Care for the End of Life: A Sourcebook for Health Care Managers and Clinicians. New York: Oxford University Press, 2000: Chapter 7.5.2.
8. Rosenfeld K, Rasmussen J. Palliative care management: A Veterans Administration demonstration project. J Palliat Med 2003;6: 831–839.
9. Stuart B, D'Onofrio C, Boatman S, Feigelman G. CHOICES: Promoting early access to end-of-life care through home-based transition management. J Palliat Med 2003;6:671–680.
10. Byock I, Twohig, JS. Expanding the realm of the possible. J Palliat Med 2003;6:311–313.
11. Rabow M, Petersen J, Schanche K, Dibble S, McPhee S. The Comprehensive Care Team: A description of a controlled trial of care at the beginning of the end of life. J Palliat Med 2003;6: 489–499.
12. Shega J, Levin A, Hougham G, Cox-Hayley D, Luchins D, Hanrahan P, Stocking C, Sachs G. Palliative Excellence in Alzheimer Care Efforts (PEACE): A program description. J Palliat Med 2003;6:315–320.
13. Poppel D, Cohen L, Germain M. The Renal Palliative Care Initiative. J Palliat Med 2003;6:321–326.
14. American Society of Clinical Oncology. Cancer care during the last phase of life. J Clin Oncol 1998;16:1986–1996.
15. Cassel C, ed. Approaching Death: Improving Care at the End of Life. Washington, DC: National Academy Press, 1997.

63

Ira Byock and Kaye Norris

A Community-Based Approach to Improving the Quality of Life's End

It takes a village to care for me. To see a group like this working as well as it does . . . I would hope would cause people to reflect on the possibilities that are there in their own communities, because it can be done. Community is possible. Relationship is possible. It's up to us to create it.—Phil Simmons, a writer and English professor living with amyotrophic lateral sclerosis (ALS), quoted on National Public Radio website

- ***Key Points***
- *Although dying is often assumed to be a medical event, illness, family caregiving, dying, and grief are primarily personal aspects of life. Each of these personal experiences of the individual and family is affected by the communities in which they live.*
- *Communities comprise people who share a stake in life—such as where and under what circumstances they live, work, or worship—and recognize a degree of commonality.*
- *The culture of a community comprises prevalent values, beliefs, assumptions, hopes, and fears, as well as patterns of behavior.*
- *People in Missoula, Montana, offered their town as a laboratory of experience to explore the meaning of living "in community" with one another with regard to advanced illness, caregiving, dying, and grieving.*
- *Research was conducted using various methodologies to obtain data on end-of-life experience and care from a broad spectrum of community members.*
- *By affirming existing values and highlighting discrepancies between what people hope for and what they do or experience, stakeholders from multiple segments of the community engaged in changing professional practice and patterns of social interaction and accelerated cultural change.*

The Personal Nature of Illness and Dying

Palliative care strives to bring the best of clinical practice to the goals of comfort and quality of life for individuals and families living with advanced illness. Toward those ends, it has become a specialty focus within the fields of medicine and nursing. Health care is often critically important in the lives of dying people. Yet, dying is fundamentally personal. Life with illness spans the entire spectrum from mundane daily activities, including basic tasks of self-care and family caregiving, to profound existential or spiritual experiences evoked by dying and grief. In caring for those whose disease has advanced beyond cure or substantial control, clinicians are wise to remember the subordinate, albeit essential, role that health care plays in lives of people who are ill. In palliative care, primacy and priority are rightfully accorded to people's personal values and goals.

What matters most to seriously ill or injured people is, almost invariably, other people. Human psychology dictates that the "who" each person experiences himself or herself to be is inextricably connected to others. Injuries and illness strike individuals, but they affect all who love the person stricken. In recognition of these features of human life, a tenant of palliative care is therapeutic focus on each patient *with his or her family.*[1–3]

Homo sapiens is a fundamentally social animal, and families and communities have always been integral features of human life.[4] Although families have traditionally been defined by marriage and blood relationships, many contemporary families are nontraditional. A suddenly incapacitated individual who is unmarried or lives alone may initially be thought to have no family yet later be found to have a close family defined by lasting bonds of friendship and love.

Similarly, communities need not be defined only by the borders of cities or towns. Communities exist within neighborhoods, places of work, and worship sites, as well as within associations formed by common interests and activities such as schools, social and service clubs, and recreation. These subcommunities form the fabric of human life. Most efforts to improve the quality of end-of-life care have focused on health care settings and health care practices.[5] To improve the quality of life for seriously ill patients and families, understanding and efforts must extend beyond the traditional confines of health care and contribute to building social capital and community responsiveness to the problems of illness, caregiving, death, and grief. It is not surprising that the recently published *Hospice Access and Values* project identified community not merely as an influence, but also as a core value for end-of-life care.[6]

One Community Offers Itself as a Laboratory of Experience

The Missoula Demonstration Project originated in 1995 when a small group of citizens in Missoula, Montana, who were concerned about the quality of end-of-life experience met to discuss ways for improving care and social support of ill people and their families. Missoula County is situated in the United States western Montana and has a population of approximately 88,000, with approximately 50,000 living within the city of Missoula. Home to a state university, Missoula has a reputation for having a strong sense of community and for being progressive and open-minded in its outlook.

A series of open meetings occurring over a handful of months drew individuals from a variety of backgrounds, including medicine, nursing, pharmacy, social work, funeral and burial services, ministry, aging services, aging advocacy, teaching, and the arts. Participants shared a belief that grassroots social change was necessary to improve quality of life for people with incurable conditions and for their families. Through these open meetings, this group of interested citizens developed a vision for using the geographic community of Missoula, Montana, as a laboratory of experience. Organizers decided to use their town to explore community interventions to improve formal, professional services and informal social support for dying persons and their families that would extend well beyond health care settings.

Under the guidance of a planning committee and founding board of directors, the Missoula Demonstration Project (MDP) was incorporated in 1996. The organization, which is now called Life's End Institute (LEI), was founded with the mission to study and improve the quality of life's end. The board of directors believed that research and community-based interventions could play complementary roles in accomplishing lasting change. Research findings have the potential for raising public and professional interest while allowing quality improvement efforts to be focused where they are needed most. Research could also track the impact of those efforts over time.

In 1997, this nascent community organization drew encouragement from an Institute of Medicine (IOM) report entitled *Approaching Death.* This influential national report endorsed "whole community" approaches to end-of-life care.[7] While emphasizing professional aspects of care, the IOM noted that "public and private policies, practices, and attitudes that help organizations and individuals" were required, including "support systems provided through workplaces, religious congregations, and other institutions to ease the emotional, financial, and practical burdens experienced by dying patients and their families." Additionally, the Institute called for "public education programs that aim to improve general awareness, to encourage advance care planning, and to provide specific information at the time of need about resources for physical, emotional, spiritual, and practical caring at the end of life."[7]

Studying end-of-life experience and care from a community perspective makes sense. Although most medical and nursing professionals encounter patients in health care settings of clinics, hospitals, or nursing homes, the people who become clinicians' patients live in the context of their families and communities. As the experiences of serious illness, dying, caregiving, grieving, and death inevitably affect each member of a person's family, each of these experiences is in part communal. All communities respond to members who are living through these difficult experiences in ways that at once reflect and shape community life. Although health care constitutes an essential component of a community's response, it cannot address the entire range of an individual's and family's needs, concerns, and challenges. Therefore, it is important to develop quality improvement programs that include both nonmedical and medical aspects of care in a community-wide context.

The term *community* often refers to a defined geographic town, city, or county and its residents. In its most general sense, the community can be defined by (1) formal associations of people that are valued by one another and (2) informal social structures and processes (discussions, activities, affiliations, and responsiveness to one another) that reflect commonalities of history, culture, interests, or perspectives that are valued by the participants.[8] Although the noun *community* conveys stability, by their very nature communities are dynamic, woven by processes and interactions of their members.

Community: A Social Compact with Entwined Self-Interests and Mutual Responsibilities

The primal social compact is founded on offering cooperation and accepting responsibility—self-interest rooted in mutual obligation.[9] The behaviors of people in communities reflect a sense of belonging and recognition of a shared "stake" in life. Although this tendency may be latent and not always obvious, when disaster strikes, such as a flood, fire, or hurricane, the sense of belonging and mutual responsibility becomes readily apparent in the behaviors and interactions of community members who are otherwise strangers.[10] Acute grief has a similar effect of revealing a shared sense of life. In the days following the death of a beloved community figure or a bus accident that claims the lives of young children or the tragedy of a school shooting, people acknowledge a commonality of grief. This impulse toward community occurs spontaneously, but it can also be cultivated.

LEI engaged the population of Missoula in exploring how people might live *in community* with one another—rather than merely in proximity to one another—with regard to issues of illness, caregiving, dying, death, and grief.[11] Questions were posed in community forums and through focus groups and surveys: What responsibilities do we have to those who are seriously ill or dying—our family members, friends, neighbors, and those we don't know? What responsibilities do we have as individuals, and collectively as a society? And what, if any, responsibilities do dying people—eventually all of us—have to those we leave behind?

Community Culture: Shared Values, Assumptions, Expectations, and Patterns of Behavior

At the heart of every community is its culture. *Culture* refers to the set of attributes that collectively characterize a community: commonly held values, attitudes, assumptions, history, expectations, hopes, fears, and customary modes of professional, social, and personal interactions. Dominant cultures, as well as subcultures, can be discerned. Culture encompasses a constellation of attributes that apply both to the community as a whole and to component subcommunities.

Cultural values, attitudes, expectations, and modes of behavior are deeply rooted and instilled individually early in childhood. They are then reinforced in the home, in schools, and in community life. The mutually reinforcing influences of values, attitudes, and expectations create a synergy that gives a local culture its power.

Yet, for all its strength and durability, culture is dynamic. Spontaneous shifts in culture tend to occur slowly. Substantial changes in attitudes and patterns of behavior can span generations; however, spurts of cultural change can occur. At times, national news, such as the death of a well-known civic figure or respected celebrity, brings media and public attention to issues and contributes to a shift in cultural expectations. Contemporary American examples include Richard Nixon's refusal of further life-prolonging treatment, Jackie Onassis's choice to be cared for at home as she died, James Michener's decision to discontinue renal dialysis and allow death to occur, and Nancy and Ronald Reagan's acceptance of his life with dementia and eventually a natural death at home. Such accounts gave rise to heightened awareness of end-of-life options and, at least transiently, increased requests for living wills and interest in home care services.

Community members' willingness (or resistance) to address end-of-life issues within formal, professional interactions as well as in informal social settings can strongly influence end-of-life outcomes. People are at once a product of their culture and participants in its ongoing evolution. Cultural attitudes, assumptions, expectations, and patterns of behavior are based in part on the collective previous experiences of its members. These attributes are malleable. Indeed, well-planned, multifaceted interventions can have mutually reinforcing effects on shaping cultural change. Because word of mouth spreads quickly within communities, a significant change in one arena, such as a hospital and nursing home program to routinely assess and treat pain, can give rise to measurable shifts in expectation on the part of patients and their families.

Life's End Institute's Research and Continuous Quality Improvement Paradigm

Missoula's whole-community approach toward improving the quality of end-of-life experience flows from a conceptual framework that supports research and program evaluation and contributes to community dialogue and action. Stewart and coworkers[12] developed a conceptual model that identifies key concepts and domains of clinical end-of-life care and related patient and family health care experiences. Using the structure-process-outcome framework pioneered by Donabedian,[13,14] the goal of the Stewart model was to integrate quality of life and quality of health care indicators (Figure 63–1).

LEI identified relevant characteristics, structures, processes, and outcomes of community life for the purposes of (1) developing an evidence base regarding current practices and patterns of behavior, (2) identifying areas in need of quality improvement, (3) determining effective interventions, and (4) supporting ongoing evaluation. Toward these ends, LEI conducted a series of quantitative and qualitative studies.

This research and quality improvement model encompasses nonclinical as well as clinical aspects of end-of-life experience. It incorporates individual experiences from surveys, interviews, chart reviews, and ethnographic research with aggregate data from regional vital statistics and national Medicare databases. This approach adapts the continuous quality improvement (CQI) model developed in manufacturing and widely used in clinical institutions, expanding the scope and response cycle of the CQI model to fit whole-community applications.[15–17] The unit of analysis and target of interventions are determined by the specific characteristic, structure, or process that is being measured or affected. For example, geographically bounded areas such as counties, health care institutions, social service agencies, or faith communities each may serve as the unit of analysis.[18] LEI's framework incorporates two dimensions of evidence that correspond to two types of interventions: individual focused and community focused.[8]

The community-focused dimension addresses environmental features, collective experiences, and common expectations. Examples of relevant community evidence include (1) a matrix of pertinent resources and services within the geographic community, such as various health care facilities, hospice and home health services, "medicab" transportation, senior housing, and meals on wheels; (2) a public survey of attitudes and behaviors regarding pain medication and related to advance directives; and (3) focused descriptions of attitudes and behaviors regarding illness, family caregiving, dying, and grief within subcommunities of workplaces, neighborhoods, congregations, and social organizations. Whole-community interventions can affect individual and family experiences in indirect but tangible ways, by creating more supportive milieus

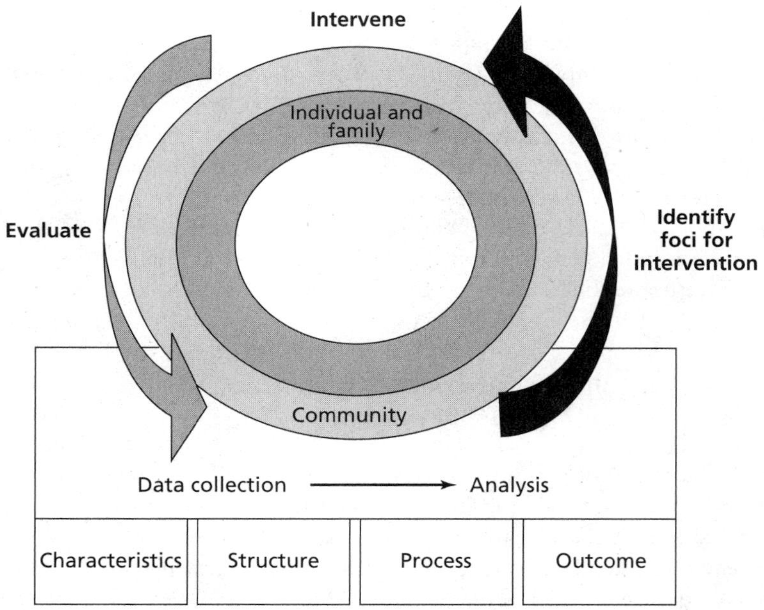

Figure 63–1. An evidence base and operational model for community-based quality improvement.

of community and subcommunity life in regard to illness, dying, caregiving, and grief.

This community-based quality improvement framework emphasizes commonly held values and expectations (including hopes and fears) and assesses the degree of concordance or variance between generally held values or hopes and experienced or observed outcomes. A community's cultural values are often deeply rooted and difficult to change. Yet preliminary findings indicated that the large majority of Missoula's population valued aging, dying, comfort and quality of life during illness, emotional and spiritual support of ill and dying people, and family support during caregiving and during grief. LEI's board of directors, researchers, and advisors recognized that other attributes of culture are more malleable and, if targeted specifically, could lead to a critical mass, or tipping point, and core cultural change.[19] By reinforcing prevailing values, correcting misconceptions, and calling attention to patterns of interaction that are inconsistent with stated values and hoped-for outcomes, it may be possible to change common behavior patterns. Community-based quality improvement efforts operate on—and test—these assumptions.

LEI crafted a platform of research that was carefully designed to examine experiences of illness, caregiving, dying, death, and grief. A set of general questions guided the research plan:

- How do people view death and dying? What is most important to them? What do they hope for—and what do they fear?
- How do people interact with one another concerning end-of-life issues?
- How do people prepare for death, dying, and caregiving?
- How do people die in Missoula? Where do they die?
- What is the quality of end-of-life care?
- How do people care for and support one another—clinically, informally, and socially—during serious illness, dying, and grief?
- How do people *perceive* care at the end of life?

A variety of methodologies were used to assess pertinent domains of personal and family experience and quality of care. Both objective and subjective data were gathered from mailed individual or family surveys, structured and semistructured interviews, surrogate after-death interviews, and medical chart reviews.[20–24] Study designs were both prospective and retrospective and gathered either epidemiological or ethnographical information. LEI's participant-observer study used an anthropological perspective that culminated in a book, *A Few Months to Live*.[25] Knowledge, attitudes, and skills among professionals were assessed by structured interviews, surveys, and standardized tests. Comprehensive community assessment enabled descriptions of patterns of care across institutions or provider groups within a community, levels of quality among available services, and aggregate personal experiences of community members (Figure 63–2).

Key Findings

Findings from the series of baseline research studies conducted during 1997–2000 informed and focused LEI's community engagement and quality improvement interventions. These studies were funded by a variety of private foundations, including the Nathan Cummings Foundation, the Robert Wood Johnson Foundation, the Arthur Vining Davis Foundations, the Kornfeld Foundation, and the Mayday Fund.

Although a detailed report of the study results is beyond the scope of this chapter, key findings that helped shape Missoula's community-based interventions are presented.

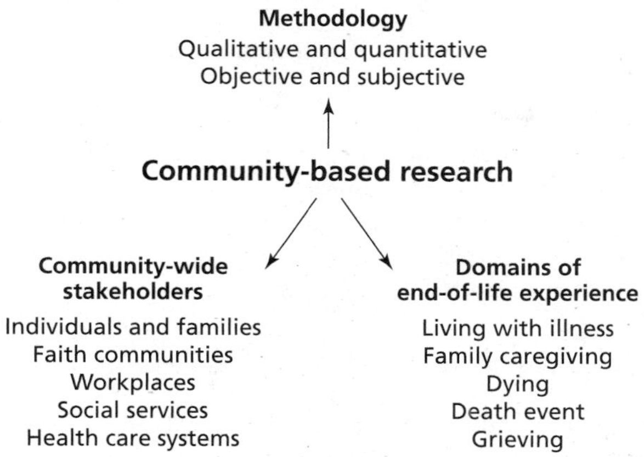

Figure 63–2. Variety and breadth of community-based research.

Values

Study data revealed overall broad agreement among the general adult population of Missoula and subcommunities of professionals with respect to values and expectations of end-of-life experience and care, albeit with some differences in frequency and intensity of attributes. For instance, there was general accord in response to the statement, "Dying is an important stage of life," in a series of surveys. Seventy-five percent of respondents from a sample of 596 members of the general public endorsed the statement. In a separate survey of 41 faith community leaders, 98% strongly agreed.[26] A subsequent survey of practicing attorneys found that 87% of those most experienced with advance directives and 83% of those less experienced concurred with this statement.[27]

Misconceptions

Misconceptions can impede the best efforts to improve people's comfort and quality of life. Fully 50% of respondents among the general public expressed some to extreme worry about dying painfully, yet significant proportions harbored beliefs that would complicate effective pain management. Thirty-two percent agreed with the incorrect statement that "Most people taking pain medicines will become addicted over time." Similarly, 36% erroneously thought that "Pain medicines should only be taken when pain is severe"; 42% agreed that "It is important to take the lowest amount of medicine possible to save larger doses for later when the pain is worse"; and 42% agreed that "People are often given too much pain medicine."

Gap Between Expectations and Outcomes

"Being able to stay in your home" was rated as important in helping to deal with one's own dying by 85% of respondents in a survey of the general public. However, in-depth chart reviews of 207 people who died "nonsudden" deaths revealed that only 22% were in a private residence during the last moments of life, and only 18% received hospice services.

"Freedom from pain" was important to 92% of community respondents, yet medical chart reviews of 207 decedents indicated that 78% experienced pain during the last week or month of their life. Eighty-eight percent of community respondents prospectively indicated that "spiritual well-being" was important during the dying process, but in a separate, retrospective study, 21% of bereaved loved ones rated the help they received from their church as the worst it could possibly be. Indeed, only 34% of faith community members in a multicongregational study said their church does a good job of providing support for families during illness. And even fewer congregants (29%) indicated that their church does a good job providing support for families at the time of death.

Although "not being a burden" to loved ones was rated as important in the dying process by 88% of general community respondents, respondents often did not engage in activities that prepare those who are likely to make decisions for them. For instance, 72% of this general public sample did not have advance directives, which allow individuals to express their own health care preferences, designate someone to speak for them, and are widely acknowledged as a way to reduce the emotional burden on families at times of medical crises. Further, 41% of this general public sample said they were unlikely to speak freely to their loved ones about death and dying. Hospice services can also reduce the family burden in caring for a dying loved one, yet 39% of surveyed local residents had never heard of hospice or had heard only a little about it.

Insufficient Preparation Among Professionals

Professionals from clinical disciplines as well as education, ministry, and law acknowledged that they have an important role to play in serving clients who are dealing with illness, death, or grief, either themselves or in their families. In each discipline, significant proportions of respondents reported less than adequate training and professional preparation to do so. Among attorneys, 36% had little or no training in advance care planning. Among member of the clergy, 34% had no training in issues related to illness and death, and 66% said that what training they did have had not prepared them well for ministry related to illness. Seventy-six percent of school teachers were either unaware of end-of-life curricula or not familiar enough to use them, and 44% were unprepared to initiate a conversation with a student about the student's serious, potentially life-threatening illness.

Even with suboptimal formal training, personal experience with advance care planning would improve professionals' ability and comfort in assisting others. However, in proportions similar to those of the general public, local professionals did not prepare for their own end-of-life experiences and care. Only 27% of physicians, 29% of attorneys, and 30% of clergy reported having named a power of attorney for health care to convey their wishes and help ensure that their preferences were followed.

In summarizing key findings to the Missoula community, LEI reported the following conclusions:

- We don't adequately prepare for end-of-life experience and care.
- Many of us have misconceptions that can adversely affect our care and increase the variance between what we hope for and what occurs.
- What we value and hope for is not always what we get.
- How we act is often inconsistent with what we value, desire, and hope to provide or receive.

Community Engagement and Quality Improvement

LEI's quality improvement strategy reinforced widely-held affirmative values and focused on identified gaps between what people value and hope for and actual outcomes—what people receive or experience. Where a gap existed between expectations and outcomes and patterns of behaviors were inconsistent with existing values and aspirations, LEI attempted to bring these patterns of professional and informal social interaction into alignment with widely held values and desired outcomes. Similarly, research data were used to identify prevalent expectations that might be raised in ways that improve the quality of care and end-of-life experiences in the community.

In summary, LEI focused on three specific targets for quality improvement: (1) formal services and care that are documented to be at variance from recognized standards for professional practice; (2) prevalent misconceptions by the general public and professionals that potentially contribute to adverse outcomes, inconsistent with widely-held values and hopes; and (3) common patterns of professional practice and informal social interaction that are incongruent with prevailing values and hopes and consequently contribute to undesirable outcomes.

Recognizing that community-wide quality improvement would not be achieved by single program or by a "top-down" approach alone, LEI chose a strategy of community engagement. Research and feedback proved essential to this approach. In addition to general public surveys and outcomes research, pertinent subcommunities provided information from their own experiences and professional practices. Once collected and analyzed, these findings were reported back. When professional groups, whether clinicians, teachers, clergy, or attorneys, reviewed their data and observed the discrepancies between what they value and hope to provide in their service and what occurs, the result was an immediate and deepened sense of ownership of the issues and expressed resolve to improve practice patterns and outcomes. Professional groups responded with education efforts and quality improvement activities by and for their members. As a center for expertise in end-of-life content, on request, LEI remained available to offer assistance to groups within Missoula, as well as to consult with other communities across the nation.

Quality Improvement Initiatives and Programs

From 1999 to 2004, a wide array of quality improvement initiatives and programs emerged from this approach to community engagement. Examples of initiatives organized by sub-communities and topic foci are presented here, with recognition that activities are rarely discrete and that overlap and synergy of efforts are desirable.

Health Care Community

A 23-member Advance Care Planning Task Force with representation from most clinical settings as well as attorneys, chaplains, disability advocates, social workers, faith community leaders, and retirees developed My Choices, an advance directive form that combines a power of attorney for health care and a living will.[28] The consistent availability of this form has bred familiarity among health care providers, who are able to more quickly locate and understand the information it contains. A companion booklet was developed to provide information about exploring and expressing one's health care preferences in situations of life-threatening illness and injury.

To further improve the accessibility of advance directives, nine Missoula organizations collaborated to develop the Choices Bank, which stores scanned advance directives on a secure Internet site (http://www.ChoicesBank.org) and makes them available to authorized individuals 24 hours per day.[28] The Choices Bank uses relatively simple and inexpensive technology, which facilitates its replication by other communities. Choices Bank evaluations to date reveal a dramatic increase in depositors' confidence that their advance directives will be found when they are needed. Not only are 82% of depositors "extremely satisfied" with the Choices Bank, but almost 80% reported that they had recommended the Choices Bank to their families and friends. What is more, 94% of depositors had discussed the health care choices they made with their families, 65% with their doctors, and 59% with close friends.

To assist patients and their doctors and nurses in assessing physical discomfort, a community-based Pain Task Force printed pain rating scales in bookmark formats. More than 4400 pain scales have been distributed throughout Missoula. Pain is now monitored as a vital sign in the two hospitals, one home health agency, and a local hospice program. Across acute and long-term care facilities and hospice and home care programs, pain management is now a routine focus for continuous quality improvement. Three of the largest local health care institutions have begun to regularly monitor performance with pain assessment and management and have developed interdisciplinary teams to evaluate and monitor pain management. The teams monitor the quality of the pain management process, including staff competency, effectiveness of treatment, and outcomes such as satisfaction, cost, readmissions, and length of stay. Both local hospitals were awarded commendations for their pain management programs by the Joint Commission on Accreditation of Health Care Organizations.

To improve spiritual care at the end of life, 12 health care institutions assessed their current services and implemented quality improvement interventions. A home health agency developed a Spiritual Care training module for all nursing staff. One hospital adapted a referral card,[29] a tool staff members can use to know when to call a spiritual advisor (see Table 63–1).

Faith Community

Fifteen local faith communities assessed their capacity to provide spiritual care at the end of life, reviewed their results, and implemented quality improvement interventions. One church formed a Health Cabinet that works with their parish nurse and includes a focus on end of life; another collated bereavement materials as a first step in addressing grief issues in their congregation; and a third started an education series on end-of-life issues. A home-based volunteer program, Caring Friends, was developed by one faith community to assist family caregivers within their congregation.

A nondenominational Caring Circles program was developed with support by parish nurses and community volunteers. Caring Circles helps family caregivers by recruiting and training teams drawn from individuals within a caregiver's network of family, friends, neighbors, coworkers, or congregants who are then prepared and coordinated in providing assistance with routine tasks such as shopping, cleaning, mowing, and cooking, as well as transportation for appointments or errands. The program informs families and Caring Circle volunteers about available resources such as hospice, topical health issue information, advance care planning, and other avenues for reducing the burden of family caregiving. The program is partially self-supported by volunteers who make and sell "Wearing Caring" jewelry. An added advantage to this strategy is that the distinctive jewelry itself provides an opportunity for the wearer to explain and promote the Caring Circle program.

Legal Community

The Wise Counsel project developed as a collaborative effort between LEI and representatives of the State Bar of Montana, the University of Montana School of Law, and the Montana Association of Legal Assistants. A national advisory panel of accomplished legal, medical, and ethics experts helped shape the research design. All four District Court judges in Missoula County signed a letter encouraging recipients to complete the Wise Counsel survey. Seventy-one percent of attorneys did so, an impressive response rate. After reviewing survey results, a statewide elder law continuing legal education seminar with the State Bar of Montana was developed, and law professors at the University of Montana included end-of-life curricula in their elder law classes.

Table 63–1
Spiritual Care Referral Card*

Spiritual Assessment

Listen for verbal clues:

- Patient refers to God or higher power
- Patient talks about church, prayer, worship, or a religious or spiritual leader
- Patient makes comments such as "It's in God's hands now," or "Why is God letting this happen?"

Look for visual clues:

- Religious or spiritual books: Bible, Torah, Koran, etc.
- Symbols in room: cross, star of David, etc.
- Articles: prayer beads, medallions, crosses, pins, etc.

Assess for religious concerns such as diet, special observations, or refusal of blood.

Listen carefully to your patients' life stories: who they are, who they have been, for this is the key to understanding their unique spirituality.

Spiritual Diagnosis

These are some cues that a patient may be experiencing spiritual distress or despair:

- Anticipatory grief
- Unable to participate in normal religious services
- Severe depression, suicidal ideation
- Concern about their relationship with God
- Feeling abandoned by God, unable to pray
- Anger toward God or established religion
- Loss of hope or spiritual beliefs

If you assess spiritual distress or despair, please contact the Chaplain right away.

Interventions

- Joining with the patient in prayer or scripture reading if you are comfortable doing so.
- Being with the patient in respectful silence can be comforting.
- Referral to the patient's own religious leader and/or hospital chaplain.

*Created by the Psychosocial/Spiritual Committee of the Palliative Care Task Force, University of Kansas Medical Center. *Source:* Malewski et al. (1999), reference 29.

School-age Education Community

Schools are a microcosm of the existing community, yet there was no system in place to support students with issues of death and bereavement. The Schools Task Force, consisting of local teachers, administrators, librarians, secretaries, counselors, parents (including those who home-schooled), and students, developed an age-appropriate bibliography of books on grief for local teachers and a literature kit and resource list for teachers and parents that featured extended activities on bereavement and coping after the death of a grandparent or other significant loss. The task force continues to collaborate with the American Hospice Foundation to conduct its annual Grief at School Workshops.

Arts Community

Community engagement employing the arts moves beyond merely placing artwork in hospitals and other clinical settings. The arts can play an active role in stimulating introspection, discussion, and community-based efforts.

In Missoula, visual and performing arts have proved to be powerful means for arousing emotions, raising awareness, and stimulating conversation, especially among those who may not otherwise seek conversation about the end of life. A variety of art forms, from paintings and photography to poetry, literature, live theater, and music, have engaged the public in exploring illness, caregiving, death, and grief. Programs have involved cultural organizations, such as museums, symphonies, and drama groups, as well as community organizations of schools, churches, and the local Area Agency on Aging.

The staged reading of a play, *Vesta,* by Bryan Harnetiaux, about an elderly woman's struggle with progressive frailty, loss of independence, and extended family dynamics, was presented to a full high school auditorium. Students invited their grandparents to attend and participated in a discussion session after the performance. A reception and exhibit of evocative self-portraits by a well-known Canadian artist, Robert Pope, created while the painter was living with progressive cancer, was hosted at the Missoula Art Museum and drew record numbers of attendees. Since then, the art museum has exhibited various works on themes of illness, dying, and grief.

In conjunction with the local University repertory theater group, LEI produced the Pulitzer Prize–winning play, *Wit,* to high attendance for five successive nights. After each performance a "talk-back session" was moderated by one or more local professionals, including chaplains, social workers, doctors, nurses, and ministers.

Participatory and experiential art activities have taken a number of forms. To assist individuals and families in honoring a deceased loved one, local artists have conducted Images and Objects of Remembrance workshops. Participants are instructed to bring photographs and small symbolic objects to transform into memorials that recall and celebrate the person who has died. Those who wish can have their image or object of remembrance displayed in a local cafe or gallery. These workshops have typically preceded Missoula's annual Festival of the Dead celebration, a week-long calendar of activities culminating in an evening, downtown parade on All Saints Day.

A collaborative project with KUFM, a public radio station, produced 32 radio programs or segments with end-of-life themes that were broadcast over 5 days. The content was varied and was tailored to a diversity of audiences listening at times throughout the broadcast day. These programs reached a potential audience of 300,000.

General Community

In recognition of the value that life review and storytelling in the experiences of seriously ill individuals and their friends and families, a group of community members joined together under the auspices of LEI as the Life Stories Task Force. They created a storytelling newspaper insert, "Everyone Has a Story, Share Yours!" which was a collection of end-of-life narratives, many both poignant and humorous, and emphasized the value of storytelling, especially as the end of life approaches. This tabloid was distributed to 20,000 households via the local daily newspaper.

The Life Stories Task Force also designed a project to elicit and help individuals record their stories with the intention of contributing a meaningful experience and enhancing the quality of life for dying persons. A short set of guidelines and suggestions were developed into a booklet, *Gathering Life Stories of the Dying* (available at http://www.lifes-end.org/gathering_life_stories.phtml). A collection of life stories is available in the public library. This task force proved so successful that members chose to develop a separate nonprofit, community-based organization called StoryKeepers, Inc. (http://www.mystorykeepers.org/mystorykeepers/). This new organization holds two workshops a year to improve skills in writing life stories and sponsors an annual storytelling festival.

LEI seeks to involve many segments of the community and people from all walks of life—because all are stakeholders.

Although it is premature to assert that the community of Missoula has been transformed, it is safe to say that the 5 years of intense activity have heightened awareness of living with illness, family caregiving, dying, and grieving. These subjects are no longer relegated to the periphery of awareness or actively avoided. Instead, they have become matters for discussion in professional groups, as well as organized social and informal discussions, and are recognized as important aspects of community life. For example, the local newspaper regularly prints editorials pertaining to end-of-life issues, the art museum continues to display exhibits that address chronic illness and loss, and philanthropic organizations as well as small businesses regularly request LEI staff to speak to their members about advance care planning and caregiving. Topics pertaining to life's end are no longer uncommon in public discourse.

Although organizations often resist change, because people's values were affirmed and achievable goals were highlighted, individuals from many walks of life and various segments of the community recognized their own and their organization's self-interest in quality improvement. Thus, resistance to LEI's efforts has been minimal.

The history of LEI is still being written. As with most community-based, nonprofit organizations, funding remains a constant challenge and the future is never secure. But whether or not LEI remains active, the process of cultural maturation concerning end-of-life issues cannot be reversed. Interest is high, and professional and cultural activities to advance peoples' values and meet their expectations will continue. This "genie" has been released and will not be forced back into the bottle.

Conclusion

Citizen and consumer efforts to improve end-of-life experience are necessary complements to initiatives in health care and can enhance general social support as well as the quality of practice among professionals in law, ministry, and education.[30] An understanding of strategic approaches that are rooted in community and culture expands the realm of effective advocacy and activism.

Community-based research and social change efforts have been successful in other areas of life. Public health interventions and campaigns have focused on a variety of social problems, including unmet needs of the chronically ill,[31] primary prevention of cardiovascular diseases,[32–35] reduction of tobacco use, preventing low birth weight,[36] eliminating child abuse,[37] and diminishing drunk driving,[38] to name a few.

Act Clinically, Think Culturally

Affirmative cultural values regarding end-of-life experience and care are prevalent and augment community-based efforts to improve the quality of life's end. Unfortunately, also common are misconceptions and low expectations regarding illness, caregiving, dying, and grief. People anticipate suffering and hope that it can be avoided or suppressed. Rarely are periods of age-related decline or the experience of dying anticipated as potentially valuable times of life.

Palliative care clinicians empirically know that these inherently difficult times are also inescapably important and can become profoundly meaningful events in the histories of patients and their families. Under conditions of comprehensive care, effective symptom management and sufficient social and family support, people have the opportunity to review their lives together and their relationships, and they have a chance to say and do the things that matter most to them. The social stature of nurses and physicians and their expertise in matters of illness and dying provide them with invaluable opportunities for cultural leadership.

Although a national crisis surrounds the ways people are cared for and the ways they die, aging and dying happen to one person and one family at a time. Palliative care providers can act clinically and culturally. In taking the best care possible of each patient and family, clinicians can contribute to the health of their communities. In so doing, they can contribute to a maturation of the culture and affirm a social covenant to care for one another through the very end of life.

REFERENCES

1. NHO Committee. A Pathway for Patients and Families Facing Terminal Disease. Arlington, VA: National Hospice Organization, 1997.
2. Last Acts Task Force. Precepts of palliative care. J Palliat Med 1998;2:109–112.
3. Cassel CK, Foley KM. Principles for Care of Patients at the End of Life: An Emerging Consensus among the Specialties of Medicine. New York: Milbank Memorial Fund, 1999.
4. Vanderpool HY. The ethics of terminal care. JAMA 1978;239: 850–852.
5. Hanson LC, Earp JA, Garrett J, Menon M, Danis M. Community physicians who provide terminal care. Arch Intern Med 1999;159: 1133–1138.
6. Jennings B, Ryndes T, d'Onofrio C, Baily MA. Access to hospice care: Expanding boundaries, overcoming barriers. Hastings Cent Rep Suppl S3–7, S9–13, S15–21 passim., 2003.
7. Field MJ, Cassell CK. Approaching Death: Improving Care at the End of Life. Washington, DC: National Academy Press, 1997.
8. Byock I., Norris K, Curtis JR, Patrick DL. Improving end-of-life experience and care in the community: A conceptual framework. J Pain Symptom Manage 2001;22:759–772.
9. McKnight J. The Careless Society: Community and Its Counterfeits. New York: Basic Books, 1996.
10. Byock I. Rediscovering community at the core of the human condition and social covenant. Hastings Cent Rep Suppl 2003; 33(2):S40–S41.
11. Atcheson R. The Missoula Experiment: How a small town learned to make dying a part of living. Modern Maturity 2000; Sep–Oct:60–62, 88.
12. Stewart AL, Teno J, Ptrick DL, Lynn J. The concept of quality of life of dying persons in the context of health care. J Pain Symptom Manage 1999;17:93–108.
13. Donabedian A. Evaluating the quality of medical care. Milbank Mem Fund Q 1996;44(3 Suppl):166–206.
14. Donabedian A. The role of outcomes in quality assessment and assurance. Qual Rev Bull 1992;18:356–360.
15. Deming W. Out of the Crisis. Cambridge, MA: Massachusetts Institute of Technology Press, 1986.
16. Berwick DM, Godfrey AB, Roessner J. Curing Health Care: New Strategies for Quality Improvement: A Report on the National Demonstration Project on Quality Improvement in Health Care. San Francisco, CA: Jossey-Bass, 1990.
17. Batalden PB, Mohr JJ. Building knowledge of health care as a system. Qual Manage Health Care 1997;5(3):1–12.

18. Robinson G, Hollister G, Hill J. Problems in the Evaluation of Community-Wide Initiatives. New York: Russell Sage Foundation, 1995.
19. Gladwell M. Tipping Point: How Little Things Can Make a Big Difference. Boston: Little, Brown, 2000.
20. Payne SA, Langley-Evans A., Hillier R. Perceptions of a 'good' death: A comparative study of the views of hospice staff and patients. Palliat Med 1996;10:307–312.
21. Byock IR, Merriman MP. Measuring quality of life for patients with terminal illness: The Missoula-VITAS quality of life index. Palliat Med 1998;12:231–244.
22. Byock IR, Teno JM, Field MJ. Measuring quality of care at life's end. J Pain Symptom Manage 1999;17:73–74.
23. Teno JM., Byock I, Field MJ. Research agenda for developing measures to examine quality of care and quality of life of patients diagnosed with life-limiting illness. J Pain Symptom Manage 1999;17:75–82.
24. Curtis JR., Patrick DL, Engelberg RA, Norris K, Asp C, Byock I. A measure of the quality of dying and death: Initial validation using after-death interviews with family members. J Pain Symptom Manage 2002;24:17–31.
25. Staton J, Shuy R., Byock I. A Few Months to Live. Washington, DC: Georgetown University Press, 2001.
26. Noris K, Strohmaier G, Asp C, Byock I. Spiritual care at the end of life: the influence of clerical training on practice [special section]. Health Progress2004; July-August:34–39.
27. Byock I, Norris K, Asp C, Tracy L. Wise counsel: a survey of attorney preparation, knowledge, and practice related to advance health care planning. J Am Geriatr Soc (in submission).
28. My Choices advance directive for health care. Available at: http://www.choicesbank.org/ (accessed March 25, 2005).
29. Malewski J, Spencer J, Thompson N. Spiritual care referral card. Created by the Psychosocial/Spiritual Committee of the Palliative Care Task Force at the University of Kansas Medical Center (now University of Kansas Hospital Authority), 1999. Available via e-mail from JMalewsk@kumc.edu.
30. Casarett DJ, Karlawish JH, Byock I. Advocacy and activism: Missing pieces in the quest to improve end-of-life care. J Palliat Med 2002;5:3–12.
31. Allen SM, Mor V. The prevalence and consequences of unmet need: Contrasts between older and younger adults with disability. Med Care 1997;35:1132–1148.
31. Lefebvre RC, Lasater TM, et al. Pawtucket Heart Health Program: The process of stimulating community change. Scand J Prim Health Care Suppl 1988;1:31–37.
33. Block L, Banspach SW, Gans K, Harris C, Lasater TM, Lefebvre RC, Carleton RA. Impact of public education and continuing medical education on physician attitudes and behavior concerning cholesterol. Am J Prev Med 1988;4:255–260.
34. Lasater TM, Carleton RA, Lefebvre RC. The Pawtucket Heart Health Program: V. Utilizing community resources for primary prevention. R I Med J 1988;71(2):63–67.
36. Flora JA., Lefebvre RC, Murray DM, Stone EJ, Assaf A, Mittelmark MB, Finnegan JR Jr. A community education monitoring system: Methods from the Stanford Five-City Project, the Minnesota Heart Health Program and the Pawtucket Heart Health Program. Health Educ Res 1993;8:81–95.
36. Koniak-Griffin D, Anderson NL, Verzemnieks I, Brecht ML. A public health nursing early intervention program for adolescent mothers: Outcomes from pregnancy through 6 weeks. Nurs Res 2000;49(3):130–138.
36. Sabol WJ, Coulton CJ, Korbin JE. Building community capacity for violence prevention. J Interpers Violence 2004;19:322–340.
38. Treno AJ, Lee JP. Approaching alcohol problems through local environmental interventions. Alcohol Res Health 2002;26: 35–40.

64

Elizabeth Ford Pitorak

Project Safe Conduct

You cannot treat a person like a textbook and expect them to live. You have to treat them like a whole person and that is what the Safe Conduct Team does. They treat the whole person.
—Daughter of a Safe Conduct patient

- ***Key Points***
- *"Safe Conduct" guides patients and their families through the cancer disease trajectory.*
- *The safe conduct team provides "safety" through times of uncertainty, confusion, and fear for patients and their families.*
- *An interdisciplinary team with expertise in end-of-life care is integrated with the acute care model, and this becomes the standard of care.*
- *The philosophies behind acute care and end-of-life care blend.*

The details of developing and implementing an integrative model of palliative care are discussed in this chapter. The concepts that contributed to the success of this program were having a well defined vision; obtaining support from top leadership; developing an extremely detailed step-by-step plan; creating an education plan; role modeling how to deliver "bad news"; creating an environment conducive to family conferences for decision-making; and establishing outcome measures for evaluation.

Project Safe Conduct, an integrative model of delivering palliative care, was a collaborative partnership between Hospice of the Western Reserve (HWR), an independent large community-based hospice, and the Ireland Cancer Center (ICC) at Case Western Reserve University and University Hospitals of Cleveland, a National Cancer Institute (NCI)-designated cancer center. The project name, Safe Conduct, is taken from concepts in Avery Weisman's *Coping with Cancer.* He coined the term *safe conduct* as "the dimension of care that guides a patient through a maze of uncertain, perplexing, and distressing events."[1] "Safe conduct" was descriptive of the envisioned role of the Safe Conduct Team (SCT), who would guide the patient and family through their disease trajectory, which could have many uncertain, perplexing, and distressing events.

In 1997, *Promoting Excellence in End-of-Life Care,* a national program office of The Robert Wood Johnson Foundation, put out a Request for Proposals. The ICC, in collaboration with HWR, submitted a letter of intent. Of the 678 letters of intent, 59 submitters were invited to write a full grant proposal; 24 had a site visit; and 4 of the 22 who received grants were cancer centers.

Normally, a formal needs assessment would be performed, but the grantees at ICC were already aware that end-of-life issues were not being addressed as much in depth as they wanted. Additionally, they realized the need for input and expertise from their colleagues at hospice. The HWR staff were extremely interested in increasing access and decreasing barriers to palliative care for those patients receiving aggressive therapy.

Vision

Throughout this chapter, the elements for success that were identified in Project Safe Conduct are discussed. The first of these was a well-defined vision that aligned the program with the missions of the individual institutions. Philosophically, both ICC and HWR agreed that cancer patients should have an opportunity for life-prolonging treatment and for exquisite care in terms of palliative care (i.e., managing pain and symptoms and addressing psychosocial, spiritual, and life closure issues). These two goals are not mutually exclusive. In fact, the Project Safe Conduct designers viewed it as their obligation to patients to acknowledge and address both. To accomplish this, an environment conducive to open communication had to be created so that staff members could simultaneously talk about both life-prolonging treatment and life closure, when appropriate, and provide aggressive pain and symptom management. This resulted in the creation of more options regarding end-of-life care. Those individual patients who chose to continue with aggressive chemotherapy until they died were also supported with palliative care via the SCT.

Goals of This Model

The overall goal was to create a seamless transition from curative to palliative or end-of-life care for persons dying of cancer and their families in the ambulatory cancer setting by integrating the principles of palliative care. To accomplish this purpose, the following four aims were identified:

- Implement pain and symptom management care paths.
- Educate providers about the same.
- Improve patient/provider communication concerning end-of-life decisions.
- Increase community awareness regarding end-of-life issues.

Two guiding principles were identified that philosophically support the rationale for developing an integrative model of palliative care. Both HWR and ICC believe that cancer patients should not be separated from their primary oncologist (and staff) at the end of their lives, because these relationships are well established, are grounded in trust, and are important psychologically to both parties. Second, the hospice model of care embraces a holistic and family-centered approach focused on enhancing the physical, emotional, social, and spiritual qualities of life. The goal was to implement this holistic approach for patients with cancer regardless of treatment, curative intent, or timeline for survival. As treatment fails, patients and families need increased support from their oncologists, who have provided their care for years. To have the capacity to do this well, oncologists need the support and counsel of trained end-of-life caregivers, in this case the SCT.

The unique innovative aspects of this model of palliative end-of-life care were twofold. First, the SCT was integrated into the standard care of the patient, whereas in other models the patient is separated from the primary oncologist and introduced to a separate team for palliative care. This model realigns the delivery of good cancer care to incorporate the simultaneous provision of palliative care. Second, the creation of a team with expertise in end-of-life care that functions in the acute cancer setting represents a combining of two entirely different philosophies of care—acute cancer and end-of-life—that is both unique and innovative.

Development of the Framework

The second element of success was an extremely detailed, step-by-step plan. In the most skeleton explanation, the SCT—composed of a nurse, social worker, and spiritual care counselor with expertise in palliative/end-of-life care—would integrate into the greater team at the ICC. This team would track the patient with the primary oncologist and integrate palliative care principles with a resulting synergistic outcome. From HWR's perspective and expertise in end-of-life care, five essential elements should be considered.

- The team would be composed of a nurse, social worker, and spiritual care counselor.
- The team would function as an interdisciplinary, not a multidisciplinary, team.
- The team would be housed at the ICC.
- All members of the team would share the same physical space.
- The unit of care would be patient and family (whomever the patient identified as family).

Initially, there was agreement on all areas except the composition of the team. The ICC researchers immediately agreed with the nurse and social worker, but questioned why a spiritual care counselor was necessary. The inclusion of this team member is extremely significant, because spiritual care is a major part of end-of-life care and is one area that distinguishes palliative care from care delivered in most acute care settings.

Collecting Baseline Data

Before beginning the project, the SCT devoted 4 months to collecting baseline data, creating care paths and documentation forms, and educating themselves as well as those other individuals who would come in contact with any aspect of the project. The study population selected was patients with stage IIIb or IV lung cancer, because the overall prognosis for these patients is poor and part of the overall goal was to determine whether hospice referral rates among appropriate patients could be improved.

Creating a Pain Care Path

The second major task for the SCT was to create a Pain Care Path, because one of goals of the ICC was to improve pain management for patients in the ambulatory cancer center. A retrospective chart review of 149 lung cancer patients who died in 1997 revealed limited documentation of pain assessment and management. In those situations in which there was documentation, no standardized protocol was followed.

The Pain Care Path is a decision tree for pain management. This standard of care also includes guidelines and supplementary forms with specific directions for implementation. The guidelines identified in the legend of the care path include pain assessment; opioid reference table; adjuvant analgesics; management of side effects; nonpharmacological interventions for psychosocial, spiritual, and physical pain; and patient/family pain education.

Of equal importance was the creation of a Pain Flow Sheet, which was designed to monitor the patient's pain management over time and to document actual practice. These two tools work well together: the Pain Care Path is "how you do it" and the Pain Flow Sheet is "how you document what you are doing." Both tools, which are extremely detailed and user friendly, can be downloaded from http://www2/edc.org/lastacts/archives/archivesJuly02/painflow.pdf and http://www2.edc.org/lastacts/archives/archivesJuly02/paincare.pdf (both accessed April 25, 2005).

The SCT and the pain consultant to the team led a mandatory meeting for all ICC nursing staff in which the principles of pain management, the Pain Care Path, and the Pain Flow Sheet were reviewed. As part of the education on pain, all ICC physicians and nurses received *A Cancer Pain Management Guide,* created by the SCT. As a result of this education, all patients at the ICC now have a Pain Flow Sheet placed in the front of their charts. When the chart is opened, the first thing in view is the Pain Flow Sheet. This serves as an objective way to determine whether patients are being assessed at every visit for pain.

Another aspect of pain management to be assessed and evaluated was the prescriptive patterns of physicians. Successful pain control was achieved using the World Health Organization's Analgesic Ladder Model and Agency for Health Care Policy and Research Pain Guidelines. Consultations with the pain specialist declined as ICC and SCT staff became increasingly skilled in implementing the Pain Care Path and protocol. Addition of a master's level nurse practitioner to the SCT further enhanced the team's ability to manage pain. Also, the Medical Director of HWR was actively involved at the weekly interdisciplinary team conferences and was instrumental in enhancing pain and symptom management with interventions such as the use of methadone for pain, specifically neuropathic pain.

At the time the SCT started working closely with the oncologists, some were immediately prescribing fentanyl patches; others routinely prescribed expensive opioids, and none used methadone. The advanced practice nurse became a major role model for the oncologists and over time gained the confidence of colleagues by her skillful and reliable interventions. The outcome was a change for the positive in prescriptive patterns.

Implementing the Education Plan

As part of the overall development plan, an extensive cross-training program was systematically created to bridge the differing cultures of aggressive cancer care and palliative care. There were many layers of professionals to be educated in end-of-life care, oncology, and Project Safe Conduct. The first was the SCT, whose members did not have a background in oncology, resulting in a knowledge deficit. Formal classes were provided to increase their general knowledge base about the lung cancer population and clinical trials. Time was spent shadowing staff in both radiation therapy and chemotherapy. An additional member of the project was the research nurse, who obtained informed consent from patients and administered the measurement tools. Her background was in oncology nursing, with limited knowledge of end-of-life care. An observational experience was done at the residential facility of HWR, where the nurse shadowed all disciplines to gain a better appreciation of the interdisciplinary team model and the blending of roles, as well as increased knowledge in palliative/end-of-life care.

A formalized education plan was implemented so that all staff members who might come in contact or work with the SCT would be oriented to the demonstration project before starting. Written information explaining the purpose of the project, identifying all core SCT members (by name, telephone and pager numbers, and how to contact them), and detailing the process of patient enrollment in the study accompanied the presentation given by the SCT members.

Members of the SCT participated in patient visits and spent one-on-one time with the medical and radiation oncologists. This provided the opportunity for SCT members to dialogue with the physicians and establish their individual preferences. Also, this time provided an opportunity to increase their knowledge base and to begin establishing rapport with the oncologists, staff, patients, and families.

Unwavering Support from Clinical and Administrative Leaders

The third and foremost reason for success was the endorsement and staunch support from the leadership of both HWR and ICC. As a kickoff to Project Safe Conduct, a day-long retreat was scheduled to discuss and launch the project and invite the oncologists to participate in the study. A psychologist from California who was knowledgeable about hospice and end-of-life care facilitated the retreat and provided support for the oncologists through some team-building activities. The unprecedented decision of the ICC Medical Director to schedule no patient appointments on the day of the retreat, so that key staff members and the oncologists could attend, was a powerful unspoken signal of the significance of this project.

From HWR, the Chief Executive Officer provided leadership support through his knowledge of palliative/end-of-life care, financial support from two large local grants for the salaries of the SCT, and in-kind support of half of the salary of the project director.

At the operational level, the Vice President of Clinical Services at ICC and the Project Director from HWR had weekly planned meetings to plan strategies for the daily implementation of the project. The Project Director oversaw every detail of the project and also developed and supervised the SCT; however, she was an outsider to the ICC system. Her counterpart at the ICC was extremely knowledgeable about the internal management system and helped the Project Director navigate through the system. This relationship was a key to success, because a marriage of two entirely different philosophies took place, and an outsider to a system was responsible for the operation of the project.

Cultural Change

Before the project was initiated, outsiders from hospice looking in at the cancer center made assumptions that "the physicians must not be talking with patients about end-of-life care and hospice." As the two systems worked beside one another, the understanding of HWR personnel changed dramatically. There were excellent oncologists at ICC who did have those conversations about end-of-life options. However, there are always patients who, despite the circumstances, respond with, "Yes, but I want to continue with chemotherapy regardless of the outcome." Certainly that is the individual patient's choice. All patients were given the option of whether to go into another clinical trial or transition into end-of-life care when the disease was not controlled. This close working relationship with the oncologists changed the hospice workers' impressions of what occurs on a daily basis at the cancer center.

Implementation Strategies

Project Safe Conduct was created as a demonstration project under The Robert Wood Johnson Foundation grant and as a research effort on the part of the ICC. Only lung cancer patients with stage IIIB or stage IV disease were eligible to enter the study. A total of 223 patients were enrolled in the study over 2 years (1999–2001). Fifty-one percent of the patients were female, and 39 percent were African American, which is representative of the demographics of Cleveland in terms of gender and race. The average length of stay with the SCT was 116 days, and at any given time there was a caseload of approximately 80 patients.

At the initial visit with the medical oncologist, the physician discussed the option of joining the clinical trial, explaining that the interventional SCT would work closely with the physician in the ongoing care and management of the patient's physical, emotional, social, and spiritual needs. If the patient agreed, during that same visit the nurse researcher obtained informed consent from the patient and administered three instruments—the FACT-L and the Missoula VITAS Quality of Life Index, both of which measure quality of life, and the Wisconsin Brief Pain Index. At the second visit, the SCT was introduced as a team so that the patient and family would become familiar with the team members. During that visit, the patient and family were introduced to the idea that family conferences would take place periodically. Also the team always asked, "How can we be of most help to you, right now, today?" Experience demonstrated that frequently there was a concern, symptom, or problem that could be addressed very quickly, immediately increasing the comfort level of the patient and family.

At every visit for chemotherapy or radiation therapy, office visit, or diagnostic test, some or all members of the SCT met with the patient and/or family, because this model focuses on the patient and family as the unit of care. Depending on the concerns of that day or week, the support and interaction of the SCT with the patient and family were very fluid and flexible. At some visits the total time was spent with the patient, whereas at others, might be with the family, because not everyone was on the same page or even the same chapter in the book at the same time. All members of the team at some point contacted those patients receiving chemotherapy over several hours during the visit.

Any time that pain medications were titrated or symptoms were treated, the advanced practice nurse called the patient at home the next day to determine the effectiveness of the intervention. All members of the team frequently interacted with patients and family members between on-site visits by telephone or e-mail.

Family Conferences: Delivering "Bad News"

One of the goals of the project was to improve communication through planned family conferences. Anyone on the larger team, including family members, could request a family conference. Sometimes the SCT held these conferences in the patients' homes, because frequently this resulted in an entirely different perspective. Family conferences were automatically scheduled at the completion of a clinical trial, because that is always a decision-making point. Typically, a computed tomography (CT) scan is scheduled to evaluate whether the cancer has responded to the therapy. The Project Director established a process that was set in motion at that time. The SCT was responsible to know the results of the CT scan and to discuss the options for treatment with the oncologist. Patients were informed that this would be a decision-making time and were encouraged to have members of their family present.

As with any topic, the level of confidence of the oncologists in delivering bad news varied greatly. Before holding the conference at which bad news would be given, the SCT usually had a meeting with the oncologist to discuss what the options were and to share with the oncologist from their perspective how prepared the patient and family were for the information. As a result of the intense work of the SCT, it was not uncommon for patients to be prepared for the news when treatment was no longer effective and the option of hospice-level care was presented. The team members were experienced in how to prepare and guide patients and families. Over time, the Project Director observed the following stages of learning and comfort displayed by the various oncologists when delivering bad news: call a member of the SCT to assist; don't leave me, keep me company; SCT take it from here; and finally, a seamless transition with the oncologist and SCT discussing the bad news with the patient and family.[2]

One of the ways senior faculty learned how to deliver bad news was by observing the SCT initiate the conversation to shift goals from cure-oriented to comfort-oriented care. The role-modeling and mentoring of senior faculty on the process of how to effectively deliver bad news and bridge the differences between palliative care and acute care was another element of success.

Team Conference

Weekly, a team conference using a hospice model took place. The Project Director, who was an advanced practice nurse with years of hospice experience, facilitated the conferences. Others in attendance were the research nurse, the SCT, the hospice physician, and the medical psychologist, who acted in a consultative role. The oncologists did not attend the weekly team conferences, although they were welcome. Their attendance was not logistically possible, because the SCT worked with more than eight oncologists and fellows who had entirely different schedules. Because the SCT was in the same building, team members could personally talk to the oncologists, e-mail them, page them, or call them by telephone.

The format for the team conference was to review any deaths that had occurred during the past week, any new admissions, and part of the active caseload and revise the plans of care with the input from all members of the team. The facilitator role-modeled how interdisciplinary teams interact and work effectively—something that takes many months to develop. New team members had to learn the roles of all other team members and how to blend their roles and still respect boundaries. Also just-in-time learning frequently took place. Having the input of a psychologist was extremely beneficial; she enhanced the management of behavioral symptoms, particularly depression. Another purpose of the team conference was to provide support to colleagues, because it was not uncommon for a team member to be visibly upset if an intervention was not as effective as anticipated or at the time of death. Debriefing, whatever the situation might be, is part of the process.

Open Access to Safe Conduct Team

In addition, patients and families could access the SCT phone line between 8:00 A.M. and 4:30 P.M., Monday through Friday. During off hours, families were directed in writing and prompted via voice message on the SCT phone line to contact their primary oncologist at all other times, as is normal practice at the ICC. During the established hours, patients and families knew that some member of the team would return their call if they did not immediately reach a team member. As a result, patients and families did not have to wait until the end of the working day, when physicians routinely return telephone calls. This open access to the team provided a certain amount of security. Because the team was monitoring these patients so closely, they were able to recognize subtle changes and encourage patients to come in to the clinic to be assessed and treated. It is likely that this careful attention to patients' symptoms prevented more complex problems from occurring.

Bereavement

If the patient was not enrolled in a hospice program, family members were referred to a bereavement center for follow-up. At the time of death, families received a bereavement card signed by all members of the team. This followed the protocol of the ICC, where the primary oncologist writes a letter to families at the time of death. The members of the SCT also attended calling hours, memorial services, funerals, or shivas whenever possible if the patient lived in the Greater Cleveland area.

Interdisciplinary Team Dynamics

Going into the project, the Project Director, who was experienced in effecting change within systems, had preconceived ideas regarding the challenges to be faced. In reality, the greatest challenge was creating and maintaining a healthy, functioning team. Although the original members of the SCT, like the Project Director, came from HWR, they never represented hospice as such. It was their knowledge and expertise in end-of-life care, not their hospice affiliation, that created their identity. The other distinguishing feature was that the SCT was an interdisciplinary team, not a multidisciplinary team. On a multidisciplinary team, members are known first by their professional identify and secondarily by their team affiliation. On an interdisciplinary team, the identity of the team supersedes the individual professional identities. Members blend roles, share information, and work together with the patient and family to develop the patient's goals.

In a period of 5½ years, the SCT has been recreated and rebuilt three times. The only persons who have remained constant on the team are the spiritual care counselor and the medical psychologist, who is a consultant to the team. The original nurse on the SCT was a home care nurse in hospice. Within a few months, it became apparent that the expectations of the role required an advanced practice nurse, because the nurse is expected to be an expert in pain and symptom management, to be capable of interfacing with oncologists as a colleague, to be able to teach pain and symptom management to staff and physicians, and ultimately to be a change agent in the system.

Any time a person on the team changed, the team dynamics immediately changed and the team building started over. To enable the SCT to work effectively as a team and to enhance the integration of the team into the cancer center, they were located in the same physical environment inside the ICC. Each time the composition of the team changed, the newly created SCT was taken off site for a day of team building.

Many factors appeared to contribute to the challenge of having a healthy functioning team. This team functioned under a palliative care model, as opposed to a palliative medicine model. The difference is that a palliative care model is flat in regard to authority, and all disciplines within their scope of practice have equal input. The other distinction is that all disciplines are involved in development of the plan of care with every patient, who determines what the goals will be, rather than being involved at the discretion of another professional. Most professionals work independently; they have not had experience working closely on an interdisciplinary team, and that is the central issue. Repeated role modeling and mentoring were the techniques used to teach the individual team members how to use a holistic approach and how to blend roles. Some professionals are never comfortable working closely on an interdisciplinary team, because their practice becomes very transparent to their colleagues.

Bridging the Gap: Creating an Interagency Interdisciplinary Team

From the beginning, there were major differences in philosophy and experience between the original SCT from HWR and the ICC staff. Therefore, a proactive plan was established to address these differences. To illustrate, a member of the SCT said, "If the patient doesn't want to eat, that's okay." That statement demonstrated lack of knowledge regarding aggressive treatments in an oncology center. The team member was responding from her own point of reference, when a patient is actively dying in a hospice program. She had no understanding of the role of nutrition for patients who are receiving aggressive treatments. This statement provided the impetus for more intense education about chemotherapy, radiation therapy, and clinical trials.

Teaching and learning took place on both sides. The SCT visited a new patient who was on the research floor, where phase I clinical trials are conducted. The patient asked, "How do I tell my children I am dying?" This led to a conversation that resulted in the patient's crying, a very appropriate reaction. The staff on the research floor interpreted the patient's crying as evidence that the SCT had upset her. The other two areas requiring education for ICC staff were pain management (discussed earlier) and a better understanding of when hospice-level care was the appropriate level of care. A gray area for the ICC staff was how to recognize when it was appropriate to refer a patient to a hospice program. After the original bumps in the road, the gap between the two cultures narrowed as the SCT integrated into the ICC and became an interagency interdisciplinary team.

Evaluation and Analysis of Data

Project Safe Conduct was a demonstration project, not a randomized controlled trial. Therefore, it is difficult to respond to frequently asked questions that could be answered only if a randomized controlled trial model had been performed. What can be shared are the processes and outcome data and the impact on complex systems. The strength of the project was that almost an entire population of lung cancer patients was studied for a period of 2 years.

The tools administered were the short and long forms of the Wisconsin Brief Pain Index (WBPI); the Missoula-VITAS Quality of Life Version 15 (MVQOL-15), which measures patients' quality of life on five dimensions; the FACT-L, which measures quality of life; and the After-Death Inventory (ADI), which measures family satisfaction.[3] In addition to using these tools, the clinical researchers tracked the length of stay in hospice for referred patients, the cost of drugs, and hospital and emergency room admissions.

Pain was present in virtually 100% of the patients at some point, and it clearly interfered with their life and well-being. Regardless of the level of pain (worst, least, or average) there was an extremely high correlation between pain and the impact on mood and sleep.

The MVQOL-15 total scores correlated with patient quality-of-life ratings in five dimensions of the patient's experience: symptoms, function, interpersonal relationships, well-being, and transcendence. A number of demographic characteristics were found to be associated with the quality of life and pain at baseline and at follow-up visits. The following subgroups of patients scored significantly lower on quality of life and higher on pain measures at baseline and at follow-up visits: young; African American; female; single, widow, divorced/separated, or unspecified marital status; and unemployed. Of these subgroups, all caught-up after 9 to 12 months except African Americans, widows, and those with unspecified marital status, who remained at high risk throughout the 1-year follow-up for selected quality of life and pain outcomes. The documentation of catch-up in the second 6-months of follow-up for the other high-risk demographic subgroups on both quality of life and pain outcomes was a positive finding. According to the statistician, it is highly likely that improvement in both quality of life and pain management was due in large part to the interventions of the SCT.

Place of Death

The most startling outcome was the shift in place of death. One of the goals of the project was to involve patients and families earlier in decision-making regarding end-of-life care. The 1997 statistics regarding lung cancer deaths for patients from the ICC were reviewed before the SCT intervention. Of the 149 deaths reviewed, 13% of patients with advanced lung cancer died with hospice support, with a median length of stay of 3 days and an average length of stay of 10 days. As of June 2001, when accrual of patients into the study was completed, 80% were dying with hospice support, with a median length of stay of 29 days and an average of 44 days. Eighteen months after the project ended, 75% of patients were dying with hospice support, with a median length of stay of 36 days and an average of 64 days. The majority of patients died in their own homes. Occasionally, patients were transferred to a hospice in-patient facility, based on the request of the patient/family when the patient had hours to days of life. These data speak to the sustainability of the intervention after the end of the demonstration project. To put these data into perspective, the national median length of stay in a hospice program is approximately 22 days and the average length of stay is 55 days, according to National Hospice and Palliative Care Organization statistics.[4]

A hospice referral is a process, not an event. Several factors contributed to moving patients to the appropriate level of end-of-life care. The members of the SCT who were experienced in palliative care knew how to guide the patient and family "through a maze of uncertain, perplexing, and distressing events" and build a trusting relationship. They were very comfortable in talking about hospice and engaging the patient and family into discussions about values, beliefs, treatment options or choices, goals, hopes, and unspoken fears. Shifting the level of care to hospice was viewed by all as an addition to the plan of care and not seen as taking everything away.

Second, the SCT was present at family conferences and provided support for the patient/family as well as the oncologist. One of the goals of the project was for the SCT to support the oncologists, especially regarding end-of-life topics. Oncologists should not be put in the position to have these conversations alone with families; they too benefited from the support of the SCT before, during, and after the news was delivered. Because of the integrative model of palliative care with the SCT, opening the conversation of end-of-life care was not viewed as withdrawing hope for these patients, but rather as part of the continuum of care at ICC. A referral to hospice was no longer seen as "giving up on" patients.

Open communication regarding palliative end-of-life care was modeled by the SCT in their daily practice with patients/families and the professional staff at the ICC. In addition, they were authorized to carry out their recommendations and interventions. This was the base for the professional staff to become comfortable with the topic and to build rapport with the patient and family. Patients were given options, and 25% chose to continue aggressive treatment until they died.

Other Comparison Data

Two other pieces of data were compared before and after the SCT intervention. The first was the number of hospital admissions and emergency room visits. Before SCT, the average number of hospital admissions or emergency room visits was 6.3 per patient. After the SCT became involved, that number decreased by 50%, to 3.1 visits per patient on average. A possible explanation for this decrease was the access patients and families had to the SCT through the team telephone number; team intervention prevented many emergency room visits.

The second piece of data was pharmaceutical costs. This information was an estimation of costs if all prescribed prescriptions for medications were filled (not including chemotherapy). Before SCT, the average daily cost per patient was $60.90, compared with $18.45 after SCT intervention. The advanced practice nurse worked very closely with the oncologists in managing pain and teaching pain management to fellows and some faculty who were less experienced. One of the outcomes of the project was a change in prescriptive patterns when doing pain management. More adjuvant medications were used, and high-cost opioids were not automatically prescribed but used only if appropriate.

Steps for Duplication of the Model of Care

Throughout this chapter, many of the essential elements of success have been identified. These elements are summarized in this section. Every system is different, so the identified steps for development of this integrative model of palliative care is the macro view; the micro aspects must be individualized according to the system.

Collaboration

- Support and buy-in from the top administrator who has control over daily operations is imperative. Do your homework well and do not attempt to implement the model until buy-in occurs.
- It is necessary to obtain buy-in not only from the top administrator, but also from the oncologists and staff who will be interacting daily with the team. The retreat off-site, where all oncologists and staff heard the same message about the project, was the beginning of buy-in for the oncologists. At all times, the message was that the oncologists do good work and the SCT is there to enhance their work and not add to it.
- Develop a steering committee, which meets every 4 months, to assist in addressing the direction of the project and developing overall strategies for implementation. The major decision-makers/implementers are at the next level.
- A trusting relationship at the decision-making/implementation level was the secret to Project Safe Conduct, beyond the more obvious ingredients. The Project Director was from HWR, and her counterpart was Vice President for Cancer Services at ICC. Those two individuals met weekly and developed a strong, trusting relationship as colleagues. The Project Director's expertise was in end-of-life care, but,

as an outsider to the ICC, she was not familiar with their system. Her counterpart had authority within the system and the ability to navigate the system. Even if both parties are from the same system, one needs clinical expertise and the other administrative authority.

Development

- Create documentation records. Numerous methods were tried by Project Safe Conduct. The final one was to have the SCT make entries in the progress notes on the patient's chart. In addition, the individual team members had their own system for tracking patients and their plans of care.
- Develop a Pain Care Path and Flow Sheet. Several weeks were devoted to development of the Pain Care Path and Flow Sheet, because that was one of the aims of the project—to improve pain management. In another system, these forms might already be in place.
- Create the Safe Conduct Team. The essential elements for the team are (1) that it is interdisciplinary, not multidisciplinary; (2) that an advanced practice nurse, not a staff RN, is part of the team; and (3) that the spiritual care counselor, social worker, and team share same physical space.
- Do as much team building as possible—go off site for a mini-retreat.
- Constantly observe the team dynamics.
- Someone outside the team, who knows team dynamics and end-of-life care, needs to facilitate the weekly conferences. During this time, role modeling and teaching always take place.

Implementation

- Educate anyone and everyone who will come in contact with the team before implementation.
- Create written information that explains the purpose, the team members and their contact numbers, and the process.
- Make appointments to meet with the staff as well as times to shadow the oncologists, the radiologists, and staff in their respective practice areas.
- Know the system, to prevent unnecessary problems.
- Most important: *integrate in, don't separate out.* When the team is working well, they should blend into the bigger team so well that they are invisible as a team.
- Enhance the care already being provided rather than creating additional work. If the staff or physicians see anything that the team does as being additional work, they will immediately reject them.

Evaluation

- The number of referrals to any hospice program was used as one measuring stick of success. If your needs assessment identifies late referrals or limited referrals as an area for improvement, this is easily measured.
- Physician surveys were done after about 6 months into the study to identify any unmet needs or problems that needed to be addressed.

Safe Conduct Team Post-project

When the Robert Wood Johnson Foundation funded Project Safe Conduct as a demonstration project, one of many questions to be answered was how the ICC planned to sustain the program after the conclusion of the grant. The outcome of the project has been a new, higher standard of care. Removal of the SCT would be interpreted as a reduction in service, because this new standard of care has now become an expectation.[5] As a result, the ICC is so committed to the SCT and the excellent work they have done that the members have been hired full-time at ICC. The cost of the team is integrated into the system and charged to the overall budget of the ambulatory ICC, with no additional fee charged to the patient/family. The Project Director, who also facilitated team conferences during the project, continues to facilitate the weekly conferences and support the team. Her time is donated as an in-kind service by HWR.

The composition of the SCT today is an advanced practice nurse with a background in palliative care, the same spiritual care counselor, and two social workers assigned according to disease entities. The target population has expanded to include patients with advanced gastrointestinal malignancies or advanced head and neck malignancies, as well as those with lung cancer stage IIIB or IV.

The number of patients followed on any given day has increased from approximately 80 during the project to a set limit of 100. With such a large census, the SCT has had to develop a system to deliver palliative care that philosophically is unchanged but permits the involvement of more patients. Table 64–1 is an example of documentation used to identify and monitor patients.

Patients are referred to the team by oncologists, radiologists, nurses, and social workers. At every appointment, some member of the team tries to meet with the patient and/or family. In addition to the information on the patient record form, a daily schedule is prepared and the team decides which member will be the primary contact, depending on the needs of that individual patient. To illustrate, if a patient is having spiritual suffering, the spiritual counselor would definitely be the primary contact. But if, during a visit, the patient begins to talk about physical pain, then the spiritual counselor would page the advanced practice nurse to see the patient during the visit. The nurse practitioner sits in on physician visits so that she can be very involved as the disease progresses. At some point during the patient's course of treatment, team members from all disciplines sit in on doctors' visits.

Table 64–1
Sample Patient Record

Last Name	First Name	Hospital No.	Physicians	Appointments	Diagnosis
Wilson	Joan	2340987	Oncologist, radiologist, pulmonologist	01/05/03—Oncologist 01/16/03—Oncologist 01/20/03—Chemotherapy 01/29/03—Radiologist 02/02/03—Oncologist 02/20/03—Oncologist 02/26/03—Radiologist, chemotherapy 03/19/03—Oncologist, chemotherapy	Stage IV NSCLC—metastases to bone, brain, mediastinum, cervical lymph nodes, liver, and adrenal glands

Today, the SCT monitors patients as they did during the project, using a holistic approach to address pain and symptoms. The SCT continues to be involved in family conferences, with some of these conferences taking place in the patient's home. The main difference is that not all team members see the patient and/or family on every visit, and the length of time spent with the patient and family may be decreased.

Conclusion

The ongoing work of the SCT has taught all participants a valuable lesson on the process of moving patients to end-of-life care when treatment no longer controls the disease—because a hospice referral is a process, not an event. The SCT practitioners used the following process as they journeyed with the patient and family: defined and interpreted information; facilitated communication; helped patients/families articulate their concerns to the physicians; offered advice about treatment options; identified and alerted patients to symptoms and changes in physical and emotional function; and were always accessible and frequently telephoned.

The clinical researchers for Project Safe Conduct astutely incorporated the following key concepts into the program design: a well-defined vision aligned with the organizations' missions; a detailed, comprehensive plan; clinical and administrative leadership endorsement and staunch support; family conferences initiated by any team member or by the patient or family; and the integration of palliative care into routine operations.

REFERENCES

1. Weisman A. Coping with Cancer. New York: McGraw-Hill, 1979:18.
2. Pitorak EF, Armour MB. Project Safe Conduct integrates palliative goals into comprehensive cancer care. J Palliat Med 2003; 6:649.
3. Byock IR, Merriman MP. Measuring quality of life for patients with terminal illness: The Missoula-VITAS quality of life index. Palliat Med 1998;12:234.
4. National Hospice and Palliative Care Organization. Hospice Facts and Figures, http://www.nhpco.org/files/public/Hospice_Facts_110104.pdf (accessed April 25, 2005).
5. Project Safe Conduct. Innovations in End-of-Life Care. July, 2002. Available at: http://www2.edc.org/lastacts/archivesJuly02/featureinn.asp (accessed April 25, 2005).

65

Eleanor Canning and Richard Payne

Harlem Palliative Care Network*

My pain is unbearable, I have no insurance, my electricity has been turned off, my family does not have enough food, and my children are sleeping on the floor.—Ms. S, a 51-year-old Spanish-speaking woman from the Dominican Republic with bilateral breast cancer

- ***Key Points***
- *The Harlem Palliative Care Network demonstrated how health care professionals were able to harness the power of collaboration among Memorial Sloan-Kettering Cancer Center, North General Hospital, and the Visiting Nurse Service of New York.*
- *This project provided a barrier-free, effective resource for patients and families needing end-of-life care, with a focus on quality of life. Key influences on end-of-life decision-making included culture and ethnicity.*
- *The project reduced pain and improved the quality of life for patients with life-limiting illness.*
- *The Harlem project also provided support and education in the advance planning process to patients, families, and professionals.*

Imagine that you are the 51-year-old, Spanish-speaking, single mother of two children, 11 and 13 years old. You have bilateral breast cancer; you are in extreme pain, and your body is distorted with edema. Your lifelong belief in spiritual healing is no longer helping to relieve the pain and fight the cancer. Your children have no bedroom furniture and are sleeping on mattresses on the apartment floor. Your family, which includes a male companion, is threatened with eviction from your East Harlem, New York, apartment. In fact, the electricity has already been turned off. You are too ill to work. Your health insurance has lapsed; your family does not have enough food. You will die in 276 days. Among other issues important to you in your care is the fact that you want to die at home.

In the summer of 2001, Ms. S was referred by her oncologist at North General Hospital (NGH) to the Harlem Palliative Care Network (HPCN), a community-based model of palliative care that was made possible by a 3-year grant from the United Hospital Fund (UHF). The UHF selected this partnership as one of six community-oriented palliative care initiatives and provided valuable financial and consultative support for the duration of the project. HPCN enjoyed additional support from the James N. Jarvie Commonweal Service, a long-time supporter of the Visiting Nurse Service of New York (VNSNY), and generous in-kind contributions from NGH, VNSNY, and Memorial Sloan-Kettering Cancer Center (MSKCC).

From 2000 until 2003, HPCN served 350 predominantly female patients, age 20 to 91 years, who were residing in East and Central Harlem and had one of the five target diagnoses: progressive cancer, congestive heart failure (CHF), chronic obstructive pulmonary disease (COPD), end-stage renal disease (ESRD), or HIV/AIDS. This chapter describes the partnership, the care model including the network, and the success of HPCN. The legacy of the HPCN is a community-based palliative care model that demonstrated reduced pain and suffering, increased the number of patients with advance planning, and improved quality of life (QOL).

*The Harlem Palliative Care Network is a community based palliative care partnership among Memorial Sloan-Kettering Cancer Center, North General Hospital, and the Visiting Nurse Service of New York.

Harnessing the Power of the Partnership

VNSNY is the preferred home care provider for both MSKCC and NGH and operates one of the largest hospice programs in New York City. VNSNY has well-developed programs to better meet the needs of the culturally and ethnically diverse populations of New York City. NGH is the primary site for serving the acute care needs of Central and East Harlem residents and provides two converted patient rooms as office space for HPCN operations. NGH has extensive knowledge of community needs and resources as well as strong relationships with community-based organizations and providers. MSKCC is an internationally renowned cancer treatment and research facility that provides patient care and clinician training on all aspects of oncology, including pain management and end-of-life care.

The UHF grant enabled the partnership to establish a core staff and begin assembling a community-based network that numbered more than 100 providers. All three partners played key roles in developing the network. Network providers were selected based on their ability to meet a category of patient need. All agencies experience capacity issues at one time or another, and for this reason HPCN sought a few providers in each category. This was not always easy or even possible.

Network members provided a variety of services and included churches, health care providers, support groups,

Table 65–1
Examples of Needs Addressed by the Harlem Palliative Care Network in Each of the Domains

Physical	Social/Emotional/ Psychological	Spiritual	Pain and Symptom Management	Advance Planning
Activities of daily living assistance	Child care	Clergy referral	Support for poorly controlled pain	End-of-life and treatment decisions
Financial	Dependent care	Support groups	Nausea/vomiting	Advance Directives
Food/meals	Legal assist	Pastoral care	Fatigue/weakness	Do-not-resuscitate (DNR) orders
Housing	Caregiver respite		Constipation	Living Will
Home care	Transportation		Sleeplessness, sleepiness, lethargy	Durable Power of Attorney (DPOA)
Hospice	Telephone reassurance		Shortness of breath	
Medical coverage	Friendly visits		Falls	
	Grief		Noncompliance with medications/treatment	
	Estrangement			
	Intentional isolation			

Table 65–2
Sample Needs, Solutions, and Possible Network Providers

Need Identified	Solution	Network Provider
Inadequate pain or symptom management	Review current prescription	Prescribing physician
No health insurance	Determine Medicaid eligibility	Social work staff at VNSNY
Inadequate pharmacy coverage	Seek subsidy	EPIC, pharmaceutical company, charitable care
Spiritual crisis	Reconnect with faith	Clergy
Hunger	Entitlements, charitable aid	Food pantries, food stamps, soup kitchens
Single parent	Guardianship	Legal Aid, Family Center
Psychological/emotional	Counseling	Family Center, HPCN staff
Isolation	Telephone reassurance, friendly visitor	Volunteers from VNSNY or local churches
Home care	Obtain physician order	VNSNY Home Care
Home hospice	Obtain physician order	VNSNY Hospice Care

EPIC, Elderly Pharmaceutical Insurance Coverage program; HPCN, Harlem Palliative Care Network; VNSNY, Visiting Nurse Service of New York

Table 65–3
Network Providers by Category

Network Member	Number	Sample Services
Churches	30	Food pantry, spiritual care, volunteer
Community-based organizations	47	Meals on Wheels, Legal Aid, Counseling
Health care providers	23	Home Care, Home Hospice pharmacy

pharmacies, pharmaceutical companies, and soup kitchens. They addressed needs in five domains: pain and symptom management, social/psychological/emotional, spiritual, physical, and advance planning. Examples of patient needs in each of these domains are presented in Table 65–1.

Examples of matching needs, solutions and network providers can be found in Table 65–2. Table 65–3 lists sample services for several categories of providers. Network members received end-of-life care education. Organized outreach included one-on-one appointments, educational presentations, and mailings to network members of current literature on palliative care designed to increase competency in end-of-life care. In addition to receiving referrals from HPCN, providers were asked to be aware of people in their community who needed palliative care and to refer those people to HPCN. The topic of advance planning was introduced within the first week after entry into the program. Multiple conversations addressed the topics of proxy, comfort, treatments, and relationships with loved ones. These conversations took place with patients and families by the HPCN staff.

Establishing a Barrier-Free Palliative Care Program

Understanding the community was the first priority. Beliefs about end of life have deep roots in culture, religion, and clinical practice patterns. HPCN sought to understand these beliefs and practice patterns, present the project's vision, and refine that vision to match the needs of the community. HPCN worked synergistically with other initiatives in the community, such as the Initiative to Improve Palliative Care for African Americans (IIPCA) and the Ziegler Professional Education Project (ZPEP), and a Nathan Cummings Foundation Grant. This initial process consumed the first 6 to 8 months of the grant and was time well spent.

First, a multidenominational clergy focus group helped to identify needs, learn about religious implications in end-of-life care, and educate clergy on palliative care. The clergy often know when a member of their congregation is facing a life-limiting illness and are in a key position to identify palliative care patients and refer them to NGH or directly to HPCN.

Second, HPCN participated in a Latino workgroup whose members reflected the growing Hispanic-Latino demographic in East and Central Harlem. The group comprised local community leaders, clergy, and medical providers and served to gather input from and effect change in the Latino community's perception of NGH. East and Central Harlem residents perceived NGH as a primarily African-American institution. A plan was adopted to infuse the community with an image of NGH as a community hospital that welcomes Hispanics and Latinos. A concrete example of the changes was a commitment on the part of the hospital to increase community outreach and to develop bilingual signage and staffing.

Third, key opinion leaders were invited to join the ongoing Community Advisory Board for HPCN. This platform provided continued community visibility for HPCN, and for palliative care in general, and feedback throughout the 3 years during which HPCN was serving the community.

Fourth, there was organized outreach to physician offices, clinics, and other community-based organizations. This outreach included one-on-one office appointments by the VNSNY Physician Relations staff, group and dinner presentations supported by pharmaceutical companies, and mailings to network members with current literature on palliative care that was designed to increase competency in end-of-life care. During the first 2 years of the project, the message of HPCN and palliative care was brought to a total of 4000 people.

Fifth, the steering committee for HPCN met regularly and consisted of decision-makers in senior clinical and business management positions at each of the three partner organizations (MSKCC, NGH, and VNSNY). Through these efforts, the steering committee concluded that this underserved community faced common progressive diseases such as cancer, heart disease, COPD, and AIDS. Many of these people died without palliative care services available to them or their caregivers and families. Rather, they died in fear and discomfort after long struggles with uncontrolled pain, unresolved grief, and other daunting symptoms. In addition to economic factors, barriers to the delivery of palliative care included lack of knowledge or clinical expertise, hesitance on the part of providers to prescribe medications that might help feed a local network of illicit drugs, and a curative culture that still undervalued symptom management and psychosocial support. On the patient's side, barriers included cultural beliefs, a distrust of the health care system, financial hardship, and a lack of insurance coverage, which impeded access to the supportive services that could improve their QOL.[1]

The staffing model for HPCN included a director, a clinical coordinator, and an administrative assistant. In the start-up months, the roles and responsibilities of program staff were blurred. As the program evolved, these roles were clarified to achieve operational efficiencies. Over the 3 years, the skill set needed to advance the project changed, and this necessitated personnel changes to be successful and develop the program.

This model relied on in-kind resources from the partners to provide administrative support for accounting, human resources, clinical leadership and strategic planning, outcome analysis, and reporting. When hiring, HPCN sought cultural and linguistic matches. The program was bilingual (English/Spanish) and produced patient education literature in both languages. HPCN was located in NGH, in two converted patient rooms on the same floor as the oncology clinic. This provided convenient access for patients in a familiar setting and ease of patient travel to HPCN during physician visits or outpatient chemotherapy sessions. The clinical coordinator was called for bedside consultations on inpatients. With a lean staff and complex cases, the network became a key partner in meeting the needs of the patients.

Table 65–6
Referral Sources

Referral source	Percent
North General Hospital	67
Community Organization	9
Visiting Nurse Service of New York	6
Patient/caregiver	6
Physicians	5
Memorial Sloan-Kettering Cancer Center	3
Other hospitals	3

Patient Care

To ensure a barrier-free environment, the admission criteria were as broad as possible. Every referral was accepted. In the rare instance in which a patient was not accepted into the program, the patient was linked to a more suitable provider. Examples of patients not enrolled in the program are persons younger than 18 years of age and those with chronic pain related to fibromyalgia. Characteristics of the enrolled patients are presented in Tables 65–4 through 65–6.

A nurse or social worker assessed each patient on referral. Data collected included demographics, information on the caregiver, proxy, diagnosis, medications and knowledge of illness, and identified barriers that made it difficult for the patient to comply with the prescribed medical regimen. Of greatest importance was how this diagnosis was affecting the QOL for the patient. A pain and symptom assessment, based on a 10-point scoring system, and the Missoula Vitas Quality of Life Index (MVQOLI) completed the initial assessment. This triad of data collection enabled the HPCN professional staff to outline a plan of palliative care designed to improve the patient's QOL in the physical, social/psychological/emotional, spiritual, and pain and symptom management domains. This interview session laid the relationship groundwork for sensitive discussions concerning advance planning.

The MVQOLI was repeated every 60 days. The pain and symptom assessment was repeated as needed, but at a minimum every 60 days. HPCN's success in advance planning, pain management, and improving QOL is discussed later.

Table 65–4
Race of Enrolled Patients

Race	Percentage
African American	74
Hispanic/Latino	14
White	6
Other	6

Table 65–5
Diagnoses of Enrolled Patients

Diagnoses	Percentage
Cancer	83
Congestive heart failure	7
End-stage renal disease	6
Acquired immunodeficiency syndrome	3
Chronic obstructive pulmonary disease	1

Social Work Versus a Nursing Model

During the first 2 years of the project, the clinical coordinator was a nurse. Review of the data after 2 years revealed that the interventions this population needed most were primarily social in nature (Table 65–7). For the remaining year, the clinical coordinator role was cast as a social worker, with a part-time nurse available to address the clinically frail patients and to collaborate with the social worker on patients with nursing needs. The average daily census was about 90 patients. This enabled all program staff to know the needs and goals of each patient and to work collaboratively when each needed the expertise of the other. A close collaborative relationship between the nurse practitioner and the physician in the oncology clinic, and the close proximity of HPCN offices to the oncology clinic, provided HPCN staff effective access to these professionals when pain and symptom management required their intervention.

Table 65–7
Needs and Linkages

Needs	Linkages ($n = 605$)	Percentage
Social/psychological/ emotional	233	39
Physical	178	29
Pain and symptom management	97	16
Spiritual	28	5
Other	69	11

The Plan of Care

A plan of care was created that linked each patient to network providers with the ability to meet that patients needs and to improve the QOL for that patient. Once the patient was socially stable, there was a sound foundation on which the medical team could build the medical plan of care. Patients' problems compete with their ability to be compliant with plans of care laid out by the medical team.

Network providers were linked to a patient to help satisfy an identified need. Sometimes it was as simple as discussing with the clinic staff the scheduling of appointments. In one case, HPCN coordinated doctor visits so the patient did not have to choose between lunch at the soup kitchen or a visit with the doctor. Patients dealing with guardianship of minor children were connected to the Legal Aid Society. Families needing counseling were connected to the Family Center. The HPCN plan of care involved the patient and family, the medical team, and, when appropriate, the Network.

Advance Planning

The HPCN model of palliative care required identifying the needs of patients concerning advance planning and meeting those needs. This process was central to the HPCN mission. Even so, we stumbled. The reasons are not surprising. Becoming comfortable with these frank discussions was a skill set that the team needed to develop. It was much easier to meet a concrete need such as pain management. During a review of the program at 9 months, the HPCN staff discovered that very few patients had become engaged in the advance planning activities. Even conversations about subjects as basic as the health care proxy were not resulting in decisions from the patients. We realized that patients do not approach advance planning in a linear fashion. After much internal discussion, the following process emerged. HPCN staff could engage the patients in discussion that naturally segued into identification of a health care proxy, completion of a living will, or creation of a do-not-resuscitate document. As this strategy was implemented, data were collected on the next 111 patients. The staff recorded strategies that the patients responded to. The ways in which patients were engaged are described in Table 65–8. Many patients eventually discussed more than one topic.

However, different topics resonated with individual patients. The clinician needed to find a common ground with the patient to introduce advance planning. Even if no document resulted from these interactions, when these patients were faced with a document to sign on admission to the hospital, their wishes had already begun to form and they were not making decisions about goals of care in a crisis. It took about eight sessions with the HPCN member to establish a relationship in which advance planning conversations were effective and not so emotionally charged for the clinicians, patients, and families.

A fair number of patients were undocumented immigrants, with better family and social support in the country of origin. Some of these patients chose to return to their country of origin for death. For some patients, HPCN assisted with funeral planning. After evaluating multiple resources and tools, HPCN

Table 65–8
Engaging the patient in the Advance Planning Process ($n = 111$)

Strategy	% of Patients
Need identified: the need for advance planning discussions was identified	93
Existing planning: patients with completed advance directive documents on referral to HPCN	7
Spoken wishes: patients articulated how they wanted the end of their life to proceed	54
Life review: an effective way to engage the patient in the advance directive discussions	74
Past experience with the illnesses of a family member, friend, or self: an effective way to engage the patient in advance planning discussions	66
Spiritual beliefs: a platform to engage the patient in the advance directive discussions	77
Meaning of the current illness or diagnosis: discussion of the current illness was an effective way to engage the patient in the advance directive discussions	69
Patients identified family/social support: and this opened up discussion about health care proxies	87
Advance planning printed information and explanations: received materials	81

HPCN, Harlem Palliative Care Network.

adopted the Five Wishes[2] document for use in patient education on end of life. This 12-page document is available in English and Spanish through the Aging with Dignity organization at their website (http://www.agingwithdignity.org).

The Outcomes and the Legacy

The HPCN model demonstrated that QOL can be improved and suffering relieved even in patients who proceed to death. Patients began to see advance directives as empowering and not as withholding of treatment. For those patients who did not complete advance directives with HPCN, the staff unanimously felt that the patient was overall prepared to make those decisions when required in urgent situations. Internal analysis of the advance planning data revealed a 39% increase in the number of patients engaged in the advance planning process (Table 65–9). In addition, the location of death was reviewed as an indicator of patient control over care at the end of life (Table 65–10).

Quality of Life

HPCN collected and acted on quality-of-life information every 60 days, using the MVQOLI. HPCN submitted multiple MVQOLIs on the first 117 patients. The tools reflected an 8-month period in the patient's life. The MVQOLI is designed to measure the subjective, experienced QOL of patients with advanced illness. Patients provide their own responses; QOL is not staff-assessed. Therefore, the data reflect the patient's experience of his or her own QOL in the five domains measured (Figure 65–1).

The instrument measures five dimensions of a person's subjective experience: symptoms (SX), functional status (F), interpersonal relations (IP), emotional well-being (WB), and transcendence (TR). Within each dimension, three types of information are elicited for patients:

1. An assessment of perceived status with respect to the experience encompassed by the dimension
2. The degree of satisfaction or dissatisfaction with the status
3. A rating of the importance of the dimension to overall QOL

A unique scoring protocol devised for the instrument allows for the weighting of each dimension based on the importance assigned to it by the patient.

Cumulative data for all patients over the 8-month period showed the following[3]:

1. On average, patient-reported QOL increased.
2. Patient-reported QOL increased during the first 60 days of care.
3. QOL remained high or continued to increase for the entire 8-month period.
4. Patients who came to HPCN with the lowest QOL showed a 50% increase in QOL scores on the MVQOLI within the first 60 days of care.
5. Improvements were seen in all domains—symptoms, function, interpersonal, well-being, and transcendent. The most dramatic improvements were seen in the emotional well-being and spiritual (transcendent) domains.

Table 65–9
Advanced planning scores

Document	On Enrollment	After Enrollment	Percent Increase
Health care proxy	43	61	30
Living will	12	30	60
Do-not resuscitate order	11	16	40
Overall	66	107	39

Table 65–10
Location of Death (First 68 Deaths)

In-hospital acute bed	31
Inpatient hospice	9
Intensive care unit	3
At home with CHHA services	7
At home with Home Hospice	9

CHHA, Certified Home Health Agency.

Pain Management

Routinely, patients were assessed for their pain levels at a minimum of every 60 days and as indicated. In addition, 48 hours after a change in the pain medication regimen, the pain score was reassessed. Patients were taught to communicate their pain to physicians and HPCN staff using the 10-point pain score. An outside evaluator for UHF found the reduction in pain scores to be significant.[3]

Sustainability

Efforts were heroic to secure additional funding for continuation of the HPCN, but to no avail. The funding after the September 11, 2001, terrorist attack in New York City was very limited. The message from funders was clear: They were

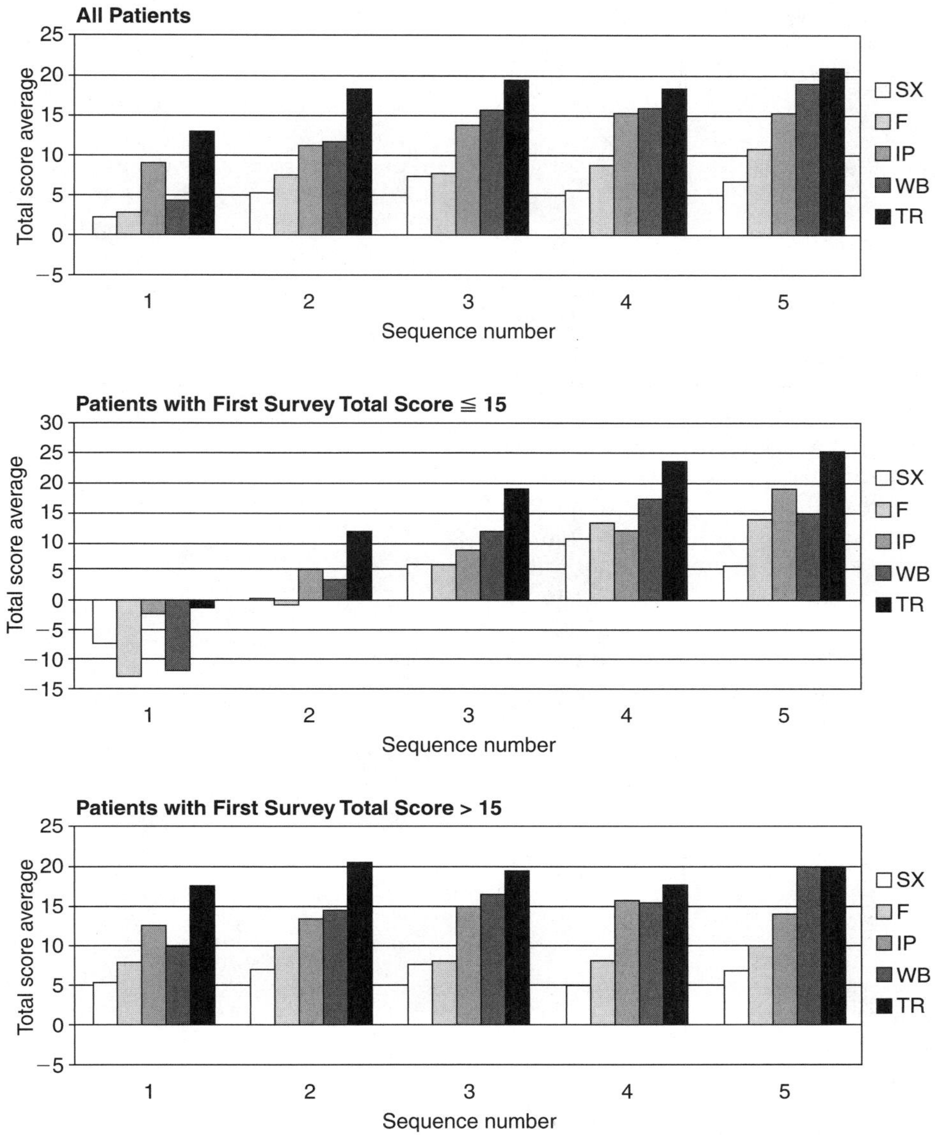

Figure 65–1. Results of administration of the Missoula Vitas Quality of Life Index (MVQOLI) at 60-day intervals to 117 patients. The instrument measures five dimensions of a person's subjective experience: symptoms (SX), functional status (F), interpersonal relations (IP), emotional well-being (WB), and transcendence (TR).

interested in programs that provided a broader reach to affect more patients. What could we take away from our HPCN work and reach more people? VNSNY Hospice Care has been successful in securing funding focused on increasing competency in palliative care and increasing the reach of programs such as HPCN. A consultation team based in VNSNY Hospice Care will lend expertise to nurses in the VNSNY Certified Home Care Agency. The team will provide an array of services that reflect the three core competencies of hospice and palliative care: advanced care planning, pain and symptom management, and counseling. In addition, the consultation team will design strategies for early introduction of palliative care and will also offer care coordination services.

The lessons learned from the HPCN model were powerful:

1. Match the staff with the ethnic backgrounds of the patients.
2. Understand the cultural implications of end-of-life decision-making.
3. Provide support for the social, psychological, and spiritual needs of the end-of-life patient to provide a steady platform for medical management of the pain and symptoms related to the terminal diagnosis.
4. Educate time and again the health professionals, clergy, and community-based agencies. Two components are essential to this education: the academic

material and the experience gaining comfort with end-of-life conversations.
5. Integrate palliative care into the medical plan of care.

Reimbursement

VNSNY is actively working with managed care organizations to make the clinical and business case for palliative care services in the hospice contracts. Palliative care at this time relies heavily on philanthropy. The data on cost savings of palliative care in health plans are mounting. There is evidence in the literature that emergency room visits are decreased, hospital stays are shortened, and pharmacy costs are decreased when palliative care is introduced.[4]

Setbacks and obstacles can be overcome if the program sets clear goals and focuses on achieving results. Although there were changes in personnel and reporting relationships, the program never lost sight of its goal to improve the QOL for Harlem residents facing life-threatening illness. The program strove to touch the lives of an increasing number of patients in need and to understand how to effectively meet those needs and overcome barriers to access.

ACKNOWLEDGMENTS

The HPCN received initial funding from the United Hospital Fund and additional support from the James Jarvie Commonweal Service. NGH, MSKCC, and VNSNY provided generous in-kind support throughout this project.

We thank others who contributed to the success of the HPCN: Terri Payne, Lisa Alvarenga, Sam Daniel, Elaine Keane, Jennifer O'Neill, Oscar Lewis, Liz Alvarado, Norma Castillo, Eno Onda, Roberto Rodriquez, Joseph Yo, Jenny Romero, Barbara Coulston, Nessa Coyle, Diane Magnuson, and Susan Hopper.

REFERENCES

1. Crawley L, Payne R, Bolden J, Payne T, Washington P, Williams S. Palliative care and end-of-life in the African-American community. JAMA 2000;284:2518–2521.
2. Five Wishes. Available at: http://www.agingwithdignity.org (accessed March 25, 2005).
3. Hopper SS. Moving Palliative Care into the Community: New Services, New Strategies. New York: United Hospital Fund, 2004.
4. Center to Advance Palliative Care. The case for hospital based palliative care. 2002. Available at: http://www.capc.org/support-from-capc/capc-publications/making-th-case.pdf (accessed April 27, 2005).

66

International Models of Excellence

PALLIATIVE CARE IN CANADA

Carleen Brenneis and Pam Brown

Canadians highly value their publically funded health care system and believe that quality end-of-life care is an imperative. Indeed, end-of-life care is consistent with the very values that resulted in the creation of a national health care system.[1] However, the current system of end-of-life and hospice palliative care in Canada has been described as a patchwork of inadequate and inequitably available services. Access to services is influenced by the diseases Canadians die from, whether they live in a city or rural area, the province in which they reside, the nature of their health insurance plans, and their personal wealth.[2] Only 5% to 10% of the 220,000 Canadians who die each year receive integrated and interdisciplinary palliative care.[3] The estimated cost of dying in Canada is approximated at $3 billion annually, with no performance indicators to suggest that resources are appropriately allocated.[4] Recent federal reports are calling for federal action to address access to palliative care services, particularly in the home.[1] The increased attention on end-of-life care and acknowledgment that services are inequitable challenge those responsible for health services delivery to develop initiatives and to address models of care for palliative care delivery.

This chapter discusses models of service delivery for palliative care in Canada. To provide context to Canada, an overview of the Canadian Health Care System is provided. The responsibilities of the federal and provincial governments and regional health authorities are described, as these three levels of government are accountable for health care delivery. The impact of the Canadian Hospice Palliative Care Association (CHPCA), in particular the consensus-based *Model to Guide Hospice Palliative Care*, is presented. Key factors influencing program development are discussed: the end-of-life care movement; the shift to community-based care; the unique needs of rural Canada;

cultural factors; and primary health care. The challenges and direction of best-practice model development is analyzed. Programs in Edmonton and Calgary are discussed as examples of integrated regional community-based programs.

Responsibility for Palliative Care

Federal Government

Health care in Canada is publicly funded and universally accessible. The Canada Health Act is federal legislation that facilitates reasonable access to health services without financial or other barriers through the five key principles of public administration, comprehensiveness, universality, portability, and accessibility.[5] While the Constitution Act of Canada (1982) defines health care as a provincial rather than federal responsibility, in practice, responsibility for health care is shared between the federal and provincial governments. The federal government can influence health care through legislation and control of financial resources. The federal government can also impact areas of health care through regulations, commissions, and activities of its various departments. For example, Health & Welfare Canada has initiated several key reports and meetings that have increased national discussion about health care and end-of-life care issues (Table 66–1).

All reports call for national initiatives to increase access to integrated palliative care services, with particular emphasis on palliative care services in the home. This is crucial to the development of palliative care in Canada because the Canada Health Act is generally viewed as a barrier to community-based palliative care.[6] The principle of "comprehensiveness," as defined in the Act, includes only health care provided in hospitals, or by physicians in any setting. Thus, each province decides which additional services, if any, will be funded. The result is that home-care coverage varies between provinces and within regions of a province. To address this inequity, the Commission on the Future of Health Care in Canada[1] specifically identified this issue and proposed that new home care transfer payments should be used to support expansion of the Canada Health Act to include medically necessary home care services, including palliative home care services to support people in their last 6 months of life.

In 2001, the federal government established the Health Canada Secrétariate on Palliative and End-of-Life Care in recognition of the need for a national action plan to ensure that all Canadians have access to quality end-of-life care. Five national working groups have been established to work on the priorities identified in a National Action Planning Workshop: Best Practices and Quality; Public Information and Education; Education of Care Providers; Research; and Surveillance. An example of improving quality of care is the Best Practice working group's initiative with the Canadian Council for Health Services Accreditation (CCHSA) to incorporate palliative and end-of-life care into recognized quality assessment and improvement processes in Canada. They plan to develop a national set of standards and to incorporate them into the existing CCHSA health service standards. Furthermore, there are plans to develop a national accreditation program for free-standing hospice organizations and volunteer-based programs, which currently have no national method of accreditation. The development and integration of national palliative care standards into the CCHSA accreditation process will challenge health care providers to ensure that they have incorporated hospice palliative care services into mainstream health care services.

The Secrétariate was influential in the development of the Employment Insurance Compassionate Care Benefit, which was launched in January 2004, to ensure that Canadians do not have to choose between keeping their jobs and caring for their families.[7] Canadians who must be absent from work to care for a gravely ill family member will be eligible to receive up to 6 weeks Compassionate Care benefit.

Provincial Government

Provinces have begun to recognize palliative care as a part of basic health care services. Some, such as Manitoba and British Columbia, acknowledge palliative care as a core health care service. Others, such as Saskatchewan and Alberta, have developed provincial guidelines for services.[8] British Columbia has developed a provincial strategy for end-of-life care.[9] Quebec has begun to integrate palliative care into its existing local community centers known as CLSC, supporting home care with a dedicated phone line and on-call physicians, nurses, and pharmacists.[10]

Barriers to accessing medications in the home are being addressed by some provinces. For example, several provinces will now cover the cost of palliative medications such as opioids and laxatives for persons who are designated as palliative by their physicians (British Columbia also provides coverage of equipment such as hospital beds and supplies). Canadian physicians have adequate access to a wide variety of analgesics for pain management and do not have to contend with the daunting regulatory impediments faced by care providers in many other countries.[11]

There is increasing recognition of the need for adequate reimbursement for family physicians to provide home visits, spend the necessary time with patient and family, work with team members, and provide 24-hour coverage.[12–14] However, only a handful of provinces have addressed palliative care codes for physician remuneration.

Regional Health Authorities

In the 1990s, most provinces in Canada partially devolved their responsibility for health care to sub-provincial regions in an effort to streamline the delivery system, making it less fragmented and more responsive to local needs. Regional Health Authorities are autonomous health care organizations with responsibility for health administration within a defined geographic region within a province or territory. They have appointed or elected boards of governance and are responsible

Table 66–1
Chronology of National Palliative and End-of-Life Care Key Events

Date	Event	Summary
1992	Palliative Care 2000 for the Cancer 2000 Task Force	Provides recommendations for priorities and coordination of cancer care. Recommends development of coordinated integrated palliative care services as a top priority.
June 1995	Special Senate Committee on Euthanasia and Assisted Suicide report *Of Life and Death*	Chaired by Senator Carstairs, recommends actions that would result in improved access to services, standards of care, and an increase in knowledge and training of professionals. Calls end-of-life care the "right of every Canadian."
June 2000	Subcommittee of the Standing Senate Committee on Social Affairs, Science and Technology tabled report *Quality End-of-Life Care: The Right of Every Canadian*	Recommends federal leadership and development of a strategy to improve care, particularly related to support for family caregivers, access to home care and pharmacare, training and education, and research and surveillance
December 2000	Blueprint for Action developed by the Quality End-of-Life Care Coalition: 24 national stakeholders join together under chairmanship of Canadian Hospice Palliative Care Association (CHPCA)	Health Canada supports the CHPCA in creation of the Quality End-of-Life Care Coalition. Blueprint identifies five key priorities from the June 2000 (above) report: availability and access; professional education; research and data collection, including surveillance; family and caregiver support; and public education and awareness
February 2001	Canadian Strategy for Cancer Control—Palliative Care Working Group Report	Palliative care chosen as one of the five areas for immediate action. Affirms palliative care as fundamental component of cancer care. Recommends improving integration of palliative care delivery within existing cancer centers and other health care systems.
March 2001	The Prime Minister of Canada appoints Senator Sharon Carstairs as Minister with Special Responsibility for Palliative Care and advisor to the Minister of Health on palliative care	
June 2001	Secretariat on Palliative and End-of-Life Care established	Coordinates Health Canada's work of a national strategy on end-of-life care. Facilitates collaboration both within federal government and with external partners.
March 2002	National Action Planning Workshop sponsored by Secretariat	150 national, provincial, territorial, and regional practitioners, plus researchers and decision-makers in end-of-life care brought together. Recommend action on availability and access to services; ethical, cultural and spiritual considerations; education and research; surveillance; support for caregivers; and public education and awareness.

(*continued*)

Table 66–1
Chronology of National Palliative and End-of-Life Care Key Events *(continued)*

Date	Event	Summary
October 2002	Senate Standing Committee on Social Affairs, Science and Technology Final Report: *The Health of Canadians—The Federal Role* (Kirby Report)	Five main recommendations about end-of-life care: (1) palliative home care program cofunded with provinces; (2) 6 weeks' employment benefits for Canadians who choose to care for palliative care family; (3) expanding tax measures for people providing care to dying family members; (4) amend Canada Labour Code to allow employees to take leave to care for family; and (5) change Treasury Board legislation to ensure job protection for its own employees caring for a loved one.
November 2002	Commission on the Future of Health Care in Canada. Report involving largest consultation ever with Canadians on Health Care (Romanov report)	Recommends new Home Care Transfer to provinces in support of expansion of the Canada Health Act for inclusion of medically necessary home care services, including palliative care. Also recommends support for informal caregivers through Human Resources Development Canada.

for funding and delivering community-based and institutional public health services within their region.[15] To date, all provinces and territories, other than Ontario and the Yukon Territory, have implemented some form of regionalization.[15] The process of regionalization has, in most areas, resulted in a decrease of acute care beds, as the community and acute care sector begin to become more integrated.

In Wilson's[16] synthesis research project, she identified that, in theory, regionalization has the potential to assist integration of end-of-life care by facilitating access and care continuity across diverse health care settings. Alternatively, regionalization could limit growth of palliative care services if particular regions do not see palliative care as a priority. The need for research to substantiate whether the theoretical benefits of regionalization are actualized is evident.

The Canadian Hospice Palliative Care Association[17] is the national nongovernmental organization that provides leadership for hospice palliative care in Canada (CHPCA, 43 Bruyère Street, Suite 131C, Ottawa, Ontario K1N, 1-877-203-4363 [toll free], info@chpca.net). Founded in 1991, its mission is to promote awareness, education, and research, advocating at a national level for policy development, resource allocation, and support for caregivers. The CHPCA board of directors is composed of the 11 provincial/territorial associations and five members-at-large. Advocacy is an important role for provincial and federal counterparts. The CHPCA chairs the Quality End-of-Life coalition, taking leadership in the advocacy role.

Historically, the terms "hospice" and "palliative care" were used in Canada in a variety of ways. The term hospice may have indicated a philosophy of care, a free-standing building, a unit in a long-term care facility, or a home-based program. New terminology in Canada was proposed in 2002. The words *hospice* and *palliative care* were combined to recognize the convergence of hospice and palliative care into one movement. The national organization for palliative care adjusted their name to include the term "hospice palliative care."[17] Their updated definition is "Hospice palliative care is aimed at relief of suffering and improving the quality of life for persons who are living with or dying from advanced illness or are bereaved." It is appropriate for any person and family living with a life-threatening illness due to any diagnosis, regardless of age and prognosis.[17] This definition calls for hospice palliative care intervention earlier in the disease trajectory for all diagnoses.

A priority of the CHPCA has been the development of national standards to guide the development of palliative and hospice care service delivery across the country. Following 10 years of extensive consensus building and collaboration across Canada, a model to guide hospice palliative care was published in 2002.[18] The model is comprised of: the values, principles and foundational concepts that underlie all aspects of hospice palliative care; a conceptual framework for the delivery of care called the "Square of Care"; and a conceptual framework to guide organizational development and function called the "Square of Organization" (Figure 66–1).

The CHPCA has also been an active partner in the establishment of palliative care as a specialty within the Canadian Nursing Association. The CHPCA Nursing Interest Group provided the venue through which nurses across Canada collaborated to

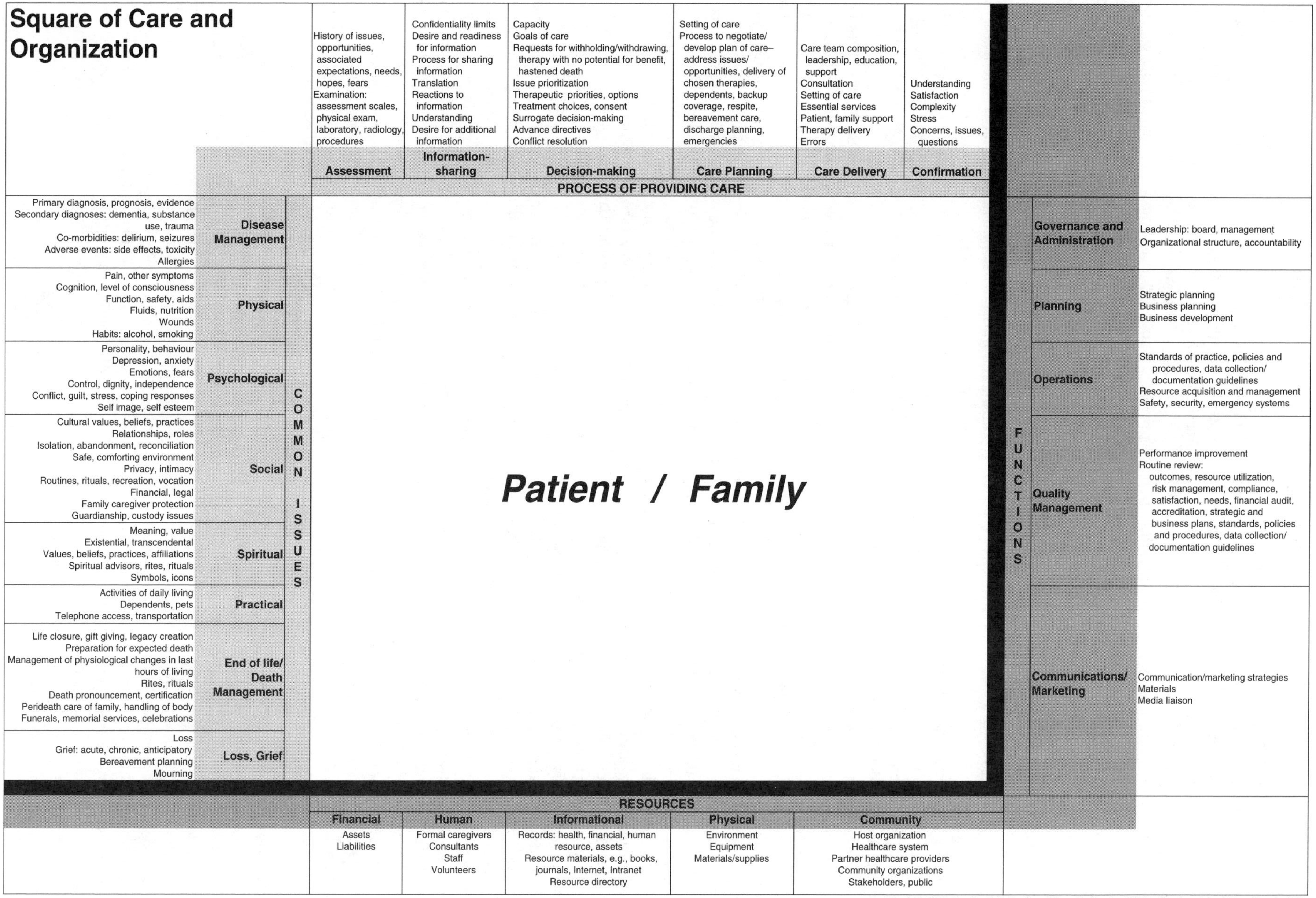

A Model to Guide Hospice Palliative Care © Canadian Hospice Palliative Care Association, Ottawa, Canada, 2002.

Figure 66–1. Square of Care and Organization.

establish the Hospice Palliative Care Nursing Standards of Practice, which were developed in 2002.[19] These standards and the CHPCA Model of Care provided the foundation for the development of palliative care nursing certification. The first sitting of the certification occurred in April 2004. More than 500 nurses are registered, the highest rate of enrollment of any certification process to date.

Forces Influencing Model Development

End-of-Life Care for All

Palliative care services in Canada developed with a specific focus on care of persons with cancer. However, the significant changes in Canada's demographics are changing attitudes. The declining birth rate, development of new technologies, and increased life expectancy have resulted in an aging population, with a burgeoning baby-boomer population that will reach retirement in the next decade.[20]

The aging of Canada's population has drawn attention to the necessity of an end-of-life care strategy that will address the needs of the increasing proportion of elderly who die every year from causes other than cancer. Currently, cancer patients receive 90% of the available palliative care services, although they only represent 25% of those who die.[21] Deaths due to progressive chronic illnesses such as congestive heart failure, chronic obstructive pulmonary disease, renal disease, and dementia will increase. Recent hospice palliative care literature is replete with articles acknowledging the benefits of the hospice palliative care approach to individuals dying from diseases other than cancer. Authors have written about the need for integration of hospice palliative care into settings such as intensive care units[22,23] and nursing homes,[24–26] and to extend palliative care to those with diseases such as end-stage renal disease, cardiorespiratory disease, neuromuscular disease, and AIDS.[27,28] It has been argued that hospice palliative care programs are providing service to a privileged minority[29]—"the ethical case for palliative care beyond cancer is resounding, and restricted practice is indefensible."[30] MacDonald[31] describes a Canadian paradox, in which we are facing growing numbers of elderly and people with chronic life-threatening illnesses during a period of continued downsizing in the health care system, while, at the same time, societal expectations for access to excellent care are rising.

Palliative care programs will be challenged to respond. Many of the characteristics of progressive chronic illnesses, such as prognostic uncertainty, do not "fit" with the admission criteria of many programs that have evolved based predominantly on a cancer model.[31] Primary care professionals and palliative care clinicians, for the most part, have not developed expertise in the management of these conditions. Human resource issues are a critical concern. Shared Care models and partnerships with other clinical specialties are beginning to be established to address care for this broader group.

The end-of-life movement has compelled Canadians to address a variety of issues such as advance directives and euthanasia. Advance directives, or living wills, are beginning to gain attention. Provinces such as Newfoundland, Alberta, and British Columbia have passed legislation to compel health care providers to follow the previously written wishes of persons in the event that they are unable to speak for themselves. The "Let Me Decide" initiative, which began in Ontario, is being replicated in nursing homes in other provinces and areas.[32]

Shift to Community-Based Care

During the initial development of palliative care in the 1970s and 1980s, health care was strongly institution based. In fact, Canada's first palliative care programs were established in tertiary hospitals. In the mid-1990s, up to 80% of total Canadian deaths occurred in hospitals. We are now beginning to see a reversal of the trend toward dying in hospital.[33,34] Growing numbers of patients, families, care providers, and planners are now advocating for increased community care and more opportunities for home deaths. The move to community-based care is seen as appropriate and fitting for palliative care.[6]

Most palliative patients do not need to be in acute care hospitals, and quality palliative care can be provided in a home or hospice setting. However, the issue of transferring the cost of care from hospitals to persons and families has not yet been adequately addressed in most settings. People cared for at home may assume responsibility for the costs of medications, supplies, additional home care services, and transportation.[6] In some provinces, persons pay a daily fee for hospice care. This fee is usually set at a rate similar to the nursing home accommodation charges.

Recent evidence suggests that dying at home may be idealized and, when family members actually have to face the challenges of care, the burden can be considerable.[35] Indeed, the shift of care from hospital to home presupposes that care providers will be available in the home. Most programs do not fund 24-hour care over the long term, and there are regional differences in availability of home support. Unless families are able to afford private funding of care providers, the burden of care falls to family and friends.[36,37] Although many Canadian palliative programs advocate for care in the home setting, there are several potential concerns to be considered. Canada has smaller family sizes, leaving fewer children to care for the wave of aging "baby boomers." Children often live far away and work outside of the home. Spouses are elderly and have their own health issues, and early discharge from acute care means more care is expected from both home care and family caregivers.[38]

There remains insufficient research into the issues and outcomes of caring for family members at home.[16,35] Since we are likely to see increasing demands for home-based care, in part because of economic pressures in the Canadian health care system, solid research investigating all aspects of such care is needed.

Palliative care needs to reflect a continuum of services that incorporates community-based options such as home care and residential hospice environments. In many communities in Canada, grass-roots, donor-based organizations have taken the initiative to develop programs, such as free-standing hospices, to address this need. As more publicly funded palliative care services are developed, collaboration and integration with the voluntary sector is paramount.

Meeting the Needs of Rural Canada

In the past 5 years, there has been an increasing awareness of the need to ensure that the health care needs of rural Canadians are reflected in national health policy and health system renewal strategies. There is a considerable body of research that indicates a marked urban–rural difference in the provision of health care and social services.[39,40] This inequity extends to the provision of palliative and hospice care.

Depending on which definition of rural is used, up to 30% of Canadians live in rural communities.[40] Ninety-five percent of Canada's territory is considered rural.[40] The rural, Northern, and Aboriginal communities that comprise rural Canada have diverse social, geographic, and economic characteristics that challenge several of the key guiding principles of hospice palliative care, in particular, the principle of access. Rural communities face an acute and persistent shortage of health care providers. Rural practitioners must function as generalists, having limited access to specialist physician services and to the full interdisciplinary team available to urban counterparts.[41,42] The restructuring and reform of health care have resulted in downsizing and closure of rural hospitals and long-term care facilities, which provided an important infrastructure for rural health services delivery. Timely access to health care service is a significant challenge. A study of referral patterns to a central palliative care service in Halifax, Nova Scotia, found that people were more likely to be referred if they were younger, receiving radiation therapy, or lived closer to the center.[43]

In their interviews with rural health personnel from six regions in Canada that were noted for their significant initiatives in rural health, MacLean and Kelley[39] identified the following themes as critical to the development of rural palliative care models:

- Be sure the philosophy, definition, and guidelines of palliative care retain and reflect the "essence and strengths of ruralness."
- Build on the strengths and experiences of people in rural areas rather than imposing a program from the outside.
- Build in flexibility and creativity to facilitate access to services.
- Ensure 24-hour access to specialist services through the most cost-efficient methods.
- Enable flexibility and "blurring" in regard to the boundaries between disciplines, job descriptions, and health care practice.
- Provide opportunities for education and integration of new information into rural practice.
- Build in social support for family caregivers and formal health care providers.
- Ensure that the rural model recognizes cultural differences.

Several recent web-based innovations in Canada will help to address some of the challenges experienced in the provision of rural palliative care. In 2001, Health Canada announced funding to support the development of the Canadian Virtual Hospice (CVH).[44] CVH goals are to facilitate, via a web-based forum, equitable distribution of mutual support, the exchange of information, communication and collaboration between and amongst healthcare professionals, researchers, the terminally ill and their families.

In December 2003 the federal government committed funding to a national outreach education and professional development initiative called the Pallium Project. The project aims to improve access, enhance quality, and provide additional capacity for palliative care in communities across Western and Northern Canada. Web-based technology is one of several strategies. Pallium is the first large-scale initiative to implement the CHPCA norms across several jurisdictions.[45]

Impact of Culture on Models of Care

Canada is a rich tapestry of cultures from around the world. The four main cultural groupings include the Aboriginal peoples, British and French "founders" of Canada, and more recently, immigrants from Asia, Africa, and other non-European nations.[46] The larger urban centers in Canada, where the "third wave" of immigrants from Asia and Africa as well as an increasing number of Aboriginal people tend to settle, are challenged to respond to the linguistic and cultural diversity.[47] Palliative care practitioners are particularly challenged by this diversity on several fronts. In regard to access, research has suggested that ethnic minorities are underrepresented in palliative care programs.[48] Access is further compromised due to the lack of translated materials and clinical assessment tools.[49] The foundations of the modern palliative care/hospice movement are based on Christian tradition and teachings and a growing recognition of the futility and indignity of continuing expensive and intrusive treatments for people who are clearly dying. Guiding palliative care principles are based on the western ethics of "truth telling" and patient autonomy.[50] These principles are often in direct conflict with the beliefs and values of many of the persons that we care for, resulting in culturally insensitive decisions and health policies.[46] Palliative care programs in Canada need to reflect cultural competence. That is, we must reflect values, behaviors, attitudes, knowledge, and skills that are respectful and inclusive of diverse cultural backgrounds.[49]

Impact of Primary Health Care

Canada is focused on the restructuring of primary health care delivery in response to a widespread call for health care reform to ensure a sustainable health care system. Over the past 2 years, $800 million was provided through the Primary Health Care Transition Fund to investigate models of primary care delivery. In 2003, the federal, provincial, and territorial governments signed a "First Ministers Accord of Primary Health Care" that included a 5-year, $16 billion commitment to improve primary health care. Primary health care is defined as a set of universally accessible first-level services that promote health, prevent disease, and provide diagnostic, curative, rehabilitative, supportive, and palliative services.[51] The effects of primary care—responsiveness, effectiveness, productivity, accessibility, continuity, and quality—are expected to be enhanced.

Primary care initiatives have the potential for positive impact on the delivery of community-based palliative care in Canada. Family physicians will continue to be key providers of these services. Strategies that discover ways to re-engage family physicians in providing quality end-of-life care are critical to the sustainability of community-based palliative care services.

Models of Palliative Care Service Delivery

Literature on model development in Canada and elsewhere remains largely in the descriptive stage. There are several challenges in regard to evaluating palliative care models in Canada. First, while there is consensus regarding the philosophy of palliative care, there is not consensus regarding the operationalization of the philosophy. There is debate regarding who should be "palliative," or when this designation should occur. Second, nationally accepted outcome indicators have not been developed or agreed upon. Much of the literature describes quality of life and satisfaction as appropriate evaluative methods for determining effectiveness of models of care, yet it is not clear what constitutes quality palliative care.[16,52,53] Therefore, there is no agreement on how to evaluate effective palliative care services. The inadequate description of services using comparable variables does not provide evidence beyond a descriptive level or allow assessment of external validity or generalizability.[54,55] The gaps in the literature make it difficult to understand what programs are currently in place across Canada, what the trends are, and what has been successful thus far.[16]

The CHPCA conceptual framework, the "Square of Care," will assist Canadian programs in developing a care model and providing a broad framework to evaluate the outcomes. The framework supports a standardized approach to ensure that all caregivers are knowledgeable and skilled, to identify gaps and opportunities for partnerships, and to ensure programs manage activities, resources and functions consistent with its approach to care delivery.[18] The challenge to programs is to use the Square of Care, ensuring that the underpinnings of model development of accessibility and continuity of care are addressed. This will involve clear definitions, common language, assessment tools, and criteria of admission that meet national and local needs.

Best Practice Model Development

It is generally agreed that service delivery models for palliative and hospice care need to include essential components such as pain and symptom management, interdisciplinary teams, consultation services, psychosocial/counseling care, spiritual care, and volunteer and bereavement programs.[53] Services to support care in the community include outpatient clinics, day care, respite care, hospice (home support, freestanding, and integrated into long-term care facilities), and community consultation teams. A seminal report to address model delivery of these components was provided by the Expert Panel of Palliative Care. Their report to the Cancer 2000 Task Force (responsible for providing recommendations on priorities and coordination for cancer to national cancer agencies) strongly recommended support of development based on regional plans. The report contained essential components such as home-based care, acute care, chronic palliative care beds, consultation services, and a tertiary, regional unit that would act as a learning and research center.[56] The development of secondary and tertiary levels of care are necessary for the collaborative management of complex cases and for the much-needed education and research development in this field.

Other authors have echoed the need for regional approaches, with primary, secondary, and tertiary levels of care based on the needs of patients and families.[18,21,57] Primary care will be central to the development of palliative care in Canada. Primary care is and will continue to be provided by family physicians in conjunction with the community interdisciplinary teams. Palliative care consultants in their secondary or tertiary roles must develop strong relationships with family practitioners and home care teams because they provide the link between various providers of care.

Clearly, the challenge today is to work within present health care systems and attain the integration and coordination of care necessary to provide the right mix of services in the "most appropriate setting." More than many other specialties, the palliative care model of care needs to be flexible and to be able to "travel" and meet the unique needs of individuals, particularly in noncancer diagnoses, where most appropriate settings of care will need to integrate with other models of care such as nephrology, pediatrics, and neurology.[57] The ideal setting for palliative care is evidently complex and varies over time.

Provinces generally report that emerging models are using generic services complemented by specialized services. Regions report working with present services, partners, and agencies to bring together the best mix of services possible. Regina Quapelle Health Region has an integrated model in which a care coordinator and interdisciplinary staff follow the client in any setting within the health care region. The Fraser Health

Authority in British Columbia has established a variety of arrangements with community-based hospice groups to establish several residential hospice environments.

For some provinces, such as Ontario, developing an integrated palliative care program in the absence of regionalization requires a unique approach to service delivery. Partnerships between organizations and across settings of care are critical. In Toronto, the Hospice Palliative Care Network was developed to formalize these partnerships. A contractual agreement between the physician group, various service providers, and government was created to address continuum-of-care needs. A computerized patient record is key to the success of the model.

This trend toward partnerships, strategic alliances, shared care models, and contractual arrangements to ensure a continuum of care from acute care to community-based options is seen in the literature. O'Connell[58] completed a comprehensive review of the literature and describes five integrated care delivery models:

1. Shared care: Sharing responsibilities between a specialist and generalist health care professionals
2. Case management/Managed care: An identified person is assigned to a person to manage their care from admission into the hospital to discharge into the community. Often part of a prospective payment system
3. Home care: Person is managed by a team of health care personnel in the community
4. Collaborative practice clinics: Groups of health care personnel who work together in community or outpatient clinic
5. Cancer centers: Incorporate support and coordination of resources, including a directory of local cancer support groups, voluntary organizations, and palliative care

All delivery models should aim to reduce costs and to enhance quality of care, communication, continuity, and patient satisfaction. O'Connell's review was limited due to the multiple interpretations of each model described, but overall she identified shared care as the preferred model because it has the potential to provide a more continuous and integrated form of care.

Rather than recommend any particular model, Wilson[16] identified four key components of end-of-life services that are essential: (1) universality: a broad range of health care and social support services need to be available to all persons who are near the end of life; (2) care coordination: care should be arranged through an end-of-life care coordinator with specialized knowledge and skills; (3) broad range of basic and advanced end-of-life support: basic services needed by most persons provided by persons who do not specialize in end-of-life care, and advanced end-of-life service needed for a small proportion of persons provided by persons who specialize in end-of-life care; and (4) care regardless of setting: services should not be limited by care setting. Care regardless of setting must be tempered with rural and cultural needs that impact plans for services, such as acute care utilization.

Rachlis[10] poses the following questions as markers of integration and innovation in hospice palliative care service delivery:

- Does your community track the number of deaths in hospitals, hospices, and homes? (If your community has more than 50% of cancer deaths occurring in hospitals, then there are not adequate palliative care services).
- Do your community's hospitals and nursing homes measure pain as a fifth vital sign?
- Do your community palliative care programs provide care to noncancer persons? These persons should make up more than 25% of the total caseload.
- Are palliative care programs available for the homeless?
- Do your community's long-term care facilities and home care services complete advance directives on all of their clients?
- What proportion of long-term care facility deaths occur in hospitals? (More than 70% should occur within the facility.)
- Do intensive care units have dedicated staff to counsel persons and their families about preference for care?
- Do ambulance dispatches and paramedics respect advance directives?

Calgary and Edmonton Model of Care

Although there is no evidence to date regarding the impact of different models of palliative care on patients' quality of life, models may be justified on other grounds, such as patient preference or cost effectiveness.[53] There have been individual studies examining aspects of integrated programs such as consultation teams and satisfaction and acute care utilization. However, the ability to research the impact of an integrated model of care is limited because these programs are relatively new and complex to describe, and the research involves linking administrative data sets.

The impact of an integrated regional community-based palliative care program on patterns of care for terminal cancer patients has been studied in the Calgary Health Region and the Capital Health Region (Edmonton), Alberta.[59] The objectives for the study were to describe, explain, and evaluate the economic consequences of introducing two comprehensive, coordinated, and integrated palliative care programs in Alberta. A before-and-after analysis of linked administrative data for cancer patients who died between April 1993 and March 2000 as residents of Calgary or Capital Health regions was completed. Cancer registry, administrative, and palliative care databases were linked, including information on utilization and cost of hospital, physician, outpatient prescriptions, and nursing home and home care data.

Shortly after the establishment of the Regional Health Authorities in Alberta, the Capital Health and Calgary Regional palliative care programs (RPCP) were created in July 1995 and October 1996, respectively. At that time, both programs presented convincing business cases for the establishment of a regional program. Regionalization provided a vehicle to develop an integrated service delivery model. The aim in both regions was to increase the access of patients to palliative care services and decrease the number of these patients dying in acute care facilities by enhancing the developing community-based service options. Services include:

- Tertiary or specialized palliative care units for those persons with complex symptoms requiring intensive interdisciplinary support (14 beds in Edmonton, 10-bed tertiary unit began after study period in Calgary)
- Hospices: end-of-life care settings for persons unable to be cared for in their home but who do not require acute care, located either freestanding or in long-term care facilities. Interdisciplinary team, 24-hour registered nursing, dedicated nurse managers, and consultants are provided. Admissions are centrally coordinated and respite care is provided if a bed is available (57 beds in Edmonton, 40 in Calgary at the time of the study).
- Palliative home care: both regions have specialized interdisciplinary home care programs to support persons in their homes. During the study period, significant investment had been made to further enhance the capacity of the home care programs to provide round-the-clock care.
- Consultants: available throughout the regions for any setting providing consultative support to primary care providers in acute care, long-term care, and community settings. Consultants are also responsible for palliative care education to primary caregivers.
- Central office to coordinate administrative, education, research, bereavement, and volunteer activities

Admission criteria for each area of the programs assist in assessing for care options. Common assessment tools are used to evaluate symptoms, cognition, and functional status. Both regions have established strong liaisons with cancer agencies that link patients to the regional palliative care services to enhance seamless care.

The results of the study are:

1. Access to palliative care was defined as referral to any part of the program, which would provide knowledgeable access to all parts of the program. Over the 7 study years, access increased from 45% to 81%. This increased coverage rate was attributed to the increase in hospice beds, consultation, and home care services (Figure 66–2).
2. People were predominantly referred to hospice palliative care services in the last month of life, with 31% of palliative home care admissions and 71% of residential hospice admissions occurring in the last month of life.
3. The percentage of time that palliative clients spend in their home is more descriptive of palliative care services than where people die. In the last study year of 1999/2000, 87% of a person's time during that year was spent at home, 12% of this while receiving palliative home care near the end of life. Time in institutional care over the year was .6% in tertiary palliative care, 7.5% in acute care,

Figure 66–2. Probability of referral to palliative care by type of service at any time in last year of life, 1993/1994 to 1999/2000 ($n = 16{,}282$). *Source:* Fainsinger et al. (2003), reference 61.

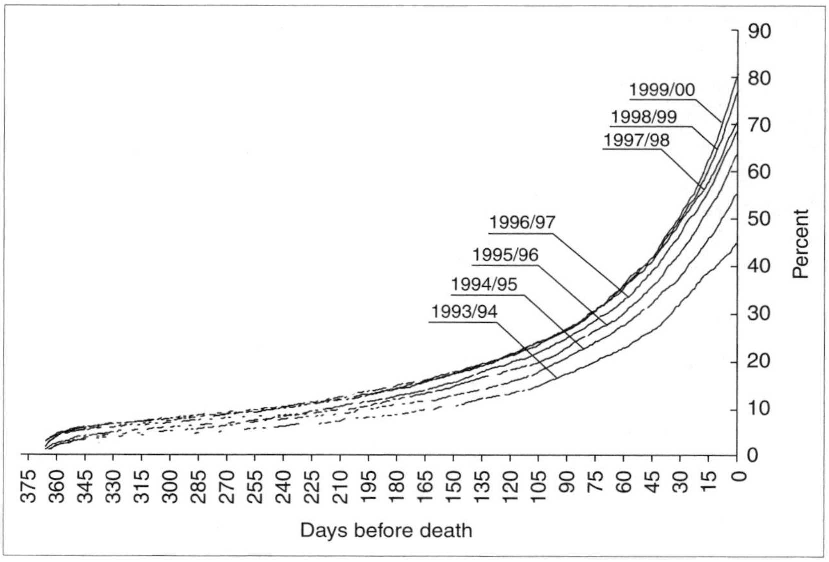

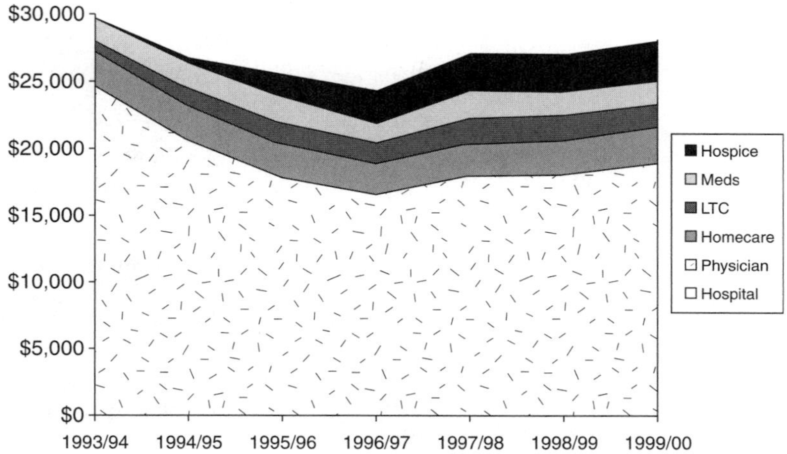

Figure 66–3. Identifiable public costs of terminally ill cancer patients in their last 365 days of life, 1993/1994 to 1999/2000 (Canadian 1999/2000 dollars).

2.4% in hospice, 3.5% in nursing home. Clearly, the majority of time is spent at home before entering specific palliative care services. The authors have identified that the time prior to entering palliative care services is an area worthy of further study.

4. Actual location of death was 37% acute care, 29% hospice, 28% home, 3% nursing home, and 3% tertiary care in the last study year of 1999/2000.
5. The integrated regional palliative care programs were implemented at no additional cost to the public sector (Figure 66–3). The number of acute care bed days per year used by palliative care persons decreased from 10.4% to 7.5%, representing a savings of 74 acute care beds/year. This has been offset by care provided in less costly settings: palliative home care increased from 7% to 12% and hospice increased from 0% to 3%, which is equivalent to 61 beds in hospice. Tertiary and nursing home and time at home remained constant.
6. Overall acute care accounts for two thirds (67%) of the cost of palliative care services provided in the last year of life, followed by physician services (10%), hospice care (8%), long-term or nursing home care (6%), home care (6%), and outpatient prescription medications (see Figure 66–3).
7. Age (older), gender (female), socioeconomic status (lower income), cancer diagnosis (breast, respiratory, buccal), and disease burden (multiple comorbidities) can significantly explain increased use of hospital and physician costs.

A community-based integrated model of palliative care service can be implemented to increase access at no additional cost to the health care system in large urban settings.

Conclusion

The Senate Subcommittee,[60] updating the 1995 special Senate report on euthanasia and assisted suicide, called their report *Quality End-of-Life: The Right of Every Canadian.* The name of this report sets the stage for public expectation for hospice palliative care services. The aging population and the prominence of the Prime Minister with Special Responsibility for Palliative Care supports the expectation of quality end-of-life care for all Canadians.

There are many components in place to enhance model development of palliative care services in Canada. The recent reports on health care, with clear expectations of palliative care services in home care, have advanced a clear rationale for universal access to competent, effective palliative care that can address the rural and cultural challenges. The national standards of hospice palliative care should guide those developing and enhancing palliative care services as we move toward national accreditation standards. Certification of palliative care for physicians and nurses is an important step in increasing the availability of palliative care within the health care structure.

Palliative care is well positioned to succeed in a community-based model of care. The call for adequate resources in these programs of care must be heeded to ensure that palliative care is widely accessible.

ACKNOWLEDGMENTS

Sandy McKinnon was an original author of the 2000 chapter on Canada. Sandy died in 2000, yet her ongoing influence on this chapter is acknowledged.

The authors would like to thank Konrad Fassbender, Linda Read Paul, and Ted Braun for editing the chapter, and to thank their many colleagues across the country who shared information: Deborah Adams, Velda Clarke, Lillian Locke, Lorena McManus, Laurie Ann O'Brien, Pat Porterfield, Judy Simpson, Anne Syme, Carolyn Taylor, and Pat Porterfield.

REFERENCES

1. Commission on the Future of Health Care in Canada. Building on values. The future of health care in Canada. Final Report. November, 2002. Available at: http://www.healthcarecommission.ca (accessed March 20, 2005).
2. End-of-life care coalition. Brief to Roy Romanow, Commissioner. Future of Health Care in Canada. April 30, 2002.
3. Subcommittee to update "Of Life and Death" of the Standing Senate Committee on Social Affairs Science and Technology. Quality End-of-Life Care: The Right of Every Canadian. Ottawa: Government of Canada, 2001.
4. Canadian Institute for Health Research. Request for Applications. Palliative and End of Life Care. Updated March 2004. Available at: http://www.cihr-irsc.gc.ca/e/15878.shtml (accessed May 10, 2005).
5. Canada Health Act, 1984, C.6, s.1,1–12. Canadian Centre for Analysis of Regionalization & Health. What is regionalization? Available at: http://www.regionalizaton.org/Regionalization/Regionalization.html (accessed April 25, 2005).
6. LaPerriere B. Overview of provincial and territorial palliative care services. A working paper prepared for invitational symposium on palliative care: Provincial and Territorial Trends and Issues in Community-Based Programming, March 23–24, 1997. Ottawa, Ontario, Canada: Health Canada Working Group on Continuing Care Policy and Consultation Branch, Health System and Policy Division, 1997.
7. Government of Canada. Employment Insurance Compassionate Care Benefit. Available at: http://www.hrsdc.gc.ca/en/ei/types/compassionate_care.shtml (accessed June 29, 2005).
8. Palliative Care: A Policy Framework. Alberta Health, December 1993.
9. Minister of Health Services, British Columbia. Discussion paper on a provincial strategy for end-of-life care in British Columbia. October 2002, http://www.healthservices.gov.bc.ca/hcc/pdf/elcpaper.pdf (accessed May 10, 2005).
10. Rachlis M. Prescription for Excellence. Toronto: HarperCollins Publishers Ltd, 2004.
11. MacDonald N, Findlay HP, Bruera E, Dudgeon D, Kramer J. A Canadian survey of issues in cancer pain management. J Pain Symptom Manage 1997;14:332–342.
12. Burge F, McIntyre P, Twohig P, Cummings I, Kaufman D, Frager G. Palliative care by family physicians in the 1990's. Can Fam Physician 2001;47:1989–1995.
13. Brenneis C, Bruera E. The interaction between family physicians and palliative care consultants in the delivery of palliative care: clinical and educational issues. J Palliat Care 1998;14: 58–61.
14. MacKenzie MR. The interface of palliative care, oncology and family practice: a view from a family practitioner. CMAJ 1998; 158:1705–1707.
15. Canadian Medical Association. CMA Policy; Regionalization (Update 2001). Ottawa, Ontario: Canadian Medical Association, 2001.
16. Wilson D. Integrated end-of-life care: a Health Canada synthesis research project. Final Report. (project #6795-15-2002/4780004). September, 2003. Available at: http://www.nursing.ualberta.ca/endoflife/hc_sum.pdf (accessed April 26, 2005).
17. Canadian Hospice Palliative Care Association. Available at: http://www.chpca.net/menu_items/faqs.htm#faz_whatis (accessed April 26, 2005).
18. Ferris FD, Balfour HM, Bowen K, Farley J, Hardwick M, Lamontagne C, Lundey M, Syme A, West P. A model to guide hospice palliative care. Ottawa: Canadian Hospice Palliative Care Association, 2002.
19. Hospice palliative care nursing standards of practice. CHPCA Nursing Standards Committee. February 2002. Available at: http://www.chpca.net/interest_groups/nurses/Hospice_Palliative_Care_Nursing_Standards_of_Practice.pdf (accessed April 26, 2005).
20. Statistics Canada 2001 Census: profile of the Canadian population by age and sex: Canada ages. Release date July 2002. Available at: http://www.12.statcan.ca/english/census01/products/analytic/index.cfm (accessed April 26, 2005).
21. Byock IR. Hospice and palliative care: a parting of the ways or a path to the future? Palliat Med 1998;1:165–176.
22. Cassell J, Buchman TG, Streat S, Stewart RM. Surgeons, intensivists, and the covenant of care: administrative models and values affecting care at the end of life. Crit Care Med 2003;31: 1551–1557.
23. Nelson JE, Danis M. End-of-life care in the intensive care unit: where are we now? Crit Care Med 2001;29(Suppl):N2–N9.
24. Froggatt KA. Palliative care and nursing homes: where next? Palliat Med 2001;15:42–48.
25. Miller SC, Mor VNT. The role of hospice care in the nursing home setting. Palliat Med 2002;5:271–277.
26. Tuch H, Parrish P, Romer AL. Integrating palliative care into nursing homes. Palliat Med 2003;6:297–309.
27. Lee KF. Future end-of-life care: partnership and advocacy. Palliat Med 2002;5:329–334.
28. Robert Wood Johnson Foundation. ESRD Workgroup final report summary on end-of-life care: recommendations to the field. Nephrology Nursing Journal: J Am Nephrol Nurses Assoc 2003(Feb);30:59–63.
29. Douglas C. For all the saints. BMJ 1992;29:304–579.
30. George R, Sykes J. Beyond cancer. In: Clark D, Hockly J, Ahmedzai S. New Themes in Palliative Care. Berkshire, UK: Open University Press, 1997:239–254.
31. MacDonald N. Palliative care—an essential component of cancer control. CMAJ 1998;158:1709–1716.
32. Molloy DW, Guyatt GH, Russo R, et al. Systematic implementation of an advance directive program in nursing homes: a randomized controlled trial. JAMA 2000;283:1437–1444.
33. Wilson D, Northcott HC, Truman C, Smith SL, Anderson MC, Fainsinger RL, Stingl M. Location of death in Canada: a comparison of 20th century hospital and nonhospital locations of death and corresponding population trends. Eval & HP 2001; 24(4):385–403.
34. Burge F, Lawson B, Johnston G. Trends in the place of death of cancer patients, 1992–1997. CMAJ 2003;168:265–279.
35. Stajduhar KI. Examining the perspectives of family members involved in the delivery of palliative care at home. J Palliat Care 2003(Spring);19:27–35.
36. Chochinov HM, Kristjanson L. Dying to pay: the cost of end-of-life care. J Palliat Care 1998;14:5–15.
37. Stajduhar KI, Davies B. Death at home: challenges for families and directions for the future. J Palliat Care 1998;14:8–14.

38. Grunfeld E, Glossop R, McDowell I, Danbrook C. Caring for elderly people at home: the consequences to caregivers. CMAJ 1997;157:1101–1105.
39. MacLean MJ, Kelley ML. Palliative care in rural Canada. Rural Social Work, Special Australian/Canadian Issue 2001;6:63–73.
40. Ministerial Advisory Council on Rural Health. Rural health in rural hands; strategic directions for rural, remote, northern and aboriginal communities. Ottawa, Ontario: Office of Rural Health, November 2002.
41. Coyte PC, Young W. Applied home care research. Int J Health Quality Assurance 1997;10:i–iv.
42. Fast JE, Keating NC, Oakes L. Conceptualizing and operationalizing the costs of informal elder care. Report to the National Health Research Development Program. Ottawa: Health Canada, 1997.
43. Johnston GM, Gibbons L, Burge FI, Dewar RA, Cummings I, Levy IG. Identifying potential need for cancer palliation in Nova Scotia. CMAJ 1998;158:1691–1698.
44. Health Canada. Canadian virtual hospice: knowledge development and support in palliative care. November 2001. Available at: http://www.hc-sc.gc.ca/english/media/releases/2001/2001_121ebk1.htm (accessed April 26, 2005).
45. Alberta Palliative Networks. Pallium–a health human resources continuing professional development (CPD) initiative in palliative care. Available at: http://www.albertapalliative.net/APN/RuralNet/pallium.html (accessed April 26, 2005).
46. Hall P, Stone G, Fiset VJ. Palliative care: how can we meet the needs of our multicultural communities? Palliat Care 1998(Summer);14:46–49.
47. Mackay B. Changing face of Canada is changing the face of medicine. CMAJ 2001(March);168:599.
48. Eve A, Smith AM, Tebbit P. Hospice and palliative care in the UK 1994–95, including a summary of trends 1990–95. Palliat Med 1997;11:31–43.
49. Bon Bernard C, Feser L. Enhancing cultural competence in palliative care: perspective of an elderly Chinese community in Calgary. J Palliat Care 2003;19:133–139.
50. Maddock I. Is hospice a western concept? In: Clark D, Hockly J, Ahmedsa S, eds. New Themes in Palliative Care. Buckingham: Open University Press 1997:195–238.
51. Health Canada. The Health Transition Fund. Sharing the learning. The health transition fund synthesis series. Primary Health Care. Ottawa, Ontario: Minister of Public Works and Government Services, 2002.
52. National Consensus Project Guidelines, 2004. Available at: http://www.nationalconsensusproject.org/Guidelines_Download.asp (accessed May 15, 2005).
53. Salisbury C, Bosanquet N, Bilkinson EK, et al. The impact of different models of specialist palliative care on patients' quality of life: a systematic literature review. Palliat Med 1999;13:3–17.
54. Critchley P, Jadad AR, Taniguchi A, Woods A, Stevens R, Reyno L, Whelan TJ. Are some palliative care delivery systems more effective and efficient than others: a systematic review of comparative studies. J Palliat Care 1999;15:40–47.
55. Emanuel EJ. Cost savings at the end of life. What do the data show? JAMA 1996;275:1907–1914.
56. Report to Cancer 2000 Task Force. The Expert Panel on Palliative Care, 1991.
57. Kristjanson L. Generic versus specific palliative care services. Final report to Health Care and Issue Division Systems for Health Directorate. Ottawa: Health Canada, 1997.
58. O'Connell B, Kristjanson L, Orb A. Models of integrated cancer care: a critique of the literature. Aust Health Rev 2000;23: 163–178.
59. Fainsinger R, Fassbender K, Brenners C, Brown P, Braun T, Neumann C, et al. Canadian Health Services Research Foundation. Final Reports. Economic Evaluation of Two Regional Palliative Care Programs for Terminally Ill Cancer Patients. Canadian Health Services Research Foundation, Ottawa, Ontario, 2002. Available at: http://www.chsrf.ca/final_research/ogc/fainsinger_e.php (accessed April 25, 2005).
60. Standing Senate Committee on Social Affairs, Science and Technology. The Health of Canadians–The Federal Role, Vol. 6, Recommendations for Reform 2002. Available at: http://www.parl.gc.ca/37/2/parlbus/commbus/senate/com-e/soci-e/rep-e/repfinnov03-e.htm (accessed April 8, 2005).
61. Fainsinger R, Fassbender K, Brenners C, Brown P, Braun T, Neumann C, et al. Canadian Health Services Research Foundation. Final Reports. Economic Evaluation of Two Regional Palliative Care Programs for Terminally Ill Cancer Patients. Canadian Health Services Research Foundation, Ottawa, Ontario, 2003. Available at: http://www.chsrf.ca/final_research/ogc/fainsinger_e.pdf (accessed May 16, 2005).

PALLIATIVE CARE IN AUSTRALIA AND NEW ZEALAND

Sanchia Aranda and Linda J. Kristjanson

. . . this source of hope—that our last moments will be guided not by the bioengineers, but by those who know who we are . . .[1]

Palliative care nursing in Australia and New Zealand shares many features of palliative care nursing as practiced elsewhere in the world. The similarities between Australasian palliative care nursing and palliative care nursing in other countries is evident in the Australasian contribution to journals such as the *International Journal of Palliative Nursing* and in the adoption of Australian palliative nursing texts by international publishers.[1a] The purpose of this chapter is to both profile palliative care in Australia and New Zealand and to provide insights into some of the key innovations in care where nurses are providing a leading role.

In developing this second edition, we have retained and updated those sections of the chapter that provide an overview of palliative care in Australia and New Zealand. This material was gained from practicing nurses in Australia and New Zealand for the first edition and has been largely updated here from website sources and published materials. In this edition, we have shifted our specific focus to the imperative to increase access to palliative care across the population. More specifically, nurses have taken a leading role in innovations featured here such as the development of models of care for noncancer populations and in provision of after-hours support. The chapter concludes with a brief look at the steps Australian palliative care nurses are taking towards advanced practice roles.

Some Essential Differences Between Australia and New Zealand

Australia and New Zealand are often considered together—consistently labeled as "down under" and far away in world consciousness. Despite being close geographically and sharing a predominantly British heritage, these countries have significantly different personalities that are important to understand before exploring palliative care developments of the two countries.

New Zealand is a small country consisting of two large islands and one smaller, sparsely populated island. The total population is 3.7 million according to the 2001 census[2] and is estimated to be 4 million in 2004 based on previous population growth. The population is unevenly spread between the two main islands, with almost 75% living on the North Island. European/Pakeha (white) make up almost 80% of the population, plus 14.5% Maori and 5.6% Pacific Islanders. The economy is predominantly agricultural. Specialist health services are likely to be confined to large cities in each of the two main islands, but most general health services are available locally. However, New Zealand's population density, 12.6 people per km^2 compared to 234.5 per km^2 in Britain, has some effect on access to health services, with those in less densely populated areas having less access to specialized services, including palliative care.[3]

In contrast, Australia is a large island continent of five states and two territories plus Tasmania, a small island state to the south of the main island. The population is approximately 20 million. According to the 2001 census (http://www.abs.gov.au), indigenous Australians make up only 2.2% of the population, although the total number of 410,003 individuals was up 16% since 1996. Australia has undergone significantly more migration than New Zealand, with 22% of the population born overseas at the 2001 census. Overseas-born Australians are predominantly from the United Kingdom and Ireland, making up 5.5% of the total population. A further 1.9% of the population was born in New Zealand, and 1.2% in Italy. However, migrants from a variety of Asian countries make up a further 4.9% of the total population, or 982,519 individuals. To illustrate the diversity, Melbourne was recently declared the world's most ethnically diverse city, with residents from more than 140 countries (http://www.melbourne.vic.gov.au).

Australia ranges from dense urban cities such as Sydney, with approximately 4 million people, through rural communities surrounding large towns, to isolated remote areas where the nearest neighbor may be a day's drive away. Although the Aboriginal population constitutes only 2.1% of the population, they make up 30% of the population of central Australia, and in some communities are the primary clients of health services.[4]

It is clear, then, that Australia and New Zealand have similarities and differences. Both countries feature a predominance of people from Anglo-Celtic origins and were populated by these settlers at a similar time, although under different circumstances—Australia was established as a penal colony and New Zealand with free settlers. Both were colonialist settlements featuring disenfranchisement of the existing population—in Australia, the native Aboriginal people, and in New Zealand, the Maori. Since that time, New Zealand has remained largely bicultural despite limited migration from other parts of the world, while Australia is considered a multicultural society. Despite the diversity of languages spoken in Australia, English is the only official language. In contrast, both English and Maori are recognized national languages in New Zealand, and significant effort has been made to maintain Maori cultural identity and influence at a national level. Resurgence in Maori nationalism over recent years has been more effective in influencing national policy than has similar indigenous nationalism in Australia.

Australian and New Zealand Models of Health and Palliative Care

Both countries have a long history of universal health insurance systems that provide basic health care to all people. This universal health care system is supplemented by a limited system of private health care, more extensive in the Australian context. There is a consistent valuing of universal access to adequate health care within the two populations despite increasing trends toward user payment for some services. User payments are more common in New Zealand, where services such as visits to the local doctor are user pay, but user copayments are increasingly common in Australia.

Both countries feature a trend toward privatization of public facilities that affects health care services, perhaps most noticeable in care of the aged. Privatization of nursing home facilities has resulted in an increased need to profit from care of the elderly, with considerable potential impact on access to palliative care services when combined with the shift toward user payments. Health care is of a high standard, with access to a range of generalist and specialist services at a level consistent with that of the United States and Europe. Most generalist services are available in rural communities, but specialist services such as radiotherapy usually require travel to a large city. In remote areas of Australia, access to health care may be limited to a regular monthly clinic by the Royal Flying Doctor Service and limited access to outreach telephone services. In some remote settings, nursing care may be provided through remote nursing stations, where nurses are expected to serve as advanced generalists attending to a range of health care concerns within the community.

Structure and Delivery of Palliative Care

Hospice and palliative care developments in Australia and New Zealand are well advanced, with services required to meet established standards of service delivery.[5,6] Models of palliative care delivery in these countries feature inpatient, home care, and hospital support teams, with New Zealand evidencing more use of palliative day care than Australia. Urban cities tend to feature all service elements, with home care provision showing the most variation. In larger rural cities, small specialist services provide support and consultancy services to generalist nurses and local doctors. Palliative care developments in both countries are notable for their lack of homogeneity, with models of care dependent on historical factors, financial support, population density, and the local community environment.

The first hospice service in New Zealand opened in 1979,[3] and there are now 37 services operating across the country (http://www.hospice.org.nz). Palliative care in New Zealand features the development of small community inpatient hospices that link strongly with local community nursing services in the provision of home care. The system is well organized through Hospice New Zealand, which facilitates communication between members and organizes the national conference (http://www.hospice.org/nz).

The first Australian hospices predate the opening of St. Christopher's in London (1969) by 79 years—the establishment by the Sisters of Charity of hospices in Sydney (1890) and Melbourne (1938). Following the global spread of modern hospice, Australia's response occurred largely through the development of community-based palliative care services, with a particular emphasis on care in the home. However, significant change is taking place in service delivery, with increased emphasis in both state and federal government health policy to improve access to palliative care by equitable service distribution across the community. New hospice inpatient developments are most likely to be located within or in close proximity to acute services in recognition of the developing role of acute palliative care and an increasing capacity to keep patients at home.

Palliative care services in both countries ascribe to the principle of supporting the patient's decision to die at home whenever possible. Australian government policy directions clearly support the care of people in their own homes.[7] This emphasis includes specific attention to respite care and 24-hour access to supportive advice. Of people receiving palliative care in Australia, approximately one third die at home.[8] Average length of stay on a home care service is approximately 102 days, and average length of stay for patients receiving inpatient palliative care is 12 days.[8] However, these figures relate only to those individuals who access specialized palliative care services. Access, including issues such as provision of after-hours care, respite services, and the spread of palliative care into areas such as aged care, is an increasing critical focus of service development efforts. In the remainder of this section, we will focus on five areas relating to access to palliative care: provision of culturally sensitive care, access in rural and remote communities, services for noncancer populations, provision of after-hours support including respite, and access to palliative care in the aged-care sector.

Cultural Issues

A key feature of New Zealand health care is its responsiveness to Maori nationalism, which calls for greater control over their own health and services compatible to cultural beliefs. Cultural safety is a feature of Maori demands for appropriate health service development, and is a concept that moves beyond cultural sensitivity, featuring both acknowledgment and respect for difference, toward implementation of strategies to promote and nurture the cultural identity of the person who is ill.[9,10] In New Zealand, nurses have taken the lead on cultural issues in health with the production of guidelines in 1992,[11] which were updated in 2002.[12] These guidelines define cultural safety as "an outcome of nursing and midwifery education that enables safe service to be defined by those who receive the service" (p.8). Ultimately this means that people of one culture feel able to use a health service provided by another culture without feeling at risk. The New Zealand Palliative Care Strategy, released in February 2001,[13] specifically details expectations for Maori and Pacific people, including development of linkages with Maori organizations, local service plans, and the employment of care coordinators in conjunction with local Maori providers.

In contrast, the Australian indigenous people remain a marginalized group, with a health status significantly below that of other Australians despite strong government programs to address indigenous issues. A long history of neglect and suffering as a result of earlier ethnocentric government policy has left a legacy of difficulties for indigenous Australians. The provision of sensitive care to dying Aboriginal and Torres Strait Islander people is beginning to feature in national consciousness, and some research in this area is emerging. The 2003 Australian palliative care conference illustrated the emerging emphasis on access to palliative care for indigenous Australians, with three conference sessions devoted to this topic with a range of indigenous and health professional speakers. Current models of palliative care delivery, with an emphasis on terminal illness, may be unsuitable for some indigenous Australians whose concept of life-death-life may not be well understood or catered for in the traditional palliative care approach.[9,14]

The National Palliative Care strategy[15] identified the need for services ". . . to cater sensitively and flexibly for the needs of Aboriginal and Torres Strait Islanders" (p.6), but did not identify specific goals or strategies, and key indigenous groups are not listed among those consulted in developing the document. More recently, Palliative Care Australia[7] released the second edition of the *Australian Service Planning Guide* for palliative care, which does not specifically address the needs of indigenous Australians or consult with key indigenous groups. However, significant government resources are being channeled into developing models for indigenous palliative care. A comprehensive needs study was commissioned by the Australian government[16] outlining a blueprint for service development. Importantly, this report recognizes the key differences in service expectations, articulates a critical role for Aboriginal health workers, and addresses the significant training and education needs of health service providers. Further work is being undertaken to develop guidelines for culturally appropriate palliative care service delivery.[17]

In a recent summary of the issues in indigenous palliative care, Dr. Olra Fried[18] demanded that services hear from indigenous Australians about what quality of life means as a way of considering how services might best be provided. She further suggested that indigenous people and mainstream service providers have differing world views, conflicting values, different ways of making important decisions, and problems with communication (both verbal and nonverbal), and that recognition of these is essential in service planning. Drawing on research work to date in Australia, Fried identified that many indigenous people ". . . feel alienated from and distrust mainstream services . . ., want to be cared for and die on their traditional country . . ." and "there are inadequate resources to support home palliative care . . ." on traditional country (p. 4). Fried's recommendations for moving forward on indigenous palliative care are to:

- Focus locally in service development.
- Develop local support and information networks.
- Provide training in palliative care for Aboriginal health workers and bereavement workers.
- Provide cross cultural training in indigenous care for non-Aboriginal workers.
- Gain Aboriginal input into service planning, development, and management.
- Make specific efforts to facilitate Aboriginal access to mainstream services.
- Maintain access to traditional healers and bush medicines for Aboriginal people receiving palliative care.

Models of care, such as the employment of an Aboriginal social worker at the Mount Isa Hospital in remote Australia offer some hope for service improvements.[19] Burns' role as a Palliative Care Aboriginal Liaison Officer helps to bridge communication between her people and mainstream services.

The large number of migrant Australians, for whom English is not a first language and cultural beliefs about death and dying differ from Western belief, creates different demands on palliative care services. The provision of palliative care for these groups is beginning to feature in national research and service delivery efforts,[20–24] with nurses often leading the call for improved service provision to people of non-English–speaking backgrounds.[25] Importantly, Kanitsaki's research has challenged a dominant palliative nursing belief in open discussion about death and dying. Participants in her studies of Italian, Chinese, and Greek Australians often perceived nurses "who attempted to discuss with them death and dying" as "negative, insensitive and transmitted to them a sense of hopelessness" (p. 39). In addition, nurses who were accepting of death and told participants they were dying were interpreted as giving up on them, producing fears that the nurses would stop caring.

Access to information about palliative care is now available in 21 languages through the website of Palliative Care Australia (http://www.pallcar.org.au); however, attempts to improve information access are just a beginning. Systematic attention to cultural safety should move beyond access to interpreters, multilingual information, and liaison with ethnic community organizations and religious groups.[9]

Improving Services for Noncancer Populations

Three projects developed from a recent National Health and Medical Research funding scheme in palliative care specifically address noncancer palliative care in the areas of heart failure, renal disease, and neurodegenerative disorders. The project in neurodegenerative disorders was developed by a national team of nurse researchers and offers some useful insights into the issues associated with palliative care for noncancer populations.

Individuals living with neurological diseases such as motor neuron disease (MND), multiple sclerosis (MS), Huntington's disease (HD) and Parkinson's disease (PD) face long-term physical and psychosocial challenges. These are all progressive diseases primarily occurring in adulthood and all are incurable. The illness trajectory for these people may be long (years or decades) and involve lengthy periods of dependency. A range of technologies and health care options may be used to ensure adequate nutrition, communication, cardiac and respiratory functioning, bowel motility, and skin integrity. All of these initiatives require learning and adjustment on the part of the individual and family. The psychological and social factors of managing living with a neurodegenerative disease are as important as physical care. Healthy recovery of family members after their eventual bereavement is also essential.

Neurodegenerative diseases have the capacity to evoke the most negative and despondent attitudes in the minds of many health care professionals. These attitudes may readily transmit to patients and their families.[26] The fact that we cannot significantly alter disease progression is sometimes interpreted to mean that there is nothing more to be done.[27] This is inaccurate and regrettable. It is precisely because we cannot reverse or even retard the disease process that everything possible must be done to alleviate symptoms and offer appropriate psychological and spiritual support. This is where a palliative approach has much to offer.

Although many of the neurodegenerative disorders are relatively rare, the symptoms that occur in association with these disorders are quite common. Symptoms such as pain, breathlessness, constipation, and insomnia are commonly encountered, and their routine management should fall within the scope of all competent practitioners.[26] Of course, more complex issues such as nutritional support using enteral feeding, respiratory function with a view to ventilator support, or management of neuropathic pain may require consultation.[3]

A team of palliative care nurses is leading a study to examine the needs of these groups of patients and their families with the aim of identifying approaches to care that may be helpful in meeting the unique needs of these populations. Results from qualitative interviews with 135 patients, family members, and key health professionals from these four disease groups revealed six common concerns: challenges of adjusting to the impact of the illness, surviving the search for essential information, gathering practical supports from many sources, bolstering the spirit, choreographing individual care, and fearing the future. Results indicate that patients and family members needing palliative support also require access to rehabilitative services, genetic counseling, and financial assistance to help them cope with the long-term needs. The role of the palliative care nurse in working with these groups of patients requires expertise in management of these unique disease symptoms, advanced skills in family counseling, and strong interpersonal skills to help patients and families navigate the rehabilitation–palliative care pathway.

Rural and Remote Communities

Nurses working in rural areas believe there is significant work needed to provide for the palliative needs of rural communities.[28] Rural and remote communities are not homogeneous; they offer various challenges to health delivery based on demographics, local culture, physical environment, and distance from health services. Rural nurses, providing palliative care as one aspect of a broader health role in the community, suffer significant professional isolation. In some settings, particularly in remote areas, the nurse may be the sole health practitioner in a community, receiving telephone support from a doctor located some distance away. The challenge is to develop sustainable models of palliative care provision in many of these communities.

The provision of palliative care to people in rural areas is a major component of government attempts to improve access to palliative care. In many rural communities, a specialist palliative nurse consultant has been employed to work with a local team of interested people to provide palliative care support to local health services. Many rural local doctors have taken up the challenge to improve their palliative care skills and work in partnership with the nurse. There is now evidence that these approaches are working.

Sach[29] undertook a major study to explore the provision of rural palliative care in Australia. This study found the role of palliative nurse consultants to be vital in the provision of quality palliative care in rural areas. The rural palliative care nurse was identified as maintaining an up-to-date knowledge of treatments and drugs that was vital for their support of local doctors. The consultative nursing role was appreciated as being in the background, supporting the family and community nurses to provide care. Despite the fact that rural palliative care services staff were likely to visit less often than city services staff, there was greater use of telephone support and community members, and innovative use of nursing support through access to specific funds available for rural health. Overall, the study found rural communities to not be disadvantaged in the quality of palliative care provided.

Since this report, a number of innovative projects have commenced that seek to redress service access issues in rural and remote communities. For example, a collaborative project between doctors and nurses in South Australia uses videophones to link specialist palliative care outreach nurses with local health services caring for patients with palliative care needs.[30] This project, while still under evaluation, enables remote clinicians to participate in multidisciplinary clinics and improves cross sector communication.

A second innovative and nurse-led project aims to implement a "Palliative Care Toolkit" that provides local community health providers with a framework for activating palliative care services when required. This framework assists the local community to work together, drawing on the existing community and health care resources to establish as-needed palliative care services. This "pop-up" model of service provision recognizes that rural and remote communities have a small number of people requiring palliative care services annually and thus require a service provision model that can be activated on demand. The toolkit is being tested in rural and remote sites in three states of Australia (Professor Kate White, personal communication, 2004). The key principles that underpin this project are sustainability, being community led, and responsiveness, and they illustrate how palliative care nurses are taking a leadership role in innovative service delivery based on the unique needs of local communities.

Models of After-Hours Service Provision

A dominant feature of Australian community palliative care service provision is 24-hour access to support. The nature of this support differs across services and between rural and metropolitan areas, and maintaining the after-hours service can place significant strain on small services in terms of small numbers of nurses sharing after-hours responsibilities. Two models of metropolitan after-hours provision have developed that address this strain. The first consists of a triage model where a related inpatient service receives calls from patients or family members at home regarding their needs. In an evaluation of this model,[31] the triage nurse was able to manage 30% (192 calls) of calls alone. The remaining 70% (437 calls) were transferred to the specialist community palliative care nurse on call. Of these, a further 43% (186 calls) were managed by the specialist nurse with telephone support. The remaining 57% (251 calls) required a home visit. Importantly, the availability of the triage nurse was significantly related to whether the call could be managed alone, suggesting improvements in training and support for the triage nurse could increase the number of calls managed in this way and further reduce burden on the specialist community palliative care nurse.

The second model consists of sharing after-hours responsibilities between specialist palliative care services and generalist community nursing services. Across Australian metropolitan areas, generalist community nursing services already offer after-hours care and are already available to visit palliative patients at home. All of these nurses are provided with basic palliative care knowledge and skills and have access to updated information about the specific palliative patients seeking after-hours support on a daily basis. In some settings, this service is supplemented by telephone support after hours by a specialist palliative care nurse, increasing the capacity of the general community nurse to meet the patients' needs.

Night respite can be another means of improving after-hours support. A recent Australian study undertaken by Kristjanson and colleagues[32] described the benefits of night respite for patients receiving a home palliative care service and their families. The investigators developed and tested a brief assessment tool to determine those patients and families most in need of night respite. Care aides were then specifically trained to provide night respite support, and 53 patients received this support over an 11-month period. Results indicated that the assessment tool was reliable and feasible for use in practice. Findings from this study revealed the types of patients most in need of night respite support were confused, agitated, or incontinent. As well, families with high levels of caretaker fatigue were particularly in need of this type of respite. Patients and family caretakers reported high levels of satisfaction with the night respite service, and 70% of patients who died during the study were able to die at home. Cost estimates indicated that the home care and night respite service was delivered for approximately one third the cost for an equivalent period of inpatient palliative care.

Palliative Care in Aged Care

During the last 2 decades, research has indicated that the proportion of people dying in Australian residential aged care facilities has steadily increased. The increased number of residents dying in residential aged care facilities has focused attention on the need for a palliative approach that may enhance the care already provided to both residents and the families. A palliative approach[33] aims to improve the quality of life for individuals with a life-limiting illness and their families by reducing their suffering through early identification, assessing and treating pain, and addressing physical, cultural, psychological, social, and spiritual needs. The palliative approach should be able to be provided by all health professionals in all settings of care, with referral to specialist palliative care services where patient needs require this.

In response to this need, in 2002, the Australian Government Department of Health and Ageing commissioned the Australian Palliative Residential Aged Care (APRAC) Project Team to develop palliative care guidelines for the residential aged care setting (http://www.apracproject.org). The interdisciplinary team was led by nurses in palliative care and aged care and includes individuals with special expertise in guideline development, dementia, and cultural issues.

The aim and scope of the guidelines is to identify evidence-based recommendations to inform a palliative approach in residential aged care facilities. The guidelines are not intended to be rigid, prescriptive pathways, for it is the needs of the individual that determine the care one receives. The guidelines prompt creative solutions appropriate to diverse settings, varied resident needs, and unique workforce characteristics of the many residential aged care facilities that exist across the country. The guidelines provide staff working in these facilities with evidence-based criteria against which their services can be monitored. The guidelines will also assist in the identification of local strengths and weaknesses in the provision of a palliative approach in residential aged care facilities, providing a mechanism by which changes in service delivery may be evaluated over time.

Advanced Practice

Advanced practice role development in Australia is in its infancy, with state nurses' boards just beginning to set frameworks for nurse practitioner endorsement. New South Wales is the most advanced in terms of nurse practitioner developments, with South Australia and Victoria having received applications for endorsement of nurse practitioners in palliative care. Karen Glaetzer became Australia's first community palliative care nurse practitioner (NP) in August 2003, the third NP in that state. Glaetzer works at the Southern Adelaide Palliative Care Service in a combined role as NP and Outreach Coordinator, with the future plan to become a full time NP. Glaetzer's role as an NP involves case management of patients identified to have complex needs, with a particular emphasis on those with difficult family/social issues, young patients with dependent children, significant mental health concerns, or serious comorbidities. To achieve endorsement, Glaetzer was required to present a portfolio addressing 10 standards set by the South Australian nurses board, including the development of relevant practice guidelines. The endorsement process also involved an interview and presentation to the board about the clinical preparation undertaken for role performance and discussion of role expectations. While there is no minimum education requirement for NP endorsement, there is an expectation that NPs will have master's degrees. Prescribing preparation has been included in NP preparation, but in South Australia, government processes to allow nurse prescribing are incomplete. For the first 5 years, Glaetzer is required to provide evidence annually of her continued maintenance of the standards (Karen Glaetzer, personal communication, April 2004). Details about the process for endorsement can be found on the following website: http://www.nursesboard.sa.gov.au. In Victoria, four community palliative care nurses have been involved in a pilot role development program over 2003 and are in the final stages of seeking endorsement. Details on the Victorian nurse practitioner projects can be obtained from the following website: http://www.nbv.org.au.

Conclusion

Palliative nursing in Australia and New Zealand continues to develop and grow. Since the first edition of this book, the leadership role of palliative care nurses in advancing the development of palliative care has become increasingly evident in practice, education, and research. This development is supported by new academic positions in palliative nursing in several states, and individuals employed in these positions are attracting research funding from state and national competitive research funding bodies. The hallmark of these academic positions is their close relationship with clinical facilities, helping to ensure that the research agenda for palliative nursing is firmly grounded in important clinical issues. As demonstrated by the work profiled in this chapter, nurses are at the forefront of developing a service system able to meet the needs of marginalized groups in our communities and are committed to sustainable models of palliative care delivery. Palliative nurses, like nurses everywhere, are being asked to demonstrate their contribution to the health and outcomes of palliative clients. We believe the important integration of research and practice developing in the Australasian context will allow palliative care nurses in Australasia to take a leadership role in advancing palliative care practice knowledge internationally.

REFERENCES

1. Nuland S. How We Die: Reflections on Life's Final Chapter. New York: Alfred A. Knopf, 1994;255.
1a. O'Connor M, Aranda S, eds., Palliative Care Nursing: A Guide to Practice, 2nd ed. Oxford: Radcliffe Medical Press, 2003.
2. New Zealand Population Census, 2001. Available at: http://www.stats.gov.nz/products_and_services/info_releases/2001_census.htm.
3. Payne S. To supplant, supplement or support? Organisational issues for hospices. Soc Sci Med 1998;46:1495–1504.
4. Fried O. Many ways of caring: reaching out to Aboriginal palliative care clients in Central Australia. Prog Palliative Care 1999;7: 116–119.
5. Standards for the Provision of Hospice/Palliative Care. Wellington: Hospice New Zealand, 1998.
6. Standards for Palliative Care Provision, 3rd ed. Canberra: Palliative Care Australia, 999.
7. Palliative Care Service Provision in Australia: a planning guide, 2nd ed. Canberra: Palliative Care Australia, 2003.
8. State of the Nation 1998: Report of National Census of Palliative Care Services. Canberra: Palliative Care Australia, 1998.
9. Prior D. Palliative care in marginalised communities. Prog Palliative Care 1999a;7:109–115.
10. Ramsden I. After Kia ora—what next? Paper presented at the Hospice New Zealand Conference, Wellington, June 24–26, 1998.
11. Ramsden I. Kawa Whakaruruhau: Guidelines for Nursing and Midwifery Education. Wellington: Nursing Council of New Zealand, 1992.
12. Guidelines for Cultural Safety: the Treaty of Waitangi, & Maori Health in Nursing and Midwifery Education and Practice. Wellington: Nursing Council of New Zealand, 2002.
13. The New Zealand Palliative Care Strategy. New Zealand Ministry of Health, Wellington, 2001.
14. Prior D. Life-death-life: Aboriginal culture and palliative care. Unpublished thesis for Master of Science, Flinders University, South Australia, 1997.
15. National Palliative Care Strategy: A Framework For Palliative Care Service Development. Publications Production Unit (Public Affairs, Parliamentary and Access Branch), Commonwealth Department of Health and Aged Care, Publications Approval Number 4065. Canberra: Commonwealth of Australia, 2000.
16. Sullivan K & Associates Pty Ltd. National Indigenous Palliative Care Needs Study. Publications Production Unit (Public Affairs, Parliamentary and Access Branch), Commonwealth Department of Health and Aged Care, Publications Approval Number 3370. Canberra: Commonwealth of Australia, 2003.
17. Indigenous Palliative Care Project. Available at: http://www.indpac.org.au (accessed March 20, 2005).
18. Fried O. Why worry about Aboriginal palliative care. Paper presented at the 7th National Australian Palliative Care Conference, Adelaide, September 9, 2003.
19. Burns H. Bridging the gap with my community. Paper presented at the 7th National Australian Palliative Care Conference, Adelaide, September 9, 2003.
20. Roddy Y. Cultural sensitivity in palliative care. Paper presented at the National Hospice and Palliative Care Conference, Melbourne, October 27–29, 1993.
21. Sforcina J. Education in diverse cultural attitudes—stereotyping or increasing cultural sensitivity. Paper presented at the National Hospice and Palliative Care Conference, Melbourne, October 27–29, 1993.
22. Cotterill D. The hospice in a multicultural society. Paper presented at the National Hospice and Palliative Care Conference, Melbourne, October 27–29, 1993.
23. Balmain V. Attitudes to death: differences between Anglo-Australian and Darwin Chinese people. Paper presented at the National Hospice and Palliative Care Conference, Melbourne, October 27–29, 1993.
24. Campbell S, Small G, Moore G. Improving palliative care in a multicultural environment. Sydney: Hope Healthcare Limited and Northern Sydney Area Health Service, 1997.
25. Kanitsaki O. Palliative care and cultural diversity. In: Parker J, Aranda S, eds. Palliative Care: Explorations and Challenges. Sydney: MacLennan & Petty, 1998:32–45.
26. O'Brien T. Neurodegenerative disease. In: Addington-Hall J, Higginson IJ, eds. Palliative Care for Non-Cancer Patients. Oxford: Oxford University Press, 2001:44–53.
27. Norris FN. Motor neuron disease. Treating the untreated. BMJ 1992;304:459–460.
28. McCarthy A, Hegney D. Rural nursing in the Australian context. In: Aranda S, O'Connor M, eds., Palliative Care Nursing: A Guide to Practice. Melbourne: Ausmed Publications, 1999:83–101.
29. Sach J. Issues for palliative care in rural Australia. Collegian 1997;4:22–27.
30. Olver I, Brooksbank M, Champion N, Keeley J, Healey T. The use of videophones to enhance palliative outreach nursing in remote areas. Paper presented at the 7th National Australian Palliative Care Conference, Adelaide, September 9, 2003.
31. Aranda S, Hayman-White K, Devilee L, O'Connor M, Bence G. Inpatient hospice triage of "after hours" calls to a community palliative care service. Int J Palliative Nurs 2001;7:214–220.
32. Kristjanson L, Cousins K, White K, Andrews L, Lewin G, Tinnelly C, Asphar D, Greene R. Evaluation of a night respite community palliative care service. Int J Pall Nurs 2004; 10(2) 84–90.
33. Finlay IG, Jones JVH. Definitions in palliative care. BMJ 1995; 311:754.

PALLIATIVE CARE IN THE UNITED KINGDOM

Andrew Knight

It is now 38 years since St. Christopher's Hospice in Sydenham, a suburb of South East London, opened its doors to patients. St. Christopher's had been long in gestation. Cicely Saunders had been thinking about, praying for, traveling (in effect, what we would call "networking"), and generally organizing her hospice for the previous 20 years. The amount of organizational effort that Saunders and her supporters put into the project that she called her "spiritual odyssey"[1] meant that it could not fail, yet they were never sure it would wholly succeed. The building itself, a large concrete and glass structure and architecturally very much of its time, proclaims a bold statement that few could ignore. Here was something new, something that would not go away.

Yet Cicely Saunders and those early pioneers did not imagine that the concept of hospice—a philosophy of care that would encompass all needs of the terminally ill patient and their family—would lead to a movement replicated around the world in hundreds of settings and cultures, and to a new form of medicine that would change forever how systems of care are delivered: palliative care.

Students of the origins of hospice are indebted to the ongoing careful work of Professor David Clark. He makes the important point "that to claim an arbitrary starting point for such a complex and far-reaching movement is unsatisfactory. Indeed it may be preferable to see the opening of St. Christopher's in 1967 as a crucial outcome of ideas and strategies . . . in which can be located the essential characteristics of the subsequent hospice movement."[2] Many of the principles of hospice care are as sound and applicable now as they were then.

Cicely Saunders's sense of a calling to undertake this work and the idea of a religious community operating outside the mainstream of the health service is prevalent throughout the decade prior to the opening of St. Christopher's.[3] It is now interesting to speculate what would have happened had she not decided, in a pragmatic way, to embrace the need to work practically within the world of modern medicine and social services. Would the movement have had so much influence? Certainly in the 1960s there was a greater openness to question the norm, to challenge tradition; and the public was beginning to become interested in alternative therapies, such as Eastern and homeopathic medicine.[4] But would politicians, administrators, and planners of health care have been so influenced by an evangelical religious community? This is not known. However, it is clear that the originators of St. Christopher's and those that followed in its wake were religiously motivated; they carried with them a religious zeal to change the way that society and, in particular, the medical establishment cared for the dying.

Would St. Christopher's have been established if it were to be proposed now, at the start of a new millennium? Many of the advisors to Cicely Saunders were religious and established figures in the church. The church in a largely secular Great Britain has much less influence and power than it did in the 1950s and early 1960s. The concept of hospice care remains hugely popular with the public, who identify with its philosophy and approach to care. Moreover, it is thought to be an essential component of the modern health care system in the United Kingdom, one that should be replicated elsewhere. Many public figures sit on hospice boards of trustees, giving voluntarily of their time. However, it is not at all clear in a modern world, where health budgets are being cut and stretched to deal with pressing needs, that another seat at the table labeled "palliative care" would be at all welcomed.

Influence of Cicely Saunders and St. Christopher's Hospice on Nursing

From the beginning, the need to publish and to spread the new principles of the care of the dying was recognized. Cicely Saunders had an article on euthanasia published in October 1959 in Britain's most widely read nursing journal, *Nursing Times.* This was the first of a seminal series of six articles, whose influence has been immeasurable, on the care of the dying. They contain advice on "should a patient know?"; pain control; mental distress in the dying; and principles of and the nursing care of the dying. It is not surprising that they can still be purchased in reprint form today, as they contain many of the founding principles of palliative care.[5] Many nurses came to know about hospice through reading these articles.

The Joint Board of Nursing Studies (later to be divided into four national boards) was formed to oversee the burgeoning number of postgraduate courses for nurses in the United Kingdom. It recognized the need to formulate a course in the "Care of the Dying Patient and their Family" in 1974—the first course appropriately being run at St. Christopher's. This course, now run by a number of colleges of nursing remains as popular as ever, containing as it does a synthesis of the subject. Known popularly as ENB 931 after its old catalogue number, it remains the touchstone course for any potential applicant to the specialty.

The impact that this new approach had on nursing throughout British hospital nursing care was considerable. The rise of a movement in the United Kingdom and the growth of hospice facilities was fired by inspired nurses wanting to practice this form of care who were frustrated by the lack of resources in the National Health Service. It was mirrored by a growing sense of professionalism in nursing and the need to formulate philosophies of care. Virginia Henderson's model 6 seemed to many to come closest to an ideal model of care and was readily taken up by the influential Royal Marsden Hospital, the United Kingdom's premier cancer hospital. However, it was not until the 1980s that a full model of care, embracing palliative and cancer care, came into being, when the Royal Marsden Hospital added palliative care to its curriculum in 1986.

The acquired immunodeficiency syndrome (AIDS) pandemic in the mid-1980s took many by surprise and challenged those who were equipped and trained to deliver palliative and cancer care to this largely dying population. The providers of mainstream hospice care were, with some notable exceptions, seen to be indifferent, fearing the difficulties of an unpredictable human immunodeficiency virus (HIV) trajectory and the effects on a largely voluntary income. Criticisms of homophobia were not unjustified. Two hospices specifically for the care of the HIV patient were formed: the London Lighthouse in North West London, and the resurrected Mildmay Mission Hospital in East London. These remain, but the focus, at least for the time being, have shifted from providing inpatient care to that of education, counseling support, and outreach work. The self-determination and questioning spirit of the HIV patient was a good foil to an apparently unquestioning elderly cancer patient. Nurses working with this group of patients learned a great deal about the care of a group of patients who questioned the status quo—lessons that have been included in palliative nursing courses.

Hospice Care Under the National Health Service

The National Health Service (NHS), promising free health care for all, was 19 years young in 1967 and still considered successful. Its modes of operation were well established and took up much of the resources and time. There was largely indifference to care of the dying. Systems of nursing, based on the traditional work-based apprentice model, were designed so that each block of extensive work practice was preceded by a (hopefully) appropriate block of classroom teaching. The Committee on Senior Nursing Staff Structure, known universally as the Salmon Report 7, refashioning nursing management and crucially introducing a tier of nursing officers that were to stay in nursing for 30 years, had yet to take effect. Matrons and assistant matrons still ruled in a world where little audit of care or questioning of practice took place. The first degree program in nursing, at Manchester University, would not appear until 1969.

The first hospices emerged into this system. Independent in nature, they relied on charitable giving and voluntary labor, raising funds to provide for capital building and staffing. At the same time, they looked to the health service, in the form of hospital boards and regional health authorities, for contractual arrangements for patients. Some, such as St. Christopher's, also received grants from the Ministry of Health for pain research.[8]

The emotional appeal of terminal care was strong. Its zealous founders were convincing in their moral arguments that society address the need to care for the dying, who were languishing without adequate pain control in hospitals. It easily captured the public's imagination, as all families would experience death; in particular, the way that the dying were cared for, good and bad, had special meaning. Catching health care planners off-guard, the spread of hospice facilities was rapid and ad hoc. Indeed, the need for hospice care and the question about the use of resources allocated to it were not carefully examined until the advent of the so-called purchaser-provider split as part of the conservative government health reforms of the 1980s.[9] To question the motivation of benefactors providing for worthy services was thought incorrect, to say the least. Although clearly the hospice movement could not exist outside, with its charitable foundations it was difficult for it to survive unchecked inside the NHS. Perhaps reluctantly, they were mutually dependent, and for hospices to survive, some growth regulation and some organizational sense had to be brought to bear. This was gradually taken up by regional, area, and local health authorities. A sense of need for hospice facilities was sought.

In 1980, the Working Group on Terminal Care produced the first report on the provision on hospice serves. Believing that a lack of specialist staff and financial resources would limit the growth of independent hospice facilities, it recommended concentrating on home care (care of the terminally ill in their own home) and day care. Fundamentally, its members held the view that the dying should not be "hidden away" from the provision of wider, hospital and community-based services.[10] However, the Working Group's prediction that the number of stand-alone services would be self-limiting was found to be false: the number of such units trebled in the next decade.[8] This also ran contrary to the recommendation of a survey by Lunt and Hillier,[11] who, in the following year, recommended that inpatient services be limited and that community services be coordinated to ensure equity of access across regions.

In 1987, 20 years after the first "modern" hospice started treating patients, the Department of Health set out its stall. In the first official circular on the subject, it firmly recommended that district health authorities gauge the need for and control the provision of hospice services.[8] It underscored the need to control hospice finances to ensure that facilities were financially secure to meet all contingencies, such as nurse salaries.

In 1990, in what was quickly to become a controversial departmental press release, the government seemed to be prepared to commit "a pound for a pound" of charitable giving. This announcement was indeed followed by a large injection of some £8 million and an unequal and divisive scramble among hospices and NHS providers of palliative care for funds. It seemed to say that monies for this health sector were limitless and, in turn, led to much ill feeling among other, apparently equally deserving, providers of health care. Deeply unpopular except among hospice providers, the scheme was dropped in 1995, and the age of earmarked monies for palliative care was over.

The 1980s had seen the beginning of health care reforms that continue to this day. Believing that the NHS was bureaucratically badly managed by ill-equipped managers who could not compete with the vested self-interests of its professionals, the conservative government finally introduced a system of general management in 1983. Writing in the report that was to carry his name, Sir Roy Griffiths, the head of a supermarket chain, famously declared that "if Florence Nightingale were carrying her lamp through the corridors of the NHS today, she would almost certainly be searching for the people in charge."[12] It was felt by commentators that with the introduction of "general management" and its business ethos, professional and clinical staff had lost out. Certainly a paradigm shift in power had taken place.

Fundamentally for the provision of hospice care, these management reforms ensured that there was now a clear demarcation between the purchasers of care, the district health authorities, and the newly formed General Practitioner fund holders, and its providers, independent hospices and charitable providers of funds, notably Macmillan Cancer Relief. Crucially, purchasers brought to bear four key components to the planning of palliative care services: an overall strategy; a service specification (of assessed need); the contracting process to allocate funds; and the need for clinical audit and quality assurance.[13]

The multidisciplinary Standing Medical Advisory and Standard Nursing Advisory and Midwifery Committees (SMAC/SNAMC), reporting in 1992, again recommended that palliative care should not be concentrated in hospice units, and that need should be assessed demographically and care delivered as an integral part of the local health service. This far-reaching report served as a blueprint for purchasers and providers alike, and by 1995, 97% of hospices had entered into a contracting relationship with health authorities.[14]

"The idea that health care services should be predicated upon a rational assessment of need rather than upon emotional pleading, political lobbying, or the vested interests of particular providers is one with which it is difficult to disagree."[8] The palliative care community was enthused at the opportunity to state the needs of their population group and lobby for a properly financed commitment based on that need. However, it became clear that the needs of the cancer patient and their families are many and include needs previously not considered by cash-strapped health authorities: psychosocial, social, and emotional. The strategy developed into one of prioritizing need and hoping that the limited resources would be shared equitably.[15]

The remaining years of the conservative governments saw the conclusion of their health care reforms. The number of general practitioner (GP) fund-holders expanded, and from 1994 were enabled to purchase palliative care services.[16]

GP fund-holding was abandoned with a change of government in May 1997. It has been replaced by, first, Primary Care Groups, and since 2000, Primary Care Trusts (PCTs), who essentially have a not dissimilar role to assess, plan, and commission a local health strategy.

In 1995, the Expert Advisory Group on Cancer published its findings on the provision of cancer services in the United Kingdom. Known universally as the Calman-Hine Report, it found a significant inequality of services—an absence in some areas, a plenitude in others. It recommended a three-tier system of primary care provision, for prevention and initial consultation; cancer units at district level for the treatment of common cancers; and cancer centers to deal with rarer cancers, covering larger populations.[17] It highlighted that palliative care should be a seamless service across all three tiers, effectively underlining the fundamental need for palliative care from diagnosis of cancer. To enable this, teams of palliative care nurses and consultants should work in cancer units and centers.

The Calman-Hine Report did much to raise the profile of cancer within the NHS, and changed the landscape of palliative care forever. It underscored its link with the provision of cancer services at a time when some were beginning to question the need for palliative care to be available for the "non-malignant" population.[18] However, palliative care was established in a mainstream area of health care and one that would assume major importance for the Department of Health.[19] A key policy in commissioning palliative care and one that developed from the work on the Calman-Hine report was the Cancer Plan.[20] The providers of palliative care had to learn how to promote their services; they had to learn a business culture. "At the dawn of the Conservative reforms of the 1990s the position was crystallized completely: join the contract culture or be condemned to obscurity. The independent hospices, after the briefest of vacillations, climbed on board and rarely looked back."[8] To enable them to do this, most independent hospices have appointed their own chief executives, with a business and financial background, and not necessarily with a health service background.

Hospices had to evolve to survive, and this was a logical step in the process. However, the appointment of chief executives as business managers meant that the tripartite management system of matron/director of nursing, medical director, and administrator became a dying model. There have been casualties, as those holding professional values in powerful positions have met managers empowered to promote business- and market-based value systems.[21] These sources of conflict have been accentuated by the formation and rise of the specialty of palliative medicine and the perception that nursing is not held in sufficient regard.[22]

The latest guidance for the specialty is that of the National Health Services' National Institute of Clinical Excellence (NICE). This Institute, a government organization for health improvement, has undertaken extensive consultation on guidance for the provision of palliative and supportive care in the United Kingdom. Their binding guidelines recommend explicit service models to the providers of cancer and palliative care services on all aspects their services undertake.[23]

The National Council for Hospice and Specialist Palliative Care Services (NCHSPCS)

Formed in 1991 as a representative and coordinating body for the hospice movement in England, Wales, and Scotland, the NCHSPCS has done much to ensure that hospices have been faithfully represented at every level. Its membership comes from national cancer charities, professional organizations, and regional representatives. Through its professionals' working parties and guidelines, it has been instrumental in affecting the practice of palliative care. Examples of this work include guidelines on ethical issues affecting palliative care, such as artificial hydration, cardiopulmonary resuscitation, and much on-going work on euthanasia. Other issues covered are guidelines for the management of the last days of life and the use of complementary therapies. Quality guidelines include the use of outcome measures in palliative care. Its work with purchasers of palliative care, ensuring that a high profile is maintained, include guidelines on contracting; needs assessment and research in palliative care; and a statement of definitions of palliative care. A full list of their publications may be obtained by visiting their website.[24]

Hospice Governance

Hospice and clinical governance is another subject on which the NCHSPCS took an early lead.[25] It helped to define the components of appropriate governance and an action plan for its introduction. It has become an established part of the way that palliative care services now manage their staff, clients, and resources; set programs to monitor and receive information on quality issues, clinical audit and evidence-based practice; and work with commissioners and assess risk management. Importantly, hospice governance systems have neatly embraced the need to bring voluntary trustees of services and staff together in a common goal. These systems have been incorporated into standard frameworks for hospices, the most notable being the accreditation program produced by the Health Quality Service, an independent charity that surveys NHS, independent hospitals and hospices, nursing homes, and clinics in the United Kingdom and mainland Europe.[26]

Settings of Care

An important piece of work undertaken by the NCHSPCS has been the gathering of information about the activities of specialist palliative care services, the Minimum Data Sets Project (MDS). In conjunction with and building on the excellent work undertaken by the Hospice Information Service, a joint organization between Help the Hospices and St. Christopher's Hospice, the MDS provides valuable information on numbers of inpatient and home care services, hospital support service, and day care, as well as how these services are used (Table 66–2).

The 10 Marie Curie Centres or hospice inpatient units are administered by a national charity, Marie Curie Cancer Care. In 2002–2003, there were some 3666 inpatient admissions. Additionally, there are thousands of nurses who care for patients in their own homes for a full working day or night shift. The presence of a Marie Curie Nurse often allows patients to remain at home. In total, they provide some one million hours of nursing care each year.

Sue Ryder Homes are administered by a national charity, the Sue Ryder Foundation, providing palliative care for patients with cancer in their homes. Several homes have visiting nurses who visit patients before and after admission.

The growth of hospice services in recent years has been considerable. In the early 1970s, The Cancer Relief Macmillan Fund began a program of capital funding to provide units within NHS hospitals, or on their grounds, with hospital authorities ensuring the responsibility for their running costs.

The number of adult inpatient hospice, community, and hospital-based services, although adequate in some areas, is variable and inequitable throughout the country. A survey undertaken by the NCHSPCS highlighted this variation.[27] In Wales and Scotland, the provision to remote communities relies largely on community teams and hospitals. Out of a total of 434 inpatient units currently providing care, there are just 34 in Wales and 46 in Scotland (see Table 66–2). There are now 51 beds per million adult population.[28]

Much is owed to these inpatient institutions. They broke new ground with their nonhierarchical teams of professionals and volunteers, incorporating patients' needs and wishes into the care that they gave. Hospice involves "a personal noninstitutional approach, promoting psychological care and physical well being through good symptom control."[29]

Table 66–2
Summary of United Kingdom Adult Inpatient Units—January 2004

	Adult Units	NHS Units	Voluntary Units	Beds	NHS Beds	Voluntary Beds
London	17	6	11	409	86	323
Midland and East England	41	12	29	584	152	432
North	62	12	50	839	98	741
South	52	12	40	805	154	651
England	**172**	**42**	**130**	**2637**	**490**	**2147**
Scotland	23	10	13	347	103	244
Wales	17	11	6	142	76	66
Northern Ireland	5	1	4	69	4	65
TOTAL	**217**	**64**	**153**	**3195**	**673**	**2522**

The voluntary units include 10 Marie Curie Hospices and 6 Sue Ryder Homes. The remainder are independent local charities including 2 exclusively for HIV/AIDS.

Table 66–3
Summary of United Kingdom Children's Inpatient Units—January 2004

	Units	Beds
London	2	8
Midland and East England	10	83
North	10	69
South	5	41
England	**27**	**201**
Scotland	1	8
Wales	1	10
Northern Ireland	1	10
TOTAL	**30**	**229**

The growth of number of hospices catering to the terminally ill child and family has been remarkable throughout the last decade and a half. There are 30 listed in the current edition of the Hospice Directory (Table 66–3).[28]

Patient statistics for 2001 reveal that 41,000 new patients were admitted to an inpatient unit. Ninety-five percent of these were suffering from cancer. There were 29,000 deaths, and the average stay was 13 days.[28]

Range of Services

The range of services offered by hospices is now considerable, the day long past when hospices cared only for the patient requiring terminal care. Johnson and colleagues reported that "our findings suggest that their [patients] management is likely to include a range of investigations and procedures that are usually associated with acute hospital care."[30] Hospices routinely admit patients who are having chemotherapy and radiotherapy for their cancer. Transfusions of blood, and rarely platelets and other blood products, and injections of bisphosphonates either as a day case or overnight inpatient admission are performed. Proponents of this rather more accommodating and enabling position feel it important that patients see hospices as places where they can be successfully treated and discharged. Critics believe that we are in danger of losing much if we forget the original binding ethos and principal aim—the holistic care of the dying—in the rush to diversify and to be seen as therapeutic, a process universally known as the "routinization and medicalization of hospice."

Much attention has been given to an integrated care pathway for the dying, in particular the Liverpool Care Pathway for the Dying Patient,[30a] a multidisciplinary framework designed to coordinate care. Its implementation in hospital, community, and care homes has meant that a focused hospice model of care can be replicated. This pathway has been incorporated into the Gold Standards Framework[33] and embraced by the NICE Guidance.[23]

Home Care

Table 66–4 illustrates the extent to which the majority of patients who receive specialist palliative care do so in their own home. In 2001, more than 150,000 patients were seen by home care teams, 3 to 4 months being the average length of time that a patient will be cared for by a team. A minimum of 60% of all cancer deaths are now cared for by these teams, with an estimated 30,000 deaths at home.[28] The MDS for 2002–2003 records the reasons for referral to a community (home care) service as pain or other symptom control 43%; psychological support 38%; caregiver support 13%; social and financial help 7%; and assessment for admission to an inpatient unit 3%. A team of clinical nurse specialists (CNS), usually with medical support, will make on average 5.3 visits per

Table 66–4
Summary of United Kingdom Community and Hospital Support Services—January 2004

	Home Care	Hospice at Home	Day Care	Hospital Support Nurses	Hospital Support Teams
London	29	9	17	5	40
Midland and East England	79	28	60	21	53
North	90	21	68	18	70
South	66	23	66	9	57
England	**264**	**81**	**211**	**53**	**220**
Scotland	52	4	223	13	28
Wales	30	7	20	4	19
Northern Ireland	10	2	4	2	14
Total	**356**	**94**	**258**	**72**	**281**

Source: NHS National Institute of Clinical Excellence (2004), reference 23.

patient; the CNS will make 79% of visits recorded; medical staff 2%; and the others being made by professions allied to medicine, social workers, and other nurses. The average length of care given to a patient in the community is 118 days, although two thirds of those cared for are on the case load for less than 3 months.[31]

"Macmillan Nurses," long a feature of the provision of specialist palliative care, are named after Macmillan Cancer Relief, which funds the first 2 to 3 years' salary of these posts in community and hospital settings, with the understanding that the health authority will pick up the costs of these posts afterwards. The principal role of these nurses remains one of personally assessing and delivering care to patients and families, and giving advice to and empowering primary caregivers. However, this has evolved to one that promotes high standards of cancer and palliative care. This is achieved by acting as a catalyst and change agent; contributing to pre- and postregistration educational curricula, and promoting and participating in clinical research and audit.[32]

The Macmillan Gold Standards Framework, a framework for community physicians and their teams caring for the palliative care patient in their own home, is now being rolled out across the United Kingdom, with more than 500 practices in 56 project areas. Based around seven "gold" standards, the program offers evidence-based advice on:[33]

- Teamwork and continuity of care
- Advanced planning
- Symptom control
- Support of patients and caregivers

Hospice at Home

Extended nursing care at home, or Hospice at Home, is a service that employs registered and auxiliary nurses in the patient's home, providing physical care and psychosocial support. Although the amount of time spent at home is small, it is thought that this type of service reinforces patients' confidence to remain in their own surroundings and in their ability to stay there. Boulstridge and colleagues[34] conclude from their retrospective study of 52 patients cared for by a Hospice at Home team that "Hospice at Home appeared to enable patients to die at home." There was a primary need for caregiver respite. Hospital admissions were mainly for appropriate specialist palliative care; 26% had been admitted for symptom control and just one patient, 2% for terminal care.

Day Care

Day centers afford the chance for patients to express their creativity, to be among others in a similar situation, to provide both a social support and the opportunity to receive symptom control as required. They can serve as an important source of respite for patients and their carers.[35,36] A questionnaire survey of 43 day centers aimed to investigate the two pervading models of day care in the United Kingdom, the "social" model and the clinical or "medical" model.[37] It showed that there were multiple reasons for admission to a day care program, but that respite for caregivers was the second most commonly cited reason. Others were psychological support, social interaction, and symptom control. An estimated 31,500 new patients attended day facilities in 2002–2003. Of the services that responded to the MDS, 19 had more than 15% noncancer patients. However, 21 services recorded that they did not have any noncancer patients. Fifty-nine percent of patients stayed with a day center for less than 3 months, while 23% stayed more than 6 months.[31]

Hospital Support Teams

Approximately 56% of cancer patients in England and Wales die in hospitals.[38] Hospital support nursing services consist of on average 2.2 nurses[31] based in hospitals, acting as a resource. Hospital support teams may have the support of a specialist doctor. Access to patients who require palliative care but who may be in a surgical, medical, or gynecological bed is vital, and a doctor facilitates this. In 2002–2003, there were an estimated 120,000 patients seen by these services.[31] An evaluation of the impact of hospital clinical nurse specialists on other doctors and nurses showed clear benefits in the support and education that they were able to provide.[39] Two important studies underline the importance of these teams. A study to evaluate whether a hospital team had an effect on the patients' symptoms showed that they benefited from being admitted to the hospital for symptom control, and that they had better symptom control for pain and anorexia,[40] while a study to assess the effect of the hospital team on cancer patients' insights, showed that those patients who received input from a team had a better insight into their diagnosis and prognosis. This enabled more open communication about impending death.[41]

Some Issues Facing the Providers of Palliative Care

Criteria for Admission to Inpatient Hospices

Criteria for admission to what is, in effect, a valuable and limited resource, has always been an important issue for hospices.[33] Admission is likely to be because the patient has symptoms in which the hospice can play an active part in treating, or because the patient is dying and the patient and/or their family believe that admission is appropriate.

A review of requests for admission are usually decided each working day by a small representative team of senior staff. They take into account the patient's physical, psychosocial, and other needs; whether they live alone and who is at home to care for them; whether there are children in the house; and what packages of care are already in place. A visit by a member of the hospice's medical staff may be necessary, but often there is little time to accomplish this. Many hospices have a businesslike understanding with their referring community or hospital-based teams, trusting their estimation of the patient's prognosis, present condition, and needs.

A study of a random sample of people who had died in 1998 investigated which terminally ill cancer patients received inpatient care in hospices and other specialist palliative inpatient units. This study interviewed families and others who knew about the last year of life. Interviews were obtained for 2074 cancer deaths. Of these, 342 had been admitted to 31 different hospices. Five factors were found to independently predict hospice inpatient care: having pain in the last year of life, having constipation, being dependent on others for activities of daily living for between 1 and 6 months before death, having breast cancer, and being under the age of 85 years. A third of patients with all five factors were admitted, compared with no patients with none of these factors. It was found that symptom severity, age, dependency level, and site of cancer played a role in determining hospice admission but had limited predictive value. The study's salutary conclusion was that "admission seems to be governed more by chance than by need."[42]

It is generally unlikely that a hospice will agree to the admission of a patient with a prognosis of longer than 3 months. In the United Kingdom, the complex social services banding procedures for estimating continuing care, residential and nursing home care mean that few hospices willingly admit patients who may require referral for this care on discharge.

Respite Care

Possibly the most common reason for admission to an inpatient unit at the end of life is the caregiver's inability to provide continuing care. Despite the increasing amounts of palliative care available, studies have highlighted the high level of anxiety experienced by caregivers.[43] The term "respite care" is a term that covers a range of services provided under the palliative care umbrella: inpatient care, day care, and hospice at home services.

The majority of hospices are able to admit for a period of 1 to 2 weeks to enable the family or caregivers to have a rest. The concept of providing this form of care is not new. Families who "battle their way through" the journey from diagnosis to death and beyond require considerable information from the palliative care team and attention to their emotional and health needs.[44] They need empowerment to undertake their role. Identification of family members who may not cope well in the bereavement period is important so that resources can be mobilized in a preventive manner. This is often achieved by the home care team, but the admission of a patient for respite care enables the caregivers to be introduced to staff who will be there to care for them later on. However, there is little evidence for the clinical effectiveness of inpatient beds for respite care.[43]

The problems associated with respite admission have been well identified. That this group of patients may be "blocking" a bed needed for a terminally ill patient taxes most inpatient units and ensures that staff carefully plan these admissions, and that restrictions are often placed on the numbers of such admissions that a unit can take at any one time. Raeside and Ellershaw, in their retrospective analysis of 34 respite admissions to St. Christopher's Hospice,[45] found that patients admitted were enabled to receive a range of services, including anesthetic referral. However, 24 (71%) died during the admission in the hospice or during a subsequent admission.

The place of day care as a means of providing support to the caregiver by ensuring that a patient achieves a regular, often weekly, day admission and break from their routine, while established and cited as the second most common reason for referral,[46] is none the less poorly evaluated.[37] The effect of the increasing amount of support at home, either provided by hospice services, national cancer charities, or local voluntary bodies is similarly probably underestimated because of inadequate sample sizes and a problem with the definition of this care.[43]

Single or Shared Accommodation

Many hospices in the United Kingdom, following a model first promoted at St. Christopher's, placed their patients in bays of two, three, and four beds. Kirk, in a search of the literature prior to undertaking his study, found no reference to room choice in a hospice "or why the people who are influential in hospice ward design chose the bed configurations they did."[47] Following criticism by the regulatory body, the Care Standards Commission,[48] and an appreciation that many patients prefer single rooms, many hospices are undertaking extensive redevelopment works to supply more single rooms. Kirk established that 21 out of 24 patients preferred a single room, especially if they had distressing symptoms such as nausea and vomiting or diarrhea. Contrary to common belief, there was no evidence to support placing patients together to share their experiences.[47] There is anecdotal evidence that placing short-term patients alongside those who are terminally ill is detrimental to their overall well-being. Many patients report being distressed and subsequently reluctant to be readmitted. Further research into the effects of placing patients for short-term admission—for example, for respite or rehabilitation—alongside those that are dying is required.

Ethnic Minorities

The need to meet the needs of all cultural and ethnic groups residing within a hospice's catchment area is recognized by a movement anxious to help hospice shed its white, middle-class image. After all, a hospice not only serves, but also depends on its local population. Information from the Hospice Information Service shows that of those cared for by palliative care services in 2001–2002, just 3% were nonwhite. That there is a poor uptake by ethnic groups was a cause of concern highlighted in the NHS Cancer Plan.[19]

The National Council for Hospice and Specialist Palliative Care Services' report, *Opening Doors*,[49] attempted to identify the extent of and reasons for low uptake of hospice and specialist palliative care services and tried to ensure that those purchasing and providing these services were aware of ways in which the service could be improved. Fountain, in his 1999 study of palliative care uptake in the city of Derby,[50] found that whereas ethnic minorities made up 9.7% of the population, they accounted for only 1.5% of the patients referred to palliative care services. The NCHSPCS report had found that the ethnic minority population had a lower proportion of elderly people and the incidence of cancer in the black and Asian communities was lower than that of the indigenous white population, a conclusion reached by other authors.[50,51]

Another concerning reason why ethnic minorities may use palliative care services less is that the services are "culturally insensitive."[52] The reluctance of GP's and other health care professionals to refer patients, the lack of information about the availability of services, and poor communication exacerbated by poor translation services were some of the reasons cited for this "insensitivity." As the authors state, it is indeed fortunate that Oliviere, among others, offers specific advice to "nurture and respect cultural difference."[53] Perhaps the best current advice is that of Sheldon, who states that an application of "the individual and whole person approach basic to palliative care, which inquires of the patient and caregiver what their goals are and makes them central, is still the most appropriate."[51] However, the providers of palliative care services still have some way to go to appeal to ethnic minorities and to not appear exclusive.

Dying from Other Diseases

The use of hospice and specialist palliative care services by patients without a cancer diagnosis is another important issue for and measure of a service that is openly diversifying and trying to shed its old image. For those with a noncancer diagnosis, palliative care is most likely to be delivered by a primary care team. Provision of specialist palliative care to this group is rare but becoming increasingly less so. In the past, few services advertised their willingness to extend their services to the noncancer patient; however, many are changing their mission statements and broad service objectives to include patients with a "life-threatening illness." However, the percentage of new patients admitted to hospice inpatient units remains very low, just 4.9%, and to home care programs, just 4.8% in 2002–2003,[31] little different to that of 1994–1995, 4%.[54] It would appear that the United Kingdom is not following reported evidence from the United States by treating and caring for a larger percentage of this group.[55] However, it is recognized that the needs of this group of patients is essentially the same as that of advanced cancer[56] and anecdotally few are now denied access to specialist palliative care. Addington-Hall and colleagues, writing one of a series of papers highlighting the need of this group, states that to answer the "question of how to meet the palliative care needs of people who die from causes other than cancer will require the qualities of imagination, innovation and dedication which have characterized the hospice movement over the past 30 years."[56] It is good to report anecdotally that nurses in home care, day care, and inpatients units do understand these needs and, using these qualities, are becoming more and more skilled in addressing them.

Cardiopulmonary Resuscitation

Cardiopulmonary resuscitation (CPR) remains a difficult issue for hospices. The debate has intensified since the publication of a joint statement from the British Medical Association, the Royal College of Nursing, and the Resuscitation Council (UK).[57] If the patient is young and wishes to receive the care and expert symptom control of a hospice and continue with active treatment, they may want and request resuscitation. The arguments against providing CPR are well documented,[58] and a complete ban on CPR in inpatient settings could be made. Hospices have not been equipped to undertake resuscitation, nursing staffs' training and experience of resuscitation may be out of date, and resuscitation may not fit with the central belief of a hospice to support but not to prolong life. However, the advent of automatic external defibrillators and the softening of attitudes towards this once-taboo area means that the debate on CPR is continuing.[59] The NCHSPCS Document[60] attempted to allay fears that nurses may have about this essentially alien, but nonetheless occasionally encountered, area of practice.

Organ Donation

The donation of organs from patients dying from cancer remains relatively rare despite recognized practice in this area for some 15 years.[61] Corneas may be removed up to 24 hours, and heart valves up to 72 hours after death,[62] and, therefore, donation need not interfere with the viewing of a patient after death and the normal grieving procedures. A study undertaken to assess how relatives reacted within the palliative care setting concluded that while the families regarded donation as separate to bereavement, it was regarded positively, and that organ donation is an acceptable issue for both families and the patient.[61]

Research in Palliative Care

The early research work of pioneers like Saunders and Hinton was important in establishing hospice/palliative care as a specialty. Research was considered one of the three "legs" supporting palliative care,[63] but there are elements of palliative care that are inherently difficult to measure.[64–66] Field and colleagues identify seven problems when attempting research in palliative care.

1. Attrition of subjects through illness progression and death
2. Ethical issues of involving the dying and bereaved when there is no perceived benefit to them
3. Health professionals who act as "gatekeepers" to subjects and caregivers
4. Use of surrogate accounts for patient experiences and opinions
5. Definitions of palliative care, quality of life, etc.
6. Selecting appropriate measures
7. Establishing appropriate outcomes of evaluation[66]

Both the number of small units delivering palliative care that are distanced geographically and actually from an academic base, and the imperative to first and foremost establish and maintain a clinical service have also meant that research has not always achieved the status that it requires in the United Kingdom.

Despite these seemingly formidable obstacles, there are now many palliative nursing academic departments in the United Kingdom. The Palliative Care Research Forum of Britain and Ireland has been in existence since 1991. In 1996, the Association of Palliative Medicine formed a science committee, and The Royal Society of Medicine created a Palliative Care Forum in 1997. The growing number of palliative medicine specialist registrar training programs and the 10 medical, nursing, multiprofessional, psychosocial, cancer, and palliative care Masters programs require that the implementation of research is addressed and that a body of knowledge continues to be assimilated. The multiprofessional journal *Palliative Medicine*, established 15 years ago and now in its 18th volume, has consistently published research from the United Kingdom and Europe, doing much to ensure the credibility and effectiveness of research among all disciplines and in all palliative care settings.

The continuing need for providers of palliative care to engage with the commissioners of health service delivery has meant that they have had to embrace their reforms and priorities to establish outcome and effectiveness measures. It is not easy to apply an evidence-based approach to palliative care for some of the reasons above, and as Higginson has noted, an absence of evidence does not mean that a service is ineffective.[67] The NICE guidance for supportive and palliative care emphasizes that "Future research should focus on determining effective solutions, rather than re-assessing need; there is a wealth of evidence on need and importance, and a relative dearth on effective solutions."[68]

However, as Clark notes, "although research has been stimulated by developments in the health service and by the development of cooperative and supportive links between researchers, the research base of palliative care is insufficiently rigorous, often failing to move beyond small-scale descriptive accounts." He optimistically concludes that "there are . . . signs that there is a sufficient volume of established researchers and research units to begin to move beyond the situation."[66]

Regulation of Hospice Services

The regulation of hospices and specialist palliative care services has long concerned nurse managers. Under the Nursing Homes Act (1984), a convenient place to lodge a facility that did not fit in with the mainstream hospital sector, hospices found that they were both overregulated and burdened by the regulations that apply to nursing homes, be they for six beds or 60. It did not reflect the comprehensive, multiprofessional work that palliative care services provide. The regulation and inspection teams were interested in inpatient facilities only, not in the important work in the community and how it impacted on these facilities. The present government undertook evidence and published its proposals for the provision and regulation of services in the independent sector. These Care Standards set up a separate regulatory body to set and inspect hospices against new, defined standards.[48] Many were looking forward to the implementation of these new standards as an opportunity to fully and appropriately demonstrate the complexities of palliative care. Some 2 years after their introduction and just when the Care Standards inspectors are coming to grips with the palliative environment, these standards are being abandoned. In the future, we will be inspected by the Health Care Commission.

User Involvement

Oliviere[69] reminds us that involving the users of palliative care was integral to its founding, and that Dame Cicely Saunders, in recounting her original vision, felt that the hospice movement should be "a voice for the voiceless." There are potential and real difficulties in transferring the concept of user involvement to palliative care, including the nature and effects of a rapidly changing disease process, patient symptoms, and concerns about their families, finances, and the future, which must take precedence. Talking openly about death and dying and the protection of patients by professionals is also paramount.[70,71] Bradburn[72] writes that user involvement in the context of palliative care requires that we listen to users' experiences, empower users to advocate on their own behalf, and work with user groups in partnership. A report into the users forum at St. Christopher's Hospice concluded that although the entire process was time-consuming, the forum for both professionals and users had been "exciting, educational and stimulating."[73] It is now understood that participation by users cannot be a token exercise, and that their input is required when considering the development of hospice services. Certainly, despite the barriers and challenges to establishing an effective means of obtaining user feedback, there are now many successful initiatives in the United Kingdom[72] to ensure that the user voice, the "voice for the voiceless," is heard.

Conclusion

It would seem appropriate to conclude that, with the advent of the NICE guidelines for palliative and supportive care,[68] our specialty, at least as far as it practiced in the United Kingdom, has "arrived" and gained its proper footing. However, despite assurances that a long-term framework for funding will be developed,[74] concerns remain that the provision of palliative care can be maintained in its present format.[75] "Agenda for Change," a grading and pay system for all clinical staff in the NHS, is just the latest package of proposals to affect how palliative care is provided. The main providers of palliative care, independent hospices in the charitable sector, are faced with the prospect of losing staff to the NHS if they are unable to meet the new terms and conditions, but of a prohibitive financial bill if they do meet them.[75] The ongoing problem of an aging nursing workforce and continued nursing shortages in the United Kingdom[76] place further pressure on the provision of care, and make it imperative that the specialty is both competitive and attractive to prospective nurses.

At this time, it appears redundant to some to again debate the name of our specialty to embrace "supportive care"[77] and to be concerned about our image. "Patients are not interested in the name of our specialty but in what we do, how compassionate we are, how well we communicate and whether we demonstrate concern for their relatives."[77] However, if we are to continue to matter to patient groups other than cancer patients and to make an impact on the potential purchasers of our care, we will have to be clear about who we are and what we stand for.[78] Although there is continuing debate in the United Kingdom, there is little ambiguity of purpose and plenty of goodwill and resolve to see that palliative care continues to grow and to assume its rightful place, remaining an influential force in nursing.

REFERENCES

1. Clark D. Cicely Saunders—Founder of the Hospice Movement: Selected Letters 1959–1999. Oxford: Oxford University Press, 2002.
2. Clark D. Originating a Movement: Cicely Saunders and the development of St. Christopher's Hospice, 1957–1967. Mortality 1998a;3:43–61.
3. Clark D. An annotated bibliography of the publications of Cicely Saunders—1958–1967. Palliative Med 1998b;12:181–193.
4. Wald FS. Hospice's path to the future. In: Strack S, ed., Death and the Quest for Meaning. Northvale, NJ: Aronson, 1997.
5. Saunders C. Care of the dying. Nursing Times reprint. London: Macmillan, 1976.
6. Henderson VA. The Nature of Nursing. Reflections After 25 Years. New York: National League for Nursing, 1991.
7. Salmon B. Ministry of Health, Scottish Home and Health Department. Report of the Committee on Senior Nursing Staff Structure. London: Her Majesty's Stationery Office, 1996.
8. Clark D, Seymour J. Reflections on Palliative Care. Buckingham: Open University Press, 1999.
9. Clark D. The Future for Palliative Care. Buckingham: Open University Press, 1993.
10. Working Party on Terminal Care [The Wilkes Report]. Report of the Working Party on Terminal Care. London: Department of Health and Social Security, 1980.
11. Lunt B, Hillier R. Terminal care: present services and future priorities. BMJ 1981;283:595–598.
12. Department of Health and Social Security. NHS Management Enquiry [The Griffiths Report] DA (83)38. London: Department of Health and Social Security, 1983.
13. Clark D, Malson H, Small N, Mallett K, Neale P, Heather P. Half-full or half-empty? The impact of health reforms on palliative care services in the United Kingdom. In: Clark D, Hockley J, Ahmedzai S, eds. New Themes in Palliative Care. Buckingham: Open University Press, 1997.
14. Standard Medical Advisory Committee/Standing Nursing and Midwifery Advisory Committee. The Principles and Provision of Palliative Care. London: Her Majesty's Stationery Office, 1992.
15. Clark D, Malson H. Key issues in palliative care needs assessment. Progr Palliative Care 1995;3:53–55.
16. Department of Health. EL(94)14. Contracting for Specialist Palliative Care Services. London: Department of Health, 1994.
17. Expert Advisory Group on Cancer [The Calman-Hine Report]. A Policy Framework for Commissioning Cancer Services: A Report by the Expert Advisory Group on Cancer to the Chief Medical Officers of England and Wales. London: Department of Health and Welsh Office, 1995.
18. Addington-Hall JM. Reaching Out Report of the Joint NCH-SPCS and Scottish Partnership Agency Working Party on Palliative Care for Patients with Non-Malignant Disease. London: National Council for Hospice and Specialist Palliative Care Services, 1997.
19. Department of Health. The NHS Cancer Plan. London: The Stationary Office, 2000.
20. NHS Executive. A policy framework for commissioning cancer services: palliative care services. EL (96) 85. London: Department of Health 1996.
21. Anning P. Have hospices lost their way? Nurs Manage 1998;5:6–7.
22. Biswas B. Medicalization: a nurse's view. In: Clark D, ed. The Future for Palliative Care. Buckingham: Open University Press, 1993.
23. NHS National Institute of Clinical Excellence. Guidance on Cancer Services. Improving Supportive and Palliative Care for Adults with Cancer. London: NICE, 2004. Available at: www.nice.org.uk
24. http://www.hospice-spc-council.org.uk (accessed March 5, 2005).
25. Tebbit P. Raising the Standard, Clinical Governance for Voluntary Hospices. Occasional Paper 18, London: National Council for Hospice and Specialist Palliative Care Services, 2000.
26. The Health Quality Service Standards for Hospice Services, 2nd ed., London: The Health Quality Service, 2004.
27. National Council for Hospice and Specialist Care Services/Department of Health. The Palliative Care Survey 1999. London: NCHSPCS/Department of Health, 2000.
28. Hospice Directory 2004. Hospice and Palliative Care Services in the United Kingdom and Ireland. London: Hospice Information, 2004. Available at: http://www.hospiceinformation.info (accessed March 5, 2005).
29. Salisbury C. What models of palliative care services have been proposed or developed in the UK, Europe, North America and Australia? In: Clark D, Seymour J, eds. Reflections on Palliative Care. Buckingham: Open University Press, 1999.
30. Johnson IS, Rogers C. Biswas C, Ahmedazi S. What do hospices do? A survey of hospices in the United Kingdom and Republic of Ireland. Br Med J 1990;306:791–793.

30a. Ellershaw J, Wilkinson S. Care of the Dying. A Pathway to Excellence. Oxford: Oxford University Press, 2003.

31. Eve A. National Survey of Patient Activity Data for Specialist Palliative Care Services (The Minimum Data Set). London: National Council for Hospice and Specialist Care Services, 2004.
32. Skilbeck J. Seymour J. Meeting complex needs: an analysis of Macmillan nurses' work with patients. Int J Pall Nurs 2002;8:574–582.
33. Thomas K. Caring for the Dying at Home. Oxford: Radcliffe Medical Press, 2003.
34. Boulstridge J, Meystre C. What do patients need to die at home? Is hospice at home the answer? Palliative Med 2001;15:543.
35. Fisher R, McDaid P. eds. Palliative Day Care. London: Arnold, 1996.
36. Hearn J, Myers K, eds. Palliative Day Care in Practice. Oxford: Oxford University Press, 2001.

37. Higginson I, Goodwin DM. Needs assessment in day care. In Hearn J, Myers K., eds. Palliative day care in practice. Oxford: Oxford University Press, 2001.
38. Office for National Statistics. Mortality Statistics. London: The Stationary Office, 2000.
39. Jack B, Oldham J, Williams A. A stakeholder evaluation of the impact of the palliative care clinical nurse specialist upon doctors and nurses within an acute hospital setting. Palliative Med 2003;17:283–288.
40. Jack B, Hillier V, Williams A, Oldham J. Hospital-based palliative care teams improve the symptoms of cancer patients. Palliative Med 2003;7:498–502.
41. Jack B, Hillier V, Williams A, Oldham J. Hospital-based palliative care teams improve the insight of cancer patients into their disease. Palliative Med 2004;18:46–52.
42. Addington-Hall J, Altmann D, McCarthy M. Which terminally ill cancer patients receive hospice in-patient care? Soc Sci Med 1998;46:1011–1016.
43. Ingleton C, Payne S, Nolan M, Carey I. Respite in palliative care: a review and discussion of the literature. Palliative Med 2003; 17:567–575.
44. Saunders C, Baines M. Living with Dying: The Management of Terminal Disease. Oxford: Oxford University Press, 1983.
45. Raeside D, Ellershaw J. What does respite care offer to cancer patients admitted to hospice? Palliative Med 1994;8:68.
46. Copp G, Richardson A, McDaid P, Marshall-Dearson DA. A telephone survey of the provision of palliative day care services. Palliative Med 1998;12:161–170.
47. Kirk S. Patient preferences for a single or shared room in a hospice. Nurs Times 2002;98:39–41.
48. Independent Health Care, National Minimum Standards. Care Standards Act. London: Department of Health, 2001.
49. National Council for Hospice and Specialist Palliative Care Services. Opening Doors: Improving Access to Hospice and Specialist Palliative Care Services by Members of the Black and Ethnic Minority Communities, Occasional Paper No. 7, London: NCHSPCS, 1995a.
50. Fountain A. Ethnic minorities and palliative care in Derby. Palliative Med 1999;13:161–162.
51. Sheldon F. Will the doors open? Multicultural issues in palliative care. Palliative Med 1995;9:9–90.
52. Randhawa G, Owens A. Palliative care for minority ethnic groups. Eur J Palliative Care 2004;11:19–22.
53. Oliviere D. Culture and ethnicity. Eur J Palliative Care 1999: 53–56.
54. Eve A, Smith AM, Tebbit P. Hospice and palliative care in the UK 1994–95, including a summary of trends 1990–95. Palliative Med 1997;11:31–43.
55. Fallon M. Palliative medicine in non-malignant disease. In: Doyle D, Hanks G, Cherny N, Calman K, eds. Oxford Textbook of Palliative Medicine, 3rd ed. London: Oxford University Press, 2004:843–847.
56. Addington-Hall J, Fakhoury W, McCarthy M. Specialist palliative care in non-malignant disease. Palliative Med 1996;12: 417–427.
57. British Medical Association, Resuscitation Council (UK), Royal College of Nursing. Decisions relating to cardiopulmonary resuscitation: a joint statement from the British Medical Association, Resuscitation Council (UK), Royal College of Nursing. J Med Ethics 2001;27:312–318.
58. Thorns A, Gannon C. The potential role for automatic external defibrillators in palliative care units. Palliative Med 2003;17: 465–467.
59. Thorns A, Ellershaw JE. A survey of nursing and medical staffs views on the use of cardiopulmonary resuscitation in the hospice. Palliative Med 1999;13:225–232.
60. National Council for Hospice and Specialist Palliative Care Services. Ethical Decision Making in Palliative Care: Cardiopulmonary Resuscitation(CPR) for People Who Are Terminally Ill. London: NCHSPCS, 1997.
61. Carey I, Forbes K. The experiences of donor families in the hospice. Palliative Med 2003;17:241–247.
62. Feuer D. Organ donation in palliative care. Eur J Palliative Care 1998;5:21–25.
63. Richards MA, Corner J, Clark D. Developing a research culture for palliative care. Palliative Med 1998;12:399–403.
64. Addington-Hall J. Research sensitivities to palliative care patients. Eur J Cancer Care 2002;11:220–224.
65. Sentiles-Monkam A, Serryn D. Conducting research in the palliative care population. Eur J Palliative Care 2004;11:23–26.
66. Field D, Clark D, Corner J, Davis C. Researching Palliative Care. Buckingham: Open University Press, 2001.
67. Higginson I. Evidence based palliative care. BJM 1999;319:462–463.
68. NHS National Institute of Clinical Excellence. Guidance on Cancer Services. Improving Supportive and Palliative Care for Adults with Cancer. London: NICE, 2004:171.
69. Oliviere D. A voice for the voiceless. Eur J Palliative Care 2000;7:102–105.
70. Oliviere D. User involvement in palliative care services. Eur J Palliative Care 2001;8:238–241.
71. Small N, Rhodes P. Too Ill to Talk: User Involvement in Palliative Care. London: Routledge, 2000.
72. Bradburn J. In: Monroe B, Oliviere D. Patient Participation in Palliative Care. Oxford: Oxford University Press, 2003.
73. Kraus F, Levy J, Oliviere D. Brief report on user involvement at St Christopher's Hospice. Palliative Med 2003;17:375–377.
74. Richards MA. Priorities on supportive and palliative care in England. Palliative Med 2003;17: 7–8.
75. Kirk S. Agenda for change: implications for the voluntary sector. Nursing Manage 2004;11:16–18.
76. Royal College of Nursing. More Nurses, Working Differently? London: RCN Publications, 2003.
77. Doyle D. Editorial. Palliative Med 2003;17:9–10.
78. Nauck F, Jaspers B. Is palliative care synonymous with end-of-life care? Eur J Palliative Care 2003;10:223.

PALLIATIVE CARE IN EUROPE

Marianne Jensen Hjermstad and Stein Kaasa

Palliative care begins from the understanding that every patient has his or her own story, relationship, and culture and is worthy of respect as an individual. This implies that palliative care should be patient-oriented, guided by the needs of the patient, taking into account his or her values and preferences, and that ethical issues are considered with cultural variation in needs and values.

In 2002, the World Health Organization (WHO) definition stated that palliative care is "an approach that improves the quality of life of patients and their families facing the problems associated with life-threatening illness, through the prevention and relief of suffering by means of early identification and impeccable assessment and treatment of pain and other problems, physical, psychosocial and spiritual."[1] These aspects are specifically emphasized in the recently released document on palliative care from the Council of Europe, Committee of Ministers: "Recommendation REC (2003) 24 of the Committee of Ministers to Member States on the Organization of Palliative Care."[2]

Palliative care should be offered at all levels in the health care system and could be regarded as an integral part of all medical services. However, based on the above, it becomes evident that palliative care has its own special characteristics that are not entirely covered by the mainstream health care system. Thus, the emergence of palliative care as a medical specialty is rapidly progressing, and palliative medicine has already been acknowledged in some countries as a specialty.

In the Nordic countries, a 2-year training program for a specialist program was started in 2003—with too many applicants. The course is composed of six 1-week slots of teaching, with working assignment in the intervals. All participants conduct a small research project and write a paper for publication, preferably for an international journal.

The scientific advances in cancer therapy have not lead to a dramatic reduction in cancer incidence. The mortality rates have remained relatively stable or slightly decreased in the western world.[3] Because palliative care goes far beyond opioid availability and pain treatment and encompasses all the key elements of the holistic nursing approach—the care needs, the suffering, and the dignity and the quality of life of patients and relatives towards the last stages of life—it seems inappropriate to draw artificial lines between disease-modifying therapy and palliative care. This becomes even more evident when we know that most cancer patients are not cured from their disease, and that palliative care should, in fact, be offered early in the stage of disease to provide the essential part of this care to all patients. Thus, the development and improvement of palliative care is an important, growing, and large public health issue across nations and cultures.

The purpose of this chapter is to present some of the European experiences with respect to the organization and delivery of palliative care, educational issues, and research.

The Situation in Europe

Due to increasing life expectancy and declining birth rates, the age distribution in many European nations is skewed toward a larger proportion of older people. Because the overall cancer incidence rises with advanced age, more people with cancer are expected in the near future. Predictions for causes of death in Europe for the next 15 years also show a changing pattern (Table 66–5), with more people living with and dying from chronic diseases.

Although different diseases present with various symptoms along the illness trajectory, epidemiological studies show that many symptoms and problems in the last year of life are similar.[4] This represents a challenge to the health care systems in the delivery of effective and adequate end-of-life care to an increasing number of people.

Europe has gone through great political changes in the last decade, economically and culturally. In spring 2004, 10 new countries became members of the European Union (EU). How to best develop palliative care across Europe is still a challenge due to the great diversity of economic, cultural, and health policy aspects, as well as the significant differences in population size, from 4.5 million in Norway to 82 million in Germany. Nevertheless, the gradually increasing medical and scientific collaboration across borders has led to the development of various models for palliative care. Some European centers are influenced by the Canadian model in Edmonton,[5] the Beth Israel Medical Center program in New York City,[6] or by the WHO project on palliative care implementation that influenced the development of palliative medicine throughout Spain.[7–9] However, directly adopting a model from another nation with a different health care system is not always feasible. An example of this is the integration of the departments of pain service and palliative medicine into one, as has been successfully done at Beth Israel in New York. The pain programs in Europe are very closely linked to anesthesiology, and, as such, not only are caring for palliative care patients but also taking care of patients with postoperative pain, chronic nonmalignant pain, chronic back pain, etc. Although pain treatment is an essential part of palliative care, the linkage between departments in Europe is more often based on cooperation and consultation services and, to some extent, translational research. Several services in Europe have begun either from pain/anesthesiology and/or oncology teams. It seems that the

Table 66–5
Predicted Causes of Death in Europe for 2020 Compared with 1990 Data

Disorder	Predicted Ranking 2020	Previous Ranking 1990
Ischemic heart disease	1	1
Cerebrovascular disease (including stroke)	2	2
Chronic obstructive pulmonary disease	3	6
Lower respiratory infections	4	3
Lung, trachea, and bronchial cancer	5	10

Source: Adapted from Murray and Lopez (1997), reference 38.

most successful programs have been able to combine the skills and knowledge across specialties.

A survey of all European countries was undertaken in 2003 to provide an overview of the national palliative care activities with respect to implementation of palliative programs, finances and funding, delivery of care through palliative care units/hospices/home care, education, specialist training, and research.[10] There has been a gradual growth in this medical field during the last 3 decades, with significant innovations in the last 10 years. The first national palliative care units (PCU) were opened in Great Britain in 1967, in Cyprus in 1974, and in Norway in 1993. Germany, France, Poland, and Finland followed before 1999; after this Romania, the Netherlands, Belgium, Hungary, Portugal, Austria, Switzerland, Slovakia, Denmark, and Luxembourg all established their units before the change of the millennium. However, the survey revealed major international as well as intranational variations with respect to most of the issues that were evaluated.

To place palliative care on the health policy agenda, strategic interventions based on evidence-based knowledge and consensus among international experts in the field are mandatory to gain the necessary influence. This can be achieved through the establishment of professional organizations, such as the European Association for Palliative Care (EAPC). The EAPC was established in 1988 with 42 members, on the initiative of Professor Ventafridda and the Floriani Foundation in Italy. The aim of the EAPC is to promote palliative care in Europe at the scientific, clinical, and social levels. In 1998, the EAPC was awarded the status of Non-Governmental Organization of the Council of Europe. The EAPC has participated in two Expressions of Interest presented to the European community for the EU 6th and 7th Framework Research Programs. As a result of this work, the issue "Innovative Research on Palliative Care in Advanced Cancer Patients" is included in the thematic priority area number 1, and as such put on the agenda for advanced research. These are great opportunities to come forward with priority topics for research.

Criteria for Excellence

There is currently no universal European consensus regarding indicators for a center of excellence in palliative care. The national models for delivery of palliative care are not identical, and they are not prioritized uniformly in each country. Because of the relatively large economic, political, and cultural diversities, for example, between the former eastern states and the rest of Europe, between the southern and northern parts of Europe, as well as within nations such as Italy, it might not be feasible to aim for the implementation of one particular model of excellence everywhere. On the other hand, there are certain criteria that should be included in all models of palliative care to ensure the sufficient comprehensive provision and quality of care. These criteria include:

Delivery and content of care:

- Inpatient professional palliative care services in PCUs or hospices
- Outpatient palliative care services or home care, organized by the PCU or through the established health care services
- Size of the unit and patient case mix
- Multidisciplinary approach
- Consultation services

Figure 66–4. The integrated palliative care model in Trondheim, Norway.

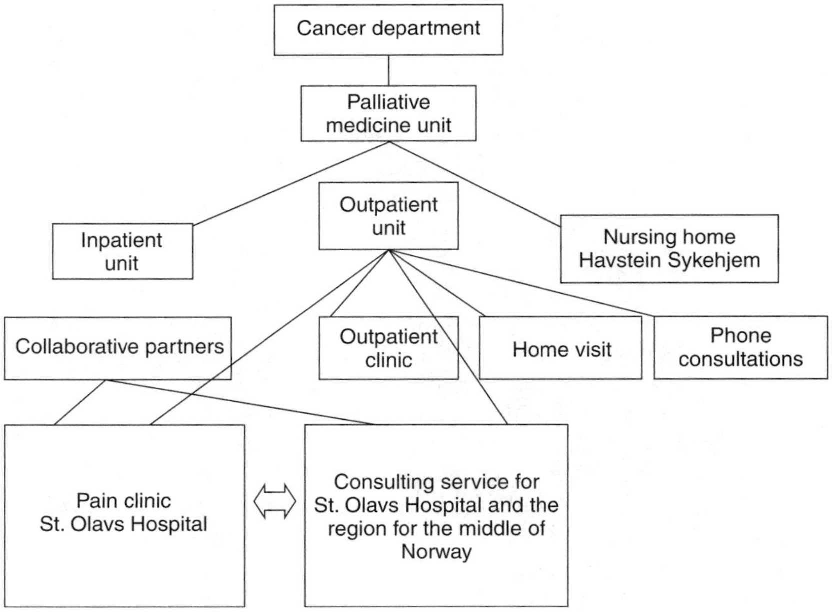

Education and advanced training:
- Basic levels, medical/nursing schools
- Continuing medical/nursing education
- Palliative medicine specialists, palliative care nurse specialists
- University chairs of palliative medicine

Research:
- Continuous evaluation of the quality of palliative care services (structure, process, delivery)
- Evidence-based knowledge to provide guidelines for treatment
- National and international multicenter studies
- Translational research to close the gap between basic sciences and clinical practice
- National and international networking

Integration of palliative medicine and care in public health care:
- Policy, advocacy, lobbying

At the University Hospital in Trondheim, a fully integrated model has been developed during the last decade (Figure 66–4). The program started with the development of a 12-bed inpatient unit (acute palliative care) and an outpatient program, including a consultation service at the various wards and departments at the University Hospital. The staff is interdisciplinary—with highly trained nurses and doctors. A close collaboration with the city of Trondheim (a 12-bed nursing home unit at Havstein) has been established as an integrated unit of the palliative care program, combined with specialist palliative care service in patients' homes in collaboration with the general practitioner's (GP) and home care nursing program in the community. The pain clinic and the palliative medicine unit are increasing their clinical, educational, and research collaborations.

EAPC Activities: An Example of International Networking

The EAPC serves as a catalyst for this work, through the steadily growing number of activities and task forces (Figure 66–5). The delivery aspects are addressed by the EAPC Task Force on Palliative Care Standards and the EAPC Task Force on Palliative Care Development in Europe. These task forces are established through initiative from the EAPC members and recommended by the board of EAPC. These working partners are time limited, with an expectation to deliver a program that can be followed up by the member states. The aim of the first one (Palliative Care Standards) is to identify the needs for some form of European standard and to create a checklist for others to follow. The second task force aims to achieve an overall vision of the care activity and development of the different palliative care teams in Europe. A new task force that was established in 2002, EAPC Task Force on Palliative Care for Children facilitates and supports the work of pediatric palliative medicine and provides a link between palliative care for adults and children.

Education and research are imperative for palliative care to become acknowledged as a medical specialty. The EAPC task forces on nursing and medical education are in the process of developing recommendations for the curricula on basic educational levels, as well as at the advanced and specialty levels.[11]

The EAPC research network was founded in 1996, based on the fact that research is a key issue for palliative care, a collaborative effort that has resulted in several scientific publications, international studies, and the organization of three research congresses—in Berlin in 2000, in Lyon in 2002, and in Stresa in 2004.

The major aims of the EAPC East project, which was established in 2001, are to support and to improve the development of palliative care and to coordinate the activities and initiatives in Eastern Europe. In most of these countries, the care is unevenly distributed and poorly developed, and drugs such as opioids are not readily accessible everywhere. In Romania, for example, a GP must write and request the drug from an oncologist, who, in turn, has to send a letter of recommendation for approval to the health authorities. An approval is valid for 3 months, but the prescription from the GP is only valid for 10 days. The drug is not in stock in all pharmacies, and if the medication needs to be changed, the entire procedure must be repeated.[12] By building a network of people and organizations interested in and working with palliative care in Eastern Europe, palliative care is put on the health policy agenda,

Figure 66–5. Overview of EAPC activities and task forces.

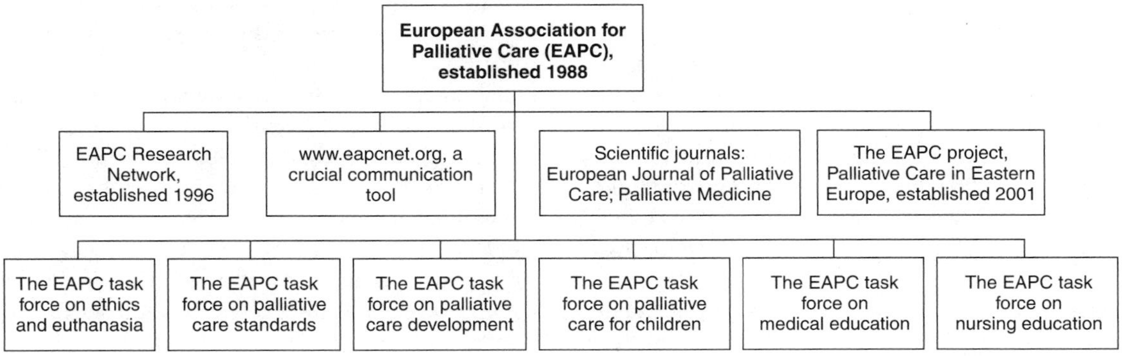

a prerequisite for funding and change of practice. The development of educational, training, and twinning projects between EAPC member institutions and Eastern European health care professionals constitutes a major part of this work, as well as the identification of national and international donors for hospice and palliative care development.

A current example is the joint European project to disseminate the recommendations from the European Council[2] for widespread use by professionals, health care administrators, politicians, and the public. The peak in this work WAS in the fall of 2004, by media campaigns, seminars, and discussions of the Council of Europe documents[2] and the recommendations from EAPC and national organizations. The work is organized through the EAPC-East office in Stockholm in collaboration with local palliative care organizations that will translate, print, and distribute the recommendations—an important tool for information and lobbying. The relevance of this work in relation to the Romanian drug example above is highlighted by the statement in the EC recommendation: "legislation should make opioids and other drugs accessible in a range of formulations and dosages for medical use."[2] The following countries are included in the project: Albania, Armenia, Azerbajdzjan, Belarus, Bosnia-Herzegovina, Bulgaria, Croatia, Czech Republic, Estonia, Georgia, Hungary, Latvia, Lithuania, Macedonia, Poland, Romania, Russia, Slovakia, Slovenia, Ukraine, and Yugoslavia.

Ethical issues are central in palliative care; the EAPC task force on Ethics and Euthanasia completed its work in 2003. The principle aim of this task force was to revise the EAPC's statement and judgment of palliative care and euthanasia. These issues created much debate; the original paper with comments[13] is found on the website: http://www.eapcnet.org/projects/ethics.asp. The guidelines have been translated into French, Italian, Hungarian, German, and Greek, with other languages in the pipeline. The EU-funded research project PALLIUM is also concerned with the elucidation of ethical principles within European palliative care services and has finalized specific country reports from a survey undertaken in 1999.[14]

Delivery of Palliative Care

Models

As pointed out earlier in this chapter, the organization and delivery of palliative care in Europe is unevenly distributed. A recent survey showed that there were no PCU beds in 35 of 53 administrative districts in one German region, while five districts had from 31 to 45 PCU beds per 1 million inhabitants.[10] The Spanish region of Catalonia has about 46% of the nation's palliative care programs but only 15% of the entire Spanish population.[15]

Palliative care is delivered through various channels, and the degree to which it is integrated, coexisting, or separated from the formal health care system varies considerably. In many countries, health professionals, as well as volunteers, private, charitable, and religious organizations, in primary care and through general hospitals carry out much palliative care. In Spain, for example, private organizations are providing home-based palliative care to a substantial number of people, and likewise through volunteers in countries such as Hungary, Italy, and France, while there is little tradition for volunteer work as a separate work force in the Nordic countries. However, with the increasing knowledge and recognition of the complexity in the symptomatology of incurable diseases, a common model of providing care in Europe has been to concentrate expertise in multiprofessional teams, who work in hospitals, inpatient units, hospices, or in the community in direct patient care or as consultants. To fully integrate palliative care into the general health care system, political guidelines from the health care authorities are prerequisites. In 2001, the Italian National Health Service passed a law saying that palliative care programs should be provided for free to patients and families, building on a previous law on hospice development that was followed by a budget allocation to the regional administrations. Several other European countries such as the United Kingdom, France, Norway, and Spain also have health policy directives on palliative care implementations.

An all-inclusive and comprehensive overview of all European centers is not possible to present. Because the statistical and reporting guidelines vary too much, it is difficult to obtain sufficient documentation to perform valid comparisons across countries at the same time, and the field is rapidly developing—maybe a quality criteria in itself! Table 66–6 presents the activities of 11 centers in Europe according to the previously mentioned criteria.

Comprehensive Care

Most studies on delivery of care uncover the importance that patients and families place on receiving a well-organized package of care.[16] Quite often these professional teams take care of the most advanced patients, with complex symptomatology and rapidly changing needs. Despite this, there is evidence that such specialized teams are effective in relieving distressing symptoms and can improve the quality of life of the patients and families towards the end of life.[16,17] Research-based knowledge from studies concerning patient preferences in relation to end-of-life care shows that up to 75% of respondents would prefer to die at home.[18] Scandinavian trials on different ways of coordinating palliative care services across the different settings of hospital, home, and community have found that a higher proportion of people can be helped to remain and to die at home as they wish to, and to spend less time in nursing homes.[19]

Most European palliative care centers have a limited number of inpatient beds, ranging from 4 to 40, as shown in Table 66–6. This is in line with the numbers in Figure 66–6, demonstrating an insufficient coverage of PCU and hospice beds on national levels in some European countries in 2003, ranging from 20 to 50 per one million inhabitants.

Table 66–6
Overview of Some European Palliative Care (PC) Centers

Country	Name	Palliative Care Unit (PCU), Size, Team Composition*	Outpatient Unit	Home Care†	Patients	Education/Training Consultation Services	Research	Specific Activities
Denmark, Copenhagen	Bispebjerg Hospital	Acute PCU, 12 beds Multidisciplinary team: doctors, nurses, social worker, physical and occupational thera-pists, psychologist, dietitians, chaplains	Yes	Yes	All cancer patients	Collaborating with the medical and nursing schools and the university Postgraduate/specialist training for nurses and doctors Consultants in other units and home care	Clinical intervention research and psycho-social research Multidisciplinary, PhD students	Continuous quality monitoring
France, Lyon	Centre de Soins Palliatif, Hospices Civils de Lyon	Acute PCU, 12 beds Multidisciplinary team: doctors, nurses, psychologist	Yes, pain clinic	In progress with another organization	99% cancer patients	Collaborating with the medical and nursing schools and the university Postgraduate training for nurses, hospital doctors and general practitioners	Clinical research on pain assessment, phase 2 and phase 4 pain studies, PhD students	Active in consensus meetings of the national palliative care development
Germany, Aachen	Department of Palliative Medicine, University Hospital of Aachen	Acute PCU, 8 beds Multidisciplinary team: doctors, nurses, psychologist, physical therapist, social worker, chaplain from hospital	Yes	PC team serves as consultants in close collaboration with home care	99% cancer patients	Collaborating with the medical and nursing schools and universities Undergraduate education with lectures and seminars, postgraduate 40-hr course, advanced PC course Involved in development of PC curriculum in Germany Consultation services for other units and home care, other professionals	Clinical drug trials, epidemiological studies, qualitative research, case reports, research on outcome and quality assurance Multidisciplinary	Political activities to advance PC, through media to inform patients, relatives, and medical staff
Hungary, Budapest	Budapest Hospice House	Acute PCU (Sept. 2004), 10 beds Multi-disciplinary team: doctors, nurses, physical therapist, social worker, psychologist, psychiatrist, bereavement counsellor	Yes, pain clinic and psycho-oncology and bereavement services	Yes	Primarily cancer patients	Continuous PC training of staff, and several courses for other professionals and the public Accredited 1-week training for nurses Organizing international courses with other former eastern European states	New psycho-oncology research program (2003), focusing on anxiety/ depression and distress, first Hungarian protocol on these issues	

(continued)

Table 66–6
Overview of Some European Palliative Care (PC) Centers *(continued)*

Country	Name	Palliative Care Unit (PCU), Size, Team Composition*	Outpatient Unit	Home Care†	Patients	Education/Training Consultation Services	Specific Research	Activities
Italy, Milan	Cure Palliative, Instituto Tumori	Acute PCU, 4 beds; day hospital, 10 beds Multidisciplinary team: doctors, nurses, social worker, physical therapists, volunteers	Yes	Yes	All cancer patients	Responsible for a school of update and education in palliative medicine, regular courses of update for nurses and doctors Pain and PC consulting service for other units	Assessment and treatment strategies for difficult cancer pain: neuropathic, chronic iatrogenic, breakthrough, bone pain, management of end-of-life care Multidisciplinary, PhD students	EAPC coordinating office located here
Netherlands, Amsterdam	VUmc	Acute PCU (Sept. 2004), 4 beds in close collaboration with hospice, 10 beds for terminally ill Multidisciplinary	Yes—multidisciplinary Anaesthesiology/pain clinic and palliative oncology clinic	PC team members serve as consultants in close collaboration with home care	90% cancer patients	Education program for medical students, regular PC pain management courses for physicians/nurses Consultation services and regional courses for professionals	Government-funded research program in PC, public health and extra—mural medicine, symptom management PhD students	Partner in Network Palliative Care Amsterdam Organized a regional helpdesk with PC help team for professionals
Netherlands, Nijmegen	UMC St. Radboud	PCU in department of oncology, 5 beds Multidisciplinary team: doctors and nurses supported by specialist nurses, psychologist	Yes—multidisciplinary through the PC team	PC team members serve as consultants in close collaboration with home care	Majority cancer patients	Continuous PC education/courses for staff Consultation services for other units and home care, other professionals	Symptom management, improvement of PC, ethics Multidisciplinary PhD students	
Netherlands, Rotterdam	Erasmus MC	Acute PCU, 11 beds Multidisciplinary team: doctors (neuro-oncologist, anaesthesiologist), specialist nurses, social worker, home care technology expert, psychiatrist, dietitians, chaplain	Yes	Yes	All cancer patients	Continuous PC education/training for oncologists, nurses, and general practitioners Educational program for nursing home physicians Postgraduate courses for medical students, oncology nurses, others Specific focus on development and implementation of intervention programs	Clinical and epidemiological research: symptom prevalence, development of clinical interventions, end-of-life decision-making, organizational aspects of PC Multidisciplinary, PhD students	Partner in Network Palliative Care Rotterdam Multidisciplinary regional PC team is coordinated for phone consultations

(continued)

Table 66–6
Overview of Some European Palliative Care (PC) Centers *(continued)*

Country	Name	Palliative Care Unit (PCU), Size, Team Composition*	Outpatient Unit	Home Care†	Patients	Education/Training Consultation Services	Research	Specific Activities
Norway, Trondheim	Seksjon lindrende behandling (SLB)	Acute PCU, 12 beds, plus 12 beds in one nursing home Multidisciplinary team: doctors, nurses, social workers, physical therapists, dietitians, chaplains	Yes	Yes	99% cancer patients	Continuous PC education and training for medical students, physicians, and nurses in collaboration with the university Regular internal education, courses, and training on basic/specialist levels Consultants in other units, home care and the nursing homes	Close link to the university, chair in palliative medicine Specific research seminars, high degree of translational research, substantial scientific publications on PC every year Multidisciplinary, several PhD students	
Spain, Barcelona	Institut Català d'Oncologia	Acute PCU, 16 beds Multidisciplinary team: doctors, nurses, social workers, psychologist, psychiatrist, physical therapist	Yes	Yes	All cancer patients	University hospital support team to serve other units Individually based continuous education and training for staff Master of PC located on site, doctors/nurses	Active research department, center based and multicenter studies Multidisciplinary research	CATLAN (Catalan multicentre cooperative group), 1998, design of studies and trials
Sweden, Stockholm	Stockholms Sjukhem (SSH)	Acute PCU, 40 beds (20 × 2) Multidisciplinary team: specialist doctors in oncology, geriatrics, algology, neurology, internal medicine, nurses, social workers, physical therapists occupational, therapists, chaplains	Yes	Yes	The PCU of the SSH has a majority of cancer patients	Continuous PC education and training for medical students, physicians, nurses in collaboration with the university One medical training position Continuous education and courses for staff members, external courses for nursing home staff, physicians in specialist training during specific 1 week courses.	Collaborating with the university, chair in palliative medicine Specific research seminars Substantial scientific publications on PC every year Multidisciplinary research, several PhD students	The Swedish Palliative Network (SPN), a web-based information service developed and based here The EAPC East Coordination Center based here The web-based research tool PANIS, a multicenter data collection system developed and based here

*No differentiation between part time and full time employment
†Defined as PC services provided out of hospital by the PC team

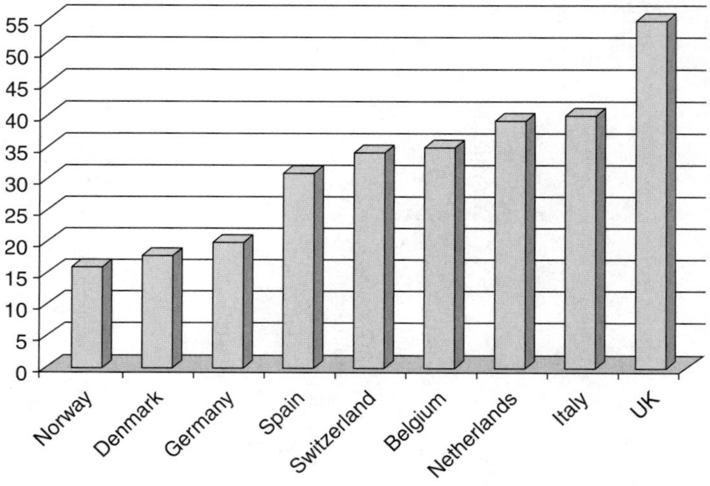

Figure 66–6. PCU and hospice beds per 1 million inhabitants in some European states.

Palliative care models encompass the provision of comprehensive care, and most centers presented in Table 66–6 also have outpatient/day care facilities and home care services. However, there is no universal way of delivering this, because the national health services are organized and reimbursed for this work in different ways. In many PCUs, the hospital palliative care teams provide direct patient care after discharge (see Table 66–6). In certain parts of Spain, private organizations have a car service to take palliative experts from the hospital to the patients' homes. In Norway, as another example, there was no tradition for physicians to leave the hospital to take care of the patients at home. The financial system was prohibitive of such activities, with no reimbursement for extramural activities. Through intense and evidence-based lobbying, however, local politicians were convinced that the hospitals, not the individual physicians, should be reimbursed for this work. Thus, the Trondheim model was implemented in one region, enabling more people to stay in their homes.[19] In the Netherlands, on the other hand, the home care services are generally well functioning, and the hospital palliative care teams basically serve as a facilitator and consultant to ease the transition between the PCU and the home. A Dutch evaluation showed that the team served the needs of the professional caregivers in a variety of settings, and that most consultations concerned physical and pharmacological problems.[20]

Some of the PCUs in Table 66–6 are closely collaborating with nursing homes, for example, in the Netherlands and Norway, as recommended by Norwegian governmental committees.[21] Extending intensive services to sites of more traditional care represents a challenge on the political, personal, organizational, economical, and educational levels. Hospitals and nursing homes often have different budgets, and cost containment might be difficult when expensive drugs, fluids, and transfusions become part of daily care. This also increases the workload for the PCU care teams with respect to direct out-of-hospital patient care, extended consultation services, continuous, and specifically designed educational programs. The increased demand for multidisciplinary teams is directly related to this.

Multidisciplinary Approach and Consultation Services

The increasing complexity of the tasks involved in palliative care makes it obvious that multidisciplinary teams are necessary in the identification and interventions to the rapidly changing needs of patients and families. Professionals in specialist palliative care settings may form relatively permanent teams, as is the case in most of the European centers presented in Table 66–6. Physicians, nurses, physical therapists, and social workers are included in most teams, supplemented by psychologists, psychiatrists, dietitians, bereavement counselors, chaplains, and others. Depending on the context of care, the individual team professionals also may serve as expert consultants for palliative patients in other hospital units, the home care service, and nursing homes. The situation may also be the opposite, with palliative care teams seeking specialist services in disciplines such as neurology, anesthesiology, and pharmacology. Continuity of care across the PCU/hospice/home care interface is more easily achieved through a multidisciplinary team composition, if the responsibilities and strategies for the care plan are agreed upon. Again, the earlier the patients are seen with this holistic interprofessional approach, the more adequately their needs might be met. Another major advantage of the multidisciplinary teamwork is the aspect of bereavement care of staff, in cases with bereavement overload, an area traditionally better managed by professions other than physicians. The increasing numbers of professions involved in palliative care is directly reflected in the membership of palliative care organizations. The German Association for Palliative Medicine was founded by 17 physicians in 1994, while there were 50% physicians and 40% nurses among the 1100 members in 2003.[10] At the EAPC 2004 Research Forum, there were 76% physicians and 11% nurses among the 449 attendants who had reported their profession, in contrast to almost 100% physicians at the first forum in 2000.

Education and Advanced Training

Rapid progress in the growth of professionals interested in palliative care began from 1995/96 and onwards. This is evidenced by the steadily increasing number of members in the EAPC, from around 7000 in 1995 to more than 50,000 in 2002 (Figure 66–7).

However, the link between academics and palliative care has only slowly progressed, by establishing palliative medicine as a formal part of the medical programs at a university level. Academic positions in this field can be found in 10 European countries (Belgium, United Kingdom, Germany, Finland, Greece, Norway, Poland, Sweden, Netherlands, Italy). Teaching in palliative medicine is on the curricula for medical students in Germany, Norway, Sweden, Finland, France, Greece, United Kingdom, Poland, Spain, and Hungary, while formal training as palliative medicine specialists can be found in United Kingdom, Romania, Poland, Germany, Norway, Sweden, Denmark, Iceland, and Finland. Specialized palliative textbooks in indigenous language are available in 12 countries. The situation is basically the same for nursing curricula, with few countries having palliative care as formal parts of the graduate or postgraduate levels or as an accredited specialization.

The recent extension of the EU has led to a more flexible employment market, with less restriction on crossing borders for work. A priority of the EU to facilitate this flexibility is the process towards more universal educational programs. Revising the different medical school curricula and the postgraduate specialist education programs to make them more standardized is an example of this.

Palliative Care Research

Palliative care had its origin in the hospice movement emerging in the United Kingdom in the late 1960s. For quite some time, it was erroneously believed that research had no priority in this context. However, the great advances in the attitudes on cancer pain and the speech by Cicely Saunders in 1965 makes it clear that this ideology was based not "only on compassion but equally on skills preferably founded on scientific evidence."[22,23] Research in the relief of distress to raise the general standard, and the collaboration with other experts in medical science, such as pharmacology, were the means to reach these goals.

The Need for Research

Research is indispensable for the further development and improvement of palliative medicine.[24] However, research is poorly embedded in this culture, partially due to the traditional focus on compassion and partially because research has relatively loose priority in routine clinical activity. The lack of scientific medicine in nursing homes and hospices further adds to this. Nevertheless, there is an increasing demand for documentation on quality and costs of care, through scientifically based evaluation of outcomes. In palliative care, there are many obstacles to the prioritization of research, methodological and clinical, in addition to the more attitudinal and ethical aspects. Based on experience, however, most patients are willing to participate in various topics of palliative care research, including randomized trials on the impact of palliative care services[25,26] and evaluation of pain programs[27] and palliative radiotherapy.[28]

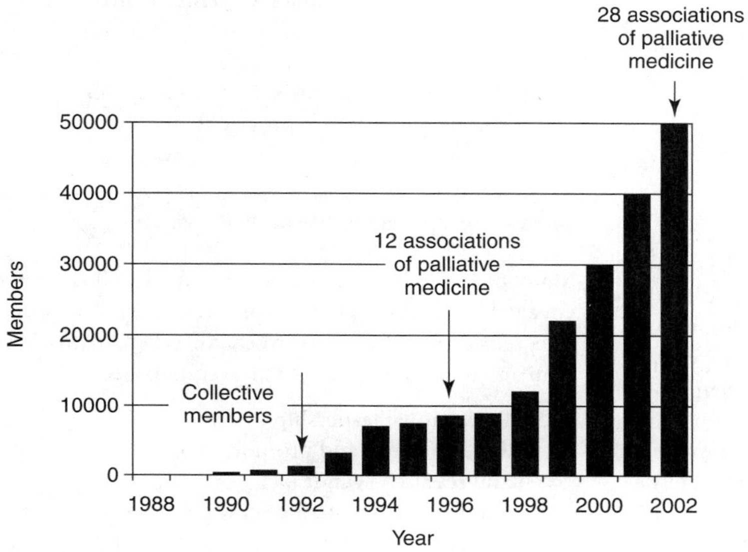

Figure 66–7. EAPC members, 1988 to 2002.

Funding still remains a major obstacle for research. A report in the United Kingdom has identified palliative care as a poorly funded area.[29] Several countries have recently reviewed their national research strategies for cancer research, and, despite the fact that about 50% of cancer patients eventually die from their disease, less than .05% of funding goes to research in palliative care.[30] On the other hand, scientific production increases the chances of receiving money for new projects. Thus, despite the difficulties involved in palliative care research, there is general consensus that the benefits of conducting research outweigh the many clinical and ethical challenges.

Evidence-based Medicine (EBM) and Palliative Care

A definition of EBM states that it is the conscientious, explicit, judged use of the best available evidence in order to offer the patient the most optimal individual care.[31] Thus, retrieving and applying the best available evidence should be an important part for every clinician in the preparation of strategies for diagnostic workup and treatment of patients.[32] As such, there should be no contradictions between the philosophy of palliative care and EBM, although this debate has been going on for decades.

Many of the decisions made in palliative care are based on inferior quality studies, clinical experience, or extrapolation from studies performed in other populations, as is often the case in pain management. Thus, the need for EBM in palliative care seems evident. Treatment of patients with a complex pathophysiology is dependent on research that focuses on the specific patient population and their problems. This includes clinical trials, as well as basic and translational research. Areas that need more in-depth studies are related to cancer and non-cancer pain and symptoms, barriers to accessing care, differences in the social, psychological, cultural and spiritual aspects of palliative care from the point of patients, relatives and caregivers (Table 66–7). One example is related to the fact that most patients in palliative care are elderly. This is in contrast to most studies in mainstream oncology, internal medicine, and even in pain treatment, where the upper age limit often is 70 to 75 years. The validity of extrapolating data from these age groups into older populations is highly questionable, and the need for appropriate research programs in the elderly is warranted.[30]

Table 66–7
Examples of Basic and Clinical Research Topics for Multidisciplinary Research

Areas	Content—Examples
Biomedical—Basic	Pain, cachexia, anorexia, and fatigue
Biomedical—Basic and clinical	Mechanisms of drug actions: variability, adverse effects
Biomedical—Clinical	Controlled clinical trials
	Symptom control/medical interventions
Psychological—Clinical	Classification of anxiety/depression
	Cognitive function
Sociological	Family
	Bereavement
	Satisfaction with care
Health care provision	Quality assurance
Philosophical	Euthanasia/patient-assisted suicide

Research Collaboration

National or international multicenter collaborative studies are prerequisites for obtaining sufficiently large samples. The EAPC research network has established particular collaborations[33,34] both in the area of clinical and basic scientific studies, including the combination of clinical data with pharmacology (phenotyping) and genetic mapping (genotyping).[35] Eleven expert working groups have been working on various topics for which a universal European consensus is warranted. An example of this is the EAPC recommendations on morphine and alternative opioids in cancer pain.[36]

Important information for palliative care providers as well as for policy makers might be gained by exploring already existing data on palliative care. This includes evaluation of different models and the huge variation in costs of care, the spending on palliative care vs. other health care, whether people die in hospices or in home care, and more. This might be facilitated through networks such as the EAPC, through channels for communication and education such as telemedicine for educational and consulting purposes in Norway, or through new national European databases such as the OICP (Italian Observatory of Palliative Care) and PANIS (Palliative Assessment Network in Sweden). The OICP is a website (http://www.oicp.org) with two main contents: a directory of all Italian palliative services and a research center with annual exclusively online surveys on palliative care issues. The PANIS network (http://www.panis.se) conducts semiannual nationwide e-mail surveys on prevalent symptoms, with rapid online feedback to attending physicians.[37]

The European Way to Promote Research

Many of the European centers presented in Table 66–6 were engaged in research activities on various levels. To successfully integrate multidisciplinary research in a palliative care program, certain criteria have to be accomplished:

- Professional leadership
- Agreement on and promotion of a clear strategy and research agenda
- Parallel development of clinic and research
- An infrastructure that ensures interaction with scientists not working in the palliative field

- Translational research
- Multicenter national and international cooperation
- Research programs at all levels: undergraduate, PhD students, postdoctoral, and researchers
- Continuous application for funding at all levels
- Dissemination of results
- Leading journals
- Conferences
- Involvement of the public

The pain and palliation research group in Trondheim, Norway is an example of a multiprofessional group that is active in international collaboration (see Table 66–6). Main areas are ethics, communication, subjective assessment, pain and opioids, and symptom palliation. Several PhD students are pursuing their dissertations in this group, and 54 scientific papers have been published over a 3½-year period. The Instituto Tumori in Milan and the Dutch university hospitals in Table 66–6 are other examples of successful collaboration between research and clinical palliative work.

An ultimate goal should be to ensure that palliative care is represented at all local and national research forums. For Europe as a whole, it is essential to promote the inclusion of palliative care research within the EU framework.

The Challenges

Although palliative care in Europe has undergone a remarkable development from its start in the 1960s to the beginning of a new millennium, there are still several challenges ahead. As we have demonstrated in this chapter, there are still major differences within Europe. During the preparation of this chapter, we inquired as to how palliative care is organized in various countries in Europe. Written responses and oral communication indicated that there is no clear definition on what is meant by a palliative care program or what a hospice is. To describe and compare programs across countries, it seems urgent to agree upon minimum criteria for developing a palliative care program at various levels of the health care system.

Therefore, EAPC is in the progress of establishing a new task force on "Centres of Excellence" in palliative care. The aim is to create a network of European countries at the university hospital level to establish common criteria of success and failure for developing a standard at all levels.

The challenges seem to be universal. These are first and foremost related to the total integration of palliative care in the general health care system both in the inpatient and outpatient sector and, as such, have huge policy implications. This includes education and specialist training at basic and advanced levels through universities and medical associations and a multidisciplinary approach. Furthermore, special national and EU research programs in palliative care are needed to take the next step towards EBM in palliation. Such programs should work toward defining relevant areas to obtain universal guidelines for treatment and delivery of care and to implement EBM. Striving for these goals is by no means in conflict with compassion—both are the cornerstones in the professional encounter with patients.

ACKNOWLEDGMENTS

The following persons have contributed to the writing of this chapter: CJ Furst, Stockholm, Sweden; M Szöllösi, Budapest, Hungary; X Gómez-Batiste, Barcelona, Spain; M Filbet, Lyon, France; M Groenvold, Copenhagen, Denmark; CC van der Reit, Rotterdam, Netherlands; C Galesloot, Nijmegen, WJJ Jansen, Amsterdam; A Rhebergen, Amsterdam, Netherlands; F de Conno, Milan, Italy; L Radbruch, Aachen, Germany.

REFERENCES

1. Davies E, Higginson IJ, eds. Better Palliative Care for Older People. WHO Geneva 2002. Available at: http://www.euro.who.int/document/E82933.pdf (accessed March 5, 2005).
2. Council of Europe website. Available at: http://www.coe.int/T/E/Social_Cohesion/Health/Recommendations/Rec(2003)24.asp# (accessed March 5, 2005).
3. Howe HL, Wingo PA, Thun MJ, Ries LAG, Rosenberg HM, Feigal EG, Edwards BK. Annual report to the nation on the status of cancer (1973 through 1998) featuring cancers with recent increasing trends. J Natl Cancer Inst 2001; 93(11):824–842.
4. Edmonds P, Karlsen S, Khan S, Addington-Hall J. A comparison of the palliative care needs of patients dying from chronic respiratory diseases and lung cancer. Palliat Med 2001;15:287–295.
5. Bruera E, Sweeney C. Palliative care models: international perspective. J Palliative Med 2002;5:319–327.
6. Portenoy R, Heller KS. Developing an integrated Department of Pain and Palliative Medicine. J Palliative Med 2002;5:623–633.
7. Stjernswärd J, Colleau SM, Ventafridda V. The World Health Organization cancer pain and palliative care program. Past, present and future. J Pain Symptom Manage 1996;12:65–72.
8. Gòmez-Batiste X, Fonals M, Roca J, Borràs JM, Stjernswärd J, Rius E. Catalonia WHO demonstration project on palliative care implementation 1990–1995: results in 1995. J Pain Symptom Manage 1996;12:73–78.
9. Gòmez-Batiste X, Porta J, Tuca A, Corrales E, Madrid F et al. Spain: The WHO Demonstration project of palliative care implementation in Catalonia: results at 10 years (1991–2001). J Pain Symptom Manage 2002;24:239–244.
10. Klaschik E. Pan-European overview. Past-present-future. Presentation at the EAPC Research Forum, Stresa, Italy, 2004.
11. European Association for Palliative Care (EAPC) Board of Directors. An overview of the EAPC task forces. EJPC 2004;11: 83–84.
12. Clark D, Wright M. Transitions in end of life care. London: Open University Press, 2003.
13. Materstvedt LJ, Clark D, Ellershaw J, Førde R, Gravgaard A-M, Müller-Busch HC, Porta I, Sales J, Rapin C-H. Euthanasia and physician-assisted suicide: a view from an EAPC Ethics Task Force. Palliative Med 2003;17:97–101.
14. Clark D, ten Have H, Janssens R. Common threads? Palliative care service development in seven European countries. Palliative Med 2000;14:479–490.

15. Centeno C, Hernansanz S, Flores LA, Rubiales AS, Lopez-Lara F. Spain: palliative care programs in Spain, 2000: a national survey. J Pain Symptom Manage 2002;24:245–251.
16. Higginson IJ, Finlay I, Goodwin DM, Cook AM, Hood K, Edwards AG, Douglas HR, Norman CE. Do hospital-based palliative teams improve care for patient and families at the end of life? J Symptom Manage 2002;23:96–106.
17. Higginson IJ, Finlay IG, Goodwin DM, Hood K, Edwards AG, Cook A, Douglas HR, Normand CE. Is there evidence that palliative care teams alter end-of-life experiences of patients and their caregivers? J Pain Symptom Manage 2003;25:150–168.
18. Higginson I, Sen-Gupta GJA. Place of care in advanced cancer: a qualitative systematic literature review of patients preferences. J Palliative Med 2000; 3:287–300.
19. Jordhøy MS, Fayers P, Saltnes T, Ahlner-Elmqvist M, Jannert M, Kaasa S. A palliative care intervention and death at home: a cluster randomised trial. Lancet 2000;356:888–893.
20. Schrijinemaekers V, Courtens A, van den Beuken M, Oyen P. The first 2 years of a palliative care consultation team in the Netherlands. Int J Palliative Nurs 2003;9:252–257.
21. Kaasa S, Breivik H, Jordhoy M. Norway: development of palliative care. J Pain Symptom Manage 2002;24:211–214.
22. Saunders C. Watch with me. Nurs Times 1965; 61:1615–1617.
23. Saunders C. A personal therapeutic journey. BMJ 1996;313: 1599–1601.
24. Kaasa S, Dale O. Pain and Palliative Research Group. Building up research in palliative care: an historical perspective and a case for the future. Clin Geriatr Med 2005;21:81–92.
25. Jordhøy MS, Kaasa S, Fayers P, Ovreness T, Underland G, Ahlner-Elmqvist M. Challenges in palliative care research; recruitment, attrition and compliance: experience from a randomised controlled trial. Palliative Med 1999;13:299–310.
26. Jordhøy MS, Fayers P, Loge JH, Ahlner-Elmqvist M, Kaasa S. Quality of life in palliative cancer care: results from a cluster randomised trial. J Clin Oncol 2001;19:3884–3894.
27. Hanks G, Robbins M, Sharp D, Forbes K, et al. The imPaCT study: a randomised controlled trial to evaluate a hospital palliative care team. BMJ 2002;87:733–739.
28. Sundstrøm S, Bremnes R, Aasebø U, Aamdal S, HatR, Brunsvig P, Johannessen DC, Klepp O, Fayers PM, Kaasa S. The effect of hypofractionated palliative radiotherapy (17Gy/2 fractions) in advanced non-small cell lung carcinoma (NSCLC) is comparable to standard fractionation for symptom control and survival. Results from a national phase II trial. J Clin Oncol 2004;22: 801–810.
29. National Cancer Research Institute. Strategic Analysis 2002. London: National Cancer Research Institute.
30. Davies E, Higginson IJ. Better Palliative Care for Older People. World Health Organization Europe, Copenhagen, Denmark, 2004.
31. Sackett D, Richardson WS, Rosenberg W, Haynes B. Evidence Based Medicine. London: Churchill Livingstone, 1996.
32. McQuay HJ, Moore A, Wiffen P. Research in palliative medicine. The principles of evidence-based medicine. In: Doyle D, Hanks G, Cherny N, Calman K. Oxford Textbook of Palliative Medicine, 3rd ed. Oxford: Oxford University Press, 2003:119–128.
33. Kaasa S, De Conno F. Palliative care research. Eur J Cancer 2001;37(Suppl 8):153–159.
34. Blumhuber H, Kaasa S, De Conno F. The European Association for Palliative Care. J Pain Symptom Manage 2002;24: 124–127.
35. Klepstad P, Cherny N, Hanks G, Radbruch L, De Conno F, Strasser F, et al. Protocol: European Pharmacogenetic Opioid Study, EPOS, 2004.
36. Hanks GW, de Conno F, Cherny N, et al. On behalf of the Research Network of the European Association for Palliative Care. Morphine and alternative opioids in cancer pain: the EAPC recommendation. BMJ 2001;84:587–593.
37. Lundstrom S, Strang P. Establishing and testing a palliative care network in Sweden. Palliative Med 2004;18:139.
38. Murray CJL, Lopez AD. Alternative projections of mortality and disability by cause 1990–2020: global burden of disease study. Lancet 1997;349:1498–1504.

PALLIATIVE CARE IN SITUATIONS OF CONFLICT

Nathan Cherny and Ora Rosengarten

We used to wonder where war lived, what it was that made it so vile. And now we realize that we know where it lives, that it is inside ourselves.

Instead of killing and dying in order to produce the being that we are not, we have to live and let live in order to create what we are.

Those who lack the courage will always find a philosophy to justify it.

—Albert Camus

Situations of political conflict are characterized by enmity and potential for, or actual, violence. Conflict of this ilk may be manifested as outright war, a cycle of terror and reprisals, or a grumbling enmity between religious, national, ethnic, or cultural groups.

Incurable, life-threatening illness is endemic, and it often occurs in places of conflict. In these circumstances, care delivery is often compromised or complicated. Situations of conflict occur in many places in the world and, at any time, a substantial proportion of the world population is involved in conflict of one sort or other. Conflicts, such as war or terror, traumatize the involved populations. Bereavement, fear, anxiety and depression become commonplace. Persistent conflicts may generate feelings of hopelessness and helplessness.

These observations are derived from our experience in working with Palestinian and Israeli patients in a Jewish hospital in Jerusalem over the past several years.

Our Context

Jerusalem is a city that has existed in a situation of conflict over the past 100 years. Historically, this has been the ancient capital of the Jewish people, and currently it is the capital of the modern state of Israel. Jerusalem, however, is also claimed by the Palestinian Arab population as their capital. Indeed, Palestinians and Jews have been in conflict over the destiny of this small strip of land between the Mediterranean and the Jordan river since the inception of the plan to reestablish a Jewish state in the area.

Attempts to achieve some form of rapprochement between the Jewish and Palestinian peoples have been intensified during the past 15 years. The breakdown of negotiations in 2000 was accompanied by a violent Palestinian uprising, characterized by a wave of terror against Israeli citizens, with subsequent restrictions on Palestinian movements and reprisals against terror organizations and their supporters. Thousands of peoples have been killed on both sides.[1,2]

In the midst of this, The Cancer Pain and Palliative Medicine Service, in the department of Oncology at Shaare Zedek Medical Center, has provided palliative care for both Israeli and Jewish patients. Shaare Zedek Medical Center is a Jewish general hospital that serves the entire population of Jerusalem. Reflecting the demographics of the city, 20% of the population are Palestinian Arabs, most of whom are Moslems.

The Cancer Pain and Palliative Medicine service is an integral part of the oncology service, based in the Oncology day hospital. The service consists of two physicians, a palliative care nurse coordinator, an education and research coordinator, three social workers (Hebrew, Arabic, Russian), a chaplain, and a liaison psychiatrist and psychologist. The service provides ambulatory and inpatient care. Community care is provided in cooperation with a number of home hospice services. Although most of the clinicians are Jewish, both the Arabic-speaking social worker and thoracic surgeon (who works very closely with the service) are Palestinian.

Uniting and Dividing Experiences

Peoples on different sides of a political conflict of this ilk share a common traumatized existence.[3] Both sides suffer from risk of violent death or injury; both sides are vexed by injustices wrought by the other. Two peoples with different readings of history and different cultures share a common home, a common homeland, and often common cities, neighborhoods and health care services.[4]

Illness is a unifying experience. The experiences of physical and psychological distress and fear of deterioration or death are universal. Similarly, the desire to care for the ill and to alleviate suffering is fundamentally universal. Indeed, even in the situation of awful conflict, heath care can provide opportunities to bridge between communities and peoples.

Nurses have a special role to play in this situation. Given the greater opportunity for intimate contact and often, greater time for dialogue and compassionate care, their role is critical. This is true both in regards to care delivery and also for the critical role of developing bonds of trust. Communication is critical to the success of this endeavor, and this will often require the use of a translator to ensure that the patient is understood and that nurses understand the care provider.

Barriers to Care in Situations of Conflict

Infrastructural Barriers

Conflicts commonly disrupt the flow of persons (patients and health care providers), the availability of care, and the delivery of health care. Often patients are unable to get to the needed health care, and health care providers may be hampered in their ability to get to their patients. Physical resources may be limited by diversion of resources for other purposes, lack of free movement of goods, or use of limited health care resources by the combatants or victims. In times of war or conflicts, medications, sterile dressings, hospital beds, and health care providers may be in short supply. Often, the cost of medications may be inflated due to the collapse of health insurance arrangements or shortage.

Bias

Both patients and health care providers may be affected by bias against persons on the other side of the conflict barrier. This bias may be generated by resentment, fear, cultural misunderstanding, or demonization. Bias may hinder patients from seeking health care that might involve contact with health care providers or other patients from the other side of the conflict divide. Similarly, bias may influence health care providers in their attitudes or in delivery of care to persons on the other side of the divide. This can be as mild as personal distaste or as severe as overt hostile neglect or sabotage of treatment.

Distrust and Enmity

Neither patients nor heath care providers are protected from the political and social environment. Both parties may carry and project distrust and/or enmity that may be manifest in the caregiver/patient interaction. Distrust and/or enmity can interfere with all aspects of care delivery. Distrust and/or enmity may also affect other relationships: patients sharing the same waiting room or adjacent hospital beds, health care providers from different sides of the conflict, or patient's family members' relationships with the health care providers.

Safety

Death or injury to health care providers is, sadly, common in war and conflict. Beneficently minded health care providers often feel naively protected by the nature of the humanitarian work that they undertake. The enmity of conflict is often such that it is stronger than any compunction about the killing of carers.[5]

Narrative: "I almost killed a patient today"

> Monday night; 11 PM. I almost killed a patient with methadone today. She was (and thankfully still is) a 68-year-old lady who came to see me from Natanya. She has a huge inoperable cancer deep in her abdomen, and even with high doses of morphine, her pain hadn't been adequately relieved.
>
> Under close supervision, I gave her two doses of methadone. Over the next 2 hours, her pain subsided. She was able to get up and walk about. She seemed to have good relief without excessive drowsiness, confusion, or sleepiness.
>
> Methadone is not widely available and, in Jerusalem, there is only one pharmacy that carries it. At 3:15 this afternoon, I wrote out a prescription and sent this lady and her husband to buy the methadone before they headed back to Natanya. To avoid parking problems, they went to the pharmacy by cab.
>
> The pharmacy is in the middle of town . . . on Jaffa road near Zion Square. Half an hour later, I was called to the emergency room. A terrorist had shot some 30 people in the center of town . . . exactly outside the pharmacy. I was quietly panicked. They didn't arrive in our emergency room. I checked with the emergency coordination center. They weren't on any of the emergency room lists. That meant that they were either alive and well or, possibly, dead but unidentified.
>
> It was a very long hour until they returned to the hospital to ask where else they could possibly get the methadone. The shooting had broken out as they approached the area, and their cab driver was diverted.
>
> Few things scare physicians more, and particularly physicians relieving pain with opioids, than almost killing a patient with a medication intended to help. I am an expert in the side effects of methadone, but this would have been a new side effect for me. These are strange and evil times.

Abuse

In some instances, health care resources are abused to facilitate violence. The harboring of combatants or weapons in hospitals or clinics and the ferrying of arms or combatants in ambulances or disguised as doctors, medics, or nurses undermines the assumption of benevolence.[6] To be respected, it is essential that the credibility of the beneficence of health care providers be maintained. Without the assumption of benevolence, ambulances, health care providers, or even patients may be submitted to justifiable suspicion, which may cause delays in genuine care delivery due to security concerns and suspicion of potentially hostile intentions.[7]

Why Provide Care in Conflict?

The ancient Rabbi Hillel stated succinctly, "If I don't look after my interests, then who will; but, if I look after my interests only, then what am I?"

Medicine is a fusion of humanity, science, and compassion. Humanity and compassion dictate that the suffering of illness must be addressed, and, when possible, relieved. This holds true for all who suffer, be they friends or foes. One need not love a foe, but their suffering can be acknowledged and should be relieved when possible. Through this process, new opportunities for understanding and for mitigating enmity can be developed.

Depersonalization and dehumanization of the enemy are common processes in conflict. Often members of the "enemy" are demonized such that they are perceived as fundamentally hostile, evil, or unworthy. These processes of depersonalization, dehumanization, and demonization are reinforced by lack of intimate contact between peoples. Perceived or real issues of fear, risk of harm, distrust, and enmity limit social contacts. All of these processes make the possibility of cooperation or conflict resolution more difficult.

Medicine has the potential to be a positive agent of change. Provision of care across lines of enmity creates the potential to reverse some of these processes. Given that suffering at the end of life is universal, there is a special opportunity for palliative care clinicians working in regions of conflict. While end-of-life care is so often ignored or neglected, palliative care emphasizes humanity and respect for human dignity in a very special way. This focus on humanity stands in stark conflict to the disregard for the value of human life that is so much part of war and terror. Through the delivery of care, there is a potential to break barriers of suspicion and hatred and to reverse the processes of depersonalization, dehumanization, and demonization.[8]

CASE STUDY

Mr. A, Husband of a Patient with Metastatic Colon Cancer

> Mr. A was a 40-year-old husband of a young Palestinian woman with metastatic colon cancer. Together they had four children and lived in East Jerusalem. In September 2000, Mr. A had been at the site of a violent clash between Palestinian protesters and the Israeli armed services. The young man who stood beside him was shot and killed, and he carried the body away from the battle scene.
>
> When Mr. A initially came with his wife to an Israeli hospital, he was full of anger at Israelis and Jews, and he had little reservation about hiding his hostility. The treating oncologist was an orthodox Jewish Israeli, Dr. S. They communicated with the help of a Palestinian social worker.
>
> For 2 years, Dr. S cared for this young family. Mrs. A underwent several lines of chemotherapy; some successful, others less so. When she developed a bowel obstruction, Dr. S arranged for a diverting colostomy and supported the family through the ordeal. The treating nurses would hold her

hands, stroke her hair, and extended the same care and support that they would to any other patient.

Slowly, enmity faded and Mr. A, his wife, and family became part of the routine in the oncology day hospital. As her illness progressed, she became increasingly dependent on help from the palliative care nurse. Because the family lived in an area that had became increasingly unsafe for Israelis, and in the absence of a Palestinian home care program, we had to make do with telephone support and hospital-based ambulatory care.

Mrs. A ultimately developed a severe pain problem with lumbosacral plexopathy. She was admitted for pain stabilization. She did not achieve adequate relief with PCA morphine, and she was switched to methadone, which provided reasonable relief. It became clear, however, that she would not be able to return home, and she died in the oncology/palliative care ward, surrounded by her family and friends and her mainly Israeli doctors and nurses.

A week after her death, her husband returned with his four children with gifts and thanks for the staff. To Dr. S he said, "You are now my brother."

Facilitating Care Delivery Across Lines of Enmity

Advertise Availability

Unless it is known that care is available irrespective of conflict, many potential patients may not seek help. Advertisement can be in the form of letters to doctors, commercial advertisements, or via the print or video media.[9]

Demilitarize Hospitals and Clinics

It is absolutely unacceptable for hospitals to be militarized by any party in the conflict. Hospitals must be respected neutral territory. When this principle is not adhered to, those in need of help may be too afraid to seek care. The abuse of hospitals either as bases for attack or as asylum for health combatants undermines impartiality and potentially invites incursion or conflict.

Ensure Care Regardless of Ability to Pay

Health care provision costs money, and, unless supported by charity, costs must be covered to ensure ongoing ability to provide care. Emergency care should be available to all who present need, irrespective of ability to pay. For patients without insurance or financial resources, providing ongoing care can present logistic challenges. Several options are possible: provision of care at cost, arranging for care to be provided by health care services across the divide of conflict, or providing subsidized or charitable care. Arranging care at lesser expense to the patient across the lines of conflict requires the development and maintenance of lines of communications with health care practitioners on the other side of the conflict. In our experience, even in the setting of political animosity and differences, this sort of humanitarian cooperation has been possible and positive.

Ensure Physical Access

Patients, their caregivers, and family members may need specific permits to enable them to reach health care facilities across lines of enmity. Members of the health care team are often able to liaise directly with the civic or military authorities to facilitate the granting of permits. In doing so, there is an element of responsibility insofar as that the clinicians need to be adequately convinced that these permits will not be abused to ferry either arms or combatants. Since the authorities at checkpoints may sometimes be hostile to the patients or their families, it is helpful to provide patients with written testimony to the fact that they are seeking health care, with a specific contact name and telephone number for verification purposes.

Provide for Cost Containment

To protect the interests of the patient and the health care provider, the clinician has a duty of care to try to contain costs of care provision as far as possible. This concern reflects itself in clinical decision-making in regard to both diagnostic investigations and therapeutics. One needs to be aware of the cost of medications and the most effective formulations to provide ongoing care. Commonly available formulations of controlled-release opioids may be prohibitively expensive, and cheaper options, such as immediate-release morphine or methadone, may be preferred.

Use Liaison Where Possible to Ensure Safety

Often patients can get adequate care without enduring all of the logistic barriers involved in crossing lines of enmity. It is often useful to liaise with physicians across the lines of enmity to evaluate the availability of care and the limits of care resources. In suggesting to a patient that they not cross lines of enmity and that they seek care locally, one must first be sure that there is a real possibility of receiving adequate care. In so doing, it is appropriate to invite open lines of communication to address any medical issues that may arise.

CASE STUDY

Mrs. FW, a Patient with Metastatic Breast Cancer

Mrs. FW, a 60-year-old Palestinian woman from a small village just outside Jerusalem, presented to an Israeli hospital with metastatic breast cancer with liver and bone metastases. She received palliative antitumor therapies in two Israeli hospitals. She was regularly reviewed in the day hospital by the palliative care service, which managed her pain with transdermal fentanyl and oral morphine.

Her condition deteriorated just as the conflict in Jerusalem worsened. Because of excessive personal risk, home hospice services were unable to attend her. The danger was understood by the patient and her family, who not only accepted this with sorry resolve, but who actively discouraged staff from placing themselves at risk.

Contact was made with a local doctor and nurse, and with the support and instruction of the palliative care service, they undertook a program of home care. When she was unable to take oral medication, a PCA pump was provided and serviced by the local medical team, with daily telephone support from the palliative care service. This arrangement was successfully maintained until the patient's death at home.

Create a Bank of Returned Medications

Returned and unused medications are usually discarded or destroyed. When there are potential patients who do not have the resources to pay for medication, this is wasteful and inappropriate. Returned medications should be stored appropriately and may be used in the care of patients who do not have resources to pay for them. In our setting, we have successfully done this with cytotoxics, analgesics and antiemetics, and other potentially expensive medications.

Use Creative Improvisation

Often, normal care structures such as home hospice services or day clinics will be unavailable or inaccessible. In such cases, the available care resources need to be evaluated to explore the possibility of some form of improvisation, which may be suboptimal, but at least fills a modicum of care needs. This may involve a compromise on care plan; for example, when a PCA could not be maintained at home because home care staff could not safely visit, we switched the patient to methadone suppositories, which were both cheap and effective. Often, family members or sometimes friends and neighbors will need to be trained to provide for care needs or even to do simple procedures such as tube feeding, suction, and wound care.

International Organizations

Several international organizations have created special infrastructures to assist in the provision of care in situations of conflict. It is very helpful to know and to develop relationships with those services and agencies active locally.

The World Health Organization (WHO)

Sponsored by the United Nations, this international organization has widely accepted and acknowledged credibility that usually crosses all lines of conflict. Indeed, WHO is mandated by its Constitution (article 2) to "furnish appropriate technical assistance and, in emergencies, the necessary aid upon the request or acceptance of Governments." In such situations, national authorities have the prime responsibility to respond to the needs of the affected population, but in protracted conflict situations, the situation can often deteriorate to a degree that undermines the capacity of the local authorities to meet the urgent public health needs. Through WHO's presence in all countries, its regional structure, its technical units and programs at headquarters, its use of the existing health partnerships (such as the well-established polio network), and its system of collaborating centres, WHO is well structured to deliver its technical advisory support to national and local authorities, sister agencies, the donor community, and international nongovernment organizations (NGOs) and local self-help groups.

Médecins Sans Frontières

Also known as Doctors Without Borders (DWB), Médecins Sans Frontières (MSF)[10] is a private, nonprofit organization at the forefront of emergency health care, as well as care for populations suffering from endemic diseases and neglect. Health care professionals working for DWB deliver emergency aid to victims of armed conflict, epidemics, and natural and man-made disasters, and to others who lack health care due to social or geographical isolation. They provide primary health care, perform surgery, rehabilitate hospitals and clinics, run nutrition and sanitation programs, train local medical personnel, and provide mental health care.

Physicians for Human Rights

Physicians for Human Rights[11] is less involved with providing actual care but contributes to health care provision in the work for protecting human rights. When the ability to provide care has been hampered by bias, malice, or draconian rule, they have been helpful as an international advocate. They provide teams of experts to investigate and expose violations of human rights.

International Medical Corps

Similar to DWB, the International Medical Corps (IMC)[12] is a global nonprofit organization dedicated to providing care in places of distress and conflict through health care training and relief and development programs. By offering training and health care to local populations and medical assistance to people at highest risk, and with the flexibility to respond rapidly to emergency situations, IMC rehabilitates devastated health care systems and helps bring them back to self-reliance.

NARRATIVE

Muhammed and Me

Dr. Muhammed Natshe is dying. A father of five, a devout Moslem, a sweet man of peace who has lived almost all of his life through the tumult of Middle East conflict. Tonight, as

I write these words, he lies in a three-bed room in Internal Medicine A at Shaare Zedek Medical Center (an Orthodox Jewish Hospital in West Jerusalem). He is weak and tired. Three of his sons were at his bedside when I bid him farewell tonight. As I left, I saw his eldest son prostrate and barefoot on his prayer mat, face to Mecca, deep in prayer.

Formerly a handsome man, with a strong resemblance to the late King Hussein of Jordan, Dr. Natshe is now withered and prematurely aged. The whites of his eyes are yellow tinged with an early jaundice from his now failing liver. His abdomen is distended with fluid and his legs are bloated by edema. His eyes are bright and his broad loving smile breaks through the misery, sadness, and fear of his current circumstances. Like many Palestinian men, he has smoked most of his adult life. Now the lung cancer that presented 9 months ago has erupted through the brief response to chemotherapy and threatens the function of his vital organs.

Today, I am Muhammed's doctor, his oncologist, and palliative medicine physician. That was not always the case. I first encountered him as a colleague. He was a highly respected general practitioner in East Jerusalem. There, close to the spectacular hubbub of the Damascus Gate of the Old City of Jerusalem, he tended to a large practice. Patients he referred were among the first Palestinians whom I treated when first I arrived in Jerusalem some 7 years ago. He was a caring and involved family doctor. I was impressed and touched by his devotion: be it visiting his patients when they were admitted to our hospital, or caring, alongside the Home Hospice Service, for his patients who were approaching their deaths.

Dr. Natshe was a general practitioner by default. He had initially wanted to be a surgeon and had, indeed, started a surgical residency at Hadassah Hospital in early 1973. Shortly after it began, his residency was interrupted by the surprise attack of the Yom Kippur War. The Jewish world was shocked and outraged at the surprise attack. Most Palestinians supported the Egyptian/Syrian alliance. Dr. Natshe took leave from Hadassah during the war and, in the aftermath, he felt too embarrassed to return to his residency in surgery. After 3 years of general practice, he applied and was accepted back to Hadassah as a radiology resident. The medical world of Israel, the West Bank, and Jordan is small, and word of Dr. Natshe's appointment quickly reached Amman. The Jordanian Medical Association dispatched a strongly worded letter of reprimand, intimating that it would be treasonous to work in an Israeli hospital. Thus, Muhammed returned to his general practice, where he worked until the toll of the lung cancer and the adverse effects of its treatment made it impossible to continue.

Faith and pragmatism: Dr. Natshe's eyes twinkle with enthusiasm as he explains his love of Islam and the word of The Prophet. He is a deeply religious man and, in the encroaching shadow of death, his faith in God's ultimate beneficence underscores his inner strength and courageous coping. His sons are dapper, deferential, and attentive to their frail father. Even in his ill-fitting hospital pajamas, I can see his tired chest rise with pride at the sight of them. He tells me that he insisted that each of them learn a trade before entering tertiary education. He has successfully assured them of short- and long-term economic opportunity. His eldest son, a part-time hairdresser, studies computer engineering at an Israeli Technical School; the second, a part-time truck driver, studies industrial chemistry at the Hebrew University. The boys speak to me in Hebrew and English. He tells them that they will need to look after their mother, as he will soon be gone.

Tomorrow, I plan to discharge Dr. Natshe back to his home in East Jerusalem. After 3 days in the hospital, his pain and vomiting are now controlled. He is very weak. I anticipate that in a week I will need to again drain his abdomen of the reaccumulating fluids that painfully distend his abdomen and compress his viscera. By then, he will probably be too weak to return to the hospital, so I will attend to him at home.

Dr. Muhammed Natshe, Palestinian physician, man of Islam, man of God, father and husband, is my colleague, my patient, and my friend. I will care for him and his family with all of the skill and devotion that I can muster. I have promised him my commitment and my service as long as it is needed. Sadly, that won't be long.

That I am a Jew, that I am Israeli, that our peoples are in conflict in an awful time of violence and hatred are irrelevant to the humanity that binds us. I will miss him when he's gone.

Behind the headlines, behind the shocking and awful images of violence, death, cruelty and humiliation . . . small acts of caring, cooperation, and love play themselves out . . . daily. This is another reality of the Intefada. Gladly, this is part of my reality; my source of hope and strength.

Conclusions

War and conflict are among the major challenges to man's humanity. The provision of palliative care in times and places of conflict is fraught with personal and infrastructural difficulty. In meeting these challenges, medicine and health care providers have the potential to be positive agents of change. The challenges are great but the potential rewards even greater.

REFERENCES

1. Blachar Y. And the doctor shall heal: the Israel-Palestinian conflict. Isr Med Assoc J 2002;4:485–486.
2. Ofran Y, Giryes SS. To be a doctor in Jerusalem: life under threat of terrorism. Ann Intern Med 2004;140:307–308.
3. Shuter J. Emotional problems in Palestinian children living in a war zone. Lancet 2002;360:1098.
4. Minear L, Weiss TG, eds. Humanitarian Action in Times of War—A Handbook for Practitioners. Boulder, CO: Lynne Rienner, 1993.
5. Siegel-Itzkovich J. David Applebaum. BMJ 2003;327:684.

6. Cohn JR, Romirowsky A, Marcus JM. Abuse of health-care workers' neutral status. Lancet 2004;363:1473.
7. Viskin S. Shooting at ambulances in Israel: a cardiologist's viewpoint. Lancet 2003;361:1470–1471.
8. Ashkenazi T, Berman M, Ben Ami S, Fadila A, Aravot D. A bridge between hearts: mutual organ donation by Arabs and Jews in Israel. Transplantation 2004;77:151–155; discussion 156–157.
9. Rees M. Amid the killing, E.R. is an oasis. Time 2003;161:36–38.
10. Doctors Without Borders. Available at: http://www.doctorswithoutborders.org (accessed March 5, 2005).
11. Physicians for Human Rights. Available at: http://www.phrusa.org (accessed March 5, 2005).
12. International Medical Corps. Available at: http://www.imc-la.com (accessed March 5, 2005).

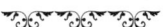

PALLIATIVE CARE IN SOUTH AMERICA

Marta H. Junin

South America occupies a territorial area of 18,678,047 square kilometers and is populated by 345 million inhabitants[1] distributed in 12 countries: Argentina, Bolivia, Brazil, Chile, Colombia, Ecuador, Guyana, Paraguay, Peru, Suriname, Uruguay, and Venezuela (Figure 66–8). There are different geographical regions with distinctive characteristics: the ocean coasts, the tallest mountain chain of the Andes, the long rivers such as the Amazon, large forests, wild jungles, prairies, lakes, deserts such as the Puna of Atacama, and islands, each one with its own cultural characteristics.

Figure 66–8. Countries of South America. *Source:* http://www.infoplease.com/atlas/southamerica.html. Copyright MAGELLAN Geographix.

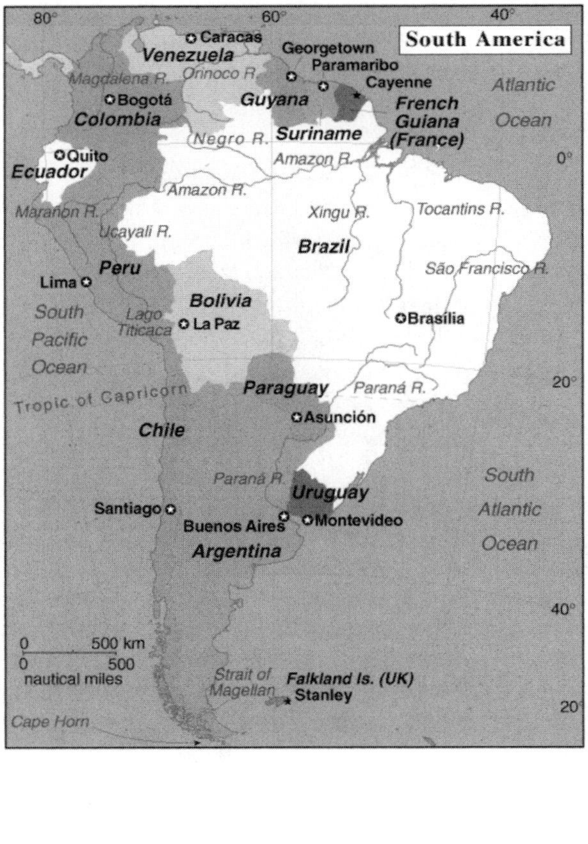

South America offers one of the more complex demographic realities from the point of view of ethnic composition, history of conquests, colonialism, and immigration. The indigenous populations over many generations have accumulated their own scientific knowledge, traditions, and holistic approaches to their lands, natural resources, and the environment. These populations are extremely vulnerable in today's society.[1]

The early indigenous populations were largely replaced at the end of the 14th and 15th centuries by Spanish and Portuguese colonization and, to a lesser extent, by the French, English, and Dutch. African slaves populated parts of the coastal regions at a later date. At the end of the 19th century to the middle of the 20th century, there was increasing European migration to South America by Spaniards, Italians, Poles, and Germans, as well as Arabian and Japanese.

The official language in the majority of South American countries is Spanish, with Portuguese spoken primarily in Brazil. Indigenous groups also have their own languages, for example, Mapuche, Quechua, Aymara, Guaraní, and Yámana. These are considered a secondary language in some countries. The South American population is mainly a mixture of races, descendants of European conquerors and American aborigines. There is a constant migration of people from areas of extreme poverty to more developed urban regions. This has resulted in problematic, uncontrolled urban growth. The large cities contain 50% of the total population. At the same time, however, there has been a large population emigration, mainly to the United States and Spain.[1]

Political and Social-Economic Situation

The government systems, after long periods of authoritarian regimes, military dictatorships, and political instability, are mainly democratic, with constitutional republics and presidents. The establishment of democratic regimes and greater societal participation in the political arena are considered important achievements in the last 2 decades. However, the return to democracy hasn't yet been sufficient to reduce the social and economic inequities that threaten a country's stability, social integration, and ability for sound government. Ways to strengthen democratic principles and practices present ongoing challenges. This is especially so in situations of economic poverty, uncertainty, and struggles between peace and violence. All of these issues affect a population's health.

The conditions and levels of social and economic development in South America are generally heterogeneous. However, these factors significantly mold the health and welfare of the population. The economic and social transformations experienced by South American countries in the 20th century have been characterized by governmental efforts to reduce inflation, increase investment, and privatize companies, all in response to recommendations of the International Monetary System.

State reform, with its emphasis on efficacy and modernization, underscores the important role of government and civil society in economic and social development. A population's health is defined by its economic situation.[1] A country's social and economic crisis presents an opportunity to promote programs with quality, efficacy, and equal access. Palliative care programs are one example.

The Health Systems

South America is a region with large income differences. At the beginning of the 21st century, large variations in life conditions were noted between countries and within countries. Differences in educational levels, technical knowledge, income, health resources and organization, health service accessibility, and other social characteristics that determined a population's state of health were also noted.

All South American countries are considered "in development" by the World Health Organization (WHO). In addition, the population is aging, with an average life expectancy of 70 years. Increasing health care needs come with age. Services such as disease prevention, recuperation, rehabilitation, and palliative care are especially important for older people. In this age group, deaths from cardiovascular diseases are the most frequent, followed by cancer.[1] For individuals suffering from advanced cancer, AIDS, cardiovascular disease, or irreversible trauma, access to palliative care is extremely important.

Resources for cancer control are not uniformly distributed in the world. More than 95% of the total resources are located in developed countries and, not surprisingly, less then 5% in the developing countries (Table 66–8).[2] Likewise, there are differences between developed and developing countries in relation to cancer diagnosis, death from cancer, and availability of treatment resources (Table 66–9).[3] Unfortunately, this means that most of the people who need palliative care live in those countries with the least resources.

In South America, there are different health systems. These are organized around three main providers that cover different percentages of the population in each country:

- The public system, with national, provincial and municipal-communal jurisdiction, supplies free clinical care through primary health centers in the community and general-specialist public hospitals for inpatients and outpatients. In some countries, the national health system provides assistance to the whole population without distinctions of race, economic situation, or religion.
- The insurance social system for working people is administered by trade unions. Employers and employees each pay a fixed fee. The cost of medical care and medicines in varying proportions are covered. Differences between the fixed fee and the actual treatment fee are paid by the patient.
- The private sector is for individuals with a good income. In this system, patients meet the total cost of their care. In some countries all non-working people are referred to this sector, with the risk that some will not be able to access health care because of lack of income. In general this health system assists a small percentage of the population.[1]

Table 66–8
Worldwide Distribution of Resources for Cancer Control

Region	Percent of All Resources
Developed countries	95.3%
Developing countries	4.7%

Table 66–9
Worldwide Difference of Availability for Cancer Control

Cancer Control	Developed Countries	Developing Countries
Cancer diagnosis	25%	12%
Cancer death	50%	80%
Cancer treatment resources	95%	5%

Overview of the Health Context and WHO Palliative Care Programs

The neoplastic diseases are the second leading cause of death in all countries of the region. Despite this figure, few resources are spent on cancer prevention measures. It is estimated that the total number of cancer cases will increase by 34% each decade. If current trends continue, by 2020 approximately one million persons in South America will need palliative care and relief from cancer pain.[4]

In response to these statistics, WHO and the Pan American Health Organization (PAHO) designated palliative care as a priority in the Cancer Relief Program. They adopted measures for the development of palliative care programs in South America that were responsive to regional needs and specific problems. Attention was paid to the different income levels, disease presentations, technical expertise, resources allocated to health organizations, and access to health services in each country.[5]

The goals of the programs are:

- That palliative care is integrated into the medical assistance models.
- That availability of resources for palliative care are evaluated.

- That opioid drugs are available for pain relief.
- That health professionals are qualified and trained.

In 2004, through the support of PAHO, there were seven model projects in palliative care. South American countries involved included Argentina, Ecuador, Chile, Colombia, and Venezuela.[6]

With a similar focus, WHO based its approach to improving palliative care in this region on three components: government policies, opioid availability, and professional education.

Government Policy

The WHO National Program against cancer[4] identified palliative care as a priority for national cancer programs. WHO requested that governments revise their policies as to how they allocate resources in cancer treatment. Most patients in developing countries with cancer present for treatment with advanced disease. Nonetheless, many developing countries assign a large proportion of their cancer resources to sophisticated treatments that have a low impact on the majority of the population. WHO recommendations are that more than half of these health care resources be directed towards palliative care, which will benefit a much greater proportion of the population. In addition, WHO suggests using the information in the program to open up discussions with regulators and institutions interested in establishing or extending palliative care services. Although palliative care professionals are aware that this approach to care offers the most holistic treatment for both patients and their families, some health authorities still think that palliative care is "second-rate" medicine, and they prefer to invest their money in newer and more expensive technology. People involved in palliative care have some responsibility for this because they have not demonstrated to the health authorities the benefit and cost-effectiveness of this work.

Despite the strong endorsement and encouragement from WHO that all countries examine their system of national cancer control programs (and if one does not exist, develop one), many countries in South America do not have such programs. As stated by WHO, "A national cancer control program is a public health program designed to reduce cancer incidence and mortality and improve quality of life of cancer patients, through the systematic and equitable implementation of evidence-based strategies for prevention, early detection, diagnosis, treatment and palliation, making the best use of available resources."[2]

Pain relief and palliative care can improve the quality of life of patients and their families. With careful planning, implementation, monitoring, and evaluation, the establishment of national cancer control programs offers the most rational means of achieving a substantial degree of cancer control, even where resources are severely limited. The establishment of a national cancer control program is recommended wherever the burden of the disease is significant. There is a rising trend of cancer risk factors, and there is a need to make the most efficient use of limited resources.[2]

Availability of and Access to Opioid Analgesics

In palliative care, one of the basic principles is the relief of pain with the use of the WHO Analgesic Ladder and the use of opioids. All the South American countries have adopted the WHO Guidelines. However, changes in legislation and regulations are urgently needed to allow adequate access to opioids.[2]

There are still some difficulties with the treatment of cancer pain in this region. The health policy does not endorse opioid analgesics. As a result, many cancer patients still die with their pain uncontrolled. Additionally, patients and their families retain many taboos related to the use of these opioids, necessitating that the palliative care teams spend much time educating the family about the use of opioids such as morphine.

There are many myths regarding palliative care, and still many health care professionals who do not know how to adequately assess and treat pain. The misplaced fear of respiratory depression or hastening death through the use of opioids remains common. Opioid phobia among regulators is illustrated through their concern that making opioids available for therapeutic use would increase the illicit drug market.

Although opioids can be easily found in the capital cities, prescriptions for controlled substances require many copies. Ready availability of opioids is not a reality for the inner-country people. These people must come to the capital city to get opioid medications for pain relief. The most frequently used opioid for pain is morphine (ampules, syrup, pills) because of its availability, effectiveness, and cost.

Morphine is available in all South American countries but the law and regulations aren't conducive to opioid use. Morphine consumption by terminally ill patients is still low in many South American countries, mainly because of insufficient medical prescription and morphine myths among health professionals and the general population. This suggests that pressure should be exerted on the government to support the teaching of palliative care in public education programs.

In many situations, opioids are available but the high cost limits their availability to only those who can pay. A comparative study among some of world's countries indicates that opioid costs in developing countries is higher than those in developed nations (medians U.S. $112 in South America vs. U.S. $53 in the United States), and in percentage in relation to monthly income per capita (medians S.A. 31% vs. U.S. 3%). In some South American countries such as Argentina, the high cost of opioid therapy can be more than 200% of the average monthly income.[7,8] This problem reflects politics where expensive and sophisticated opioid preparations such as ampules and controlled-release oral morphine are available, whereas cheaper preparations such as immediate-release oral morphine tablets or elixir are not available.

Many countries, in their eagerness to prevent opioid misuse, have adopted laws and regulations resulting in restrictions that have affected the medical use of opioids; for example, imposing limits on the doses and days of treatment allowed per patient. A comparative study of a group of Latin American countries indicated that none abided by the principles of drug availability. Indeed, some of them have included articles to forbid the use of control drugs or the administration of opioids to minors; yet children develop painful cancers and will die of their cancer.[9]

For many years, the Pain and Policy Studies Group (PPSG), WHO Collaborating Center for Policy and Communications in Cancer Care, and University of Wisconsin in the United States, have given advice and technical support to PAHO and South American countries to find a solution to the problem of guaranteeing the availability of opioids analgesics for the whole population.[10,11] Their guidelines offer tools to help governments and health workers identify barriers in laws and regulations that make access to the tools of palliative care (for example, opioids) impossible or difficult to obtain.

PPSG and PAHO have designed a workshop for governments, drugs regulators, and palliative care professionals. During this experience, the representatives of both groups identify specific problems of each country and find solutions.[10] They have developed two workshops: in the Andean region—in Quito 2000—which includes Bolivia, Chile, Colombia, Ecuador, Peru, and Venezuela; for the South region MERCOSUR—South Common Market—including Argentina, Brazil, Paraguay, and Uruguay—in Montevideo, 2002. In both workshops, questionnaires indicated that in countries where communication between government representatives and health professionals was good, palliative care was more developed. Argentina, Colombia, Chile, and Brazil were examples where there was good communication and there were fewer problems with opioid availability.[12–14]

South America uses less than 1% of the world's morphine consumed for medical purposes.[15] Some of the reasons are restrictions or excessive bureaucracy in the importation process of drugs, which increase the final cost of the product; legislation and restrictive control that impose maximum limits in the daily doses; delivery systems that are insufficient to make availability of these drugs uncomplicated in the rural area; health staff that are uneducated in the use of opioids for the relief of pain; concerns about addiction; and reticence to prescribe or store opioid drugs because of concern about legal liability if the drugs are stolen. In addition, there is a lack of authorized pharmacists for the preparation and delivery of opioid drugs. This was the description and consensus of the participants in both the Quito and Montevideo Workshops.[12,13]

Strategies were developed by PPSG of Wisconsin for implementation of the WHO Guidelines[16] to eliminate those barriers that hinder the provision of opioid analgesics to patients in South America:

- Organization of a symposium similar to Quito and Montevideo in all the countries. In addition, to organize a meeting with representatives of several professional groups working in pain relief, oncology, and palliative care, along with control and regulation drug authorities. The purpose of the meeting would be to discuss and develop national policies to improve opioid availability for the relief of pain.
- To set up a committee with representatives from pain and palliative care organizations to study the WHO Guidelines in relation to their own situation in each country. They would collaborate with the PAHO regional officers in developing a proposal for national policy reform in relation to these guidelines.
- Diffusion via the media and by scientific publications of the WHO Guidelines through government and nongovernment organizations (NGOs).

There are still many problems regarding adequate availability and access to potent analgesics in South American countries. This region is still challenged by poverty, lack of education and training, and barriers at the regulatory, legal, and administrative levels. Governments are concerned with such problems as lack of infrastructure, difficulty gaining access to care centers, and improving control of acute infections and vaccinations, and many have yet to place opioid availability on their priority list.

Because improving access to opioids is an international effort, we are all affected to some degree by the decisions and actions taken by others. We need to become aware that opioid availability is not just a local issue, but, rather, one with no borders. All stakeholders in this process, including patients, professionals, multilateral organizations, the pharmaceutical industry, policy makers, and health care professionals, need to be included in the development of strategies to improve this situation.[8]

Education

There are educational needs for the general public, health professionals, legislators, and regulators. In many South American countries, there is lack of community information and education programs about palliative care and insufficient and nonsystematic education activities for health professionals. Examples are nonaccreditation of services and noncertification of professionals in palliative care.[13]

In some South American countries, there are regional and local initiatives for professional palliative care education, however, standards in training are lacking. Training is generally done by the professional, on her/his own initiative, and it is generally theoretical, with few opportunities for clinical practice. At the moment, a fundamental change is occurring in palliative care education opportunities. A variety of training systems have been implemented, including university or nonuniversity courses, single discipline or interdisciplinary methodology, distance-education systems, or activities with a marked clinical emphasis. These diverse types of learning methods facilitate the professional's ability to acquire or complete his or her pain and palliative care education. In addition, topics on pain treatment, palliative care, and mourning are being included at the undergraduate level in medicine, social work, and psychology, and in nursing schools and universities. In some university hospitals, access to the palliative care approach is possible for all health care students. There are lectures or modules on palliative care available to all students in the last year of their training. This surely is an important way to improve patients' access to palliative care in the future. At a postgraduate level, activities are carried out at the main educational centers.[17] The current focus on palliative care in the educational system gives hope for real change in the future.

One of the main obstacles to palliative care team members' training is the high cost of medical and nursing education. Nevertheless, in recent years, several Latin American programs have generated free education resources for professionals training in symptom control and palliative care, WHO Guidelines Spanish translation, and medical and nursing scholarships. Financial support is given mainly by NGOs to individuals who are willing to travel abroad for training in palliative care and for leaders to attend major scientific conferences.

The nurse's education in pain relief and palliative care is one of the basic principles in the priority ladder on pain control by WHO.[18] This is taken into account in many South American countries by the coordinators of nursing training programs to include these issues in undergraduate, service education and postgraduate levels.

The Historical Perspective and Current Status of Palliative Care

During the early 1980s, due to the influence of the Hospice Movement and WHO's Cancer Pain Program, modern palliative care concepts began to spread in an organized manner across South America. The development was unlike that in Europe or North America, because social, cultural, and economic characteristics made it difficult to follow those models exactly.

The historical context of palliative care was similar in many South American countries, with a lack of support from governments and health authorities. The palliative care movement began with small, motivated groups of health professionals working with terminally ill patients in public and private institutions. This movement coincided in some countries with the beginnings of democracy and ending of dictatorships and years of violence. Progress was slow, largely due to lack of financial support. However, once links were established with European and North American centers or universities, physicians and nurse leaders gained an opportunity to receive palliative care experience in more developed services and programs outside of South America.

Eventually, palliative care units were established in public hospitals, with programs that provide hospital-based care to terminally ill patients. In some cases, close and collaborative relationships were built between the oncology departments and palliative care services. During these early stages, support from the international palliative care community and NGOs was invaluable. Advice on educational, philosophical, and organizational skills was sought from experienced palliative care practitioners in the United Kingdom and the United States.[19]

The experience of Chile in the 1990s shows what can be achieved with important support from national health administrators. It began with the development of several interdisciplinary palliative care teams organized as "local programs" in their respective health centers. Later, each one of these teams was consolidated as a "motor team"—the driving force of the future national program. The aim was to create awareness in the health sector about palliative care. Up until this time, there was little awareness. These pioneer groups became the National Committee. The committee reviewed the international literature and similar programs in other countries and organized standards. A high level of interest and financial support from the Health Ministry regarding "Pain Relief and Palliative Care National Programs" was officially recognized for cancer patients. Primary health services and public hospitals introduced a consulting team for inpatients and for patients cared for in the ambulatory setting. Today these centers cover 70% of the Chilean territory.[17]

Ministries of Health need to invite health institutions to form an advisory committee to draft national quality standards for palliative care and to create a national network. The message is: "If you have a poor community, then you must introduce palliative care programs to provide the majority of the population access to this health care." In some countries, there are national laws that guarantee access to palliative care throughout the health system, but these laws have little real impact on practice.[19]

In 1991, the First Palliative Care Latin American Meeting took place in Argentina. The participants recommended that national associations of palliative care be created. Today almost all of the South American countries have their own scientific Palliative Care Association. Prior to the formation of these organizations, palliative care teams could only count on support from the Anesthesiology Association for the Study of Pain, oncology societies, and the experience of neighboring countries. The Latin American Association of Palliative Care was created in 2000. The last Congress took place in Montevideo, Uruguay in April 2004, with the participation of professionals from all Latin American countries.

The Palliative Care Teams

The Palliative Care South America teams are made up of doctors from different specialties, registered and practical nurses, pharmacists, psychologists, social workers, spiritual or religious representatives, and volunteers. The coordinator is generally a doctor. The number of team members varies according to availability of resources. The teams work in a similar way to other teams throughout the world, but in many cases without enough resources and government support. The team's activities are symptom control, psychosocial support to the patient and the family, bereavement support, education and training, and clinical research. The team members are available via a 24-hour telephone-contact service.

Different models have been developed including general hospital units, consulting teams for inpatients and patients in the ambulatory setting, and, when possible, home care. Some teams do not see patients at home because of lack of government funding. There is already a movement to provide such care with the support of NGOs. However, some palliative care services have only informal support from the national health system, because palliative care is not recognized as a specialty and is still considered to be unimportant. Plans for future development include improvement of home care public programs specific for palliative care from the hospitals. Some teams that provide private care already exist, but there are few health institutions similar to a hospice. In some places, there are charitable, nongovernment associations designed to provide clinical care to hospital inpatients and outpatients. These only exist in large institutions in the main cities of some countries, but not in rural areas. In general, palliative care teams do not exist in rural communities.

The frequency of use of a specialized palliative care team varies, and is dependent on recognition by the patient's primary physician of the need for input from such a team. In some cases, general doctors are struggling to address a patient's concerns regarding end-of-life care, but the physician in charge of the patient has primary influence on that patient's care.

In many hospitals in South America, the concept of teamwork is not evident. Professionals work more as individuals within a group, each with his or her own tasks and objectives. Doctors may fear losing their patients, as they would also lose the patients' fees. Therefore, there is an element of understandable competition among colleagues. Conversely, the atmosphere among nurses is more passive. The doctors' competition and the nurses' passivity appear to block interprofessional communication, which, in turn, can affect patient care. The concept of interdisciplinary teamwork is poorly developed in most centers, and the nurse tends to have a low status. Encouraging communication between the two groups and the development of interdisciplinary palliative care training programs is important to enhance the understanding of the role of the other.

Today there are many registered teams, including pediatric teams, working in different parts of South America. Some areas have many teams, others few. There is an increasing interest by health professionals in improving knowledge in their respective regions and in creating new palliative care centers. The challenge is to work with the local community as well as governmental and other agencies.

The Nurse's Role in Palliative Care Teams

The number of interdisciplinary teams working in palliative care is expanding in all regions of South America. Nursing interventions in outpatient, home care, and inpatient hospital settings are increasing day by day, and nurses have independent roles in this area. There are specific characteristics and substantial differences between the role of palliative care nursing and those in other medical specialties.

In all care settings, registered nurses working in palliative care assume key roles in the following areas: patient and family assessment; provision of direct care such as hygiene, comfort, wound dressings, and other treatment; management of distressing symptoms; monitoring the therapeutic effect and side effects of the opioid analgesics; administration of medicines and other procedure regimens; liaison with related services, particularly local doctors; referral and coordination of volunteers; provision of patient and family resources; professional and community education; and provision of bereavement support are all part of their role. One of the most important nursing tasks is family support, education, and training on various aspects of symptom management. Without appropriate education, care of the terminally ill patient by the family at home becomes impossible. The nurse supervises home care through visits or telephone support. In addition to these responsibilities, the nurse participates in multidisciplinary patient consultations, takes an active part in the assessment, diagnosis, treatment, and decision-making processes with the patient and family, and actively participates in the palliative care team meetings.[17]

In many South American countries, working conditions are difficult. Hospital wards are overcrowded and understaffed, often with many patients per nurse. This situation causes a high level of stress. The nurse's status is relatively low, and nursing is not a profession that many people enthusiastically pursue. There are few nurses working full-time in palliative care, and many work part-time. In addition, interprofessional communication is not on an equal level. Multidisciplinary–interdisciplinary workshops have been encouraged, and palliative care is one of the first disciplines in medicine-nursing to be taught in such a collaborative fashion. Nurses now have a voice in medical meetings, and they are beginning to be recognized for what they can offer, and not just as handmaids to doctors. Another innovation in nursing is the use of interactive teaching sessions rather than the traditional didactic methods common in unidisciplinary nursing and medical teaching.

Nurses working in rural areas believe there is significant work to be done to help them provide for the palliative needs of the community. Rural and remote communities are not homogeneous; they offer various challenges to health care delivery based on demographics, local culture, physical environment, and distance from health services. Rural nurses providing palliative care in the community suffer significant professional isolation. But interestingly, people living in these regions do not have the profound negative beliefs and thoughts about death and dying as seen in large cities. In some settings, particularly in remote areas, the nurse may be the sole health practitioner in a community, receiving telephone support from a doctor located some distance away. The challenge is to find sustainable models of palliative care provision in many of these communities without specialist services and technological advances.

It is important to understand the different levels of nurse training that exist in South American countries: those with a doctoral or master's degree in nursing, those with a college or university degree, licensed nurses, and auxiliaries.[17] There is a lack of consistent inclusion of palliative care in undergraduate curricula across the countries. In general, a discrete module in the form of an elective is offered to a small group of students. This situation is changing, as there are more and more nursing colleges and universities that include palliative care content in the curriculum at all levels of undergraduate programs. Palliative care team staff are commonly involved in the provision of theoretical and practice education to the students, at their personal initiative.

The demand for palliative care education has increased. There are education programs available to prepare nurses for their role in some government institutions. These courses range from 1 day to 50-/100-hour programs on different aspects of palliative care. Nurses with experience and knowledge set up palliative nursing inservice programs for their unit and for nurses from surrounding hospitals. All of them have benefited from the work in presentation and teaching skills.

Access to postgraduate palliative care education is often a product of geography, with more educational opportunities in large urban centers than elsewhere. There is an increasing emphasis on the provision of specialist courses via distance education. In some cases, this is supported by information technology such as teleconferencing and Internet delivery. These approaches overcome some of the access issues. Currently there are no postregistration diplomas or master's-degree nursing programs in South American countries, nor are such programs available to other health care professionals.

One recommendation is that postregistration continuing education should be structured in such a way as to ensure the development of nurses prepared for clinical nursing roles in specialist areas. Also recommended is that links with higher-education institutions be developed to accredit such courses for nurses, and that all courses be subjected to a joint professional and academic validation and accreditation.[17]

In the area of palliative care nursing research, the aim is to develop knowledge to sustain and to guide nursing practices. However, health research in South America is primarily carried out by medical doctors, with minimal nurses' participation in these projects. The overall number of nurses involved in research is very low. The reasons for this scant nursing participation in research include inadequate training at an undergraduate level on the principles of clinical research, the need to work two or three jobs because of low wages, and the limited number of grants available for nursing research. However, some institutions have generated initiatives as fellowships for nursing research, including participation in presenting work guidelines, explaining patient informed consent, gathering information personally or by phone, entering statistical data for future analysis, and presenting and discussing results in quantitative and qualitative research.[17]

Sociocultural, Religious, and Spiritual Issues Influencing Palliative Care

In spite of South America's cultural diversity, the predominant religion is Catholicism. Most people have a deep faith, so the spiritual aspect of care is very important to terminally ill patients. A patient who realizes that he or she is dying may lean heavily on religion, as does the family. As a result, most patients prefer to spend their last days at home, surrounded by relatives. In addition, the presence of a spiritual assistant at the hour of death and confession to a Catholic priest may be very important at this time. In South American cultural groups, many patients think that illness is a punishment of God and that only God can grant salvation, relief, and even healing.

Nurses have a hard humanistic role to carry out in accordance with Catholic principles. They are the first and the last contact when the patient consults at a health institution, and they usually hear and are exposed to all the family problems, worries, anxieties, feelings, and grief. Nurses recognize the need for appropriate palliative care education to respond appropriately to the patient's religious needs.

Some people in rural areas have adopted a stoic attitude in the face of painful experiences. In villages far away from large cities there is also a strong influence of folk medicine, quackery, and popular herbal alternative treatments not prescribed by medical doctors. All of these beliefs and practices hinder dying persons from accepting medical treatments such as pain and symptom control.

In addition, both health care professionals and the general public see morphine as synonymous with death. Its safe and effective use needs to be seen to be believed and be understood. To change popular myths about opioids, the palliative care associations need to offer professional health care education and training in all regions of the countries. The educational role of nurses is crucial because they are especially sensitive and aware of the importance of the relief of pain.

In South America's multicultural environment, the lower social status of most patients in relation to doctors makes it difficult for them to communicate fears, needs, and queries, and, as a result, almost impossible for them to understand the implications of treatment. In most instances, there are nurses acting in an advocacy-and-treatment translator's role. Direct and honest communication between patients and doctors is rare. Constraints on the doctor's time make meaningful explanations difficult. In addition, the relatives may see the doctor first and tell the doctor not to tell the patient about a diagnosis and prognosis. A "conspiracy of silence" isolates the patient early on, denying the opportunity to attend to "unfinished business," and imprisons him or her in a lonely world of silence and secrecy in which all treatment choices are denied.

The concept of the strong family support network in South America is currently under threat. It still exists, but the culture is changing. More women go out to work as opposed to working at home, and more families are becoming isolated from the larger family unit. The move away from the village to the cities continues as people search for work. There are reports of patients with advanced cancer being abandoned by their families because financial resources are so drained, or because family members cannot cope with their own terrible suffering and feeling of impotence at the sight of someone they love in uncontrollable pain.[17]

Sometimes relatives are not caregivers of terminally ill patients because patients are frequently sent to hospitals far away from their homes. This also means that family doctors are not involved in this type of care; rather, the main responsibility for terminal care remains on the hospital doctors and nurses where the patient has been admitted. Even though these doctors and nurses are improving their knowledge and skills in palliative care, the challenge is still great because most patients and families do not participate in the decision-making process.

When the hospital is near to the patient's home, in keeping with the family structure and South American traditions, a relative is required to stay at the health center when the patient is admitted. The relatives are involved in the training program during this period. The training given is as follows: importance of cleanliness and hygiene at the personal and family level, wound care and dressing, how to feed the patient, pain treatment, use of morphine, patient's medication including the patient's timetable at home, and how to keep the patient occupied. The team staff are acutely aware of the patient's needs and transmit this to the family.

Traditionally in South American countries people died at home, but the situation is changing. Because most of the patients who come to a palliative care service arrive from the rural areas of the country or from surrounding towns, they prefer to stay in the hospital. Acute care beds are used for palliative care, where some patients feel safer because of staff presence. They have added spiritual and psychological support from the palliative care team. Most of these patients do not have a home care service to ensure that they will be cared for in their homes.

There are regional differences in availability of home support. In some South American countries, palliative care can be provided in the home through national, provincial, and municipal programs, but community-based palliative care programs for the whole population are still a challenge in most countries. Although many patients would prefer to die at home, there are multiple reasons to explain why the majority of patients nowadays die in hospitals in these countries. These reasons include low educational level, lack of socioeconomic resources, fears harbored by relatives about the development of the disease and end of life, past bad experiences, lack of relatives, and difficulty in symptom control. An educational family program must be established with the aim of helping the family become aware of their importance and role in the care of the patient at home. Palliative care teams keep in touch with relatives by phone to offer help in case of unexpected home events. The availability and accessibility of comprehensive and coordinated home care services are pivotal in making death at home a realistic option.

Inpatient hospices are not yet the chosen place to die for most individuals. Two reasons contributing to this are the lack of such hospices and the stigma and fear sometimes associated with this type of institution in South American culture.

Ethical Issues Influencing End-of-Life Care

Because of cultural barriers existing in South American countries, most doctors have difficulty in communicating with patients regarding their cancer disease and terminal status. The doctor usually informs the family, but the relatives often desire to protect the patient from knowing the truth. The patient progressively loses his or her autonomy, and the family makes decisions without the patient's explicit consent. Freedom of choice is compromised for patients due to:

- A patriarchal–protective presence of family members in medical decision-making
- A paternalistic attitude toward patient care on the part of physicians
- The strong influence exerted by the Catholic church on public debate
- A lack of communication skills among health care professionals

In recent years, increasing attention has been given to patient self-determination and autonomy, especially in decisions surrounding the end of life. The challenge of addressing South American attitudes to truth-telling within a multicultural society is experienced by some countries. "Truth with tenderness," with patients determining how much they wish to know and who should have access to their information, is the goal of communication. Ideally, communication regarding goals of care should include discussions about the use of hydration, antibiotics, and artificial feeding, as well as the potential use of cardiopulmonary resuscitation. Palliative care has initiated a change from the long-established practice of not telling a patient his or her diagnosis to one that respects the patient's right to know and facilitates open communication. The concept of patient autonomy is just starting to emerge in some South American countries.

In large cities, one of the problems confronting palliative care doctors is the high expectations of both professionals and the public regarding the preservation of life at all costs, especially when the dying person is in the intensive care unit (ICU). Health care technology is used indiscriminately, and patients with advanced cancer are often dying alone in ICUs, wired up to every possible machine and with no nurse in attendance. Outside the ward, the patient's family, denied access to the bedside, wait for the inevitable. Both family and patient therefore suffer the final stage of separation alone, at a time when they most need to be united.

Discussions about resuscitation or the benefit- versus-burden of admitting a patient to an ICU if chances for improvement are small or nonexistent are held infrequently in South American countries. Most patients have difficulty addressing these subjects, and few palliative care teams broach them. In addition, the use of living wills and other advance directives are still uncommon, and such documents do not carry much legal weight. Some palliative care teams, however, appear to be making inroads in addressing these issues.

Communicating diagnosis and prognosis to the patient, and recognition of the ethical responsibility of obtaining informed consent from the patient regarding treatment and other important decisions, appear to be occurring more frequently and to be approached with less discomfort. In recent years, interest in ethical issues at the end of life has increased. The need for ongoing discussion of ethical issues and for continuing education in palliative care and ethical dilemmas for physicians in training and nurses who provide end-of-life care is evident. Some nurses express feelings of guilt and unethical practice when asked by a doctor to sedate a patient, and some feel that they are being asked to practice euthanasia by following medical orders.

In an attempt to change this situation, the palliative care team must run workshops and support groups for families and patients, where they can speak about subjects such as feelings, the myths of morphine, doubts and fears about death, and any worries that the family or the patient have. All those involved in end-of-life care, including patients and families, also need to understand the difference between palliative sedation for intractable symptoms at end of life and physician-assisted suicide or euthanasia.

Overall, in South American countries, there is a growing consensus that end-of-life issues must be discussed more fully, including the country's position regarding euthanasia and physician-assisted suicide.[19]

In addition, there is consensus that access to high-quality palliative care must be promoted through government policies that provide resources for a competent multidisciplinary palliative care workforce across South America.[20] We have come a long way, but we still have a long way to go.

Palliative Care in South America: Weaknesses and Strengths

Weaknesses

Government Policy:

- Lack of recognition of palliative care needs in the national and regional health programs
- Difficulties in all the health sectors: public, private, and social-security, with insufficient fulfillment of palliative care requests
- Lack of institutional financial support because palliative care programs are not a priority
- Failure to uphold the WHO recommendations in practice regarding cancer relief and palliative care

Availability of and Access to Opioids Analgesics:

- Lack of suitable legislation; bureaucracy; passivity and inequality regarding the prescription; availability and allocation of opioids
- Excessive cost, inefficiency in the management and administration of analgesic drug supplies
- Common popular and professionals' attitudes regarding morphine prescription and myths
- Economic difficulties of the poor population to pay for the treatment, and lack of government analgesic provision

Education:

- Absence of informative and educative programs about palliative care benefits for the community
- No systematic training activities for the health professionals before and after graduation
- Little and expensive palliative care advance education
- No master, specialized degree, or diploma levels in palliative care education
- Misconceptions about the use of morphine and other strong opioids by health professionals
- Difficulty accessing palliative care education for health professionals in rural areas
- Lack of professional training about how to listen and how to communicate bad news
- Limited academic connection among palliative care professionals

The Palliative Care Team:

- Absence of palliative care standards, professional certification, and systematic service accreditation
- Lack of an operational network of palliative care providers among different cities, regions, and countries
- Unequal interprofessional communication
- Lack of professionals trained in palliative care
- Insufficient financial support of palliative care teams
- Low salaries, and sometimes none, for palliative care professionals
- Difficulties in guaranteeing volunteer work and charitable funding
- Few researcher opportunities due to a low priority given to research in the culture, and a lack of time, rigorousness in the scientific methodology, resources, and industry support

The Nurse's Role in the Palliative Care Team:

- Medical community unaware of the importance of the nurse's role in the interdisciplinary palliative care team and as agent of change in society
- Widespread acceptance in the medical community of the paternalistic attitude of the physicians
- Palliative care training needs not considered in order to achieve safe practices
- Many eligible patients, yet few nurses with training in palliative care
- Low nurse status in relation to other health professionals
- Lack of participation in clinic updates and research with colleagues and others members of the team

Sociocultural, Religious, and Spiritual Issues:

- High level of distressing, unbearable pain and low expectations in unrelieved oncological patients
- Difficulty of communication between rural population and palliative care centers in big cities because of large distances
- Barriers to access of palliative care teams because of economic problems in needy populations
- Family need to work as an obstacle to taking care of the patient at home
- Rural population's beliefs about folkloric/chamanes medicine and use of traditional complementary therapies in symptom control more frequently than use of traditional medicine
- Religious and family obstacles about end-of-life decision-making
- Difficulties in management of spiritual suffering associated with chronic, advanced, and progressive disease by health professionals

Ethical Issues Influencing End-of-Life Care:

- Difficulties about end-of-life decision-making: terminal sedation vs. euthanasia, truth and bad news communication, silence conspiracy vs. patient autonomy, diagnosis and prognosis disclosure
- Inequality in the distribution of health resources
- Futility in the end-of-life ICUs in many hospitals
- Failure to address issues surrounding death and dying
- Lack of palliative care quality-of-life standards

Strengths

Government Policy:

- Some countries in the beginning of the development of palliative care national or regional policy
- Integration of the different health professions and scientific societies creating organization rules and standards, with government agreement

Availability of and Access to Opioids Analgesics:

- Availability of analgesic opioid but with restrictions to access for the whole population
- Opioid consumption increased over the last few years

Education:

- Some educational activities for health professionals before and after graduation but not systematic training.
- A few palliative care training opportunities for professionals together with experienced palliative care teams locally and abroad
- Nongovernmental organizations' support of palliative care advanced-education programs
- Human resources of health care with specific training in palliative care, not many but goods.

The Palliative Care Team:

- An increase in palliative care teams with active assistance programs for adults and children, most of them in public hospitals
- Support of the initiatives and programs by international organizations, with the agreement of leaders
- Exchange of experiences and resources with other regional groups or countries
- No governments, local associations, or foundations that promote and practice palliative care
- Possibility to work in an interdisciplinary way in some cities and regions
- An increasing use of rules and symptom-control protocols
- There are associations of palliative care that coordinate scientific activities in most South American countries.

The Nurse's Role in the Palliative Care Team:

- Historical hierarchical position of the nurse in the interdisciplinary palliative care team
- More closeness to the patient than most health professionals
- Maintain sensitivity in the face of family needs
- Ability to communicate with people of different social and cultural status
- Ability to creatively adapt to lack of resources

Sociocultural, Religious, and Spiritual Issues:

- Change of attitudes relating to palliative care in people and professionals: "cure" attitude vs. "care" attitude
- Family inclusion in care of the patient at home and in the hospital setting
- Increased family, friends', or neighbors' role in providing care to ease the process of adaptation
- Patient's and families' satisfaction with the palliative care team's assistance at home

- Volunteers and social networks for providing resources locally
- Acceptance and approval of palliative care by different religions, with official recognition, especially by the Catholic church

Ethical Issues Influencing End-of-Life Care:
- There are more hospital ethical committees collaborating with palliative care teams regarding the difficulties in end-of-life decision-making.

Challenges of Palliative Care in South America

Government Policy:
- Integrate palliative care programs into national, provincial, municipal, and regionals health systems.
- Implement palliative care teams, services, or units in all countries according to individual needs.
- Establish rules, standards, handbooks, and team directories, by professional team leaders, according to international guidelines, with regional and cultural adaptations.
- Ensure governmental and nongovernmental institutions work together to identify communities' palliative care needs and, by integrating resources, determine the most effective care delivery.
- Improve distribution of health resources.
- Detect and resolve obstacles blocking implementation of palliative care programs.
- Develop regional strategies and communication among South American countries, and request international support.

Availability of and Access to Opioid Analgesics:
- Include universal availability and allocation of recommended opioid analgesic with free access for the whole population.
- Enact laws that assure coverage of treatment for palliative care patients.
- Decrease the cost of the opioids.

Education:
- Distribute information about palliative care throughout the population.
- Determine attitudes regarding morphine prescription and myths and carry out popular education related to findings.
- Assure systematic palliative care training activities for health professionals both before and after graduation, with inclusion in the curriculum.
- Provide masters, specialized degree, and diploma levels in palliative care professionals' education.
- Provide exchange of professionals with training in palliative care for education programs in developing countries.

The Palliative Care Team:
- Develop communication between government and institutions' administrators to implement and consolidate palliative care programs, using community resources.
- Design own palliative care standards, professionals' certification, and systematic services accreditation.
- Include palliative care in the early stages of patient assistance[21] to improve care management and to provide services complementary with other medical specialities.[22]
- Eliminate interprofessional communication barriers in the team.
- Include psychotherapists with training in palliative care team support to avoid burn-out situations.
- Develop a supportive group that includes volunteers and charitable funding to support palliative care teams.
- Create an operational network of palliative care providers among different cities, regions, and countries.
- Increase opportunities for researchers to work together.
- Create palliative care associations throughout South America.

The Nurse's Role in the Palliative Care Team:
- Achieve standards of training in palliative care and relief of pain for all nursing levels.
- Include palliative care in schools' and universities' nursing curriculum.
- Create awareness of the nurse's role in the interdisciplinary palliative care team and as change agent in the society.
- Increase the nurse's participation in clinic update and research with colleagues and other members of the team.

Sociocultural, Religious, and Spiritual Issues:
- Adapt international models to the South American multicultural/sociopolitical environment, reality, and resources, and define each country's own palliative care model.
- Respect culture values in different ethnic groups and be aware of the need for cross-cultural palliative care teams appropriate for aboriginal culture of South America.
- Establish volunteers and social networks to provide resources.
- Make communities aware of their rights to increase requests for palliative care's efficient services.

- Develop palliative care in all places with own resources, even in poor countries and among marginalized communities.
- Emphasize the important role of the family in providing care in places with few palliative care human resources.

Ethical Issues Influencing End-of-Life Care:

- Provide widespread information to the population about end-of-life decision-making in relation to incurable diseases.
- Ensure greater participation of palliative care professionals in the discussion about euthanasia.
- Collaborate with authorities and legislators to advance knowledge about palliative care's objectives and scopes.
- Institutions need to demand that health professionals assure ethical and quality palliative care for patients.
- People must demand respect for human rights and ethical basic principles from health professionals, including autonomy, beneficence, nonmaleficence, and justice.

Conclusions

Palliative care as a medical discipline began to grow throughout South America in the mid-1980s thanks to the pioneer initiatives of multiprofessional health teams, working with a holistic approach to promote the care of dying people. These first initiatives were supported by the enthusiasm of their leaders and were able to prosper with few available resources, both inside and outside of the hospital setting. At that time, institutional recognition was either partial or nonexistent. The teams were small and the job was hard; however, they have grown a lot and been an instrument of change in bettering citizens' quality of life. Many difficulties still remain, and the need to provide skilled and compassionate care for seriously ill and dying patients is now being recognized as a major challenge in most South American countries.

In recent years, WHO has proposed providing more palliative care at the time of diagnosis for patients in developing countries. The reasons behind this are that by the time many patients get to the doctor, it is either too late in the course of their disease, the country/institution is unable to offer a curative therapy, or the patient is unable to access curative options. Therefore, they need a great deal more palliative care. It means that the allocation of resources in their countries and in their institutions should not be focused necessarily on diagnostic and curative oncological procedures and therapies, but rather, on issues such as adequate access to and availability of opioids and other medications.[4]

The developing countries need technological and financial support to develop palliative care programs that cover the patients with advanced and progressive disease and family needs. International and nongovernmental organizations play an important role in this process and must offer assistance as much as possible. In a sense, WHO and PAHO can cause a stir in the development of new programs and in the consolidation of the existing ones.

Because of the great diversity of resources in South American health systems, there are many different methods that exist for providing palliative care. Integrating resources from public sectors and nongovernmental organizations can facilitate the implementation of programs, the promotion of palliative care services, and the provision of research and education opportunities. There are also scientific associations of palliative care in almost all countries.

In South America, there is evidence of growth in palliative care initiatives to improve availability of opioid analgesics for the treatment of cancer pain, as well as more educational opportunities for physicians, nurses, social workers, psychologists, and, at the community level, volunteers.

There is still a great need to develop national health policies that promote and implement palliative care as an effective way of assisting people suffering from advanced and terminal disease. The social and economic crises of South American countries is a good opportunity to encourage programs of great medical-social importance, verifiable cost-effectiveness, evident user satisfaction, and efficiency. High-quality palliative care programs meeting these criteria have been proven effective.

Such policies also must increase undergraduate and postgraduate education opportunities and research on palliative care topics, including ethics. There is also a need to promote home care as a low-cost option, making it an important resource for developing and poor countries. Active participation by the entire health care system, by members of community groups, and, most importantly, by patients and families, is needed.

Today, the majority of people in South American cities die in hospitals, and care must be provided in this setting. But it is also important not forget the Latin American tradition that identifies relatives as the main caregivers. This means active participation of families in care, even in the hospitals. When models of palliative care are being designed, one must also consider the diverse needs of a multicultural society.

Palliative care's aim has been a model of care based on the concept of an interdisciplinary, multiprofessional team: nurses, physicians, social workers, psychologists, religious care providers, pharmacists, physio/occupational therapists, and volunteers. In South American countries, palliative care strongly highlights nurses' roles, and they are beginning to be considered as important members of the team. However, we must also remember that the doctor's role was traditionally hierarchical, and physicians maintained a paternalistic relationship with other team members—though this situation is beginning to change.

South American nurses are the front line in their respective teams, fighting against the difficulties in providing palliative care. There has been much personal effort by each nurse to improve her or his own scientific knowledge and professional skills. However, in this region, there is still much to be done to allow dying people to live with dignity until the end of their lives. We, the South American nurses, have assumed this commitment.

REFERENCES

1. Pan American Health Organization. Health in the Americas, Vol I & II. Scientific and Technical Publication No. 587. Washington, DC: Author, 2002.
2. De Lima L, Esser S, Steigerwald I. Pain relief and palliative care programs: the WHO and IAHPC Approach in developing countries. Pain Pract 2003;3:92–96.
3. De Lima L. Palliative Care in Developing Countries: Challenges and Resources. 2nd Congress of the Latin American Association of Palliative Care. Montevideo, Uruguay, March 2004.
4. World Health Organization. Cancer Control Programs: Policies and Managerial Guidelines, 2nd ed. Geneva: WHO, 2002.
5. Pan American Health Organization. Framework for a Regional Project on Cancer Palliative Care in Latin America. Washington, DC: PAHO, 1997.
6. DeLima L, et al. Development of palliative medicine in Latin America. In: M Gómez Sancho, ed. Palliative Care Advances, Vol. III. Las Palmas de Gran Canaria, Spain: Gabinetede Asesoramiento y Formación Sociosanitaria, 2003.
7. Sweeney C, Palmer JL, De Lima L, Bruera E. Potent analgesics are more expensive for patients in developing countries: a comparative study. International Association for the Study of Pain, 10th World Congress on Pain, San Diego, CA, 2002.
8. De Lima L. Opioid availability in Latin America as a global problem: a new strategy with regional and national effects. J Palliative Med 2004;7:97–103.
9. De Lima L, Bruera E. The role of international treaties in the opioid availability process: relationship between international narcotics control boards, national governments, the pharmaceutical industry and physicians. Prog Palliative Care 2000;8:2.
10. World Health Organization Collaborating Center for Symptom Evaluation. Cancer Pain Release 2000;13(1). Madison, WI: University of Wisconsin. Available at: http://www.whocancerpain.wisc.edu/eng/13-1/whoccpc.html (accessed April 27, 2005).
11. World Health Organization. Achieving Balance in National Opioids Control Policy: Guidelines for Assessment. Geneva: WHO, 2001.
12. WHO-PAHO. First Meeting of Andean Region about Opioids Availability and Palliative Treatment: Quito's Activities Inform. Washington, DC: Pan American Health Organization, 2001.
13. WHO-PAHO. First Mercosur Meeting about opioids availability and Palliative Treatments. Participants Consensus Summary. Washington, DC: PAHO, 2002.
14. Joranson D. Improving availability of opioid pain medications: testing the principle of balance in Latin America. J Palliative Med 2004;7:105–114.
15. United Nations. Narcotic Drugs: Estimated World Requirements for 2002 and Statistics for 2000. UN Document No. E/INCB/2001/2. New York: United Nations, 2001. Available at: http://www.unodc.org/unodc/en/publications/report_incb_2001-02-28_1.html (accessed April 27, 2005).
16. World Health Organization Collaborating Center for Symptom Evaluation. WHO: new gyidelines to evaluate national opioid policy. Cancer Pain Release 2001;14(1). Madison, WI: University of Wisconsin. Available at: http://www.whocancerpain.wisc.edu/eng/14_1/action.html (accessed April 27, 2005).
17. Cullen CM, Vera MM. South America: Argentina. In Ferrell B, Coyle N, eds. Textbook of Palliative Nursing. New York: Oxford University Press, 2001;797–801.
18. World Health Organization Collaborating Center for Symptom Evaluation. Building nursing competency in pain control and palliative care. Cancer Pain Release 1999;12(3). Madison, WI: University of Wisconsin. Available at: http://www.whocancerpain.wisc.edu/eng/12_3/competency.html (accessed Aril 27, 2005).
19. The International Observatory on End-of-Life Care—Countries A–Z-Argentina. Available at: http://www.eolc-observatory.net (accessed March 13, 2005).
20. Materstvedt LJ, et al. Euthanasia and physician-assisted suicide: a view from a European Association for Palliative Care Ethic Task Force. Palliative Med 2003;17:97–101.
21. Bertolino M, Heller KS. Promoting quality of life near the end of life in Argentina. J Palliative Med 2001;4:423–430.
22. Eisenchlas J, Junin M, De Simone G. Oncology-palliative care interface audit on expectations and communication in patients who received palliative chemotherapy. Argentinian Association of Palliative Care Bulletin 2002;3:35–36.

X

"A Good Death"

67

Richard Steeves and David Kahn

Understanding a Good Death: James's Story

A good death is as difficult to define as a good life in that the former is, or should be, an extension of the latter. What makes life enjoyable and worth living does not change when a person is dying. But while most of us are concerned with how to make our lives as good as possible, we rarely think about what might make our deaths good. We might consider the details of dying while reading serious fiction, however, we are unlikely to think of them in the context of our daily experience. But to paraphrase an old saw, there is nothing like the prospect of death to focus a person's attention. The dying want their deaths and what remains of their lives to be as good as possible. They count on palliative care nurses to do as much as possible to ensure this goodness. Of course, there may come a time for any patient when death will seem preferable to life. For example, an 87-year-old man dying of lung cancer, who was an informant in our study of cancer patients in hospice, stated: "I'm going downhill now and I don't like it. It just gets harder to breathe. I can see that eventually I'll be far enough down that hill that it will be better to be at the bottom and dead then still sliding down." The goal of palliative care is to ensure that this desire for the bottom of the hill is not inevitable even though finally reaching that bottom may be.

The goal of palliative care nurses is to attend to the symptoms that are part of the disease from which their clients are dying: pain, fatigue, nausea, constipation, depression and/or anxiety, dry mouth, and so on. The ideal is to work quickly and carefully, attending the specifics of each problem as soon as they arise. Clinical practice with suffering and dying people takes place in the immediate present. Often there is little time to step back and look at the situation from a broader and longer temporal perspective. The desire for this broader view is probably chief among the impetuses that lead us into doing research.

In our research, we have the luxury of stepping back from the immediate demands of alleviating symptoms into a more distanced position of participant-observer, if such a thing is possible. In this role, we watch and interview and consider the dying of patients from as many points of view as possible: patient, family, and clinicians, as well as our own. The result of these observations is a text, the written account of what we have seen and been told. These texts naturally take the form of narratives or stories of dying. Our approach is in keeping with the narrative turn of recent social science, which is predicated on the belief that narratives of illness and other forms of suffering provide access to the private and cultural life-worlds of individuals.[1–7] This turn or trend toward narrative has been put to good use in understanding the experience of death, dying, and bereavement.[8–11]

Our hope is that our contribution of stories and their analysis will further the goals of theory and research and in so doing improve practice. However, dying is as complex and ambiguous and as relatively inexplicable as living; therefore these narratives often raise more questions than can be answered given the current state of knowledge about death and dying. But our narratives may afford their readers an opportunity to step back and view the phenomenon from a perspective that is longer in time, broader in framework, and deeper in reflection than might otherwise be available. In this regard, we present the narrative below, James's story,* which is one of more than a hundred we have collected in our research on suffering and making meaning of suffering at the end of life. This narrative, which takes the point of view of a husband caring for his dying wife, is typical of many of our stories in terms of themes, timing and events. However, the specific details of an individual's experience are unique as lived.[2]

CASE STUDY

James's Story

December 7

James, a man in his early 80s, is caring for his wife, Marti, who is dying of a neurological disease of which he can never remember the name. When I first meet him, Marti has been in the hospice program for 3 or 4 months. She is almost completely paralyzed. Each morning James bathes her in bed, transfers her to a wheelchair, and brings her to the kitchen. He cooks breakfast and feeds her, then turns her chair so she can look out the window or watch television. She is unable to speak, but he has learned to interpret the sounds she can make and the small slow gestures she can make with her hands. But mostly she communicates with her eyes and her smile, both of which are bright and expressive. James says he appreciates having the hospice aide come and bathe her twice a week, because then he can make the 27-mile trip to the nearest supermarket for groceries—they live deep in the country.

More than once, doctors have suggested that James put Marti in a nursing home, but he refuses. "So impersonal, and if she go in a nursing home, well, we gonna lose everything anyway, 'cause nursing home's still gonna take the house—they take everything. It just wipe out the little saving you got, just like that."

James is proud of his independence. "I always made it on my own. Lot of people tell me, they say what a wonderful job I do with her . . . but you see, I just try to do the right thing. Now, when I came up, it was during the Depression, and people didn't have nothin', and my daddy and them had that land, but they ain't had no money. We had plenty of food, but as far as money and clothes, you got what you could get. And people didn't have less or no more than you had, so couldn't nobody help nobody . . . but just as soon as I could, I got me a job and went to work and helped taking care of the others. I've been takin' care of family before I got married."

James and Marti were part of the diaspora of African Americans from the south to north that started in the 1930s and continued through the 1950s. He and Marti married in rural Virginia—to which they returned when Marti became ill—but moved north while they were both young. She went to Philadelphia and he to Brooklyn. They agreed that the first one to find good prospects would send for the other. In a few months, Marti lied and said she had found him a good job. She missed him too much. He was not angry when he arrived and there was no job. Things worked out in Philadelphia anyway.

January 3

James says Marti has been doing better since Christmas. She has her good days and bad, but lately she has been a little stronger. The changes are subtle, he says, but because he is here and sees her every day, he notices them. She raises her arms now to help with dressing and is able to bring a cup to her mouth more often.

He tells me about the work he has to do around the house. He purees all of Marti's food now. He had never been a cook but has learned recently. It is also clear that he keeps an immaculate house. He said he had always worked outside the house and had to learn housekeeping from scratch. But cleaning "came natural" to him. He wants a spotless house. It is also very important to him that Marti is clean and has a fresh nightgown and has her hair combed every morning.

February 15

Marti is a little weaker now. A few weeks ago, she was able to take a step or two with James's help, but now she will not try. She can no longer swallow her medications, and James is applying transdermal patches. As I watch him feed her a pureed lunch, I cannot see much change in her condition.

In Philadelphia in the 1960s and 1970s, James and Marti organized a floating poker game with a group of friends. The game would move from house to house two or three times a week, and locals and neighbors would be invited. Whoever was

*Names have been changed to ensure confidentiality. The use of first names reflects the relationships established and how the participants wanted to be addressed and written about. The appropriate university committee for the protection of human subjects approved the procedures of the research study from which this narrative evolved.

hosting the game would skim 10% from the pots. Soon, James was making wine in his basement and selling it by the glass at the games. Marti didn't drink, but she was a great poker player. She developed a reputation, and soon people who knew her skills would not sit at the same table with her. As they grew older, James became more religious. He stopped drinking and playing cards, joined the church, and even became a deacon. Marti refused to join the church and was organizing poker games in the country even from her wheel chair. James said he was worried about her soul, but when he said this in front of her, she would grin and her eyes would twinkle.

James explains how Marti came to be in the hospice program. "We done spent thousands and thousands of dollars [on Marti's medical care]. But now, we certainly was blessed when this doctor one day said, 'James, I'm gonna tell you the truth. There's no man that I know of that has been trying to do more for their wife than you. You are two nice people. But if things keep on going like it going, I don't know . . . there's such a thing as nursing homes, you know that, don't you?' But I said I seen too much going on in 'em. Nursing home, that gonna be the last result. So, then, he said, 'Yeah, I know what you saying. But, if there ever was two people need any help, it's y'all, 'cause you ain't eligible for Medicaid. So there's a company I'm gonna try to contact and see what I can do for y'all.' That's how we got in the hospice."

James says his age makes it difficult for him to do all the work that needs to be done in the house and around his two acres. But he does some things he believes keep him healthy. He keeps strands of copper wire, and when he has cramps, wraps that area of his body with the wire. At night, he drinks vinegar and takes a quinine pill to help him sleep and stay well. He prays for Marti to be healed, but that does not seem to him to be working. But his prayers that he stay well and strong do seem to be working. He believes his "powers" are strong enough for himself but not for her.

His friends admire how he is helping his wife and refusing to put her in a nursing home, and they are helping him financially. He makes money by fattening calves on his two acres over the summer. A friend gives him deep discounts on the calves and on the hay he needs to feed them before the grass comes in. Another friend has told him what he must do to raise the cattle so they can be sold to a kosher butcher at a premium price. Yet another friend has told him he will fix his car for the price of the parts. Even the local itinerant barber who serves the black community will come to his house and cut his hair at discount.

James and Marti have always been in the flea market trade. They used to buy broken bicycles at the dump, fix and paint them, then sell them at market. Marti is too sick to go now, and James misses the money and the fun. He says in private that when Marti "passes" he will take all her clothes and sell them at the flea market, because that is what she would want.

March 2

Marti is doing about the same, but their granddaughter-in-law, the wife of a grandson they raised because their oldest son had deserted his family, has just died of cancer. James's brother is dying of liver cancer, and James is trying to arrange a trip to New Jersey to see him one last time. His challenge is to find somebody he can trust to stay with Marti, and that someone has to be willing to do it for room and board.

March 25

Marti doesn't look as well today. James says she is having a down day. She sleeps most of the time I am there, opening her eyes occasionally, looking around, trying to wipe her eyes with a napkin, then sleeping some more. James is going to call hospice and have them come out and take a look at her.

This week has been awful for them. Their next-door neighbors to the south were Marti's older sister (near 90) and her son. In the middle of the night, James was awakened by heavy traffic on their dirt road and looked out to see fire trucks and his sister-in-law's house on fire. The place burned to the ground, and both she and her son died. Marti was not told immediately. James called hospice and asked someone to come out because he worried about how she might react. So the day after the fire, the hospice nurse and social worker came out. James says that Marti did not seem to react: "She didn't make no expression, you know, she didn't output no sorrowness or no surprise or no nothing. I was afraid to take a chance on this. This was her sister. But she still didn't, so then we discover it must be rough inside. But something wrong with her output." He decided her disease was preventing her from expressing how she felt inside.

I ask James how he is handling all these deaths. He says, "I don't care how often death come around, he's a stranger."

April 12

Marti seems unchanged. She recovered a little from being withdrawn but not completely. As I am visiting, the hospice nurse is visiting as well. As she leaves, she says to Marti, "See you next week." Marti shakes her head, no. The nurse says, "I hope to see you at least." Out of James's hearing, the nurse tells me that patients know when their death is coming and she does not expect to see Marti next week.

A few years ago, when Marti was fairly well, James was teasing her about being a month younger than she is. James says Martha told him, "Well, when the both of us get old, and I've died of old age, and you come to my funeral all dressed up in your finest clothes, I wouldn't bother going home and changing because you will be joining me soon."

June 1

Marti did not die that week, she died on the 24th of May, 6 weeks later. James tells me the whole story of her decline. Six years ago she gave up walking on her own. For another 2 years she could feed herself. But for the last 4 years, he has been feeding her. Each step down was very gradual.

In retrospect, James believes Marti started to die the week her sister died in the fire. "Laurie [the hospice nurse] was away on her vacation when Marti passed. She wasn't doing good, just wouldn't half eat. These worldly things she wouldn't pay no attention to. You tell her something like when the house burned down . . . she didn't do nothing. She just held her chin. I said, you understand what I'm saying? She said, 'Uh huh,' shaking her head yeah."

At the time, James accepted the nurse's interpretation that Marti could not express herself but was feeling the pain inside. Later in the day when he moved Marti in her wheel chair out to the kitchen, he did not put her in her usual spot by the window because the burning embers of her sister's house were the center of the view. But Marti insisted. She stared out the window but did not seem moved. James says, "Something tell me she was giving up. I just believe as time goes on, you start to giving up the worldly things, when you're coming near the time to go. Because you be giving up the world, gradually giving up all the worldly things."

Marti had responded with no emotion when James told her about the death of her granddaughter-in-law, and even when he had shown her a picture of her new great granddaughter. She smiled briefly and went back to staring out the window.

One day Marti refused to eat. She would turn away from the spoon James offered. When he insisted, she would take the food in her mouth and spit it back out when he turned his back. James called Laurie and asked her to come out. Two days later, Laurie came and examined Marti and said it was close to the end and presented James with some choices. James says, "Laurie told me maybe we can have IV come in. You have a nurse come in here and give her fluid and do this and do that, right here at home, and we don't have to put her in the hospital or nursing home. I said, Laurie, I know how you feel about these places. But sometime you come to a time you have to do what you got to do. I'm mighty afraid this is the time for the hospital. I'm not talking about the nursing home. I am just talking about hospital because it's round the clock. They are with you 24 hours."

Laurie calls Marti's doctor and arranges to have her admitted, then calls the ambulance. James busies himself with packing her nightgowns and medications. He says, "Laurie comes, tapping me on the shoulder. She says, 'You know what, James?' I said, What? 'Marti decided that she don't want to go to the hospital.' I said, Oh, no. Are you sure you understood what she said? Because you are not with her every day, maybe you misunderstood. She said, 'No, I'm sure.' I said, 'Wait a minute, let me go back in there.' The ambulance people is all at the bed, you know, for to take her out and put her on the stretcher. Before I could get in there, Laurie said, 'James, Marti's passing now . . . she's on her way out.' I said, 'Now you got to be kidding.' Boy, I goes in there, I put my hand on top of her head, I just pat on it, you know, then that was it."

Discussion

Narratives are not reality. What we actually experience is more complex and nuanced than any story about experience can hope to capture. However, listening to the stories of others may be as close as we will ever come to being able to understand experiences not our own. In fact, nursing is developing a tradition of using narratives to understand illness. Nurses began to write about this approach starting in the early 1990s.[12–15] Narratives provide to nurses who are trying to understand and to treat suffering at the end of life an opportunity to see palliative care in as much of its complexity as possible, the nonlinear, nonrational, and contradictory complexity of experience as it appears in narrative. The story of James and Marti can stand alone in portraying that complexity, but a few comments might also be helpful. James and Marti can be seen as experiencing this death on a number of different levels, as a political/economic event, as a spiritual event, and as an aesthetic event.

Political/Economic Aspects of Marti's Death

For James, the politics of his situation are manifest at the most basic level and the highest level. James and Marti seemed to have always participated in an underground economy. From legitimate participation in flea markets to illegal wine and gambling ventures, they found a way to supplement their incomes (while having fun). Now, when James needs help, his friends are generous. He receives deep discounts and free labor. The itinerant barber probably has no business license and no formal training and makes his living below the view of official bureaucracies, but he is no swindler and is willing to help a friend in need.

James and Marti have Social Security and own a home, and thus are not eligible for Medicaid. James is savvy enough to realize that he would have to spend enough of his assets to become poor before he could receive more government help. The idea of spending his money on a nursing home would be an anathema to James's sense of financial responsibility. He would be spending too much for a service he does not believe provides quality.

Hospice is the kind of service James can appreciate. He increases his benefits in terms of having a team to help with symptom control and in medication costs. As with most caregivers, his own economic contribution to Marti's care has been both considerable and invisible to any official agency. Research has also confirmed James's situation in that the burden of caregiving was always very high and increased tremendously in the last stages of Marti's life, which is typical of many families.[16–19]

His recounting of Marti's doctor's referral to hospice makes it sound as though it was a "social" referral. James and Marti needed the help. They were good, hardworking people. The doctor saw them as deserving, and thus referred them to hospice. Of course, this is not the way it is supposed to happen. The standards should be objective and not based on how much a physician likes a family. And of course, this is James's story of what happened and does not necessarily actually reflect what the doctor was thinking, what he did in terms of the paperwork, or even what he actually said to James. We all make sense of conversations based on what we want to hear and believe. Marti was in the hospice program for a little under a year with a neurodegenerative disease, the progression of which is very difficult to predict.

That nursing homes are seen as not good options for the dying elderly, and that an elderly man believes he must spend himself into poverty to receive help keeping his wife in a nursing home are failures of the system. Or at least they are failures if one believes that having options for good care at the end of life is something we owe every citizen and not just those who can pay. James wants Marti to die in the hospital, where, in his experience, she will receive excellent round-the-clock care. He does not question the right for Marti to be there. Hospitals are for the sick, and Marti is dying, which is as sick as one can be. The hospice nurse who comes to make the transfer offers James other options, such as increased home therapy. Her motives, we would guess, are first to offer James as wide a range of options as possible. However, as a hospice nurse, she must also keep in mind that hospitalization is the most expensive care Marti can receive and hospice will have to pay for it. Comfortable deaths at home are prized by hospices, who are rewarded for them, but a well-attended death in a hospital is prized by James.

The lesson for palliative care nurses in this part of James's story is one we already know but need to keep ourselves reminded of. There are none better than us, palliative care nurses, at knowing when and how the system does not work. We have an obligation to be politically active on behalf of the people whose lives are so deeply affected by this system of rules and regulations. Families suffering the loss of a loved one are perhaps more vulnerable than at any other time and need professionals advocating for them when they are struggling to care for themselves and their family member.

Spiritual Aspects of Marti's Death

Nurses and other clinicians have long recognized that dying is a spiritual event for most people.[20–23] James is a religious man, but, interestingly, he does not use the occasion of his wife's illness to think about what is arguably the central question in all religions, why must human beings suffer? Or maybe because he is religious, he does not need to consider this question. He does, however, test the power of prayer with Marti's illness. When he prays for his own health, his prayers are effective, but when he prays for Marti's health, these prayers do not work. He says his powers are limited. It is as though the power of prayer lies within James and not in God. He does not entertain the idea that his prayer for Marti to be healed is not answered because it is not God's will that she continue to live. He does not seem to believe that the power of prayer lies in the prayer itself or in the goal of the prayer, but lies in the one who is praying. This is both an assumed position of great power and of great vulnerability. If he has the power to keep himself well, what is wrong with him that he cannot heal his wife? Is his faith not as strong as the disease it must overcome? James does not seem to be dismayed by his lack of power; he treats it as a fact he must accept.

After James told us that Marti seemed to be losing interest in life, we began to wonder if she was depressed. Marti showed signs of anhedonia and dysthymia. She was more withdrawn and less communicative. Our conviction is that depression is a disease and should be treated aggressively when it is discovered, both because the disease can cause damage to bodily organs (the changes in the brain caused by depression are well documented) and because it causes unnecessary suffering. Because someone is nearing the end of life does not mean that he or she should not be treated for depression—just as we would not let a diabetic's blood sugar wildly fluctuate just because he or she is in a hospice program. But treating Marti's depression, if indeed she was depressed, could have spiritual ramifications. James believes that Marti was giving up the things of this life in order to move on to the next life. In his mind, she was starting a spiritual journey, not becoming depressed. If Marti were treated with an antidepressant and became more involved in life, would James have appreciated this backward step in her spiritual journey? Of course, Marti might not have seen it as a spiritual journey and may have appreciated something that would lighten her mood. Sometimes what is spiritual and what is medical are confused and confusing. Nurses' responsibilities are not easily defined or carried out in this area, but they cannot be denied.

Aesthetic Aspects of Marti's Death

Art is the conscious molding of the raw experiences of life into something that is important, meaningful, and has the potential of enlightening us in some way. Ceremonies such as weddings, graduations, baptisms, and funerals can be, if done with originality and care, art forms. These rituals are culturally constructed to make them beautiful and give them all the meaning and portent that beauty implies. To some degree, births and deaths can fall into this category. But one could argue that art implies an artist, someone controlling and creating the experience for an audience, and what is possible to be controlled often seems very little in birth and death. However, there are parts of death and birth over which nurses do have control, and we contend that nurses can and will be judged on the aesthetic qualities of these events. An older person dying of cancer being coded in a busy, noisy emergency department may well be remembered by the family as an ugly death, as might the sudden exsanguination of a patient who has no platelets secondary to a terminal disease. On the other hand, most of us who have worked in palliative care have heard family members tell us, weeks after an expected death in a quiet room with family all in attendance, that the death was beautiful.

On its most basic level, the qualities used to make aesthetic judgments are boundaries, rhythm, and clarity [these are adapted from Aquinas].[24–25] In terms of boundaries, artistic or aesthetic narratives have beginnings, middles, and endings.[26] While it is true that some of the boundaries of James's story are established by his telling and our rendition of it, much of the experience fits well into a self-contained story. The story of Marti's dying starts rather vaguely. Marti has been sick for a long time and has progressively become more debilitated. James never says that her disease is incurable and never says that Marti is dying, but the fact seems to be a given. The story can be said to have started when Marti is referred to hospice, even though James does not acknowledge that the hospice program is for the dying, he was surely told that it was. As with most stories we tell about ourselves, the beginning is not as clearly delineated as the ending.

As the narrative progresses, James does not use the dominant metaphor, the one we heard in most of the interviews, that of a struggle or a war. We often heard that a patient and family were fighting against the disease and trying to overcome it. Often the caregiver and the patient were proud of how hard they struggled against death and did not give up. For James, the metaphor was one of a journey or a passage rather than a fight. He talks about Marti's "passing" and "moving on." When he does use the term "giving up," he is referring to her relinquishing one world for another, not refusing to fight. For James, the narrative of Marti's death was a long, slowly played-out journey.

James has some fairly strong ideas about the elements that should be in the middle of the narrative. The narrative should not be about the slow decline of their financial status and their ability to be independent. The story should have James and Marti as the major characters. James does not believe that other caregivers should play a major role, although he appreciates all the help he receives. Finally, he wants the ending of the narrative to play out at home and not in a nursing home. Nursing homes are too ugly—uncaring, impersonal, and expensive—for Marti. But the final act of the story should take place in the hospital. James holds that narratives about expected deaths should end in the hospital where people are ready to deal with such things. The fact that Marti appeared to decide otherwise was, however, not a great disappointment to him. If someone else besides Marti had decided she should die at home or in a nursing home, James would probably not have been so contented.

This "choice" by Marti leads to the second criteria for an aesthetic death, rhythm. Marti dies when she should in James' narrative, much the opposite of the Colonel in Gabriel Garcia Marquez's great novel, *One Hundred Years of Solitude*, who, when asked as a old man why he is still alive, says "A man dies when he can, not when he should." Marti moves slowly toward death, and her death is the last in a series that, for James, are precursors and rehearsals. As in a well-wrought play, Marti, as the central figure, watches others die before her, each one seemingly making her own death a little more inevitable. The final node in this narrative rhythm is the death of Marti's sister. We, of course, do not see the rhythm of the narrative from Marti's point of view, but James understands his sister-in-law's death as a precursor. Whether her sister's death is the occasion for Marti to move toward the other world or merely an opportunity for her to demonstrate that she has already started that movement, is not clear in James's story. However, the rhythm of the narrative is demonstrable in terms of the Marti's slow decline and the spacing of the deaths leading up to her own climatic one.

The third aesthetic criterion is clarity, our translation of the Aquinas' *claritas*. By this we mean a sense that things generally happened in a meaningful way. That is, Marti's death was not random or arbitrary or contingent (although a contingent death might fit well with a postmodern aesthetic). Not that Marti was supposed to die. Her death was tragic and sad. But there was a sense of the inevitable about it. Marti did not die because of something done or left undone by James or anyone else. She did not die from a medical mistake, or because James did not call the ambulance in time. An aesthetically satisfying story does not leave the listener with anger or guilt. Instead, one is left with a sense of clarity. That is, the sadness is deep and profound, but the reasons are clear and not confused with regrets about what was done or left undone.

Palliative care is, to a great degree, about helping people create a narrative about a death that has as many aesthetic qualities as possible. James directed (in the sense that one directs a play or movie) Marti's dying for the most part. But at the very end, the hospice nurse stepped in and, while she did not change anything that happened, she changed the narrative by offering James a way of looking at the event. The nurse interpreted the narrative in such a way that gave Marti the power to decide her own time and manner of dying. The nurse orchestrated, to some degree, the meaning of the event. Whether we as palliative care nurses want the responsibility of orchestrating a death or not, we often have it. We have to learn the rhythm of the narrative to know when it is time for the dying person to stay home and when it is time to call the ambulance.

What is aesthetically satisfying to one family may not be to another. For many families, the narrative should end at home and not in the hospital, where the dying person would be surrounded by strangers. James wanted Marti to die in the hospital where she would receive around-the-clock expert care. That was the ending he intended. Should James have been able to dictate this part of the narrative? Certainly. But how much should he be able to dictate? What if Marti had been in excruciating pain at the end of life and James had wanted her to receive a morphine dosage aimed at not only stopping the pain but at helping her pass to the next world? Luckily, Marti did not die in pain, and we are not suggesting that medical treatments, such as the titration of morphine, be dictated by the aesthetic sensibilities of the family alone. We are arguing that nurses and physicians must realize that this sense of aesthetics should be a part of the considerations.

Summary

In this presentation of James's story and our discussion of it, we have carefully avoided defining a good death or predicting or prescribing how to achieve one. The complexity of the experience prevents our doing so. Offering prescriptions would be denying the differences that make stories meaningful. What we mean by this is that there are no general cases; there are no theoretical lives; living is never done in the abstract. This seems obvious, but it may sometimes be lost in the science of our practice. Usually we base our interventions on what works most of the time for most people. This is the essence of science-based nursing practice. We do things to help our patients based on a high probability that it will work, and that probability is based on an abstraction. It is based on looking at many cases and generalizing about what usually happens. Necessarily, the specifics of individuals must be lost in the process of making general statements.

Thus, there is a tension between the goals of science, producing abstract general knowledge that can be acted upon with some confidence of success, and the notion that narratives are unique and cannot be prescribed. Our goal has been to bridge this gap and reduce the tension through the use of narratives. A narrative approach to understanding palliative care can rescue the individual particularities of life from being lost in our practice and, at the same time, offer some abstractions to guide clinicians, such as the elements of aesthetics, and an attention to political and economic and spiritual issues. Listening to James and Marti's story—their move to the urban north, the floating poker games and bootlegging, their cows and flea markets and network of friends—makes it impossible to see them as anything but a real couple with a complex life that is uniquely theirs. Recognizing this "suchness" of their lives cannot help but make us care for them in a different way.

ACKNOWLEDGMENT

The authors acknowledge the financial support of the National Institute of Nursing Research (R15 NR02482 and R01 NR04693) and the National Institute of Aging (R01 NR03517), National Institutes of Health.

REFERENCES

1. Beverly J. Testimonio, subalternity, and narrative authority. In: Denzin NK, Lincoln YS, eds. Handbook of Qualitative Research, 2nd ed. Thousand Oaks, CA: Sage, 2000: 555–566.
2. Cohen MZ, Kahn DL, Steeves RH. Hermeneutic Phenomenological Research: A Practical Guide for Nurse Researchers. Thousand Oaks, CA: Sage, 2000.
3. Kleinman A. The Illness Narratives: Suffering, Healing and the Human Condition. New York: Basic Books, 1988.
4. Meier A. Narrative in psychotherapy theory, practice, and research: a critical review. Counseling and Psychotherapy Research 2002; 2:239–251.
5. Neimeyer RA, Levitt H. Coping and coherence: a narrative perspective. In: Snyder C, ed. Perspective on Coping. New York: Wiley, 2001.
6. Polkinghorne DE. Narrative Knowing and the Human Sciences. Albany: State University of New York Press, 1988.
7. Sandelowski M. Telling stories: narrative approaches in qualitative research. Image 1991;23:161–166.
8. Kahn DH, Steeves RH. Grief and bereavement in the elderly. Nursing care of the elderly. In: Swanson EA, Trip-Reimer T, eds., Life Transitions in the Older Adult. New York: Springer, 1999.
9. Shapiro ER. Grief in interpersonal perspective: theories and their implications. In: Stroebe MS, Hansson RO, Stroebe W, Schut H, eds., Handbook of Bereavement Research. Washington, DC: American Psychological Association, 2001.
10. Steeves RH. The rhythm of bereavement. Fam Community Health 2002;25:1–10.
11. Neimeyer RA. Reauthoring life narratives: grief therapy as meaning construction. Isr J Psychiatry Relat Sci 2001;38: 171–183.
12. Gregory D, Longman A. Mothers' suffering: sons who died of AIDS. Qualitative Health Res 1992;2:334–357.
13. Newman MA, Moch SD. Life patterns of persons with coronary heart disease. Nursing Sci Q 1991;4:161–167.
14. Steeves RH. Patients who have undergone bone marrow transplantation: their quest for meaning. Oncol Nurs Forum 1991;19: 899–905.
15. Thompson JL. Exploring gender and culture with Khmer refugee women: reflections on participatory feminist research. Adv Nurs Sci 1991;13:30–48.
16. Casarett DJ, Hirschman KB, Crowley R, Galbraith LD, Leo M. Caregivers' satisfaction with hospice care in the last 24 hours of life. Am J Hospice Palliative Care 2003;20:205–210.
17. Haley WE, LaMonde LA, Han B, Narramore S, Schonwetter R. Family caregiving in hospice: effects of psychological and health functioning among spousal caregivers of hospice patients with lung cancer or dementia. Hospice J 2001;15:1–18.
18. Newton M, Bell D, Lambert S, Fearing A. Concerns of hospice patient caregivers. ABNF J 2002; 13:140–144.
19. Weitzner MA, McMillan SC. The Caregiver Quality of Life Index-Cancer (CQOLC) Scale: revalidation in a home hospice setting. J Palliative Care 1999;15: 13–20.
20. Burton LA. The spiritual dimension of palliative care. Semin Oncol Nurs 1998;14:121–128.
21. Driscoll J. Spirituality and religion in end-of-life care. J Palliative Med 2001;4:333–335.
22. McLain CS, Rosenfeld B, Breitbart W. Effect of spiritual well-being on end-of-life despair in terminally-ill cancer patients. Lancet (NA ed.) 2003;361:1603–1607.
23. Smith D. Spiritual perspectives in end of life care. In: Poor B, Poirrier GP, eds., End-of- Life Nursing Care. Sudbury, MA: Jones and Bartlett Publishers, 2001:201–209.
24. Aquinas T. Selected writings, McInerny R, trans. New York: Penguin Books,1998.
25. Eco E. The Aesthetics of Thomas Aquinas, Brendin H, trans. Cambridge, MA: Harvard University Press, 1988.
26. Aristotle: Poetics, McLeish K, trans. The New York Theater Communication Group, 1999.

APPENDIX *Rose Virani and Stacey Pejsa*

Palliative Care Resource List

Bibliographies/References/Texts

American Journal of Nursing, Palliative Nursing Series
http://www.AJNonline.com
City of Hope Pain/Palliative Care Resource Center
http://prc.coh.org
End-of-Life Nursing Education Consortium (ELNEC) Series
http://www.aacn.nche.edu/ELNEC/ELNECSeries.htm
Journal of the American College of Surgeons, Palliative Care in Surgery Series
http://www.facs.org/cqi/jacsarticles.html
Mary Ann Liebert, Inc.—Unipac Series
http://www.liebertpub.com/publication.aspx?pub_id=119

- *UNIPAC One*: The Hospice/Palliative Medicine Approach to End-of-Life Care
- *UNIPAC Two*: Alleviating Psychological and Spiritual Pain in the Terminally Ill
- *UNIPAC Three*: Assessment and Treatment of Pain in the Terminally Ill
- *UNIPAC Four*: Management of Selected Non-pain Symptoms in the Terminally Ill
- *UNIPAC Five*: Caring for the Terminally Ill-Communication and the Physician's Role on the Interdisciplinary Team
- *UNIPAC Six*: Ethical and Legal Decision Making When Caring for the Terminally Ill
- *UNIPAC Seven*: The Hospice/Palliative Medicine Approach to Caring for Patients with HIV/AIDS
- *UNIPAC Eight*: The Hospice/Palliative Medicine Approach to Caring for Pediatric Patients

Oxford University Press
http://www.oup-usa.com

- Lynn J, Schuster JL, Kabcenell A. *Improving Care for the End of Life: A Sourcebook for Health Care Managers and Clinicians* (© 2001).
- Armstrong-Dailey A, Zarbock S. *Hospice Care for Children*, 2nd edition (© 2002).
- Doyle D, Hanks G, Cherny NI, Calman K. *Oxford Textbook of Palliative Medicine*, 3rd edition (© 2004).

Shaare Zedek Cancer Pain and Palliative Care Reference Database
http://www.chernydatabase.org

Guidelines

Agency for Healthcare Research and Quality (AHRQ) Pain Guidelines (formerly Agency for Health Care Policy and Research [AHCPR])
http://www.ahrq.gov
National Comprehensive Cancer Network (NCCN)—palliative care clinical practice guidelines
http://www.nccn.org
National Consensus Project for Quality Palliative Care
http://www.nationalconsensusproject.org
World Health Organization (WHO)
http://www.who.int/en

Journals/Newsletters

American Journal of Hospice & Palliative Care
http://www.pnpco.com
Americans for Better Care of the Dying Exchange Newsletter
http://www.abcd-caring.org/newslettermain.htm
Cancer Care News Newsletter
http://www.cancercare.org
The European Journal of Palliative Care
http://www.ejpc.co.uk
International Association for Hospice and Palliative Care
http://www.hospicecare.com
International Journal of Palliative Nursing
http://www.markallengroup.com/healthcare.ijpn
Journal of Hospice and Palliative Nursing
http://www.jhpn.com
Journal of Pain and Palliative Care Pharmacotherapy
http://www.haworthpress.com
Journal of Pain and Symptom Management
http://www.elsevier.com

Journal of Palliative Care
http://www.ircm.qc.ca/bioethique/english
Journal of Palliative Medicine
http://www.liebertpub.com
Journal of Psychosocial Oncology
http://www.haworthpress.com
Journal of Supportive Oncology
http://www.supportiveoncology.net
National Comprehensive Cancer Network (NCCN) News
http://www.nccn.org
National Hospice and Palliative Care Organization (NHPCO) Newsline
http://www.nhpco.org
Oncology Nursing Form (ONF)
http://www.ons.org
Pain: Clinical Updates
http://www.iasp-pain.org
Palliative & Supportive Care
http://journals.cambridge.org
Palliative Medicine
http://www.arnoldpublishers.com/journals
Psycho-Oncology
http://www.wiley.com
Progress in Palliative Care
http://www.leeds.ac.uk/lmi
Southern California Cancer Pain Initiative (SCCPI) Newsletter
http://sccpi.coh.org
Supportive Care in Cancer
http://www.springerlink.org

Organizations and Websites (Patient, Professional, and State Pain Initiatives)

AARP (formerly known as the American Association of Retired Persons)
http://www.aarp.org/life/endoflife
About Herbs, Botanicals & Other Products
http://www.mskcc.org/aboutherbs
Agency for Healthcare Research and Quality Clinical Practice Guidelines
http://www.ahcpr.gov/clinic/cpgarchv.htm
Aging With Dignity
http://www.agingwithdignity.org
American Academy of Hospice and Palliative Medicine (AAHPM)
http://www.aahpm.org
American Academy of Pain Medicine (AAPM)
http://www.painmed.org
American Academy of Pediatrics (AAP)
http://www.aap.org
American Alliance of Cancer Pain Initiatives
http://www.aacpi.org
American Association for Therapeutic Humor
http://www.aath.org
American Board of Hospice & Palliative Medicine
http://www.abhpm.org
American Cancer Society (ACS)
http://www.cancer.org
American Geriatrics Society (AGS)
http://www.americangeriatrics.org
American Holistic Nurses Association
http://www.ahna.org
American Hospice Foundation
http://www.americanhospice.org
American Medical Association (AMA)
http://www.ama-assn.org
American Nurses Association (ANA)
http://www.ana.org
American Pain Foundation
http://www.painfoundation.org
American Pain Society (APS)
http://www.ampainsoc.org
American Society for Bioethics and Humanities
http://www.asbh.org
American Society of Clinical Oncology (ASCO)
http://www.asco.org
American Society of Law, Medicine and Ethics
http://www.aslme.org
American Society for Pain Management Nursing (ASPMN)
http://www.aspmn.org
Americans for Better Care of the Dying (ABCD)
http://www.abcd-caring.org
Approaching Death: Improving Care at the End of Life
http://www.nap.edu/readingroom/books/approaching
Association for Death Education and Counseling (ADEC)
http://www.adec.org
Association of Oncology Social Work (AOSW)
http://www.aosw.org
Association of Pediatric Oncology Nurses (APON)
http://www.apon.org
Before I Die: Medical Care and Personal Choices
http://www.thirteen.org/bid
Beth Israel Medical Center, Department of Pain Medicine and Palliative Care
http://stoppain.org
Candlelighters Childhood Cancer Foundation
http://www.candlelighters.org
Caregiver Network
http://www.caregiver.ca/index.html
Caregiver Regional Resources
http://www.caregiver911.com
Catholic Health Association of the United States
http://www.chausa.org
Center to Advance Palliative Care
http://www.capc.org
Center for Applied Ethics and Professional Practice (CAEPP)
http://caepp.edc.org
Center for Palliative Care (Harvard Medical School)
http://www.hms.harvard.edu/cdi/pallcare
Center for Palliative Care Studies (formally known as Center to Improve Care of the Dying)
http://medicaring.org
Center for Practical Bioethics
http://www.midbio.org
Children's Hospice International (CHI)
http://www.chionline.org
Children's Project on Palliative/Hospice Services (CHIPPS)
http://www.nhpco.org
City of Hope Pain/Palliative Care Resource Center (COHPPRC)
http://prc.coh.org

Compassion in Dying Federation
http://www.compassionindying.org
The Compassionate Friends, Inc. (TCF)
http://www.compassionatefriends.org
Department of Health and Human Services, Healthfinder
http://www.healthfinder.gov
Dying Well: Defining Wellness Through the End of Life
http://www.dyingwell.org
http://www.dyingwell.com
Edmonton Regional Palliative Care Program
http://www.palliative.org
Education for Physicians on End-of-Life Care Project (EPEC)
http://epec.net/EPEC/webpages/index.cfm
The End of Life: Exploring Death in America
http://www.npr.org/programs/death
End-of-Life Care for Children
http://www.childendoflifecare.org
End-of-Life Nursing Education Consortium (ELNEC)
http://www.aacn.nche.edu/ELNEC
End-of-Life Physician Education Resource Center (EPERC)
http://www.eperc.mcw.edu
European Association for Palliative Care (EAPC)
http://www.eapcnet.org
FACCT: Foundation for Accountability Family Caregiver Alliance (Markle Foundation)
http://www.markle.org/resurces/faact/index.php
Family Caregiver Alliance
http://www.caregiver.org
Grief.Net
http://www.griefnet.org
Growth House, Inc.
http://www.growthhouse.org
GROWW: Grief Recovery Online for All Bereaved
http://www.groww.org
Gundersen Lutheran
http://www.gundluth.org/eolprograms
Hospice Association of America
http://www.hospice-america.org
Hospice Foundation of America
http://www.hospicefoundation.org
Hospice Net
http://hospicenet.org
Hospice and Palliative Nurses Association (HPNA)
http://www.hpna.org
Hospice Resources.Net
http://www.hospiceresources.net
International Association for the Study of Pain (IASP)
http://www.iasp-pain.org/
The International Work Group on Death, Dying and Bereavement
http://www.wwdc.com/death/iwg/iwg.html
Life's End Institute (Missoula Demonstration Project)
http://www.missoulademonstration.org
Mayday Pain Project
http://www.painandhealth.org
Medical College of Wisconsin, Center for the Study of Bioethics
http://www.mcw.edu/bioethics
Medical College of Wisconsin Palliative Care Center
http://www.mcw.edu/pallmed
Missoula Demonstration Project (Dying Well)
http://www.dyingwell.org
National Association for Home Care (NAHC)
http://www.nahc.org
National Cancer Institute (NCI)
http://www.nci.nih.gov
National Consensus Project (NCP)
http://www.nationalconsensusproject.org
National Hospice and Palliative Care Organization (NHPCO)
http://www.nhpco.org
The National Institute of Aging
http://www.nia.nih.gov
National Institute of Health
http://www.nih.gov
National Prison Hospice Association
http://www.npha.org
National Public Radio (NPR)
http://www.npr.org
Not Dead Yet
http://www.notdeadyet.org
On Our Own Terms
http://www.thirteen.org/onourownterms
Oncology Nursing Society (ONS)
http://www.ons.org
Open Society Institute Project on Death in America
http://www.soros.org/initiative/pdia
Oregon Health Sciences University, Center for Ethics in Health Care
http://www.ohsu.edu/ethics
Palliative Care: One Vision, One Voice
http://www.palliativecarenursing.net
Patient Education Institute
http://www.patient-education.com
Pediatric Pain
http://pediatricpain.ca
Promoting Excellence in End-of-Life Care
http://www.promotingexcellence.org
The Robert Wood Johnson Foundation (RWJF)
http://www.rwjf.org
Southern California Cancer Pain Initiative (SCCPI)
http://sccpi.coh.org/
Supportive Care of the Dying
http://www.careofdying.org
University of Wisconsin Pain and Policy Studies Group
http://www.medsch.wis.edu/painpolicy
Wisconsin Cancer Pain Initiative
http://www.medsch.wisc.edu/painpolicy/

Position Statements

American Nurses Association (ANA)
http://www.ana.org
- Active Euthanasia
- Assisted Suicide
- Foregoing Nutrition and Hydration
- Nursing and the Patient Self-Determination Acts
- Nursing Care and Do-Not-Resuscitate (DNR) Decisions
- Pain Management and Control of Distressing Symptoms in Dying Patients

American Nursing Leaders
http://www.dyingwell.com/downloads/apnpos.pdf
- Advanced Practice Nurses Role in Palliative Care

American Society of Pain Management Nurses (ASPMN)
http://www.aspmn.org
- Assisted Suicide
- End-of-Life Care

Hospice and Palliative Nurses Association (HPNA):
http://www.hpna.org
- Artificial Nutrition and Hydration in End-of-Life Care
- Complementary Therapies
- Evidence-Based Practice
- Legalization of Assisted Suicide
- Pain
- Palliative Sedation at End of Life
- Providing Opioids at the End of Life
- Shortage of Registered Nurses
- Value of the Nursing Assistant in End-of-Life Care
- Value of Nursing Certification
- Value of Professional Nurse in End-of-Life Care

Oncology Nursing Society (ONS):
http://www.ons.org
- Cancer Pain Management
- The Nurse's Responsibility to the Patient Requesting Assisted Suicide
- ONS and Association of Oncology Social Work Joint Position on End-of-Life Care
- Use of Complementary and Alternative Therapies in Cancer Care

Reports

Center for Palliative Care Studies
- Living Well at the End of Life: Adapting Health Care to Serious Chronic Illness in Old Age—http://medicaring.org/whitepaper
- Medicare Beneficiaries' Costs and Use of Care in the Last Year of Life—http://medicaring.org/educate/download/medpac.doc

Institute of Medicine
- Approaching Death: Improving Care at the End of Life—http://www.iom.edu/report.asp?id=12687
- Improving Palliative Care for Cancer—http://www.iom.edu/report.asp?id=12684
- When Children Die: Improving Palliative and End-of-Life for Children and their Families—http://www.iom.edu/report.asp?id=4483

National Hospice and Palliative Care Organization (Children's International Project on Palliative/Hospice Services-ChIPPS)
- A Call for Change: Recommendations to Improve the Care of Children Living with Life-Threatening Illness—http://www.nhpco.org/files/public/ChIPPSCallforChange.pdf

Promoting Excellence in End-of-Life Care
- Advanced Practice Nursing: Pioneering Practices in Palliative Care—http://www.promotingexcellence.org/apn

Robert Wood Johnson Foundation
- Disparities at the End of Life—http://www.rwjf.org/newsroom/featureDetail.jsp?featureID=152&type=3
- Means to a Better End—http://www.rwjf.org/files/publications/other/meansbetterend.pdf
- Precepts of Palliative Care—http://www.sgna.org/resources/statements/statment10b.html
- Precepts of Palliative Care for Children, Adolescents and Their Families—http://www.apon.org/files/public/last_acts_precepts.pdf

Research Instruments

Brown University Center Toolkit of Instruments To Measure End-of-Life Care (TIME)
http://www.chcr.brown.edu/pcoc/toolkit.htm

Center to Improve Care of the Dying/Toolkit of Instruments to Measure End of Life
http://www.gwu.edu/~cicd/toolkit/toolkit.htm

City of Hope Pain/Palliative Care Resource Center
http://prc.coh.org (refer to Research Instruments section)

Edmonton Assessment Tools
http://www.palliative.org/PC/ClinicalInfo/AssessmentTools/AssessmentToolsIDX.html

Patient-Reported Outcome and Quality-of-Life Instruments Database
http://www.proqolid.org

Promoting Excellence in End-of-Life Care
http://www.promotingexcellence.org/tools/index.html

State of the Art Review of Tools for Assessment of Pain in Nonverbal Older Adults
http://prc.coh.org (refer to Pain in the Elderly section)

Supportive Care of the Dying
http://www.careofdying.org

Videos

Applied Vision
http://www.appliedv.com/catalog.htm

Aquarius Productions, Inc.
http://www.aquariusproductions.com

City of Hope Pain/Palliative Care Resource Center
http://prc.coh.org (refer to End-of-Life/Palliative Care section for extensive video listings)

Fanlight Productions
http://www.fanlight.com

Initiative for Pediatric Palliative Care (IPPC)
http://www.ippcweb.org

PBS Home Video
http://www.pbs.org

Lippincott Williams & Wilkins Electronic Media Division
http://www.lww.com

INDEX

Page numbers followed by *f* indicate figures; those followed by *t* indicate tabular material; those followed by *c* indicate case studies.